15048 WS
700
RU1

D1348799

Child and Adolescent Psychiatry

Child and Adolescent Psychiatry

Edited by

Michael Rutter

CBE, MD, FRCP, FRCPsych, FRS, FMedSci
Professor of Developmental Psychopathology
Social, Genetic and Developmental Psychiatry Research Centre
Institute of Psychiatry
London

Eric Taylor

MA, MB, FRCP, FRCPsych, FMedSci
Professor of Child and Adolescent Psychiatry
Department of Child and Adolescent Psychiatry
Institute of Psychiatry
London

Blackwell
Science

First published 1976
Second edition 1985
Reprinted as paperback 1987, 1990, 1991
Third edition 1994
Reprinted 1995
Reprinted as paperback 1995, 1998, 2000
Fourth edition 2002
Reprinted 2003 (twice)
Reprinted 2004

ISBN 0-632-05361-5

A catalogue record for this title is available from the British Library

Library of Congress Cataloging-in-Publication Data

Child and adolescent psychiatry / edited by Michael Rutter, Eric Taylor.— 4th ed.
        p. ; cm.
    Includes bibliographical references
    and index.
    ISBN 0-632-05361-5 (printed case)—ISBN 0-86542-880-8 (pbk.)
    1. Child psychiatry.   2. Adolescent psychiatry.   I. Rutter, Michael, 1933–
    II. Taylor, Eric A.
    [DNLM: 1. Mental Disorders—Adolescence.   2. Mental Disorders—Child.
    3. Adolescent Behavior.   4. Developmental Disabilities.   WS 350 C53503 2002]
    RJ499 .C486 2002
    618.92′89—dc21

                                                    2001037921

Set in 9/12 Sabon by SNP Best-set Typesetter Ltd., Hong Kong
Printed and bound in Great Britain at CPI Bath

For further information on Blackwell Science, visit our website:
www.blackwellpublishing.com

Contents

CONTENTS

Contributors

Adrian Angold BSc, MB BS, MRCPsych
Associate Professor of Psychiatry and Behavioral Science, Center for Developmental Epidemiology, Box 3454, Duke University Medical Center, Durham, NC 27710, USA

Anthony Bailey BSc, MB BS, MRCPsych, DCH
MRC Clinical Scientist and Consultant Psychiatrist, Social, Genetic and Developmental Psychiatry (SGDP) Research Centre, Institute of Psychiatry, 5 Windsor Walk, London SE5 8BB

Sue Bailey MB, ChB, FRCPsych
Consultant Adolescent Forensic Psychiatrist, Adolescent Forensic Service, Mental Health Services of Salford NHS Trust, Bury New Road, Prestwich, Manchester M25 3BL

Jacqueline Barnes BSc, MSc, PhD
Senior Lecturer in Psychology, Leopold Muller Centre for Child and Family Mental Health, Paediatrics and Child Health, Royal Free & University College Medical School, University College London, Rowland Hill Street, London NW3 2PF

Kathryn J. Bennett PhD
Associate Professor, Department of Clinical Epidemiology and Biostatistics, Room 3V4D, Canadian Centre for Studies of Children at risk, McMaster University, 1200 Main St W, Hamilton, Ontario L8N 3Z5, Canada

Molly Benson BA
Doctoral Student in Clinical Psychology, Department of Psychology, University of Vermont, Burlington, VT 05405, USA

Sarah H. Bernard MD, MRCPsych, DRCOG
Consultant Psychiatrist, Learning Disabilities Team, Children's & Adolescents Department, The Maudsley Hospital, Denmark Hill, London SE5 8AZ

Colin D. Binnie MD, MA, FRCP
Professor of Clinical Neurophysiology, Department of Clinical Neurophysiology, Division of Neurosciences, Guy's, King's & St Thomas' School of Medicine, King's College Hospital, Denmark Hill, London SE5 9RS

Dorothy V.M. Bishop MA, DPhil
Wellcome Principal Research Fellow, and Professor of Developmental Neuropsychology, Oxford Study of Children's Communication Impairments, Department of Experimental Psychology, University of Oxford, South Parks Road, Oxford OX1 3UD

Dora Black MB, BCh, FRCPsych, FRCPCH, DPM
Honorary Consultant Child and Adolescent Psychiatrist, Traumatic Stress Clinic, London WIT 4PL

Malgorzata Borzyskowski FRCP, FRCPsych
Consultant Neuro-Developmental Paediatrician, Guy's and St. Thomas' Trust, Newcomen Centre, Guy's Hospital, London SE1 9RT

Stewart G. Boyd MD
Consultant Clinical Neurophysiologist, Department of Clinical Neurophysiology, The Hospital for Sick Children, Great Ormond Street, London WC1N 9NX

Margaret Boyer BA
Doctoral Student in Clinical Psychology, Department of Psychology, University of Vermont, Burlington, VT 05405, USA

David Brent MD, MS Hyg
Academic Chief, Child and Adolescent Psychiatry and Professor of Psychiatry, Pediatrics and Epidemiology, University of Pittsburgh School of Medicine, Western Psychiatric Institute and Clinic, 3811 O'Hara Street, Suite 112, Pittsburgh, PA 15213, USA

Kevin Browne PhD, CPsychol
Professor of Forensic & Family Psychology, University of Birmingham, Edgbaston, Birmingham B15 2TT and Advisor to the World Health Organisation Regional Office for Europe, Copenhagen

R. Brumback MD
Professor and Chairman Department of Pathology, Creighton University School of Medicine, St Joseph Hospital, 601 N. 30th Street, Omaha, NE 68131, USA

Stephen J. Ceci PhD
The Helen L. Carr Professor of Developmental Psychology, Department of Human Development, Cornell University, Ithaca, NY 14853, USA

P. Lindsay Chase-Lansdale PhD
Professor of Developmental Psychology, School of Education and Social Policy Faculty Fellow, Institute for Policy Research, Northwestern University, 2040 Sheridan Road, Evanston, IL 60208-4100, USA

Graham Clayden FRCP, FRCPCH
Reader and Consultant Paediatrician, St Thomas' Hospital, Lambeth Palace Road, London SE1 7EH

Donald J. Cohen MD (deceased)
Director, Child Study Center, Yale University School of Medicine, 230 South Frontage Road, New Haven, CT 06520-7900, USA

Nancy J. Cohen PhD, CPsych
Director of Research, Hincks-Dellcrest Institute, 114 Maitland Street, Toronto, Ontario M4Y 1E1, Canada

Bruce E. Compas PhD
Professor of Psychology, Medicine, and Pediatrics, Department of Psychology, University of Vermont, Burlington, VT 05405, USA

Elisabeth Dykens PhD
Professor of Psychology, University of California Los Angeles, Neuropsychiatric Institute, 760 Westwood Plaza, Los Angeles, C A 90024, USA

Felton Earls MD
Professor of Social Medicine, Project on Human Development in Chicago Neighborhoods, Harvard Medical School, 1430 Massachusetts Avenue, 4th floor, Cambridge, MA 02138, USA

Melinda Edwards BSc, DipClinPsych
Consultant Clinical Psychologist, Guy's and St. Thomas' Trust, Bloomfield Centre, Guy's Hospital, London SE1 9RT

Ivan Eisler MA, PhD, CPsychol
Senior Lecturer in Clinical Psychology and Course Chair MSc in Family Therapy, Psychotherapy Section, Institute of Psychiatry, De Crespigny Park, Denmark Hill, London SE5 8AF

Robert E. Emery PhD
Professor, Director of Clinical Training, and Director of the Center for Children, Families and the Law, Department of Psychology, Gilmer Hall, Box 400400, University of Virginia, Charlottesville, VA 22904-4400, USA

Anne Farmer MD, FRCRsych
Professor of Psychiatric Nosology, Social, Genetic and Developmental Psychiatry (SGDP) Research Centre, Institute of Psychiatry, De Crespigny Park, Denmark Hill, London SE5 8AF

Stanka A. Fitneva MA
Advanced Doctoral Candidate, Department of Human Development, Cornell University, Ithaca, NY 14853, USA

Eric Fombonne MD
Professor of Child and Adolescent Psychiatry, McGill University, and Director of Child and Adolescent Psychiatry, Montreal Children's Hospital, 4018 Ste-Catherine West, Montreal, Québec H3Z 1P2, Canada

Ruth Friedman MA, PhD
Legislative Associate, Democratic Staff, House Committee on Education and the Workforce, US House of Representatives, 1107 Longworth House Office Building, Washington, D.C. 20515, USA

M. Elena Garralda MD, MPhil, FRCPsych, FRCPCH
Professor of Child and Adolescent Psychiatry, Faculty of Medicine, Imperial College, St Mary's Campus, Norfolk Place, London W2 1PG

Scott T. Gaynor PhD
Assistant Professor of Psychology, Western Michigan University, Department of Psychology, 1903 West Michigan Avenue, Kalamazoo, MI 49008-5439, USA

Tiejo van Gent MD
Head of the Department for the Deaf and Hard of Hearing, Academic Centre for Child and Adolescent Psychiatry (Curium), Oegstgeest, The Netherlands, and Associate Professor of Child and Adolescent Psychiatry, University of Leiden, The Netherlands

Livia L. Gilstrap MA
Advanced Doctoral Candidate, Department of Human Development, Cornell University, Ithaca, NY 14853, USA

Danya Glaser MB, DCH, FRCPsych
Consultant Child and Adolescent Psychiatrist, Department of Psychological Medicine, Great Ormond Street Hospital for Children, London WC1N 3JH

Robert Goodman PhD, FRCPsych, MRCP
Professor of Brain and Behavioural Medicine, Department of Child and Adolescent Psychiatry, Institute of Psychiatry, De Crespigny Park, Denmark Hill, London SE5 8AF

Jonathan Green MB BS, FRCPsych
Senior Lecturer and Honorary Consultant in Child and Adolescent Psychiatry, University of Manchester and Manchester Children's University Hospitals, Academic Department of Child and Adolescent Psychiatry, Booth Hall Children's Hospital, Blackley, Manchester M9 7AA

Renzo Guerrini MD
Professor of Paediatric Neurology, Department of Neurology, The Hospital for Sick Children, Great Ormond Street, London WC1N 9NX

Jennifer Gutstein BA
315 College Road, Bronx, NY 10471, USA (formerly Research Assistant, Columbia University, 1051 Riverside Drive, Unit 78, NY 10032, USA)

Caryn Harper MS
Faculty Associate, Department of Neurology, University of Texas Southwestern Medical Center at Dallas, Exchange Park, Suite 13350, 6303 Forest Park, Dallas, TX 75390-9119, USA

Richard Harrington MB, ChB, MD, FRCPsych
*Professor of Child and Adolescent Psychiatry, University of
Manchester, Department of Child & Adolescent Psychiatry,
Royal Manchester Children's Hospital Pendlebury,
Manchester M27 4HA*

Jennifer Havens MD
*Assistant Professor of Clinical Psychiatry, Columbia University
College of Physicians & Surgeons, Children's Hospital of New York
Presbyterian, Room 619 North, 3959 Broadway, New York,
NY 10032, USA*

Martin Herbert PhD, FBPS
*Emeritus Professor of Clinical and Community Psychology, Exeter
University, School of Psychology, Exeter University, Exeter*

Isobel Heyman MB BS, PhD, MRCPsych
*Consultant Child Psychiatrist, Department of Child and Adolescent
Psychiatry, Institute of Psychiatry, De Crespigny Park, Denmark Hill,
London SE5 8AF*

Thomas V. Hicks BA
*Doctoral Student in Clinical Psychology, Department of Psychology,
University of Vermont, Burlington, VT 05405, USA*

Jonathan Hill BA, MBBChir, MRCP, MRCPsych
*Professor of Child and Developmental Psychiatry, University of
Liverpool, University of Child Mental Health, Mulberry House,
Royal Liverpool Children's Hospital, Alder Hey, Eaton Road,
Liverpool L12 2AP*

Peter Hill MA, MB, BChir, FRCP, FRCPsych, FRCPCH
*Professor of Child and Adolescent Psychiatry, Department of
Psychological Medicine, Great Ormond Street Hospital for Children,
London WC1N 3JH*

Peter Hindley BSc, MRCPsych, CACDP Stage III
*Consultant and Senior Lecturer in Child and Adolescent Psychiatry,
Department of Psychiatry, St Georges Hospital Medical School,
Cranmer Terrace, London, SW17 0RE*

Alison E. Hipwell BSc, MA, PhD, ClinPsyD
*Assistant Professor, Pittsburgh Girls Study, Western Psychiatric
Institute and Clinic, 4415 Fifth Avenue, Suite 134, Pittsburgh, PA
15213, USA*

Chris Hollis MB BS, BSc, PhD, DCH, MRCPsych
*Professor of Child & Adolescent Psychiatry, Developmental
Psychiatry Section, Division of Psychiatry, South Block, E Floor,
Queen's Medical Centre, Nottingham NG7 2UH*

Patricia Howlin BA, MSc PhD, FBPS
*Professor of Clinical Psychology, St Georges Hospital Medical
School, Psychology Department, Cranmer Terrace,
London SW17 0RE*

Joyce S. Hunter DSW
*Assistant Clinical Professor, Psychiatric Social Work, Department
of Psychiatry, College of Physicians & Surgeons, and Assistant
Professor of Public Health, Sociomedical Sciences, Columbia
University, New York; Director, Community Liaison Program,
HIV Center for Clinical and Behavioral Studies, New York State
Psychiatric Institute, Unit 29, 1051 Riverside Drive, New York,
NY 11104, USA*

Brian W. Jacobs MA, MRCP, DCH, FRCPsych
*Consultant Child and Adolescent Psychiatrist, Children's Department,
The Maudsley Hospital, Denmark Hill, London SE5 8AZ*

Michael Jellinek MD
*Professor of Psychiatry and of Pediatrics, Harvard Medical School,
and Chief, Child Psychiatry Service, Massachusetts General Hospital,
Bullfinch 351, Fruit St, Boston, MA 02114, USA*

Rachel Klein PhD
*Professor of Psychiatry, New York University, Child Study Center,
550 First Avenue, New York, NY 10016, USA*

Brian Konik BA
*Doctoral Student in Clinical Psychology, Department of Psychology,
University of Vermont, Burlington, VT 05405, USA*

R. Channi Kumar MD, PhD, FRCPsych (deceased)
*Professor of Perinatal Psychiatry, Section of Perinatal Psychiatry,
Institute of Psychiatry, De Crespigny Park, Denmark Hill,
London SE5 8AF*

Jonna Kuntsi BSc, MSc, PhD, CPsychol
*Lecturer, Social, Genetic and Developmental Psychiatry (SGDP)
Research Centre, Institute of Psychiatry, De Crespigny Park,
Denmark Hill, London SE5 8AF*

Lisa Laumann-Billings PhD
*Postdoctoral Fellow, Prevention Research Center for Family and
Child Health, University of Colorado Health Sciences Center,
1825 Marion Street, Denver, Colorado 80218, USA*

James F. Leckman MD
*Neison Harris Professor of Child Psychiatry, Pediatrics and
Psychology, Room I-265 SHM, Child Study Center, Yale University
School of Medicine, 230 South Frontage Road, New Haven, CT
06520-7900, USA*

Michael Little BA, PhD
*Researcher, Chapin Hall Center for Children at the University
of Chicago and Researcher, Dartington Social Research Unit,
Warren House, Dartington, Totnes TQ9 6EG*

Peter Loader MB BS, FRCPsych
*Senior Lecturer in Child and Adolescent Psychiatry, Guy's, Kings'
& St. Thomas' School of Medicine, Honorary Consultant in
Child and Adolescent Psychiatry, South London and Maudsley
NHS Trust, Department of Child and Adolescent Mental Health,
35 Blackprince Road, London SE11 6JJ*

Catherine Lord PhD
*Professor and Director of University of Michigan Autism &
Communicative Disorders Center (UMACC), 1111 Catherine Street,
Ann Arbor, MI 48109, USA*

Maureen Marks DPhil, CPsychol, AFBPS, MBPAS
*Senior Lecturer, Sections of Perinatal Psychiatry and Psychotherapy,
Institute of Psychiatry, De Crespigny Park, Denmark Hill,
London SE5 8AF*

Peter McGuffin MB, PhD, FRCP, FRCPsych, FMedSci
*Professor of Psychiatric Genetics and Director, Social, Genetic and
Developmental Psychiatry (SGDP) Research Centre, Institute of
Psychiatry, De Crespigny Park, Denmark Hill, London SE5 8AF*

Claude Ann Mellins PhD
*Assistant Professor of Clinical Psychology, Department of Psychiatry,
Columbia University, and Research Scientist, HIV Center for Clinical
and Behavioral Studies, New York State Psychiatric Institute, PO Box
15, 1051 Riverside Drive, New York, NY 10032, USA*

Enrico Mezzacappa MD
*Assistant Professor of Child Psychiatry, Department of Psychiatry, The
Children's Hospital, Boston, MA, USA*

Helen Minnis MD, PhD
*Specialist Registrar and Research Fellow, Department of Child and
Adolescent Psychiatry, Caledonia House, Yorkhill NHS Trust,
Glasgow G3 8SJ*

Janette Moore MSc, MRCPsych
*Social, Genetic and Developmental Psychiatry (SGDP) Research
Centre, Institute of Psychiatry, De Crespigny Park, Denmark Hill,
London SE5 8AF*

David A. Mrazek MD, FRCPsych
*Chair of Psychiatry and Psychology, Mayo Clinic, 200 First St SW,
Rochester, MN 55905, USA*

Michael Neve MA, PhD
*Senior Lecturer in the History of Medicine, Wellcome Trust Centre for
the History of Medicine, University College London, Euston House, 24
Eversholt Street, London NW1 1AD*

A. Rory Nicol MPhil, FRCP, FRCPsych, FRCPCH
*Visiting Professor, WHO Collaborating Centre, Institute of Psychiatry,
De Crespigny Park, Denmark Hill, London, SE5 8AF*

Anula Nikapota FRCPsych
*Honorary Senior Lecturer, Institute of Psychiatry, London, and
Consultant in Child and Adolescent Psychiatry, Lambeth Child and
Adolescent Community Mental Health Service, South London and
Maudsley NHS Trust, 19 Brixton Water Lane, London SW2 1NN*

Thomas G. O'Connor PhD
*Senior Lecturer, Department of Child and Adolescent Psychiatry and
Social, Genetic and Developmental Psychiatry (SGDP) Research
Centre, Institute of Psychiatry, De Crespigny Park, Denmark Hill,
London SE5 8AF*

David Offord MDCM, FRCP(C)
*Director, Canadian Centre for Studies of Children at Risk McMaster
University, & Hamilton Health Sciences Corporation,
1200 Main St W, Hamilton, Ontario L8N 3Z5, Canada*

Joanna Pearse RMN, CQSW, DipFT
*Family and Systemic Psychotherapist, The Maudsley Hospital,
South London and Maudsley NHS Trust, Denmark Hill,
London SE5 8AZ*

Daniel S. Pine MD
*Chief, Section on Development and Affective Neuroscience, Mood
and Anxiety Disorders Program, National Institute of Mental Health,
9000 Rockville Pike, Building 1, Room B3-10, Bethesda, Maryland
20892, USA*

Ronit Pressler MD
*Chadburn Lecturer in Clinical Neurophysiology, Department of
Clinical Neurophysiology, Division of Neurosciences, Guy's,
King's & St Thomas' School of Medicine, King's College Hospital,
Denmark Hill, London SE5 9RS*

Judith L. Rapoport MD
*Chief, Child Psychiatry Branch, Bldg 10 National Institute of Mental
Health, 10 Center Drive, MSC 1600, Bethesda, MD 29892, USA*

Paula K. Rauch MD
*Director, Child Psychiatry Consultation Service, Massachusetts
General Hospital, 55 Fruit Street, Boston, MA 02114, USA*

Alan Rushton BA, CQSW, PhD
*Senior Lecturer in Social Work, Section of Social Work and Social Care,
Health Services Research Department, The David Goldberg Centre,
Institute of Psychiatry, De Crespigny Park, London SE5 8AF*

Michael Rutter CBE, MD, FRCP, FRCPsych, FRS, FMedSci
*Professor of Developmental Psychopathology, Social, Genetic and
Developmental Psychiatry (SGDP) Research Centre, Institute of
Psychiatry, De Crespigny Park, Denmark Hill, London SE5 8AF*

Seija Sandberg MD
*Consultant and Senior Lecturer, Department of Psychiatry and
Behavioural Sciences, Royal Free and University College Medical
School, Wolfson Building, 48 Riding House Street,
London W1N 8AA*

Paramala Santosh MD, MRCPsych
*Lecturer, Department of Child and Adolescent Psychiatry,
Institute of Psychiatry, De Crespigny Park, Denmark Hill, London
SE5 8AF*

Russell Schachar MD, FRCP(C)
*Professor, Department of Child Psychiatry, The Hospital for Sick
Children, University of Toronto, Toronto, M5G 1X8, Canada*

Stephen Scott BSc, FRCP, MRCPsych
*Senior Lecturer and Consultant in Child and Adolescent Psychiatry,
Institute of Psychiatry, De Crespigny Park, Denmark Hill,
London SE5 8AF*

Joseph Sergeant PhD
Professor of Clinical Neuropsychology, Department of Clinical Psychology, Faculty of Psychology, University of Amsterdam, Roetersstraat 15, 1018 WB Amsterdam, The Netherlands

David Shaffer MB BS, FRCP, FRCPsych
Irving Philips Professor of Child Psychiatry, Columbia University, College of Physicians & Surgeons, New York State Psychiatric Institute, Division of Child Psychiatry, 722 West 168th Street, New York, NY 10032, USA

Emily Simonoff MD, MRCPsych
Professor of Child and Adolescent Psychiatry, Department of Child and Adolescent Psychiatry, Guy's, Kings' & St Thomas' Medical Schools, The Munro Centre, Kings College London, 66 Snowsfields, London SE1 3SS

David H. Skuse MD, FRCP, FRCPsych, FRCPCH
Professor of Behavioural Sciences, Behavioural Sciences Unit, Institute of Child Health, 30 Guilford Street, London WC1N 1EH

Margaret J. Snowling PhD, DipClinPsych, FBPsS
Professor of Psychology, Department of Psychology, University of York, Heslington, York YO10 5DD

Alan Stein MB BChir, FRCPsych
Professor of Child and Adolescent Psychiatry, Section of Child and Adolescent Psychiatry, Department of Psychiatry, University of Oxford, Warneford Hospital, Oxford OX3 7JX

Hans-Christoph Steinhausen MD, Dipl Psych, PhD
Professor and Head of Department of Child and Adolescent Psychiatry, University of Zurich, Neumuensterallee 9, Postfach CH-8032 Zurich, Switzerland

Susan E. Swedo MD
Chief, Pediatrics and Developmental Neuropsychiatry Branch, MSC 12 Building 10, National Institute of Mental Health, 10 Center Drive, Bethesda, MD 20892, USA

Rosemary Tannock PhD
Senior Scientist, Brain and Behavior Research Program, The Hospital for Sick Children and Associate Professor of Psychiatry, University of Toronto, Toronto, M5G 1X8, Canada

Eric Taylor MA, MB, FRCP, FRCPsych, FMedsci
Professor of Child and Adolescent Psychiatry, Department of Child and Adolescent Psychiatry, Institute of Psychiatry, De Crespigny Park, Denmark Hill, London SE5 8AF

Trevor Turner MD FRCPsych
Honorary Senior Lecturer at St Bartholomew's and The Royal London School of Medicine and Dentistry, Honorary Senior Research Fellow at the Wellcome Trust Centre for the History of Medicine at UCL, Department of Psychological Medicine, William Harvey House, St Bartholomew's Hospital, London EC1A 7BE

Jan Van der Ende MS
Research Psychologist, Erasmus Medical Center/Sophia Children's Hospital, Rotterdam, The Netherlands

Frank C. Verhulst MD, PhD
Professor and Director of Child and Adolescent Psychiatry, Erasmus Medical Center/Sophia Children's Hospital, Rotterdam, The Netherlands

Fred Volkmar MD
Professor of Child Psychiatry, Pediatrics and Psychology, Yale University School of Medicine, New Haven, CT 06520, USA

V. Robin Weersing PhD
Postdoctoral Fellow, Child Psychiatry, Western Psychiatric Institute Clinic, 3811 O'Hara Street, Suite 112, Pittsburgh, PA 15213, USA

Warren A. Weinberg MD
Professor of Neurology and Pediatrics, Director of Pediatric Behavior Neurology Program, Division of Pediatric Neurology, Department of Neurology, University of Texas Southwestern Medical Center at Dallas, 6303 Forest Park, Suite 13.350, Dallas, TX 75235-9119, USA

William Yule MA, DipPsychol, PhD, FBPsS, C. Psychol
Professor of Applied Child Psychology, Department of Psychology, Institute of Psychiatry, De Crespigny Park, Denmark Hill, London SE5 8AF

Kenneth J. Zucker PhD, CPsych
Psychologist-in-Chief, Centre for Addiction and Mental Health, and Head, Child and Adolescent Gender Identity Clinic, Child Psychiatry Program–Clarke Division, 250 College St, Toronto, Ontario M5T 1R8, Canada

Preface to the Fourth Edition

The rate of change in child and adolescent mental health has accelerated in the years between the third and fourth editions of this book. Nearly every chapter has had to be completely rewritten and reconceptualized to take account of substantial research and clinical advances; the preparation of this volume has correspondingly been an exciting and encouraging (albeit challenging) task. In this preface, we pick our some of the main factors that are driving this development.

This edition differs from its predecessors in seven main respects. First, it reflects real gains in empirical knowledge and conceptual understanding. These are evident in all chapters throughout the book. Second, there is an extended range of chapters on measurement issues, a field in which considerable progress has been made. Third, we have sought to balance 'academic' advances with an equally detailed attention to clinical skills and clinical application. That is evident through the book but is also indexed by new chapters on diagnostic formulations and on the applied science aspects of clinical assessment. Fourth, we have endeavoured to introduce a greater developmental orientation; again, this is reflected both in many individual chapters and in a new chapter on this consideration. Fifth, we have sought to pay greater attention to sociocultural and ethnic issues and have added two chapters dealing specifically with these features. Sixth, there is greater attention to genetic findings and their implications, with a detailed discussion of misunderstandings about supposed genetic determinism and the possible misuse of genetics, as well as the huge clinical potential that is likely to follow genetic advances. Finally, the trend for an increasing international, and interdisciplinary, authorship that has applied over the first three editions has been further extended. This reflects not only the wide distribution of centres of excellence in the field of mental health but also the increasing cooperation and collaboration among such centres.

The gains in knowledge over the last few years have been driven both by the accumulation of scientific research and by changes in the wider society. One research development with high impact has been the advance of the methodology of assessment. Reliable instruments for data capture, and agreed criteria for disorders, have made knowledge more public. This in turn is driving both an increase in replicable findings about disorders and an increase in the practical application of quantitative measures to clinical assessment. Many clinics, for example, now apply schemes of assessment that were originally worked out for research purposes.

Advances in basic scientific knowledge have also provided some influential changes in the field. The pervasiveness and impact of genetic contributions to disorder have been increasingly recognized: twin and adoptive studies have clarified both the genetic and the environmental influences on the common problems of mental health, and an increasing range of uncommon single-gene influences have been identified. The mapping of the human genome and the use of molecular chemistry to clarify the modes of expression of genetic variations have added an immediate relevance to genetic investigations and it seems certain that these will continue. Of course, the application of this knowledge to the clinic is for the most part confined to the advice and explanations that clinicians provide. Indeed, it is necessary to caution against a narrowly deterministic notion of how genes influence psychopathology. Even for the simplest genetic influences, their expression is strongly influenced by the actions of other genes and by interactions with the environment. The relationships between genotype and phenotype will need a great deal more understanding, and for the multifactorial disorders with which psychiatry usually deals their complexity may baffle our understanding for some time to come.

The rapid development of neuroimaging techniques is also full of promise for the future, and the chapter on physical investigations has correspondingly been expanded substantially. The availability of techniques (such as magnetic resonance) that do not depend upon ionizing radiation has allowed their application to young people, and the psychiatry of childhood has therefore started to be changed by the understanding of the brain that has informed adult psychiatry for decades. For this, as for genetic advances, the major immediate impact has been intangible: it has created a climate of opinion in which the disorders of mental health are seen in the context of neurobiology. The use of psychotropic drugs for young people has increased considerably in most countries over the last ten years. This increase is not primarily because new and more satisfactory drugs have been introduced but, rather, it has arisen as a result of an increased professional readiness to prescribe, and this in turn may follow as much from beliefs about causality as from improved knowledge of indications. Indeed, there may be a risk of a professional and practical division between a biologically oriented psychiatry and a group of disciplines focusing on psychosocial influences. Any such split would weaken understanding and practice. The authors in this volume come from a wide range of professional disciplines, but all have been at pains to bring together different perspectives and indicate how different approaches can fit together.

Developmental psychopathology, still a young science, is making it possible for clinicians to make more informed judgements about the future course of disorder and the influences upon it that need to be assessed. The impact of deprivation and adversity is better understood, and advice to social work agencies and law courts has changed accordingly. The psychological understanding of what is altered in the neurodevelopmental disorders has pressed on, and has been one of the agents of change in the ascertainment and treatment of pervasive developmental disorders. The increased recognition of depressive disorders in young people owes a good deal to the clarification of their longitudinal course. The developmental issues involved in psychopathology have received increased attention in this edition, both in disorder-oriented chapters and in a new chapter bringing them together.

The increase in randomized controlled clinical trials is making the foundations of treatment ever more explicit. For the most part, it is still the case that evidence for any one disorder comes from a number of small trials with varying methodology. Indeed, the differences are so substantial that it has not yet been possible to base all treatment recommendations on systematic and quantitative meta-analytic reviews. Rather, authors have made critical narrative reviews about the evidence base and their recommendations are based on clinical expertise as well as the published literature. Nevertheless, it is plain from the chapters on treatments and services that evaluative research is increasingly the basis of guidelines.

Many of the factors driving change have been social and economic rather than scientific. Health care purchasers have become more organized, better informed, and increasingly concerned to contain the costs of health care. The results, whether in managed care or publicly funded services, includes pressure on providers to follow agreed guidelines and even detailed protocols in management regimes. This can have advantages: treatment recommendations should of course be explicit and challengeable, and there are too many areas noted in this volume where common clinical practices still fall well short of good practice guidelines. But there are dangers if protocols are applied mechanically and without sufficient consideration of individual variability. It remains the case that treatment should be focused on the individual, not the disorder. Our authors have correspondingly emphasized the principles underlying assessment and treatment rather than a set of rules, and they have borne in mind the great variety of ways in which health care is organized. Furthermore, protocols that are not based on sound evidence are very likely to be counterproductive, and the chapters of this book have striven to indicate the extent to which recommendations are based on public and reliable evidence and therefore the confidence that can be placed in them.

The information revolution has combined with other forms of social change to make a different relationship between the consumers and the providers of health care. In principle, there is everything to welcome in the increasingly active and well-informed participation of families in treatment decisions. But the heterogeneity and volume of health information available, for instance on television and the Internet, brings its own problems. Myths spread as quickly as truths. Our authors have often found it hard to recommend sources of health information for the public that are clear, accessible and authoritative. The problem of improving the quality as well as the quantity of public information about mental health remains unsolved. The need for authoritative and integrative texts for professionals remains strong.

The changing face of child and adolescent psychiatry is reflected in changes of authors for a good number of the chapters, and we should like to take this opportunity of expressing our deep gratitude, not only to the contributors to this edition but to those who created the previous three editions. Most especially, we are personally as well as editorially indebted to Lionel Hersov for his wise and supportive editorship over the whole of the earlier history of this work and for his contribution to its success.

Acknowledgements

We are most appreciative of the authors' expertise and effort, and of their constructive responsiveness in dealing with the many editorial suggestions on possible new material that needed adding, topics that required strengthening, extended international coverage that was desirable, clarifications that would help readability and integrations across chapters. We note with great sadness the premature deaths of Channi Kumar and Donald Cohen during the course of producing the book. Both were at a peak in their careers. The world is much indebted to Channi Kumar for his pioneering work in developing and championing the field of perinatal psychiatry, and to Donald Cohen for his bridging of psychoanalysis and biological research, as well as for his international leadership in child and adolescent psychiatry as a whole.

The production of the book has been very much a team effort, and we have been fortunate in having such a good team to work with. Special thanks are due to Rachel Mawhood who exercised overall administrative responsibility for the complex enterprise of checking chapters prior to submission to the publishers, and to Gill Rangel who had the comparable responsibility for the task of checking and collating proofs (as well as much detailed work on individual chapters prior to submission). Both stages needed to run smoothly to a tight timetable and it was crucial to keep an eagle eye for inconsistencies or inaccuracies. We are also most grateful to Alice Emmott for her efficiency in translating the manuscripts into the printed page. Authors will be well aware of the care with which these multiple tasks were undertaken. Thanks also go to Angela Cottingham for her professionalism in preparing the index. Expert referees who commented on individual chapters were very helpful, but must remain anonymous. The editorial team also owes much to Jenny Wickham who had the main responsibility for dealing with several individual chapters but who also played a full role as a member of a cohesive, effective administrative team. We would also like to express particular thanks to David Shaffer for most helpful guidance and suggestions on authors during the planning stage of the book.

Michael Rutter
Eric Taylor

Preface to the First Edition

These are exciting times for anyone working in the field of child psychiatry. A wider understanding of child development now throws a clearer light on deviations from the normal pattern; knowledge of the nature and causes of psychiatric disorders in childhood is steadily increasing; new and effective methods of treatment are evolving; and clinical and education services for children with mental disorders are growing in scope and sophistication. The first academic departments of child psychiatry in the United Kingdom are now established to meet the needs for teaching and research and to add to the existing body of knowledge. A serious concern to raise training standards in the specialty has led to recommendations on the range of content of training and a national exercise to visit and appraise all training schemes is under way.

For these reasons the time seemed ripe for a new and different textbook of child psychiatry. Our aim has been to provide an accurate and comprehensive account of the current state of knowledge through the integration of research approaches and findings with the understanding that comes from clinical experience and practice. Each chapter scrutinizes existing information and emphasizes areas of growth and fresh ideas on a particular topic in a rigorous and critical fashion, but also in practical vein to help clinicians meet the needs of individual children and their families.

In planning the book we had to decide how to choose authors of individual chapters. Obviously we wanted colleagues who had made important contributions in their fields of interest and who could write with authority and knowledge. We were fortunate in our choice and we are deeply indebted to all of them. We also decided that it would be appropriate to invite contributions from those who had worked at The Bethlem Royal and The Maudsley Hospital or its closely associated postgraduate medical school, The Institute of Psychiatry. Over the years 'The Maudsley' has played a major role in training psychiatrists from all parts of the world and members of its staff have been among the leaders in both research and clinical practice. The fact that we have all worked at the same institution has produced some similarities: a firm acceptance of the value of interdisciplinary collaboration; an intense interest in new ideas and creative thinking; a commitment to the integration of academic and clinical approaches; a concern for empirical findings; and a belief in the benefits that follow from open discussion between people who hold differing views. As all of us work with children we have a common concern with developmental theories and with the process of development. However, as will also be apparent, we do not share any single theoretical viewpoint. A variety of theoretical approaches are represented in the chapters which also reflect a differing emphasis on biological, sociocultural, behavioural and psychodynamic aetiologies and formulations.

It is also fitting that this book should be based on The Joint Hospital as it has player such an important part in the development of child psychiatry. Children with psychiatric disorders were first seen at The Bethlehem Royal Hospital as long ago as 1800 and Henry Maudsley was unusual among the psychiatrists of his day in appreciating the importance of psychiatric disorders arising in childhood. In his *Physiology and Pathology of Mind*, published in 1867, he included a 34-page chapter on 'Insanity of early life'. The Maudsley Hospital first opened its doors just over half a century ago, children have always been included among its patients and the Children's Department became firmly established during those early years. Since then, and especially with the first British academic appointment in child psychiatry at the Institute of Psychiatry in the 1950s, it has trained many child psychiatrists who now practise in all parts of the globe.

The book is organized into five sections. The first eight chapters review different influences on psychological development in childhood and are followed by three that discuss the foremost developmental theories. A third section describes some of the crucial issues in clinical assessment and the fourth deals systematically with the various clinical syndromes and their treatment. The final section comprises six chapters that bring together knowledge on some of the main therapeutic approaches. We have sought to include most of the topics and issues that are central to modern child psychiatry, but there has been no attempt to cover all known syndromes and symptoms. Instead, the focus has been on concepts and methods with special emphasis on those areas where development of new ideas or knowledge has been greatest.

We hope that the book's contents will be of interest and use to all those professionally concerned with the care, study and treatment of children with psychiatric disorders. We will be satisfied if, in the words of Sir Aubrey Lewis, it also helps the psychiatrist in training to acquire 'reasoning and understanding' and fits him 'to combine the scientific and humane temper in his studies as the psychiatrist needs to'.

M. Rutter
L. Hersov

1

Classification: Conceptual Issues and Substantive Findings

Eric Taylor and Michael Rutter

Uses and abuses of classification

A classification is more like a language than a collection of objects. It supports communication and provides an aid to thinking about complex problems. The virtues of a good scientific classification are clarity, comprehensiveness, acceptability to users and fidelity to nature; a scheme should change as understanding alters. Each class in the scheme is a concept, not a thing. Its value is in relating individual cases to others, and a scientifically powerful class will do so in ways that are important to the user and include a good deal of meaning. When a case is assigned to a powerful class, many predictions follow.

Students of mental health face a remarkably broad collection of phenomena, the sort of classification they need will vary for different purposes, and therefore any one scheme is bound to be a compromise. Early attempts at classifying children's disorders were strongly based on psychoanalytic theory (Freud 1965; Group for the Advancement of Psychiatry 1966). However, this was theory without strong empirical foundations and it soon became evident that different practitioners used the concepts in rather different ways. The reliability among raters was found to be very low for diagnoses based on theoretical concepts (Rutter *et al.* 1969); by contrast, reasonable agreement could be reached on the description of what mental problems were actually being presented. The overriding need for clarity in communication therefore gave rise to a change of approach. Modern schemes, which can be taken to date from DSM-III (American Psychiatric Association 1980) and ICD-9 (World Health Organization 1977, 1978) are founded mostly, though not exclusively, on descriptions of patterns of symptomatology. However, they are not intended to end there. The classic instance of psychiatric classification is Kraepelin's distinction between schizophrenia and manic-depressive psychosis; it was justified by the prediction from symptom pattern to developmental course. The justification of child psychiatric classes is their ability to predict significant aspects of course, causes and response to intervention (Rutter 1965, 1978). As understanding develops, these aspects are likely to play a stronger part in the definition of concepts of disorder.

Research purposes

Researchers into the psychopathology of young people need good diagnostic schemes for several purposes. They often need groups of children that are reasonably homogeneous with respect to what is being investigated. The replicability of their group definitions will affect the use that others can make of their results. They are also likely to be interested in the testable predictions that derive from a classification. In mature sciences, a classification can itself be a scientific tool, as in cladistics where the relations of bodily structure among animals are a means for studying evolutionary descent. This is occasionally the case in psychopathology, when similarities between obsessions and stereotypies led to trials of a treatment for one condition in the other, or similarities between the symptoms of mania and attention deficit hyperactivity disorder (ADHD) led to cross-disorder neurochemical studies. For all these purposes, precision and replicability are the key requirements. Often it will not matter very much if many cases are left unclassified, so long as those that are classified are done so accurately but researchers also want their conclusions to guide practice, and therefore they wish to choose classes that practitioners will recognize and use.

Clinical purposes

Practitioners need to know how to apply research findings to an individual case, so a widely accepted classification scheme is indispensable. For them, a scheme leaving many cases unclassified has serious drawbacks because it cuts the bridge between their practice and the research that should inform it. Indeed, if research definitions have drifted too far from clinical ones, it may be quite misleading to generalize lessons from strictly defined research groups to broader and vaguer clinical ones. They have other needs for classification: for example, in communication between clinicians, statistical record-keeping and audit, for which homogeneity of groups in severity and responsiveness to intervention may be more important than homogeneity with respect to cause. In communication with users and carers, they may use an implicit system of classification that is based upon lay as well as scientific concepts; as when the idea of a minimal brain dysfunction, although discredited scientifically, supposedly is still found useful in explanation.

Abuses

Classifications, like other useful tools, can be abused. Critics have attacked the abuses of psychiatric categorization from various points of view. The critiques are important to heed because they carry lessons for practice. They caution, for example, that it is possible to reify a diagnosis and exaggerate the power of the concept. Psychiatric categories may come to be regarded by long familiarity as things rather than as concepts. This would occur if, for example, a teacher protests that an inattentive and impulsive child does not 'really' have ADHD because the cause lies in the social situation; or if children with a disproportionate difficulty in learning to read were to be denied specific educational help on the grounds that they did not 'really' have a specific learning disability because there was no evidence of neurological abnormality. It needs to be kept in mind that psychiatric diagnoses are usually descriptive, not explanatory. 'ADHD' is a description of the behaviour of a child who is inattentive and impulsive, not a disease that explains why the child behaves in that way.

A diagnostic label may also be misleading by lumping unlike things together. For example, it has been noted several times that tricyclic antidepressants are very frequently prescribed for children with major depressive disorders in spite of the evidence base that indicates that they are usually ineffective in depressed children. The practice seems to be maintained by the use of the diagnostic concept derived from adult psychopathology without sufficient recognition of a crucial age difference with respect to tricyclic medications.

Another adverse effect of diagnosis is the obscuring of assumptions that are involved. Sonuga-Barke (1998) has re-emphasized the psychopathologist's fallacy—that because a child has been brought as a patient there must be something wrong with him or her. Impulsiveness, for example, is not necessarily an organismic dysfunction; it may, under some conditions of reward, represent an adaptive adjustment to the environment. Therefore one needs to keep in mind the full range of problems that present; for example, to classify social stressors as well as behavioural patterns.

Similarly, a diagnosis may hide heterogeneity. Children with a disorder are not all the same. To take just one example of this truism, the intelligence of children with Down syndrome (which is not usually inherited) still shows strong genetic influences, because the differences of intelligence within children who have Down syndrome are marked and are partly determined by the same factors that determine intelligence in the general population. The corresponding caution is that disorders are the subject of classification, not people. Descriptors, such as 'the autistic' or 'the brain damaged', seem to imply that all affected people are similar and that the disorder represents all that is important about the individual. This serves to reinforce false overgeneralization and stereotyping; phrases such as 'people with autism' are to be preferred.

Other problems in developing classifications, such as cultural dependence, will be considered throughout this chapter. The recognition of abuses is not a reason to abandon classification. It would be impossible to do so if we are to maintain the possibility of learning and teaching about disorder. However, it does underline the need to appreciate the strengths and the weaknesses of particular classificatory schemes. This chapter describes scientific issues in identifying and arranging the taxons (which

are the units of a scheme of classification and may be categories or dimensions), and in assigning individual cases to the taxons, and some practical issues in the application of their results.

Types of classification

Categories and dimensions

The choice of a categorical or a dimensional system of ordering has generated much debate (Sonuga-Barke 1998). A thoroughgoing categorical arrangement is often described, although only by its detractors, as a medical model. This is a highly misleading view of medicine, which incorporates dimensional as well as categorical approaches. One example would be that of blood pressure, which is a dimension distributed continuously in the population; elevated blood pressure (hypertension) is a diagnostic category, but it is based on the quantitative idea of the degree of elevation that entails significant risk and at which treatment is justified. Another example is that of anaemia; not only are levels of haemoglobin continuously distributed, but the level that is judged to be a problem to treat will depend upon other factors, such as the cause and the society in which it is encountered.

Nevertheless, it is plain that there are many constraints on clinicians' thinking that favour a set of categories. The output from many clinical encounters is a set of categorical decisions: a child either is, or is not, prescribed a drug; or admitted into a treatment programme; or taken into care. It is therefore convenient, though obviously not essential, for diagnostic thinking to fall into the same mode. The convenience may be more apparent than real. It invites an immediate abuse, in which the treatment is determined directly and exclusively by the diagnosis. This possibility becomes all too real in some types of practice. The need of busy clinicians for simple rules of thumb, and the wish of some purchasers of health care to restrict treatment to mechanically defined groups and protocols, can lead to a lack of careful planning of care for the individual case.

It is sometimes said that categorical thinking is inherent in the human mind. It arises in the first months of life (Blewitt 1994); in adults it is deeply rooted, to the extent that formless sets of stimuli are often perceived as consisting of component categories, and categorical thinking characterizes the lay theories through which non-experts perceive psychological abnormality (Schoeeman et al. 1993). Even if this is the natural tendency of the mind, especially when coping with complex information under pressure to make decisions, it is not necessarily the best approach. Artificial intelligence can increasingly be used to assist in handling complex information sets, and need not be constrained by human infirmity.

Categories have other practical advantages (Klein & Riso 1996); a single term, if carefully chosen, carries a great deal of meaning very conveniently and will be much more tractable in communication with parents and teachers than a large set of dimensional scores. These advantages have ensured that diagnostic schemes are mostly categorical; and dimensional ordering is for the most part either secondary or rather tentative and speculative (e.g. Appendix B of DSM-IV: American Psychiatric Association 1994).

Dimensional thinking has been more attractive to contemplative researchers, especially those dealing with graded environmental stressors, be they physical or psychosocial. However, dimensional liability is also a key feature in genetic thinking, despite the fact that individual alleles are either present or absent (see McGuffin & Rutter, Chapter 12). Which type of thinking maps most helpfully on to the causes of disorder is not obvious, and may well differ for different kinds of psychopathology. Nevertheless, throughout medicine, even when dealing with categorical disease states, dimensional risk factors are the rule rather than the exception.

The distinctions between categories and dimensions should not be exaggerated. Generally, each can be translated into the other. A category can be expressed as a set of dimensional scores, and a profile of dimensional scores is a category. Indeed, the degree to which an individual case fits a category can itself be a dimensional construct, and should perhaps be considered as such more often. Sometimes it is preferable to use both ways of thinking about a single domain. IQ is better conceived as a dimension when the purpose is to predict educational achievement; but low IQ (e.g. below 50) is better thought of categorically when the purpose is to consider whether structural disorder of the brain is likely to be present (see below). Hypertension is conveniently regarded as a diagnostic category when the purpose is to select cases for treatment; as a dimension when analysing the physiological reasons for changes in blood pressure; and as a category again when considering the different factors determining variations in the most severely affected cases at the top of the range.

Another conceptual problem arises because an undoubtedly discrete cause may give rise to a continuum of problems at the level of behavioural expression. For example, the two genes known to give rise to tuberous sclerosis can both be associated with a very wide range in the severity and type of the resulting psychological disorder. This is not strange; their effects in giving rise to physical changes, such as the characteristic malformations in the brain, vary greatly between individuals. It would have been quite wrong to conclude from the continuously distributed range of severity of psychological disorder associated with tuberous sclerosis that the underlying cause would also be graded in severity.

In spite of the difficulties involved, the testing of assumptions about the nature of the underlying problems is important. For example, it is likely to guide research strategy in investigating a genetic contribution to disorder (see McGuffin & Rutter, Chapter 12). One classic research strategy has been to examine distributions of cases along a continuum of severity to see if there is a discontinuity between normality and pathology, such as a bimodal distribution. Most rating scales, for example, have indicated that hyperactive behaviour is distributed continuously, with progressively fewer cases at successively higher levels of definition and no sign of a 'hump on the graph' (Taylor et al. 1991). This is technically and conceptually problematic. The power of

tests for mixed distributions is low (Meehl 1995) and even very large numbers of cases can fail to give unequivocal answers. Random error in the measurement of properties will blur the sharpness of any distinctions based upon them. Severity in itself may not be the grounds for definition of a separate category. For example, the identification of a poor-outcome subgroup in early onset schizophrenia is based upon a qualitative difference—the presence of neurocognitive changes—rather than on the severity of 'schizophrenic symptoms' (see Hollis, Chapter 37).

Some investigators have compared the effect size of a continuous measure with a categorical one in predicting an external association such as outcome. For example, Fergusson & Horwood (1995) argued on this basis that a dimensional measure of disruptive behaviour in childhood gave a better prediction of adolescent outcome than a discrete category of childhood disorder. This may say more about the power of alternative statistical methods than about taxonomy; and it ignores the possibility that a strongly predictive category of antisocial behaviour may be present, but one that is based upon the type of problems rather than the severity of disruptiveness. This was, for example, the conclusion of Bergman & Magnusson (1997) in another longitudinal study, predicting antisocial outcome, that included a wider range of possible predictors, physiological as well as behavioural. Moffitt (1993) also concluded, from analysis of the longitudinal course of a population cohort of boys, that an antisocial outcome in adult life was characteristic, not so much of the boys who had been the most disruptive adolescents, but those who had had the combination of early onset and neurodevelopmental impairments.

Another research strategy has been to examine the distribution of cases against a measure of presumed aetiology and to seek a point of discontinuity; for example, in comparing successive levels of definition of hyperactivity against measures of neurodevelopmental delay and reporting that the putative risk factor was more common only in the most severe subgroup of 'hyperkinetic disorder' (Taylor et al. 1991). This strategy shares the limitations of the first, and entails the further doubt of whether the risk factor chosen is truly causative. It may become more feasible as more specific causes are discovered—such as molecular genetic abnormalities. Other genetic strategies have already been elegantly employed in twin designs. Eaves et al. (1993) went beyond the definition on the basis of single cut-off scores, and applied a latent class analysis to ADHD symptoms in a comparison of monozygotic and dizygotic twins. They successively fitted models assuming different numbers of classes, and found the best fit with a model of three separate classes. Gjone et al. (1996) addressed a similar question by comparing group heritability with individual heritability of ADHD symptoms in a twin study using multiple regression techniques (De Fries & Fulker 1988). Their conclusion was different. The extent to which cotwins show a regression to the mean in their scores did not function differently at the extremes of the distribution. This was in keeping either with a more dimensional view—with heritability similar across the whole continuum—or with a single, very common category. The issues are not resolved, even for this rather well-studied condition; and indeed the method can require troublesomely large numbers. But genetic strategies such as these, especially when they can be applied to test hypothesized qualitative distinctions of severity, seem to offer encouraging future advances.

In short, the choice of dimensions against categories is complex, hard to resolve, and likely to be different for different conditions. Mixed classification systems are likely to develop, in which some types of problems are subclassified by severity and others by type. For the moment, there are so many uncertainties about whether dimensional or categorical arrangements better represent nature that a deeper pathogenetic understanding will be needed before the question is resolved.

Multiaxial classification systems

Categorical classifications can be based on allotting cases to the single category they best fit, or on multiple categorization—a case may be simultaneously classified in several ways. Powerful classifications, such as those of botany, aim for a set of mutually exclusive categories that are collectively exhaustive. Every case then falls into one, and only one, class. This would be an idealized view of medicine, because in practice multiple diseases are often present in the same person—sometimes because one kind of adversity tends to entail others. It can be a good discipline to try to fit multiple problems into a single pattern, but it is also important to detect a secondary disease even when it is masked by a more obvious one.

One kind of multiplicity is obviously necessary; different domains of problems need different classifications. It makes no sense to ask whether a child has asthma or intellectual retardation. They constitute problems of different types, and are best considered on separate axes. Field trials of early versions of the International Classifications of Disease (ICD) (Rutter *et al.* 1969; Tarjan *et al.* 1972) indicated that many disagreements between clinicians were of this type and, correspondingly, that reliability among diagnostic raters could be increased if they were not asked to choose between, say, autism and severe intellectual retardation, but were allowed to choose both, one on an axis of psychiatric disorder and the other on one of intellectual ability. This not only increases agreement, but provides a richer conceptualization and an opportunity to code and examine the extent to which, in this example, intellectual ability modifies the course and treatment response of autism.

A multiaxial system embodies this conceptual refinement; it differs from a multicategory system in that every axis needs a coding (even if the coding is of 'no abnormality'). Axes of psychiatric syndromes, somatic diseases, psychosocial stressors and severity of impairment have been incorporated in the multiaxial version of ICD-10 (WHO 1992, 1993). Specific learning disabilities and intellectual impairments are dealt with in rather different ways by DSM-IV and ICD-10 (in which they are independent axes); the important feature is that both, in different ways, allow the clinician to record, systematically and separately, the extent to which both general and specific learning impairments are present.

Multiaxial systems of classification have become the norm in child/adolescent psychiatry for five main reasons. First, they avoid false dichotomies resulting from having to decide between two diagnoses that do not, in any meaningful sense, constitute alternatives. The example given of autism or mental retardation illustrates the point. The first gives information on the clinical syndrome whereas the second describes the level of intellectual impairment. Secondly, because there has to be a coding on each and every axis, the classification provides information that is both more complete and less ambiguous. Thus, in a multicategory system the absence of a coding of mental retardation could mean that the child had normal intelligence, or that the child was mentally retarded but the clinician did not consider that it was relevant to the referral problem, or that the diagnosis was omitted by error. Such an ambiguity could not arise with a multiaxial system. Thirdly, it avoids artefactual unreliability resulting from differing theoretical assumptions. Thus, psychosocial adversity would be coded as present by both the clinician who viewed it as the main cause and by the clinician who saw it as only a minor contributor. The same would apply to somatic conditions such as cerebral palsy or diabetes. Fourthly, it provides a means by which to note systematically, not only the presenting clinical picture, but also possible causal factors (or factors likely to influence prognosis or response to treatment) and degree of overall psychosocial impairment. Finally, because of these features it represents a style of thinking that is much closer to most clinician's preferred style of conceptualization than is the case with a system that forces everything into the Procrustean bed of a diagnosis based only on symptom pattern.

Handling of comorbidity: single vs. multiple category systems

Another kind of multiplicity is provided by the co-occurrence of two different types of symptom pattern, such as major depression and conduct disorder. The key issue is whether, in reality, these represent varied manifestations of the same disorder, the simultaneous presence of two conditions that happen to have arisen in the same individual quite independently, the fact that the two disorders share some of their risk factors, or some mechanism by which one disorder creates a risk for the other (Caron & Rutter 1991; Rutter 1997). Such comorbidity (meaning the situation in which two or more separate and independent disorders are present in the same person) is almost the rule in the field of psychopathology (Angold *et al.* 1999). It complicates the diagnostic process throughout medicine. On the other hand, the reasons for the associations among disorders can also provide valuable clues to the understanding of pathogenesis.

The presentation of several patterns of disturbance by the same person may not be caused only by comorbid disorders; and in practice the term 'comorbidity' is often applied more broadly, to all the possible reasons for apparent associations between disorders. Comorbidity is less common in epidemiological studies than in clinic surveys, because referral and other biases play a part in generating—or obscuring—associations in clinic attenders. It has long been known that comorbid disorders will always be misleadingly frequent in clinic groups, if either condition can lead to referral (Berkson 1946). However, it is plain that overlap is very common in epidemiological series, even if less dramatically so than at clinics, so these kinds of bias cannot be the whole story. Sometimes the overlap stems from imperfections in the definitions of disorder, so that the same criteria are common to more than one condition, as when symptoms of overactivity are included in the definitions both of mania and of ADHD. Sometimes an apparent association arises because of a lack of clarity about the boundaries of disorders. Obsessive-compulsive symptomatology may, for example, sometimes arise only in the course of a depressive disorder and remit with it. Similarly, the complications of a disorder may sometimes, and misleadingly, appear as a separate problem; people with long-standing obsessive-compulsive disorder may become depressed as a reaction to their predicament. Sometimes an association between disorders arises because they are both consequences of an underlying, and more fundamental psychopathological liability. For example, autistic and hyperactive features are quite commonly found together in children with diffuse disease or disorder of the brain. Evidence can be quite conflicting about the reasons for associations, and they may vary from one centre to another. For example, there is an undoubted link between Tourette disorder and ADHD, but some investigators find that this reflects genetic cosegregation, others that it does not (see Leckman & Cohen, Chapter 36).

However, comorbidity can also arise because one disorder represents an early manifestation of the other; this seems to be the case with generalized anxiety and depressive disorder (Silberg *et al.*, 2001), and with oppositional/defiant disorder and conduct disorder (Lahey *et al.* 1999; Eaves *et al.*, 2000). In this circumstance, at the point of transition, both 'disorders'—actually both manifestations of the same disorder—may co-occur. Alternatively, the presence of one disorder may, through its effects, provide a risk mechanism for another condition. Possibly, this is one reason why antisocial behaviour predisposes to depressive symptomatology. Antisocial individuals act in ways that create interpersonal and social stress situations (Robins 1966; Champion *et al.* 1995).

Fuller consideration of the reasons for comorbidity and investigational strategies are provided by Caron & Rutter (1991) and Rutter (1997). Classification schemes need to be able to change to reflect advancing knowledge, and to be flexible enough to accommodate the differing reasons for the coexistence of mental disorders.

In the meanwhile, classification systems have to have rules on how to deal with comorbidity. Both ICD-10 and DSM-IV accept the need to be able to make multiple diagnoses if it is clear that the individual truly does have two or more separate conditions. After all, in most circumstances, it cannot be supposed that the presence of one disorder protects against others, although that can happen. Accordingly, someone with, say, autism or schizophrenia, will sometimes develop some other mental disorder if they experience the risk factors for it. It is necessary to be able to record that that is the case. A strict single category system would be unworkable and neither of the main systems have such a requirement.

Nevertheless, there is a dilemma on how to classify when there is uncertainty on whether or not the two conditions are truly separate and independent. ICD-10 and DSM-IV differ somewhat in their approach (see Rutter & Taylor, Chapter 2). Both provide for a hierarchical approach in a few instances (see below) and both provide a few mixed categories when there is good evidence that they both represent a single disorder (e.g. mixed episode of mania and depression). However, ICD-10 has rather more mixed categories (e.g. mixed anxiety and depressive disorder and depressive conduct disorder). The rationale is that the weight of evidence suggests either that there is something distinctive about the admixture, as compared with the situation when either condition occurs on its own, or that the same disorder commonly gives rise to this admixture of symptoms. It provides an economical way of communicating and it is a practice that is common in medicine. However, it has two possible disadvantages. First, the overall placement of the combination category in the classification system carries messages that may be misleading. Thus, in ICD-10, mixed anxiety and depression is classified as a variety of anxiety disorder, although the evidence suggests that it is more likely to represent a mood disorder (see Harrington, Chapter 29). Depressive conduct disorder is classified as a variety of conduct disorder which does seem to be better justified in that research findings suggest that conduct disorder has much the same set of correlates and much the same outcome, irrespective of the co-occurrence of depression (Rutter *et al.* 1970), although there are some differences (Simic & Fombonne, 2001). On the other hand, the evidence is inconsistent on whether the presence of conduct disorder alters the meaning of the depression (Fombonne *et al.*, 2001a,b). Secondly, it limits finer distinctions, such as between the subvarieties of anxiety disorder that may be associated with either conduct disorder or major depression.

The availability of mixed categories in ICD-10 is quite limited, however, and the bigger difference from DSM-IV lies in the approach to mixed symptom patterns that are not covered by a combination category. ICD-10 is not entirely explicit in how they should be dealt with but the implicit expectation is a profile recognition or prototypic approach. Thus, if the main picture is one of severe depression, but there are marked obsessional features that ebb and flow with fluctuations in the depression, the mood disorder only would be the expected diagnosis. By contrast, DSM-IV would code obsessional disorder in addition (if the criteria were met) unless the *content* was mood-specific (as, for example, with a guilty rumination). The ICD-10 prototypic approach probably closely approximates ordinary clinical practice. The main problem is that it has proved difficult to make prototypes sufficiently explicit that they will always be used in the same way. For example, Asperger syndrome has been conceptualized on the basis of clinical case descriptions (see

Lord & Bailey, Chapter 38) but this has led to rather varied diagnostic sources on both the history of the concept and the experience of the clinicians using it.

With DSM-IV the mixture of two or more symptom patterns leads to the coding of as many diagnoses as there are patterns. This has the advantage of not requiring hierarchical judgements about which pattern is primary when in reality it may be very hard to tell, and it also succeeds in retaining a good deal of information when many patterns are present and no single category would convey them all. On the other hand, there are practical drawbacks to such a scheme. It encourages an unchallenged assumption that they are indeed independent patterns and that each can be dealt with in the same way as if there were no other problems. Alternatively, after multiple diagnoses are made, the clinician may then after all resort to a superordinate single-category way of thinking in which every possible profile has its own place. The coexistence of many diagnoses can be confusing and work against the key purposes of clarity and understanding how the research literature may apply to a particular child. It does not allow for the possibility of artefactual associations (see below). Furthermore, it is cumbersome, and perhaps impossible, for a clinician to review the presence or absence of every possible category and clinicians vary a good deal in their willingness to record symptom patterns that are not the main presentation (Rutter *et al.* 1975).

Hierarchical classification systems

Most classification schemes make some use of hierarchies based on a view that some conditions are fundamental and that, if others are present, they are likely to derive from the fundamental condition. The implication is that the former includes and accounts for the latter. Foulds (1976), for example, presented rating scale data from adult psychiatric inpatients to argue that the symptoms of people with schizophrenia usually included depression and anxiety; that those of people with depression did not usually include those of schizophrenia but did include anxiety; whereas people with anxiety did not usually show either depression or schizophrenia and were therefore at the bottom of a hierarchy of schizophrenia–depression–anxiety. There are evident dangers of circular reasoning, but with care the predictions can be tested. Clearly, this type of prediction would be unlikely to give a complete account of child psychopathology; but could be practical within groups of children sharing risk factors, such as diffuse brain damage, or with problems in a particular domain, such as hyperactivity (Taylor 1986).

Thus, DSM-IV excludes the diagnosis of generalized anxiety disorder if it occurs exclusively during a mood disorder, or a psychotic disorder (such as schizophrenia) or a pervasive developmental disorder (such as autism), and ICD-10 does so if the criteria for a panic disorder or an obsessive-compulsive disorder are met. Both DSM-IV and ICD-10 exclude the diagnosis of autism if Rett disorder is present, and exclude the diagnosis of

reactive attachment disorder if a pervasive developmental disorder is present. The general assumption that severe and pervasive mental disorders may often give rise to secondary symptom patterns is well based. The problem is that the evidence to justify hierarchies is generally rather thin and neither DSM-IV nor ICD-10 is consistent in its approach.

Polythetic/monothetic classes

Almost all medical classifications are polythetic. That is, cases are defined on the basis of having many, but not all, of a list of specified attributes in common. That is because variability in manifestation is a general biological feature, even with diseases solely caused by one major gene. In the neuropsychiatric arena, such variability is evident in marked degree with conditions such as tuberous sclerosis or the fragile X anomaly (see Skuse & Kuntsi, Chapter 13). There is similarly great variability in the manifestations of autism, as shown by the genetic findings (see Lord & Bailey, Chapter 38). The phenotype extends from severe handicap to quite subtle disturbances of social function. It would not therefore be reasonable to require that the disorder in any particular individual had to have *all* the diagnostic features. The trouble is that, in the absence of a diagnostic test of some kind, there are real difficulties in deciding both how varied the manifestations could be and where and how the boundaries should be drawn. Latent class analyses may help but what are really required are external validators (see below).

Lumping, splitting and empirical justification

There can be no one answer to the question of whether it is better to have a relatively small number of well-validated diagnoses or, rather, a large number that provides finer clinically useful distinctions that lack adequate empirical justification. Much depends on the purpose to which the classification is to be put. The most crucial distinction is between classifications to facilitate communication, and those designed to test out the meaningfulness of new ways of grouping and splitting disorders (Stengel 1959). The latter have been crucial in the identification of new syndromes (see Rutter & Taylor, Chapter 2, for examples). It would make no sense to confine researchers to the prevailing classifications. On the other hand, researchers have to communicate their findings to others and it would be equally unhelpful to have a proliferation of 'private' classifications.

Subclassification using dimensions

There are many examples in medicine of dimensional approaches being used as a supplement to a categorical classification. For example, respiratory physicians make more use of dimensional measures of lung function in considering clinical management and prognosis than they do of whether or not the criteria for chronic bronchitis or emphysema are met. Similarly, oncologists regularly grade the degree of malignancy of tumours and cardiologists measure the degree of occlusion of coronary arteries and the degree of exercise tolerance. The multiaxial system in child psychiatry (World Health Organization 1996) provides a similar facility with respect to degree of social impairment and intellectual level and DSM-IV provides a means of coding the severity of disorders, as well as the extent to which a disorder is in remission. Similarly, in dealing with schizophrenia it is helpful to differentiate between positive and negative symptoms (see Hollis, Chapter 37). Some of these further differentiations, both categorical and dimensional, have become standardized and quantified in ways that are used routinely, but others are still in the course of development. However, what is clear is that there is an important place for functional subclassification that falls somewhere between overall diagnostic classifications and individual diagnostic formulations (see Rutter & Taylor, Chapter 2).

ICD-10 and DSM-IV

ICD-10 (World Health Organization 1992, 1993) and DSM-IV (American Psychiatric Association 1994) constitute the two major psychiatric classifications used throughout the world. Their predecessors (ICD-9 and DSM-III) were very different from one another and strenuous efforts were made to bring ICD-10 and DSM-IV much closer together. Those efforts were successful in all sorts of important ways that constituted a major step forward in achieving better international understanding and communication. Nevertheless, there are some differences. Mention has already been made of the difference in approach to comorbidity and an equally important difference is that DSM-IV has one scheme that is designed for both research and routine clinical usage, whereas ICD-10 has two separate but interlinked schemes for these two rather different purposes, the research version being closer to DSM-IV.

There is something to be said in support of deliberate differences when evidence is lacking to decide which of two alternatives is to be preferred. Further research comparing the two systems should provide for an empirically based choice in the future. For example, the two schemes differ in the rules to be followed in the diagnosis of ADHD. The symptom lists are almost identical but the two systems have different requirements for pervasiveness across situations, whether all problems or only some need to be present, and on the use of exclusion criteria in relation to comorbidity. The consequence is that hyperkinetic disorder in ICD-10 is a subcategory of ADHD in DSM-IV, the grounds for translating one into the other are reasonably clear, and the research findings to compare the two should be informative. The two schemes also differ in how they deal with emotional disorders with an onset in childhood. ICD-10 makes a distinction between separation anxiety that represents an exaggeration or prolongation of a normal stage of emotional development (operationally defined as requiring an onset before age 6 years and absence of a generalized anxiety disorder) whereas DSM-IV makes the diagnosis solely on the basis of symptom pattern without regard to either age of onset or generalized anxiety. Whether or not the developmental approach of ICD-10 is helpful remains uncertain. Research could resolve the issue but, unfortunately, researchers tend to have an allegiance to one scheme over the other rather than a commitment to test the validity of different diagnostic approaches.

In addition to these deliberate differences, there are other minor differences which, although trivial in themselves and seemingly inadvertent in their origins, have been found to have major implications (Kendell 1991) as shown, for example, by the findings with respect to post-traumatic stress disorder (PTSD). A difference between the two schemes in relation to just one item (numbing of general responsiveness) had a dramatic effect on concordance between the two schemes (Andrews & Slade 1998).

Culture-specific categories

There are many syndromes that have been particularly, or exclusively, associated with particular cultures or populations. 'Brain fag' in West African students and both 'koro' and 'latah' in Indonesia constitute well-known examples. Such syndromes continue to have a controversial status. Both ICD-10 and DSM-IV have appendices dealing with them but neither provides a satisfactory solution for their handling. Clearly, some represent culturally influenced variations in the manifestations of well-validated disorders (see Rutter & Nikapota, Chapter 16). Thus, there are variations in the terms people use to describe depressive feelings (Kleinman & Good 1985) and in the significance attached to anxiety and to oppositional behaviour in childhood (Weisz et al. 1993). It is important that clinicians are aware of these variations if they are to avoid mistaken references (Bhugra & Bhui 2000; Canino & Bravo 2000; Cohen & Kasen 2000). However, it is also possible that there could be disorders that are truly different and found only in certain populations if they derive from risk factors that are confined to those populations. Empirical findings that could test that possibility are largely lacking.

Validation of diagnostic categories

Basis for diagnosis

The first systematic attempt to bring some sort of order into the classification of child psychopathology was provided by Hewitt & Jenkins's (1946) factor analysis of symptoms and linking of factors with differences in psychosocial circumstances. Their differentiation of emotional disturbance and disruptive behaviour, both on the grounds of intercorrelations among symptoms (that is, they 'hung together' in ways that separated the two), and different correlations with family features, has been amply confirmed in numerous subsequent studies. In the last few decades, more sophisticated multivariate analyses have led to the derivation of a much larger number of syndromes based on symptom profiles (Achenbach & Edelbrock 1978; Achenbach 1988, 1995). They bear some resemblance to the diagnostic categories in modern psychiatric classifications but it is not evident that the multivariate dimensions have any strong advantages over the latter and they have not led to much research testing diagnostic validation. Nevertheless, what the two have in common is the use of groupings based on patterns of symptomatology. The Washington University group were pioneers in the development of systematic rules for psychiatric diagnosis in the adult field (Feighner *et al.* 1972) and Cantwell (1975) extended the model to child psychiatry.

Both DSM-IV and ICD-10 have adopted this phenomenological approach. Without doubt it has aided comparability across centres in diagnostic usage. However, real comparability requires both the use of standard diagnostic instruments and application of diagnostic criteria (see Angold, Chapter 3; Cantwell 1988). A greater problem has come from the assumption that diagnoses should be based only on cross-sectional patterns of symptomatology, as if this was an end in itself. It is not enough that diagnoses differ in symptomatology; if those differentiations are to have any meaning they must be validated by criteria that are *external* to the symptomatology and which have clinical meaning and utility (Rutter 1965, 1978; Rutter & Gould 1985; Cantwell & Rutter 1994).

Clinicians sometimes assume that an ideal classification should be based on aetiology; however, that is not so. Most successful medical diagnoses are based instead on the underlying pathophysiology that gives rise to the clinical syndrome. Thus, diabetes is defined in terms of the metabolic abnormality and not which pattern of susceptibility genes is present. Similarly, ischaemic heart disease is based on the process of occlusive atheroma and not on the presence of key risk factors, such as high cholesterol levels, smoking or genetic liability. The key consideration is that most disorders are multifactorial and cannot therefore be classified on the basis of a single main cause. Elucidation of causal factors is important because it is likely to lead to an understanding of the basic pathophysiology (Rutter & Plomin 1997). However, it needs to be recognized that there may be more than one causal route to the same syndromic endpoint (Rutter 1997). The consequence of these considerations is that the goal must be the identification of the underlying pathophysiology of mental disorders, rather than finding the single main cause. We are a long way from reaching that goal at the moment. For the same reason, there cannot be any one validating test against some hypothetical gold standard. Instead, there has to be recourse to multiple validating approaches with the hope, and expectation, that when they all point in the same direction, it is likely that the diagnosis has some meaningful discriminative validity. Accordingly, we summarize such evidence briefly before seeking to draw conclusions on the current state of play on diagnostic validity. When the research findings were reviewed in previous editions (Rutter & Gould 1985; Cantwell & Rutter 1994), or elsewhere, we simply refer to these reviews but we note the main new findings.

Biological findings

In many respects, the clearest biological distinction is between severe mental retardation (IQ below 50), mild mental retardation (IQ 50–69) and the range of normal intelligence (Rutter & Gould 1985; Cantwell & Rutter 1994; Simonoff *et al.* 1996). Individuals who are severely retarded have a much reduced fecundity and life expectancy, the great majority show gross neuropathological abnormalities of the brain, and most have either clinical brain disorders (such as cerebral palsy or epilepsy) or marked congenital abnormalities. Their social class background is generally similar to that of the general population. By contrast, most people with mild retardation show a normal fertility pattern and a normal life expectancy, but to a marked extent they are disproportionately likely to come from a socially disadvantaged background. The genetic influences are more likely than in the case of severe retardation to reflect many genes operating as part of a multifactorial liability, and thus constitute the end of a continuum on the dimension reflecting normal variations in intelligence. Nevertheless, a substantial minority (the precise proportion is not known) have the same major genetic mutations as those found with severe retardation. That would be so, for example, with Down syndrome, tuberous sclerosis, fragile X and Williams syndrome. Accordingly, the validation is more accurately expressed in terms of a two-group differentiation that is roughly indexed by IQ level, rather than in terms of a severe vs. mild retardation split (see Volkmar & Dykens, Chapter 41).

Autism is differentiated from the broad run of other psychiatric disorders by its reduced life expectancy, mainly as a result of deaths associated with epilepsy (Isager *et al.* 1999), and by the high rate of epilepsy (about 25%). It does not differ from mental retardation in either respect but it does differ with respect to the age of onset of epilepsy (Rutter 1970; Gillberg & Steffenburg 1987; Volkmar & Nelson 1990). In autism, the peak is in late adolescence/early adult life, whereas in mentally retarded individuals it is in early childhood (Richardson & Koller 1992), as it is also in individuals of normal intelligence (Cooper 1965). Neuropathological studies are few, but the findings do not reflect the gross pathology that is typical of severe retardation (see Lord & Bailey, Chapter 38). Also, whereas small head size is associated with mental retardation, a larger than normal head size is more characteristic of autism (Woodhouse *et al.* 1996; Fombonne *et al.* 1999).

Biological findings are distinctly less helpful in differentiating among other disorders. Abnormalities on both structural and functional imaging are found in many cases of autism (see Lord & Bailey, Chapter 38), schizophrenia (see Hollis, Chapter 37), hyperkinetic disorder (see Schachar & Tannock, Chapter 25) and obsessive-compulsive disorder (see Rapoport & Swedo, Chapter 35), for example, and the findings provide a substantial case for a neural basis for the disorders, at least as a contributory factor in aetiology. Much the same applies to the positive findings with respect to neurodevelopmental impairment. Three main problems arise with any use of these findings for validation. First, the specifics of the abnormalities found are rather inconsistent within diagnoses (Bailey *et al.* 1996, with respect to autism; Eliez & Reiss 2000, with respect to magnetic resonance imaging findings across a range of disorders). Secondly, the associations have only limited diagnostic specificity. Thirdly, there have been rather limited direct comparisons across diagnostic groups. We do not know, for example, whether the findings in relation to autism might not apply also to, say, anxiety disorders or tics. Accordingly, the most that can be said is that the biological findings suggest that neural abnormalities are particularly likely to be found in some of the most severe psychiatric disorders, and there are a few pointers to possible diagnostic specificity, but the findings provide at best only weak evidence of diagnostic validation.

To some extent, similar problems apply to the associations between neurodevelopmental impairment—as indexed by motor delay and language impairment—and schizophrenia (McDonald *et al.* 2000). Thus, although the associations are weaker, those seem to apply also to bipolar psychoses (although probably not to other forms of emotional or behavioural disturbance; Cannon *et al.*, in press). The associations between schizophrenia and obstetric complications or congenital anomalies are weaker (Byrne *et al.* 2000; Kendell *et al.* 2000) and even less 'diagnosis-specific. Life-course-persistent antisocial behaviour differs from that which is adolescence-limited in its association with neurodevelopmental impairment (Moffitt *et al.* 1996; Rutter *et al.* 1998; Moffit *et al.*, 2001).

Drug response

It might be expected that drug responses would help greatly in diagnostic validation but, regretfully, they do not. The generally marked beneficial response to neuroleptics in the case of schizophrenia constitutes a partial exception (see Hollis, Chapter 37). Although these classes of drugs carry some benefits in other disorders (see Heyman & Santosh, Chapter 59), their efficacy in schizophrenia is substantially greater. Several problems arise with respect to the use of drug response as a diagnostic validator. First, and most importantly, most drugs have several distinct therapeutic actions. For example, tricyclics have independent effects on disorders as diverse as depression, ADHD and nocturnal enuresis (see Heyman & Santosh, Chapter 59). Secondly, in many cases the therapeutic effects fall far short of the dramatic. There are substantial benefits at the group level but these are not sufficiently great at the individual level to help much in diagnosis. Most especially, the fact that someone who is depressed does not return to a normal mood following administration of antidepressants by no means rules out the diagnosis of depression. Marked individual variations in drug response are common throughout medicine. Thirdly, many drugs appear to affect behaviours rather than diagnosis-specific pathophysiologies. Thus, the effects of stimulants on inattention/overactivity are qualitatively much the same, albeit quantitatively less marked, in individuals who do not have ADHD as in those who do (see Schachar & Tannnock, Chapter 25; Heyman & Santosh, Chap-

ter 59). There had been a hope that the response might nevertheless help in differentiating ADHD from restlessness/inattention caused by high anxiety. Early studies indicated a lesser effect of stimulants in the presence of high anxiety (see Schachar & Tannock, Chapter 25) but this was not found in the recent US multicentre trial (March *et al.* 2000).

Genetic/family study findings

Findings from twin, adoptee and family studies have been crucial in establishing some very important differences among diagnostic groups. Schizophrenia tends to breed relatively true, with associations that extend to schizotypal and paranoid disorders but not much wider than that (see Hollis, Chapter 37; Kendler *et al.* 1995). The same applies to autism and its broader phenotype (Bolton *et al.* 1994, 1998; Bailey *et al.* 1995; see also Lord & Bailey, Chapter 38). There is no evidence of any genetic association between schizophrenia and autism. Affective disorders similarly show a substantial familial loading for depression, but also for generalized anxiety disorders, with twin data suggesting a substantial shared genetic liability (Kendler 1996). Twin data also raise queries about whether prepubertal depression is the same disorder as major depression starting in adolescence or adult life (see Harrington, Chapter 29; Thapar & McGuffin 1994; Silberg *et al.* 1999, 2001). The findings are not clear-cut on whether bipolar disorders and unipolar depression are genetically distinct (see Harrington, Chapter 29; Silberg & Rutter, in press), but they may be. Some overlap is, of course, to be expected because some cases of unipolar depression are bound to represent bipolar disorders that have not yet included a manic episode. The heritability of bipolar disorder is clearly much greater than that of the ordinary run of unipolar disorder, but whether this reflects a different condition or a more severe variant of the same disorder is the unresolved query.

Attention deficit disorders with hyperactivity clearly stand out as having a substantively higher heritability than that for other disorders involving disruptive behaviour (Thapar *et al.* 1999). On the other hand, to an important extent, they share the same genetic liability (Eaves *et al.*, 2000; Nadder *et al.*, in press), but the findings also raise queries about the validity of a qualitatively distinct diagnosis of ADHD, because the heritability of hyperactivity seems much the same throughout its range (Levy *et al.* 1997) and because of the shared genetic liability with other disorders of behaviour. However, from a genetic perspective there is no justification for differentiating between oppositional/defiant disorder and conduct disorder (Eaves *et al.*, 2000).

The genetic findings on Tourette syndrome are mainly of interest in relation to validity because they suggest some overlap with both multiple chronic tics and obsessive-compulsive disorder. Genetic findings on other disorders (see chapters throughout the book) all indicate a significant genetic component but they are less informative on discriminative diagnostic validity, apart from the findings in adults (Kendler *et al.* 1992) suggesting that the specific phobias may be relatively distinct from generalized anxiety and from panic disorder. Rett syndrome is probably distinctive through its association in some cases with a specific genetic mutation (Amir *et al.* 1999) but to date there have been no studies testing for its association with other psychiatric conditions.

Psychosocial risk factors

On the whole, there is relatively little diagnostic specificity with respect to the psychopathological risks associated with psychosocial stress and adversity (see Friedman & Chase-Lansdale, Chapter 15; Sandberg & Rutter, Chapter 17). However, there are two important exceptions. First, severe institutional deprivation in the early years of life has a relatively specific association with syndromes involving disinhibited attachment (see O'Connor, Chapter 46; Rutter *et al.*, 2001). Secondly, severe and acute stress experiences of an exceptional kind are particularly likely to lead to post-traumatic stress disorder phenomena (see Yule, Chapter 32). There is also some tendency for psychological loss stresses to lead to depression and danger-type stresses to lead to anxiety (see Sandberg & Rutter, Chapter 17). Family conflict, discord and hostility are also more likely to lead to antisocial behaviour than to emotional disturbance; the same applies to social disadvantage (Rutter *et al.* 1970). Within antisocial disorders, life-course-persistent varieties show a stronger association in serious family adversities than that found with adolescence-limited varieties (Rutter *et al.* 1998).

Cognitive correlates

Autism stands out from other psychiatric disorders both because of its particularly strong association with general cognitive impairment and its relatively specific association with theory of mind deficits (see Lord & Bailey, Chapter 38). ADHD is also relatively distinctive, but to a much lesser degree, through its association with mild cognitive impairment (Fergusson *et al.* 1993; see also Schachar & Tannock, Chapter 25). To a lesser extent, schizophrenia is also associated with a slightly below average IQ before the onset of the psychosis (Tarrant & Jones 2000).

Epidemiology

The two epidemiological features that are of greatest value with respect to diagnostic validity are age of onset and sex ratio. Interestingly, they go together to a considerable extent. Thus, disorders involving neurodevelopmental delay, such as developmental disorders of language, autism, ADHD, and life-course-persistent antisocial behaviour, characteristically begin early in life and are much more common in males. Emotional disorders beginning in adolescence, such as depression and eating disorders, by contrast, tend to be much more common in females (see Rutter & Taylor, Chapter 2). Antisocial behaviour beginning in adolescence also differs from earlier onset varieties

in having a much weaker male preponderance (Moffitt *et al.*, 2001). Rett syndrome is unique in being confined—or almost confined—to females (see Lord & Bailey, Chapter 38).

Course of disorder

The long-term course of disorders also helps sort out diagnostic distinctions. The plateau of developmental progress and loss of purposive motor skills associated with Rett syndrome (see Lord & Bailey, Chapter 38) makes it quite distinct. Adult outcome findings (Rutter 1995) are relevant in showing the major continuities between depression in childhood/adolescence and recurrent depression in adult life (Harrington *et al.* 1990; Weissman *et al.* 1999a,b; Fombonne *et al.*, 2001a,b); similarly, strong continuities between antisocial behaviour, including conduct and oppositional/defiant disorders, and personality disorders in adult life (Rutter *et al.* 1998); the strong persistence of autism (see Lord & Bailey, Chapter 38); the relatively strong persistence of schizophrenia (see Hollis, Chapter 37), of obsessive-compulsive disorders (see Rapoport & Swedo, Chapter 35), and of tics/Tourette syndrome (see Leckman & Cohen, Chapter 36). There are fewer data on anxiety disorders but, although there is some overlap with depression, specific phobias seem somewhat distinct (see Klein & Pine, Chapter 30).

Summary of validity inferences

Putting together the evidence discussed above, it is possible to arrive at a threefold division of disorders into those that are reasonably well-validated; those with pointers suggesting possible validity; and those where the evidence indicates that the categorical subdivisions are probably invalid.

The first group clearly contains autism and autism spectrum disorders (considered together), schizophrenia and schizophrenic spectrum disorders (again as a grouping), depressive disorders, hyperkinetic behaviour as a feature that differentiates it from other disorders of disruptive behaviour, oppositional and conduct disorders (considered together) and Rett syndrome. A range of contrasting approaches all provide good evidence of discriminative validity. The same applies to the distinction between the usually severe mental retardation that is associated with gross neuropathology and the usually mild retardation that is not.

The second cluster of possibly valid syndromes includes obsessive-compulsive disorder, eating disorders (pooling anorexia and bulimia nervosa), tics and Tourette syndrome, specific phobias, post-traumatic stress disorder, disinhibited attachment disorder, bipolar affective disorders, and the distinction between life-course-persistent and adolescent-linked antisocial behaviour. As briefly noted above, in each instance there is some evidence of discriminative validity but it is either less consistent or it spans fewer research approaches. From a practical point of view, these provide sufficient grounds for retaining the diagnostic category, even though there are important questions to be tackled.

The third cluster of probably invalid categories is less easy to deal with, if only because of the usual problem of knowing how much weight to attach to a lack of evidence of a meaningful difference, when new research could change that situation completely. Nevertheless, it is important to be aware that our usage of prevailing classifications means that we are making distinctions that, at least currently, lack substance. That applies to most of the detailed subclassifications, such as those among anxiety disorders or those among pervasive developmental disorders (PDD), Rett syndrome apart. It definitely does not mean that we should necessarily switch to some broader category. Thus, although there is no good evidence that the distinction between, say, autism and Asperger syndrome or atypical autism means much, the evidence on discriminative validity applies to the more narrow category of autism and not to the broader category of PDD. Also, up to now it has proved quite difficult to provide either a clear conceptualization or precise application of the criteria for the broader category. The issue is the one that pervades psychiatry: namely, uncertainty on the boundaries of a syndrome when the defining pathophysiology is unknown. It should be added that this uncertainty applies in some (often major) degree to most of the conditions for which there is no evidence of validity.

A second group of probably invalid categories includes syndromes that are clinically striking but for which the external correlates provide little support for basic differences from other diagnostic categories. Selective mutism and conversion reactions fall into that group. In both cases, the distinctiveness of the clinical picture and the particular therapeutic challenges it presents probably warrant the retention of the category. However, the same might have been said of school refusal (Hersov 1977) and that no longer has a place in most classification schemes (Elliott 1999). Then there are categories that derive from theoretical concepts but which lack satisfactory diagnostic criteria that would allow the testing of validity. Inhibited attachment disorder (see O'Connor, Chapter 46) is a diagnosis of that type and many would argue that borderline personality disorder is too (see J. Hill, Chapter 43). Certainly, subdivisions among personality disorders remain rather unsatisfactory. It should be added that epidemiological findings indicate that there are quite a few children with psychosocial impairment but whose mental health problem does not fulfil any particular diagnostic category. Moreover, they have a mental health outcome, at least in the short term, that is as poor as those with a diagnosis (Angold *et al.* 1999). Evidently, there is a need for some sort of residual psychopathological category.

Finally, it is necessary to return to the uncertainties when deciding between categorical and dimensional approaches. ADHD disorders well illustrate this dilemma (see Schachar & Tannock, Chapter 25). Most of the biological validity evidence, such as the neuroimaging findings and associations with motor and language problems, applies to a relatively narrow diagnos-

tic category, but most of the genetic findings point to a dimensional liability (Levy *et al.* 1997). Of course, it may well be that there is both a qualitatively distinct disorder and a risk dimension, which look similar but which differ in their pathophysiology.

Agreement on clinical psychiatric diagnoses

Diagnostic ratings by experienced clinicians show at least a modest concordance. Limited agreement within panels of independent clinicians has been found over the years: for DSM-III (Mattison *et al.* 1979; Mezzich *et al.* 1985; Prendergast *et al.* 1988) and for ICD-9 (Gould *et al.* 1988; Prendergast *et al.* 1988; Remschmidt 1988). Field trials for DSM-IV reported better agreement, but on the basis of self-selected pairs of psychiatrists who made diagnoses on selected patients. The shortcomings of this strategy were pointed out by Rutter & Shaffer (1980), who noted that one would expect clinicians working together to have similar diagnostic practices. Further work needs to be carried out before the language of child psychiatry becomes sufficiently explicit to sustain scientific progress.

On the other hand, good diagnostic agreement can be achieved by independent research teams that have agreed supplementary criteria in advance (Prendergast *et al.* 1988). This satisfactory agreement is comparable with that obtained by studies in which two clinicians from the same centre rated cases with fuller information (Stroeber *et al.* 1981; Werry *et al.* 1983). The conclusion seems to be that training can improve diagnostic reliability to a satisfactory level, so the goal of an adequate system is not impossibly distant. The increased clarity of diagnostic rules in ICD-10 has been reported to increase interrater reliability, though the overall accuracy still leaves much to be desired (Steinhausen & Erdin 1991). Other procedures that have been reported to enhance reliability are the use of a standard coding form after interview (Beitchman *et al.* 1989) and the use of a multiaxial system (Skovgaard *et al.* 1988).

Clinical diagnosis and formulation

The clinical diagnosis is made for purposes of convenient and economical communication, for statistical recording and purposes of audit. Diagnosis is seldom the automatic generator of a plan for management. A child with autism and repetitive self-injury should not be treated in the same way as a person with autism who does not show challenging behaviour; a child with ADHD who is socially competent and valued should not receive the same management as one who is severely impaired in social role performance. Pervasive variables, such as IQ and peer relationships, are important predictively, even if their lack of discriminative validity means that they do not enter into current definitions. The diagnosis is just one of several aspects of the case that guide decision-making. It functions like a map for navigators, to help them know what they are likely to encounter. Ignoring it is like going to sea without a map; relying upon it to dictate treatment is more like the action of a navigator who never looks at the ocean to spot approaching vessels or the danger of icebergs. There is a potential danger in the development of treatment protocols or payment plans that are based solely upon diagnosis: they may inhibit the process of tailoring services to individual needs.

The product of assessment should therefore be not only a categorization, but a full clinical formulation. The point is so important that a separate chapter (see Rutter & Taylor, Chapter 2) considers the development of clinical formulations that bring out what is individual and special about the problems faced by a child. The clinical formulation encompasses more information than the diagnosis. It is a convenient way of combining dimensional with categorical information, and it allows for the inclusion of information that may determine clinical decision-making even if it does not enter into the diagnosis. It should include a problem list, a description of the child's profile of disturbance on the major types of behavioural change, cognitive abilities and impairment, strengths and weaknesses in the family and school environment, and any relevant risk factors.

A formulation can also indicate uncertainties or missing information, and the possible needs for review. It allows, for instance, judgements to be recorded about the confidence with which different aspects of the case have been assessed. This in turn directs the clinician's attention towards re-evaluations that may need to be made in the management of a case, and avoid perseveration on an initially erroneous judgement. It allows for plans to be made for the management of a case falling short of diagnostic criteria. Rather similarly, it allows a case to be detected as having a definite problem even if the exact nature of the problem does not fit current diagnosis.

Another function of the clinical formulation is to record judgements about the developmental significance of clinical findings. The 'psychosocial' axis of the ICD refers to stressors that may affect the child. Reliability for research purposes is enhanced if one codes only their presence or absence rather than their role in aetiology. The formulation of the case can and should include judgements concerning the impact of those stressors upon the child's development (see Sandberg & Rutter, Chapter 17).

The clinical formulation also permits the clinician to record judgements about the weight to be given to different aspects of the case. For example, within a multicategory scheme such as DSM-IV, it will be commonplace for a referred child to receive several diagnoses. Serious errors of judgement could be made if it were assumed that each diagnosis had the same significance as it would have in a non-comorbid case and that each diagnosis could be treated independently. A child with autism who is afraid of going out of doors may have come to that state through a very different route from one with simple social phobia and may need a different approach in treatment.

Conclusions

The development of agreed and reasonably reliable diagnostic schemes has been essential for beginning a scientific understanding of child mental health problems. Cross-sectional symptom patterns have been the foundation for this advance. Succeeding chapters describe the considerable progress that has been made in the accuracy and reliability with which symptoms are elicited. Several sources of developing knowledge can now be expected to have a great impact on the details and the principles of classifications. Advancing knowledge of patterns of inheritance is likely to lead to some redefining of the boundaries of disorder. The long-term process of mapping genotypes to phenotypes will probably produce new diagnostic entities and lead to some regrouping of old ones. Advances in neuropsychological understanding about the bases of a disorder may lead to altered views about what constitute its key features. New treatments will call for new categorizations of the groups of patients to whom they are relevant. The nosological study of comorbid groups will clarify how the overlap of different symptom patterns should be handled. Developmental psychopathology will produce knowledge about the interaction of risk and protective factors that allow a richer classification of the factors operating on a child and the developmental tracks that children may take. These foreseeable advances have in common the increasing integration of other sources of information with current symptomatology as the basis of classification. It seems certain that sound classification will remain a necessary condition for progress.

References

Achenbach, T.M. (1988) Integrating assessment and taxonomy. In: *Assessment and Diagnosis in Child Psychopathology* (eds M. Rutter, A.H. Tuma & I.S. Lann), pp. 300–343. Guilford Press, New York.

Achenbach, T.M. (1995) Developmental issues in assessment, taxonomy, and diagnosis of child and adolescent psychopathology. In: *Developmental Psychopathology*, Vol. 1. *Theory and Methods* (eds D. Cicchetti & D. Cohen), pp. 57–80. John Wiley, New York.

Achenbach, T.M. & Edelbrock, C.S. (1978) The classification of child psychopathology: a review and analysis of empirical efforts. *Psychological Bulletin*, 85, 1275–1301.

American Psychiatric Association (1980) *Diagnostic and Statistical Manual of Mental Disorders*, 3rd edn. American Psychiatric Association, Washington, DC.

American Psychiatric Association (1994) *Diagnostic and Statistical Manual of Mental Disorders (DSM-1V)*, 4th edn. American Psychiatric Association, Washington, DC.

Amir, R.E., van den Veyver, I.B., Wan, M., Tran, C.Q., Francke, U. & Zoghbi, H.Y. (1999) Rett syndrome is caused by mutations in X-linked MECP2, encoding methyl-CpG-binding protein 2. *Nature Genetics*, 23, 185–188.

Andrews, G. & Slade, T. (1998) Depression, dysthymia and substance use disorders: sources of dissonance between ICD-10 and DSM-IV. *International Journal of Methods in Psychiatric Research*, 7, 116–120.

Angold, A., Costello, E.J., Farmer, E.M., Burns, B.J. & Erkanli, A.

(1999) Impaired but undiagnosed. *Journal of American Academy of Child and Adolescent Psychiatry*, 38, 129–137.

Bailey, A., Le Couteur, A., Gottesman, I. *et al.* (1995) Autism as a strongly genetic disorder: evidence from a British twin study. *Psychological Medicine*, 25, 63–77.

Bailey, A., Phillips, W. & Rutter, M. (1996) Autism: towards an integration of clinical, genetic, neuropsychological and neurobiological perspectives. *Journal of Child Psychology and Psychiatry*, 37, 89–126.

Beitchman, J.H., Kruidenier, B., Clegg, M., Hood, J. & Corradini, A. (1989) Diagnostic interviewing with children: the use and reliability of the diagnostic coding form. *Canadian Journal of Psychiatry*, 34, 283–290.

Bergman, L.R. & Magnusson, D. (1997) A person-oriented approach in research on developmental psychopathology. *Development and Psychopathology*, 9, 291–319.

Berkson, J. (1946) Limitations of the application of fourfold table analysis to hospital data. *Biometrics*, 2, 47–49.

Bhugra, D. & Bhui, K. (2000) *Cross-Cultural Psychiatry: a Practical Guide.* Arnold, London.

Blewitt, P. (1994) Understanding categorical hierarchies: the earliest levels of skill. *Child Development*, 65, 1279–1298.

Bolton, P., Macdonald, H., Pickles, A. *et al.* (1994) A case–control family history study of autism. *Journal of Child Psychology and Psychiatry*, 35, 877–900.

Bolton, P.F., Pickles, A., Murphy, M. & Rutter, M. (1998) Autism, affective and other psychiatric disorders: patterns of familial aggregation. *Psychological Medicine*, 28, 385–395.

Byrne, M., Browne, R., Mulryan, N. *et al.* (2000) Labour and delivery complications and schizophrenia: case–control study using contemporaneous labour ward records. *British Journal of Psychiatry*, 176, 531–536.

Canino, G. & Bravo, M. (2000) The translation and adaptation of diagnostic instruments for cross-cultural use. In: *Diagnostic Assessment in Child and Adolescent Psychopathology* (eds D. Shaffer, C.P. Lucas & J.E. Richters), pp. 285–298. Guilford Press, New York.

Cannon, M., Caspi, A., Moffitt, T.E. *et al.* (in press) Evidence for early, specific, pan-developmental impairment in schizophreniform disorders: results from a longitudinal birth cohort. *Archives of General Psychiatry.*

Cantwell, D. (1975) A model for the investigation of psychiatric disorders of childhood: its application in genetic studies of the hyperkinetic syndrome. In: *Explorations in Child Psychiatry* (ed. E.J. Anthony), pp. 57–59. Plenum Press, New York.

Cantwell, D. (1988) DSM-III studies. In: *Assessment and Diagnosis in Child Psychopathology* (eds M. Rutter, A.H. Tuma & I.S. Lann), pp. 3–36. Guilford Press, New York.

Cantwell, D.P. & Rutter, M. (1994) Classification: conceptual issues and substantive findings. In: *Child and Adolescent Psychiatry: Modern Approaches*, 3rd edn. (eds M. Rutter, E. Taylor & L. Hersov), pp. 3–21. Blackwell Scientific Publications, Oxford.

Caron, C. & Rutter, M. (1991) Comorbidity in child psychopathology: concepts, issues and research strategies. *Journal of Child Psychology and Psychiatry*, 32, 1063–1080.

Champion, L., Goodall, G.M. & Rutter, M. (1995) Behavioural problems in childhood and stressors in early adult life: a 20-year follow-up of London school children. *Psychological Medicine*, 25, 231–246.

Cohen, P. & Kasen, S. (2000) The context of assessment: culture, race, and socioeconomic status as influences on the assessment of children. In: *Diagnostic Assessment in Child and Adolescent Psychopathology* (eds D. Shaffer, C.P. Lucas & J.E. Richters), pp. 299–381. Guilford Press, New York & London.

Cooper, J.E. (1965) Epilepsy in a longitudinal survey of 5000 children. *British Medical Journal*, 1, 1020–1022.

De Fries, J.C. & Fulker, D.W. (1988) Multiple regression analysis of twin data: aetiology of deviant scores versus individual differences. *Acta Geneticae Medicae et Gemellologiae*, 37, 205–216.

Eaves, L., Siberg, J., Hewitt, J.K. *et al.* (1993) Genes, personality, and psychopathology: a latent class analysis of liability to symptoms of attention-deficit hyperactivity disorder in twins. In: *Nature, Nurture and Psychology* (eds R. Plomin & G.E. McLearn), pp. 285–303. APA Books, Washington, DC.

Eaves, L.J., Rutter, M., Silberg, J.L., Shillady, L., Maes, H. & Pickles, A. (2000) Genetic and environmental causes of covariation in interview assessments of disruptive behavior in child and adolescent twins. *Behavior Genetics*, 30, 321–334.

Eliez, S. & Reiss, A.L. (2000) MRI neuroimaging of childhood psychiatric disorders: a selective review. *Journal of Child Psychology and Psychiatry*, 41, 679–694.

Elliott, J.G. (1999) School refusal: issues of conceptualisation, assessment, and treatment. *Journal of Child Psychology and Psychiatry*, 40, 1001–1012.

Feighner, J.P., Robins, E., Guze, S.B., Woodruff, R.A., Winokur, G. & Munoz, R. (1972) Diagnostic criteria for use in psychiatric research. *Archives of General Psychiatry*, 26, 57–63.

Fergusson, D.M. & Horwood. L.J. (1995) Prevalence and comorbidity of DSM-III-R diagnosis in a birth cohort of 15 year olds. *Journal of the American Academy of Child and Adolescent Psychiatry*, 32, 1127–1134.

Fergusson, D.M., Horwood. L.J. & Lynskey, M.T. (1993) The effects of conduct disorder and attention deficit in middle childhood on offending and scholastic ability at age 13. *Journal of Child Psychology and Psychiatry*, 34, 899–916.

Fombonne, E., Rogé, B., Claverie, J., Courty, S. & Fremolle, J. (1999) Microcephaly and macrocephaly in autism. *Journal of Autism and Developmental Disorders*, 29, 113–119.

Fombonne, E., Wostear, G., Cooper, V., Harrington, R. & Rutter, M. (2001a) The Maudsley long-term follow-up of child and adolescent depression. I. Psychiatric outcomes in adulthood. *British Journal of Psychiatry*, 179, 210–217.

Fombonne, E., Wostear, G., Cooper, V., Harrington, R. & Rutter, M. (2001b) The Maudsley long-term follow-up of child and adolescent depression. II. Suicidality, criminality and social dysfunction in adulthood. *British Journal of Psychiatry*, 179, 218–223.

Foulds, G.A. (1976) *Hierarchical Nature of Personal Illness.* Academic Press. London.

Freud, A. (1965) *Normality and Pathology in Childhood.* International Universities Press, New York.

Gillberg, C. & Steffenburg, S. (1987) Outcome and prognostic factors in infantile autism and similar conditions: a population-based study of 46 cases followed through puberty. *Journal of Autism and Developmental Disorders*, 17, 273–287.

Gjone, H., Stevenson, J. & Sundet, J.M. (1996) Genetic influences on parent-reported attention-related problems in a Norwegian general population twin sample. *Journal of the American Academy of Child and Adolescent Psychiatry*, 35, 588–596.

Gould, M.S., Shaffer, D., Rutter, M. & Sturge, C. (1988) UK/WHO Study of ICD-9. In: *Assessment and Diagnosis in Child Psychopathology* (eds M. Rutter, A.H. Tuma & I.S. Lann), pp. 37–65. Guilford Press, New York.

Group for the Advancement of Psychiatry (1966) *Psychopathological Disorders in Childhood: Theoretical Considerations and a Proposed Classification (Research Report no. 62)*, pp. 229–230. Group for the Advancement of Psychiatry, New York.

Harrington, R., Fudge, H., Rutter, M., Pickles, A. & Hill, J. (1990)

Adult outcomes of childhood and adolescent depression. I. Psychiatric status. *Archives of General Psychiatry*, 47, 465–473.

Hersov, L. (1977) School refusal. In: *Child and Adolescent Psychiatry: Modern Approaches* (eds M. Rutter & L. Hersov), pp. 455–486. Blackwell Scientific Publications, Oxford.

Hewitt, L.E. & Jenkins, R.J. (1946) *Fundamental Patterns of Maladjustment: the Dynamics of Their Origin*. Michigan Child Guidance Institute, Illinois.

Isager, T., Mouridsen, S.E. & Rich, B. (1999) Mortality and causes of death in pervasive developmental disorders. *Autism*, 3, 7–16.

Kendell, R.E. (1991) Relationship between the DSM-IV and the ICD-10. *Journal of Abnormal Psychology*, 100, 297–301.

Kendell, R.E., McInneny, K., Juszczak, E. & Bain, M. (2000) Obstetric complications and schizophrenia: two case–control studies based on structures obstetric records. *British Journal of Psychiatry*, 176, 516–522.

Kendler, K.S. (1996) Major depression and generalised anxiety disorder: same genes (partly) different environments—revisited. *British Journal of Psychiatry*, 168 (Suppl. 30), 68–75.

Kendler, K.S., Neale, M.C., Kessler, R.C., Heath, A.C. & Eaves, L.J. (1992) The genetic epidemiology of phobias in women: the interrelationship of agoraphobia, social phobia, situational phobia, and simple phobia. *Archives of General Psychiatry*, 49, 273–281.

Kendler, K.S., Neale, M.C. & Walsh, D. (1995) Evaluating the spectrum concept of schizophrenia in the Roscommon family study. *American Journal of Psychiatry*, 152, 749–754.

Klein, D.N. & Riso, L.P. (1996) Psychiatric disorders: problems of boundaries and comorbidity. In: *Basic Issues in Psychopathology* (ed. C.G. Costello), pp. 19–66. Guilford Press, New York.

Kleinman, A. & Good, B. (1985) *Culture and Depression: Studies in the Anthropology and Cross-Cultural Psychiatry of Affect and Disorder*. University of California Press, Berkeley.

Lahey, B.B., Applegate, B., Barkley, R.A. *et al.* (1999) DSM-IV field trials for oppositional defiant disorder and conduct disorder in children and adolescents. In: *DSM-IV Sourcebook*, Vol. 4 (eds T.A. Widiger, A.J. Frances, H.A. Pincus *et al.*), pp. 661–681. American Psychiatric Association, Washington D.C.

Levy, F., Hay, D.A., McStephen, M., Wood, C. & Waldman, I. (1997) Attention-deficit hyperactivity disorder (ADHD): a category or a continuum? Genetic analysis of a large-scale twin study. *Journal of the American Academy of Child and Adolescent Psychiatry*, 36, 737–744.

March, J.S., Swanson, J.M., Arnold, L.E. *et al.* (2000) Anxiety as a predictor and outcome variable in the multimodal treatment study of children with ADHD (MTA). *Journal of Abnormal Child Psychology*, 28, 527–541.

Mattison, R., Cantwell, D.P., Russell, A.T. & Will, L. (1979) A comparison of DSM-III in the diagnosis of childhood psychiatric disorders B. II. Inter-rater agreement. *Archives of General Psychiatry*, 36, 1217–1222.

McDonald, C., Fearon, P. & Murray, R. (2000) Neurodevelopmental hypothesis of schizophrenia 12 years on: data and doubts. In: *Child Onset of 'Adult' Psychopathology: Clinical and Research Advances* (ed. J.L. Rapoport), pp. 193–220. American Psychiatric Press, Washington D.C.

Meehl, P.E. (1995) Bootstrap taxometrics: solving the classification problem in psychopathology. *American Psychologist*, 50, 266–275.

Mezzich, A.C., Mezzich, J.E. & Coffman, G. (1985) Reliability of DSM-III vs. DSM-II in child psychopathology. *Journal of the American Academy of Child Psychiatry*, 24, 273–280.

Moffitt, T.E. (1993) Adolescence-limited and life-course-persistent antisocial behavior: a developmental taxonomy. *Psychological Review*, 100, 674–701.

Moffitt, T.E., Caspi, A., Dickson, N., Silva, P. & Stanton, W. (1996) Childhood-onset versus adolescent-onset antisocial conduct in males: natural history from ages 3–18 years. *Development and Psychopathology*, 8, 399–424.

Moffitt, T.E., Caspi, A., Rutter, M. & Silva, P.A. (2001) Sex differences in antisocial behavior: Conduct disorder, delinquency, and violence in the Dunedin Longituclinal Study. Cambridge University Press, Cambridge.

Nadder, T.S., Silberg, J.L., Rutter, M., Maes, H.H. & Eaves, L.J. (in press) Genetic effects on the variation and covariation of ADHD and ODD/CD symptomatologies across informant and occasion of measurement. *Psychological Medicine*.

Prendergast, M., Taylor, E., Rapoport, J.L. *et al.* (1988) The diagnosis of childhood hyperactivity: a US–UK cross-national study of DSM-III and ICD-9. *Journal of Child Psychology and Psychiatry*, 29, 289–300.

Remschmidt, H. (1988) German study of ICD-9. In: *Assessment and Diagnosis in Child Psychopathology* (eds M. Rutter, A.H. Tuma & I.S. Lann), pp. 66–83. Guilford Press, New York.

Richardson, S. & Koller, H. (1992) Vulnerability and resilience in adults who were classified as mildly mentally handicapped in childhood. In: *Vulnerability and Resilience in Development* (eds B. Tizard & V. Varma), pp. 102–122. Jessica Kingsley Publishers, London.

Robins, L. (1966) *Deviant Children Grown Up*. Williams & Wilkins, Baltimore.

Rutter, M. (1965) Classification and categorization in child psychiatry. *Journal of Child Psychology and Psychiatry*, 6, 71–83.

Rutter, M. (1970) Autistic children: infancy to adulthood. *Seminars in Psychiatry*, 2, 435–450.

Rutter, M. (1978) Diagnostic validity in child psychiatry. *Advances in Biological Psychiatry*, 2, 2–22.

Rutter, M. (1995) Relationship between mental disorders in childhood and adulthood. *Acta Psychiatrica Scandinavica*, 91, 73–85.

Rutter, M. (1997) Comorbidity: concepts, claims and choices. *Criminal Behaviour and Mental Health*, 7, 265–285.

Rutter, M. & Gould, M. (1985) Classification. In: *Child and Adolescent Psychiatry: Modern Approaches*, 2nd edn (eds M. Rutter & L. Hersov), pp. 304–319. Blackwell Scientific, Oxford.

Rutter, M. & Plomin, R. (1997) Opportunities for psychiatry from genetic findings. *British Journal of Psychiatry*, 171, 209–219.

Rutter, M. & Shaffer, D. (1980) DSM-III: a step forward or back in terms of classification of child psychiatric disorder? *Journal of the American Academy of Child Psychiatry*, 19, 371–394.

Rutter, M., Lebovici, S., Eisenberg, L. *et al.* (1969) A triaxial classification of mental disorders in children. *Journal of Child Psychology and Psychiatry*, 10, 41–61.

Rutter, M., Tizard, J. & Whitmore, K. (eds) (1970). *Education, Health and Behaviour*. Longmans, London.

Rutter, M., Shaffer, D. & Shepherd, M. (1975) *A Multiaxial Classification of Child Psychiatric Disorders*. WHO, Geneva.

Rutter, M., Giller, H. & Hagell, A. (1998). *Antisocial Behaviour by Young People*. Cambridge University Press, Cambridge.

Rutter, M., Kreppner, J., O'Connor, T., & on behalf of the English and Romanian Adoptees (ERA) Study Team (2001) Specificity and heterogeneity in children's responses to profound institutional privation. *British Journal of Psychiatry*, 179, 97–103.

Schoeeman, T.J., Segerstrom, S., Griffin, P. & Gresham, D. (1993) The psychiatric nosology of everyday life: categories in implicit abnormal psychology. *Journal of Social and Clinical Psychology*, 12, 429–453.

Silberg, J. & Rutter, M. (in press) Nature–nurture interplay in the risks associated with parental depression. In: *Children of Depressed Parents: Mechanisms of Risk and Implications for Treatment* (eds

S.H. Goodman & I.A. Gotlib) American Psychological Association, Washington D.C.

Silberg, J., Pickles, A., Rutter, M. *et al.* (1999) The influence of genetic factors and life stress on depression among adolescent girls. *Archives of General Psychiatry*, **56**, 225–232.

Silberg, J., Rutter, M. & Eaves, L. (2001) Genetic and environmental influences on the temporal association between earlier anxiety and later depression in girls. *Biological Psychiatry*, **49**, 1040–1049.

Simic, M. & Fombonne, E. (2001) Depressive conduct disorder: symptom patterns and correlates in referred children and adolescents. *Journal of Affective Disorders*, **62**, 175–185.

Simonoff, E., Bolton, P. & Rutter, M. (1996) Mental retardation: genetic findings, clinical implications and research agenda. *Journal of Child Psychology and Psychiatry*, **37**, 259–280.

Skovgaard, A.M., Isager, T. & Jorgensen, O.S. (1988) The reliability of child psychiatric diagnosis: a comparison among Danish child psychiatrists of traditional diagnoses and a multiaxial diagnostic system. *Acta Psychiatrica Scandinavica*, **77**, 469–476.

Sonuga-Barke, E.J. (1998) Categorical models of childhood disorder: a conceptual and empirical analysis. *Journal of Child Psychology and Psychiatry*, **39**, 115–133.

Steinhausen, H.C. & Erdin, A. (1991) The inter-rater reliability of child and adolescent psychiatric disorders in the ICD-10. *Journal of Child Psychology and Psychiatry*, **32**, 921–928.

Stengel, E. (1959) Classification of mental disorders. *Bulletin of the World Health Organization*, **21**, 601–663.

Stroeber, M., Green, J. & Carlson, G. (1981) Reliability of psychiatric diagnosis in hospitalized adolescents: inter-rater agreement using DSM-III. *Archives of General Psychiatry*, **38**, 141–145.

Tarjan, M.D., Tizard, J., Rutter, M. *et al.* (1972) Classification and mental retardation: issues arising in the Fifth WHO Seminar on Psychiatric Diagnosis, Classification and Statistics. *American Journal of Psychiatry*, **128** (Suppl.), 34–45.

Tarrant, C.J. & Jones, P.B. (2000) Biological markers are precursors to schizophrenia: specificity, predictive ability, and etiological significance. In: *Child Onset of 'Adult' Psychopathology: Clinical and Research Advances* (ed. J. Rapoport), pp. 65–102. American Psychiatric Press, Washington D.C.

Taylor, E. (1986) Subclassification and diagnosis. In: *The Overactive Child: Clinics in Developmental Medicine* No. 97 (ed. E. Taylor), pp. 174–191. MacKeith Press/Blackwell Scientific Publications, London/Oxford.

Taylor, E., Sandberg, S., Thorley, G. & Giles, S. (1991) *The Epidemiology of Childhood Hyperactivity. Maudsley Monograph No. 33.* Oxford University Press, Oxford.

Thapar, A. & McGuffin, P. (1994) A twin study of depressive symptoms in childhood. *British Journal of Psychiatry*, **165**, 259–265.

Thapar, A., Holmes, J., Poulton, K. & Harrington, R. (1999) Genetic basis of attention deficit and hyperactivity. *British Journal of Psychiatry*, **174**, 105–111.

Volkmar, F.R. & Nelson, D.S. (1990) Seizure disorders in autism. *Journal of the American Academy of Child and Adolescent Psychiatry*, **29**, 127–129.

Weissman, M., Wolk, S., Goldstein, R. *et al.* (1999a) Depressed adolescents grown up. *Journal of the American Medical Academy*, **281**, 1707–1713.

Weissman, M., Wolk, S., Wickramaratne, P. *et al.* (1999b) Children with prepubertal-onset major depressive disorder and anxiety grown up. *Archives of General Psychiatry*, **56**, 794–801.

Weisz, J.R., Suwanlert, S., Chaiyasit, W., Weiss, B., Achenbach, T.M. & Eastman, K.L. (1993) Behavioral and emotional problems among Thai and American adolescents: parent reports for ages 12–16. *Journal of Abnormal Psychology*, **102**, 395–403.

Werry, J., Methren, R.J., Fitzpatrick, J. & Dixon, H. (1983) The inter-rater reliability of DSM-III in children. *Journal of Abnormal Psychology*, **11**, 341–354.

Woodhouse, W., Bailey, A., Rutter, M., Bolton, P., Baird, G. & Le Couteur, A. (1996) Head circumference in autism and other pervasive developmental disorders. *Journal of Child Psychology and Psychiatry*, **37**, 665–671.

World Health Organization (1977) *Manual of the International Statistical Classification of Diseases, Injuries and Causes of Death* (9th revision), Vol. 1. WHO, Geneva.

World Health Organization (1978) *Manual of the International Statistical Classification of Diseases, Injuries and Causes of Death* (9th revision), Vol. 2. WHO, Geneva.

World Health Organization (1992) *The ICD-10 Classification of Mental and Behavioural Disorders: B. Clinical Descriptions and Diagnostic Guidelines.* WHO, Geneva.

World Health Organization (1993) *The ICD-10 Classification of Mental and Behavioural Disorders: B. Diagnostic Criteria for Research.* WHO, Geneva.

World Health Organization (1996) *Multiaxial Classification of Child and Adolescent Psychiatric Disorders: The ICD-10 Classification of Mental and Behavioural Disorders in Children and Adolescents.* Cambridge University Press, Cambridge.

Clinical Assessment and Diagnostic Formulation

Michael Rutter and Eric Taylor

Initial questions regarding referral

Any clinical appointment will have been initiated by someone making a referral and usually that will involve some form of focused question, although the extent to which this is made explicit is likely to vary among referrals. In the case of children and younger adolescents, it will be rather unusual for the young people themselves to have initiated referral, but that may sometimes be the case. Although the clinician is likely to wish to organize the initial assessment around the question as to whether the child has a clinically significant disorder and, if there is such a disorder, what its nature is, that may or may not be the question that is uppermost in the mind of the person making the referral. The main concern may be what the family or school should do about a particular behaviour that is causing concern in that setting. Alternatively, there may be questions over particular administrative decisions, such as whether the school the child is attending is most appropriate, whether there is a need for exclusion from school, or whether the child should be removed from the family. In other cases, the referral may be to request an opinion that is relevant to a court case involving either child care or the child's responsibility for some criminal act or possible need to respond to such an act with some form of therapeutic intervention. In yet other cases, there may be an implicit query as to the meaning of the child's behaviour—perhaps as to whether or not it represents an early manifestation of some serious mental disorder (such as schizophrenia or autism) that is thought to run in the family. Another possibility is that the main problem concerns disturbed family function that happens to have involved the child in some way (Shepherd *et al.* 1971). If so, there is the need to understand why this child has been referred at this time in this way. It is quite common, too, for different people to have quite discrepant views as to what is the problem and what needs to be done about it. Thus, the father and mother may be at loggerheads over this, their views may be different from those of the child, and all of these may differ from the perspectives of the school, the social services or the family doctor.

Because of all of these uncertainties, and the wide range of possibilities, it is crucial for any assessment to begin with some procedures designed to clarify questions about the referral (Kanner 1957; Rutter 1975). Who initiated the referral? Why was the referral made? Why was the referral made now? Whose problem is it? What are the key concerns or questions to which people want a response? Are there administrative decisions that hang on the assessment and, if so, what are they?

To some extent, these questions can be clarified through obtaining relevant reports in advance of the interview for diagnostic assessment. This needs to be done through discussion with the family and with their approval. However, it is desirable to have available at the time of the first interview relevant reports from the school, from any social agencies that have been involved, from previous medical assessments, and from psychological and educational evaluations.

As well as clarifying the reasons for referral, the initial assessment needs to be planned in such a way as to provide information on how the members of family interact with one another and how they deal with each others' concerns. The aim is to identify possible strengths and limitations in the family and to understand their ways of functioning in order that this may be taken into account in planning therapeutic interventions.

Observations of the family

Observations need to begin with the ways in which the communications—either by letter or telephone call—were dealt with prior to the first interview (Cox & Rutter 1985). Who took the lead? What was the style used? What implications might there be for either the parents' attitudes towards their children or towards professionals. Similar questions need to be considered in relation to observations in the waiting room. If the availability of chairs provided open choice, how did the family choose to sit? What was the style of interactions among family members while waiting to be seen and how did they respond to meeting the clinicians? How did they spend their time in waiting and what were they doing when the clinician went to collect them for interview?

Regardless of how later stages of the assessment are to be undertaken, it is usually informative to have a brief meeting with the family all together in order to clarify these sort of issues and also to explain how the assessment will be organized and who will be seeing who for what purpose. Similar queries to those posed in relation to the waiting room arise with respect to the seating in the interview room. If the aim is to assess family interaction, it is crucial that the interview questions be addressed to the family as a whole, rather than singling out individual family members for their views. Often it may be better to put the query in the form of a questioning statement of a general kind, rather than a specific enquiry. Thus, the clinician may say something like: 'I wonder how much you talked together about coming to see me today?' or there could be a general question such as 'Have you had a family discussion about the reasons for coming here today?' Many parents are likely to have the cultural expectation that they, rather than the child, should answer the clinician's questions and, in interpreting how they respond, it is important to take that into account. Nevertheless, direct questions to the child in this initial family session may make him or her feel put on the spot and, thereby, uncomfortable. Again, a more general style of bringing the whole family into the interview may be preferable (see Eisler, Chapter 9, for a fuller discussion of family interviewing). For example, if someone has responded with a firm answer on expectations or the reasons for coming, the interviewer might say something like: 'I wonder whether everyone in the family sees things in this way?' It is helpful to note how much the parents provide the child with 'space' to express his or her own views. How do the parents react if the child puts things in oppositional or confrontational ways? How do members of the family react when someone is expressing feelings of distress, anger or resentment? What are the patterns of eye to eye gaze among family members? What are their facial expressions and body gestures? Although it is usually a mistake to move quickly into interpretations, it may be helpful to make observations or express reactions as a means of getting the family to talk about the situation. Thus, the clinician may say things such as, 'That appears to be a very difficult situation' or 'It feels as if that was awkward for you to talk about' or 'It sounds as if that came as a bit of a surprise to you'.

Depending on how the interview progresses, it may be appropriate to move on to direct questions about some aspect of the referral. For example, if the school or social services initiated the referral, the family may be asked how they felt about whatever it was that precipitated the referral. Was that something that they, too, were concerned about or did they see it rather differently? Similarly, if the parents have initiated referral because they were worried about some aspect of the child's behaviour or emotional state, it may be important to ask the child directly whether this was something he or she was concerned about.

Younger children should not be expected to sit still during the interview and the interviewer needs to decide in advance what toys or play materials will be made available for the children. The interview provides the opportunity of seeing what the children decide to do and also whom they talk to or whom they turn to during the interview. How do the parents respond if the child seems distressed or is behaving in a disruptive way? Again, it is necessary to recognize that there may be culturally influenced expectations as to how the parents should behave. If the clinician wants the parents to be able to respond to the child it may be appropriate to say that directly by indicating 'It's okay if you want to respond to (*child's name*) while we're talking' or 'By all means go to (*child's name*) if you'd feel more comfortable doing that'.

Interview with the child

Angold (Chapter 3) describes the approaches to be used in inter-

viewing children. As he notes, interviews with older children and adolescents can follow rather similar approaches to those used with adults, but various adaptations are needed with young children. Several points warrant emphasis in that connection. First, it is usually helpful to be able to assess children's behaviour, styles of social interaction and ways of talking, in several contrasting situations. Thus, it is usually desirable to have an opportunity of seeing the child with the rest of the family. Psychological testing will provide the quite different stimulus of a series of structured tasks requiring the child's engagement and attention. Psychological testing should always include a careful description of the child's behaviour and social interactions, as well as test performance (see Sergeant & Taylor, Chapter 6). The interview with the child will be different yet again in providing a dyadic interaction opportunity but of a much less structured kind. Particularly at the beginning of the interview, the style needs to be such as to encourage the child to express his or her own concerns and this needs to proceed to a more systematic approach to specific behaviours and feelings.

Ceci *et al.* (Chapter 8) describe some of the considerations that apply particularly to the interviewing of young children. On the whole, free descriptions in answer to open questions provide accounts of behaviour that are most accurate and least prone to distortion. On the other hand, these tend to be very lacking in detail and, almost always, it will be necessary to follow with more specific questions. As Angold (Chapter 3) points out, however, it is important that this be done in a way that does not provide a lead to specific answers. People of all ages are open to the influence of suggestion but this is particularly the case with younger children (see Ceci *et al.*, Chapter 8).

Variations in the style of child interview and observation are needed when the child has some handicap in their communication and social skills and when the clinical issues require a focus on particular forms of behaviour that may not be tapped adequately in an ordinary interview. The Autism Diagnostic Observation Schedule (ADOS) provides an example of the former (DiLavore *et al.* 1995; Lord *et al.* 1989, 2000). This was developed as a set of social/communicative situations that provide a 'press' or expectation for either social/communicative responses or overtures. A generic version of the test with four modules adapted to children of different communicative levels is now available (Lord *et al.* 2000). It was initially developed primarily for research purposes but specialized clinics are now increasingly using it for clinical assessments. Even if the standardized half-hour assessment is not used clinically, the principles are certainly relevant to any form of clinical diagnostic interview with children or adults for whom the diagnosis of some form of pervasive developmental disorder has been raised (see Lord & Bailey, Chapter 38). There is a similar need to adapt interview approaches for children with seriously impaired hearing or vision (see Hindley & van Gent, Chapter 50).

The need to consider how assessments should be adapted for particular purposes is exemplified by the approaches needed for the assessment of possible attachment disorders (see O'Connor, Chapter 46). The concept of these disorders is that they are characterized by pervasive problems in selective attachment. The disinhibited variety of attachment disorder might be thought to comprise a relative lack of selective attachments, and the inhibited variety both a lack of security provided by established selective attachments and by various abnormal features. So far as the disinhibited variety is concerned, there are two features that particularly require attention. The first concerns the child's response to a stranger and the degree to which this lacks the normal wariness, plus the extent to which there is an inadequate appreciation of social boundaries and an unusual degree of physical closeness or contact before a relationship has been established. In addition, there may be a lack of selectivity in going to the principal caregivers for security or comfort and it is important that the child's response to family members be observed, as well as the response to a stranger. It might be thought that the Strange Situation (Ainsworth *et al.* 1978) ought to be the most appropriate way of determining whether or not there is an inhibited attachment disorder, but it has severe limitations for this purpose. On the face of it, the category of 'disorganized' attachment might seem to be the nearest equivalent of a clinical diagnostic concept. However, it seems that the category of disorganized attachment occurs much more frequently than would be expected for the diagnosis of inhibited attachment disorder (van Ijzendoorn *et al.* 1999). It is clinically appropriate to base assessments on the way the child responds to reunions after separation, but the Strange Situation procedure was designed only for very young children and it is not likely to have the same meaning in older ones. What is needed clinically is a form of assessment that provides the opportunity to assess the child's reaction to strangers (the clinicians fill that role), responses to separations from and reunions with the parents (taking the child to be seen on his or her own and returning later serves that purpose); and the child's use of the parents as a secure basis (a joint family interview is useful in that connection).

Whatever the age of the child, and whatever the clinical issue, it is important that the interview combines an appropriate degree of structure and standardization (which is essential for comparability across children) and sensitivity to the unexpected and to the individual issue. The latter have been most studied in relation to the interviewing of parents in a clinical setting (Cox *et al.* 1981; Rutter *et al.* 1981) in which one of the most striking findings was the very high frequency of clinically significant information of an unusual kind that would be most unlikely to have been picked up by confining questioning only to predetermined topics. The same consideration certainly applies to interviews with children. It is very important for clinicians to be sensitive to the cues provided by children and these will need to be followed through in whatever way seems most appropriate to the individual situation. This need applies even more to what children say about their psychosocial circumstances than it does to what they say about psychopathology (see below).

Parental interview

Angold (Chapter 3) outlines in some detail the approach that needs to be taken when interviewing parents. The main focus in Chapter 3 is on the assessment of psychopathology and the additional point that needs to be made here is that, in planning therapeutic interventions, several other features need to be considered. To begin with, it is essential to determine what it is about the child's behaviour or feelings or social interactions that is of the greatest concern to the parents. It may not necessarily be the feature that the clinician considers to be of the greatest psychopathological importance but, ordinarily, it is sensible that early therapeutic interventions be recognized by the parents as addressing their concerns. In addition, it is important to find out how the parents, and other people, have tried to deal with the concern. How have they tried to respond and what success or otherwise have their approaches achieved? If adequate use is to be made of this in therapeutic planning, it will be essential to move beyond a general answer (such as admonish the child, or comfort him or her, or try to be understanding) and, instead, obtain a more detailed sequential account of *how* this has been done. What did they do and what was the child's response? If certain approaches did not work, did they persist (and if so, for how long and under what circumstances) or did they keep changing? A closely related issue is the impact that the child's disturbance has had on them and on the rest of the family.

In dealing with the development of the disorder, attention needs to be paid to possible predisposing factors in life circumstances or physical state. Before proceeding with specific questioning, it is usually better to elicit the parents' views on what might have been important. There is then the functional analysis of the behaviour that is causing concern (see Herbert, Chapter 53). In other words, what are the features that seem to make the behaviours of concern more likely or less likely to occur? What circumstances seem to improve the situation? Questions regarding the degree to which behaviours are situation-specific or pervasive are important, not only for their implications with respect to severity (see Angold, Chapter 3) but also in terms of features in the environment that may act as a risk or protective factor.

There are important advantages in making sure that children are seen with their parents for part of the diagnostic assessment. However, people do not behave, or talk, in the same way when seen on their own as when seen as part of a family group. Accordingly, it is usually desirable for part of the assessment time to be spent in seeing the child on his or her own and similarly for the parents to be seen separately. Not only may this provide information that would not be obtained quite so readily in a family setting, but it also makes explicit a concern to pay attention to family members as individuals as well as part of a group. Some clinicians prefer to conduct the whole of the diagnostic assessment interview in a conjoint family setting but, in our view, this has disadvantages with respect to information gathering. A similar decision needs to be made as to whether both parents should be seen together or whether there should be some time with each parent separately. Our usual practice is to follow parental preferences in the first instance but to be alert to cues that suggest that it may be necessary to see parents on their own for a brief period in addition. However, it should be noted that one study (Cox *et al.* 1995) showed that families did not respond well to a change of style from family to individual, or vice versa, when making the transition from diagnostic assessment to therapeutic intervention.

School reports

It is always desirable to obtain a school report, preferably in advance of the first interview with the family, but after obtaining their agreement that the school may be contacted. Children may well behave differently at school from the way they do at home and it is important to obtain an account of scholastic functioning; educational difficulties are frequently associated with psychopathology. There are some advantages in using a standard questionnaire as part of the reporting from school (see Verhulst & Van der Ende, Chapter 5). However, a questionnaire is never adequate on its own: it is crucial for teachers to be able to express their own concerns which may involve features that are outside the coverage of the questionnaire; it is important to consider changes over time and not just present behaviour; and it is important to find out how school has dealt with difficulties and how the child has responded to whatever actions were taken. There may be specific queries that arise out of the diagnostic assessment and, when that is the case, it may be useful for a member of the clinical team to contact the school directly in order to discuss the points that have arisen. Particularly when there seems to be a major discrepancy between the accounts of the child's behaviour at home and at school, visits to both settings to observe what is happening may be informative.

Psychological testing

Sergeant & Taylor (Chapter 6) provide an account of both the approach that needs to be taken to psychological testing and of its role in the overall diagnostic assessment. As they note, a key part of the psychological evaluation concerns the psychologist's observation of the child's behaviour in relation to the tasks that have been given and in relation to the social encounter with the psychologist. This is important because of the information that it provides about the child's psychological functioning generally, and not just because of its importance in relation to the interpretation of the psychological test findings.

So far as the latter are concerned, it is essential in all cases to consider whether the scores are consistent with the account of the child's performance given by the parents and by the school and in keeping with the clinician's observations of the child. Of course, it is to be expected that there will not be perfect agreement across all assessments but, if there are major discrepancies, that always has to be a matter for further study. If the child's performance during standardized testing was markedly better or markedly worse than that expected on that basis of other people's reports, what is the explanation? Does it reflect differences in the cognitive demands in the several situations, or does it reflect social features of the situation? What are the implications for the situational factors that seem to facilitate better performance?

A crucial part of any psychological assessment concerns the evaluation of the likely validity of the findings. Attention needs to be paid to the extent to which it was possible to engage the child in the relevant tasks, noting whether disturbed behaviour may have interfered with task performance. Particularly in the case of young children for whom there is a query regarding possible severe mental retardation, it is important to note how the child dealt with the situation as a whole, and with the task presented. A clear enquiring curiosity about the environment, a systematic problem-solving approach, and initiative combined with imagination in dealing with test materials, would all raise questions about the validity of a very low test score. Obviously it is necessary to consider whether overall task performance has been constrained because of specific difficulties in functions such as language, motor coordination or vision. In terms of the predictive validity of scores, consideration also needs to be given to the possibility that current cognitive functioning has been impaired as a result of severely disadvantageous rearing experiences that no longer apply. In short, test scores provide invaluable information but they need to be interpreted in relation to the assessment as a whole.

Medical examination and testing

The considerations that apply to medical examination and possible testing are discussed by Bailey (Chapter 10). The principles that should underlie decision-making on this issue are those that apply in any clinical assessment. The most fundamental requirement is that a thoughtful and systematic history-taking should be used as a guide to the possibility that somatic problems may be relevant to the psychopathology that has been the focus of the referral. When there is nothing in the history to suggest the presence of a possibly relevant somatic condition, it is sufficient to measure the child's height and weight, and to undertake a screening neurodevelopmental examination that does not require the child to undress fully. Questions should be asked to determine pubertal status but, unless it appears likely to be specifically relevant, there is no need to undertake a physical examination for this purpose.

When the child has a possible global or specific developmental delay, or a disorder such as autism (see Lord & Bailey, Chapter 38) or hyperkinetic disorder (see Schachar & Tannock, Chapter 25), a rather fuller assessment is necessary (see Bailey, Chapter 10; Volkmar & Dykens, Chapter 41). This needs to be guided by leads provided in the history but routine assessment for somatic conditions (such as tuberous sclerosis or chromosomal abnormalities) for which there may not be leads in the history, and which have a significant association with psychopathology, need to be covered by the appropriate screening examinations and tests. It is important to bear in mind the possibility of relevant general medical conditions, as well as those directly involving the central nervous system (see Goodman, Chapter 14). Possible endocrine problems in relation to the differential diagnosis of eating disorders should be considered (see Steinhausen, Chapter 34). Appropriate medical assessments are essential when there are symptoms affecting somatic functions, because this could result from somatic disease. Early studies of so-called hysterical conversion reactions in both children (Caplan 1970) and adults (Slater 1965) have shown the relatively high frequency with which these were wrongly diagnosed as psychogenic in origin, as shown by the clear emergence of underlying physical disease of a directly pertinent kind during the course of follow-up. With proper clinical assessment, such misdiagnoses nowadays should be much less common, but clinicians need to be aware of the possibility (see Mrazek, Chapter 48).

Presence/absence of clinically significant psychopathology

Because most psychiatric disorders do not include pathognomonic qualitatively abnormal features that cannot be found in normal children or adolescents, a key basic question has to be whether the severity or nature of psychopathology is such as to be clinically significant. Necessarily, that query comprises two somewhat different issues. First, there is the question of whether the problems being considered are causing significant suffering for the individual or significant distress for others. Secondly, there is the question of whether the psychopathology is such as to fall outside the normal range of behaviour, or which carries with it a significant likelihood of recurrent or chronic malfunction. Clinical intervention will sometimes be indicated when the answer to one of the questions is in the affirmative but in the negative to the other. Thus, a serious grief reaction following the death of a loved one is quite common in normal individuals but it may warrant offering appropriate counselling (see Black, Chapter 18), even though it may not be a psychiatric disorder in the normal sense of the word. Similarly, many parents present at health clinics with their child's difficulties in eating or sleeping, which are essentially normal, but are yet causing major family disruption. Appropriate guidance and help may well be needed in such circumstances (see Stein & Barnes, Chapter 45).

Angold (Chapter 3) considers the features that need to be considered when deciding whether emotional disturbance amounts to a clinically significant disorder. The question is an important one because anxiety, depression and fears are a normal part of the human condition that most people experience at some time. The considerations to be taken into account include: whether there has been a substantial change from the person's usual mental state; whether the intensity of the emotions goes beyond the range of normal variation; whether the person is able to control the unpleasant emotions by means of distraction or engagement in pleasurable activities; whether the emotions intrude into and interfere with normal life functioning; and whether the emotions are pervasive across situations. Somewhat similar criteria

apply to overactivity/inattention but with the difference that, because these are usually first manifest in the preschool years, there will not usually be a recognizable change from any previous normal pattern. The assessment of disruptive behaviour is rather less straightforward because the child may not perceive that there is a need to control such behaviour.

From the time of the Isle of Wight studies (Rutter *et al.* 1970) onwards, the degree to which psychopathology gives rise to impairment of psychosocial functioning has been a key consideration in the assessment of clinical significance. There was a further impetus to use such a criterion from the epidemiological evidence that some forms of symptomatology, particularly specific phobias, were present in what seemed to be an absurdly high proportion of the population if impairment was not taken into account (Bird *et al.* 1990; Bird 1999). This has appeared a reasonable approach because, if psychopathology is not impairing functioning, there would not seem to be much need for intervention. Epidemiological findings have been consistent in showing that there are substantial differences among different forms of psychopathology in the extent to which there is associated impairment. Quite a few children show psychosocial impairment associated with psychopathology but without the required number of symptoms to fulfil the criteria for a specific diagnosis (Angold *et al.* 1999b). When this is the case, intervention may well be justified. The presence of marked symptoms in the absence of impairment is most frequently seen in relation to specific phobias (Simonoff *et al.* 1997). Conversely, it is rather unusual for there to be multiple symptoms of depression without there being any impairment (Pickles *et al.*, 2001). However, the diagnosis here is made not just on the severity of negative mood, but also on associated phenomena such as self-depreciation, feelings of guilt, feelings of hopelessness about the future, and suicidal thoughts or actions. The need to consider associated symptomatology constitutes a key element in diagnosis.

Thus, clinically significant developmental disorders of language need to be differentiated from normal variations in language development on the basis of the breadth of affected language functions (e.g. including understanding as well as use of spoken language), impaired use of language-related skills in make-believe play, difficulties in the control of motor movements associated with spoken language (as with drooling), and associated socioemotional or behavioural problems (Rutter 1987). Although certainly a useful criterion to employ, there are both logical and practical problems associated with giving it too high a priority. First, from a medical perspective, it would seem foolish to say that a person did not have a disorder because they were not impaired if there were signs or symptoms (or test findings) indicating an obviously pathological condition. Thus, someone with diabetes, whose condition has been shown by the appropriate laboratory tests, would still be diagnosed as having diabetes even if functioning was unimpaired because symptoms were well controlled by diet or the use of insulin. The same would clearly apply in the case of schizophrenia that was well controlled by appropriate medication. In these instances, however, the abnormality is evident in terms of qualitatively abnormal findings, as evident either by history or present status, or both. The second concern is that a person may cope successfully with their disorder to the extent that symptoms are not manifest because the situations that elicit them have been avoided. There will not be psychosocial impairment if the person's life is so organized that the issues do not arise. This most obviously applies in the case of certain phobias. Thirdly, the degree to which there is psychosocial impairment will inevitably be influenced by social circumstances. Many decades ago Wootton (1959) pointed to the absurdity of rates of disorders going up and down according to fluctuations in the employment rate. She noted too the major difficulties in basing a diagnosis of psychiatric disorder on the extent to which it caused problems for other people. This has been a problematic issue in deciding whether conduct disorders should be regarded as psychiatric conditions (Hill & Maughan 2001). In this case, what is a persuasive argument in favour of regarding it as a disorder is the extensive evidence of impaired personal functioning in both childhood and adult life, including an increased risk of suicide and of other forms of psychopathology.

Although qualitative abnormalities are not a feature of most psychiatric disorders in childhood or adolescence, they are present in some. For example, the pattern of socioemotional deficits shown by individuals with autism is one that would be abnormal at any age (see Lord & Bailey, Chapter 38). The same applies to the thought disorder, negative symptoms, and delusions/hallucinations found in schizophrenia (see Hollis, Chapter 37). The situation is not quite so clear-cut with obsessive-compulsive phenomena but, although ruminations and minor checking behaviour may be regarded as falling within the normal range of variation, that is not the case with overt compulsive rituals of a marked kind (see Rapoport & Swedo, Chapter 35). Somewhat similar considerations apply to Tourette syndrome and chronic multiple tics (see Leckman & Cohen, Chapter 36). Particular care needs to be taken in eliciting detailed descriptions of such qualitatively abnormal features because, if people have not experienced these phenomena, they may interpret the questions as referring to the more normal features that are within their experience (see Angold, Chapter 3).

Duration and timing of disorder

Classification systems have often used duration of disorder as a key criterion by which to determine whether or not psychopathology is clinically significant. For example, DSM-IV (American Psychiatric Association 2000) has specified a minimum duration of 2 weeks for a major depressive disorder, 1 month for a generalized anxiety disorder, 6 months for a conduct disorder or a generalized anxiety disorder, and 2 years for a dysthymic disorder (but no duration is specified for anorexia nervosa). It is immediately obvious that there is an essentially arbitrary nature to the choice of these time periods. Thus, most clinicians would regard 2 weeks as a rather short period of time

for a major depressive disorder, and it is noteworthy that the research diagnostic criteria specify 4 weeks, rather than 2 (Mazure & Gershon 1979). Also, 2 years seems an incredibly long time to require a dysthymic disorder to last in order to regard it as meeting criteria. A further problem is that, even with high quality research interviewing that involves a specific focus on personalized timing, the reliability of the timing of onset of disorder has proved rather poor (Angold et al. 1996). In all probability, this is not mainly because people find it difficult to remember some clearly identifiable time when a disorder began, but rather because many disorders do not have a clear-cut onset. Frequently, symptomatology builds up over time with several points at which new symptoms become apparent and/or when psychosocial impairment first becomes evident (Rutter & Sandberg 1992; Sandberg et al., 2001). Clearly, it is important for clinicians to obtain as good an account as possible of how psychopathology developed over time and to seek to identify times that might be conceptualized as either an onset of disorder or a clear worsening of disorder. However, from a clinical perspective it is less appropriate to follow DSM-IV rules about duration in a slavish fashion than it is to decide that the symptoms constitute something that manifestly falls outside the range of normal variation for that person and which either involves qualitative abnormalities or has interfered with psychosocial functioning to a substantial extent.

Nature of the mental disorder

If the assessment has indicated that there is a significant psychopathological disorder, the next question is what form it takes, and what diagnosis or diagnoses may be applied to it (see Taylor & Rutter, Chapter 1). ICD-10 (World Health Organization 1992) and DSM-IV (American Psychiatric Association 2000) adopt different approaches to this issue. Both accept the frequency with which mixed patterns of symptomatology occur but they deal with them in different ways.

DSM-IV takes the line that, in most cases, good well-validated empirical evidence is lacking on how to decide on the precedence to be given among differing patterns of symptomatology. Accordingly, rather than make arbitrary decisions on some hierarchy, for the most part the clinician is expected to diagnose as present any pattern that meets the criteria for a diagnosis. The inevitable consequence of this approach is that comorbidity (the co-occurrence of two or more supposedly separate disorders) is exceedingly common (Caron & Rutter 1991; Angold et al. 1999a). Indeed, it is quite frequent for individuals to receive three or four or even more diagnoses. The merit of this approach is that it provides a means of noting the mixed patterns of psychopathology without having to invoke hierarchical rules for which there is a lack of good supporting evidence. The disadvantage is that it implies that a high proportion of patients have multiple separate conditions. Common sense indicates that that is not likely to be true with most children in community clinics.

ICD-10, by contrast, takes the line that, ordinarily, one should assume that there is just one condition, unless there are good grounds for supposing the true occurrence of several. What this means in practice is that the clinician is expected to consider the psychopathology as a whole and then decide which diagnosis constitutes the 'best fit' to the pattern seen in the individual case. There is little doubt that this conceptualization is likely to be valid, but the problem lies in the lack of good empirical bases for many types of decision-making that are required.

Two particularly common examples may be used to illustrate the dilemmas. Numerous studies have shown the high frequency with which anxiety symptomatology and depression symptomatology co-occur (see Harrington, Chapter 29; Klein & Pine, Chapter 30) and the same applies to the overlap between oppositional/defiant behaviour and conduct problems (see Earls & Mezzacappa, Chapter 26). In both cases, research findings clearly point to the need to take a developmental perspective. Longitudinal studies have shown that a common sequence is for anxiety disorders in middle childhood to lead on to depressive disorders in adolescence or early adult life (Kovacs et al. 1989; Weissman 1990; Orvaschel et al. 1995; Wickramaratne & Weissman 1998). Twin studies in both children (Thapar & McGuffin 1997) and adults (Kendler 1996) have shown that to a very considerable extent anxiety and depression share the same underlying genetic liability. This is probably indexed to a considerable extent by the personality trait of neuroticism (Kendler 1996). That does not necessarily mean that anxiety disorders and depressive conditions should be regarded as synonymous because both involve environmental, as well as genetic, risk factors. There is some evidence in both children and adults (see Sandberg & Rutter, Chapter 17) that they are associated with rather different forms of precipitating stress experiences (psychological loss predominating in the case of depression and threat in the case of anxiety). Longitudinal twin data (Silberg et al., 2001) are informative in showing that early anxiety problems are associated with postpubertal depression and that a shared genetic liability is important in that link. The diagnostic problem at the time of clinic assessment, however, has to focus on the slightly different issue of overlapping symptomatology at the same point in time. Regardless of which diagnostic convention is followed, it is important for the clinician to assess the relative importance of anxiety and depression in relation to the clinical picture as it presents at that time. It will be necessary to take account of both sorts of psychopathology in deciding how to intervene therapeutically but, in so far as medication is used, it is clear that antianxiety drugs are not a good way of treating depression, but that antidepressants may be effective in reducing anxiety as well as depressive phenomena (see Harrington, Chapter 29).

Somewhat comparable issues arise with respect to oppositional/defiant conduct problems. The two frequently co-occur, but longitudinal studies show the frequency with which oppositional/defiant behaviour in early childhood leads on to conduct disorders in later childhood or adolescence (Hinshaw et al. 1993). Because transitions in psychopathology tend to take

place over lengthy periods of time, it follows that it is likely that there will be many instances in which the child has a mixture of the two types of problem behaviour but below the threshold for each, because one disorder is gradually being taken over by the other. That is exactly what the field studies for DSM-IV showed (Lahey et al. 1998). Moreover, twin studies have shown that the two forms of symptomatology share the same genetic liability to a very considerable extent (Eaves et al., 2000). The implication is that, in reality, these are probably somewhat different manifestations of the same basic psychopathology, rather than two different conditions with different causes and different implications for treatment (see Earls & Mezzacappa, Chapter 26). Similar issues arise with respect to the evidence that overactivity/inattention in early childhood carries with it a substantially increased risk for later antisocial behaviour (Rutter et al. 1998a). These associations extend well beyond the diagnostic boundaries, at least of hyperkinetic disorder as conceptualized in ICD-10. It is noteworthy that the strong genetic component in hyperactivity seems to apply across a broad range (to a dimensional variation in this characteristic) and not just to an extreme disorder (Thapar et al. 1999). There may well be good grounds for retaining a concept of hyperkinetic disorder as a separate categorical condition (see Schachar & Tannock, Chapter 25) but there is also a need to recognize the prognostic importance of patterns of overactivity and inattention that fall short of the diagnostic criteria for that disorder. Again, the clinical need, regardless of which set of diagnostic conventions are followed, is for the clinician to try to decide the meaning and mechanisms underlying the mixed pattern of symptomatology. Twin data indicate that both forms of symptomatology share a common genetic liability to a considerable extent (Nadder et al., in press), even though oppositional/defiant and conduct problems are, to an important extent, separate from hyperactivity (Nadder et al., 2001).

The need to sort out meaning and mechanisms goes well beyond decisions on which diagnostic conventions to follow. A more basic hypothesis-testing approach to diagnostic assessment is fundamental to the diagnostic enterprise. For example, although not well reflected in either of the two main classification systems, it is important to differentiate among the various causes of faecal soiling (Rutter 1975). This may arise, for example, because the child has failed to gain bowel control. Alternatively, control may well have been achieved and maintained, with the disorder lying in the deposition of faeces in inappropriate places, rather than in any lack of or loss of control. A third possibility is that there has been faecal retention leading to gross distension of the bowel and partial blockage. In these circumstances, faecal soiling may arise because there has been an overflow of faeces stemming from the prior distension. In order to differentiate among these possibilities, careful assessment is needed of whether or not the faeces are normal in form and consistency; whether there is a history of previous normal bowel control; whether the soiling has been preceded by patterns of retention or other abnormalities in bowel functioning; and whether the deposition of faeces is essentially random, according to where the child happens to be at the time that the bowels are opened, rather than selectively placed in situations having psychological meaning. Clearly, the therapeutic interventions need to be chosen on the basis of the type of disorder represented by the soiling (see Clayden *et al.*, Chapter 47).

A decision tree approach may also be very useful in the assessment of developmental disorders of language (see Bishop, Chapter 39). When the diagnostic issue concerns some pattern of psychopathology associated with the language delay, it is helpful to tackle the decision-making in stepwise fashion (Rutter 1985). Thus, it is usually best to begin by determining the child's overall level of cognitive functioning, going on to consider whether language skills are significantly below those of other aspects of cognitive functioning. The question then is whether the psychopathology shown is outside the range of normal behaviour expected in relation to the child's overall mental age and overall level of language functioning. If it is outside that range, rather than move on straight away to consider the complete list of possible psychiatric diagnoses, it is generally helpful to question whether the behaviours are of a kind that might be found in any child (the usual run of emotional problems and disorders of disruptive behaviour, etc.) or whether the pattern is qualitatively different in a way that is associated with pervasive developmental disorders. It is then easier to move on to a consideration of which particular diagnostic concept best fits the picture in the light of that decision.

The possibility that the disorder is not represented at all in the current classification system should also be considered. As Kanner aptly put it in the title of one of his papers on differential diagnosis, 'The children haven't read those books' (Kanner 1969). The point that he was making was that there is a most imperfect match between the neat diagnostic descriptions given in textbooks and the clinical presentations seen in referred patients. The usual explanation will be that the person has a somewhat atypical variety of a well-recognized well-validated disorder. Nevertheless, the last half century has seen the recognition for the first time of several disorders of considerable importance. Kanner's (1943) identification of autism is the most striking example, but it is closely followed by the identification of Rett syndrome (Rett 1966; Hagberg *et al.* 1983). Both Asperger syndrome (Asperger 1944) and Wolff's concept of schizoid disorder of childhood (Wolff & Chick 1980; Wolff 1995) constitute other variants within the realm of what might be regarded as autism-spectrum disorders. 'New' conditions are by no means restricted to this group of pervasive developmental disorders. Russell's (1979) identification of bulimia nervosa and Meadow's (1977) account of the Munchausen by proxy syndrome constitute other important examples of a very different kind. The concept of attachment disorders (see O'Connor, Chapter 46) constitutes yet another example. More recent, and therefore less validated, examples are also provided by the quasi-autistic pattern seen in some children who have experienced profound institutional deprivation (Rutter *et al.* 1999a); the social abnormalities that have been found to be associated with severe developmental disorders of receptive language

(Howlin *et al.* 2000; Mawhood *et al.* 2000); and the autistic-like patterns seen with some cases of congenital blindness (Brown *et al.* 1997). Not all of these patterns of psychopathology constitute well-validated syndromes but the general point remains: clinicians must always be on the alert for unusual patterns that do not fit existing diagnostic conventions.

In some cases, the clinical question may refer to a particular phenomenon rather than a pattern of psychopathology. For example, during the 1980s there was some excitement over reports that autistic children who could not speak could nevertheless communicate at a high level when given assistance through a range of techniques that came to be called 'facilitating communication'. The children were said to communicate by guiding someone else's arm to point to letters to spell out words, or some other comparable means of communicating via another person, called a facilitator. The key to sorting out the validity of these claims (in the individual case just as much as in the studies of groups) lay in setting up a situation in which the information available to the child and the information available to the facilitator was different. When this was done it became apparent that the communications were being determined by the facilitator rather than the handicapped child (Rutter *et al.* 1998b). Comparable issues arise in relation to the diagnosis of selective mutism (see Bishop, Chapter 39), a syndrome characterized by a high degree of selectivity in circumstances of talking. In both instances, as in experimental studies more generally, the need is to design a situation in which children can and do succeed but do so in ways that are informative on the mechanisms involved. Thus, in the case of selective mutism, the need is to be able to demonstrate that the children can use spoken language in particular circumstances, just as much as showing that they do not use spoken language in other situations.

Psychosocial assessment

Psychosocial risks are important in the development of psychopathology (see Friedman & Chase-Lansdale, Chapter 15; Sandberg & Rutter, Chapter 17). It is important therefore that the diagnostic assessment provides an efficient, reliable and valid means of assessing the presence of psychosocial risk factors. However, it should not be seen as exclusively related to questions of causation. In planning psychological interventions (when indicated) it is important to identify possible protective mechanisms, as well as risk features. Moreover, it is necessary to assess risk and protective factors, not only in terms of what is happening within the family, but also what is happening within the peer group, school and community (Rutter *et al.* 1998a; Shonkoff & Phillips 2000). Furthermore, the psychosocial assessment needs to include both past experiences and current circumstances. On the whole, most early experiences do not have enduring effects that are independent of later psychosocial circumstances (Clarke & Clarke 2000). Nevertheless, profoundly depriving experiences can have major sequelae that persist long after children have ceased to suffer deprivation and have had good rearing experiences in a well-functioning family (Rutter *et al.*, in press, a). Similarly, there may be enduring effects of seriously abusive experiences (see Emery & Laumann Billings, Chapter 20; Glaser, Chapter 21). The same applies to some instances of very severely traumatic experiences in relation to persisting post-traumatic stress disorder (see Yule, Chapter 32).

A key consideration with respect to all these experiences, risk and protective, is the need to appreciate that the experiences cannot be thought of as impinging on a passive organism. Children, and adults, think and feel about what they experience and the cognitive/affective sets that they develop (or internal working models) may be very important in determining the consequences of such experiences. What this means is that the assessment needs to determine both how children have coped with their experiences (see Compas *et al.*, Chapter 55) and what they have thought about what has happened to them and how they view their current experiences.

Research over recent decades has made it abundantly clear that genetic factors play an important part in the origins and persistence of all forms of behaviour, including all forms of psychopathology (Rutter *et al.* 1999b,c; see McGuffin & Rutter, Chapter 12). The findings are of major clinical importance for several rather different reasons. They show the importance of recognizing the influence of genetic susceptibilities with respect to individual differences in the liability to psychopathology. That means, amongst other things, that any adequate diagnostic assessment will need to include systematic questioning with respect to a family history of psychopathology. Particular attention needs to be paid to disorders in parents and in siblings, not just because they are the closest relatives with respect to genetic inheritance, but also because mental disorders in the immediate family will involve environmentally mediated, as well as genetically mediated, psychosocial risks (Rutter 1989). Thus, parental mental disorder is associated with a substantially increased risk of family discord and family breakdown, and also focused hostility on individual children (Rutter *et al.* 1997). It is important to assess the ways in which parental mental disorder impinges on the family and not just be content with recognizing its presence. The risks may also involve physical risk factors in relation to substances that cross the placental barrier during pregnancy. Thus, high levels of alcohol ingestion in the early months of pregnancy may lead to the neurodevelopmental abnormalities associated with fetal alcohol syndrome (Spohr & Steinhausen 1996; Stratton *et al.* 1996). There may also be effects from taking recreational drugs or prescribed medications (Singer *et al.* 1997; Delaney-Black *et al.* 2000; see also Marks *et al.*, Chapter 51). The extent to which there is enquiry about mental disorders occurring in second- and third-degree relatives needs to be guided by the particular clinical problem. However, it should be routine to ask about the occurrence of major mental disorders or developmental problems in both sides of the family. Genetic testing (using cytogenetic and molecular genetic methods) is not part of routine assessment but it is important in some circumstances (see Skuse & Kuntsi, Chapter 13) and could become more generally applicable in the future.

Research methods that provide systematic standardized assessments of psychosocial features are too time-consuming for use in most clinics. Nevertheless, they do provide helpful guides on how such routine clinical assessments should be undertaken. As with the assessment of psychopathology, the agreement between the reports of parents and children tends to be modest to moderate at best (Rutter *et al.* 1970; Achenbach *et al.* 1987; Simonoff *et al.* 1997; Borge *et al.*, 2001). That is partly because parents will not know about the full range of children's experiences outside the home, partly because their perspectives may not be the same, and partly because some disorders may be relatively situation-specific (Cox & Rutter 1985). The implication is that some assessment of psychosocial risk and protective experiences needs to be obtained from both parents and children. The classification of psychosocial experiences developed by the World Health Organization (van Goor-Lambo *et al.* 1990) provides some guidance on the range of experiences that need to be considered and there are standardized interviews that cover most of the relevant experiences (Sandberg *et al.* 1993). However, the research findings from studies that have used designs that can separate environmental from genetic mediation (Rutter *et al.*, in press, b) suggest that the experiences carrying the greatest psychopathological risk mainly concerns marked negativity in close personal relationships, a lack of continuity in personalized caregiving, a lack of appropriate learning experiences, and participation in social groups with a deviant ethos, attitudes or styles of behaviour (Rutter 2000a). Although not much investigated in genetically sensitive designs, it is likely that parental monitoring and supervision of children's behaviour are also important in relation to antisocial problems (Rutter *et al.* 1998a; but see Stattin & Kerr 2000 with respect to the role of children's disclosures). In relation to all these experiences, it is necessary to determine the ways in which such experiences impinge on the individual child, and are responded to, and not just the experiences as they affect the family as a whole. Although excessive claims have been made about the preponderant importance of child-specific experiences (Rutter *et al.* 1999a; Reiss *et al.* 2000), it is the risks as they affect the individual child that are important, even if they impinge similarly on other children in the same family.

In that connection, the research evidence suggests that it is often useful to make direct comparisons among children in the family with respect to features such as whether one is more likely to be criticized than others, or is more frequently favoured, or is more likely to be involved in relevant risk or protective experiences in the family (Carbonneau *et al.*, 2001 & submitted). In addition, research has shown how much can be inferred from the ways in which a parent talks about the children. This was first demonstrated in the Camberwell Family Interview (Brown & Rutter 1966; Rutter & Brown 1966) but has been developed as a much briefer assessment in relation to the 5-min speech sample (Magaña *et al.* 1986). The implication is that it is important to have a time during the assessment when parents are asked neutral questions about their children, not just questions focusing on problems. Thus, it is helpful to get parents to talk about what their children are like as individuals, how easy they are to be friendly and affectionate with, what is their most striking individual characteristic, etc. The same, of course, applies similarly to the ways in which children talk about their parents and about their siblings.

Diagnostic formulation

Diagnoses serve the important role of providing a succinct summary of the key clinical features that are held in common with disorders experienced by others (see Taylor & Rutter, Chapter 1). This is a most important purpose and one that is central to communication among clinicians, just as much as among researchers. Multiaxial systems of classification can go somewhat further because they serve to classify relevant psychosocial situations that may have played a part in either causation or which may be pertinent with respect to therapeutic planning, as well as intellectual level and a level of adaptive functioning. By considering the information included across a complete range of axes, quite a lot of clinically relevant information can be summarized succinctly.

Nevertheless, that is not quite the same thing as developing hypotheses about causal processes and hypotheses about therapeutic interventions. For example, suppose it has been found that the child has cerebral palsy. As outlined by Goodman (Chapter 14) there is good epidemiological evidence that this is associated with a substantial increase in psychopathological risk in groups of children with this condition. However, the risk could come about through several different routes, each of which have different implications for intervention. Thus, in some instances, the main risk may derive from the electrophysiological disturbance associated with frequent, poorly controlled epileptic attacks. In other cases, the risk may stem from impaired cognitive skills and from the educational difficulties to which they may give rise. In some cases there may be relatively direct neural effects of brain dysfunction, as exemplified in so-called frontal lobe syndromes exhibiting social disinhibition that sometimes occur after severe head injuries (Rutter *et al.* 1983). In yet other cases, the psychopathological risk may derive from the child's negative self-image as a result of his or her physical limitations, or perhaps from parental overprotection that came about as a way of dealing with a physically handicapped child. In yet other cases, the cerebral palsy may be a relatively incidental finding that has no particular relevance to the mental disorder. When dealing with a single case, it is difficult to have hard evidence to enable a choice between these alternatives, but it is important for the clinician to have a view on the likely importance of different mechanisms.

Closely comparable issues arise with respect to psychosocial risk factors. If the mother is alcoholic, did the psychopathological risk derive from the child's *in utero* exposure to high levels of alcohol, from the genetic susceptibility, or from the family disruption and poor parenting to which the alcoholism may have given rise. In considering causal processes, crucial distinctions

need to be drawn between distal and proximal risk processes (Rutter *et al.* 1998a) and also between influences on the initiation of the child psychopathology and the processes that are currently maintaining it. Thus, poverty and social disadvantage are associated with an increased risk of mental disorders in childhood, but most of the risks seem to be indirectly mediated. The overall disadvantageous social circumstances do not, in themselves, cause psychopathology but they do make good parenting more difficult and the main risks stem from the parenting problems (Conger *et al.* 1992, 1993). In the same sort of way, parental loss and parent–child separations are associated with an increased risk of antisocial behaviour but, again, this seems to be largely because of the associated family discord and conflict (Rutter 1971; Fergusson *et al.* 1992). Furthermore, although family conflict is associated with an increased risk of psychopathology, it seems that this largely comes about when the conflict leads to negativity that is focused on that particular child (Reiss *et al.* 1995). In these examples, the global family situation needs to be thought of as a risk indicator, rather than an immediate risk mechanism. It is implicated in the causal processes but largely because it predisposes to other psychosocial features that constitute a more direct psychopathological risk. It is by no means easy to make these distinctions in the individual case, or even at a group level, but it is important when trying to decide how best to intervene.

The distinction between initiatory or provoking risk factors and factors concerned with the maintenance of a disorder is somewhat different. For example, an extremely traumatic experience may precipitate a post-traumatic stress disorder (see Yule, Chapter 32) but some individuals recover quite quickly whereas others go on suffering for several years afterwards. In most cases, the difference between recovery and persistence is likely to lie less in the severity of the initial experience than in how the person thinks about that experience and how they have dealt with it. The original traumatic experience cannot be taken away but the person may be helped to deal better with both the thought patterns and emotional reactions to which the experience gave rise. In other cases, it may be helpful to differentiate between the factors that played a major part in the timing of the onset of disorder and those that were responsible for the increased liability that led to the disorder occurring at all (see Sandberg & Rutter, Chapter 17). Thus, severely threatening life events (such as psychological loss or humiliation) may precipitate the onset of a depressive reaction or the initiation of a particular behaviour such as a suicidal act (see Shaffer & Gutstein, Chapter 33). On the other hand, the overall susceptibility to disorder may have more to do with the associated chronic psychosocial adversity than with the time-limited acute event itself. One of the important findings in life events research is the high frequency with which seriously negative events derive out of chronic psychosocial adversity. Both are important but they may serve a somewhat different risk role.

Clearly, the proximal risk mechanisms involved with the maintenance disorder must play a major part in determining the therapeutic hypotheses that constitute the basis for planning treatment. However, several other matters have to be taken into account. To begin with, it is necessary to consider possible protective mechanisms, as well as risk processes (Rutter 1990). As in the broader consideration of features associated with resilience (Rutter 1999, 2000b), such possible protective processes may reflect a quite diverse range of features. Thus, the strengths may lie in the child's temperamental qualities and/or coping skills (Sandler *et al.* 2000), in the presence of a particularly good close relationship in or outside the family, of compensating good experiences at school or in the peer group, or in a possible change of pattern in family functioning. Thus, if one parent is particularly under stress, the other parent may be encouraged to take a greater role in parenting. The point is that the clinician needs to think broadly about the child's psychosocial situation in order to identify possible strengths and protective possibilities.

In planning any intervention, it is as necessary to decide which features are modifiable as it is to determine which are the risk and causal mechanisms. Thus, it is necessary to decide whether the intervention should focus primarily on working with the child, the parents, the family as a whole, the school, or trying to change other aspects of the broader environment. Of course, the treatment strategy may involve more than one of these avenues. One aspect of deciding about openness to modifiability concerns different perceptions of the child and of what needs to be done. Part of the same issue concerns a decision on what are realistic goals. The aim must be to provide relief for the child's suffering in the first instance, but restoration of full normality may not be a realistic goal (for example, only rarely would it be so in the case of autism; see Lord & Bailey, Chapter 38). Similarly, the intervention may not necessarily focus on the hypothesized basic causal process. Again, to use the example of autism, there would be general acceptance that this is a neurodevelopmental disorder but, equally, the evidence suggests that behavioural/educational interventions working with parents and teachers currently provides the best opportunities for reducing handicaps, even though autism has clearly not been caused by the lack of such experiences.

Another decision concerns whether or not to use medication and, if medication is used, how it should be employed and when it should be introduced. There are no drugs that are curative for child psychiatric disorders but there are several conditions for which medication has been shown to produce worthwhile benefits. These include depressive disorders (see Harrington, Chapter 29), obsessive-compulsive disorders (see Rapoport & Swedo, Chapter 35), tics and Tourette syndrome (see Leckman & Cohen, Chapter 36), schizophrenia (see Hollis, Chapter 37) and hyperkinetic disorders (see Schachar & Tannock, Chapter 25). They may also provide symptomatic benefits in other disorders. Decisions on drug usage are influenced, among other things, by the severity of overall impairment and the particular pattern of symptomatology. Thus, stimulants seem to work less well when hyperactivity is accompanied by marked anxiety (see Schachar & Tannock, Chapter 25), and antidepressants are more likely to be effective when the depression is accompanied

by vegetative symptoms, such as sleep and appetite disturbance, and psychomotor retardation (see Harrington, Chapter 29). In most cases, medication needs to be combined with some form of psychological or educational intervention. Although medication brings marked benefits, it does not restore normality by itself and steps may be needed to help the child and/or family cope more effectively and deal with any life situations or circumstances that provide psychopathological risk. Such interventions may only involve guidance or counselling of some kind but, in other cases, more intensive psychological intervention may be indicated. Decisions should be guided by what seem to be risk features, either in the psychosocial situation or the child's style of thinking, or perhaps of behaviour. It should be added, however, that the use of medication will carry psychological messages and that, unless carefully handled, these can undermine the psychological intervention (see Craighead *et al.* 1981 for an example in relation to dieting). The implication is not that different forms of intervention should not be combined, but rather that the clinician needs to present the combination in an appropriate way.

However, it should not be thought that drugs will only influence somatic features and not cognitions. The use of antidepressants in adult depression makes it clear that this is not the case (see Harrington, Chapter 29). Equally, it should not be supposed that psychological treatments cannot influence somatic functioning. The effects of psychological treatments in obsessive-compulsive disorder, in terms of their effects on functional imaging findings, negate that expectation (Baxter *et al.* 1992). Nevertheless, in relation to hypotheses about maintaining factors, the clinician will wish to take decisions on the appropriate choice, and mixture, of therapeutic interventions. It is important that this is done in a way that will indicate whether the therapeutic hypothesis is correct or needs modification as a result of the response to intervention.

Research findings are not as helpful as one might wish in the choice of which particular kind of psychological treatment to use. Although the evidence is reasonably consistent that focused goal-orientated interventions work better than more general open-ended ones (Rutter 1982), that would seem to suggest that the specifics of the treatment are important and that general support is not enough. On the other hand, although the range of comparisons remains more limited than one would like, the evidence does not indicate that, for any disorder, one particular style of psychological treatment is clearly generally better than others. Moreover, even when treatment is given by experienced clinicians with an investment in more intensive treatments, studies with both young people (Le Grange *et al.* 1992) and adults (Wallerstein 1986) have shown that skilled counselling may be as effective as more intensive psychological interventions that are designed to get more into the heart of the psychological problem. Although it should certainly not be supposed that simple treatments are always to be preferred, the findings do indicate that more complicated and intensive ones are not necessarily better. Decisions on the particular form of psychological intervention need to be guided by the nature of the psychological difficulties, the personal characteristics and preferences of the individual child and family, and the preferences of the clinician in terms of skills, experience and preferred mode of working. Nevertheless, cost–benefit considerations are important and the choice of a more prolonged treatment over a shorter one always needs to be justified.

Conclusions

In this chapter, we sought to bring together some of the main considerations that should guide the approach to diagnostic assessment and the planning of treatment. Research findings are informative in providing guidance on some of the methods of assessment that work better than others and undoubtedly indicate the value of a systematic approach to the degree of standardization. But it is essential to be responsive to the individual needs and circumstances of each patient, to pick up cues and adapt assessment procedures accordingly. With respect to both diagnosis and the planning of treatment, it is also important to adopt a problem-solving hypothesis-generating, and hypothesis-testing, style. The gathering of factual data on psychopathological signs and symptoms and on risk and protective circumstances constitutes the essential basis. On this basis, it is important to seek to tell a 'story' about causal processes and to use that 'story' to plan a treatment strategy and to do so in a way in which the response to treatment indicates whether or not the therapeutic hypothesis was correct.

References

Achenbach, T.M., McConaughy, S.H. & Howell, C.T. (1987) Child–adolescent behavioural and emotional problems: implications of cross-informant correlations for situation specificity. *Psychological Bulletin*, **101**, 213–232.

Ainsworth, M.D.S., Blehar, M.C., Waters, E. & Wall, S. (1978) *Patterns of Attachment: a Psychological Study of the Strange Situation*. Erlbaum Associates, Hillsdale, NJ.

American Psychiatric Association (2000) *Diagnostic and Statistical Manual of Mental Disorders (DSM-IV)*, 4th edn. American Psychiatric Association, Washington D.C.

Angold, A., Erkanlis, A., Costello, E.J. & Rutter, M. (1996) Precision, reliability and accuracy in the dating of symptom onsets in child and adolescent psychopathology. *Journal of Child Psychology and Psychiatry*, **37**, 657–664.

Angold, A., Costello, E. & Erkanli, A. (1999a) Comorbidity. *Journal of Child Psychology and Psychiatry*, **40**, 55–87.

Angold, A., Costello, E., Farmer, E.M.Z., Burns, B.J. & Erkanli, A. (1999b) Impaired but undiagnosed. *Journal of the American Academy of Child and Adolescent Psychiatry*, **38**, 129–137.

Asperger, H. (1944) Die 'Autistischen Psychopathen' im Kindesalter. *Archiv für Psychiatrie und Nervkrankheiten*, **117**, 76–136. Translated in: *Autism and Asperger Syndrome* (ed. U. Frith), pp. 37–92. Cambridge University Press, Cambridge.

Baxter, L.R., Schwartz, J.M., Bergman, K.S. *et al.* (1992) Caudate glucose metabolic rate changes with both drug and behavior therapy for obsessive-compulsive disorder. *Archives of General Psychiatry*, **49**, 681–689.

Bird, H. (1999) The assessment of functional impairment. In: *Diagnostic Assessment in Child and Adolescent Psychopathology* (eds D. Shaffer, C.P. Lucas & J.E. Richters), pp. 209–229. Guilford Press, New York.

Bird, H.R., Yager, T., Staghezza, B., Gould, M., Canino, G. & Rubio-Stipec, M. (1990) Impairment in the epidemiological measurement of childhood psychopathology in the community. *Journal of the American Academy of Child and Adolescent Psychiatry*, **29**, 796–803.

Borge, A., Samuelsen, S. & Rutter, M. (2001) Observer variance within families: confluence among maternal, paternal and child ratings. *International Journal of Methods in Psychiatric Research*, **10**, 11–21.

Brown, G. & Rutter, M. (1966) The measurement of family activities and relationships: a methodological study. *Human Relations*, **19**, 241–263.

Brown, R., Hobson, R.P., Lee, A. & Stevenson, J. (1997) Are there autistic-like features in congenitally blind children? *Journal of Child Psychology and Psychiatry*, **38**, 693–703.

Caplan, H. (1970) *Hysterical 'conversion' symptoms in childhood*. MPhil dissertation, University of London.

Carbonneau, R., Eaves, L.J., Silberg, J.L., Simonoff, E. & Rutter, M. (submitted) Assessment of the within-family environment in twins: absolute versus differential ratings, and relationship with conduct problems.

Carbonneau, R., Rutter, M., Simonoff, E., Silberg, J.L., Maes, H.H. & Eaves, L.J. (2001) The twin inventory of relationships and experiences (TIRE): psychometric properties of a measure of the nonshared and shared environmental experiences of twins and singletons. *International Journal of Methods in Psychiatric Research*, **10**, 72–85.

Caron, C. & Rutter, M. (1991) Comorbidity in child psychopathology: concepts, issues and research strategies. *Journal of Child Psychology and Psychiatry*, **32**, 1063–1080.

Clarke, A.M. & Clarke, A.D.B. (2000) *Early Experience and the Life Path*. Jessica Kingsley, London.

Conger, R.D., Conger, K.J., Elder, G.H., Lorenz, F.O., Simons, R.L. & Whitbeck, L.B. (1992) A family process model of economic hardship and adjustment of early adolescent boys. *Child Development*, **63**, 526–541.

Conger, R.D., Conger, K.J., Elder, G.H. & Lorenz, F.O. (1993) Family economic stress and adjustment of early adolescent girls. *Developmental Psychology*, **29**, 206–219.

Cox, A. & Rutter, M. (1985) Diagnostic appraisal and interviewing. In: *Child and Adolescent Psychiatry: Modern Approaches* (eds M. Rutter & L. Hersov), 2nd edn, pp. 233–248. Blackwell Scientific Publications, Oxford.

Cox, A., Rutter, M. & Holbrook, D. (1981) Psychiatric interviewing techniques. V. Experimental study: eliciting factual information. *British Journal of Psychiatry*, **139**, 29–37.

Cox, A., Hemsley, R. & Dare, J. (1995) A comparison of individual and family approaches to initial assessment. *European Child and Adolescent Psychiatry*, **4**, 94–101.

Craighead, L.W., Stunkard, A.J. & O'Brien, R.M. (1981) Behaviour therapy and pharmacotherapy for obesity. *Archives of General Psychiatry*, **38**, 763–768.

Delaney-Black, V., Covington, C., Templin, T. *et al.* (2000) Teacher-assessed behavior of children prenatally exposed to cocaine. *Pediatrics*, **106**, 782–791.

DiLavore, P.C., Lord, C. & Rutter, M. (1995) The Pre-linguistic Autism Diagnostic Observation Schedule. *Journal of Autism and Developmental Disorders*, **25**, 355–379.

Eaves, L.J., Rutter, M., Silberg, J.L., Shillady, L., Maes, H. & Pickles, A. (2000) Genetic and environmental causes of covariation in interview assessments of disruptive behavior in child and adolescent twins. *Behavior Genetics*, **30**, 321–334.

Fergusson, D.M., Horwood, L.J. & Lynskey, M.T. (1992) Family change, parental discord and early offending. *Journal of Child Psychology and Psychiatry*, 33, 1059–1073.

van Goor-Lambo, G., Orley, J., Poustka, F. & Rutter, M. (1990) Classification of abnormal psychosocial situations: preliminary report of a revision of a WHO scheme. *Journal of Child Psychology and Psychiatry* 31, 229–241.

Hagberg, B., Aicardi, J., Dias, K. & Ramos, O. (1983) A progressive syndrome of autism, dementia, ataxia and loss of purposeful hand use in girls: Rett syndrome—report of 35 cases. *Annals of Neurology*, 14, 471–479.

Hill, J. & Maughan, B., eds. (2001) *Conduct Disorders in Childhood and Adolescence*. Cambridge University Press, Cambridge.

Hinshaw, S.P., Lahey, B.B. & Hart, E.L. (1993) Issues of taxonomy and comorbidity in the development of conduct disorder. *Development and Psychopathology*, 5, 31–49.

Howlin, P., Mawhood, L. & Rutter, M. (2000) Autism and developmental receptive language disorder: a follow-up comparison in early adult life. II. Social, behavioural and psychiatric outcomes. *Journal of Child Psychology and Psychiatry*, 41, 561–578.

van Ijzendoorn, M.H., Schuengel, C. & Bakermans-Kranenburg, M.J. (1999) Disorganized attachment in early childhood: meta-analysis of precursors, concomitants, and sequelae. *Development and Psychopathology*, 11, 225–249.

Kanner, L. (1943) Autistic disturbances of affective contact. *Nervous Child*, 2, 217–250.

Kanner, L. (1957) *Child Psychiatry*, 3rd edn. Chas. C. Thomas, Springfield, IL.

Kanner, L. (1969) The children haven't read those books: reflections on differential diagnosis. *Acta Paedopsychiatrica*, 36, 2–11.

Kendler, K.S. (1996) Major depression and generalised anxiety disorder: same genes (partly) different environments—revisited. *British Journal of Psychiatry*, 168 (Suppl. 30), 68–75.

Kovacs, M., Gatsonis, S., Paulauskas, S.L. & Richards, C. (1989) Depressive disorders in childhood. IV. A longitudinal study of comorbidity with and risk for anxiety disorders. *Archives of General Psychiatry*, 46, 776–782.

Lahey, B.B., Applegate, B., Barkley, R.A. *et al.* (1998) DSM-IV field trials for oppositional defiant disorder and conduct disorder in children and adults. In: *DSM-IV Sourcebook* (eds T.A. Widiger, A.J. Frances, H.A. Pincus *et al.*), pp. 627–657. American Psychiatric Association, Washington D.C.

Le Grange, D., Eisler, I., Dare, C. & Russell, G.F.M. (1992) Evaluation of family treatments in adolescent anorexia nervosa: a pilot study. *International Journal of Eating Disorders*, 12, 347–357.

Lord, C., Rutter, M., Goode, S. *et al.* (1989) Autism Diagnostic Observation Schedule: a standardized observation of communicative and social behavior. *Journal of Autism and Developmental Disorders*, 19, 185–212.

Lord, C., Risi, S., Lambrecht, L. *et al.* (2000) The Autism Diagnostic Observation Schedule–Generic: a standard measure of social and communication deficits associated with the spectrum of autism. *Journal of Autism and Developmental Disorders*, 30, 205–223.

Magaña, A.B., Goldstein, M.J., Karno, M. & Miklowitz, D.J. (1986) A brief method for assessing expressed emotion in relatives of psychiatric patients. *Psychiatric Research*, 17, 203–212.

Mawhood, L., Howlin, P. & Rutter, M. (2000) Autism and developmental receptive language disorder: a comparative follow-up in early adult life. I. Cognitive and language outcomes. *Journal of Child Psychology and Psychiatry*, 41, 547–559.

Mazure, C. & Gershon, E.S. (1979) Blindness and reliability in lifetime psychiatric diagnosis. *Archives of General Psychiatry*, 36, 521–525.

Meadow, R. (1977) Munchausen syndrome by proxy: the hinterland of child abuse. *Lancet*, ii, 343–345.

Nadder, T., Silberg, J.L., Rutter, M., Maes, H.H. & Eaves, L.J. (2001) Comparison of multiple measures of ADHD symptomatology: a multivariate genetic analysis. *Journal of Child Psychology and Psychiatry*, 42, 475–486.

Nadder, T., Silberg, J.L., Rutter, M., Maes, H.H. & Eaves, L.J. (in press) Genetic effects on the variation and covariation of ADHD and ODD/CD symptomatologies across informant and occasion of measurement. *Psychological Medicine*.

Orvaschel, H., Lewinsohn, P.M. & Seeley, J.R. (1995) Continuity of psychopathology in a community sample of adolescents. *Journal of the American Academy of Child and Adolescent Psychiatry*, 34, 1525–1535.

Pickles, A., Rowe, R., Simonoff, E., Foley, D., Rutter, M. & Silberg, J. (2001) Child psychiatric symptoms and psychosocial impairment: relationships and prognostic significance. *British Journal of Psychiatry*, 179, 230–235.

Reiss, D., Hetherington, M., Plomin, R. *et al.* (1995) Genetic questions for environmental studies: differential parenting and psychopathology in adolescence. *Archives of General Psychiatry*, 52, 925–936.

Reiss, D., Neiderhiser, J.M., Hetherington, E.M. & Plomin, R. (2000) *The Relationship Code: Deciphering Genetic and Social Influences on Adolescent Development*. Harvard University Press, Cambridge, MA.

Rett, A. (1966) Uber ein eigenartiges himatrophisches Syndrom bei Hyperammonamie in Kindesalter. *Weiner Medizinische Wochenschrift*, 116, 723–726.

Russell, G.F.M. (1979) Bulimia nervosa: an ominous variant of anorexia nervosa. *Psychological Medicine*, 9, 429–448.

Rutter, M. (1971) Parent–child separation: psychological effects on the children. *Journal of Child Psychology and Psychiatry*, 12, 233–260.

Rutter, M. (1975) *Helping Troubled Children*. Penguin Books, Harmondsworth.

Rutter, M. (1982) Psychological therapies: issues and prospects. *Psychological Medicine*, 12, 723–740.

Rutter, M. (1985) Infantile autism. In: *The Clinical Guide to Child Psychiatry* (eds D. Shaffer, A. Erhardt & L. Greenhill), pp. 48–78. Free Press, New York.

Rutter, M. (1987) Assessment of language disorders. In: *Language Development and Disorders* (eds W. Yule & M. Rutter), pp. 295–311. Blackwell Scientific Publications, Oxford.

Rutter, M. (1989) Psychiatric disorder in parents as a risk factor in children. In: *Prevention of Psychiatric Disorders in Child and Adolescent: the Project of the American Academy of Child and Adolescent Psychiatry* (eds D. Shaffer, I. Philips, N. Enver, M. Silverman & V. Anthony). *OSAP Prevention Monograph 2*, pp. 157–189. Office of Substance Abuse Prevention, US Department of Health and Human Services, Rockville, MD.

Rutter, M. (1990) Psychosocial resilience and protective mechanisms. In: *Risk and Protective Factors in the Development of Psychopathology* (eds J. Rolf, A.S. Masten, D. Cicchetti, K.N. Neuchterlein & S. Weintraub), pp. 181–214. Cambridge University Press, Cambridge & New York.

Rutter, M. (1999) Resilience concepts and findings: implications for family therapy. *Journal of Family Therapy*, 21, 119–144.

Rutter, M. (2000a) Psychosocial influences: critiques, findings, and research needs. *Development and Psychopathology*, 12, 375–405.

Rutter, M. (2000b) Resilience reconsidered: conceptual considerations, empirical findings and policy implications. In: *Handbook of Early Childhood Intervention* (eds J.P. Shonkoff & S.J. Meisels), pp. 651–682. Cambridge University Press, New York & Cambridge.

Rutter, M. & Brown, G. (1966) The reliability and validity of measure of family life and relationships in families containing a psychiatric patient. *Social Psychiatry*, **1**, 38–53.

Rutter, M. & Sandberg, S. (1992) Psychosocial stressors: concepts, causes and effects. *European Journal of Child and Adolescent Psychiatry*, **1**, 3–13.

Rutter, M., Tizard, J. & Whitmore, K. (1970) *Education, Health and Behaviour*. Longmans, London (reprinted 1981, F.A. Krieger, Melbourne).

Rutter, M., Cox, A., Egert, S., Holbrook, D. & Everitt, B. (1981) Psychiatric interviewing techniques. IV. Experimental study: four contrasting styles. *British Journal of Psychiatry*, **138**, 456–465.

Rutter, M., Chadwick, O. & Shaffer, D. (1983) Head injury. In: *Developmental Neuropsychiatry* (ed. M. Rutter), pp. 83–111. Guilford Press, New York.

Rutter, M., Maughan, B., Meyer, J. *et al.* (1997) Heterogeneity of antisocial behavior: causes, continuities, and consequences. In: *Nebraska Symposium on Motivation*, Vol. 44, *Motivation and Delinquency* (series ed. R. Dienstbier; volume ed. D.W. Osgood), pp. 45–118. University of Nebraska Press, Lincoln, NB.

Rutter, M., Giller, H. & Hagell, A. (1998a) *Antisocial Behavior by Young People*. Cambridge University Press, New York & London.

Rutter, M., Maughan, B., Pickles, A. & Simonoff, E. (1998b) Retrospective recall recalled. In: *Methods and Models for Studying the Individual* (eds R.B. Cairns, L.R. Bergman & J. Kagan), pp. 219–242. Sage, Thousand Oaks, CA.

Rutter, M., Andersen-Wood, L., Beckett, C. *et al.* (1999a) Quasi-autistic patterns following severe early global privation. *Journal of Child Psychology and Psychiatry*, **40**, 537–549.

Rutter, M., Silberg, J., O'Connor, T. & Simonoff, E. (1999b) Genetics and child psychiatry. I. Advances in quantitative and molecular genetics. *Journal of Child Psychology and Psychiatry*, **40**, 3–18.

Rutter, M., Silberg, J., O'Connor, T. & Simonoff, E. (1999c) Genetics and child psychiatry. II. Empirical research findings. *Journal of Child Psychology and Psychiatry*, **40**, 19–55.

Rutter, M., Kreppner, J., O'Connor, T. & the E.R.A. Research Team (2001) Specificity and heterogeneity in children's responses to profound privation. *British Journal of Psychiatry*, **179**, 97–103.

Rutter, M., Pickles, A., Murray, R. & Eaves, L. (2001) Testing hypotheses on specific environmental causal effects on behavior. *Psychological Bulletin*, **127**, 291–324.

Sandberg, S., Rutter, M., Giles, S. *et al.* (1993) Assessment of psychosocial experiences in childhood: methodological issues and some illustrative findings. *Journal of Child Psychology and Psychiatry*, **34**, 879–897.

Sandberg, S., Rutter, M., Pickles, A., McGuinness, D. & Angold, A. (2001) Do high-threat life events really provoke the onset of psychiatric disorder in children? *Journal of Child Psychology and Psychiatry*, **42**, 523–532.

Sandler, I., Tein, J.-Y., Mehta, P., Wolchik, S. & Ayers, T. (2000) Coping efficacy and psychological problems of children of divorce. *Child Development*, **71**, 1099–1118.

Shepherd, M., Oppenheim, B. & Mitchell, S. (1971) *Childhood Behaviour and Mental Health*. University of London Press, London.

Shonkoff, J.P. & Phillips, D.A. (2000) *From neurons to neighborhoods. The Science of Early Childhood Development*. National Academy Press, Washington, D.C.

Silberg, J., Rutter, M. & Eaves, L. (2001) Genetic and environmental influences on the temporal association between earlier anxiety and later depression in girls. *Biological Psychiatry*, **49**, 1040–1049.

Simonoff, E., Pickles, A., Meyer, J. *et al.* (1997) The Virginia twin study of adolescent behavioral development: influences of age, sex and impairment in rates of disorder. *Archives of General Psychiatry*, **54**, 801–808.

Singer, L., Arendt, R., Farkas, K., Minnes, S., Huang, J. & Yamashita, T. (1997) Relationship of prenatal cocaine exposure and maternal postpartum psychological distress to child developmental outcome. *Development and Psychopathology*, **9**, 473–489.

Slater, E. (1965) The diagnosis of 'hysteria'. *British Medical Journal*, **1**, 1395–1399.

Spohr, L. & Steinhausen, C., eds (1996) *Alcohol, Pregnancy and the Developing Child*. Cambridge University Press, Cambridge.

Stattin, H. & Kerr, M. (2000) Parental monitoring: a reinterpretation. *Child Development*, **71**, 1072–1085.

Stratton, K., Howe, C. & Battaglia, F. (1996) *Fetal alcohol syndrome: Diagnosis, Epidemiology, Prevention, and Treatment*. National Academy Press, Washington, D.C.

Thapar, A. & McGuffin, P. (1997) Anxiety and depressive symptoms in childhood: a genetic study of comorbidity. *Journal of Child Psychology and Psychiatry*, **38**, 651–656.

Thapar, A., Holmes, J., Poulton, K. & Harrington, R. (1999) Genetic basis of attention deficit hyperactivity. *British Journal of Psychiatry*, **174**, 105–111.

Wallerstein, R.S. (1986) *Forty-Two Lives in Treatment: a Study of Psychoanalysis and Psychotherapy*. Guilford Press, New York.

Weissman, M. (1990) Evidence for comorbidity of anxiety and depression: family and genetic studies of children. In: *Comorbidity of Mood and Anxiety Disorders* (eds J.D. Maser & C.R. Cloninger), pp. 349–378. American Psychiatric Press, Washington, D.C.

Wickramaratne, P. & Weissman, M.M. (1998) Onset of psychopathology in offspring by developmental phase and parental depression. *Journal of the American Academy of Child and Adolescent Psychiatry*, **37**, 933–942.

Wolff, S. (1995) *Childhood and Human Nature: the Development of Personality*. Routledge, London.

Wolff, S. & Chick, J. (1980) Schizoid personality in childhood: a controlled follow-up study. *Psychological Medicine*, **10**, 85–100.

Wootton, B. (1959) *Social Science and Social Pathology*. George Allen & Unwin, London.

World Health Organization (1992) *The ICD-10 Classification of Mental and Behavioural Disorders*. World Health Organization, Geneva.

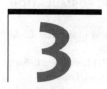

Diagnostic Interviews with Parents and Children

Adrian Angold

The purposes of the diagnostic interview

The clinical interview is the primary diagnostic tool in child and adolescent psychiatry, as in the rest of clinical medicine. Its first purpose is to collect information that will assist in the tasks of making a diagnosis and formulating and implementing a treatment plan. With the official adoption of more fully defined phenomenologically based official psychiatric nosologies (World Health Organization 1992, 1993; American Psychiatric Association 1994) and the introduction and increasingly widespread use of structured interviews, the diagnostic process has become more consistent over the last 20 years. Phenomenological diagnosis requires that information be collected in a coherent and consistent fashion, and thus sets the predominant style of the interview. The basic format is one of *sensitive guidance* by the clinician, rather than a free format in which parents or children simply play or discuss whatever occurs to them. The clinician guides, organizes and structures the collection of information in a way that is sensitive to the child's and parent's problems and concerns. This approach is very different from that of the 'nondirective' interviewer, who attempts to act as a sympathetic observer or sounding board and 'interprets' the material presented by the respondent. It has been shown that even supposedly 'nondirective' interviews are more directed than was once thought (Truax 1966, 1968), because the use of 'uh huh's' and the timing of reflections on what the patient has said, serve as strong indicators of the clinician's real interests.

However, a good interview also aims to achieve several other objectives apart from discovering the 'facts' about a patient. A diagnostic interview is often the initial contact between child or parent and clinician, and then it is the first step in establishing a treatment alliance with the clinical team. The same clinician may provide psychotherapy for one or more family members later on, so the diagnostic interview also represents a first step in the formation of a therapeutic relationship. All too frequently the initial diagnostic assessment is the only contact an individual or family has with the clinical team, as many never return for treatment. With this in mind, it is important to avoid increasing the barriers to future treatment-seeking by providing a good experience of psychiatric services. For all these reasons, and because of the need to ask about emotionally sensitive material, the clinician should approach the task of collecting information in such a way as to assure the family of a genuine interest in their problems and sympathy with their difficulties. Under the best circumstances, the product of such interviews is not only much relevant information, but also the family leaving the office with a sense that something important about their problems has been understood by someone who cares and is willing (and perhaps able) to help. The respondent's behaviour in the interview is another important source of diagnostic information. Thus, the art of good clinical interviewing lies in the ability to combine the efficient collection of reported information, an observant eye, and the projection of interest and concern about the child's problems.

The need for multiple informants

Until the late 1960s, in both clinical practice and research, interviews and questionnaires directed to a parent or teacher about a child's behaviour and *observation* of the child's behaviour were the predominant methods of assessment in child and adolescent psychiatry. Verbal information from the child was typically regarded as being only supplemental, or material for psychodynamic interpretation (Lapouse 1966). In standard texts, much more attention was paid to playing with the child than to the collection of information through direct questioning. In 1968, a key transitional paper reported on the reliability and validity of the Isle of Wight interview with the child (Rutter & Graham 1968). Here the behaviour of the child in a face-to-face interview was examined directly, but it is notable that not much was made of the factual content of what the child said. Herjanic *et al.* (1975) answered the question 'are children reliable reporters' of factual information in the affirmative, on the basis of findings from the use of an early structured interview.

Since then, a great deal of work has confirmed the importance of children's self-reports as a source of factual information, with the result that fact-finding (as opposed to interpretative) interviews with both parents and children are now regarded as being of equal weight in the diagnostic process, at least from late childhood to late adolescence. The one exception is in the evaluation of attention deficit hyperactivity disorder (ADHD) symptoms, where child reports have been found to be of little help (Loeber *et al.* 1991). Even here the growth of interest in ADHD in adolescence and adulthood has led to the development of new measures in this area, as in the recent revisions of the Conners' rating scales (Conners 1997). This emphasis on the factual content of the history given by the child does not imply that clinical observation of the child's behaviour is not of great value; it is, as we shall see later.

Disagreement among informants and implications for combining information from multiple informants

Until the 1980s, agreement between child and parent reports of symptomatology was widely regarded as being a test of the *validity* of *child* reports (Rutter & Graham 1968; Herjanic *et al.* 1975). However, subsequent research using all sorts of measures soon showed that only low levels of agreement among informants (correlation coefficients around 0.3 for agreement among children, parents and teachers) could be expected (Reich *et al.* 1982; Stanger & Lewis 1993). It is now considered that low levels of agreement amongst different informants about the child's clinical state are to be expected and do not invalidate the reports of any of them. Rather, each key informant (typically, child, parent and teacher) is seen as presenting a particular view of the child's problems. Indeed, it is precisely because agreement among informants is low that multiple informants are needed. Were agreement very high, taking the history from more than one informant would be redundant.

The problem is that disagreement among informants means that one has to decide how to weight the information from each informant in arriving at a diagnosis. Because it is uncommon for informants to invent fictitious symptoms (though sometimes they do, and it is as well to be on the lookout for inconsistencies that may tip one off here), the simple rule of regarding a symptom as being present if any informant reports it usually suffices well enough. When symptoms are combined to make diagnoses, the usual procedure is to 'ignore' the source, and to add up all positive symptoms from any source. Thus, a diagnosis of a major depressive episode (which requires the presence of at least five symptoms) might be made on the basis of three relevant symptoms being reported by the child (say, depressed mood, anhedonia and excessive guilt), with two other relevant symptoms (perhaps sleep and appetite disturbances) being reported by the parent. Though some interview developers have recommended 'reconciliation' discussions involving the interviewer, the parent and the child to clear up discrepancies between their reports, such discussions are problematic in several ways. First, to achieve their purpose, one informant must modify his or her story, but that means admitting being wrong, or at least uninformed. Requiring such admissions at the start of the therapeutic process will often not be helpful, although confronting individuals with different perceptions of their behaviour may be an important part of the therapeutic strategy beyond the initial diagnostic stage. Secondly, it offers a chance for family members to become engaged in arguments with one another—again, something not helpful to the initial phenomenological diagnostic process. Thirdly, the knowledge that such a discussion will occur could cause informants (e.g. drug-using adolescents) to withhold important information that they did not wish other informants (such as their parents) to hear about. Finally, in most research applications, one wishes to assure informants that what they say will not be revealed to anyone else, in which case a 'reconciliation' interview is ruled out.

There are also situations in which consideration of the differences between informants' reports may be of interest. Another way of saying that different informants present different 'views' of a child's problems is that different informants provide information about different *aspects* of the child's emotions and behaviour, even when each provides that information using the 'same' scale. Looked at in this way, it comes as no surprise that sometimes the correlates of reports of child psychopathology from different informants differ. For instance, the enormous increase in the rate of depression in girls during puberty seems to be accounted for by changes in *self*-reports of depressive symptoms, while parent reports do not change very much (Angold *et al.* 1991). An even more striking example is provided by the substantial differences in patterns of genetic and environmental effects resulting from the analysis of ratings of the 'same' phenomena by different reporters (mothers, fathers, teachers and children) in the Virginia Twin Study of adolescent behavioural development (Eaves *et al.* 1997). Such differences raise a number of interesting scientific questions about exactly what different informants are telling us about, but in everyday clinical practice, the usual 'either/or' combination rule suffices for the most part. However, it is worth noting an important exception—the case in which parental reports are uncorroborated by any other source, including the clinician's observation of the child. Here, the possibility of Münchausen syndrome by proxy should come to mind (Schreier 1997).

Implications of comorbidity for diagnostic interviewing

Research over the last decade or so has demonstrated beyond doubt that diagnostic comorbidity (the presence of symptoms meeting criteria for multiple diagnoses) is extremely common (Angold *et al.* 1999a), so the task of the assessment is not to find the *single* diagnosis that best accounts for all the symptoms. Rather the question is *which* disorders can the child be said to suffer from, no matter how many they may be. As far as assessment is concerned this means that once one has decided that the child is depressed, one cannot then skip over the assessment of, say, disruptive behaviour, because a depressed child is also very likely to be oppositional, or conduct disordered, or a substance abuser as well.

Potential problems with using children younger than 9 as key informants

After the age of 9, the diagnostic interview with the child proceeds along much the same lines as is familiar from interviews with adults, as far as its structure is concerned. However, substantial differences in the case-mix to be expected in child psychiatric clinics and adult clinics (and in the child and adult general populations for that matter) have a substantial effect on the content of a typical child evaluation. In children, for instance, psychotic disorders are rare, but attention deficit/hyperactivity problems are common. Although it is possible to demonstrate increased rates of forgetting in younger children in formal memory tests (Brainerd & Ornstein 1991; Ornstein *et al.* 1992) it seems that rates of forgetting are not markedly different, at least from the age of 6 to adulthood. Even 3-year-olds have been shown to be capable of remembering some events that occurred as much as a year before the interview (Pillemer & White 1989), though many such memories contain erroneous elements. In both adults and children, there is a tendency to conflate memories of repeated events into 'scripts' that provide a generalized memory of such events (Nelson *et al.* 1983; Saywitz 1987), incorporating features from a number of specific instances. Though there have been concerns about the accuracy with which children and adolescents can *date* events and the onsets of symptoms in their lives, there is little evidence that after the age of 9 they are any worse than adults at this task (Angold *et al.* 1996a). The adult literature suggests that it is easier to recall that something happened than when it happened, and major events are more likely to be remembered than minor events. The work of Cannell *et al.* (1977) in relation to the adult household survey suggests high rates of forgetting minor health problems (like headaches) over periods as short as 1 week, and substantial under-reporting of even major events by 1 year.

Before the age of 8 or 9, 'adult-style' diagnostic interviews work very poorly. The problem is that younger children are incapable of providing the detailed information about onset, timing, duration and co-occurrence of symptoms that are required to meet standard criteria for a full diagnosis. However, we should also remember that older children and adults also often have difficulty with providing this sort of information (Breton *et al.* 1995; Schwab-Stone *et al.* 1994; Angold *et al.* 1996a), so the problem is one of degree, rather than kind. Nevertheless, children 8 years old and younger can describe fears and worries, mood states and covert antisocial behaviours (such as substance use, lying or stealing) that may not be apparent to any adults. If questioned sensitively and carefully, and without leading, they can often provide sufficient detail to help with diagnostic evaluation. Children themselves may also be the only available sources of information about physical and sexual abuse, though here particularly careful interviewing is needed (Steward & Steward 1996; Bruck *et al.* 1998; see also Ceci *et al.*, Chapter 8). Progress has also been made in developing approaches to collecting information from children that go beyond the 'adult-style' question and answer formats, such as the MacArthur Story-Stem Battery (Warren *et al.* 1996, 2000) in which the interviewer uses toys to act out the beginnings of stories which the child is then asked to complete. The videotapes of these interactions can then be scored to provide indices of a variety of internal states. The Berkeley Puppet Interview (Measelle *et al.* 1998) employs two puppets to express two moods/states, and the child then indicates the puppet most like him- or herself, thereby providing self-report assessments of perceived academic functioning, social relationships, depression, anxiety and aggression/hostility. Some simpler 'questionnaires with pictures' have also shown promise with preschool-age children in relation to

the assessment of depression and anxiety (Martini *et al.* 1990; Ialongo *et al.* 1993). However, none of these methods is capable of yielding all the information necessary for a DSM-IV (American Psychiatric Association 1994) or ICD-10 (World Health Organization 1992, 1993) diagnosis, and there is no general agreement about how such information should be incorporated into the overall diagnostic assessment. A great deal of work needs to be carried out to place the diagnosis of younger children on an equal footing with that of later childhood.

From the age of 3 until the teenage years, there is an increase in the amount of information provided in free recall situations. Though younger children provide less information, they are no less accurate in their recall than older children and adults. The use of open questions is therefore the starting point for good interviewing, whether of children or adults about their children.

When closed questions, and especially forced-choice question formats are used, younger children (including preschool-age children) can usually provide more information than in the free recall situation (Ornstein *et al.* 1992). However, they are also more likely to provide *erroneous* information (Bruck *et al.* 1998). This is not to say that closed questions do not have an important place in the clinical interview, but they are best used to fill in the gaps in the information provided in response to open questions, or to clarify confusion, rather than constituting the basic approach. While preschool-age children are more likely to incorporate erroneous material introduced through repeated questioning, suggestion and leading questioning than older children, such techniques also induce reporting errors in older children, and even adults. There is no place for such techniques in psychiatric interviewing at any age (Bruck *et al.* 1998).

The need for a structured approach to diagnostic interviewing

It should be noted that structured interviews were originally developed because researchers were aware that clinicians unaided by such instruments tended to operate in an idiosyncratic fashion (Cantwell 1988; Gould *et al.* 1988; Remschmidt 1988), and to adopt inefficient decision rules in coming to a diagnosis. It was also apparent that there was a tendency to focus on a particular set of problems without giving adequate weight to an exploration of the full range of symptomatology. Both of these problems are typical of unstructured medical decision-making in general. Other general human information processing characteristics that may endanger the diagnostic process include 'illusory correlation' (Chapman & Chapman 1967), in which the expectation that a correlation exists between two phenomena leads to the imputation of the presence of a second phenomenon from the observed presence of the first. People also appear to have great difficulty identifying correlations when they really do exist in the phenomena that they are observing (Chapman & Chapman 1971). Thus, the observation that a child had made a suicide attempt might lead a clinician who believes that such actions are related to depression to assume that the child must be depressed, and to interpret any hint of sadness as confirming this supposition. This latter tendency to weight information that fits in with expectations is also called the 'confirmatory bias' (Tversky & Kahneman 1974). Its corollary is that information that does not fit in with expectations tends to be ignored (thus our clinician might fail to take a careful history of behaviour problems, which would be a serious mistake, because suicidality is also strongly related to conduct problems). Confirmatory bias has also been identified as a real problem in the collection of evidence of abuse from young children (Bruck *et al.* 1998).

The 'representativeness heuristic' (Tversky & Kahneman 1974) may also bias clinical judgements when a child has the characteristics of a particular group (say, children with conduct disorder), leading the clinician to impute to the child other characteristics of conduct-disordered children, which actually do not apply to that individual (see Achenbach 1985 for a basic introduction to the application of decision-making analysis to the assessment of psychopathology; Sox 1987; Dawes 1988 for more advanced treatments). That these effects occur in ordinary clinical practice is indicated by Costello's (1982) examination of diagnostic case conferences at a major child psychiatric centre (described in Cantwell 1988), whereas Bird *et al.* 1992) found that clinicians were less likely to assign certain comorbid diagnoses than a computer algorithm incorporating the DSM-III diagnostic rules, when both made diagnoses based on the same information. In arguing that a structured *approach* to diagnostic interviewing is necessary, I do not mean to imply that the use of any recognized structured interview is mandatory, although I do believe that the growing practice of using such interviews in clinical situations is to be applauded. Rather, I mean that good diagnostic practice demands the adoption of an organized, coherent, repeatable interview structure that avoids the information collection biases inherent in the unstructured diagnostic process. In this the psychiatric history is no different from the history taken in any other branch of medicine. As a variety of structured interviews have been developed to deal with these problems, they provide helpful information about ways that individual clinicians can develop their own structured approach to diagnostic interviewing.

Review of the current status of structured diagnostic psychiatric interviews for child and adolescent disorders

All structured diagnostic interviews seek, by whatever means, to achieve the following goals (which should also be the goals of every diagnostician):
1 structure information coverage, so that all interviewers will have collected all relevant information from all subjects;
2 define the ways in which relevant information is to be collected;
3 make a diagnosis only after all relevant confirmatory and disconfirmatory information has been collected; and
4 structure the process by which relevant confirmatory and

disconfirmatory information is combined to produce a final diagnosis.

Goals **1**, **3** and **4** are achieved by all the major diagnostic interviews in rather similar ways; all cover at least the most common DSM or ICD diagnoses, and all have a set of rules, often computer algorithms, for combining the information collected to make diagnoses. However, goal **2**, defining how the information is to be collected, has led to two quite different approaches to structured interviewing. These two methods have been dubbed 'interviewer-based' (or sometimes 'investigator-based') and 'respondent-based' (Angold *et al.* 1995). Respondent-based interviews have often been referred to as being 'highly structured', while interviewer-based interviews have been called 'semistructured'. These are misnomers, because the issue is not *how much* structure is present, but *what* is structured.

Interviewer-based and respondent-based interviews

Interviewer-based interviews

In an interviewer-based interview, the *mind of the interviewer* is structured. In essence, the interview schedule serves as a guide to the interviewer to help him or her determine whether a symptom is present; the interviewer makes that decision on the basis of information collected from the patient or other respondent. Definitions of symptoms are provided, and the interviewer is expected to question until he or she can decide whether a symptom meeting this definition is present. This group of interviews includes the Anxiety Disorders Interview Schedule (ADIS; Silverman & Nelles 1988; Silverman & Rabian 1995), the Child and Adolescent Psychiatric Assessment (CAPA; Angold & Costello 2000), the Child Assessment Schedule (CAS; Hodges *et al.* 1982; Hodges 1993), the paper and pencil (not the computerized) versions of the Diagnostic Interview Schedule for Children and Adolescents (DICA; Reich 2000) and its close relative, the Missouri Assessment of Genetics Interview for Children (MAGIC), the Interview Schedule for Children and Adolescents (ISCA; Sherrill & Kovacs 2000), the various versions of the Kiddie Schedule for Affective Disorders and Schizophrenia (K-SADS; Ambrosini 2000), and the Pictorial Instrument for Children and Adolescents (PICA-IIIR; Ernst *et al.* 2000). All of these interviews, except the PICA-IIIR, make a wide range of DSM-IV diagnoses, and have components for assessing psychosocial impairment resulting from psychiatric symptoms and disorders. The PICA-IIIR is unusual in that it provides a series of pictures meant to illustrate particular forms of psychopathology around which the interview is structured. However, it is suitable for use only by clinicians and has been little tested. The DICA has also been used with children younger than 6 years, although special training is required for its administration in such situations. Interviewers are instructed to ignore the usual questioning format laid out in the schedule and use their own questions. The result is that much of the usual structure of the DICA is jettisoned, with unknown results for reliability or validity. Various other interviews exist for specialized purposes (such as the

Autism Diagnostic Interview, ADI; Lord *et al.* 1994), but they will not be discussed further here.

Among interviewer-based interviews there are two subtypes: glossary-based and non-glossary-based. The K-SADS-P IVR and the CAPA (and the ADI) are glossary-based. They provide detailed written symptom definitions and rules for coding level of symptom severity and impairment resulting from symptomatology. The MAGIC provides a detailed *procedural* glossary (as opposed to the *definitional* glossaries of the CAPA and K-SADS-P IVR), which is a mine of information on good interviewing technique. The other interviews mentioned above (including various other versions of the K-SADS) provide much less definitional information to guide the interviewer and can be regarded as being non-glossary-based. More detailed comparisons among the members of this group of interviews can be found in Angold & Fisher (1999).

Respondent-based interviews

In a respondent-based interview, it is the *questions* put to the *respondent* that are structured; prescribed questions are asked verbatim in a preset order, and the interviewee's responses are recorded with a minimum of interpretation or clarification by the interviewer. Thus, although one knows exactly what has been asked in each interview, there is no control over differences in how subjects interpret questions or respond to them. It has been shown that, in the case of 'bizarre' phenomena (such as obsessive-compulsive symptoms), respondents' thresholds for answering questions about them in the affirmative are much lower than is helpful (far more cases are identified than really exist; Breslau 1987).

There are two types of respondent-based interviews: pure verbal interviews and pictorial interviews. The former are like adult diagnostic interviews, and most of the interviewer-based interviews, in that they rely solely on verbal questioning without visual aids. The pictorial interviews involve showing children cartoon pictures intended to illustrate the questions being asked. The Diagnostic Interview Schedule for Children (DISC; Shaffer *et al.* 1999, 2000) is the most widely used pure verbal interview. The current version is the DISC-IV. A great advantage of the respondent-based approach is that it lends itself easily to computerization. Questions are arranged in unvarying logical sequences in such an instrument, with stem questions followed by sequences of further questions contingent upon the answers to the stems. Software is available to allow the presentation of such interviews on a personal computer. Computerization can be achieved at two levels. Computer-*assisted* psychiatric interviews (CAPI) employ an interviewer to read questions from the screen and enter the appropriate codes into the computer as the interview progresses. The machine takes the interviewer to the appropriate stem questions, and stores the responses in a database. There is no need for bulky interview schedules to be copied and carried around, and data entry is completed during the interview. Furthermore, the computer will not accidentally skip parts of the interview, or vary the order of its presentation.

The next level of computerization is referred to as computer-*administered* survey interviewing (CASI). Here no interviewer is used at all; digitized audio recordings of the questions (sometimes even with digitized video of an interviewer) are played back by the computer as the written form of the question is displayed. The respondent enters a response to the question, which is saved to the database. The DISC has become progressively more complex over the last 20 years (largely because of the ever-increasing complexity of the DSMs), and the DISC-IV is now expected to be completed in its CAPI format, because it is really too difficult to administer it effectively in a paper-and-pencil format. There is also a CAPI version of the DICA, but this differs from paper-and-pencil version of the interview in being fully respondent-based (Reich *et al.* 1995).

The advantage of computerizability is somewhat offset from a clinical perspective by the fact that clinicians find the task of completing a long respondent-based interview rather tedious. If they go off interview to follow-up on particular clinical leads in their own way, the strengths of a respondent-based interview are vitiated. In general, the interviewer-based format is more suitable for clinical use by clinicians. However, we have reached the point where it is feasible to have parents and children complete a diagnostic interview, such as the DISC, before they see a clinician at all. The possible output from the DISC is almost infinitely flexible, and requires only programming to allow the production of reports tailored to particular clinical needs that can be generated immediately the interview is finished. Equipped with such a report, a clinician familiar with one of the interviewer-based interviews would then be starting with a very respectable initial diagnostic formulation to guide further elucidation of the clinical status of the child.

The Children's Interview for Psychiatric Symptoms (ChIPS; Weller *et al.* 2000) was designed as a screening tool covering 20 DSM-IV Axis 1 disorders. 'Cardinal questions' concerning symptoms most often seen in children with a particular disorder are asked at the beginning of each section. If the answers to these screening questions are in the negative, then the rest of that section is skipped.

The pictorial interview that makes the nearest approach to a DSM diagnosis is the Dominic-R (Valla *et al.* 2000), which is intended for use with 6–11-year-olds. Pictures representing psychopathology relevant to seven diagnoses are shown to the child, and questions about whether each symptom is present are read at the same time. Because no frequency, duration or onset data are collected, it is not yet clear how such information should be combined with diagnostic information from other sources. However, this should not be seen as a criticism of the measure, rather it shows how limited our understanding of psychopathology in younger children really is.

Interview time frames

One very important difference among the interviews considered here is the wide range of time frames they cover. The K-SADS interviews, the ADIS, the CAS, the Dominic and the ISCA all focus on the child's 'current' status, though the definition of 'current' is largely unspecified. The K-SADS-PL and K-SADS-E also explore lifetime histories of 'worst' episodes, while the ISCA also provides for assessment of lifetime disorder, and an 'interim' version provides an assessment of current status plus the child's status in the interim between the current assessment and the last assessment, for use in follow-up studies. The DICA and MAGIC adopt a lifetime time frame as their standard format. Here there is always a lifetime focus, but for some disorders an additional shorter time frame is also included. For instance, in the depression section, the MAGIC asks about the 'past month' as well as whether the child has 'ever' had symptoms. The CAPA covers a 'primary period' of 3 months, but also asks whether certain uncommon symptoms (such as suicide attempts) have ever occurred, and a version that provides lifetime coverage of major episodes of certain disorders is also available. The full DISC-IV can be used to assess either the last month or the last year, and also offers a module to determine whether certain syndromes that did not occur during the preceding year had occurred at any point since the age of 5.

Reliability and validity of structured diagnostic interviews

Table 3.1 shows the results of studies of the *test–retest* reliabilities (kappas) of diagnoses measured by the instruments considered in this chapter. It can be seen that all do a reasonably good job, and that there is not much to choose between them, so far as test–retest reliability of diagnosis is concerned. These reliability coefficients are similar to those reported for psychiatric interviews with adults. Reliabilities for scale scores derived from these interviews are typically rather better than they are for diagnosis, and it is important to remember that some of the unreliability of diagnostic measures is a product of the diagnostic system itself, with its numerous details relating to onset dates, durations of symptoms and the like—information that humans do not remember very well, no matter what their age. One often sees reports of *interrater* reliabilities in the interview literature. However, interrater reliability is not a very useful index of interview performance. With respondent-based interviews it tests nothing but whether one interviewer can read aloud adequately while another fills in a form containing the answers to the questions. In an interviewer-based interview the questions are not fixed, and so different interviewers could use different questions to elicit the same information. As the interrater reliability paradigm uses multiple raters to score the same videotaped interview, this major source of potential unreliability is eliminated, with the result that the interrater reliability is likely to substantially overestimate the reliability of the interview in actual use.

A problem with the test–retest assessment of reliability is that it requires that the interview be repeated within a short period of time. With both questionnaires and interviews one finds that fewer symptoms are endorsed at the second interview than at the first (Angold *et al.* 1996b; Lauritsen 1998; Lucas *et al.* 1999;

Table 3.1 Test–retest reliabilities (kappas) of diagnoses in clinical samples from the instruments considered in this chapter (where available).

	MDD	Dysthymia/minor depression	Any depression	GAD/OAD	Separation anxiety disorder	Simple phobia	Social phobia	Any anxiety disorder	PTSD	ADHD	CD	ODD	SA/D
K-SADS-P	0.54	0.70						0.24					
K-SADS-P IIIR	0.77	0.89						0.72		0.91		0.46	
K-SADS-PL current	0.90			0.78				0.80	0.67	0.63		0.74	
K-SADS-PL lifetime	1.0			0.78				0.60	0.60	0.55	0.83	0.77	
CAS	1.0	0.85	0.83	0.38				0.72		0.43			
DICA			0.90					0.76		1.0		0.61	
CAPA child only	0.90	0.85	0.82	0.79				0.64	0.64		0.55		1.0
ISCA child only				0.82	0.81								
ADIS combined P & C				0.64	0.64	0.84	0.73	0.75					
DISC-IV combined P & C	0.65			0.58	0.51	0.86	0.48			0.62	0.55	0.59	

Abbreviations: ADHD, attention deficit hyperactivity disorder; ADIS, Anxiety Disorders Interview Schedule; CAPA, Child and Adolescent Psychiatric Assessment; CAS, Child Adolescent Schedule; CD, Conduct disorder; DICA, Diagnostic Interview Schedule for Children and Adolescents; DISC-IV, Diagnostic Interview Schedule for Children-IV; GAD, generalized anxiety disorder; ISCA, Interview Schedule for Children and Adolescents; K-SADS, Kiddie Schedule for Affective Disorders and Schizophrenia; MDD, major depressive disorder/episode; OAD, overanxious disorder; ODD, oppositional/defiant disorder; PTSD, post-traumatic stress disorder; SA/D, substance abuse or dependence.

Piacentini *et al.* 1999). There are many possible explanations for this effect (Jensen *et al.* 1992), but current evidence suggests that the results of the first interview are probably the most accurate representation of reality. The usual interpretation of test–retest reliability statistics—such as Cohen's kappa for categorical data (such as diagnoses) and the intraclass correlation coefficient (ICC) for continuous data (such as scale scores)—involves the supposition that the relationship between scores at the first interview and those at the second involves two components: agreement and random error. The presence of a *consistent difference* between first and second interviews indicates that such statistics underestimate the 'true' (and unmeasurable) reliability of both interviews and psychopathology scales. Despite enormous efforts on the part of interview developers, it cannot be said that the reliability of diagnostic interviews has increased much over the years. We now have a fairly mature interview technology, and new developments leading to major increases in reliability are unlikely to occur. The current arsenal of diagnostic interviews probably offers as good reliability as can be achieved with this approach.

The problem with trying to assess the validity of psychiatric interviews is that there is no non-interview test for most psychiatric disorders. The structured interview itself has become the closest approximation we have to a 'gold-standard'. So how are we to 'validate' the diagnoses obtained from such interviews? This is a version of a very old problem in psychology; one that led to the concept of *construct validity*. The key idea is that the validity of an instrument for the measurement of a psychological construct resides not in some single agreement coefficient with one external standard, but in the instrument's performance within the *nomological net* of theory and empirical data concerning the construct or constructs that the instrument purports to measure (Jenkins 1946; Anastasi 1950; Gulliksen 1950; Peak 1953; Cronbach & Meehl 1955; Weitz 1961; Wallace 1965; Novick 1985; Anastasi 1986). As Gulliksen (1950) remarked, 'at some point in the advance of psychology it would seem appropriate for the psychologist to lead the way in establishing good criterion measures, instead of just attempting to construct imperfect tests for attributes that are presumed to be assessed more accurately and more validly by the judgement of experts.'

Structured interviews were developed because of the poor psychometric properties of unaided clinical diagnosis, so comparisons with clinical judgement are a flawed test of diagnostic interview validity. In considering the validity of any interview, we should take a construct validation approach, and describe what we currently know about it in relation to the nomological net pertaining to child and adolescent psychiatric diagnosis. So far, only the developers of the CAPA have explicitly laid out the evidence for the validity of the CAPA using this approach, but most of the interviews considered here can point to similar chains of evidence. To give a flavour of the sort of evidence relevant to construct validation, the following findings have been adduced as construct validators of the CAPA.

1 Diagnostic rates and age and gender patterns of disorder given by the CAPA are consistent with those found using other interviews.

2 Patterns of diagnostic comorbidity are consistent with those found by other interviews.

3 Symptomatic diagnoses are associated with psychosocial impairment.

4 Parent and child reports of psychopathology on the CAPA are related to parent and teacher reports of problems on well-established scales for detecting psychopathology.

5 Children with CAPA-identified disorders use more mental health services than children without diagnoses.

6 CAPA-diagnosed children tend to come from families with a history of mental illness.

7 There is genetic loading for a number of CAPA scales scores and diagnoses.

8 CAPA diagnoses show consistency over time.

9 CAPA diagnoses predict negative life outcomes (Angold & Costello 2000).

10 Different CAPA diagnoses are differentially related to the physiological changes of puberty (Angold *et al.* 1999b).

The need is for a change from concentration on single correlation coefficients, describing the interview's level of agreement with 'experts' as evidence of validity, to concentration on comparisons of the information collection properties of different measures. In deciding which interview will be best for any clinical or research application, the key question is 'Which collects the information I want in the way that I want to collect it in a reasonably reliable and efficient manner?' A second useful question is 'Is there any strong reason (practical or based on research on the instrument's properties) why I should *not* use this instrument?' The current evidence certainly does not support the notion that any single interview is 'best' for all applications. It is worth bearing in mind that low 'validity' coefficients may also be the product of the *diagnostic system*. A perfect measure of an invalid diagnosis will still produce an invalid diagnosis, so some of the problems with validity typically attributed to our interviewing technology should probably be placed at the door of the nosologies instantiated by the interviews (Robins 1985).

Clinical interviewing style

Open and closed questions

The distinction between open and closed questions is not absolute, but open questions are those that offer the chance to provide a wide range of answers or free-recall descriptions of phenomena, while closed questions call for one of a limited set of responses. For example, an open question response to being told by a child that he or she had received a bad school report might be 'how did you feel about your bad grades?', whereas 'did your bad grades make you feel unhappy?' would be a closed question. If a child had just admitted to stealing, responding with 'tell me more about that' involves an open question, whereas 'what did you steal' is a closed question. Basically, closed questions call for a yes/no answer or a date, frequency, duration, or other quite specific piece of information, while open questions give the opportunity for the child to provide a description of his or her behaviour and feelings.

The work of Cox and Rutter and their colleagues offers some direct guidance on the best ways to use these different sorts of questions with adults and, in the light of the literature on children's memory cited above, there is little reason not to use a similar approach with children. In general, most factual information was collected when a systematic approach that relied heavily on open questions was used. Furthermore, this approach was also conducive to parental expressions of emotion, because it involved less talking on the part of the interviewer and gave more time for parents to discuss their concerns. A non-interventionist approach resulted in the provision of less relevant information, while challenging interpretations and a confrontational style proved less effective in eliciting emotions (Cox *et al.* 1981a–c; Hopkinson *et al.* 1981; Rutter & Cox 1981; Rutter *et al.* 1981). This is not to say that closed questions do not have an important place in the clinical interview, but they should be used to fill in the gaps in the information provided in response to open questions, or to clarify confusion, rather than constituting the basic approach. Sometimes it seems as though it might be quicker to ask a set of specific questions, especially when working through a set of diagnostic criteria; however, this is rarely the case. If open questions are well thought out, respondents will often provide much of the necessary information spontaneously, so that only a few follow-up questions need be asked. Thus, open questions may actually save time, and simultaneously avoid a barrage of closed questions that may seem to respondents to reflect the clinician's needs more than their own.

Leading questions

Leading questions are sometimes confused with closed questions, but whereas the latter are a necessary part of interviewing technique, leading questions have almost no place at all in psychiatric interviewing, for the simple reason that one can never believe the answer to such a question, especially in the case of young children. A leading question is one that directly suggests its answer. For example, to return to the child with problems at school, a response like 'I expect that made you feel pretty unhappy, didn't it', places the child in the position of having to disagree with the interviewer if he or she really did not care about his or her grades. We have already noted that young children may be prone to respond with what they believe is being demanded of them, so we can expect agreement, even if the child was, in fact, angry or completely unconcerned. On the other hand, such a question provides a golden opportunity for an oppositional adolescent to demonstrate how wide of the mark the interviewer was, regardless of his or her actual feelings about school.

Double and multiple questions

A double question asks about two different things at the same

time. Consider the question, 'When you got your school report were you worried, or angry, or didn't you care?' Such a question will often draw an answer like 'yes' or 'no', but one cannot tell what that answer refers to—it could refer any combination of worrying, anger or insouciance. The operation of the recency effect means that it is quite likely that the response refers to the last part of the question, but the only way to be sure is to ask specific questions about worrying, anger and not caring. As this could have been done in the first place, the multiple question has only served to waste time. Double and multiple questions also place an increased load on the cognitive capacities of the respondents, because they must remember several options in order to choose among them. Thus, double and multiple questions join leading questions as major interviewing sins.

Though multiple questions cause problems, the same cannot be said of 'redundant' questions: questions that contain two presentations of the same item, as in 'Did you feel angry about your report . . . did it make you angry at all?' The adult survey literature (Cannell *et al.* 1977, 1992) suggests that such redundancy can actually be helpful, and the same may be true in interviewing children, though this issue does not appear to have been studied specifically.

Multiple choice questions

Multiple choice questions are a subset of closed questions that have a place when regular open and closed questions fail to provide an adequate answer. For instance, if one asks about the frequency of temper tantrums, and the child says he or she 'doesn't know', a question like 'Well, is it every day, once a week or once a month?' can be helpful. However, such multiple choice questions may not include the proper range of choices. What is the right answer if tantrums actually occur only a couple of times a year, or if they occur many times a day? It is usually necessary to ask a supplementary question or two to clarify these points, so multiple choice questions are relatively inefficient, though they may be the only way to get the necessary information. They also have a second drawback in that, like multiple questions, they require the child to hold the available choices in memory before selecting among them. It has already been noted that the multiple choice format leads to the reporting of more incorrect information in younger children.

Repeated questions

Asking the 'same' question with some rewording can be helpful in allowing increased time and cognitive processing to be allocated to providing an appropriate answer. However, frequently repeated questioning, especially when combined with leading questions or other suggestive techniques, and failure to pay attention to disconfirmatory information also appears to be a good way to generate *false* reports. Indeed, in the sexual abuse arena, some authors have suggested that the retraction of previously made accusations is a typical part of the process of dealing with having been abused (hence, such retractions appear almost to become confirmatory evidence). However, studies of *confirmed* sexual abuse have found that such retractions are uncommon (occurring in 3–8% of cases) (Bruck *et al.* 1998). As with other sorts of statements, inconsistency in the reporting of abuse by a particular informant should lead one to question the accuracy of those reports.

Inappropriately worded questions

In most circumstances, it is best to use simple words and short sentences. It is also important to be on the alert for possible misunderstanding. Here again the open question approach, with its emphasis on getting descriptions of experiences and behaviour, helps to ensure that both interviewer and interviewee are talking about the same thing.

Organizing the interview

So far, we have examined some basic interviewing techniques. The next question is how to organize these into a coherent interview in a clinical setting.

Beginning the interview

The first task is to get the interviewee into a conducive situation: somewhere quiet, private and undistracting. The presence of large numbers of interesting toys should be avoided in interviews with children.

The child often does not know why he or she is talking to the interviewer, as parents may have told the child that he or she is going to the dentist or some other fiction. The first step, then, is to clarify why the child thinks he or she is seeing you, and to allay fears that injections or extractions are just around the corner. Even if the child has a reasonable notion of where he or she is, his or her ideas about why he or she is there may differ dramatically from the actual reasons for referral. The next step is to explain why you think that the child is there, to explain the purpose of the interview, and to give a brief description of what it will be like. Similarly, parents who have come at the behest of another agency may have only a dim understanding of why they are there, so, again it is helpful to outline what the purpose of the visit is at the beginning.

As an immediate barrage of questions about emotionally loaded topics is likely to be very off-putting, it is usually best to begin with some questions that allow the respondent to describe the family situation, the things the referred child enjoys doing and is good at, and what his or her social life is like. If the child is aware that he or she has problems, a brief description of how he or she sees those problems can be helpful. By this point, both the respondent and the interviewer should have a fairly good idea of what to expect from one another, so the interviewer can formulate a plan for the rest of the interview. If it has become clear that some topics are a source of discomfort or avoidance, it is best to steer away from these at the start, and to begin with less threatening material, allowing a sense of trust to develop. On the other hand, some respondents (especially parents) are keen to get right down to a description of what bothers them most. In either case, following the respondent's leads and exploring his or her problems in the order in which they come up is a good strategy. However, in being sensitive to the respondent's ordering of the material, it is important not to allow the interview to become incoherent. Once a topic (such as symptoms of depression) has been begun, it is usually best to continue with it until all the necessary information has been collected. Otherwise it is very likely that important questions will be forgotten in jumping from topic to topic. There is nothing wrong with telling the respondent that you will come back to a different topic later (as long as you do).

Those just beginning work in child and adolescent psychiatry usually do not know what all the relevant symptoms are, and here the use of a simple checklist (for the interviewer, not the respondent) based on the DSM or ICD criteria can be very helpful. However, these criteria give no guidance as to how to turn them into suitable questions, and familiarity with a well-structured interview helps to fill this gap. If the respondent has previously completed a symptom checklist, it is a good idea to have looked it over before starting the interview. It is vital that the diagnostic criteria are not allowed to become a straitjacket for the interview. It is all too easy to emerge with more or less accurate diagnoses but little idea of what the child is actually like. Much goes into good treatment planning besides the diagnosis.

Common child psychopathology is divided into two broad domains: emotional and behavioural disorders, and the next two sections discuss some general principles for assessing symptoms in these areas.

Emotional disorders

The central distinctions to be made here are between *moods* or *affects*, *thoughts* and *behaviours*, and *impairments* secondary to the first three. The distinction between moods and thoughts is the most difficult to maintain in practice, largely because English does not clearly distinguish between them in everyday speech. For instance, it is usual to ask whether someone 'felt' guilty rather than whether they 'had guilty thoughts', though the latter is more accurate. When interviewing one must use everyday language, but it is important to be clear that while 'feeling guilty' may be evidence of a depressive disorder, it is not the same thing as depressed mood. It is quite possible to have an overdeveloped sense of guilt without depressed mood and vice versa. Thus, some common questions like 'Did you feel bad about that?' must be treated with caution, because an affirmative response could refer either to a mood state (as in 'That made me feel unhappy'), or a cognitive state (as in 'That induced the thought that I had done something bad or wrong'). Similarly, worrying (a cognitive symptom) must be distinguished from anxiety (a mood state). While at first these distinctions may seem to be splitting psychopathological hairs, they are diagnostically important, and of direct relevance to treatment; consider, for example, cognitive therapy for depression, which focuses directly on thought processes, rather than the mood state itself.

When is an emotional 'symptom' abnormal?

One problem with emotional symptoms is that they are often extremes of normal emotions. This presents no problem when someone reports that they have been depressed all day, every day, for 2 months, and that before that they were of a cheerful disposition. Unfortunately, things are not always so simple. In the absence of a detailed epidemiological literature describing how much time the average child spends feeling depressed, or worrying, it is necessary to have some general rules of thumb for deciding what is abnormal.

1 *Look for changes in state or failure to make normal developmental progress.* A description of a marked change in state, especially if it is of relatively acute onset, is strong evidence for the pathological status of a symptom. However, it has to be said that in developmental psychopathology, acute onsets are the exception rather than the rule. Symptoms may also have begun years before the child presents for help. However, if care is taken to get adequate descriptions, and the respondent is encouraged to think hard about whether and when a change occurred, it is usually possible to determine whether a symptom represents a change from some previous state.

Some symptoms represent the inappropriate continuation of a state that is normal in earlier life. Separation anxiety is the paradigmatic example here. Most children show separation and stranger anxiety in their second year, and many are unhappy about leaving their parents on first going to school. However, much more independence is expected of teenagers, and in a 12-year-old a wish to sleep with her parents, because she is afraid to sleep alone, would be distinctly abnormal.

2 *How long do bouts of the symptom last, and how often do they occur?* Most people worry or feel depressed sometimes, but these are evanescent phenomena. They are only symptomatic when present for an inordinate amount of time. Once again, we lack data on how much worrying is normal, but can determine how much time (average length of bout of worrying $\times$ number of bouts per week) has been spent worrying and make a common sense judgement about whether this is pathological.

3 *Is the symptom intrusive into other thoughts and activities?* A symptom that disappears as soon as something comes along to take an individual's mind off it, is unlikely to be of psychopathological import, so it is important to ask whether symptoms intrude into, or interfere with, other activities. Worrying that interferes with concentrating on schoolwork represents a problem, whereas worries that disappear as soon as there is a job to be done probably do not.

4 *Is the symptom controllable?* If a child can get rid of a symptom by thinking about, or doing, something else, then one can usually be fairly sure that it is not psychopathologically significant. Intrusiveness and uncontrollability are very closely related ideas and, in general, both will be reported in relation to important symptoms.

5 *Is the symptom generalized across more than one activity?* A 'symptom' that is restricted to a single activity (such as worrying about a maths test just before it, but only then) is usually not a marker for a clinically relevant problem. In the case of specific phobias, a child who is frightened of dogs only when a dog is barking at them, is unlikely to encounter many problems, while the child who is afraid of dogs whenever he or she is out in the street, regardless of the presence of a dog, can be regarded as being symptomatic.

Behavioural problems

An overlapping set of considerations is of primary relevance for behaviour problems. Some undesirable behaviours are normal (such as disobedience or lying) when they occur at low frequency, and should only be regarded as 'symptoms' when they occur often. In such cases, frequency, controllability and generalization are relevant, but bout duration and intrusiveness are not. Until recently, information about the frequency of oppositional/defiant disorder (ODD) symptoms in the community have not been available, so clinicians have had no choice but to rely on their own judgement in determining whether such symptoms were present. Angold & Costello (1996) recently presented general population norms for ODD symptoms in 9–14-year-olds and, based on 90th percentile cutpoints, suggested that these symptoms should be regarded as 'often' occurring as follows. *Spitefulness and vindictiveness* and *blaming others* should occur at least once every 3 months; *being touchy or easily annoyed, losing temper, arguing with adults, and defying or refusing adults' requests* should occur at least twice a week; and *being angry and resentful* or *deliberately annoying others* should occur at least four times per week. Now we can expect that, at other ages, different normative values would be more appropriate, and it is to be hoped that such norms will be forthcoming. However, it is also important to consider some other characteristics of antisocial behaviours.

1 *Response to admonition.* Here, two levels of non-response may be discerned; some children simply do not do as they are told, while others actively challenge their admonisher (for instance by swearing at, or hitting, a teacher).

It is also worth noting that clinical experience indicates that many children with marked attentional and activity problems are poor reporters of their behaviour in this respect. It is not uncommon for such children to report that they are not fidgety and have no difficulty remaining seated when told to do so, despite the fact that they have spent most of the interview wandering around the office, in the face of repeated requests that they should sit down. They may also seem to be unaware of their social skills defects, so it is important to get detailed descriptions of how they interact with their reported 'best friends'.

2 *In what situations did the behaviour occur?* Three general settings may be distinguished as: (a) home; (b) school; and (c) elsewhere. Determining where problematic behaviour occurs has important treatment implications, and also seems to have some prognostic importance, in that pervasively disturbed children appear to have more persistent problems and do worse in young adulthood.

3 *Was the child usually alone or in company when performing antisocial acts?* Such information is helpful in determining the degree to which the child's social environment may be contributing to his or her antisocial behaviour.

4 *Who was the victim of the antisocial acts?* Here distinctions may be made between (a) community property (as in vandalizing park benches); (b) the property of individuals not known to the child (as in shoplifting); and (c) the property of individuals known to the child (as in stealing from mother's purse).

Many types of antisocial acts are considered abnormal whenever they occur (armed robbery, for instance), and are not at all uncommon in some psychiatric settings (such as substance abuse treatment programmes), so it is important to ask teenagers about these sorts of activities. In many areas, it is also common for teenagers, and even younger children, to carry weapons, and to use them, so it is worth asking about this as well. In countries where guns are freely available, it is also important to know whether the child has access to guns, especially if the child is at risk of making a suicide attempt. Parents should then be advised to eliminate the child's access to weapons (preferably by removing them from the house).

Delusions, hallucinations and other symptoms of serious psychopathology that may be confused with normal phenomena

Children and adolescents may manifest all the symptoms characteristic of adult disorders such as schizophrenia or bipolar disorders. Disorders involving hallucinations and delusions are uncommon in childhood, but both become more common in adolescence. In childhood especially, great care must be taken in establishing the presence of delusions and hallucinations, because a number of other phenomena can easily be confused with these very serious symptoms. In particular, hypnogogic hallucinations (vivid true hallucinations occurring when falling asleep) and hypnopompic hallucinations (vivid true hallucinations occurring on waking up) are normal phenomena. In general, hallucinations occurring only when the child is in bed should not be regarded as evidence of the presence of major disorders, even if the child insists that he or she was not falling asleep or waking up when they occurred. Care also needs to be taken not to mistake eidetic imagery, imaginary companions, elaborated fantasies, perceptual illusions, seizure phenomena, drug-induced experiences, subcultural beliefs, and hallucinations accompanying toxic encephalopathies, for manifestations of delusional or hallucinatory psychopathologies.

Déjà vu, jamais vu, derealization and depersonalization are states that most people experience from time to time, but sometimes occur in schizophrenia, schizo-affective states and bipolar disorders. Once again, it is important to get a clear description of the phenomena, and to pay particular attention to how often they occur and how long they last. Derealization and deperson-

alization are also common effects of certain drugs (such as cannabis and LSD) and the possibility of drug use should be investigated when these states are reported. Premonitions of events are also often described by quite normal people, and should only be regarded as being psychotic phenomena when they clearly fall outside the normal range of experiences for the cultural group to which the child belongs. In most cases, consideration of the overall clinical picture will ensure that these phenomena are interpreted appropriately.

Many of these psychopathological distinctions are relatively subtle, and parents can usually provide only very limited descriptions of such phenomena. Here (as with adults), there is no substitute for the direct face-to-face mental status evaluation of the child, supplemented by longer term clinical evaluation.

Impairment of psychosocial functioning

Psychiatric disorders impact on a person's ability to function at their highest level in the psychosocial environment, and it is vital to assess the degree to which such functioning is impaired. Here the main areas of concern are school (or work) performance and behaviour, peer relationships, social and spare-time activities, and relationships within the family. Relying solely on symptom ratings and DSM-III for diagnosis has been found to lead to ridiculously high rates of diagnosis in epidemiological studies using respondent-based interviews and one strategy for producing more sensible estimates has been to require some degree of psychosocial impairment to be present if a diagnosis is to be made (Bird *et al.* 1988). In clinical settings, most patients have some degree of impairment, so the issue of using impairment as a measure of severity looms larger there. The same may be said of glossary-based interviewer-based interviews (CAPA or K-SADS-P IVR) that do not require the use of additional impairment criteria to compensate for symptomatic overdiagnosis.

Several approaches have been adopted to the measurement of impairment (reviewed in Costello *et al.* 1998). The first is to consider the patient's overall level of functioning, by combining information about symptomatology and psychosocial impairment into a single rating. The Children's Global Assessment Scale (Shaffer *et al.* 1983; Bird *et al.* 1987) and the Columbia Impairment Scale (Bird *et al.* 1993, 1996) are the best examples. These instruments, based on the DSM-IIIR Axis V, provide simple, reliable scales, and can be coded after all the symptom information about the child has been gathered.

More molecular assessments of impairment are available from the Social Adjustment Inventory for Children and Adolescents (SAICA; John *et al.* 1987), which is a 20-min interview schedule that includes ratings of a number of psychosocial problems. It also includes items that are ordinarily regarded as conduct problems, and usually covered in the exploration of symptomatology. However, it is quite possible to use the non-symptom items alone, although the usual scoring system does not adopt this approach. The same applies to the more extensive Child and Adolescent Functional Assessment Scale (Hodges *et* al. 1998). When the developmental impairment of younger children and those with mental retardation is at issue, the Vineland Adaptive Behaviour Scales (Sparrow et al. 1984; Sparrow & Cicchetti 1989; Cicchetti et al. 1991) are without peer, although some scales also include what, from a psychiatric perspective, are better regarded as being symptoms rather than impairments.

An alternative approach is provided by the CAPA and DISC-IV, which calls for separate ratings of psychosocial impairment, secondary to psychiatric symptomatology, in a number of domains. In this case, the symptom ratings are separated out from the impairment ratings and the contributions of particular symptom areas to the overall degree of impairment are assessed. This can be helpful with children with multiple problems, because it gives an idea of which areas of symptomatology are most responsible for any psychosocial difficulties, and this may help in deciding where to begin as far as treatment is concerned.

The K-SADS-P adopts a somewhat different approach by including aspects of psychosocial functioning in a number of the ratings of specific symptoms (Chambers et al. 1985). The strength of this combined technique is that it provides an overall clinical summary of how 'disturbed' the child is, and it is widely used in both clinical practice and research. However, because symptoms and psychosocial impairments are conflated in the ratings, it is impossible to look at each dimension separately.

Lifetime histories

Two studies (Orvaschel et al. 1982; Fendrich et al. 1990) have found that the kappas for child reports of known depressive episodes reported on between 6 months and 2 years later were around 0.6. Fendrich et al. (1990) also present evidence of reasonable stability for diagnoses of conduct disorder, attention deficit disorder and substance abuse, but poor stability for anxiety diagnoses. However, it is important to remember that the usual form of instability is failure to recall a previous episode; few symptoms are 'invented'. The use of scripts means that a series of events may be conflated into a single memory, so very accurate dating may not be attainable. However, recent work in the survey literature suggests that attempts to 'decompose' such memories into a series of more specific instances can be surprisingly successful. Likewise, tying the onsets of symptoms to events, such as birthdays and school terms, can also lead to finer-grained dating than seemed possible at the beginning of the interview. It is usually possible to determine the age by which a symptom was definitely present, which is certainly better than nothing. In general, the further back in time one goes the more information is lost although, for events of major significance, the degree of decrement after the first year may be small. It is also important to remember that in adults, for most memories, there is a 'brought forward' effect, by which events are remembered as having happened more recently than was the case, although there are exceptions to this rule, as in the case of memories for certain developmental milestones in one's children (Hart et al. 1978), and there is no reason to suppose that this is not the case in children too. In fact, the situation may be more complicated

than this in children because it has been found that the age at which children and adolescents were interviewed about their depressive psychopathology had a significant effect on the rates at which they reported depressive symptoms and the reported timing of their first episodes and worst episodes of dysphoria, with girls around the age of 16 reporting earlier episodes than either younger or older girls (Angold et al. 1991). This age group also reported a higher level of current symptoms, so it may be that the finding from adults that being currently depressed increases the chance of reporting a previous depression holds in children too. As long as these caveats are borne in mind, a lifetime history is well worth taking, but it must be remembered that negative responses are not as reliable as positive ones.

Special interviewing situations

Children with limited understanding: the young and the mentally retarded

Any interview is an exercise in verbal skills, and it is important to be sensitive to verbal limitations in those being interviewed. Young children are unlikely to provide much information in a free-recall setting, and the same is true of the mentally retarded. These groups also have shorter attention spans, and usually cannot be expected to sit for 2 h of interview without breaks. However, they may well be the only available sources of information about their inner lives.

The temptation for the clinician when dealing with individuals who can provide only limited detail in response to open-ended questions is to ask a lot of closed questions, and this often leads to the use of leading questions in order to make it 'easier' for the individual to respond. However, these groups are particularly likely to respond to such questioning by supposing that they are expected to agree with the interviewer, and mistakenly trying to oblige in this way. While there may be no way around the need to ask greater numbers of closed questions, every attempt should be made to get as good descriptions as possible of the phenomena that the child is referring to, so as to avoid confusion. It is also important to try to check that the words that the child is using to describe their inner world are being used in the same way that we would use them. Thus, a 4-year-old's 'worry' might be our 'frightened' or 'depressed'. It can be helpful to find situations in which one can be fairly sure that a child was feeling a particular emotion (like sadness), and then ask whether the feeling they are talking about now is the same as that. In fact, this problem is not qualitatively different from the general issue of making sure that both parties in the interview mean the same thing, but it is quantitatively more demanding.

Additional tools may be helpful in getting descriptions of events that occurred; using play-like materials, such as puppets, toy houses, or photographs of individuals involved in events may be useful. Drawing is also a time-honoured modality in child psychiatry, and can be useful here. The aim is to provide a focus for cognitively reconstructing the situation to be remembered. However, it is important to recognize that the aim, in this case, is to help the child to remember and not to make interpretations. The degree to which these aids generate misleading, as well as accurate information has not been adequately tested.

Investigation of abuse

Now that greater attention is being paid to the problems of physical and sexual abuse, an increased load has been placed upon the clinical interview, and a new set of demands are being made on the 'evidence' collected. In collecting material that may be called into evidence it is particularly important that leading questions or other 'suggestive' strategies should be avoided because, in some well-publicized cases, such material has led to children's testimony being rejected (Cole & Loftus 1987). In dealing with issues that may be frightening or embarrassing, or about which the child may have been threatened should he or she ever reveal what happened, there is naturally a wish to make it as easy as possible to give a full description. Furthermore, as most young children lack an adequate anatomical vocabulary to describe sexual abuse, the use of anatomically 'correct' dolls or pictures to allow children to demonstrate what happened has become fashionable, and has received research support (Steward & Steward 1996). However, some have argued that such dolls (with their obvious protuberances and orifices) themselves suggest certain forms of play that may then be misinterpreted as evidence of sexual abuse (King & Yuille 1987). Indeed, experimental studies have found that, while the use of props such as dolls can increase accurate positive reports, they can also increase the incidence of problematic reports (reports of things known not to have happened) (Ornstein et al. 1997; see also Ceci et al., Chapter 8). Case reviews of sexual abuse records have suggested that fabrications of stories of sexual abuse are rare, and that such fabrications are usually begun by an adult when they occur (Jones 1985).

The definitive answers to the best way to collect evidence of abuse are still some way off, but at present an acceptable approach seems to be to use ordinary good interviewing strategies as far as possible and to supplement these with descriptions using anatomically correct dolls or pictures when necessary, always bearing in mind that the child must understand that one is asking 'What actually happened' rather than 'What can you do with these dolls' (Steward & Steward 1996). As defence lawyers are almost certain to make the claim that evidence of abuse was obtained by the use of leading questions and techniques that relied on the child's supposed suggestibility, it is important to be sure that this was not the case, and the best way of doing this is to record (preferably on videotape) exactly what happened in the interview. When this is not possible, it is important to record both the *questions asked* and the answers obtained (see Bruck *et al.* 1998 for helpful discussions of the implications of memory development research for children's testimony; Leippe &

Romanczyk 1987 on juror's reactions to child witnesses; also Ross *et al.* 1987; Ornstein *et al.* 1997).

Children who 'don't know'

All child psychiatric clinicians have been faced with children who resolutely 'don't know'. In such cases, persistence can make a huge difference, particularly with information about duration, frequency and the timing of symptom onsets. It may also be the case that some children really do not know how to answer questions like 'How have you been feeling lately?', because they are unfamiliar with describing their feelings. In such cases, more focused questions (such as 'Have you been feeling miserable?') can help by providing a series of categories that children can use to describe their feelings. Thus, the ubiquitous 'boredom' of adolescence may be reducible to a number of more sharply focused states, when a framework for more accurate descriptions is offered.

The psychodynamic interview

Psychodynamic psychotherapy uses an interview format as its central modality. However, the aims of such interviews are rather different from those of the diagnostic clinical interview. The emphasis is not on collecting 'facts' in an efficient manner, but on engaging the child in an exploration of his or her own inner world and attempting to understand how that world combines fantasy and reality in relation to experience and behaviour. It is therefore usual for the therapist to be much less active and to allow the child to play and draw quite freely. The therapist provides interpretations that represent attempts to understand the meaning of the child's experiences within the framework of psychodynamic theory. This is not the place to explore the intricacies of psychodynamic technique, but it should be borne in mind that these differences in aim and practice mean that a psychodynamically orientated interview is unlikely to provide the best means of collecting the information necessary to make a phenomenological diagnosis; that is not its purpose. Although the phenomenological interview is not the best method for psychodynamic interpretation, it is important that a sense of trust and understanding be generated in such interviews, so as not to compromise later psychodynamic work. Many of the techniques involved in a good phenomenological interview may be seen as laying the groundwork for psychodynamic therapy and there is no reason to see the two as being in opposition (see Jacobs, Chapter 58, for a discussion of some further aspects of psychodynamic psychotherapy).

Projective testing

The aim of projective testing is to provide a child with an ambiguous stimulus, and then to use the responses to indicate underlying problems. At the simple end of the spectrum, children have been asked for years what their 'three magic wishes' would be, and it has been shown that the magic wishes of psychiatrically referred children differ in content from those of normal controls (Winkley 1982) in frequently containing wishes related to real problems. However, it has not been shown that these same problems could not have been uncovered by simply asking the child about his or her problems in a straightforward way. The same applies to the standardized scoring schemes developed for the Thematic Apperception Test (TAT; Winter 1999) or the Rorschach Inkblot Test (Exner & Weiner 1995), and herein lies the issue with projective testing in general. In a thorough review of the literature on the subject, Gittelman-Klein (1978) concluded that there was no evidence that such testing revealed any information that was either not already known to the clinicians before testing or could not have been discovered by the simpler means of asking about it directly. If the aim is to explore a child's fantasy life, particularly as part of psychodynamically orientated play therapy or psychotherapy, then projective techniques clearly have an important part to play, and Winnicott's (1971) famous interactive squiggle game and talking about drawings can certainly serve to initiate and maintain psychotherapeutic interactions.

Observations of behaviour

Observation of the child's behaviour is a central focus of the diagnostic interview. Indeed, with some very disturbed children, it may contribute the most significant material. All clinicians associated with the child should make a point of keeping in mind a checklist of the behavioural areas outlined below, so that the child's behaviour can be compared across the various settings or 'stimulus conditions' provided by the clinic. Such observations should begin in the waiting room, which may offer an opportunity to observe the child's initial mode of interaction with completely unfamiliar adults and peers. A number of dimensions should be considered, including separation responses, physical appearance, motor behaviour, form and content of speech, the quality of social interactions, affective behaviour, level of consciousness and developmental level. Although this section concentrates on observation of the child, it is also important to bear in mind that an interview with a parent about the child also provides an opportunity to conduct a mental status examination of the parent. As parental psychiatric disorders are major risk factors for child psychiatric disorders, such an evaluation is important for the development of a full diagnostic formulation. Child psychiatric disorders also have significant impacts on parents' lives, emotionally, socially and financially (Angold *et al.* 1998), and the clinician should also take care to find out whether such impacts are present in each case.

Separation responses

The younger the child, the more likely he or she is to protest against separation from parents, so the interviewer may also need to engage parents in helping the child to separate, and this provides an opportunity to observe parental responses. During the interview a child will often become more anxious, and ask to see his or her parents. If this anxiety seems likely to disrupt the interview, then a quick visit to the parents will usually settle things down for a while. Sometimes the level of anxiety is such that a child simply cannot be interviewed when the parents are absent, in which case there is no alternative to conducting the interview with them in the room. Other children who have experienced multiple caregivers will separate with undue ease, and may end up trying to sit on the interviewer's knee and shower him or her with kisses. A firm, but friendly, attempt to get the child to adopt more suitable seating usually has the desired effect.

Physical appearance

The physical appearance of the child may provide indications of abuse (e.g. bruising) or neglect (such as dirty, ill-fitting clothes or signs of malnourishment). Signs of genetic abnormalities (such as low-set ears) or other deformities should also be looked for (see A. Bailey, Chapter 10). Sometimes oddities of dress, hairstyle or make-up may be helpful in identifying deviant subculture membership, or even psychosis.

Motor behaviour

A number of motor abnormalities that may have psychiatric significance may be observed. The most common example is the restlessness, fidgetiness and distractibility of hyperactivity, which needs to be distinguished from manic motor excitement. Depression may be accompanied by motor slowness and underactivity and, in very rare cases, primary obsessional slowness may occur in severe obsessive-compulsive disorder. Obsessive-compulsive disorders may manifest as compulsive acts or rituals, which must be distinguished from motor stereotypies, tics and mannerisms. Potentially self-injurious behaviour such as head-banging or self-biting may occur (usually in mentally retarded subjects), and catatonic states may even more occasionally be observed. The clinician should also be on the alert for medication-induced movement disorders (such as the tremor of lithium intoxication or the choreo-athetoid movements of tardive dyskinesia), and symptoms and signs of drug or alcohol use.

Form of speech

Speech disorders, such as stuttering, cluttering and articulation defects, should be noted if they occur, because they may require specialist treatment. A number of psychiatric disorders also produce abnormalities in the form of speech, such as the low volume mumbling of some socially anxious or depressed individuals, the slowness of speech of psychomotor retardation, manic pressure of speech, and the prosodic abnormalities that may occur in some psychotic states or autism. Vocal tics may occur alone or in combination with motor tics.

Content of speech

A range of speech content abnormalities may be observed, including the neologisms, incoherence and poverty of content that may occur in schizophrenia, and manic flight of ideas. Unusual grammatical forms (such as the pronominal inversions of autistic children) may occur, and verbal stereotypies and the occurrence of self-directed speech should also be watched for.

Social interaction

An interview is a social interaction, and can provide a good deal of information about a child's social abilities. Both verbal and non-verbal social functioning should be considered.

How readily does the child provide information? Does the child engage in normal reciprocal social communication with good articulation of both verbal and non-verbal interchanges? Are the child's overtures and responses appropriate to the interview situation or is the child overly withdrawn, overly friendly or socially inappropriate or odd? Is the pattern of eye contact unusual in any way? Does the child maintain an appropriate social distance? Is the child unusually disinhibited, aggressive or oppositional during the interview? Is there unusual preoccupation with idiosyncratic special interests? What is the overall quality of the rapport between the interviewer and the child?

Affective behaviour

Though many children are shy, anxious or sullen at the beginning of an interview, most 'warm up' after a little while and it then becomes possible to determine whether there are signs of affective dysfunction.

Does the child smile and laugh appropriately and show a normal range of facial expressions and emotional responses? Are there any signs of overly expansive mood? Is the predominant facial expression one of sadness or anxiety? Are there any visible signs of autonomic disturbance, such as sweating or hyperventilation? Is the child frequently tearful, irritable, suspicious or perplexed? Is affective behaviour appropriate to the material being discussed, and does the child show a full range of affective responses? Is the child's mood abnormally labile?

Level of consciousness

In most circumstances, clouding of consciousness will be obvious. However, on rare occasions, previously unrecognized *absences* can be spotted by a careful interviewer.

Developmental level

A full developmental assessment requires expertly administered standardized testing, but a brief evaluation of a child's verbal, reading, writing, mathematical and drawing abilities can indicate the presence of obvious delays or deficits.

How long should the interview last?

This chapter has indicated that diagnostic interviews are intensive and extensive data-gathering exercises. They cannot therefore be completed in a few minutes. A proper psychiatric assessment cannot be encompassed within the frame of a typical paediatric consultation. With good interviewing skills, a full diagnostic interview can usually be completed in an hour and sometimes much less, but when substantial comorbidity is present considerably longer than this may be needed. Allowance also needs to be made for the poor attention spans of many disturbed children (and many of their parents), and it is better to allow breaks during the interview than to plough ahead in the face of waning attention. As elsewhere in medicine, the failure to take a good history, and conduct an adequate examination, leads to diagnostic and treatment mistakes. Indeed, in psychiatry, which relies much less on laboratory studies than many other branches of medicine, it is even more critical to spend the necessary time and effort to learn how to interview proficiently, and then to apply this learning to every patient.

Family interviews

So far, this chapter has considered interviews mostly from the perspective of gathering reported 'facts' from multiple informants, using more or less structured approaches. However, in clinical practice it is important to be aware that information of a different sort can be obtained from interviews involving more than one family member. Given the difficulty of getting whole families to turn up for clinical assessments, such interviews will often involve only one parent and the child, but that is still a very useful combination. Here the focus is on observing how family members interact with one another, and the ways in which symptoms are manifested in such interactions. As a starting point, the clinician needs to provide a structure within which interactions can be observed, and the information collected in separate interviews with the parent and child is helpful here, because it will have indicated the key issues that have resulted in a clinic appointment. The fact that the parent and child often have not reported the same things provides one starting point. One can simply ask each informant why the other mentioned something that they did not (in the clinical setting one rarely guarantees confidentiality among family members). The aim here is not specifically to 'reconcile' reports (though that may be a useful by-product), but to observe how the family deals with the conflict implicit in the question. A well-known pattern often seen in families with children with behavioural problems is for disagreements to escalate into angry coercive exchanges (Patterson 1981). Such patterns are susceptible to amelioration by family behavioural techniques (Patterson & Reid 1973; Patterson *et al.* 1981). It will often be the case that information collected in family interviews will have an important place in the design of the eventual treatment plan, regardless of the diagnosis.

If both parents are present, it is also important to keep an eye on the interactions between the parents (and each parent's apparent mental state), because the child's problems are often associated with parental and interparental problems, which may themselves merit specific treatment. Similarly, when the patient's siblings are also present, it is helpful to compare their behaviour with the referred child's. The ostensible patient may not be the only one with problems (or even the greatest problems).

More structured tasks that the mother and child or whole family are required to work together on can also be very revealing; for instance, in identifying the withdrawal, negativity and hostility often displayed by depressed parents towards their children (Zahn-Waxler et al. 1990). For research purposes, a huge variety of observational coding schemes is available but, in the clinical setting, straightforward observations of the characteristics of interactions still have an important place in the overall diagnostic assessment.

An interview with the family also provides a rather different sort of setting for the child than the highly formalized one-on-one diagnostic interview with the clinician. It is important to observe whether the child behaves differently in these two settings, and any others that may be encountered in the clinic; such as interactions during psychological testing. Sometimes a child whose behaviour was well under control in the one-on-one structured interview or testing setting manifests far more disturbed behaviour with the family. If it turns out that a similar pattern is manifested at school, then interventions aimed at providing more structured interactions at home and at school may be warranted. Different phases of the assessment process are often conducted by different individuals, and here again it is important to evaluate the degree of consistency of behaviour with different individuals across situations. If there is considerable variation across settings and individuals it is important to try to identify the characteristics of those settings and individuals that are associated with problematic as opposed to adaptive behaviour.

Cultural and subcultural variations in behaviour

Any assessment of type and severity of psychopathology, no matter how structured or unstructured, relies upon explicit or implicit suppositions about the limits of 'normality' and the borders of pathology. As the vast majority of empirical research on psychopathology has been conducted in the USA and Western Europe, most of the constructs familiar to clinicians dealing with child and adolescent psychopathology have been derived from clinical experience with children from those areas. Although there has been rather little cross-cultural research on psychopathology, there are indications that there are national differences in patterns of presentation. For instance, Thai parents report lower levels of conduct problems in their children

than do Western European or American parents. Thus, a given level of conduct disturbance may be more deviant (compared with the rest of the population) in a Thai child than a Dutch child. In such a circumstance it is easy to imagine that a Thai parent, aware that the child was highly deviant within his or her culture, could seem to be making a fuss over nothing as far as a Dutch psychiatrist used to Dutch norms was concerned. A second example concerns sleep patterns. Nearly all of the literature on sleep and its disorders concerns sleep patterns typical in the industrialized West, but there are many populations where sleeping continuously for 8h at a fixed time each day would be regarded as being highly abnormal (Worthman & Melby, in press). Indeed we have only to consider what 'good British parents' thought of as a proper bedtime for a 2-year-old in the 1950s and the typical practice of parents today, to realize that 'good parenting' is a moving target, not a fixed pattern of practice.

Even within cultures there are subgroup differences in what is regarded as being appropriate parental behaviour. For instance, in the areas of the rural southeastern USA where much of my research is conducted, many well-adjusted parents of well-adjusted children, heeding the biblical injunction not to 'spare the rod and spoil the child' are willing to take a belt to their child for serious infractions of discipline. My experience is that few British social workers would be comfortable with such behaviour. However, such disciplinary practices were pretty much universal in the West until the second half of the twentieth century, and it is by no means apparent that reductions in the use of physical discipline in many quarters have led to reductions in child psychiatric morbidity. The point here is not to encourage the use of corporal punishment, but to emphasize that as clinicians and researchers we need to remain aware that the boundaries of individual and family pathology are to some extent culturally determined, and that we should not make the mistake of labelling all differences from today's middle-class, Caucasian, industrialized Western norms of behaviour as 'pathology'. By that standard, most of our own great grandparents bordered on being child abusers.

Future directions

It is my opinion that structured psychiatric interviews for parents and children aged 9 and above are now probably as good as they can be. Many years of work have gone into producing the interviews we have today, and there is little evidence that recent enormous efforts to further 'improve' such measures have had much effect on their reliability, although they have succeeded in making some interviews much longer than they used to be. As we learn more about psychopathology we need to modify our measures' content to reflect what we need to measure, but the basic principles used to design new or revised modules will remain the same (and will work just as well or poorly as they do now). What is needed is to extend the range of structured assessments down to younger ages. There is startlingly little research on preschool psychopathology, for instance, and it was only in 2000 that the first structured parent report diagnostic interview specifically designed for use with this age group became available. A good deal of work still needs to be carried out to determine what forms of information from the child and caretakers other than parents can usefully be integrated into diagnostic assessments.

Now that a range of very extensive diagnostic measures is available, it is time to move them out of the research field and into ordinary clinical practice. It seems odd that the unstructured clinical interview has been almost entirely supplanted for research purposes because of its well-documented inadequacies as a data-gathering and diagnostic procedure, but continues to be the main assessment tool in clinical practice, where good phenomenological assessment is of the greatest importance. All clinicians dealing with psychopathology can benefit from training on an interviewer-based structured interview (particularly one of the glossary-based interviews), and it is to be hoped that such training will soon become part of all training programmes for clinicians who deal with child psychopathology (as it is already in some). However, it must be admitted that the time to conduct a full psychiatric assessment is not always available, and when that is the case it would be helpful to have shorter interviews available to serve as screening tools. At the time of writing, work is happily beginning on a version of the DISC to fulfil this function. The idea here is not to encourage slavish dependence on any particular structured interview or other assessment technique, but to use the strengths of standardized interviews to underpin further explorations of the nature and meaning of psychopathology by clinicians with a solid understanding of the principles of good interviewing and the phenomenological approach to psychiatric diagnosis. Methodologically, we have come a long way in the last 30 years, and it is time to bring the benefits of methods first derived for research purposes to all of our patients and clients.

References

Achenbach, T.M. (1985) *Assessment and Taxonomy of Child and Adolescent Psychopathology*. Sage Publications, Beverly Hills, CA.

Ambrosini, P.J. (2000) Historical development and present status of the schedule for affective disorders and schizophrenia for school-age children (K-SADS). *Journal of the American Academy of Child and Adolescent Psychiatry*, 39, 49–58.

American Psychiatric Association (1994) *Diagnostic and Statistical Manual of Mental Disorders (DSM-IV)*, 4th edn. American Psychiatric Press, Washington, DC.

Anastasi, A. (1950) The concept of validity in the interpretation of test scores. *Journal of Psychology and Educational Measures*, 10, 67–78.

Anastasi, A. (1986) Evolving concepts of test validation. *Annual Review of Psychology*, 37, 1–15.

Angold, A. & Costello, E.J. (1996) Toward establishing an empirical basis for the diagnosis of Oppositional Defiant Disorder. *Journal of the American Academy of Child and Adolescent Psychiatry*, 35, 1205–1212.

Angold, A. & Costello, E.J. (2000) The Child and Adolescent Psychi-

atric Assessment (CAPA). *Journal of the American Academy of Child and Adolescent Psychiatry*, 39, 39–48.

Angold, A. & Fisher, P.W. (1999) Interviewer-based interviews. In: *Diagnostic Assessment in Child and Adolescent Psychopathology* (eds D. Shaffer, C.P. Lucas & J.E. Richters), pp. 34–64. Guilford Press, New York.

Angold, A., Weissman, M.M., John, K., Wickramaratne, P. & Prusoff, B.A. (1991) The effects of age and sex on depression ratings in children and adolescents. *Journal of the American Academy of Child and Adolescent Psychiatry*, 30, 67–72.

Angold, A., Prendergast, M., Cox, A., Harrington, R., Simonoff, E. & Rutter, M. (1995) The Child and Adolescent Psychiatric Assessment (CAPA). *Psychological Medicine*, 25, 739–753.

Angold, A., Erkanli, A., Costello, E.J. & Rutter, M. (1996a) Precision, reliability and accuracy in the dating of symptom onsets in child and adolescent psychopathology. *Journal of Child Psychology and Psychiatry*, 37, 657–664.

Angold, A., Erkanli, A., Loeber, R., Costello, E.J., Van Kammen, W. & Stouthamer-Loeber, M. (1996b) Disappearing depression in a population sample of boys. *Journal of Emotional and Behavioral Disorders*, 4, 95–104.

Angold, A., Messer, S.C., Stangl, D., Farmer, E.M.Z., Costello, E.J. & Burns, B.J. (1998) Perceived parental burden and service use for child and adolescent psychiatric disorders. *American Journal of Public Health*, 88, 75–80.

Angold, A., Costello, E.J. & Erkanli, A. (1999a) Comorbidity. *Journal of Child Psychology and Psychiatry*, 40, 57–87.

Angold, A., Costello, E.J. & Worthman, C.M. (1999b) Pubertal changes in hormone levels and depression in girls. *Psychological Medicine*, 29, 1043–1053.

Bird, H.R., Canino, G., Rubio-Stipec, M. & Ribera, J.C. (1987) Further measures of the psychometric properties of the Children's Global Assessment Scale. *Archives of General Psychiatry*, 44, 821–824.

Bird, H.R., Canino, G., Rubio-Stipec, M. *et al.* (1988) Estimates of the prevalence of childhood maladjustment in a community survey in Puerto Rico: The use of combined measures. *Archives of General Psychiatry*, 45, 1120–1126.

Bird, H.R., Gould, M.S. & Staghezza, B.M. (1992) Patterns of diagnostic comorbidity in a community sample of children age 9 through 16 years. Presented at the Annual Meeting of the Society for Research in Child and Adolescent Psychopathology, Sarasota.

Bird, H.R., Shaffer, D., Fisher, P.W. *et al.* (1993) The Columbia impairment scale (CIS): pilot findings on a measure of global impairment for children and adolescents. *International Journal of Methods in Psychiatric Research*, 3, 167–176.

Bird, H.R., Andrews, H., Schwab-Stone, M. *et al.* (1996) Global measures of impairment for epidemiologic and clinical use with children and adolescents. *International Journal of Psychiatric Research*, 6, 295–307.

Brainerd, C. & Ornstein, P.A. (1991) Children's memory for witnessed events: the developmental backdrop. In: *The Suggestibility of Children's Recollections* (ed. J. Doris), pp. 10–20. American Psychological Association, Washington, D.C.

Breslau, N. (1987) Inquiring about the bizarre: false positives in Diagnostic Interview Schedule for Children (DISC) ascertainment of obsessions, compulsions, and psychotic symptoms. *Journal of the American Academy of Child and Adolescent Psychiatry*, 26, 639–644.

Breton, J.-J., Bergeron, L., Valla, J.-P., Lepine, S., Houde, L. & Gaudet, N. (1995) Do children aged 9–11 years understand the DISC version 2.25 questions? *Journal of the American Academy of Child and Adolescent Psychiatry*, 34, 946–956.

Bruck, M., Ceci, S.J. & Hembrooke, H. (1998) Reliability and credibility of young children's reports: from research to policy and practice. *American Psychologist*, 53, 136–151.

Cannell, C.F., Marquis, K.H. & Laurent, A. (1977) A summary of studies of interviewing methodology. *Vital and Health Statistics: Series 2*, 69, 1–78.

Cannell, C.F., Miller, P.V. & Oksenberg, L. (1981) Research on interviewing techniques. *Sociological Methodology*, 12, 389–437.

Cantwell, D.P. (1988) DSM-III studies. In: *Assessment and Diagnosis in Child Psychopathology* (eds M. Rutter, A.H. Tuma & I.S. Lann), pp. 3–36. Guilford Press, New York.

Chambers, W.J., Puig-Antich, J., Hirsch, M. *et al.* (1985) The assessment of affective disorders in children and adolescents by semistructured interview: Test–retest reliability of the Schedule for Affective Disorders and Schizophrenia for School-age Children, Present Episode Version. *Archives of General Psychiatry*, 42, 696–702.

Chapman, L.J. & Chapman, J.P. (1967) Genesis of popular but erroneous psychodiagnostic observations. *Journal of Abnormal Psychology*, 74, 271–280.

Chapman, L.J. & Chapman, J.P. (1971) Associatively based illusory correlation as a source of psychodiagnostic folklore. In: *Readings in Personality Assessment* (eds D. Goodstein & R.I. Lanyon), pp. 558–579. John Wiley, New York.

Cicchetti, D.V., Sparrow, S.S. & Carter, A.S. (1991) Development and validation of two Vineland Adaptive Behavior Screening Instruments. Paper presented at the Annual American Psychological Association, San Francisco, CA.

Cole, C.B. & Loftus, E.F. (1987) The memory of children. In: *Children's Eyewitness Memory* (eds S.J. Ceci, M.P. Toglia & D.F. Ross), pp. 178–208, Springer-Verlag, New York.

Conners, C.K. (1997) *Conners' Rating Scales Revised: Instruments for Use with Children and Adolescents*. Multi-Health Systems, North Tonawanda, NY.

Costello, E.J., Messer, S.C., Reinherz, H.Z., Cohen, P. & Bird, H.R. (1998) The prevalence of serious emotional disturbance: a re-analysis of community studies. *Journal of Child and Family Studies*, 7, 411–432.

Cox, A., Holbrook, D. & Rutter, M. (1981a) Psychiatric interviewing techniques. VI. Experimental study: eliciting feelings. *British Journal of Psychiatry*, 139, 144–152.

Cox, A., Hopkinson, K. & Rutter, M. (1981b) Psychiatric interviewing techniques. II. Naturalistic study: eliciting factual information. *British Journal of Psychiatry*, 138, 283–291.

Cox, A., Rutter, M. & Holbrook, D. (1981c) Psychiatric interviewing techniques. V. Experimental study: eliciting factual information. *British Journal of Psychiatry*, 139, 27–37.

Cronbach, L.J. & Meehl, P.E. (1955) Construct validity in psychological tests. *Psychological Bulletin*, 52, 281–302.

Dawes, R.M. (1988) *Rational Choice in an Uncertain World*. Harcourt Brace Jovanovich, New York.

Eaves, L.J., Silberg, J.L., Maes, H.H. *et al.* (1997) Genetics and developmental psychopathology. II. The main effects of genes and environment on behavioral problems in the Virginia Twin Study of adolescent behavior development. *Journal of Child Psychology and Psychiatry*, 38, 965–980.

Ernst, M., Cookus, B.A. & Moravec, B.C. (2000) Pictorial instrument for children and adolescents (PICA-III-R). *Journal of the American Academy of Child and Adolescent Psychiatry*, 39, 94–99.

Exner, J.E.J. & Weiner, I.B. (1995) *The Rorschach: a Comprehensive System*, Vol. 3, *Assessment of Children and Adolescents*, 2nd edn. John Wiley & Sons, New York.

Fendrich, M., Weissman, M.M., Warner, V. & Mufson, L. (1990) Two-year recall of lifetime diagnoses in offspring at high and low risk for major depression: the stability of offspring reports. *Archives of General Psychiatry*, 47, 1121–1127.

Gittelman-Klein, R. (1978) Validity of projective tests for psychodiagnosis in children. In: *Critical Issues in Psychiatric Diagnosis*, (eds R.L. Spitzer & D.F. Klein), pp. 141–166. Raven Press, New York.

Gould, M.S., Shaffer, D., Rutter, M. & Sturge, C. (1988) UK/WHO study of ICD-9. In: *Assessment and Diagnosis in Child Psychopathology* (eds M. Rutter, A.H. Tuma & I.S. Lann), pp. 37–65. Guilford Press, New York.

Gulliksen, H. (1950) Intrinsic validity. *American Psychologist*, 5, 511–517.

Hart, H., Bax, M. & Jenkins, S. (1978) The value of a developmental history. *Developmental Medicine and Child Neurology*, 20, 442–452.

Herjanic, B., Herjanic, M., Brown, F. & Wheatt, T. (1975) Are children reliable reporters? *Journal of Abnormal Child Psychology*, 3, 41–48.

Hodges, K. (1993) Structured interviews for assessing children. *Journal of Child Psychology and Psychiatry*, 34 (1), 49–68.

Hodges, K., McKnew, D., Cytryn, L., Stern, L. & Kline, J. (1982) The Child Assessment Schedule (CAS) Diagnostic Interview: a report on reliability and validity. *Journal of the American Academy of Child Psychiatry*, 21, 468–473.

Hodges, K., Wong, M.M. & Latessa, M. (1998) Use of the child and adolescent functional assessment scale (CAFAS) as an outcome measure in clinical settings. *Journal of Behavioral Health Services and Research*, 25, 325–336.

Hopkinson, K., Cox, A. & Rutter, M. (1981) Psychiatric interviewing techniques. III. Naturalistic study: eliciting feelings. *British Journal of Psychiatry*, 138, 406–415.

Ialongo, N., Edelsohn, G., Werthamer-Larsson, L., Crockett, L. & Kellam, S. (1993) Are self-reported depressive symptoms in first-grade children developmentally transient phenomena? A further look. *Development and Psychopathology*, 5, 433–457.

Jenkins, J.G. (1946) Validity for what? *Journal of Consulting and Clinical Psychology*, 10, 93–98.

Jensen, P.S., Shaffer, D., Rae, D. *et al.* (1992) Attenuation of the Diagnostic Interview Schedule for Children (DISC 2.1): sex, age and IQ relationships. Paper presented at the 39th Annual Meeting of the American Academy of Child and Adolescent Psychiatry, Washington, D.C.

John, K., Davis, G.D., Prusoff, B.A. & Warner, V. (1987) The Social Adjustment Inventory for Children and Adolescents (SAICA): testing of a new semistructured interview. *Journal of the American Academy of Child and Adolescent Psychiatry*, 26, 898–911.

Jones, D.P.H. (1985) *Reliable and fictitious accounts of sexual abuse in children*. Seventh National Conference on Child Abuse and Neglect, Chicago, IL.

King, M. & Yuille, J.C. (1987) Suggestibility and the child witness. In: *Children's Eyewitness Memory* (eds S.J. Ceci, M.P. Toglia & D.F. Ross), pp. 24–35. Springer-Verlag, New York.

Lapouse, R. (1966) The epidemiology of behavior disorders in children. *American Journal of Disfunctional Children*, 111, 594–599.

Lauritsen, J.L. (1998) The age–crime debate: assessing the limits of longitudinal self-report data. *Social Forces*, 77, 127–154.

Leippe, M.R. & Romanczyk, A. (1987) Children on the witness stand: a communication/persuasion analysis of jurors' reactions to child witnesses. In: *Children's Eyewitness Memory* (eds S.J. Ceci, M.P. Toglia & D.F. Ross), pp. 155–177. Springer-Verlag, New York.

Loeber, R., Green, S.M., Lahey, B.B. & Stouthamer-Loeber, M. (1991) Differences and similarities between children, mothers, and teachers as informants on disruptive child behavior. *Journal of Abnormal Child Psychology*, 19, 75–95.

Lord, C., Rutter, M. & LeCouteur, A. (1994) Autism Diagnostic Interview—revised: a revised version of a diagnostic interview for caregivers of individuals with possible pervasive developmental disorders. *Journal of Autism and Developmental Disorders*, 24, 659–685.

Lucas, C.P., Fisher, P., Piacentini, J. *et al.* (1999) Features of interview questions associated with attenuation of symptom reports. *Journal of Abnormal Child Psychology*, 27, 429–437.

Martini, D.R., Strayhorn, J.M. & Puig-Antich, J. (1990) A symptom self-report measure for preschool children. *Journal of the American Academy of Child and Adolescent Psychiatry*, 29, 594–600.

Measelle, J.R., Ablow, J.C., Cowan, P.A. & Cowan, C.P. (1998) Assessing young children's views of their academic, social, and emotional lives: an evaluation of the self-perception scales of the Berkeley Puppet Interview. *Child Development*, 69, 1556–1576.

Nelson, K., Fivush, R., Hudson, J. & Lucariello, J. (1983) Scripts and the development of memory. In: *Trends in Memory Development Research: Contributions to Human Development* (ed. M.T.H. Chi), pp. 52–70. S. Karger, Basel.

Novick, M.R. (1985) *Standards for Educational and Psychological Testing*. American Psychological Association, Washington, D.C.

Ornstein, P.A., Baker-Ward, L., Gordon, B.N. & Merritt, K.A. (1997) Children's memory for medical experiences: implications for testimony. In: *Applied Cognitive Psychology* (eds A. Ornstein & G. Davies), pp. 87–104. John Wiley & Sons, Chapel Hill.

Ornstein, P.A., Gordon, B.N. & Larus, D.M. (1992) Children's memory for a personally experienced event: implications for testimony. *Applied Cognitive Psychology*, 6, 49–60.

Orvaschel, H., Puig-Antich, J., Chambers, W., Tabrizi, M.A. & Johnson, R. (1982) Retrospective assessment of prepubertal major depression with the Kiddie-SADS-E. *Journal of the American Academy of Child Psychiatry*, 21, 392–397.

Patterson, G.R. (1981) *Coercive Family Process*. Castalia Publishing, Eugene, OR.

Patterson, G.R. & Reid, J.B. (1973) Intervention for families of aggressive boys: a replication study. *Behaviour Research and Therapy*, 11, 383–394.

Patterson, G.R., Chamberlain, P. & Reid, J.B. (1981) A comparative evaluation of parent training procedures. *Behavior Therapy*, 13, 638–650.

Peak, H. (1953) Problems of objective observation. In: *Research Methods in the Behavioral Sciences* (eds L. Festinger & D. Katz), pp. 243–300. Dryden Press, New York.

Piacentini, J., Roper, M., Jensen, P. *et al.* (1999) Informant-based determinants of symptom attenuation in structured child psychiatric interviews. *Journal of Abnormal Child Psychology*, 27, 417–428.

Pillemer, D.B. & White, S.H. (1989) Childhood events recalled by children and adults. *Advances in Child Development and Behavior*, 21, 297–340.

Reich, W. (2000) Diagnostic interview for children and adolescents (DICA). *Journal of the American Academy of Child and Adolescent Psychiatry*, 39, 59–66.

Reich, W., Herjanic, B., Welner, Z. & Gandhy, P.R. (1982) Development of a structured psychiatric interview for children: agreement on diagnosis comparing child and parent interviews. *Journal of Abnormal Child Psychology*, 10, 325–336.

Reich, W., Cottler, L., McCallum, K., Corwin, D. & VanEerdewegh, M. (1995) Computerized interviews as a method of assessing psychopathology in children. *Comprehensive Psychiatry*, 36, 40–45.

Remschmidt, H. (1988) German study of ICD-9. In: *Assessment and Diagnosis in Child Psychopathology* (eds M. Rutter, A.H. Tumain & I.S. Lann). Guilford Press, New York.

Robins, L.N. (1985) Epidemiology: reflections on testing the validity of psychiatric interviews. *Archives of General Psychiatry*, 42, 918–924.

Ross, D.F., Miller, B.S. & Moran, P.B. (1987) The child in the eyes of the jury: assessing mock jurors' perceptions of the child witness. In: *Children's Eyewitness Memory* (eds S.J. Ceci, M.P. Toglia & D.F. Ross), pp. 142–154. Springer-Verlag, New York.

Rutter, M. & Cox, A. (1981) Psychiatric interviewing techniques. I. Methods and measures. *British Journal of Psychiatry*, 138, 273–282.

Rutter, M. & Graham, P. (1968) The reliability and validity of the psychiatric assessment of the child. I. Interview with the child. *British Journal of Psychiatry*, 114, 563–579.

Rutter, M., Cox, A., Egert, S., Holbrook, D. & Everitt, B. (1981) Psychiatric interviewing techniques. IV. Experimental study: four contrasting styles. *British Journal of Psychiatry*, 138, 456–465.

Saywitz, K.J. (1987) Children's testimony: age-related patterns of memory errors. In: *Children's Eyewitness Memory* (eds S.J. Ceci, M.P. Toglia & D.F. Ross), pp. 6–52. Springer-Verlag, New York.

Schreier, H.A. (1997) Factitious presentation of psychiatric disorder: when is it Munchausen by proxy? *Child Psychology and Psychiatry Review*, 2, 108–115.

Schwab-Stone, M., Fallon, T., Briggs, M. & Crowther, B. (1994) Reliability of diagnostic reporting for children aged 6–11 years: a test–retest study of the Diagnostic Interview Schedule for Children—Revised. *American Journal of Psychiatry*, 151, 1048–1054.

Shaffer, D., Gould, M.S., Brasic, J. *et al.* (1983) A children's global assessment scale (CGAS). *Archives of General Psychiatry*, 40, 1228–1231.

Shaffer, D., Fisher, P.W. & Lucas, C.P. (1999) Respondent-based interviews. In: *Diagnostic Assessment in Child and Adolescent Psychopathology* (eds D. Shaffer, C.P. Lucas & J.E. Richters), pp. 3–33. Guilford Press, New York.

Shaffer, D., Fisher, P., Lucas, C.P., Dulcan, M.K. & Schwab-Stone, M.E. (2000) NIMH Diagnostic Interview Schedule for Children version IV (NIMH DISC-IV): description, differences from previous versions, and reliability of some common diagnoses. *Journal of the American Academy of Child and Adolescent Psychiatry*, 39, 28–38.

Sherrill, J.T. & Kovacs, M. (2000) Interview schedule for children and adolescents (ISCA). *Journal of the American Academy of Child and Adolescent Psychiatry*, 39, 67–75.

Silverman, W.K. & Nelles, W.B. (1988) The Anxiety Disorders Interview Schedule for Children. *Journal of the American Academy of Child and Adolescent Psychiatry*, 27, 772–778.

Silverman, W.K. & Rabian, B. (1995) Test-retest reliability of the DSM-III-R childhood anxiety disorders symptoms using the Anxiety Disorders Interview Schedule for Children. *Journal of Anxiety Disorders*, 9, 139–150.

Sox, H.C. Jr (1987) Decision analysis: a basic clinical skill? *New England Journal of Medicine*, 316 (5), 271–272.

Sparrow, S.S. & Cicchetti, D.V. (1989) The Vineland Adaptive Behavior Scales. In: *Major Psychological Assessment Instruments* (ed. C.S. Newmark), pp. 199–231. Allyn & Bacon, Needham Heights, MA.

Sparrow, S., Balla, D. & Cicchetti, D. (1984) *Vineland Adaptive Behavior Sales: Interview Edition Expanded Form Manual*. American Guidance Service, Circle Pines, MN.

Stanger, C. & Lewis, M. (1993) Agreement among parents, teachers, and children on internalizing and externalizing behavior problems. *Journal of Clinical Child Psychology*, 22, 107–115.

Steward, M.S. & Steward, D.S. (1996) Interviewing young children about body touch and handling. *Monographs of the Society for Research in Child Development, Serial No. 248*, 61, 1–236.

Truax, C.B. (1966) Reinforcement and non-reinforcement in Rogerian psychotherapy. *Journal of Abnormal Psychology*, **71**, 1–9.

Truax, C.B. (1968) Therapist interpersonal reinforcement of client self-exploration and therapeutic outcome in group psychotherapy. *Journal of Counseling Psychology*, **15**, 225–231.

Tversky, A. & Kahneman, D. (1974) Judgement under uncertainty: heuristics and biases. *Science*, **185**, 1124–1131.

Valla, J.-P., Bergeron, L. & Smolla, N. (2000) The Dominic-R: a pictorial interview for 6- to 11-year-old children. *Journal of the American Academy of Child and Adolescent Psychiatry*, **39**, 85–93.

Wallace, S.R. (1965) Criteria for what? *American Psychologist*, **20**, 411–417.

Warren, S.L., Emde, R.N. & Sroufe, A. (2000) Internal representations: predicting anxiety from children's play narratives. *Journal of the American Academy of Child and Adolescent Psychiatry*, **39**, 100–107.

Warren, S.L., Oppenheim, D. & Emde, R.N. (1996) Can emotions and themes in children's play predict behavior problems? *Journal of the American Academy of Child and Adolescent Psychiatry*, **35**, 1331–1337.

Weitz, J. (1961) Criteria for criteria. *American Psychologist*, **16**, 228–231.

Weller, E.B., Weller, R.A., Fristad, M.A., Rooney, M.T. & Schecter, J. (2000) Children's interview for psychiatric syndromes (ChIPS). *Journal of the American Academy of Child and Adolescent Psychiatry*, **39**, 76–84.

Winkley, L. (1982) The implications of children's wishes—research note. *Journal of Child Psychology and Psychiatry*, **23**, 477–483.

Winnicott, D.W. (1971) *Therapeutic Consultations in Child Psychiatry*. Hogarth Press, London.

Winter, D.G. (1999) Linking personality and 'scientific' psychology: the development of empirically derived Thematic Apperception Test measures. In: *Evocative Images: the Thematic Apperception Test and the Art of Projection* (eds L. Gieser & M.I. Stein), pp. 107–124. American Psychological Association, Washington D.C.

World Health Organization (1992) *ICD-10: the ICD-10 Classification of Mental and Behavioral Disorders: Clinical Descriptions and Diagnostic Guidelines*. World Health Organization, Geneva.

World Health Organization (1993) *The ICD-10 Classification of Mental and Behavioural Disorders: Diagnostic Criteria for Research*. World Health Organization, Geneva.

Worthman, C.M. & Melby, M. (in press) Toward a comparative developmental ecology of human sleep. In: *Adolescent Sleep Patterns: Biological, Social, and Psychological Influences* (ed. M.A. Carskadon). Cambridge University Press, New York.

Zahn-Waxler, C., Iannotti, R.J., Cummings, E.M. & Denham, S. (1990) Antecedents of problem behaviors in children of depressed mothers. *Developmental Psychopathology*, **2**, 271–291.

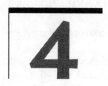

Case Identification in an Epidemiological Context

Eric Fombonne

Introduction

This chapter addresses the issues raised by the assessment of psychopathology within a broader, epidemiological context. The principles underlying the clinical assessment of children in a clinical context are addressed in a preceding chapter (Rutter & Taylor, Chapter 2). The focus here is on the use of assessment methods within studies requiring the investigation of large samples of children seen in their natural home and school environments.

Some achievements of 40 years of epidemiological research in child psychiatry are reviewed briefly. Attention is paid to the design of surveys and to prevalence findings on global psychiatric morbidity (findings on specific disorders are discussed in other chapters). In the second section, key concerns are addressed regarding: the definition and assessment of child psychopathology in relation to the differentiation between normal and abnormal development; the use of dimensional or categorical approaches to case definition; the need to use impairment measures and to combine data from multiple informants; the need to take into account the high rates of comorbidity between disorders; and the implications of pervasiveness or situational specificity of behaviours in estimating rates and risk associations for psychiatric disorders. The third section addresses more specialized issues pertaining to psychometric theory and the measurement of performances of instruments; the assessment of special groups, such as young children or those from different cultural backgrounds; the use of computerized assessments and the development of clinical databases useful for clinical epidemiology.

Epidemiological investigations of child psychopathology

Conceptual/methodological issues

Child psychiatric epidemiology started in the mid-1960s with the British Isle of Wight surveys (Rutter *et al.* 1970, 1976). Prior to this landmark study, there had been few investigations of rates of psychopathology in general population samples. The survey by Lapouse & Monk (1958) is a notable exception. It emphasized the high prevalence of fears and worries and the discrepancies in rates of problems according to the informant. Most knowledge at the time relied on observations drawn from

clinical case series. Behaviours were interpreted and theoretical inferences were made without having a proper calibration system allowing a focus on those behaviours that discriminated best between children seen in clinics and non-referred children. Epidemiology, with its focus on general population samples and on comparisons between individuals with or without disorders, provided an obvious tool for the empirical investigation of child psychopathology.

The Isle of Wight surveys had key design characteristics that provided a model for surveys in the years after (Rutter 1989). A two-phase design was used with a systematic questionnaire screening of a large sample, followed by in-depth assessments administered in a subsample selected according to their positive and negative results at screening. Multiple informants were used at both phases, involving parents, teachers and children. The value of asking children direct questions was established and interviews subsequently replaced the old indirect techniques (projective tests and free play) as investigation tools. Questionnaires and diagnostic interviews of known reliability and validity were employed to gather data. Caseness was defined according to both a recognizable behavioural pattern and evidence of impairment in the child's functioning. The surveys also adopted longitudinal approaches to measure prospectively risk factors and chart the natural history of disorders, and behavioural measures were related to neurological and educational risk factors. These methodological advances have been developed further in the series of surveys conducted since.

The planning of epidemiological studies requires precise methods to ascertain 'cases' of the disorder under study (Verhulst & Koot 1995). This implies two related activities. First, a definition of 'caseness' must be adopted at the outset. Its nature should be shaped by the goals of the survey. A survey of autism to identify representative cases for inclusion in genetic studies will require detailed phenotypic assessments, precise diagnostic subtyping and exclusion of autistic syndromes associated with known medical disorders. If, on the other hand, the goal of the study is to generate estimates of special educational needs for service planning, then a less detailed and broader approach to 'caseness' such as the 'triad of impairments' (Wing & Gould 1979) may be sufficient. Following the adoption of the most appropriate concept of the disorder, decisions must be made about the choice of various assessment procedures and instruments. Guidelines to select instruments are provided in Appendix 1.

Secondly, once a case definition has been established, case

identification methods are selected. This involves sampling techniques that aim to provide a sample that will allow inferences about rates and correlates of disorders in the target population. Adequate sampling techniques are mandatory in order to provide unbiased estimates of the rates and the risk factors associated with disorders. The drawing of a sample requires the availability of a sampling frame and of sampling units covering the population of interest (Boyle 1995). In child psychiatry, surveys have often relied upon school rosters (Fombonne 1994) because, with compulsory education, they provide comprehensive sampling frames. Alternatively, households may be used as sampling units (Bird et al. 1988; Meltzer et al. 2000). These will still miss a small proportion of children, such as homeless or street children (Bird et al. 1988) or children from families who migrate seasonally for employment reasons. Children in long-term residential facilities may also be overlooked. The extent to which these sampling limitations will bias findings will depend on the strength of the association between a psychiatric disorder and these psychosocial circumstances.

Sampling techniques vary from simple random sampling to more complex stratified or cluster sampling strategies that aim to increase the precision of estimates, while optimizing survey resources and reducing costs. In selecting children for inclusion in the study sample, it is crucial to note the probability for each child to be selected, so that subsequently these probabilities can be used to weight the figures (usually with weights that are the inverse of the sampling fraction) for extrapolation to the target population. This allows oversampling of some subgroups without distortion of the final estimates provided that proper weights are devised and applied. The analysis of two-phase or more complex survey designs is discussed by Pickles (1998) and by Dunn et al. (1999).

Methods for dealing with missing data are crucial and have been addressed more efficiently in recent surveys. Survey participation rates have generally been high, often well over 80%. Bias in the estimates of prevalence and risk associations might result, nevertheless, if those who do not participate have higher rates of disorders, more severe disorders or disorders arising through different mechanisms. Empirical findings indicate that it should be expected that non-respondents will differ systematically from respondents (Cox et al. 1977). Fombonne (1994), in a French survey, found that behavioural disturbance was some 60% higher among non-participants than participants, but it was possible to correct for this bias in the final prevalence estimation. Similarly, attrition bias in longitudinal studies may attenuate predictions regarding the persistence of disorders over time (Boyle et al. 1991). However, it will be possible to correct for non-respondents' levels of psychopathology, when there are data on them either from records or from earlier points of data collection.

Missing data can also occur at the item level with respondents omitting items on a checklist or failing to answer all questions in an interview. This may jeopardize data collection (if incomplete screens are deemed ineligible for further interview) or analysis (if incomplete interviews are not dealt with separately). Sophis-

ticated statistical techniques are available to take account of missing data according to the reasons that they are missing (Kalton 1983; Little & Rubin 1987).

Findings from cross-sectional epidemiological surveys

Epidemiological surveys to assess prevalence usually rely on cross-sectional methods. Numerous prevalence surveys have now been conducted across the world (Brandenburg et al. 1990; Canino et al. 1995; Verhulst & Koot 1995; Bird 1996; Roberts et al. 1998). Table 4.1 presents the main results of some selected recent surveys. The rates for specific disorders are discussed in the chapters dealing with them. Some key findings from longitudinal investigations are noted in Rutter, Chapter 28; Rutter, Chapter 19; and Taylor & Rutter (Chapter 1).

The rates of disorder in Table 4.1 results underscore the most important finding, that psychopathology in young people is common, most studies estimating the prevalence to be between 10 and 20%. Verhulst & Koot (1995) reviewed 49 surveys and computed an average rate of 12.9%. Emotional disturbances and disorders of disruptive behaviour are equally common (with rates of 6–8%; see Table 4.1). It should be noted that many of these surveys will not have included neurodevelopmental disorders, such as autism, and may not have picked up psychotic disorders with an onset in late adolescence.

Community samples have also shown that only a small proportion (typically between 10 and 30%) of children with disorders have had contact with specialist mental health services. Thus, in the recent British nationwide survey of 10 000 5–15-year-olds (Meltzer et al. 2000), 27% of children with a psychiatric disorder had been in contact with specialist health care services and 30% had had no contact with any sort of professional. Similar figures have been reported in other studies (Offord et al. 1987; Costello & Janiszewski 1990; Zahner et al. 1992; Leaf et al. 1996). Disorders involving disruptive behaviour (Verhulst & Koot 1992; Meltzer et al. 2000), and those that are severe or of long duration (Whitaker et al. 1990), are more likely to be referred. However, contextual factors (such as parental psychopathology) and family features also influence referral (Jensen et al. 1990). The findings indicate the need for caution in extrapolating from clinical samples or experience. Children seen in clinics often differ in systematic ways from non-referred children with comparable levels of psychopathology. Epidemiological findings are needed for the development of psychopathological models.

Issues in case definition

Normality and disorder

All epidemiological surveys have shown the high frequency of individual items of emotional or behavioural difficulties (Rutter et al. 1970; Shepherd et al. 1971; Achenbach & Edelbrock

Table 4.1 Prevalence findings from recent epidemiological surveys.

Authors/year	Site	Age	N	Instruments/diagnosis	Period	Prevalence		
						Any emotional disorder	Any behavioural disorder	Any disorder
Vikan (1985)	North Trøndelag, Norway	10	1510	Isle of Wight interview/ICD-9	3 months	—	—	5.4
Anderson et al. (1987)	Dunedin, New Zealand	11	925	DISC-C/DSM-III	1 year	7.3	11.6	17.6
Offord et al. (1987)	Ontario, Canada	4–16	2679	Structured interview/DSM-III like	6 months	—	—	18.1
Bird et al. (1988)	Puerto Rico	4–16	777	DISC/DSM-III	6 months	—	—	17.9
Esser et al. (1990)	Mannheim, Germany	8	1444	Clinical interview/ICD-9	6 months	6.0	6.0	16.2
Morita et al. (1990)	Gunma prefecture, Japan	12–15	1999	Isle of Wight interview/ICD-9	3 months	—	—	15.0
Jeffers & Fitzgerald (1991)	Dublin, Ireland	9–12	2029	Isle of Wight interview/ICD-9	3 months	—	—	25.4
Fergusson et al. (1993)	Christchurch, New Zealand	15	986	DISC/DSM-III-R	—	—	—	22.1 [C] 13.0 [P]
Lewinsohn et al. (1993)	Oregon, USA	16–18	1710	K-SADS/DSM-III-R	Current	—	1.8	9.6
Fombonne (1994)	Chartres, France	6–11	2441	ICD-9/Isle of Wight module	3 months	5.9	6.5	12.4
Costello et al. (1996)	Great Smokey Mountains, North Carolina, USA	9,11,13	4500	CAPA/DSM-III-R	3 months	6.8	6.6	20.3
Verhulst et al. (1997)	Nationwide, the Netherlands	13–18	780	DISC C & P/DSM-III-R	6 months	—	7.9 [CorP] 0.9 [C & P]	35.5 [CorP] 4.0 [C & P]
Simonoff et al. (1997)	Virginia, USA	8–16	2762	CAPA/DSM-III-R	3 months	8.9	7.1	14.2
Steinhausen et al. (1998)	Zurich, Switzerland	7–16	1964	DISC-P/DSM-III-R	6 months	—	6.5	22.5
Breton et al. (1999)	Quebec, Canada	6–14	2400	Dominic-DISC2/DSM-III-R	6 months	—	—	19.9 [P] 15.8 [C]
Meltzer et al. (2000)	Nationwide, England and Wales	5–15	10438	DAWBA/ICD-10	3 months	4.3	5.8	9.5

C, based on child as informant; P, based on parent as informant.

1981). However, whereas some have a strong association with psychiatric disorders, others do not. Thus, in the Isle of Wight survey, thumb-sucking, nail-biting and bilious attacks all had very weak associations with psychiatric disorders (Rutter *et al.* 1970). Similarly, item scores for *asthma* and *allergy* have been removed from the computation of the total score of the Child Behaviour Checklist after consistent evidence that these were not associated with psychiatric referral. By contrast, the symptom of *depressed mood* has been shown to account for much of the variance in comparisons of matched samples of non-referred and referred children (Achenbach & Edelbrock 1981; Fombonne 1992).

However, continuities and discontinuities between individual symptoms and disorders may involve crucial transitions. Thus, depressed mood is experienced by about a third of adolescents in the general population (Petersen *et al.* 1993) but the rate of depressive disorder is only about 5% (see Harrington, Chapter 29). Similarly, some half of female adolescents diet but anorexia nervosa occurs in less than 1% (Fombonne 1995; see also Steinhausen, Chapter 34). The situation with substance use and abuse (see Rutter, Chapter 28; Weinberg *et al.*, Chapter 27) and with disruptive behaviour (see Earls & Mezzacappa, Chapter 26) is directly comparable. Many problem behaviours have a continuous distribution in the population and quantitative, rather than qualitative, deviance often defines psychopathology.

Categories and dimensions

Because of this, most epidemiological studies use a mixture of dimensional and categorical approaches. The former are needed both to assess symptom severity and to allow the adoption of different cut-offs for different purposes. The latter is required for clinical decision-making with respect to individual diagnosis and service planning (see Taylor & Rutter, Chapter 1). The issues are not specific to psychopathology; rather, they apply throughout most of medicine (as exemplified by asthma, hypertension, anaemia, diabetes and occlusive coronary artery disease—all of which have dimensional parallels). It is sometimes assumed that dimensional measures are synonymous with questionnaires and categorical ones with interview assessments, but that is not so. All standardized interviews (see Angold, Chapter 3) provide for various forms of quantification of severity or numbers of symptoms. Conversely, most questionnaires (see Verhulst & Van der Ende, Chapter 5) provide the means for deriving categories from dimensional scores.

The most appropriate choice of measure constitutes a crucial step in any epidemiological study (Table 4.2). Choice should be driven by the main purposes of the study. Questionnaires have all the advantages of economy and simplicity and may be the first preference if the goal involves only group differences and trends. They will almost always be used in the first screening phase of multistage studies. However, they are less suitable for individual diagnosis or for the assessment of uncommon disorders involving qualitative departures from normality. Standardized interviews have the opposite set of strengths and weaknesses. The chief decision issue with interviews is whether to use an investigator-based interview that obtains descriptions of behaviour that are rated using a standardized research-driven concept or a respondent-based approach that obtains yes/no answers to carefully structured questions. As Angold (Chapter 3) discusses, each has its own merits and researchers will need to consider carefully which is most likely to meet the needs for the particular investigation to be undertaken. A further decision is needed on whether to choose a broad-based measure designed to tap all the common varieties of psychopathology or rather to use one or more focused instruments. The former will meet most needs but is less suitable for uncommon or unusual disorders, such as autism, schizophrenia or Tourette syndrome. Whatever the particular choice of instrument, investigators will usually need to test their chosen set of measures and data collection procedures in pilot studies of adequately sized samples to determine the procedural feasibility and its acceptability by respondents. Pilot studies should be analysed carefully using quantitative methods whenever appropriate.

Impairment

The importance of including impaired functioning in case definition was well shown in Bird *et al.*'s (1988) general population epidemiological study. The prevalence of psychiatric disorder was 50% if assessed on the basis of symptoms alone, without taking account of impairment, but 18% if the latter was required for case definition (Bird *et al.* 1988). Similar results have been found in other studies (Bird *et al.* 1996; Simonoff *et al.* 1997).

The need to assess functional impairment is now generally accepted, but it has proved more difficult to define and measure it in a valid fashion. Impairment is related to concepts of role performance that reflect the individual's adaptation into his social environment (Bird 1999). This must be related to developmental level and sociocultural context. Typically, impairment resulting from psychopathology is assessed in four domains: interpersonal relationships; academic/work performance; social and leisure activities; and ability to enjoy and obtain satisfaction from life. These need to be evaluated with respect to functioning at home, school and in the community.

In earlier epidemiological surveys (Rutter *et al.* 1970), and in most classification schemes (World Health Organization 1992; American Psychiatric Association 1994), the assessment of impairment was largely left to a global clinical judgement by the interviewer. In the early 1980s, instruments were developed to address this issue with the development of the Children's Global Assessment Scale (Shaffer *et al.* 1983). This instrument was shown to have adequate psychometric properties but it still relied on an experienced clinician, and did not specify how impairment data should be obtained. Further developments of this scale led to a simplified non-clinician version (Bird *et al.* 1996; Bird 1999). Another instrument, the Columbia Impairment Scale (CIS; Bird *et al.* 1993), was devised to be completed by both parent and adolescent respondents; it has the advantage of being brief and providing scores for specific domains. Preliminary data suggest that it is a useful measure with the parent CIS having consistently better validity than the children's version. Other instruments, such as the Social Adjustment Inventory for Children and Adolescents (John *et al.* 1987) and the Child and Adolescent Functional Assessment Scale, were reviewed by Bird (1999).

The issues to be addressed still include: (i) the differentiation between impairment and psychiatric symptoms (for example, aggression to peers is both a symptom of conduct disorder and a reflection of impaired functioning with respect of peer relationships); (ii) how to determine causal connections between symptoms and impairment (preliminary findings suggest that informants found this difficult (Bird 1999) and interrater agreement was low (Sanford *et al.* 1992)); and (iii) the difference between impairment and symptom severity. Pickles *et al.* (2001) found that depressive symptoms predicted later depression equally well with and without the presence of impairment; by contrast, the predictive power of conduct symptoms was increased in the presence of impairment. Angold *et al.* (1999a) found, in a community study, that over a fifth of children showed impairment even though their number of symptoms fell below specified cut-offs for diagnosis. These impaired children with subthreshold disorders were likely later to be referred to services. Conversely, disorders without impairment tended to have a good outcome (Costello *et al.* 1999). The findings from the Ontario study tell much the same story (Sanford *et al.* 1992).

Diagnostic interviews now include separate measures of impairment associated with disorders and symptoms (Angold & Costello 2000; Shaffer *et al.* 2000; see also Angold, Chapter 3). However, research is still needed on the origins of impairment; it cannot be presupposed that they will necessarily be the same as for symptoms.

Age of onset

Age of onset is a definitional feature of several disorders. Enuresis cannot be diagnosed before the age of 5, attention deficit hyperactivity disorder (ADHD) symptoms must exist before age 7 and Asperger syndrome is differentiated from highfunctioning autism by the absence of a significant language delay by the age of 3. Age of onset is usually assessed retrospectively. However, the interrater and retest reliabilities of age of onset have been found to be poor outside the last 3 months for disorders with a recent onset and outside 1 year for those with a longer duration (Angold *et al.* 1996). Imperfect measurement of onset and offset of disorder can therefore influence prevalence estimates which are contingent upon specific time periods.

Age of onset also indexes differential outcomes. Moffitt (1993) found that conduct disorders with an adolescent onset differed from early-onset conduct problems, with the latter more likely to be associated with neuropsychological impairments and with a worse long-term outlook. Similarly, adolescent-onset depression is associated with a particularly strong risk of recurrence in adult life (Weissman *et al.* 1999a; Fombonne *et al.*, 2001) whereas the course and correlates of depression beginning before puberty is rather different (Harrington *et al.* 1997; Rende *et al.* 1997; Weissman *et al.* 1999b). The timing of onset is also crucial in order to explore the direction of causal effects in patterns of comorbidity (see Rutter, Chapter 28). The demonstration that ADHD is a risk factor for later conduct disorder, but that the reverse does not apply (Taylor *et al.* 1996; Taylor 1999), and that dysthymic disorder is a gateway to major depressive disorders (Kovacs *et al.* 1994), provide examples of this issue. Retrospective assessment of age of onset is also an issue in adult studies (Kessler *et al.* 1999), particularly as accurate assessment of this variable can influence results from familial studies (Schurhoff *et al.* 2000) and from studies of secular trends (Simon & Von Korff 1992). One way to avoid the problem of unreliability in the timing of onsets is to use lifetime prevalence estimates (Lewinsohn *et al.* 1993). These have the advantage of avoiding the problem of unreliability in the timing of onset and are probably the best approach for disorders present at the time of assessment. Doubts arise over the reliability and validity of reports of past disorders that are no longer present. Such doubts probably apply less to disorders in childhood than in adult life because time spans are shorter and because multiple instruments are available.

Comorbidity

The high frequency of co-occurrence of two supposedly separate forms of psychopathology was noted in the Isle of Wight studies over 30 years ago (Rutter *et al.* 1970). However, it is only in the last 15 years that it has received much conceptual attention and empirical study (Achenbach 1991a; Caron & Rutter 1991; Hinshaw *et al.* 1993; Nottelman & Jensen 1995; Rutter 1997; Angold *et al.* 1999b;). In their thorough review of the topic, Angold *et al.* (1999b) concluded that artefacts cannot account entirely for the frequency and patterns of comorbidity, and that mechanisms underlying comorbid presentations should be studied more systematically, preferably with epidemiological samples. The classification issues associated with comorbidity are discussed by Taylor & Rutter (Chapter 1) and the use of longitudinal data to study causal mechanisms is discussed by Rutter (Chapter 28) in relation to depression and substance abuse. Several research findings show how comorbidity may carry meaning. For example, the results of a family study of depression changed once comorbidity in the probands was properly taken into account (Merikangas *et al.* 1998) and a trend emerged for a positive drug response to tricyclic antidepressants in noncomorbid depressed subjects when results from a clinical trial were stratified according to the presence or absence of comorbid conduct disorder (Hughes *et al.* 1990).

However, in order to undertake research using comorbidity it is necessary that the epidemiological studies methods of measurement are adequate for dealing with the assessment of psychopathology that involves comorbid patterns.

Situation and multiple informant specificity

From the Isle of Wight studies onwards, it has been evident that the agreement on childhood psychopathology between different informants is typically low, and is only moderate at best. Thus, in an epidemiological survey of 6–11-year-olds, only a quarter of children scoring above the cut-off on at least one screening measure were scoring above threshold on both parent and teacher questionnaires (Fombonne 1994). In a meta-analysis of 119 studies, Achenbach et al. (1987) found that the agreement was best (≈0.60) when the pairs of informants had similar roles in relation to the child (such as with mother–father or teacher–teacher) whereas the mean correlation fell to the 0.20s for other types of pairs (such as parent–child or parent–teacher).

There are many possible reasons for this low agreement between informants. These include: random error in measurement; different perceptions of behaviour according to the perspective of the observer; different frames of reference; and variations in the child's behaviour according to both setting and interpersonal features. The relative importance of these different possibilities is not known. However, it is clear that multiple informants are essential for any adequate epidemiological study. That is partly because each informant contributes uniquely to the measurement of psychopathology, as well as contributing to shared variance; because when studying the correlates of disorder it is necessary to go across informants, or use composite ratings, in order to avoid halo effect artefacts; and because of the importance of differentiating between situation-specific and pervasive disorders (Schachar et al. 1981).

That leaves open the crucially important, but largely unresolved question of how to combine the data from different informants and from different settings. Although there is some evidence that different informants have different strengths, only rarely will it be desirable to adopt a hierarchical approach in which the report of one informant is automatically given precedence over those of others. Nevertheless, child self-reports are particularly important for the assessment of mood disturbances (see Harrington, Chapter 29). Conversely, they are of very limited use for the assessment of hyperactivity (see Angold, Chapter 3; Schachar & Tannock, Chapter 25). On the whole, teachers are better at the assessment of disruptive behaviour than they are of depressed mood. As the findings from Verhulst et al. (1997) show dramatically (see Table 4.1), prevalence findings are often hugely affected by how multiple ratings are dealt with.

Clinical interviewers usually use their 'best' judgement in order to weigh the symptoms endorsed by each informant, resolving discrepancies by personal rules derived from a combination of experience and theoretical predictions. This is likely to result in different clinicians combining data in different ways.

Another approach is trying to seek to resolve discrepancies between informants through a conjoint interview involving different informants (such as parent and child). This might be helpful in eliminating some errors brought about by miscomprehension and 'reconciling' the informants (Angold et al. 1999b). However, the method is far from free of problems, most especially in giving rise to delicate situations that threaten to broach confidentiality. Nevertheless, this judgement method is recommended for the use of some diagnostic interviews, such as the Kiddie Schedule for Affective Disorders and Schizophrenia (K-SADS; Ambrosini 2000), in order to allow the generation of a single unique score for each symptom rating.

A third commonly used approach uses computer generation of diagnoses based on predefined algorithms. The method has the advantage of accuracy and speed. However, the algorithms must deal with differences in reporting by informants according to specified rules. Usually, a symptom is counted as positive when it is reported by at least one informant: the so-called 'or' rule (Bird et al. 1992). This technique typically leads to high numbers of generated diagnoses.

For dimensional assessments, Achenbach (1991b) has revised the data collected through his set of questionnaires in order to solve this cross-informant problem. Based on systematic analyses of the Child Behaviour Checklist (CBCL), the Teacher Report Form (TRF) and the Youth Self Report (YSR), he identified common syndromes on each of these questionnaires, and core syndromes that appeared consistent across sex and age subgroups. He then selected a set of cross-informant core syndromes that spanned at least two instruments. These were subsequently scaled with the relevant normative sample. This approach does not resolve the problem of how to combine data from discrepant informants but it helps in increasing the interpretability of a profile of scores for a given child (Achenbach 1991b, 1995). More sophisticated statistical techniques are available to researchers to deal with the measurement problems associated with multiple data sources and discrepancies between informants (see below).

Measurement

At the core of medicine, and of any scientific enquiry, is measurement theory (see also Sergeant & Taylor, Chapter 6). In essence, this specifies the relationship between a conceptual construct and empirical measures. With respect to psychopathology, the construct cannot be directly observed, as through a pathognomonic test. There is a good deal of evidence for some of the key psychiatric diagnostic concepts, such as autism or schizophrenia (see Taylor & Rutter, Chapter 1). Nevertheless, there has to be an empirical means of going from observables (whether those be signs or symptoms), to the postulated diagnostic entity. Child psychiatry research has progressed tremendously in that direction over the last two decades. Far from being a question mattering uniquely to researchers, the same measurement considerations and needs apply to everyday clinical practice. In that sense, the choice is not between measuring or not (or between research and clinical practice), but rather between measuring with known and replicable procedures or not.

Concepts of validity and reliability

Two major properties, validity and reliability, are examined in the evaluation of assessment procedures (instruments or simple clinical judgement) for which Fig. 4.1 provides a convenient representation. Data collected as part of clinical or research assessments can be seen as empirical indicators of the underlying (unobserved) constructs of interest.

Reliability is the tendency of measures to yield consistent results over repeated trials. Reliability concerns the replicability of measures and the extent to which each measurement is affected by random error. Reliability can therefore be examined empirically (see bottom level on Fig. 4.1). Typical procedures to estimate reliability are the test–retest paradigm, interrater agreement, and techniques based on correlations between subsets of instruments (split-half reliability) or among items composing a questionnaire (internal consistency). The reliability of the measurement is assessed within each procedure by specific statistics, such as the kappa coefficient for categorical measurements (Spitzer & Fleiss 1974), the intraclass correlation coefficient for quantitative scores (Bartko 1976) and other statistics (e.g. Cronbach's (1951) alpha coefficient). Reliability is a necessary condition, but not a sufficient one, for validity. If empirical indicators are unduly contaminated by random error (so that measurements cannot be replicated), then the question of their relationship to the constructs that they are purported to tap cannot be assessed meaningfully. On the other hand, high replicability does not necessarily mean good validity.

Validity concerns the crucially important relationship between the empirical observables and the postulated latent construct (in this case diagnosis) as represented by the connections between the bottom and top levels on Fig. 4.1. Several types of validity have been described. *Content* validity is concerned with the extent to which an instrument is representative of the universe of indices that are related to the concept measured. It is usually assessed by reliance on experts or on agreement with established instruments tapping the same concept. *Criterion-related* validity is the most empirical form of validity. It allows

an index to be compared to an independent external criterion thought to assess the same concept. This can be either *concurrent* or *predictive*.

Construct validity is the most elusive and theoretical type of validity. It concerns the extent to which individual items or measures intercorrelate or group together to produce derived higher order constructs. Factor analysis has often been used for this purpose in the field of psychopathology. Thus, numerous factor analyses of questionnaires have consistently identified separate dimensions (or constructs) of psychopathology (such as attention problems, conduct symptoms or emotional disturbances). These tend to map onto a broad bipartite division into internalizing/emotional problems and externalizing/disruptive behaviours (Achenbach & Edelbrock 1978; Elander & Rutter 1995). Consistency of these factor analyses results has been taken as evidence of the construct validity of these psychopathology dimensions.

Diagnostic reliability

Since the first collaborative efforts sponsored by the World Health Organization to improve diagnosis in psychiatry, reliability studies have been undertaken to examine interrater agreement and to improve the definition, and thereby the diagnostic reproductibility of disorders (Rutter *et al.* 1969, 1975). In the late 1970s, with the development of research diagnostic criteria (Spitzer *et al.* 1978) and of standardized diagnostic interviews, emphasis was placed on the development of operational diagnostic criteria. This was embodied in the DSM-III (American Psychiatric Association 1980) and its successors and in the clinical and research versions of ICD-10 (World Health Organization 1992, 1993). Studies of the reliability of child psychiatric diagnoses have been conducted with various schemes and instruments, giving rise to broadly similar overall conclusions (Rutter *et al.* 1988; Shaffer *et al.* 1999).

The concept of reliability involves three rather different potential sources of error or variability: *information* variation (features to do with how data are collected); *interpretation* variance (how data are weighted and put together); and *criterion* variance (how algorithms are used to produce diagnoses). These need to be assessed in different ways. The first may be examined through test–retest studies to examine the extent to which the same answers are obtained on two consecutive occasions. On the whole, the findings have been of moderate to good reliability that is higher for symptom dimensions than for categorical diagnoses (Shaffer *et al.* 1999). It is affected, however, by the tendency for informants to report less psychopathology on the second occasion (Piacentini *et al.* 1999; Shaffer *et al.* 1999). This is more pronounced with highly structured interviews but can be reduced somewhat by attention to details of wording of questions and interview organization (Lucas *et al.* 1999).

Interpretation variance can be assessed by determining the extent to which two informants agree (see above), or two investigators agree on their ratings of behavioural descriptions (Strober *et al.* 1981; Werry *et al.* 1983; Gould *et al.* 1988; Pren-

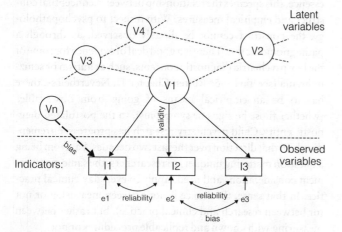

Fig. 4.1 Measurement model.

dergast *et al.* 1988), or two different diagnostic instruments give the same answer. Typically, this form of variance is greater — particularly across informants and across instruments.

Criterion variance needs to be evaluated by comparing different ways of putting the data together. Standardization aims to keep this to a minimum but it is clear that different systems often give different answers (see, for example, the findings with respect to age of onset in ADHD (Applegate *et al.* 1997), number of symptoms in antisocial diagnoses (Lahey *et al.* 1994) or diagnostic algorithms in autism (Volkmar *et al.* 1994)).

Diagnostic validity

Diagnostic validity concerns the extent to which a diagnostic construct truly reflects a syndrome that is different from others. The testing of validity therefore requires research that examines correlates of diagnosis with respect to basic features that are external to the behaviours that define the hypothesized diagnostic construct (Rutter 1978). Such correlates might include genetic influences, neuropathology, biological indices, course and response to specific treatments. The evidence on such validity is discussed by Taylor & Rutter (Chapter 1).

From a measurement perspective, validity concerns the extent to which empirical measures tap the crucial features that provide the basis of the diagnostic construct: the vertical connections between the top level (the latent construct) and the bottom level (empirical measures) in Fig. 4.1. The main measurement issue concerns the possible operation of biases in those vertical connections (expressed as Vn in Fig. 4.1).

The main, possibly biasing factor considered up to now has been the mental state of the informant. Thus, there has been concern that a depressed mother might over-report psychopathology in her child (Brewin *et al.* 1993). To test that possibility it is necessary to determine whether maternal depression alters the pattern of associations between maternal reports of child psychopathology and teacher or child reports (Chilcoat & Breslau 1997). The key statistic here relates to pattern differences and not to correlations as such. Thus, with respect to maternal depression the issue is whether a difference in child psychopathology is found on maternal reports that is not evident on reports from others. If there is, a bias is suggested. The weight of evidence from a range of studies indicates that there is some biasing effect, although not a great one. Recently, attention has broadened to consider whether depression in one parent alters the rating of the *other* parent by virtue of its influence on the overall family context (Borge *et al.*, 2001). Preliminary findings suggest that possibly it may, although further research is needed to investigate the matter. A comparable rating bias concern was raised with respect to possible *contrast* effects in parental ratings of twins. Thus, it was hypothesized that parents, in their ratings, might exaggerate differences between dizygotic (non-identical) twins. Again, the test involves pattern effects in relation to the others. Such contrast effect biases have been found with respect to parental ratings of hyperactivity but, interestingly, not of other forms of disruptive behaviour (Simonoff *et al.* 1998).

Other examples of such possible rating biases concern the effects of a person's current social situation and mental state on their retrospective rating of negative childhood experiences (Maughan & Rutter 1997). Findings suggest that there is a slight tendency for people who are doing well to *under*-report past adversities but no tendency for people who are doing well to *over*-report. Obviously, to test this possibility, it is necessary to have longitudinal data involving contemporaneous measurement of the adverse experiences. Yet another example concerns the possibility that people with a mental disorder may over-report comparable disorders in relatives (Kendler *et al.* 1991; Rende & Weissman 1999). In all these examples the tests have involved some form of pattern difference that involves comparisons among different informants. Usually, the biases found have been small, but equally they have not been zero. The implication is that investigators need to use multiple informants and need to test for such possible biases, statistically correcting for them when required.

Latent variable models

Historically, researchers tended to deal with these measurement problems either by choosing what seemed to be the 'best' informant or alternatively by combining the ratings in some way (such as by adding them together or counting a report of a behaviour if it comes from just one of a number of informants). Such composite strategies have the advantage of simplicity and, for this reason, they continue to have a worthwhile place in research. However, they fail to make use of all the data, they do not deal quantitatively with possible biases, and they do not remove random measurement error. Latent variable models were developed to deal with these issues (see Fergusson 1995, 1997 for clear descriptions of the rationale and the assumptions involved). In brief, multivariate statistics are used to *infer* the latent construct (which can be either dimensional or categorical) that underlies the associations among a variety of behavioural measures. The focus is on the variance that is *shared* across measures — in effect putting to one side that which is unique to just one measure on the ground that, whatever its intrinsic importance, it is not measuring that which is common across measures. This 'special' element is not 'thrown away' but, rather, it can be isolated and examined in its own right.

Latent variable methods have another key feature: they take into account prior probabilities. For example, let us take a child in a longitudinal study who has three positive ratings, one negative, and then two more positive ones and compare him with a child who has six negative ratings. Intuition and common sense tells one that the fourth rating of the first child is much more likely to be a false negative than the fourth rating of the second child. In coming to that judgement, we use what we know about the findings at other data points. Latent variable methods do the same but in a quantitative mathematical fashion. Although certainly not a 'cure-all' for measurement problems, latent variable methods have very considerable strengths and are likely to be employed more in the future. The main 'health warnings' regarding their use is that there should be caution if the shared variance among measures is very low (because the latent construct will tap so little of the individual differences in the psychopathology of interest; see Simonoff *et al.* 1998 for an example), and that there needs to be an awareness that modelling methods will sometimes discard features because their effects fall short of statistical significance, even though the evidence limits tell one that there might be a substantial true effect (see Rutter *et al.* 1999, 2001 for a discussion of the matter in relation to genetic modelling).

Applications of latent construct measures in child psychiatry include studies of the impact of maternal depression on ratings of child psychopathology (Boyle & Pickles 1997a,b), the cross-informant correlations of behavioural reports (Fergusson & Horwood 1987a,b), or the adult outcomes of antisocial behaviour (Zoccolillo *et al.* 1992).

Cut-offs, sensitivity and specificity

Dimensional measurements (whether by questionnaire or interview) lead to total scores ranging from a minimum (usually implying normality) to a maximum (mostly implying psychopathology). For both clinical and research reasons, investigators may want to transform these scores into categories (e.g. inferred normality vs. inferred disorder). Note that the category has to be inferred, rather than measured directly (unless of course there is a pathognomonic test, which there is not so far for any child psychiatric disorder). The measurement question concerns the probability that any given score on a measure means that the psychopathology warrants a 'caseness' designation—in other words, what score provides the best discrimination between cases and non-cases as assessed in some other way. All cut-offs, of course, result in some degree of misclassification. Figure 4.2 depicts a fairly common situation in which scores among normals (non-cases) are plotted next to those with a disorder (cases). Any cut-off will partition a sample into four groups, designated false and true positives and false and true negatives. Various indices can be used to summarize the data in this situation (see Appendix 1). A Receiving Operating Characteristics (ROC)

analysis provides a convenient way of assessing this trade off mathematically in order to select an optimal threshold (Fombonne 1991; see also Verhulst & Van der Ende, Chapter 5). It simply plots sensitivity on one axis of a graph and specificity on the other and uses the resulting curve to identify the best cut-point. However, it does more in that it takes into account the prevalence of the disorder, the severity of cases under detection, and the consequences of all types of misclassification errors (Hsiao *et al.* 1989; Fombonne 1991).

ROC analyses have been a huge help in decision-making with respect to using scores to infer categories. However, two points require emphasis. First, measurement error is the rule rather than the exception and its influence must always be recognized in any interpretation of data. Scores above a cut-off point that has been empirically set by ROC analyses do not mean that a disorder is definitely present. All they indicate is that, using the particular measures in question, the probability of a good differentiation between caseness and normality is optimal; but it is a probability and not a certainty. A mechanical use of instruments to provide diagnoses should be proscribed.

Secondly, the various properties of sensitivity, specificity, positive predictive value and so forth (see Appendix 2) are context-specific and *not* inherent qualities of the instrument. A cut-off that works well in a clinical context may not be at all satisfactory in a community survey. That is because probabilities are greatly influenced by population base rates for the disorder being measured. For example, Berument *et al.* (1999), in their analysis of the Autism Screening Questionnaire (ASQ) found that the score that best differentiated autism from other spectrum disorders was much higher than that which was best differentiating autism from uncomplicated mental retardation or developmental language disorders. Some instruments are much more valid than others and attention needs to be paid to their technical properties. Nevertheless, the measuring device has no absolute intrinsic validity. Rather, its validity will fluctuate according to the goals and context of the assessment.

Norms

Reference to normative data is implicit in the assessment of psychopathology. However, it was only in the late 1950s that systematic surveys of children's behaviours and emotions were undertaken on large samples of non-referred children (Lapouse & Monk 1958, 1959). The epidemiological surveys of child psychiatric disorders that followed helped to promote knowledge of normative behaviour at different ages with the useful development of standardized questionnaires for use with multiple informants (Rutter *et al.* 1970; Achenbach & Edelbrock 1981; Verhulst & Koot 1995; see also Verhulst & Van der Ende, Chapter 5). Increasingly, data from large representative samples of non-referred children have been used to calibrate measures in order to provide the best identification of probably psychopathology. Verhulst & Van der Ende (Chapter 5) summarize both the research approaches and the findings for a range of measures. Much has been achieved, yet some care is needed in

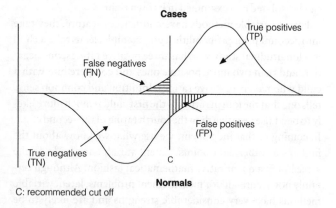

C: recommended cut off

Fig. 4.2 Distribution of scores in normals and cases.

using these norm-referenced assessments. Not all standardizations have used fully representative general population samples. There must be reservations about generalizability when convenience samples have been used.

Norms are derived from particular regional or national samples and the query is whether it is justifiable to extrapolate to other regions or countries. For example, a 10–15-point difference in mean CBCL total scores has been reported among American, Australian (Achenbach *et al.* 1990a), French (Stanger *et al.* 1994) and Puerto Rican children (Achenbach *et al.* 1990b). The question is whether these differences reflect true regional differences in psychopathology or rating tendencies that have been influenced by cultural contextual features. Both possibilities have to be considered seriously but their differentiating requires the use of external validators of some kind. The Isle of Wight–Inner London comparison indicated that a true difference in rate of psychopathology was likely (Rutter & Quinton 1977) whereas the UK–Hong Kong comparison with respect to hyperactivity suggested a rating difference effect (Leung *et al.* 1996). Investigators are well advised to be cautious about assumptions that one set of norms can be generalized to different populations.

Similar issues concern extrapolations from one large representative population to subgroups within. For example, are associations between social class and behavioural disturbance (Achenbach & Edelbrock 1981; Fombonne 1992) a true reflection of valid differences or a contextual rating bias effect? The same applies to age and gender differences. An automatic assumption that subgroup norms should be used or that any differences from total population norms are necessarily valid should be resisted. As ever, external validation is essential.

Norms apply to one particular point in time. Evidence has accumulated that there have been secular changes in the incidence of various psychosocial disorders (Rutter & Smith 1995; Fombonne 1998a,b) and of individual behavioural problems. Achenbach & Howell (1993) compared two large representative samples of American youth surveyed 13 years apart and found increased scores on 46 of 118 behavioural problems and on all scale scores (the mean total score increasing from 18 to 24.2) in the most recent birth cohorts. Periodic recalibration of instruments is necessary in child psychopathology just as it is for other measures, such as psychometric tests (Flynn 1987; Fuggle *et al.* 1992) or physical indices such height, weight, head circumference and pubertal maturation (Fredriks *et al.* 2000).

Assessment of young children

Epidemiological investigations of preschool samples have been surprisingly few (Earls 1980; Richman *et al.* 1982; Pianta & Castaldi 1989; Pianta & Caldwell 1990; Cohen & Bromet 1992; van den Oord *et al.* 1995; Lavigne *et al.* 1996). Nevertheless, studies have shown that psychiatric disorders starting in the preschool years show a high degree of persistence over time and that their course is systematically associated with identifiable risk and protective factors. For example, a difficult tempera-

ment in the child interacts with characteristics of family dysfunction to increase the risk of psychopathology 5 years later (Maziade *et al.* 1987); and a shy inhibited style of interaction predicts later onset of anxiety disorders in childhood (Kagan *et al.* 1998). Evidence has accumulated that developmental disorders usually identified in the early years have short (Stevenson *et al.* 1985) and long-term consequences (Mawhood *et al.* 2000) with respect to psychosocial disturbances and functioning. Long-term follow-up of birth cohorts have also shown continuities between preschool behaviour and adult psychopathology (Caspi *et al.* 1996). Thus, identification of preschool problems is important, especially because early intervention might be more effective in the case of some disorders (Rogers 1998).

However, there are particular challenges in the assessment of preschool-age children (Mayes 1999). Infants and toddlers present with disturbances that tend to be closely associated with somatic development. Thus, feeding and sleeping difficulties are common in this age group (see Stein & Barnes, Chapter 45). It is also an age when the effects of prenatal/perinatal risk factors may be particularly marked. As implied in Winnicott's (1965) remark that 'there is no such thing as a baby', infants' behaviour is closely intertwined with interactions with their caregivers. Accordingly, it is necessary to consider the extent to which any disturbance reflects psychopathology in the child rather than difficulties in a dyadic relationship (see O'Connor, Chapter 46). Specific developmental delays, such as language or social relationship, are first evident in the preschool years and call for a multifaceted developmental assessment (see Bishop, Chapter 39; Lord & Bailey, Chapter 38). The American Academy of Child and Adolescent Psychiatry (1997) has issued guidelines on standards of practice for the assessment of infants and toddlers. Very few dimensional measures assessing behavioural/emotional deviance have been properly validated for children below the age of 4. Current diagnostic schemes have acknowledged limitations for use with very young children (Emde *et al.* 1993). Scales such as the Temperament and Atypical Behaviour Scale (TABS; Bagnato *et al.* 1999) and classifications such as the Zero to Three Diagnostic Classification (Zero to Three 1994) have been developed for infants and toddlers but they are based on particular conceptual frameworks and are closely linked to intervention strategies. The value of these measures and systems remains to be established.

Cultural and ethnic minorities issues

Most industrialized societies today are multicultural, multiethnic and multilingual, which has important implications for clinical practice (see Rutter & Nikapota, Chapter 16; Rutter & Taylor, Chapter 2). It also has implications for the assessment of psychopathology by means of standardized interviews or questionnaires, as noted a quarter of a century ago by Warwick & Lininger (1975). It would be a mistake to exaggerate the methodological difficulties. Rating scales have usually been found to function in much the same way across cultures (Verhulst & Achenbach 1995; Weisz & Eastman 1995; Crijnen *et al.*

1999) with, for example, comparable gender differences (Achenbach *et al.* 1990a; Stanger *et al.* 1994; Crijnen *et al.* 1999).

Nevertheless, three issues require attention. First, there is a concern to ensure linguistic equivalence (see Verhulst & Van der Ende, Chapter 5). This is usually accomplished by a series of back-translations from one language to the other by independent bilingual translators who are familiar with the psychopathological concepts. The last specification is important to ensure that the appropriate words are selected to tap the intended meaning. This is relevant, too, in relation to the need to ensure equivalence between American and British versions of instruments. The problem does not mainly lie in there being different words for the same thing in the two countries; most people are aware of these. The main hazard is provided by words that are the same but have a different meaning in the two countries. For example, 'quite' adds emphasis in the USA, but usually reduces emphasis in the UK, although in certain contexts the reverse applies. The problem of moving across languages is even greater and it is crucial that the translators appreciate the intended meaning in relation to psychopathology. Issues in relation to the translation of diagnostic interviews for Hispanics were described by Canino & Bravo (1999) and examples of translation inaccuracies and of their effects on deviance scores were noted by Woodward *et al.* (1989).

Secondly, there is the question of conceptual and perceptual equivalence. Thus, Weisz *et al.* (1988) reported differences between Thai and American adults in their concern over particular behaviours; Lee (1991) queried whether a morbid fear of fatness had the same implications for anorexia nervosa in Hong Kong as it does in Western societies; and King & Bhugra (1989) posed the same question with respect to questions on dieting when used in cultures where this is part of religious practice. It cannot be claimed that there is an adequate database to show either the importance of these concerns or how they are best dealt with, but investigators need to be alert to their possible effects on measurement. They are likely to have effects because most ratings involve an explicit or implicit comparison with some norms, the behaviours being normal at a low level but abnormal at some higher level.

Thirdly, there is diagnostic equivalence. As Taylor & Rutter (Chapter 1) note, some cultures have syndromes that appear to have no obvious equivalent in other cultures, although systematic evidence on this is largely lacking. From a measurement perspective, perhaps the key point is that when different cultures express the same disorder through differently expressed manifestations, there needs to be caution in the application of diagnostic algorithms. For example, there is evidence that cultures vary in the extent to which they express depression in reports of feelings of misery; some are more likely to report these in terms of somatic complaints (Kleinman & Good 1985). Similar issues arise with respect to age variations, as reflected in the different role given to irritability in the diagnosis of depression in childhood and in adult life (American Psychiatric Association 1994). Once more, there is at least as much of a danger of wrongly assuming an age (or cultural) difference as of overlooking a real difference. The arbitration has to lie in empirical studies, most of which are still waiting to be undertaken.

Computerized assessments

Modern technology has allowed many assessment procedures to be computerized. For example, Berg *et al.* (1992) compared the reliability, concurrent and criterion validity of two standard and computer-assisted procedures to collect data using two common psychopathology scales, the Rutter A2 scale and the CBCL. Psychometric properties were similar with the two procedures, suggesting that computer-assisted technologies might be used more extensively in routine practice.

There are numerous advantages to computerization: it eliminates observer bias; it ensures that all respondents receive precisely the same instructions and questions; by having a voice read aloud the questions it avoids illiteracy problems; it allows more complex and flexible skip and branching patterns than possible with paper-and-pencil procedures; immediate checking of the consistency and range of responses is possible; and it provides error-free computation of scores with or without reference to existing norms. Data are readily stored in a format that allows for further analysis and computer storage also makes the data collection procedure less vulnerable to errors such as accidental loss of data, theft, or inadvertent disclosure of confidential materials.

Several structured diagnostic interviews already have computerized versions. The role of the computer does, however, vary considerably. Computers are sometimes used to assist interviewers in their task of conducting the interview. In this instance, the interviewer still performs a face-to-face interview and records the answers of the respondent on a (usually laptop) computer as the interview proceeds. This procedure has both the advantage and disadvantage of allowing some degree of interviewer judgement. Fully computerized diagnostic interviews tend to be highly structured, with restricted response options. Computer-aided administration is particularly useful in helping the interviewer to follow complex skip rules and to track respondent's answers that require follow-up questions in the course of the interview. The Diagnostic Interview Schedule for Children (NIMH DISC-IV; Shaffer *et al.* 2000) is typical of such interviews devised for large-scale epidemiological surveys. The Development and Well-Being Assessment (DAWBA; Goodman *et al.* 2000), used in the UK National Survey of Child Mental Health (Meltzer *et al.* 2000) provides another example, with the additional feature that space is allocated to record respondents' descriptions verbatim as well, so allowing a subsequent overarching clinical interpretation of all structured data and the addition of open-ended commentaries. However, this procedure detracts somewhat from the greater efficiency of the computerized interviews—a major 'selling' point. In other developments, computers are used to replace interviewers fully. Some sound versions of diagnostic interviews have now been developed for full self-administration, using headphones or speakers. The Voice DISC

Appendix 1 Selecting an instrument.

	Interview	Questionnaire
Purpose	Screening/diagnosis	Screening/assessment
Main use	Epidemiological/clinical	Epidemiological/clinical
Reliability	Test–retest	Test–retest
	Interrater	Split-half, internal consistency
Validity	Content, discriminant, concurrent, predictive	Content, discriminant, concurrent, predictive
	Cross-cultural	Factorial/construct validity Cross-cultural
Coverage/content	Diagnostic categories	Psychopathological constructs
	Number of disorders	Number of items
Method	Face-to-face interview	Self-report (usually) or other informant (parent, teacher, clinician)
Response format	Yes/No (respondent-based)	Interval
		Likert scaling
	All informants' descriptions (investigator-based)	Visual analogue
Completion time	Long (hours)	Brief (minutes)
Informant	Subject	Subject (over 10 years)
	Parent	Parent, teacher
	Other	Clinician, interviewer, other
Time frame	Current (last 3 or 6 months)	Current, last week
	Last year	Last 3–12 months
	Lifetime	
Age assessed	Depends on informant and content	Depends on informant and content
Training	Required:	None (self-administered) or minimal
	detailed for investigator-based	(interviewer-assisted)
	limited for respondent-based	
	Availability of training packages	Literacy requirement
	Availability of manual	Availability of manual
Version	Paper-and-pencil	Paper-and-pencil
	Computer-assisted	Computer administered
	Computer administered	
Data entry	Laborious (unless computerized)	Easy (optical forms)
Scoring	Diagnostic algorithms	Norms, centiles, cut-offs
Costs	High	Low
Repeat assessments	Modularity of the interview	Easy, demonstrated sensitivity to change
	Scale scores available	
Extra features		
Other domains	Personal and family details, impairment, burden, etc.	Personal and family details, scholastic achievement, etc.
Suitability for longitudinal studies	Adult diagnostic interviews	Parallel adult forms
Observational assessments	Companion observational schedule	Parallel observational scale
Cultural context	Availability in other languages	Availability in other languages
	Validity in different populations	Validity in different populations

(Shaffer *et al.* 2000) and a substance abuse module of the Child and Adolescent Psychiatric Assessment (CAPA; Angold & Costello 2000) are examples of such developments, which totally eliminate interviewer costs.

Investigator-based interviews have been, for obvious reasons, less amenable to computerization, although some attempts have been made, such as with the Diagnostic Interview Schedule for Children and Adolescents (DICA; Reich 2000). One diagnostic interview relying on displays of pictures or cartoons to elicit symptomatic data has been released in computerized form

(Interactive Dominic Questionnaire; Valla *et al.* 2000) but data are still needed on its basic properties.

Computerized interviewing does not usually decrease the time needed to administer the interview, but it can lead to substantial savings in terms of interviewer time (and costs) by eliminating that used for coding and interpretation. Successful use has been achieved in recent epidemiological surveys (Patton *et al.* 1999; Meltzer *et al.* 2000).

It is possible, too, that computerized interviews may be better at eliciting potentially embarrassing personal information because it eliminates the interpersonal context. Reich *et al.* (1995) found that children enjoyed the computerized DICA-R interview, preferring it over a personal interview and said that they would tell things to the computer that they would not tell to a person. Survey research has shown that rates of at-risk behaviours involving sexual contacts and use of addictive substances were three times higher when questions were asked via audio-computerized methods than when asked face-to-face (Turner *et al.* 1998). Similar results have been found regarding suicidal behaviours (Reich *et al.* 1995).

It is too early to draw firm conclusions on the merits and demerits of computerized interviews. Clearly, they have very important advantages for some purposes and there is no doubt that they will be used more in the future. However, for some purposes their chief advantage of eliminating the need for interviewers may be a disadvantage just because it eliminates personal contact. The structural format, too, will be limiting in relation to the eliciting of important unexpected information (see Rutter & Taylor, Chapter 2).

Multiaxial systems and recording clinical data

Epidemiological investigations have contributed much to our knowledge and the use of standardized methods has played an important role in ensuring their success, as has attention to the measurement and sampling issues discussed in this chapter. However, many of the same principles also apply to databases used for clinical monitoring and clinical research (World Health Organization 1996). A good example of such a clinical data recording system is the Item Sheet that has been in place at the Maudsley Hospital for over half a century and which records diagnoses, symptoms, demographic details, psychosocial features, test findings, details of referral and rating of clinical outcome. As a result, a large computerized database has been available to facilitate clinical research. Examples of its use are the study of specific problem behaviours (Thorley 1987; Wannan & Fombonne 1998; Moore & Fombonne 1999); the sampling of subjects for long-term follow-up studies (Harrington *et al.* 1990; Fombonne *et al.*, 2001); patient comparisons between centres in different countries (Duyx & van Engeland 1993); the investigation of trends over time in specific behavioural problems and of their causes (Fombonne 1998a); and the study of comorbid patterns (Simic & Fombonne, 2001). More streamlined data recording systems could easily achieve the same goals if a core set of variables was defined. Also, centres could decide to add on, for specific groups of patients of interest, or for defined periods of time, more exhaustive data recording procedures, because databases can easily be managed on modularity principles. Progress in information technology has made it easy and cheap to set up such databases and to exchange data when appropriate. Indeed, the need to audit services and to be accountable of services activity for the health service will make such systems increasingly mandatory in most countries. Timely recognition of these needs and of the usefulness of these databases will help mental health professionals to influence these information systems in a way that might be more clinically relevant and useful for their own research and practice.

Appendix 2

Hypothetical data from a screening study.

	Cases D	Normal $\bar{D}$	
Test positive (T+)	a	b	a+b
Test negative (T–)	c	d	c+d
	a+c	b+d	a+b+c+d=N

D, diseased; $\bar{D}$, non-diseased.
True positives, TP=a; True negatives, TN=d; False negatives, FN=c; False positives, FP=b.
Sensitivity (or rate of true positives, RTP): Se=a/a+c=p (T+/D).
Specificity (or rate of true negatives, RTN): Sp=d/b+d=p (T–/$\bar{D}$).
Rate of false negatives: RFN=c/a+c=p (T–/D).
Rate of false positives: RFP=b/b+d=p (T+/$\bar{D}$).
Prevalence: P=a+c/N=p(D).
Positive predictive value: PPV=a/a+b=p(D/T+).
Negative predictive value: NPV=d/c+d=p($\bar{D}$/T–).

This table provides the results of a hypothetical screening study (see also Fig. 4.2). Several proportions are used to summarize the data: sensitivity (proportion of cases above the threshold); and specificity (proportion of non-cases below the threshold). These two proportions can be regarded as indices of the criterion of validity of the instrument. Both proportions vary inversely and changes in the proposed cut-off to improve sensitivity would normally result in decreased specificity, and vice versa.

Another proportion of importance is the positive predictive value which expresses the probability that a subject with a positive screening has a disorder. The proportion varies as a function of the sensitivity and the specificity of the instrument, but also with the prevalence of the disease in the population:

$$PPV = (P \times Se) / (P \times Se) + [(1-P) + (1-Sp)].$$

It can be shown that the PPV associated with an excellent instrument (sensitivity = specificity = 90%) is very good (79%) if the prevalence of the disorder is high (P=0.3), but poor (8%) when the prevalence falls to a low value of 1%. This reminds us that intrinsically good instruments might have poor performances, depending on the context of their use.

References

Achenbach, T. (1991a) 'Comorbidity' in child and adolescent psychiatry: categorical and quantitative perspectives. *Journal of Child and Adolescent Psychopharmacology*, 1, 271–278.

Achenbach, T.M. (1991b) *Integrative Guide for the 1991 CBCL/4–18, YSR and TRF Profiles*. Department of Psychiatry, University of Vermont, Burlington, VT.

Achenbach, T.M. (1995) Diagnosis, assessment, and comorbidity in psychosocial treatment research. *Journal of Abnormal Child Psychology*, **23**, 45–65.

Achenbach, T.M. & Edelbrock, C.S. (1978) The classification of child psychopathology: a review and analysis of empirical efforts. *Psychological Bulletin*, **85**, 1275–1301.

Achenbach, T.M. & Edelbrock, C.S. (1981) Behavioral problems and competencies reported by parents of normal and disturbed children aged 4 through 16. *Monographs of the Society for Research in Child Development*, **46**, 1–82.

Achenbach, T.M. & Howell, C.T. (1993) Are American children's problems getting worse? A 13-year comparison. *Journal of the American Academy of Child and Adolescent Psychiatry*, **32**, 1145–1154.

Achenbach, T., McConaughy, S. & Howell, C. (1987) Child–adolescent behavioral and emotional problems: implications of cross-informant correlations for situation specificity. *Psychological Bulletin*, **101**, 213–232.

Achenbach, T.M., Hensley, V.R., Phares, V. & Grayson, D. (1990a) Problems and competencies reported by parents of Australian and American children. *Journal of Child Psychology and Psychiatry*, **31**, 265–286.

Achenbach, T.M., Bird, H.R., Canino, G., Phares, V., Gould, M.S. & Rubio-Stipec, M. (1990b) Epidemiological comparisons of Puerto Rican and US mainland children: parent, teacher, and self-reports. *Journal of the American Academy of Child and Adolescent Psychiatry*, **29**, 84–93.

Ambrosini, P. (2000) The historical development and present status of the Schedule for Affective Disorders and Schizophrenia for School-Aged Children (K-SADS). *Journal of the American Academy of Child and Adolescent Psychiatry*, **39**, 49–58.

American Academy of Child and Adolescent Psychiatry (1997) Practice parameters for the psychiatric assessment of infants and toddlers (0–36 months). *Journal of the American Academy of Child and Adolescent Psychiatry*, **36**, 21S–36S.

American Psychiatric Association (1980) *Diagnostic and Statistical Manual of Mental Disorders: DSM-III*. American Psychiatric Association, Washington, D.C.

American Psychiatric Association (1994) *Diagnostic and Statistical Manual of Mental Disorders: DSM-IV*. American Psychiatric Association, Washington, D.C.

Anderson, J.C., Franz, C.P., Williams, S., McGee, R. & Silva, P.A. (1987) DSM-III disorders in preadolescent children. *Archives of General Psychiatry*, **44**, 69–76.

Angold, A. & Costello, E.J. (2000) The Child and Adolescent Psychiatric Assessment (CAPA). *Journal of the American Academy of Child and Adolescent Psychiatry*, **39**, 39–48.

Angold, A., Erkanli, A., Costello, E. & Rutter, M. (1996) Precision, reliability and accuracy in the dating of symptom onsets in child and adolescent psychopathology. *Journal of Child Psychology and Psychiatry*, **37**, 657–664.

Angold, A., Costello, E., Farmer, E., Burners, B. & Erkanli, A. (1999a) Impaired but undiagnosed. *Journal of the American Academy of Child and Adolescent Psychiatry*, **38**, 129–137.

Angold, A., Costello, E. & Erkanli, A. (1999b) Comorbidity. *Journal of Child Psychology and Psychiatry*, **40**, 57–87.

Applegate, B., Lahey, B.B., Hart, E.L. *et al.* (1997) Validity of the age-of-onset criterion for ADHD: a report from the DSM-IV field trials. *Journal of the American Academy of Child and Adolescent Psychiatry*, **36**, 1211–1221.

Bagnato, S., Neisworth, J. & Salvia, J. (1999) *Early childhood indicators of developmental dysfunction*. Paul H. Brookes, Baltimore, MD.

Bartko, J.J. (1976) On various intraclass correlation reliability coefficients. *Psychological Bulletin*, **83**, 762–765.

Berg, I., Lucas, C. & McGuire, R. (1992) Measurement of behaviour difficulties in children using standard scales administered to mothers by computer: reliability and validity. *European Child and Adolescent Psychiatry*, **1**, 14–23.

Berument, S.K., Rutter, M., Lord, C., Pickles, A. & Bailey, A. (1999) Autism screening questionnaire: diagnostic validity. *British Journal of Psychiatry*, **175**, 444–451.

Bird, H.R. (1996) Epidemiology of childhood disorders in a cross-cultural context. *Journal of Child Psychology and Psychiatry*, **37**, 35–49.

Bird, H. (1999) The assessment of functional impairment. In: *Diagnostic Assessment in Child and Adolescent Psychopathology* (eds D. Shaffer, C. Lucas, J. Richters), pp. 209–229. Guilford Press, New York.

Bird, H.R., Canino, G., Rubio-Stipec, M. *et al.* (1988) Estimates of the prevalence of childhood maladjustment in a community survey in Puerto Rico. *Archives of General Psychiatry*, **45**, 1120–1126.

Bird, H.R., Gould, M.S. & Staghezza, B. (1992) Aggregating data from multiple informants in child psychiatry epidemiological research. *Journal of the American Academy of Child and Adolescent Psychiatry*, **31**, 78–85.

Bird, H., Shaffer, D., Fisher, P. *et al.* (1993) The Columbia Impairment Scale (CIS): pilot findings on a measure of global impairment for children and adolescents. *International Journal of Methods in Psychiatric Research*, **3**, 167–176.

Bird, H., Andrews, H., Schwab-Stone, M. *et al.* (1996) Global measures of impairment for epidemiologic and clinical use with children and adolescents. *International Journal of Methods in Psychiatric Research*, **6**, 1–13.

Borge, A., Samuelsen, S. & Rutter, M. (2001) Observer variance within families: confluence among maternal, paternal and child ratings. *International Journal of Methods in Psychiatric Research*, **10**, 11–21.

Boyle, M. (1995) Sampling in epidemiological studies. In: *The Epidemiology of Child and Adolescent Psychopathology* (eds F. Verhulst & H. Koot), pp. 66–85. Oxford University Press, Oxford.

Boyle, M.H. & Pickles, A.R. (1997a) Influence of maternal depressive symptoms on ratings of childhood behavior. *Journal of Abnormal Child Psychology*, **25**, 399–412.

Boyle, M.H. & Pickles, A. (1997b) Maternal depressive symptoms and ratings of emotional disorder symptoms in children and adolescents. *Journal of Child Psychology and Psychiatry*, **38**, 981–992.

Boyle, M.H., Offord, D.R., Racine, Y.A. & Catlin, G. (1991) Ontario Child Health Study follow-up: evaluation of sample loss. *Journal of the American Academy of Child and Adolescent Psychiatry*, **30**, 449–456.

Brandenburg, N.A., Friedman, R.M. & Silver, S.E. (1990) The epidemiology of childhood psychiatric disorders: prevalence findings from recent studies. *Journal of the American Academy of Child and Adolescent Psychiatry* **29**, 76–83.

Breton, J.J., Bergeron, L., Valla, J.P. *et al.* (1999) Quebec child mental health survey: prevalence of DSM-III-R mental health disorders. *Journal of Child Psychology and Psychiatry*, **40**, 375–384.

Brewin, C.R., Andrews, B. & Gotlib, I.H. (1993) Psychopathology and early experience: a reappraisal of retrospective reports. *Psychological Bulletin*, **113**, 82–98.

Canino, G. & Bravo, M. (1999) The translation and adaptation of diagnostic instruments for cross-cultural use. In: *Diagnostic Assessment in Child and Adolescent Psychopathology* (eds D. Shaffer, C. Lucas & J. Richters), pp. 285–298. Guilford Press, New York.

Canino, G., Bird, H., Rubio-Stipec, M. & Bravo, M. (1995) Child psychiatric epidemiology: what we have learned and what we need to learn. *International Journal of Methods in Psychiatric Research*, 5, 79–92.

Caron, C. & Rutter, M. (1991) Comorbidity in child psychopathology: concepts, issues and research strategies. *Journal of Child Psychology and Psychiatry*, 32, 1063–1080.

Caspi, A., Moffitt, T.E., Newman, D.L. & Silva, P.A. (1996) Behavioral observations at age 3 years predict adult psychiatric disorders: longitudinal evidence from a birth cohort. *Archives of General Psychiatry*, 53, 1033–1039.

Chilcoat, H.D. & Breslau, N. (1997) Does psychiatric history bias mothers' reports? An application of a new analytic approach. *Journal of the American Academy of Child and Adolescent Psychiatry*, 36, 971–979.

Cohen, S. & Bromet, E. (1992) Maternal predictors of behavioural disturbance in preschool children: a research note. *Journal of Child Psychology and Psychiatry*, 33, 941–946.

Costello, E.J. & Janiszewski, S. (1990) Who gets treated? Factors associated with referral in children with psychiatric disorders. *Acta Psychiatrica Scandinavica*, 81, 523–529.

Costello, E., Angold, A., Burns, B., Erkanli, A., Stangl, D. & Tweed, D. (1996) The Great Smoky Mountains Study of Youth: functional impairment and serious emotional disturbance. *Archives of General Psychiatry*, 53, 1137–1143.

Costello, E., Angold, A. & Keeler, G. (1999) Adolescent outcomes of childhood disorders: the consequences of severity and impairment. *Journal of the American Academy of Child and Adolescent Psychiatry*, 38, 121–128.

Cox, A., Rutter, M., Yule, B. & Quinton, D. (1977) Bias resulting from missing information: some epidemiological findings. *British Journal of Preventive and Social Medicine*, 31, 131–136.

Crijnen, A.A.M., Achenbach, T.M. & Verhulst, F.C. (1999) Problems reported by parents of children in multiple cultures: the Child Behavior Checklist syndrome constructs. *American Journal of Psychiatry*, 156, 569–574.

Cronbach, L. (1951) Coefficient alpha and the internal structure of tests. *Psychometrika*, 16, 297–334.

Dunn, G., Pickles, A., Tansella, M. & Vazquez-Barquero, J. (1999) Two-phase epidemiological surveys in psychiatric research. *British Journal of Psychiatry*, 174, 95–100.

Duyx, J. & van Engeland, H. (1993) Factoranalyse van de Maudsley Psychiatric Child Rating Scale: Een replicatiestudie. *Tijdschrift Voo Psychiatrie*, 35, 303–309.

Earls, F. (1980) Prevalence of behavior problems in 3-year-old children. *Archives of General Psychiatry*, 37, 1153–1157.

Elander, J. & Rutter, M. (1995) Use and development of the Rutter Parents' and Teachers' Scales. *International Journal of Methods in Psychiatric Research*, 5, 1–16.

Emde, R., Bingham, R. & Harmon, R. (1993) Classification and the diagnostic process in infancy. In: *Handbook of Infant Mental Health* (ed. C. Zeanah), pp. 225–235. Guilford Press, New York.

Esser, G., Schmidt, M.H. & Woerner, W. (1990) Epidemiology and course of psychiatric disorders in school-age children: results of a longitudinal study. *Journal of Child Psychology and Psychiatry*, 31, 243–263.

Fergusson, D. (1995) A brief introduction to structural equation models. In: *The Epidemiology of Child and Adolescent Psychopathology* (eds F. Verhulst & H. Koot), pp. 122–145. Oxford University Press, Oxford.

Fergusson, D.M. (1997) Structural equation models in developmental research. *Journal of Child Psychology and Psychiatry*, 38, 877–887.

Fergusson, D. & Horwood, L. (1987a) The trait and method components of ratings of conduct disorder. I. Maternal and teacher evaluations of conduct disorder in young children. *Journal of Child Psychology and Psychiatry*, 28, 249–260.

Fergusson, D. & Horwood, L. (1987b) The trait and method components of ratings of conduct disorder. II. Factors related to the trait components of maternal and teacher ratings of childhood conduct disorder. *Journal of Child Psychology and Psychiatry*, 28, 261–272.

Fergusson, D.M., Horwood, L.J. & Lynskey, M.T. (1993) Prevalence and comorbidity of DSM-III-R diagnoses in a birth cohort of 15-year-olds. *Journal of the American Academy of Child and Adolescent Psychiatry*, 32, 1127–1134.

Flynn, J. (1987) Massive IQ gains in 14 nations: what IQ tests really measure. *Psychological Bulletin*, 101, 171–191.

Fombonne, E. (1991) The use of questionnaires in child psychiatry research: measuring their performance and choosing an optimal cut-off. *Journal of Child Psychology and Psychiatry*, 32, 677–693.

Fombonne, E. (1992) Parent reports on behaviour and competencies among 6–21-year-old French children. *European Child and Adolescent Psychiatry*, 1, 233–243.

Fombonne, E. (1994) The Chartres study. I. Prevalence of psychiatric disorders among French school-aged children. *British Journal of Psychiatry*, 164, 69–79.

Fombonne, E. (1995) Eating disorders: time trends and explanatory mechanisms. In: *Psychosocial Disorders in Young People: Time Trends and Their Causes* (eds M. Rutter & D. Smith), pp. 616–685. Wiley, Chichester.

Fombonne, E. (1998a) Increased rates of psychosocial disorders in youth. *European Archives of Psychiatry and Clinical Neuroscience*, 248, 14–21.

Fombonne, E. (1998b) Suicidal behaviours in vulnerable adolescents: time trends and their correlates. *British Journal of Psychiatry*, 173, 154–159.

Fombonne, E., Wostear, G., Cooper, V., Harrington, R. & Rutter, M. (2001) The Maudsley long-term follow-up of child and adolescent depression. I. Psychiatric outcomes in adulthood. *British Journal of Psychiatry*, 179, 210–217.

Fredriks, A.M., van Buuren, S., Burgmeijer, R.J. *et al.* (2000) Continuing positive secular growth change in the Netherlands, 1955–97. *Pediatric Research*, 47, 316–323.

Fuggle, P.W., Tokar, S., Grant, D.B. & Smith, I. (1992) Rising IQ scores in British children: recent evidence. *Journal of Child Psychology and Psychiatry*, 33, 1241–1247.

Goodman, R., Ford, T., Richards, H., Gatward, R. & Meltzer, H. (2000) The Development and Well-Being Assessment: description and initial validation of an integrated assessment of child and adolescent psychopathology. *Journal of Child Psychology and Psychiatry*, 41, 645–656.

Gould, M., Rutter, M., Shaffer, D. & Sturge, C. (1988) UK/WHO study of ICD-9. In: *Assessment and Diagnosis in Child Psychopathology* (eds M. Rutter, A. Tuma & I. Lann), pp. 37–65. David Fulton, London.

Harrington, R., Fudge, H., Rutter, M., Pickles, A. & Hill, J. (1990) Adult outcomes of childhood and adolescent depression. I. Psychiatric status. *Archives of General Psychiatry*, 47, 465–473.

Harrington, R., Rutter, M., Weissman, M. *et al.* (1997) Psychiatric disorders in the relatives of depressed probands. I. Comparison of prepubertal, adolescent and early adult onset cases. *Journal of Affective Disorders*, 42, 9–22.

Hinshaw, S., Lahey, B. & Hart, E. (1993) Issues of taxonomy and comorbidity in the development of conduct disorder. *Development and Psychopathology Special Issue: Toward a Development Perspective on Conduct Disorder*, 5, 310–349.

Hsiao, J., Bartko, J. & Potter, W. (1989) Diagnosing diagnoses. *Archives of General Psychiatry*, 46, 664–667.

Hughes, C., Sheldon, H., Preskorn, S. *et al.* (1990) The effect of concomitant disorder in childhood depression on predicting treatment response. *Psychopharmacological Bulletin*, 26, 235–238.

Jeffers, A. & Fitzgerald, M. (1991) *Irish Families Under Stress*, 2. Eastern Health Board, Dublin.

Jensen, P., Bloedau, L. & Davis, H. (1990) Children at risk. II. Risk factors and clinic utilization. *Journal of the American Academy of Child and Adolescent Psychiatry*, 29, 804–812.

John, K., Gammon, G.D., Prusoff, B.A. & Warner, V. (1987) The Social Adjustment Inventory for Children and Adolescents (SAICA): testing of a new semistructured interview. *Journal of the American Academy of Child and Adolescent Psychiatry*, 26, 898–911.

Kagan, J., Snidman, N. & Arcus, D. (1998) Childhood derivatives of high and low reactivity in infancy. *Child Development*, 69, 1483–1493.

Kalton, G. (1983) *Compensating for Missing Data*. Institute for Social Research, Ann Arbor, MI.

Kendler, K., Silberg, J., Neale, M., Kessler, R., Heath, A. & Eaves, L. (1991) The family history method: whose psychiatric history is measured? *American Journal of Psychiatry*, 148, 1501–1504.

Kessler, R., Mroczek, D. & Belli, R. (1999) Retrospective adult assessment of childhood psychopathology. In: *Diagnostic Assessment in Child and Adolescent Psychopathology* (eds D. Shaffer, C. Lucas & J. Richters), pp. 256–284. Guilford Press, New York.

King, M. & Bhugra, D. (1989) Eating disorders: lessons from a cross-cultural study. *Psychological Medicine*, 19, 955–958.

Kleinman, A. & Good, B. (1985) *Culture and Depression: Studies in the Anthropology and Cross-Cultural Psychiatry of Affect and Disorder*. University of California Press, Berkeley, CA.

Kovacs, M., Akiskal, H., Gatsonis, C. & Parrone, P. (1994) Childhood onset dysthymic disorder: clinical features and prospective naturalistic outcome. *Archives of General Psychiatry*, 51, 365–374.

Lahey, B.B., Applegate, B., Barkley, R.A. *et al.* (1994) DSM-IV field trials for oppositional defiant disorder and conduct disorder in children and adolescents. *American Journal of Psychiatry*, 151, 1163–1171.

Lapouse, R. & Monk, M. (1958) An epidemiologic study of behaviour characteristics in children. *American Journal of Public Health*, 48, 1134–1144.

Lapouse, R. & Monk, M. (1959) Fears and worries in a representative sample of children. *American Journal of Orthopsychiatry*, 29, 803–818.

Lavigne, J.V., Gibbons, R.D., Christoffel, K.K. *et al.* (1996) Prevalence rates and correlates of psychiatric disorders among preschool children. *Journal of the American Academy of Child and Adolescent Psychiatry* 35, 204–214.

Leaf, P.J., Alegria, M., Cohen, P. *et al.* (1996) Mental health service use in the community and schools: results from the four-community MECA Study — Methods for the Epidemiology of Child and Adolescent Mental Disorders Study. *Journal of the American Academy of Child and Adolescent Psychiatry*, 35, 889–897.

Lee, S. (1991) Anorexia nervosa in Hong Kong: a Chinese perspective. *Psychological Medicine*, 21, 703–711.

Leung, P.W.L., Luk, S.L., Ho, T.P., Taylor, E., Mak, F.L. & Bacon-Shone, J. (1996) The diagnosis of prevalence of hyperactivity in Chinese schoolboys. *British Journal of Psychiatry*, 168, 486–496.

Lewinsohn, P.M., Hops, H., Roberts, R.E., Seeley, J.R. & Andrews, J.A. (1993) Adolescent psychopathology. I. Prevalence and incidence of depression and other DSM-III-R disorders in high school students. *Journal of Abnormal Psychology*, 102, 133–144.

Little, R.J.A. & Rubin, D.B. (1987) *Statistical Analysis with Missing Data*. Wiley, New York.

Lucas, C.P., Fisher, P., Piacentini, J. *et al.* (1999) Features of interviews questions associated with attenuation of symptom reports. *Journal of Abnormal Child Psychology*, 27, 429–437.

Maughan, B. & Rutter, M. (1997) Retrospective reporting of childhood adversity: some methodological considerations. *Journal of Personality Disorders*, 11, 19–33.

Mawhood, L., Howlin, P. & Rutter, M. (2000) Autism and developmental receptive language disorder: a comparative follow-up in early adult life. I. Cognitive and language outcomes. *Journal of Child Psychology and Psychiatry*, 41, 547–549.

Mayes, L.C. (1999) Addressing mental health needs of infants and young children. *Child and Adolescent Psychiatric Clinics of North America*, 8, 209–224.

Maziade, M., Cote, R., Boutin, P., Bernier, H. & Thivierge, J. (1987) Temperament and intellectual development: a longitudinal study from infancy to four years. *American Journal of Psychiatry*, 144, 144–150.

Meltzer, H., Gatward, R., Goodman, R. & Ford, T. (2000) *The Mental Health of Children and Adolescents in Great Britain*. The Stationery Office, London.

Merikangas, K.R., Mehta, R.L., Molnar, B.E. *et al.* (1998) Comorbidity of substance use disorders with mood and anxiety disorders: results of the International Consortium in Psychiatric Epidemiology. *Addictive Behaviors*, 23, 893–907.

Moffitt, T.E. (1993) Adolescence-limited and life-course-persistent antisocial behavior: a developmental taxonomy. *Psychological Review*, 100, 674–701.

Moore, J. & Fombonne, E. (1999) Psychopathology in adopted and nonadopted children: a clinical sample. *American Journal of Orthopsychiatry*, 69, 403–409.

Morita, H., Suzuki, M. & Kamoshita, S. (1990) Screening measures for detecting psychiatric disorders in Japanese secondary school children. *Journal of Child Psychology and Psychiatry*, 31, 603–617.

Nottelmann, E. & Jensen, P. (1995) Comorbidity of disorders in children and adolescents: developmental perspectives. In: *Advances in Clinical Child Psychology* Vol. 1 (eds T. Ollendick & R. Prinz), pp. 109–155. Plenum Press, New York.

Offord, D.R., Boyle, M.H., Szatmari, P. *et al.* (1987) Ontario Child Health Study. II. Six-month prevalence of disorder and rates of service utilization. *Archives of General Psychiatry*, 44, 832–836.

van den Oord, E., Koot, H., Boomsma, D., Verhulst, F. & Orlebeke, J. (1995) A twin–singleton comparison of problem behaviour in 2–3-year-olds. *Journal of Child Psychology and Psychiatry*, 36, 449–458.

Patton, G.C., Coffey, C., Posterino, M., Carlin, J.B., Wolfe, R. & Bowes, G. (1999) A computerised screening instrument for adolescent depression: population-based validation and application to a two-phase case–control study. *Social Psychiatry and Psychiatric Epidemiology*, 34, 166–172.

Petersen, A., Compas, B., Brooks-Gunn, J., Stemmler, M., Ey, S. & Grant, K. (1993) Depression in adolescence. *American Psychologist*, 48, 155–168.

Piacentini, J., Roper, M., Jensen, P. *et al.* (1999) Informant-based determinants of symptom attenuation in structured child psychiatric interviews. *Journal of Abnormal Child Psychology*, 27, 417–428.

Pianta, R. & Caldwell, C. (1990) Stability of externalizing symptoms from kindergarten to first grade and factors related to instability. *Developmental Psychopathology*, 2, 246–258.

Pianta, R. & Castaldi, J. (1989) Stability of internalizing symptoms from kindergarten to first grade and factors related to instability. *Developmental Psychopathology*, **1**, 305–316.

Pickles, A. (1998) Psychiatric epidemiology. *Statistical Methods in Medical Research*, 7, 235–251.

Pickles, A., Rowe, R., Simonoff, E., Foley, D., Rutter, M. & Silberg, J. (2001) Child psychiatric symptoms and psychosocial impairment: relationship and prognostic significance. *British Journal of Psychiatry*, **179**, 230–235.

Prendergast, M., Taylor, E., Rapoport, J.L. *et al.* (1988) The diagnosis of childhood hyperactivity: a US–UK cross-national study of DSM-III and ICD-9. *Journal of Child Psychology and Psychiatry*, **29**, 289–300.

Reich, W. (2000) Diagnostic Interview for Children and Adolescents (DICA). *Journal of the American Academy of Child and Adolescent Psychiatry*, **39**, 59–66.

Reich, W., Cottler, L., McCallum, K., Corwin, D. & Eerdewegh, V. (1995) Computerized interviews as a method of assessing psychopathology in children. *Comprehensive Psychiatry*, **36**, 40–45.

Rende, R. & Weissman, M. (1999) Assessment of family history of psychiatric disorder. In: *Diagnostic Assessment in Child and Adolescent Psychopathology* (eds D. Shaffer, C. Lucas & J. Richters), pp. 230–255. Guilford Press, New York.

Rende, R., Weissman, M., Rutter, M., Wickramaratne, P., Harrington, R. & Pickles, A. (1997) Psychiatric disorders in the relatives of depressed probands. II. Familial loading for comorbid non-depressive disorders based upon proband age of onset. *Journal of Affective Disorders*, **42**, 23–28.

Richman, N., Stevenson, J. & Graham, P. (1982) *Pre-School to School: a Behavioural Study*. Academic Press, London.

Roberts, R.E., Attkisson, C.C. & Rosenblatt, A. (1998) Prevalence of psychopathology among children and adolescents. *American Journal of Psychiatry*, **155**, 715–725.

Rogers, S. (1998) Empirically supported comprehensive treatments for young children with autism. *Journal of Clinical Child Psychology*, **27**, 168–179.

Rutter, M. (1978) Diagnostic validity in child psychiatry. *Advances in Biological Psychiatry*, 2, 2–22.

Rutter, M. (1989) Isle of Wight revisited: twenty-five years of child psychiatric epidemiology. *Journal of the American Academy of Child and Adolescent Psychiatry*, **28**, 633–653.

Rutter, M. (1997) Comorbidity: concepts, claims and choices. *Criminal Behaviour and Mental Health*, 7, 265–285.

Rutter, M. & Quinton, D. (1977) Psychiatric disorder: ecological factors and concepts of causation. In: *Ecological Factors in Human Development* (ed. H. McGurk), pp. 173–187. North-Holland, Amsterdam.

Rutter, M. & Smith, D.J., eds (1995) *Psychosocial Disorders in Young People: Time Trends and Their Causes*. Wiley, Chichester.

Rutter, M., Lebovici, L., Eisenberg, L. *et al.* (1969) A tri-axial classification of mental disorders in childhood. *Journal of Child Psychology and Psychiatry*, **10**, 41–61

Rutter, M., Tizard, J. & Whitmore, K. eds (1970) *Education, Health and Behaviour*. Robert E. Krieber Publishing, New York.

Rutter, M., Shaffer, D. & Shepherd, M. (1975) *An Evaluation of a Proposal for a Multiaxial Classification of Child Psychiatric Disorders*. World Health Organization Monograph. World Health Organization, Geneva.

Rutter, M., Tizard, J., Yule, W., Graham, P. & Whitmore, K. (1976) Research report: Isle of Wight studies, 1964–74. *Psychological Medicine*, **6**, 313–332.

Rutter, M., Tuma, A. & Lann, I., eds (1988) *Assessment and Diagnosis in Child Psychopathology*. David Fulton, London.

Rutter, M., Silberg, J., O'Connor, T. & Simonoff, E. (1999) Genetics and child psychiatry. I. Advances in quantitative and molecular genetics. *Journal of Child Psychology and Psychiatry*, **40**, 3–18.

Rutter, M., Pickles, A., Murray, R. & Eaves, L. (2001) Testing hypotheses on specific environmental causal effects on behavior. *Psychological Bulletin*, **127**, 291–324.

Sanford, M.N., Offord, D.R., Boyle, M.H., Peace, A. & Racine, Y.A. (1992) Ontario Child Health Study: social and school impairments in children age 6–16 years. *Journal of the American Academy of Child and Adolescent Psychiatry*, **31**, 60–67.

Schachar, R., Rutter, M. & Smith, A. (1981) The characteristics of situationally and pervasively hyperactive children: implications for syndrome definition. *Journal of Child Psychology and Psychiatry*, **22**, 375–392.

Schurhoff, F., Bellivier, F., Jouvent, R. *et al.* (2000) Early and late onset bipolar disorders: two different forms of manic depressive illness? *Journal of Affective Disorders*, **58**, 215–221.

Shaffer, D., Gould, M.S., Brasic, J. *et al.* (1983) A children's global assessment scale (CGAS). *Archives of General Psychiatry*, **40**, 1228–1231.

Shaffer, D., Lucas, C. & Richters, J. (1999) *Diagnostic Assessment in Child and Adolescent Psychopathology*. Guilford Press, New York.

Shaffer, D., Fisher, P., Lucas, C.P., Dulcan, M.K. & Schwab-Stone, M.E. (2000) NIMH Diagnostic Interview Schedule for Children, Version IV (NIMH DISC-IV): description, differences from previous versions, and reliability of some common diagnoses. *Journal of the American Academy of Child and Adolescent Psychiatry*, **39**, 28–38.

Shepherd, M., Oppenheim, B. & Mitchell, S. (1971) *Childhood Behaviour and Mental Health*. University of London Press, London.

Simic, M. & Fombonne, E. (2001) Depressive conduct disorder: symptom patterns and correlates in referred children and adolescents. *Journal of Affective Disorders*, **62**, 175–185.

Simon, G. & Von Korff, M. (1992) Re-evaluation of secular trends in depression rates. *American Journal of Epidemiology*, **135**, 1411–1422.

Simonoff, E., Pickles, A., Meyer, J.M. *et al.* (1997) The Virginia Twin Study of Adolescent Behavioral Development: influences of age, sex, and impairment on rates of disorder. *Archives of General Psychiatry*, **54**, 801–808.

Simonoff, E., Pickles, A., Hervas, A., Silberg, J.L., Rutter, M. & Eaves, L. (1998) Genetic influences on childhood hyperactivity: contrast effects imply parental rating bias, not sibling interaction. *Psychological Medicine*, **28**, 825–837.

Spitzer, R.L. & Fleiss, J.L. (1974) A re-analysis of the reliability of psychiatric diagnosis. *British Journal of Psychiatry*, **125**, 341–347.

Spitzer, R., Endicott, J. & Robins, E. (1978) Research diagnostic criteria: rationale and reliability. *Archives of General Psychiatry*, **35**, 773–782.

Stanger, C., Fombonne, E. & Achenbach, T.M. (1994) Epidemiological comparisons of American and French children: parent reports of problems and competencies for ages 6–21. *European Child and Adolescent Psychiatry*, **3**, 16–28.

Steinhausen, H.C., Metzke, C.W., Meier, M. & Kannenberg, R. (1998) Prevalence of child and adolescent psychiatric disorders: the Zurich Epidemiological Study. *Acta Psychiatrica Scandinavica*, **98**, 262–271.

Stevenson, J., Richman, N. & Graham, P. (1985) Behaviour problems and language abilities at three years and behavioural deviance at eight years. *Journal of Child Psychology and Psychiatry*, **26**, 215–230.

Strober, M., Green, J. & Carlson, G. (1981) Reliability of psychiatric diagnosis in hospitalised adolescents: interrater agreement using DSM-III. *Archives of General Psychiatry*, **38**, 141–145.

Taylor, E. (1999) Developmental neuropsychopathology of attention deficit and impulsiveness. *Development and Psychopathology*, 11, 607–628.

Taylor, E., Chadwick, O., Heptinstall, E. & Danckaerts, M. (1996) Hyperactivity and conduct problems as risk factors for adolescent development. *Journal of the American Academy of Child and Adolescent Psychiatry*, 35, 1213–1226.

Thorley, G. (1987) Factor study of a psychiatric child rating scale: based on ratings made by clinicians on child and adolescent clinic attenders. *British Journal of Psychiatry*, 150, 49–59.

Turner, C., Ku, L., Rogers, S., Lindberg, L., Pleck, J. & Sonenstein, F. (1998) Adolescent sexual behavior, drug use, and violence: increased reporting with computer survey technology. *Science*, 280, 867–873.

Valla, J., Bergeron, L. & Smolla, N. (2000) The Dominic-R: a pictorial interview for 6- to 11-year-old children. *Journal of the American Academy of Child and Adolescent Psychiatry*, 39, 85–93.

Verhulst, F.C. & Achenbach, T.M. (1995) Empirically based assessment and taxonomy of psychopathology: cross-cultural applications—a review. *European Child and Adolescent Psychiatry*, 4, 61–76.

Verhulst, F. & Koot, H. (1992) Child psychiatric epidemiology: concepts, methods and findings. In: *Developmental Clinical Psychology and Psychiatry Series* (ed. A. Kazdin). Sage Publications, Newbury Park, CA.

Verhulst, F. & Koot, H. (1995) *The Epidemiology of Child and Adolescent Psychopathology*. Oxford University Press, Oxford.

Verhulst, F. & Van Der Ende, J. (1997) Factors associated with child mental health service use in the community. *Journal of the American Academy of Child and Adolescent Psychiatry*, 36, 901–909.

Verhulst, F., van der Ende, J., Ferdinand, R. & Kasius, M. (1997) The prevalence of DSM-III-R diagnosis in a national sample of Dutch adolescents. *Archives of General Psychiatry*, 54, 329–336.

Vikan, A. (1985) Psychiatric epidemiology in a sample of 1510 10-year-old children. I. Prevalence. *Journal of Child Psychology and Psychiatry*, 26, 55–75.

Volkmar, F.R., Klin, A., Siegel, B. *et al.* (1994) Field trial for autistic disorder in DSM-IV. *American Journal of Psychiatry*, 151, 1361–1367.

Wannan, G. & Fombonne, E. (1998) Gender differences in rates and correlates of suicidal behaviour amongst child psychiatric outpatients. *Journal of Adolescence*, 21, 371–381.

Warwick, D. & Lininger, C. (1975) *The Sample Survey: Theory and Practice*. McGraw-Hill, New York.

Weissman, M., Wolk, S., Goldstein, R. *et al.* (1999a) Depressed adolescents grown up. *Journal of the American Medical Association*, 281, 1707–1713.

Weissman, M., Wolk, S., Wickramaratne, P., Goldstein, R., Adams, P. & Greenwald, S. (1999b) Children with prepubertal-onset major depressive disorder and anxiety grown up. *Archives of General Psychiatry*, 56, 794–801.

Weisz, J. & Eastman, K. (1995) Cross-national research on child and adolescent psychopathology. In: *The Epidemiology of Child and Adolescent Psychopathology* (eds F. Verhulst & H. Koot), pp. 42–65. Oxford University Press, Oxford.

Weisz, J.R., Suwanlert, S., Chaiyasit, W., Weiss, B., Walter, B.R. & Anderson, W.W. (1988) Thai and American perspectives on over- and under-controlled child behavior problems: exploring the threshold model among parents, teachers, and psychologists. *Journal of Consulting and Clinical Psychology*, 56, 601–609.

Werry, J.S., Methven, R.J., Fitzpatrick, J. & Dixon, H. (1983) The interrater reliability of DSM-III in children. *Journal of Abnormal Child Psychology*, 11, 341–354.

Whitaker, A., Johnson, J., Shaffer, D. *et al.* (1990) Uncommon troubles in young people: prevalence estimates of selected psychiatric disorders in a non-referred adolescent population. *Archives of General Psychiatry*, 47, 487–496.

Wing, L. & Gould, J. (1979) Severe impairments of social interaction and associated abnormalities in children: epidemiology and classification. *Journal of Autism and Developmental Disorders*, 9, 11–29.

Winnicott, D. (1965) *The Maturational Process and the Facilitating Environment*. Hogarth Press, London.

Woodward, C.A., Thomas, H.B., Boyle, M.H. & Links, P.S. (1989) Methodologic note for child epidemiological surveys: the effects of instructions on estimates of behavior prevalence. *Journal of Child Psychology and Psychiatry* 30, 919–924.

World Health Organization (1992) *The ICD-10 Classification of Mental and Behavioural Disorders: Clinical Descriptions and Diagnostic Guidelines*. World Health Organization, Geneva.

World Health Organization (1993) *ICD-10 Classification of Mental and Behavioural Disorders: Diagnostic Criteria for Research*. World Health Organization, Geneva.

World Health Organization (1996) *Multiaxial Classification of Child and Adolescent Psychiatric Disorders*. Cambridge University Press, Cambridge.

Zahner, G.E., Pawelkiewicz, W., DeFrancesco, J.J. & Adnopoz, J. (1992) Children's mental health service needs and utilization patterns in an urban community: an epidemiological assessment. *Journal of the American Academy of Child and Adolescent Psychiatry*, 31, 951–960.

Zero to Three (1994) *Diagnostic Classification DC:0–3: Diagnostic Classification of Mental Health and Developmental Disorders of Infancy and Early Childhood*. National Center for Clinical Infant Programs, Washington, D.C.

Zoccolillo, M., Pickles, A., Quinton, D. & Rutter, M. (1992) The outcome of childhood conduct disorder: implications for defining adult personality disorder and conduct disorder. *Psychological Medicine*, 22, 971–986.

Rating Scales

Frank C. Verhulst and Jan Van der Ende

Introduction

Over the last 30 years or so, many rating scales have been developed to assess general child/adolescent psychopathology. Their number and variety creates a potential problem because of the uncertainties about generalizing findings from one study to another if different instruments have been used. In this chapter we consider the purposes for which such rating scales may be used, discuss their psychometric properties, note their similarities and differences, and outline the criteria by which to judge which instrument best suits a particular purpose.

The evaluation of rating scales does not result in a static conclusion. Many of the scales have developed over time in terms of content, age span covered, the production of parallel versions for parents, teachers and adolescents themselves, the means of administration and scoring, and the availability of standardized data.

Specific rating scales are referred to in the text by their abbreviations. Table 5.1 and Appendix 1 give the full name, author(s) and relevant information for each scale. Our focus is exclusively on scales to measure general psychopathology; those for specific disorders/behaviours and for psychosocial features are considered in the relevant chapter elsewhere in the book.

Our evaluation of general scales is based on four key assumptions:

1 that diagnoses are hypothesized latent constructs, the validity of which need empirical testing (see also Fombonne, Chapter 4; Taylor & Rutter, Chapter 1);

2 as follows from the first assumption, we do not regard agreement with a clinical diagnosis as the ultimate test of the validity of a rating scale;

3 that no single measure is ever a perfect index of the construct that it aims to tap (see Fombonne, Chapter 4); and

4 that the value of any rating scale needs to be considered in relation to the purposes to which it is to be put.

It is most unlikely that any one scale will be optimal for all purposes. To give an obvious example, the type of measure needed to examine changes over a short time (such as in a trial of treatment) is scarcely likely to be the same as that needed to assess continuing liability (as in a genetic study).

Issues specific to scales for child psychopathology

Age-relatedness

Many problem behaviours, such as temper tantrums or separation anxiety, are common and therefore statistically normal at a young age, but much less frequent and more likely to indicate psychopathology at older ages. Clinical significance has to take into account the child's developmental level. For young people within the normal range for cognitive and physical development, comparisons with normative samples of children of the same age (and sex) provide guidelines for evaluating behaviours. If the ages of children to be studied differ substantially from those in the standardization sample for the scale, valid comparisons are not possible.

Some rating scales employ the same version for different age groups. This has the considerable advantage that scores obtained for children at one age can be compared directly with scores obtained for the same children at a later age. Provided that there are age-standardized norms, comparisons can also be made on the relative levels of problems at different ages.

Other scales use different versions for different age groups. These have the advantage that behaviours relevant for one age group but not for another are included only in the age-relevant version. For example, alcohol and drug use, truancy or vandalism are applicable in adolescence but not in the preschool period. However, a disadvantage is that in the transition from one age group to another, there is loss of continuity of item and scale scores. This is especially problematic for longitudinal studies.

Informant and situational specificity

For both statistical and clinical reasons, it is necessary to obtain information from different informants that cover behaviour in different settings, such as home and school (see Fombonne, Chapter 4; Rutter & Taylor, Chapter 2).

Instead of viewing low agreement among different informants (the usual picture—Achenbach *et al.* 1987) as a nuisance, or systematically discarding one source of information, it is important to regard each informant as a potentially valid source of information. Each informant has their own unique, and potentially valid, contribution to the formation of an overall picture of the child's functioning (Verhulst *et al.* 1994, 1997; Van der Valk *et al.* in press). Even disagreement among informants can be valuable (Jensen *et al.* 1999). An example of the potential value of information from different sources is the finding that children who are hyperactive at home *and* at school have a poorer prognosis than children who are hyperactive only at home *or* at school (Schachar *et al.* 1981).

Most rating scales for the assessment of child/adolescent psychopathology have parallel versions for parents and teachers. Some rating scales have versions for adolescents' self-reports, although sometimes the self-report version is not parallel to the parent and teacher versions and may tap other domains, such as personality (e.g. Behavioral Assessment System for Children (BASC); Millon Adolescent Clinical Inventory (MACI); Minnesota Multiphasic Personality Inventory (MMPI)). The advantage of rating scales with parallel parent, teacher and self-report versions is that the scores across the different informants can be compared. The Achenbach System of Empirically Based Assessment (ASEBA; Achenbach & Rescorla 1999) is an example of a rating scale with versions for parents, teachers and self-reports that yield scale scores that can be compared.

Dimensional nature of child/adolescent problem behaviours

The construction of rating scales is usually based on psychometric principles. The basic premise is that most problem behaviours in children and adolescents constitute quantitative variations rather than present/absent categories. To identify quantitative gradations, multiple items are rated by the respondent using standardized procedures. The items of rating scales are then usually aggregated into subscales. Thus, items can be grouped to derive scale scores for domains such as 'hyperactivity', 'anxiety', or 'oppositional' behaviour.

This quantitative approach allows assessment of the degree to which one child's behaviour differs from that of comparable children of the same age and sex in the normative samples. The quality of normative samples used varies considerably. Some scales have large representative standardization samples from the general population [e.g. ASEBA; Conners' Rating Scales–Revised (CRS-R); Devereaux Scales of Mental Disorder (DSMD); MACI; others use samples of convenience [e.g. Revised Behavior Problem Checklist (RBPC); Paediatric Symptom Checklist (PSC); Strengths and Difficulties Questionnaire (SDQ)].

The advantage of using quantitative scores is that they contain more statistical information than categories (Streiner & Norman 1998; Goldberg 2000). This is because they use data across the whole range and not just around a particular cut-off point and because they avoid the major problems of classification error for scores just above and below that point. Thus, if a categorical diagnosis is made if a score is above, say, 10, scores of 10 and 11 are treated as radically different although the difference between them is as likely to be caused by measurement error as to the presence/absence of a disorder. All measures

include error (see Fombonne, Chapter 4). By focusing on the consistency of answers across many items, measurement error is reduced (Streiner & Norman 1998). The reliability of dimensional measures therefore tends to be greater than that for categories (Shaffer *et al.* 1999a). Nevertheless, if needed for decision-making purposes, it is a straightforward matter to transform dimensions into categories (see Fombonne, Chapter 4). Conversely, for most diagnostic categories, it is usual to bring in dimensional considerations (e.g. symptom severity or degree of impairment).

Overview of generic rating scales

We searched the literature for psychometrically sound rating scales for the assessment of general child/adolescent psychopathology (excluding those designed for very limited purposes such as the Achenbach, Conners, Quay questionnaire, ACQ; Achenbach *et al.* 1991). We contacted the authors and/or publishers and requested information on the format, administration, scoring and interpretation of questionnaires. Where appropriate, we sought feedback from the authors and/or publishers to detect any errors in the factual information we provided in the text.

Detailed information on individual questionnaires is available elsewhere (Maruish 1999; Shaffer *et al.* 1999b). Accordingly, we focus on the principles and quality criteria to be employed in the valuation of any rating scale. Table 5.1 provides an overview of the scales considered and Appendix 1 gives a more comprehensive description of each.

Item content

The content of an instrument is chosen on the basis of what it is intended to measure. Generic instruments seek to tap a broad range of psychopathology, using items likely to be relevant for all common types of mental disorder and giving priority to those that apply to several disorders and not just one.

For scales that have been developed over many years through successive revisions, empirical information obtained from earlier versions (for instance on content coverage or on the discriminative validity of specific items) is incorporated into the newer versions. Examples are the ASEBA (Achenbach & Rescorla 1999) and the CRS-R (Conners 1997). In CRS-R, Conners included items that were modelled on the DSM-IV criteria (American Psychiatric Association 1994).

Item response scaling

Most scales have items that can be scored on a 3-point scale (0, 1 and 2), but some use 4-point scaling (0, 1, 2 and 3), and a few use a 2-point 'true/false' scoring approach such as the MMPI-A (Butcher *et al.* 1992). From a psychometric point of view, some argue that the higher the number of scoring categories within the range of 2–10, the better the reliability will be (Streiner &

Table 5.1 Overview of generic rating scales for the assessment of psychopathology.

Instrument	Acronym	Current authors	Informants	Age range	Number of items	Time in minutes	Item scaling	Norms	Derivation of scales	Scales†
Achenbach System of Empirically Based Assessment	ASEBA*	T.M. Achenbach, L.A. Rescorla	Parent Teacher Self	2–3 4–18 2–5 5–18 11–18	100 140 100 136 137	20	0–2	Normal Clinical	Empirical	Activities, Social, School, Total competence Score, Withdrawn, Somatic Complaints, Anxious/Depressed, Social Problems, Thought Problems, Attention Problems, Delinquent Behaviour, Aggressive Behaviour, Internalizing, Externalizing, Total Problem Score
Behavioral Assessment System for Children	BASC*‡	C.R. Reynolds, R.W. Kamphaus	Parent Teacher	2½–5 6–11 12–18 2½–5 6–11 12–18	105 138 126 109 148 138	10–20	0–3	Normal Clinical	Empirical	Aggression, Hyperactivity, Conduct Problems, Anxiety, Depression, Somatization, Attention Problems, Atypicality, Withdrawal, Adaptability, Leadership, Social Skills, Externalizing Problems, Internalizing Problems, Adaptive Skills, Behavioural Symptoms Index
Child Symptom Inventories	CSI	K.D. Gadow, J. Sprafkin	Parent Teacher Self	3–5 6–12 13–18 3–5 6–12 13–18 12–18	108 97 120 87 77 79 120	10–15	0–3 0–1	Normal Clinical	A priori	ADHD-inattentive type, ADHD-hyperactive-impulsive type, ADHD-combined type, Oppositional/Defiant Disorder, Conduct Disorder, Generalized Anxiety Disorder, Social Phobia, Separation Anxiety, Specific Phobia, Obsessive-Compulsive Disorder, Post-traumatic Stress Disorder, Motor Tic Disorder, Vocal Tic Disorder, Tourette's Disorder, Major Depressive Disorder, Dysthymic Disorder, Autistic Disorder, Asperger's Disorder, PDD not otherwise specified, Schizophrenia, enuresis, encopresis
Conners' Rating Scales–Revised	CRS-R	C.K. Conners	Parent Teacher Self	3–17 3–17 12–17	80 59 87	15–20	0–3	Normal	Empirical	Oppositional, Cognitive Problems/Inattention, Hyperactivity, Anxious-Shy, Perfectionism, Social Problems, Psychosomatic, Conners' Global Index, Restless-Impulsive, Emotional Lability, ADHD Index, DSM-IV Symptoms subscales, DSM-IV Inattentive, DSM-IV Hyperactive-Impulsive
Devereux Scales of Mental Disorders	DSMD	J.A. Naglieri et al.	Parent Teacher	5–12 13–18 5–12 13–18	111 110 111 110	15	0–5	Normal Clinical	Empirical	Conduct, Attention, Anxiety, Depression, Autism, Acute Problems, Internalizing, Externalizing, Critical Pathology

Instrument	Abbrev.	Author	Informant	Age range	No. of items	No. of scales		Norm	Derivation	Scales/Indices
Eyberg Child Behavior Inventory	ECBI	S.M. Eyberg	Parent	2–16	36	5	0–6	Normal	A priori	Total Intensity Score, Total Problem Score
Sutter–Eyberg Student Behavior Inventory–Revised	SESBI-R		Teacher	2–16	36		0–1			
Millon Adolescent Clinical Inventory	MACI§	T. Millon	Self	13–19	160	30	0–1	Clinical	A priori	Eating Dysfunctions, Academic Non-compliance, Alcohol Predilection, Drug Proneness, Delinquent Disposition, Impulsive Propensity, Anxious Feelings, Depressive Affect, Suicidal Ideation (only Clinical Indices)
Minnesota Multiphasic Personality Inventory–Adolescent	MMPI-A[d]	J.N. Butcher et al.	Self	14–18	478	60	0–1	Normal	A priori	Hypochondriasis, Depression, Hysteria, Psychopathic Deviate, Masculinity–Femininity, Paranoia, Psychasthenia, Schizophrenia, Mania, Social Introversion
Pediatric Symptom Checklist	PSC	M.S. Jellinek, J.M. Murphy	Parent / Self	2–16 / 11–16	35 / 35	5	0–2	–	A priori	Total Problem Score
Revised Behavior Problem Checklist	RBPC	H.C. Quay, D.R. Peterson	Parent / Teacher	5–18 / 5–18	89 / 89	20	0–2	Normal / Clinical	Empirical	Conduct Disorder, Socialized Aggression, Attention Problems–Immaturity, Anxiety–Withdrawal, Psychotic Behaviour, Motor Tension–Excess
Revised Rutter Scales	Rutter	M. Rutter	Parent / Teacher	3–5 / 6–16 (Parent); 3–5 / 6–16 (Teacher)	43, 50 (Parent); 41, 59 (Teacher)	6	0–2	–	A priori	Emotional Difficulties, Conduct Difficulties, Hyperactivity/Inattention, Prosocial, Total Difficulties
Strengths and Difficulties Questionnaire	SDQ	R. Goodman	Parent / Teacher / Self	4–16 / 4–16 / 11–16	25 / 25 / 25	5	0–2	–	A priori	Conduct Problems, Emotional Symptoms, Hyperactivity, Peer Problems, Prosocial Behaviour

* For ASEBA and BASC adaptive behaviour are listed in addition to problem scales.
† If scales differ by informant, only parent scales indicated; if scales differ by age, only scales for broadest age range; see Appendix 1 for more complete information.
‡ The BASC includes a self-report personality inventory, which is not listed in this overview.
§ The MACI and MMPI-A include personality scales, which are not listed in this overview.

Norman 1998). However, with untrained raters (such as parents) and with relative phenomena (such as degree of misery or overactivity) raters tend to use scores only in the middle range. For example, Achenbach, Conners and Quay (Achenbach *et al.* 1991) developed a new scale (ACQ) which included items that originated from the three authors' original scales, choosing a 4-point item scoring format. However, it was found that the ACQ items that had counterparts on the Child Behaviour Checklist (CBCL; Achenbach 1991a) discriminated less well between clinically referred and non-referred children than the original CBCL items which have a 3-point scoring format. Whatever the theoretical psychometric advantages of many scoring points, 3-point scales are usually to be preferred. The psychometric advantages are better obtained through many items rather than through many scoring points.

Composition of scales

Empirical vs. a priori approaches

Two main approaches, the *empirical* and the *a priori*, may be used to select and group items. Empirical approaches employ multivariate statistical techniques, such as factor analysis or principal components analysis, to identify sets of problems that tend to occur together, and thereby make up syndromes. Each syndrome can be quantified by summing the scores of the items that compose the syndrome. This 'from the ground up' approach starts with empirical data derived from informants, without any assumptions about whether the syndrome reflects predetermined diagnostic categories.

The empirical-quantitative approach forms the basis of most of the rating scales listed in Table 5.1. It is not always clear from the description of the derivation of scales whether the authors used general population samples or clinical samples to compute their syndrome scales. For the construction of the scales for the ASEBA (Achenbach & Rescorla 1999) and the RBPC (Quay & Peterson 1996), scores derived from large clinical samples were used.

It remains a matter of controversy what kind of samples are needed to create the scales. Achenbach (1991b) has been a strong proponent of the use of clinical samples as the data source for multivariate analyses, because they yield items with frequencies high enough to be retained in reliable factor analyses or principal component analyses. Also, the use of clinical samples will result in scales that relate to aggregations of problems as encountered in clinical practice. Others, especially those who use rating scales in general population samples, argue that syndrome scales should be based on data derived from general population samples, because the factor structure should reflect the underlying structure of problems in the samples to be studied. Before using a factor structure in samples that are essentially different from the ones from which the factor structure was derived, it is important to test the applicability of the factor structure (De Groot *et al.* 1994, 1996; Koot *et al.* 1997).

The second approach is to take the diagnostic categories of one of the two international classification systems as the basis for the syndromes to be scored with the rating scales. This a priori or consensus approach is a 'from the top down' method because it starts with experts' assumptions about which disorders exist and which symptoms are relevant for them.

The a priori approach formed the basis of the Child Symptom Inventories (CSI; Gadow & Sprafkin 1998). Like the DSM categories, the CSI syndromes can be scored as present vs. absent by using cutpoints that are based on DSM criteria. For computing the so-called Symptom Criterion score, the authors transformed the original 0–3 item scale into a 2-point present-vs.-absent category by combining the scores 0 and 1 indicating the absence of the symptom, and the scores 2 and 3 indicating the presence of the symptom. Unlike DSM, the syndromes can also be scored as dimensions using the so-called Symptom Severity scoring by retaining the original 4-point item scoring format.

The advantage of the empirical approach is that it does not start from unvalidated assumptions about the disorders; yet it can help to improve existing knowledge about nosology. Because the empirical approach starts with data derived from representative samples, its intrinsic validity is appealing. However, a disadvantage is that the empirically based syndrome scales vary as a function of the item content, the number of items, the statistical technique that was used to compute the syndromes, and the samples used to derive the data. As a consequence, the content and the number of scales differ across the different instruments.

An advantage of the a priori approach is that despite the lack of validity of most DSM and ICD (World Health Organization 1992) diagnostic categories, they represent a system that is widely accepted. This facilitates communication across researchers and clinicians.

Although the empirical and a priori approaches converge, they do not converge to a degree that one approach can replace the other (Edelbrock & Costello 1988; Jensen *et al.* 1993; Kasius *et al.* 1997). Both approaches are needed and can be combined. For example, the revision of the CBCL (Achenbach & Rescorla 2001), will make it possible to score the items on two sets of scales. One involves empirically derived scales, and the other scales related to DSM categories. Both sets can be scored quantitatively and categorically by imposing cutpoints to each scale (Achenbach & Rescorla 2000).

Overall index of psychopathology

If the main purpose is to decide only whether an individual has some form of psychopathology, syndrome scales may not be needed. The sum of the scores for all items (the total problem score) usually serves as a general indicator of the overall level of psychopathology. Most scales have this option in addition to syndrome scores. One, the 35-item PSC (Jellinek *et al.* 1986), designed for primary care settings, can only yield a total problem score.

Externalizing and internalizing scales

For some purposes, a level of precision that is intermediate between the fine-grained syndrome level and the crude total problem score may be desirable. For those purposes, a number of instruments use two broad band groupings: 'externalizing' and 'internalizing'. Externalizing reflects interpersonal and societal norm conflicts, whereas internalizing reflects internal distress. These groupings are usually determined through second-order factor analyses of the correlations among the syndrome scale scores. Some rating scales, such as the CBCL (Achenbach 1991a), the DSMD (Naglieri *et al.* 1994) and the BASC (Reynolds & Kamphaus 1992), can be scored in this way.

Weighting of items

It might be thought that simple summation of all items will lose valuable information, because some items are more important than others and should be weighted accordingly. Differential weighting using weights derived from factor analyses or regression analyses may yield greater precision in that sample. However, applying weights to new samples does not usually increase precision (Wainer 1976). Because the use of differential weighting contributes relatively little, except added complexity, all rating scales considered here use non-weighted summation scoring.

Percentiles and T-scores

The various subscales of the same instrument have different mean scores in normative samples because of differences in the number of items of each scale, and resulting differences in mean scores. Because each scale is scored on a different metric, comparisons across syndrome scales are difficult. How can a score of 20 on a syndrome scale (e.g. of aggression) with a scoring range between 0 and 40, be compared with a score of 10 on a syndrome scale (e.g. of depression) with a scoring range between 0 and 20? They are measured on different yardsticks so any comparison would require transforming the raw scores into scores that have a similar metric.

One approach is the use of *percentiles*. A percentile is the percentage of individuals who score below a certain value. The height and weight charts used to assess the physical development of children provide a well-known example. Percentiles can be computed on the basis of questionnaire scores for a representative normative sample of children whose scores are ranked from the highest to the lowest. The advantage of percentiles is that they are easy to interpret. For instance, if a boy received a score on the aggression scale corresponding with the 90th percentile, this means that only 10% of normal boys of the same age obtain higher aggression scores.

A second approach to transforming scores into ones that can be compared across scales with different metrics is the use of *T-scores*. A T-score is a score with a mean of 50 and a standard deviation of 10. A T-score of 50 will correspond with the 50th percentile. The advantage of both percentiles and T-scores is that they allow us to determine where an individual's score stands in relation to scores of individuals of the same sex and age. The utility of both percentiles and T-scores depends on the size and the representativeness of the reference samples.

Most instruments listed in Table 5.1 have data on reference samples and provide T-scores, including the ASEBA, BASC, CRS-R, DSMD, MMPI-A and the RBPC. Some instruments provide T-scores based on representative clinical samples in addition to T-scores based on normative samples. This is true for the ASEBA and the RBPC. T-scores based on clinical samples enable us to determine where an individual's score stands in relation to scores of individuals of the same sex and age who are referred for mental health services.

The MACI (Millon 1993) uses what the authors call 'base rate' scores that (arbitrarily) take account of the base rates of certain disorders in clinical samples.

Psychometric qualities of rating scales

Reliability

Any measurement is affected by both random and systematic error. The ratio of variability among subjects (true score variation) to the total measurement variability (the sum of subject variability, random error and systematic error) is called reliability. In practice, reliability refers to the replicability of measurement.

It is important to know the degree to which the same informants provide similar results on different occasions (see also Fombonne, Chapter 4). The time intervals used for assessing the *test–retest reliability* should be short enough to expect that the subject's behaviour will not have changed. In case of teachers as informants it is possible to assess the level of agreement between scores obtained from two teachers—*interrater reliability*.

Because parents are such a central source of information on their child's functioning, it is also helpful to know the degree of agreement between scores from fathers and mothers. Because reliability involves variation in assessments of the same phenomena, *interparent agreement* should not be treated as a reliability measure. Because ratings by mothers and fathers are based on somewhat different samples of the child's behaviour, interparent agreement is not expected to be as high as test–retest or interinterviewer reliability.

Scores obtained through repeated measurements can be affected both by their rank ordering and by differences in level so it is important that reliability measures reflect both. Pearson correlation coefficients are often used as reliability measures but they are affected only by differences in rank ordering of the correlated scores, whereas *t*-tests are affected only by differences in mean scores (level of the trait). A measure that is affected both by differences in the rank ordering and mean scores is the *intraclass correlation coefficient* (ICC; Shrout & Fleiss 1979). When evaluating the psychometric qualities of an instrument, it is important to be aware of the kind of reliability measure that is reported.

Reliability is often wrongly treated as an intrinsic characteristic of a measure. Reliability is highly linked to the population to which the measure is applied, and to the procedure with which the reliability was tested.

For most scales listed in Table 5.1, data on test–retest reliability are reported and, where appropriate, data on interrater reliability or interparent agreement. Reliability measures for these instruments are usually favourable for broad measures such as total problem scores. For some individual syndrome scales, reliability may be lower, and in fact problematic in some instances.

A somewhat different measure, also referred to as reliability, is the instrument's index of *internal consistency*, often presented as coefficient alpha, or Cronbach's alpha (Schmitt 1996). Alpha is a function of the interrelatedness of the items in a test. Internal consistency does not tell us anything about the degree to which an instrument will give us the same results over different occasions, such as the reliability measures discussed so far.

There is yet another problem with internal consistency in those instances where the scales are derived through principal components analysis. Because principal components analysis aims at arriving at scales with intercorrelated items, it is not surprising that measures of internal consistency for such scales are very high. In fact, measures of internal consistency for such scales are redundant as they do not give much new information. In most instances it is found that the shorter the scale, the lower the internal consistency.

Validity

Validity refers to the degree to which an instrument measures what it is designed to measure (see also Fombonne, Chapter 4). The most basic form of validity is *content validity*, meaning that the items tap the behaviours thought to be relevant because they map onto prevailing diagnostic concepts or because empirically they differentiate between clinically referred and non-referred children (if that is the purpose of the scale). The latter criterion may result in the conclusion on the scale of some rarely occurring, but usefully discriminatory, items. Thus, the CBCL has items dealing with self-harm, pica and faecal soiling.

Construct validity refers to the extent to which scores are related to external validating criteria, such as aetiology, outcome or response to treatment. Construct validation is an ongoing process of interrelated procedures through which we try to learn more about the construct. In this way, each new study can strengthen what Cronbach & Meehl (1955) called the 'nomological network' of interrelated procedures intended to reflect the underlying construct. Instruments used in many studies, such as the CRS (Wainwright 1996) and the CBCL (Vignoe et al. 1999), thereby have an advantage.

Concurrent validity concerns the associations (or correlations) between the scores on one instrument with those on other instruments designed to measure similar constructs. Why this should be carried out; if a good measure already exists, why

bother to test another one? It is usually performed because the instrument used as the criterion is too long or expensive. This may be the case when a brief and inexpensive rating scale is compared with a more time-consuming and expensive clinical interview. For example, the Youth Self-Report (YSR; Achenbach 1991d), an inexpensive and easy to administer self-report questionnaire, was correlated with the Semistructured Clinical Interview for Children and Adolescents (SCICA; McConaughy and Achenbach 1994), an interview that has to be given by a trained clinician (Kasius 1997). The intercorrelation between the two was 0.62, comparable to the mean correlation of 0.60 found for pairs of similar informants using the same scale (Achenbach et al. 1987).

Criterion-related validity refers to the relationship of a measure to another measure that is regarded as the 'gold standard'. For brief rating scales, this type of validity can be called *predictive validity*. The external reference criterion usually takes the form of a comprehensive definitive clinical diagnostic evaluation, but it is very dubious whether this should be viewed as a 'gold standard' in view of the uncertainties over the validity of such assessments. Questionnaire scores have been tested against DSM diagnoses derived from standardized interviews (e.g. Grayson & Carlson 1991; Kasius et al. 1997; Gadow & Sprafkin 1998), or with DSM diagnoses derived through unstandardized clinical procedures (Naglieri & Pfeiffer 1999).

Because of doubts about the superiority of one approach over others, these studies are really testing *concurrent* validity. This view is supported by Boyle et al. (1997) who compared the associations with external validators of a rating scale (the Ontario Child Health Study scales) and a psychiatric interview (the revised version of the Diagnostic Interview for Children and Adolescents; DICA). They concluded that validity differences between the two procedures were small and, where present, showed a somewhat better performance for the rating scales than the interview.

Referral status is used for many rating scales to test the criterion-related validity by testing the ability of an instrument to discriminate between children and adolescents who are referred for mental health services and those who are non-referred (ASEBA, CRS-R, RBPC, DSMD, Rutter, SDQ, CSI). Referral status is not an infallible morbidity criterion either, because some children and adolescents are referred for reasons other than being truly disordered. Equally, it is known that many disordered children and adolescents in the general population do not receive professional help for their problems. When an instrument is tested against referral status as the criterion, this may result in an underestimate of its ability to discriminate between disordered and normal children or adolescents.

Other validity issues

Measuring change

Because rating scales may be used to test changes over time, it is important that they are sensitive to such changes. Few tests of this feature have been undertaken with most scales. The CRS-R and earlier versions of the CRS have been shown to be sensitive to the effects of drug treatment of hyperactive children, supporting the validity of the hyperactivity construct (Conners 1999). The CBCL was found to be sensitive to change and to be useful for evaluating the clinical significance of therapeutic intervention (Kendall *et al.* 1999). The manual of the CBCL and related instruments (Achenbach 1991a–d) and a number of studies with the CBCL (Crijnen *et al.* 1997, 1999; Stanger *et al.* 1997) showed that the CBCL captures age differences in scores in cross-sectional as well as in longitudinal studies. However, these usually span longer time periods than used in trials of interventions.

Drop in scores on re-administration

A well-known, but poorly understood, phenomenon is that re-administration of a rating scale usually results in a decrease in scores (see Fombonne, Chapter 4). By testing differences in mean scores over time in test–retest analyses, the magnitude of differences in mean scores on re-administration can be determined; however, such information is available for very few scales. For the original version, as well as for the Dutch translation of the CBCL, it was found that for some scales re-administration resulted in a small but significant decrease in scores across intervals of 1–2 weeks (Achenbach 1991a; Verhulst *et al.* 1996). In a separate study, a decrease in CBCL scores was found over a 2-year period but this was not maintained at a 4-year follow-up (Verhulst & Althaus 1988; Verhulst *et al.* 1990). This decrease in levels of problems has also been reported for standardized interviews, both for adult and child psychiatric disorders (Edelbrock *et al.* 1985; Helzer *et al.* 1985).

The reason for this decline in scores on re-assessment is not known, so it is not clear how it should be dealt with. Case–control intervention comparisons should be robust to this bias because the decline should affect both, provided measures are taken at the same time intervals. The bias is more problematic in simple group longitudinal studies. Although not done routinely, it may be advisable to ask each respondent who completes a rating scale to indicate whether the same rating scale had been completed earlier.

Short vs. long rating scales

Most rating scales take between 10 and 20 min to complete. For screening and early assessment procedures in which a global impression of the child's functioning is needed, to be followed by more extensive assessment in a later phase for those who have elevated problem scores, a very brief rating scale is sometimes desirable. Another situation in which there is often a need for a very brief rating scale is when one teacher has to complete rating scales for many children in one classroom.

A number of rating scales in their standard format are relatively brief, such as the Eyberg Child Behaviour Inventory (ECBI), PSC, Revised Rutter Scales, and the SDQ. The ECBI and the PSC only provide an overall measure of dysfunctioning, whereas the other rating scales allow more differentiation and can be scored on syndrome scales.

The CRS-R has abbreviated versions in addition to the longer standard forms. The short parent form is approximately one-third of the length of the long form, and covers only four scales instead of the 14 scales in the long form. Although the correlations among the four scales of the short form and the corresponding scales of the long form are reported to be very high, there are no comparisons between the short and the long versions with respect to validation against external measures (Conners 1997). Also, it is clear that the short form gives a much less differentiated picture of the child's problems.

There are few studies that directly compare short vs. long rating scales. One study compared the short SDQ with the much longer CBCL (Goodman & Scott 1999). Scores from the SDQ and CBCL were equally able to discriminate psychiatric from non-psychiatric comparison children. As judged against a semistructured parent interview, the SDQ was better than the CBCL at detecting inattention and hyperactivity, and did equally well at detecting internalizing and externalizing problems.

For measuring psychopathology in adults, the General Health Questionnaire (GHQ; Goldberg & Williams 1988) is used with different numbers of items varying from the full 60 to 12. The shorter versions perform rather well in discriminating between psychiatric cases and normal individuals (Goldberg *et al.* 1997), and some even advocate the use of only four items of the GHQ to detect cases (Jacobsen *et al.* 1995).

The use of extremely brief rating scales with only a few items, questions the rationale for using a rating scale at all. Why not just pose two questions to parents: 'Do you think your child has a problem?', and 'Do you or other people have a problem with your child?' The fact that very short rating scales do not perform much worse than the longer versions in detecting psychiatric cases also reflects the lack of specificity of psychopathology, and casts doubt on the usefulness of mass screening if the initial screening is not followed by more extensive evaluation.

Measures of accuracy of a rating scale

Rating scales applied to populations not known to have psychiatric conditions can be regarded as *screening tests*, whereas the same rating scales applied to populations known to have symptoms can be termed *diagnostic tests* (Weiss 1998). The underlying rationale for the use of a test is identical for both screening and diagnostic tests. The rationale is that among individuals to whom the test is administered, the monetary, physical and psychological costs of the condition along with the cost of the test and the errors that arise when the test does not classify individuals accurately, will be exceeded by the costs of the condition had the test not been carried out.

Sensitivity, specificity and predictive value

The usefulness of a test depends on its accuracy. This can be assessed in several different ways: by sensitivity, specificity, positive and negative prediction. The meaning of these terms, and how to measure them is described by Fombonne (Chapter 4). As he points out, sensitivity and specificity do not reflect an intrinsic quality of a test; they will vary with the samples on which they were based and with the critical values chosen. Robins (1985) showed how the sensitivity of a test for the presence of a psychiatric disorder was higher in a patient sample than in a general population sample (such tests usually detect severe cases more readily than mild ones), but specificity will be higher in general population than in patient samples. Cutpoints are chosen by making compromises among several considerations. Any cutpoint chosen is a trade-off between sensitivity and specificity.

The relationship between sensitivity and specificity can also be expressed by a Receiver Operating Characteristic (ROC) curve. The ROC curve is constructed by plotting the sensitivity on the vertical axis, against the false positive rate (100-specificity) on the horizontal axis. The use of ROC curves has two advantages. The curve readily shows the trade-off between sensitivity and specificity, and so indicates the optimal scoring range for choosing the cutpoint that provides the best match with the aims of the user. The area under the curve (AUC) can be computed and used as an index for the criterion-related validity of a test. The AUC can be conceptualized as the probability of correctly identifying a randomly chosen pair of individuals (one who has the disorder, one who does not have the disorder). The AUC ranges between 0.5, which indicates that the test does not add to the chance probability of correctly classifying individuals, and 1.0 which would indicate a perfect test. The AUC enables us to compare the discriminative power of different rating scales (Kresanov et al. 1998).

We can also express the accuracy of a test as the extent to which being categorized as 'test positive' or 'test negative' actually predicts the presence of the disorder. This may be an important method by which to determine the probability that an individual has a certain disorder, given the results of a test.

Predictive value is much influenced by prevalence. In a sample with relatively few disordered individuals, the positive predictive value (PV+) of even a very specific test will be low, meaning that a 'positive' result will yield many false positives. If the same test was used in a sample with a much higher prevalence, the PV+ would be much higher. This makes screening for very rare disorders, such as autism, using rating scales in community settings unattractive. Although the problem of low base rates for predicting rare conditions, even with highly valid tests, was observed long ago (Meehl & Rosen 1955), Clark & Harrington (1999) showed that few child mental health professionals who regularly use questionnaires to screen for mental disorders were aware of this problem. A technique that can be used to overcome low base rates problems is *sequential screening* (Derogatis & Lynn 1999; see epidemiological applications below).

For some rating scales in Table 5.1, the authors specify the sensitivity and specificity (ASEBA, Rutter, SDQ, PSC, CSI); they are usually satisfactory and in the same range as rating scales for adult psychiatric disorders. However, the relative nature of these measures makes it imperative for the potential user to judge these values against the background of the specific purpose for which the rating scales is intended.

Scoring procedures and interpretation

The scoring procedures and the interpretation of the results of a rating scale should be easy to follow and understandable. Most rating scales have scoring forms or graphic displays that describe the scores relative to the norms. Computerized scoring and profile printouts in graphic form have many advantages. The majority of rating scales listed in Table 5.1 have the option of using computerized scoring, including the ASEBA, CRS-R, BASC, DSMD, CSI, MMPI-A and the MACI. Rating scales are developed to assist in determining the likelihood that the subject does or does not have the specific problem the instrument is designed to identify. Use for any other purpose (e.g. assigning a diagnosis based solely on the instrument's results) only serves to undermine the integrity of the instrument (Maruish 1999, p. 16).

Translation

There is a growing need for translations of psychometrically sound rating scales, mostly from English into other languages. This comes from researchers and clinicians in various countries, but also from researchers and clinicians who work in major metropolitan areas with their multiethnic multilanguage character.

There are no generally accepted guidelines for gauging the adequacy of translation, although there is an increasing awareness of the many difficulties in the faithful translation of instruments (Weisz & Eastman 1995; Streiner & Norman 1998; Canino & Bravo 1999; see also Fombonne, Chapter 4). To ensure optimal accuracy in translations, some authors advise repetition of the translation-back-translation procedure (Weisz & Eastman 1995), whereas others emphasize the importance of field testing (Canino & Bravo 1999). However, even very accurate translations may result in linguistic nuances that need explicit reporting.

The CBCL (Achenbach 1991a), the CSI (Gadow & Sprafkin 1998), the CRS-R (Conners 1997), the DSMD (Naglieri et al. 1994) and the Revised Rutter Scales have all been translated into multiple languages.

Accurate translation is the first step towards using an existing instrument in different cultural settings. The second step is the testing of the instrument's psychometric properties in these other contexts, including the reliability and validity. In particular, the determination of the factorial structure needs to be determined in case empirically derived syndromes are used. The third step is the derivation of reference scores, both in representative normative and clinical samples. The last step is the testing of the generalizability of the results by comparing population norms (Crijnen *et al.* 1997, 1999), and by comparing the factor structure across different cultural settings.

Advantages and disadvantages of rating scales

One of the great advantages of rating scales over clinical interviews is that they can be applied in a flexible, easy to administer and economic way. Administration time is usually modest— some 10–20 min. Rating scales are also characterized by great flexibility in the way they can be administered: in person, by telephone or by mail. Administration can be facilitated by using computer-assisted client entry programs. Some rating scales, such as the ASEBA, CRS-R, and the BASC have a computer-assisted client entry program.

Rating scales need not be administered by expensive clinically trained professionals. This means that they can be routinely administered in (mental) health settings at intake, or can be used in large-scale epidemiological surveys. Thanks to their practicality, many rating scales also have good data on reliability and validity.

Rating scales also have a number of disadvantages, some of which are shared by other measurement procedures. They are limited to the informant's perspective. Characteristics of the informant and the tendency toward response biases are sources of variation in ratings (Briggs-Gowan *et al.* 1996; Fergusson 1997; Sawyer *et al.* 1998). Scales are limited to the structured scores for standardized items. Information that may be relevant but that is not covered by the items of the scale will be missed. It is not possible to explore the informant's responses and subjective experiences, nor is it possible to observe behaviour directly. Misunderstandings and ambiguous answers that may be clarified in a clinical interview are missed when using questionnaires. Slight changes in the wording of instructions, or the wording of the items themselves, may have large effects that limit comparability (Woodward *et al.* 1989). Despite these limitations, one study that directly compared the validity of a rating scale against a structured interview in the ability to predict external criteria did not find the rating scale to be less valid (Boyle *et al.* 1997). Many of these problems can be prevented by unambiguous wording of items and instructions. For instance, before having a respondent complete a screening questionnaire, we must have an indication of the respondent's reading skills.

Use of rating scales as screening instruments

Because rating scales are relatively inexpensive and easy to administer, they are often thought of as handy tools for screening large populations both for research and community health pur-

poses. The medical meaning of screening refers to the examination of asymptomatic or non-referred people in order to classify them as likely or unlikely to have the disease that is the object of screening (Morrison 1998). People who appear likely to have the disease are investigated further to arrive at a final diagnosis. Those people who are then found to have the disease are treated. When the application of early diagnosis and treatment is organized within large groups, this is described as mass screening or population screening. It is not readily evident that psychiatric conditions meet all the criteria for being subjected to screening programmes (Derogatis & Lynn 1998).

First, screening is a method originally developed for detecting highly specific medical target conditions that are either present or absent, such as phenylketonuria or breast cancer or HIV. Medical screening usually has a narrow focus, and is able to use a single test with a high degree of diagnostic precision. In contrast, psychiatric disorders lack specificity and do not have a highly accurate diagnostic test.

The second concern is that most child and adolescent psychiatric disorders are not characterized by an asymptomatic or benign period in which detection can be reliably and validly performed. Moreover, most conditions lack a clear-cut well-delineated onset (see Sandberg & Rutter, Chapter 17). If subthreshold psychopathology is accepted as a risk factor for the persistence or recurrence of psychopathology, then the early detection of problems could be advantageous. The moderate to strong continuity of problem behaviour from childhood or adolescence into young adulthood supports this view (Ferdinand *et al.* 1995; Verhulst & Van der Ende 1995; Hofstra *et al.* 2000). It has been found that high levels of parent reported problem behaviours in non-referred children from the general population were not only predictive of referral for mental health services as recorded in a psychiatric case register in the year following the assessment, but they were almost equally strong predictors of referral for up to 5 years later (Laitinen-Krispijn *et al.* 1999). Earlier detection and subsequent treatment may improve the prognosis or reduce the period of suffering.

The third factor that makes it not readily evident that mass screening is helpful is that is has not been definitively demonstrated that treatment or prevention of child and adolescent disorders at the stage before disorder is manifest is beneficial (see Brent, Chapter 54).

We do not advocate the use of rating scales, or any other assessment procedure, in mass population screening to detect whether or not a certain psychiatric condition is present. However, if precision in individual diagnosis is not required, as in epidemiological studies in which the error can be taken into account, or if early assessment is just one component in decision making, then there is a place for the use of rating scales.

Application of rating scales in screening procedures and early assessment

Epidemiological application of screening procedures

Epidemiology, with its emphasis on large-scale measurements, has an evident need for assessment procedures that are accurate, practical and economical. When the first child psychiatric epidemiological studies were planned, the lack of such assessment procedures was the driving force for developing the first generation of brief rating scales. The first version of the Rutter scales proved their value in the Isle of Wight study (Rutter *et al.* 1970).

Multistage/multimethod sampling

Epidemiological measures for large-scale descriptive or aetiological studies need to be brief and inexpensive. Especially when investigating conditions with low base rates, it is problematic to assess many individuals who do not have a disorder with elaborate procedures. Therefore, it is advantageous to use a multistage sampling approach (Dohrenwend & Dohrendwend 1982; Verhulst & Koot 1992; Derogatis & Lynn 1998).

In stage 1, a rating scale is applied to the total sample in which the base rate of a disorder is relatively low. Individuals with high problem scores are designated cases or 'screen positives'. All others are designated non-cases or 'screen negatives'. The advantage here is that although a low base rate has a bad effect on positive predictions, its impact on negative predictions is far less.

In stage 2, all 'screen positives' (thereby an enriched sample with a higher prevalence rate, so avoiding the problematic effect of low base rates) and a random sample of the 'screen negatives' from stage 1, are assessed using more elaborate procedures, such as a clinical interview. The results of the interviews will confirm or disconfirm 'caseness' as determined in stage 1.

For some purposes this two-stage approach may be sufficient. However, if greater precision is desirable, a third assessment procedure can be introduced, preferably using other indices of malfunctioning. This may be a measure of social impairment or some alternative method, such as the use of records.

Either total problem scores or specific syndrome scale scores can be used in these ways. Some individuals who score above the cutpoint of a specific syndrome scale may score below the cutpoint for the total problem score and vice versa. Because selection of individuals based solely on one strategy may miss cases that would have been identified by the other strategy, it may be advantageous to combine both approaches. By doing so not only will the number of cases identified by the procedure be raised (a higher sensitivity), but the number of normal individuals misclassified as disordered will also be raised (lower specificity). This need not be a problem if a higher specificity in the stage 2 assessment is achieved.

Specific questionnaires, generic questionnaires, or both?

When information about only one disorder (such as depression) is sought, it is possible to use a brief questionnaire in stage 1 that is focused only on the condition of interest. However, if a specific selection strategy in stage 1 is chosen, it is important that the stage 2 assessments cover a much broader range of psychopathology otherwise problems that are associated with depression (such as conduct problems or substance abuse; see Rutter, Chapter 28) will be missed.

A question that may arise is whether it is better to use one generic rating scale or multiple specific rating scales at the initial stage of assessment. Most generic rating scales have the option of using the total problem score, the specific syndrome scales, or both, to score each individual. A disadvantage of using multiple instruments that only assess one area (such as depression, anxiety, or hyperactivity) is that each instrument has its own metric and norms, making comparisons difficult, and there may be considerable overlap in the items across the various instruments. Accordingly, we do not advocate the general use of multiple focused scales for sceening purposes. An exception when this might be a preferred option is when it is important to detect disorders not well encompassed by syndrome scores and which might not be picked up by a high total score. This might apply, for example, to obsessive-compulsive disorders, Tourette syndrome and anorexia nervosa.

Combining information from multiple informants

For all the reasons discussed here and by Fombonne (Chapter 4) all stages of epidemiological assessment need to be based on multiple informants. The key issue is how best to combine this information. Each strategy for combining the results from multiple informants has its consequences for the sensitivity and specificity of the assessment procedure. If any positive result is accepted, the sensitivity of the procedure will be higher than when all tests need to be positive. The more restrictive the criterion, the lower the sensitivity will be, and the more disturbed the individuals who are selected (Verhulst *et al.* 1994).

There is another way to combine information from different informants by treating the data from rating scales as continuous scores. The problem that different scores will have different metrics can be overcome by transforming the scores for each version into standard scores (z-scores) with a mean of 0 and a standard deviation of 1. It is now possible to compute each individual's mean z-score across the different informant versions of rating scales. By applying a cutpoint to the frequency distribution of this mean score, we can determine the individuals who score above this cutpoint and who may be selected for further evaluation (Verhulst *et al.* 1997).

Clinical applications of rating scales

The application of rating scales need not to be confined to community samples, but can also be applied in routine clinical practice to assist in decision-making. Many countries have financial or other constraints on the services that can be provided to children and adolescents with mental health problems. Rating scales can help in ensuring that professionals' valuable time is used in the most efficient and productive way. At the time of referral, decisions are needed on whether assessment at this particular clinic is the most appropriate way of proceeding; if it is, what sort of diagnostic assessment should be undertaken, what type of treatment should be provided for how long, what type and degree of improvement should be expected with intervention, and what should be done after treatment?

Clinical practice can benefit from a standardized approach to these various decisions. When decisions are based on explicit rules and procedures, we may improve our ways of helping young people. The series of steps that need to be taken from first contact with the clinic to the time of case closure should be based on an adequate database, and at each point decisions need to be taken on what is needed for that purpose. Clearly, it would not be feasible for everyone to have the fullest evaluation from the most experienced clinicians at all stages. Rather, some sort of filter, or process of triage, is needed to decide which cases need the most extensive and specialized assessments and treatments.

Rating scales can have a useful role in this process. For example, they may be mailed to parents, teachers or the adolescents themselves before first attendance. Many clinicians combine this contact with a request to the family to outline their main concerns and questions that they want addressed. This combination of standardized measurement and open-ended enquiry can be useful in guiding the form of the initial (fuller) evaluation, and it may also assist decisions on which part of the clinical service should be involved.

Once a comprehensive formulation has been made (questionnaires can never provide that), rating scale data can aid in the selection of the key targets for intervention. It has been found that interventions that are effective under research conditions are often much less so under typical clinical conditions (Weisz *et al.* 1992). If standardized assessments are used systematically to identify the target problems that should be matched with the most appropriate treatment, it may be possible to improve the efficacy of interventions in routine practice. Similarly, by monitoring the effects of interventions, it should be possible to decide whether the treatment is being effective or whether a change needs to be considered. Rating scales can have a valuable role in this monitoring because they are quantified and provide measures that are comparable from case to case. The same advantages apply to the assessment of outcome.

How to select a rating scale

In our review of generic rating scales we were more impressed by the similarities among the various scales than we were with their differences. Most cover a roughly similar content, although their extensiveness varies, most have evidence of reliability and validity, most are user-friendly and most can be scored in a comprehensive way. However, there are some differences that may be relevant for some purposes. Answers to a series of questions may help in making a choice of which scale to use.

1 Do I need multiple informants? The ASEBA, CSI, CRS-R and the SDQ have versions for parents, teachers and self-report on problems.

2 Do I need a rating scale for early assessment/screening, or do I need one for more extensive evaluation, and will the instrument be completed for one individual or for many individuals by the same informant? Most scales take 10–20 min to complete. The ECBI, PSC, Revised Rutter Scales and the SDQ are much shorter. However, only the Revised Rutter Scales and the SDQ can be scored on specific syndrome scales and not only on a global index of malfunctioning. The CRS-R has both short and long forms.

3 Do I need to assess problems only, or do I need to assess competence as well? The ASEBA, BASC, the Revised Rutter Scales and the SDQ have scales for adaptive functioning.

4 Do I want to obtain ratings that can be scored on DSM-orientated scales, on empirically derived scales, or both? Five instruments have empirically derived scales (ASEBA, BASC, CRS-R, DSMD, RBPC), whereas the other seven have a priori derived scales. The new version of the ASEBA will have both options: the same rating scale can be scored on empirically derived scales as well as on DSM-orientated scales.

5 Are translations of the instrument available in the languages I need? The most widely used scales (ASEBA, CRS-R, Revised Rutter Scales) have the advantage that they are translated in different languages. This is not only an advantage for cross-cultural research but also for the assessment of children from different cultures living in our present day pluriform societies.

6 Are there local norms available for the instrument or not? The ASEBA is probably the instrument with the largest number of normative data from different countries.

7 Do I want to compare my findings with those from others? The most widely used instruments (ASEBA, CRS-R, Revised Rutter Scales) have the most well-documented and published findings with which new findings can be compared.

Challenges and prospects for the future

It is hard to imagine that any future rating scale would be much better than the ones that already exist, or that this new instrument would solve the problems that are probably inherent in the assessment of child psychopathology. Rather than designing new instruments, the challenge for the future lies in the improvement of the construction and, especially, the use of scales. This may come from the application of modern statistical techniques (such as structural equation modelling) and from genetic studies that aim at constructing phenotypes that are more genetically informative. Also, the development of parallel scoring of the same instrument on both empirical and DSM-orientated scales may be a step towards more informative diagnostic information.

There is an increasing need for more standardized assessment of child psychiatric conditions and for evaluation of treatment. Rating scales can be valuable in clinical practice where research standards are increasingly adopted. Future directions then include the development of methodologies, including the use of rating scales, that will enhance clinical decision making.

Appendix 1

Description of generic screening questionnaires

Achenbach System of Empirically Based Assessment (ASEBA)

The ASEBA (Achenbach 1991a–d, 1992, 1999; McConaughy & Achenbach 1994; Achenbach & Rescorla 1999) are rating scales for assessing psychopathology, social competence and adaptive behaviours. There are separate forms for different ages and for parents, teachers and self-reports. The forms for parents are: the Child Behavior Checklist/2–3 (CBCL/2–3) for ages 2–3 years; and the Child Behavior Checklist/4–18 (CBCL/4–18) for ages 4–18 years. The forms for teachers are: the Caregiver–Teacher Report Form (C-TRF) for ages 2–5 years; and the Teacher's Report Form (TRF) for ages 5–18 years. The self-report form, the Youth Self-Report (YSR), is for ages 11–18 years. The items for assessing psychopathology are rated on a 3-point scale ranging from 'Not true' to 'Very true or often true'. The items of the CBCL/4–18, TRF and YSR are scored on the eight scales listed in Table 5.1 for ages 4–11 and 12–18 years, although the number of items per scale varies slightly across informants. The items of the CBCL/2–3 and C-TRF are scored on separate scales. For the CBCL/2–3 these scales are Anxious/Depressed, Withdrawn, Sleep Problems, Somatic Complaints, Aggressive Behaviour and Destructive Behaviour. For the C-TRF these scales are Anxious/Obsessive, Depressed/Withdrawn, Fears, Somatic Problems, Immature, Aggressive Behaviour, and Attention Problems. The CBCL/4–18, TRF, YSR, CBCL/2–3 and C-TRF can be scored on the composite scales of Internalizing, Externalizing and Total Problems. CBCL/4–18, TRF and YSR norms for different gender and age groups 4–11 and 12–18 years are based on a representative sample of children who were not referred for mental health services or did not attend special classes in the year prior to data collection. Rating scales can be scored using hand scoring profiles or computer scoring profiles. The computer scoring profiles also gives the level of agreement between informants. Computer software for administering the rating scales is available. The CBCL is translated into nearly 60 languages. The bibliography of published studies using ASEBA (Vignoe *et al.* 1999) lists over 3000 studies.

Behavioral Assessment System for Children (BASC)

The BASC (Reynolds & Kamphaus 1992; Kamphaus *et al.* 1997; Kamphaus *et al.* 1999) are rating scales for assessing psychopathology, self-perceptions and personality. There are separate forms for different ages and for parents, teachers and self-reports (only for perceptions and personality). The Parent Rating Scale (PRS) forms are for ages 2½–5, 6–11 and 12–18 years. The Teacher Rating Scale (TRS) forms are for ages 2½–5, 6–11 and 12–18 years. The self-report forms, the Self-Report of Personality (SRP), are for ages 8–11 and 12–18 years (not listed in Table 5.1). The items of the PRS and TRS are rated on a 4-point scale ranging from 'Never' to 'Almost always'. The items are scored on the scales listed in Table 5.1, with scales and number of items per scale varying slightly across ages and informants. The PRS cannot be scored on the scales Learning Problems, Study Skills, and on the composite scale School Problems. The SRP assesses personality traits; therefore they are not listed here (Reynolds & Kamphaus 1992). Norms for different gender and age groups are based on a representative sample, except for the SRP which was based on convenience samples. Rating scales can be scored using hand scoring profiles or computer scoring profiles. Computer software for administering the rating scales is available.

Child Symptom Inventories (CSI)

The CSI (Gadow & Sprafkin 1996, 1997a,b, 1998, 1999) are rating scales for assessing psychopathology. There are separate forms for different ages and for parents, teachers and self-reports. The forms for parents and teachers are: the Early Childhood Inventory-4 (ECI) for ages 3–5 years, the Child Symptom Inventory-4 (CSI) for ages 6–11 years, the Adolescent Symptom Inventory-4 (ASI) for ages 12–18 years. The self-report form is the Youth's Inventory-4 (YI) for ages 12–18 years. Most items are rated on a 4-point scale ranging from 'Never' to 'Very often'. Some items are rated with only 'No' or 'Yes'. The items of the CSI are scored on scales representing DSM-IV categories (see Table 5.1). Scales and number of items per scale vary slightly across ages and informants. Norms for different gender and age groups 3–5, 6–11 and 12–18 years are based on samples of children who did not receive special education services. Rating scales can be scored using hand scoring profiles or computer scoring profiles.

Conners' Rating Scales–Revised (CRS-R)

The CRS-R (Conners 1997; Conners *et al.* 1997, 1998a,b) are rating scales for assessing psychopathology. There are separate forms for different ages and for parents, teachers and self-reports. The form for parents is the Conners' Parent Rating Scale (CPRS-R:L) for ages 3–17 years. The form for teachers is the Conners' Teacher Rating Scale (CTRS-R:L) for ages 3–17 years. The self-report form is the Conners/Wells Adolescent Self-Report of Symptoms (CASS:L) for ages 12–17 years. These forms also exist in short versions for parents (CPRS-R:S), teachers (CTRS-R:S) and self-report (CASS:S). The items are rated on a 4-point scale ranging from 'Not true at all' to 'Very much true'. The items of the CRS-R are scored on the scales in Table 5.1, although scales and number of items per scale vary slightly across ages and informants. The CTRS-R:L does not have a Psychosomatic scale. The items of the CASS:L are scored on different scales than the scales of the CPRS-R:L and the CTRS-R:L. The items of the CASS:L are scored on Family Problems, Emotional Problems, Conduct Problems, Cognitive Problems/Inattention, Anger Control Problems, Hyperactivity, ADHD Index, DSM-IV Symptoms, DSM-IV Inattentive, and DSM-IV Hyperactive-Impulsive. Norms for different gender and age groups 3–5, 6–8, 9–11, 12–14 and 15–17 years are based on representative samples. Rating scales can be scored using hand scoring profiles or computer scoring profiles. Computer software for administering the CRS-R is available. An annotated bibliography (Wainwright 1996) lists over 450 studies.

Devereux Scales of Mental Disorders (DSMD)

The DSMD (Naglieri et al. 1994) are rating scales for assessing psychopathology. There are separate versions for different ages and for parent and teachers. The parent and teacher forms are for ages 5–12 and 13–18 years. The items are rated on a 5-point scale ranging from 'Never' to 'Very frequently'. The rating scales are scored on the scales in Table 5.1, although scales and number of items per scale vary slightly across ages and informants. The scale Attention is for ages 5–12 years only, and the scale Delinquency is for ages 13–18 years only. Norms for different gender and age groups 5–11 and 12–18 years are based on a representative sample of children who did not receive special education services. Rating scales can be scored using hand scoring profiles and computer scoring profiles.

Eyberg Child Behaviour Inventory (ECBI) and Sutter–Eyberg Student Behaviour Inventory–Revised (SESBI-R)

The ECBI and SESBI-R (Eyberg & Pincus 1999) are rating scales for assessing disruptive behaviours. There are separate forms for different informants. The form for parents is the ECBI for ages 2–16 years. The form for teachers is the SESBI-R for ages 2–16 years. The items are rated on a 7-point Intensity scale, and on a Problem scale with 'True' or 'False' answering categories. Norms for different gender groups are based on a representative sample. The rating scale is hand scored.

Millon Adolescent Clinical Inventory (MACI)

The MACI (Millon 1993) is a rating scale for assessing personality and psychopathology. There is only a self-report for ages 13–19 years. The items are rated with 'True' or 'False' answering categories. The items of the MACI are scored on scales indicating personality traits and scales indicating psychopathology. Only the psychopathology scales are listed in Table 5.1. Norms for different gender and age groups 13–15 and 16–19 years are based on a representative sample. Rating scales can be scored using hand scoring profiles.

Minnesota Multiphasic Personality Inventory–Adolescent (MMPI-A)

The MMPI-A (Butcher et al. 1992) is a rating scale for assessing personality and psychopathology. There is only a self-report for ages 14–18 years. The items are rated on 'True' or 'False' answering categories. The items of the MMPI-A are scored on scales indicating personality traits and scales indicating psychopathology. Only the psychopathology scales are listed in Table 5.1. Norms for different gender groups are based on a representative sample. Rating scales can be scored using hand scoring profiles.

Paediatric Symptom Checklist (PSC)

The PSC (Jellinek et al. 1979, 1986; Jellinek & Murphy 1988; Pagano et al., 2000) are rating scales for assessing psychopathology. There are separate versions for different parents and self-reports. The form for parents is for ages 2–16 years. The self-report form is for ages 11–16 years. The items are rated on a 3-point scale ranging from 'Never' to 'Often'. The items of the PSC can only be scored on a Total Problem scale. The rating scale is hand scored. A form for teachers is currently being tested.

Revised Behaviour Problem Checklist (RBPC)

The RBPC (Quay & Peterson 1996) is a rating scale for assessing psychopathology. There is a single form for both parents and teachers for ages 5–18 years. The items are rated on a 3-point scale ranging from 'Not a problem' to 'Severe problem'. The items of the RBPC are scored on the scales in Table 5.1. Norms for different gender and age groups 5–8, 9–11 and 12–13 years are based on samples of children who did not receive special education services. Rating scales can be scored using hand scoring profiles.

Revised Rutter Scales (Rutter)

The Revised Rutter Scales (Rutter et al. 1970; Rutter 1976; Elander & Rutter 1996a,b; Hogg et al. 1998) are rating scales for assessing psychopathology and prosocial behaviour. There are separate versions for ages 3–5 and 6–16 years, and for parents and teachers. The items are rated on a 3-point scale ranging from 'Does not apply' to 'Certainly applies'. The items of the Revised Rutter Scales are scored on the scales in Table 5.1. Rating scales can be scored using hand scoring sheets.

Strengths and Difficulties Questionnaire (SDQ)

The SDQ (Goodman 1997; Goodman et al. 1998; Goodman & Scott 1999) are rating scales for assessing psychopathology and prosocial behaviour. There are separate forms for parents and teachers for ages 4–16 years. The self-report form is for ages 11–16 years. The items are rated on a 3-point scale ranging from

'Not true' to 'Certainly true'. The items of the SDQ are scored on the scales in Table 5.1. Cutpoints for discriminating between normal and clinical cases based on community and clinical samples are available. Rating scales can be scored using hand scoring sheets.

References

Achenbach, T.M. (1991a) *Manual for the Child Behavior Checklist/4–18 and 1991 Profile*. Department of Psychiatry, University of Vermont, Burlington, VT.

Achenbach, T.M. (1991b) *Integrative guide for the 1991 CBCL/4–18, YSR, and TRF profiles*. Department of Psychiatry, University of Vermont, Burlington, VT.

Achenbach, T.M. (1991c) *Manual for the Teacher's Report Form and 1991 Profile*. Department of Psychiatry, University of Vermont, Burlington, VT.

Achenbach, T.M. (1991d) *Manual for the Youth Self-Report and 1991 Profile*. Department of Psychiatry, University of Vermont, Burlington, VT.

Achenbach, T.M. (1992) *Manual for the Child Behavior Checklist/2–3 and 1992 Profile*. Department of Psychiatry, University of Vermont, Burlington, VT.

Achenbach, T.M. & Rescorla, L.A. (1999) *Mental Health Practitioners' Guide for the Achenbach System of Empirically Based Assessment (ASEBA)*. Department of Psychiatry, University of Vermont, Burlington, VT.

Achenbach, T.M. & Rescorla, L.A. (2000) *Manual for the ASEBA Preschool Forms and Profiles*. Department of Psychiatry, University of Vermont, Burlington, VT.

Achenbach, T.M. & Rescorla, L.A. (2001) *Manual for the ASEBA School Age Forms and Profiles*. Research Center for Children, Youth and Families. University of Vermont, Burlington, VT.

Achenbach, T.M., McConaughy, S.H. & Howell, C.T. (1987) Child/adolescent behavioral and emotional problems: implication of cross-informant correlations for situational specificity. *Psychological Bulletin*, 101, 213–232.

Achenbach, T.M., Howell, C.T., Quay, H.C. & Conners, C.K. (1991) National survey of problems and competencies among 4- to 16-year-olds: parents' reports for normative and clinical samples. *Monographs of the Society for Research in Child Development*, 56, 1–131.

American Psychiatric Association (1994) *Diagnostic and Statistical Manual of Mental Disorders*, 4th edn. American Psychiatric Association, Washington D.C.

Boyle, M.H., Offord, D.R., Racine, Y.A., Szatmari, P., Sanford, M. & Fleming, J.E. (1997) Interview versus checklists: adequacy for classifying childhood psychiatric disorder based on parent reports. *Archives of General Psychiatry*, 54: 793–799.

Briggs-Gowan, M.J., Carter, A.S. & Schwab-Stone, M. (1996) Discrepancies among mother, child and teacher reports: examining the contributions of maternal depression and anxiety. *Journal of Abnormal Psychology*, 24, 749–765.

Butcher, J.N., Williams, C.L., Graham, J.R. *et al.* (1992) MMPI-A (Minnesota Multiphasic Personality Inventory–Adolescent): manual for administration. *Scoring and Interpretation*. University of Minnesota Press, Minneapolis.

Canino, G. & Bravo, M. (1999) The translation and adaptation of diagnostic instruments for cross-cultural use. In: *Diagnostic Assessment in Child and Adolescent Psychopathology* (eds D. Shaffer, C.P. Lucas & J.E. Richters), pp. 285–298. Guilford Press, New York.

Clark, A. & Harrington, R. (1999) On diagnosing rare disorders rarely: appropriate use of screening instruments. *Journal of Child Psychology and Psychiatry*, 40, 287–290.

Conners, C.K. (1997) *Conners' Rating Scales: Revised Technical Manual*. Multi Health Systems, North Tonawanda, New York.

Conners, C.K. (1999) Conners' Rating Scales: Revised. In: *The Use of Psychological Testing for Treatment Planning and Outcomes Assessment* (ed. M.E. Maruish), 2nd edn, pp. 467–495. Lawrence Erlbaum, Mahwah, NJ.

Conners, C.K., Wells, K.C., Parker, J.D.A., Sitarenios, G., Diamond, J.M. & Powell, J.W. (1997) A new self-report scale for asessment of adolescent psychopathology: factor structure, reliability, validity, and diagnostic sensitivity. *Journal of Abnormal Child Psychology*, 25, 487–497.

Conners, C.K., Sitarenios, G., Parker, J.D.A. & Epstein, J.N. (1998a) Revision and restandardization of the Conners Teacher Rating Scale (CTRS-R): factor structure, reliability, and criterion validity. *Journal of Abnormal Psychology*, 26, 279–291.

Conners, C.K., Sitarenios, G., Parker, J.D.A. & Epstein, J.N. (1998b) The revised Conners' Parent Rating Scale (CPRS-R): factor structure, reliability, and criterion validity. *Journal of Abnormal Psychology*, 26, 257–268.

Crijnen, A.A.M., Achenbach, T.M. & Verhulst, F.C. (1997) Comparisons of problems reported by parents of children in 12 cultures: total problems, externalizing, and internalizing. *Journal of the American Academy of Child and Adolescent Psychiatry*, 36 (9), 1269–1277.

Crijnen, A.A.M., Achenbach, T.M. & Verhulst, F.C. (1999) Problems reported by parents of children in multiple cultures: the Child Behavior Checklist Syndrome Constructs. *American Journal of Psychiatry*, 156, 569–574.

Cronbach, L.J. & Meehl, P.E. (1955) Construct validity in psychological tests. *Psychological Bulletin*, 52, 281–302.

De Groot, A., Koot, H.M. & Verhulst, F.C. (1994) The cross-cultural generalizability of the CBCL cross-informant syndromes. *Psychological Assessment*, 6 (3), 225–230.

De Groot, A., Koot, H.M. & Verhulst, F.C. (1996) Cross-cultural generalizability of the Youth Self-Report and Teacher's Report Form cross-informant syndromes. *Journal of Abnormal Child Psychology*, 24 (5), 651–664.

Derogatis, L.R. & Lynn, L.L. (1999) Psychological tests in screening for psychiatric disorder. In: *The Use of Psychological Testing for Treatment Planning and Outcomes Assessment* (ed. M.E. Maruish), 2nd edn, pp. 41–79. Lawrence Erlbaum, Mahwah, NJ.

Dohrenwend, B.P. & Dohrenwend, B.S. (1982) Perspectives on the past and future of psychiatric epidemiology. *American Journal of Public Health*, 72, 1271–1279.

Edelbrock, C. & Costello, A.J. (1988) Convergence between statistically derived behavior problem syndromes and child psychiatric diagnoses. *Journal of Abnormal Child Psychology*, 16, 219–231.

Edelbrock, C.S., Costello, A.J., Dulcan, M.K., Kalas, R. & Conover, N.C. (1985) Age differences in the reliability of the psychiatric interview of the child. *Child Development*, 56, 265–275.

Elander, J. & Rutter, M. (1996a) Use and development of the Rutter parents' and teachers' scales. *International Journal of Methods in Psychiatric Research*, 6, 63–78.

Elander, J. & Rutter, M. (1996b) An update on the status of the Rutter parents' and teachers' scales. *Child Psychology and Psychiatry Review*, 1, 31–35.

Eyberg, S. & Pincus, D. (1999) *ECBI: Eyberg Child Behavior Inventory and SESBI-R: Sutter-Eyberg Student Behavior Inventory-Revised Professional Manual*. Psychological Assessment Resources, Odessa, FL.

Ferdinand, R.F., Verhulst, F.C. & Wiznitzer, M. (1995) Continuity and change of self-reported problem behaviors from adolescence into young adulthood. *Journal of the American Academy of Child and Adolescent Psychiatry*, **34**, 680–690.

Fergusson, D.M. (1997) A brief introduction to stuctural equation models. In: *The Epidemiology of Child and Adolescent Psychopathology* (eds F.C. Verhulst & H.M. Koot), pp. 122–145. Oxford Medical Publications, Oxford.

Gadow, K.D. & Sprafkin, J. (1996) *Early Childhood Inventories Manual*. Checkmate Plus, Stony Brook, NY.

Gadow, K.D. & Sprafkin, J. (1997a) *Adolescent Symptom Inventory 4 Screening Manual*. Checkmate Plus, Stony Brook, NY.

Gadow, K.D. & Sprafkin, J. (1997b) *ADHD Symptom Checklist-4 Manual*. Checkmate Plus, Stony Brook, NY.

Gadow, K.D. & Sprafkin, J. (1998) *Child Symptom Inventory 4 Screening manual*. Checkmate Plus, Stony Brook, NY.

Gadow, K.D. & Sprafkin, J. (1999) *Youth's Inventory 4 Manual*. Checkmate Plus, Stony Brook, NY.

Goldberg, D. (2000) Plato versus Aristotle: categorical and dimensional models for common mental disorders. *Comprehensive Psychiatry*, **41** (Suppl. 1), 8–13.

Goldberg, D.P. & Williams, P. (1988). *A User's Guide to the GHQ*. NFER-Nelson, Windsor.

Goldberg, D.P., Gater, R., Sartorius, N. *et al.* (1997) The validity of two versions of the GHQ in the WHO study of mental illness in general health care. *Psychological Medicine*, **27**, 191–197.

Goodman, R. (1997) The Strengths and Difficulties Questionnaire: a research note. *Journal of Child Psychology and Psychiatry*, **38**, 581–586.

Goodman, R. & Scott, S. (1999) Comparing the Strengths and Difficulties Questionnaire and the Child Behavior Checklist: is small beautiful? *Journal of Abnormal Child Psychology*, **27**, 17–24.

Goodman, R., Meltzer, H. & Bailey, V. (1998) The Strengths and Difficulties Questionnaire: a pilot study on the validity of the self-report version. *European Child and Adolescent Psychiatry*, **7**, 125–130.

Grayson, P. & Carlson, G.A. (1991) The utility of a DSM-III-R based checklist in screening child psychiatric patients. *Journal of the American Academy of Child and Adolescent Psychiatry*, **30**, 669–673.

Helzer, J.E., Robins, L.N., McEvoy, L.I. *et al.* (1985) A comparison of clinical and Diagnostic Interview Schedule diagnoses: physician re-examination of lay-interviewed cases in the general population. *Archives of General Psychiatry*, **42**, 657–666.

Hofstra, M.B., Van der Ende, J. & Verhulst, F.C. (2000) Continuity and change of psychopathology from childhood into adulthood: a 14-year follow-up study. *Journal of the American Academy of Child and Adolescent Psychiatry*, **39**, 850–858.

Hogg, C., Rutter, M. & Richman, N. (1998) Emotional and behavioural problems in children. In: *Child Psychology Portfolio* (ed. I. Sclare), pp. 1–13. NFER-Nelson, London.

Jacobsen, B.K., Hasvold, T., Høyer, G. & Hansen, V. (1995) The General Health Questionnaire: how many items are really necessary in population surveys? *Psychological Medicine*, **25**, 957–961.

Jellinek, M.S. & Murphy, J.M. (1988) Screening for psychosocial disorders in pediatric practice. *American Journal of Diseases in Children*, **142**, 1153–1157.

Jellinek, M., Evans, N. & Knight, R.B. (1979) Use of a behavior checklist on a pediatric inpatient unit. *Journal of Pediatrics*, **94**, 106–115.

Jellinek, M., Murphy, J.M. & Burns, B. (1986) Brief psychosocial screening in outpatient pediatric practice. *Journal of Pediatrics*, **109**, 371–378.

Jensen, P.S., Salzberg, A.D., Richters, J.E. & Watanabe, H.K. (1993) Scales, diagnoses and child psychopathology. I. CBCL and DISC relationships. *Journal of the American Academy of Child and Adolescent Psychiatry*, **32**, 397–406.

Jensen, P.S., Rubio-Stipec, M., Canino, G. *et al.* (1999) Parent and child contributions to diagnosis of mental disorder: are both informants always necessary? *Journal of the American Academy of Child and Adolescent Psychiatry*, **38**, 1569–1579.

Kamphaus, R.W., Huberty, C.J., DiStefano, C. & Petoskey, M.D. (1997) A typology of teacher-rated child behavior for a national US sample. *Journal of Abnormal Child Psychology*, **25**, 453–463.

Kamphaus, R.W., Petoskey, M.D., Cody, A.H., Rowe, E.W. & Huberty, C.J. (1999) A typology of parent-rated child behavior for a national US sample. *Journal of Child Psychology and Psychiatry*, **40**, 607–616.

Kasius, M.C. (1997) *Interviewing children: development of the Dutch version of the semistructured clinical interview for children and adolescents (SCICA) and testing of the psychometric properties*. Unpublished doctoral thesis: Erasmus University, Rotterdam, The Netherlands.

Kasius, M.C., Ferdinand, R.F. & Van den Berg, H. & Verhulst, F.C. (1997) Associations between different diagnostic approaches for child and adolescent psychopathology. *Journal of Child Psychology and Psychiatry*, **38**, 625–632.

Kendall, P.C., Marrs-Garcia, A., Nath, S.R. & Sheldrick, R.C. (1999) Normative comparisons for the evaluation of clinical significance. *Journal of Consulting and Clinical Psychology*, **67**, 285–299.

Koot, H.M., Van den Oord, E.J.C.G., Verhulst, F.C. & Boomsma, D.I. (1997) Behavioral and emotional problems in young preschoolers: cross-cultural testing of the validity of the Child Behavior Checklist/2–3. *Journal of Abnormal Child Psychology*, **25** (3), 183–196.

Kresanov, K., Tuominen, J., Piha, J. & Almqvist, F. (1998) Validity of child psychiatric screening methods. *European Child an Adolescent Psychiatry*, **7**, 85–95.

Laitinen-Krispijn, S., Van der Ende, J., Wierdsma, A.I. & Verhulst, F.C. (1999) Predicting adolescent mental health service use in a prospective record-linkage study. *Journal of the American Academy of Child and Adolescent Psychiatry*, **38**, 1073–1080.

Maruish, M.E. (1999) *The Use of Psychological Testing for Treatment Planning and Outcomes Assessment*, 2nd edn. Lawrence Erlbaum, Mahwah, NJ.

McConaughy, S.H. & Achenbach, T.M. (1994) *Manual for the Semistructured Clinical Interview for Children and Adolescents*. Department of Psychiatry, University of Vermont, Burlington, VT.

Meehl, P.E. & Rosen, A. (1955) Antecedent probability and the efficiency of psychometric signs, patterns, or cutting scores. *Psychological Bulletin*, **52**, 194–216.

Millon, T. (1993) *The Millon Adolescent Clinical Inventory Manual*. NCS, Minneapolis, MN.

Morrison, A.S. (1998) Screening. In: *Modern Epidemiology* (eds K.J. Rothman & S. Greenland), pp. 499–518. Lippincott-Raven, PA.

Naglieri, J.A. & Pfeiffer, S.I. (1999) Use of the Devereux Scales of Mental Disorders for diganosis, treatment planning, and outcome assessment. In: *The Use of Psychological Testing for Treatment Planning and Outcomes Assessment* (ed. M.E. Maruish), 2nd edn, pp. 535–561. Lawrence Erlbaum, Mahwah, NJ.

Naglieri, J.A., LeBuffe, P.A. & Pfeiffer, S.I. (1994) *Devereux Scales of Mental Disorders*. Psychological Corporation, San Antonio, TX.

Pagano, M.E., Cassidy, L.J., Murphy, J.M., Little, M. & Jellinek, M.S. (2000) Identifying school-age children at risk: the Pediatric Symptom Checklist as a self-report measure. *Psychology in the Schools*, **37**, 91–106.

Quay, H.C. & Peterson, D.R. (1996) *Revised Behavior Problem Checklist*. Psychological Assessment Resources, Odessa, FL.

Reynolds, C.R. & Kamphaus, R.M. (1992) *Manual for the Behavior Assessment System for Children*. American Guidance Service, Circle Pines, MN.

Robins, L.N. (1985) Epidemiology: reflections on testing the validity of psychiatric interviews. *Archives of General Psychiatry*, **42**, 918–924.

Rutter, M. (1967) A children's behaviour questionnaire for completion by teachers: preliminary findings. *Journal of Child Psychology and Psychiatry*, **8**, 1–11.

Rutter, M., Tizard, J. & Whitmore, K. (1970) *Education Health and Behaviour*. Longman, London. (Reprinted 1981, Krieger, Melbourne.)

Sawyer, M.G., Streiner, D.L. & Baghurst, P. (1998) The influence of distress on mothers' and fathers' reports of childhood emotional and behavioral problem. *Journal of Abnormal Child Psychology*, **26**, 407–414.

Schachar, R., Rutter, M. & Smith, A. (1981) The characteristics of situationally and pervasively hyperactive children: implications for syndrome definition. *Journal of Child Psychology and Psychiatry*, **22**, 375–392.

Schmitt, N. (1996) Uses and abuses of coefficient alpha. *Psychological Assessment*, **8**, 350–353.

Shaffer, D., Fisher, P.W. & Lucas, C.P. (1999a) Respondent-based interviews. In: *Diagnostic Assessment in Child and Adolescent Psychopathology* (eds D. Shaffer, C. Lucas & J. Richters), pp. 3–33. Guilford Press, New York.

Shaffer, D., Lucas, C.P. & Richters, J.E. (1999b) *Diagnostic Assessment in Child and Adolescent Psychopathology*. Guilford Press, New York.

Shrout, P.E. & Fleiss, J.L. (1979) Intraclass correlations: uses in assessing rater reliability. *Psychological Bulletin*, **86**, 420–428.

Stanger, C., Achenbach, T.M. & Verhulst, F.C. (1997) Accelerated longitudinal comparisons of aggressive versus delinquent syndromes. *Development and Psychopathology*, **9**, 43–58.

Streiner, D.L. & Norman, G.R. (1998) *Health Measurement Scales: a Practical Guide to Their Development and Use*. Oxford University Press, Oxford.

Van der Valk, J., Van den Oord, E., Verhulst, F.C. & Boomsma, D. (2001) Using parental ratings to study the etiology of 3-year-old twins' problem behaviours: different views or rater bias? *Journal of Child Psychology and Psychiatry*, **42**, 921–931.

Verhulst, F.C. & Althaus, M. (1988) Peristence and change in behavioral/emotional problems reported by parents of children aged 4–14: an epidemiological study. *Acta Psychiatrica Scandinavica*, **77** (Suppl. 339), 1–28.

Verhulst, F.C. & Koot, H.M. (1992) *Child Psychiatric Epidemiology*. Sage Publications, Newbury Park.

Verhulst, F.C. & Van der Ende, J. (1995) The eight year stability of problem behavior in an epidemiologic sample. *Pediatric Research*, **38**, 612–617.

Verhulst, F.C., Koot, H.M. & Berden, G.F.M.G. (1990) Four-year follow-up of an epidemiological sample. *Journal of the American Child and Adolescent Psychiatry*, **29**, 440–448.

Verhulst, F.C., Koot, H.M. & Van der Ende, J. (1994) Differential predictive value of parents' and teachers' reports of children's problem behaviors: a longitudinal study. *Journal of Abnormal Child Psychology*, **22**, 531–546.

Verhulst, F.C., Van der Ende, J. & Koot, H.M. (1996) *Handleiding voor de CBCL/4–18 (Manual for the CBCL/4–18)*. Afdeling Kinder-en Jeugdpsychiatrie, Sophia Kinderziekenhuis/Academisch Ziekenhuis Rotterdam. Erasmus University, Rotterdam, The Netherlands.

Verhulst, F.C., Dekker, M. & Van der Ende, J. (1997) Parent, teacher and self-reports as predictors of signs of disturbance in adolescents: whose information carries the most weight? *Acta Psychiatrica Scandinavica*, **96**, 75–81.

Verhulst, F.C., Van der Ende, J., Ferdinand, R.F. & Kasius, M.C. (1997) The prevalence of DSM-III-R diagnoses in a national sample of Dutch adolescents. *Archives of General Psychiatry*, **54**, 329–336.

Vignoe, D., Bérubé, D.L. & Achenbach, T.M. (1999) *Bibliography of Published Studies Using the Child Behavior Checklist and Related Materials: 1999 Edition*. Department of Psychiatry, University of Vermont, Burlington, VT.

Wainer, H. (1976) Estimating coefficients in linear models: it don't make no nevermind. *Psychological Bulletin*, **83**, 231–217.

Wainwright, A. (1996) *Conners' Rating Scales: Over 25 Years of Research — an Annotated Bibliography*. Multi-Health Systems, Toronto.

Weiss, N. (1998) Clinical epidemiology. In: *Modern Epidemiology* (eds K.J. Rothman & S. Greenland), pp. 519–528. Lippincott-Raven, PA.

Weisz, J.R. & Eastman, K.L. (1995) Cross-national research on child and adolescent psychopathology. In: *The Epidemiology of Child and Adolescent Psychopathology* (eds F.C. Verhulst & H.M. Koot), pp. 42–65. Oxford Medical Publications, Oxford.

Weisz, J.R., Weiss, B. & Donenberg, G.R. (1992) The lab versus the clinic: effects of child and adolescent psychotherapy. *American Psychologist*, **47**, 1578–1585.

Woodward, C.A., Thomas, H.B., Boyle, M.H., Links, P.S. & Offord, D.R. (1989) Methodologic note for child epidemiological surveys: the efforts of instructions on estimates of behavior prevalence. *Journal of Child Psychology and Psychiatry*, **30**, 919–924.

World Health Organization (1992) Mental disorders. *Glossary and Guide to Their Classification in Accordance with the Tenth Revision of International Classification of Diseases*, 10th edn. World Health Organization, Geneva.

6

Psychological Testing and Observation

Joseph Sergeant and Eric Taylor

Introduction

The approach of a psychologist to assessing a case is that of an investigator. The first step is to understand and clarify the problem being presented, and from then on the process of assessment is a succession of formulating hypotheses about the nature of the problem, testing them, and modifying the formulation and the intervention plan accordingly. From this perspective, a 'test' is any systematic and quantified way of describing behaviour. It may be as highly standardized as an IQ test, or it may be developed and used for the unique problems of an individual case. The rating scale and interview approaches described by Verhulst & Van der Ende (see Chapter 5) and Angold (see Chapter 3) are tests in this sense; so are psychophysiological measures and naturalistic observations. It is important for the assessor to think broadly and creatively about the process of assessment, and to bring together different sources of evidence (see Rutter & Yule, Chapter 7).

The more narrow and traditional definitions of psychological tests concentrate on those procedures and instruments that have been standardized through psychometric refinement, have demonstrated satisfactory reliability, and are known to be valid in giving descriptions of an individual child in relation to the rest of the population or in predicting a specified criterion. Such tests can bring power to clinical inferences, because they allow one to know the accuracy with which a test can be generalized to other circumstances—whether, for instance, it will give the same result if administered again. Some clinical problems lend themselves very well to the use of such batteries: for example, whether a child who is failing to make school progress has an impairment of intellectual function. IQ scales then include a good (but not complete) description of a range of functions. Even then, the essential rationale remains that of testing a falsifiable hypothesis. However, many clinical problems require one to go beyond the boundaries of standardized tests. The assessor will then consult the research literature for suitable measures as well as compendia of established tests (Sattler 2001).

This volume describes many clinical uses of psychological tests and systematic observational schemes. They include contributing to psychiatric diagnosis, as of disorders in the autism spectrum (see Lord & Bailey, Chapter 38); to neurological diagnosis, as in the early stages of dementing disorders (see Goodman, Chapter 14); resolving differences when there are discrepant accounts of a child's competence or problems, as in the case of hyperactivity (see Schachar & Tannock, Chapter 25);

and differentiating between the various possible causes of a clinical problem, such as reading (see Snowling, Chapter 40). They contribute strongly to decisions outside the mental health services, for instance in helping to determine special needs in education (see Howlin, Chapter 68). Most of them give rise to one or more of a key set of objectives for the assessment process: describing a child's behaviour or cognitive performance relative to that of other children; predicting the future; determining profiles of performance to indicate whether one ability is out of keeping with others; analysing the reasons for discrepancy between different reports; explaining a behaviour change or cognitive alteration by reference to another level of description; and tracking changes over time.

The development of psychological testing and observation has been a process of making mental assessments more reliable and closer to what they seek to measure. Test developers start from concepts of the mental function they wish to assess. They seek to make the assessments *quantitative*, so that individuals can be ordered according to level of function they show; *standard*, so that the ways assessments are made are constant; *referenced*, so that children can be ordered with respect to the population they come from; and *explicit*—for example, in interrater reliability and stability—so that the strengths and limitations of inferences based upon them can be known.

All these are aspirations of other types of assessment too. Investigators developing rating scales (see Verhulst & Van der Ende, Chapter 5) and standardized interviews (see Angold, Chapter 3) have also made explicit their reliability and validity and established normative values. The characteristic quality of tests is that they are also *operational*. That is to say, they seek to obtain more objective data than can be obtained through the filter of descriptions made by people who are already in a relationship with the child. They specify what procedures are to be carried out—for example, what task the child is asked to do—and provide explicit ways of scoring the child's responses.

Observational methods are not usually so well operationalized (although they can be) and they may be conducted in naturalistic as well as in controlled settings. However, they do provide either control or careful description of the stimulus setting, they substitute a professional observer of known reliability for the involved parent or teacher, and correspondingly they are able to record behaviour more accurately and more precisely. Further, they may be necessary to interpret the validity of test results.

Tests of cognition

Descriptions of individual differences

The key concept in the minds of early developers of cognitive tests was 'intelligence' (Binet 1905). There were already many and varying definitions even by that time; but the main notions were the capacity to learn from experience and the ability to adapt successfully to changing environmental demands. More recently, Gregory (1981) has succinctly described intelligence as the creation and understanding of successful novelty.

The tests that were developed therefore used problems that would be novel to a child being tested. They were intended at first for educational purposes. If one knows only that a child is failing in school, there is no way of distinguishing ability from motivation or previous learning experiences. The use of an IQ scale aims to control for previous learning by giving quite unfamiliar and culture-fair problems, and for motivation by providing a standard setting with distractions minimized. If this is successful—and the extent to which it is successful is an empirical question—then a poor score suggests low aptitude.

The study of individual differences in test scores proved to be very productive. Scores were stable over time (see below) and predicted quite well to real-world measures such as examination grades. In turn, the technology of IQ testing altered concepts of intelligence. Long familiarity with IQ scores has led most clinicians tacitly to accept that intelligence is what an IQ score measures, and that it is an important aspect of mental function. This is in some contrast to developing theories of cognitive functioning, which largely reject a unified intellectual capacity, and propose a variety of independent (but cooperating) systems for processing information, or a hierarchy of competencies (Sternberg & Kaufman 1988). Furthermore, the advent of cognitive paradigms in experimental psychology in the 1960s generated a different approach to information processing. This work was theory driven (Broadbent 1971) and could predict human performance in relation to task demands, stimuli, temporal characteristics and the effect of higher order control systems (Sanders 1983). In contrast to the psychometric approach in IQ development (where norms and standardization are key issues), cognitive psychologists showed that task performance on tests and paradigms depended upon whether the task demands were continuously varying or held constant (Shriffrin & Schneider 1977). From this emerged the concept of *controlled* and *automatic* processing, whereby attentional allocation and resource deployment depended upon whether the task was new or old. Later work showed that cognitive resources not only depended upon this distinction but also upon whether in a double task, the child was required to perform attentional switches (Allport & Styles 1997).

The tension between 'cognitive' and 'IQ' approaches is pervasive. It is one of the reasons that some practitioners have abandoned intellectual testing in their work with children. Yet the practical value of tests is substantial. IQ tests have evolved through several generations since the original work of Binet and Simon to the modern test batteries described below. The most influential consist of a range of different, short puzzles that require a variety of intellectual operations to solve them. They are given on a one-to-one basis, the child sitting with the examiner in a quiet and distraction-free room. The examiner takes care to establish a rapport with the child, explains what will happen and allays worries about the situation. This usually entails going through the same process with the parent, and explaining why the child is being seen separately from them. General encouragement to performance is given, but not feedback about whether individual answers are correct.

Standardized scores for each subtest are calculated on the basis of the child's performance and age. The scores show a Gaussian distribution in the population, not because this reflects a fundamental truth about the population but because the tests have been developed in order to give such a distribution. Statistical methods of taxonomy—especially, factor analysis—have been applied to them so that the results from the variety of items can be reduced to a small number of factor scores, and ultimately to a single score, the IQ. The standardization of the tests ensures that these scaled scores will have a mean of 100 and a standard deviation of 15. The IQ score therefore gives an estimate of the individual's deviation from the population mean. The main such test 'batteries' are described below. It is also possible to use the individual subtests as measures of more specific processes, though caution is needed in this. The reliability of an individual subtest is considerably less than that of the scales based on several subtests. Correspondingly, there needs to be a large difference between one subtest score and what is expected from other scores before one can conclude that poor performance on what that subtest measures is a robust description of the child's ability. Even scale scores can be influenced by many factors, and a trained psychologist's judgement is needed to interpret them.

Stability of individual differences

Early in the development of IQ tests, longitudinal studies followed individuals with regular testing from infancy into adult life: after the age of about 6 years there were high correlations between test scores at different times, typically of the order 0.8 over 5-year periods (Bayley 1949). The prediction is substantial but incomplete, and individuals can show considerable difference between successive administrations. Nevertheless, Moffitt *et al.* (1993) have analysed trajectories of intellectual development in a longitudinal study of a birth cohort, and have stressed that continuity of individual differences is the rule. When a child has departed from the previous trajectory at a testing point, then he or she is likely to return to the previous level at subsequent testing points. Most change over time is unpredictable and seldom shows evidence of systematic increase or decline.

At the individual level, it is not possible to regard IQ as a fixed capacity. As most change is random, then a child who is far removed from the mean when first tested is likely to be closer to the mean on subsequent testing. This can be quantified for the group—for instance, if the correlation between two age points is 0.7, then children will regress almost half the distance towards the mean at subsequent testing. This cannot be taken to the individual level, and clinicians should remember that there is change as well as continuity in test scores. When decisions have to be based upon IQ tests (e.g. recommendations about suitable schools) the psychologist should retest and not base judgements on outdated information.

Test scores also predict other qualities of children. Some of these are important only at the extremes of the range. An IQ less than 50, for example, predicts quite strongly that there will be structural abnormalities of the brain, that there will be a much higher prevalence than normal of known medical causes of intellectual retardation, that independent life will not be reached in adulthood, that fertility will be reduced, and so on. For reasons such as these, the categories of intellectual handicap are an important classification of clinical cases and constitute one of the axes of the ICD-10 diagnostic scheme.

Profile analysis

It can be of great help in assessing a case to know that different abilities are out of keeping with one another. For instance, for a child who is failing in school and scoring poorly on IQ tests, it may be very illuminating to know that all the depression of the scores can be accounted for by one factor, such as processing speed. A specific rather than a global impairment is suggested. It helps the child and family to understand the problem, and it suggests strategies to teachers: in this instance, perhaps to relax time pressure.

The distinction of global and specific delays is not exclusive. A child with global delay may still have an extra problem in one type of function, such as language (see Bishop, Chapter 39). Detecting a specific problem in the presence of a global one would be very difficult in the absence of quantified tests for a range of functions.

It is important to remember that this practical value does not depend on acceptance of any one theory. Even those who reject the idea of a unified concept of intelligence, and prefer to think of a number of specific intelligences, will find it valuable to describe children in terms of their strengths and weaknesses. An investigator who is trying to establish whether a particular function is impaired will need to establish whether it is impaired by comparison with other functions. IQ is convenient as a summary description of some of those functions. Its value therefore does not depend upon supposing that it indexes an underlying entity. Indeed, judgement is often needed in deciding exactly what one is controlling for, and therefore on the exact tests to be used. If the aim is to measure short-term memory, then one would want to say that it is (or is not) disproportionate to scores on IQ tests that do not place much load on memory. One is controlling for other aspects of test performance. If memory tests were included in the IQ measure that is used as a control, one would be in danger of controlling out the main subject of study.

Analysis of impaired function

Psychological testing is also used in a more explanatory way. The aim then is to clarify a known problem by reference to a more fundamental level of description. An example would be the testing of a child with poor reading. Not only can the severity of the reading problem be quantified and its severity be shown to be out of proportion to general cognitive development, but it can also be shown to be associated with a finding of specific problems in phonological processing or word recognition (see Snowling, Chapter 40).

The process of understanding a dysfunction often takes the investigator to the research literature, selecting tests from experimental psychology that may not have much normative data. Caution is needed when applying tests, whose validity is known only at the group level, to individuals. This is all the more true when a test is given repeatedly with systematic variation in the way it is given. Experimental control of one aspect of a test is, in theory, a powerful way of analysing a deficit. For example, it might be highly relevant to know that a child had poor performance on a continuous performance test (CPT) of attention when given without incentives, yet a normal performance when correct responses were rapidly rewarded. Experimental tests are often set up in this way for comparing groups. For assessing individuals, the reliability between two administrations of the test should ideally be known. Without this knowledge, test results should be seen as aids to making a clinical formulation, not as direct providers of diagnostic information. Nevertheless, the suggestions made from analysing problems in this way are often illuminating, and can be tested by the consequences of actions based on them.

Descriptions of outcome

Clinicians often wish to quantify change over time—both the natural course of disorder and the response to treatment. Accurate quantification helps not only in detecting subtle differences (e.g. whether attention has improved during a course of stimulant medication) but also in allowing for the fact that the child is maturing over the period of observation. Cognitive tests standardized for different ages are therefore very valuable. They can, however, be confounded by the effects on test scores of repeating the test. 'Practice' effects are of various kinds. First, and simplest, the child may remember from one administration to another what the answers were, so that memory rather than problem-solving is being tested on the second occasion. This kind of practice effect is perhaps the easiest for the clinician to manage. Some tests have alternative forms available, so that the second presentation can be of different material but of comparable difficulty. For a well-standardized scale, such as the Wechsler, the effects of repeated testing are known and can be allowed for, both by specifying the minimum time between administrations for them to be valid and by providing tables for the probable limits of practice effects. For less well-standardized tests, even the simple effects of practice may be unknown.

A second kind of practice effect is more fundamental: the child has acquired an insight into how to do tests of this type. For instance, an effective strategy for coding one set of symbols into another may only have been worked out by the end of the first test administration, but is available right from the start of a second. This is best detected by the observation of the alert examiner, who will be noting the way that the child is carrying out the test as well as recording the score.

A third kind of practice effect, particularly affecting attentional performance, is a shift from automatic to controlled processing in the same test. Some tests evoke both automatic and controlled processing, so that the effects of repetition are complex. For example, the Stroop test (see Executive Function, below) is based upon an interference effect between an overlearned and automatic process—reading words such as red, blue, green and yellow—and the controlled process of inhibiting the reading and naming the colour in which they are printed. With repetition the inhibition may become automatic. The converse of the Stroop effect is the phenomenon that controlled attention is independent of past learning and depends upon the child being able to meet changing relations within the task. For example, in one version of the CPT, the letter that has to be identified as a target changes from trial to trial. This places demands upon the child that are different from the version of the CPT in which the target remains constant over the entire series of trials. In the first case there is clearly demanded controlled attention. In the second case the child may learn the target–non-target relations and become swifter in performance as the task progresses. If sufficient trials are given in the constant target condition, a relatively automatic process of detection will develop, which is called an automatic attention response. Thus analysis of the task demands of what is apparently the same test, the CPT, can involve quite different attentional processes, each of which are of interest in themselves. These subtle differences may point to quite different types of deficits in attention, and may vary in different ways over time.

For all these reasons, one should record in detail the previous testing history of the child. Even when carrying out an initial assessment, it is important to find out whether the child has had any previous exposure to the test so that possible practice effects can be allowed for.

Cognitive tests and test batteries

Tests differ in the psychological functions measured and the cognitive theories that underlie them. For example, the Wechsler scales (see below) derive from a psychometric approach. Subscales are derived from factor analysis, and items are chosen partly for the strength of their loadings on specific factors. The aim is to give an economical description of a range of performance scores, and the scales are not necessarily to be reified into specific mental modules. By contrast, more recent scales such as the Kaufman (see below) were developed to reflect more explicitly the theoretical distinctions between different types of cognitive function that have come from experimental psychology. Many cognitive tests are available, and we mention only a few: they are chosen to indicate the range of purposes and methods, and the considerations that enter into the choice of test. To go more deeply into the existing tests, the reader may consult a recent review (e.g. Sparrow & Davis 2000) or text book (e.g. Sattler 2001).

Intellectual functions

The Wechsler Intelligence Scales are the most popular of all the comprehensive and general-purpose test batteries. The Wechsler Preschool and Primary Scale of Intelligence-Revised (WPPSI-R) (Wechsler 1989) is standardized for ages 3–7 years; the Wechsler Intelligence Scale for Children–Third Edition (WISC-III) (Wechsler 1991) for ages 6–16 years; and the Wechsler Adult Intelligence Scale–Third Edition (WAIS-III) (Wechsler 1997) for ages 16–74 years. The extensive data available about them, their translation into a number of languages, and the existence of norms for some countries outside the USA (e.g. for Wechsler 1992a) are all substantial advantages. Each subtest is standardized to a mean of 10 and standard deviation of 3 and has a range of 3 standard deviations on either side of the mean. The two subscales—verbal and performance IQ—and the full scale IQ have means of 100 and standard deviations of 15. The standardization allows quantitative inferences to be made about the significance of discrepancies between the scales and the reliability of differences between two administrations. Figures for judging the reliability of subtest scores on items such as memory have also been published (Ryan et al. 2000).

These are, of course, statistical considerations. A 'significant' discrepancy means that it is likely to be a reliable description of that child's performance but it does not in itself imply a pathological cause. Further, a 'verbal-performance' distinction is about the type of information that is being presented, not the way it is being handled. Many practitioners prefer to base their interpretations on a four-factor solution: verbal comprehension, perceptual organization, freedom from distractibility and processing speed. These roughly correspond to some clinical distinctions, e.g. groups of children with attention deficit hyperactivity disorder (ADHD) tend to have low scores on 'freedom from distractibility', and children with language disabilities tend to score poorly on 'verbal comprehension' (Wechsler 1991). However, the match cannot be pushed too far; there is considerable overlap between groups, and individual diagnosis on this basis should not be attempted.

The Wechsler scales have been criticized on various grounds—most pervasively, for lacking a clear theoretical rationale (some perceive this as a strength). Individual items have been criticized for including emotionally laden material, information derived from education, and language-driven instructions. These could reduce its fairness to children from adverse backgrounds or whose native language is different from that of the tester. The corresponding advantage is that it does include important aspects of linguistic and social intelligence for use in groups to whom they are appropriate. The 3-standard deviation range (either side of the mean) makes it somewhat insensitive to differences at the extremes of the range.

Other tests are also available, some of which avoid some of the disadvantages and are preferred in some situations. The Stanford–Binet Test, Fourth Edition (SB-IV) (Thorndike *et al.* 1986) has the longest pedigree of any test. The norms are good, and extend from age 2 years to adulthood. It shares many of the limitations of the Wechsler, and the linguistic demands of test presentation are considerable. It does have a potential advantage in assessing differences at the top end of the IQ range, and is sometimes used by those assessing gifted children. A version has also been developed for children with visual impairment (Perkins–Binet Test of Intelligence for the Blind; Davis 1980).

The Leiter International Performance Scale–Revised (Roid & Miller 1997) avoids much of the dependence upon language to understand tests—which are presented with pantomime and simple practice items. Its norms extend from age 2 to 20 years and it yields standard scores on scales of reasoning, visualization, attention and memory. It is therefore popular in assessing children with communication problems. Raven's Progressive Matrices (PM) (Court & Raven 1995) are suitable from age 5 years to adult life. Like the Leiter, the tests can be presented with virtually no spoken language; like the Leiter, they are untimed. PM testing is quicker, but less comprehensive, than most other tests of intellectual function. Both these tests are useful in assessing children with hearing impairment. The Hiskey–Nebraska Test of Learning Aptitude (Hiskey 1966) is particularly intended for hearing-impaired children and has been standardized for them (ages 3–17 years).

The Kaufman Assessment Battery for Children (Kaufman & Kaufman 1983) is firmly based on cognitive theory, and especially on the distinction between sequential processing (involved in processing information that is ordered in time or space) and simultaneous processing (in which several pieces of information are integrated and processed as a whole) (Luria 1980). In practice most 'simultaneous' tasks are visuoperceptual, and most 'sequential' tasks are verbal or motor; so the theoretical distinctions may be confounded in practice. Other items are derived from Piagetian theory and from Luria's notions of high-level planning ability (especially decision-making and hypothesis evaluation). The test was standardized on 2000 children in the USA. It covers ages 2–12 years (and the Kaufman Adult and Adolescent Intelligence Test extends the range to adult life). It has been translated into several languages, though not yet standardized for other cultures. Its exclusion of verbal abilities and specific knowledge has made it of particular interest to those working with children with communication disorders. It gives not only Sequential Processing and Simultaneous Processing scales but also a Mental Processing Composite that is equivalent to an IQ score.

The Cognitive Assessment Scale (Naglieri & Das 1997) is another attempt to combine psychometric credibility with satisfying psychological theory, and yields subscales of planning, attention, simultaneous and successive processes, as well as

a Full Scale. It was standardized on 2200 children in the USA, and its validity was tested in several criterion groups. It is too early to assess its full value, and especially the extent to which it will prove culture-fair.

The British Ability Scales (Cook 1988) also include items that are based on current cognitive theories of attention, information processing and memory. The test battery was standardized on 1700 children in the UK, which has made it popular in this country. It covers ages 2–6 years in one form, and 6–18 years in another. It yields scales of verbal (often interpreted as 'crystallized') and non-verbal (often interpreted as 'fluid') reasoning and spatial ability; there is a general conceptual ability scale (corresponding to IQ) and another general measure from which verbal test scores have been excluded ('special non-verbal composite').

Neuropsychological tests

Neuropsychological test batteries base their component tests on theories rather different from those informing IQ tests—those of brain–behaviour relationships (Korkman 1999). Their emphasis in the past has been on those tests that are similar to the adult neuropsychological tests that have shown themselves sensitive to localized neurological disorders, e.g. the Halstead–Reitan battery (Reitan & Wolfson 1993) and Luria Nebraska (Golden 1987). Scepticism has often been expressed about the extent to which this localization is relevant to the problems shown by children with brain abnormalities, for whom the psychological consequences are characterized by plasticity and compensation and by global rather than specific outcomes (Taylor 1991). More recent development of neuropsychological batteries aim to give a broader description of the strengths and weaknesses of cognitive function. The NEPSY (Korkman *et al.* 1997), for example, includes scores for language and communication, sensorimotor functions, visuospatial abilities, learning and memory, and executive functions such as attention and planning. It therefore represents something of a compromise between the psychometrically based tests such as the Wechsler (with their advantage of comprehensiveness) and the more experimental neuropsychological tests (with their advantage of close and detailed analysis of a specific function).

The study of brain–behaviour relationships in cognition is currently undergoing a rapid and exciting change. The correlation of psychological test performance with underlying alterations of the brain has been thrown into revolution by the advent of modern neuroimaging (see Bailey, Chapter 10). Some tests have shown surprisingly strong associations, e.g. tests of attention with size of frontal structures and basal ganglia (Castellanos 1997). It is too soon to know how far this process will go, but it seems to give promise of understanding which functions are carried out in a modular way by particular brain structures, and which (and how) are served by the cooperative working of several brain structures. Such tests are likely to play an increasingly large part in the future of assessing children psychologically.

The most common neuropsychological functions assessed are the following.

Language

The verbal IQ of the Wechsler can give a general guide. More detailed analyses of language function are available, such as the Clinical Evaluation of Language Fundamentals–Third Edition (CELF-3; Semel *et al.* 1995). Language assessments can make distinctions about types of language impairment, e.g. comprehension, expression and pragmatic use, and quantify the degree of any impairment (see Bishop, Chapter 39).

Memory

Brief tests stressing memory are found in the Wechsler Memory Scales, Binet Short-Term Memory, and the Kaufman tests. More detailed assessment, with some normative data, are provided by the Rivermead Behavioural Memory Test (Wilson *et al.* 1985) which includes useful tests of new learning with non-verbal and motor as well as verbal components; the California Verbal Learning Test–Children's Version (Delis *et al.* 1993; Elwood 1995) and the Wide Range Attention and Memory and Learning Test (Sheslow & Adams 1990).

Visuospatial skills

Visuospatial processing is included in all the main test batteries. Specific tests are available, but usually add rather little by way of superior standardization or making finer distinctions. However, a motor-free visual perception test may be useful in assessing perceptual processes more specifically (Aliotti & Rajabiun 1991) and the Bender–Gestalt Test (Piotrowski 1995) offers a complementary emphasis on visuomotor integration—though its initial purpose of detecting brain damage would no longer be seen as a valid rationale.

Attention

A large experimental literature has not yet translated itself into well-standardized tests (Sergeant *et al.* 1999). It has been conceptually and practically difficult to distinguish between attention on a test and ability at the test when the only measure available is test performance. Experimental tests are usually presented under strict timing control (usually with a computer) and with manipulation of experimental parameters. Standard automated versions of the CPT are available with age norms (Conners 2000). Simple counts of number of errors will reflect processes other than attention, but analysis of different patterns of error is feasible and may give clues to the presence of such 'attentional' problems as overrapid and impulsive responding (see Schachar & Tannock, Chapter 25). Computer batteries exist for tests of attention (de

Sonneville *et al.* 1999) and executive functioning (Robbins *et al.* 1998).

Attention is a behavioural as well as a cognitive construct. Observation of children's behaviour during testing (see below) is probably the main source of evidence on which judgements about attention are based.

Executive functioning

Since the 1970s, cognitive neuroscientists have stressed study of the active, planning and evaluative systems of cognitive performance (Broadbent 1971; Posner 1978; Shallice 1982; Sanders 1983). Various tests are intended to measure the high-level functions of planning, inhibiting immediate or inappropriate reactions, decision-making and organization. For the most part their standardization is weak. They include the Stroop Colour–Word Test (Stroop 1935), in which a conflict of information is set up (e.g. the word 'blue' being printed in red colours), so that successful completion of the test requires one to suppress an 'obvious' but wrong response. Like many neuropsychological tests, it is dependent upon a wide variety of processes. Colour perception and reading ability influence performance (Semrud-Clickeman *et al.* 2000; Tannock *et al.* 2000). The interference score derived from the Stroop may not simply reflect a sole process, such as inhibition. Unlike many neuropsychological tests, the Stroop controls for some of the processes: it contains separate information on colour naming and reading.

Other 'executive function' tests are intended to test aspects of problem-solving, e.g. the Trail Making and Wisconsin Card Sort Tests (WCST; Berg 1948), especially when an abstract element of thinking before response is required, e.g. Tower of London (TOL; Shallice 1982). A set of tests of this type is available as the CANTAB (Cambridge Neuropsychological Test Automated Battery; Lowe & Rabbitt 1998; Robbins *et al.* 1998; Luciana & Nelson 2000). These computerized tests include set-shifting, working memory, pattern recognition, inhibition and planning. There are developmental trends on these tasks, which have been followed (for example) from age 4–8 years by Luciano & Nelson (1998), but they do not yet have the kind of standardization that would allow for secure inferences about individual children. Tests of planning and organization are embodied in tests such as the Behavioural Assessment of Dysexecutive Syndrome (BADS; Wilson *et al.* 1996), which have been applied essentially to adults with disorders such as schizophrenia but have a face validity for neurodevelopmental disturbances in childhood. (Evans *et al.* 1997; Krabbendam *et al.* 1999). Tests of inhibition are operationalized as 'stop' tests, in which a response to a stimulus has to be interrupted after another stimulus has indicated that one should not respond; 'go–no go' tests, in which standard signals call for a response but others require the response to be withheld; and 'delay' tests, in which a stimulus calls for a response to be emitted only after a period of a few seconds has elapsed (Rubia *et al.* 1999).

Some of these tests are very prone to the practice effect mentioned above. For instance, a child's performance on the

TOL requires careful clinical observation. In the beginning of such a task, the child has to 'catch on' to the sort of planning that is required, so thoughtful reflection is needed before carrying out a sequence of permissible moves. As time passes, the child learns which moves are required or, in the WCST, learns when hearing 'no' that the principle for sorting cards has been changed. Once the child has caught on to what 'the trick' is, the test no longer measures planning or control over perseveration in the same way. If one repeats the TOL or WCST with the same child, reliability will be found to be low, because the child is often able to recall 'the trick'. Hence in clinical practice, careful inspection of the performance of the child over time is required to assess at what point planning may have been measured and at what point the trick has been applied. Scores on such tests may over- or underestimate the child's planning ability.

Executive function tasks are sometimes supposed to draw on a common working memory (Baddeley & Hitch 1974). This assumption has been modified: there may be specific and distinguishable working memory domains (Baddeley 1990). Indeed, Kimberg & Farrach (1993) have argued that performance on the TOL, Stroop and WCST may be managed by separate working memory systems. If this proves to be correct, it would emphasize that the terms 'executive functioning' and 'working memory' are not homogeneous. This being the case, practical neuropsychological assessment must examine different features of these concepts (Pennington & Ozonoff 1996). A flexible rather than a fixed test battery approach would seem more appropriate to answer issues such as which type of working memory is deficient in children with learning disabilities. If one does not apply sufficiently comprehensive testing with sufficient flexibility to meet the case at hand, one may be replacing one 'wastepaper basket' term with another. In summary, choosing a 'working memory' task may result in greater heterogeneity than one might expect, but may still validly reflect cognitive-neuropsychological processing. Clinicians should not be surprised when the apparent cross-reliability between tests is not found to be high.

Motor abilities and adaptive function

The organization and coordination of motor tasks is a difficulty for children referred with problems related to dyspraxia. Clinical neurological examination is usually the key tool for assessment. It aims to uncover patterns of incoordination (such as cerebellar ataxia, motor overflow or ideomotor apraxia) as well as underlying causes (such as mild cerebral palsy). Standardized tests of various kinds are available, and are used when the level of incoordination needs to be quantified more precisely (when a test battery of a wide range of fine and gross motor coordination, such as the Henderson & Sugden (1992) Movement ABC, based on the Lincoln Oseretsky, is suitable); or when a specific problem is detected (as by the Fogs tests; Szatmari & Taylor 1984, concentrating on the observation of associated and redundant movements during specified effortful motor tasks).

Quantified motor tests have a particular place in the assessment of the development of younger children, for whom tasks involving complex communication and symbolic understanding are not appropriate. The Griffiths Scales of Mental Development (Griffiths 1970) contain a range of tasks requiring motor skills, and locomotor development constitutes some of the scales of the Revised Denver Developmental Screening Test (Frankenburg & Dodds 1967; Frankenburg et al. 1986)

Griffiths and Denver scales also include items that relate to self-care and independence skills. Quantifying these kinds of 'adaptive function' are important in assessing the needs of children with global learning disabilities (see Bernard, Chapter 67). The Vineland Adaptive Behaviour Scales (Sparrow et al. 1984) are widely used for this purpose, and have a practical advantage in that information can be acquired by parental report as well as by direct examination of the child's abilities.

Achievement tests

It is often useful to quantify the level of academic achievement— for instance, in reading or mathematics—that a child has attained. Schools do so for many purposes—to assess pupils, teachers and whole school systems—and the methods vary with the aims.

The most common aim in clinical practice is diagnostic—to determine whether the degree of difficulty in (say) reading is above and beyond that which can be attributed to any global cognitive impairment. If there is a specific problem, then detecting it helps in giving advice to young people and their families, and (in many school systems) leads to administrative decisions about provision of special help and placement in special units. For this purpose, the tester is seeking evidence of a discrepancy between achieved scores and those predicted from the age and IQ of the child. In order to do this, one should not rely on impressionistic statements that the child is below expectation, or that the child is so many years behind his or her peers (because the significance of, say, a 2-year discrepancy will be very different at the age of 8 to that at 14 years), or arbitrary statistics such as the ratio of reading age to mental age. These fail to achieve the precision that is the point of quantifying. Regression formulae or expectancy tables should be used to predict the expected level of attainment from age and IQ (Yule 1967) and identify those with an extreme difference between that and the observed level, such as 2 standard errors of prediction below expectation (see Snowling, Chapter 40). The best scales to use for this purpose will be those that have been developed and standardized alongside IQ scales. A tester using the Wechsler Intelligence Scales will usually choose the Wechsler Objective Reading and Numerical Dimensions (Wechsler 1992b, 1996); one using the Kauffman will opt for the Kaufman Test of Educational Achievement (Kaufman & Kaufman 1985).

In educational practice, simple achievement tests are helpful in screening to detect children whose progress is untypical. This is a part of routine good practice in schools, but nationally standardized tests are also valuable as reference points. For this purpose, the prime consideration will be to choose a test with the best national standardization. The Wide Range Achievement Test (Jastak & Wilkinson 1984) is extensively used and provides both a brief screen and a more comprehensive version analysing types of errors in reading decoding, reading comprehension, mathematics applications, mathematics computation, and spelling. The Neale tests of reading (Neale 1997) are reasonably quick to administer and widely used.

Teachers are often disappointed with the results of psychological testing because they are hoping for a prescriptive approach to guide curriculum and classroom practice for the individual child. There is still a considerable gap between the description of abilities that comes from testing and the decisions about the most helpful remedial approaches. For this reason, many educationists emphasize the approach of curriculum-based assessment (Tucker 1985). This is criterion-based rather than based on what is average for the population; the aim is simply to describe whether or not a young person has mastered what they are expected to learn. The test items should be drawn directly from the curriculum, and assessment is closely bound up with teaching. Such tests are indicative of the level reached rather than diagnostic of the reasons for any impairment.

Social and emotional understanding

Standardized self-reports are valuable tools in an assessment of social and emotional function (see Angold, Chapter 3). Further questions often arise as to how far an abnormality of social behaviour is based on a failure to understand social situations and the expectations of others. Research approaches to this issue can be adapted to the assessment of individuals. 'Theory of mind' tests describe the extent to which individuals can understand situations involving the motives and understanding of other people—the extent, for instance, to which they appreciate what will embarrass other people or how they will understand deception. Carefully constructed false-belief tasks have been found to show good test–retest reliability and internal consistency (Hughes et al. 2000). They are therefore suitable for individual assessment. The recognition of faux pas has also been assessed with a test showing predictive validity in distinguishing groups of people with and without Asperger disorder (Baron-Cohen et al. 1999). Heavey et al. (2000) have presented an Awkward Moments Test: an advanced theory of mind task, developed to approximate the demands of real-life mentalizing in able individuals with autism. Excerpts of films showing characters in social situations are presented, with participants required to answer questions on characters' mental states and on control, non-social questions.

Projective tests are still widely used, in spite of having fared poorly against empirical tests of reliability and validity. The lack of structure, and the difficulty of making quantitative sense out of the enormous number of possible responses, has worked against their utility. When clear and explicit rules for administration and scoring have been applied, then progress can be made. The presentation of projective test materials has been

used as the key operational manipulation in several experimental means of eliciting responses. For example, 'communication deviance' can be scored from responses to Thematic Apperception Test material, and was predictive of breakdown in young people at risk for schizophrenia (Doane et al. 1981). A specified scoring system for the Rorschach has been introduced (Exner & Weiner 1994), although even the most recent evaluations (Jorgensen et al. 2000; Wood et al. 2000) have had to conclude that the test is unsuitable for scientifically based assessment. However, the principle that has survived the individual tests is that of providing a standard set of stimuli to elicit the behaviours for professional observation—a principle taken up under 'Observational approaches', below.

Cognitive testing in very young children

Several test batteries describe the cognitive abilities of very young and preverbal children: the most commonly used are probably the Bayley Scales of Infant Development, now in their second edition (Bayley 1993). Other tests, such as the Merrill Palmer (Stutsman 1931), are sometimes used but have less satisfactory normative data. The same tests are used to describe the competencies of older children with severe mental retardation. The two uses, however, raise rather different issues.

There are at present serious limitations to the predictive value of cognitive testing when one tries to predict from infancy to later childhood. This can be a pressing clinical issue, because it would often be very useful to know whether a baby with a risk factor for later cognitive development (such as a very low birth weight) is in fact specifically vulnerable. Remedial education could then be started very early for the high-risk group in the hope of preventing the later sequelae. The hope has not yet been translated into reality, partly because of a lack of strong predictors from infancy to cognitive abilities in later childhood. The difficulty does not arise from lack of measures for infant development, nor from lack of reliability in those tests (Bayley 1993). Indeed, there is a respectable measure of agreement between different types of developmental assessment when carried out in children aged 1 year (Raggio et al. 1994). Rather, the problem seems to be that the abilities that are assessed in early development (such as sensorimotor coordination) have rather little to do with the symbolic cognitive operations that are assessed in later childhood.

The situation is improving with further research. More recently developed measures for infants, such as those of visual information processing and means–ends problem-solving show significant correlations with IQ in later childhood (Slater 1995). They have clarified some of the reason for poor predictiveness of traditional tests. For example, habituation to sensory stimuli at the age of 4–8 months is not a stable trait. It does not predict similar measures taken at the age of 3 years. It does, however, predict developmental quotients at the age of 3 years quite well (McCall & Carriger 1993). The apparent paradox—that an unstable test can have predictive validity—emphasizes that a test such as habituation indexes different psychological functions at different ages.

The new generation of tests in infancy may well come to be applicable on a routine clinical basis, though at present it is difficult to achieve robust and reliable descriptions of individuals because of marked fluctuations in scores depending on the state of the infant. Nevertheless, the prediction of later impairment is still rather too weak to be a basis for selecting children for intervention. Practically, the best predictors of cognitive outcome in very high-risk groups remain neurological signs, or neuroimaging tests of the extent to which the physical structure of the brain has been altered by perinatal hazards (Stewart *et al.* 1999).

The assessment of older children at very low levels of function raises different issues. Nearly all such children have diffuse structural abnormalities of the brain, and the cognitive consequences are complex. The tests are highly predictive of later cognitive functioning at this extreme of the range. However, individual tests have rather little in common. Gould (1977), for example, found very little association between measures of social maturity, visuospatial skills not involving symbolic concepts, and level of language comprehension in an epidemiological study of young people with severe disability. The discrepancies probably reflect the true situation of the children, and underline the importance of understanding the range of strengths and weaknesses that they present.

Special testing situations

Every child needs individual consideration; the tests and observations to be used will need to reflect not only the presenting problems, but the effect that testing is having on the children, their developmental level and ability to understand test expectations, and their willingness to comply with them. The length and difficulty of tests need to be taken into account: if difficult items are presented too early in the course of an assessment, or if children are asked to persist for too long at test items that are too hard for them, then they may become demotivated. The extent to which tests are giving a valid description of the individual needs always to be considered; the issues involved in doing so are described by Rutter & Yule (Chapter 7).

The clinician is often confronted with situations where for one reason or another the standard approach to testing needs to be modified considerably. For example, sensory or motor impairments can have their own influence on cognitive tests. At the simplest, the professional making the assessment needs to check that children do indeed have the spectacles or hearing aids that they may need for adequate performance; and to be alert throughout the assessment for signs that a superficially cognitive difficulty (for example, of detecting fine differences between pictures) may be caused by a sensory impairment (in this instance, diminished visual acuity). Sometimes, more meaningful scores may be obtained by special procedures. For example, inability to follow spoken instructions may be bypassed by the choice of a test (such as Raven's Progressive Matrices) where very little such instruction is needed, or by a test battery (such as the Leiter) that is designed to be fair to children with sensory impairments—and therefore covers a narrower range of intellectual skills. Children with severe motor disability may need to be helped to a signalling system before their cognitive strengths and weaknesses can be fairly assessed, and reliance may have to be placed on tests (such as Raven's Matrices) where the answer is a choice from a limited range of alternatives and can be indicated through many different kinds of motor response. Clumsy children may obtain low scores on tests where speed of reaction is being assessed, merely because their motor responses take longer, and it may be wise to discount such tests in making the overall cognitive assessment. Very shy children, or those with selective mutism, may need to write down their responses or whisper them without eye contact with the tester. Care must be taken to indicate the limits of confidence that there may be in non-standard testing; but creative use of cognitive test materials has sometimes been able to show the presence of high ability in children whose sensory or motor impairments have previously prevented the abilities from being shown, and this rightly guides formulation of their special needs in education.

Observational approaches

As already indicated, observation of behaviour is always an important part of psychological testing. Observation can also be applied in many situations where testing is not feasible, and its reliability and validity need be no less.

The most explicit schemes of observation provide an experimental control of the environment and give standard stimuli to evoke informative behaviour. In a clinic or laboratory setting, specific tasks are imposed on the child and defined types of response are elicited. For example, Ainsworth's Strange Situation Test (see O'Connor, Chapter 46) has been the foundation of attachment research. In clinics it is seldom appropriate for it to be used in its exact experimental form, but observations of children reacting to a contrived separation and reunion are used extensively to inform judgements about the nature of the children's attachment to their parents.

The Autism Diagnostic Observational Schedule (ADOS; Lord *et al.* 2000; see Lord & Bailey, Chapter 38) is a good example of an observational scheme that is based on specified operations by the examiner (for example, providing a variety of standard stimuli and social presses) and explicit descriptions of the behavioural responses that are to be made. It was originally introduced for research purposes, and its high interrater and test–retest reliability, and its ability to discriminate well between autistic people and people with different diagnoses, have led to its adoption in clinical practice.

Kagan (1997) has reviewed an extensive series of studies based on the direct observation of young children's behavioural reaction to the standardized presentation of unfamiliar stimuli. Four-month-old infants who show a low threshold for becoming distressed and motorically aroused to unfamiliar stimuli are more likely than others to become fearful and subdued during early childhood; whereas infants who show a high arousal threshold are more likely to become bold and sociable. Observed inhibition in this method has made predictions to later anxiety, even though only a small proportion of children maintain a consistently inhibited or uninhibited phenotype through their childhood (Kagan *et al.* 1998). Clinical application so far has been limited by the variability that individual children show over time on the measure.

Several observational schemes for inattentive and overactive behaviours have been presented; they have been reviewed by Luk (1985). In general, they have made rather less use of careful control of what social presses are imposed by the examiner, but specify the expectations that are on the child (e.g. by observation during psychological testing). The schemes have mostly been used in research, e.g. to describe the alteration in spontaneous activities of children in classrooms (Schachar *et al.* 1986), playroom and testing situations (Luk *et al.* 1987), controlled settings with parents (Kalverboer 1971) and interview with a psychiatrist (Dienske *et al.* 1985). In these studies they discriminate well between children with ADHD and healthy controls, and predict to questionnaire and interview measures. They gain something in 'ecological validity' by being based on naturally occurring events, but correspondingly lose the clarity of interpretation that comes from experiment.

Attempts to combine both sets of virtues have involved the careful description of a limited set of frequently occurring events (e.g. mother giving an instruction to child) so that the child's reactions to those events can be clearly specified (Dunn & Kendrick 1980; Bates *et al.* 1985). Very large amounts of data are sometimes generated, so that analysis may become very complex. The techniques have therefore been limited to research applications, but the conclusions about process may well give good ideas to clinicians about what to look for; e.g. when interviewing and observing families, to note especially sequences in which the child has been asked to do something and has in fact done it, so as to record the consequence of compliance.

Most of these clinical applications of observational techniques are based on ratings that take into account the function and purpose of the behaviour. These qualitative ratings can be very reliable, but usually require training of the raters to make them so. They are needed because molecular descriptions of acts are usually rather unilluminating without their context. It is not only the speed of an action that determines whether it is impulsive, but whether it is too rapid to allow appraisal of the situation; therefore it depends on the amount of uncertainty in what response should be made. It is not just whether a child points at an object that is important in his or her appraisal of it; it is also whether that pointing includes the social function of indicating it to somebody else.

In some situations, however, systematic observation is trying to quantify a rather simple act. The frequency of tics may be important to note, so as to gauge the impact of a treatment; or the number of times a child strikes him- or herself may be an important dependent variable for understanding how different contingencies affect the self-injury. There is then a choice of techniques: recording during a set interval how often the behaviour has happened, or sampling brief periods over a session to record whether or not it has occurred at each point. The decision will depend on the properties of the behaviour. If it fluctuates considerably over time (as tics may) then the counting of events during one time period may be seriously unrepresentative, and short intervals scattered throughout a longer period may be substantially more reliable. If the behaviour is infrequent then a succession of very short samples may not elicit enough events for a reliable estimate.

Clinical applications of observational analysis

Clarifying rater and source effects

In clinical practice, observation is sometimes used as the gold standard when there is discrepancy between sources of information. For example, a parent may say that a child is well-behaved but cannot concentrate, while a teacher says that the same child is able to concentrate but chooses not to; so the clinician decides to go to the classroom to decide for him- or herself. The simple question of 'who is correct?' often underestimates the complexity of what the professional observer strives to do. In the first place, the method has important limitations as well as strengths. It may be based on a very atypical period of observation; the observer may alter the behaviour unknowingly, and allowance needs to be made for this.

In the second place, the observer is not only trying to establish who is right but the reasons for the discrepancy. It will probably be very useful for the observer to check with the real life rater whether they are giving different meanings to the same behaviour, or referring to different behaviours shown on different occasions by the same child. In the above example, both parent and teacher may be observing the same thing—a high level of off-task activity; whether it is construed as disability or choice may stem from the significance attached to the observations. The raters' accounts might be strongly coloured by their own personal circumstances or their relationship with the child. It may then be useful to explore what different actions would result from the theoretical expectations—how, for example, parents might provide incentives to test the idea that motivation would alter performance; or how the teacher might test the idea of a disability by presenting materials to be learned in a simplified and clearer way.

The third and most fundamental reason for regarding 'who is correct?' as an oversimplified question is that different accounts by different observers can reflect important situational influences. The reasons underlying situational differences in behaviour can be crucial clues to the nature of a child's problems. For example, a child may be referred because of a massive recent deterioration in school performance; no emotional problems are apparent, and the first working hypothesis, of cognitive impairment, is provisionally disconfirmed by good performance at the clinic on tests of intellectual aptitude and executive dysfunction. This does not mean that there is 'no real problem'. The next set of hypotheses should then relate to the reasons for the discrepancy: is it associated with the kind of test that is performed, the place it is carried out in, or the contingencies attending the way it is carried out? In one such example, the next step was to arrange for academic tasks (solving mathematics problems) and an attentional task (deleting the 'e's from a prose passage) to be performed in three settings: the clinic; the regular classroom; and the same classroom during a visit from the clinic psychologist. Both tasks were performed much less well in the classroom than the clinic, but the performance at school was as good as in the clinic when the psychologist was seen to be present. The discrepancy between school and clinic appeared not to lie in the precise nature of the tests used in the different settings, nor in the generic qualities of the settings, but in the degree to which the child received the attention of an adult. The provisional recommendation was therefore for enhanced monitoring in the classroom, and indeed intermittent individual attention from an aide quickly led to a resumption of good academic progress. The finding also led to another set of hypotheses about why performance should have been selectively affected—whether adult attention was providing monitoring or safety or warmth of interest—and therefore to reinvestigation of psychosocial stresses (in this case, a neighbourhood feud had spilled into the school setting). The general point is that the interactions between child traits and environments can often be understood from the effects of contrasting environmental circumstances. A functional analysis of a behaviour problem—which is often the purpose of making observations in natural settings—requires specification of the antecedents and consequences of the behaviour in the environment (see Herbert, Chapter 53).

It follows that the observations carried out at a school or home visit should not only focus on the child but also on the qualities of the environment. At school, one should note not only the child's scholastic behaviour and relationships with peers and teacher but also the organization of the classroom. In elementary class, can the child see a record of their achievement (such as a points system), and are examples of their good work on display? Do they know the activity to engage in, and are they in a position where their activity can readily be monitored by the teacher? Is the atmosphere of class and school one of safety and constructive activity? At home, is there a cognitively stimulating environment with toys or books? Are there rules for conduct and can caregivers tell what children are doing? What is the affective tone in exchanges between parents and children and between siblings?

Naturalistic observations can be distorted by the accidents of what salient events happen to take place during the visit, and it can be hard to be sure of the sequence of events in an escalating situation: did the child protest at an instruction about behaviour or was the instruction in response to the beginning of rebellion? It is therefore helpful, when possible, to give particular notice to how the child reacts to contrived or independent events. For example, transitions between activities in the classroom are a high-risk point for disruptive behaviour, so in investigating this problem the teacher can be asked to introduce an activity change. Similarly, at home, the parent would be asked to introduce a press for an unwelcome activity (such as 'tidy up your toys now') so that the nature and consequences of compliance can be seen. As ever, it is necessary to check whether the sequence of behaviours that has been observed has been typical of what would normally occur in that situation.

Observational analyses of some clinical problems extend to a quasi-experimental use of specified procedures. A closely specified challenge can be inserted into a period of naturalistic observation. For example, intellectually impaired children who show challenging behaviours may have learned them in diverse ways (see Volkmar & Dykens, Chapter 41). Some may have learned to continue injuring themselves because the behaviour has been rewarded by the attention of others, some because self-injury serves to help them escape from unwelcome tasks, and some because the self-stimulation involved is inherently rewarding to them. It may not be obvious which of these apply in a particular situation, and the consequences matter a good deal. If a behavioural programme involves withdrawing contingent attention through a time-out procedure (see Herbert, Chapter 53) and if the true rewarder in the situation is escaping from school work, then the time-out may be a strong reward and perpetuate the problem. Accordingly, it is possible to introduce escape or contingent attention as consequences of self-injury during an extended period of observation and examine the effects (Sturmey et al. 1988). The method is laborious because of the need for repetition of observations, and it is not always possible to be certain that these 'analogue observations' are representative of real life; but it can be a helpful guide to practice in difficult and refractory situations.

Clarifying discrepancies between test scores

Discrepancies between performance scores on tests may be illuminating in clarifying the nature of a problem—for instance, in detecting specific learning disorders. However, interpretation is often uncertain because of the imperfect reliability in test scores and the corresponding uncertainties about how far apparent differences are clinically meaningful. Observation is then a useful means of helping to determine the validity of test scores. For example, it may be apparent that a poor score on one subtest was associated with an uninterested and uncooperative attitude towards it. The tester may then do much more than usual by way of coaxing a good performance, or repeating it on another occasion—with, of course, the note that it was obtained in nonstandard ways; and may interpret the difference as secondary to motivational factors.

Observation may suggest new functions to be tested. For example, a boy was referred for assessment some years after an episode of severe encephalitis. Even after apparent neurological recovery, he was quite unable to cope with the classwork in his academically orientated school. Extensive testing of intellectual function showed no deficit: although premorbid testing was not available, he tested in the superior or very superior range on all tests given. The possibility of a breakdown in his confidence was entertained, but incidental observation and the description of his family both emphasized how muddled and disorganized he could be in simple everyday tasks, such as getting his outdoor clothes to go home—even though all tests relating to dyspraxia, attention and memory had shown better than average scores. He was therefore observed while carrying out several simple tasks simultaneously; and there was a marked disability in doing this that was not present when he was asked to carry them out successively. It appeared that he had an executive type of dysfunction in which the allocation of effort to tasks was uncontrolled. Statistical significance on this would have been hard to obtain, in that it would have required larger number of observations than could be obtained feasibly. Accordingly, the testing of the hypothesis was by the response to intervention. The result was in a sense encouraging, because careful breaking down of academic tasks into components helped performance of them substantially. But the disability remained, the burden of the intervention on teachers in a mainstream school was unsustainable, and specialist education was sought.

Examining relationships between functions

Systematic observation may assist in disentangling the relationships between different psychological processes, especially when they are hard to detect by rating scales and interviews. For example, an adolescent with Tourette disorder was referred because of recurrent transient episodes of great distress, but found it hard to describe the changes of his mood and the reasons for them, and the relationship between them and his tics was correspondingly difficult to formulate. Psychophysiological recordings of skin conductance and heart rate were carried out simultaneously with event recording of tics, and showed consistent marked increases immediately after bouts of tics—interpreted (in discussion with him) as indicating increased emotionality (associated with a distressed feeling that he had failed to control them and would be in trouble). This is not a usual pattern; more commonly, in our experience, children report a sense of tension as they strive to suppress the tics and even a sense of relief after a bout is finished. For him, it suggested an approach to treatment in which he practised coping skills while watching videos of himself during tics and was praised by parents for his courage in ignoring adverse comments by others. Although the tics continued a poorly controlled and fluctuating course, he described himself as less distressed and better able to cope with perceived teasing.

Description of outcome

Observed behaviour is often less vulnerable than cognitive tests to repeated administration. A lack of standardization may not be a serious problem for this purpose, because children act as their own controls. Observation is particularly helpful when rating scales do not give the fineness of discrimination that is sometimes required. For example, rating scales made by teachers and parents for a boy of 6 years who had started on stimulant medication indicated that he was quieter and possibly more withdrawn in social situations. The question therefore arose of whether this was an adverse effect or an acceptable part of the package of drug action. It was possible that the behavioural descriptions described a more clinging and dependent style of interaction, or a lack of spontaneous interactions. Attachment behaviour was therefore observed by ratings during separation and reunion, analogous to the Strange Situation Test, and peer behaviour in a playroom situation with neighbourhood friends; both were recorded on and off medication by a clinical student who was blind to the treatment condition. Attachment measures did not show a change. Observations of approaches to peers and shared play with peers indicated that they were actually higher during medication. The description of quietness was confirmed, but it related to a diminution of loudness of speech and disinhibited behaviour, rather than to a lack of spontaneity. The conclusion was that the social change was unlikely to be harmful and did not constitute an indication for stopping medication. Conversely, clinical observation that a medicated child is socially unspontaneous, or perseverative in attention, may be crucial in detecting an adverse effect that is not apparent in everyday monitoring at school, where perseverativeness may be confused with enhanced attention.

Inferences from tests and observations

In the course of this chapter we have described tests and observational methods that can provide incremental knowledge by which a clinician can conclude that working hypotheses about the nature of children's problems are supported or rejected. This is an approach, not a diagnostic protocol. The way in which a clinician should organize tests to come to evidence-based decisions is guided by judgement and a clear sense of the questions that need to be answered. In other areas of medicine, there has been a considerable body of research on how clinicians gather and evaluate information. This knowledge base has not been applied systematically to child mental health issues, so this section briefly mentions some of the cognitive heuristics that are useful to bear in mind.

One common cognitive heuristic is *representativeness*. By this is meant that incoming information is processed primarily on the similarity it has with a particular class of information. For example, the clinician seeks to place incoming data (such as symptoms and signs) into a limited number of classes (syndromes). Psychiatrists and clinical psychologists are trained to detect symptoms that could be part of a prototype (Genero & Cantor 1987). A bias can arise if symptom variance is underestimated. Clinicians may overestimate the extent to which the symptoms agree with the prototype or syndrome, seeking confirmatory instances and not disproof. For training purposes, the use of distinctive prototypes is a good starting point, but needs to be varied to show the full range of cases involved in the syndrome (Horowitz *et al.* 1979). The clinician then learns to make sure that the assessment is comprehensive, and has not stopped at the recognition of a prototype but has gone on to understand what is out of keeping with the prototype and what further problems are present.

Once a first impression has been formed, it can be hard to change it. 'Anchoring' refers to the potential problem that perceptions can become rigid as a result of the initial impression that one has made of a client. Friedlander & Stockman (1983) found that pathology that appeared late in a series of interviews had much less impact on diagnostic decisions than when it appeared early in the series. In short, we need to stay alert to new information that should force us to revise and review the case.

Prior conceptions have been shown to influence the interpretation which diagnosticians place on test results. An illusory association is constructed between a test result and a diagnosis, which can be hard to change. A study that neatly illustrates the problem of erroneous diagnostic observation was conducted over 30 years ago by Chapman & Chapman (1967). Novices tried to match responses on a projective test (Draw-a-Person) with a set of contrived symptoms. In one sense, they were successful, in that they produced the same associations between responses and symptoms as the experts, but in the experimental design the symptoms had been contrived so as to have no actual association with the responses at all. Apparent reliability between raters was achieved, but the validity of their ratings was zero.

Similarly, Golding & Rorer (1972) repeatedly presented to subjects an individual Rorschach response and asked them to predict what symptom was associated with the response. They were given immediate feedback on their decision and informed of the actual symptoms of the patient—which of course did not necessarily correspond. Despite this there persisted a strong illusion of an association between the Rorschach response and the actual symptoms of the patient. The remedy for the clinician is to remain open to the empirical reality of the case in spite of the temptations to theoretical overconfidence.

Fischoff & Lichtenstein (1978) discussed how prediction of events was influenced by the knowledge that the event had occurred. This effect has been confirmed by Arkes *et al.* (1981). They showed that trained physicians, when required to diagnose one of four possible illnesses, were just as susceptible to hindsight bias as had been found by Fischoff when using students. Those who knew the actual diagnosis overestimated the likelihood that they would have been able to predict the correct diagnosis had they been asked to do so beforehand. Even experienced clinicians have also been shown to suffer from this bias when dealing with patients who later commit suicide (Goggin & Range 1985). Systematic evaluation of one's practice is an essential way of counteracting misleading subjective impressions.

Another important consideration in the interpretation of tests is the application of understanding about base rates (see Rutter & Yule, Chapter 7). The significance that clinicians attach to an abnormal test result can be influenced by a variety of factors, one being the frequency with which they encounter it. Most clinicians work on the basis of the frequency with which they see the combination of a clinical problem and an abnormal test result, rather than the *relative* frequencies of an abnormal test in the presence or absence of the problem. For example, if clinicians are asked to judge the likelihood of pneumonia from an X-ray, a preliminary diagnosis can be given. When they are further provided with information on the sensitivity and specificity of the test and the prevalence of the disease and asked to estimate the predictive value (positive and negative), the prevalence tends to be ignored in their estimations (Casscells *et al.* 1978). Clinicians generally use frequency as a major principle guiding retrieval of information, so it is important that they school themselves to base their judgements about the significance of a test on the relative frequency.

Another important cognitive heuristic is *comprehensiveness*. This is intended to overcome one of the common errors in judgement—to focus too narrowly on one aspect of a complex case. Problem behaviour does not come packed in neat parcels. Comorbidity, correlated dimensions, and associated features have become much better recognized over the last 15 years and are dealt with by Fombonne (see Chapter 4), Verhulst & Van der Ende (see Chapter 5), Rutter (see Chapter 19) and Taylor & Rutter (see Chapter 1). This development implies that the assessment procedure must be sufficiently comprehensive in order to detect correlated dimensional problems, at the least, and to be aware that exceptions can occur that require probing for noncorrelated conditions. For example, the clinician can use a standardized diagnostic interview that covers at least the most common presenting problems.

Comprehensive problem definition implies that the clinical problem as presented needs to be assessed at a variety of levels, including clinical syndrome; severity of impairment; somatic condition; personality; cognitive performance; social skills; and emotional processing (to name but a few). The problem then arises of how to square comprehensiveness with the costs of assessment? It is obvious that choices will have to be made. One policy (not recommended here) is to assess only that which is necessary for a particular treatment. One confirms a hypothesis, but rejects none of the alternatives and misses fundamental explanatory factors. Part of this issue can be solved by using 'screeners' for covering a wide range of pathology and psychological dysfunctioning.

The cognitive heuristics discussed above clearly spell out the message that empirical support for one's hunches is required. They also have a second message: searching only to confirm a hunch exposes one to finding only what one expects. For most of the possible biases mentioned above, the remedy is the adoption of an investigative and hypothesis-testing approach, with a critical willingness to revise hypotheses about the nature of a problem that do not fit the data (see Rutter & Yule, Chapter 7).

Conclusions

In this chapter we have attempted to indicate the use of tests, tasks and observation in the diagnostic process. Further, we have touched on the cognitive biases which operate in the interpretation of the psychological assessment. We note that one of the major differences between classical psychometric tests and cognitive tasks is that the latter are theory driven. From the neuropsychological perspective, cognitive tests are linked to complex brain networks and not specific brain loci.

While cognitive heuristics have their dangers, when conditions are met and they are applied, these heuristics can be effective tools in clinical work. It seems likely that the future will bring an increase in their clinical use, especially as neurodevelopmental disorders are seen to depend strongly upon alterations of cognitive processing. However, their very strength can lead to their application in inappropriate conditions. It is this last point where the expert can excel the novice in detecting whether the cognitive heuristics are producing answers that are acceptable. This in turn is determined by the theoretical position, model or hypotheses being generated. Tests and observations are simply means to assess whether the assumptions and hypotheses about a case are being met. This requires insight into when or when not to use a test or task for a particular purpose and under which state they may or may not be applied. Consequently, child psychiatrist and psychologist need to work hand in hand in developing the rules and criteria for which tests can be applied to test specific aims. Standardized batteries depend for their application not on a slavish philosophy of assessment but on a critical definition of purpose, conditions, intervening variables and criteria. This places clinical diagnostics into the realm where it belongs: of critical cognitive processing.

References

Aliotti, N.C. & Rajabiun, D.A. (1991) Visual memory development in preschool children. *Perceptual and Motor Skills, 73*, 792–794.

Allport, D.A. & Styles, E.A. (1997) Shifting intentional set: exploring the dynamic control of tasks. In: *Attention and Performance XV* (eds C. Umlita & M. Moscovitch), pp. 421–452. Erlbaum, Hillsdale.

Arkes, H.R., Wortman, R.L., Saville, P.D. & Harkness, A.R. (1981) Hindsight bias among physicians weighting the likelihood of diagnoses. *Journal of Applied Psychology, 66*, 252–254.

Baddeley, A.D. (1990) *Human memory: Theory and Practice*. Erlbaum, Hillsdale.

Baddeley, A.D. & Hitch, G.J. (1974) Working memory. In: *The Psychology of Learning and Motivation*, Vol. VIII (ed. G. Bower), pp. 49–90. Academic Press, New York.

Baron-Cohen, S., O'Riordan, M., Stone, V., Jones, R. & Plaisted, K. (1999) Recognition of faux pas by normally developing children and children with Asperger syndrome or high-functioning autism. *Journal of Autism and Development Disorders, 29*, 407–418.

Bates, J.E., Maslin, C.A. & Frankel, K.A. (1985) Attachment security, mother–child interaction and temperament as predictors of behaviour-problem ratings at age three years. *Monographs of the Society for Research in Child Development, 50* (1–2), 167–193.

Bayley, N. (1949) Consistency and variability in the growth of intelligence from birth to 18 years. *Journal of Genetic Psychology, 75*, 165–196.

Bayley, N. (1993) *Bayley Scales of Infant Development Manual*, 2nd edn. Psychological Corporation, San Antonio, TX.

Berg, E.A. (1948) A simple objective test for measuring flexibility in thinking. *Journal of General Psychology, 39*, 15–22.

Binet, A. (1905) A propos de la mesure de l'intelligence. *Annee Psychologique, 11*, 69.

Broadbent, D.E. (1971) *Decision and Stress*. Academic Press, New York.

Casscells, W., Schoenberger, A. & Graboys, T.B. (1978) Interpretation by physicians of clinical laboratory results. *New England Journal of Medicine, 299*, 999–1001.

Castellanos, F.X. (1997) Toward a pathophysiology of attention-deficit/hyperactivity disorder. *Clinical Paediatrics, 36*, 381–393.

Chapman, L.J. & Chapman, J.P. (1967) Genesis of popular but erroneous psychodiagnostic observations. *Journal of Abnormal Psychology, 72*, 193–204.

Conners, C.K. (2000) *Conners' Continuous Performance Test II Computer Program for Windows*. International Psychology Services, Hurstpierpoint, UK.

Cook, J. (1988) An investigation of the validity of the British Ability Scales with respect to the Wechsler Intelligence Scale for Children–Revised and the wide range achievement test: revised on a group of Canadian children. *British Journal of Educational Psychology, 58* (2), 212–216.

Court, J.H. & Raven, J. (1995). *Manual for Raven's Progressive Matrices and Vocabulary Scales*. Oxford Psychologists Press, Oxford.

Davis, C.J. (1980) *Perkins–Binet Tests of Intelligence for the Blind*. Perkins School for the Blind, Watertown, MA.

Delis, D.C., Kramer, J.H., Kaplan, E. & Ober, B.A. (1993) *California Verbal Learning Test: Childrens Version*. Psychological Corporation, San Antonio, TX.

Dienske, H., de Jonge, G. & Sanders-Woudstra, J.A. (1985) Quantitative criteria for attention and activity in child psychiatric patients. *Journal of Child Psychology and Psychiatry, 26*, 895–915.

Doane, J.A., West, K.L., Goldstein, M.J., Rodnick, E.H. & Jones, J.E. (1981) Parental communication deviance and affective style: predictors of subsequent schizophrenia spectrum disorders in vulnerable adolescents. *Archives of General Psychiatry, 38*, 679–685.

Dunn, J. & Kendrick, C. (1980) Studying temperament and parent–child interaction: comparison of interview and direct observation. *Developmental Medicine and Child Neurology, 22* (4), 484–496.

Elwood, R.W. (1995) The California Verbal Learning Test: psychometric characteristics and clinical application. *Neuropsychological Review, 5*, 173–201.

Evans, J.J., Chua, S.E., McKenna, P.J. & Wilson, B.A. (1997) Assessment of the dysexecutive syndrome in schizophrenia. *Psychological Medicine, 27*, 635–646.

Exner, J.E. Jr & Weiner, I.B. (1994) *The Rorschach. A Comprehensive System*, Vol. 3, *Assessment of Children and Adolescents*, 2nd edn. Wiley, New York.

Fischoff, B. & Lichtenstein, S. (1978) Don't attribute this to the Reverend Bayes. *Psychological Bulletin, 85*, 239–243.

Frankenburg, W.K. & Dodds, J.B. (1967) The Denver Developmental Screening Test. *Journal of Pediatrics, 71*, 181–191.

Frankenburg, W.K., van Doorninck, W.K., Liddell, T.N. & Dick, N.P. (1986) *Revised Denver Prescreening Developmental Questionnaire (R-PDQ)*. DDM/Test Agency, High Wycombe, UK.

Friedlander, M.L. & Stockman, S.J. (1983) Anchoring and publicity effects in clinical judgement. *Journal of Clinical Psychology*, **39**, 637–643.

Genero, N. & Cantor, N. (1987) Exemplar protypes and clinical diagnosis: toward a cognitive economy. *Journal of Social and Clinical Psychology*, **5**, 59–78.

Goggin, W.C. & Range, L.M. (1985) The disadvantage of hindsight in the perception of suicide. *Journal of Social and Clinical Psychology*, **3**, 232–237.

Golden, C.J. (1987) *Luria Nebraska Neuropsychological Battery: Children's Revision*. Western Psychological Services, Los Angeles, CA.

Golding, S.L. & Rorer, L.G. (1972) Illusory correlation and subjective judgement. *Journal of Abnormal Psychology*, **80**, 249–260.

Gould, J. (1977) The use of the Vineland Social Maturity Scale, the Merrill–Palmer Scale of mental tests (non-verbal items) and the Reynell Developmental Language Scales with children in contact with the services for severe mental retardation. *Journal of Mental Deficiency Research*, **21**, 213–226.

Gregory, R.L. (1981) *Mind in Science: A History of Explanations in Psychology and Physics*. Weidenfeld & Nicholson, London.

Griffiths, R. (1970) *The Abilities of Young Children*. Child Development Research Centre, London.

Heavey, L., Phillips, W., Baron-Cohen, S. & Rutter, M. (2000) The Awkward Moments Test: a naturalistic measure of social understanding in autism. *Journal of Autism and Development Disorders*, **30**, 225–236.

Henderson, S.E. & Sugden, D.A. (1992) *Movement Assessment Battery for Children (Movement ABC)*. Psychological Corporation, London.

Hiskey, M.S. (1966) *The Hiskey–Nebraska Test of Learning Aptitude*. Union College Press, Lincoln, NB.

Horowitz, L.M., Inouye, D. & Siegelman, E.Y. (1979) On averaging judges' ratings to increase their correlation with an external criterion. *Journal of Consulting and Clinical Psychology*, **47**, 453–457.

Hughes, C., Adlam, A., Happe, F., Jackson, J., Taylor, A. & Caspi, A. (2000) Good test–retest reliability for standard and advanced false: belief tasks across a wide range of abilities. *Journal of Child Psychology and Psychiatry*, **41**, 483–490.

Jastak, S. & Wilkinson, G.S. (1984) *Wide Range Achievement Test–Revised*. Jastak, Wilmington, DE.

Jorgensen, K., Anderson, T.J. & Dam, H. (2000) The diagnostic efficiency of the Rorschach Depression Index and the Schizophrenia Index: a review. *Assessment*, **7**, 259–280.

Kagan, J. (1997) Temperament and the reactions to unfamiliarity. *Child Development*, **68**, 139–143.

Kagan, J., Snidman, N. & Arcus, D. (1998) Childhood derivatives of high and low reactivity in infancy. *Child Development*, **69**, 1483–1493.

Kalverboer, A.F. (1971) Observation of exploratory behaviour of preschool children alone in the presence of the mother. *Psychiatria Neurologia Neurochirurgia*, **74**, 43–57.

Kaufman, A.S. & Kaufman, N.L. (1983) *Kaufman Assessment Battery for Children*. American Guidance Service, Circle Pines, MN.

Kaufman, A.S. & Kaufman, N.L. (1985) *Kaufman Test of Educational Achievement*. American Guidance Service, Circle Pines, MN.

Kimberg, D.Y. & Farrach, M.J. (1993) A unified account of impairments following frontal lobe damage: the role of working memory in complex organised behaviour. *Journal of Experimental Psychology: General*, **122**, 411–428.

Korkman, M. (1999) Applying Luria's diagnostic principles in the neuropsychological assessment of children. *Neuropsychology Review*, **9**, 89–105.

Korkman, M., Kirk, U. & Kemp, S. (1997) *NEPSY*. Psychological Corporation, San Antonio, TX.

Krabbendam, L., de Vugt, M.E., Derix, M.M. & Jolles, J. (1999) The behavioural assessment of the dysexecutive syndrome as a tool to assess executive functions in schizophrenia. *Clinical Neuropsychology*, **13**, 370–375.

Lord, C., Risi, S., Lambrecht, L. *et al.* (2000) Autism diagnostic observation schedule–generic: a standard measure of social and communication deficits associated with the spectrum of autism. *Journal of Autism and Developmental Disorders*, **30**, 205–223.

Lowe, C. & Rabbitt, P. (1998) Test–retest reliability of the CANTAB and ISPOCD neuropsychological batteries: theoretical and practical issues. Cambridge Neuropsychological Test Automated Battery, International Study of Post-Operative Cognitive Dysfunction. *Neuropsychologica*, **36**, 915–923.

Luciana, M. & Nelson, C.A. (1998) The functional emergence of prefrontally-guided working memory systems in four- to eight-year-old children. *Neuropsychologia*, **36**, 273–293.

Luciana, M. & Nelson, C.A. (2000) Neurodevelopmental assessment of cognitive function using CANTAB: validation and future goals. In: *Functional Neuroimaging in Child Psychiatry* (eds M. Ernst & J.M. Rumsey), pp. 379–397. Cambridge University Press, Cambridge.

Luk, S.L. (1985) Direct observation studies of hyperactive behaviours. *Journal of the American Academy of Child Psychiatry*, **24**, 338–344.

Luk, S.L., Thorley, G. & Taylor, E. (1987) Gross overactivity: a study by direct observation. *Journal of Psychopathology and Behavioural Assessment*, **9**, 173–182.

Luria, A.R. (1980) *Higher Cortical Functions in Man*, 2nd edn. Basic Books, New York.

McCall, R.B. & Carriger, M.S. (1993) A meta-analysis of infant habituation and recognition memory performance as predictors of later IQ. *Child Development*, **64**, 57–59.

Moffitt, T.E., Caspi, A., Harkness, A.R. & Silva, P.A. (1993) The natural history of change in intellectual performance: who changes? How much? Is it meaningful? *Journal of Child Psychology and Psychiatry*, **34**, 455–506.

Naglieri, J.A. & Das, J.P. (1997) *Cognitive Assessment System*. Riverside Publishing, Itasca, IL.

Neale, M.D. (1997) *Neale Analysis of Reading Ability: Second Revised British Edition*. NFER-Nelson, Windsor.

Pennington, B.F. & Ozonoff, S. (1996) Executive functions and developmental psychopathology. *Journal of Child Psychology and Psychiatry*, **37**, 51–87.

Piotrowski, C. (1995) A review of the clinical and research use of the Bender–Gestalt Test. *Perceptual and Motor Skills*, **81**, 1272–1274.

Posner, M.I. (1978) *Chronometric Explorations of Mind*. Hillside, Erlbaum.

Raggio, D.J., Massingale, T.W. & Bass, J.D. (1994) Comparison of Vineland Adaptive Behavior Scales: Survey Form age equivalent and standard score with the Bayley Mental Development Index. *Perceptual and Motor Skills*, **79**, 203–206.

Reitan, R.M. & Wolfson, D. (1993) *The Halstead–Reitan Neuropsychology Test Battery: Theory and Clinical Interpretation*. Neuropsychology Press, Tuscon, AZ.

Robbins, T.W., James, M., Owen, A.M. *et al.* (1998) A study of performance on tests from the CANTAB battery sensitive to frontal lobe dysfunction in a large sample of normal volunteers: implications for theories of executive functioning and cognitive aging. Cambridge Neuropsychological Test Automated Battery. *Journal of the International Neuropsychological Society*, **4**, 474–490.

Roid, G.H. & Miller, L.J. (1997) *Leiter International Performance Scale-Revised: Examiner's Manual*. Stoelting, Wood Dale, IL.

Rubia, K., Overmeyer, S., Taylor, E. *et al.* (1999) Hypofrontality in attention deficit hyperactivity disorder during higher-order motor control: a study with functional MRI. *American Journal of Psychiatry*, **156**, 891–896.

Ryan, J.J., Arb, J.D. & Ament, P.A. (2000) Supplementary WMS-III tables for determining primary sub-test strengths and weaknesses. *Psychological Assessment*, **12**, 193–196.

Sanders, A.F. (1983) Towards a model of stress and performance. *Acta Psychologica*, **53**, 61–97.

Sattler, J.M. (2001) *Assessment of Children: Cognitive Applications*, 4th edn. Sattler, San Diego.

Schachar, R., Sandberg, S. & Rutter, M. Agreement between teachers' ratings and observations of hyperactivity, inattentiveness and defiance. *Journal of Abnormal Child Psychology*, **14**, 331–345.

Semel, E., Wiig, E.H. & Secord, W.A. (1995) *Clinical Evaluation of Language Fundamentals*, 3rd edn. Psychological Corporation, San Antonio, TX.

Semrud-Clickeman, M., Steingard, R.J., Filipek, P., Biederman, J., Bekken, K. & Renshaw, P.F. (2000) Using MRI to examine brain–behaviour relationships in males with attention deficit disorder with hyperactivity. *Journal of the American Academy of Child and Adolescent Psychiatry*, **39**, 477–484.

Sergeant, J.A., Oosterlaan, J. & van der Meere, J.J. (1999) Information processing and energetic factors in attention deficit hyperactivity disorder. In: *Handbook of Disruptive Behavior Disorders* (eds. H.C. Quay & A. Hogen), pp. 75–104. Plenum Press, New York.

Shallice, T. (1982) Specific impairments of planning. *Philosophical Transactions of the Royal Society of London, B*, **298**, 199–209.

Sheslow, D. & Adams, W. (1990) *Wide Range Assessment of Memory and Learning*. Jastak, Wilmington, DE.

Shriffrin, R.M. & Schneider, W. (1977) Controlled and automatic human information processing. II. Perceptual learning, automatic attending, and a general theory. *Psychological Review*, **84**, 127–190.

Slater, A. (1995) Individual differences in infancy and later IQ. *Journal of Child Psychology and Psychiatry*, **31**, 69–112.

de Sonneville, L.M.J., Visser, M. & Licht, R. (1999) Attention and information processing in 4- and 5-year-old children: results of a computerised assessment technique. In: *Cognitive Ergonomics, Clinical Assessment and Computer Assisted Learning: Computers in Psychology* (eds. B.P.L.M. den Brinker, P.J. Beek, A.N. Brand, S.J. Maarse & L.J.M. Mulder), Vol. 6, pp. 204–217. Swets & Zeitlinger, Lisse.

Sparrow, S.S. & Davis, S.M. (2000) Recent advances in the assessment of intelligence and cognition. *Journal of Child Psychology and Psychiatry*, **36**, 117–131.

Sparrow, S.S., Balla, D.B. & Cicchetti, D.V. (1984) *The Vineland Adaptive Behavior Scales*. American Guidance Service, Circle Pines, MN.

Sternberg, R.J. & Kaufman, J.C. (1988) Human abilities. *Annual Reviews of Psychology*, **49**, 479–502.

Stewart, A.L., Rifkin, L., Amess, P.N. *et al.* (1999) Brain structure and neurocognitive and behavioural function in adolescents who were born very preterm. *Lancet*, **9165**, 2653–2657.

Stroop, J.R. (1935) Studies of interference in serial verbal reactions. *Journal of Experimental Psychology*, **18**, 643–662.

Sturmey, P., Carlsen, A., Crisp, A.G. & Newton, J.T. (1988) A functional analysis of multiple aberrant responses: a refinement and extension of Iwata *et al.*'s 1982 methodology. *Journal of Mental Deficiency Research*, **32**, 31–46.

Stutsman, R. (1931) *Mental Measurement of Preschool Children*. World Books, New York.

Szatmari, P. & Taylor, D.C. (1984) Overflow movements and behaviour problems: scoring and using a modification of Fogs' test. *Developmental Medicine and Child Neurology*, **26**, 297–310.

Tannock, R., Martinussen, R. & Frijters, J. (2000) Naming speed and stimulant effects indicate effortful semantic processing deficits in attention deficit hyperactivity disorder. *Journal of Abnormal Child Psychology*, **28**, 237–252.

Taylor, E. (1991) Developmental neuropsychiatry. *Journal of Child Psychology and Psychiatry*, **32**, 3–47.

Thorndike, R.L., Hagen, E.P. & Sattler, J.M. (1986) *Stanford–Binet Intelligence Scale*, 4th edn. Riverside Publishing, Chicago, IL.

Tucker, J.A. (1985) Curriculum-based assessment: an introduction. *Exceptional Children*, **52**, 199–204.

Wechsler, D. (1989) *Wechsler Preschool and Primary Scale of Intelligence–Revised*. Psychological Corporation, San Antonio, TX.

Wechsler, D. (1991) *Wechsler Intelligence Scale for Children Manual*, 3rd edn. Psychological Corporation, San Antonio, TX.

Wechsler, D. (1992a) *Manual for the Wechsler Intelligence Scale for Children*, 3rd edn. Psychological Corporation, London.

Wechsler, D. (1992b) *Wechsler Objective Reading Dimensions (WORD)*. Psychological Corporation, London.

Wechsler, D. (1996) *Wechsler Objective Numerical Dimensions (WOND)*. Psychological Corporation, London.

Wechsler, D. (1997) *Wechsler Adult Intelligence Scales (WAIS)*. Psychological Corporation, London.

Wilson, B.A., Cockburn, J. & Baddeley, A. (1985) *The Rivermead Behavioral Memory Test*. Thames Valley Test Company, Reading, UK; National Rehabilitation Services, Gaylord, MI.

Wilson, B.A., Alderman, N., Burgess, P.W., Emslie, H.C. & Evans, J.J. (1996) *The Behavioural Assessment of the Dysexecutive Syndrome*. Thames Valley Test Company, Hempton, Bury St Edmunds.

Wood, J.M., Lilienfeld, S.O., Garb, H.N. & Nezworski, M.T. (2000) The Rorschach test in clinical diagnosis: a critical review, with a backward look at Garfield (1947). *Journal of Clinical Psychology*, **56**, 395–430.

Yule, W. (1967) Predicting reading ages in Neale's Analysis of Reading Ability. *British Journal of Educational Psychology*, **37**, 252–256.

7 Applied Scientific Thinking in Clinical Assessment

Michael Rutter and William Yule

Concepts of applied science

Both clinical psychology and clinical psychiatry (together with the rest of medicine) aspire to being applied sciences (Shapiro 1957; Kennedy & Llewelyn 2001; Rutter 1975; Yule 1989; see also Taylor & Rutter, Chapter 1). This does not mean that clinical practice only involves the use of scientific methods and scientific knowledge; interpersonal skills, and social sensitivity, are also crucially important. Intuition and experience constitute key elements in assessment, as well as in the planning and undertaking of treatment. Moreover, there are many points during the clinical process when either ethical considerations or value judgements have to be made. The current debate on whether tricyclic medication or selective serotonin uptake inhibitors should be the drug of first choice in treating depression in adults well illustrates the considerations that have to go into the interpretation of empirical findings (Barbui & Hotopf 2001; Thompson 2001). Findings on efficacy are fundamental but the choice of drug needs to be influenced also by side-effects, patient acceptability, and cost.

The concept of an applied science does not mean that practice has to be based just on 'facts'. It is a common misunderstanding that science is an enterprise defined by its production of factual knowledge. Rather, science constitutes a way of thinking and a set of approaches that is concerned with solving problems — with formulating hypotheses, putting these together in an integrated and cohesive notion of how nature might operate (a theory) and in finding ways of putting those ideas to the test. Scientific study does provide immensely useful findings but knowledge is always partial. It has been said that of the 'facts' learned during training, a third will prove to be true, a third will subsequently be shown to be wrong, and a further third will be found to be irrelevant. More importantly, scientific advances mean that during the course of a professional lifetime, clinical practice will change, and will need to change, as a result of the understanding and clinical opportunities that derive from research (Rutter 1998, 1999, 2000).

First and foremost, clinical training has to involve the acquisition of a large amount of factual knowledge because of the basic requirement that clinicians must function in ways that are both safe and effective. However, there are two other needs that are almost as important. First, training involves a considerable focus on experimental psychology, neurophysiology, neuroscience and biology. In addition, psychiatric training includes systematic learning about pharmacology, neurology and internal medicine as they impinge on the workings of the brain and the functioning of the mind. This is not primarily because such knowledge is of immediate clinical importance: indeed, rather little is. Rather, it is because it provides a rich source of ideas about the ways in which nature operates and which might apply to clinical problems. It is likely, if not actually certain, that much of this knowledge will lead to clinical advances during the course of people's working years.

Secondly, in the course of their clinical lifetime, people will need to practise on the basis of new knowledge derived from research since they completed their formal training. They will have to cope with a flood of claims and counterclaims and an essential part of training is to enable people to understand enough about research for them to evaluate research evidence and its clinical implications — not just on the basis of the hyperbole of the evangelists, but on the basis of their own assessment of the quality of the evidence and of how it might, or should, alter what they do clinically. This applies, not just to psychologists and psychiatrists, but to nurses, social workers and psychotherapists; indeed to all clinicians.

These broad issues pervade the whole of this book. In this chapter, we concentrate on the narrower issue of how the concept of clinical psychology and psychiatry as applied sciences impinges on clinical assessment as applied to children and adolescents. We argue that the key defining feature is the use of experimental concepts and stratagems in the planning and undertaking of clinical assessment. The starting point has to be some type of clinical question. That is so whether the assessment is designed to lead to diagnosis, to the design of treatments, or to their evaluation (Mash & Terdal 1981). Psychiatrists are irritated by referrals that simply say, 'This is John Brown. Please see and advise.' Psychologists, equally, take exception to requests that just state that the referral is for 'IQ testing' or 'tests of language'. That is not to say that there is not a place for screening assessments of various kinds. Some form of medical screening is desirable in all clinical referrals, and some medical investigations should be undertaken as a routine (see Bailey, Chapter 10). For example, assessments of hearing and vision, and screening for chromosomal abnormalities, should be part of the routine in the case of all children referred for serious developmental disorders. In the same way, the high frequency with which psychopathology is associated with scholastic retardation and/or cognitive deficits means that screening for them should be a routine matter in clinical assessment.

This may be carried out through obtaining information from schools, or clinics may choose to undertake some form of screening testing.

Nevertheless, a clinical question should constitute the starting point for most referrals for clinical assessment—either psychological or psychiatric. An applied scientific approach, we suggest, involves several key elements. First, there is a need to identify the key clinical issues. Those may be implicit or explicit in the clinical question posed but the starting point, nevertheless, needs to be a reconsideration and reconceptualization of those clinical issues. The second, and most basic step, constitutes the translation of the clinical issues into testable questions. These necessarily involve a consideration of alternative hypotheses and a decision on how one hypothesis may be pitted against another (Rutter et al., 2001). Naturally, that requires a knowledge of the range of possible stratagems that may be employed for this purpose. This is the essence of experimental thinking.

For this testing to be undertaken satisfactorily, the clinician needs to consider how to ensure that the testing will be based on high-quality data that are relevant to this individual and which have the appropriate meaning in relation to the clinical issues being considered. Some of the key technical issues that concern psychometric testing, the development of diagnostic interviews, the construction of questionnaires, and the use of medical testing and investigations, are considered in other chapters and will not be discussed further here (see Sergeant & Taylor, Chapter 6; Angold, Chapter 3; Verhulst & Van der Ende, Chapter 5; Bailey, Chapter 10). The main principles apply to clinical work with all age groups but the assessment of children involves, in addition, the need to adopt a developmental perspective. This requires a good understanding of developmental psychology (Rutter & Rutter 1993) and of developmental psychopathology (Rutter & Sroufe 2000).

Fombonne (see Chapter 4) discusses how all of these need to be put together for case identification and Rutter & Taylor (see Chapter 2) consider how this fits into an overall approach to clinical assessment and diagnostic formulations. Here we focus more narrowly on the special considerations with respect to data quality as they apply to experimental or applied scientific approaches in clinical evaluation.

Hypothesis testing almost always requires some form of quantification. That is because the essence of an experiment lies in the manipulation of one variable, under controlled conditions, to determine if, in a systematic and regular fashion (as shown across a range of varying conditions) this causes another variable to 'move'. This can only be carried out if there is a way of determining that the initial 'manipulation' truly involves a substantial change in the first variable and if the predicted change in the second variable is robust to the extent that it exceeds the variations that may be expected by chance. Occasionally, this may involve some qualitative categorical alteration, rather than a quantified dimensional change but, either way, quantification (of the presence/absence variety or of a point on a continuum variety) has occurred.

In both psychology and psychiatry, there has been much debate in recent years with respect to the merits and demerits of quantitative and qualitative approaches (Rutter, 2001). This is a false dichotomy and the polarization between the two research approaches has been unhelpful. Qualitative researchers have rightly been critical of the mindless application of quantitative methods before determination of the meaning of the phenomena to be assessed. Some form of qualitative analysis will almost always need to proceed the application of quantitative methods (see Rutter & Nikapota, Chapter 16, for a consideration of this issue in relation to social group comparisons). On the other hand, hypothesis testing requires quantitative research. The main reason that this is so derives from epidemiological considerations. First, because almost all psychopathology is multifactorial in origin, even in relation to a single case, it is crucial to be able to test whether a particular effect is a consequence of one factor rather than another (see below). For obvious reasons, that can only be done if there is adequate quantitative measurement of both the risk factors and the psychopathology. Secondly, all human groups (whether they involve members of the general population or patient samples) are very heterogeneous. For good reason, qualitative studies (which tend to be quite intensive) need to use relatively small samples. That is perfectly acceptable for the purpose of gaining a better understanding of what is happening, such understanding being used to generate testable hypotheses. On the other hand, it is not acceptable for testing hypotheses, because small heterogeneous samples inevitably mean uncertainty as to whether the findings refer to the psychopathological defining feature of the sample or to some other source of heterogeneity. Most research questions require a *combination* of qualitative and quantitative methods and the same applies to the assessment of individual cases. They have a different mix of strengths and limitations and both approaches are required.

In considering clinical assessment, we turn first to diagnosis. Apart from the applied scientific methods we advocate, four other approaches to diagnosis are possible and we need to consider whether their use now means that experimental methods are no longer needed in diagnosis, even if they are needed in other aspects of clinical work.

First, there are the *algorithmic approaches* based on standardized diagnostic instruments. Thus, both DSM-IV (American Psychiatric Association 1994) and the research version of ICD-10 (World Health Organization 1993) have formulae that generate diagnoses once the specified set of criteria have been met. Moreover, computer programs have been written to enable people to do this entirely through computer software without the need for the manual counting of numbers of particular sorts of symptoms, duration and other inclusionary and exclusionary specifications. Undoubtedly, this has been a most useful advance but two basic problems remain. There is the key question of the validity of the data that are read into the algorithm. The agreement among different instruments and among different algorithms has been found to be only moderate (Volkmar et al. 1992; Farmer et al. 1993; McGuffin & Farmer, in press). As we discuss below, experimental approaches can be helpful in testing the validity of the basic data. Very few psychiatric diagnoses have an unambiguous external validating criterion and, hence, it is most unlikely that the precise algorithmic criteria will ultimately prove to be fully valid (see Taylor & Rutter, Chapter 1).

Secondly, diagnoses may be determined by *pattern recognition*. The late Jack Tizard, a most important mentor for both of us, often remarked that he saw this approach as the one that was most different between medicine and clinical psychology. He expressed amazement at the surprising ability of good medics to recognize rare and unusual syndromes that they had seen only once before some 30 years ago or indeed may never have seen, relying only on textbook descriptions. It is certainly true that this constitutes a key part of medical training and, at its very best, works well. Moreover, this human skill is one in which the top level minds can often defeat supercomputers despite the immensely greater capacity of the computer to test vast numbers of possibilities very swiftly. It was this pattern recognition skill that enabled chess masters to defeat supercomputers at chess for a long time. The skill, it is true, does not involve experimental thinking at all in the ordinary sense. However, it would be a grave error to think that this is how most medical diagnoses are made (let alone psychiatric ones). Rather, diagnosis consists of putting together very complex sets of data, weighting different elements appropriately, and considering possible interactions among risk and protective factors. There is no question that computers are usually very considerably better at this than are human minds. That is why computer diagnoses have come to have an increasingly important role in medical diagnoses. For them to work really satisfactorily, of course, there must be some external diagnostic criterion and, when that comes in the field of psychopathology, computers are likely to play an increasing part there as well. On the other hand, as we discuss below, ending up with the 'correct' diagnosis is not all that clinical assessment is about and hypothesis-testing approaches are likely to continue to be important for a long time to come.

A third approach is provided by *quantified* diagnostic methods that are based on the well-justified assumption that many disorders (in medicine as a whole and not just in psychopathology) represent extremes on some continuously distributed liability dimension. Thus, just as hypertension may be diagnosed on the basis of a blood pressure above a certain predetermined and specified level, so mental retardation may be diagnosed by an IQ score below some particular criterion point. Similarly, depressive disorder may be diagnosed by a depression symptom score above a certain threshold on some standardized measure. Unquestionably, this approach has considerable utility but very few diagnoses can be made on the basis of a single dimension. It is usual to need to consider patterns of symptoms and to assess functional consequences. At a more basic level, however, it is essential to determine whether the test score (whatever the test may be) has the meaning that is required for its use in diagnosis. Just as it is necessary to check whether a high blood pressure may reflect excessive alcohol consumption, smoking, exercise or anxiety, so it is crucial to test whether a low IQ score reflects a limited cognitive capacity rather than a lack of engagement in the task, negativism, the distorting effect of psychopathology or situational features. That is where experimental thinking needs to come in.

Finally, diagnoses may rest on some *qualitative* abnormality that is a necessary requirement for the diagnosis, even though it may not be a sufficient one. There are examples among mental disorders where a particular abnormality is both a necessary and sufficient feature. For example, this applies to chromosome abnormalities (as with Down syndrome) and with other entirely genetic disorders (such as the fragile X anomaly or Huntington disease). However, these account for a tiny proportion of mental disorders. The situation is quite different with multifactorial disorders. Nevertheless, even with them, it may possibly turn out that one or more genetic mutations are a necessary basis for the diagnosis, even though they are not a sufficient one (because the disorder requires the operation of other genetic or environmental risk factors). Certainly, molecular genetics has the potential to deliver diagnostic tests of this kind (see McGuffin & Rutter, Chapter 12) but it is most uncertain whether genetic factors will operate in this way (as a necessary risk factor) for most forms of psychopathology. Also, it needs to be appreciated that many diagnostic tests in internal medicine involve a crucial experimental element. Most diagnoses are based on an abnormal pathophysiology that relates to function, rather than to a fixed feature that is independent of circumstances. Thus, the glucose tolerance test for diabetes, the exercise tolerance test for cardiac function, the various sensitivity tests for allergies and tests of respiratory function, all involve determining changes of some kind in response to a particular stimulus, but not to other stimuli. As we discuss below, this is similarly true of most psychological tests.

In short, an experimental way of thinking is likely to continue to have a central role in clinical assessment for many years to come. Its operation is central to the whole of biology and medicine and not something that is peculiar to mental disorders or psychopathology. Moreover, it is a need that applies to both clinical psychology and clinical psychiatry. It was for that reason that the authorship of this chapter combines disciplines. In the remainder of this chapter, we consider various different applications of applied scientific thinking in clinical assessment. The examples we use span both psychometric testing and psychiatric diagnostic methods because we wish to emphasize the generality of the application of the concepts we discuss. However, we have deliberately chosen more examples from psychology than psychiatry because, quite mistakenly, it is often assumed that, with well-established psychological tests, experimental thinking is not needed. Nothing could be further from the reality.

It should be added that the current trend to encourage the use of well-designed assessment and treatment protocols in order to ensure high standards in service delivery will not obviate the need for an applied scientific approach. There is much to be said for the use of standardized approaches but, as Kanner (1958) emphasized years ago, the problems that children present at the clinic do not adhere to textbook descriptions. The systematic standardized protocols provide an excellent starting point, but clinicians need to appreciate the extent and importance of individual differences. This will often require the undertaking of individually tailored scientifically based assessments of the kind we describe here.

Obtaining valid psychometric test scores

Psychological tests vary considerably in the extent to which standardization data on appropriate populations have shown them to have adequately high reliability and validity. Other things being equal, a clinician will want to use instruments for which there is the best data demonstrating high reliability and validity. However, a differentiation needs to be made between a reliable and valid *instrument* and a reliable and valid *assessment* (Berger & Yule 1972). The latter concerns the qualities of the testing of a particular child under particular circumstances.

Although written 30 years ago, Berger & Yule's (1972) suggestions with respect to the testing of young disabled children with a possible language disorder are relevant. They argued that motivation is important in all testing and the tests constructed for use with children need to incorporate items that will arouse and maintain their interest. This is particularly the case with disabled children who may have experienced frequent failure and may therefore be unwilling to participate in, and persist with, items that they perceive as difficult. The clinician may choose to deviate somewhat from the prescribed order of testing procedures, and to intersperse simpler items among those likely to tax the child. It is usually wise to begin testing at a point much below the level at which a child is thought to be capable in order to provide the child with sufficient successes to encourage him or her to attempt more difficult tasks. Clark & Rutter (1979) showed that this was particularly important with some autistic children who tended to move into a stereotyped pattern of responses if they encountered a series of items that they could not deal with. Also, if the child appears to enjoy a particular task and is unwilling to attempt others, it is often a good idea to allow the child to work at what they like on condition that they attempt other tasks later. Similarly, it may, in some circumstances, be appropriate to allow the child to respond in a non-standardized way that provides the same information. Thus, Clark & Rutter (1979) described an example of a 'negativistic' child who became amenable to testing when allowed to say what the answer was, rather than to point to the correct solution. Board forms of Raven's Coloured Progressive Matrices (Raven *et al.* 1990) have also been devised to allow disabled children to demonstrate their choice by picking up the piece that provides the correct answer, rather than to use pointing (which some autistic individuals do not do well). Comparable adaptations of tests have also been devised for children with severe impairments of hearing or vision (see Hindley & van Gent, Chapter 50).

Sometimes, it is appropriate for parents to be present during the assessment in order to allow the child to be more at ease and also to help as a translator of instructions and responses. This is a two-edged sword, however, and it is most important that parents appreciate the importance of allowing the tester to obtain the child's response without parental help. Certain items on cognitive tests require the child to complete the task correctly within prescribed time limits, and some give bonus points for rapid solutions. Particular care needs to be exercised when using these timed items with disabled children. Those with motor coordination problems, or those who are highly distractable, are most likely to be penalized with timed tests. Special considerations also apply to the testing of children who lack speech, or whose understanding of speech is limited. It is essential to differentiate between items failed because the child could not perform the task and items 'failed' because the child did not know what task it was they were supposed to perform. When this is in doubt, instructions should be given in some form (such as mime or demonstration) that avoids the use of spoken language.

These principles played a major part in Stutsman's (1948) development of the Merrill–Palmer scales many years ago. It was appreciated that young and disabled children often get tired, distracted or oppositional. That is why the test was devised to take account of circumstances in which items are refused or have to be omitted for some reason. Standardization of the test is now out of date and lacks qualities that are now regarded as essential. Nevertheless, the approach has many advantages and it may well be that modern day test construction pays inadequate attention to the realities of young children's engagement and interest and lacks adequate steps for dealing with items refused.

Clinicians need to be very sensitive to the fact that the more that they depart from standard test administration procedures, the more cautious they must be in the interpretation of test findings. Nevertheless, for reasons discussed below, adequate psychometric testing requires determination of the tasks that the child can perform as well as those leading to failure. The meaning of the test score is crucially dependent on this mixture of passes and failures and on the ability to determine the features that go along with each. When we started in clinical practice, some four decades ago, it was very common for psychologists to report that disabled children (especially those with autism) were 'untestable'. As Berger & Yule (1972) commented, this is simply a statement that the psychologist has failed in his or her endeavour and it says nothing about the child except that he or she was difficult to test. The challenge with such difficult children is to use the reports of others, and the psychologist's own observations, to think of ways in which the child may be induced to be engaged in the relevant tasks and to persist at them. It will readily be appreciated that finding how to do this will provide invaluable information on the features that affect the child's behaviour as well as bringing about a means for obtaining a valid test assessment.

One particular concern that occupies a major place in the literature on cognitive testing is the desire to develop and use culture-free or culture-fair psychological tests. There are both good and bad aspects of this concern. The positive side is that it is appropriate, indeed essential, to use forms of assessment that are not biased because of an individual's particular experiences or lack of experiences—in exactly the same way that it is essential to use tests that are not biased by a person's disabilities in vision, hearing or language. The negative side is that the concept seems to presuppose that it would be possible to devise a pure measure of innate cognitive capacity that is not open to the influence of experience. Theoretically, this is nonsense. Intelligence, just like other psychological qualities, is multifactorially determined and its development will be influenced by experiences as well as by genetic background. The concept is also misleading because, in so far as constitutional features are strongly operative, they set a reaction range and not a particular level of performance. Also, psychological tests are measures of performance and not of some hypothesized internal quality as it might be if the child's experiences had been different.

That does not mean that the issue of the effects of culture on test performance can be ignored: on the contrary. However, what it does mean is that it may be more appropriate to examine the positive effects of culture directly rather than try to devise tests that are free of them. The example of the Brazilian street vendors mentioned by Rutter & Nikapota (see Chapter 16) is illuminating. What was important in studying their mathematical skills was to devise ways of testing that were relevant to the particular circumstances in which they had to function in real life. A highly unusual clinical example was provided by a young man seen by one of us some 40 years ago. He originated from an isolated rural community in one of the smaller Caribbean islands and on coming to London encountered a form of life that was entirely different to anything he had ever experienced before. He lacked family ties and emotionally he rather 'fell apart', ultimately being admitted to hospital with what seemed a psychotic-like disorder. Formal psychological testing gave rise to a score in the mentally retarded range but this seemed out of keeping with his behaviour as observed on the ward. It was appreciated that he was virtually unschooled and that the test tasks might well have a quite different meaning for him than for other people in the standardization sample. He was a fisherman by trade and, after some discussion with staff in the occupational therapy department, it was decided to give him the run of the materials in that department with a request that he construct the type of fishing basket that he used in the Caribbean. The result was spectacular. To begin with, he came into his own emotionally and became highly engaged in the task. From our point of view, we observed with awe his skill in using an unfamiliar set of materials to make a complicated basket involving a sleeve that went into its interior. The rationale was that the fish swam down this sleeve that had a very large opening and swam out of the narrower end into the middle of the basket and was thereby caught, because it was much more difficult for the fish to find the entrance to the interior end of the sleeve. It rapidly became obvious that, although this task could not give rise to a cognitive 'score', he clearly was not mentally retarded. The circumstance was a highly unusual one, but the general principle has a wider application. That is, as with the Brazilian street vendors, it may be worthwhile to make positive use of the cultural variations (rather than avoid them) and to seek ways of tapping skills, rather than finding failures, although, as always, it is the pattern of the two that is most informative.

Two other issues warrant mention. First, it is necessary to differentiate between the use of psychological assessment to consider performance in a person from a quite different background who is going to return to that background, and the rather different issues with respect to someone from a very different culture who is going to need to live in an industrialized country with all the usual expectations about schooling, jobs and the like. The former case might, for example, be relevant with respect to a clinical referral from abroad in relation to a child living in circumstances quite different from those of London (where we practise). The second point is that when there has been a very major change in life circumstances, test findings may have a quite different meaning with respect to their predictions for future performance. For example, in the children adopted into UK families from Romanian orphanages, the shift from profound deprivation to somewhat above-average family environment was followed by major cognitive gains (Rutter *et al.* 1998a; O'Connor *et al.* 2000).

Determining the validity of a test score

There are three main ways in which the validity of a score may be assessed in an individual case. First, use may be made of the psychologist's own observations of the child's motivation and persistent engagement in the tasks involved in the test. It is not always easy to differentiate between task failure and a lack of adequate engagement but careful observation of the child's performance, together with information from parents and teachers on the child's response to tasks, will usually provide an adequate lead. Other things being equal, if task failure occurs on tasks that obviously interest the child and attract adequate engagement, it is much more likely that the failure reflects lack of competence than if a child has only made a half-hearted attempt to do what was required.

The second approach is provided by an internal analysis of the pattern of task passes and fails. The basic assumption, or hypothesis, underlying the test is that success or failure reflects task difficulty rather than extraneous features such as distraction, anxiety or motivation. Accordingly, it is necessary to examine the pattern of item responses to determine if there is a reasonably consistent hierarchy with successes on easier items and failures on more difficult ones. Some tests, such as Raven's Progressive Matrices (Court & Raven 1995), build this in to the test construction so that there is a systematic progression from easy items to more difficult ones, back to easy ones and on to more difficult ones, and so forth. This is not usual in other tests but, nevertheless, there is a means of assessing the association with the task difficulty by going across subtests. There should always be caution about the validity of an overall score that is made up of a mixture of passes and failures on both more difficult and easier items. This will usually require further testing in order to determine what explains the pattern. Consistency across different tests or across separate testing occasions can also be helpful. When the test findings do not show a consistent pattern of response to task difficulty, an experimental approach will be needed in order to pit against each other alternative hypotheses about the reasons for these discrepancies.

The third approach is provided by examining the consistency between the test findings and other assessments of performance that derived from observations by the clinician or reports from parents or teachers. From a psychiatric perspective, it has been our practice always to use observations and reports in order to come up with a clinical expectation of test performance level (whether this be in relation to general intelligence or language or scholastic attainment) *before* hearing about test findings. It is only by having some sort of quantified other assessment that it is possible to determine whether there is a discrepancy to be explained. However, in doing this it is essential not to be content with some overall impression but rather to have thought through carefully what it is in the observations or reports that give rise to the expectation. This may be, for example, reports or observations of problem-solving skills outside the test situation, or it may involve the child's level of curiosity and organized exploration of the environment, or it may involve the style of approach to problem-solving (e.g. whether it is random trial and error or systematic and organized). The observations may involve the extent to which the child attempts, and succeeds, in finding out how toys and how sold objects 'work' or it may involve complexity in play (Rutter 1985a).

As Berger & Yule (1972) emphasize, it is never acceptable to leave discrepancies between test findings and parental reports unexplained; their existence is *always* an indication for a critical hypothesis-testing study of possible reasons for the discrepancy. The reasons may lie in the nature of the task (e.g. the child having more cues at home than in the controlled test situation), or in the parent's or teacher's interpretation (or misinterpretation) of the child's behaviour, or in the nature of the cognitive skills being assessed. If the parental report suggests marked skills or deficits on clinically important abilities that have not been tapped by standardized tests, other tests should be used to sample the additional functions. In cases where the child seems able to perform the task at a higher level at home than he or she does in the clinic, and when no reasons in the nature of the task seem to explain this discrepancy, the psychologist should seek to repeat observations in the home (or in the school if that is relevant) in order to determine the explanation for the discrepancy. Psychological assessment is complete only when this has been accomplished and when it has given rise to an explanation for the discrepancy.

An example of this kind arose with respect to a clinical referral of a boy who had suffered a very severe head injury. The school that the boy had attended both before and after the injury had concluded that the boy, of previously superior intelligence, had been left mentally retarded by the injury. To everyone's surprise, standardized testing, by contrast, showed that his overall IQ was still well above the population mean (although not as high as it is likely to have been before the injury). Observations in the classroom and of the boy coping with work at home

seemed to indicate that he was indeed performing poorly. One possibility was that the successful test performance was a function of the tasks being very short. Accordingly, a different set of tasks was constructed that required more prolonged persistence. The boy performed equally well on these and that explanation could be ruled out. It was similarly possible to rule out the possibility that his failures reflected undue distraction by extraneous stimuli. Eventually, it appeared that the key feature involved the requirement for initiative and individual decision-making in more open-ended tasks. This provided important clues as to how he might be helped to improve his school learning.

A very different example was provided by a young girl who had been referred because of puzzlingly variable uncooperative behaviour. Her school record made it clear that she was of above average intelligence and therefore it was a surprise to find that on standardized cognitive testing her score was only about 80. However, the psychologist also reported that although the girl had been cooperative throughout the testing, had spoken appropriately and seemed to be engaged in the tasks, her behaviour did not seem normal in that she appeared not quite 'with it'. This contrasted with her style of interaction when seen by the psychiatrist and a discussion of possibilities led to an arrangement whereby the next time that the child seemed to be behaving in the reported somewhat unusual fashion, an EEG was to be performed instantly. Interestingly, when this was carried out, it showed that she was in petit mal status. At first sight, it seemed impossible that she could be functioning as well as she was (albeit below her best) while having a continuous set of minor epileptic seizures. However, a careful examination of the EEG record showed that there were very brief breaks and apparently these were enough to enable her to function. Subsequent cognitive testing both within and outside periods of petit mal status confirmed the low average functioning in the one and the superior functioning in the other.

A further example is provided by a girl referred because of acquired aphasia with epilepsy (see Bishop, Chapter 39). Standardized testing showed that her understanding of spoken language was negligible but her parents reported that, despite her virtually complete loss of use of spoken language, she seemed to understand surprisingly well what was said to her. Both our observations in the clinic and parental reporting suggested that this might be because of her use of non-language information to guess correctly what was being communicated. Systematic observation, using situations that varied according to the level of possible other information that was available to the girl, confirmed that this was indeed the case. Once more, the resolution of the discrepancy provided an important lead as to how best to help her.

A more structured experimental design was needed to investigate several cases of supposed 'facilitated communication' in autistic individuals, seen at a time before this concept became fashionable. Although the details were slightly different in each case, what they had in common was that in all ordinary circumstances the young people were performing at an extremely low level, whether assessed on the basis of standardized test performance or spontaneous behaviour at home or at school. By contrast, when cognitive performance was assessed by any means involving the mediation of a facilitator (in two cases a parent but in the third case a therapist) a surprisingly high level of knowledge or understanding was shown. In each case, it was necessary for the child to rest their hand on the arm of the facilitator (or vice versa) and to use a system of pointing to letters or spelling out words on a kind of simplified typewriter. Observations confirmed that the reports of performance using this type of facilitation were indeed correct and there was every reason to suppose that the facilitator was not consciously manipulating what the child was doing. It quickly became apparent that the challenge was to account for the successes with facilitation, rather than the failures without it. Furthermore, it was clear that nothing would be gained by structuring the circumstances so that there could be failure with the facilitated task. That was because it would be easy to account for such failure on the basis of motivational influences. Instead, it was decided that the way ahead lay in tackling head-on the two main alternatives—that the correct answers derived from the facilitator or that they derived from the child. This led to the stratagem of so organizing the task that one or other of them would have to give the right answers to the wrong questions. The need to undertake this testing was fully explained but the precise details of how this was to be carried out were not revealed in advance (by agreement with those concerned). The child and the facilitator were each given the same set of questions but they were in a different order, without this being obvious to either of them. In all three cases, replicated testing showed that the answers reflected the questions as evident to the facilitator and not those evident to the child. Subsequent systematic studies of small groups of young people showing facilitated communication used a broadly comparable strategy with much the same results (Montee *et al.* 1995; Bebko *et al.* 1996).

These four rather different examples illustrate the range of ways in which an experimental, or quasi-experimental, approach to hypothesis testing in relation to the validity of a test score may be undertaken. The facilitated communication example approximates to a single case research investigation (Yule & Hemsley 1977); the epilepsy example involved the use of testing outside the psychological domain; and the other two examples required only variations in a more 'ordinary' exploratory clinical approach. In all four cases, however, it was necessary to ask questions about the validity of the test findings, to pose alternative explanations, and to devise means of differentiating among these alternatives.

Exploring reasons for situational variation in behaviour

It is a commonplace in both research and clinical practice to find that children's behaviour in one situation is not the same as that in another, or that their behaviour with one person differs from that with another. It is necessary in both research and clinical practice to develop hypotheses with respect to possible causes of the variation, and to devise means to test which explanation or explanations are valid. Apart from the usual need to consider how hypothesis testing may be undertaken, there is clearly a requirement to have adequate measures of both the child's behaviour and the situational or interpersonal circumstances. In addition, it is necessary to check that the apparent situational variation is real. The alternative is that the behaviour is actually similar across situations but that it is being perceived differently by different people. Again, the approach may be illustrated by giving a few varied examples.

The first example concerned a request from a particular school in relation to an apparent 'epidemic' of hysterical attacks in the classroom (McEvedy *et al.* 1966; Moss & McEvedy 1966; Benaim *et al.* 1973). This was a new phenomenon in an otherwise well-functioning school and it was also noteworthy that this was only occurring in some lessons and with some teachers. Observations showed that the behaviour of one girl constituted the usual initiator of similar behaviour in others. Also, it became apparent that the ways in which different teachers responded to what was happening made quite a difference to whether it spread. The details in both cases provided the lead on how the school might deal with the situation and the limited 'epidemic' soon came to an end.

Another quite different circumstance in which explanations of situational variation are needed concerns reports that a child's behaviour is influenced by diet. Thus, it is relatively common to have reports that, for example, children are more hyperactive when they have ingested foods that contain additives or when they have eaten particular foods, such as chocolate. The approach needed is reasonably straightforward in principle, although often very difficult in practice. The first need is to consider alternative hypotheses for the apparent variation in behaviour. In most cases, the two chief contenders are chance variations and the influence of other features. Thus, the clinician needs to consider whether the variation might be caused by the fact that at the times when behaviour is worse the child is in a different situation, or is tired or excited for reasons unconnected with the content of the food. Sometimes, careful history-taking makes it evident that the supposed connection with foods is so inconstant and weak that it is most unlikely to represent a causal effect. However, quite often, it is necessary to go on to some more systematic documenting of temporal relationships. In most cases, a key step is to identify specific time-limited behaviours that can serve as an index of the behavioural disturbance that is at issue. The parents may then be asked to keep a careful daily diary of the occurrence of such behaviours, together with possible circumstances or precipitants (other than food) that might be relevant. It is only when procedures of this kind provide evidence that indicates a strong case for an association with particular foods that it is justified to undertake the more searching experimental testing of the hypothesis. Basically, this requires going to a very simple diet and then experimentally adding, one by one, in blind fashion, different types of food substance (Egger *et al.* 1985; Carter *et al.* 1993). Single case studies of this kind are arduous and demanding and are not to be engaged in lightly. Nevertheless, they do have a place and the results have shown that, although most claims that specific foods have a predictable worsening effect on behaviour cannot be substantiated, they have proved valid in some instances and have led to effective and worthwhile therapeutic interventions.

Similar issues may arise in relation to parental responses to a 'problem' behaviour. For example, some years ago, one of us saw a young mother who was at her wits' end because her toddler would not sleep through the night. She had received conflicting advice from family and friends. One big issue was whether she should allow the child to have a nap in the middle of the day. Some people advised her to ensure that he did *not* have a nap; she should keep him awake so that he was sufficiently tired at the end of the day to go to sleep promptly. Others urged her to let the child have a nap when he wanted, on the grounds that to prevent it would merely make him irritable and oppositional. The mother was asked to keep a systematic sleep diary over a period of several weeks. A simple statistical test showed that on days when he was kept awake he would not settle at night, whereas on days when he had a nap, he slept through the night. This had seemed counterintuitive but data settled the issue.

Another example of the same kind was provided by a child who had been placed in a residential unit after a series of foster and adoptive placements had broken down. The unit had a good reputation for preparing children to move on to new families but, in this case, they were faced with what seemed to be unpredictable aggression. The main concern was over infrequent severe outbursts, but minor episodes were more common. On the principle that low-frequency high-amplitude behaviours can often be understood by looking at high-frequency low-amplitude equivalents, all episodes of aggression were systematically charted. The next step was to examine the temporal pattern in order to relate it to possible precipitants. It quickly became apparent that aggression was particularly likely to follow his sessions with the art therapist who was undertaking 'life story work' with him. It appeared that he was not yet ready to face the pain of his past, and a different approach proved more effective with him. Individual differences, as ever, are crucial.

Very comparable issues arise with respect to the possibility that mood disturbances are a function of phases in the menstrual cycle or that a marked change in a child's behaviour represents some fundamental alteration in their physical condition. For example, a consultation was sought by a residential institution for young people with autism in relation to a particular child who had shown a marked escalation in quite dangerous aggressive and destructive behaviours. They were concerned that it might reflect some unusual form of epileptic disturbance or some neurological deterioration. Again, careful history-taking from staff at the institution and from parents led to several alternative possibilities that needed to be considered. There had been marked changes of staff, the young person was now primarily looked after by someone new, and there had been possibly important changes in schedule and expectations. The problem required, again, selecting the key behaviours that gave the prime cause for concern with respect to the changes and a recording system was instigated, being planned jointly with staff, to test out the various possibilities. In this particular case, the evidence showed that the variations were related fairly systematically to changes in the institution and that when these were modified in ways that seemed likely to be helpful, there was a substantial reduction (although not elimination) of the aggressive and destructive behaviour. In another somewhat similar referral, the approach taken was similar but the answer was rather different. In the second case, the variations in behaviour seemed likely to be a function of a cyclical mood disturbance. This is not easy to gauge in non-verbal autistic individuals but appropriate medication proved helpful. It is often said that, if you want to understand a behaviour, introduce experimental changes to alter it. Hypothesis testing in assessment has a two-way relationship with therapeutic intervention: each can inform the other.

Sometimes the need is to check the validity of the referrer's perception of the problem. When working with teachers on part of a school-based clinical intervention project, concern was expressed over an apparently highly intelligent 6-year-old who 'never settled to do any work'. The teacher was helped to define and operationalize what she meant by 'work', and then to undertake a simple binary on/off task observation every fifth minute for 1 hour each morning. The results showed that the boy was on-task 60% of the time. This led to a redefinition of the problem and a focus on reinforcing his on-task behaviour, which was plentiful. Soon he was working at a level above the average for the class.

Reports that a child's behaviour is much worse at school than at home, or vice versa, are extremely common and clinicians need to decide whether systematic investigation is indicated or whether the evidence from research, together with the particular findings in this case, provide enough leads to indicate some of the likely features and therefore some of the elements that might constitute a focus for intervention. The hypothesis generation requires a knowledge of what might be relevant in the school environment as judged from studies of school effectiveness (Maughan 1994; Mortimore 1995, 1998), together with psychopathological evidence of the possible importance of features such as structure, group instruction, task demands and so forth. Similarly, hypotheses about relevant features in the family and in the home need to be guided by evidence from observational studies that have systematically investigated different features (Patterson 1982). It is usually helpful when focusing on situational variation to try to identify situations and circumstances that have comparabilities across the settings showing variation. It may then be most appropriate to move to a functional analysis of the behaviours in that situation (see below).

Functional analysis of behaviour

Systematic approaches to functional analysis of behaviour developed as an intrinsic element of the development of behavioural methods of treatment (see Herbert, Chapter 53).

However, in a more general sense, they are inherent in all forms of clinical assessment. In seeking to understand the nature of disturbed behaviour that has constituted the basis for referral, it is necessary to develop and test hypotheses about alternative explanations. For example, with respect to faecal soiling, it may have arisen because the child has failed to gain control of bowel function that ordinarily arises in childhood, or it may arise because the bowel has become blocked through impaction and there is seepage of faecal material around the blockage, or the child may have no blockage, have full control of bowel function, but for psychological reasons is depositing faeces in inappropriate places (Rutter 1975; see also Clayden *et al.*, Chapter 47). Various predictions follow from these alternatives. Thus, the form and consistency of the bowel motions is likely to be normal in the first and third alternatives but abnormal in the second. Also, the spatial deposition of faeces is likely to be relatively haphazard in the first two possibilities but systematic and psychologically meaningful in the third. Of course, there may be a combination of features and there are also other possibilities. The basic point, however, is that the clinician needs to adopt an experimental approach to the development and testing of clinical hypotheses.

Similar issues arose with respect to school non-attendance in which the main alternatives lie between avoidance of school as part of truancy associated with an antisocial propensity and avoidance of school for emotional reasons associated either with separation anxiety in relation to the family or fear of some aspect of the school situation (Hersov 1960a,b; Eysenck & Rachman 1965). In the same sort of way, these alternatives give rise to predictions about the details of the function of school non-attendance.

Functional analysis needs to be applied to the somewhat different issue of predisposing circumstances and immediate provoking stimuli or controlling contingencies. It can be important to determine the extent to which disruptive behaviours or emotional disturbance are most likely to arise when children are tired or hungry, when they are being required to do things that they do not want to do, when they are unable to communicate their needs or wishes (a particular issue in relation to autism, see Rutter 1985b; Howlin & Rutter 1987), or when maternal depression is associated with increased family discord or impaired parenting, or when father goes away from home on work, or when it is an anniversary of some particularly stressful situation. The analysis with these issues is broadly comparable to those already considered in relation to situational variations.

The more detailed 'blow-by-blow' sequential analysis of the circumstances most likely to provoke a particular behaviour or cut it short requires a careful systematic attention to particular episodes of behaviour. The well-based assumption is that, although there are major individual differences in children's liability to show different forms of psychopathology, there are also important situational influences on whether such psychopathology is manifest and how long it continues. The issues are well illustrated in the pathways involved in substance use and abuse (see Rutter, Chapter 28) or suicidal behaviour (see Shaffer & Gutstein, Chapter 33) or antisocial behaviour (Rutter *et al.* 1998b; see also Earls & Mezzacappa, Chapter 26). Such a behavioural analysis needs to be guided by both what research has shown as likely features to influence behaviour and what seems to be happening with this particular individual. A hypothesis-testing approach is obviously the way to proceed.

However, an important caveat is that the most important feature may not be what parents or teachers do after a particular behaviour has occurred but, rather, what they do to avoid it happening in the first instance. Thus, skilled parenting may have less to do with efficient disciplinary methods or social problem-solving strategies or coping techniques than with an accurate picking up of social cues and an appropriate use of diversionary tactics. This was well illustrated in one study of children's and parents' behaviour negotiating a supermarket (Holden 1983) and in other studies of parenting strategies (Gardner *et al.* 1999).

Ordinarily, functional analysis of behaviour tends to be thought of in terms of the features in the immediate situation that influence the occurrence of behaviours. However, precisely the same issues and approaches are relevant in relation to the possibility that the key influences on behaviour derive from meaningful connections with some past experiences. At one time, psychoanalytic psychotherapies were largely predicated on this basis; that the origins of mental disorders lay in internal thought processes in relation to past experiences, real or imagined. These approaches have become outmoded, at least as applied in their original form, because theoretical assumptions have not proved valid, because it became obvious that there was a need to take the immediate life situation into account, and because therapeutic methods lacked efficacy as compared with other forms of intervention. Nevertheless, the general notion that past experiences may have contemporary relevance is valid as shown, for example, by the persistence of post-traumatic stress disorder symptoms in some cases (see Yule, Chapter 32), by the long-term sequelae of sexual abuse in some circumstances (see Glaser, Chapter 21), or by the ways in which the experience of past relationships influences people's approach to current ones (Cassidy & Shaver 1999). However, if these possible connections with past experiences are to be used in clinical assessment (as they should be) it is important that ways be found of translating the notion into some form of testable hypothesis to which experimental thinking may be applied in putting the hypothesis to test.

Analysing test score discrepancies

Throughout the history of psychological testing, there has been an interest in the inferences that may be drawn from discrepancies between scores on two different tests or subtests. Thus, there has been a wish to draw conclusions about brain function when large differences have been found between verbal and performance subscores on the Wechsler scales, or from instances when performance on some skill such as language or reading is markedly lower than that expected of the child's age and overall level of intelligence. Three rather different issues have to be considered in relation to the topic of score discrepancies (Yule 1989). First, there is a need to appreciate the relatively wide confidence limits that surround most subtest scores. That is to say, it is very common for a child to obtain some particular score on one testing occasion and a somewhat higher, or lower, score on a subsequent occasion. The method of dealing with this is a straightforward statistical one requiring no hypothesis testing. With many tests (such as the Wechsler scales) tables are provided on the reliability (the likelihood that the same pattern would be found consistently over repeated testing) of different sized discrepancies. These data indicate whether the pattern is truly characteristic of the child, but they do not indicate whether it is statistically unusual.

The answer to this second, although closely related, question requires data on frequency of discrepancies in the general population of different sizes. Again, statistical tables are available for many tests and the findings generally show that discrepancies have to be quite large for them to be regarded as statistically rare.

The third question concerns the clinical meaning to be attached to a statistically unusual discrepancy. This immediately raises a base rate problem when trying to use a relatively common finding (a large discrepancy) to predict a rare phenomenon (such as brain damage) (Yule 1989). The key consideration is that differences between groups may provide a misleading expectation of the meaning of a finding in an individual case, unless attention is paid to base rates (Meehl & Rosen 1955). Thus, in the Isle of Wight survey (Rutter *et al.* 1970) verbal performance discrepancies of 25 points or greater on the Wechsler Intelligence Scale for Children (WISC) were twice as common in children with neurological disorders as in controls (14 vs. 7.5%). However, when the base rate of neurological disorders (6.4 per 1000) was taken into account, this translated into a chance of only 1 in 60 that a child with a large V–P discrepancy would have a neurological disorder (Yule 1989). The practical point is that even when there is a very strong association between features (one of which is rare), false positive predictions will be usual simply because normality is much more common than the abnormal disorder being predicted.

Some assistance is provided by paying attention to patterns made up of several different indices. For example, longitudinal studies have shown that various social abnormalities, developmental delays and attentional deficits all predict the later development of schizophrenia (Rutter & Garmezy 1983). Each of these is relatively common in the general population and of very little use for individual prediction. However, the combination of all three is much rarer, but is fairly common in the abnormal group. The findings in this instance are still, even in combination, not sufficiently distinctive to be of value in individual diagnosis, but the principle is one of utility. It is always worthwhile to consider whether there are several different indices that could be put together in this way and, if there are, whether data are available on the frequency of particular pattern occurrences.

A further problem concerns the supposed purity of the function being tapped by a particular test or subtest. Research findings are clear-cut in indicating that most tests reflect a wider range of skills than might be anticipated from the name or description of the test. Thus, most of the so-called non-verbal tests on the Wechsler Scales actually are influenced to some extent by language and language-related skills. Accordingly, care needs to be taken before assuming that an unusually high or low score is indeed measuring what it purports to measure. In many instances, a full understanding of this is not crucial in the clinical assessment of an individual case. Nevertheless, occasionally it is important, and the appropriate single case design means to investigate the meaning of unusual talents or deficits, as illustrated by studies of idiot savants (Hermelin 2001). These are individuals who have highly precocious skills in one narrow area that enable them to perform at levels well above those achieved by most people in the general population, despite the fact that their own level of overall intelligence is in the retarded range. A high proportion of such individuals show autism. One of the questions that needs to be addressed is whether their unusually high level of performance in their special talent constitutes some trick of rote learning or whether it is based on the same sorts of cognitive processes employed by more generally talented individuals. The style of investigation has involved setting the tasks in ways that allow, or prevent, different rule-based strategies, or different sources of information, to be used. Very similar strategies are relevant for the investigation of particular severe deficits.

A further issue concerns the clinical implications of marked discrepancies (giving rise to either skills or deficits). There has often been a wish to jump from test findings to inferences about brain lesions. Thus, for example, tests may be labelled as 'left hemisphere' or 'right hemisphere' tests (Prior 1979) or tests of frontal lobe function (Prior & Hoffman 1990). Sergeant & Taylor (see Chapter 6) point to the many problems involved in such inferences. So far as childhood is concerned, a crucial consideration is that lateralized or localized lesions incurred in early life do not lead to the same patterns of psychological functions that they do when the lesion has been incurred in adult life (see Goodman, Chapter 14; Vargha-Khadem *et al.* 1992; Rutter 1993). Particular genetic conditions can and do give rise to relatively distinctive psychological profiles in some instances (see Skuse & Kuntsi, Chapter 13) but there is rather less specificity to the supposed cognitive and behavioural phenotypes than sometimes claimed. They are real, and clinically important, but attention needs to be paid to individual variability as well as to syndrome specificity.

A rather different clinical implication has been that the identification of particular test score patterns may indicate which form of intervention is likely to be most effective in this child—giving rise to so-called 'prescriptive teaching'. The intention is clearly laudable and, in the future, it may prove possible to use test findings in this way (Sternberg 1997; Sternberg *et al.* 1998). However, this remains a field in which claims rather outstrip accomplishments and caution is needed in moving from test findings to the planning of intervention strategies. On the other hand, if a hypothesis-testing single case approach is followed (Berger 1994) it can be clinically worthwhile. The difficulty remains as to whether it is better to build on areas of strength, or concentrate attention to countering areas of weakness, or of finding ways to circumvent the difficulties.

Designing assessments to elicit specific psychological features

For many years *projective tests* used to comprise a major part of the psychological assessment in many clinics. The basic idea was that by presenting people with ambiguous visual stimuli, such as inkblots, as in the Rorschach test, or pictures, as in the Thematic Apperception Test, the meaning that individuals read into these ambiguous stimuli could be used to tap their innermost thoughts, of which they might not even be aware. Furthermore, it was thought that responses could lead to relatively strong diagnostic inferences. Such tests have now largely fallen out of regular usage because empirical findings have shown that the tests have many problems in interpretation and do not give rise to reliable diagnoses as assessed in other ways (Klein 1986). Nevertheless, the basic strategy of using tasks or situations to tap particular realms of behaviour, rather than to rely simply on their occurrence in unstructured situations, or to rely on reporting, remains clinically useful. The well-established clinical assessment tools of this kind are not projective in quite the same sense as the ambiguous pictures. Several different examples may serve to illustrate the approach. In each case, research findings were used to hypothesize the sorts of tasks or settings that might be expected to elicit the relevant behaviours and the tests were constructed in ways designed to isolate the specific psychological features of interest.

Ainsworth's 'Strange Situation procedure' is an example (Ainsworth 1967; Ainsworth *et al.* 1978). It was designed to use very brief separation and reunion episodes to tap qualities of security or insecurity in selective dyadic attachments (see O'Connor, Chapter 46). It was originally developed in Uganda, then further tested and developed in the USA and subsequently used in many different countries. Although it is not without its critics (Lamb *et al.* 1984), it has proved a remarkably robust measure of certain important attachment qualities. It has been important, however, that studies of abnormal groups of various kinds indicated the need to modify the scoring procedures in order to pick up qualities that were not captured by the original scoring system (Main & Solomon 1990; van Ijzendoorn *et al.* 1995). It does not pick up so clearly some of the key unusual features associated with attachment disorders in institutionally deprived children (see O'Connor, Chapter 46) and because of that, and because of the very limited age range to which it is applicable, it is not a tool that can be recommended for ordinary clinical use. Nevertheless, the principles are applicable and it may be that further developments using methods that are more appropriate to tapping variations in attachment behaviour in older children (Waters *et al.* 1995; Cassidy & Shaver 1999) may give rise

to tools that could be used for individual clinical assessment, although that point has not yet been reached.

The Autism Diagnostic Observation Schedule (ADOS) (Lord *et al.* 2000) provides a rather different example. It arose out of an appreciation that it was not particularly informative simply to observe possibly autistic individuals in an unstructured fashion and, at least with younger children, it was not possible to interview them in the ordinary way. Accordingly, various situations providing 'presses' for various forms of social initiatory, socially responsive behaviours, types of play or types of communication, were devised. Empirical research findings showed that it was not particularly useful to score whether or not the children performed particular actions in relation to these situations but the findings also indicated that standardized ratings of social and communicative behaviour were possible. Settings tapped a rich variety of behaviour, the ratings were reasonably reliable, and they had reasonable diagnostic differential validity. The half an hour or so period of observation is not sufficient on its own to give rise to a diagnosis, but the evidence does show that it contributes in a most valuable way to diagnosis when combined with parental reports as also obtained using standardized interviews such as the Autism Diagnostic Interview (Lord *et al.* 1994). Training is required for the use of this assessment but it has come increasingly to be used as part of ordinary clinical assessments in tertiary care clinics that see a large number of children with possible autism spectrum disorders.

It has been a universal experience that the kind of structured diagnostic interviews that are appropriate for older children do not work so well with very young children. Accordingly, a variety of interview techniques, using pictures and play stimuli, have been developed (see Angold, Chapter 3). Similarly, in an attempt to avoid direct, possibly leading, questions about experiences of sexual abuse, there has been the development of play-based interviews using anatomically explicit dolls (see Glaser, Chapter 21). In each case, it seems likely that the 'props' have been useful in getting the children engaged and in stimulating them to talk about relevant experiences. On the other hand, there is the twin risk that the props themselves may bias the information given because of the particular leads they provide. The remedy does not lie in either an uncritical acceptance of these approaches or an equally uncritical dismissal of their use. Rather, it is necessary to approach their use in an empirical way. In so doing, it will not be appropriate to rely on any overall statistic of reliability or validity. Rather, in relation to the situations in which they are used, it will be important to consider rates of false positives and false negatives and also to consider which of these is the more important in the circumstance in which they are to be used (see Fombonne, Chapter 4).

A range of psychometric tests to assess different functions have been devised (see Sergeant & Taylor, Chapter 6) and some of these include the element of response to particular stimuli; e.g. the continuous performance test, in which one of the key aims is to assess children's task performance in circumstances that have, or do not have, distracting stimuli (Rosvold *et al.* 1956; Conners

2000). Portable galvanic skin response (GSR) measures are also available to provide biofeedback to anxious children when they face feared situations.

Assessment approaches, of a quasi-experimental kind, have also been developed to assess both patterns of family interaction and patterns of social cue perception. For example, Goldstein *et al.* (Goldstein 1995) developed a method in which different family members were interviewed separately, differences among them in their perceptions of joint behaviour were identified, and the family was then brought together for a videotaped session in order to discuss these revealed differences. The idea was to provide a standardized stimulus that provided a potential for conflict in order to see how the family dealt with disagreements and differences. Video clips have also been developed to tap people's ability to identify different social cues and to assess the extent to which their interpretations of behaviour (as, for example, in relation to hostility or anxiety) were consonant with those of other people (Roeyers *et al.* 2001). Brown & Rutter (1966) (Rutter & Brown 1966) used parental interviews to tap the emotions expressed when parents talked about their children in response to neutral questions. This gave rise to a measure that came to be called 'expressed emotion' and subsequently to modifications based on a 5-min speech sample (Magaña *et al.* 1986) either in response to a request that parents simply talk unprompted about their children or talk in response to a series of neutral questions about their qualities (Sandberg *et al.* 1993). In each case, the development is hypothesis-based in the sense that standardized stimuli have been devised in order to elicit particular forms of behaviour in ways that are meant to be unbiased. In each case, in addition to the usual matters of standardization, reliability and the like, there is the key question of the extent to which the behaviour in these standard situations is or is not representative of behaviours shown in the more ordinary circumstances of life.

It is clear from numerous studies that these approaches have real value, but equally they also have important limitations. For the most part, the procedures are ones largely confined to research use at the moment, although at least some of them have the potential for development into procedures that might be applied in ordinary clinical assessment.

Conclusions

Throughout the last century, clinical psychology has paralleled clinical medicine in its aspiration that clinicians should be 'scientist-practitioners'; such a concept has had its critics but it is interesting that a recent British survey showed a continuing general endorsement of the evidence-based scientist-practitioner model (Kennedy & Llewelyn 2001). These authors emphasized, as we have done, the range of diverse approaches to scientific enquiry and the importance of a critical pragmatic approach to the integration of research into practice, as well as the need for a high degree of responsiveness to the cultural and institutional contexts of practice. We agree. There are important

ways in which psychology and psychiatry differ but they agree in showing the need for, and value of, a style of applied scientific thinking in approaching clinical assessment. Deliberately, we have referred to applied scientific thinking, rather than experimental designs, because the range of applications is so broad, extending from something that is little more than thoughtful questioning clinical enquiry, to a scientific investigation that approximates to a piece of research that can be applied to individual cases. This is not the whole of clinical assessment, as we have striven to emphasize, but it is an important, we would argue, essential, part of what is involved and it is an aspect that draws as heavily on the clinicians' creative and innovative skills as on their academic knowledge.

References

Ainsworth, M.D.S. (1967) *Infancy in Uganda: Infant Care and the Growth of Love.* Johns Hopkins University Press, Baltimore, MD.

Ainsworth, M.D.S., Blehar, M.C., Waters, E. & Wall, S. (1978) *Patterns of Attachment: A Psychological Study of the Strange Situation.* Erlbaum, Hillsdale, NJ.

American Psychiatric Association (1994) *Diagnostic and Statistical Manual of Mental Disorders (DSM-1V)*, 4th edn. American Psychiatric Association, Washington, D.C.

Barbui, C. & Hotopf, M. (2001) Amitriptyline vs. the rest: still the leading antidepressant after 40 years of randomised controlled trials. *British Journal of Psychiatry*, 178, 129–144.

Bebko, J.M., Perry, A. & Bryson, S. (1996) Multiple method validation study of facilitated communication. II. Individual differences and subgroup results. *Journal of Autism and Developmental Disorders*, 26, 19–42.

Benaim, S., Horder, J. & Anderson, J. (1973) Hysterical epidemic in a classroom. *Psychological Medicine*, 3, 366–373.

Berger, M. (1994) Psychological tests and assessment. In: *Child and Adolescent Psychiatry, Modern Approaches* (eds M. Rutter, E. Taylor & L. Hersov), 3rd edn, pp. 94–109. Blackwell Science, Oxford.

Berger, M. & Yule, W. (1972) Cognitive assessment in young children with language delay. In: *The Child with Delayed Speech* (eds M. Rutter & J.A.M. Martin), pp. 120–135. Spastics International Medical Publications, London.

Brown, G.W. & Rutter, M. (1966) The measurement of family activities and relationships: A methodological study. *Human Relations*, 19, 241–263.

Carter, C.M., Urbanowicz, M., Hemsley, R. *et al.* (1993) Effects of a few food diet in attention deficit disorder. *Archives of Disease in Childhood*, 69, 564–568.

Cassidy, J. & Shaver, P.R. (1999) *Handbook of Attachment: Theory, Research and Clinical Applications.* Guilford Press, New York.

Clark, P. & Rutter, M. (1979) Task difficulty and task performance in autistic children. *Journal of Child Psychology and Psychiatry*, 20, 271–285.

Conners, C.K. (2000) *Conners' Continuous Performance Test II Computer Program for Windows.* International Psychology Services, Hurstpierpoint, UK.

Court, J.H. & Raven, J. (1995) *Manual for Raven's Progressive Matrices and Vocabulary Scales.* Oxford Psychologists Press, Oxford.

Egger, J., Carter, C.M., Graham, P.J., Gumley, D. & Soothill, J.F. (1985) Controlled trial of oligoantigenic treatment in the hyperkinetic syndrome. *Lancet*, 1, 540–545.

Eysenck, H.J. & Rachman, S.J. (1965) The application of learning theory to child psychiatry. In: *Modern Perspectives in Child Psychiatry* (ed. J.G. Howells), pp. 104–169. Oliver & Boyd, Edinburgh.

Farmer, A.E., Jones, I., Williams, J. & McGuffin, P. (1993) Defining schizophrenia: operational criteria. *Journal of Mental Health*, **2**, 209–222.

Gardner, F.E.M., Sonuga-Barke, E.J.S. & Sayal, K. (1999) Parents anticipating misbehaviour: an observational study of strategies parents use to prevent conflict with behaviour problem children. *Journal of Child Psychology and Psychiatry*, **40**, 1185–1196.

Goldstein, M. (1995) Transactional processes associated with relatives' expressed emotion. *International Journal of Mental Health*, **24**, 76–96.

Hermelin, B. (2001) *Bright Splinters of the Mind*. Jessica Kingsley, London.

Hersov, L.A. (1960a) Persistent non-attendance at school. *Journal of Child Psychology and Psychiatry*, **1**, 130–136.

Hersov, L.A. (1960b) Refusal to go to school. *Journal of Child Psychology and Psychiatry*, **1**, 137–145.

Holden, G.W. (1983) Avoiding conflict: mothers as tacticians in the supermarket. *Child Development*, **54**, 233–240.

Howlin, P. & Rutter, M. (1987) *Treatment of Autistic Children*. Wiley, Chichester.

van Ijzendoorn, M.H., Juffer, F. & Duyvesteyn, M.G. (1995) Breaking the intergenerational cycle of insecure attachment: a review of the effects of attachment-based interventions on maternal sensitivity and infant security. *Journal of Child Psychology and Psychiatry*, **36**, 225–248.

Kanner, L. (1969) The children haven't read those books: reflections on differential diagnosis. *Acta Paedopsychiatrica*, **36**, 2–11.

Kennedy, P. & Llewelyn, S. (2001) Does the future belong to the scientist practitioner? *Psychologist*, **14**, 74–78.

Klein, R.G. (1986) Questioning the clinical usefulness of projective psychological tests for children. *Journal of Developmental and Behavioral Pediatrics*, **7**, 378–382.

Lamb, M.E., Thompson, R.A., Gardner, W., Charnov, E.L. & Estes, D. (1984) Security of infantile attachment as assessed in the 'Strange Situation': its study and biological interpretation. *Behavioral and Brain Sciences*, **7**, 127–171.

Lord, C., Risi, S., Lambrecht, L. *et al.* (2000) The ADOS-G (Autism Diagnostic Observation Schedule–Generic): a standard measure of social and communication deficits associated with the spectrum of autism. *Journal of Autism and Developmental Disorders*, **30**, 205–223.

Lord, C., Rutter, M. & Le Couteur, A. (1994) Autism Diagnostic Interview–Revised: a revised version of a diagnostic interview for caregivers of individuals with possible pervasive developmental disorders. *Journal of Autism and Developmental Disorders*, **24**, 659–685.

Magaña, A.B., Goldstein, M.J., Karno, M. & Miklowitz, D.J. (1986) A brief method for assessing expressed emotion in relatives of psychiatric patients. *Psychiatric Research*, **17**, 203–212.

Main, M. & Solomon, J. (1990) Procedures for identifying infants as disorganized/disorientated during the Ainsworth Strange Situation. In: *Attachment in the Preschool Years: Theory, Research and Intervention* (eds M.T. Greenberg, D. Cicchetti & E.M. Cummings), pp. 121–160. University of Chicago Press, Chicago.

Mash, E.J. & Terdal, L.G. (1981) *Behavioral Assessment of Childhood Disorders*. Guilford Press, New York.

Maughan, B. (1994) School influences. In: *Development Through Life: a Handbook for Clinicians* (eds M. Rutter & D. Hay), pp. 134–158. Blackwell Scientific Publications, Oxford.

McEvedy, C.P., Griffith, A. & Hall, T. (1966) Two school epidemics. *British Medical Journal*, **2**, 1300–1302.

McGuffin, P. & Farmer, A.E. (2001) Polydiagnostic approaches to measuring and classifying psychopathology. *American Journal of Medical Genetics*, **105**, 39–41.

Meehl, P.A. & Rosen, A. (1955) Antecedent probability and the efficiency of psychometric signs, patterns or cutting scores. *Psychological Bulletin*, **52**, 194–216.

Montee, B.B., Miltenberger, R.G., Wittrock, D. *et al.* (1995) An experimental analysis of facilitated communication. *Journal of Applied Behavioral Analysis*, **28**, 189–200.

Mortimore, P. (1995) The positive effects of schooling. In: *Psychosocial Disturbance in Young People: Challenges for Prevention* (ed. M. Rutter), pp. 333–363. Cambridge University Press, New York.

Mortimore, P. (1998) *The Road to Improvement: Reflections on School Effectiveness*. Swets and Zeitlinger, Lisse, The Netherlands.

Moss, P.D. & McEvedy, C. (1966) An epidemic of overbreathing among schoolgirls. *British Medical Journal*, **2**, 1295–1300.

O'Connor, T., Rutter, M., Beckett, C., Keaveney, L., Kreppner, J. & the E.R.A. Study Team. (2000) The effects of global severe privation on cognitive competence: extension and longitudinal follow-up. *Child Development*, **71**, 376–390.

Patterson, G. (1982) *Coercive Family Process*. Castalia Publishing Company, Eugene, OR.

Prior, M. (1979) Cognitive abilities and disabilities in infantile autism: a review. *Journal of Abnormal Child Psychology*, **7**, 357–380.

Prior, M. & Hoffmann, W. (1990) Neuropsychological testing of autistic children through an exploration with frontal lobe tests. *Journal of Autism and Developmental Disorders*, **20**, 581–590.

Raven, J.C., Court, J.H. & Raven, J. (1990) *Coloured Progressive Matrices*. Oxford Psychologists Press, Oxford.

Roeyers, H., Buyss, A., Ponnet, K. & Pichal, B. (2001) Advancing advanced mind-reading tests: empathic accuracy in adults with a pervasive developmental disorder. *Journal of Child Psychology and Psychiatry*, **42**, 271–278.

Rosvold, H.E., Mirsky, A.F., Sarason, I., Bransome, E.D. Jr & Beck, L.H. (1956) A continuous performance test of brain damage. *Journal of Consulting Psychology*, **20**, 343–350.

Rutter, M. (1975) *Helping Troubled Children*. Penguin Books, Harmondsworth, Middlesex.

Rutter, M. (1985a) Infantile autism. In: *The Clinical Guide to Child Psychiatry* (eds D. Shaffer, A. Erhardt & L. Greenhill), pp. 48–78. Free Press, New York.

Rutter, M. (1985b) The treatment of autistic children. *Journal of Child Psychology and Psychiatry*, **26**, 193–214.

Rutter, M. (1993) An overview of developmental neuropsychiatry. In: *The Brain and Behaviour: Organic Influences on the Behaviour of Children* (eds F.M.C. Besag & R.T. Williams), pp. 4–11. *Special Supplement to Educational and Child Psychology*, 10.

Rutter, M. (1998) Practitioner review: routes from research to clinical practice in child psychiatry—retrospect and prospect. *Journal of Child Psychology and Psychiatry*, **39**, 805–816.

Rutter, M. (1999) Autism: two-way interplay between research and clinical practice. *Journal of Child Psychology and Psychiatry*, **40**, 169–188.

Rutter, M. (2000) Research into practice: future prospects. In: *Speech and Language Impairments in Children: Causes, Characteristics, Intervention and Outcome* (eds D.V.M. Bishop & L. Leonard), pp. 273–290. Psychology Press, Hove, East Sussex.

Rutter, M. (2001) Family influences on behaviour and development. Challenges for the future. In: *Retrospect and prospect in the psychological study of families* (eds J. McHale & W. Grolnick), pp. 321–351. Erlbaum, Mahwah, NJ.

Rutter, M. & Brown, G. (1966) The reliability and validity of measures of family life and relationships in families containing a psychiatric patient. *Social Psychiatry*, 1, 38–53.

Rutter, M. & Garmezy, N. (1983) Developmental psychopathology. In: *Socialization, Personality, and Social Development*, Vol. 4, *Mussen's Handbook of Child Psychology* (ed. E.M. Hetherington), 4th edn, pp. 775–911. Wiley, New York.

Rutter, M. & Rutter, M. (1993) *Developing Minds: Challenge and Continuity Across the Lifespan*. Penguin Books, Harmondsworth, Middlesex.

Rutter, M. & Sroufe, A. (2000) Developmental psychopathology: concepts and challenges. *Development and Psychopathology*, 12, 265–296.

Rutter, M., Graham, P. & Yule, W. (1970) A neuropsychiatric study in childhood. *Clinics in Developmental Medicine* 35/36. Heinemann/SIMP, London.

Rutter, M. & the English and Romanian Adoptees Study Team (1998a) Developmental catch-up, and deficit, following adoption after severe early global privation. *Journal of Child Psychology and Psychiatry*, 39, 465–476.

Rutter, M., Giller, H. & Hagell, A. (1998b) *Antisocial Behaviour by Young People*. Cambridge University Press, Cambridge.

Rutter, M., Pickles, A., Murray, R. & Eaves, L. (2001) Testing hypotheses on specific environmental causal effects on behaviour. *Psychological Bulletin*, 127, 291–324.

Sandberg, S., Rutter, M., Giles, S. *et al.* (1993) Assessment of psychosocial experiences in childhood: methodological issues and some illustrative findings. *Journal of Child Psychology and Psychiatry*, 34, 879–897.

Shapiro, M.B. (1957) Experimental method in the psychological description of the individual psychiatric patient. *International Journal of Social Psychiatry*, 3, 89–103.

Sternberg, R.J. (1997) Educating intelligence: infusing the Triarchic Theory into school instruction. In: *Intelligence, Heredity and Environment* (eds R.J. Sternberg & E.L. Grigorenko), pp. 343–362. Cambridge University Press, New York.

Sternberg, R.J., Torff, B. & Grigorenko, E.L. (1998) Teaching triarchically improves school achievement. *Journal of Educational Psychology*, 90, 374–384.

Stutsman, R. (1948) *Merrill–Palmer scale of mental tests: preprints of Part III, mental measurement of pre-school children*. Stoelting Co., Chicago IL.

Thompson, C. (2001) Amitriptyline: still efficacious but at what cost? *British Journal of Psychiatry*, 178, 99–100.

Vargha-Khadem, F., Isaacs, E., Van der Werf, S., Robb, S. & Wilson, J. (1992) Development of intelligence and memory in children with hemiplegic cerebral palsy: the deleterious consequences of early seizures. *Brain*, 115, 315–329.

Volkmar, F.R., Cicchetti, D.V., Bregman, J. & Cohen, D.J. (1992) Three diagnostic systems for autism: DSM-III, DSM-III-R, and ICD-10. *Journal of Autism and Developmental Disorders*, 22, 483–492.

Waters, E., Vaughn, B.E., Posada, G. & Kondo-Ikemura, K., eds. (1995) Caregiving, cultural and cognitive perspectives on secure-base behaviour and working models: new growing points of attachment theory and research. *Monographs of the Society for Research in Child Development*, 60,

World Health Organization (1993) *The ICD-10 Classification of Mental and Behavioural Disorders: Diagnostic Criteria for Research*. World Health Organization, Geneva.

Yule, W. (1989) An introduction to clinical investigation in clinical child psychology. In: *An Introduction to Clinical Child Psychology* (eds S.J.E. Lindsay & G.E. Powell), pp. 28–50. Gower, Aldershot.

Yule, W. & Hemsley, D. (1977) Single case methodology in medical psychology. In: *Contributions to Medical Psychology* (ed. S. Rachman), Vol. 1, pp. 211–229. Pergamon, London.

Children's Testimony

Stephen J. Ceci, Livia L. Gilstrap and Stanka A. Fitneva

Introduction

Every day courts, social services, mental health professionals and law enforcement personnel are faced with the difficult job of deciding whether to believe a child's report of abuse or neglect. It can be devilishly difficult to sort out the truth in such cases, and it is becoming increasingly common for courts to look to the field of developmental psychology for help. The relationship between research, practice and the law is complicated (see Little, Chapter 71). Consider the following case, which illustrates some unfortunately typical ingredients in such cases, and by implication suggests some areas of need that developmental psychologists might address.

Children's testimonial behaviour in the real world

Case of State of New Jersey v. D.G.

In the State of New Jersey v. D.G., the defendant was an enlisted man in the US Navy. He married a woman who had two children previously. One of her children, Michelle, was four and a half years old at the time of the alleged abuse. Michelle claims that her stepfather asked her to accompany him on an errand one day, and during it he took her to an empty house that the family was planning to move into.

'Michelle stated that the defendant . . . laid down next to her and proceeded to place his hands under her shirt. Defendant touched and squeezed her breasts, fondled her vagina, and kissed her on the mouth. He then pulled off her shirt and pants, removed his own pants and climbed on top of her. Michelle testified that the defendant put his 'dinky' into her and then that he cleaned up the 'wet stuff' on the bed with a towel. He then told her to clean herself up and get dressed. The pair then proceeded to a pizza place and then returned to the great-grandmother's house.' (State of NJ v. D.G. 1999, WL 64702)

Three weeks later, while Michelle was playing with two girls, her 'Aunt Sandy' found her lying on the bed with these girls who had their pants down to their knees and one of them had her hand down Michelle's pants. Aunt Sandy testified that she 'freaked out' and called the girls bad names. She ordered Michelle to sit alone and told her she was very upset with her.

Aunt Sandy testified that she took her daughters to the bathroom, washed them, and attempted, in her word, to 'deprogram' them. One of these girls told Aunt Sandy that Michelle wanted to 'lick her pee-pee'.

Forty-five minutes after being scolded and isolated, Aunt Sandy returned to Michelle and questioned her. Although she purported to have calmed down by then, she said that Michelle still seemed nervous. At first, Michelle allegedly blamed the behaviour on Aunt Sandy's two daughters; however, after more questioning she stated that her stepfather did those things to her. Michelle testified that Aunt Sandy asked her: 'What made you do this? Did anybody ever do anything like this to you to make you do this?' Michelle replied that her stepfather stuck his 'thing' in her and then 'peed on the bed', wiping it up with a towel. Michelle begged Aunt Sandy not to tell her mother. (Michelle's mother testified for the prosecution that the stepfather was 'a fanatic about towelling himself off after intercourse even after ejaculating inside her'.)

Several days after the incident with the two daughters of Aunt Sandy, Michelle was interviewed by a female detective trained to conduct sex abuse investigations. Her Aunt Sandy accompanied her to this interview. During this interview, however, Michelle failed to make a disclosure about her stepfather, saying only that he touched her 'boobies'. After frequent failed attempts to get Michelle to talk, the detective sensed that she was scared and was holding back. She stopped the videotaped interview because Michelle's nose began to bleed and brought her to a bathroom to stop the bleeding. Then the detective asked Aunt Sandy to reassure Michelle about talking to her. Aunt Sandy put Michelle on her lap and told her to tell the detective the truth. Approximately 7 minutes later, the videotape was turned back on and the interview proceeded. Now on video Michelle proceeded to claim the stepfather had put his penis into her vagina.

The following week, Michelle was examined by a paediatrician who specialized in sexual abuse. Although he found no physical evidence that was diagnostic of sexual trauma to Michelle's genitalia (not unusual, even in cases of known sexual penetration), this paediatrician did report that Michelle demonstrated with an anatomically detailed doll that she had been raped, plus she told him that the stepfather had rubbed his penis against her 'private'. Based on Michelle's doll use and her oral description of events, the paediatrician concluded there was a 'high likelihood that sexual abuse had occurred'.

Michelle alleged that her mother beat her in an attempt to get her to recant her allegations. She was sent to live out of state with her biological father. When Michelle returned from his home, however, she accused him of raping her in a similar manner (e.g. including the wiping off with a towel). When examined again by the paediatrician, Michelle recanted her allegation against her stepfather but made three different allegations of sexual abuse against her biological father. In the following 6 months, Michelle told her Aunt Sandy, a social worker and an investigator that she had been lying about her stepfather. To confuse matters even more, Michelle recanted her recantations at various times.

Just before the case came to court, Michelle met with the prosecutor and detective and told them her stepfather did not rape her, but after further questioning she told them that her mother had urged her to deny the rape. During the trial, Michelle's testimony changed somewhat from her prior statements. A child abuse expert testified that it is not unusual for abused children to change their statements, especially when they believe that others will not believe them or will criticize them. The jury convicted the stepfather; he was sentenced to a 7-year term of imprisonment.

The case of State of New Jersey v. D.G. illustrates many of the challenges facing those who must interview alleged child victims. Should we believe Michelle's claims of abuse, or her recantations, or her recantations of her prior recantations? And was Michelle's behaviour with anatomical dolls diagnostic of abuse? These are a few of the questions that courts turn to developmental psychology for answers. In this chapter we will briefly review the relevant scientific research from the field of children's testimonial competence. We will address each of the following six topics: historical research on suggestibility; recent trends in suggestibility research; whether statement consistency is diagnostic of an accurate report; the use of anatomical dolls in interviewing; boundary conditions beyond which children are hypothesized not to be suggestible; and conclude with the application of suggestibility findings for forensic interviewers.

Historical research on suggestibility

Scientific researchers have examined the question of children's testimonial competence for more than a century, since a study by W.S. Small (1896). Small first asked several students to come to the front of the classroom and smell a clear liquid in a bottle that was an essence familiar to children of that era. After these children announced their answers (claiming it was a familiar fragrance), Small asked the rest of the class to raise their hands if and when they could smell the same fragrance when he sprayed it into the air in front of their classroom. In actuality, the bottle he sprayed contained only distilled water, yet many children claimed to smell its fragrance after seeing classmates' hands raised. Small repeated this practice with sounds, sights (apparent movement of a toy), and other stimuli, and he tested children both in classroom groups as well as individually. He concluded that young children were highly suggestible, particularly when they were in groups. We will return to this claim below as it con-

nects historical research with both more modern research and with actual testimonial situations of past and present.

From the beginning, the dominant view among researchers has been that young children are suggestible—more so than older children and adults. With a few notable exceptions, early scientific studies reported that young children are vulnerable to a variety of suggestive techniques and pressures, such as leading questions, peer pressure, repeated questioning, the tendency to perceive conditions as conforming to expectancies created by adults, and the need to comply with adults' wishes.

One of the earliest scientific researchers of children's suggestibility was Alfred Binet, the French psychologist best known as the father of the modern IQ test. Binet's (1900) book on suggestibility continues to have a role in modern discussions of the topic. Indeed, although Binet's experimental methods may now appear relatively primitive, he reached several conclusions that have continued to be echoed by later research.

First, Binet concluded that young children were highly suggestible. Like others after him (Lipmann 1911; Dale *et al.* 1978), Binet argued that suggestibility reflects the operation of two different factors: cognitive and social. The first factor, which he called 'auto-suggestion', develops within the child without outside influence because it fulfils his or her expectation of what it supposed to happen. In one of Binet's experiments, five lines of increasing length were presented to children of ages 7–14, followed by a series of 'target' lines that were of the same length as the longest (final) line of the series. Children tended to be influenced by the expectation of ever-increasing lines; their reproductions of the target line were systematically too long because they expected that it would be longer than the line that had preceded it. Binet questioned the children after the study and found that many knew that the lines they had drawn were incorrect; they were able to redraw them more accurately on demand. Binet claimed that this demonstrated that children could escape the influence of auto-suggestions.

Binet's second factor was the desire to conform to the expectations or pressures of an interviewer, and thus reflected a form of mental obedience to another. For example, Binet showed that children sometimes asserted that they witnessed non-existent events that they were led to expect. Binet reported that one of the external forces that could affect children's responses was the examiner's language. In one of his studies, he showed children between the ages of 7 and 14 years a poster that contained six everyday items. He asked children a series of questions, some of which were misleading (e.g. implying that a button was affixed to a poster with thread rather than glue). He found that these children often went along with the erroneous suggestion (e.g. claiming to have seen the thread). Some children were asked for their free recall—to write down everything they observed, without being aided by specific questions. These children were the most accurate, although they recalled very little. Other children were asked direct questions about the objects (e.g. 'How is the button attached to the board?') These children, although not as accurate as children in free recall, were significantly more accurate than children who were asked leading questions that suggested an inaccurate answer (e.g. 'Wasn't the button attached by a thread?') who in turn were more accurate than children asked highly misleading and suggestive questions that assumed factually incorrect information (e.g. 'What was the colour of the thread that attached the button to the board?'). Binet did not test questions that were correctly leading (e.g. 'Wasn't the button glued?'). Subsequent research has demonstrated that such questions are answered with the highest degree of accuracy.

All modern commentators agree on this relationship between the nature of questioning and accuracy: free recall is the most accurate (although yielding the sparsest recollections); followed by responses to direct non-leading questions; then by responses to leading questions suggesting an inaccurate answer; and finally by misleading questions (Cunningham 1988; Ceci & Bruck 1993; Ceci & Friedman 2000).

Binet also noted that children's answers to questions are often characterized by exactness and confidence, regardless of their accuracy level. Even among adults, there is low correlation between an eyewitness's confidence and accuracy (Bothwell *et al.* 1987). When the children in Binet's study were later asked if they had made any mistakes, they did not correct their inaccurate responses to misleading questions. Binet concluded that the children's erroneous responses and subsequent high confidence reflected gaps in their memories, which they attempted to fill in order to please the experimenter. Once an erroneous response was given, Binet surmised that it became incorporated into their memory. This assumption on his part was based on the fact that, in contrast to the auto-suggestion study, in which children could later re-draw the line correctly, children in this study were unable later to correct their wrong answers.

Finally, Binet concluded that children are more suggestible in groups than when alone. When a group of three children was shown the same six everyday objects, asked a series of misleading questions, and told to call out the answer to each question as quickly as possible, children who responded second and third were more likely to give the same answer as the first respondent—even if that answer was inaccurate.

The late seventeenth century Swedish witch trials present an interesting analogue to Binet's finding of group conformity effects. Sjoberg (1995) analysed the statements given to parish priests by 809 children and reported that they were more likely to claim to have witnessed celestial apparitions, witches flying on brooms, and so forth, if they gave their testimony to the parish priest after waiting in line with other witnesses outside the rectory to attend prayer meetings. Sjoberg believes this was because they were influenced by other witnesses who also were waiting in line. 'Only 59% of the children testifying at other places than prayer meetings were sure about the real life quality of their experiences of the witches' sabbath whereas as many as 91% were sure about it after standing in line with others at prayer meetings. The differences were significant.'

Other early twentieth century researchers reached results consonant with Binet's, and drew further conclusions that continue to find support. The Belgian psychologist J. Varendonck, a contemporary of Binet's, conducted a number of experiments on children's suggestibility with the specific intent of demonstrating the unreliability of children's testimony and so enabling him to provide expert testimony in a murder case (Varendonck 1911). In one study, 7-year-old children were asked about the colour of a teacher's beard. Sixteen of 18 children provided a response, whereas only two said they did not know. The teacher in question did not have a beard. In another demonstration, a teacher from an adjoining classroom came into Varendonck's classroom and, without removing his hat, talked in an agitated fashion for approximately 5 minutes. (Keeping one's hat on when entering a room was uncommon then because it was considered a sign of rudeness in that society.) After this teacher had left the classroom, the children were then asked in which hand that teacher had held his hat. Only 3 of the 27 students claimed that the hat was not in his hand.

Varendonck, as well as other researchers in this early period, emphasized one of the points found by Binet, that questioning by influential adults could lead children to make false statements. According to the German psychologist William Stern, children viewed such suggestive questions as imperatives (Stern 1910). Further, both Varendonck and Stern provided early support for the proposition that repeat questioning can have a particularly powerful effect. Stern concluded that a child was likely to remember his or her answers to earlier questions better than the underlying events themselves.

Research by Lipmann (1911) and colleagues (e.g. Piaget 1986) in the same period, also suggested that very young children often have difficulty distinguishing fantasy from reality. More generally, researchers in the 1920s and 1930s consistently found that younger children were more suggestible than older ones (Otis 1924; Messerschmidt 1933; Burtt 1948). At the same time, scientists also recognized that even adults can be suggestible to a significant degree (for details, see Loftus 1979).

For several reasons, this early research is of limited usefulness in analysing issues of forensic significance. Most obviously, although some of the early researchers, including Binet and Varendonck, had forensic use in mind, the subject matter of the questions they posed bore little resemblance to the subject matter of statements that children give in actual cases. In the early experiments, children were often asked leading questions about details that they likely regarded as peripheral and of little significance, such as the colour of a strange man's beard in one of Varendonck's (1911) studies, which of several lines was longer in Binet's (1900) study, or whether they smelled a non-existent fragrance when a liquid was sprayed in front of the classroom that in reality was distilled water in Small's (1896) study.

'. . . . Most research on children as eyewitnesses has relied on situations that are very different from the personal involvement and trauma of sexual abuse. Researchers have used brief stories, films, videotapes, or slides to simulate a witnessed event. A few have used actual staged events, but these events—for example, a man tending plants—are also qualitatively different from incidents of child abuse. The children are typically bystanders to the events, there is no bodily contact between the child and adult, and it is seldom even known whether the events hold much interest for the children. Of even more importance, the questions the children are asked often focus on peripheral details of the incident like what the confederate was wearing, rather than on the main actions that occurred, or more to the point, whether sexual actions were committed.' (Goodman & Clarke-Stewart 1991)

In contrast to laboratory research, in actual forensic investigations—most of which involve abuse of the child herself—the child is usually questioned about central, bodily actions, often experienced rather than merely witnessed, and frequently associated with embarrassment, fear and pain.

Thus, whatever the early experiments might show about the reliability of children under the conditions of the experiments, they lack *external* or *ecological validity* for the context of principal contemporary significance. That is, they cannot be relied on with confidence to show how suggestible children are in the real-world context of interest—when a child makes an allegation of abuse. Nevertheless, this brief historical review indicates that recent research findings on the suggestibility of children is not a modern departure from earlier understandings; on the contrary, it fits in squarely with what has been the dominant view for a full century.

Defining suggestibility

Traditionally, suggestibility has been defined as 'the extent to which individuals come to accept and subsequently incorporate postevent information into their memory recollections' (Gudjonsson & Clark 1986; see also Powers *et al.* 1979). This definition implies that:

1 suggestibility is an unconscious process;

2 suggestibility results from information that was supplied *after* an event; and

3 suggestibility is thought to influence reports via incorporation into the memory system, not through social pressure to lie or conform to expectations.

This traditional conceptualization and demonstration of suggestibility is too restrictive to aid in understanding real case studies like that presented at the beginning of this chapter. Therefore, many researchers have broadened the definition of suggestibility to encompass what is usually connoted by its lay usage. Suggestibility is defined as the degree to which the encoding, storage, retrieval and reporting of events can be influenced by a range of internal and external factors. By adding 'reporting' to the definition, we broaden the definition of suggestibility to include false reporting. False reporting implies that it is possible to accept information while fully conscious of its divergence from the originally perceived event, as in the case of acquiescence to social demands, lying or efforts to please loved ones. This broadened definition of suggestibility does not necessarily involve the alteration of the underlying memory; a child may still remember what actually occurred but choose not to report it for motivational reasons. By removing 'postevent' from the definition, we imply that suggestibility can result from the provision of information either before (e.g. in the form of expectations or stereotypes) or after an event.

Thus, this broader conceptualization of suggestibility accords with both the legal and everyday uses of the term, to connote how easily one is influenced by subtle suggestions, expectations, stereotypes and leading questions that can unconsciously alter memories, as well as by explicit bribes, threats and other forms of social inducement that can lead to the conscious alteration of reports without affecting the underlying memory.

Recent trends in suggestibility research

Beginning in the late 1970s, there was a resurgence of interest in the area of children's suggestibility, which has continued to the present. This virtual explosion of research was fuelled by various factors: a dramatic increase of reports of child abuse and increasing recognition of the commonness of abuse; greater receptivity by courts to expert psychological testimony; increased focus of social scientists on socially relevant issues; and increasing interest in the study of eyewitness testimony of adults (Ceci & Bruck 1993). Thus, researchers became increasingly concerned by the frequency with which children failed to report abuse, by the fact that when they did allege abuse the reports were met with scepticism and also, later, by the possibilities for contamination of their reports. Although virtually all researchers agree that these two possibilities exist, they disagree about the likelihood of each occurring. Additionally, there is vigorous disagreement in interpretation of the recent studies, with some seeing them as supporting the view that children are highly suggestible, and others seeing these studies as evidence for children's resistance to suggestions.

Lyon (1999) has termed the group of researchers who emphasize children's suggestibility the 'New Wave'. In contrast to the so-called New Wave research, those who focus on children's testimonial strengths have reported studies showing that, in the absence of strongly suggestive questioning techniques, preschool-age children are capable of providing courts with highly accurate recollections. In response to this claim, researchers have provided evidence that actual front-line interviewers routinely employ highly suggestive techniques when questioning young children, leading to the expectation that potential suggestibility errors may occur (Ceci & Friedman 2000). Below, we briefly review some of the studies that are used by each of these camps to bolster their competing claims.

Rather than attempt a full summary of modern research on suggestibility, we begin by discussing four illustrative studies conducted by Goodman *et al.* We have chosen Goodman because she is the scholar most favoured by child advocates and critics of the so-called New Wave research. Yet, her studies provide strong evidence that children, especially young children, *are* suggestible to a significant degree—even about abuse-related questions.

Paediatric examination study

In a study by Saywitz *et al.* (1991), girls whose genitalia and anus were touched during a paediatric examination were much more likely to report that touching in response to doll-aided directed questioning than in response to open-ended questions. In fact many studies have found that young children provide little information to open-ended questions although the information they do provide tends to be highly accurate. This highlights the potential benefits of directed questioning. However, in the Saywitz *et al.* study, although the vast majority of girls whose genitalia had *not* been touched during the exam correctly denied a genital touch, during directed questioning one out of 35 (2.86%) did answer affirmatively when asked about a genital touch, and two out of 36 girls (5.56%) answered affirmatively when asked about an anal touch. Thus, directed questioning can also lead to false allegations of touching.

A common finding in the literature is that directed questioning elicits both more accurate details and more inaccurate details (Ceci & Friedman 2000). We could conclude, as Saywitz *et al.* did, that 'although there is a risk of increased error with doll-aided direct questions, there is an *even greater risk* that not asking about vaginal and anal touch leaves the majority of such touch unreported' (Saywitz *et al.* 1991, emphasis added). However, the data on young children's suggestibility in the face of directed questioning suggest a more conservative approach to its use that acknowledges both the potential benefits and the potential risks.

Delayed inquiry study

Goodman *et al.* (1989) asked 3–6-year-olds to play a game with a strange man for approximately 5 minutes. During this time, the man did not engage in any behaviours that were sexually provocative. Four years later, 15 of these same children, now between 7 and 10 years old, were re-interviewed and asked what they could recall of their prior experience with the strange man. To create an 'atmosphere of accusation', the interviewers said such things as: 'Are you afraid to tell? You'll feel better once you've told.' Goodman & Clarke-Stewart wrote that 'the children were more resistant to abuse-related than to non-abuse-related suggestions'. Nevertheless, these children were quite susceptible to abuse-related questioning: five of the 15 children agreed with the interviewer's false suggestion that the stranger had kissed them or hugged them, two out of the 15 agreed that they had their photo taken by the stranger, and one child even agreed she had been given a bath by him. Goodman & Clarke-Stewart acknowledged that some of these errors 'might lead to suspicion of abuse' (Goodman *et al.* 1989).

Trailer study

Rudy & Goodman (1991) conducted a study in which pairs of 4- and 7-year-olds were left in a trailer with a strange adult. One child watched while the adult played games with the other, helped her dress in a clown's costume, lifted her onto a desk, and took two photographs of her. Each child was asked various types of questions 10–12 days later, some of which involved actions that might be of special concern in child abuse investigations, such as, 'How many times did he spank you?' and 'Did he put anything into your mouth?' Rudy & Goodman reported that the 7-year-olds 'did not make a single commission error to the specific abuse questions'. The authors concluded that 4-year-old participants made very few commission errors (3%), while the 4-year-old bystanders evidenced a slightly higher, but still low, error rate (7%) (Rudy & Goodman 1991).

Mount Sinai study

Eisen *et al.* (1998) conducted an experiment involving 108 children between the ages 3 and 15 who were examined as part of a 5-day assessment period for children with suspected histories of abuse at Chicago's Mount Sinai Hospital. The important focus of this experiment was of increasing ecological validity by studying children who were actually involved in abuse investigations. The authors expressed the view that, because of various problems that they suffered, this group could be more suggestible than the children typically involved in suggestibility studies. 'It is also possible', they wrote, 'that abused children are hypervigilant regarding abusive actions or abuse suggestions and, as a result, would be more resistant to such questioning than non-abused children' (Eisen *et al.* 1998). On the first day of their stay, children received a medical check-up. On the second day, the children were given an anogenital examination, and swabbed for culture. On the fifth day, the children were interviewed, and the interview included misleading or other suggestive questions. Eisen *et al.* concluded:

'Despite performing more poorly than their older counterparts, the 3–5-year-olds still demonstrated *relatively good resistance* to misleading information in answering abuse-related questions. When presented with misleading questions related to abusive or inappropriate behaviour by the doctor and/or nurse (e.g. 'How many times did the doctor kiss you?'), 3–5-year-olds answered 79% of the questions without making commission errors.' (Eisen *et al.* 1998, emphasis added.)

The unstated implication is that this group made commission errors in answering 21% of misleading abuse-related questions. Furthermore, the authors pointed out that 'approximately 40% of the errors made by the 3–5-year-olds in response to misleading abuse-related questions were produced by only 6 of the 29 children in this group.' Thus, although the group's proportion of commission errors to misleading abuse-related questions was relatively low on average, some children were more suggestible than others. 'If such children were interviewed in an abuse investigation', the authors acknowledged, 'a false accusation could potentially result' (Eisen *et al.* 1998). Children in the older groups did substantially better, but still answered a fairly sizeable percentage of the misleading abuse-related questions incorrectly, 16% for the 6–10-year-olds and 9% for the 11–15-year-olds.

These studies by Goodman *et al.* are each important for understanding children's intellectual development and in revealing the underlying mechanisms of suggestibility and memory. As we have shown, it has been understood since the time of Binet (1900) that a child's free recall tends to be more accurate than his or her responses to suggestive questioning. However, free recall also tends to be extremely sparse. When asked for free recall, children usually give correct but very brief answers, and they often omit important details. This is especially so for very young children, and it is especially true in the abuse context because of the possibility of embarrassment and threats from the alleged perpetrator. One response of researchers such as Goodman has been to emphasize the potential value of suggestive or other directed questioning in securing disclosure of abuse. Abuse investigators have used more directive and focused approaches, including leading and repeated questions, in an attempt to secure useful information from the child and some modern research highlights the potential value of these techniques.

Consider the study by Saywitz *et al.* (1991), discussed above. When girls whose paediatric examinations had included an exterior vaginal and anal examination were asked for their free recall, only 8 of 36 (22%) correctly mentioned the vaginal touch and only 4 of 36 (11%) mentioned the anal touch. Directed questioning with the aid of anatomically correct dolls raised these numbers to 31 (86%) and 25 (68%), respectively. Thus, directed questioning will often be more effective than requests for free recall in prompting disclosures of abuse.

On the other hand, there is risk of creating false positives by suggestive questioning. Although the four studies we reviewed used suggestive questions ('Did the doctor touch you there?' 'How many times did he spank you?' 'Did he put anything into your mouth?' 'How many times did the doctor kiss you?'), they did not use highly suggestive techniques, such as repeating the suggestive questioning over time (Poole & White 1993, 1995), coercion or peer pressure. This is a point that the authors recognized. In three of the four studies, the suggestive techniques employed were embedded in neutral or supportive interviews. These studies therefore provide weak tests of young children's vulnerability to suggestion. Even in this research, however, the evidence shows that error rates for false claims range between 3 and 40%. They do not indicate how high these error rates might go in the presence of a web of motives, strong suggestions, threats and inducements. As we will now show, such highly suggestive techniques can produce much higher error rates.

Impact of highly suggestive techniques

As we have indicated, the studies described above may underestimate the susceptibility of young children when confronted with stronger suggestions. To test this hypothesis, a number of attempts have been made to design and conduct studies that incorporate stronger forms of suggestions—including suggestive techniques that have been used by investigators in some well-publicized child abuse cases (see Ceci & Bruck 1995 for review

of several well-publicized cases). Among these stronger forms of suggestion that research has shown to be detrimental are repetition of question within the same interview (Poole & White 1993), stereotype inducement (Leichtman & Ceci 1995), guided imagery (Ceci *et al.* 1994), peer pressure and selective reinforcement. Numerous studies have shown that when exposed to these forms of suggestion the error rates of children can be very high, sometimes exceeding 50%. Moreover, this phenomenon holds true even when the questions concern events that supposedly affect the child him- or herself as opposed to events to which he or she was supposedly a bystander; even when the questions are central, rather than peripheral to the supposed event; and even when the questions concern abuse-related matters. For the sake of brevity and symmetry with the research we have already reviewed, we will present below only a subset of evidence that falls into this category.

Garven *et al.* (1998) used strong suggestions (e.g. reinforcing answers that were consistent with interviewers' hunches and invoking pressure to conform) based on tactics used in the McMartin daycare sexual abuse case. These researchers found a 57% false claim rate as to various behaviours in which an adult had supposedly engaged, vs. only a 17% error rate when weaker suggestions were used. In a follow-up publication (Garven *et al.* 2000), these researchers found between 35 and 52% false claims—including statements that the adult had tickled the child's tummy or had kissed the child on the nose—in response to strong suggestions, vs. 13–15% when these were not used. The following exchange in their study is an example of a combination of conformity pressure with positive reinforcement:

I: The other kids say that Paco took them to a farm.
   Did Paco take you to a farm?

C: Yes.

I: Great. You're doing excellent now.

Other researchers who have used these stronger suggestive techniques also have reported high error rates for claiming a strange man 'put something yucky into their mouths' during a visit to a science exhibit (Poole & Lindsay 1996), took off their clothes and kissed them (Lepore & Sesco 1994), or touched them inappropriately (Rawls 1996).

Studies focusing on repeated questions include a study by Bruck *et al.* (1995) in which 3-year-olds were repeatedly asked strongly suggestive questions about a doctor touching their anogenital regions (e.g. 'Can you show how Dr Emmett touched your vagina?'). Among children whom the doctor did not touch, fully 50% falsely claimed the doctor had inserted objects into their anogenital cavities. After a third exposure in a period of a week to an anatomically correct doll, one 3-year-old child reported that her paediatrician had tried to strangle her with a rope, insert a stick into her vagina and hammer an earscope into her anus. Similarly, Steward *et al.* (1996) interviewed children aged 3–6 years three times after a paediatric clinic visit. With each interview, children's false reports of anal touching increased; by the final interview, which took place 6 months after the initial visit, more than one-third of the children in this study falsely reported anal touching.

Poole & White (1991) interviewed 4-, 6- and 8-year-olds and adults immediately and 1 week following a staged encounter with a man. Another group of subjects were interviewed only once, after a delay of 1 week. Some of the repeated questions were open-ended ones (e.g. 'What did the man look like?'), whereas others were closed or yes/no ones (e.g. 'Did the man hurt Melanie?'). Poole & White reported that the 'repeat-interview' 4-year-olds were significantly more likely than the 'single-delayed' ones to give a false affirmative answer to the closed question while the repetition of the open-ended questions did not result in more errors. Collapsing across age and gender of subjects, those in the repeat condition were significantly more likely to report that the man hurt Melanie (60%) than were those in the single interview condition (33%).

Finally, in a study by Rawls (1996), 30 5-year-olds and seven 4-year-olds participated in a series of benign play events with a male adult. Over the course of four interviews, the children were asked both open-ended questions such as 'Where were you with X?' and 'What sort of things did you do with him?', and closed questions such as 'Do you know why he touched that part of your body?' Rawls reported that nearly one-quarter of her sample falsely claimed the man inappropriately touched them, with three of the children (10%) falsely reporting genital touching, two (7%) falsely reporting anal touching, and two additional children reporting mutual adult–child touching (e.g. claiming the adult pretended to rub cream into their bodies). The authors stated that 'reports of mutual undressing without touching were also common, although this often reflected a confusion between dress-up items and ordinary clothes.' Similarly, in the so-called Monkey Thief study, Bruck et al. (1997) found that over half of the youngest children made false claims of witnessing a theft of food in their daycare facility when they were exposed to repeated suggestions and pressures. (For additional examples of false claims—involving bodily touching or witnessing a bicycle theft—see Cassel & Bjorklund 1996; Ornstein et al. 1997).

Taken together, the above studies indicate that if very young children are subjected to questioning techniques that are *highly* suggestive, their rates of making false claims, even on abuse-related questions, may be very high. However, these studies are of limited utility for forensic purposes unless children are in fact exposed to these techniques in the real world of abuse investigation. Elsewhere, we have provided evidence that front-line interviewers use, on average, 8–10 suggestive utterances per interview (questions such as 'He forced you to do that, didn't he?' (Lamb et al. 1996; see Ceci & Friedman 2000 for review of this evidence).

Since this article has been in draft, Warren et al. (2000) have presented a paper, based on interview transcripts with child protective service workers in a southern state of the USA, that in their view provides some support for the contention that the most egregiously suggestive practices are used only rarely by front-line interviewers of children. The interviews they analysed contained far fewer egregious practices than the studies we listed above. But their data revealed that some particularly suggestive techniques, although usually constituting a small part of the interaction in any given interview, are quite common in that they appear in most interviews at least once. Even a single occurrence of such a technique is capable of derailing the entire interview. Perhaps most strikingly, the interviewers in Warren et al.'s analysis invoked negative consequences such as telling the child, 'You haven't told us anything' in 28 of the 42 (67%) interviews. In 40 (95%) of the interviews, the interviewer repeated a question, in an attempt to elicit a new answer, even though the child had unambiguously answered the question in the immediately preceding portion of the interview. In five (12%) of the interviews the interviewer told the child about information received from another person. In 37 (88%) of the interviews the interviewer invoked positive consequences on at least one occasion for an answer, although the researchers report that this occurred mainly in the context of the early rapport-building part of the interview. In 14 (33%) of the interviews the interviewer invited the child to speculate about past events or to use imagination or solve a mystery.

Taken together, the data on practices employed by front-line interviewers indicates that highly suggestive techniques are very common.

Is statement consistency diagnostic?

Consistency of a child's report is often one of the most important criteria used by professionals in evaluating the reliability of children's allegations of abuse (Conte et al. 1991), whereas inconsistency in young children's reports lowers their credibility in the eyes of mock jurors (Ross et al. 1990; Leippe et al. 1992). Several studies have found that when preschool-age children are interviewed twice about an event, about 30% of the information they recall is consistent across interviews, and it tends to be highly accurate (Fivush & Schwarzmueller 1998; Fivush & Shukat 1995). However, accuracy rates when suggestive questioning is used may differ from those of Fivush et al. in which there was no suggestive questioning. Perhaps repeated opportunities to reminisce are an advantage if the interviewer avoids using suggestive questioning. We turn to this possibility next.

Based on two findings from a recent study by Bruck et al. (in press) that: (i) the length of children's narratives remained the same with repeated interviews; and (ii) the number of their new reminiscences during each new interview were greater for false than true narratives, one would predict that the same details are more likely to be repeated in true compared to false narratives. This was tested directly in analyses that included spontaneous as well as prompted utterances.

We examined how frequently children reported an event in one interview that had been reported in a previous interview. Thus, we examined consistency of utterances beginning at the third interview (because the first interview was a baseline interview that was of necessity not included, so the first comparison was between the second and third interviews), asking whether these details had been mentioned in any previous interview. Similarly, we examined how many utterances in the fourth interview had been mentioned in previous interviews, and how many in the fifth interview had been mentioned in any of the previous interviews. Numerators were then divided by the total number of utterances in each interview. This measure reflects the proportion of details in each interview that had already been provided by the child in previous interviews.

It was discovered that the true reports were more consistent than the false reports. Summing over the third, fourth and fifth interviews, consistency rates were 67% for true reports about negative events, 50% for true reports about positive events, 30% for false reports about negative events, and 25% for false reports about positive events. The consistency in narratives increased between the third (35%) and fourth interviews (47%), with no change between the fourth and fifth interview (47%).

In summary, repeated suggestive questioning takes a toll on children's accuracy, with increasing errors over time and the consistency of false reports exceeding that of true reports.

Is intercourse positioning with anatomic dolls diagnostic?

Anatomically detailed dolls are frequently used by professionals when they interview young children about suspected sexual abuse. It is thought that the dolls facilitate disclosure by providing props that help young children describe complex and embarrassing events as well as providing them with the appropriate non-verbal cues to facilitate memory retrieval (Boat & Everson 1996). These techniques, which have been especially designed to overcome language, memory and motivational (e.g. embarrassment) problems when interviewing children about sexual abuse, may be potentially suggestive. However, existing data indicate that the dolls do not facilitate accurate reporting (Goodman & Aman 1990) and it also appears that the use of dolls increases errors for younger children (3- and 4-year-olds) when asked to demonstrate certain events that never happened (Gordon et al. 1993) or when they are asked to use the dolls to act out an experienced medical procedure (Goodman et al. 1997).

Recent studies by Bruck et al. (1995, 1997) give examples of the potential suggestion inherent in doll use when interviewing about genital touch. Three- and 4-year-old children had a medical examination, with some of the children receiving a routine genital examination. The children were then interviewed about the examination. During the interview they were given an anatomical doll and told, 'Show me on the doll how the doctor touched your genitals.' A significant proportion of the children who had not been touched (particularly the girls) showed touching on the doll. Furthermore, when children who had received a genital examination were asked the same question, a number of children (particularly the girls) incorrectly showed that the doctor had inserted a finger into their genitals; the paediatrician did not do this. Next, when the children were given a stethoscope and a spoon and asked to show what the doctor did or might do with these instruments, some children incorrectly showed that

he used the stethoscope to examine their genitals and some children inserted the spoon into the genital or anal openings or hit the doll's genitals; none of these actions occurred. We concluded that these false actions were the result of implicit suggestions (communicated through a number of requests that the child use the dolls to show and talk about touching of the genitals and buttocks) that it is permissible to show sexualized behaviours. Also, because of the novelty of the dolls, children were drawn to insert fingers and other objects into their cavities.

A number of recent studies have raised concerns about the use of dolls with young children, who generally have difficulty with symbolic representations. Deloache et al. have argued that because young children exhibit general problems in symbol-referent relations, they therefore may have difficulty in using dolls as symbols of self and colleagues. Some of Deloache's work confirms this prediction. In these studies (Deloache & Marzolf 1995; Uttal et al. 1995), a sticker was first placed on a child or on a researcher, then the child was asked to use a doll to show where the sticker was placed. Children between the ages of 2.5 and 3.5 years made many errors when they used a doll to show where the sticker was placed on their own body. However, they were much more accurate when asked to represent one doll with another doll or when the sticker was placed on the research assistant and the child showed on his or her own body where the sticker had been placed. From these findings, Deloache concluded that children do poorly when they have to use dolls as a symbol of a person.

Although there is concern about the use of dolls with 3-year-old children, the results of a study by Saywitz et al. (1991) suggest that these concerns do not extend to 5- and 7-year-old girls. In their study, half of the children had received a genital examination and the other half had received a scoliosis examination in which the child's genitals were not touched by the doctor. When questioned several weeks later, most of the children in this study who had received a genital examination made omission errors (they failed to report genital or buttock touching when they were asked for a verbal report of their examination, or they failed to show on the dolls what had actually happened). However, when the experimenter pointed to either the genitalia or buttocks of the doll and asked a direct question, 'Did the doctor touch you here?', a substantial majority of the children now correctly assented to buttock or genital touching, thus reversing their earlier omission error. In contrast to the Bruck et al. findings, children who received the scoliosis examination (with no genital touching) never made false reports of genital touching (errors of commission) in either the verbal free recall or the doll enactment conditions. For this group, errors of commission were very low when the experimenter pointed to the genital or anal region of the doll and asked, 'Did the doctor touch you here?'

In summary, the dolls in the Saywitz et al. study of older children did not promote false reports of touching, and when used in a very directive manner, they reduced children's resistance to talk about anogenital touching, and reversed their former false denials.

Are there boundaries beyond which children are not suggestible?

There is still some controversy regarding the boundary conditions for younger children's greater suggestibility. Some argue that suggestibility is diminished or even non-existent when the act in question concerns a significant action, or when the child is a participant as opposed to a bystander, or when the report is a free narrative (Goodman *et al.* 1990; Fivush 1993). The strongest claim of this sort is that children are not suggestible about personally experienced central actions, especially those that involve their own bodies.

While it is probably true that children are somewhat less prone to false suggestions about actions to their own bodies as opposed to neutral non-bodily acts, the literature clearly does not support the strong view that bodily acts are impervious to suggestion. There are numerous demonstrations of how suggestive interviewing procedures can lead children to make inaccurate reports about events involving their own bodies and at times these reports have been tinged with sexual connotations. As noted earlier, young children have made false claims about 'silly events' that involved body contact (e.g. Did the nurse lick your knee? Did she blow in your ear?), and these false claims persisted in repeated interviewing over a 3-month period (Ornstein *et al.* 1992). Young children falsely reported that a man put something yuckie in their mouths (Poole & Lindsay 1995). Three-year-olds falsely alleged that their paediatrician had inserted a finger or a stick into their genitals (Bruck *et al.* 1995). Preschool-age children falsely alleged that some man touched their friends, kissed their friends on the lips and removed some of the children's clothes (Lepore & Sesco 1994). Studies of children who have undergone a radiological procedure (a voiding cystourethrogram) accord with this claim (Goodman *et al.* 1997). These children have their bladders pumped with fluid and are encouraged to urinate on the table in front of the medical staff. Later, they are asked suggestive questions about whether they were kissed during the procedure, etc., and the results indicate that children are suggestible about such matters.

Additional examples are provided by research by Goodman *et al.* In one study, 3-year-olds gave false answers 32% of the time to questions such as, 'Did he touch your private parts?', whereas 5-year-olds gave false answers 24% of the time (Goodman *et al.* 1990). In response to questions such as, 'How many times did he spank you?', 3-year-olds gave false answers 24% of the time, while 5-year-olds gave false answers only 3% of the time (Goodman & Aman 1990). When 3–4-year-olds were interviewed about events surrounding an inoculation, there was an error rate of 23% on questions such as, 'How many times did she kiss you?' and 'She touched your bottom didn't she?'. Many of these children replied 'yes' even though these events did not occur.

Taken together, one can safely conclude that, compared to older children, young children, and specifically preschool-age children, are at a greater risk for suggestion about a wide variety of topics, including those containing sexual themes.

Conclusions

Notwithstanding the above conclusion, it is clear that children—even preschool-age children—are capable of accurately recalling much that is forensically relevant. For example, in many of our own studies, children in the control group conditions recalled events flawlessly. This indicates that the absence of suggestive techniques allows even very young preschool-age children to provide highly accurate reports, although they may be sparse in the number of details. There are a number of other studies that highlight the strengths of young children's memories (see Goodman *et al.* 1992; Fivush 1993 for a review). What characterizes many such studies is the neutral tone of the interviewer, the limited use of misleading questions (for the most part, if suggestions are used, they are limited to a single occasion) and the absence of the induction of any motive or stereotype for the child to make a false report. When such conditions are satisfied, it is a common (although not universal) finding that children are relatively immune to isolated suggestive influences, particularly about sexual details.

An important implication of the studies that focus on the strength of children's reports is that although children are generally accurate when they are interviewed by a neutral experimenter, who asks few leading questions, and when they are not given any motivation to produce distorted reports, there are occasionally a few children who do give bizarre or sexualized answers to some leading questions. For example, in the Saywitz *et al.* (1991) study of children's reports of their medical examinations, one child, who never had a genital exam, falsely reported that the paediatrician had touched her buttocks and on further questioning claimed that it tickled and that the doctor used a long stick. In a study of children's recollection of their visit to a laboratory (Rudy & Goodman 1991), one young child claimed that he had seen bones and blood in the research trailer (see Goodman *et al.* 1992 for additional examples). Thus, young children occasionally make spontaneous, strange and unfounded allegations, and the individual difference factors that may contribute to these bizarre narratives are unknown. However, as Goodman *et al.* point out, many of these allegations can be understood by sensibly questioning the child and parents further. Still, interviewers must be especially cautious when dealing with younger children because they are disproportionately suggestible to deviation from the ideal neutral interview. This leaves three important questions.

1 What is it about younger children that makes them more susceptible than older children?

2 Why do some children provide spontaneous elaborate false reports?

3 What do these findings tell us about who should interview and what types of training interviewers should be given?

Why younger children may be more susceptible to suggestive interviewing

Not a great deal is known about factors that lead some children to create embellished false narratives and colleagues to resist this tendency. Despite vigorous research activity on this issue, there is much that we know does not account for variation among children. For example, differences in intelligence (above the borderline retarded threshold level) do not appear to discriminate between children who develop false narratives and those who do not; nor do a variety of personality attributes, such as need for compliance, need for closure, and dissociation. The few factors that have been found to be associated with false narratives are source monitoring ability (keeping track of the source of memories) and memory strength. In general, younger children lack well-developed source monitoring skills, and this may be a major reason why they produce more false narratives than older children and adults. If a child learns about an event from a story read to them, or even through a dream, they are more likely to later believe that they learned of it through actual participation. Similarly, younger children's memories are weaker and fade quicker than older children's memory traces, and this, too, may be a reason they create more false narratives. In studies of individual differences among children of the same age, these same factors appear to be associated with differences in false narratives. Children who have stronger memories are more resistant to suggestions about those memories.

Interviewer training and selection

There is not a great deal of data on who should interview, although people prone to emphasizing their own authority or who have an ingrained bias or expectation as to the outcome of an interview which cannot be dissuaded by training are probably not ideal candidates. Some data on the effectiveness of specific interviewer training programmes has emerged (Warren *et al.* 1999), but more research needs to be carried out in this area. The types of interviewer behaviours that should be encouraged, however, have received attention and we have discussed many of those: open-ended questioning; the use of directed questioning with caution and only in the most neutral manner; avoiding any stereotype induction; minimizing motivation to provide specific answers; and not introducing information or preferences to the child.

It is important to note that both areas of research have contributed to a growing body of knowledge that is beginning to influence the training of forensic interviewers. These findings have resulted in texts that provide interviewers with clear real-world recommendations on interviewing (Ceci & Bruck 1995; Poole & Lamb 1998). Changes in interviewer behaviour to more open-ended questioning helps both victims of child abuse and victims of false accusations.

References

Binet, A. (1900) *La Suggestibilité*. Schleicher Frères, Paris.

Boat, B.W. & Everson, M.D. (1996) Concerning practices of interviewers when using anatomical dolls in child protective services investigations. *Child Maltreatment*, 1(2), 96–104.

Bothwell, R.K., Deffenbacker, K.A. & Brigham, J.C. (1987) Correlation of eyewitness accuracy and confidence: optimality hypothesis revisited. *Journal of Applied Psychology*, 72, 691–695.

Bruck, M., Ceci, S.J., Francoeur, E. & Renick, A. (1995) Anatomically detailed dolls do not facilitate preschoolers' reports of a pediatric examination involving genital touching. *Journal of Experimental Psychology: Applied*, 1, 95–109.

Bruck, M., Hembrooke, H. & Ceci, S. (1997) Children's reports of pleasant and unpleasant events. In: Recollections of trauma: Scientific evidence and clinical practice, (eds J.D. Read & D.S. Lindsay), pp. 199–219. Plenum Press, New York.

Bruck, M., Ceci, S.J., & Hembrooke, H. (in press) The nature of children's true and false narratives. *Developmental Review*.

Burtt, H.E. (1948) *Applied Psychology*. Prentice Hall, Englewood Cliffs, NJ.

Cassel, W. & Bjorklund, D. (1996) Developmental patterns of eyewitness memory, forgetting, and suggestibility: an ecologically based short term longitudinal study. *Law and Human Behavior*, 19, 507–532.

Ceci, S.J. & Bruck, M. (1993) The suggestibility of the child witness: a historical review and synthesis. *Psychological Bulletin*, 113, 401–432.

Ceci, S.J. & Bruck, M. (1995) *Jeopardy in the Courtroom: a Scientific Analysis of Children's Testimony*. American Psychological Association, Washington, D.C.

Ceci, S.J. & Friedman, R.D. (2000) The suggestibility of children: scientific research and legal implications. *Cornell Law Review*, 86, 101–182.

Ceci, S.J., Loftus, E.F., Leichtman, M.D. & Bruck, M. (1994) The role of source misattributions in the creation of false beliefs among preschoolers. *International Journal of Clinical and Experimental Hypnosis*, 62, 304–320.

Conte, J.R., Sorenson, E., Fogarty, L. & Rosa, J.D. (1991) Evaluating children's reports of sexual abuse: Results from a survey of professionals. *American Journal of Orthopsychiatry*, 61(3), 428–437

Cunningham, J.L. (1988) Contribution to the history of psychology. XLVL. The pioneer work of Alfred Binet on children as eyewitnesses. *Psychological Reports*, 62, 272–283.

Dale, P.S., Loftus, E.F. & Rathburn, L. (1978) The influence of the form of the question on eyewitness testimony of preschool children. *Journal of Psycholinguistic Research*, 7, 269–277.

DeLoache, J.S. & Marzolf, D.P. (1995) The use of dolls to interview young children: Issues of symbolic representation. *Journal of Experimental Child Psychology*, 60, 155–173.

Eisen, M.L., Goodman, G.S., Qin, J. & Davis, S.L. (1998) Memory and suggestibility in maltreated children: new research relevant to evaluating allegations of abuse. In: *Truth in Memory* (eds S. Lynn & K. McConkey), pp. 163–188. Guilford Press, New York.

Fivush, R. (1993) Developmental perspectives on autobiographical recall. In: *Child victims, child witnesses: Understanding and improving testimony* (eds G.S. Goodman & B.L. Bottoms), pp. 1–24. Guilford Press, New York.

Fivush, R. & Schwarzmueller, A. (1998) Children remember childhood: Implications for childhood amnesia. *Applied Cognitive Psychology*, 12, 455–473.

Fivush, R. & Shukat, J. (1995) Content, consistency, and coherence of early autobiographical recall. In: *Memory and testimony in the child witness* (eds M.S. Zaragoza, J.R. Graham, G.C.N. Hall, R. Hirschman & Y.S. Ben-Porath), pp. 5–23. Thousand Oaks, CA: Sage.

Garven, S., Wood, J.M., Malpass, R.S. & Shaw, J.S., III. (1998) More than suggestion: the effect of interviewing techniques from the

McMartin Preschool case. *Journal of Applied Psychology*, **83**(3), 347–359.

Garven, S., Wood, J.M. & Malpass, R.S. (2000) Allegations of wrongdoing: the effects of reinforcement on children's mundane and fantastic claims. *Journal of Applied Psychology*, **85**(1), 38–49.

Goodman, G.S. & Aman, C. (1990) Children's use of anatomically detailed dolls to recount an event. *Child Development*, **61**(6), 1859–1871.

Goodman, G.S. & Clarke-Stewart, A. (1991) Suggestibility in children's testimony: implications for child sexual abuse investigations. In: *Suggestibility of Children's Recollections* (ed. J.L. Doris), pp. 92–105. American Psychological Association, Washington, D.C.

Goodman, G., Wilson, M.E., Hazan, C. & Reed, R.S. (1989) Children's testimony nearly four years after an event. Paper presented at the annual meeting of the Eastern Psychological Association, Boston MA.

Goodman, G.S., Rudy, L., Bottoms, B. & Aman. C. (1990) Children's concerns and memory: issues of ecological validity in the study of children's eyewitness testimony. In: *Knowing and Remembering in Young Children* (eds R. Fivush & J. Hudson), pp. 249–284. Cambridge University Press, New York.

Goodman, G.S., Batterman-Faunce, J.M. & Kenney, R. (1992) Optimizing children's testimony: Research and social policy issues concerning allegations of child sexual abuse. In: *Child abuse, child development and social policy* (eds D. Cicchetti & S. Toth). Ablex, Norwood, NJ.

Goodman, G.S., Quas, J.A., Batterman-Faunce, J.M., Riddlesberger, M.M. & Kuhn, G. (1997) Children's reactions to and memory for a stressful event: influences of age, anatomical dolls, knowledge, and parental attachment. *Applied Developmental Science*, **1**, 54–75.

Gordon, B.N., Ornstein, P.A., Nida, R.E., Follmer, A. *et al.* (1993) Does the use of dolls facilitate children's memory of visits to the doctor? *Applied Cognitive Psychology*, **7**(6), 459–474.

Gudjonsson, G.H. & Clark, N.K. (1986) Suggestibility in police interrogation: A social psychological model. *Social Behaviour*, **1**, 83–104.

Lamb, M.E., Hershkowitz, I., Sternberg, K.J. *et al.* (1996) Effects of investigative utterance types on Israeli children's responses. *International Journal of Behavioral Development*, **19**, 627–637.

Leichtman, M.D. & Ceci, S.J. (1995) The effects of stereotypes and suggestions on preschoolers' reports. *Developmental Psychology*, **31**, 568–578.

Leippe, M.R., Manion, A.P. & Romanczyk, A. (1992) Eyewitness persuasion: How and how well do fact finders judge the accuracy of adults' and children's memory reports? *Journal of Personality and Social Psychology*, **63**(2), 181–197.

Lepore, S.J. & Sesco, B. (1994) Distorting children's reports and interpretations. *Applied Psychology*, **79**, 108–120.

Lipmann, O. (1911) Pedagogical psychology of report. *Journal of Educational Psychology*, **2**, 253–260.

Loftus, E.F. (1979) *Eyewitness Testimony*. Harvard University Press, Cambridge, MA.

Lyon, T.D. (1999) The New Wave in Children's Suggestibility Research: A Critique. *Cornell Law Review*, **84**, 1001–1081.

Messerschmidt, R. (1933) The suggestibility of boys and girls between the ages of six and sixteen. *Journal of Genetic Psychology*, **43**, 422–437.

Ornstein, P.A., Gordon, B.N. & Larus, D.M. (1992) Children's memory for a personally experienced event: *Implications for testimony*. *Applied Cognitive Psychology*, **6**, 49–60.

Ornstein, P.A., Shapiro, L., Clubb, P. & Follmer, A. (1997) The influence of prior knowledge on children's memory for salient medical experiences. In: *Memory for Everyday and Emotional Events* (eds N. Stein, P.A. Ornstein, T. Trabasso & C. Brainerd), pp. 83–112. Erlbaum, Mahwah, NJ.

Otis, M. (1924) A study of suggestibility in children. *Archives of Psychology*, **11**, 5–108.

Piaget, J. (1986) *Judgment and Reasoning in the Child*. Harcourt Brace & Co., New York.

Poole, D.A. & Lamb, M.E. (1998) *Investigative interviews of children: a guide for helping professionals*. American Psychological Association, Washington, D.C.

Poole, D.A. & Lindsay, D.S. (1995) Interviewing preschoolers: Effects of nonsuggestive techniques, parental coaching, and leading questions on reports of nonexperienced events. *Journal of Experimental Child Psychology*, **60**, 129–154.

Poole, D.A. & Lindsay, D.S. (1996) Interviewing preschoolers: effects of nonsuggestive techniques, parental coaching, and leading questions. *Journal of Experimental Child Psychology*, **60**, 129–154.

Poole, D.A. & White, L.T. (1991) Effects of question repetition on the eyewitness testimony of children and adults. *Developmental Psychology*, **27**, 975–986.

Poole, D.A. & White, L.T. (1993) Two years later: effects of question repetition and retention interval on the eyewitness testimony of children and adults. *Developmental Psychology*, **29**, 844–853.

Poole, D.A. & White, LT.. (1995) Tell me again and again: stability and change in the repeated testimonies of children and adults. In: *Memory and Testimony in the Child Witness* (eds M.S. Zaragoza, J.R. Graham, C.N. Gordon, R. Hirschman & Y. Ben-Porath), pp. 24–43. Sage Publications, Thousand Oaks, CA.

Powers, P., Andriks, J.L. & Loftus, E.F. (1979) Eyewitness accounts of females and males. *Journal of Applied Psychology*, **64**, 339–347.

Rawls, J.M. (1996) How question form and body-parts diagrams can affect the content of young children's disclosures. Paper presented at the NATO Advanced Study Institute, Recollections of trauma: Scientific research and clinical practice. Port de Bourgenay, France. *Lawtalk*, April 1996, pp. 28–29.

Ross, D.F., Dunning, D., Toglia, M. & Ceci, S.J. (1990) The child in the eyes of the jury. *Law & Human Behavior*, **14**, 5–23.

Rudy, L. & &. Goodman, G.S. (1991) Effects of participation on children's reports: implications for children's testimony. *Developmental Psychology*, **27**, 527–538.

Saywitz, K.J., Goodman, G.S., Nicholas, E. & Moan, S.F. (1991) Children's memories of a physical examination involving genital touch: implications for reports of child sexual abuse. *Journal of Consulting and Clinical Psychology*, **59**(5), 682–691.

Sjoberg, R. (1995) Child testimonies during an outbreak of witch hysteria, Sweden 1670–71. *Journal of Child Psychology and Psychiatry*, **36**, 1039–1051.

Small, W.S. (1896) *Suggestibility of Children*. 13 Pedagogical Seminar.

Stern, W. (1910) Abstracts of lectures on the psychology of testimony and on the study of individuality. *American Journal of Psychology*, **21**, 270–282.

Steward, M., Steward, D.S., Farquahar L. *et al.* (1996) Interviewing young children about body touch and handling. *Monographs of the Society of for Research in Child Development*, **61**, (4–5: Serial no. 248).

Uttal, D., Schreiber, J.C. & DeLoache, J.S. (1995) Waiting to use a symbol: The effects of delay on children's use of models. *Child Development*, **66**(6), 1875–1889.

Varendonck, J. (1911) Les témoignages d'enfants dans un procès retentissant. *Archives de Psychologie*, **11**, 129–171.

Warren, A.R., Woodall, C.E., Thomas, M. *et al.* (1999) Assessing the effectiveness of a training program for interviewing child witnesses. *Applied Developmental Science*, **3**, 128–135.

Warren, A., Garven, S., Walker, N., Woodall, E. (2000) *Setting the record straight*. Paper presented at the Biennial Meeting of the American Psychology-Law Society, New Orleans, LA.

Family Interviewing: Issues of Theory and Practice

Ivan Eisler

Introduction

Conjoint family interviews, whether as part of assessment or treatment, have become a standard part of child psychiatric practice. A well-conducted family interview will provide the clinician with an important source of information about the family and opportunities for intervention that are not available when family members are seen on their own. Like other clinical interviews, the family interview will generally have a mixture of objectives—making an engagement with the members of the family, obtaining information and observing family process for purposes of assessment and making therapeutic interventions.

The family interview has a number of distinct features in comparison with an individual interview, which gives it both strengths as well as certain weaknesses. It offers the opportunity to observe family members in direct interaction, which can give unique insights into the way the family is currently functioning and the way it is organized around the presenting problem. The family interview is also well suited to explore the perceptions and meanings that different family members hold about the problem, which can lead to new understandings of the part it might be playing in their lives. If the family members experience the clinician as someone who has a real interest in their different points of view and takes each of them seriously, the opening up of different perspectives in this way can be an important starting point for the process of therapeutic change. On the other hand, as Cox (1994) has argued, the family interview is not ideally suited for the gathering of historical data about the individual (or family) and its 'public' nature may make it more difficult, and sometimes inappropriate, to discuss issues that family members may feel are private or awkward to talk about in the family context.

A useful framework for thinking about the family interview (both in terms of understanding the observed family process and also as a way of framing some of the specific techniques and interventions that may be used by the clinician when seeing the family) is provided by family systems theory. Before outlining this theoretical framework, an important caveat needs to be made.

Clinicians sometimes assume that the principal reason for a family assessment is to identify dysfunctional patterns of family functioning, which may be the underlying cause of the child's problem and which need to be corrected if the child is to be helped. Over the years a variety of theoretical family models (see Jacobs & Pearse, Chapter 57) have been put forward to explain

the development of a range of disorders from schizophrenia (Bateson *et al.* 1956; Lidz *et al.* 1957), through anorexia nervosa (Palazzoli 1974; Minuchin *et al.* 1975) to conduct disorder (Patterson 1982). These models, based on careful clinical observations, are often very persuasive and have been highly influential, leading to important developments in family therapy (Dare *et al.* 1995). Paradoxically, alongside the growing evidence for the effectiveness of family interventions for most child and adolescent disorders (Alexander & Parsons 1973; Patterson *et al.* 1982; Russell *et al.* 1987; Henggeler & Borduin 1991; Joanning *et al.* 1992; Kazdin *et al.* 1992; Borduin *et al.* 1995; Webster-Stratton & Hammond 1997; Eisler *et al.* 1997, 2000; see also reviews by Carr 2000a,b), there is also increasing evidence that many of the theoretical models, such as Bateson's double-blind theory (Bateson *et al.* 1956) or Minuchin's model of the Psychosomatic Family (Minuchin *et al.* 1978) are flawed (Olson 1972; Kog *et al.* 1985; Eisler 1995a).

While it is undoubtedly true that relationships within the family, the emotional climate and the patterns of family interaction are an important part of the complex matrix that contributes to the development and/or maintenance of individual psychopathology, the evidence that specific family factors or particular forms of family organization are directly associated with certain disorders is not very persuasive. Poor family functioning, family discord, inadequate parenting or neglect are generally higher in clinical samples than in control groups (Sawyer *et al.* 1988; Friedman *et al.* 1997; Beavers & Hampson 2000) but this is likely to be a reflection of a complex interaction over time between the effect of the family environment, personality and temperamental characteristics of the child, the impact of the developing disorder on the family, resilience factors as well as mediating genetic factors (Fergusson & Lynskey 1996; Rutter 1999). This is highlighted by behavioural genetic research showing the differential impact of the family environment on children within the same family (Dunn & Plomin 1990; Reiss *et al.* 1995; Rutter *et al.* 1999).

When observing a family in the clinic setting it is all too easy to forget the complexity of the interaction that has led to the current situation and to jump to the conclusion that the observed pattern of family functioning can provide the explanation of why the child has problems. Such a conclusion is not only diagnostically simplistic but also therapeutically unhelpful as it reinforces feelings of guilt and blame which family members, and parents in particular, are likely to experience (Reimers & Treacher 1995). The clinician needs to be sensitive to the fact that inviting the whole family to attend together may be interpreted by them as an indication that the family is seen as the source of their child's problem.

Family systems theory

The idea that the family can be thought of as a *system* may seem at one level self-evident, as clearly the family is an entity that is more than just a collection of individuals. Members of a family are intimately connected, they have a shared history, they may share certain beliefs and values, they take on particular roles and they find themselves responding to one another in predictable ways. The connectedness of the elements of the system and the notion that what happens in one part of the system has an effect on the rest of the system fits well with our notion of the family, but accords less well with how we think of individuals. It seems to take away from the value that we attach to individuals, their individual feelings, beliefs and their ability to make choices about individual actions.

A similar tension arises when we consider individual development as being part of an evolving family system. If children as well as parents are considered 'merely' as elements in the system, how do we account, for instance, for the differences in power between parents and children to influence the evolving system? Even though we may readily accept that parents and children influence each other mutually, we still want to emphasize that it is primarily parents who socialize their children, and not vice versa. While at a theoretical level it may be possible to integrate the essentially linear notions of individual development and growth with the systems notion of circular causality (Minuchin 1988), in practice there is always likely to be a tension between the two perspectives. There is a danger therefore that we either concentrate on the individual without taking sufficient account of the family context, or that we focus on the family to the extent that we lose sight of the needs of individual members and, in particular, the child (Strickland-Clark *et al.* 2000).

It is beyond the scope of this chapter to discuss family systems theory in detail but the following are the key features (for more detailed accounts see Gorell Barnes 1985; Eisler 1993; Dallos & Draper 1999).

The social context of behaviour

Individual behaviour and individual personal characteristics need to be viewed in the social context in which they occur. It is a familiar observation that individuals will behave differently in the different contexts in which they find themselves. At the simplest level, every behaviour is both a response to the previous behaviour and, at the same time, a stimulus for the next element of behaviour in the sequence (such sequences often being recursive, so that behaviours may be mutually reinforcing). The way in which even a simple sequence of behaviours evolves is complex, as it depends on the meaning attached to the observed behaviour as well as the anticipation of future response(s). For instance, an

anxious child may complain of feeling sick before going to school, which may evoke a worried response from the child's mother which in turn may reinforce the child's anxiety. Mother's response will have been determined not only by her perception of the situation but also by her anticipation of how others (father, school, etc.) are likely to respond. If father perceives the child's behaviour as manipulative and/or views mother's worried response as something that is fuelling the anxiety in the child, he may try to play down the urgency of the situation. Mother may see this as father's lack of understanding (or lack of concern) and she may respond by highlighting the seriousness of the situation, which will have an effect on both the father's and the child's further response. Each of the behaviours is only fully comprehended when both the preceding behaviours and anticipated responses are taken into account. In fact, without knowing the social context, it is difficult to know what meaning to attach to a particular behaviour.

Patterns of interactions in families

Over time families develop a set of patterns of interactions which become relatively stable. These patterns are connected to the beliefs, perceptions and expectations that different members of the family have, some of which may be shared and may also become relatively fixed (Byng-Hall 1986; Papp & Imber-Black 1996). Some patterns are related to the structure or the hierarchical organization of the family and the different roles that the family members take on, reflecting family beliefs, often strongly influenced by cultural or specific family traditions, about the nature of family life, gender roles, parenting tasks, etc. Subtler patterns of family process, of which family members themselves may not be always aware, can be observed in the moment-to-moment interaction in the family. When a family discussion is observed, relatively stable patterns can be observed of who-speaks-to-whom, turn-taking, interruptions, etc. (Lennard & Bernstein 1969). More complex patterns, e.g. in the way that a family handles disagreement or conflict, will also be characteristic of a particular family (Minuchin *et al.* 1978; Street & Foot 1984); so that, for instance, when a teenage daughter and her father start having a disagreement, mother will step in and diffuse the argument. In families with an ill child, the symptomatic behaviour will often take on a central role in the process of family transactions to the point where much of what happens seems to revolve around the symptomatic behaviour in a way that may both reinforce the symptom and in turn be maintained by it.

Stability and change in families

The family system evolves through alternating periods of stability and periods of change in response to the changing developmental needs of its members and/or external pressures. The stability and predictability of the family environment is an important aspect of family life, as it provides the context in which the individual developmental needs of its members are met. For instance, the child's need for dependence and attachment require a degree of stability and constancy in the family but, as the child develops, the family must find ways of meeting his or her needs for independence and separation as well (Langmeier & Matějček 1975; Byng-Hall 1991; Eisler 1993). Thus, as the family evolves through the predictable stages of the family life cycle (Carter & McGoldrick 1989), it needs to be able to adapt and change its habitual style of functioning. These transitional points in the family life cycle (whether in response to developmental changes or to unpredictable events, such as bereavement or family break-up, migration, major societal change, etc.) create pressure on individual family members and may lead to increased psychological morbidity (Hetherington 1989; Sartorius 1996; Gorell Barnes *et al.* 1998; Ritsner & Ponizovsky 1999). The way the family adapts may be a crucial factor in determining the extent of individual vulnerability to such pressures (Walsh 1997).

Current systems theory (von Foerster 1981; Hoffman 1990; Dallos & Draper 1999) emphasizes that the clinician, in exploring the family system, is never a passive detached observer looking in on the system, but has an active role observing him- or herself in interaction with the family. This has important implications for thinking about the way family interviews are conducted and how descriptions of interaction are made, which will be discussed later on in the chapter. It is best illustrated by an example. Clinical accounts of families often include descriptions of 'overprotective' parental behaviour (Levy 1939; Minuchin *et al.* 1978). Such a label is limited, in that it does not take into account the interaction between the parent's protective behaviour and the child's dependent behaviour and often ignores the context in which it occurs (e.g. a serious illness in the child). Equally importantly, it assumes that the clinician is a detached observer who is simply describing a behaviour and is not influenced by his or her own relationship with the family. However, the parent who is described as 'overprotective' is probably also being experienced by the clinician as someone who is reluctant to heed the advice to give the child more independence, thereby frustrating the well-meant efforts of the clinician. The description of overprotectiveness therefore has to be seen both as a reflection of the observed parent–child relationship and also of the relationship between the clinician and the family.

Social and cultural context of the family

Earlier family therapy texts tended to treat the family as a normative entity and took little account of the enormous diversity of family life and the role of the wider social and cultural context in which the family is placed. These issues are noted also in Jacobs & Pearse (Chapter 57) and will not be discussed in detail here. However, it is important to stress that awareness and sensitivity to cultural and social diversity of families is a crucial factor in how we as clinicians relate to families, the language that we use, the meanings that we attach to our observations of family interaction, as well as the choice of therapeutic interventions

and our expectations of the effect that these might have on the family (Lau 1984; Hodes 1985; Messent 1992; Wieselberg 1992; Gorell Barnes 1994, 1998).

The other aspect of the wider social context that the clinician needs to keep in mind is the family's position in relation to other professionals or agencies. Often there is a network of helpers within health, education or social services, with whom the family has an ongoing relationship. These relationships have an important bearing on what the family expects of us, how the family members present themselves and how they experience our interventions. At times the network of professional relationships can become quite disabling, creating a sense of neediness and helplessness, which is met with further provisions of support, making any resources that the family itself has more and more invisible (Cooklin *et al.* 1983; Imber-Black 1988; Boyd-Franklin 1989). Exploring the relationship that the family has with the professional network can therefore be an important part of understanding how the family is functioning.

Practical aspects of family interviewing

How and when clinicians use family interviews in their clinical practice varies considerably. This is largely determined by theoretical preferences, although factors such as the age of the child, the nature of the presenting problem or other factors, such as research or training needs, may also have a role. Different considerations may also apply, depending on whether one is thinking of the family interview as part of engagement, assessment or treatment, although clearly the distinction between the three is somewhat arbitrary. An assessment interview is a starting point for the development of a treatment alliance but, at the same time, enquiring sympathetically about the problem, clarifying its nature and asking how it affects different family members is also a very powerful therapeutic intervention in its own right. By the same token, however thorough the initial diagnostic assessment interview has been, during the process of treatment new information and new connections will emerge, adding to or changing the initial conclusions that were reached during the assessment stage. For the purposes of this discussion the distinction between engagement, assessment and treatment is useful, because it may help to clarify some of the ideas of when and how it may be useful to include family interviews in clinical practice.

The family interview as a context for engagement in treatment

For the systemically orientated clinician, the family interview is both the principal assessment instrument as well as the main context for therapeutic interventions. Most family therapy texts therefore assume that a family interview will also be where the engagement and the negotiation of the treatment contract takes place. Not all clinicians use the family interview to this extent, seeing it perhaps primarily as just one of the components of a comprehensive assessment and would not necessarily think of inviting the whole family to the first meeting. However, there will be many instances when it is useful to start by seeing the family together. Children and adolescents seldom seek psychiatric help for themselves and how they are to be engaged in the treatment process has to be considered alongside of how one engages the parents. For young children, being seen together with the parents, at least initially, may feel less threatening than being seen on their own. There may also be advantages, as will be discussed later, in seeing a reluctant child or adolescent in the context of a family meeting, as it may be possible to engage them even without them taking a particularly active part.

Whether the family is initially seen in a conjoint interview or separately may make a difference to their expectation of future treatment and perhaps also to their perception of why they are being asked to attend as a family. In a randomized study in which a conjoint family assessment was compared with separate parent and child assessments, Cox *et al.* (1995) found that there was a significantly higher failure rate of attendance for subsequent appointments if the mode of contact (conjoint or separate) was changed after the initial assessment. There is also evidence that families in which both parents attend the first interview are more likely to continue in treatment than when only the mother attends (LeFave 1980). Engaging the whole family may be more difficult where there is hostility, criticism or generally poorer family functioning (Szmukler *et al.* 1985; Dare *et al.* 1990; Hampson & Beaver 1996a), particularly if the style of treatment does not provide sufficient structure and containment (Hampson & Beaver 1996b).

The family interview as part of assessment

In one sense the case for including conjoint family interviews in a comprehensive assessment is the most obvious. The family interview certainly provides an ideal opportunity to assess the patterns of relationships, the emotional climate of the family and a chance to see the way in which the family has become organized around the symptomatic behaviour of the child. However, to argue that such information can only be obtained by seeing the family together would be to overstate the case. A number of studies have shown that, when global measures of family functioning are used (family or marital satisfaction, family competence, family health, etc.), self-report measures correlate highly with clinical ratings of observed interaction in both clinical (Miller *et al.* 1994; Hayden *et al.* 1998; Beavers & Hampson 2000) and non-clinical samples (Stevenson-Hinde & Akister 1995). Ratings on individual subscales showed moderate but significant correlations both between individual family members' self-reports and between self-report and observer rating, with the exception of ratings of affective expressiveness and behavioural control (Miller *et al.* 1994; Stevenson-Hinde & Akister 1995). Comparisons have also been made of ratings of Expressed Emotion (one of the most widely used measures of family atmosphere) from individual and family interviews (Szmukler *et al.* 1987; Hodes *et al.* 1999) showing a moderate to strong correlation of ratings between the two settings.

The above studies suggest that while conjoint family interviews may provide a richer and, in some cases, more meaningful picture of family functioning, if the principal aim is to assess the overall level of family functioning, individual interviews should provide a reasonably accurate picture. Indeed, in some instances, individuals may be more willing to report negative aspects of family functioning when they are interviewed on their own (Haynes *et al.* 1981).

The question of whether to include conjoint family interviewing in an overall assessment cannot be answered simply on the basis of comparing the quality of information obtained from individual or family interviews but must also depend on the context and the purpose for which the assessment is made and how the information is to be used. Where the primary aim is to provide a detailed considered assessment on which important decisions about the child might be made (e.g. for a Court report), a combination of family and individual interviews would be advisable. In such cases an open-ended unstructured family interview could be usefully supplemented by one of several available structured family interviews and clinical rating scales that have been developed based on well-defined theoretical models of family functioning: the McMaster Model of Family Functioning (Epstein *et al.* 1978; Bishop *et al.* 1980; Miller *et al.* 2000); the Beavers Systems Model of Family Functioning (Beavers & Hampson 1990, 2000); or the Olson Circumplex model (Olson *et al.* 1989; Olson 1990, 2000). These measures are well researched and have satisfactory psychometric properties (see also Grotevant & Carlson 1989; Kerig & Lindahl 2001 for reviews of family assessment measures). Research and/or training needs might be additional factors weighing in support of the use of such measures.

The potential disadvantage of such an approach is that the assessment of family functioning can easily become a search for family dysfunction. All too often there is at least an implicit assumption that the primary aim of family assessment is to uncover areas of poor functioning, that can be corrected by providing treatment for the family. The evidence that well-functioning families benefit more from family therapy than poorly functioning families (Hampson & Beavers 1996a) suggests that correcting family dysfunction may not be a necessary ingredient of effective family interventions.

The above points highlight the importance for family assessment to focus at least as much on family strengths, family resources and family competencies as on areas of poor functioning. While assessing strengths and resources is an important aspect of any comprehensive diagnosis, it is particularly important if the aim is to engage the family in treatment. A family assessment that is a prelude to (or perhaps more accurately the initial phase of) family treatment is above all a way of answering questions of *how best to work with the family*; questions about *whether or how the family might need to change* should come second. The manner in which we engage the family in this process and the nature of the evolving therapeutic relationship is probably more important than whether the family is seen together or separately.

The family interview as part of treatment

The different ways in which family interviews are used in the context of treatment are discussed in detail in Jacobs & Pearse (Chapter 57) so only some general points will be made here. If one assumes that the impact of a clinical interview experience is directly related to how 'new' the experience is, then clearly the family interview, in exploring a multiplicity of perspectives, always has the potential of having a significant impact on the family and, as Tomm (1987a) pointed out, affords considerably more therapeutic opportunities than clinicians sometimes realize. Positive results have been reported following single session interventions with the family (Boyhan 1996; Campbell 1999; Hampson *et al.* 1999). Because one of the aims of the family interview is to gain access to the different perceptions of individual family members, there are always opportunities for new meanings and new perspectives to emerge. Not all family members will have the same knowledge and understanding of the problem and some may be involved for the first time in discussing the problem openly. Some connections, particularly ones that are linked with the non-verbal processes occurring in families, may have been outside of the awareness of all the family members. The fact that the family interview is an experience shared with other family members means that sometimes even seemingly trivial things occurring during the interview can have quite a powerful effect.

One should not automatically assume that these effects are necessarily always experienced as positive by the family. The process of bringing out unspoken or hidden meanings into the open may sometimes be quite painful for them (Gorell Barnes 1998). This may be particularly true if the family feels judged or criticized, or if the interview itself becomes acrimonious or hostile and is dominated by mutual criticisms among family members. Some of these issues will be addressed in more detail later in the chapter.

How the family is most effectively involved in the treatment process varies depending on the type of problem (Carr 2000b), although there is also evidence that how families respond to treatment may be dependent on an interaction between type of family organization and therapeutic style. Hampson & Beavers (1996b) found that families rated as high on general family functioning responded best to an open collaborative therapeutic style, whereas disorganized families, with unclear internal boundaries, were more likely to do well when the therapist adopted a less open and more directive style. This was particularly true for families where there was open conflict and hostility.

Who should be included in the family interview?

To some extent this will depend on the specific aim of the particular interview and the subsequent plans for how the family should be involved in treatment. In general, it is useful to start by inviting all members of the family living in the household. This provides the fullest picture of the family, both in the way that dif-

ferent family members might be affected (e.g. a 'non-problem' sibling who may be sidelined by the amount of attention that is demanded by the 'problem' child in the family) but, more importantly, the presence of siblings often makes it easier to see some of the family strengths and resources that would otherwise remain hidden.

While one ought not to be rigid about who should come to the family meeting, it is important not to accept too readily that certain members of the family should be excluded, either because the family feels it would not be appropriate for them to attend, or because there is a view that they would refuse anyhow. Often the apparent unwillingness or inability to attend, e.g. because of work commitments on the part of father, turns out to be more to do with his sense that he would not be able to help anyhow and when the clinician stresses his or her belief that father has an important part to play in helping the child, the initial reluctance is usually readily overcome. If a family is being seen as part of ongoing treatment it can sometimes be helpful to see different subgroupings of the family (parents, siblings) on different occasions as this may allow different perspectives to emerge (Eisler 1995b; Gustafsson *et al.* 1995).

Who should be seen when divorced or step-families are involved may be more difficult to decide. It is usually best to start, as one does with intact families, by inviting the existing household. Inviting divorced parents to subsequent meetings may be useful, although care needs to be taken that this is not interpreted as signalling to the children that the aim of such a meeting is to re-create the old family (Robinson 1990). Where the parents have new partners, and where there may be complex step-family arrangements, it is important to take care not only in who is being invited but also in the way in which the invitation is made. Asking the family to help clarify who has what role in relationship to the children (for the purpose of knowing who should be coming to the family meetings) is often useful in helping to clarify boundaries and in exploring where the family is in the process of its life cycle transition. Such clarification can help to provide a greater sense of coherence for the children affected by the family break-up and this in itself may be an important part of helping them to adjust to the transition (Gorell Barnes *et al.* 1998).

Engaging the family and observing family process

It is important at the start of the initial meeting with the family to engage all family members in an age-appropriate way. This requires relating to all family members in a way that makes it clear that their different viewpoints are valued and that the reason they have been asked to come as a family is because they are seen as a resource for helping to deal with the problem, rather than being seen as its cause. It is useful to start by asking relatively low-key social questions about schools, jobs, interests that the children might have, how far the family had to travel for the appointment and so on. This phase of the interview should generally be unhurried and relaxed, making sure that all the family members are included in the interchanges in a way that is appropriate for their age. Although the primary goal during this phase is to allow the family to feel more at ease and to get a sense that they are being taken seriously, it also provides the therapist with an opportunity to make initial observations about patterns of interaction and the structure of the family. Who speaks to whom, how family members respond to one another, who is attended to, who finds it easy or difficult to join in the conversation, how disagreements or conflicts are handled, how the children are helped to settle down, etc., will all provide important initial impressions about the family. If the family is being interviewed in a room with a one-way screen or video cameras it is important, during this initial phase, to point these out to the family and explain the role of the observing team, stressing issues of confidentiality.

While much of the initial family interview is likely to be concerned with obtaining information about the nature and history of the problem, the ways in which the family has tried to tackle the problem, and so on, the presence of the whole family makes this a different kind of exercise from individual history-taking. Asking the views of different family members requires the family to reflect on the problem and on their relationship to the problem in new ways, especially if the questions are formulated in a relational manner (as will be described in the following section). Thus, although the focus remains primarily on the presenting problem, the clinician is beginning to collect information about the way the family may be organized in relationship to the problem. The clinician may develop certain hypotheses about the nature of these links which will lead to further questions and the response to these will provide further evidence about the usefulness or otherwise of such hypotheses. This information comes both in the form of the verbal response to the question but also from the non-verbal responses of the different family members.

Specific interview techniques

It is beyond the scope of this chapter to cover in depth the variety of techniques that have been developed for interviewing families (Palazzoli *et al.* 1980; Penn 1982; Tomm 1987a,b, 1988; Burnham 1986; Dallos & Draper 1990; l'Abate 1994). The following provides a brief outline of some of the different styles of questioning that have proved useful in family interviews. Tomm (1988) suggests the following classification.

Lineal questions

These are questions that are asked to orientate the clinician in determining what the problem is, what the family sees as the nature or the cause of the problem, etc. All interviews will include some questions of this type: 'What is the problem that you have come with?', 'How long has it been going on for?', etc. The disadvantage of lineal questions is that they tend to elicit a rather automatic response. Families tend to have a preferred, and often well-rehearsed, way of presenting their problem which may be quite fixed and expresses not only their belief about the nature of

the problem but also often connects with feelings of helplessness, guilt, blame and resentment. This preferred 'story' may be shared by some, though not necessarily all, family members. Tomm (1988) argued that lineal questions, particularly if they are the only type of questions asked, may invoke defensiveness and guilt or lead to criticism among family members.

Circular questions

These differ from lineal questions not only in form but also in their underlying assumption. They are questions that make the assumption that individual problems are connected or embedded in patterns of relationships, and the aim of these questions is therefore to illuminate or make visible what these patterns are. So for instance, instead of simply asking 'What is the problem?', one might ask 'How would different people in the family describe your problem?', 'Who worries about it?', 'Who else worries?', 'When people get worried about how unhappy you are, does it make you more or less depressed?' Other questions might require family members to describe what they make of behaviours that they observe, or speculate about thoughts and feelings of other family members. For instance, instead of asking just about the duration of the problem, the therapist might ask, 'When did your family first notice that you had a problem?' or 'What effect did it have on you when your parents started talking about the problem?' Additional questions might be asked about the way different people in the family responded to the problem and what interactions this might lead to; 'When your mother shows her worry, what does your father do?'

Asking circular questions around the problem often starts to provide a basis for describing the problem in a more contextual way and also allows for alternative descriptions to be heard. For instance, the family might explain that 'Mum is the one that worries most, because she's at home much more, whereas dad is always at work and doesn't really know what's going on', implying that the father, perhaps, cares less than the mother does about the child. Asking the question 'How much time does your father spend worrying about you when he is at work?', 'What is the difference between the way he shows his worry and the way your mother shows hers?' may elicit an alternative description, namely that father feels quite isolated and excluded but prefers not to show this because he fears that he will be told once more that he does not really understand. The unexpected nature of these questions and the sometimes surprising responses may provide both the clinician and the family with alternative ways of viewing the problem, or may bring out a new aspect of behaviour that had not been part of the family's awareness. This can open up new options for the family to act on in search of new solutions.

Strategic questions

These are questions that are used with the primary aim of influencing the family in a particular way rather than to obtain information and are analogous to giving instructions but, because they are formulated as a question, this may not always be immediately apparent. 'Why do you let your mother speak for you?' is as much a statement which implies that it would be better for the adolescent to speak for him- or herself, as a question asking for an explanation. Challenging interventions of this kind can be useful at times but should be used sparingly, as they can induce feelings of guilt and they may also undermine the therapeutic relationship with the family (Tomm 1988).

Reflexive questions

These are questions that are also intended to influence the family but are less directive, instead requiring family members to reflect on how things might be different under changed circumstances, or if they took a different course of action: 'What would happen if you were able to hide your worry when your daughter got depressed?', 'If your mother didn't try to help next time you have a row with your father which one of you would be more likely to find a way of ending the argument; who would be the one to suggest a compromise solution?' Reflexive questions will typically introduce an alternative way of framing a particular behaviour, opening up new possibilities and challenging the assumptions that may underlie a particular pattern of behaviour. They may address an emotion or an aspect of behaviour that is not being expressed overtly and may only be guessed at. They may include an implicit assumption: 'What will you argue about with your mother when you are no longer bulimic?' — implying both that there will be change and that arguments between adolescents and parents are normal. Reflexive questions, like circular questions, assume that behaviours and the meanings that we attach to them are part of the relational context of the family and that there may be more than one meaning that might be attached to a particular behaviour. The aim is for the family to reflect on this context and to explore the way in which thoughts, feelings and behaviours of different family members connect and how they might change. The following example provides an illustration.

During an interview with a family with a daughter suffering from bulimia the therapist noted the critical tone of mother's voice when she described the bulimic behaviour of her daughter. The daughter would mostly turn away from her mother but occasionally would snap back, which would evoke a very defensive response from her mother. After this happened several times the therapist turned to the daughter: 'When your mother talks about your bulimia are you more aware of her irritation or of her worry about you?' to which the daughter replied, 'I know she's very worried but her irritation drowns that out.' At which point mother joined in: 'I know I sound terribly critical but I'm so worried and I can't stop myself.' Acknowledging mother's anxiety made it possible to also talk about her being critical without it sounding as if the therapist was criticizing her for being critical. The pattern of criticism–irritation–defensiveness–criticism was broadened to include mother's anxiety and both mother's and daughter's sense of guilt.

It is important for the clinician to be able to use a range of interview styles with families and to have a repertoire of different types of questions. Circular questions, for instance, can be extremely useful in illuminating patterns of relationships in the family and this in itself may be an important and powerful part of the therapeutic process. However, such questions are most usefully applied when the interviewer has a clear hypothesis about the nature of the family relationships and the part played by the symptomatic behaviour in the family organization (Burnham 1986). When the interviewer has a clear focus, one question will naturally lead to the next one, helping to confirm or disconfirm the particular hypothesis. If, however, such questions are used without a clear focus they are more likely to create confusion and a sense of alienation (Reimers 1999; Strickland-Clark et al. 2000).

Using genograms

Constructing a family tree is a useful way of enquiring about family history, family beliefs, patterns of relationship over time but also to assess some of the strengths and resources that the family might have, which they themselves may have lost sight of (for detailed discussions of the use of genograms see McGoldrick & Gerson 1985; Bloch et al. 1994). This is best performed when an opportunity presents itself, arising spontaneously from a conversation with the family, e.g. about the extended family or a piece of family history that the family themselves have mentioned. 'I need to have a clear picture of who fits where, perhaps you could help me draw a family tree so that I can see this', could be a way of introducing the idea. It is important that the way in which the discussion about the family is conducted highlights that one is enquiring about the family primarily because one is interested in having a better understanding of the wider family context and in particular of the family strengths, resources and resilience, rather than because one is searching for family pathology.

One should enquire not only about individuals and events from the family history but also about the nature of the relationships, looking for patterns across generations in dealing with relevant life cycle transitions, identifying important beliefs and values that the family holds, etc. Enquiring about differences between traditions and beliefs on the mother's and father's side of the family, and which of these and how they have been incorporated into their own family, can provide a useful starting point for a discussion amongst family members. If there are younger children in the family they can be asked to help in drawing the family tree and encouraged to ask questions about the details of the families of their parents of which they are unsure.

When techniques such as genograms are used during family interviews a degree of caution is needed. It is all too easy to read into a genogram far more than is actually warranted and relatively trivial matters may be included and interpreted as giving the 'true' picture of the family. It is therefore particularly important not to try and interpret the meaning of such patterns too readily and it is generally more useful to ask the family what they themselves make of the patterns that they have identified.

Tracking and responding to the interaction process

Awareness and sensitivity to the processes within the family are important, not only as ways of assessing the nature of the relationships within the family, but also as an important part of the process of joining the family and introducing change (Minuchin & Fishman 1981). For instance, if one notices that questions directed towards an adolescent are repeatedly answered by one or other of the parents, one might want to check out how readily such a pattern might change. This might be done non-verbally, by fixing the adolescent's gaze more intently next time one asks a question, or leaning forward so that it is more difficult for someone else to join in the conversation. Alternatively, one could ask a question or comment in a way that draws attention to what is happening; 'I have noticed that you often let your mother speak for you; it is as if you thought she has better answers than you do.' When commenting on family process it is always important to recognize that the same phenomenon can be described in a number of ways: ranging from neutral (questions addressed to the daughter are more likely to be answered by the mother than by the daughter herself); through ascribing agency to one or other participant in the interaction (mother speaks for daughter; daughter lets mother speak for her); to overtly critical (mother behaves in an intrusive way; daughter cannot be bothered to answer any questions). Even quite neutral comments may appear critical to family members and the clinician therefore has to be careful in choosing an appropriate style of comment or question. Andersen (1987) recommended that reflections of this kind are best done in a tentative way rather than being pronouncements or authoritative interpretations that are likely to come across as being judgemental.

Interviewing families with young children

All too often when a family with young children is seen, the children become passive participants of a discussion between the adults. Even very young children can be effectively included in family interviews, provided they are engaged in an age-appropriate way. This can be aided through providing toys, drawing materials, etc., and using creative and play techniques in a similar way that they would be used in individual interviews with a child. Engaging a child effectively is often very reassuring for parents, who may feel unsure whether bringing the child to a psychiatric setting is the right thing to do. The choice of language in talking to parents about their child's problems is also important with young children present as it may be difficult for the child to understand what is being said. Often it is better to ask the parents to explain things to the child, rather than the clinician doing this directly as this may be both less threatening for the child and also reinforces the sense that the parents are the experts in their own child.

With very lively active children the first task is to create a working environment in which what family members have to say can be attended to. This is best achieved by actively collaborating with the parents. Asking the parents for advice on how best to occupy young children 'so that we can also talk' will both reinforce the parents' sense that they are being taken seriously and also may make it easier for the child to join in spontaneously at some point during the interview. Little is gained from trying to talk to the parents until one has assisted them to help the children settle down and play in a way that both the parents and the clinician are comfortable with. Children are often reluctant attendees in a psychiatric setting and may not be too keen to take part in discussions at first. Making it clear at the start of the session that everyone in the room will have an opportunity to have their say, while stressing that it is also fine to sit and listen, is important for some children, to avoid making them feel that they are being put on the spot. When the pressure on them to join in is removed, children will often join in spontaneously. Joining with a child in creative play or talking about a drawing he or she has made can also provide an opportunity for the child to have his or her voice heard in the session (see also Dare & Lindsey 1979; Larner 1996; Wilson 1998).

A similar situation can sometimes arise with an adolescent who may be reluctant to talk, while the parents may have an expectation that the 'experts' will succeed where they themselves have been unable to get through. While sometimes such an adolescent may be more willing to talk when seen individually this is, by no means, always the case. The advantage of a family interview is that even a reluctant or unwilling participant can be included in an interview through indirect means. Making it clear that the therapist respects the adolescent's right not to speak can avoid an unhelpful battle. This can be done in a way that respects the adolescent's autonomy while at the same time making sure that he or she is not being simply ignored. One might say: 'I often find that young people, when they come here, feel that its best for them not to say too much at first, which is fine, but if you want to say how things are from your point of view I would obviously be interested to know. I do need to know your parents' views about things as well but I want to make sure that we don't simply ignore you, so I will check from time to time whether you want to add something.'

Problems and pitfalls of family interviews

Personal and intimate issues

There will always be areas and topics that are either too difficult or inappropriate to raise in the context of a family interview. The distinction between difficult and inappropriate may sometimes be obvious (e.g. discussing the sexual relationship of the parents in the presence of their children) but more often than not the two tend to get blurred. Often the reluctance to talk about certain topics in the presence of the whole family is either to protect other family members from painful feelings or to avoid the re-opening of a disagreement or a confrontation. The appropriateness or otherwise of discussing specific topics will vary from family to family, which will be determined partly by their social, cultural and religious background, but may also be idiosyncratically connected to specific aspects of their own family history and beliefs. Sometimes the uncertainty that the interviewer feels about whether or how to raise a particular topic may be as much to do with his or her own feelings and attitudes on the subject as they are to do with the family themselves. It is important that it is always made clear to the family that they have a choice about what is to be discussed. Asking questions that help to clarify what the family find appropriate, or asking for permission to talk about a certain subject, will often make it possible to talk about the issue without the discomfort that would otherwise accompany it or prevent the discussion altogether.

As clinicians we are sometimes driven by a quest for 'complete' information in order to make sure that we have not missed anything important. This may be justified from an assessment perspective, but clinically it is sometimes more important to respect that families maintain control over the flow of information. It is also important to recognize that the fact that a particular area has not been addressed directly does not automatically mean that the clinical interventions are less effective. In a study that compared two forms of family intervention in anorexia nervosa—conjoint family therapy and a separated family therapy in which the parents were seen as a couple, and the adolescent was seen separately by the same therapist—it was found (Eisler *et al.* 2000) that the conjoint family therapy produced more individual psychological change than did the separated therapy. This was in spite of the fact that some of the areas for which this was true (e.g. psychosexual adjustment) the topics were seldom addressed directly in the conjoint family interviews.

Unequal relationships with family members

With some families the clinician may find it difficult to maintain an equal relationship with all family members. This is particularly true with families where there is an open dispute between family members and where simply being sympathetic to an account from one person may give the impression that one is taking sides. For instance, the parents may have a disagreement as to how best to respond to the difficult behaviour of their child. The clinician may feel more sympathetic to one or the other of the parents, not necessarily because of believing that that parent's approach is better or more effective but more because of the way he or she perceives the parents overall. Strictly speaking, it is never possible to be entirely neutral, as any act implies that one has taken a certain position and even the overt expression of neutrality itself implies that one is preferring the *status quo* and does not take into account that different family members (children, adults, men, women) are not in equal positions with respect of being able to bring about change. A recognition of this is of particular importance when working with families where there is abuse or violence (Goldner *et al.* 1990; Glaser & Frosh 1993).

Critical or hostile interactions may be difficult to contain

Interviewing families where there is open conflict, hostility or frequent criticism is particularly difficult. Studies of family therapy have shown that such families are more likely to drop out of treatment (Szmukler *et al.* 1985) and are less likely to benefit from conjoint family therapy (Hampson & Beavers 1996a; Eisler *et al.* 2000). There is some evidence that with this type of family a relatively structured directive style of interviewing may lead to a better therapeutic outcome than when a more open collaborative interview style is used, whereas the reverse seems to be the case with other types of families (Hampson & Beavers 1996b). Criticism and hostility are often accompanied by feelings of guilt and self-blame (Besharat *et al.* 2001) and conjoint family interviews that are unable to provide sufficient containment may reinforce such feelings. In such cases it is sometimes better not to see the whole family together, or at least to postpone conjoint meetings to a time when the family is well engaged and some of the painful feelings have been addressed in separate sessions.

It has been a recurrent theme in this chapter that one of the risks of inviting the whole family for conjoint family interviews is that it will be understood by the family as suggesting that they are the cause of the problem. Even when it has been made clear that the purpose of seeing the family is to help them rediscover their own resources as a family, feelings of guilt and blame are very easily re-ignited. A number of studies have shown that even when family interventions are effective they may be perceived as blaming by the family (Squire-Dehouck 1993; Reimers & Treacher 1995).

Confidentiality, boundaries and family secrets

As mentioned earlier, when interviewing families, issues arise around confidentiality and boundaries that are different, to some extent, from individual interviews with patients or parents. Family interviews, by definition, are more 'public' than individual interviews. This is not only because of the presence of more people in the room but also because family interviews are often conducted with other people observing through one-way screens or using a video link. This is partly to do with the history of the development of family therapy, which places strong emphasis on the importance of the observing team providing an outside perspective (Palazzoli *et al.* 1978; Hoffman 1981; Boscolo *et al.* 1987), partly with the development of a variety of intervention techniques that make use of the different views held within the team (Papp 1980; Andersen 1987), and also with the way in which family therapy training has developed through trainees being supervised 'live' (Liddle *et al.* 1988). There is some empirical evidence that the input of the observing team enhances the efficacy of family interventions (Green & Herget 1989a,b) but it is also clear that families often find the experience unpleasant or at least uncomfortable, particularly if not enough thought has been given to how such devices should be introduced to the family (Howe 1989; Reimers & Treacher 1995). Reimers & Treacher (1995) found that much of the negative effect on the family of having an invisible team behind the screen could be mitigated by introducing the team members to the family at the beginning of the first session.

Getting informed consent for having an observing team or using a video is part of good practice but it is also a useful way of emphasizing that we respect the family's boundaries and their right to act as gatekeepers to the amount of intrusion that they will allow as part of the clinical process. Demystifying the process by introducing the members of the team to the family and perhaps showing the children how the camera works, can also help in making the family feel more at ease and facilitate the engagement process.

Respecting boundaries within the family is no less important. There are a number of contexts where the clinician needs to be particularly aware of confidentiality issues when seeing families. One is when interviewing a family with an adolescent who may quite appropriately feel that there are aspects of his or her life that he or she does not want to talk about in front of parents. The difficulty arises when the issues of privacy and confidentiality concern behaviours that are potentially risky or dangerous (e.g. self-harm), or symptoms that are clearly of clinical significance and may need to be discussed with others. The clinician will need to be both sensitive to the internal family boundary issues while at the same time making it clear that in some cases issues of safety or health might override issues of confidentiality. For instance, an adolescent girl suffering from anorexia may be reluctant to talk about the absence of her periods in front of her father or brother but at the same time this may be part of the general picture of her trying to hide the seriousness of her illness from the family. The clinician may therefore agree to discuss this in an individual meeting, while making it also clear that her parents need to know the extent of her illness in order to be able to help her. If the adolescent is seen on her own it is important to re-state the confidentiality of the individual interview as well as its limits.

It is sometimes assumed that there is an advantage in seeing adolescents on their own as a way of promoting the process of individuation/separation from the family. While it is possible to use individual sessions to address such issues, there is always the danger that the therapist gets co-opted into a parental role and the adolescent's independence may become largely illusory (e.g. as would be the case of the adolescent who is always brought by a parent who then sits in the waiting room while the adolescent is seen individually). If, instead, the individual sessions are combined with, or replaced by, family meetings in which one regularly checks on the appropriateness of what is being discussed in the family context, the issue of separateness/independence is addressed much more directly.

Another type of situation sometimes arises, particularly with families with younger children, when sensitive issues for the family or family secrets are touched on. While one should not assume that anything that is difficult for the family to talk about should be avoided, one also has to respect that when and how a family talk about such issues may determine whether it has been a useful experience for them or not (Karpel 1980). This is particularly important to bear in mind with families with quite young children, as the clinician can sometimes be too 'skilful' in helping the children to talk about things that they actually would rather not say, with the child then perhaps feeling disloyal to the family. It is therefore important that one emphasizes that as clinicians we have to be free to ask even the most awkward questions but the family always has the right not to discuss any particular issues if they feel that the time, the place or the constellation of people in the room is not right.

Conclusions

The conjoint family interview is undoubtedly a valuable part of clinical practice in child psychiatry, regardless of the theoretical orientation that the clinician adopts. Seeing the whole family together provides valuable information that would otherwise be inaccessible to the clinician, about patterns of interaction and family function which the family may not necessarily be always aware of and therefore not always be able, or willing, to provide information on. The aim of this chapter has been to emphasize, both in the account of the theoretical framework and in the account of some of the interviewing techniques, the interactive nature of the task. The clinician interviewing the family is not a neutral detached observer but is an active participant entering into a relationship with the family which inevitably contributes to the picture that he or she forms about the family. This has implications not only for the way that the clinician conducts family interviews and the judgements drawn from them, but also for the effect that the interview is likely to have on the family.

References

l'Abate, L. (1994) *Family Evaluation: A Psychological Approach*. Sage, Thousand Oaks, CA.

Alexander, R. & Parsons, B. (1973) Short-term behavioural interventions with delinquent families: impact on family process and recidivism. *Journal of Abnormal Psychology*, 81, 219–225.

Andersen, T. (1987) The reflecting team: dialogue and metadialogue in clinical work. *Family Process*, 26, 415–428.

Bateson, G., Jackson, D.D., Haley, J. & Weakland, J.H. (1956) Towards a theory of schizophrenia. *Behavioural Science*, 1, 251–265.

Beavers, R. & Hampson, R.B. (1990) *Successful Families: Assessment and Intervention*. W.W. Norton, New York.

Beavers, R. & Hampson, R.B. (2000) The Beavers systems model of family functioning. *Journal of Family Therapy*, 22, 128–143.

Besharat, M.A., Eisler, I. & Dare, C. (2001) The self- and other-blame scale (SOBS): the development and reliability of an observational measure of guilt and blame in families. *Journal of Family Therapy*, 23, 208–223.

Bishop, D., Epstein, N., Keitner, G., Miller, I. & Zlotnick, C. (1980) *The McMaster Structured Interview for Family Functioning*. Brown University Family Research Program, Providence, RI.

Bloch, S., Hafner, J., Harari, E. & Szmukler, G.I. (1994) *The Family in Clinical Psychiatry*. Oxford University Press, Oxford.

Borduin, C., Mann, B., Cone, L. & Henggeler, S. (1995) Multisystemic treatment of serious juvenile offenders: long-term prevention of criminality and violence. *Journal of Consulting and Clinical Psychology*, 63, 569–578.

Boscolo, L., Cecchin, G., Hoffman, L. & Penn, P. (1987) *Milan Systemic Family Therapy*. Basic Books, New York.

Boyd-Franklin, N. (1989) *Black Families in Therapy: a Multisystems Approach*. Guilford Press, New York.

Boyhan, P.A. (1996) Client's perception of single session consultations as an option to waiting for family therapy. *Australian and New Zealand Journal of Family Therapy*, 17, 85–96.

Burnham, J. (1986) *Family Therapy*. Tavistock, London.

Byng-Hall, J. (1986) Family scripts: a concept which can bridge child psychotherapy and family therapy thinking. *Journal of Child Psychotherapy*, 12, 3–13.

Byng-Hall, J. (1991) The application of attachment theory to understanding and treatment in family therapy. In: *Attachment Across the Family Life-Cycle* (eds C.M. Parkes, J. Stevenson-Hinde & P. Marris), pp. 199–215. Routledge, London.

Campbell, A. (1999) Single session interventions: an example of clinical research in practice. *Australian and New Zealand Journal of Family Therapy*, 20, 183–194.

Carr, A. (2000a) Evidence-based practice in family therapy and systemic consultation. I. Child focused problems. *Journal of Family Therapy*, 22, 29–60.

Carr, A. (2000b) *What Works for Children and Adolescents?: A Critical Review of Psychological Interventions with Children, Adolescents and Their Families*. Routledge, London.

Carter, B. & McGoldrick, M. (1989) *The Family Life-Cycle: a Framework for Family Therapy*, 2nd edn. Allyn & Bacon, Boston.

Cooklin, A., Miller, A.C. & McHugh, B. (1983) An institution for change: developing a family day unit. *Family Process*, 22, 453–468.

Cox, A. (1994) Diagnostic appraisal. In: *Child and Adolescent Psychiatry: Modern Approaches* (eds M. Rutter, E. Taylor & L. Hersov), 3rd edn, pp. 34–50. Blackwell Scientific Publications, Oxford.

Cox, A., Hemsley, R. & Dare, J. (1995) A comparison of individual and family assessment approaches to initial assessment. *European Child and Adolescent Psychiatry*, 4, 94–101.

Dallos, R. & Draper, R. (1999) *An Introduction to Family Therapy: Systemic Theory and Practice*. Open University Press, Buckingham.

Dare, C. & Lindsey, C. (1979) Children in family therapy. *Journal of Family Therapy*, 1, 253–269.

Dare, C., Eisler, I., Russell, G.F.M. & Szmukler, G.I. (1990) The clinical and theoretical impact of a controlled trial of family therapy in anorexia nervosa. *Journal of Marital and Family Therapy*, 16, 39–57.

Dare, C., Eisler, I., Colahan, M., Crowther, C., Senior, R. & Asen, E. (1995) The listening heart and the Chi square: clinical and empirical perceptions in the family therapy of anorexia nervosa. *Journal of Family Therapy*, 17, 19–45.

Dunn, J. & Plomin, R. (1990) *Separate Lives: Why Siblings Are So Different*. Basic Books, New York.

Eisler, I. (1993) Families, family therapy and psychosomatic illness. In: *Psychological Treatments in Human Disease and Illness* (eds S. Moorey & M. Hodes), pp. 42–62. Gaskill, London.

Eisler, I. (1995a) Family models of eating disorders. In: *Handbook of Eating Disorders: Theory, Treatment and Research* (eds G.I. Szmukler, C. Dare & J. Treasure), pp. 155–176. Wiley, London.

Eisler, I. (1995b) Combining individual and family therapy in the treatment of adolescent anorexia nervosa. In: *Treating Eating Disorders* (ed. J. Werne), pp. 217–257. Jossey–Bass, San Francisco.

Eisler, I., Dare, C., Russell, G.F.M., Szmukler, G.I., Dodge, E. & le Grange, D. (1997) Family and individual therapy for anorexia nervosa: a 5-year follow-up. *Archives of General Psychiatry*, 54, 1025–1030.

Eisler, I., Dare, C., Hodes, M., Russell, G.F.M., Dodge, E. & le Grange, D. (2000) Family therapy for adolescent anorexia nervosa: the results of a controlled comparison of two family interventions. *Journal of Child Psychology and Psychiatry*, 41, 727–736.

Epstein, N., Bishop, D. & Levin, S. (1978) The McMaster model of family functioning. *Journal of Marriage and Family Counseling*, 4, 19–31.

Fergusson, D.M. & Lynskey, M.T. (1996) Adolescent resiliency to family adversity. *Journal of Child Psychology and Psychiatry*, 37, 281–292.

von Foerster, H. (1981) *Observing Systems*. Intersystems Publications. Seaside CA.

Friedman, M., McDermut, W., Wolomon, D., Ryan, C., Keitner, G. & Miller, I. (1997) A comparison of psychiatric and nonclinical families. *Family Process*, 36, 357–367.

Glaser, D. & Frosh, S. (1993) *Child Sexual Abuse*, 2nd edn. University of Toronto Press, Buffalo, NY.

Goldner, V., Penn, P., Sheinberg, M. & Walker, G. (1990) Love and violence: gender paradoxes in volatile attachments. *Family Process*, 29, 343–364.

Gorell Barnes, G. (1985) Systems theory and family therapy. In: *Child Psychiatry: Modern Approaches* (eds M. Rutter & L. Hersov), 2nd edn, pp. 216–229. Blackwell Scientific Publications, Oxford.

Gorell Barnes, G. (1994) Family therapy in the 1990s. In: *Child and Adolescent Psychiatry: Modern Approaches* (eds M. Rutter, E. Taylor & L. Hersov), 3rd edn, pp. 946–967. Blackwell Scientific Publications, Oxford.

Gorell Barnes, G. (1998) *Family Therapy in Changing Times*. Macmillan, Basingstoke.

Gorell Barnes, G., Thompson, P., Daniel, G. & Burchardt, N. (1998) *Growing Up in Step-Families*. Clarendon Press, Oxford.

Green, R.J. & Herget, M. (1989a) Outcomes of systemic/strategic team consultation. I. Overview and one-month results. *Family Process*, 28, 37–58.

Green, R.J. & Herget, M. (1989b) Outcomes of systemic/strategic team consultation. II. Three-year follow-up and a theory of 'emergent design'. *Family Process*, 28, 419–437.

Grotevant, H.D. & Carlson, C.I. (1989) *Family Assessment: a Guide to Methods and Measures*. Guilford Press, New York.

Gustafsson, P.A., Enquist, M.-L. & Karlsson, B. (1995) Siblings in family therapy. *Journal of Family Therapy*, 17, 317–327.

Hampson, R.B. & Beavers, W.R. (1996a) Measuring family therapy outcome in a clinical setting: families that do better or do worse in therapy. *Family Process*, 35, 347–361.

Hampson, R.B. & Beavers, W.R. (1996b) Family therapy and outcome: relationships between therapist and family styles. *Contemporary Family Therapy*, 18, 345–370.

Hampson, R., O'Hanlon, J., Franklin, A., Pentony, M., Fridgant, L. & Heins, T. (1999) The place of single session family consultations: five years experience in Canberra. *Australian and New Zealand Journal of Family Therapy*, 20, 195–200.

Haynes, S.N., Jensen, B.J., Wise, E. & Sherman, D. (1981) The marital intake interview: a multimethod criterion validity assessment. *Journal of Consulting and Clinical Psychology*, 49, 379–387.

Hayden, L.C., Schiller, M., Dickstein, S. *et al.* (1998) Levels of family assessment: I. Family, marital, and parent–child interaction. *Journal of Family Psychology*, 12, 7–22.

Henggeler, S. & Borduin, C. (1991) *Family Therapy and Beyond: A*

Multisystemic Approach to Treating Behavior Problems of Children and Adolescents. Brooks Cole, Pacific Grove, CA.

Hetherington, M.E. (1989) Coping with family transitions: winners, losers and survivors. *Child Development*, **60**, 1–14.

Hodes, M. (1985) Family therapy and the problem of cultural relativism. *Journal of Family Therapy*, 7, 261–272.

Hodes, M., Dare, C., Dodge, E. & Eisler, I. (1999) The assessment of expressed emotion in a standardised family interview. *Journal of Child Psychology and Psychiatry*, 40, 617–625.

Hoffman, L. (1981) *Foundations of Family Therapy: a Conceptual Framework for Systems Change.* Basic Books, New York.

Hoffman, L. (1990) Constructing realities: an art of lenses. *Family Process*, **29**, 1–12.

Howe, D. (1989) Client experience of counselling and treatment interventions: a qualitative study of family views of family therapy. *British Journal of Guidance and Counselling*, 24, 367–375.

Imber-Black, E. (1988) *Families and Larger Systems: a Family Therapist's Guide Through the Labyrinth.* Guilford Press, New York.

Joanning, H., Quinn, W., Thomas, F. & Mullen, R. (1992) Treating adolescent drug abuse: a comparison of family systems therapy, adolescent group therapy and family drug education. *Journal of Marital and Family Therapy*, 18, 345–356.

Karpel, M.A. (1980) Family secrets. I. Conceptual and ethical issues in the relational context. II. Ethical and practical considerations in therapeutic management. *Family Process* 19, 295–306.

Kazdin, A.E., Siegel, T. & Bass, D. (1992) Cognitive problem-solving skills training and parent management training in the treatment of antisocial behavior in children. *Journal of Consulting and Clinical Psychology*, 60, 733–747.

Kerig, P. & Lindahl, K. (2001) *Family Observational Coding Systems: Resources for Systemic Research.* Lawrence Erlbaum, Mahwahl, NJ.

Kog, E., Vandereycken, W. & Vertommen, H. (1985) The psychosomatic family model: A critical analysis of family interaction concepts. *Journal of Family Therapy*, 7, 31–44.

Langmeier, J. & Matějček, Z. (1975) *Psychological Deprivation in Childhood.* Halstead, New York.

Larner, G. (1996) Narrative child family therapy. *Family Process*, 35, 423–440.

Lau, A. (1984) Transcultural issues in family therapy. *Journal of Family Therapy*, 6, 91–112.

LeFave, M.K. (1980) Correlates of engagement in family therapy. *Journal of Marital and Family Therapy*, 6, 75–81.

Lennard, H.L. & Bernstein, A. (1969) *Patterns of Human Interaction.* Jossey–Bass, San Francisco, CA.

Levy, D.M. (1939) Maternal overprotection. *Psychiatry*, 2, 99–128.

Liddle, H.A., Breunlin, D.C. & Schwartz, R.C. (1988) *Handbook of Family Therapy Training and Supervision.* Guilford Press, New York.

Lidz, T., Cornelison, A., Fleck, S. & Terry, D. (1957) The intrafamilial environment of schizophrenic patients. II. Marital schism and marital skew. *American Journal of Psychiatry*, 114, 241–248.

McGoldrick, M. & Gerson, R. (1985) *Genograms in Family Assessment.* W.W. Norton, New York.

Messent, P. (1992) Working with Bangladeshi families in the East End of London. *Journal of Family Therapy*, 14, 287–304.

Miller, I.W., Kabacoff, R.I., Epstein, N. *et al.* (1994) The development of a clinical rating scale for the McMaster Model of family functioning. *Family Process*, 33, 53–69.

Miller, I.W., Ryan, C.E., Keitner, G.I., Bishop, D.S. & Epstein, N.B. (2000) The McMaster Approach to Families. Theory, assessment, treatment and research. *Journal of Family Therapy*, 22, 168–189.

Minuchin, P. (1988) Relationships within the family: a systems perspective on development. In: *Relationships Within Families: Mutual Influences* (eds R.A. Hinde & J. Stevenson-Hinde), pp. 7–26. Clarendon Press, Oxford.

Minuchin, S. & Fishman, H.C. (1981) *Family Therapy Techniques.* Harvard University Press. Cambridge, MA.

Minuchin, S., Baker, L., Rosman, B.L., Liebman, R., Milman, L. & Todd, T.C. (1975) A conceptual model of psychosomatic illness in childhood. *Archives of General Psychiatry*, 32, 1031–1038.

Minuchin, S., Rosman, B.L. & Baker, L. (1978) *Psychosomatic Families: Anorexia Nervosa in Context.* Harvard University Press, Cambridge, MA.

Olson, D.H. (1972) Empirically unbinding the double bind: review of research and conceptual reformulations. *Family Process*, 11, 69–94.

Olson, D.H. (1990) *Clinical Rating Scale for the Circumplex Model.* Family Social Science, University of Minnesota, St. Pauls, MN.

Olson, D.H. (2000) The Circumplex Model of Marital and Family Systems. *Journal of Family Therapy*, 22, 144–167.

Olson, D.H., Russell, C.S. & Sprenkle, D.H. (1989) *Circumplex Model: Systemic Assessment and Treatment of Families.* Haworth Press, New York.

Palazzoli, M.S. (1974) *Self Starvation: From the Intrapsychic to the Transpersonal Approach to Anorexia Nervosa.* Chaucer Publishing, London.

Palazzoli, M.S., Boscolo, L., Cecchin, G. & Prata, G. (1978) *Paradox and Counterparadox.* Jason Aronson, New York.

Palazzoli, M.S., Boscolo, L., Cecchin, G. & Prata, G. (1980) Hypothesizing–circularity–neutrality: three guidelines for the conductor of the session. *Family Process*, 19, 3–12.

Papp, P. (1980) The Greek Chorus and other techniques of paradoxical therapy. *Family Process*, 19, 45–58.

Papp, P. & Imber-Black, E. (1996) Family themes: transitions and transformations. *Family Process*, 35, 5–20.

Patterson, G. (1982) *Coercive Family Process.* Castalia, Eugene, Oregon.

Patterson, G., Chamberlain, P. & Reid, J. (1982) A comparative evaluation of a parent-training program. *Behaviour Therapy*, 13, 636–650.

Penn, P. (1982) Circular questioning. *Family Process*, 21, 267–280.

Reimers, S. (1999) 'Good morning, Sir!', 'Axe handle': talking at cross-purposes in family therapy. *Journal of Family Therapy*, 21, 360–376.

Reimers, S. & Treacher, A. (1995) *Introducing User Friendly Family Therapy.* Routledge, London.

Reiss, D., Hetherington, E.M., Plomin, R. *et al.* (1995) Genetic questions for environmental studies: differential parenting and psychopathology in adolescence. *Archives of General Psychiatry*, 52, 925–936.

Ritsner, M. & Ponizovsky, A. (1999) Psychological distress through immigration: the two-phase temporal pattern? *International Journal of Social Psychiatry*, 45, 125–139.

Robinson, M. (1990) *Family Transformation Through Divorce and Remarriage.* Routledge, London.

Russell, G.F.M., Szmukler, G.I., Dare, C. & Eisler, I. (1987) An evaluation of family therapy in anorexia nervosa. *Archives of General Psychiatry*, 44, 1047–1056.

Rutter, M. (1999) Resilience concepts and findings: implications for family therapy. *Journal of Family Therapy*, 21, 119–144.

Rutter, M., Silberg, J., O'Connor, T. & Simonoff, E. (1999) Genetics and child psychiatry. I. Advances in quantitative and molecular genetics. *Journal of Child Psychology and Psychiatry*, 40, 3–18.

Sartorius, N. (1996) Recent changes in suicide rates in selected Eastern

European and other European countries. *International Psychogeriatrics*, 7, 301–308.

Sawyer, M.G., Sarris, A., Baghurst, P.A., Cross, D.G. & Kalucy, R. (1988) Family assessment device: reports from mothers, fathers and adolescents in community and clinic a families. *Journal of Marital and Family Therapy*, 14, 287–296.

Squire-Dehouck, B. (1993) *Evaluation of conjoint family therapy vs. family counselling in adolescent anorexia nervosa patients: a two-year follow-up study*. MSc Dissertation, University of Surrey.

Stevenson-Hinde, J. & Akister, J. (1995) The McMaster Model of Family Functioning: observer and parental ratings in a nonclinical sample. *Family Process*, 34, 337–347.

Street, E. & Foot, H. (1984) Training family therapists in observational skills. *Journal of Family Therapy*, 6, 335–346.

Strickland-Clark, L., Campbell, D. & Dallos, R. (2000) Children's and adolescent's views on family therapy. *Journal of Family Therapy*, 22, 324–341.

Szmukler, G.I., Eisler, I., Russell, G.F.M. & Dare, C. (1985) Parental Expressed Emotion', anorexia nervosa and dropping out of treatment. *British Journal of Psychiatry*, 147, 265–271.

Szmukler, G.I., Berkowitz, R., Eisler, I., Leff, J. & Dare, C. (1987) 'Expressed Emotion' in individual and family settings: a comparative study. *British Journal of Psychiatry*, 151, 174–178.

Tomm, K. (1987a) Interventive interviewing. I. Strategizing as a fourth guideline for the therapist. *Family Process*, 26, 3–13.

Tomm, K. (1987b) Interventive interviewing. II. Reflexive questions as a means to enable self-healing. *Family Process*, 26, 167–183.

Tomm, K. (1988) Interventive interviewing. III. Intending to ask lineal, strategic or reflexive questions. *Family Process*, 27, 1–15.

Walsh, F. (1997) The concept of family resilience: crisis and challenge. *Family Process*, 35, 261–281.

Webster-Stratton, C. & Hammond, M. (1997) Treating children with early onset conduct problems: a comparison of child and parent training interventions. *Journal of Consulting and Clinical Psychology*, 65, 93–109.

Wieselberg, H. (1992) Family therapy and ultra-orthodox Jewish families: a structural approach. *Journal of Family Therapy*, 14, 305–330.

Wilson, J. (1998) *Child-Focused Practice: a Collaborative Systemic Approach*. Karnac Books, London.

10 Physical Examination and Medical Investigations

Anthony Bailey

Introduction

The presenting problems seen by individual clinicians vary considerably, reflecting differences in disease prevalence, the organization of psychiatric and paediatric services and the particular interests and expertise of practitioners. The relative importance of the medical history, physical examination and investigations naturally also varies from patient to patient. Some readers may anticipate that this chapter will be irrelevant to their daily practice, whereas neuropsychiatrists may bemoan a lack of detail. In charting a course between Scylla and Charybdis, the overarching objectives are to remind practitioners of the importance of assessing and treating the whole patient, of the need consciously to question the significance of historical information and any physical findings, and to highlight some of the recent developments in investigations, particularly in genetics and neuroimaging.

One of the initial goals is to identify any biological factors that may underlie the referral disorder, as well as to assess growth, nutritional status and general health. In many general child psychiatry outpatient services, identifiable biological factors may be infrequent. However, worldwide these factors are as relevant now as ever, both because of the increasing impact of environmental (particularly infectious) agents on children's health, and because of the advances in identifying genetic influences on developmental and psychiatric disorders, with the associated implications for diagnosis and management. Thus, in the last 5–10 years, HIV and tuberculosis have had a devastating effect upon children in the developing world. Recent wars, political upheavals and changed attitudes have also coincided with an increased incidence of sexually transmitted diseases (with the associated risk of vertical transmission), substantial transnational movement of refugees and a growth in international adoption—all trends that require continuing vigilance for infectious diseases. In parallel there has been a worldwide increase in the non-medicinal use of drugs by the young, with all the attendant psychiatric, social and physical risks.

Previous chapters deal with assessment of psychopathology and the family environment and the measurement of cognitive deficits and developmental delays. Nevertheless, this information will often not be adequate to identify somatic ('organic') aetiologies. This is an important goal because identification of causal influences is necessary to provide optimal treatment, specific advice on prognosis and likely complications and, occasionally, genetic counselling or screening of at-risk relatives. In ordinary outpatient practice, the amount of detail that it is necessary to obtain from the history, physical examination and investigations will vary according to the nature of the presenting complaint and local circumstances. Thus, this chapter is structured according to the nature of the presenting difficulties and the level of examination and investigation that they require. By necessity, this approach is illustrative rather than exhaustive; the goal is to encourage clinicians to go through a problem-solving approach with each case that they assess. The strategy outlined here is not intended for tertiary services dealing with unusual cases, or for research.

General child psychiatry cases

In most individuals presenting with one of the common disorders of behaviour or emotions, there are unlikely to be aetiological somatic conditions. The starting point is for clinicians first to satisfy themselves that the disorder is what it seems; in other words, are the history and symptomatology typical, the age and nature of onset in keeping with the provisional diagnosis, as well as the clinical course and response to treatment. Usually the clinical picture will be straightforward, but clinicians need to be alert to mention of any physical abnormalities (particularly neurological symptoms such as gait disturbance, clumsiness, or visual changes), an unusual or partial clinical picture, or impairments that seem disproportionate to the degree of symptomatology. These aspects of the history may require clarification to establish if they signify a somatic disorder. On the rare occasion that suspicions are aroused, bodily systems should be reviewed as this will usually provide some of the most obvious pointers to neurological dysfunction or systemic disease (see Edgeworth *et al.* 1996).

Next, the clinician needs to consider whether there is any history suggestive of cognitive impairments in the form of mental retardation, specific developmental delays, chronic difficulties with school work or deteriorating school performance. Again, cognitive difficulties indicate the need for a much more probing history and thorough physical examination (see below). It is not uncommon for mild mental retardation to go undetected until middle childhood and many children first come to attention because of behavioural problems, often associated with poor school performance. Consequently, when patients do not have routine psychometric assessment, the clinician will need to take sufficient history to exclude cognitive difficulties.

A further step is to enquire about any pertinent environmental aetiological factors; drug and alcohol abuse are particularly relevant. Children at increased risk for substance abuse include those with parents who abuse drugs or alcohol, who are in dysfunctional or divorced families, who are subject to abuse and who are under- or overcontrolled by their parents (Belcher & Shinitzky 1998; Milberger *et al.* 1999). It is important always to enquire directly about drug and alcohol abuse, especially in those who smoke. That is because young people who use drugs or alcohol often do not seek help for these problems but are seen because of associated difficulties, such as school underachievement, delinquency, teenage pregnancy and depression (Belcher & Shinitzky 1998). Indeed, alcohol abuse is one of the few factors associated with eventual suicide in adolescents who self-harm (Hawton *et al.* 1993). Identifying drug and alcohol abuse can require clinical acumen, knowledge of familial and individual risk factors, as well as familiarity with the locality. The clinician will also want to establish whether there is any possibility that the child has been subject to abuse; if so, a full physical examination is indicated to search for signs of old and fresh injuries, malnourishment and general neglect. A detailed examination to determine if there is any evidence of sexual abuse should be performed by clinicians (usually paediatricians or police surgeons) with the relevant training and experience.

Before proceeding to the physical examination, the clinician needs to consider several further issues. First, are there any medical conditions relevant to the psychiatric disorder? For instance, behavioural problems are not uncommon amongst children and adolescents with chronic conditions such as diabetes (see Mrazek, Chapter 48), and some drug treatments, such as high-dose steroids, can lead directly to mental state changes. Secondly, in areas of the world where serious infectious diseases are endemic the clinician should enquire directly about relevant symptomatology. That is not because these diseases are common causes of behavioural difficulties (although they are occasionally implicated), but because the physician's concern is with the health of the whole individual, and ensuring that a child receives treatment for tuberculosis, malaria or other serious diseases is a crucial aspect of clinical management. Thirdly, the clinician needs to consider whether the young person's behaviour may itself lead to medical complications. Thus, the drug-using adolescent is at increased risk for contracting a variety of infectious diseases, as well as for criminal behaviour. HIV and hepatitis B may be acquired from contaminated needles and individuals may also be exposing themselves to sexually transmitted infections. The earlier adolescents initiate sexual activity the less likely they are to use a condom and the more likely they are to have unprotected sex with multiple partners; the risks are not trivial because one in every eight adolescents aged between 13 and 19 in the USA has had a sexually transmitted disease (Rome 1999). Part of overall management is to ensure that at-risk individuals are subsequently screened for sexually transmitted and other infectious diseases. Finally, it may be relevant to enquire about medical problems in other family members; e.g. a family history of thyroid disease may be linked to an adolescent onset of anxiety disorder.

A psychiatric diagnostic assessment should always include a physical examination, albeit sometimes limited in scope. Often an appropriate examination will have been undertaken by referrers, and repetition will not advance the diagnostic process. Nevertheless, if the history suggests an unexpected somatic condition, clinicians should search specifically for the relevant signs. In some settings, not all children will be seen initially by medical staff and the need then is to ensure that an appropriate physical examination has either already been undertaken or can be arranged in a timely manner. It is also helpful to ensure that non-medical staff have some basic training in the features of the history and mental state that indicate a possible organic aetiology and are able routinely to measure height, weight and head circumference.

Clinicians usually begin the physical examination as soon as they meet a patient, whether or not this is performed consciously. An abnormal facial appearance is often most obvious when first seen. Similarly, the patient's language or speech may raise the possibility of neurological or cognitive impairments, and abnormal movements may be noted in the waiting area that the patient is later able to suppress. How the patient rises from a chair, their gait, and possibly stair climbing, can all be observed *en route* to the interview or examination room. Whether the patient looks well or ill, obese or malnourished, well cared for or unkempt should also guide the extent of the subsequent examination.

It is worth paying some attention to the environment for the physical examination proper. If this is to be satisfactory then the room needs to be warm, well lit (but able to be blacked out) and private. In addition to the usual medical equipment, a fixed rule for measuring height, accurate weighing scales, a non-stretchable tape measure, a vision testing chart and a Wood light should be available. A parent or chaperone should usually accompany children and adolescents.

When there is no suspicion from the history or mental state that the child has a somatic condition, when there is no evidence of cognitive deficits and when the patient's appearance has not caused concern, what should be the minimum physical examination? All patients should have height, weight and head circumference measured and these percentiles plotted. One reason for measuring growth is to identify any deviations from normal which in combination with behavioural difficulties, cognitive deficits or physical signs raise the possibility of an underlying syndrome. Another reason is to detect suboptimal development associated with systemic disease or malnutrition. Unless cooperation is limited, growth should usually be measured at the beginning of the examination because some abnormalities may not be apparent until charted, and these should always prompt a search for recognized associations. Clinicians should also be aware that there have been significant upward secular trends in height, weight and head circumference in the developed world over the last century, but there are considerable vagaries in the extent to which growth charts are based on up-to-date data.

If growth parameters are abnormal, the clinician needs to consider the possible underlying causes and also whether the combination of particular behaviours and abnormal growth may signify a syndrome. Short stature and/or microcephaly should both prompt the clinician to review whether there is clear evidence that intelligence is in the normal range; when there is doubt, consideration should be given to psychometric testing. Abnormal growth parameters should also lead to a full physical examination. In the absence of mental retardation or cognitive difficulties, the usual causes of suboptimal growth in developing and developed regions are quite different. In developed countries short stature is usually constitutional, and chronic illness is a much more frequent cause of short stature than are hormonal abnormalities. An appropriate history should already have alerted the clinician to impaired growth as a consequence of feeding difficulties (see Stein & Barnes, Chapter 45). Worldwide, malnutrition is the most common cause of growth retardation and is frequently compounded by parasitic infections; these infect over 3.5 billion people (Albonico et al. 1999), and intestinal helminths are the main disease burden in children aged 5–14 years (World Bank 1993). The other major cause of impaired growth or weight loss in the developing world is tuberculosis, which is the leading cause of death as a result of infectious disease: a problem exacerbated by the HIV pandemic and drug resistance (Zumla et al. 1999). Clinicians working in areas where parasitic and other infectious diseases are endemic will usually be familiar with their presentation, but a high index of suspicion is also required by those working with exposed immigrant communities, refugees and international adoptees.

Tall stature is usually either constitutional or linked with obesity. However, it is also a feature of several syndromes associated with behavioural disturbance and/or learning difficulties. By and large, clinicians are less aware of the significance of increased as opposed to decreased growth and several syndromes that are not uncommon can easily be missed, especially if they are not associated with obvious cognitive difficulties. Thus, if the diagnosis of Klinefelter syndrome, which affects approximately 1 in 800 males, is not made prenatally, it is very unlikely to be made at all during the first decade (Abramsky & Chapple 1997). Affected males show increased growth and weight associated with eunuchoid proportions, delayed or incomplete puberty and small testes and penis; most individuals are eventually karyotyped for hypogonadism or infertility. Klinefelter syndrome is associated with an increased rate of learning disabilities, poor impulse control and a range of psychiatric disorders (Rovet et al. 1996; Smyth & Bremner 1998). 47XYY syndrome affects approximately 1 in 1000 males, about half of whom are diagnosed because of developmental delay or behavioural problems (Abramsky & Chapple 1997; see also Skuse & Kuntsi, Chapter 13). The additional Y chromosome causes increased growth, and body, head and craniofacial dimensions are greater than in control and male relatives (Grön et al. 1997). Children with Sotos syndrome show prenatal onset of excessive size with significantly increased growth in infancy. They have a relatively large span and large hands and feet as well as macrocephaly.

Obesity is usually a consequence of excess calorie intake and insufficient exercise, and often it becomes a problem during adolescence. Much less frequently it signifies a congenital or acquired syndrome. Because many of these disorders are characterized by hypogonadism and delayed puberty, obesity should always prompt a full physical examination. Some of the congenital syndromes include major malformations that should already have aided their identification.

Small head size may be a familial or ethnic trait, and may be proportionate to height. Similarly macrocephaly may also be a normal variant and often has a familial basis (Lorber & Priestley 1981). An estimate of pubertal status can usually be obtained from the history from parents and/or the young person. There is considerable variation in the timing of normal puberty, but the physical changes are considered delayed if not evident before 13 years in girls or 14 years in boys, and precocious when seen before 8 years in girls or 9 years in boys. If the history raises the possibility of abnormal timing then the patient should have a full physical examination. The differential diagnosis of disorders of pubertal timing is complex, although some causes are linked with psychiatric and/or cognitive difficulties.

In patients for whom there is no a priori reason (from the history, mental state examination, cognitive testing and measurement of growth) to suspect a concomitant somatic disorder, it is difficult to justify a full physical examination that includes complete undressing. What should the physician do? First, the clinician should check the patient's face and hands for any evidence of obvious dysmorphic features that may signify a perturbation in development. Secondly, there needs to be an examination to identify any signs of drug use. The arms should be examined for evidence of intravenous or subcutaneous drug injection in the form of needle tracks, abscesses, areas of hyperpigmentation, or scar tissue from healed abscesses. Long-term stigmata of oral or nasal ingestion of drugs are minimal, with the exception of inhalation of solvents from a bag which may produce a circumoral rash. Pupillary constriction or dilatation and tachycardia may be seen acutely with many drugs. The clinician should then ensure as a minimum that there are no localizing neurological abnormalities, no evidence of gait abnormalities (an early sign in most progressive neurological disorders) or significant co-ordination problems, and no visual impairments detectable with a testing chart or hearing difficulties to whispered voice. When young people are assessed who have not had routine developmental surveillance or access to medical services, the physical examination should include undressing and examination of all bodily systems.

Sometimes patients will refuse an examination or be extremely unco-operative. A flexible discussion with the patient and their family, the co-opting of doctors with whom the patient has a rapport, or an attempt at a different time or in a different place will usually be successful. Neither should the utility of repeating an examination be overlooked. That situation is most likely to arise if the diagnosis remains uncertain, the clinical picture deteriorates or the disorder is unusually resistant to appropriate treatment. In these circumstances, signs may be detected that were previously overlooked or whose significance was not appreciated initially.

There is currently no evidence to suggest that routine medical investigation of all child psychiatry patients makes clinical or economic sense. In the absence of symptoms or signs, are there any other indications for routine screening investigations? First, depending on local circumstances, clinicians will want to consider whether a urine screen for drugs should be routine in newly presenting adolescents or only in those with identifiable risk factors (see Weinberg *et al.*, Chapter 27). Urinalysis should not be restricted to any reported drug of abuse because multiple drug abuse is common. Some drugs, such as cannabis, may appear in the urine for several weeks after consumption, the psychostimulant methylenedioxymethamphetamine (MDMA) or 'ecstasy' disappears within 24 h whereas hallucinogens—such as lysergic acid diethylamide (LSD)—will not be detected by urinalysis at all. Secondly, international adoptees are at especial risk of infectious diseases and if they have not had an infection screen at time of entry into the country (Hostetter 1999), the clinician should consider which infectious agents should be excluded. Thirdly, if it is planned to administer psychotropic medication, renal and liver function should be checked (also thyroid function if lithium is to be administered) and, if administration of drugs with cardiac effects is anticipated, then a baseline electrocardiogram (ECG) should be obtained (see Heyman & Santosh, Chapter 59).

Individuals with disorders that involve specific cognitive deficits or developmental delays

In neurodevelopmental disorders, such as attention deficit disorder (ADHD), some form of abnormal brain function is likely to be present, but the association with identifiable medical conditions is much weaker than in individuals with mental retardation. Parents will sometimes wonder whether obstetric or neonatal difficulties were a factor in aetiology, and clinicians will occasionally be faced with the need to differentiate between possible obstetric causes of psychopathology and a suboptimal obstetric history that is a consequence of a genetic susceptibility.

The first task is to clarify whether these difficulties are manifestations of a more pervasive abnormality. Thus, it is essential that a comprehensive developmental history is obtained in all areas of functioning to establish whether the child has a general or specific cognitive difficulty or evidence of motor dysfunction. Also, language delay and symptoms of inattention and overactivity are common in children with pervasive developmental disorders. There should be no diagnostic confusion with cases of clear-cut autism, but it is not unusual for children with milder variants of pervasive developmental disorders (such as Asperger syndrome) to receive an initial diagnosis of ADHD, 'communication disorder' or dyspraxia. Thus, the clinician needs to obtain an adequate history of social development. Secondly, these difficulties are usually developmental in origin and the clinician

should be particularly alert to symptoms that arise later in childhood in case they are the initial manifestations of either progressive neurological disorders or abuse.

The next task is to obtain a detailed obstetric and neonatal history. Illegal drug use during pregnancy is now a considerable problem in some communities and should be enquired about in at-risk groups. Drug use is linked with suboptimal pregnancy outcome (Loebstein & Koren 1997), an increased risk for perinatal acquisition of HIV (Belcher & Shinitzky 1998) and subsequent child abuse (Jaudes *et al.* 1995). Similarly, fetal alcohol syndrome now affects at least 2.8 in 1000 live births (Sampson *et al.* 1997) and an alcohol history should be obtained routinely in these cases. It has been suggested that even in the absence of a suggestive pattern of craniofacial dysmorphism (see below), symptoms such as hyperactivity and language delay may be consequences of alcohol use during pregnancy; so-called fetal alcohol effects (Weinberg 1997). When alcohol use was not obviously excessive, the clinician needs to be cautious about assuming an aetiological role when genetic vulnerability may be more relevant. It should also not be forgotten that parental alcohol abuse is an ongoing risk factor for injury, poisonings and medical hospitalizations.

Language difficulties are more common amongst twins than singletons and the rate of multiple births in the developed world has increased significantly over the last two decades, in part because of infertility treatment (D'Souza *et al.* 1997). Currently, there is no clear evidence of an increased risk of psychopathology associated with assisted reproduction. Nevertheless, conception by subzonal injection of spermatozoa appears to have been associated with a skewed sex ratio and a slightly elevated rate of major malformations (Patrat *et al.* 1999) and twins conceived by *in vitro* fertilization are at significantly higher risk for prematurity and associated neonatal morbidity and mortality than spontaneously conceived twins (Moise *et al.* 1998). Indeed twins and other multiples are a vulnerable group, as twinning is associated with prematurity, low birth weight and increased perinatal mortality, as well as an elevated rate of congenital anomalies (Myrianthopoulos 1976). The rate of cerebral palsy is also increased, particularly when a comultiple suffers a fetal or neonatal death (Petterson *et al.* 1998). Thus, when assessing twins (or singleton survivors) clinicians need to obtain a thorough history of the obstetric course and neonatal period. Quite how one interprets a history of obstetric adversity that is not a clear cause of brain damage is problematic in both singletons and twins. Clinicians may need to reassure parents that mild obstetric difficulties are not likely to be aetiological factors.

The role of genetic influences in the causation of ADHD and specific developmental delays has been increasingly recognized (see McGuffin & Rutter, Chapter 12; Schachar & Tannock, Chapter 25), and the clinician should enquire directly about whether other family members are affected by similar difficulties, although the absence of a family history does not preclude genetic influences in complex disorders. Rarely, postnatal environmental aetiologies may need to be considered in the genesis of these difficulties. Thus, paediatric autoimmune neuropsychiatric disorders associated with streptococcal infection (PAN-DAS) have been suggested to represent a distinct clinical entity from rheumatic fever (Garvey *et al.* 1998; see also Rapoport & Swedo, Chapter 35). Affected children show motor hyperactivity, new problems with attention and impulsivity, clumsiness, choreiform movements and emotional lability. The validity of the syndrome as a separate entity remains somewhat uncertain (Garvey *et al.* 1998) and the streptococcal-induced disease remain largely a clinical diagnosis because investigations provide only ancillary evidence (Thatai & Turi 1999).

Interpreting the significance of symptoms of inattention and overactivity and developmental delay depends on knowledge about the child's overall level of cognitive functioning. Accurate diagnosis and optimal management requires comprehensive psychometric assessment and ideally the clinician should be aware of the findings before conducting a physical examination. In practice, this will often not be possible and if evidence of mental retardation subsequently becomes available the clinician should consider whether further examination is warranted.

In terms of the physical examination, several causes of abnormal growth associated with learning difficulties are noted above. The full fetal alcohol syndrome is associated with pre- and/or postnatal growth deficiency (and usually mental retardation). Short stature is also a minor disease manifestation of neurofibromatosis 1 (NF1)—the most common single gene disorder to affect the nervous system—with about one-third of patients having a height at or below the third percentile (North 1998). The rate of mental retardation in NF1 patients is only slightly elevated, but specific learning disabilities affect between 30 and 60% of children. Head circumference is also increased.

In patients with a neurodevelopmental disorder a more thorough physical examination should be conducted that includes undressing, attention to dysmorphic features and examination of all bodily systems. Most children dislike undressing in front of strangers and only the area to be examined should be exposed at any one time, unless there is a concern about disproportion. The examiner should also be able to make full use of humour and any available props.

The major skin and eye manifestations of NF1 to look out for include *café au lait* spots, axillary freckling, cutaneous neurofibromas and iris hamartomas (Lisch nodules). Particular attention should be paid to the neurological examination and handedness noted; language delays are sometimes early manifestations of neuromuscular disorders and the clinician is quite likely to identify neurological soft signs. These refer to a heterogeneous collection of motor delays and problems with coordination that do not indicate a localized abnormality in the central nervous system.

When the age of onset and clinical picture is typical, there is no evidence of mental retardation, and growth parameters and the physical examination are unremarkable, there are no indications for routine blood or urine tests. When the history is atypical, cognitive difficulties are more widespread than anticipated

or there are dysmorphic features or other physical signs, a high-resolution karyotype should be obtained and any suspected single gene or other disorders tested for specifically. Occasionally, the assessment will reveal that the child has mental retardation or a progressive disorder. Although there is some evidence that at a population level an allele of the dopamine D4 receptor gene (LaHoste *et al.* 1996) and a variant of the dopamine transporter gene (Cook *et al.* 1995) may confer a modest increased risk for ADHD, testing for these alleles is not currently useful at an individual level. Similarly, a potential susceptibility locus for language disorder has been localized to chromosome 7 (Fisher *et al.* 1998; Lai *et al.* 2000) and there is evidence for a susceptibility locus for reading difficulties on chromosome 6p (Cardon *et al.* 1994; Grigorenko *et al.* 1997; Fisher *et al.* 1999), but the potential clinical application of these findings awaits further study. Although there has been much research interest in the use of structural and functional neuroimaging in elucidating the brain basis of language and reading disorders, these investigations are not currently indicated in straightforward cases. The clinician should ensure, however, that children with developmental language delay have their hearing tested by a trained audiologist. If treatment with stimulant medication is planned it is important that baseline growth parameters, blood pressure and full blood count are obtained and regularly monitored.

Mental retardation and autism

Both types of disorder are dealt with in this section because autism is frequently accompanied by mental retardation (although identifiable aetiological factors are much more common in mentally retarded individuals who do not have autism). Whether child psychiatrists assess children with severe mental retardation will depend on individual working practices and expertise, but all clinicians can expect to see mildly retarded individuals, although their cognitive difficulties may not have been identified previously. The approach of the clinician, at least with respect to mentalretardation, is somewhat different from that outlined above. That is because the starting assumption is that an identifiable cause for general cognitive impairment *can* be found in roughly half of all cases of mental retardation.

The overall approach to these disorders is to obtain a systematic history of potential aetiological factors, to conduct a careful and comprehensive physical examination in order to identify physical signs that might suggest specific causes or syndromes, and to choose investigations judiciously, based either on available evidence or what is known about the probability of individual factors. It is difficult to acquire this range of skills—particularly in physical examination—from reading alone and the training of child psychiatrists should include the opportunity to gain paediatric experience, particularly in developmental surveillance and genetic clinics. Often a specific aetiology will not be identifiable in individual cases, but an understanding of the most likely cause may be sufficient to answer the family's questions. Several studies suggest that a diagnosis or cause of mental retardation can be identified in 40–60% of cases (Curry *et al.* 1997) and with advances in molecular and cytogenetics and in neuroimaging this rate is likely to increase. Nevertheless, common and distinctive syndromes, such as trisomy 21, will have been identified at birth or shortly thereafter, and the rate of identifiable aetiologies in cases presenting to most child psychiatrists is likely to be somewhat lower.

The history will often indicate probable aetiological factors and consequently needs to be particularly thorough, especially when there are no initial clues as to the most likely aetiology. Exposure to drugs, toxins and radiation during pregnancy must be asked about directly. Maternal infections should also be recorded and, even if there was no significant history during pregnancy, congenital infection should be suspected if there was intrauterine growth retardation, prematurity or a history of neonatal jaundice, hepatosplenomegaly, purpura or rashes. Congenital malformations should be noted.

Medical advances over the last decade have led to improved survival rates for extremely premature and very low birth weight babies, but there has been little change in their neurodevelopmental outcome (Hack & Fanaroff 1999). These infants are at particular risk for cerebral palsy, mental retardation and visual impairments (Lorenz *et al.* 1998). With respect to the aetiology of cerebral palsy, the current consensus is that in most cases the critical events occur in the fetus before the onset of labour or in the newborn after delivery (MacLennan 1999 for the International Cerebral Palsy Task Force). Spastic quadriplegia and, less commonly, dyskinetic cerebral palsy, are the only subtypes that appear to be associated with acute hypoxic intrapartum events. If the clinician suspects that a developmental disorder is linked to prior perinatal difficulties, reviewing the obstetric and paediatric notes may be informative, but the possibility that obstetric difficulties are a consequence of abnormal development should not be overlooked. When children are adopted or fostered it may be difficult to obtain details of pregnancy and early development, but this information will occasionally be relevant. Some internationally adopted children will have come from countries where there is an increased risk for vertical transmission of HIV and syphilis (as well as for infection with HIV by unscreened blood and its products) and in these circumstances more thorough screening investigations are warranted.

With respect to infancy and early childhood, the physician needs to obtain a detailed developmental history and not forget to enquire about signs that may have resolved, such as hypotonia (an early sign of Prader–Willi syndrome) and mild paresis. Severe postnatal infections, such as meningitis and encephalitis, seizures and any associated cognitive decline should also be documented. Children with disabilities are also at risk of secondary complications from their behaviour and any history of pica (potentially leading to lead exposure) and severe self-injury should be noted.

The family history is particularly important in identifying genetic causes of mental retardation. Relatives with psychiatric or medical disorders linked to the patient's condition should be identified, as well as individuals who might benefit from examination, testing or possibly genetic counselling. The usual starting point is a three-generation pedigree of family members, including an enquiry about consanguinity. Attention should be paid to the presence of learning difficulties, developmental delays and mental retardation, psychiatric disorders and neurological and other medical disorders. Identifying whether the mother has had any miscarriages, stillbirths or neonatal deaths may also be pertinent, as many genetic syndromes show quite variable phenotypic expression and a congenital abnormality in another pregnancy may be related to a milder phenotype in the index child — the holoprosencephaly spectrum providing a clear example (Gorlin *et al.* 1990).

Occasionally, the physical examination may be challenging because of limited co-operation, potentially necessitating a piecemeal or opportunistic approach. With respect to measurement of growth, the association of many mental retardation syndromes with short stature has already been noted. Prader–Willi syndrome (Khan & Wood 1999) is the most common genetic mental retardation syndrome associated with obesity and physical signs include infantile hypotonia, short stature, severe obesity, hypogonadism, and small hands and feet. Microcephaly arising on the basis of *in utero* infection may also be accompanied by eye signs such as retinopathy, cataracts, corneal scarring and micopthalmia and by hearing impairment and cerebral palsy. Otherwise, obtaining newborn and postnatal head circumference measurements may help to differentiate a prenatal from postnatal (e.g. HIV, Rett syndrome) onset of microcephaly. Increased head circumference is found in some individuals with fragile X syndrome (De Vries *et al.* 1998), autism (Kanner 1943; Bailey *et al.* 1993; Woodhouse *et al.* 1996) and is characteristic of Sotos syndrome. Increased head circumference may also be secondary to much rarer conditions, such as the mucopolysaccharidoses. Delayed or incomplete puberty is a feature of Klinefelter, Prader–Willi and Turner syndromes, whereas precocious puberty is sometimes seen in children with neurofibromatosis, tuberous sclerosis, and occasionally as a sequelae of meningitis or encephalitis.

A comprehensive head-to-toe examination of individuals with mental retardation is always necessary, particularly to identify minor anomalies that might lead to specific syndrome diagnosis, or help to date the onset of a developmental problem (Curry *et al.* 1997; Battaglia *et al.* 1999). In this section, the dysmorphic features that the examiner should search for are covered in detail, as most psychiatrists have no particular training in their identification and usually they are not brought together in standard texts. There is a deliberate focus on abnormal facial structures as these provide the most frequent clues to specific syndrome diagnosis. Photographs of dysmorphic features are available in standard texts (Gorlin *et al.* 1990; Jones 1997) and computerized databases (Winter & Baraitser 2000).

The skin should be examined for evidence of phakomatoses. The earliest skin lesion in tuberous sclerosis is the depigmented, ash leaf shaped macule, which is most easily seen under a Wood ultraviolet light. Fibroangiomatous naevi occur principally in the nasolabial folds and on the cheeks but these may not be apparent until 4–7 years of age. The skin should also be examined for hypo- or hyperpigmentation and naevi, looseness or oedema, absent or excessive facial or body hair, telangiectases and haemangiomas. A malar flush is usually seen in homocystinuria and a photosensitive eruption is common in Hartnup disease.

The shape of the skull should be noted and the forehead inspected for prominent supraorbital ridges or frontal bossing. The examiner should consider whether the face is particularly round, broad, triangular or flat and note any excessive subcutaneous tissue or coarseness. Facial structure should be examined to establish whether the jaw is unusually prominent or receding and whether there is malar or maxillary hypoplasia. The ears should be inspected for signs of malformation, abnormal vertical position or posterior rotation. Inspection of the hair may reveal displacement of the parietal whorl, unusual hair loss, or altered form or brittleness of the hairs.

The examiner should assess whether the nose is particularly short, small or unusually prominent and also note whether the nostrils are properly formed, or are hypoplastic or anteverted. Whether the nasal bridge is unusually low, high or prominent should be considered as well as whether the nasal bridge and nasal root are unusually broad.

The overall size and shape of the mouth, lips and philtrum should be assessed and the possibility of hypotonia considered. The size of the tongue and any irregularities in its shape and the presence of frenula should be observed. The height and width of the palate can also be assessed and the alveolar ridges examined for hypertrophy and lead lines. The examiner should consider whether the right number of teeth are present in the right position and whether their form or size is abnormal.

Eye abnormalities are found in association with all the major chromosomal aberrations, with many inborn errors of metabolism and with congenital infections. During embryonic development the eyes move medially; many syndromes and diseases are associated with an increased distance between the orbits (hyperteleorism) or, less commonly, a decreased distance (hypoteleorism). Many facial features may produce the appearance of hyperteleorism and when the abnormality is suspected interpupillary distance can be measured and compared with published norms (Hall *et al.* 1989; Jones 1997). The slant and length of the palpebral fissures should be assessed, any prominence or retraction of the eyeballs noted, and the eyes examined for congenital ptosis. Whether the medial canthi are laterally displaced should be considered and any epicanthal folds noted. The sclera should be inspected for abnormal pigmentation and the cornea for abnormal size, clouding, opacity or deposits. Defects, unusual patterning or colouration of the iris may also be noted. Brushfield spots may be seen in both Klinefelter and Down syndrome; and Lisch nodules, pigmented hamartomas of the iris, are seen in the majority of patients with neurofibromatosis.

A thorough fundoscopic examination of the eye requires pupillary dilatation. Whether this is a worthwhile procedure must be decided on the basis of the fundal findings without mydriasis, and the abnormalities detected in the remainder of the examination. A darkened room will normally ensure a reasonable view. Cataracts and lens dislocation may be noted and the retina should be examined for abnormal pigmentation, chorioretinitis and the macular changes seen in storage diseases, such as a cherry red spot or grey colouration. The optic nerve should be examined for atrophy.

The length of the neck should be noted and any abnormal formation of the thorax, such as pectus excavatum or carinatum. The spine should be examined for evidence of scoliosis, kyphosis, vertebral defects and sacral dimples.

The examiner should consider whether the limbs are in proportion to body size and look for fixed deformities of the joints; any joint hyperextensibility should also be recorded. The hands and feet should be carefully examined, paying attention to their overall size, absence or duplication of any fingers or toes or their partial fusion. The examiner may also assess whether the fingers or thumb are unusually long or short and whether there is metacarpal or metatarsal hypoplasia. The thumb and big toe should be inspected to determine if they are unusually broad, and the examiner should determine if any digits are either bent or permanently flexed. The pattern of creases on the fingers, palms and soles should be checked and the nails examined for unusual formation, in particular hypoplasia or hyperconvexity.

A thorough examination of the bodily systems is always necessary and particular attention paid to the presence of heart murmurs, hepatosplenomegaly and anomalies or hyper- or hypoplasia of the external genitalia. Mental retardation is frequently accompanied by sensory impairments and all affected individuals should have audiometry and a thorough assessment of visual acuity.

Sometimes the physical examination will reveal structural abnormalities of uncertain significance and then the next steps are to refer to appropriate atlases and texts and measure possible minor anomalies with reference to population norms (Hall *et al.* 1989). Consultation with clinical genetics colleagues may also be necessary; indeed many clinical genetics laboratories will not order expensive specific cytogenetic investigations unless a clinical geneticist has reviewed the child.

The approach to the investigation of a child with developmental delay varies considerably. A recent survey of consultant community paediatricians found that the typical number of investigations ordered varied from 0 to 15 (Gringras 1998) with the associated costs ranged from £0–1181. At the level of tertiary neurology/developmental paediatric services a comprehensive set of investigations may be routine (Majnemer & Shevell 1995; Battaglia *et al.* 1999) with considerable costs, particularly for neuroimaging and neurophysiological investigations. The current consensus (Curry *et al.* 1997) is that the choice of investigations should be based on the information available from the history and physical examination.

Several different types of abnormality illustrate the general approach. Children with a history or signs of prenatal infection can be tested for immunological evidence of the common aetiological agents: toxoplasmosis, rubella, cytomegalovirus, herpes simplex and syphilis—the so-called TORCHES screen. These tests are usually most informative when conducted early in life, prior to postnatal infection or vaccination. Some individuals with congenital infections will be asymptomatic at birth, with mental retardation or neurological abnormalities, such as seizures, sensorineural hearing loss, microcephaly or motor problems, appearing at a later age. Although a TORCHES screen is still relevant in older individuals, the interpretation of positive findings is not straightforward. Unlike many causes of mental retardation, the relative importance of infectious aetiologies is subject to secular trends. There has been a recent dramatic increase in the prevalence of sexually transmitted diseases amongst young women in some countries, with the attendant risk of congenital infection. For instance, the rate of syphilis amongst girls age 15–17 years increased 126-fold in the Russian Federation between 1988 and 1996 (Tichonova et al. 1997). In high-risk areas a search should be made for Hutchinson teeth, interstitial keratitis, eighth nerve deafness, Clutton joints and rhagades. There is also an argument for routine screening for syphilis in children with mental retardation in endemic areas. The venereal disease reference laboratory test (VDRL) and the rapid plasma reagin flocculation test (RPR) are indirect antigen tests which are sensitive, inexpensive and easy to perform, but false positives occur in 1–2% of the general population. Accordingly, positive findings should be followed by a sensitive and specific test for treponemal antigen, such as the fluorescent treponemal antibody absorption test (FTA-ABS) and the micro-haemagglutination assay for antibody to Treponema pallidum (MHA-TP). Similar issues with respect to screening arise when clinicians know that there has been a recent upsurge in one of the other infectious aetiologies. Because detailed local knowledge is not usually available when children are internationally adopted, children with mental retardation should routinely have a comprehensive infection screen (Hostetter 1999).

Severe kernicterus is another relatively easily identified cause of mental retardation. Rhesus incompatibility will usually have been investigated in the postnatal period, but if this was excluded the possibility of glucose-6-phosphate dehydrogenase (G6PD) deficiency should be considered, especially as further episodes of haemolysis may be precipitated by a variety of chemicals and drugs. Prolonged jaundice accompanied by feeding difficulties, a hoarse cry and subsequent hypotonia strongly suggests congenital hypothyroidism and the face should be examined for myxoedema and a protruding tongue. Affected infants will occasionally have escaped detection by newborn screening.

Some children may have dysmorphic features that suggest a syndrome that can be tested for specifically, or are strongly suggestive of a chromosomal abnormality:
• fragile X syndrome is characterized by a long face, prominent jaw, thickening of the nasal bridge and large ears;
• Prader–Willi syndrome by a narrow bifrontal diameter, almond-shaped palpebral fissures, narrow nasal bridge and a downturned mouth;
• velocardiofacial syndrome by palatal anomalies, a long narrow face, narrow palpable fissures, flat cheeks, prominent nose, small ears and mouth and a retruded chin;
• Sotos syndrome by increased head circumference, frontal bossing, antimongoloid slant and a prominent jaw; and
• fetal alcohol syndrome by microcephaly, short palpebral fissures, a long smooth philtrum, a thin vermilion border, epicanthal folds and a flat midface.

However, these physical phenotypes often change with development, further complicating recognition:
• the typical fragile X faces may not be apparent until after childhood;
• the face in Sotos syndrome becomes longer in adolescence with disproportionate prominence of the chin; and
• fetal alcohol syndrome is difficult to recognize at birth and may also become less obvious after puberty.

Developmental changes in physical and behavioural phenotypes are one of the key reasons for comprehensive serial evaluations of individuals, as this increases the likelihood of a specific diagnosis being made. Regular photographic records of patients may be particularly helpful in aiding recognition of an emerging physical phenotype.

Children may show clinical features, such as encephalopathic or acidotic states, unusual odours, poor growth or dysmorphic features, that will suggest the need for targeted metabolic investigation (Curry et al. 1997). Neuroimaging is indicated in patients with micro- or macrocephaly or unusual skull shape, and when there are seizures, neurological signs or loss of psychomotor skills. Magnetic resonance imaging (MRI) is now the procedure of choice except when it is necessary to visualize intracranial calcification (e.g. in congenital toxoplasma or tuberous sclerosis) or visualization of the skull is required (as in the various craniosynostosis syndromes).

There will be many children, however, who are not dysmorphic, show no growth abnormalities, and do not have features suggesting either a metabolic abnormality or the likelihood of a central nervous system problem visualizable with neuroimaging. Traditionally, many of these children would have had a comprehensive screen for mental retardation. The current consensus (Curry et al. 1997) has been to move away from a routine screen, when there are no clinical indicators of particular disorders, to a more restricted approach. In part that consensus derives from the very low detection rate associated with routine administration of tests such as plasma amino acid chromatography (Curry et al. 1997). The current view is that, in the absence of pointers to specific disorders, children with developmental delay should routinely have a karyotype at the 500 band level. That is because chromosomal abnormalities are the single most common known cause of mental retardation and, increasingly, it has been appreciated that they may not always be associated with obvious dysmorphology (Curry et al. 1996).

Knight et al. (1999) have recently reported that 7% of children with unexplained moderate to severe mental retardation and normal routine karyotypes have subtelemeric chromosomal rearrangements detectable using a multiprobe fluorescent in situ hybridization (FISH) protocol. If these findings are replicated by others, screening for submicroscopic telomeric chromosomal rearrangements should probably also become routine. Because the fragile X syndrome is such a common cause of unexplained mental retardation, laboratory testing is relatively inexpensive and the diagnosis has implications for patient management and genetic advice, *FMR1* testing should also be considered in most patients with unexplained mental retardation (Curry *et al.* 1997).

The advice to move to a limited screen in the absence of pointers to disease is geared towards clinicians with expertise in the assessment of children with mental retardation, who are expected to recognize indications for specific tests. Clinicians who do not consider themselves expert must decide whether to refer on for a more expert assessment or, in situations where this is impractical, to conduct a traditional screen. In addition to a TORCHES screen and karyotyping this would typically include a routine urine examination for unusual colour, odour or sediment; tests for protein, glucose, ketones and occult blood and measurement of specific gravity and pH. The urine should also be examined for metachromatic granules and tested for the presence of mucopolysaccharides (if the Lesch–Nyhan syndrome is suspected in boys, uric acid should also be measured) and the amino acid, organic acid and sugar composition of the sample determined. Haematological investigations include a full blood count with red cell indices, and microscopic examination of a blood film for vacuolated lymphocytes and metachromatic inclusions. Biochemical investigations on blood includes measurement of thyroxine (T_4), thyroid-stimulating hormone (TSH), calcium and phosphate; and plasma amino acid chromatography. In those areas where lead remains an environmental hazard, serum levels should routinely be estimated.

If the course of the disorder is progressive, or there is clinical evidence of a particular disorder but screening tests are negative, then further investigation should be conducted by a centre with expertise in inborn errors of metabolism and progressive neurological disorders. If an aetiology for mental retardation is eventually identified, then optimal care will be provided if the child is seen by a doctor with experience in the underlying disorder. As new aetiologies are recognized and diagnostic testing improves, clinicians should also consider re-examination and testing for young people under their care. This is especially important when disorders are genetically determined because of the potential implications for relatives.

A rather similar approach applies to the assessment of children with autism. A variety of studies suggest that an identifiable medical disorder of aetiological significance occurs in only a small minority of patients (Rutter *et al.* 1994; Barton & Volkmar 1998; Skjeldal *et al.* 1998; Fombonne 1999); chromosomal abnormalities, fragile X and tuberous sclerosis being the most frequently identified disorders. As with mental retardation, a thorough history and comprehensive head-to-toe examination of all cases — including a search for depigmented lesions with a Wood light — is necessary to identify any pointers to identifiable aetiologies. When the history and physical examination are unremarkable, routine investigation should be confined to karyotyping and *FMR1* testing. If there are clinical indications of seizure activity an electroencephalogram (EEG) should also be performed. Because macrocephaly is found in a minority of individuals with idiopathic autism, the finding in isolation is not an indication for neuroimaging.

Loss of skills

The extent to which children who lose skills present to child psychiatrists depends upon their age, which skills are lost and the nature of any associated symptomatology. In early childhood, development may first slow or reach a plateau before there is frank loss of skills but this pattern will only be recognized if a detailed developmental history is taken. Establishing the child's developmental trajectory may require repeat assessments of psychological and physical development.

Infants and toddlers with metabolic disorders will usually present to paediatricians with poor feeding or acute illnesses. Girls with Rett syndrome may occasionally be seen initially by child psychiatrists when there is a presumption of autism, although that confusion should now be much less common (see Lord & Bailey, Chapter 38). Some parents of children with autism are worried about their development from shortly after birth, but most are identified as showing abnormalities or delays in the second year of life. About one-quarter to one-third of children with autism lose speech in the first years of life (Rogers & DiLalla 1990) often accompanied by or preceded by changes in social behaviour. The history of uninterrupted motor development and the previous acquisition of only a very small vocabulary are important in differentiating autism from disintegrative psychosis, which usually has an onset after age 2 and involves the loss, not just of language, but also of motor and self-help skills and bowel/bladder control. The final outcome is usually indistinguishable from profound mental retardation and autism (Hill & Rosenbloom 1986), although deterioration can continue with more severe motor dysfunction and the development of seizures and localized neurological signs (Corbett *et al.* 1977). The age of onset and the usual lack of an association with seizures are also important features differentiating autism from Landau–Kleffner syndrome (see Bishop, Chapter 39), which affects previously healthy children who lose language comprehension and expression over a period of weeks or months, usually (but not always) accompanied by epileptic seizures. The peak age of onset occurs at 3–8 years.

Geography and the family and social history will usually indicate the likelihood of HIV encephalopathy rather than the other causes of early developmental slowing and loss seen by neuropsychiatrists. The pandemic of HIV has now made progressive neurological disorder a very significant presenting problem in Sub-Saharan Africa and Southeast Asia (Oleske & Czarniecki 1999). Infants acquire HIV from their mothers during pregnancy or delivery, or postnatally through breastfeeding (Giaquinto *et al.* 1998). Children with HIV-associated progressive encephalopathy usually develop neurological symptoms in the first 2–3 years of life (see Havens *et al.*, Chapter 49). There is loss of developmental milestones or cognitive abilities and progressive symmetric motor deficits; sometimes loss or impairment of language and social adaptation skills may be the first signs of encephalopathy. Some children have a more insidious illness, with non-progressive cognitive and motor deficits and slowed developmental progression.

In children with early loss of skills the physical examination needs to be particularly comprehensive, both with respect to a search for dysmorphic features and the neurological examination. In terms of growth parameters, an important clinical sign differentiating Rett syndrome from idiopathic autism is the deceleration in head growth leading eventually to acquired microcephaly. When Rett syndrome is suspected clinically it is possible to test directly for mutations in the MECP2 gene (Amir *et al.* 1999), which are found in 75% to 90% of sporadic cases and 50% of familial cases (Shahbazian & Zoghbi 2001) as well as in male relatives with profound mental retardation (Orrico *et al.* 2000). Childhood disintegrative disorder has been linked to cerebral lipidoses, mucopolysaccharidoses, leukodystrophies and other neurological conditions (see below). These children should usually be investigated by a paediatric neurologist as screening tests may be negative and more focused specific testing indicated. Landau–Kleffner syndrome is associated with spike and wave discharges originating in auditory cortex; these abnormalities may sometimes only be seen during slow wave sleep. Often MRI will not reveal structural abnormalities.

In older children with progressive neurological disorders, loss of skills may not be the presenting complaint; rather, individuals may be seen because relatively non-specific psychiatric symptomatology or psychosis are the first signs of dementia. The early identification of affected individuals will usually rely on obtaining a detailed history of school performance, and this should be a routine part of the psychiatric history. Any decline should prompt a detailed enquiry about those neurological difficulties that may not be volunteered, particularly gait, co-ordination and visual difficulties. The extreme psychological consequences of physical or sexual abuse will occasionally need to be differentiated from somatic conditions, and this requires a thorough history and a high index of suspicion. Often observation in an inpatient setting may help to differentiate such psychological reactions from somatic disorders. Abuse may also constitute a risk factor for brain injury or infection.

Location and disorders in other relatives will often provide clues to the most likely aetiological factors underlying progressive disorders; a number of different aetiologies are outlined that illustrate some general principals. AIDS is now the leading cause of presenile dementia, characterized by cognitive impairment ranging in intensity from memory dysfunction to global dementia, motor disabilities, involuntary and slowed movements and behavioural abnormalities such as psychosis and depression. Outside endemic areas, drug-abusing adolescents, sexually abused children (Hammerschlag 1998) and individuals who may have been exposed to unscreened blood products are at most risk.

Wilson disease (Bacon & Schilsky 1999; Schaefer & Gitlin 1999) is an autosomal recessive disorder of copper metabolism for which an effective therapy is available; consequently the challenge is to make the diagnosis before end organ damage and to identify potentially at-risk siblings. Wilson disease is usually symptomatic in adolescents and young adults and the majority of patients show neurological/psychiatric disorders (Cuthbert 1998). Common psychiatric manifestations include abnormal behaviour, personality change, a schizoaffective picture, depression and cognitive impairment.

Huntington disease is an autosomal dominant disorder and so the presence of other affected family members substantially narrows the diagnostic possibilities, although psychological disturbance may be a consequence of an abnormal family environment. Juvenile onset occurs in about 5% of cases, usually via paternal inheritance. Affected individuals may first become withdrawn or show emotional disturbances or changes in personality.

X-linked adrenoleukodystrophy is a peroxisomal disorder associated with abnormal accumulation of very long chain fatty acids (VLCFA) (Smith *et al.* 1999). The commonly recognized form affects boys between 4 and 8 years of age and begins with signs and symptoms of ADHD followed by intellectual, behavioural and neurological deterioration; progression is slower with an adolescent presentation. Juvenile onset metachromatic leukodystrophy may also present with emotional or schooling difficulties.

When progressive neurological disorders are suspected, examination of the motor system is particularly critical and early gait ataxia may be detected during tandem walk. Thus, the early neurological findings in AIDS include gait ataxia (which may be mild), hyperreflexia and weakness of the lower limbs. In Wilson disease, four types of movement disorder are seen: parkinsonian, pseudosclerotic, dystonic and choreic (Cuthbert 1998). Copper is deposited in the cornea and the basal ganglia at the same time and a slit lamp examination of the cornea should be undertaken for Kayser–Fleischer rings (a brown–green discolouration in the limbic area of the cornea). Hepatomegaly or splenomegaly may also be found. The abnormal movements in Huntington disease also include chorea, akinesia and rigidity. In X-linked adrenoleukodystrophy the disease process targets the white matter of the central nervous system, the adrenal cortex and the gonads. In patients with adrenal failure increased skin pigmentation may be noted in skin folds, in addition to pyramidal and extrapyramidal signs. In metachromatic leukodystrophy the examiner may detect nystagmus, hypertonia and intention tremor as well as ataxia.

Specific investigations are available to detect these diverse disorders. In endemic areas, testing for HIV should be routine in the assessment of children with onset of cognitive difficulties, depression or psychosis. Available tests either measure antibodies to HIV-1 or HIV-2 or detect the virus directly. Enzyme-linked immunosorbent assay (ELISA) to detect antibody is readily available and cheap, but this test will not detect antibodies within 3 months of infection and is not useful in children less than 24 months of age. HIV DNA can be screened by polymerase chain reaction (PCR) and culture; but the growth characteristics of viral strains from different countries may differ and laboratories should be alerted to the country of origin of the child (Hostetter 1999). In parallel with the worldwide spread of HIV, the prevalence of other sexually transmitted diseases has increased and infected children should also be tested for syphilis. When available, baseline neuroimaging studies are usually performed as screening for encephalopathy and to detect secondary neurological complications. HIV is rapidly becoming the most common cause of basal ganglia calcifications in children (States *et al.* 1997) and is unique to vertically infected children, thus computed tomography (CT) is the imaging modality of choice for evaluating the symptomatic HIV-infected child. Both CT and MRI will reveal atrophy in 57–86% of children (States *et al.* 1997).

In Wilson disease hepatic copper is not incorporated into ceruloplasmin or excreted into bile and accumulates in the hepatocyte cytoplasm, eventually resulting in cellular necrosis and leakage of copper into plasma. A 24-h urine collection to detect elevated urinary copper levels is the most cost-effective screen. The level of ceruloplasmin-bound copper and total copper are decreased, as is ceruloplasmin oxidase activity. Serum ceruloplasmin levels are also decreased, as non-copper-containing ceruloplasmin has a shorter half-life. Measurement of hepatic copper by biopsy, together with the other tests, allows a definitive diagnosis. Molecular genetic studies enable early diagnosis of affected presymptomatic siblings and treatment with zinc salts to reduce copper absorption. Nevertheless, this is complicated because more than 60 mutations and polymorphisms in the gene have been identified (Bacon & Schilsky 1999) and many patients have different mutations in each copy of their gene: compound heterozygotes (Gasser 1997). Particular mutations are frequently found in members of a specific population or ethnic group and screening of family members by haplotype analysis is possible (Cuthbert 1998).

In Huntington disease (Huntington's Disease Collaborative Research Group 1993) a CAG expansion in a protein-coding region of the gene results in an abnormal protein. Repeat length explains about 50–60% of the variance in age at onset, with lengths of >60 or 70 CAG triplets frequently resulting in juvenile onset (Trottier *et al.* 1994). Definitive diagnosis is by detection of the expanded triplet repeat using PCR. Neuroimaging may demonstrate caudate atrophy and hypometabolism. There is also the possibility of presymptomatic genetic testing (see Simonoff, Chapter 66). In the cerebral form of leukodystrophy, cerebral demyelinating lesions usually start in the spleenium of the corpus callosum and show a slow progression; symmetrical demyelinating lesions in the parieto-occipital regions can be detected by MRI. A total of 200 genetic mutations have been reported with the majority of kindreds having private mutations (Smith *et al.* 1999).

There is still much uncertainty about the scale of the problem presented by new variant Creutzfeldt–Jakob prion disease (Collinge 1999). These brain diseases are associated with accumulation of an abnormal isoform of a host encoded glycoprotein known as prion protein. A new variant prion protein that can be passed from cattle infected with bovine spongiform encephalitis (BSE)—mainly acquired through the consumption of feed containing animal products—to humans and other animals has been recognized since 1986, initially in the UK, but now also in mainland Europe. Infection probably occurs via the food chain and infected individuals probably also have a high innate sensitivity to BSE. In the early stages the disorder predominantly presents with psychiatric symptoms. These include particularly depression, and also anxiety, withdrawal, aggression/irritability, first rank symptoms, hallucinations, delusions, forgetfulness and suicidal ideation. There is also pain in the limbs or joints, or painful or unpleasant paraesthesia or dysaesthesia (Will *et al.* 1999). Obvious neurological symptoms subsequently develop, including gait and motor disturbance and dementia. Diagnosis usually awaits the onset of these neurological abnormalities. The prion protein can be detected in tonsils and other lymphoreticular tissue, and other tests include immunoassay for 14-3-3 protein (Will *et al.* 2000). So far all identified cases have been associated with homozygosity for methionine at codon 129 of the prion protein gene, highlighting the role of genetic influences on susceptibility. Because of the long incubation period of the prion diseases (mean of 12 years in kuru), it is unclear whether the number of cases will ever reach epidemic proportions.

Psychosis and acute behavioural change

Many children present to child psychiatrists with acute changes in their behaviour. When not obvious, an organic aetiology will need to be considered if the symptomatology is atypical, there are no psychological stressors or relevant family history or the disorder is subsequently refractory to adequate treatment. Additionally, these young people may be at increased risk for acquiring other diseases because of their behaviour. A comprehensive history is the most important part of the assessment and should establish the time course and severity of symptoms, as well as highlighting unusual features and possible aetiological factors. Depression, mania and schizophrenia are rare before puberty and a marked behavioural change in a prepubertal child should raise the possibility of a somatic condition or physical or sexual abuse. In addition to eliciting psychiatric symptoms, the physician will also need to gather information about the individual's overall level of functioning, including school reports and any deterioration in self-help skills. The most puzzling cases will often require admission and in these circumstances planned investigations, particularly to identify progressive neurological impairments, should usually be discussed with neurological colleagues.

Young people with an acute brain syndrome (Lishman 1998) with impairments in consciousness, thinking and memory and disturbances of perception, emotion and motor behaviour will usually be seen by paediatricians, or in the emergency department. When there are hallucinations or irrational behaviour, however, patients may be sent initially to psychiatric services. Consequently, the mental state examination must include a cognitive assessment, and any evidence of an acute organic syndrome should lead to a focused search for underlying causes (including use of drugs). Ideally, this should be in a paediatric setting where there are the appropriate resources for rapid investigation and resuscitation.

A preliminary physical examination will need to establish whether the child is acutely unwell or pyrexial, detect any neurological impairments (which are often evident in progressive disorders) or evidence of an underlying disease process. In the absence of pyrexia and obvious pointers to underlying aetiology, a routine screen for a severe change in behaviour or psychosis should include:

- a full blood count and erythrocyte sedimentation rate (ESR);
- urea, electrolytes and glucose;
- calcium and phosphate;
- alkaline phosphatase, aspartate transaminase and albumin;
- T_4 and TSH; and
- a routine urinalysis (including porphyrins and metachromatic granules) and a urine toxicology screen.

Many clinicians will now undertake an MRI scan routinely following the first episode of psychosis. An EEG should also be performed if there is a suspicion of epilepsy. Subsequent tests should be guided by the clinical course, but clinicians should also consider the possibility of conditions such as cerebral systemic lupus erythematosis as well as the progressive disorders outlined above.

Worldwide cerebral infections may present with behavioural change or cognitive decline, and clinicians in the relevant areas will need to be alert to the key features of these disorders. A change in temperament of a child with a primary tuberculosis complex should arouse suspicion of tuberculous meningitis. Many parasitic organisms invade the central nervous system producing focal seizures, signs of space-occupying lesions, encephalopathies or behavioural change; these include: hydatid cyst disease, malaria, schistosomiasis, tapeworms, toxocariasis and trichinosis. Where measles remains endemic, the virus can also cause a progressive central nervous system disorder (subacute sclerosing panencephalitis) that begins several years after measles infection (Roos 1998).

Somatizing disorders

The tendency to experience and communicate somatic distress and symptoms in the absence of organic pathology is common in childhood. Symptoms undergo a developmental sequence and are usually monosymptomatic initially. Recurrent abdominal pain and, less frequently, headaches are the most prominent complaints prepubertally, whereas limb pain or aching muscles, fatigue and neurological symptoms increase with age (Fritz *et al.* 1997). The disorders are more common in girls and in non-Western clinical settings (Chandrasekaran *et al.* 1994; see also Rutter & Nikapota, Chapter 16). They are also associated with childhood sexual abuse (Friedrich & Schafer 1995; Kinzl *et al.* 1995). Pain and neurological symptoms do not fit with any local anatomical or physiological process, whereas fatigue is usually present to a pathological degree and can rarely be objectively confirmed (Jordan *et al.* 1998).

The initial goal is to rule out diagnosable medical disease. The history is particularly important in differentiating physical disease from somatic symptoms and requires an accurate description of the nature and timing of the problem, direct questioning about associated symptoms that might suggest an organic condition and a wide-ranging search for precipitating or maintaining factors. The clinician should then attempt to elicit physical signs and note whether growth and pubertal status are appropriate for the child's age. The investigation of individual disorders should be undertaken by a physician with the relevant expertise, in order that any underlying pathology is not missed. The psychiatrist must search for diagnosable psychiatric disorders, particularly depression and panic disorder. All the involved professionals need to establish a collaborative therapeutic alliance with the patient, making symptom palliation, coping and rehabilitation the focus of the clinical enterprise (Barsky & Borus 1999).

Anorexia and bulimia

Anorexia and bulimia are disorders in which abnormal behaviours adversely affect the patient's physical health (see Steinhausen, Chapter 34). The history should include the patient's view about their weight and shape, details of their diet, the frequency and severity of any vomiting and purging, the amount of exercise they take, the chronology of weight change and, in females, the pattern of menstruation. The physical examination has several purposes. The patient's current weight and height should be measured and the percentage of expected body weight or body mass index (BMI; Wt/H^2) calculated. The extent of emaciation in patients with weight loss should be noted, pubertal status assessed and a search made for the complications of malnutrition, vomiting, purging and medication abuse (Becker *et al.* 1999).

Measuring endocrine and metabolic disturbances provides a means of monitoring the course of the disorder and the findings can be explained to patients and parents, who may doubt the severity of the condition. Serum potassium may be decreased and bicarbonate elevated from vomiting or diuretic abuse, whereas a non-anion gap acidosis is associated with laxative use. Decreased sodium is usually a consequence of excess water intake or inappropriate antidiuretic hormone secretion. A full blood count may reveal leucopenia, neutropenia, anaemia and thrombocytopenia. Amenorrhoea is a consequence of decreased pulsatility of gonadotrophin-releasing hormone which leads to low oestradiol/testosterone levels. Bone loss can be assessed by bone densitometry. If tricyclic antidepressants are being contemplated, an ECG should be performed as prolongation of the QT interval is a contraindication to their use.

Investigations

There have been remarkable advances in the investigation of neuropsychiatric disorders since the last edition of this textbook. Genetic testing and structural and functional neuroimaging deserve especial mention, both because of the progress to date and the potential for substantial future developments. Chromosomal abnormalities constitute the largest identifiable cause of mental retardation syndromes and are even more common in aborted fetuses and preimplantation embryos (Delhanty et al. 1997; Munne et al. 1999). There is now improved detection of some of the subtle chromosomal abnormalities linked with developmental difficulties, as typified by the microdeletion syndromes. The physical and behavioural phenotypes and the underlying genetic basis of Prader–Willi and Angleman syndromes (Khan & Wood 1999), 22q deletion syndrome (Basset & Chow 1999)—which encompasses velocardiofacial syndrome and DiGeorge syndromes—and Williams syndrome (Bellugi et al. 1999) nicely illustrate the complex pathways between genetic predisposition and phenotypic expression, including the role of genetic imprinting (see Skuse & Kuntsi, Chapter 13).

Improved detection of these syndromes and other chromosomal abnormalities has depended upon recent advances in cytogenetics. FISH combines molecular genetic and conventional karyotype banding approaches. It involves the binding of specific DNA probes to denatured chromosomes, hybridization being detected using fluorescently labelled molecules linked to the probes. FISH can detect deletions, duplications and translocations of specific chromosomal regions with sufficient sensitivity to detect intragenic rearrangements (Ekong & Wolfe 1998). Specific probes are now available to detect Prader–Willi, Angelman, velocardiofacial, Williams, Smith–Magenis and Dieker syndrome microdeletions, but the requesting clinician must still specify the syndrome/chromosomal region. Another important development is a multiprobe FISH protocol to detect subtelomeric microdeletions when there is no knowledge about which chromosome might be affected (Knight et al. 1997). A further advance is spectral karyotyping (SKY; Schröck et al. 1997): the colour differentiation of all chromosomes based on the simultaneous hybridization of 24 chromosome-specific painting probes. This research tool can identify subtle translocations and those that involve regions with similar traditional banding patterns.

In terms of psychopathology linked with single gene disorders, identification of the unusual patterns of inheritance associated with expansion of trinucleotide repeats represents a significant advance (Margolis et al. 1999). Of most relevance to child psychiatry are the mechanisms underlying the fragile X syndrome (and related conditions); an X-linked condition that is the most common genetic cause of severe cognitive deficit (De Vries et al. 1998; Kaufmann & Reiss 1999). The disorder arises from an expansion of a long CGG repeat in the FMR1 gene, leading to hypermethylation of an adjacent genomic region and consequent loss of gene transcription. The CGG repeat expansion can be detected by either Southern blotting or PCR. The FMR1 protein is absent in males with a fully methylated mutation and an antibody test is a rapid and cheap means of screening in mentally retarded males and male neonates, although it will not differentiate between normal and premutation alleles (De Vries et al. 1998).

Recent progress in identifying genes for relevant Mendelian disorders includes tuberous sclerosis 1 (van Slegtenhorst et al. 1997), most cases of Rett syndrome (Amir et al. 1999) and Wilson disease (Bull et al. 1993; Tanzi et al. 1993; Petrukhin et al. 1994). Testing individuals for mutations in such disorders can be useful when symptoms or signs are equivocal, or to detect at-risk relatives when effective treatments are available. Often, however, de novo analysis for specific mutations is difficult if either the gene is large or there are many different mutations. In these situations, knowledge about the most frequent mutations in a particular population may be helpful, or family members can be screened using haplotype analysis (Bacon & Schilsky 1999). In the future, methodologies that screen the entire coding system of genes may make it practical to consider direct molecular genetic testing (Saugier-Veber et al. 1998).

For many childhood psychiatric disorders, however, a complex genetic predisposition is thought to be relevant (Rutter et al. 1999). Although there are promising developments in this area, none so far is useful at the individual level. In autism there is overlap in the linkage findings from several whole genome scans (see Lamb et al. 2000; Maestrini et al. 2000 for reviews), particularly on chromosome 7 (IMGSAC 1998). There has also been progress in respect to ADHD and language-related disorders (see above). The extent to which testing for individual susceptibility genes will be clinically relevant in the future will depend upon the magnitude of the gene's effect, the degree of genetic heterogeneity (whether an identified gene is implicated in a particular family), whether there is epistasis (interactions between genes), and how phenotypic expression relates to particular loci (Turner et al. 2000). Paradoxically, as knowledge about susceptibility loci increases, the recognition that complex genetic influences are not implicated in individual cases may indicate the need for further investigation. Keeping abreast of the rapid developments in genetic testing can be problematical and HTTP://www.genetests.org provides a regularly updated list of available investigations.

Neuroimaging

Over the last decade there have been considerable advances in the ability to visualize brain structure and function. The main clinical use of neuroimaging is in the detection and investigation of neurological disorders, but in the future clinical applications may extend to idiopathic childhood psychiatric disorders. The detail of the physics and practical aspects of neuroimaging are beyond the scope of this chapter and interested readers are referred to several excellent books (Orrison et al. 1995; Lewis & Higgins 1996; Frackowiak et al. 1997; Ernst & Rumsey 2000).

A brief summary of the main methodologies is included in Appendix 1. The detailed findings in child psychiatry have been frequently reviewed (Bailey & Cox 1996; Filipek 1999; Santosh 2000; Overmeyer & Taylor, in press) and the findings in individual disorders are also covered in the relevant chapters.

Neuroimaging has had most clinical impact in epileptology, investigation of mental retardation and assessment of progressive neurological disorders. The imaging of intractable epilepsy nicely illustrates the potential of multiple imaging approaches when there are neurodevelopmental and metabolic abnormalities as well as secondary pathology. Structural MRI is clinically useful in the investigation of temporal lobe epilepsy, demonstrating hippocampal sclerosis and atrophy in intractable complex partial seizures, often removing the need for invasive or expensive presurgical investigations (Cross et al. 1993; Cook 1994). Magnetic resonance spectroscopy (MRS) can also detect pathology by measuring the changes in N-acetylaspartate : creatinine + choline ratios associated with neuronal loss or damage (Gadian et al. 1994; Cross et al. 1997). In many cases of intractable epilepsy, ictal technetium-99 HMPAO single photon emission CT (SPECT) will demonstrate areas of hyperperfusion predictive of the seizure focus, whereas interictal studies can show unilateral hypoperfusion (Cross et al. 1997), which is also visualized using FDG-PET (Gaillard et al. 1995). Metabolic abnormalities may also be detectable when there are no focal cerebral structural abnormalities and ligands to benzodiazepine receptors are claimed to further increase the sensitivity of positron emission tomography (PET) studies (Muzik et al. 2000).

Structural MRI has also been invaluable in identifying areas of cortical dysgenesis in patients with intractable partial seizures, particularly those associated with mental retardation (Palmini et al. 1991; Brodtkorb et al. 1992; Wolf et al. 1995). The dysplastic lesions can be intrinsically epileptogenic, as demonstrated by electrocorticography, magnetoencephalography (MEG) and the results of surgery (Palmini et al. 1995; Morioka et al. 1999), but surgical outcome studies also indicate that structural abnormalities may extend beyond the visualized boundaries of cortical dysplasia (Palmini et al. 1994). Immunocytochemical studies of surgically resected tissue suggest that the epileptogenicity of these dysplastic lesions is in part a consequence of decreased numbers of gamma-aminobutyric acid (GABA) -ergic neurones (Spreafico et al. 1998) and recent advances in MRS editing techniques now allow non-invasive measurement of brain GABA, glutamate and glutamine levels, with some evidence that seizure frequency in patients with complex partial seizures is inversely related to brain GABA levels (Petroff et al. 1999). Analyses of quantitative relationships between cortical surface areas and volumes in cerebral dysgenesis (Sisodiya & Free 1997) offers another approach to identification of presumed abnormal connectivity in the absence of visual abnormalities.

Severe and intractable cases of epilepsy sometimes benefit from surgery, but this requires establishing whether eloquent cortex is affected and clarifying language lateralization. Increas-

ingly functional MRI (fMRI) is being used for presurgical mapping of cortical function and language laterality (Stapleton et al. 1997; Bookheimer et al. 1999), with a reduced risk of morbidity and mortality compared to traditional methods. The excellent temporal and good spatial resolution of MEG is also useful in the presurgical evaluation of Landau–Kleffner syndrome: an acquired aphasia secondary to a focal epileptogenic lesion affecting speech cortex. MRI (and CT) are typically normal (Sobel et al. 2000). Spike and spike-wave discharges originate in intraperisylvian regions (Paetau et al. 1999; Sobel et al. 2000) and may be triggered by environmental sounds (Paetau et al. 1999). Multiple subpial transection is claimed to be an effective treatment in unilateral cases (Morrell et al. 1995) and MEG can identify sources precisely, and also those individuals with a unique unilateral pacemaker and spread to the opposite hemisphere (Paetau et al. 1999).

Structural brain abnormalities are found in a significant proportion of individuals with mental retardation (Curry et al. 1997). These patients often have epilepsy (see above) and MRI has revealed the full range of neuronal migration disorders and dysgenetic lesions, as well as other gross developmental abnormalities visualizable by CT. MRI is also the modality of choice for detecting lesions associated with cerebral palsy: that applies to common (Truwit et al. 1992) and rare (Kuzniecky et al. 1993) migration disorders; vascular lesions, such as periventricular leukomalacia; localized cortical necrosis; multicystic encephalomalacia; and basal ganglia injury (Krägeloh-Mann et al. 1995).

There are some contradictory results in the fields of epileptology and mental retardation, but the convergence of findings is impressive. This contrasts with the discrepant findings from many neuroimaging studies of childhood psychiatric disorders (see Lord & Bailey, Chapter 38). As the field matures, current methodological difficulties are likely to be overcome, but it is too soon to gauge the future role of neuroimaging in routine clinical practice. One of the aims of this work is to identify the impaired neural systems underlying complex neurodevelopmental disorders. The obstacles are the weaknesses of current explanatory models (which are largely derived from animal work and lesion studies in adults) and the limited availability of histopathological and post-mortem neurochemistry data. These findings are necessary to link genetic and molecular biology findings with the macroscopic phenomena visualized by structural and functional imaging.

Findings from several disorders illustrate the range of conceptual problems. Measuring the size of brain structures in vivo has a long history. Recently, for instance, the caudate nucleus has been the subject of scrutiny in ADHD (Filipek 1999; Overmeyer & Taylor, in press). Nevertheless, there are no post-mortem studies against which to judge these findings, and although these abnormal frontostriatal interactions are considered to partly underlie some behavioural abnormalities in ADHD, there is no clear consensus about whether the effects lateralize, and if so to which side. Measures of planum temporale asymmetry in individuals with specific reading difficulties are similarly contradictory (Bailey & Cox 1996; Filipek 1999) and the rationale underlying this measure is uncertain when nearly 40% of the general population do not show the supposedly 'normal' pattern of asymmetry. Even in autism (for which there is some limited post-mortem data), contradictions abound. Thus, claims of specific hypoplasia of cerebellar vermal lobules VI and VII (Courchesne *et al.* 1988) have not been consistently replicated (reviewed by Filipek 1999). Also the predicted macroscopic correlates of increased cell packing density in the hippocampus and related structures (Kemper & Bauman 1998) are unclear, which complicates the interpretation of unchanged (Filipek *et al.* 1992; Piven *et al.* 1998), decreased (Aylward *et al.* 1999) and increased (Abell *et al.* 1999; Howard *et al.* 2000) measures of medial temporal structures. Although establishing age-appropriate norms for human brain development (Giedd *et al.* 1996) should aid interpretation, the underlying conceptual problem will persist: there is not a universal relationship between size of a structure and either pathology or function.

In the longer term, functional imaging is likely to transform our understanding of the brain basis of developmental psychopathology. There may also be scope for clinical applications: e.g. in complex cases in which symptomatology is compatible with several different diagnoses; when there are also severe psychosocial stressors; in clinically mild cases who may pass standard cognitive tests using alternative neural pathways; and in monitoring treatment response. For disorders such as hyperactivity, in which there are strong psychopharmacological effects, it is already possible to visualize differential responses to medication during functional imaging (Vaidya *et al.* 1998). However, it seems probable that most psychiatric disorders arise on the basis of several cognitive (and emotional) deficits, and clinically specific diagnostic approaches will likely require a heterogeneous functional test battery. Clinical utility will also demand considerable standardization of tasks, stimulus presentation parameters and data analysis.

There are also conceptual challenges in the interpretation of functional imaging data. Cognitive studies using PET and fMRI rely upon subtraction paradigms in which brain activity generated by a control task is subtracted from that evoked by the task of interest. The resulting image is a difference image, not a response to a physically presented stimulus. If the underlying disorder involves the use of qualitatively different processing strategies (Rubia *et al.* 1999), unusual processing of control stimuli will be most evident if there is also a baseline task in addition to control and probe tasks. Subtraction approaches also assume that cognition is serial and non-interactive. Cognitive processes that are interactive or which are similar in their anatomical distribution but differ in their order or time course will not be properly differentiated using subtraction methodology (see Sergent *et al.* 1992, for a fuller discussion of this issue). Consequently, complementary methods with adequate temporal resolution, such as EEG or MEG, are also necessary. However, all of these approaches assess function at the level of large populations of neurones which ultimately constrains the

neurophysiological models that can be tested. A final challenge is to understand the developmental processes that lead to abnormal localization of activation in older children and adolescents. Whereas such abnormalities may represent localized dysfunction, they may also be a consequence of abnormal input, possibly earlier in development, and while appropriate tasks may identify current input abnormalities, identifying developmental precursors will ultimately require studies of infants and young children.

Appendix 1

Computerized tomography (CT)

Computerized tomography is an X-ray technique that isolates a plane of interest in the subject by blurring out adjacent planes. It produces a series of sectional images, usually transverse to the long axis of the subject, which reflect the radiographic density of tissues in the plane of sectioning. The technique was a major innovation in modern imaging and, although now largely superseded by MRI, it remains the modality of choice for visualizing calcification and the skull.

Positron emission tomography (PET) and single photon emission computed tomography (SPECT)

Positron emission tomography and single photon emission computed tomography are techniques in which radioactive isotopes linked to tracers cross the blood–brain barrier and emit gamma radiation while decaying. PET uses isotopes of carbon, nitrogen, oxygen and fluorine which emit a positron when they decay. After travelling a few millimetres the positron collides with an electron, producing two high energy photons which travel in opposite directions. By detecting both photons outside the head their origin can be pinpointed to a within slice resolution of 5–6 mm. Depending on the property of the tracer to which the isotope is attached, it is possible to calculate increases in absolute regional cerebral blood flow or glucose metabolism associated with neuronal activity, or image neurotransmitter synthesis, the distribution and occupancy of receptors and the density of neurotransmitter transporters. The various isotopes have short half-lives necessitating manufacture on-site using expensive cyclotron or particle accelerators. The short half-life of the isotopes enables several activation studies to be conducted during one scanning session, with the administration of a series of cognitive tasks and the 'subtraction' of one image from another to identify statistically significant brain activity associated with cognitive components.

A variety of statistical techniques are available for analysing data produced by brain activation studies, but statistical parametric mapping (SPM) using the general linear model (Friston *et al.* 1995) is particularly widely used. In order to compare groups of subjects, regions of interest can be delineated, or the functional images can be co-registered with structural images or plastically transformed (Friston *et al.* 1995) onto a standard brain shape (Talairach *et al.* 1967).

SPECT uses radioactive isotopes such as iodine and technetium, which have a comparatively long half-life (thus not requiring expensive on-site generation) and hence involve greater radiation exposure. They decay with emission of a single photon that has relatively low energy and thus the technique is less sensitive than PET. Although only relative blood flow and semi-quantitative indices of receptor binding can be calculated, these will be adequate for many purposes. The exposure to ionizing radiation largely precludes the use of PET and SPECT in children for research into the brain correlates of cognition.

Magnetic resonance imaging (MRI)

Magnetic resonance imaging is based on the capacity of organic tissue placed in a magnetic field to absorb energy from radio waves and then re-emit this energy in proportion to the mobile hydrogen ion concentration (Wolbarst 1993). The magnetic resonance image is a map of signal strengths across a defined section of tissue and the signals are influenced by the tissue environment in which the protons are situated. The technique does not involve ionizing radiation and there is a very wide choice in scanning parameters, which can emphasize the contrast between different tissue types, with new approaches being developed continuously. Diffusion tensor imaging also has the potential to identify the direction and confluence of white matter tracts (Jones *et al.* 1999). Unlike CT, MR images can be generated in any plane and spatial resolution is excellent.

Functional magnetic resonance imaging (fMRI)

Functional MRI refers to a fast imaging method for indirectly visualizing regional changes in brain activity by detecting local haemodynamic changes. Following brain activation there is a disproportionate increase in blood flow resulting in increased oxygenation of venous blood compared with the resting state. The increased MRI signal from oxygenated blood compared to the inactive state can be visualized by appropriate choice of pulse sequence (blood oxygen level dependent effect, BOLD; Kwong *et al.* 1992; Ogawa *et al.* 1992). Signal intensity is measured in arbitrary units and it is usually necessary to compare two activation states with each other. The haemodynamic response lags behind brain activity and this delay is taken into account in data analysis.

Most published studies have presented alternating blocks of contrasting stimuli and correlated measured signal intensity from each point (voxel) in the image with the time course of stimulus presentation to detect statistically significant differences in activation between the two stimulus types. It is now possible to interleave different types of stimuli and analyse the correlation between single trials and blood flow changes (event-related fMRI; Buckner *et al.* 1996) allowing new classes of behavioural paradigms to be tested.

Other methods of visualizing haemodynamic changes are also available. fMRI data can be combined with structural MRI images to provide excellent localization of activation and fMRI data analysis techniques have built upon those developed to analyse PET data. Regardless of imaging sequence, the main practical problems are minimizing subject movement during the experiment and correction for any movements during statistical analysis. The lag between neuronal activity and haemodynamic response ultimately constrains the time resolution of fMRI approaches, but this is a rapidly developing field with continuing improvements in temporal resolution and quantification of data.

Magnetic resonance spectroscopy (MRS)

Magnetic resonance spectroscopy is a method for detecting the presence and amount of different molecules in tissue, either *in vivo* or *in vitro*. The technique detects differences in how atoms with an odd number of protons (e.g. hydrogen, carbon, fluorine, sodium, potassium, phosphorus) resonate in a magnetic resonance scanner. The resonant frequency is affected by the local magnetic field surrounding the nucleus (the chemical shift) and thus the same atom in different chemical compounds produces a distinctive peak in a frequency spectrum. In child psychiatry most interest has focused on the study of membrane phospholipids and the levels of N-acetylaspartate (NAA), a compound largely found in neurones.

Electroencephalopathy (EEG) and magnetoencephalography (MEG)

Electroencephalopathy and magnetoencephalography are the only currently available techniques that directly detect the activity of populations of neurones with millisecond time resolution. The primary source of signals are postsynaptic potentials in activated cortical dendrites that are generally orthogonal to the cortical surface. EEG detects the induced extracellular volume currents, regardless of their orientation, which spread passively throughout the head. MEG detects the minute magnetic fields that wrap around the currents flowing along dendrites, but only neurones in sulci (or whose dendritic fields are parallel to the skull) produce a magnetic field detectable outside the head.

The chief advantages of MEG over EEG are the lack of signal distortion by the skull and scalp and the ability to model the underlying current source. In addition to 'resting' brain activity, the potentials induced by physical stimuli or cognitive tasks can be recorded to permit computation of the underlying neural sources with no requirement for subtraction methods. The data from EEG and MEG can be combined with anatomical data from structural MRI to constraint calculations of underlying neural generators.

References

Abell, F., Krams, M., Ashburner, J. *et al.* (1999) The neuroanatomy of autism: a voxel based whole brain analysis of structural scans. *Neuroreport*, **10**, 1647–1651.

Abramsky, L. & Chapple, J. (1997) 47,XXY (Klinefelter syndrome) and 46,XYY: estimated rates of and indication for postnatal diagnosis with implications for prenatal counselling. *Prenatal Diagnosis*, 17, 363–368.

Albonico, M., Crompton, D.W.T. & Savioli, L. (1999) Control strategies for human intestinal nematode infections. *Advances in Parasitology*, 42, 277–341.

Amir, R.E., Van den Veyver, I.B., Wan, M., Tran, C.Q., Francke, U. & Zoghbi, H.Y. (1999) Rett syndrome is caused by mutations in X-linked MECP2, encoding methyl-CpG-binding protein 2. *Nature Genetics*, 23, 185–188.

Aylward, E.H., Minshew, N.J., Goldstein, G. *et al.* (1999) MRI volumes of amygdala and hippocampus in non-mentally retarded autistic adolescents and adults. *Neurology*, 53, 2145–2150.

Bacon, B.R. & Schilsky, M.L. (1999) New knowledge of genetic pathogenesis of hemochromatosis and Wilson's disease. *Advances in Internal Medicine*, 44, 91–116.

Bailey, A.J. & Cox, T. (1996) Brain imaging in child and developmental psychiatry. In: *Brain Imaging in Psychiatry* (eds S. Lewis & N. Higgins), pp. 301–315. Blackwell Science, Oxford.

Bailey, A., Luthert, P., Bolton, P., Le Couteur, A., Rutter, M. & Harding, B. (1993) Autism and megalencephaly (Letter). *Lancet*, 341, 1225–1226.

Barsky, A.J. & Borus, J.F. (1999) Functional somatic syndromes. *Annals of Internal Medicine*, 130, 910–921.

Barton, M. & Volkmar, F. (1998) How commonly are known medical conditions associated with autism? *Journal of Autism and Developmental Disorders*, 28, 273–278.

Bassett, A.S. & Chow, E.W.C. (1999) 22q11 deletion syndrome: a genetic subtype of schizophrenia. *Biological Psychiatry*, 46, 882–891.

Battaglia, A., Bianchini, E. & Carey, J.C. (1999) Diagnostic yield of the comprehensive assessment of developmental delay/mental retardation. *American Journal of Medical Genetics*, 1, 60–66.

Becker, A.E., Grinspoon, S.K., Klibanksi, A. & Herzog, D.B. (1999) Eating disorders. *New England Journal of Medicine*, 340, 1092–1098.

Belcher, M.E. & Shinitzky, H.E. (1998) Substance abuse in children. *Archives of Paediatrics and Adolescent Medicine*, 152, 952–960.

Bellugi, U., Lichtenberger, E., Mills, D., Galaburda, A. & Korenberg, J.R. (1999) Bridging cognition, the brain and molecular genetics: evidence from Williams syndrome. *Research News*, 22, 197–207.

Bookheimer, S.Y., Dapretto, M. & Karmarkar, U. (1999) Functional MRI in children with epilepsy. *Developmental Neuroscience*, 21, 191–199.

Brodtkorb, E., Nilsen, G., Smevik, O. & Rinck, P.A. (1992) Epilepsy and anomalies of neuronal migration: MRI and clinical aspects. *Acta Neurologica Scandanavica*, 86, 24–32.

Buckner, R.L., Bandettini, P.A., O'Craven, K.M. *et al.* (1996) Detection of cortical activation during averaged single trials of a cognitive task using functional magnetic resonance imaging. *Proceedings of the National Academy of Science*, 93, 14878–14883.

Bull, P.C., Thomas, G.R. & Rommens, J.M. (1993) The Wilson disease gene is a putative copper transporting P-type ATPase similar to the Menkes gene. *Nature Genetics*, 5, 327–337.

Cardon, L.R., Smith, S.D., Fulker, D.W., Kimberling, W.J., Pennington, B.F. & DeFries, J.C. (1994) Quantitative trait locus for reading disability on chromosome 6. *Science*, 266, 276–279.

Chandrasekaran, R., Goswami, U., Sivakumar, V. & Chitralekha, J. (1994) Hysterical neurosis: a follow-up study. *Acta Psychiatrica Scandanavica*, 89, 78–80.

Collinge, J. (1999) Variant Creutzfeldt–Jakob Disease. *Lancet*, 354, 317–323.

Cook, M.J. (1994) Mesial temporal sclerosis and volumetric investigations. *Acta Neurologica Scandanavica*, 152, 109–114.

Cook, E.H. Jr, Stein, M.A., Krasowski, M.D. *et al.* (1995) Association of attention-deficit disorder and the dopamine transporter gene. *American Journal of Human Genetics*, 56, 993–998.

Corbett, J., Harris, R., Taylor, E. & Trimble, M. (1977) Progressive disintegrative psychosis of childhood. *Journal of Child Psychology and Psychiatry*, 18, 211–219.

Courchesne, E., Yeung-Courchesene, R., Press, G., Hesselink, J.R. & Jernigan, T.L. (1988) Hypoplasia of cerebellar vermal lobules Vl and Vll in autism. *New England Journal of Medicine*, 318, 1349–1354.

Cross, J.H., Jackson, G.D., Neville, B.G.R. *et al.* (1993) Early detection of abnormalities in partial epilepsy using magnetic resonance. *Archives of Disease in Childhood*, 69, 104–109.

Cross, J.H., Gordon, I., Connelly, A. *et al.* (1997) Interictal $^{99}Tc^m$ HMPAO SPECT and ^{1}H MRS in children with temporal lobe epilepsy. *Epilepsia*, 38, 338–345.

Curry, C.J., Sandhu, A., Frutos, L. & Wells, R. (1996) Diagnostic yield of genetic evaluations in developmental delay/mental retardation. *Clinical Research*, 44, 130A.

Curry, C.J., Stevenson, R.E., Aughton, D. *et al.* (1997) Evaluation of mental retardation: recommendations of a consensus conference. *American Journal of Medical Genetics*, 72, 468–477.

Cuthbert, J.A. (1998) Wilson's disease: update of a systemic disorder with protean manifestations. *Gastrointestinal Disorders and Systemic Disease*, 27, 655–681.

D'Souza, S.W., Rivlin, E., Cadman, J., Richards, B., Buck, P. & Lieberman, B.A. (1997) Children conceived by *in vitro* fertilisation after fresh embryo transfer. *Archives of Disease in Childhood*, 76, F70–F74.

De Vries, B.B.A., Halley, R.J.J., Oostra, B.A. & Niermeijer, M.F. (1998) The Fragile X syndrome. *American Journal of Medical Genetics*, 35, 579–589.

Delhanty, J.D.A., Harper, J.C., Ao, A., Handyside, A.H. & Winston, R.M.L. (1997) Multicolour FISH detects frequent chromosomal mosaicism and chaotic division in normal preimplantation embryos from fertile patients. *Human Genetics*, 99, 755–760.

Edgeworth, J., Bullock, P., Bailey, A., Gallagher, A. & Crouchman, M. (1996) Why are childhood brain tumours still being missed? *Archives of Disease in Childhood*, 74, 148–151.

Ekong, R. & Wolfe, J. (1998) Advances in fluorescent *in situ* hybridisation. *Analytical Biotechnology*, 9, 19–24.

Ernst, M. & Rumsey, J.M., eds (2000) *Functional Neuroimaging in Child Psychiatry*. Cambridge University Press, Cambridge.

Filipek, P.A. (1999) Neuroimaging in the developmental disorders: the state of the science. *Journal of Child Psychology and Psychiatry*, 40, 113–128.

Filipek, P.A., Richelme, C., Kennedy, D.N. *et al.* (1992) Morphometric analysis of the brain in developmental language disorder and autism (Abstract). *Annals of Neurology*, 32, 475.

Fisher, S.E., Vargha-Khadem, F., Watkins, K.E., Monaco, A.P. & Pembrey, M.E. (1998) Localisation of a gene implicated in a severe speech and language disorder. *Nature Genetics*, 18, 168–170.

Fisher, S.E., Marlow, A.J., Lamb, J. *et al.* (1999) A quantitative-trait locus on chromosome 6p influences different aspects of developmental dyslexia. *American Journal of Human Genetics*, 64, 146–156.

Fombonne, E. (1999) The epidemiology of autism: a review. *Psychological Medicine*, 29, 769–786.

Frackowiak, R.S.J., Friston, K.J., Frith, C.D. *et al.*, eds (1997) *Human Brain Function*. Academic Press, London.

Friedrich, W.N. & Schafer, L.C. (1995) Somatic symptoms in sexually abused children. *Journal of Paediatric Psychology*, 20, 661–670.

Friston, K.J., Holmes, A.P., Worsley, K.J., Poline, J.P., Frith, C.D. & Frackowiak, R.S.J. (1995) Statistical parametric maps in functional imaging: a general linear approach. *Human Brain Mapping*, **2**, 189–210.

Fritz, G.K., Fritsch, S. & Hagino, O. (1997) Somatoform disorders in children and adolescents: a review of the past 10 years. *Journal of the American Acadamy of Child and Adolescent Psychiatry*, **36**, 1329–1338.

Gadian, D.G., Connelly, A., Duncan, J.S. *et al.* (1994) ^{1}H magnetic resonance spectroscopy in the investigation of intractable epilepsy. *Acta Neurologica Scandinavica*, **152**, 116–121.

Gaillard, W.D., White, S., Malow, B. *et al.* (1995) FDG-PET in children and adolescents with partial seizures: role in epilepsy surgery evaluation. *Epilepsy*, **20**, 77–84.

Garvey, M.A., Giedd, J. & Swedo, S.E. (1998) PANDAS: the search for environmental triggers of paediatric neuropsychiatric disorders—lessons from rheumatic fever. *Journal of Child Neurology*, **13**, 413–423.

Gasser, T. (1997) Advances in genetics of movement disorder: implications for molecular diagnosis. *Journal of Neurology*, **244**, 341–348.

Giaquinto, C., Ruga, E., Giacomet, V., Rampon, O. & D'Elia, R. (1998) HIV: mother-to-child transmission, current knowledge and on-going studies. *International Journal of Gynaecology and Obstetrics*, **63**, S161–S165.

Giedd, J.N., Vaituzis, A.C., Rajapakse, J.C. *et al.* (1996) Quantitative MRI of the temporal lobe, amygdala and hippocampus in normal human development: ages 4–18. *Journal of Comparative Neurology*, **366**, 223–230.

Gorlin, R.J., Cohen, M.M. & Levin, L.S. (1990) *Syndromes of the Head and Neck. Oxford Monographs on Medical Genetics No 19* (3rd edn). Oxford University Press, Oxford.

Grigorenko, E.L., Wood, F.B., Meyer, M.S. *et al.* (1997) Susceptibility loci for distinct components of developmental dyslexia on chromosomes 6 and 15. *American Journal of Human Genetics*, **60**, 27–39.

Gringras, P. (1998) Choice of medical investigations for developmental delay: a questionnaire survey. *Child Care Health and Development*, **24**, 267–276.

Grön, M., Pietila, K. & Alvesalo, L. (1997) The craniofacial complex in 47,XYY males. *Archives of Oral Biology*, **42**, 579–586.

Hack, M. & Fanaroff, A.A. (1999) Outcomes of children of extremely low birth weight and gestational age in the 1990s. *Early Human Development*, **53**, 193–218.

Hall, J.G., Froster-Iskenius, U.G. & Allanson, J.E. (1989) *Handbook of Normal Physical Measurements*. Oxford Medical Publications, Oxford.

Hammerschlag, M.R. (1998) Sexually transmitted diseases in sexually abused children: medical and legal implications. *Sexually Transmitted Infections*, **74**, 167–174.

Hawton, K., Fagg, J., Platt, S. & Hawkins, M. (1993) Factors associated with suicide after parasuicide in young people. *British Medical Journal*, **306**, 1641–1644.

Hill, A.E. & Rosenbloom, L. (1986) Disintegrative psychosis of childhood: teenage follow-up. *Developmental Medicine and Child Neurology*, **28**, 34–40.

Hostetter, M.K. (1999) Infectious diseases in internationally adopted children: findings in children from China, Russia and Eastern Europe. *Advances in Paediatric Infectious Diseases*, **14**, 147–161.

Huntington's Disease Collaborative Research Group (1993) A novel gene containing a trinucleotide repeat that is expanded and unstable on Huntington's disease chromosomes. *Cell*, **72**, 971–983.

Howard, M.A., Cowell, P.E., Boucher, J. *et al.* (2000) Convergent neuroanatomical and behavioural evidence of an amygdala hypothesis of autism. *NeuroReport*, **11**, 2931–2935.

The International Molecular Genetics Study of Autism Consortium. A full genome screen for autism with evidence for linkage to a region on chromosome 7q. *Human Molecular Genetics* (1998) **7**, 571–578.

Jaudes, P.K., Ekwo, E. & Van Voorhis, J. (1995) Association of drug abuse and child abuse. *Child Abuse and Neglect*, **19**, 1065–1075.

Jones, D.K., Simmons, A., Williams, S.C.R. & Horsfield, M.A. (1999) Non-invasive assessment of axonal fiber connectivity in the human brain via diffusion tensor MRI. *Magnetic Resonance Medicine*, **42**, 37–41.

Jones, K.L. (1997) *Smith's Recognisable Patterns of Human Malformation*, 5th edn. W.B. Saunders, Philadelphia.

Jordan, K.M., Landis, D.A., Downey, M.C., Osterman, S.L., Thurm, A.E. & Jason, L.A. (1998) Chronic fatigue syndrome in children and adolescents: a review. *Journal of Adolescent Health*, **22**, 4–18.

Kanner, L. (1943) Autistic disturbances of affective contact. *Nervous Child*, **2**, 217–250.

Kaufmann, W.E. & Reiss, A.L. (1999) Molecular and cellular genetics of fragile X syndrome. *American Journal of Medical Genetics (Neuropyschiatric Genetics)*, **88**, 11–24.

Kemper, T.L. & Bauman, M. (1998) Neuropathology of infantile autism. *Journal of Neuropathology and Experimental Neurology*, **57**, 645–652.

Khan, N.L. & Wood, N.W. (1999) Prader–Willi and Angelman syndromes: update on genetic mechanisms and diagnostic complexities. *Current Opinion in Neurology*, **12**, 149–154.

Kinzl, J.F., Traweger, C. & Beibl, W. (1995) Family background and sexual abuse associated with somatization. *Psychotherapy and Psychosomatics*, **64**, 82–87.

Knight, S.J.L., Horsley, S.W., Regan, R. *et al.* (1997) Developmental and clinical application of an innovative fluorescence *in situ* hybridisation technique which detects submicroscopic rearrangements involving telomeres. *European Journal of Human Genetics*, **5**, 1–8.

Knight, S.J.L., Regan, R., Nicod, A. *et al.* (1999) Subtle chromosomal re-arrangements in children with unexplained mental retardation. *Lancet*, **354**, 1676–1681.

Krägeloh-Mann, I., Petersen, D., Hagberg, G., Vollmer, B., Hagberg, B. & Michaelis, R. (1995) Bilateral spastic cerebral palsy: MRI pathology and origin—analysis from a representative series of 56 cases. *Developmental Medicine and Child Neurology*, **37**, 379–397.

Kuzniecky, R., Andermann, F., Guerrini, R. & CBPS Multicenter Collaborative Study (1993) Congenital bilateral perisylvian syndrome: study of 31 patients. *Lancet*, **341**, 601–612.

Kwong, K.K., Belliveau, J.W., Chesler, D.A. *et al.* (1992) Dynamic magnetic resonance imaging of human brain activity during primary sensory stimulation. *Proceedings of National Academy of Sciences, USA*, **89**, 5675–5679.

LaHoste, G.J., Swanson, J.M., Wigal, S.B. *et al.* (1996) Dopamine D4 receptor gene polymorphism is associated with attention deficit hyperactivity disorder. *Molecular Psychiatry*, **1**, 121–124.

Lai, C.S., Fisher, S.E., Hurst, J.A. *et al.* (2000) The SPCH1 region on human 7q31: genomic characterization of the critical interval and localization of translocations associated with speech and language disorder. *American Journal of Human Genetics*, **67**, 357–368.

Lamb, J., Moore, J., Bailey, A. & Monaco, A. (2000) Autism: recent molecular genetic advances. *Human Molecular Genetics*, **9**, 861–868.

Lewis, S. & Higgins, N. (1996) *Brain Imaging in Psychiatry*, 1st edn. Blackwell Science, Oxford.

Lishman, W.A. (1998) *Organic Psychiatry: the Psychological Consequences of Cerebral Disorder*, 3rd edn. Blackwell Science, Oxford.

Loebstein, R. & Koren, G. (1997) Pregnancy outcome and neurodevelopment of children exposed in utero to psychoactive drugs: the Motherisk experience. *Journal of Psychiatry and Neuroscience*, **22**, 192–196.

Lorber, J. & Priestley, B.L. (1981) Children with large heads: a practical approach to diagnosis. *Developmental Medicine and Child Neurology*, **23**, 494–504.

Lorenz, J.M., Wooliever, D.E., Jetton, J.R. & Paneth, N. (1998) Quantitative review of mortality and developmental disability in extremely premature newborns. *Archives of Paediatric and Adolescent Medicine*, **152**, 425–435.

Maestrini, E., Paul, A., Monaco, A. & Bailey, A. (2000) Identifying autism susceptibility genes. *Neuron*, **28**, 19–24.

Majnemer, A. & Shevell, M.I. (1995) Diagnostic yield of the neurologic assessment of the developmentally delayed child. *Journal of Paediatrics*, **127**, 193–199.

Margolis, R.L., McInnis, M.G., Rosenblatt, A. & Ross, C.A. (1999) Trinucleotide repeat expansion and neuropsychiatric disease. *Archives of General Psychiatry*, **56**, 1019–1031.

MacLennan, A. (1999) A template for defining a casual relation between acute intrapartum events and cerebral palsy: international consensus statement. *British Medical Journal*, **319**, 1054–1059.

Milberger, S., Faraone, S.V., Biederman, J., Chu, M. & Feighner, J.A. (1999) Substance use disorders in high-risk adolescent offspring. *American Journal of Addiction*, **8**, 211–219.

Moise, J., Laor, A., Armon, Y., Gur, I. & Gale, R. (1998) The outcome of twin pregnancies after IVF. *Human Reproduction*, **13**, 1702–1705.

Morioka, T., Nishio, S., Ishibashi, H. *et al.* (1999) Intrinsic epileptogenicity of focal cortical dysplasia as revealed by magnetoencephalography and electrocorticography. *Epilepsy Research*, **33**, 177–187.

Morrell, F., Whisler, W.W., Smith, M.C. *et al.* (1995) Landau–Kleffner syndrome: treatment with subpial intracortical transection. *Brain*, **118**, 1529–1546.

Munne, S., Magli, C., Cohen, J. *et al.* (1999) Positive outcome after preimplantation diagnosis of aneuploidy in human embryos. *Human Reproduction*, **14**, 2191–2199.

Muzik, O., da Silva, E.A., Juhasz, C. *et al.* (2000) Intracranial EEG versus flumazenil and glucose PET in children with extratemporal lobe epilepsy. *Neurology*, **54**, 171–179.

Myrianthopoulos, N.C. (1976) Congenital malformations in twins. *Acta Geneticae Medicae et Gemellologiae*, **24**, 331.

North, K.N. (1998) Neurofibromatosis in childhood. *Seminars in Paediatric Neurology*, **5**, 231–242.

Ogawa, S., Tank, D.W., Menon, R. *et al.* (1992) Intrinsic signal changes accompanying sensory stimulation: functional brain mapping with magnetic resonance imaging. *Proceedings of National Academy of Sciences, USA*, **89**, 5951–5955.

Oleske, J.M. & Czarniecki, L. (1999) Continuum of palliative care: lessons from caring for children infected with HIV-1. *Lancet*, **354**, 1287–1290.

Orrico, A., Lam, C., Galli, L. *et al.* (2000) MECP2 mutation in male patients with non-specific X linked mental retardation. *FEBS Letters*, **481**, 285–288.

Orrison, W.W., Jr., Lewine, J.D., Sanders, J.A. & Hartshorne, M.F. (1995) *Functional Brain Imaging*. Mosby, St. Louis.

Overmeyer, S. & Taylor, E. (in press) Neuroimaging in Hyperkinetic Children and Adults: An Overview. *Paediatric Rehabilitation*.

Paetau, R., Granström, M.-L., Blomstedt, G., Jousmaki, V., Korkman, M. & Liukkonen, E. (1999) Magnetoencephalography in presurgical evaluation of children with the Landau–Kleffner Syndrome. *Epilepsia*, **40**, 326–335.

Palmini, A., Andermann, F., Olivier, A. *et al.* (1991) Focal neuronal migration disorders and intractable partial epilepsy: a study of 30 patients. *Annals of Neurology*, **30**, 741–749.

Palmini, A., Gambardella, A., Andermann, F. *et al.* (1994) Operative strategies for patients with cortical dysplastic lesions and intractable epilepsy. *Epilepsia*, **35**, S57–S71.

Palmini, A., Gambardella, A., Andermann, F. *et al.* (1995) Intrinsic epileptogenicity of human dysplastic cortex as suggested by corticography and surgical results. *Annals of Neurology*, **37**, 476–486.

Patrat, C., Wolf, J., Epelboin, S. *et al.* (1999) Pregnancies, growth and development of children conceived by subzonal injection of spermatozoa. *European Society of Human Reproduction and Embryology*, **14**, 2404–2410.

Petroff, O.A.C., Behar, K.L. & Rothman, D.L. (1999) New NMR measurement in epilepsy: measuring brain GABA in patients with complex partial seizures. *Advances in Neurology*, **79**, 939–945.

Petrukhin, K., Lutsenko, S., Chernov, I. *et al.* (1994) Characterization of the Wilson disease gene encoding a P-type copper transporting ATPase: genomic organisation, alternative splicing, and structure function prediction. *Human Molecular Genetics*, **3**, 1647–1656.

Petterson, B., Blair, E., Watson, L. & Stanley, F. (1998) Adverse outcome after multiple pregnancy. *Baillière's Clinical Obstetrics and Gynaecology*, **12**, 1–17.

Piven, J., Bailey, J., Ranson, B.J. & Arndt, S. (1998) No difference in hippocampus volume detected on magnetic resonance imaging in autistic individuals. *Journal of Autism and Developmental Disorders*, **28**, 105–110.

Rogers, S. & DiLalla, D. (1990) Age of symptom onset in young children with pervasive developmental disorders. *Journal of the American Academy of Child and Adolescent Psychiatry*, **29**, 863–872.

Rome, E.S. (1999) Sexually transmitted diseases: testing and treating. *Adolescent Medicine: State of the Art Reviews*, **10**, 231–241.

Roos, K.L. (1998) Pearls and pitfalls in the diagnosis and management of central nervous system infectious diseases. *Seminars in Neurology*, **18**, 185–196.

Rovet, J., Netley, C., Keenan, M., Bailey, J. & Stewart, D. (1996) The psychoeducational profile of boys with Klinefelter syndrome. *Journal of Learning Disabilities*, **29**, 180–196.

Rubia, K., Overmeyer, S., Taylor, E. *et al.* (1999) Hypofrontality in attention deficit hyperactivity disorder during higher-order motor control: a study with functional MRI. *American Journal of Psychiatry*, **156**, 891–896.

Rutter, M., Bailey, A., Bolton, P. & Le Couteur, A. (1994) Autism and known medical conditions: myth and substance. *Journal of Child Psychology and Psychiatry*, **35**, 311–322.

Rutter, M., Silberg, J., O'Connor, T. & Simonoff, E. (1999) Genetics and child psychiatry. I. Advances in quantitative and molecular genetics. *Journal of Child Psychology and Psychiatry*, **40**, 3–18.

Sampson, P.D., Streissguth, A.P., Bookstein, F.L. *et al.* (1997) Incidence of fetal alcohol syndrome and prevalence of alcohol-related neurodevelopment disorder. *Teratology*, **56**, 317–326.

Santosh, P.J. (2000) Neuroimaging in child and adolescent psychiatric disorders. *Archives of Disease in Childhood*, **82**, 412–419.

Saugier-Veber, P., Martin, C., Le Meur, N. *et al.* (1998) Identification of novel L1CAM mutations using fluorescence-assisted mismatch analysis. *Human Mutation*, **12**, 259–266.

Schaefer, M. & Gitlin, J.D. (1999) Genetic disorders of membrane transport. IV. Wilson's disease and Menkes disease. *American Journal of Physiology*, **276**, G311–G314.

Schröck, E., Veldman, T., Padilla-Nash, H. *et al.* (1997) Spectral karyotyping refines cytogenetic diagnostics of constitutional chromosomal abnormalities. *Human Genetics*, **101**, 255–262.

Sergent, J., Zuck, E., Levesque, M. & MacDonald, B. (1992) Positron emission tomography study of letter and object processing: empirical findings and methodological considerations. *Cerebral Cortex*, 2, 68–80.

Shahbazian, M.D. & Zoghbi, H.Y. (2001) Molecular genetics of Rett syndrome and clinical spectrum of MECP2 mutations. *Current Opinion in Neurology*, 14, 171–176.

Sisodiya, S.M. & Free, S.L. (1997) Disproportion of cerebral surface areas and volumes in cerebral dysgenesis: MRI-based evidence for connectional abnormalities. *Brain*, 120, 271–281.

Skjeldal, O.H., Sponheim, E., Ganes, T., Jellum, E. & Bakke, S. (1998) Childhood autism: the need for physical investigations. *Brain Development*, 20, 227–233.

van Slegtenhorst, M., de Hoogt, R. Hermans, C. *et al.* (1997) Identification of the tuberous sclerosis Gene TSC1 on chromosome 9q34. *Science*, 277, 805–808.

Smith, K.D., Kemp, S., Braiterman, L.T. *et al.* (1999) X-linked adrenoleukodystrophy: genes, mutations, and phenotypes. *Neurochemical Research*, 24, 521–535.

Smyth, C.M. & Bremner, W.J. (1998) Klienefelter syndrome. *Archives of Internal Medicine*, 158, 1309–1314.

Sobel, D.F., Manug Aung & Horoshi Otsubo, Smith, M.C. (2000) Magnetoencephalography in children with Landau–Kleffner Syndrome and acquired epileptic aphasia. *American Journal of Neuroradiology*, 21, 301–307.

Spreafico, R., Battaglia, G., Arcelli, P. *et al.* (1998) Cortical dysplasia: an immunocytochemical study of three patients. *Neurology*, 50, 27–36.

Stapleton, S.R., Kiriakopoulos, E., Mikulis, D. *et al.* (1997) Combined utility of functional MRI, cortical mapping and frameless stereotaxy in the resection of lesions in eloquent areas of brain in children. *Paediatric Neurosurgery*, 26, 8–82.

States, L.J., Zimmerman, A. & Rutstein, R.M. (1997) Imaging of paediatric central nervous system HIV infection. *Neuroimaging Clinics of North America*, 7, 321–339.

Talairach, J., Szikla, G., Tournoux, P. *et al.* (1967) *Atlas d'Anatomie Stereotaxique Du Telecephale*. Masson, Paris.

Tanzi, R.E., Petrukhin, K., Chernov, I. *et al.* (1993) The Wilson disease gene is a copper transporting ATPase with homology to the Menkes Disease Gene. *Nature Genetics*, 5, 344–350.

Thatai, D. & Turi, Z.G. (1999) Current guidelines for the treatment of patients with rheumatic fever. *Drugs*, 57, 545–555.

Tichonova, L., Borisenko, K., Ward, H., Meheus, A., Gromyko, A. & Renton, A. (1997) Epidemics of syphilis in the Russian federation: trends, origins and priorities for control. *Lancet*, 350, 210–211.

Trottier, Y., Biancalana, V. & Mandel, J.L. (1994) Instability of CAG repeats in Huntington's disease: relation to parental transmission and age of onset. *Journal of Medical Genetics*, 31, 377–382.

Truwit, C.L., Barkovich, A.J., Koch, T.K. & Ferreiro, D.M. (1992) Cerebral palsy: MR findings in 40 patients. *American Journal of Neuroradiology*, 13, 67–78.

Turner, M., Barnby, G. & Bailey, A. (2000) Genetic clues to the biological basis of autism. *Molecular Medicine Today*, 6, 238–244.

Vaidya, C.J., Austin, G., Kirkorian, G. *et al.* (1998) Selective effects of methylphenidate in attention deficit hyperactivity disorder: a functional magnetic resonance study. *Neurology*, 95, 14494–14499.

Weinberg, N.Z. (1997) Cognitive and behavioural deficits associated with parental alcohol use. *Journal of the American Academy of Child and Adolescent Psychiatry*, 36, 1177–1186.

Will, R.G., Stewart, G., Zeidler, M., Macleod, M.A. & Knight, R.S.G. (1999) Psychiatric features of new variant Creutzfeldt–Jakob disease. *Psychiatric Bulletin*, 23, 264–267.

Will, R.G., Zeidler, M., Stewart, G.E. *et al.* (2000) Diagnosis of new variant Creutzfeldt–Jakob disease. *Annals of Neurology*, 47, 575–582.

Winter, R.M. & Baraitser, M. (2000) *The London Dysmorphology Database* (CD-ROM). Oxford University Press, Oxford.

Wolbarst, A.B. (1993) *Physics of Radiology*. Appleton & Lange, Norwalk, CT.

Wolf, H.K., Wellmer, J., Muller, M.B., Wiestler, O.D., Hufnagel, A. & Pietsch, T. (1995) Glioneuronal malformative lesions and dysembryoplastic neuroepithelial tumors in patients with chronic pharmacoresistant epilepsies. *Journal of Neuropathology and Experimental Neurology*, 54, 245–254.

Woodhouse, W., Bailey, A., Bolton, P., Baird, G., Le Couteur, A. & Rutter, M. (1996) Head circumference and pervasive developmental disorder. *Journal of Child Psychology and Psychiatry*, 37, 665–671.

World Bank (1993) *World Development Report: Investing in Health*. Oxford University Press, New York.

Zulmla, A., Mwaba, P., Squire, S.B. & Grange, J.M. (1999) The tuberculosis pandemic: which way now? *Journal of Infection*, 38, 74–79.

11 Clinical Neurophysiology

Colin Binnie, Stewart Boyd, Renzo Guerrini and Ronit Pressler

Introduction

As a non-invasive, inexpensive and repeatable means of assessing cerebral function, the electroencephalogram (EEG) is an invaluable diagnostic aid in child psychiatry. Nevertheless, it presents many complexities, not least because of the changes in the EEG occurring throughout childhood and adolescence as a result of maturation. The EEG is of most value in epilepsy and the various cerebral degenerative diseases. Its utility as a 'soft' sign of cerebral dysfunction in a wider range of disorders is more questionable.

Evoked potentials (EPs) elicited by sensory stimulation serve two purposes: assessment of sensory function (e.g. hearing in children with communication difficulties); and the detection, and sometimes identification of, cerebral disease involving the afferent pathways in the brainstem and white matter and projection areas.

Standard clinical neurophysiological techniques in children

Electroencephalogram (EEG)

Origins of the EEG

The EEG is a recording of cerebral electrical activity from the scalp. It mainly comprises the averaged synchronous postsynaptic potentials from radially orientated cortical neurones. The ongoing activity of the spontaneous EEG is rhythmic in character, reflecting synchronous oscillatory processes involving many neurones. Several sources of rhythmic neuronal activity are known. Individual neurones or groups of interconnected cells can display rhythmic discharge. There are also anatomically discrete pacemakers, or distributed systems of interacting neurones (see Steriade *et al.* 1990 for review). Rhythmic activity may be suppressed, e.g. by brainstem projections which desynchronize the EEG (increased frequency and reduced amplitude) during arousal. Conversely, functional deafferentation during sleep promotes synchrony, reflected in increased EEG amplitude and reduced frequency, and by an increase of synchronous transients, such as spikes.

Evoked potentials (EPs) are recorded from the scalp when a brief sequence of synchronous neuronal events is elicited by a sudden transitory stimulus. Various other transient EEG phenomena, both normal and pathological, also owe their synchronicity to a triggering event.

Recording the EEG

Like other bioelectrical signals, such as the electrocardiogram (ECG), the EEG is picked up by electrodes and amplified to drive a display, formerly a chart recorder but nowadays usually a computer screen. The signal is smaller than the ECG, of the order of 10–200 μV. Consequently, the recording is more liable to artefacts, from biological sources such as the eyes and scalp muscles, and from electrical interference. These can be reduced by meticulous technique. Electrode preparation and application are crucial. Low stable electrode potentials and contact resistances reduce susceptibility to physical interference, and the promotion of co-operation and relaxation in the subject helps to minimize biological artefact. These may be difficult to achieve in children, especially infants and those who are mentally retarded or disturbed. The importance of skill on the part of the technologist is reflected in the difference between the technical quality of children's EEGs obtained in routine departments and those recorded in specialized paediatric units.

Sometimes it is impossible to obtain an EEG without sedation or even anaesthesia, and it is then necessary to consider whether the clinical value of the investigation justifies such measures. Preschool-age children will usually take a sedative antihistamine syrup (e.g. trimeprazine (alimemazine) 2–4 mg/kg), and older patients can be sedated with short-acting barbiturates (e.g. secobarbital 100–150 mg). Before the last resort of general anaesthesia, which precludes a waking EEG, intramuscular droperidol may be tried.

Normal EEG phenomena in childhood and adolescence

For descriptive purposes, continuous *ongoing activity* is distinguished from *transients*. Ongoing EEG activities are classified into four frequency bands:
1 *delta*, below 4 c/s;
2 *theta*, from 4 up to 8 c/s;
3 *alpha*, from 8 up to 14 c/s; and
4 *beta*, from 14 c/s upwards.

The EEG changes from birth, throughout childhood and adolescence, stabilizing as the adult pattern at about 22 years. The main feature of the waking adult EEG is usually the alpha rhythm: α frequency activity, at about 9–10 c/s, with an amplitude of 50–100 μV seen symmetrically at the back of the head. The *alpha rhythm* is best developed in quiet wakefulness with closed eyes; it is attenuated by eye opening and disappears in drowsiness. *Beta activity*, usually at about 18–25 c/s is of lower amplitude, usually some 10–20 μV, again symmetrical, and most prominent over the frontal regions. *Gamma activity* describes fast components above 40 c/s. It is a term that was used early in the history of EEG, then abandoned, and more recently re-introduced because of interest in high-frequency components in intracranial recordings and also claims of significant changes in gamma activity in various psychiatric disorders. *Theta activity* may be inconspicuous but is always present, generally with a bitemporal maximum, increasing in drowsiness. Particularly in young adults, theta activity of half the alpha frequency may be seen posteriorly intermixed with the alpha rhythm and showing a similar response to eye opening (this is 'slow alpha variant'). Delta activity is not usually obvious in the mature waking EEG.

Changes in sleep are classified into five stages, by a system described by Dement & Kleitman (1957).

- *Stage I*. In drowsiness the alpha rhythm is replaced by theta and/or beta activity; slow lateral eye movements appear. Auditory stimuli elicit sharp transients at the vertex.
- *Stage II*. Delta activity appears, beta activity increases further and spindle-shaped bursts of activity at about 14 c/s appear with a frontal preponderance (*sleep spindles*). Arousal now produces more complicated waveforms near the vertex, typically 'K-complexes': a sharp wave, a delta wave and a spindle.
- *Stages III and IV*. These are distinguished by increasing amounts of delta activity, and a possible disappearance of spindles in stage IV.
- *REM*. After the first 90 min of sleep, episodes occur in which the EEG is of low amplitude, resembling stage I, but accompanied by rapid lateral eye movements, seen as oculographic artefacts, which give this stage the name of REM sleep. REM appears to accompany dreaming.

The EEG of the full-term waking newborn mainly consists of diffuse activity in the delta range with amplitudes of 50–100 μV. Two sleep patterns may be distinguished: in 'quiet sleep', bursts of delta activity are separated by 6–10 periods of relatively low amplitude ('*tracé alternant*'); whereas in 'active sleep', probably corresponding to adult REM, continuous delta activity is seen with ripples of superimposed faster rhythms.

The first year of life sees a gradual increase in EEG frequency and the emergence of a responsive posterior theta rhythm which reaches about 6 c/s by 12 months and will attain a low alpha frequency of about 8 c/s by the age of 3 years. From 3 to 12 months a Rolandic rhythm of 6–7 c/s is seen. A transitional state between waking and sleep appears at about 6 months, with dominant theta activity. From this time the classical sleep stages are distinguishable and much the same criteria apply as in adults. Spindles appear at about 2 months and vertex sharp transients and K-complexes in the middle of the first year.

In early childhood the alpha rhythm gradually emerges, increasing in frequency and responsiveness, but its frequency shows considerable variability, both between subjects and between published normative series. A dominant frequency of 8–9 c/s may be expected by the age of 5 years, but underlying the alpha rhythm large amounts of theta and delta activity remain. The theta activity takes on the characteristics of a slow alpha variant and the delta becomes intermittent and focal over the posterior temporal regions. The further evolution of the waking EEG though late childhood and adolescence involves quantitative rather than qualitative change. The slow alpha variant and posterior delta activity become more limited in extent and less in amount, the posterior slow waves usually disappearing entirely by the age of 22 years, and slow alpha variant a few years later. Drowsiness in early childhood produces an EEG dominated by theta activity with a frontal maximum, a picture which can easily be misinterpreted as abnormal if the reduced level of arousal is not recognized. Slow activity in sleep shows a posterior maximum up to 3 years of age, thereafter non-REM sleep patterns are not unlike those of adults. REM sleep is characterized by persisting slow activity to the age of 5 years but resembles the mature pattern thereafter.

The EEG changes with age and state of awareness, but a further source of intersubject variance is simply that the EEGs of individuals differ considerably one from another. EEG characteristics are genetically influenced to a major degree. The records of monozygotic twins are more similar than those of dizygotic twins, both on visual assessment (Lennox *et al.* 1945) and using quantitative measures (Dümermuth 1968; Stassen *et al.* 1988). These similarities extend to changes on hyperventilation and in sleep (Vogel 1958). Various unusual or arguably abnormal EEG features (see below) are also genetically determined (Doose & Gerken 1973).

Pathological EEG phenomena

Clinical EEG interpretation is based on subjective judgements which are complicated by the difficulty of defining normality at different ages. Maturation is accompanied by a reduction of the slower components, whereas drowsiness and cerebral dysfunction both produce slowing; thus, it may be difficult to distinguish between the effects of immaturity, drowsiness and pathology. Currency has been given to statements to the effect that some 15% of normal children have abnormal EEGs. Such a statement defies logical thought. Normality is largely a statistical concept: findings that are common in health are normal. However, rare variants found mainly in healthy subjects must also be regarded as normal. Conversely, changes within the normal range may be pathological for the individual concerned. Reporting of normal maturational phenomena as abnormalities is probably the most common single cause of misinterpretation in electroencephalography. Slow alpha variants or posterior temporal slow waves are usually phase-locked to the ongoing alpha activity. Consequently, these slow components take off and end with an exaggerated sharpened alpha wave of opposite polarity. Misinterpretation of this single common normal phenomenon results in innumerable children being misdiagnosed as suffering from epilepsy.

Another important consideration is that the EEG reflects cerebral function, and structural abnormality is manifest only in functional changes. Cerebral dysfunction produces in the EEG a rather limited range of abnormal phenomena, of uncertain pathophysiology.

Ongoing activities

Amplitude reduction. The most unequivocal sign of cerebral dysfunction is reduction in amplitude of normal activities. This may result from neuronal loss and from suppression of neuronal activity by toxic or metabolic factors. Extreme amplitude reduction is therefore found in brain death, after barbiturate overdose, during profound surgical hypothermia, in the terminal stages of various dementias, and immediately after a convulsive seizure. Amplitude reduction may also result from impaired conduction from the cortex to the scalp, e.g. because of an intervening subdural haematoma. Reduction in EEG amplitude may occur at the onset of an epileptic seizure (an 'electrodecremental event'), involving yet another mechanism, desynchronization of neuronal activity.

Some healthy adolescents constitutionally have low amplitude EEGs and other children exhibit a marked voltage reduction when anxious or hyperaroused; thus minor amplitude reduction may not be recognizable as abnormal unless also asymmetrical. An asymmetry greater than 50% in normal activities will generally reflect disease on the side where the amplitude is less.

Slowing. An increase in slower components of the EEG is seen in many cerebral disorders. Minor changes in ongoing frequencies may be recognized as pathological only if they are also asymmetrical. As low-frequency activity may reflect cerebral dysfunction, it might be expected to be of greater amplitude over the more disturbed hemisphere; however, the opposite will be found if the underlying pathology also leads to amplitude reduction. Slowing is a non-specific abnormality which can reflect various pathological processes including cerebral hypoxia, oedema, raised intracranial pressure, cerebral inflammatory or degenerative processes, and intoxications.

Excess beta activity. The amount of beta activity varies greatly between children. Beta activity is, moreover, increased in spontaneous drowsiness and by many sedative drugs, notably barbiturates and benzodiazepines. Excess beta activity is rarely pathological, but if very prominent may raise the possibility that the patient is consuming non-prescribed drugs.

Altered responsiveness. When the dominant rhythm over the postcentral region is slowed, whether or not still within the alpha range, it often shows a reduced responsiveness to eye opening or alerting. However, some normal subjects exhibit only minimal alpha blocking, and most will show reduced reac-

tivity when drowsy. Poor responsiveness cannot reliably be regarded as pathological unless it is also asymmetrical (less response on the more abnormal side), or is seen in a subject whose EEG was previously responsive in the same behavioural state.

Localized abnormalities

Amplitude reduction and slowing may be bilateral or asymmetrical. Essentially similar disturbances can be more localized. Amplitude reduction over a small area may involve all components of the EEG, or the higher frequencies selectively. Global reduction of amplitude generally reflects gross hypofunction or destruction of underlying cortical neurones.

Localized slow activities apart from so-called 'rhythms at a distance' (see below) generally reflect structural abnormality in the underlying cortex. Note that it is not cerebral lesions but dysfunctional neurones that generate abnormal EEG activity, so slowing may be seen around the periphery of a space-occupying lesion but not over its centre where amplitude reduction may be detected. Localized slowing may present as abnormal activity in the lower alpha, theta or delta ranges, or combinations of these.

Another important category of abnormal phenomena which may be localized, epileptiform activity, is considered in a later section.

Rhythms at a distance

Structurally normal cortex may generate abnormal activities in response to altered afferents from deep structures; these are termed 'rhythms at a distance'.

Frontal intermittent rhythmic delta activity. Frontal intermittent rhythmic delta activity (FIRDA) occurs over the frontal regions, usually bilateral and synchronous. The frequency is 1.5–2.5 c/s, and the waveform typically sinusoidal or sawtoothed. The rhythmic bursts typically last 2–5 s. It is dependent on arousal level, being absent in the fully alert subject and below stage I of sleep. FIRDA can occur in metabolic and toxic disorders, status epilepticus, and occasionally postictally, and in association with abnormalities of the diencephalon. It may occur with thalamic tumours and with obstruction of the aqueduct. However, the most common pathological correlate of FIRDA is diffuse disease involving grey and white matter (Gloor *et al.* 1968).

Bitemporal theta activity. In early drowsiness theta activity may increase over the temporal regions but in various states causing pathological drowsiness bilateral rhythmic temporal or frontotemporal theta activity occurs. It occurs under much the same circumstances as FIRDA. It must not be confused with the very prominent frontotemporal theta activity of drowsiness seen in preschool-age children.

Posterior slow activity. As noted above, posterior temporal slow activity is a normal finding in the young, disappearing in the early twenties. Posterior temporal slow waves may exceed the norm for the child's age, as a non-specific abnormality after such cerebral insults as trauma, cerebrovascular accidents and severe hypoglycaemia. The slow activity may be of greater amplitude on the side of greater cerebral abnormality, but in general it shares with maturational posterior temporal slow activity a tendency to predominate over the non-dominant hemisphere. Sometimes there is evidence of brainstem dysfunction as the immediate cause of posterior slow activity.

Very slow delta waves (> 1 s duration) are sometimes seen over the occipital regions, particularly in children, in association with mass lesions in the posterior fossa, and also with haemorrhage from the vertebrobasilar system.

Rhythmic, usually bilateral, posterior slow activity at about 3/s is seen in some children with absence seizures. It may represent a variant of spike-and-wave activity (see below), as on overbreathing it often acquires a notched waveform and spreads more widely before being replaced by typical generalized spike-and-wave discharges.

Epileptiform activity

Cerebral electrical activity changes during epileptic seizures and becomes characteristically spiky. Waves of sharp outline standing out from the background rhythms and lasting less than 70 ms are 'spikes'. Those lasting 70–200 ms are termed 'sharp waves'. Spikes are often followed by delta waves to form 'spike-and-wave' complexes, which may occur in runs as 'spike-and-wave activity'. Any of these can be generalized or focal. Spikes and sharp waves are, according to the latest approved terminology of the International Federation of Societies for Clinical Neurophysiology (Noachtar et al. 1999) 'clearly distinguished from background activity, with a pointed peak', which makes sense to experienced electroencephalographers but clearly lacks objectivity. In practice, an epileptiform pattern is whatever an experienced electroencephalographer says it is—not a satisfactory criterion.

Sharp waveforms occur in the interictal state (between overt seizures) in most people with epilepsy. Similar phenomena are also found in some patients with other cerebral disorders without seizures. There is no agreement as to a suitable collective term to describe this category of phenomena, but 'epileptiform activity', used here, acknowledges the association with epilepsy underlying the concept, while stressing that the term refers to the waveform, not a diagnosis.

Interpretative difficulties are increased by the occurrence in normal subjects of various sharp waveforms, unrelated to epilepsy. The most important of these in paediatrics are 6 and 14/s positive spikes which occur in short bursts at these two distinctive frequencies. At the focus the spike components are positive, a distinctive feature as most spikes are negative. Positive spikes occur in 20–30% of adolescents and young adults during drowsiness and light sleep. An increased incidence has been claimed in conditions ranging from behaviour disorders to allergies, but they contribute nothing to the diagnosis of epilepsy.

These and other spiky phenomena which are normal or of little diagnostic significance are distinguishable by characteristic morphology, topography or circumstances of occurrence.

'Periodicity'

Various pathological EEG phenomena occur at more or less constant intervals. The most dramatic example is provided by stereotyped complexes of slow waves, spikes, and sharp waves occurring every 10–20 s in subacute sclerosing panencephalitis. Periodic phenomena appear in various conditions; if these have any common feature, it is probably diffuse dysfunction of both white and grey matter.

Other transients

Triphasic complexes comprise three waves of alternating polarity, some or all of which lie in the delta range. Typically, the first and third components are frontonegative but the whole complex spreads across the head from front to back with a small time lag. This phenomenon is a sign of severe diffuse cerebral dysfunction, usually associated with metabolic disorder and typically with hepatic encephalopathy.

Paroxysmal lateralized epileptiform discharges (PLEDS) are stereotyped sharp waves or complexes of sharp waves repeating at intervals of about 1 s. They generally show a localized maximum but appear widely over one hemisphere. Occasionally, the phenomenon is bilateral, although usually asynchronous. PLEDS are seen in a variety of conditions, both acute and chronic, but always associated with localized structural disease and possibly more generalized cerebral dysfunction; examples include rapidly growing tumours, cerebrovascular accidents, herpes simplex encephalitis, cerebral abscess and following head injury.

Activation procedures

Various measures may be used to 'activate' the EEG to increase the yield of clinically significant findings. Hyperventilation, probably by reducing cerebral blood flow, slows the EEG especially in the young. Children from the age of 3 years can be persuaded to overbreathe, if necessary with the help of a toy windmill. Background rhythms are slowed, posterior slow activity increases, and rhythmic bifrontal delta activity appears. Various abnormalities may be increased, epileptiform activity in particular, and generalized spike-and-wave discharges may occur, notably in children with absences. Bifrontal delta activity on overbreathing in young people is normal, but often misinterpreted, sometimes resulting in unnecessary administration of antiepileptic drugs or neuroimaging investigations.

Photic stimulation by discrete flashes elicits visual evoked potentials (see below). Repetitive flashes at 4–30/s or more produce a rhythmic response at the back of the head, termed photic following. In some people, most of whom have epilepsy, generalized epileptiform discharges are elicited by flicker at certain frequencies, most readily at 18/s. Between these extremes, other anomalous responses may be observed, some of which are genetically determined but of little clinical significance.

Some confusion has resulted in the literature from some authors attaching the term 'photosensitivity' to all anomalous photic responses, and others confining it to the triggering of generalized spike-and-wave activity (the 'photoconvulsive response' of Bickford *et al.* 1952). Generally accepted current terminology follows that of Waltz *et al.* 1992 who distinguished four grades of 'photoparoxysmal response', of which only type 4, generalized spikes or spike-and-wave activity, is strongly associated with epilepsy. However defined, photosensitivity is considerably more common in children than in adults. Some 20% of children with epilepsy show a type 4 photoparoxysmal response. The diagnostic specificity of this phenomenon is disputed. Various authors have reported photosensitivity in as many as 15% of normal children but have generally failed to distinguish clearly between the different types of anomalous responses.

Photosensitivity in a child with epilepsy has practical significance. In most cases it lends support to the classification of the epilepsy as idiopathic. However, various non-idiopathic conditions which may be accompanied by photosensitivity should be ruled out (severe myoclonic epilepsy, late-infantile ceroid lipofuscinosis). More importantly, some 40% of photosensitive patients with epilepsy have no spontaneous seizures, all attacks being precipitated by visual stimuli. Thus, seizure control may be achieved without drugs, by practical measures to avoid provocative stimuli. Further, some 30% of children with photosensitive epilepsy use visual stimuli to induce seizures. The most easily recognized manoeuvre is to wave the outspread fingers of one hand in front of the eyes while staring at a bright light. However, the majority of children use a more subtle method involving a slow eye-closure with lid fluttering, itself easily mistaken for a seizure or a tic. EEG and video may be required to establish the occurrence of self-induction, and should be considered in any therapy-resistant photosensitive child. Monitoring in a well-lighted environment may facilitate self-induction, whereas recording in a dark environment will be accompanied by cessation of both the self-inducing behaviour and its EEG correlates.

Sleep has a profound effect on epilepsy, and many seizure types show a marked dependence on the sleep–wake cycle. In general, epileptiform activity occurs more readily in sleep than in waking, particularly focal discharges. Recording of the EEG during sleep, induced if necessary by sedative drugs, therefore plays an important part in the diagnostic EEG investigation of epilepsy.

Evoked potentials

Evoked potentials are responses to stimulation. An abrupt stimulus, such as a click, produces a synchronous volley in the afferent pathways of the cord and/or brainstem and thalamic radiations, followed by a more complex sequence of events when the signal reaches the specific and non-specific cortical projection areas. These phenomena have a fairly constant time course following each stimulus, whereas the waves of the ongoing EEG occur randomly in time. Therefore if the average of the signals following repeated stimulus presentations is calculated, the random activity tends to zero and the constant response to the stimulus is unmasked. Registration of EPs thus requires a special recorder containing a computer to average signals, and control the stimulators.

EPs consist of a sequence of waves, or 'components', identified by their latency and polarity. Normative values are published, but minor differences in technique and instrumentation result in substantial differences between laboratories; every department should obtain its own local reference data, a difficult achievement in paediatric practice as different norms apply to each age group.

Auditory evoked potentials

Auditory EPs are divided into early, middle latency and late. The early components, arising from the VIIIth nerve, cochlear nucleus and brainstem pathways, are termed brainstem auditory EPs (BAEPs). They are elicited by a click and, being of low amplitude, may be detected only after many stimuli; difficult children will often need sedation. The BAEPs are designated by the roman numerals I–VII and occur within 10 μs after the stimulus. BAEPs are recorded between bilateral mastoid or earlobe electrodes and the vertex. Wave I arises from the peripheral part of the ipsilateral cochlear nerve and may persist even when the brainstem or the proximal part of the nerve is damaged. Wave II is often inconspicuous and originates in the proximal part of the nerve and the cochlear nucleus. The other components arise in the brainstem and are recorded remotely from the vertex. The most robust is wave V which persists close to the subjective auditory threshold and can be used for audiometry. Waves I, III and V are present at birth. The latencies of BAEPs are the most stable of all EPs within and between subjects but diminish with maturation, virtually attaining the adult values by 3 years of age. Conduction velocity in the brainstem is assessed by measurement of the peak to peak latencies of waves I–III or I–V (the latter is typically about 4 μs).

Middle latency auditory evoked potentials (MLAEPs) occur in the 10–50 μs after the stimulus. Five waves are distinguished, of which only those at 16–20 μs and 27–33 μs are sufficiently consistent to be of clinical value. Asymmetries may provide evidence of hemisphere lesions.

Long latency auditory evoked potentials (LLAEPs) comprise a negative wave at about 100 μs and a 180-μs latency positive component. Their amplitude and latency are unstable, as they are influenced by vigilance, cognitive processes and drugs. Formerly they were used for audiometric testing, but have been superseded by BAEPs. However, abnormal or absent LLAEPs may offer evidence of hemispheric lesions.

Visual evoked potentials

Visual stimuli, flashes of light or reversing black and white patterns, elicit potentials both from the retina (the electroretinogram; ERG) and from the cortex (visual evoked potentials; VEPs).

The ERG to white flash is characterized by two waves: a and b. The a-wave arises from the receptor layers of the retina, and is followed by the b-wave which probably originates in the Müller cells. Some small faster waves appear superimposed upon the b-wave: the oscillatory potentials. Later components, the c- and d-waves, are of little clinical significance. By changing the intensity and colour of the flash or the state of light adaptation, it is possible to distinguish rod and cone components of the ERG. Ideally, electroretinography requires corneal electrodes; these are not tolerated by children, so supraorbital electrodes are used. Paediatric ERG is therefore rather crude, and may be limited to establishing whether a response is present, as a check on retinal function which greatly aids the interpretation of abnormal VEPs. If necessary, the examination can be performed under general anaesthesia. The flash ERG is detectable after the first week of life, but is smaller and of greater latency than in adults. The mature pattern is attained by the age of 1–2 years.

The VEPs to a diffuse flash of light comprise up to seven waves, within 250 µs of the stimulus, of which the most consistent are N70, P100 and P160. The intersubject variation of latency and amplitude is considerable. For clinical purposes, absence of response and interocular asymmetries of latency or amplitude are considered. In infants the earliest wave is positive at 170–190 µs, followed by a negative at 220–240 µs. An adult waveform is attained by 4–6 years but the P100 still has a latency of 110–130 µs.

Responses to patterned stimuli may appear more physiological than those elicited by diffuse flash, and indeed pattern VEPs generally prove of greater clinical value. For routine purposes the stimulus used is the sudden reversal of the black and white squares of a checkerboard. The pattern VEPs comprise three main waves: N75, P100 and N145, of which P100 is the most prominent. Pattern VEP studies require good co-operation and ocular fixation by the subject and are difficult before the age of 6 years, by which time the potentials resemble those of adults. Only limited normative data are available for infancy and early childhood. Latencies are much greater than in adults.

Somatosensory evoked potentials

Somatosensory evoked potentials (SEPs) are elicited by electrical shocks applied to peripheral nerves. The ascending impulses can be traced along the limbs, the brachial plexus and spinal cord, to the cortex. In the present context only cortical potentials are relevant, and for simplicity only latencies from median nerve stimulation will be cited.

The first short latency cortical potentials comprise a parietal N20–P27 complex, and the frontocentral P22 and N30 potentials; all are recorded contralateral to the stimulus, but the N30

often extends to the ipsilateral frontal area. Responses to right- or left-sided stimuli are of equal amplitude and latency, and asymmetries reflect pathology of the underlying pathways. The short latency SEPs include two later components: the P45 and N60 potentials, neither of which is studied for clinical purposes.

Auditory and visual EPs show a reduction in latency from infancy to adulthood, with increasing conduction velocity caused by myelination and increase in fibre diameter. However, in the case of SEPs a second factor comes into play; the lengthening of the neural pathways with growth, delaying and desynchronizing the afferent volleys. In the preschool period the net effect is a reduction in latency, thereafter latencies again increase and the waveforms are widened. Comparison of the findings to normative values is simplified by correcting latencies for limb length or height, but again it is essential that each laboratory collects its own set of reference data.

Event-related potentials

The EPs described above are generated as a direct consequence of a stimulus. However, there are some, termed event-related potentials (ERPs), that are associated with endogenous or cognitive events. These include potentials preceding a voluntary movement, the Bereitschaftspotential (BP), and potentials 'evoked' when a stimulus is omitted from a regular series of stimuli. In psychiatry special attention has been directed to the P300, a positive wave with a latency of 250–450 µs, related to decision-making or recognition of a stimulus relevant to a particular task (for a review see Picton 1988; and for details of maturation of ERPs Picton *et al.* 1984).

Selection and interpretation of clinical neurophysiological results in a clinical setting

Clinical neurophysiological investigations have been used in psychiatric disorders ever since the introduction of EEG, although clinicians have often found it difficult to relate the findings to the specific clinical context. However, with a better understanding of the significance of particular EEG findings and the development of newer techniques, such as EPs, combined neurophysiological investigations now offer improved prospects of obtaining clinically meaningful data. Nevertheless, it is important to understand the strengths and limitations of particular investigations. For example, many clinicians request visual or auditory EPs in the expectation that they will reveal whether the child 'sees' or 'hears'. Although conventional EP testing can indicate whether the pathways are functioning appropriately, it will not determine what use the child is able to make of the sensory information. To take two extreme cases, an infant may have normal short-latency EP findings yet not respond normally as a result of severe impairment of cortical activity, while a bright child with a severe visual pathway problem and grossly impaired EP findings may have learned ploys of head movement, etc. that allow the child to use residual visual function to the full.

Table 11.1 Stages in the selection and interpretation of clinical neurophysiological investigations.

What is the clinical question?

Can it be addressed by clinical neurophysiological investigation and if so which procedure is most likely to be useful?

Are the findings normal or abnormal?

What does this mean in the clinical context?

What further investigations might be helpful?

Does the combination of neurophysiological and other findings suggest a specific diagnosis or process?

Are repeat investigations likely to be helpful and after what interval?

Clinical neurophysiological investigations in paediatric psychiatry have been used in two ways.

1 As additional 'clinical signs', evaluated as components of a pattern of signs in a particular clinical context. For a neurophysiological finding to be useful clinically, it should fulfil the criteria that it is a definite abnormality, and found consistently in a large proportion of cases with a particular condition, allowing patients to be clearly distinguished. They may also be used to check on the presence or absence of known complications of a particular condition (e.g. infantile spasms in Down syndrome).

2 As tools to elucidate specific underlying mechanisms of 'mental retardation' or 'psychiatric disease'. Before a finding can be used to illustrate some more fundamental aspect of disordered function, there should be supporting evidence that it is likely to be relevant.

Discussion in this chapter focuses on conventional clinical neurophysiological investigations because quantitative methods have often failed to fulfil their promise and have not entered routine practice (Nuwer 1988a,b). Some research techniques offer particular insights into psychophysiological processes and are reviewed in the appropriate specialist chapters. Selection and interpretation of such investigations should be considered as a continuing clinical process of reappraisal between clinicians and neurophysiologists (Table 11.1).

If the diagnosis is secure, then neurophysiological investigations are not usually relevant, but may be helpful in the management and understanding of the cases. When there are specific questions relating to aspects of management, such as episodic alterations in behaviour, then appropriately selected neurophysiological investigations may help clarify the nature of the problem, within the limitations of the tests as described above. Prior discussion with the clinical neurophysiologist will facilitate the selection of relevant tests.

When the diagnosis is in doubt, and particularly where there is concern about progressive organic disorder, then investigations at an early stage may suggest the nature of the problem. Investigations in clinical neurophysiology should not be undertaken on a purely speculative basis, but there may be clinical hints which will repay further consideration if supported by neurophysiological findings. As Batten disease (see below) is the most common neurodegenerative (central nervous system) disease, it is useful to combine flash ERG/VEP studies with EEG recording.

If there is continuing clinical uncertainty, then repeating the investigations after an interval, determined by the tempo of the clinical condition, may indicate whether the process is progressive.

Special techniques

Polygraphic recordings

The term 'polygraphy' is used to refer to the simultaneous recording of several physiological signals. This technique provides very useful information on the relationships between behavioural phenomena and physiological variables (Tassinari & Rubboli 1997). To exploit effectively the possibilities of polygraphy, recordings must be tailored to the patient's clinical presentation. The main points of polygraphic semiology consist in the correlations of EEG events with the other physiological functions monitored and their temporal relationship. Polygraphic recordings are usually carried out using an EEG apparatus with some channels used for other biological signals. The two main clinical applications in children are seizures and sleep disorders. Polygraphic recordings of the sleep–wake cycle is termed 'polysomnography' and is particularly important in studying the relationship between sleep and epilepsy. The main variables that can be monitored are EEG, electromyographic activity, electro-oculogram, ECG, respirogram, blood pressure, movement and micturition. Recordings with simultaneous surface EMG acquisition from multiple muscles are of particular interest for studying the various epileptic motor manifestations in children, including myoclonus, spasms, tonic seizures, atonic phenomena and tonic–clonic activity, all easily misdiagnosed on the basic of clinical evidence only.

Jerk-locked computerized EEG averaging is a special technique which is used to detect the cortical potentials associated with EMG activity. EEG averaging triggered by the EMG potential permits extraction of low-voltage cortical potentials from the background EEG activity. This technique allows characterization of different types of myoclonus, according to the presence or absence of a cortical potential and to its temporal relationships with the EMG activity. Non-epileptic disorders that may be diagnosed with the help of polysomnography or other prolonged nocturnal recordings include sleep apnoea, with oxygen desaturation and cessation of airflow, and night terrors arising from deep sleep.

Long-term EEG monitoring

There are serious limitations to the routine EEG investigation of known or possible epilepsy. The clinical and electrophysiological manifestations of epilepsy are intermittent; a single routine recording may fail to show epileptiform activity, which may indeed occur only during seizures. The relevance of interictal discharges to specific clinical events may be uncertain; spikes in the EEG of a mentally retarded child with episodes of aggressive behaviour do not indicate that these attacks are epileptic. Finally, clinical and electrophysiological observations of seizures in the EEG laboratory offer little guide as to their frequency and significance in daily life. These problems can be addressed by long-term monitoring of EEG and behaviour. Two methods are available: continuous EEG recording by telemetry with behavioural observation by video recording, and ambulatory monitoring of the EEG in the patient's everyday environment with a portable recorder. These technologies are not alternatives and have different applications.

Telemetry

Routine EEG recording limits the patient's activity and will not be tolerated by a lively child for much more than an hour. Moreover, limiting activity may prevent the observation of subtle ictal phenomena, or the effects of behaviour and environment on seizures. Greater mobility is achieved by telemetering the EEG through a long flexible cable, or by a radio link.

Simultaneous video recording is important. Subtle clinical and electrophysiological ictal events are often identifiable only by comparison of EEG and behaviour. Thus, a momentary arrest of activity may be shown to be a seizure because it consistently coincides with an EEG change. Conversely, apparent subclinical discharges may prove to be ictal because of associated but inconspicuous clinical events.

Some misunderstanding surrounds the significance of the 'negative ictal EEG'. All epileptic seizures involve abnormal neuronal discharge, but this may not be recorded from the scalp. Ictal EEG changes may be entirely absent or consist not of 'epileptiform activity', but rather of a minor change in ongoing rhythms. Some seizure types, such as absences, are consistently accompanied by epileptiform activity. Some are usually associated with other changes, such as bitemporal theta activity during a complex partial seizure. Simple partial seizures, particularly with psychic or viscerosensory symptoms, often produce no EEG change. Interpretation of an apparently negative ictal EEG depends on the nature of the seizure and correlation in time of EEG and behaviour to detect subtle changes.

Ambulatory monitoring

Ambulatory recorders permit recording outside the EEG laboratory. Formerly, audio cassettes were used as the recording medium but these have been superseded by solid state digital devices, such as flash cards. Each runs for 24 h between technical checks. Recording quality of cassettes was inferior to that of telemetry, and this increased the difficulty of distinguishing EEG activity from artefact, which may be abundant in an actively moving child. Solid state devices are more satisfactory, but there remain difficulties in correlating the EEG findings with behaviour in the absence of synchronized video registration.

Ambulatory monitoring is no substitute for video EEG telemetry, e.g. for detecting subtle seizures or deciding whether particular events are epileptic. However, it is invaluable for investigating a known EEG phenomenon in a particular situation, e.g. to determine the frequency of absence seizures during school.

Brain mapping and dipole modelling

As the EEG and EPs are distributed over a three-dimensional surface and change with time, ideally they should be presented using a five-dimensional display system. As this is not practical they are usually demonstrated in two dimensions as voltage–time curves. However, by adopting a stylized two-dimensional scalp outline and sacrificing information about changes in time, the distribution of the electrical field can be displayed as an isopotential contour map. This can highlight features of both EEGs and EPs which are not easily recognized in conventional displays. Mapping has, for instance, shown that the negative Rolandic spike of benign childhood epilepsy is typically accompanied by a mid-frontal positive wave—an unusual distribution, as dipolar fields with simultaneous positive and negative foci are rarely recognizable in the scalp EEG. Minor variations in the topography of this phenomenon appear to be clinically significant. The technique depends critically on the skill of the user who must first identify those momentary salient features of field distribution which justify closer inspection.

Mapping is also applied to quantitative results of EEG analysis, e.g. the total electrical power or the ratio between the amounts of activities in two frequency bands. Temporal information is again lost, as the analysis presents a time average of some EEG feature over one or more epochs, typically of many seconds. This user-friendly way of presenting quantitative information is fraught with problems. The values plotted at each site represent, not the cerebral activity of that region, but the difference between the electrode and a reference. For instance, if the reference is obtained jointly from both ears and the patient has a temporal delta focus, a map may show maximum delta power in the contralateral central region. Any but the most sophisticated user, who hardly needs the help of mapping, is likely to interpret the map as showing an abnormality incorrectly localized and over the wrong hemisphere.

Interest in this long-established technique has been recently increased by developments in computer graphics. There is great appeal in the apparent demystification of the EEG and EPs by the substitution of simple coloured maps for long and complex chart tracings. It must be hoped that the present misuse of this potentially valuable technique will prove a temporary aberration (Binnie & MacGillivray 1992).

Another approach to display of EEG topography, of equal potential value and no less open to abuse, is equivalent dipole modelling. A source generating an electrical field must produce one site, or pole, that is maximally negative and another that is most positive (a dipole). A dipole may be described by its location, orientation, and the changing potential difference it generates between its two poles as a function of time. If such a generator were present within the brain it is possible from considerations of biophysics to predict the field that it would produce on the scalp (the so-called 'forward solution'). The electrical field over the scalp at any instant in time will be maximally negative at one site and most positive at another; it is possible by means of suitable computer programs to estimate with greater or less reliability the characteristics of a hypothetical dipole, or dipoles that could produce such a field (the 'inverse solution'). When the EEG field is strikingly dipolar, the Rolandic spike providing a good example, such a dipole or dipoles may usefully summarize the electrical field. The danger in the use of dipole modelling is the belief that because a particular dipole or group of dipoles could produce the observed field, such dipole generators actually exist. This misconception is seen particularly in studies of temporal lobe epilepsy. Interictal discharges from mesial temporal structures propagate to involve lateral temporal neocortex. The resulting widespread field can be represented by a deep temporal dipole which, almost inevitably, will be located in or somewhere adjacent to mesial temporal structures, notably the hippocampus. It may then be claimed that dipole modelling has identified a mesial temporal source of the discharges—erroneously of course, as even if the epilepsy is in fact of mesial temporal origin, the signals used for the modelling arise from lateral neocortex. The more sophisticated workers recognize that dipole modelling merely provides a useful method of synoptic representation of complex electrical fields, the more naïve persist in the belief that they are identifying physiological generators and that dipole modelling is useful for locating such sources, e.g. in presurgical assessment of epilepsy.

EEG findings in psychiatric disorders

Pervasive developmental disorders

Autism

Clinical neurophysiological abnormalities have been reported more often in autism than in any other psychiatric condition in childhood (Small 1987), but usually simply as evidence of an organic basis for the condition. The criteria for definition of autism, degrees of severity at the time of testing, EEG recording conditions (sleep or wakefulness), and the EEG abnormalities described have all varied widely (Tuchman 1994). This complicates interpretation of the findings, but slow activity or discharges, generalized or in a variable focal distribution, will be found in around 30–45% in single recordings (Small 1975; Tsai et al. 1985). The percentage was much higher when multiple recordings and sleep recordings were used. There is a relationship between IQ and the likelihood of finding EEG abnormalities, the more severely affected children being more likely to show changes (Small 1975).

Epilepsy is quite frequent in children with autism (see Lord & Bailey, Chapter 38). Major attacks are the most common seizure type but complex partial seizures also occur. In cases where there is doubt over whether a particular behaviour is ictal, evidence of persistent EEG foci with changes during the episodic behaviour should identify children who might respond to anticonvulsants.

Lewine et al. (1999) suggested that epileptiform discharges in children with autism spectrum disorders might be clinically relevant, even in the absence of manifest seizures. They performed a magnetoencephalographic (MEG) study in 50 children with an autism spectrum disorder involving regression after 30 months. Only 16 of the 50 children had been diagnosed as having autism as such, and 15 had experienced epileptic seizures; 41 had epileptiform abnormalities during sleep (simultaneous surface EEG could detect abnormalities in only 34 of them). Multiple subpial transections (Morrell et al. 1989) with or without small topectomies, aimed at reducing the amount of discharges, were claimed to lead to a reduction of autistic features and improvement in language skills in 12 of 18 cases, despite the multifocal origin of the EEG abnormalities. However, the authors pointed out that surgery was not the only option, as steroid treatment led to an improvement in autistic features in some cases. Also, surgery was accompanied by speech and behaviour therapy.

Performing an EEG recording including at least the transition from wakefulness to sleep and at least 15–20 min of slow wave sleep is strongly advised. Epilepsy with continuous spike-wave during slow-wave sleep (CSWS; Patry et al. 1971) may be ruled out if the initial sleep is not accompanied by activation of frequent epileptiform discharges. However, there is evidence that discharges vary from night to night so that a single sleep recording cannot definitely rule out CSWS or atypical benign partial epilepsy (Deonna 1991; Tuchman et al. 1991).

EP studies, particularly of the auditory system, have been widely used to test various hypotheses concerning putative defects in acquisition and/or processing of sensory information. Between one-third and one-half of autistic patients show impairment of function in the auditory pathways, particularly through the upper brainstem (Thivierge et al. 1990; Wisniewski et al. 1991). However, it remains difficult to assess the clinical relevance of this finding and routine BAEP studies are not indicated.

Rett syndrome

There is a clustering of EEG features in Rett syndrome which may evolve with the clinical stages of the disease (Glaze & Frost 1985). EEG development is normal until about 18 months of age, when there is often loss of sleep spindles and normal rhythmic activities. Discharges appear, solely or especially during sleep (Hagberg et al. 1983), mostly over the parasagittal and centrotemporal regions whether or not clinical seizures have occurred (Robb et al. 1989; Aldrich et al. 1990). In the later stages, repetitive bursts of slow components are seen during sleep (Hagne et al. 1989) but, in our own experience, this is rather variable. In some girls, discharges are related to obsessive finger tapping and can also be elicited by passive finger tapping by the EEG technician during recording; it was found in one-third of the cases seen by Robb *et al.* (1989). In fact, these EEG discharges appear to be giant SEPs which originate from a hyperexcitable sensorimotor cortex. Studies of the C-reflex at rest show that stimulation of the median nerve produces a giant SEP and a cortical reflex myoclonic jerk (Guerrini *et al.* 1998a).

Episodic hyperventilation and apnoea during waking, sometimes leading to cyanosis or even to loss of consciousness (Lugaresi *et al.* 1985), has also been studied. Elian & Rudolf (1991) found bursts of high-amplitude slow waves associated with apnoea and faster activities during hyperventilation or normal breathing. Although the breathing pattern is normal during sleep, Nomura *et al.* (1984) found abnormalities of tonic and phasic components of sleep and of incremental increase in percentage REM sleep with increasing age. Evoked potentials showed variable abnormalities in nine girls aged 10–12 years investigated by Bader *et al.* (1989a,b).

Other disorders

EEG abnormalities have been found in about 35% of children with symptoms of hyperactivity, impulsive behaviour and inattention (Cantwell 1980). These include diffuse non-specific changes, excessive slow activity and epileptiform activity (Satterfield *et al.* 1974); also reduced amounts of well-organized alpha waves (Shetty 1973). However, the interpretation of neurophysiological findings in these disorders is complicated by differences in both clinical classification and methodology. There are no specific clinical implications.

Young people with depression may have reduced REM latency and increased REM time, similar to depressed adults (Emslie *et al.* 1990). However, it has been suggested that this may be accounted for, in part, by methodological problems and the effects of treatment (Thaker *et al.* 1990). The abnormalities associated with depression seem to occur less frequently in prepubertal patients, but may be expressed at a younger age when there is familial evidence for depression and abnormal sleep in a parent (Dahl *et al.* 1991; Giles *et al.* 1992).

In children with, or at high risk of, schizophrenia, non-specific EEG changes (Waldo *et al.* 1978), excessive fast activity and lack of alpha waves (Itil *et al.* 1974, 1976) and abnormalities in event-related potentials (Strandburg *et al.* 1991) have been reported. Abnormalities in these disorders are mainly of academic interest and there are no indications for routine clinical neurophysiological studies.

Mental retardation

Associations between particular conditions and neurophysiological findings have usually been of more immediate clinical assistance than efforts to define the nature of changes related to 'mental retardation'. Many children with mental retardation have normal EEGs; in most others, abnormalities are non-specific and inconstant. In a small number of conditions, neurophysiological findings are sufficiently distinctive and consistently associated to suggest the diagnosis. Unusual neurophysiological features shared by retarded siblings can also be used to help delineate a recognizable syndrome (Baraitser & Winter 1992).

Down syndrome

Infantile spasms are not uncommon in Down syndrome (Gregoriades & Pampiglione 1966) and the EEG features are similar to those associated with other conditions. The notion that other forms of seizures are rare in children with Down syndrome has been discarded. Guerrini *et al.* (1990) suggested that reflex seizures are common (20% of their series) in children with Down syndrome and epilepsy, and speculated that this might be related to increased cortical excitability. The risks of neurological deficit resulting from cervicomedullary compression seem to be less than originally feared, but in those cases where further investigation seems warranted, SEPs are a useful component of the assessment (Pueschel *et al.* 1987).

Angelman syndrome

The EEG in Angelman syndrome shows a distinctive pattern consisting of three different elements each comprising high-amplitude rhythmic activities of delta and theta frequencies, with other sharp theta components appearing over the occipital region, usually enhanced by, or only seen on, eye closure. They are found in variable proportions in the same or in serial records (Boyd *et al.* 1988). These EEG changes are not present at birth but develop in the first year of life (Bower & Jeavons 1967) and are seen during both wakefulness and sleep. The abnormalities are most striking in younger children and the amplitude of these changes tends to decrease with age, although this is not invariable.

Many patients present with episodes of decreased alertness with hypotonia and mild jerking lasting days or weeks, described as non-convulsive status epilepticus with diffuse slow spike-and-wave complexes (Viani *et al.* 1995). Almost all patients with Angelman syndrome also exhibit quasi-continuous multifocal rhythmic cortical myoclonus at about 11 Hz, mainly involving the hands (Guerrini *et al.* 1996).

Severity of epilepsy, but not the EEG pattern, appears to vary according to the genetic classes of Angelman syndrome (Minassian *et al.* 1998). Whereas slow spike-and-wave complexes or notched slow waves are present irrespective of the genetic mechanism involved, patients with large deletions have much more severe epilepsies, in which generalized seizure types are largely predominant. The epilepsy phenotype is relatively milder in patients with loss-of-function mutations or methylation imprint abnormalities.

By contrast, no striking EEG changes are seen in Prader–Willi syndrome, the other condition associated with mental retardation and the same chromosome deletion, but of the paternal inherited 15q region (see Skuse & Kuntsi, Chapter 13). Conventional clinical EP investigations have not shown clinically useful changes in either condition.

Malformations of the cerebral cortex

Abnormal cortical development is increasingly recognized as a cause of human epilepsy and mental retardation (Guerrini *et al.* 1996). Abnormal neuronal proliferation and differentiation can result in hemimegaloencephaly (HME) and the focal dysplasia of cerebral cortex described by Taylor *et al.* 1971. In HME one cerebral hemisphere is enlarged and structurally abnormal. The clinical spectrum is wide, ranging from early onset epileptic encephalopathies to patients with normal cognitive level and mild epilepsy. Several EEG patterns have been described in children with refractory seizures in infancy, including 'burst-suppression' (Paladin *et al.* 1989). The abnormalities may be bilateral but this does not affect outcome following hemispherectomy (Doering *et al.* 1999). In focal dysplasia, histological abnormalities involve a smaller area. Patients usually develop intractable partial epilepsy. Focal status epilepticus or epilepsia partialis continua are relatively frequent. The interictal EEG often shows focal rhythmic epileptiform discharges but epileptiform discharges may be totally absent from the scalp EEG.

Disorders affecting neuronal migration are characterized by abnormal neuronal positioning. Horizontal lamination is impaired, while radial organization is still recognizable. Several malformations, almost all highly epileptogenic, belong to this category, including the syndrome of X-linked bilateral periventricular nodular heterotopia (BPNH) and the so-called agyria–pachygyria band spectrum. The latter designates a subgroup of migration abnormalities for which the genetic basis is beginning to be elucidated. Classical lissencephaly is characterized by absent (agyria) or decreased (pachygyria) convolutions. All patients have early developmental delay and severe mental retardation; several syndromes have been described, of which the Miller–Dieker syndrome is the best known. About 80% of affected children have infantile spasms. Lissencephaly has been shown to be associated with striking patterns of high-amplitude rhythmic activity in the EEG (Gastaut *et al.* 1987). In older children, widespread slow activity may be the only feature (Hakamada *et al.* 1979). In subcortical band heterotopia a thin band of white matter separates the cortex from the heterotopic grey matter; cognitive impairment and epilepsy are again the major manifestations. There appears to be a close correlation between the thickness of the heterotopic band and the degree of pachygyria and the likelihood of developing Lennox–Gastaut syndrome (Barkovich *et al.* 1994). A malformation originating during late neuronal migration is Aicardi syndrome, which is thought to be caused by an X-linked gene with lethality in the hemizygous male. In this highly epileptogenic malformation, specific electroclinical features change little, if at all, over time and include early onset of intractable infantile spasms and partial seizures. A typical EEG feature of Aicardi syndrome, attributable to agenesis of the corpus callosum and multiple epileptogenic cortical areas, is the so-called 'split brain pattern' consisting of bilateral asynchronous hemispheric discharges.

The best-known cortical malformation originating after completion of neuronal migration is four-layered polymicrogyria, in which horizontal neuronal lamination usually persists. Seizures, poorly controlled in about 65% of patients, often occur as Lennox–Gastaut-like syndromes. Polymicrogyria may be unilateral, producing a syndrome of hemiparesis, mild mental retardation and epilepsy. Almost all seizure types and several epileptic syndromes may be observed, including sleep-related electrical status epilepticus, evolving towards spontaneous remission (Guerrini *et al.* 1998b).

Reading disorders

Clinical neurophysiological findings have been used by various groups to support organic models of dyslexia and other less well-defined disorders. Conners (1978) noted that whereas many studies had reported EEG abnormalities in dyslexic children, the nature of these abnormalities varied between the different studies and that strict definitions of dyslexia were not used. It is worth bearing these strictures in mind when considering subsequent claims for more subtle abnormalities which often depend on finding differences between the patient and normal populations using increasingly complex statistical measures. Some studies have used small numbers of subjects and a few have not incorporated a control group. There is as yet no consensus despite numerous studies of dyslexics as to whether there are characteristic features in the EEG. For example, many EEG investigations of dyslexia have shown coherence differences between the two hemispheres, but methodological difficulties (French & Beaumont 1984) were not always appreciated in the older studies. Galin *et al.* (1992) have reviewed criteria for selection and methods in this difficult area of research, stressing the importance of examining dyslexic and normal readers during both silent and oral reading.

Language disorders

Acquired dysphasia (Landau–Kleffner syndrome)

Landau & Kleffner (1957) described six children (including siblings) with acquired dysphasia who had discharges in their EEGs and who improved with anticonvulsant treatment. An association between a prompt improvement in the EEG with treatment and a satisfactory clinical outcome continues to be reported (Lerman *et al.* 1991), but individual cases may be left with severe language deficits (van Dongen *et al.* 1989).

The nature of the relationship between the discharges and the dysphasia is much debated. The two main hypotheses are that the discharges and the dysphasia are epiphenomena related to a single underlying cause, or that the dysphasia is a direct consequence of focal discharges. On reviewing the condition, Deonna (1991) cited the absence of structural pathology and improvement with anticonvulsant treatment in favour of the latter explanation, a view supported by MEG studies (Paetau *et al.* 1991). The elegant study of Seri *et al.* (1998) has added solid evidence to this pathophysiological interpretation. These authors studied spike-triggered auditory evoked responses in a group of children with Landau–Kleffner syndrome and observed that spikes over the left hemisphere were associated with a greater reduction in the amplitude and increased latency of the N1 component than spikes occurring in the contralateral hemisphere. Spike-related abnormal processing of the auditory information may therefore play a substantial part in the language dysfunction of Landau–Kleffner syndrome. Cole *et al.* (1988) reported that EEG discharges were generalized, bilateral, multifocal or with shifting predominance, but with a mainly temporal distribution in 85% of cases, and unilateral and again predominantly temporal in the remaining 15%.

Although Landau & Kleffner defined the eponymous syndrome as one of acquired dysphasia, other evidence (Maccario *et al.* 1982) suggested that it may also present as a developmental language disorder.

Developmental language disorder

In common with many disorders, estimates of the prevalence of EEG abnormalities in children with developmental language disorder (DLD) is complicated by the fact that the condition is heterogeneous and that children are much more likely to have an EEG if seizures are suspected. In a survey of 237 DLD children without evidence of autism, Tuchman *et al.* (1991) found that EEGs had been carried out on all 19 with epilepsy but on only 66 (30%) without seizures. EEG abnormalities, mainly epileptiform changes, were found in 63% of those with seizures and 20% of those without. Both the proportion and the type of EEG changes were similar to those seen in a comparison group of 314 children with autism, but they were very variable.

Such findings make it difficult to devise definitive guidelines for identifying children with dysphasia who might benefit from anticonvulsant medication. However, most patients with the Landau–Kleffner syndrome show continuous temporal or bitemporal discharges during sleep at some stage. It would therefore seem reasonable to consider the diagnosis in those children where the EEG during sleep shows frequent or continuous discharges predominantly in the temporal regions, and to adopt a more sceptical approach when the discharges are only sporadic and mainly extratemporal. In patients in whom speech disturbance is clearly episodic (and occurring several times per week), ictal recording may be warranted.

Neurological disorders with psychiatric consequences

Epilepsy

EEG and the classification of the epilepsies

Epileptic disorders are described in terms of syndromes, and within the general framework of a classification of the epilepsies (Commission on Classification & Terminology of the Inter-national League Against Epilepsy 1989). The classification distinguishes generalized epilepsies, in which seizures apparently arise in both hemispheres, and partial (or 'localization-related') epilepsies in which seizure onset is in a circumscribed cortical area. A division is also made between symptomatic epilepsies in patients with structural brain disease, cryptogenic epilepsies in which the pathology is presumed but unproven, and idiopathic epilepsies arising in an intact brain. These criteria are reflected in the EEG.

In idiopathic generalized epilepsies, both ictal and interictal discharges are generalized often with a frontal emphasis, as typified by the bilateral spike-and-wave activity in absences. Partial epilepsies are accompanied by focal discharges, both at seizure onset and in the interictal state. These are not, however, necessarily detectable in the scalp EEG (see above). Both partial seizures and focal discharges may spread to surrounding cortical areas, involve homologous regions of both hemispheres, or become generalized. In some patients the secondarily generalized phenomena may dominate the picture and the underlying focal elements pass undetected. In symptomatic generalized epilepsies, both multifocal and generalized interictal discharges are usually found, against a diffusely abnormal background, reflecting the generalized cerebral pathology.

EEG features of epilepsy syndromes of childhood and adolescence

Many epileptic syndromes are described in childhood and all present characteristic EEG features. Those seen in the neonatal period will not be considered here.

The association of epileptic spasms with the EEG pattern termed 'hypsarrhythmia' characterized by diffuse high-voltage irregular slow waves with multifocal sharp waves and spikes has been called either West syndrome or infantile spasms. However, spasms *per se* only represent a special type of epileptic seizure and although in infants they are usually associated with the hypsarrhythmic EEG pattern to form a syndrome, they may also occur well beyond infancy. The current view (Commission on Paediatric Epilepsy of the International League against Epilepsy 1992) is that West syndrome results from the association of the hypsarrhythmic EEG pattern and epileptic spasms, therefore representing a subgroup of infantile spasms. In this sense, the term 'epileptic spasms' only applies to a type of seizures, irrespective from the age at which they occur. During spasms of West syndrome there is usually a reduction of amplitude often with the appearance of fast activity, preceded by an initial high-voltage slow wave with or without a spike. In some instances the ictal EEG consists of high-amplitude slow waves and spikes. In many patients this condition subsequently evolves into the Lennox–Gastaut syndrome. Although epileptic spasms beyond the nosological limits of West syndrome may have several different underlying aetiologies, they are likewise associated with brain malformations (Dulac *et al.* 1994).

Febrile convulsions are seizures, usually tonic–clonic, occurring with fever. Postictal slowing of background activity reflects the length of the seizure, but except where gross cerebral pathology is present, the EEG is of little value for predicting the subsequent development of epilepsy.

The Lennox–Gastaut syndrome is a form of symptomatic or cryptogenic generalized epilepsy presenting in mid-childhood and characterized by atonic and axial tonic seizures, atypical absences, myoclonic jerks and generalized tonic–clonic as well as partial seizures. The EEG is grossly abnormal with features of symptomatic generalized epilepsy but, in particular, slow spike-and-wave EEG activity (at less than 2.5/s) is among the diagnostic criteria of the syndrome.

Benign myoclonic epilepsy in infancy presents after 6 months of age with single generalized myoclonic seizures. The waking EEG contains occasional spike-and-wave discharges, increasing during sleep. By contrast, severe myoclonic epilepsy in infancy (Dravet et al. 1992) is characterized by generalized or unilateral febrile clonic attacks beginning in the first year of life with subsequent appearance of myoclonic and partial seizures. The EEG is normal initially but later develops fast generalized spike-and-wave discharges, often early photosensitivity and focal abnormalities.

Myoclonic astatic epilepsy of early childhood is included amongst the generalized epilepsy syndromes which may be either symptomatic or cryptogenic (Commission on Classification & Terminology of the International League Against Epilepsy 1989) in that a subset of children present with developmental delay and resistant seizures. However, recent studies have shown that the clinical and EEG pattern and outcome presented by some children is consistent with a specific form of idiopathic generalized epilepsy (Guerrini et al. 1994). Epilepsy onset is in, or soon after, late infancy, usually with generalized tonic–clonic seizures. Children later develop additional seizure types including violent myoclonic jerks causing drop attacks, and episodes of absence status with mild erratic myoclonus. The interictal EEG is initially normal or contains excess theta activity. Subsequently, irregular fast spike-and-wave activity appears. Many patients are photosensitive.

Absence seizures occur in various forms of idiopathic generalized epilepsy. Childhood absence epilepsy appears at 6–7 years, with typical absence seizures but without myoclonus. The EEG shows classical 3/s spike-and-wave activity against a normal background. Despite very frequent seizures, prognosis is good; three-quarters of the patients become seizure-free, but the remainder continue to suffer absences or develop tonic–clonic seizures at puberty or in early adult life. Patients who are at risk of persisting seizures usually have atypical features, including slow spike-and-wave discharges, slow background activity or mental retardation. Their inclusion in the category of idiopathic childhood absence epilepsy is questionable.

Epilepsy with myoclonic absences differs from the above in that the seizures are accompanied by rhythmic myoclonic jerks which are synchronous with the spike component of spike-and-wave discharges. The prognosis is less favourable with respect to response to treatment, subsequent development of other seizure types and cognitive level. The EEG findings are similar to those in childhood absence epilepsy; however, absences are of longer duration.

Juvenile absence epilepsy presents at puberty. The seizures are generally less frequent than in the childhood syndrome, but most of the patients also develop tonic–clonic seizures. All types of absence seizure occur. The EEG shows spike-and-wave activity typically slightly faster than 3/s.

Benign partial epilepsy of childhood with centrotemporal spikes (also called Rolandic epilepsy) is characterized by focal seizures with somatosensory symptoms often starting in the face or mouth, mainly during sleep. Prognosis for seizure control is good, and the condition usually remits at an age of about 16 years. The EEG shows frequent centrotemporal spikes or sharp waves of high amplitude (sometimes exceeding $300\,\mu V$) often followed by a slow wave. Twenty per cent of patients also show generalized spikes and waves or multiple spikes and waves which are activated during slow wave and REM sleep. Typically, the discharges have a dipolar distribution, being negative in the central region with a positivity in the mid-frontal area. A liability to Rolandic spikes is genetically determined, and many children with this EEG abnormality have no overt seizures. Rolandic epilepsy is traditionally not considered to be associated with any neuropsychological deficits. However, several studies have reported impaired visuomotor co-ordination (Heijbel & Bohman 1975), attention problems (Piccirilli et al. 1994), auditory–verbal memory (Croona et al. 1999), deficits in performance IQ, visual perception, short-term memory and behavioural problems (Weglage et al. 1997). Weglage et al. (1997) assessed the behavioural status of 40 children with centrotemporal spikes with and without obvious seizures and compared them with 20 matched controls. Patients had significantly more problems in the subscales social problems, delinquent behaviour and compulsive behaviour. Cognitive deficits may be closely related to psychological impairments occurring in association with the frequent, but apparently subclinical, discharges (Binnie et al. 1992; see below).

Benign partial epilepsy of childhood with occipital foci is accompanied by interictal posterior–temporal–occipital spike-and-wave activity or sharp waves. The seizures are characterized by visual symptoms in older children (Gastaut 1982) and by version with vomiting and occasionally hemiconvulsions in smaller children (Ferrie et al. 1997). Prognosis of this type of epilepsy appears to be invariably good in early onset cases but less uniformly good when onset is in late childhood.

Epilepsy with continuous spike waves during slow-wave sleep is probably underdiagnosed, presenting as a progressive neuropsychological deterioration, affecting language, memory and attention span. This condition may appear in children with brain damage or be cryptogenic. The typical features are onset of rare nocturnal partial motor seizures at preschool age, followed by the appearance of intractable atypical or atonic absences at school age. Prolonged sleep EEG recording is required to recognize the syndrome: spike-and-wave activity present during the greater part of slow-wave sleep. The condition is self-limiting, remitting by the age of 10 years but the prognosis for cognitive function is often poor, especially if the sleep-related electrographic abnormalities have persisted for a long time. Several discrete mild subsyndromes with deterioration of specific neuropsychological functions may sometimes be recognized upon thorough clinical observation or neuropsychological assessment (Veggiotti *et al.* 1999). Ongoing diurnal cognitive effects of discharges occurring during sleep should be distinguished from instantaneous disruption of cognition at the time of the abnormal EEG activity, known as transitory cognitive impairment (TCI; see below).

A specific condition often accompanied by CSWS is the Landau–Kleffner syndrome. Again there is cognitive deterioration, particularly affecting language, but epilepsy occurs in only two-thirds of the patients and is rarely severe. The EEG shows diffuse, or focal, usually bilateral spike-and-wave discharges, in waking and marked activation during sleep. This syndrome is considered more fully below.

Chronic progressive epilepsia continua of childhood may be caused either by a discrete cerebral lesion or by more diffuse Rasmussen encephalitis. In the former case, focal EEG discharges usually occur against a normal background. In Rasmussen syndrome the picture is variable but typically there is a marked diffuse abnormality of background activity and often bilateral discharges. The encephalitic process is usually unilateral and the EEG is asymmetrical, but progressive destruction of one hemisphere may reduce all EEG activities, so that the discharges are paradoxically of greater amplitude on the unaffected side.

Juvenile myoclonic epilepsy is a syndrome with a strong genetic background, with irregular bilateral myoclonic jerks generally worse within an hour of waking. The EEG shows both ictal and interictal irregular fast multiple spike-and-wave discharges and many patients are photosensitive. Later tonic–clonic seizures may appear, especially upon sleep deprivation. Medication is effective but often needs to be lifelong.

Another syndrome of adolescence continuing into adulthood is 'epilepsy with tonic–clonic seizures on awakening'. It is debatable whether this is an independent syndrome or just part of the same spectrum as juvenile myoclonic epilepsy. The background EEG activity is often abnormal and various types of generalized spike-and-wave discharges occur. Despite the name, the distinguishing characteristic is a marked dependence of seizure occurrence on wake–sleep rhythms and disturbances of sleep. Some patients do indeed have seizures on awakening; in others attacks occur in the late evening or after sleep deprivation.

A recently defined epilepsy syndrome which is at particular risk of being misdiagnosed as a parasomnia, a psychiatric disorder or a form of sleep-related paroxysmal dystonia is nocturnal frontal lobe epilepsy (see also section on sleep disorders). This condition may occur in isolated patients or show an autosomal dominant pattern of inheritance (Scheffer *et al.* 1994). Mutations of the neuronal nicotinic acetylcholine receptor alpha-4 subunit gene has been identified in some families (Steinlein *et al.* 1995). The disorder, usually beginning in childhood, is charac-terized by clusters of brief nocturnal motor seizures with tonic and hyperkinetic manifestations, typically appearing during drowsiness or upon awakening. Interictal EEGs are usually unhelpful. Good control is achievable with drug treatment. Behaviour disorders and epilepsy are also prominent in an apparently unrelated condition where there is ring formation of chromosome 20. Interictal EEG abnormalities are usually prominent and often frontal, and prolonged episodes resembling non-convulsive status are associated with EEG abnormalities which some authors consider distinctive (Inoue *et al.* 1997; Kobayashi *et al.* 1998).

The progressive myoclonic epilepsies of childhood and adolescence include various unrelated disorders with the common clinical features of myoclonus, other types of seizure, progressive mental deterioration and variable neurological symptoms. Various specific neurodegenerative conditions fall in this group, and some have characteristic EEG features. However, in general the EEG shows bursts of spikes, spike-and-wave activity and multiple spikes and slow waves, with slowing of ongoing activity and disruption of sleep patterns.

EEG investigation of children with epilepsy

It is a truism that epilepsy is a clinical diagnosis, to which the EEG can add only confirmatory evidence. In general the EEG is of greater value in identifying syndromes than for establishing, or excluding, epilepsy. Thus, slow spike-and-wave activity is among the diagnostic criteria of the Lennox–Gastaut syndrome, and (without an adequate history) benign childhood epilepsy is often first identified by the EEG finding of Rolandic spikes. If in a particular clinical context the EEG excludes the only plausible syndrome, another diagnosis should be considered. For instance, if a child reported to be inattentive overbreathes for 3 mins hard enough to produce EEG slowing, and does not exhibit spike-and-wave activity, active absence epilepsy can be excluded, and some other explanation should be sought.

Using the EEG as a screening test for epilepsy without adequate clinical evidence is rarely helpful, particularly in children with 'soft signs' of organic cerebral disease. Thus, only an ictal EEG will establish an epileptic basis for episodic behavioural disturbances in a disabled, presumably brain-damaged child; interictal epileptiform discharges are without diagnostic significance in this context. Some scenarios will be briefly considered.

'Routine' investigation of newly diagnosed epilepsy

The EEG may help to identify the syndrome, with implications for management and prognosis. Significant unexpected findings sometimes arise, e.g. photosensitivity or frequent unrecognized seizures. If a waking record does not provide the information required, a sleep tracing should always be obtained; this increases the yield of abnormal findings, especially in partial epilepsies, and may be crucial to early identification of benign childhood epilepsy, or CSWS.

Screening of children with an increased risk or doubtful evidence of epilepsy

Abnormal findings should be interpreted cautiously. Spiky EEG phenomena unrelated to epilepsy (6 and 14/s positive spikes, for instance) should be ignored. Rolandic spikes, photosensitivity and generalized spike-and-wave activity may reflect a genetic liability, rather than an active seizure disorder. However, such findings justify further enquiry, which may reveal previously unrecognized ictal events related to visual stimuli: myoclonus in proximity to a television set, self-inducing behaviour, etc.

During apparently subclinical EEG discharges, unexpected ictal events may be detected. If the child sits upright with outstretched arms during recording, momentary loss of muscle tone may be shown to accompany the discharges. Psychological tests administered under EEG monitoring often detect TCI associated with seemingly subclinical discharges. TCI has been found in about 50% of patients with epilepsy during both generalized and focal discharges (Aarts *et al.* 1984; Binnie *et al.* 1990). These findings may have clinical implications in a child with psychiatric manifestations or learning difficulties as TCI can impair day-to-day psychosocial function, such as school performance (Kasteleijn-Nolst Trenité *et al.* 1988), driving a car (Kasteleijn-Nolst Trenité *et al.* 1987) and behaviour (Binnie *et al.* 1992; Marston *et al.* 1993). Technically, such events are epileptic seizures and they are subclinical only in the sense that conventional methods of observation fail to detect the clinical manifestations.

Investigation of episodic abnormal behaviour

The only reliable method of establishing that a particular episodic behaviour is epileptic is by demonstrating ictal EEG changes. This applies equally to children with known epilepsy and to those without. The dangers of misinterpreting an interictal EEG abnormality in this context were noted above. The practicalities of capturing an ictal EEG depend on the frequency, nature and circumstances of occurrence of the episodes (see section on long-term EEG monitoring). It must be recognized, however, that even intensive monitoring may not solve the problem. If the seizures are infrequent they are unlikely to be captured at all and, if of certain types, may not produce ictal EEG changes. Referral for EEG investigation of episodic behavioural disorder should be selective and not viewed as a panacea for this common problem. Equally, it is important that every effort be made to distinguish epileptic from non-epileptic seizures, bearing in mind that these may coexist. 'Uncertainty or equivocation on the physician's part can be disabling' (Stores 1999). A relaxed pragmatic approach, suggesting that the nature of the attacks is unimportant will not lead to effective management, as the recognition and specific treatment both of epilepsy and of non-epileptic attacks are equally essential.

Neurodegenerative disease

Clinical neurophysiological findings can help identify individuals who may be suffering from a neurodegenerative disease, as a number of distinctive patterns have been associated with various conditions (Boyd & Harden 1997). They may also suggest that the child does *not* have a neurodegenerative disorder by demonstrating some other process leading to a decline in behaviour or performance, notably non-convulsive status epilepticus.

Subacute sclerosing panencephalitis

The association between subacute sclerosing panencephalitis and periodic complexes in the EEG is probably one of the best-known electroclinical associations. Despite this, cases are still missed, often because of a failure to consider the condition. This may be because of an unusual presentation such as visual disturbance (8.75% of a series of 80 children, Pampiglione & Harden 1986)) or because behavioural disturbances or fits initially suggest other conditions. The EEG complexes themselves may not be striking or their significance may be dismissed because of the presence of normal activities, including alpha rhythm.

Batten disease

Distinctive neurophysiological findings in the different forms have been useful in helping to identify affected children. In the juvenile form, the child presents at around 5–6 years of age with visual symptoms and may be referred to the psychiatrist if no ophthalmic cause is found. By this time the ERG is usually absent and the flash VEP is poorly formed or absent. The EEG shows runs of sharp waves and slower components at around 2/s in about 50% of cases.

Variant forms of this group of disorders are not infrequent and Santavuori *et al.* (1991) has emphasized the wider spectrum of clinical presentation. In one case, a girl presenting with a progressive dementia without any other clinical features was eventually shown to have Batten disease on biopsy following the unexpected finding of a small ERG.

Sleep disorders

Sleep disorders in children have been characterized as both underdiagnosed and undertreated (Stores 1990). A comprehensive classification of diagnostic criteria, including neurophysiological findings, was published in 1990 (Thorpy 1990). Technical aspects of making polysomnographic recordings in infants, children and adolescents have also been reviewed (Guilleminault & Philip 1992; Hoppenbrouwers 1992; Keenan 1992). However, most of these disorders, including night terrors (Guilleminault & Silvestri 1982), are rarely associated with seizures or with EEG abnormalities. Different disorders may be associated with particular phases of sleep (Table 11.2).

Epileptic disorders manifesting as abnormal movements during sleep, especially frontal lobe seizures, are also difficult to

Table 11.2 Electroencephalogram (EEG) and polysomnographic features in some sleep disorders of infancy, childhood and adolescence. (After Thorpy 1990; see text for epileptic and mental disorders.)

Disorder	Typical age of onset	Polysomnographic features	EEG features
Dyssomnias			
Intrinsic sleep disorders			
Idiopathic insomnia (childhood-onset insomnia)	Birth	Sleep spindles may be poorly formed. and somnograms difficult to score. Long periods of REM sleep without eye movements	Varied, minor non-specific abnormalities are common
Narcolepsy	Second decade. Peak incidence 14 years	Short sleep latency. Sleep-onset REM can be associated with hypnogogic hallucinations	Often features of drowsiness. Eye opening may increase alpha activity
Recurrent hypersomnia (Kleine–Levin syndrome)	Adolescence	High sleep efficiency. Reduced stage III and IV sleep	Low-voltage slow activity or diffuse alpha activity
Idiopathic hypersomnia (NREM narcolepsy)	Adolescence	Normal	Normal
Obstructive sleep apnoea	Any age	Complex and varied. Some have initial central apnoea followed by obstruction (mixed type). Short sleep latency; occasionally sleep-onset REM	Normal
Central alveolar hypoventilation	Idiopathic: adolescence Acquired: any age	Periods of oxygen desaturation worse in REM sleep. Frequent arousals, body movements	Normal
Restless legs syndrome	Any age (mostly in middle age)	Sustained tonic EMG activity alternates between legs, occurs in antagonistic muscles during flexion and extension of legs	Normal (wake) EMG and nerve conduction studies usual in young subjects
Extrinsic sleep disorders			
Adjustment sleep disorder (transient psychological insomnia)	Any age	Very variable	Normal
Limit-setting sleep disorder (childhood insomnia)	2–3 years variable	Normal	Normal
Sleep-onset association disorder	6 months	Normal	Normal
Food allergy insomnia (food intolerance)	In first to second year	Frequent arousals. No preceding EEG change	Normal
Nocturnal eating (drinking) syndrome	6 months	Normal except for increased waking	Normal
Stimulant-dependent sleep disorder (stimulant sleep suppression)	Adolescence	↑ Sleep and REM latency. ↓ Total sleep and REM time. Rebound on stimulant withdrawal; MSLT may then resemble narcolepsy	Normal
Circadian rhythm sleep disorders. Irregular sleep–wake pattern	Variable	Paucity of information	↓ Sleep spindles and K-complexes ±changes associated with underlying cerebral condition
Delayed sleep phase syndrome	Adolescence	↑ Sleep latency. Some ↓ REM latency	Normal
Non-24-h sleep–wake syndrome	Variable. Usually blind infant/child	Paucity of information	↓ Sleep spindles and K-complexes ±changes associated with any underlying cerebral problem

Continued

Table 11.2 *continued*

Disorder	Typical age of onset	Polysomnographic features	EEG features
Parasomnias *Arousal disorders*			
Confusional arousals (sleep drunkenness)	< 5 years	Arousals from slow wave sleep, especially first third of night	Slow activity during episode, otherwise normal
Sleepwalking	4–8 years	Begins in stage III or IV sleep	Normal*
Sleep terrors (night terrors)	Childhood	Especially in stage III or IV sleep	Normal*
Sleep–wake transition disorders Rhythmic movement disorder (head-banging, body-rocking)	Usually < 1 year	Episodes in drowsiness or (mainly) light sleep	Normal*
Parasomnias usually associated with REM sleep Nightmares	Any age 3–6 years	Abrupt awakening from REM sleep, ↑ REM duration and density	Normal
Sleep paralysis	Adolescence	Loss of tone, ↓ EMG activity, H reflex studies; ↓ anterior horn cell excitability as in REM sleep	Slow activity and/or pendular eye movements during episode
Other parasomnias Bruxism (tooth grinding)	10–20 years	↑ Masseter and temporalis activity; stage II sleep	Normal
Sleep enuresis	Primary from infancy. Secondary any age	Episodes in all sleep stages, also wakefulness	Occasionally associated with epilepsy, discharges may be found
Nocturnal paroxysmal dystonia	Variable	Episodes mainly in stage II, but also in stage III or 4 sleep. EEG desynchronization; no discharges	Normal*
Infant sleep apnoea (apparent life-threatening event)	First days to weeks of life	Usually no abnormalities. Prematures; AS > QS	*Rarely* associated with localized discharges†
Benign neonatal sleep myoclonus	First week of life	EMG bursts lasting 40–30 μs, usually in QS	Normal*
Psychiatric sleep disorders Psychosis	Adolescence	Very variable	(See text)
Mood disorders (depressive disorder)	Childhood and adolescence	Typically ↓ delta and ↑ REM sleep Short REM latency. ↑ density REM. Findings in children and adolescents less marked, cf. adults	Normal
Anxiety disorder	Any age	Mild changes. ↑ Sleep latency, ↑ stage I and II sleep	Normal

Abbreviations: AS, active sleep; EMG, electromyogram; MSLT, multiple sleep latency test; NREM, non-rapid eye movement; QS, quiet sleep; REM, rapid eye movement.

* Normal: Useful contribution by excluding other conditions in differential diagnosis.

† Watanabe *et al.* (1982).

recognize (Stores *et al*. 1991) and often have to be considered in the differential diagnosis (Fish & Marsden 1994).

A summary of polysomnographic and EEG findings in sleep disorders seen mainly in childhood and adolescence is shown in Table 11.2.

Future developments

The history of clinical neurophysiological investigations in psychiatry and psychology has been one of high hopes succeeded by disappointment as each technique in turn proved unable to sustain the expectations placed upon it. It is to be hoped that some of the lessons have now been learnt, and that the importance of careful definition of the type of disorder being investigated and equally careful patient selection will lead to much greater progress. The experience with EEG and latterly EPs should be borne in mind when considering the claims of topographic mapping and ERPs. The need to establish reliable norms, and proper caution in establishing the limits and strengths of any new technique, are fundamental, as is the need to discriminate between individual and group differences from 'normal'. Despite this need for caution, there has been some progress in developing relevant clinical protocols (Byrne *et al*. 1999).

Conventional techniques, used carefully and in combination both with each other and with other methods of investigation are still capable of providing valuable insights into psychological processes both in normal children and in those with psychiatric disease. This is likely to be enhanced by improved applications of the powerful mathematical tools provided by digital signal processing, although the importance of ensuring that the signals obtained from the patient are of the highest quality must never be forgotten. Current interest in high-frequency components of EEG signals may lead to striking new insights into how different regions of the brain communicate, particularly when combined with other techniques, such as transcranial magnetic stimulation, but as yet there are no specific clinical associations. A similar situation pertains to the use of other techniques, such as magnetoencephalography (Baumgartner 2000); despite a large literature on localization of function obtained with this technique, its place in the investigation of brain disorders remains unclear, compounded by the limited availability of the facility in many countries. While it may find a role in the non-invasive localization of epileptic foci in children undergoing presurgical evaluation (Minassian *et al*. 1999), at present it seems unlikely to supersede EEG entirely. There is also much interest in combining MRI with simultaneous MEG/EEG recording as a means of overcoming the inherent limitations of each method when used alone (Dale *et al*. 2000), but much basic research still needs to be carried out.

Rather than being superseded by other techniques, it seems more likely that clinical neurophysiological investigations will continue to provide unique information on the function of the nervous system. While new techniques of data collection and manipulation may prove useful, cross-reference to other investigations and other methods of studying the nervous system are also likely to be fruitful. As a consequence, the quality and relevance of this information seems likely to improve markedly as a result of improvements in its interpretation and in our confidence concerning its clinical and biological significance.

References

Aarts, J.H.P., Binnie, C.D., Smith, A.M. & Wilkins, A.J. (1984) Selective cognitive impairment during focal and generalised epileptiform EEG activity. *Brain*, **107**, 293–308.

Aldrich, M.S., Garofalo, E.A. & Drury, I. (1990) Epileptiform abnormalities during sleep in Rett syndrome. *Electroencephalography and Clinical Neurophysiology*, **75**, 365–370.

Bader, G.G., Witt-Engerstrom, I. & Hagberg, B. (1989a) Neurophysiological findings in the Rett syndrome. I. EMG, conduction velocity, EEG and somatosensory evoked potential studies. *Brain and Development*, **11**, 102–109.

Bader, G.G., Witt-Engerstrom, I. & Hagberg, B. (1989b) Neurophysiological findings in the Rett syndrome. II. Visual and auditory brainstem, middle and late evoked responses. *Brain and Development*, **11**, 110–114.

Baraitser, M. & Winter, R. (1992) *The London Neurology Database*. Oxford University Press, Oxford.

Barkovich, J.A., Guerrini, R., Battaglia, G. *et al.* (1994) Band heterotopia. Correlation of outcome with MR imaging parameters. *Annals of Neurology*, **36**, 609–617.

Baumgartner, C. (2000) Clinical applications of magnetoencephalography. *Journal of Clinical Neurophysiology*, **17**, 175–176.

Bickford, R.G., Sem-Jacobsen, C.W., White, P.T. & Daly, D. (1952) Some observations on the mechanism of photic and photo-metrazol activation. *Electroencephalography and Clinical Neurophysiology*, **4**, 275–282.

Binnie, C.D. & MacGillivray, B.B. (1992) Brain mapping: a useful tool or a dangerous toy? *Journal of Neurology, Neurosurgery and Psychiatry*, **55**, 527–529.

Binnie, C.D., Channon, S. & Marston, D. (1990) Learning disabilities in epilepsy: neurophysiological aspects. *Epilepsia*, **31** (Suppl. 4), 2–8.

Binnie, C.D., de Silva, M. & Hurst, A. (1992) Rolandic spikes and cognitive function. *Epilepsy Research Supplement*, **6**, 71–74.

Bower, B.D. & Jeavons, P.M. (1967) The 'happy puppet' syndrome. *Archives of Disease in Childhood*, **42**, 298–302.

Boyd, S.G. & Harden, A. (1997) Clinical neurophysiology of the central nervous system. In: *Paediatric Neurology* (ed. E.M. Brett), 3rd edn, pp. 747–821. Churchill Livingstone, Edinburgh.

Boyd, S., Harden, A. & Patton, M.A. (1988) The EEG in the early diagnosis of the Angelman (happy puppet) syndrome. *European Journal of Pediatrics*, **147**, 508–513.

Byrne, J.M., Connolly, J.F., MacLean, S.E., Dooley, J.E., Gordon, K.E. & Beattie, T.L. (1999) Brain activity and language assessment using event-related potentials: development of a clinical protocol. *Developmental Medicine and Child Neurology*, **41**, 740–747.

Cantwell, D.P. (1980) Drug and medical intervention. In: *Handbook of Minimal Brain Dysfunction: a Critical Review* (eds H.E. Rie & E.D. Rie), pp. 000–000. Wiley, New York.

Cole, A.J., Andermann, F., Taylor, L. *et al.* (1988) The Landau–Kleffner syndrome of acquired epileptic aphasia: unusual clinical outcome, surgical experience, and absence of encephalitis. *Neurology*, **38**, 31–38.

Commission on Classification and Terminology of the International

League Against Epilepsy (1989) Proposal for revised classification of epilepsies and epileptic syndromes. *Epilepsia*, 30, 389–399.

Commission on Pediatric Epilepsy of the International League against Epilepsy (1992) Workshop on infantile spasms. *Epilepsia*, 33, 195.

Conners, C.K. (1978) Critical review of 'electroencephalographic and neurophysiological studies in dyslexia'. In: *Dyslexia: an Appraisal of Current Knowledge* (eds A.L. Benton & D. Pearl), pp. 251–264. Oxford University Press, New York.

Croona, C., Kihlgren, M., Lundberg, S., Eeg-Olofsson, O., Eeg-Olofsson, K.E. (1999) Neuropsychological findings in children with benign childhood epilepsy with centrotemporal spikes. *Development Medicine and Child Neurology*, 41, 813–818.

Dahl, R.E., Ryan, N.D. & Birmaher, B. *et al.* (1991) Electroencephalographic sleep measures in prepubertal depression. *Psychiatry Research*, 38, 201–214.

Dale, A.M., Liu, A.K., Fischi, B.R. *et al.* (2000) Dynamic statistical parametric neurotechnique mapping: combining fMRI and MEG for high resolution of cortical activity. *Neuron*, 26, 55–67.

Dement, W. & Kleitman, N. (1957) Cyclic variations in EEG during sleep and their relation to eye movements, body motility, and dreaming. *Electroencephalography and Clinical Neurophysiology*, 9, 673–690.

Deonna, T.W. (1991) Acquired epileptiform aphasia in children (Landau–Kleffner syndrome). *Journal of Clinical Neurophysiology*, 8, 288–298.

Doering, S., Cross, H., Boyd, S., Harkness, W. & Neville, B.G. (1999) The significance of bilateral EEG abnormalities before and after hemispherectomy in children with unilateral major hemisphere lesions. *Epilepsy Research*, 34, 65–73.

van Dongen, H.R., Meulstee, J., Blauw-van Mourik, M. & van Harskamp, F. (1989) Landau–Kleffner syndrome: a case study with a 14-year follow-up. *European Neurology*, 29, 109–114.

Doose, H. & Gerken, H. (1973) On the genetics of EEG-anomalies in childhood. IV. photoconvulsive reaction. *Neuropaediatrie*, 4, 162–171.

Dravet, C., Bureau, M., Guerrini, R., Giraud, N. & Roger, J. (1992) Severe myoclonic epilepsy in infants. In: *Epileptic Syndromes in Infancy, Childhood and Adolescence* (eds J. Roger, C. Dravet, M. Bureau, F.E. Dreifuss, P. Wolf & A. Perret), 2nd edn, pp. 75–88. John Libby Eurotext, London.

Dulac, O., Chugani, H.T. & Dalla Bernardina, B. eds. (1994) *Infantile Spasms and West Syndrome*. W.B. Saunders, London.

Dümermuth, G. (1968) Variance spectra of electroencephalograms in twins: a contribution to the problem of quantification of EEG background activity in childhood. In: *Clinical Electroencephalography of Children* (eds P. Kellaway & I. Petersén), pp. 119–154. Almquist & Wiksell, Stockholm.

Elian, M. & Rudolf, N.D. (1991) EEG and respiration in Rett syndrome. *Acta Neurologica Scandinavica*, 83, 123–128.

Emslie, G.J., Rush, A.J., Weinberg, W.A., Rintelmann, J.W. & Roffwarg, H.P. (1990) Children with major depression show reduced rapid eye movement latencies. *Archives of General Psychiatry*, 47, 119–124.

Ferrie, C.D., Beaumanoir, A., Guerrini, R. *et al.* (1997) Early onset occipital seizure susceptability syndrome. *Epilepsia*, 38, 285–293.

Fish, D.R. & Marsden, C.D. (1994) Epilepsy masquerading as a movement disorder. In: *Movement Disorders 3* (eds. C.D. Marsden & S. Fahn), pp. 346–358. Butterworth, Oxford.

French, C.C. & Beaumont, J.G. (1984) A critical review of EEG coherence studies of hemisphere function. *International Journal of Psychophysiology*, 1, 241–254.

Galin, D., Raz, J., Fein, G., Johnstone, J., Herron, J. & Yingling, C. (1992) EEG spectra in dyslexic and normal readers during normal and silent reading. *Electroencephalography and Clinical Neurophysiology*, 82, 87–101.

Gastaut, H. (1982) A new type of epilepsy: benign partial epilepsy of childhood with occipital spike-waves. *Clinical Electroencephalography*, 13, 13–22.

Gastaut, H., Pinsard, N., Raybaud, C.L., Aicardi, J. & Zifkin, B. (1987) Lissencephaly (agyria-pachygyria): clinical findings and serial EEG studies. *Developmental Medicine and Child Neurology*, 29, 167–180.

Giles, D.E., Roffwarg, H.P., Dahl, R.E. & Kupfer, D.J. (1992) Electroencephalographic sleep abnormalities in depressed children: a hypothesis. *Psychiatry Research*, 41, 53–63.

Glaze, D.G., Frost, J.D., el Hibri, H.Y. & Percy, A.K. (1985) Rett's syndrome: polygraphic electroencephalographic–video characterization of sleep and respiratory patterns during sleep and wakefulness. *Annals of Neurology*, 18, 417–418.

Gloor, P., Kalabay, O. & Giard, N. (1968) The electroencephalogram in diffuse encephalopathies: electroencephalographic correlates of grey and white matter lesions. *Brain*, 91, 779–802.

Gregoriades, A. & Pampiglione, G. (1966) Seizures in children with Down's syndrome. *Electroencephalography and Clinical Neurophysiology*, 21, 307.

Guerrini, R., Genton, P., Bureau, M., Dravet, C. & Roger, J. (1990) Reflex seizures are frequent in patients with Down's syndrome and epilepsy. *Epilepsia*, 31, 406–417.

Guerrini, R., Dravet, C., Gobbi, G., Ricci, S. & Dulac, O. (1994) Idiopathic generalized epilepsies with myoclonus in infancy and childhood. In: *Idiopathic Generalized Epilepsies: Clinical, Experimental and Genetic Aspects* (eds A. Malafosse, P. Genton, E. Hirsch, C. Marescaux, D. Broglin, & R. Bernasconi), pp. 267–280. John Libbey Eurotext, London.

Guerrini, R., Andermann, F., Canapicchi, R., Roger, J., Zifkin, B.G. & Pfanner, P., eds. (1996) *Dysplasias of Cerebral Cortex and Epilepsy*. Lippincott-Raven, New York.

Guerrini, R., De Lorey, T.M., Bonanni, P. *et al.* (1996) Cortical myoclonus in Angelman syndrome. *Annals of Neurology*, 40, 39–48.

Guerrini, R., Bonanni, P., Parmeggiani, L., Santucci, M., Parmeggiani, M. & Sartucci, F. (1998a) Cortical reflex myoclonus in Rett Syndrome. *Annals of Neurology*, 43, 472–479.

Guerrini, R., Genton, P., Bureau, M. *et al.* (1998b) Multilobar polymicrogyria, intractable drop attack seizures and sleep-related electrical status epilepticus. *Neurology*, 51, 504–512.

Guilleminault, C. & Philip, P. (1992) Polygraphic investigation of respiration during sleep in infants and children. *Journal of Clinical Neurophysiology*, 9, 48–55.

Guilleminault, C. & Silvestri, R. (1982) Disorders of arousal and epilepsy during sleep. In: *Sleep and Epilepsy* (eds M.B. Sterman, M.N. Shouse & P. Passouant), pp. 513–529. Academic Press, New York.

Hagberg, B., Aicardi, J., Dias, K. & Ramos, O. (1983) A progressive syndrome of autism, dementia and loss of purposeful hand use in girls: Rett's syndrome—a report of 35 cases. *Annals of Neurology*, 14, 471–479.

Hagne, I., Witt-Engerström, I. & Hagberg, B. (1989) EEG development in Rett syndrome: a study of 30 cases. *Electroencephalography and Clinical Neurophysiology*, 72, 1–6.

Hakamada, S., Watanabe, K., Hara, K. & Miyazaki, S. (1979) The evolution of electroencephalographic features in lissencephaly syndrome. *Brain and Development*, 1, 277–283.

Heijbel, J. & Bohman, M. (1975) Benign epileppsy of children with centrotemporal EEG foci: intelligence, behaviour and school adjustment. *Epilepsia*, 16, 679–687.

Hoppenbrouwers, T. (1992) Polysomnography in newborns and young infants: sleep architecture. *Journal of Clinical Neurophysiology*, **9**, 32–47.

Inoue, Y., Fujiwara, T., Matsuda, K. *et al.* (1997) Ring chromosome 20m and non-convulsive status epilepticus: a new epileptic syndrome. *Brain*, **120**, 939–953.

Itil, T.M., Hsu, W., Saletu, B. & Mednick, S. (1974) Computer EEG and auditory evoked potential investigations in children at high risk for schizophrenia. *American Journal of Psychiatry*, **131**, 892–900.

Itil, T.M., Simeon, J. & Coffin, C. (1976) Qualitative and quantitative EEG in psychotic children. *Diseases of the Nervous System*, **37**, 247–252.

Kasteleijn-Nolst Trenité, D.G., Riemersma, J.B., Binnie, C.D., Smit, A.M. & Meinardi, H. (1987) The influence of subclinical epileptiform EEG discharges on driving behaviour. *Electroencephalography and Clinical Neurophysiology*, **67**, 167–170.

Kasteleijn-Nolst Trenité, D.G.A., Bakker, D.J., Binnie, C.J., Buerman, A. & Van Raaij, M. (1988) Psychological effects of subclinical epileptiform discharges: scholastic skills. *Epilepsy Research*, **2**, 111–116.

Keenan, S.A. (1992) Polysomnography: technical aspects in adolescents and adults. *Journal of Clinical Neurophysiology*, **9**, 21–31.

Kobayashi, K., Inagaki, M., Sasaki, M., Sugai, K., Ohta, S. & Hashimoto, T. (1998) Characteristic EEG findings in ring 20 chromosome as a diagnostic clue. *Electroencephalography and Clinical Neurophysiology*, **107**, 258–262.

Landau, W.M. & Kleffner, F.R. (1957) Syndrome of acquired aphasia with convulsive disorder. *Neurology*, **7**, 523–530.

Lennox, W.G., Gibbs, E.L. & Gibbs, F.A. (1945) The brain wave pattern, an hereditary trait. Evidence from 74 'normal' pairs of twins. *Journal of Heredity*, **36**, 233–243.

Lerman, P., Lerman-Sagie, T. & Kivity, S. (1991) Effect of early corticosteroid therapy for Landau–Kleffner syndrome. *Developmental Medicine and Child Neurology*, **33**, 257–260.

Lewine, J.D., Andrews, R., Chez, M. *et al.* (1999) Magnetoencephalographic patterns of epileptiform activity in children with regressive autism spectrum disorders. *Pediatrics*, **104**, 405–418.

Lugaresi, E., Cirignotta, F. & Montagna, P. (1985) Abnormal breathing in the Rett syndrome. *Brain and Development*, **7**, 329–333.

Maccario, M., Hefferen, S.J., Keblusek, S.J. & Lipinski, K.A. (1982) Developmental dysphasia and electroencephalographic abnormalities. *Developmental Medicine and Child Neurology*, **24**, 141–155.

Marston, D., Besag, F., Binnie, C.D. & Fowler, M. (1993) Effects of transitory cognitive impairment on psychosocial functioning of children with epilepsy: a therapeutic trial. *Developmental Medicine and Child Neurology*, **35**, 574–581.

Minassian, B., DeLorey, T., Olsen, R.W. *et al.* (1998) The epilepsy of Angelman syndrome due to deletion, disomy, imprinting center and UB3A mutations. *Annals of Neurology*, **43**, 485–493.

Minassian, B.A., Otsubo, H., Weiss, S., Elliott, I., Rutka, J.T. & Snead, O.C. III (1999) Magnetoencephalographic localization in pediatric epilepsy surgery: comparison with invasive intracranial electroencephalography. *Annals of Neurology*, **46**, 627–633.

Morrell, F., Whisler, W.W. & Black, T.P. (1989) Multiple subpial transection. a new approach to the surgical treatment of focal epilepsy. *Journal of Neurosurgery*, **70**, 231–239.

Noachtar, S., Binnie, C.D., Ebersole, J., Maugiere, F., Sakamoto, A. & Westmoreland, B. (1999) A glossary of terms most commonly used by clinical electroencephalographers and proposal for the report form for the EEG findings. In: *Recommendations for the Practice of Clinical Neurophysiology: Clinical Neurophysiology (Supplement 52)* (eds G. Deuchl & A. Eisen), pp. 21–40. Elsevier, Amsterdam.

Nomura, Y., Segawa, M. & Hasegawa, M. (1984) Rett syndrome: clinical studies and pathophysiological consideration. *Brain and Development*, **6**, 475–486.

Nuwer, M.R. (1988a) Quantitative EEG. I. Techniques and problems of frequency analysis and topographic mapping. *Journal of Clinical Neurophysiology*, **5**, 1–44.

Nuwer, M.R. (1988b) Quantitative EEG. II. Frequency analysis and topographic mapping in clinical settings. *Journal of Clinical Neurophysiology*, **5**, 45–86.

Paetau, R., Kajola, M., Korkman, M., Hamalainen, M., Granstrom, M.L. & Hari, R. (1991) Landau–Kleffner syndrome: epileptic activity in the auditory cortex. *Neuroreport*, **2**, 201–204.

Paladin, F., Chiron, C., Dulac, O., Plouin, P. & Ponsot, G. (1989) Electroencephalographic aspects of hemimegalencephaly. *Developmental Medicine and Child Neurology*, **37**, 377–383.

Pampiglione, G. & Harden, A. (1986) SSPE: neurophysiological findings in 80 cases. In: *Subacute Sclerosing Panencephalitis: a Reappraisal* (eds F. Bergamini, C.A. Defanti & P. Ferrante), pp. 98–105. Elsevier, Amsterdam.

Patry, G., Lyagoubi, S. & Tassinari, C.A. (1971) Subclinical 'electrical status epilepticus' induced by sleep in children. A clinical and electroencephalographic study of six cases. *Archives of Neurology*, **24**, 242–252.

Piccirilli, M., D'Alessandro, P., Sciarma, T. *et al.* (1994) Attention problems in epilepsy: possible significance of the epileptogenic focus. *Epilepsia*, **35**, 1091–1096.

Picton, T.W., ed. (1988) *Human Event Related Potentials: EEG Handbook Revised Series*, Vol. 3. Elsevier Biomedical Division, Amsterdam.

Picton, T.W., Stuss, D.T., Champagne, S.C. & Nelson, R.P. (1984) The effects of age on human event-related potentials. *Psychophysiology*, **21**, 312–325.

Pueschel, S.M., Findley, T.W., Furia, J., Gallagher, P.L., Scolla, F.H. & Penzullo, J.C. (1987) Atlantoaxial instability in Down syndrome: roentgenographic, neurologic and somatosensory evoked potential studies. *Journal of Pediatrics*, **110**, 512–521.

Robb, S.A., Harden, A. & Boyd, S.G. (1989) Rett syndrome: an EEG study in 52 girls. *Neuropediatrics*, **20**, 192–195.

Santavuori, P., Rapola, J., Nuutila, A. *et al.* (1991) The spectrum of Jansky–Bielschowsky disease. *Neuropediatrics*, **22**, 92–96.

Satterfield, J.H., Cantwell, D.P., Saul, R.E. & Yusin, A. (1974) Intelligence, academic achievement, and EEG abnormalities in hyperactive children. *American Journal of Psychiatry*, **131**, 391–395.

Scheffer, I.E., Bhatia, K.P., Lopes-Cendes, I. *et al.* (1994) Autosomal dominant frontal epilepsy misdiagnosed as sleep disorder. *Lancet*, **343**, 515–517.

Seri, S., Cerquiglini, A. & Pisani, F. (1998) Spike-induced interference in auditory sensory processing in Landau–Kleffner syndrome. *Electroencephalography and Clinical Neurophysiology*, **108**, 506–510.

Shetty, T. (1973) Some neurological electrophysiological and biochemical correlates of the hyperactive syndrome. *Pediatric Annals*, **29**, 29–38.

Small, J.G. (1975) EEG and neurophysiological studies of early infantile autism. *Biological Psychiatry*, **10**, 355–397.

Small, J.G. (1987) Psychiatric disorders and EEG. In: *Electroencephalography: Basic Principles, Clinical Applications and Related Fields* (ed. E. Niedermeyer), 2nd edn, pp. 526–527. Urban & Schwarzenburg, Baltimore.

Stassen, H.H., Lykken, D.T., Propping, P. & Bomben, G. (1988) Genetic determination of the human EEG. *Human Genetics*, **80**, 165–176.

Steinlein, O.K., Mulley, J.C., Propping, P. *et al.* (1995) A missense mutation in the neuronal nicotinic acetylcholine receptor a4 subunit is associated with autosomal dominant nocturnal frontal lobe epilepsy. *Nature Genetics*, **11**, 201–203.

Steriade, M., Gloor, P., Llinas, R.R., Lopes da Silva, F.H. & Mesulam,

M.-M. (1990) Basic mechanisms of cerebral rhythmic activities. *Electroencephalography and Clinical Neurophysiology*, **76**, 481–508.

Stores, G. (1990) Sleep disorders in children. *British Medical Journal*, **301**, 351–352.

Stores, G. (1999) Practitioner review: recognition of pseudoseizures in children and adolescents. *Journal of Child Psychology and Psychiatry*, **40**, 851–857.

Stores, G., Zaiwalla, Z. & Bergel, N. (1991) Frontal lobe complex partial seizures in children: a form of epilepsy at particular risk of misdiagnosis. *Developmental Medicine and Child Neurology*, **33**, 998–1009.

Strandburg, R.J., Marsh, J.T., Brown, W.S., Asarnow, R.F., Guthrie, D. & Higa, J. (1991) Reduced attention-related negative potentials in schizophrenic children. *Electroencephalography and Clinical Neurophysiology*, **79**, 291–307.

Tassinari, C.A. & Rubboli, G. (1997) Polygraphic recordings. In: *Epilepsy: a Comprehensive Textbook* (eds J. Engel, Jr. & T.A. Pedley), pp. 897–917. Lippincott-Raven, Philadephia.

Taylor, D.C., Falconer, M.A., Bruton, C.J. & Corsellis, J.A.N. (1971) Focal dysplasia of the cerebral cortex in epilepsy. *Journal of Neurology, Neurosurgery and Psychiatry*, **34**, 369–387.

Thaker, G.K., Wagman, A.M., Tamminga, C.A. (1990) Sleep polygraphy in schizophrenia: methodological issues. *Biological Psychiatry*, **28**, 240–246.

Thivierge, J., Bedard, C., Cote, R. & Maziade, M. (1990) Brainstem auditory evoked responses and subcortical abnormalities in autism. *American Journal of Psychiatry*, **147**, 1609–1613.

Thorpy, M.J., ed. (1990) *International Classification of Sleep Disorders: Diagnostic and Coding Manual*. American Sleep Disorders Association, Rochester.

Tsai, L.Y., Tsai, M.C. & August, G.J. (1985) Brief report of EEG diagnoses in the subclassification of infantile autism. *Journal of Autism and Developmental Disorders*, **15**, 339–344.

Tuchman, R.F. (1994) Epilepsy, language and behavior: clinical models in childhood. *Journal of Child Neurology*, **9**, 95–102.

Tuchman, R.F., Rapin, I. & Shinnar, S. (1991) Autistic and dysphasic children. II. Epilepsy. *Pediatrics*, **88**, 1219–1225.

Veggiotti, P., Beccaria, F., Guerrini, R., Capovilla, G. & Lanzi, G. (1999) Continuous spike-and-wave activity during slow-wave sleep: syndrome or EEG pattern? *Epilepsia*, **40**, 1593–1601.

Viani, F., Romeo, A., Viri, M. *et al.* (1995) Seizure and EEG patterns in Angelman's syndrome. *Journal of Child Neurology*, **10**, 467–471.

Vogel, F. (1958) *Über die Erblichkeit des Normalen EEG: Zwillingsuntersuchungen 1958*. Thieme, Stuttgart.

Waldo, M.C., Cohen, D.J., Caparulo, B.K., Young, J.G., Prichard, J.W. & Shaywitz, B.A. (1978) EEG profiles of neuropsychiatrically disturbed children. *Journal of the American Academy of Child Psychiatry*, **17**, 656–670.

Waltz, S., Christen, H.-J. & Doose, H. (1992) The different patterns of the photoparoxysmal response: a genetic study. *Electroencephalographical and Clinical Neurophysiology*, **83**, 138–145.

Watanabe, K., Hara, K., Hakamada, S. *et al.* (1982) Seizures with apnea in children. *Pediatrics*, **79**, 87–90.

Weglage, J., Demsky, A., Pietsch, M. & Kurlemann, G. (1997) Neuropsychological, intellectual, and behavioral findings in patients with centrotemporal spikes with and without seizures. *Developmental Medicine and Child Neurology*, **39**, 646–651.

Wisniewski, K.E., Segan, S.M., Miezejeski, C.M., Sersen, E.A. & Rudelli, R.D. (1991) The Fragile (X) syndrome: neurological, electrophysiological and neuropathological abnormalities. *American Journal of Medical Genetics*, **38**, 476–480.

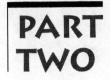

PART TWO

Influences on Psychopathology

12 Genetics of Normal and Abnormal Development

Peter McGuffin and Michael Rutter

Introduction

The climate of opinion has changed markedly since McGuffin & Gottesman (1985) noted the comparative neglect of genetics, and in some quarters overt hostility, among child psychiatrists. Why have views changed, and will a new-found interest in genetics ultimately be of benefit to child psychiatry? The answer to the first question could lie in the major advances in the understanding of the causation of medical diseases brought about by molecular genetics. That might suggest that child psychiatry is merely following fashion, but if we ask why that fashion has become so widespread in biomedical sciences, the answers are not trivial. A genetic approach to human health is seen to offer new benefits in terms of predicting illness, refining diagnosis and classification and ultimately discovering new methods of prevention and treatment.

As a counterbalance to such optimism, it needs to be pointed out that the promise of genetics has sometimes been oversold, particularly when findings stray from the pages of scientific journals into the popular media. Thus, in addition to hearing about the discovery of 'genes for' particular diseases, it is now not uncommon to hear about scientists discovering 'the gene for' traits such as aggression, homosexuality or feminine intuition. This cannot be wholly blamed on poor journalism. Geneticists quite often use a misleading shorthand that gives a quasi-deterministic impression of what genes do. Genes, of course, are not strictly 'for' anything other than to replicate themselves. Furthermore, most behaviours, and indeed most common traits and disorders, involve an interplay between the environment and a collection of genes, rather than just a single locus.

Patterns of transmission

Finding that a trait or disorder is familial is a necessary first step before embarking on genetic studies. However, finding familiality does not provide sufficient evidence that genes play a part. We resemble our relatives because of a combination of the genes that we share with them and of environmental effects that we have in common. Shared environmental effects may include socioeconomic status which may in turn be reflected in indices of social deprivation. However, other factors aggregate in families including cultural values that may be reflected in, for example, religious persuasion, substance use, hobbies and interests or even career choice. Shared environment also includes the pos-

sibility of physical contagion and exposure to the same infectious agents. Therefore, traits or disorders may be strongly familial, but mainly or entirely non-genetic. Edwards (1960) pointed out that traits resulting from a family environment may even simulate Mendelian traits; this is borne out by a study of career choice. McGuffin & Huckle (1990) showed that not only is attending medical school highly familial (a not too surprising finding) but also that the 'trait' passed nearly all of the tests for autosomal recessive inheritance when modern statistical techniques were applied.

The other side of the coin is that genetic effects have sometimes being overlooked when familiality is less obvious or striking. A good example is childhood autism where some authors in the past doubted any important genetic contribution because the recurrent risks of strictly defined autism in the siblings of autistic patients was so low in absolute terms—about 3% (Rutter 1966; Hanson & Gottesman 1976). However, this has to be compared with the general population risk using the same narrow criteria, which is in the region of 5–10 per 10 000 (Rutter 2000a). Hence, the relative risk of autism in siblings, sometimes denoted by the symbol λ_s (Risch 1990), is some 50–100 times that of the general population.

Another source of confusion is that clinicians and researchers sometimes attempt a straightforward separation of disorders into familial and 'sporadic', with the latter being those cases where no other members of the family are affected. Even with single gene disorders, this is less straightforward than it looks. A 'sporadic' case of autosomal dominant disorders, such as Huntington disease or tuberous sclerosis, may arise because of a fresh mutation or because the diagnosis was missed in the parental generation. For example, a parent carrying the Huntington disease mutation may have died of some other cause before developing the disorder and a parent with tuberous sclerosis may have a mild form of the disorder with just skin lesions and no epilepsy or mental retardation. In either case, the offspring of such individuals will be at the same 50% risk as they would if a family history had been detected. Similarly, a high proportion of cases of rare recessive disorders present as 'chance isolates' (when neither parents nor more distant relatives are affected), but where both parents turn out to be heterozygous carriers.

A further problem about using a family history positive/ negative dichotomy when it comes to more complex traits and diseases is that the probability of classifying the subject as family history positive increases with the number of relatives on which there is available information. Therefore, a common trait that affects, say, 10% of the general population, but which actually shows no true familial aggregation will, by chance, result in anyone with five relatives having a 41% probability of being classified as 'family history positive' (McGuffin *et al.* 1987a). Therefore, there is no substitute for carrying out family studies in which the numbers of affected and unaffected relatives are actually counted and compared with some appropriate control group.

Family study methods

Family studies have been carried out extensively in adult psychiatry but their application in child psychiatry is more recent. For most child psychiatric disorders, the precise relative risks (λ) of recurrence in siblings or other categories of relatives remain uncertain. In part, this reflects difficulties in defining *ascertainment* or the method of selecting families for inclusion in a study. Ascertainment of a family takes place via index cases or *probands*. The most common method of doing this is via a consecutive series of patients referred to a clinic or hospital. All probands fulfilling diagnostic criteria must be included in the study *independently*. That is, no consideration is given to whether there is prior information about other members of the family being affected. If a disorder is rare, it is likely that no family will be ascertained more than once (*single ascertainment*) but if a disorder is comparatively common in the same clinic or treatment facility that sees many patients, some families will only be sampled a single time whereas others will contain more than one proband and be counted more than once. This is referred to as *multiple incomplete* ascertainment. If it is possible to study an entire population and hence count every case as a proband, this is described as *complete* ascertainment.

Accurate ascertainment is important for the use of statistical methods of segregation analysis to infer the mode of transmission. In practice, diseases in humans fall into two groups: those where inferring mode of transmission is straightforward and where there is a simple regular Mendelian pattern of transmission; and those where the pattern of transmission is more complicated and where there is not a straightforward correspondence between genotype and phenotype. Most Mendelian disorders are decidedly uncommon, and sometimes exceedingly rare. Several thousands of such disorders have been listed (OMIM 2000) and hundreds of these are of relevance to psychiatry, usually because they cause mental retardation, but sometimes because they result in relatively specific behavioural phenotypes (see Skuse & Kuntsi, Chapter 13). The disorders include fragile X mental retardation (FRA-XMR1; X-linked), phenylketonuria (autosomal recessive) and tuberous sclerosis (autosomal dominant) which exists in two forms (Sampson 2000). However, taken together, such single genes affect only 1% or less of the population. By contrast, common disorders such as childhood depression, attention deficit hyperactivity disorder (ADHD) and conduct disorder show familial aggregation, but do not show simple Mendelian patterns of transmission and

almost certainly have complex inheritance in the sense of involving multiple genes as well as environmental effects. One apparent exception to the 'rare equals simple, common equals complex' rule is childhood autism, for which the narrowly defined form of the disorder has a population frequency of under 1 in 1000, but where the recurrence risk in relatives is far too low to invoke Mendelian mechanisms. More recently it has been found that a 'lesser variant' of autism is found more frequently than narrowly defined autism in the relatives of autistic probands (Bolton *et al.* 1994; Bailey *et al.* 1998) and so it may be that there is a spectrum of autistic behaviours in the general population that are far more common than was once thought (Rutter 2000a). Indeed, many psychiatric disorders that used to be considered categories may be based on dimensions that show no clear line of demarcation between disease and normality.

Models of inheritance for complex traits

At the most basic level, the problem in the inheritance of complex traits is how to reconcile irregular segregation ratios with Mendelian inheritance. The simplest way to deal with this is to invoke the notion of *penetrance*. This is defined as the probability of manifesting a trait given a certain genotype. For regular Mendelian traits, the penetrance is always either 0 or 1. For example, if we consider a trait at a locus where there are two alternative genes or alleles *a* and *A*, there are three possible genotypes:

aa, aA, AA.

Each of these is associated with a penetrance depending upon the mode of transmission. With a recessive trait where *a* is recessive with respect to *A*, the penetrances of these genotypes are 0, 0 and 1, respectively. With a dominant trait the penetrances are 0, 1 and 1, respectively. Departures from Mendelian segregation can be explained in terms of penetrances that take values between 0 and 1. Thus, suppose we are dealing with a dominant trait with incomplete penetrance, we might find that some of those who do not carry the allele *A* (those who have genotypes aa) manifest the trait. These are true sporadics (they show the trait but do not carry the genotype) and they have a penetrance, $0 < f_1 < 1$. Rather than everyone with genotypes *aA* and *AA* manifesting the trait, only proportions $0 < f_2 < 1$ and $0 < f_3 < 1$ can be identified as affected.

In general, genes tend to arrive at an equilibrium within the population as dictated by the Hardy–Weinberg law. This means that if *a* has a frequency of p and *A* has a frequency of q (= 1 − p), the population tends to a steady state where the total population frequency is:

$$p^2 + 2pq + q^2.$$

This means that we are dealing with a disease or complex trait with penetrances as described above of f_1, f_2 and f_3, the total population frequency of the trait (Kp) is given by:

$$Kp = f_1 p^2 + f_2 2pq + f_3 q^2.$$

This is sometimes called the *general* single major locus (SML) model. It has the obvious attractions of relative economy and simplicity, and a good deal of effort has been expended with adult psychiatric disorders, such as schizophrenia and bipolar affective disorder, in exploring models of this type. It turns out that neither schizophrenia (McGue *et al.* 1983) nor bipolar disorder (Craddock *et al.* 1996) can adequately have their inheritance explained by SML models. The general SML model remains of both theoretical and practical importance in the application of linkage analysis (see below) to complex traits, but the inheritance of most psychiatric disorders is more plausibly explained by models involving multiple genes.

As we have noted earlier, there are two types of phenotypic variation, quantitative and categorical. Traditionally, psychiatrists like other medical practitioners have attempted to classify disorders as present or absent. Thus, a child psychiatrist may categorize a child as being affected or unaffected by a particular disorder. However, with many common disorders, such as those categorized by symptoms of anxiety, depression or antisocial behaviour, symptoms of at least a mild degree are highly prevalent, and it may be difficult to define a clear-cut point at which the level or intensity of symptoms differentiate those who are 'affected' from those who are 'unaffected'. Current classification schemes, such as DSM-IV (American Psychiatric Association 1994) or ICD-10 (World Health Organization 1993) have sought to deal with the difficulty by producing explicit definitions in the form of operational criteria. These facilitate good interrater agreement, but may give an overoptimistic view of the ease with which we can distinguish between children who are 'ill' and those who (despite having some symptoms) are 'well'.

In fact, the value of taking both a dimensional and a categorical approach has well-been recognized in epidemiological research in child psychiatry (Rutter & Garmezy 1983). This is not peculiar to child psychiatry. The notion of an underlying continuum of *liability* to disorder has long been recognized by geneticists attempting to study other common complex diseases (Falconer 1965; Reich *et al.* 1972). Where a disorder is contributed to by several (or perhaps many) genetic loci, as well as environmental factors acting additively, it can be reasonably assumed that liability follows a normal distribution, where only those individuals whose liability at sometime exceeds a certain threshold can be classified as affected. Relatives of affected individuals will tend to have an increased mean liability compared with the general population and hence a high proportion of relatives will lie beyond the threshold.

The first application of a model of this type in psychiatry was for schizophrenia (Gottesman & Shields 1967). Here the model helped explain certain phenomena that were not explained by earlier attempts to apply SML models, e.g. why the risk in relatives increases with the severity of the disorder in the proband as well as increasing with the number of relatives already affected. This is because more severe cases or individuals from families containing several affected individuals will tend to be at more extreme positions on the continuum of liability. The threshold model approach also allows the calculation of a useful index of how familial a disorder is. If we know the frequency of a disorder in the general population and the frequency in a particular category of relatives it is possible to estimate the *correlation in liability*. (The statistically minded reader may be aware that this is effectively the same thing as a tetrachoric correlation.)

The relationship between severity and liability can be extended further to include the idea of multiple thresholds (Reich *et al.* 1972). It is assumed that there are two or more clinical forms of the disease that are contributed to by the same genetic and environmental factors, hence they can be ordered on the same continuum of liability where one form of disorder is common and less severe (the broad form) while the other is less common and more severe (the narrow form). Patients with either type of illness will have higher rates of the disorder in their relatives than is found in the population generally, but a greater proportion of relatives affected will occur among those with patients with the narrow form of the disorder. This type of model has been put forward to explain the familial coaggregation of multiple tics (the broad form) and Tourette syndrome (Pauls *et al.* 1981). More recently this has been applied to some twin study data and offered as an explanation for why co-occurring conduct disorder and ADHD appears to be more familial than ADHD alone (Thapar *et al.*, 2001).

Classic methods of study

As we have already discussed, genetic traits are necessarily familial, but familiality does not necessarily indicate genetic influences. Traits and disorders may cluster in families, because of shared genes, shared environment or a combination of the two. Estimating the extent to which each of these contribute may not be straightforward but, fortunately, two 'experiments of nature' come to our assistance.

Twin studies

Twins are of two main types: monozygotic (MZ) or identical twins who have all of their genes in common; and dizygotic (DZ), non-identical or fraternal twins who, on average across all loci, share half of their genes. Similarities in members of twin pairs also result from the environments that they share. If we accept the *equal environment assumption* (EEA) that MZ and DZ twins share their environment to roughly the same extent, then any greater similarity in MZ than DZ twins should reflect genetic effects. It is therefore of importance to consider whether EEA usually holds or whether it is, on the contrary, frequently violated. In practice, when researchers have asked adult twins or the parents of younger twins direct questions about environmental sharing during childhood, MZ twins tend to report more sharing than DZ twins, with respect to having the same friends, being in the same class at school or dressing alike (Thapar & McGuffin 1994) and this is so even when studies are restricted to same sex DZ twins (McGuffin *et al.* 1996). A simple test of whether this is problematic for EEA is to explore whether these types of environmental sharing influence similarity in the trait that is under investigation. For example, Thapar & McGuffin (1994) found that their measures of shared environmental effects had no significant relationship to twin similarity with respect to depressive symptoms in childhood. On the other hand, other studies have shown significant effects within MZ pairs for environmental features such as stressful life events and family negativity (Rutter *et al.* 1999b, 2000b). This violation of the EEA is to be expected whenever there are important environmental effects on a disorder and when individual differences in experiencing such environments are genetically influenced. That applies to both disruptive behaviour and the more common forms of unipolar depression but is much less likely to apply to autism, schizophrenia and bipolar disorder.

Another method of testing whether greater environmental sharing of MZ than DZ twins in childhood invalidates inferences from twin studies is to consider the pattern of similarity in relation to the twins' or their parents' own assumptions about zygosity as compared with a more objective methods of assessing zygosity. In a classic study of this type (Scarr & Carter-Saltzman 1979), a surprisingly high proportion (around 40%) of 400 adolescent pairs were mistaken about their true zygosity. On tests of cognitive ability, DZ twins who thought that they were identical were no more alike than DZ pairs who were correct about their zygosity. Similarly, MZ pairs who incorrectly believed themselves to be non-identical showed only slightly greater differences than MZ pairs who were not mistaken about their zygosity.

As we will discuss in more detail later, one of the reasons that the equal environment assumption is likely to be an oversimplification is that genes can have an influence on the behaviours that individuals carry out in shaping and selecting their environments. Therefore, it may be that variations in experience are systematically related to the trait being studied (Rutter *et al.* 1999b). More complicated methods of analysis, using multivariate methods, can be devised to take this into account (Slutske *et al.* 1997).

A more radical method of trying to overcome the possibility that MZ twins experience greater environmental sharing that DZ twins is to concentrate upon twins who have been separated early in life and then reared apart. Unfortunately, monozygotic twins reared apart are rare, their degree of separation is often incomplete and the method of ascertainment, e.g. by advertisement in the media, may introduce its own biases. The scarcity of reared apart twins makes this design of limited use in studying disorders, but the results have proved to be interesting in studies of continuous traits within the normal range, such as IQ and personality. The approach has been used most recently by Bouchard (1998) to study cognitive ability and various aspects of personality.

We have noted that twins and their parents may be mistaken about zygosity. Fortunately for researchers, objective and reliable methods are available and the best approach is to use a combination of several highly polymorphic DNA markers. This can

now be carried out relatively cheaply and efficiently. Nevertheless, in very large-scale studies involving hundreds or thousands of twins the expense may be prohibitive and therefore many researchers use questionnaire measures that have been 'calibrated' against the results of DNA genotyping. Typically, questionnaires can give agreement in the region of 90–95% with genotyping results and, in practice, experienced twin researchers can assign zygosity on appearance with sometimes even better accuracy (McGuffin *et al.* 1991). However, the use of a more objective method remains desirable in overcoming other potential sources of bias which could occur if the same researcher was assigning both diagnosis and zygosity.

Finally, attention to method of ascertainment is important in twin studies. This is particularly so in studies of disorders that includes treated cases. Simply asking for twins to be referred from hospital or clinics tends to result in a bias in the direction of 'conspicuous' pairs who are both MZ and concordant. This can be avoided by ascertaining via a hospital register which lists consecutively all new patients who are twins or by matching national or regional twin registers against registers of treated cases. Increasingly in childhood traits and disorders twin studies are being carried out on samples that are epidemiologically based. For example, in some parts of the UK it is possible to identify all of the twins in a particular area via community paediatric registers, while in the USA some states note twin births on their birth registers.

For continuous traits, twin similarity is expressed as a correlation (preferably the intraclass correlation) but for present/absent traits, concordance rates are reported. It is sometimes a source of confusion that these can be reported in more than one way. The most common way of reporting concordance rates are as *pairwise* and *probandwise*. Probandwise concordance is the number of affected cotwins divided by the total number of cotwins, whereas pairwise concordance is simply the number of pairs, both having the same diagnosis divided by the total number of pairs. These two concordance rates often turn out to be different if the method of ascertainment has been truly systematic. This is because ascertainment from a register ensures that every proband is included in a study series independently. Consequently, some twin pairs may appear twice where both are affected and both appear on the register as a proband. The aim here is not to inflate the MZ concordance rates spuriously; in fact, it is quite the reverse as twin series ascertained in a non-systematic way have inevitable bias, for the reasons mentioned earlier.

Adoption studies

Adoption studies provide the other mainstay of psychiatric genetics in an attempt to disentangle genes and environment. Adoption studies have been highly influential in convincing sceptics that there is a genetic contribution to adult psychiatric disorders, particularly schizophrenia (Gottesman 1991). There are three main designs.

1 *Adoptee studies.* The adopted-away offspring of affected parents are studied and compared with control adoptees.

2 *Adoptee's family study.* The index cases are adopted individuals who have developed the disorder under study. The rates of illness are then compared in their biological and adoptive relatives or with the rates in the relatives of control adoptees.

3 *Cross-fostering study.* The rates of illness in adoptees who have affected biological parents and were raised by unaffected adopting parents are compared with the rates in the offspring of normal parents brought up by affected adopting parents.

Despite the obvious appeal of adoption studies designs, a major drawback is that adoption is in many senses an abnormal event. The rates of psychopathology tend to be somewhat higher in adoptees than in the general population (Maughan & Pickles 1990). There is a tendency for adoptees to be born to unmarried teenage mothers who, in turn, are less likely than average to receive good obstetric care (Maughan & Pickles 1990; DeFries *et al.* 1994). A further complication is that the placement of adoptees is not random. On the one hand, there is a tendency with some adoption agencies to seek a good 'match' for physical social or ethnic characteristics between an adoptee and prospective parents and, on the other, adopting parents tend to be better educated and have more social advantage than average, as well as having unusually low rates of antisocial behaviour (Rutter *et al.* 1999b). The restriction in range of environmental conditions does create a problem for estimating the strength of genetic influences (Stoolmiller 1999).

Estimation of heritability and beyond

The contributors to complex traits (phenotypes resulting from multiple, genetic and environment effects) can be reduced to a simple basic formula:

$$\text{Phenotype} = \text{additive genes} + \text{shared environment} + \text{non-shared environment}.$$

Here we use the term *additive* genes because the simplest kind of model is one where scores on some continuous measure (such as height or IQ) result from simple addition of the phenotypic values contributed by genes at different loci. When considering present/absent or threshold traits, the genetic contribution to liability would be considered in the same way. There are obviously two sources of resemblance between relatives, additive genes and *shared environment* and one source of difference, *non-shared environment*. However, it should be noted that the non-shared environmental effect includes everything that is left over once the additive genetic and shared environmental components have been accounted for, and it therefore includes measurement error and random effects. Non-shared environment is therefore also sometimes referred to as *residual* environment. The proportion of variation in a phenotype explained by additive genetic affects is called the *heritability*, usually denoted as h^2, and the proportion of variance contributed by common environment is usually given the symbol c^2.

Estimates of h^2 and c^2 can be obtained for particular traits if we have measures on pairs of MZ and DZ twins or on the biological and non-biological relatives of adoptees. This is now

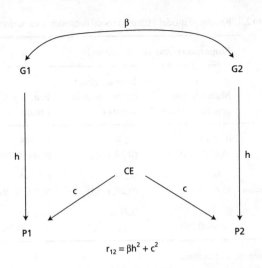

Fig. 12.1 A simple univariate path model: The expected value of the correlation, r_{12} between phenotypes P1 and P2 is the sum of the connecting paths via the common environment (CE) and the genotypes G1 and G2. The correlation β between genotypes is 1 for monozygotic twins and 0.5 for dizygotic twins.

most commonly performed using the structural equation modelling (Neale & Cardon 1992). Path analysis is used to derive the expected values for correlations (or covariances) between pairs of relative phenotypes for models such as the simple univariate one based on analysis of MZ and DZ data illustrated in Fig. 12.1.

A widespread application of genetic model fitting in childhood traits and disorder has been one of the major trends in recent research in the field. Although the details are complicated, the overall idea is straightforward. Essentially, the process involves a repetitive search for values of the model parameters that give the optimum fit. To carry this out the researcher provides the computer program with the relevant data and starting values for the parameters that are effectively his or her best guess what the 'correct' value should be. This information determines the initial value of a mathematical function supplied by the investigator, the form of which depends upon the model being tested. Typically, the mathematical function is either a χ-square or a log likelihood. The optimization routine on a computer program then calculates 'improved' estimates of the values that provide better fit (either an increase in the likelihood or a decrease in the χ-square). Iteration then ceases when either the maximum likelihood or the minimum χ-square is obtained yielding the 'best bet' estimates of the model parameters.

The standard approach is to start out with a full model containing, e.g. additive genetic (A), shared environment (C) and non-shared environmental (E) components and then attempt to fit a reduced model, such as an AE or a CE model, to see whether a more parsimonious explanation of the data can be achieved without worsening the fit. An illustration of model fitting on some data from child and adolescent twins examining social cognitive ability as measured by questionnaire is given in Table 12.1. Despite its obvious advantages, it should be noted that the model fitting approach will sometimes involve the dropping of

Table 12.1 Results of model fitting on social cognition examining differences across sexes in all twins. (Adapted from Scourfield *et al.* 1999.)

Model	Proportion of variance explained					$\chi^2_{(df)}$	P	AIC
	Male additive genetic variance	Male unique environmental variance	Female additive genetic variance	Female unique environmental variance	Female non-additive genetic variance			
I	0.7440 (0.67, 0.80)	0.256 (0.20, 0.33)	0.7264 (0.44, 0.79)	0.2736 (0.21, 0.35)	0.0000 (0.00, 0.33)	$6.912_{(10)}$	0.7	−13.088
II	0.7440 (0.67, 0.80)	0.256 (0.20, 0.33)	0.7264 (0.44, 0.79)	0.2736 (0.21, 0.35)	—	$6.912_{(11)}$	0.8	−15.088
III	0.7350 (0.68, 0.78)	0.2650 (0.22, 0.32)	0.7350 (0.68, 0.78)	0.2650 (0.22, 0.32)	—	$7.089_{(13)}$	0.9	−18.911

(df), degrees of freedom.

effects that fall short of statistical significance but which, in reality, are valid and important (Rutter *et al.* 1999b).

Uses and abuses of 'heritability'

We need to stress that heritability is no more than an estimate of the proportion of population variance explained by additive genetic affects, and therefore it has no meaning at an individual level. Moreover, an estimate of heritability is only applicable to the population from which the estimate is derived. Other populations may show greater overall variance or different proportions of the variance that can be explained by genetic and environmental effects. This means that heritability may differ for a trait, not just between different populations, but that it may also change over historical time. For example, if height is influenced by both genes and an environmental factor such as nutrition, heritability is necessarily less in the situation where there is large variability in access to adequate nutrition than where all growing children receive an adequate diet.

It must also be pointed out that finding that a disorder or trait is heritable does not mean that it cannot be altered by non-physical methods. Thus, there is no incompatibility between twin study evidence that depressive disorder is substantially influenced by genes and the clinical trial evidence that depression responds well to cognitive behavioural therapy.

Unfortunately, debates about heritability often centre upon the issue of what is the 'correct' estimate without taking these caveats into account. This has been particularly true of contentious areas, such as analyses of the proportion of variance in IQ that is explained by genes (McGue 1997). Such debates are inevitably of the 'more heat than light' variety. Although it is of interest that there is a substantial genetic contribution to a trait such as cognitive ability, or a disorder such as depression, it matters less whether the heritability in the samples studied was actually, say, 0.4 rather than 0.6.

Nevertheless, it may be of some value to differentiate between disorders with very high heritability (say, 70% or greater) as estimated from a range of different samples, and those with only moderate heritability (say, 30–60%). The first group includes autism (Rutter 2000a), schizophrenia (McGuffin *et al.* 1994), bipolar affective disorder (Craddock & Jones 1999) and ADHD. Although these are multifactorial disorders subject to environmental as well as genetic influences, the high heritability (together with other biological findings; see, e.g. Hollis, Chapter 37) suggests that identification of susceptibility genes is likely to provide leads on causal neural mechanisms (see below). The second group includes the more common varieties of unipolar depression (Sullivan *et al.* 2000), oppositional/defiant and conduct disorders that do not include hyperactivity (Rutter *et al.* 1998), and probably anxiety disorders (see Klein & Pine, Chapter 30). These too are likely to involve some form of neural substrate but the lower heritability suggests that it is more likely to comprise indirect dimensional risk factors (such as temperament) and the operation of nature–nurture interplay. Of course, there is no sharp dividing line between these two groups, and the implications are probable rather than definite. It should be added that there are other child psychiatric disorders for which the heritability is much less certain, either because of inconsistencies in findings, concerns over ascertainment, the need to consider multiphase causal pathways, and/or doubts over the boundaries of the phenotype. Eating disorders, tics, drug dependency and obsessional disorders probably all fall in this uncertain category.

Changes over time

Not only may heritability change over historical time, but, for many traits, it varies over a lifetime. One of the first studies to indicate changes during early development was the Louisville twin project (Wilson 1978). A large variety of measures was carried out on twin and other siblings at frequent intervals from the ages of 3 months to 6 years. Before the age of 18 months, the overall MZ and DZ correlations on measures of cognitive ability showed only small differences, although MZ pairs showed a striking similarity in their profile of mental development over time. By contrast, DZ pairs became less similar during their preschool years so that by the age of 6 the intraclass MZ correlation had stabilized at 0.85 and the DZ correlation at 0.63. More recent work on twins of different age groups (McGue *et al.* 1993) showed that MZ–DZ differences in twin correlations for measures of IQ increase a little further in late adolescence and early adult life, and even into old age (McClearn *et al.* 1997). This suggests that genetic influences on the trait increase as we grow older. This may seem surprising from a common sense viewpoint, because as we grow older we accumulate more experiences and tend to be exposed to an increasing variety of environments. The explanation, almost certainly, is that two of the ways in which genetic influences operate are through effects on susceptibility to environmental risks and on the likelihood of experiencing such risks (through gene–environment interaction and correlations, respectively; see below). Although in reality these involve genes and environment working together, they appear as a purely genetic effect in most traditional forms of analysis (Rutter *et al.* 1999b).

Some psychopathological phenomena also show changes in heritability during development. The familial aggregation of depressive disorder in adults has received considerable attention and there is reasonably consistent evidence that early onset of unipolar depression is associated with high degree of familiality, a finding which is striking in some (Weissman *et al.* 1986), but not all, studies (McGuffin *et al.* 1987b). It might therefore be predicted that very early onset of depressive disorders or symptoms in childhood would be associated with even greater familial effects. As it turns out there have now been four twin studies showing that genetic influence on depression is stronger in adolescents than in younger children (Thapar & McGuffin 1994; Murray & Sines 1996; Eley & Stevenson 1999; Silberg *et al.* 1999). There has been some support from a family study (Harrington *et al.* 1997) which found that family loading did not vary substantially according to age of onset of depression in childhood and adolescents, but that early onset did seem to be associated with a history of antisocial problems in relatives in addition to depression alone.

Gene–environment correlation

Thus far we have considered genes and environment as coacting in an additive fashion but have indicated that this may not always be the case. In fact, it seems likely that there will be situations in which genes and environment are positively correlated (or show covariance). There are at least three different possible mechanisms by which this can arise (Plomin *et al.* 2000).

Passive gene environment correlation results from parents not just passing on genes to their children, but also rearing them and therefore helping create their early environment. Parents may pass on susceptibility genes for a disorder such as depression, but also influence the child's environment by their own behaviour. For example, studies of families where one parent is mentally ill found that parental psychopathology tends to be associated with increased family discord and conflict (Quinton & Rutter 1988). Interestingly, this may result in differences and outcome in the children as there is often a tendency for one child to bear the brunt of the family's upset (Rutter *et al.* 1997b),

which might actually result in negative gene environment correlations. There is comparatively little work published to date attempting to detect gene–environment correlation using model fitting approaches, but there is a suggestion that passive gene–environment correlation may occur with respect to the occurrence of depression and provision of adverse parenting (Kendler *et al.* 1997). This is potentially important because if gene–environment correlation is simply ignored in model fitting but does actually exist, the result is an overestimate of the genetic contribution to variation in liability.

Active gene–environment correlation describes situations where individuals of a particular genotype will tend to seek out a particular sort of environment. For example, it could be that individuals with a higher innate ability for intellectual and scholastic tasks will tend to find themselves in cognitively more stimulating environments than those who are innately less able. Over the course of a lifetime, this will tend to increase so that a gene–environment correlation is induced. This could explain, at least in part, the apparent increase in heritability of cognitive ability with increasing age.

Gene–environment correlation can be explored using adoption designs. Psychopathology in the biological parent is used as an index of the genetic risks and rearing environment of the adopting parents as indexing the environmental risks. In a study of antisocial behaviour in adopted-away children who were at high genetic risk, O'Connor *et al.* (1998) found that the children experienced increased negative parenting from their adoptive mothers which in turn derived from the children's own disruptive behaviour. This finding represents a third source of correlation between genes and environment sometimes called *evocative* because the individual genetically influenced phenotype plays a part in evoking (or perhaps in this case provoking) an environmental response.

Some of the difficulties posed by gene–environment correlations and some possible solutions to unravelling them have been explored in recent twin studies. Three different studies on children (Kendler & Karkowski-Shuman 1997; Thapar *et al.* 1998; Silberg *et al.* 1999) showed an overlap between the liability to depression and to report negative life events. These suggest that there may be ways in which some individuals behave that predispose them to encounter negative experiences. However, it is difficult to distinguish between the phenomena of actually encountering unpleasant events and merely showing a tendency to remember and report negative experiences. Furthermore, family data on adults, although they show a tendency for family loading for depression and for unpleasant events to cluster together (McGuffin *et al.* 1988), it may be partly or even totally explained by the same events impinging upon more than one family member.

Gene–gene interactions

The other category of non-additive effects is termed *interactions*. Gene–gene interactions occur at single loci where there is dominance. Again, we can consider a single locus with two alleles *a* and *A* contributing to some phenotype that can be measured on a continuous scale. The effects would be additive if the value on the continuous measure of the heterozygote *Aa* were mid-way between that of the homozygotes *aa* and *AA*. Deviations from such additive affects are termed *dominance deviations*. The presence of dominance variance in traits resulting from multiple genes presents complications in estimating heritability. This is because the effect of dominance variation in contributing to similarities between relatives is less straightforward than it is for additive variance. For example, covariance between MZ twins, because they share all of their genes, is the sum of the additive and the dominance variance. On the other hand, for DZ twins or full siblings, the genetic covariance is the sum of half the additive variance plus one-quarter of the dominance variance. The reason for half of the additive variance contributing to the covariation is straightforward because, averaged across all loci, DZ twins or siblings share half of their genes. Why it is a quarter of dominance variance is less obvious and proof of this requires some algebra (Falconer & Mackay 1996) (but a quick explanation is that the probability of a pair of siblings sharing two alleles identical by descent at a given locus is one-quarter: 0.5×0.5). Dominance variation should be suspected if the MZ correlation for a trait is more than double that of the DZ correlation. Sibling correlations will also be higher than a parent offspring correlations in the presence of dominance (again a proper proof requires algebra, but a quick explanation is that a parent offspring pair can never have two alleles at a given locus identical by descent and therefore *dominance variation* does not contribute to parent offspring covariation).

If the aim is simply to estimate how much of a trait is contributed by any type of genetic effect, these subtleties are sometimes ignored and researchers content themselves with estimating *broad heritability*, also sometimes referred to as a degree of genetic determination (Falconer & Mackay 1996).

Gene–gene interactions *between* loci, *epistasis*, can also occur. This is when two or more loci have multiplicative effects. It has been suggested for example that in schizophrenia, the large difference in concordances between MZ twins (over 40%), DZ and other categories of first-degree relatives (10–15%) and a rapid fall-off in pairs of second-degree or more distant relatives (around 3–4%) suggest a small number of loci acting together in a multiplicative fashion (Risch 1990). A similar and indeed even more dramatic difference in relative concordance rates is found in childhood autism moving from MZ twins to siblings to more distant relatives; again statistical model fitting exercises suggest that epistasis may be present (Pickles *et al.* 1995). One of the great challenges for current molecular genetic studies attempting to locate and identify the genes involved in complex disorders is in detecting susceptibility loci where there are interactions rather than merely additive coactions.

Gene–environment interactions

Although the term *gene environment interaction* is sometimes used in a rather loose way to mean any form of genetic–

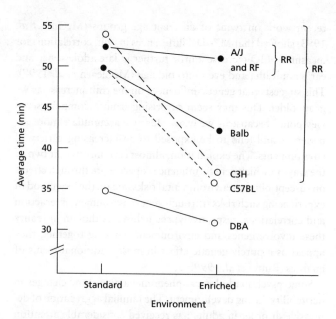

Fig. 12.2 Average time required to reach food for six inbred mouse strains reared in two different environments. RR = reaction range. Data from Henderson (1970).

environmental interplay, the strict meaning of the term interaction denotes non-additive effects (Rutter & Silberg, in press). The biological reality of gene–environment interaction has been amply demonstrated in laboratory animals, where it is possible to breed genetic homogenous strains and experimentally rear them in differing environments. The results from one such classic experiment (Henderson 1970) are summarized in Fig. 12.2. Mice reared in an enriched environment do better than those in a standard environment on a timed task involving food finding. However, some strains (A/J and RF in the figure) showed only modest improvement whereas other strains, such as C3H, show a marked improvement under a purely additive model. All would be expected to show a parallel improvement in the performance of their tasks, whereas in fact this is not the case and even the rank order of the phenotypes changes from one environment to the next. This experiment also demonstrates another aspect of a complex trait which is that genes do not determine or fix the phenotypes but rather prescribe a *reaction range* (Gottesman 1963) so that what is actually observed at a point in time is a dynamic interplay between the relevant genes and the relevant environmental stimuli.

Because such environmental manipulations are not possible in humans, gene–environment interactions have been more difficult to demonstrate, but natural experiments, such as adoption studies, provide evidence that they exist. For example, Cadoret *et al.* (1995) studied adoptees with and without a biological predisposition to antisocial behaviour (with and without a biological antisocial parent). They showed that adverse circumstances associated with rearing, plotted on a linear scale, had a direct relationship with adult antisocial behaviour only in those adoptees with a biological predisposition but had negligible effect on those without an antisocial biological parent.

Assortative mating

Another complication that needs to be considered is that one of the basic assumptions of a simple model is the existence of a 'random mating population'. In practice there is evidence that people select their mates in a non-random fashion so that there is a tendency for like to pair with like. This is referred to as assortative mating or homogamy. Positive correlations between spouses tend to be particularly high (at 0.3 or more) for IQ and for antisocial behaviour, but there is also a tendency for couple resemblance for some personality traits and disorders, such as affective disorder, schizophrenia and alcoholism, to be greater than would be expected by chance (Plomin et al. 2000). There are broadly two types of mechanism to account for this. The first is social homogamy where pairing off of couples tends to occur because of opportunity, as, for example, because both are in the same class at school or college, or work in the same place of employment. However, opportunity will also be influenced by styles of social life (Pawlby et al. 1997a,b) and by their 'currency' in the marriage market (Engfer et al. 1994). Thus, the strong tendency for antisocial individuals to mate with others showing the same behaviour probably reflects both their peer group and who is willing to live with them. The second is phenotypic homogamy whereby men and women have a direct preference for mates who are similar to themselves. Taking IQ as an example, it is plausible that both types of mechanisms operate.

Over the course of time, assortative mating for a heritable trait has the tendency to increase the genetic contribution (Falconer & Mackay 1996). However, somewhat paradoxically, assortative mating causes an underestimate of heritability in twin studies. This is because it increases the genetic similarity of DZ but not of MZ pairs.

Locating and detecting genes

So far, we have discussed genetic effects in a quantitative and somewhat abstract way. However, human genetics has changed in a most dramatic fashion over the past 20 years with the introduction of molecular genetic approaches that enable specific genes involved in disease to be located and identified. Having identified genes, we can study their structure, sequence, and investigate the variations in the proteins that they encode for that are involved in the causation of pathology. This whole process, called *positional cloning* (Collins 1992), has had a revolutionary effect in improving understanding of the biological underpinnings of single gene disorders and, more recently, complex multigene disorders. The vital first step in bringing about this modern era of *positional cloning* was the introduction of improved marker maps of the human genome (the 23 pairs of chromosomes) based upon new methods for reliable genotyping of DNA polymorphisms.

Before the introduction of molecular genetic methods, attempts to map genes had to rely on what are now termed classical genetic markers. A genetic marker, by definition, is a characteristic that has simple Mendelian transmission and two or more common alleles. Classical markers include ABO, Rh and other blood types, HLA antigens, various protein polymorphisms found in the blood and various red cell enzymes. By the early 1980s a few dozen such markers were known and only some had had their chromosome locations assigned, so that carrying out linkage studies aiming to detect and identify disease genes was definitely a pursuit for optimists only. Even with very good collaboration among several laboratories, it would be difficult to study more than about 30 markers in a single disease (McGuffin et al. 1983), whereas about 10 times that number of markers is required to carry out a systematic search throughout the genome using a linkage study design (see below).

The first type of marker to provide a solution was restriction fragment length polymorphisms (RFLPs) (Botstein et al. 1980). Markers of this type are detected by first digesting DNA using bacterial enzymes of a class called endonucleases. These are also known as restriction enzymes because each enzyme in this class has a site of cleavage of DNA molecules that is restricted to a certain sequence of DNA. If these sequences are changed by mutation (e.g. by the deletion or insertion of a single nucleotide where restriction site is lost) such changes bring about variations in the length of DNA fragments which result after DNA is digested using a particular restriction enzyme. Fragments of different size can then be separated by electrophoresis, probed with a radio-labelled short sequence of DNA (an oligonucleotide) that has a complementary based sequence to the target RFLP and then blotted on to filter paper before exposure on to X-ray film. This process, known as Southern blotting (Southern 1975), had a revolutionary effect and led to the first nearly complete marker map being published in 1987 (Donis-Keller et al. 1987).

Although RFLPs remain important mapping tools in certain circumstances, they have now largely been superseded for systematic mapping studies by a category of markers called microsatellites or short sequence repeat polymorphisms (SSRPs). SSRPs consist of repeated sequences of di-, tri- or tetra-nucleotides, with the most common being dinucleotide repeats of cytosine-adenosine (CA). Apart from the fact that these are abundant throughout the genome and therefore allow the possibility of very dense marker maps consisting of thousands of markers, CA repeats or other SSRPs can be genotyped using rapid semiautomated high throughput methods. These depend first on amplifying the DNA using the polymerase chain reaction (PCR). Here, oligonucleotides are constructed, called 'primers', that recognize opposite ends of each of the two strands of double stranded DNA. DNA is 'melted' into its two single strands by heating it in a machine called a thermocycler. The primers then attach to the single strands and, in the presence of a thermostable enzyme, *Taq* polymerase initiate the reaction where two new strands of complementary DNA are formed. Cooling then takes place and the strands of DNA reanneal, after which the whole reaction is repeated multiple times. During PCR two, then four, then eight (and so on) copies are produced. By incorporating a fluorescent label in the primers, the resultant amplified fragments of DNA can be detected and again, are separated on a gel according to length, where length is dictated by the number of dinucleotide (or tri- or tetra-nucleotide) repeats. Microsatellite markers tend to be highly polymorphic with many alleles and are therefore particularly useful in mapping studies.

Currently, huge efforts are being invested in a 'third generation' of DNA markers, single nucleotide polymorphisms (SNPs) and a large-scale collaboration is taking place between industry and academic centres in an attempt to produce an extremely fine-scale map of the human genome based upon about 100 000 such markers. SNPs occur as a result of a single base change on average about every 1000 base pairs throughout the genome. They can be detected efficiently within known genes using methods such as denaturing high-performance liquid chromatography (DHPLC; O'Donovan et al. 1998) and a variety of other methods including direct sequencing. Methods are currently being developed and refined for very rapidly genotyping thousands of SNPs. These use oligonucleotides placed on to microarrays ('SNPs on chips') (Southern 1975; Asherson et al. 1998).

Linkage

The starting point for positional cloning is the discovery of where genes are within the genome, going on to take advantage of knowledge about their position to study the genes themselves and the ways in which their allelic variation may affect protein structure or expression. Positional information is gained by two types of related, but somewhat different approaches: linkage and association. Linkage is the phenomenon whereby pairs of loci in close proximity on the same chromosome fail to follow Mendel's law of independent assortment. For example, if we consider two bi-allelic loci with alleles A, a and B, b, a double heterozygote parent of the type Aa Bb whose partner is homozygous at both loci, aa bb will, in the case of independent assortment have offspring of the types Aa Bb, aa Bb, aa Bb, aa bb, occurring with equal probability. This is because, if the loci are on different chromosomes or are far apart on the same chromosome, during meiosis in the germ line cell of the double heterozygote parent, the alleles of the two loci will remain together half the time and for the other half will cross-over (or recombine). However, if the two loci are close together on the same chromosomes, a different pattern is seen. This depends on the *linkage phase*, that is whether A is on the same chromosome as B rather than b. But let us suppose that A and B are on the same chromosome (a and b on the other member of the homologous or paired chromosome). Offspring of the type Aa, Bb and bb, bb (non-recombinants) will outnumber offspring of the types aa, Bb (recombinants).

The number of non-recombinant offspring divided by the total number of offspring is called the recombination fraction and has a maximum value of 0.5 because in independent assortment, the average numbers of recombinant and non-recombinant offspring are equal. Over small distances, the size of the recombination fraction is roughly proportional to the physical distance between the two loci. For example, recombi-

nation that occurs 1 time in 100, a unit of recombination which defines a linkage map distance of 1 centimorgan (cM) corresponds approximately to a physical distance of one million bases (1 Megabase).

It is therefore the aim in linkage studies to attempt both to detect recombination fractions of less than 0.5 and to estimate their size. In experimental plants and animals, this is relatively straightforward because mating can be performed experimentally. Unfortunately, humans pose greater problems and, inevitably, the statistical methods become more complicated. The standard approach for detecting linkage and estimating recombination for Mendelian traits in humans is lod score analysis (Morton 1955). Logarithm of the odds (lod) scores use odds ratios to compare the likelihood of linkage (a recombination fraction <0.5) with the likelihood of no linkage (a recombination fraction =0.5). A curve can be plotted for values of the recombination fraction between 0 and 0.5 and its peak can be taken as the maximum likelihood (or best bet) estimator of the recombination fraction. By convention, a lod score of 3 or greater is considered as proof of linkage while odds of −2 or less is accepted as excluding linkage. A lod of 3 corresponds to odds in favour of linkage of 1000 : 1, but it can also be shown to be the equivalent of a χ-square of 13.8 with one degree of freedom giving a nominal one tailed P-value of 1×10^{-4}. This may sound excessively conservative but the original reasoning of Morton (1955) was that the prior probability of two loci being found in linkage was low and, when this is taken into account, a lod score of 3 corresponds to a reliability of 95% and hence is equivalent to the conventional cut-off level for statistical significance of 0.05.

The lod score method can be adapted to non-Mendelian traits by invoking the general SML model that we discussed earlier in the chapter. The main difficulty about doing this is that the parameters defining the model for a given trait need to be specified correctly. Where these are mis-specified, at best the recombination fraction will be estimated incorrectly and at worst linkage will fail to be detected when it is actually present (Clerget-Darpoux 1991). A common method of attempting to overcome this problem of false negatives in linkage analysis of complex traits is to try out several models, but this then introduces the problem of multiple testing and increases the risk of false positives. Nevertheless, providing that this problem is taken into account, maximizing a lod score over multiple models has been shown to be a useful approach (Abreu et al. 1999).

Despite the difficulties, applying lod score approaches to complex traits has resulted in considerable success in some complex disorders, e.g. Alzheimer disease (Sandbrink et al. 1996), but has been confusing with no definite loci identified so far in other disorders, such as schizophrenia (Riley & McGuffin 2000). The reason for this varied picture almost certainly depends upon whether the simplifying assumptions that need to be made about a complex trait are realistic. These assumptions are first that a major gene is involved in the transmission of at least some forms of the disorder and, secondly, that at least within families containing two or more affected individuals homogeneity can be assumed. That is, even if the disorder as a whole is genetically heterogeneous, affected relatives can be assumed to be carrying the same major gene. Thirdly, there is the assumption that, even if the mode of transmission is not known precisely, it can be specified approximately. As it turns out, Alzheimer disease exists in some comparatively rare early onset forms where the pattern of transmission complies fairly closely to autosomal dominance. In other adult psychiatric disorders, such as schizophrenia and bipolar disorder, although a large number of families containing multiple affected individuals have now been studied and although some linkage findings replicate across more than one centre (including loci on chromosomes 6p, 8q, 13q and 22q), there are no apparent major gene effects. In other words, no locus so far implicated in schizophrenia appears to be necessary or sufficient to cause the disorder, so that it seems likely that major gene forms are rare or non-existent. Therefore, although highly heritable in the vast majority of cases, schizophrenia is oligogenic (resulting from the effects of several genes) or polygenic (resulting from many genes). It has been suggested that this will be the rule rather than the exception for the majority of complex traits and disorders (Plomin et al. 1994). There has therefore recently been a tendency in complex diseases to focus on nuclear families containing affected sibling pairs rather than on extended multiplex pedigrees.

There are several attractions of the affected sibling pair approach. Nuclear families containing just one pair of affected individuals are likely to be more common than extended multiplex families and therefore arguably more representative, as well as easier to collect. In addition, using affected sibling pairs requires no assumptions about the mode of transmission of the disorder. This is because for any given marker locus, the expectation of sharing zero, one or two alleles is one-quarter, one-half and one-quarter, respectively. Significant departure from expectation in the direction of increased allele sharing in affected sibling pairs indicates that the marker is linked with a susceptibility gene contributing to the disease.

Systematic genome searches using closely spaced microsatellite markers have been useful in identifying loci conferring susceptibility to physical diseases, such as insulin-dependent diabetes (Cordell & Todd 1995), and have now been employed by several groups in childhood autism (see review by Lamb et al. 2000; also Lord & Bailey, Chapter 38) with fairly consistent evidence of linkage with a susceptibility locus on chromosome 7 and suggestive evidence elsewhere, particularly on chromosomes 13 and 15. One of the recurrent problems in such studies has been how to decide if a replication really does confirm a previous positive finding if the locus is not in precisely the same spot on the chromosome. In that connection, it is important to appreciate that there is substantial chance variation in the location estimate (Roberts et al. 1999), but also that the length of a peak may help in deciding whether it is a true or false finding (Terwilliger et al. 1997).

Sibling pair linkage approaches can also be applied to quantitative traits (Haseman & Elston 1972). Here the idea is that the degree of similarity between siblings for phenotypic scores depends upon the degree of allele sharing at a quantitative

trait locus (QTL). This approach has been elaborated (Fulker & Cardon 1994) and used to locate a gene contributing to a reading disability on the short arm of chromosome 6 (Cardon et al. 1994). This has subsequently been supported by other studies (Grigorenko et al. 1997; Fisher et al. 1999; Gayan et al. 1999).

Alternative approaches for mapping QTLs include variance components analysis in pedigrees, taking into account other types of relative pairs in addition to siblings (Amos 1994). However, such methods depend on the QTLs having relatively large effects, that is being able to explain at least 10% of the total variance. For QTLs where the effect size is smaller than this, the sample needed to detect linkage may be enormous, running into several thousand sibling pairs (Fulker & Cardon 1994). Similarly, for dichotomous phenotypes, such as the presence or absence of a disease, affected sibling pair approaches are only really efficient at detecting moderately large effects (a locus contributing a relative risk of 3 or more). Sample size requirements become very large for loci contributing a relative risk of 2 or less (Risch & Merikangas 1996).

Allelic association

Because of the problems of detecting small effects using affected sibling pairs or QTL linkage approaches, there has been increasing interest in using allelic association to detect genes involved in complex traits. The standard approach to allelic association simply compares allele frequencies in a sample of cases affected by a disorder and a sample of ethnically matched controls. This case–control design can be easily extended to quantitative traits by selecting 'cases' as having an extreme score on a quantitative measure, comparing them with controls who have either average score or, preferably in terms of maximizing power, low scores. The attraction of case–control studies, in addition to the simplicity of design, is that they have long been known to be capable of detecting genes of small effect contributing as little as 1% variance (Edwards 1965; McGuffin & Buckland 1991). Allelic association arises for three main reasons (Edwards 1991).

1 The marker locus itself may have some causative role in the disease or trait. This is sometimes referred to as pleiotropy (a gene having two or more apparently different effects).

2 The marker itself may not have a direct role, yet be very closely linked to a gene that does, so that the association is undisturbed over many generations of recombination. This is known as linkage disequilibrium. Except in special circumstances, such as recently founded populations, linkage disequilibrium will only occur between loci that are very close together, the distance apart being around 1 cm or less.

3 Population stratification arises when there has been a recent admixture of populations that have different distributions of a particular trait, as well as different frequencies of polymorphisms. Let us suppose, for example, that there is a wave of immigration of a particular ethnic group who on average are markedly taller than the indigenous population. It is likely with a highly polymorphic marker, such as a DNA microsatellite, that the populations also show differences in marker allelic frequency. Therefore, an association study, which simply compares allelic frequencies in samples drawn from the tallest vs. the shortest sections of the population without taking ethnic origin into account, might find an association. Such an association would be unlikely to have anything to do with the biological basis of stature and will be more likely to reflect the frequency of alleles in tall people in the immigrant population.

In an attempt to overcome spurious associations arising because of population stratification, family-based association studies using 'internal controls' have been developed. One such approach is to apply the transmission disequilibrium test (TDT; Spielman *et al.* 1993) which uses trios of affected individuals and both of their parents. At least one of the parents has to be heterozygous at the marker locus for the test to be applied. The TDT has been elaborated in various ways to include multi allelic markers (Sham 1998) and continuous traits (Page & Amos 1999). However, it has been pointed out that provided proper matching of cases and controls is carried out, the classic case–control design is both more efficient (Morton & Collins 1998) and more powerful (Page & Amos 1999) than the TDT or similar tests.

Because allelic associations of the biologically informative kind only arise when the polymorphism is actually in a susceptibility locus or QTL, or very close to it, allelic association studies have an additional disadvantage compared with linkage studies. This is that thousands rather than hundreds of markers would be required to perform a whole genome scan attempting to find disease susceptibility loci or the QTLs underpinning a continuous trait. To date, no whole genome scan has been undertaken using allelic association/disequilibrium approaches but, as we have discussed earlier, non-gel-based methods of performing very high-throughput genotyping using microarrays are now being developed to facilitate such studies.

In the meantime, an alternative approach has been put forward based on DNA pooling (Daniels *et al.* 1998). This uses microsatellite markers and instead of initially genotyping all subjects individually, the DNA from cases is pooled and the DNA from controls is also pooled and the results compared. It relies on the assumption that all cases can be combined on the basis of homogeneity (which may be a problem in some circumstances; Rutter 2000a). Any differences from the two groups that emerge at this initial screen stage can then be checked using individual genotyping. So far, the approach has been used in searching whole chromosomes for genes that may be involved in cognitive ability (Fisher *et al.* 1999; Hill *et al.* 1999). Such rapid screening methods would also be useful in following up positive findings on regions of interest identified by linkage studies. Indeed, it is becoming increasingly obvious that linkage and association are complementary strategies that need to be employed in studying complex diseases and traits rather than 'either' or' alternatives.

The reason for this is that association studies are 'short-sighted', presenting difficulties in searching large stretches of

Table 12.2 Comparing some of the main features of linkage and association studies.

Linkage	Association
Cosegregation of markers and disorder in families	Comparison of allele frequencies in case and control populations or in families using 'internal controls'
Capable of detecting only comparatively large gene effects (e.g. odds ratio of >2 or variance explained of >10%)	Capable of detecting small effects (e.g. odds ratios of <2 or variance explained of as little as 1%)
Detection possible over fairly large distance (e.g. 10–15 cm)	Detection possible only over small distances (<1 cm)

genome but, on the other hand are more capable than linkage of detecting small effects and of locating the genes precisely (Morton & Collins 1998) while linkage is 'far-sighted' but can only detect large effects. For example, Morris *et al.* (2000) followed up the findings which originally came from linkage analysis in multigenerational families of a gene contributing to reading disability located on chromosome 15 (Smith *et al.* 1983; Grigorenko *et al.* 1997). Closely spaced microsatellite markers were studied in a two-stage family-based linkage disequilibrium mapping design, identifying a small region containing a number of potential candidate genes.

Some of the more important features of linkage and association are compared and contrasted in Table 12.2.

Candidate genes

The most direct approach to detecting allelic association is to focus on polymorphisms in or very close to genes that encode for proteins that are thought to be involved in the biochemical bases of the trait. So far, in psychiatry, as with most common diseases, potential candidate genes have been identified by indirect roots, e.g. by knowledge of the mode of action of a drug which has shown to be beneficial in treating the disorder. However, it is likely in the future that with the sequencing of the entire human genome, now close to completion, and the subsequent inevitable identification of all genes, that candidates will be identified by a combination of positional methods and computer searching of databases. For example, the region on chromosome 15 implicated by the linkage disequilibrium mapping study of Morris *et al.* (2000) of reading disability contains 20 known genes in the publicly accessible databases of which three are known to be involved in the regulation of neurotransmission and one is a member of the same gene family as a dyslexia candidate gene in the region identified by other groups on chromosomes 6p.

Some interesting results in child psychiatry have recently been produced using a pharmacologically driven search for candidates. It is known that methylphenidate is beneficial in controlling symptoms of ADHD and this works at least in part by argumenting dopaminergic transmission. Therefore, candidate gene association studies in ADHD have mainly concentrated on candidates that encode for proteins involved in dopamine pathways. There is now fairly consistent evidence of an association with a common variant in the dopamine *DRD4* receptor gene and somewhat less consistent, but nevertheless suggestive, evidence of an association with a polymorphism in the dopamine transporter (*DAT1*) gene (Thapar *et al.* 1999).

Impact of genetics on child psychiatry

Research developments

In the early days of psychiatric genetics, it was important to use twin and adoptee studies to quantify the strength of genetic influences on the underlying liability to each type of psychiatric disorder. That was because, at the time, there was a considerable scepticism about the suggestion that genetic factors might play *any* significant part. That day has passed and it is now abundantly clear that genetic factors play a part in most, or perhaps all, forms of psychopathology, and a good deal is known on those for which genetic influences are strongest. There was also a time when there was an equal degree of scepticism over the suggestion that genetic factors could play a part in influencing individual differences in behaviours giving rise to environmental risk exposure. Again, it is now clear that genetic factors play a part in relation to individual differences in all human behaviour, and not just liability to disorder. Thus, genetic factors influence the likelihood that someone will experience divorce, stressful life events or maladaptive parenting (Plomin 1994; Jockin *et al.* 1996). The findings have important implications for the research designs that must be used to test for environmentally mediated risks (Rutter *et al.*, 2001b). The case has now been made and should be accepted. Although it is true that there are still traits for which there are few data on heritability, there is limited value in carrying out further studies to obtain that information alone. More interesting and potentially important topics are:

1 nature–nurture interplay;
2 continuities between normality and disorder;
3 phenotypic definition;
4 comorbidity; and
5 continuities/discontinuities over the course of development.

Gene–environment interactions in both directions may be important. For example, genetic factors may moderate sensitivity to environmental stressors—as suggested by findings with respect to both life events with relation to depression (Silberg *et al.*, 2001) and adverse parenting in relation to antisocial behaviour (Crowe 1974; Cadoret *et al.* 1995). Alternatively, if genetic and environmental factors operate through independent routes, it may be that genetic influences are least when environmental conditions are worst, as suggested by a finding from one study (still to be replicated) regarding the effects of socioeducational disadvantage on intelligence (Rowe *et al.* 1999). As dis-

cussed earlier, dimensional traits may provide good indicators of the liability to a disorder, but sometimes the role of genetic factors at the extreme end of a distribution may differ from those affecting variation within the normal range. This appeared to be the case in one study of language levels at age 2 years (Dale *et al.* 1998), although again the finding has still to be replicated.

One of the important findings with respect to many serious psychiatric disorders has been that the genetic liability extends well beyond the traditional diagnostic category involving major handicap. For example, this has been evident with both autism (see Lord & Bailey, Chapter 38) and Tourette syndrome (see Leckman & Cohen, Chapter 36). Quantitative genetic studies can be very helpful in defining the boundaries of these extended phenotypes. Comorbidity, the co-occurrence of supposedly separate psychiatric disorders (Caron & Rutter 1991; Rutter 1997; Angold *et al.* 1999), is widespread in psychiatry. Cross-twin, cross-trait analyses of twin data, especially when combined with longitudinal data, can be very helpful in sorting out the possible meaning of such patterns. For example, findings both with adults (Kendler 1996) and children (Thapar & McGuffin 1997) suggest that, to a considerable extent, the liability to both anxiety and depressive symptoms or disorders may derive from the same genes. It also seems that the overlap between ADHD and conduct disturbance to a considerable extent reflects shared genetic liability (Nadder *et al.* 2001). One of the oddities with respect to several areas of psychopathology is that, as mentioned earlier in this chapter, even disorders showing high continuities over time (such as depression or antisocial behaviour) may show marked age-related changes in heritability (and see also Harrington, Chapter 29; Earls & Mezzacappa, Chapter 26). Quantitative genetic analyses of longitudinal data can be very helpful in sorting out how this happens. They can also be informative with respect to the different phases in the development of drug dependence. For example, the influences on first taking drugs, moving on to using them regularly and heavily, and then becoming dependent, may not be identical (Vanyukov & Tarter, 2000).

Molecular genetics research is still at an early stage in psychiatric disorders but this is also true for much of the rest of internal medicine, in that it is proving difficult to identify susceptibility genes for multifactorial disorders. That is partly because it is generally the case that each susceptibility gene has only a tiny effect (although the accumulation of effects of several genes can be quite great), because genetic effects may be most evident in environmental high-risk groups if genetic effects operate through susceptibility to environmental stressors, and because gene–gene interactions may be important. The problems are immense but they are ultimately tractable. The solutions lie in several different developments.

1 Technological advances, such as the availability of SNPs and the use of DNA pooling.
2 Better use of clinical, quantitative genetic, and biological data to define phenotypes.
3 Pooling of data from several different studies using the same standardized methods will enable much larger samples to

be investigated. However, in doing this it will be important to appreciate that often there will be differences among populations in the specific allelic variations, or even the genes, that predispose to disorder, and that there may also be ethnic variations in the strength of effect of susceptibility genes (Rutter, 2001).

4 Rather than survey the total population, greater leverage on the identification of susceptibility genes may be afforded by a focus on high-risk groups. This will be particularly important when the genetic influences operate through effects on environmental susceptibility.

5 An iterative interaction among genetic research, psychosocial research and biological research will be helpful. Too often, each of these has operated in isolation. Each should provide leads for what needs to be done in one of the others and, as genetics is informative on both environmental risk factors and biological risk mechanisms, it will be equally important for molecular genetics research to take on the lessons that come from research in these other two fields.

Mode of operation of genetic risk factors

Non-geneticists sometimes assume that identification of important genetic influences on mental disorder automatically equates with genetic determinism. Nothing could be further from the truth. One of the important findings from genetic research is the multiplicity of ways in which genetic factors may operate (Rutter, 2001). For example, even with wholly genetic Mendelian disorders (which are likely to account for a trivial proportion of child psychiatric disorders) the effects may be on neural functioning that almost inevitably results in a particular psychiatric disorder (Huntington disease would be an example of this kind); alternatively, when the genes operate through susceptibility to some aspect of the environment, whether or not functional impairment results may be entirely dependent on the environmental factor (phenylketonuria is the obvious example here); or the neural effects may be direct and wholly genetic but yet clinical outcome immensely varied for reasons that are as yet ill-understood (tuberous sclerosis is an example of this kind).

With multifactorial disorders, the modes of operation of genetic influence are even more varied. Genetic risk factor could operate through the creation of a relatively direct risk for the disorder even though the effects are probabilistic and require additional environmental risk factors. It is not known if this is the case with any psychiatric disorder but it could turn out to be so for schizophrenia or autism. A second possibility is that the genes may have relatively direct effects (through their influence on proteins) on part functions that, when combined with other functions, serve to make up the disorder. That could turn out to be the case with elements of dyslexia (see Snowling, Chapter 40). Thirdly, genes may influence temperamental (or other) dimensions that, in themselves, do not constitute the disorder, but which serve indirectly to increase the risk of disorder when combined with other risk factors. That is thought to be the case with respect to the role of neuroticism and the increased risk of affective and anxiety disorders (Kendler 1996) and it could be the

case with respect to sensation-seeking or novelty-seeking and the risk for ADHD (see Schachar & Tannock, Chapter 25). The implication here, however, is that personality feature involves no direct risk for disorder even though, in some circumstances, it may predispose to it. Thus, novelty-seeking could foster behaviours as varied as creative science, risky sports such as rock climbing, or antisocial behaviour.

A fourth alternative is that the genes may act through their role in increasing (or decreasing) environmental risk exposure—this coming about through passive, active or evocative gene–environment correlations (Rutter *et al.* 1997a). The genes, of course, do not cause the environmental risks directly; rather, they do so through their effects on behaviour. People's behaviour does much to shape and select environments that they experience.

Fifthly, genes may exert their effects through influences on susceptibility to environmental risks; that is gene–environment interactions. Molecular genetic studies in internal medicine have begun to document specific genetic risks in relation to features as varied as infections, allergies, immune responses, head injury and cigarette smoking (see Rutter 2000b). The findings from quantitative genetics in the field of psychopathology indicate that it is highly likely that the same will be found there.

It is clear that evidence of high heritability, or even of specific susceptibility genes, of itself provides no information on the nature of risk processes. Genetic findings provide a hugely helpful lead but they constitute the beginning, and not the end, of research into causal mechanisms. An important future goal is sorting out how nature–nurture interplay predisposes to, or protects from, psychopathology.

Another important misconception is that genes can be subdivided into those that are inherently 'bad' and those that are inherently 'good'. To begin with, the same genetically influenced behavioural trait may have both risk and protective functions. For example, an anxious emotionally hyper-responsive temperament constitutes a risk for anxiety disorders but a protection against antisocial behaviour. Many genes have effects on several different functions and these may involve both adaptive and maladaptive consequences. Sometimes the concept of 'good' and 'bad' genes is extrapolated to the potential to identify genetically high-risk and low-risk individuals, with the assumption that genetic profiling of fetuses should enable parents to choose which pregnancies to proceed with. The possibility raises important ethical issues (Rutter 1999) but it would not in any case be practical. Diseases derive from the action of multiple genes and the strong likelihood is that everyone carries important susceptibility genes for some undesirable outcome. It would be necessary to balance an increased risk for one disorder against a reduced risk for another one. In any case, whether or not a particular genetic susceptibility would actually lead to disease would depend in part on environmental risks. The risks are both probabilistic and contingent on circumstances. It should be added that the genetic risks are also not universal across individuals and across populations. Thus, the strength of the risk for Alzheimer disease associated with *APOE-4* varies across ethnic groups (Farrer *et al.* 1997). It is also the case that some simple single gene disorders, such as phenylketonuria, result from several different mutations in the same gene whereas others, such as spino-cerebellar ataxia, result from mutations in several distinct genes. The practical consequence is that, even in these relatively straightforward examples, it is easier to be sure that a person has a susceptibility gene than that he or she has not.

Potential for clinical practice from gene identification

Understanding the neurobiology of mental disorder

At least with respect to highly heritable neurodevelopmental disorders such as autism, schizophrenia and ADHD, the greatest benefit that is likely to come from molecular genetic research is the leads that will be provided for biological studies that could delineate the causal neural processes that constitute the biological underpinning of the conditions (Rutter & Plomin 1997; Rutter 2000a, 2001). Up to now, the findings from biological research have been frustratingly inconclusive on the specifics and have not been much help in delineation of diagnosis-specific pathophysiology or even non-specific brain processes that truly mediate psychopathological risk, albeit risk that spans several diagnoses (see Hollis, Chapter 37; Lord & Bailey, Chapter 38; Schachar & Tannock, Chapter 25). The identification of susceptibility genes will not, on its own, provide an answer but the determination of what the genes 'do' is likely to do much to provide the leads that are greatly needed to redirect biological studies. It has to be appreciated that determination of gene effects is far from straightforward and the research enterprise is likely to take quite a long time and will certainly involve areas of science that go beyond molecular genetics. Experimental gene 'knockout' and 'insertion' studies in species such as the mouse (genetically remarkably similar to humans) is going to be an essential first step (Wicker *et al.* 1995; Sibilia & Wagner 1996; Flint 1999). The need is to have a model that reflects the genetic alterations and which gives rise to a behavioural picture that recreates essential components of the human condition. That has not proved at all easy to do in the field of internal medicine and it will be even more difficult with mental disorders. This needs to be followed by research into the structure and interplay among proteins, proteomics (Pandey & Mann 2000). That requires entry into the burgeoning field of protein chemistry and so-called functional genomics. However, even that will not be the end because there is a need then to determine how these effects on proteins lead on to the clinical picture. That is likely to involve study of the interplay between genes and the environment, bringing in the field of molecular genetic epidemiology. This will need to lead on to a model, or series of possible models, of what might be the basic pathophysiology and the process by which it leads to the disorder (Rutter 2000a).

Although it is necessary to appreciate the long haul ahead, it is equally important to appreciate that molecular genetic findings may well constitute the key that will open the door to biological studies that will at last provide an understanding of the biological processes underlying mental disorder, and of the ways in which they relate to environmental risk factors. That understanding is certainly going to have implications for both prevention and intervention and it is a safe prediction that it will alter clinical practice, even though it is not possible to predict quite what changes will occur.

Pharmacogenetics

The same research process should also be helpful in providing leads for the development of more effective pharmacological interventions. Some effective drug treatments are already available in child psychiatry (see Heyman & Santosh, Chapter 59; and other chapters on specific disorders) but there are conditions, such as autism, where one might expect to find benefits from drug treatment but where, so far, these have proved quite minor (see Lord & Bailey, Chapter 38). Even when effective drugs are available, it is evident, as it is throughout psychiatry and internal medicine more generally, that there is marked individual variability in people's response to drugs. We know a good deal about which groups of drugs tend to benefit which groups of patients but we know much less about what differentiates those within those groups who do and do not respond. Molecular genetic findings could help greatly in that connection—the growing field of pharmacogenetics (Evans & Relling 1999).

Nature–nurture interplay

Throughout this chapter we have emphasized the fact that child psychiatric disorders are multifactorial in origin. This means not only the involvement of both genetic and environmental risk factors, but also that the causal processes often derive from an interplay between the two, stemming from gene–environment coactions, correlations and interactions. Although the importance of this interplay has been evident from quantitative genetic studies, as well as implied from epidemiological findings (Rutter & Silberg, in press), the study of such interplay has been constrained by both limitations on identifying factors where the risks are truly environmentally mediated and that genetic risks could not be assessed at the individual level. The former difficulty has been diminished by the development of research strategies that can test environmental risk hypotheses (Rutter *et al.*, 2001b) and the findings have been successful in identifying environmentally mediated risk processes, albeit at a more general level than one would wish (Rutter, 2000b).

The identification of individual susceptibility genes will allow the identification of genetic risks in the individual and that should greatly facilitate both the identification of environmental risks, and the interplay between the two (Plomin & Rutter 1998). The major practical problem that lies ahead is that there will usually be many susceptibility genes and partialling out specific genetic effects will depend on identification of all, or at least most, of the relevant genes and not just a few of them. That constitutes quite a challenge and will not be achieved easily.

Nevertheless, ultimately there is no doubt that much of the potential of molecular genetics will lie in its value for studying nature–nurture interplay. It should also help in determining whether the causal neural processes that underlie environmentally mediated risks are the same as those that underlie genetic risks. For example, in so far as institutional rearing predisposes to inattention/overactivity (Rutter et al., in press) or quasi-autistic patterns (Rutter et al. 1999a), does it do so by affecting the same neural processes as 'ordinary ADHD' and 'ordinary autism' or is the pathophysiology quite different?

In considering environmental influences it will be essential to go beyond psychosocial factors to include physical risks, such as those deriving from maternal alcohol consumption, obstetric–perinatal complications, and minor developmental aberrations (Rutter 2000a,b).

Psychiatric diagnosis

Because psychiatric diagnosis has lacked an external validating criterion, such as some physiological test, it has proved very difficult to establish what the true boundaries, criteria and demarcations should be. The identification of susceptibility genes will be of some use in that connection (Farmer & Owen 1996; Rutter & Plomin 1997). Thus, for example, it will enable determination of which social and communicative abnormalities are part of the same genetic liability as autism and which are caused by something quite different. The same applies to schizotypy and schizophrenia (see Hollis, Chapter 37) and obsessive-compulsive phenomena and Tourette syndrome (see Leckman & Cohen, Chapter 36). Those constitute major advantages but this approach to diagnosis works best when there is a major gene that *directly* causes the disease and that applies to only a tiny proportion of psychiatric disorders. Moreover, it is necessary to appreciate that most medical diagnoses are *not* based on a primary cause; rather, they are based on a unifying pathophysiology (see Taylor & Rutter, Chapter 1). The consequence is that the real progress in psychiatric diagnosis will come from the understanding of the underlying neurobiological processes, rather than from identification of the susceptibility genes as such (Owen et al. 2000).

Genetic screening

Some people have expressed high expectations of what could be achievable in the future through genetic screening. The 'Star Wars' scenario is that once we have identified all the relevant susceptibility genes (that is certainly going to take a long while) each person could be given their genetic profile that would specify whether or not they will develop one or another of a range of disorders. However, it will not actually work like that, because disease liability is not influenced by just one gene but rather by several genes. In theory, genetic research could provide that information but whether or not it will do so remains uncertain. More crucially, however, even when the full picture of genetic liability is available, the prediction of disease outcome will still depend on whether or not the individual encounters particular environmental hazards. The ways in which multifactorial disorders function will not lend them easily to a deterministic approach. On the other hand, through provision of an understanding on the mechanisms underlying nature–nurture interplay, genetic research should provide invaluable leads on which environmental manipulations could *lower* the risk of a disease outcome which does constitute a really important potential.

Genetic counselling

Much the same considerations apply to genetic counselling (Scourfield et al. 1999; see also Simonoff, Chapter 66). Molecular genetic findings will be helpful because predictions of genetic liability can be made on an individual basis, and not just on the basis of population averages. Unfortunately, the situation with respect to multifactorial disorders is much complicated by the fact that the risks are probabilistic and not deterministic, and are contingent on future life circumstances. Genetic advances will help the field of genetic counselling but the range of skills involved in this important speciality is going to be rather broader than is the case today. Genetic counsellors will have to have a good understanding of clinical diagnosis and of environmental risk processes.

Ethical issues

We need to end this chapter with a recognition that there will be crucial ethical issues arising as a result of genetic advances in the future. Although these are many and various, they should be manageable if properly dealt with (Farmer & McGuffin 1998; Rutter 1999). Nevertheless, history tells us that scientific findings have often been misused in ways that misrepresent the science and ignore ethical issues. Society as a whole will need to ensure that this does not happen and researchers have a special responsibility in that connection. Several concerns need highlighting.

First, concern has been expressed that an excessive focus on the priorities of molecular genetic research could result in a seriously damaging neglect of research into environmental risk mechanisms. As we have pointed out, although that is a risk that requires attention, genetic findings are clear-cut in pointing to the need for research into both environmental and genetic risk factors, and most especially on their interplay. A related concern is that genetic research will encourage a misleading genetic determinism that will impair policy initiatives and practical innovations to deal with serious environmental hazards (Rose 1995). Again, that is a risk but, once more, it arises out of a *mis*understanding of the messages of genetic research. This is sometimes linked with a concern that genetic advances will lead to a 'medicalization' of social problems, with a consequent excessive use of drug treatments, to the neglect of interventions focusing on psychosocial risk factors. In that connection, one of the key messages of genetic research is that genetic factors are *not* just concerned with disease. They concern the whole of human behaviour and carry no implications one way or the other with respect to medicalization. On the other hand, although nothing to do with genetics, it has to be said that the risk of excessive use of drug treatments given by community practitioners who lack expertise in their use is real, because such treatments can be viewed as cheap, undemanding and saving of time (Zito *et al.* 2000). Another often expressed concern is that genetic findings may increase psychiatric stigma. Although anything could happen, we see that as a curious expectation because the existing stigma arises in considerable part because of an attitude that mental disorders arise because people are acting irresponsibly, not coping when they should, and not trying hard enough, and it seems to us likely, at least if biological findings are responsibly handled, that evidence of contributory biological propensities could well reduce stigma, rather than increase it (Farmer & McGuffin 1998).

A rather greater concern is that genetic information could be used to disadvantage individuals with respect to health or life assurance, or employment (Royal Society 1997). It has to be said that that is a definite risk and it is appropriate, and necessary, that governments throughout the industrialized world are considering what legislation is needed to avoid the misuse of genetic data in this way. However, the probabilistic contingent nature of genetic risks in relation to multifactorial disorders means that the main problem comes from a misuse and misunderstanding of genetics, rather than from genetic findings as such.

Conclusions

The section of this chapter that has sought to look into the future is substantially longer than that in most other chapters. That is because the field of genetics is one of the fastest moving fields of research and because many of these advances are so recent that practitioners will have undergone their main training at a time when much of this was not even on the horizon. As a consequence, there is the twin danger of people underestimating how useful genetic findings are going to be and also overestimating the attendant risks. We have tried to convey something of the excitement and high potential of genetics while at the same time being realistic about how much remains to be done (see Rutter, in press). Of all the chapters in this volume, this is the one most likely to require major revision by the time the next edition appears.

References

Abreu, P.C., Greenberg, D.A. & Hodge, S.E. (1999) Direct power comparisons between simple LOD scores and NPL scores for linkage analysis in complex diseases. *American Journal of Human Genetics*, 65, 847–857.

American Psychiatric Association (1994) *Diagnostic and Statistical Manual of Mental Disorders*, 4th edn. American Psychiatric Association, Washington D.C.

Amos, C.I. (1994) Robust variance-components approach for assessing genetic linkage in pedigrees. *American Journal of Human Genetics*, 54, 535–543.

Angold, A., Costello, E. & Erkanli A. (1999) Comorbidity. *Journal of Child Psychology and Psychiatry*, 40, 55–87.

Asherson, P., Curran, S. & McGuffin, P. (1998) Molecular genetics: approaches to gene mapping. *Central Nervous System*, 1, 18–22.

Bailey, A., Palferman, S., Heavey, L. & Le Couteur, A. (1998) Autism: the phenotype in relatives. *Journal of Autism and Developmental Disorders*, 28, 381–404.

Bolton, P., Macdonald, H., Pickles, A. *et al.* (1994) A case–control family history study of autism. *Journal of Child Psychology and Psychiatry*, 35, 877–900.

Botstein, D., White, R.L., Skolnick, M. & Davis, R.W. (1980) Construction of a genetic linkage map in man using restriction fragment length polymorphisms. *American Journal of Human Genetics*, 32, 314–331.

Bouchard, T.J. Jr (1998) Genetic and environmental influences on adult intelligence and special mental abilities. *Human Biology*, 70, 257–279.

Cadoret, R.J., Yates, W.R., Troughton, E., Woodworth, G. & Stewart, M.A.S. (1995) Genetic–environmental interaction in the genesis of aggressivity and conduct disorders. *Archives of General Psychiatry*, 52, 916–924.

Cardon, L.R., Smith, S.D., Fulker, D.W., Kimberling, W.J., Pennington, B.F. & DeFries, J.C. (1994) Quantitative trait locus for reading disability on chromosome 6. *Science*, 266, 276–279.

Caron, C. & Rutter, M. (1991) Comorbidity in child psychopathology: concepts, issues and research strategies. *Journal of Child Psychology and Psychiatry*, 32, 1063–1080.

Clerget-Darpoux, F. (1991) The uses and abuses of linkage analysis in neuropsychiatric disorder. In: *The New Genetics of Mental Illness* (eds P. McGuffin & R. Murray), pp. 44–57. Butterworth-Heinemann, London.

Collins, F.S. (1992) Positional cloning: let's not call it reverse anymore. *Nature Genetics*, 1, 3–6.

Cordell, H.J. & Todd, J.A. (1995) Multifactorial inheritance in type 1 diabetes. *Trends in Genetics*, 11, 499–504.

Craddock, N. & Jones, I. (1999) Genetics of bipolar disorder. *Journal of Medical Genetics*, 36, 585–594.

Craddock, N., Rees, M., Norton, N., Feldman, E., McGuffin, P. & Owen, M. (1996) Association between bipolar disorder and the VNTR polymorphism in intron 2 of the human serotonin transporter gene (HSERT). *Psychiatric Genetic Abstracts*, 6, 147.

Crowe, R.R. (1974) An adoption study of antisocial personality. *Archives of General Psychiatry*, 31, 785–791.

Dale, P.S., Simonoff, E., Bishop, D.V.M. *et al.* (1998) Genetic influence on language delay in two-year-old children. *Nature Neuroscience*, 1, 324–328.

Daniels, J., Holmans, J., Williams, N. *et al.* (1998) A simple method for analysing microsatellite allele image patterns generated from DNA pools and its application to allelic association studies. *American Journal of Human Genetics*, 62, 1189–1197.

DeFries, J.C., Plomin, R. & Fulker, D.W. (1994) *Nature and Nurture During Middle Childhood*. Blackwell Science, Oxford.

Donis-Keller, H., Green, P., Helms, C. *et al.* (1987) A genetic linkage map of the human genome. *Cell*, 51, 319–337.

Edwards, J.H. (1960) The simulation of mendelism. *Acta Genetica*, 10, 63–70.

Edwards, J.H. (1965) The meaning of the associations between blood groups and disease. *Annals of Human Genetics*, 29, 77–83.

Edwards, J.H. (1991) The formal problems of linkage. In: *The New Genetics of Mental Illness* (eds P. McGuffin & R. Murray), pp. 58–70. Butterworth–Heinemann, Oxford.

Eley, T.C. & Stevenson, J. (1999) Exploring the covariation between anxiety and depression symptoms: a genetic analysis of the effects of age and sex. *Journal of Child Psychology and Psychiatry*, **40**, 1273–1284.

Engfer, A., Walper, S. & Rutter, M. (1994) Individual characteristics as a force in development. In: *Development Through Life: a Handbook for Clinicians* (eds M. Rutter & D.F. Hay), pp. 79–111. Blackwell Scientific Publications, Oxford.

Evans, W.E. & Relling, M.V. (1999) Pharmacogenomics: translating functional genomics into rational therapeutics. *Science*, **286**, 487–491.

Falconer, D.S. (1965) The inheritance of liability to certain diseases, estimated from the incidence among relatives. *Annals of Human Genetics*, **29**, 51–76.

Falconer, D.S. & Mackay, T.F. (1996) *Introduction to Quantitative Genetics*, 4th edn. Longman, Harrow.

Farmer, A. & McGuffin, P. (1998) Ethics and psychiatric genetics. In: *Ethics and Psychiatry* (ed. S. Block), 3rd edn, pp. 479–493. Oxford University Press, Oxford.

Farmer, A. & Owen, M.J. (1996) Genomics: the next psychiatric revolution? *British Journal of Psychiatry*, **169**, 135–138.

Farrer, L.A., Cupples, L.A., Haines, J.L. *et al.* for the APOE & Alzheimer Disease Meta Analysis Consortium (1997) Effects of age, sex, and ethnicity on the association between apolipoprotein E genotype and Alzheimer disease. *Journal of the American Medical Association*, **278**, 1349–1356.

Fisher, P.J., Turic, D., McGuffin, P. *et al.* (1999) DNA pooling identifies QTLs for general cognitive ability in children on chromosome 4. *Human Molecular Genetics*, **8**, 915–922.

Flint, J. (1999) The genetic basis of cognition. *Brain*, **122**, 2015–2031.

Fulker, D.W. & Cardon, L.R. (1994) A sib-pair approach to interval mapping of quantitative trait loci. *American Journal of Human Genetics*, **54**, 1092–1103.

Gayan, J., Smith, S.D., Cherny, S.S. *et al.* (1999) Quantitative-trait locus for specific language and reading deficits on chromosome 6p. *American Journal of Human Genetics*, **64**, 157–164.

Gottesman, I.I. (1963) Genetic aspects of intelligent behavior. In: *The Handbook of Mental Deficiency: Psychological Theory and Research* (ed. N. Ellis), pp. 346–347. McGraw-Hill, New York.

Gottesman, I.I. (1991) Schizophrenia genesis. *The Origins of Madness.* W.H. Freeman, New York.

Gottesman, I.I. & Shields, J. (1967) A polygenic theory of schizophrenia. *Proceedings of the National Academy of Sciences, USA*, **58**, 199–205.

Grigorenko, E.L., Wood, F.B., Meyer, M.S. *et al.* (1997) Susceptibility loci for distinct components of developmental dyslexia on chromosomes 6 and 15. *American Journal of Human Genetics*, **60**, 27–39.

Hanson, D.R. & Gottesman, I. (1976) The genetics, if any, of infantile autism and childhood schizophrenia. *Journal of Autism and Schizophrenia*, **6**, 209–233.

Harrington, R., Rutter, M., Weissman, M. *et al.* (1997) Psychiatric disorders in the relatives of depressed probands. I. Comparison of prepubertal, adolescent and early adult onset cases. *Journal of Affective Disorders*, **42**, 9–22.

Haseman, J.K. & Elston, R.C. (1972) The investigation of linkage between a quantitative trait and a marker locus. *Behaviour Genetics*, **2**, 3–10.

Henderson, N.D. (1970) Genetic influences on the behavior of mice can be obscured by laboratory rearing. *Journal of Comparative Physiology and Psychology*, **72**, 505–511.

Hill, L., Asherson, P., Ball, D. *et al.* (1999) DNA pooling and dense marker maps: A systematic search for genes for cognitive ability. *NeuroReport*, **10(4)**, 843–848.

Jockin, V., McGue, M. & Lykken, D.T. (1996) Personality and divorce: a genetic analysis. *Journal of Personality and Social Psychology*, **71**, 288–299.

Kendler, K.S. (1996) Major depression and generalised anxiety disorder: same genes, (partly) different environments—revisited. *British Journal of Psychiatry*, **168** (Suppl. 30), 68–75.

Kendler, K.S. & Karkowski-Shuman, L. (1997) Stressful life events and genetic liability to major depression: genetic control of exposure to the environment? *Psychological Medicine*, **27**, 539–547.

Kendler, K.S., Sham, P.C. & MacLean, C.J. (1997) The determinants of parenting: an epidemiological, multi-informant, retrospective study. *Psychological Medicine*, **27**, 549–563.

Lamb, J.A., Moore, J., Bailey, A. & Monaco, A.P. (2000) Autism: recent molecular genetic advances. *Human Molecular Genetics*, **9**, 861–868.

Maughan, B. & Pickles, A. (1990) Adopted and illegitimate children growing up. In: *Straight and Devious Pathways from Childhood to Adulthood* (eds L. Robins & M. Rutter), pp. 36–61. Cambridge University Press, New York.

McClearn, G.E., Johansson, B., Berg, S. *et al.* (1997) Substantial genetic influence on cognitive abilities in twins 80 or more years old. *Science*, **276**, 1560–1563.

McGue, M. (1997) The democracy of the genes. *Nature*, **388**, 417–418.

McGue, M., Gottesman, I.I. & Rao, D.C. (1983) The transmission of schizophrenia under a multifactorial threshold model. *American Journal of Human Genetics*, **35**, 1161–1178.

McGue, M., Bouchard, T.J. Jr & Iacono, W.G. (1993) Behavioral genetics of cognitive ability: a life-span perspective. In: *Nature, Nurture and Psychology* (eds R. Plomin & G.E. McLearn), pp. 59–76. American Psychological Association, Washington, D.C.

McGuffin, P. & Buckland, P. (1991) Major genes, minor genes and molecular neurobiology of mental illness: a comment on 'quantitative trait loci and psychopharmacology' by Plomin, McLearn and Gora-Maslak. *Journal of Psychopharmacology*, **5**, 18–22.

McGuffin, P. & Gottesman, I.I. (1985) Genetic influences on normal and abnormal development. In: *Child and Adolescent Psychiatry: Modern Approaches* (eds M. Rutter & L.A. Hersov), 2nd ed, pp. 17–33. Blackwell Scientific Publications, Oxford.

McGuffin, P. & Huckle, P. (1990) Simulation of Mendelism revisited: the recessive gene for attending medical school. *American Journal of Human Genetics*, **46**, 994–999.

McGuffin, P., Festenstein, H. & Murray, R. (1983) A family study of HLA antigens and other genetic markers in schizophrenia. *Psychological Medicine*, **13**, 31–43.

McGuffin, P., Farmer, A.E., Gottesman, I.I. (1987a) Is there really a split in schizophrenia? The genetic evidence. *British Journal of Psychiatry*, **150**, 581–592.

McGuffin, P., Katz, R. & Bebbington, P. (1987b) Hazard, heredity and depression: a family study. *Journal of Psychiatric Research*, **21**, 365–375.

McGuffin, P., Katz, R. & Bebbington, P. (1988) The Camberwell Collaborative Study. III. Depression and adversity in the relatives of depressed probands. *British Journal of Psychiatry*, **152**, 775–782.

McGuffin, P., Katz, R., Rutherford, J. (1991) Nature, nurture and depression: A twin study. *Psychological Medicine*, **21**, 329–335.

McGuffin, P., Asherson, P., Owen, M. & Farmer, A. (1994) The strength of the genetic effect: is there room for an environmental influence in the aetiology of schizophrenia? *British Journal of Psychiatry*, **164**, 593–599.

McGuffin, P., Katz, R., Watkins, S. & Rutherford, J. (1996) A hospital-based twin register of the heritability of DSM-IV unipolar depression. *Archives of General Psychiatry*, **53**, 129–136.

Morris, D.W., Robinson, L., Turic, D. *et al.* (2000) Family-based association mapping provides evidence for a gene for reading disability on chromosome 15q. *Human Molecular Genetics*, **9**, 843–848.

Morton, N.E. (1955) Sequential tests for the detection of linkage. *American Journal of Human Genetics*, **7**, 277–318.

Morton, N.E. & Collins, A. (1998) Tests and estimates of allelic association in complex inheritance. *Proceedings of the National Academy of Science, USA*, **95**, 11389–11393.

Murray, K.T. & Sines, J.O. (1996) Research report: parsing the genetic and nongenetic variance in children's depressive behavior. *Journal of Affective Disorders*, **38**, 23–34.

Nadder, T.S., Silberg, J.L., Rutter, M., Maes, H.H. & Eaves, L.J. (2001) Comparison of multiple measures of ADHD symptomatology: a multivariate genetic analysis. *Journal of Child Psychology and Psychiatry*, **42**, 475–486.

Neale, M.C. & Cardon, L.R. (1992) *Methodology for Genetic Studies of Twins and Families*. Kluwer Academic, Dordrecht.

O'Connor, T.G., Deater-Deckard, K., Fulker, D., Rutter, M. & Plomin, R. (1998) Early adolescence: antisocial behavioral problems and coercive parenting. *Developmental Psychology*, **34**, 970–981.

O'Donovan, M.C., Oefner, P.J., Roberts, S.C. *et al.* (1998) Blind analysis of denaturing high-performance liquid chromatography as a tool for mutation detection. *Genomics*, **52**, 44–49.

OMIM Online (2000) National Center for Biotechnology Information. http://www.ncbi.nlm.nih.gov/entrez/query.fcgi?db=OMIM.

Owen, M.J., Cardno, A.G. & O'Donovan, M.C. (2000) Psychiatric genetics: back to the future. *Molecular Psychiatry*, **5**, 22–31.

Page, G.P. & Amos, C.I. (1999) Comparison of linkage-disequilibrium methods for localization of genes influencing quantitative traits in humans. *American Journal of Human Genetics*, **64**, 1194–1205.

Pandey, A. & Mann, M. (2000) Proteomics to study genes and genomes. *Nature*, **405**, 837–846.

Pauls, D.L., Cohen, D.J., Heimbuch, R. & Kidd, K.K. (1981) Familial pattern and transmission of Gilles de la Tourette syndrome and multiple tics. *Archives of General Psychiatry*, **38**, 1091–1093.

Pawlby, S.J., Mills, A., Taylor, A. & Quinton, D. (1997a) Adolescent friendships mediating childhood adversity and adult outcome. *Journal of Adolescence*, **20**, 633–644.

Pawlby, S.J., Mills, A. & Quinton, D. (1997b) Vulnerable adolescent girls: opposite-sex relationships. *Journal of Child Psychology and Psychiatry*, **38**, 909–920.

Pickles, A., Bolton, P., Macdonald, H. *et al.* (1995) Latent-class analysis of recurrence risks for complex phenotypes with selection and measurement error: a twin and family history study of autism. *American Journal of Human Genetics*, **57**, 717–726.

Plomin, R. (1994) *Genetics and Experience: the Interplay Between Nature and Nurture*. Sage Publications, Thousand Oaks, CA.

Plomin, R. & Rutter, M. (1998) Child development, molecular genetics and what to do with genes once they are found. *Child Development*, **69**, 1223–1242.

Plomin, R., DeFries, J.C., McClearn, G.E. & McGuffin, P. (2000) *Behavioral Genetics*, 4th edn. Worth, New York.

Plomin, R., Owen, M.J. & McGuffin, P. (1994) The genetic basis of complex human behaviours. *Science*, **264**, 1733–1739.

Quinton, D. & Rutter, M. (1988) *Parenting Breakdown: the Making and Breaking of Inter-generational Links*. Avebury, Aldershot.

Reich, T., James, J.W. & Morris, C.A. (1972) The use of multiple thresh-olds in determining the mode of transmission of semi-continuous traits. *Annual Human Genetics*, **36**, 163–186.

Riley, B.P. & McGuffin, P. (2000) Linkage and associated studies of schizophrenia. *American Journal of Medical Genetics*, **97**, 23–44.

Risch, N. (1990) Linkage strategies for genetically complex traits. II. The power of affected relative pairs. *American Journal of Human Genetics*, **46**, 229–241.

Risch, N. & Merikangas, K. (1996) The future of genetic studies of complex human diseases. *Science*, **273**, 1516–1517.

Roberts, S.B., MacLean, C.J., Neale, M.C., Eaves, L.J. & Kendler, K.S. (1999) Replication of linkage studies of complex traits: an examination of variation in location estimates. *American Journal of Human Genetics*, **65**, 876–884.

Rose, S. (1995) The rise of neurogenetic determinism. *Nature*, **373**, 380–382.

Rowe, D.C., Jacobson, K.C. & van den Oord, J.C.G. (1999) Genetic and environmental influences on vocabulary IQ: parental education level as a moderator. *Child Development*, **70**, 1151–1162.

Royal Society (1997) Human genetics: uncertainties and the financial implications ahead. *Philosophical Transactions of the Royal Society of London: Biological Sciences* (ed. R.N. Anderson), **352**, 1035–1114.

Rutter, M. (1966) *Children of Sick Parents*. Oxford University Press, Oxford.

Rutter, M. (1997) Comorbidity. *Concepts, Claims and Choices: Criminal Behaviour and Mental Health*, **7**, 265–285.

Rutter, M. (1999) Genes and behaviour: health potential and ethical concerns. In: *Inventing Heaven? Quakers Confront the Challenges of Genetic Engineering* (eds A. Carroll & C. Skidmore), pp. 66–88. Sowle Press, Reading.

Rutter, M. (2000a) Genetic studies of autism: from the 1970s into the Millennium. *Journal of Abnormal Child Psychology*, **28**, 3–14.

Rutter, M. (2000b) Psychosocial influences: critiques, findings, and research needs. *Development and Psychopathology*, **12**, 375–405.

Rutter, M. (2001) Child psychiatry in the era following sequencing the genome: commentary. In: *Attention, Genes and ADHD* (eds D. Hay & F. Levy), pp. 225–248. Brunner-Routledge, Hove, UK.

Rutter, M. (in press) Nature, nurture and development: from evangelism through science towards policy and practice. *Child Development*.

Rutter, M. & Garmezy, N. (1983) Developmental psychopathology. In: *Socialization, Personality, and Child Development*, Vol. 4. *Mussen's Handbook of Child Psychology* (ed. E.M. Hetherington), 4th edn, pp. 775–911. Wiley, New York.

Rutter, M. & Plomin, R. (1997) Opportunities for psychiatry from genetic findings. *British Journal of Psychiatry*, **171**, 209–219.

Rutter, M. & Silberg, J. (in press) Gene-environment interplay in relation to emotional and behavioral disturbance. *Annual Review of Psychology*, **53**.

Rutter, M., Dunn, J., Plomin, R. *et al.* (1997a) Integrating nature and nurture: implications of person–environment correlations and interactions for developmental psychology. *Development and Psychopathology*, **9**, 335–364.

Rutter, M., Maughan, B., Meyer, J. *et al.* (1997b) Heterogeneity of antisocial behavior: causes, continuities, and consequences. In: *Nebraska Symposium on Motivation*, Vol. 44. *Motivation and Delinquency* (eds R. Dienstbier & D.W. Osgood), pp. 45–118. University of Nebraska Press, Lincoln, NE.

Rutter, M., Giller, H. & Hagell, A. (1998) *Antisocial Behaviour by Young People: the Main Messages from a Major New Review of the Research*. Cambridge University Press, New York.

Rutter, M., Andersen-Wood, L., Beckett, C. *et al.* & the English & Romanian Adoptees (ERA) Study Team (1999a) Quasi-autistic patterns following severe early global privation. *Journal of Child Psychology and Psychiatry*, **40**, 537–549.

Rutter, M., Silberg, J., O'Connor, T. & Simonoff, E. (1999b) Genetics and child psychiatry. I. Advances in quantitative and molecular genetics. *Journal of Child Psychology and Psychiatry*, **40**, 3–18.

Rutter, M., Kreppner, J., O'Connor, T.G., & the English & Romanian Adoptees (ERA) Study Team (2001a) Specificity and heterogeneity in children's responses to profound privation. *British Journal of Psychiatry*, **179**, 97–103.

Rutter, M., Pickles, A., Murray, R. & Eaves, L. (2001b) Testing hypotheses on specific environmental causal effects on behavior. *Psychological Bulletin*, **127**, 291–324.

Rutter, M., Roy, P. & Kreppner, J. (in press) Institutional care as a risk factor for inattention/overactivity. In: *Hyperactivity Disorder* (ed S. Sandberg), 2nd ed. Cambridge University Press, Cambridge.

Sampson, J.R. (2000) Tuberous sclerosis complex: molecular genetic insights into pathogenes. *Brain Pathology*, **10**, 600.

Sandbrink, R., Hartmann, T., Master, C.L. & Beyreuther, K. (1996) Genes contributing to Alzheimer's disease. *Molecular Psychiatry*, **1**, 27–40.

Scarr, S. & Carter-Saltzman, L. (1979) Twin method: defense of a critical assumption. *Behavior Genetics*, **9**, 527–542.

Scourfield, J., Neilson, M., Lewis, G. & McGuffin, P. (1999) Heritability of social cognitive skills in children and adolescents. *British Journal of Psychiatry*, **175**, 559–564.

Sham, P. (1998) *Statistics in Human Genetics*. Arnold, London.

Sibilia, M. & Wagner, E.F. (1996) Transgenic animals. *European Review*, **4**, 371–392.

Silberg, J., Pickles, A., Rutter, M. *et al.* (1999) The influence of genetic factors and life stress on depression among adolescent girls. *Archives of General Psychiatry*, **56**, 225–232.

Silberg, J., Rutter, M., Neale, M. & Eaves, L. (2001) Genetic moderation of environmental risk for depression and anxiety in adolescent girls. *British Journal of Psychiatry*, **179**, 116–121.

Slutske, W.C., Heath, A.C., Dinwiddie, S.H. *et al.* (1997) Modeling genetic and environmental influences in the etiology of conduct disorder: a study of 2682 adult twin pairs. *Journal of Abnormal Psychology*, **106**, 266–279.

Smith, S.D., Kimberling, W.J., Pennington, B.F. & Lubs, H.A. (1983) Specific reading disability-identification of an inherited form through linkage analysis. *Science*, **219**, 1345.

Southern, E.M. (1975) Detection of specific sequences among DNA fragments separated by gel electrophoresis. *Journal of Molecular Biology*, **98**, 503–517.

Spielman, R.S., McGinnis, R.E. & Ewens, R.J. (1993) Transmission test for linkage disequilibrium: the insulin gene region and IDDM. *American Journal of Human Genetics*, **52**, 506–516.

Stoolmiller, M. (1999) Implications of the restricted range of family environments for estimates of heritability and nonshared environment in behavior–genetic adoption studies. *Psychological Bulletin*, **125**, 392–409.

Sullivan, P.F., Neale, M.C. & Kendler, K.S. (2000) The genetic epidemiology of major depression: review and meta-analysis. *American Journal of Psychiatry*, **157**, 1552–1562.

Terwilliger, J.D., Shannon, W.D., Lathrop, G.M. *et al.* (1997) True and false positive peaks in genomewide scans: applications of length-biased sampling to linkage mapping. *American Journal of Human Genetics*, **61**, 430–438.

Thapar, A. & McGuffin, P. (1994) A twin study of depressive symptoms in childhood. *British Journal of Psychiatry*, **165**, 259–265.

Thapar, A. & McGuffin, P. (1997) Anxiety and depressive symptoms in childhood: a genetic study of comorbidity. *Journal of Child Psychology and Psychiatry*, **38**, 651–656.

Thapar, A., Harold, G. & McGuffin, P. (1998) Life events and depressive symptoms in childhood: shared genes or shared adversity? A research note. *Journal of Child Psychology and Psychiatry*, **39**, 1153–1158.

Thapar, A., Holmes, J., Poulton, K. & Harrington, R. (1999) Genetic basis of attention deficit hyperactivity. *British Journal of Psychiatry*, **174**, 105–111.

Thapar, A., Harrington, R. & McGuffin, P. (2001) Examining the Comorbidity of ADHD-related behaviours and conduct problems using a twin study design. *British Journal of Psychiatry*, **179**, 224–229.

Vanyukov, M.M. & Tarter, R.E. (2000) Genetic studies of substance abuse. *Drug and Alcohol Dependence*, **59**, 101–123.

Weissman, M.M., Merikangas, K.R., Wickramaratne, P. *et al.* (1986) Understanding the clinical heterogeneity of major depression using family data. *Archives of General Psychiatry*, **43**, 430–434.

Wicker, L.S., Todd, J.A. & Peterson, L.B. (1995) Genetic control of autoimmune diabetes in the NOD mouse. *Annual Review of Immunology*, **13**, 179.

Wilson, R.S. (1978) Synchronies in mental development: an epigenetic perspective. *Science*, **202**, 939–948.

Wilson, R.S. (1985) The Louisville twin study: developmental syndromes in behavior. *Child Development*, **56**, 298–316.

World Health Organization (1993) *The ICD-10 Classification of Mental and Behavioural Disorders: Diagnostic Criteria for Research*. World Health Organization, Geneva, Switzerland.

Zito, J.M., Safer, D.J., dos Reis, S., Gardner, J.F., Botes, M. & Lynch, F. (2000) Trends in the prescribing of psychotropic medications to preschoolers. *Journal of the American Medical Association*, **283**, 1025–1030.

13 Molecular Genetic and Chromosomal Anomalies: Cognitive and Behavioural Consequences

David H. Skuse and Jonna Kuntsi

Introduction

Behavioural phenotypes are the psychological equivalent of the somatic or physiological manifestations of a syndrome that has a genetic aetiology. There is no consensus about how they should be defined. Flint (1996) suggested they constitute 'behaviour(s), including cognitive processes and social interaction style, that [are] consistently associated with, and specific to, a syndrome which has a chromosomal or a genetic aetiology'. He added 'where there is little doubt that the phenotype is a consequence of the underlying anomaly', but others feel that additional definition is too restrictive (Hodapp 1997; Finegan 1998). Dykens & Cassidy (1995) suggested behavioural phenotypes should be characterized as 'the heightened probability [that] people with a given syndrome will exhibit certain behavioural sequelae relative to those without the syndrome' (see also Volkmar & Dykens, Chapter 41). Hodapp (1997) emphasized the point that genetic disorders should not be considered to have uniform effects, either on behaviour or on somatic aspects of the phenotype. There is great variability in the expression of even the most 'characteristic' features of a syndrome. The remaining genotype of the affected individual will modify the behavioural expression of the anomaly, as will developmental trends, and the impact of the environment in which the child is raised. Thus, it is unusual for a genetic disorder to be associated with a pattern of behaviour that is specific to that condition, especially in the context of mental retardation. However, it is not unusual for two or more genetic disorders to lead to outcomes that are not shared by others with equivalent learning difficulties (Hodapp 1997).

Opinions are divided between those who regard the study of behavioural phenotypes as being generally worthwhile, and those who have their doubts. A few moments reflection indicates that there are many problems with the concept. First, is the term to be restricted only to disorders in which a genetic anomaly has been identified? Many conditions appear to have a genetic origin, as well as characteristic behavioural features, but the nature of the genetic deficit is not known. Should the clinical manifestations of such conditions be classified as behavioural phenotypes? Secondly, is it likely that any specific cognitive or behavioural features will be consistently found associated with a genetic anomaly, unless they are part of the syndrome's definition? The genetic background of the individual will inevitably modify phenotypic expression; if there is no specificity in the

narrow sense, the behavioural phenotype may be so vague as to be virtually meaningless. Thirdly, because behaviour is modified by experience, any phenotype is likely to vary in intensity for that reason alone, independent of genotype. How then should we differentiate between the direct effects of the genetic anomaly and the indirect influence of the circumstances of upbringing? Finally, how is it possible in studies of humans, as opposed to model systems (Skuse 2000a), to clarify the mechanisms that link genetic anomalies to behaviour, and to show they are causally related to cognitive or behavioural manifestations?

The term 'behavioural phenotype' is used here for a typical style of behaviour that occurs in association with conditions in which a genetic anomaly has been demonstrated in a substantial proportion of cases. To include features of a disorder in which a genetic anomaly is only suspected, but where it has not been demonstrated, is liable to cause confusion. The danger is a widening of the concept to include the cognitive and behavioural features of all conditions that are highly heritable (such as autism or attention deficit hyperactivity disorder; ADHD) irrespective of whether any aetiological chromosomal or genetic anomaly is known. The term will therefore be restricted to conditions in which a genetic deletion/mutation or at least a chromosomal anomaly has been identified. Of course, conditions that have not met this criterion to date could meet it in the future, if a genetic cause for the syndrome is identified. A case in point is Rett syndrome, for which no genetic aetiology was known until the discovery that a mutation in the gene *MECP2* can lead to the onset of the condition in a minority of cases (Amir *et al.* 1999). Behavioural phenotypes may occur as a consequence of sporadic events, such as a mutation, or of a chromosomal rearrangement that has not been inherited, as well as those that are heritable.

Why study behavioural phenotypes?

The concept of behavioural phenotypes has clinical value. For many parents it is perplexing to be faced with a child who has a genetic disorder with easily identifiable somatic manifestations, such as short stature and facial dysmorphology, who also displays disturbed behaviour that is inexplicably starkly different from that of their siblings. To be able to reassure parents that features such as the hyperphagia of Prader–Willi syndrome

(Cassidy 1992) or the self-injury associated with Lesch–Nyhan syndrome (Nyhan 1997), are characteristic of the disorder may be helpful in alleviating unwarranted guilt. Parents need to be reassured that behavioural manifestations of the condition are not their fault, nor are they a result of wilfulness on the part of the child; yet often they are manageable.

Another reason for interest in behavioural phenotypes is the hope that by understanding how they arise from a genetic anomaly, they can facilitate location of genes that influence specific behavioural patterns. Much genetic research to date has been 'top-down' in its approach to quantitative genetic analysis of complex traits (see McGuffin & Rutter, Chapter 12). We commonly use linkage or association strategies to track down naturally occurring alleles of candidate genes in a 'wild-type' population. Alleles are stable alternative forms of the same gene that differ in their identified DNA sequence at a particular location. Different forms of the same gene (so-called polymorphisms) may have functionally different effects upon the phenotype. On the other hand, if those alleles are naturally occurring variations and thus widely distributed in the population at large they are likely to have only a minor influence upon the phenotype of the individual. This is so, simply because alleles with a more dramatic effect could reduce fitness and so would be selected against during evolution.

There is the prospect of genes that influence the development of brain systems that regulate the cognitive skills and behaviour. Importantly, such genes are unlikely to account for individual differences in the normal distribution of traits such as intelligence, personality or talents. The genes that are disrupted or lost in conditions that have a behavioural or cognitive phenotype may, however, be important in predisposing toward specific learning difficulties or psychiatric illness, in a (probably very small) proportion of individuals with those disorders. Identifying such genes may be rather easier than locating susceptibility loci from linkage or association studies. Identification of a behavioural phenotype implies that disruption to a particular gene, or a set of genes at a particular locus, consistently leads to specific cognitive or behavioural consequences. Having shown this, it is a fair assumption that the genetic locus in question regulates the development of a cognitive or behavioural system. The next stage of an investigation would be to show that targeted disruption of the locus in an animal model may also lead to cognitive or behavioural deficits. If so, the role of that locus in brain development and function becomes open to direct study (Skuse 2000a).

The investigation of behavioural phenotypes provides an indirect route to understanding the development of neurobehavioural systems that are dysfunctional in a range of neurodevelopmental disorders and specific learning difficulties, both in childhood and adulthood. There is an important related point: occasionally, a particular genetic mutation, or deletion, is associated with a behavioural phenotype that looks like a known disease, such as autism or schizophrenia. The finding should not be taken to imply the genetic locus has any direct part to play in the predisposition of individuals from the general population to develop that disorder. Major psychiatric disorders are likely to have a multigenic aetiology. Predispositions are not caused by mutations in single genes. If they were, the individuals carrying those mutations would probably have such reduced fertility that they would be eliminated in the course of evolution.

Rather, the discovery that a behavioural phenotype resembles a known disorder provides a key with which it may be possible to unlock the secrets of the development of a particular cognitive or behavioural brain system which, if disrupted, may lead to a conventionally identifiable disorder. (Of course, we should not assume all instances of the disorder are necessarily going to be associated with dysfunction of that system.) Cases of the disorder that are identified from the general population are likely to have a multigenic or polygenic aetiology. Particular configurations of functional gene variants will usually be required to cause its full manifestations. These will act epistatically (synergistically) to increase the risk of a disease phenotype becoming manifest. Environmental risk factors may also play a part in tipping the balance toward disease. However, we may gain valuable information about how the systems that maintain—for example, normal social cognition—have evolved by studying the impact of a known genetic mutation on brain development and function.

Genetic mechanisms leading to behavioural phenotypes

We normally have 46 chromosomes in every cell of our body, with the exception of germ cells in the testis and ovary. Each chromosome has both a long and a short arm (in some cases the short arm is much abbreviated). These arms are joined by a region known as the centromere, which is essential for normal cell division to take place and which does not contain expressed genetic material. At the end of each is a cap of repetitive DNA sequences known as the telomere. Autosomes are numbered from 1 to 22, approximately in descending order of their size. There are two sex chromosomes. The X chromosome is moderately large, and possesses about 1000 genes. It lies between autosomes 7 and 8 in magnitude. The Y chromosome consists of relatively little genetic material, and has only 30–40 expressed genes (D.C. Page, personal communication). Our genotype comprises the set of 30 000–40 000 protein-coding genes that are expressed at some time or another from our genome. Not all are switched on all the time, and different tissues will express different combinations of genes. How the regulation of switching on and off during development is achieved is still a matter of speculation. Each gene is defined by characteristic sequences of DNA. In general, at any one genetic locus there will be a pair of genes, one of which was inherited from our mother and the other from our father. Most, but not all genes, are concerned with the production of proteins; others have regulatory functions. The outward manifestation of our genetic constitution comprises our phenotype.

Our chromosomal constitution can be visualized under a microscope, after appropriate preparation. Chromosomes can be seen in dividing cells, and blood cells are the usual source for cytogenetic investigations after they have been induced to divide by chemical treatment. T lymphocytes are stained and otherwise manipulated to make their nuclear material visible. The complement of chromosomes visualized in this way is known as our karyotype. Banding patterns, effectively dark and light stripes of differing widths, can be recognized by cytogeneticists and provide useful information about gross structure.

Mutations and polymorphisms

A germ-line mutation that occurs in the DNA of cells that produce gametes (sperm or eggs) is inherited by the cells of subsequent generations. Any change in a DNA sequence is a mutation. Most such changes are neutral, with no effect on the phenotype. This is because most of the human genome consists of material that is not transcribed by the machinery that reads the genetic code. Not all genes that are transcribed are subsequently translated into a protein product, and even within the coding regions a base change may only lead to the substitution of one synonymous codon for another. There is redundancy within the system and many synonyms in the genetic code, so the protein product may ultimately not be affected at all by nucleotide substitutions. These neutral mutations will, nevertheless, lead to DNA polymorphisms, which are alternative forms of DNA sequence within a population. Such polymorphisms (which may or may not affect the function of the gene, such as the speed of its translation) are important for tracking down genes in families or populations, but they are individually unlikely to have other than a subtle effect on the phenotype.

Mutations have sometimes been thought to imply alterations in gene product that are detectable by some phenotype change. Inevitably, the evidence for such change will depend on the sensitivity of the measures used to detect it. It should not be taken to imply disease as such. In complex disorders, the phenotype will be influenced by the interaction of a range of polymorphisms (each of which may be regarded as a 'mutation') on different chromosomes. Each of these may be insufficient to produce a disease phenotype in its own right, but generally they act in combination (either additively or synergistically) to increase susceptibility to disease. In other words, the genotype at any given locus may affect the probability of disease but yet not fully determine the outcome. Environmental factors also have a crucial part to play.

Mendelian inheritance

The term Mendelian inheritance is used to describe conditions directly caused by inherited single mutant genes. Homozygotes have two copies of the mutant allele, but heterozygotes only one. Recessive conditions are seen only in the homozygote. If the mutation in just one allele is associated with a phenotype, the condition is said to be dominant. In most syndromes that result from simple Mendelian mechanisms, phenotypic manifestations are variable. Genes often have multiple different (pleiotropic) effects. For example, children with untreated phenylketonuria have distinctive skin and hair colour as well as mental retardation (Simonoff *et al.* 1996), but this is a single-gene disorder. The 'classic' presentation of genetic syndromes may be rather more variable in the general population than is ascertained by the study of cases from a specialist referral centre. Diagnostic criteria for syndromes that are inherited in a simple Mendelian fashion are usually uncontentious. It is a straightforward matter to establish which clinical features are caused directly by the genetic disorder (such as mental retardation) and which are indirect (such as temper tantrums precipitated by frustration).

Chromosomal anomalies

Some behavioural phenotypes are not associated with abnormalities in a particular gene, but with numerical or structural abnormalities in a chromosome. These relatively gross genetic anomalies affect the expression of several or even many genes. Numerical abnormalities are associated with either the loss of one of a pair of chromosomes completely, or with the aberrant formation of more than one copy of a chromosome (as in trisomy 21, or 47,XXY). Structural anomalies are more subtle, and usually involve microdeletions of a few thousand nucleotide bases or, more rarely, the loss of a substantial part of a chromosome (such as the short arm of an X chromosome). Structural anomalies may sometimes be associated with the doubling or tripling of segments of a chromosome; lengthening it. They can also result from the aberrant translocation of a part of one chromosome onto another.

Such anomalies may occur during the formation of the sperm or egg; they may occur during formation of the zygote, when the egg and sperm fuse; or they can occur after cell division begins in early embryonic development. In the first situation, the abnormality is going to be represented in every somatic cell. If the structural problem occurred later, in just a proportion of developing cells, the individual will be a mosaic for the abnormality, with some cells showing it, and colleagues not. The distribution of the affected cells will be clonal (rather than random), reflecting the original population of normal or abnormal cells from which they were derived. If the affected cells are not capable of functioning to a certain minimal degree of efficiency, they could be selected against as the tissue develops over time, and would not then be represented. Somatic mosaicism for genetic anomalies may explain, to some degree, the phenotypic variability associated with a chromosomal anomaly such as Turner syndrome. For example, in about 5% of individuals with that phenotype there is both an abnormal set of cells with just 45 chromosomes (they lack a second X chromosome), and also an entirely normal set with a 46,XX constitution just like other females (Jacobs *et al.* 1997). The degree of phenotypic severity varies with the proportion of normal cells to abnormal cells.

Structural chromosomal anomalies

Structural abnormalities include deletions of part of the long or short arms, which may be terminal or within the arm (interstitial). Gene dosage is usually a delicate affair, and if it is interfered with in a major way (e.g. by monosomy or triploidy) a phenotype results.

Spontaneous breaks in chromosomal material can occur during the formation of the germ cells, or during recombination which occurs normally only during meiosis. The germ cells contain just 23 chromosomes, and if any of these are broken they can be repaired. However, sometimes if two breaks have occurred the joins may mismatch, resulting in a 'translocation' of material from one chromosome to another. If such breaks have damaged genetic material, phenotypes may result even though there is no net loss of genetic material. If there is a net gain or loss of genetic material, chromosomal structural abnormalities are known as 'unbalanced'. Other forms of break include loss of material from within the q or p arm (interstitial), or from the end of the arm (terminal). Material may be turned around within the arm (paracentric inversion), or between arms (pericentric). Rarely, there is a normal complement of chromosomes but one pair derives from maternal or paternal origin. Obviously, cells that contained all three copies will have been lost. Rather more frequently, a small area of one chromosome within the long or the short arm derives from maternal or paternal origins on both copies. This may not cause any problems provided the region does not contain an imprinted locus, containing a gene that is expressed systematically from either a maternal or a paternal allele.

Numerical chromosomal anomalies

Numerical chromosomal abnormalities include too few and too many chromosomes. Complete duplication or erasure of a chromosome is only possible with the sex chromosomes, and chromosome 21. So, for instance, there are duplications of the sex chromosomes (e.g. XXX, XYY, XXY), and there is monosomy (45,X, but never 45,Y).

Imprinted genes

A few genes are systematically different in their activity, depending on whether they have been inherited from the mother or from the father—genomic imprinting (Tilghman 1999). There is consequently monoallelic expression; that is to say, the gene is expressed from only one of the pair of alleles, but it is important to note this may only be detected in certain tissues, or at certain periods of development. There is no alteration in the underlying DNA sequence. The existence of imprinted genes in a region may be revealed when the only active copy is mutated or lost because of a structural abnormality of the chromosome containing it. Alternatively, that chromosome, or region of a chromosome, may show uniparental disomy, both copies of the gene in question (and part of the surrounding genome) having been inherited

from just one parent. In general, the clinical phenotypes that result from abnormalities involving imprinted loci tend to be severe.

It is important to bear in mind that the phenotypic manifestations of our genotype will depend in part on epigenetic phenomena, such as genomic imprinting, and in part on the interaction over time of our genotype with the environment. Epigenetic mechanisms are factors that can be transmitted to progeny cells following cell division, but which are not directly attributable to the DNA sequence of the genome (Strachan & Read 1999). They tend to be influences that alter the expression of genes, and by definition do not alter the underlying nucleotide sequence itself. Imprinting is a good example of an epigenetic mechanism (Petronis et al. 2000).

Trinucleotide expansion repeats and anticipation

Dominant conditions sometimes result in phenotypes that become more severe in successive generations—the phenomenon of anticipation (McInnis 1996). This is exemplified by the fragile X syndrome (Turner et al. 1997) and by Huntington disease (Huntington's Disease Collaborative Research Group 1993). Trinucleotide repeat expansions have been proposed as its biological basis (Margolis et al. 1999). Trinucleotide repeats are triplets of nucleotides, usually cytosine, guanine and arginine. These are designated CGG, CAG, and so on. The repeats may occur within genes, or they may be found in regions of DNA that lie between genes. If they lie actually within genes they may be in transcribed sequences (exons), or within DNA sequences that are excised by the RNA-making machinery (introns). Expansions occur in the course of DNA replication (Margolis et al. 1999) and the repeats grow in length as they are passed from one generation to the next.

For reasons that we do not understand, there are proportionately more neurological than other diseases caused by expansion of CTG, CGG, CAG or GAA repeats (Weatherall 1999). The conditions caused by the expansion are associated with considerable phenotypic heterogeneity because of variability in the length of the repeat sequences, and in the degree to which they disrupt transcription and function of the genes with which they are associated. Conditions associated with this phenomenon include fragile X syndrome (CGG repeats), Huntington chorea and other conditions associated with CAG repeat expansions such as dentatorubral pallidoluysian atrophy, and myotonic dystrophy (CTG repeats).

Genetically complex disorders

Many psychiatric problems in childhood or adulthood, and specific learning difficulties such as dyslexia, are likely to be genetically complex (see McGuffin & Rutter, Chapter 12). While a substantial heritability can be demonstrated by twin studies (Rutter et al. 1999) their genetic predisposition reflects the contribution of many different genes. One of the greatest challenges facing psychiatric genetics is to understand how such multigenic diseases result in behavioural or cognitive phenotypes.

Complex disorders, especially in psychiatry, have a number of characteristics in common. First, people with the phenotype may not have inherited any susceptibility alleles but manifest the disorder because of non-genetic causes (*phenocopies*). Secondly, the probability that someone who is carrying a susceptibility allele or alleles will actually develop the disorder will vary according to influences such as age, sex, environment and other genes. For example, boys are substantially more susceptible to autism or Tourette syndrome, but the former usually has its onset before 2 years of age, whereas the latter usually first manifests in middle childhood. We do not know why this is so. Schizophrenia, on the other hand, has its onset in later adolescence or adulthood. In all three diseases it is indisputable that some form of genetic susceptibility is inherited, but the relative roles of genes and environment in influencing phenotypic expression are unclear.

The greatest progress in understanding how a complex genetic predisposition results in a disease has been with type 1 diabetes. It serves as a paradigm for psychiatric geneticists, although it is a disease that is characterized by an unambiguous phenotype that is easily recognized. Unfortunately, the same cannot be said for most psychiatric disorders. A decade ago, Todd first showed that the development of this autoimmune condition was largely caused by an interaction between the environment and alleles at many different loci (Todd 1991; Mein *et al.* 1998). More recently Todd (1999) has demonstrated that susceptibility to the disorder is almost incredibly widespread in the general population, with up to 30% of us possessing susceptibility alleles. It is unlikely that predisposition to psychiatric disorders will be any less prevalent.

Genetic or locus heterogeneity

Many conventionally specified disorders that are highly heritable (ADHD is an example) could theoretically be caused by mutations in any one of a variety of genes, all of which result in apparently identical phenotypes. *Genetic heterogeneity* could come about because a range of specific genes is required for a common biochemical pathway or cellular structure. When trying to identify cases of psychiatric disorder to study genetically we would like them all to have the same genetic predisposition! Unfortunately, in practice, we have no way of knowing this, both because of genetic heterogeneity and also *allelic heterogeneity*. In the latter condition, different mutations (or polymorphisms) at the *same* locus produce the same, or a very similar, phenotype. Such allelic heterogeneity occurs archetypically in the inherited disorders of haemoglobin. Weatherall (1999) commented that the study of the genetic predisposition to autoimmune disease such as insulin-dependent diabetes type 1 is helping us understand complex mechanisms. However, when it comes to psychiatric disease 'we are dealing with a level of complexity that is infinitely greater than that which underlies the phenotypic diversity of the monogenic diseases. So, it may be a

very long time before we are in a position to use this information in clinical practice.'

Quantitative trait loci

Most commentators do not use the term 'behavioural phenotype' to indicate the consequences of variation in so-called quantitative trait loci (QTL). These are non-Mendelian characteristics, which reflect variation at a number of loci, and such variation may be very common in the general population. QTL can be thought of as influencing the quantity of a phenotype, and are likely to be important in the determination of complex traits such as intelligence. The haplotype at a locus may be influential in determining a QTL, rather than the variation of one or other allele. A haplotype is a set of alleles that are on the same small segment of the chromosome, and which tend to be transmitted down the generations as a block because they are so very close together. Very little is known about how QTL actually contribute to variation in psychological abilities or disabilities, although there has been some interesting work tracking down loci that apparently contribute to genetic susceptibility to dyslexia (Grigorenko *et al.* 1997; Fisher *et al.* 1999; Gayan *et al.* 1999).

Epistasis

Most contemporary data analysis and statistical modelling strategies for genome scanning investigations assess the significance of only the main effects of potential trait loci, meaning the average effect of a gene above those of all other genes with which it may or may not interact. Consequently, the influence of key genes on neurodevelopment may be missed, because their effect could only be detected within a framework that accommodates epistasis (Frankel & Schork 1996). *Epistasis* is relevant to gene mapping efforts for complex traits and is said to occur when the combined effect of two or more genes on a phenotype could not have been predicted as the sum of their separate effects. To date, there has been relatively little discussion of epistasis in the child psychiatric genetic literature, although its potential importance was pointed out by Rutter (Rutter 1994a). It seems likely that all the common child psychiatric disorders with reasonably high heritability, such as ADHD and autistic spectrum disorder, are caused by the additive or interactive effects of alleles at a small number of genes rather than to a single mutation at a major gene locus.

Using behavioural phenotypes to identify genes that influence cognition and behaviour

Biologically meaningful phenotypic markers

Genetic modelling might be facilitated if a discriminating biological trait was closely correlated with the liability to develop the disease. For example, schizophrenia researchers have become interested in defects in smooth pursuit eye movements, which may be found in the first-degree relatives of those with the disorder (Lencer *et al.* 1999). There may be a genetic link between eye-tracking problems or inhibition of the P50 auditory evoked response to repeated auditory stimuli and liability to develop schizophrenia (Adler *et al.* 1999). Although this notion has been explored in connection with adult psychiatry, it has not been used in child psychiatric genetic research to date. What we are seeing here, it seems, are the phenotypic effects of one aspect of the polygenic predisposition to a major mental illness. Whether there is any such specificity between susceptibility alleles and phenotypic features that fall short of the full phenotype in other highly heritable disorders, such as autism, is still open to question. One might anticipate that there would be (Skuse 2000b) but the evidence is against it at present (Pickles *et al.* 2000).

In both linkage and association studies (see McGuffin & Rutter, Chapter 12), the aim is to find a measure of dysfunction that is closely and causally linked to the genetic anomaly. Realistically, no cognitive or behavioural feature is likely to be unique to a single genetic disorder, nor is that feature likely to be found in all instances of the disorder. By what means, then, is the choice of marker made? The difficulty in using gross behavioural measures (e.g. hyperactivity, self-injury, impulsiveness, clumsiness) or personality characteristics (e.g. aloofness or a tendency to express anxiety) is that these features are found in association with many genetic disorders and have low specificity. Broad cognitive measures, such as IQ, are little better. Ideally, one wishes to find phenotypic markers that are unlikely to have been substantially modified by experience, and which are aetiologically linked to the genetic anomaly. The choice of a phenotype to designate someone who is presumably at high risk of possessing the genotype of interest requires the identification of phenotypic features that reliably discriminate those with the genotype from those without it. It is very difficult, even in family studies of individuals at known genetic risk—let alone in an association study of a population sample—to make this discrimination on the grounds of cognitive or behavioural characteristics.

Turner syndrome, with the classic 45,X karyotype, is associated with a gross genetic anomaly and, in most non-mosaic cases, with a striking phenotype. Affected individuals are known to have cognitive deficits including a relatively specific problem with visuospatial skills. Ross *et al.* (1997) used discriminant function analysis to find what set of neurocognitive tests could distinguish reliably between a sample of females with the condition and a comparison group who were matched for age, height, IQ and socioeconomic status. The best discrimination identified just 45% of the 45,X females as belonging to the case group, although only 3% of comparison females were so identified. Such heterogeneity in cases of genetic anomalies with cognitive or behavioural phenotypes is likely to be the rule rather than the exception. Few investigations of the sensitivity and specificity of the behavioural and neurocognitive profile of such disorders have been published. Why is the result of this study so

important? Because if we want to link the behavioural or cognitive features to a genetic anomaly we must know who in our patient sample possesses the genetic anomaly and who does not.

Contrast this picture with the study of a family reported by Vargha Khadem *et al.* (1998), known as the KE family. This family had previously generated considerable excitement when Gopnik (1990) claimed that they had a fundamental language disorder involving a mutation in a single gene that affected a component of Universal Grammar (in the Chomskyian sense) which was inherited in a simple autosomal dominant fashion, with full penetrance. The locus of the gene that is mutated in this family (*SPCH1*) has since been mapped to an interval in 7q31 (Fisher *et al.* 1999) and then identified and cloned. This precise mapping was possible because, fortunately for the investigators, members of the family with the mutation could be distinguished reliably from those who did not. It is rather unusual for a behavioural phenotype to characterize carriers of the mutation so precisely. Yet, failure to take account of variability in the genetically modified population can make interpretation of data for deletion mapping very difficult indeed.

Limitations of the behavioural phenotype approach

It is often very difficult to discover how the genotype of an individual with a naturally occurring genetic anomaly contributes to the behavioural manifestations of that condition. Conceptual flaws in study design and interpretation are widespread. The key point is related to Bayesian statistical theory. In other words, given the phenotype, what is the probability that this individual has the genotype of interest? Bayesian statistics is used in genetic counselling, where the risk of carrier status can be calculated given certain parameters and assumptions about the mode of inheritance of the condition of interest. It is quite a different matter, to take a condition that is not inherited in any simple Mendelian fashion, and to infer from some aspects of the phenotype that a particular genotype is present. We may be able to do this fairly successfully with the physical features of Down syndrome, for example, but we certainly could not infer trisomy 21 from the cognitive profile of Down syndrome alone. This is not only because there is variability within the Down syndrome population but, more importantly, because only a very small proportion of individuals with that degree of mental retardation will have trisomy 21.

Take Williams syndrome as an example. A few years ago Frangiskakis *et al.* (1996) claimed to have discovered that deletion of the *LIMK1* gene, in the Williams syndrome critical region of chromosome 7, led to visuospatial deficits in affected children. The implication was that *LIMK1* was involved in the development of areas of the brain that were important for visuospatial abilities. A series of children with Williams syndrome in whom the gene was deleted had such deficits, and colleagues with a partial phenotype and no visuospatial deficits did not have the gene deleted on the affected chromosome 7. The variability of the visuospatial phenotype within Williams syndrome was not known, and so the extent to which it correlated in general with the size of the microdeletion was not known. Furthermore, visuospatial deficits are found in a substantial minority of the general population, for reasons that probably have nothing to do with *LIMK1*. Accordingly, in some children the deficits could have been a chance finding, and the lack of deficit could have also been a chance finding for an equivalent reason. In other words, a drop in visuospatial IQ of 20 points in a child who was, in the absence of Williams syndrome, destined to have a verbal IQ of 100 and a non-verbal IQ of 120, would result in apparent absence of deficit. Failure to take account of these variables is probably why successes such as those claimed by Frangiskakis *et al.* (1996) have subsequently been countered by other data (Tassabehji *et al.* 1999).

Variation in behavioural phenotypic manifestations may be either relatively direct, resulting from the genetic anomaly itself, or indirect, arising for instance from the impact of the genetic anomaly upon the affected child's social immaturity. A condition that results in very small stature may be associated with a tendency for both adults and peers to treat the exceptionally short child according to the age they appear, rather then their chronological age (Gilmour & Skuse 1996), possibly evoking such immaturity in behaviour functioning.

Once an alleged behavioural phenotype has been described, subsequent studies have often failed to confirm the stereotypes proposed by the clinical observer who first described the behavioural, or cognitive dysmorphology of a condition with a known or suspected genetic aetiology. Take, for instance, Prader–Willi syndrome, which is characteristically associated with hyperphagia (Cassidy 1984). It is possible nowadays to make the diagnosis on the basis of molecular tests, rather than relying on the presence of the full clinical phenotype (Mann & Bartolomei 1999). Although many clinicians believe that hyperphagia is an invariable feature of the condition, that is not the case (Gilmour *et al.*, 2001), although the reasons for the variability have yet to be defined, and may not have a genetic origin.

One of the most common complicating features of any study of behavioural phenotypes is ascertainment bias. Cases of any condition with a distinctive behavioural characteristic are more likely to be detected if that characteristic is present. Thus, the key behavioural features are likely to be more common in an identified clinical population than in unidentified cases from the general population. Examples could be hyperphagia in Prader–Willi syndrome or autistic features in association with fragile X syndrome. On the other hand, if it can be demonstrated that the reason for ascertainment is never, or hardly ever, the cognitive or behavioural features, such bias would not apply. Many studies also fail to take account of the need to recruit comparison subjects: both to find out the degree to which the behavioural feature of interest is directly linked to the genetic anomaly rather than associated with some other non-specific factor, such as low IQ; and to control for the possibility that the behavioural feature is linked to some other specific characteristic of that syndrome, so confounding the relationship of interest.

In a study of behavioural phenotypes in children, the interpretation of cognitive or behavioural data is complicated by developmental considerations. A comprehensive account will include factors such as whether all features manifest at all ages, or whether various manifestations are developing in an invariable progression, and whether the progressive change in the cognitive and behavioural picture is itself genetically programmed (rather than depending on the influence of environmental contexts). Genes are switched on and off over time, according to both an internal clock as well as in response to environmental influences (Skuse 2000a). Their effects will depend on their pattern of expression during any given period of development. The natural history of genetically specified disorders with relatively circumscribed cognitive deficits (e.g. early stages of Huntington chorea; Lawrence *et al.* 1998) shows how dysfunction can develop in later life; it is by no means always present during infancy, or even childhood. In Huntington chorea there appears to be a deficit in inhibitory control mechanisms that are under the influence of striatofrontal circuits. Individuals with Huntington chorea also demonstrate a remarkably specific failure to recognize the facial expression of disgust (Gray *et al.* 1997). On the other hand, remarkable talents in certain cognitive skills may also be observed to develop over time in disorders with a strong genetic component, such as the enhancement of certain visuospatial skills in some boys with autism (Hermelin *et al.* 1999).

In summary, the concept of 'behavioural phenotypes' is fraught with difficulties, and falsely implies that there are characteristic patterns of behaviour that are specific to particular chromosomal anomalies. This assumption is hardly, if ever, justified. For instance, Hodapp (1997) reviewed the notion of 'total specificity' and quoted Flint & Yule (1994) as judging only the self-mutilation in Lesch–Nyhan syndrome, the hyperphagia of Prader–Willi syndrome, and the hand-wringing of Rett syndrome as being unique to that syndrome. There are no data on the uniqueness of the Lesch–Nyhan phenotype, but the Prader–Willi phenotype is certainly not unique (Skuse *et al.* 1997; Gilmour *et al.*, 2001), although the Rett phenotype might be (Mount *et al.*, 2001). To a limited extent, one may tell from genetic variation within a syndrome, as indexed by the degree of mosaicism for the aberrant cell line or the extent of a microdeletion, what degree of behavioural anomaly will arise in later life. However, precise prognostication is likely to be impossible for the great majority of conditions currently regarded as having 'behavioural phenotypes'. Nevertheless, the study of genotype–phenotype correlations should lead to the identification of genes that influence the development of cognitive brain systems. This will be greatly facilitated by the study of animal models. In some cases the cognitive brain systems will be important for the integrity of psychological domains that, if disrupted, lead to phenotypes resembling common conditions such as autism or ADHD. Accordingly, it should be possible, by a 'bottom-up' approach, to work out how those systems normally operate, so gaining insights that could lead to the development of new treatments.

In this section we review some of the most widely recognized and more common genetic disorders that are associated with cognitive or behavioural characteristics that could be considered to constitute a phenotype. In most instances the phenotype has been reasonably well characterized, and in some cases there has been considerable work published on these aspects of the syndrome. However, for a variety of reasons, not always connected with the rarity or otherwise of the condition, there is rather little information available. We review a selection of intensively researched and less well-investigated syndromes. A summary of the findings is shown in Tables 13.1–13.3. These also give the reference number for the putative genetic aetiology of the disorders, which can be accessed from the Online Mendelian Inheritance in Man website (HTTP://www3.ncbi.nlm.nih.gov/Omim).

Behavioural phenotypes associated with single gene mutations

Duchenne muscular dystrophy

This X-linked condition comprises a range of muscular dystrophies with associated degrees of handicap from mild to severe.

Genetic anomaly

Muscular dystrophies are X-linked myopathies that result from mutations on the dystrophin gene, lying on the short arm of the X chromosome at Xp21.2. This gene encodes a protein that is involved in cytoskeletal development. There are many possible mutations (usually deletions) of exons (transcribed segments) in the huge dystrophin gene, which is the largest gene yet discovered on the human genome.

Cognitive and behavioural phenotype

There is a mild to moderate degree of mental retardation in one-quarter to one-third of cases (Bresolin *et al.* 1994) and, rarely, there is familial segregation with schizophrenia in families (Zatz *et al.* 1993).

Genotype–phenotype relationships

The dystrophin gene is expressed in the brain, but deletions that remove the brain-specific promoter are compatible with normal intelligence (Bushby *et al.* 1995). Recently, Bardoni *et al.* (1999) found evidence that deletions in the Dp140 regulatory sequences are specifically linked to cognitive impairments. This finding is compatible with previous work (Moizard *et al.* 1998) and therefore may be reliable.

Kallman syndrome

Kallman syndrome is a sex-linked condition in which affected males have anosmia because of agenesis of the olfactory lobes, and hypogonadism which is secondary to a deficiency of

Table 13.1 Syndromes with behavioural phenotypes.

	Single gene mutations				Microdeletion and duplication syndromes				Sex chromosome aneuploides	
	Duchenne muscular dystrophy	Tuberous sclerosis	Fragile X female carriers (full mutation)	Neurofibromatosis type 1	Williams syndrome	Prader–Willi syndrome	Smith–Magenis syndrome	Velocardio-facial syndrome	Turner syndrome	Klinefelter syndrome (47,XXY)
Sex ratio Chromosome	M only Xp21.2	M=F 50% 9q34; 50% 16p13.3	F only Xq27.3	M=F 17q11.2	M=F 7q11.23	M=F 15q11–q13	?M=F 17p11.2	M=F 22q11	F only X	M only X
Genes implicated in the phenotype (up to three) (OMIM number)	DMD (310200)	TSC1 (191100); TSC2 (191092)	FMR-1 (309550)	NF1 (162200)	ELN (130160); LIMK1 (601329); ?RFC2 (600404)	SNRPN (182279); NDN (602117)	RNU3 (180710)	?COMT (116790); ?TMVCF (602101); ?CLTD (601273)	SHOX/ PHOG (312865); ?CGF1 (300082)	?
Mouse behavioural phenotype described	+			+	−	+		+	+	
Deficits in gross or fine motor skills	+	+	+	+	+	+		+	+	+

Table 13.2 Cognitive characteristics.

	Single gene mutations			Microdeletion and duplication syndromes					Sex chromosome aneuploides	
	Duchenne muscular dystrophy	Tuberous sclerosis	Fragile X female carriers (full mutation)	Neuro-fibromatosis type 1	Williams syndrome	Prader–Willi syndrome	Smith–Magenis syndrome	Velocardio-facial syndrome	Turner syndrome	Klinefelter syndrome (47,XXY)
General learning difficulties	+ 25–30%	+ 50–60%	+ up to one third	+ 30–45%	+ 55% severe, 40% moderate, 5% borderline to low average	+ mostly borderline to moderate	+ mild to severe; majority moderate	+ 90%+	− (VIQ normal, PIQ slightly below average)	− (VIQ slightly below average, PIQ average)
Verbal–non-verbal skills discrepancy	NV>V	?	−	V>NV	V>NV	NV>V	?	V>NV	V>NV	NV>V
Deficits in speech production	+	+	?	+	−	+	+	+	−	+
Impairment in verbal fluency	+	?	−	?	−	+	?	?+	−	+
Reading/writing difficulties	+	+	−	+	+	+	?	+	−	+
Visuospatial deficits	+	?	+	+	+	+	?	+	+	−
Numeracy deficits	+	+	+	+	+	+	?	+	+	+

Abbreviations: PIQ, performance IQ; VIQ, verbal IQ; ?, some evidence for phenotype, but inconclusive; blank, no evidence for phenotype.

Table 13.3 Behavioural and emotional problems.

	Single gene mutations				Microdeletion and duplication syndromes				Sex chromosome aneuploides	
	Duchenne muscular dystrophy	Tuberous sclerosis	Fragile X female carriers (full mutation)	Neuro fibromatosis type 1	Williams syndrome	Prader–Willi syndrome	Smith–Magenis syndrome	Velocardio facial syndrome	Turner syndrome	Klinefelter syndrome (47,XXY)
Behaviour problems										
impulsivity	NA									
overactivity	NA	+		+	+	–	+	+		
self injury							+			
obsessive-compulsive behaviours					+	+	+			
social interaction problems	+	+	+	+	+	+		+	+	+
Emotional problems										
anxiety	+	?+	+	+	+	+			+	
depression	+	?+	+	+		+		+		
Autistic features	+	+							+	
Schizotypal features	+							+	–	

hypothalamic gonadotrophin-releasing hormone (GnRH). Hardelin *et al.* (1992) described additional phenotypic features including renal agenesis, and mirror movements of the hands, as well as pes cavus, a high-arched palate and cerebellar ataxia.

Genetic anomaly

The *KAL1* gene is located just proximal to the pseudoautosomal region at the tip of the short arm of the X chromosome. It escapes inactivation on the X chromosome in the female, although it is a pseudogene, and non-functional, on the Y chromosome in the male. Mutations in or loss of the single-expressed *KAL1* gene in males results in the phenotype of Kallman syndrome. There are also rare autosomal dominant and recessive forms of the disorder (*KAL2* and *KAL3*).

Cognitive and behavioural phenotype

Kallman syndrome has behavioural correlates. In about 85% of cases there are mirror movements, which comprise involuntary, non-suppressible movements of the contralateral upper limb. They are provoked by voluntary movement that is intended to be unilateral, and are maximal in distal hand and finger muscles (Krams *et al.* 1999). Interestingly, they are seen only among Kallman patients with the X-linked form of the disorder. Recent evidence has attributed these movements to abnormal development of the ipsilateral corticospinal tract (Krams *et al.* 1999).

The fact that affected individuals have both impaired development of the olfactory system and delayed sexual maturation links the two aspects of our everyday functioning to the same genetic system, in which the Kallman gene plays a part (Rugarli 1999). There is, as yet, no mouse model of the disorder. Affected individuals may have mental retardation, but this is usually mild. They have a range of odd social behaviours, some of which may be attributable directly to the loss of the Kallman gene, others to the loss of contiguous genes in cases where there has been a microdeletion, and yet others to the endocrinological abnormalities found in association with the syndrome.

Genotype–phenotype relationships

Is the Kallman gene dosage sensitive? Female carriers of the Kallman mutation have one functioning copy of the gene (as do normal males) yet are reported to have partial or complete anosmia, a key phenotypic feature of the condition. On the face of it, this finding is hard to explain; it suggests that although males can manage perfectly well with one copy of the gene, females need to have two functioning copies. Quinton *et al.* (1996) described a range of mutations at the *KAL* locus, but these did not correspond in any obvious way to phenotypic variability.

Tuberous sclerosis

Tuberous sclerosis is heterogeneous in both genetic and phenotypic terms (Harrison & Bolton 1997). The condition is charac-terized by lesions in many parts of the body, including the brain. Indeed, the name of the syndrome refers to the potato-like growths seen in the brains of affected individuals which develop in early fetal life and appear to be static (Gomez 1995). The syndrome's phenotypic heterogeneity is probably caused in part by the seemingly random distribution of the areas of abnormal cell proliferation (Flint 1996). Epilepsy is common, affecting 60–80% of cases (Webb *et al.* 1996). The prevalence of tuberous sclerosis is estimated to be about 1 in 10 000 (Osborne *et al.* 1991).

Genetic anomaly

The condition is inherited in an autosomal dominant fashion. Approximately 60% of cases are caused by a spontaneous mutation, in one of two genes. These include the *TSC1* gene on chromosome 9q34, which encodes a protein known as hamartin. The *TSC2* gene lies on chromosome 16p13.3 and codes for tuberin. It is now known that there is an interaction of these two proteins at every stage of the cell cycle, and both seem to play a part in attenuating cell proliferation (Cheadle *et al.* 2000).

Cognitive and behavioural phenotype

About 50–60% of people with tuberous sclerosis have mental retardation, although precise estimates are hard to obtain because of lack of standardized IQ assessments (Harrison & Bolton 1997). There is some suggestion that mental retardation may be more common among affected males than females (Clarke *et al.* 1996). The number of tubers and the type and age of onset of epilepsy seem to be associated with the risk for mental retardation. Little is known about the exact nature of specific cognitive deficits in tuberous sclerosis, but problems such as dyspraxia, dyscalculia and visuomotor disturbance have been observed in affected individuals without general cognitive impairment (Jambaque *et al.* 1991). Harrison *et al.* (1999) conducted a detailed neuropsychological assessment of seven individuals with tuberous sclerosis and nine matched controls. Although all the patients had IQ scores in the normal range, five of them showed significant specific cognitive impairments. The individuals with tuberous sclerosis were particularly likely to perform poorly on a spatial planning task and a task involving cognitive shift, whereas none of them showed impairment on tests of semantic or phonological fluency or on tests of spatial span capacity.

Epidemiological studies indicate an association between tuberous sclerosis and pervasive developmental disorders. Compared to the general population, the risk of autism and atypical autism is 200–1000 times greater in individuals with tuberous sclerosis. Conversely, the risk of tuberous sclerosis is 100–300 times higher in individuals with autism (Wing & Gould 1979; Osborne *et al.* 1991; Hunt & Shepherd 1993; Gillberg *et al.* 1994; Smalley 1998). A neuroimaging study of a clinic sample of individuals with tuberous sclerosis obtained evidence of an association between localized, structural abnormalities in the brain and the development of pervasive developmental disorders (Bolton & Griffiths 1997). The association between tuberous sclerosis and pervasive developmental disorders was related to the presence of tubers in the temporal lobes.

Fragile X syndrome

Fragile X syndrome is often quoted as being the single most common form of inherited mental handicap after Down syndrome, but it is probably far less common than was once thought. In the general population its prevalence is between 1.5 and 2.5 per 10 000 males (DeVries *et al.* 1997; Turner *et al.* 1997). In a large population of children at schools for those with learning difficulties, the prevalence could be as high as 1.3% (DeVries *et al.* 1997), with no difference in prevalence between those with mild and those with moderate to severe mental retardation.

Genetic anomaly

The mutation underlying the disease is a CGG triplet repeat expansion occurring within an untranslated portion of the *FMR1* gene. The clinical severity of the disorder, which is far greater in males than females, is substantially more marked if there are more than 200 CGG repeats, for this is associated with transcriptional silencing of the gene. Expansions in the number of CGG repeats occur exclusively during female transmission of FRAX A.

Cognitive and behavioural phenotype

Females with fragile X syndrome have a more variable clinical picture than affected males. They are said to show similar difficulties in social interaction, including shyness, gaze avoidance and poor modulation of interpersonal communication (Lachiewicz & Dawson 1994; Sobesky *et al.* 1996). They may also be more prone to sadness, and even depression (Thompson *et al.* 1994), and have poor attention skills (Franke *et al.* 1999).

Both males and females can have a degree of cognitive and behavioural abnormality that is related to the degree to which the trinucleotide CGG repeat is methylated, and hence the amount of fragile X protein that is produced (Tassone *et al.* 1999). If no FMR1 protein is produced there will be moderate to severe mental disability; this situation is found virtually exclusively in males, for females have two copies of the *FMR1* gene, and even if one is mutated the other can compensate to a degree in certain circumstances. If the male is a mosaic, or if his full mutation is only partially methylated, the IQ deficit will be less marked. The phenotype in females depends on the inactivation pattern of the X chromosome. If the normal X is the active one, in any particular clone of cells, the functions of those cells will be relatively unimpaired and the corresponding phenotypic feature will not be found (Wolff *et al.* 2000). The full mutation (fM) is associated with deficits in short-term visual memory, visuospatial skills,

visuomotor co-ordination, the processing of sequential information, and in executive function skills. Attention deficits and hyperactivity are found in most cases of both referred and non-referred subjects (Baumgardner *et al.* 1995). It has been suggested that many such problems with activity and sensory stimuli may relate to anomalies in the posterior cerebellar vermis and caudate nucleus (Reiss *et al.* 1995). However, the neuropsychological deficits are associated with rather non-specific brain changes on magnetic resonance imaging (MRI), especially within the temporal cortex and hippocampus. However, there is no simple relationship between neuropsychological test performance, CGG triplet repeat lengths and structural brain abnormalities (Merenstein *et al.* 1996).

The notion current some years ago that fragile X syndrome is commonly associated with autism has not been supported by more recent rigorous analyses (Dykens & Volkmar 1997). The consensus seems to be that a minority of fragile X males do have classical autism (from 15 to 25%; McCabe *et al.* 1999) but the majority show behavioural characteristics that could be regarded as 'autistic-like' in character. These include gaze avoidance, shyness, social anxiety and withdrawal. Some of them could be regarded as having an autistic spectrum disorder, or the broader autistic phenotype (LeCouteur *et al.* 1996). A proportion is found to have stereotypies, impulsivity and be oversensitive to certain perceptual experiences. In contrast to males with classical autism, they are able to recognize facial expressions and emotions in others (Turk & Cornish 1998).

Genotype–phenotype relationships

Flint (1999) commented that the mutation in the *FMR1* gene was detected 10 years ago (Verkerk *et al.* 1991) and was the first of the trinucleotide repeat expansions to be discovered and yet we still do not know its physiological function. He argued that research has told us nothing about how the mutation results in mental retardation. We do know that the protein is associated with ribosomes, and it is believed to bind to specific RNAs and to regulate their expression so as to ensure that neurones develop correctly (Inoue *et al.* 2000). We also have a mouse model of fragile X, and these mice have certain of the features of the human condition including macro-orchidism and impaired spatial learning abilities. However, the degree of learning impairment in the mouse has not been as marked as is found in humans. The reason appears to be related to the strain of mouse used in the investigation (Dobkin *et al.* 2000). Despite this range of knowledge, we still know nothing specific about what the gene actually does.

Mental retardation associated with thalassaemia

Inherited disorders of haemoglobin are the most common monogenic disorders worldwide and amongst the most intensively studied. Weatherall & Clegg (1999) estimated that 6–7% of the global population are carriers. They serve as a paradigm of our state of knowledge about the relationship of molecular pathology and the associated clinical phenotype (Weatherall 1999). The major phenotypic differences can be attributed to the actions of mutational variability at a single locus (Higgs 1993), and the interactions of this locus with two other major modifying loci. Yet, the complexity of the genetic mechanisms involved is far greater than was initially anticipated (Weatherall 1999).

Genetic anomaly

There are two syndromes in which mental retardation is associated with α thalassaemia, which occur in European rather than tropical populations (Wilkie *et al.* 1990a,b). One is associated with structural rearrangements of the short arm of chromosome 16, including microdeletions, and constitutes an aspect of a contiguous gene syndrome in which variable numbers of genes are deleted, each of which may have rather specific functions (Weatherall 1999). The other disorder is X-linked, and is known as ATR-X syndrome. It is associated with a mild form of α thalassaemia, a characteristic facial appearance, profound developmental delay, neonatal hypotonia and genital abnormalities. The mutated gene is *ATR-X*. This syndrome is of particular interest because the effects of the single gene mutation are pleiotropic and it was one of the first disorders in which mutations of a putative transcriptional regulator have been described (Gibbons *et al.* 1995). *ATR-X* is widely expressed in the brain, heart and in skeletal muscles, and is very likely to have a key role in the regulation of other genes. Mutations of transcription factors are likely to result in complex phenotypes, and potentially such mutations may account for a small proportion of behavioural phenotypes (Skuse 2000a).

Rett syndrome

Rett syndrome is a progressive neurodevelopmental disorder of females, which occurs in no more than 1 per 10000–15000 live female births (Hagberg *et al.* 1993). It is devastating in its consequences upon normal development.

Genetic anomaly

Interest in the genetic aetiology of the syndrome was heightened recently when two families possessing more than one affected member were studied. As the condition is manifest only in females, the X chromosome is the likely location of the susceptibility locus, probably the long arm (Willard & Hendrich 1999). Males with a mutation in the gene usually cannot survive beyond birth. The variability in the female phenotype suggests the gene is likely to be subject to X inactivation, and thus is like fragile X syndrome in this respect. The female expression pattern will depend on whether the X chromosome carrying the abnormal gene is active in critical tissues, especially the brain, and some reports have suggested skewing of X inactivation does occur in females with the syndrome or their mothers (Kirchgessner *et al.* 1995; Sirianni *et al.* 1998). Amir *et al.* (1999) reported

that there are mutations in a gene known as *MECP2* in a proportion of Rett females, a gene that is involved in transcriptional regulation of other genes, which appears to have very widespread influence. Genes that are targets of MeCP2 protein in the brain need to be identified. An important lesson from this research is that although the key mutation may be in *MECP2*, it is the failure of this regulatory gene to act normally on other genes that causes the symptoms of Rett syndrome (Willard & Hendrich 1999). We already know from studies of females with ring X chromosomes, in which functional disomy of X-linked genes may occur (Dennis *et al.*, 2000), that impaired dosage regulation of such genes can result in a severe cognitive and behavioural phenotype (Kuntsi *et al.*, 2000).

Behavioural phenotype

Although affected girls appear to be quite normal for the first few months after birth, there is a failure to gain new skills during early infancy and subsequent deterioration between the ages of 1 and 4 years. There is progressive loss of speech, purposeful hand use, microcephaly and epilepsy (Hagberg *et al.* 1993). Following this period of loss of skills, various behavioural and cognitive features become evident which, taken together, are quite characteristic of the clinical features of the syndrome (Mount *et al.*, 2001). They include breathing difficulties and involuntary movements, especially 'hand-wringing' or washing movements, and a jerky truncal ataxia. Interest has been heightened by the fact that a number of affected girls display autistic-like behaviours, and some commentators think it could be regarded as a subtype of autism (Gillberg 1994; Rutter 1994b). Given the degree of mental retardation associated with the condition, and the fact that autistic features are rather more common among moderate to severely mentally retarded individuals (Bailey *et al.* 1995), a comparison between Rett syndrome and mentally retarded comparisons was clearly needed. Mazzocco *et al.* (1998) conducted such a study, and concluded that the autistic features of Rett syndrome are not simply a consequence of severe mental retardation.

Genotype–phenotype relationships

It is too early to know if the Rett mutation that has been identified will be associated with a phenotype that differs to any significant extent from the majority of cases that do not share this mutation. We may learn more from the study of an animal homologue of the disorder. Mice in which the mecp2 gene has been knocked out have been produced (Chen *et al.* 2001). Such mice have a behavioural phenotype but unlike humans they are only viable if they contain only a small proportion of cells with the mecp2 mutation. As the severity of the human phenotype varies according to whether the X chromosome containing the Rett gene is inactivated or not, the chimeric mouse model could be a parallel to the presumed human mosaicism for the mutation, based upon the pattern of X inactivation.

Behavioural phenotypes associated with chromosomal deletions and duplications

Spontaneously occurring chromosomal aberrations can provide a useful pointer to the existence and location of genes that are important in the development of normal cognition and behaviour, although to date the study of such anomalies has been mainly in the study of cancers (Strachan & Read 1999). Abnormalities of chromosomes that can be observed under the microscope are known as cytogenetic abnormalities. Several important discoveries were made simply because rare cytogenetic abnormalities in a few patients led to the 'disease' gene. These included dystrophin (MIM 310200), retinoblastoma (MIM 180200) and neurofibromatosis 1 (MIM 162200). Central to this approach is the need to identify a candidate gene, and discovering the correct candidate can be very time consuming.

Even microdeletions can disrupt a large number of genes, any one of which could be the candidate of interest. Once the Human Genome Project is completed the task should be rather easier because it will be possible to use unique markers (short sequences of DNA) to define the boundaries of the deleted or reduplicated segment. It should then be a straightforward matter to look up which genes are known to be expressed in the candidate region. If we are interested in genes that are expressed in the brain, there are ways of discovering whether our candidate is expressed in fetal brain. However, merely finding that a gene is expressed in the brain at some time during fetal development does not actually tell us as much as might at first appear, for up to 70% of all genes in the human genome are probably expressed in fetal brain at some time (Andrew Copp, personal communication).

Chromosome abnormalities can occur in all the cells of the body if they originated in the germ-line, or during formation of the zygote. Alternatively, they may come about as a consequence of some acquired insult, such as exposure to a carcinogen. Structural abnormalities do not always result in disruption to genetic function; they may be benign.

Microdeletion and duplication syndromes

Williams syndrome

Williams syndrome is a rare sporadic disorder with an incidence estimated to be about 1 in 20 000 live births (Perez Jurado et al. 1996). The condition is associated with a relatively distinctive cognitive profile. Affected individuals have both a superficial facility with language and with facial recognition, but they possess poor visuospatial skills (Bellugi et al. 1999).

Genetic anomaly

In over 90% of cases, there is a submicroscopic deletion of one copy of chromosome 7. The region of chromosome 7 most commonly deleted contains the following genes, the list of which is not exhaustive:

1 homologue of the drosophila gene frizzled (fzd3);
2 the syntaxin 1 A gene (STX1A);
3 the elastin gene (ELN), which accounts for some aspects of the physical phenotype, especially the associated cardiac anomaly supravalvular aortic stenosis (SVAS);
4 the LIM-kinase gene (LIMK1);
5 WSCR1;
6 RCF2; and
7 GTF21 (Bellugi et al. 1999).

In total at least 20 genes may be deleted, including a number of highly repetitive DNA sequences. The deletion arises because occasionally recombination occurs between misaligned repeat sequences either side of the critical region (Baumer et al. 1998) during gamete formation. The replication factor C2 (RFC2) and syntaxin 1 A (STX1A) genes have also been mapped to the Williams syndrome critical region. The extent of the deletion is variable, but the classic Williams syndrome phenotype is associated with deletion of ELN, and usually LIMK1 too. Although it was reported that haploinsufficiency for LIMK1, which is widely expressed in the brain, was likely to be responsible for the non-verbal cognitive deficits (Frangiskakis et al. 1996), subsequent research has suggested this is unlikely. Patients with hemizygosity for this gene may not have any detectable cognitive deficits. Furthermore, it appears that LIMK1, STX1A and RFC2 are not dosage sensitive.

Cognitive and behavioural phenotype

The overall IQ of patients with Williams syndrome is low, on average about 60, but this disguises a discrepancy between verbal and non-verbal abilities. Non-verbal abilities are much more seriously impaired (Udwin et al. 1987). One of the most difficult tasks for affected individuals is pattern construction, such as the block design subtest of the Wechsler scales (Wechsler 1986, 1992). Verbal fluency is similar in quantitative terms to normal age-matched individuals, although it is qualitatively abnormal (Bellugi et al. 1999). In contrast to children with fragile X syndrome, those with Williams syndrome do not have social deficits of an autistic character. Indeed, it is often said that their social interactions are relatively unimpaired in character. They are described as outgoing, with good eye contact, and they may be friendly and have good empathic skills (Gosch & Pankau 1997; Dykens & Rosner 1999). However, it would be a mistake to assume their social interactions are normal. Rather, the abnormality is of a different character to that found in conditions where the impairment to social skills is autistic-like. Children with Williams syndrome are often strikingly disinhibited and relate indiscriminately to unfamiliar children and adults, which may put them at social risk (Davies et al. 1997; Dykens & Rosner 1999). The social disinhibition found in association with this syndrome, as occurs in many cases of ADHD of unknown origin, is correlated with poor performance on standard tests of attention. There is also overactivity, impulsivity and anxiety.

Several research groups have examined the Williams syndrome cognitive phenotype (Howlin *et al.* 1998; Jarrold *et al.* 1998; Bellugi *et al.* 1999). Their current view is that the discrepancy between relatively preserved verbal skills and poor non-verbal abilities, previously reported as being common in the condition, has been exaggerated. Nevertheless, there continues to be considerable interest in their odd use of language (Karmiloff-Smith *et al.* 1997; Sacks 1995). Paterson *et al.* (1999) reassessed the claim that the uneven cognitive profile of children with Williams syndrome provides evidence for an innate inherited faculty for understanding and using grammatical constructions (Pinker 1994). In its simplest form, the theory of modularity, based upon a superficial study of the Williams syndrome cognitive and behavioural phenotype, predicts that innately specified modules are impaired at birth as a consequence of the genetic disorder. Only those modules of ability that are linked to the genetic anomaly will be impaired, others will be spared. Paterson *et al.* (1999) showed that some language skills are poor among toddlers with Williams syndrome, whereas some numerosity skills are relatively good. Yet in adulthood the opposite pattern of discrepancies is observed. Hence, they concluded, neither numerosity nor language skills can be innately specified modules, or the same pattern of impairment would have been present since infancy. Some would argue the evidence for a radical shift in the cognitive phenotype of Williams syndrome during development is not as strong as was claimed (Bishop 1999). Others might feel it is naïve to imagine that genetically specified cognitive modules would be laid down at birth and would be unchanging over time, in any event.

Some earlier reports suggested a selective preservation of face recognition abilities in Williams syndrome (Bellugi *et al.* 1988; Udwin & Yule 1991), despite the visuospatial deficits. On closer inspection it appears that face processing in individuals with Williams syndrome is in fact atypical. Karmiloff-Smith (1997) obtained preliminary evidence suggesting that individuals with Williams syndrome perform well only on those face processing tasks that require feature-by-feature componential analysis. More recently, Deruelle *et al.* (1999) compared configural and local processing of faces in children with Williams syndrome to that of both age- and mental age-matched controls. Inverted faces are in general harder to recognize than faces presented upright, which is taken as a sign of configural processing. The control children showed the normal inversion effect for faces (and not for houses), but no such effect was observed in the Williams syndrome group. On a matching-to-sample task the control children showed a bias toward a configural mode of face and geometrical shape processing, whereas the children with Williams syndrome did not show any bias. These results not only suggest an impairment in configural processing of faces in Williams syndrome, but also indicate that this impairment may generalize to other visual objects too. Other studies using visuospatial tasks similarly indicate difficulties in performing part integration tasks in Williams syndrome (Bihrle *et al.* 1989; Bertrand *et al.* 1997).

Brain development of Williams syndrome subjects has been investigated, both *in vivo* with the aid of MRI scans and at postmortem. So far, there have not been any published attempts to link variations in genotype with variations in brain phenotype, although that is clearly an interesting and potentially valuable line of enquiry. The cognitive profile is but a crude measure of changes that occurred in brain development because of haploinsufficiency for the gene(s) responsible. It is certainly possible that rather more extensive abnormalities will be found in the brains of Williams syndrome individuals with partial deletions than would be suspected from their cognitive abilities. Neuroanatomical studies have contrasted Williams syndrome subjects with normal and with Down syndrome controls (Bellugi *et al.* 1999). There seems to be relative preservation of the anterior cortical areas, and enlargement of neocerebellar areas, together with preservation of the mesial temporal lobe. Galaburda *et al.* (1994) studied Williams syndrome brains at autopsy and reported microencephaly and relatively small volumes of occipital and posterior parietal areas of several brains.

Finally, anxiety may be a common feature of the syndrome, although the reasons for this are not clear. Dykens & Rosner (1999) reported 'anticipatory anxiety' in over 50% of a sample of both children and adults. They also showed that up to 95% had persistent or marked fears that lasted up to 6 months or more. Others had phobic symptoms too. In a minority of cases these fears could be connected to the hyperacusis that is characteristic of the syndrome.

Gene–phenotype relationships

Frangiskakis *et al.* (1996) claimed, in a sophisticated piece of research, that hemizygosity for a specific gene was responsible for the impairment in visuospatial constructive cognition in Williams syndrome. They identified two families with 13 members who had a partial Williams syndrome phenotype, associated with one of two differing deletions of limited extent that incorporated both the *ELN* and the *LIMK1* genes. These individuals did not suffer from the general cognitive impairment usually associated with the syndrome; instead, they had a marked deficiency only in visuospatial constructional abilities. On the basis that targeted disruption of protein kinases in mice results in impaired spatial learning (Ashkenas 1996), the investigators hypothesized that *LIMK1*, which is widely expressed in human cerebral cortex, was of particular significance for this aspect of the phenotype. Individuals from the families with the partial phenotypes who had the typical cognitive profile were found to have a microdeletion that incorporated this gene, as did 62 individuals with classic Williams syndrome. In a further sample who had only the cardiac anomaly (SVAS), which is thought to be associated with deletion of the elastin gene, there was no such abnormal profile. *ELN* is not expressed in the brain.

Whereas the findings were undoubtedly appealing, and were claimed to herald the discovery of the first human gene to be associated with a specific cognitive ability, subsequent studies have failed to support this conclusion. Tassabehji *et al.* (1999) pointed out that for most genes a 50% decrease in gene dosage has no phenotypic effect, which is obvious when we consider the large number of recessive characteristics we harbour in our genome. Secondly, they suggest mouse knockouts are of limited relevance to human cognitive function. Certainly, the spatial deficits seen in mice with protein kinase knockouts are of quite a different character to the visuoconstructional problems found in individuals with Williams syndrome. Finally, Tassabehji *et al.* (1999) drew attention to the confounding issue of genetic background when interpreting phenotypes in limited samples of (wild-type) individuals. They reported an intensive investigation of three individuals who, despite deletion of one copy of the *LIMK1* gene, did not have the impairment in pattern-construction that would have been predicted from the Frangiskakis *et al.* (1996) report. Why would this anomalous result be found? Tassabehji *et al.* (1999) claimed that ascertainment of Williams syndrome is not influenced by the associated cognitive impairment, and that almost every individual with the physical phenotype has the typical cognitive profile. Biased ascertainment remains, however, an important consideration to be firmly excluded. The jury is out on whether the gene responsible for the fascinating cognitive profile of the condition has yet to be discovered. However, it would be conceptually muddled to claim that because the disorder is associated with impaired visuospatial abilities, the critical gene is responsible for the specific development of such skills. Visuospatial deficits are found in association with a variety of microdeletion syndromes (Skuse 1999), although not with Down syndrome which is a favourite comparison group in Williams syndrome investigations.

Prader–Willi syndrome

Prader–Willi syndrome is a distinctive disorder, associated with a genetic anomaly on the long arm of chromosome 15, in which hyperphagia, mild to moderate mental retardation and obesity combine with a typical developmental history. In the great majority of cases there is no inherited predisposition, but a sporadic event during meiosis leads to the failure to express the paternal copy of some as yet unidentified critical gene, or set of genes. There is debate about the true incidence of the condition. Donaldson *et al.* (1994) suggested that former estimates of 1 in 10 000 births were too high, because of overdiagnosis of Prader–Willi syndrome. Unless a molecular investigation is confirmatory, caution should be exercised in making the diagnosis (Chu *et al.* 1994). Using molecular techniques in combination with the clinical diagnostic criteria developed by Holm *et al.* (1992), a more accurate prevalence rate may now emerge.

Genetic anomaly

This disorder is associated with structural rearrangements of the long arm of chromosome 15. The anomalies include deletions, translocations, inversions and supernumerary marker chromosomes, as well as uniparental disomy. Such anomalies can be found not only among patients with Prader–Willi syndrome but also those with the much rarer condition, Angelman syndrome.

Deletion or disruption of the Prader–Willi/Angelman critical region (PWACR) within the 15q11-q13 region may result in either Prader–Willi or Angelman syndrome, when the affected homologue is paternal and maternally inherited, respectively. This parent-of-origin effect has been explained as a consequence of oppositely imprinted genes within this region (Feil & Kelsey 1997). Occasionally, there is inheritance of a cytogenetically detectable interstitial duplication of proximal 15q. Those that do not contain the PWACR are not associated with any specific phenotype, and are equally likely to be maternally or paternally inherited. Duplications that are maternal in origin, and include the PWACR, are associated with developmental delay and speech difficulties in all probands (Browne *et al.* 1997).

Submicroscopic duplications of this region could also exist, and they may account for some cases of developmental delay and/or learning difficulties, despite an apparently normal karyotype. A report by Bundey *et al.* (1994) demonstrated that the presence of a *de novo* duplication of part of the long arm of the chromosome 15 of maternal origin was associated with autism and severe mental retardation. Other reports of autism in association with duplications of this region have recently been made (Cook *et al.* 1997), as well as with a microdeletion in 15q11-12 (Schroer *et al.* 1998). In all cases reported to date, the abnormality has been maternally derived, whether it was a duplication or deletion of the region. Interestingly, the results of linkage studies are also consistent with involvement of the long arm of chromosome 15 in the predisposition to childhood autism (Maddox *et al.* 1999).

Prader–Willi syndrome is probably not the result of a deficit in a single gene, as there have been seven genes (and candidate genes) identified in the Prader–Willi syndrome region, all of which appear to be brain-specific (Nicholls *et al.* 1998; Nicholls 1999). The function of these genes is unknown, but one that has been identified, *IPW*, does not even code for a protein and is therefore similar to two other imprinted non-translated RNAs, H19 and Xist. Potentially then, the phenotype arises from deficits in all these genes, but it is not known how the genetic defect causes intellectual impairment. Mice that have chromosomal deletions in the equivalent region to the PWACR, or uniparental disomy for the region, or imprinting mutations, have a severe phenotype leading to early postnatal death (Gabriel *et al.* 1999; Tsai *et al.* 1999).

Behavioural phenotype

Dysmorphic features include a disproportionately narrow forehead, almond-shaped eyes, downturned mouth and abnormally shaped ears (Cassidy 1992; Holm *et al.* 1993). There is hypogonadism in 90–100% (Butler 1990; Cassidy 1992). Small hands and feet are found in 70% of typical cases and hypopigmentation in 40% (Holm *et al.* 1992). A squint occurs in 60–70% and scoliosis in 40–60% (Cassidy 1992).

Ninety-seven per cent of Prader–Willi syndrome affected individuals have an IQ below 70 (Butler 1990), with an average IQ of about 60, in the moderate retardation range (Dykens *et al.*

1992). Cognitive strengths and weaknesses may be uneven. For example, visual processing skills could be relatively strong (Curfs *et al.* 1991; Holm *et al.* 1992; Taylor 1992), although that finding is not consistent (Gabel *et al.* 1986). There may be deficits in attention, perceptual–motor integration and motor control too—all of which exacerbate the Prader–Willi syndrome group's poorer performance on IQ testing. Dykens *et al.* (1992) suggested sequential processing was relatively weak whereas attainment and achievement were relatively strong. Although just under half of children with Prader–Willi syndrome attend a mainstream elementary school, by secondary school age the proportion in mainstream education may drop. Whether this shift is because of a developmental decline in IQ is uncertain. Dykens *et al.* (1992) reported that in contrast to Down syndrome, there was no evidence of IQ decline in Prader–Willi syndrome on the basis of both cross-sectional and longitudinal data. Dykens & Cassidy (1995) found no relationship between IQ and maladaptive behaviour.

Poor muscle tone (hypotonia) is evident in almost 100% of infants with Prader–Willi syndrome. Between 90 and 100% have feeding problems and failure to thrive (Butler 1990; Cassidy 1992). The feeding problems appear to be caused by hypotonia, with poor sucking and gagging reflexes (Holm *et al.* 1992). Tube feeding is often necessary (Ehara *et al.* 1993) until 10–18 months, after which weight gain increases dramatically. Motor milestones are delayed to approximately twice the equivalent age of normal children (Butler 1990; Cassidy 1992).

The most distinctive feature of Prader–Willi syndrome is hyperphagia; 80–90% of children become hyperphagic, which often results in obesity (Cassidy 1992), although this outcome is not inevitable, but depends in part on parental management style (Holland *et al.* 1995). Its onset occurs at an average age of 2 years (Butler 1990), and in most cases before the child is 6 years old (Holm *et al.* 1993; Holland *et al.* 1995). A number of studies have attempted to identify the physiological basis of this appetite disorder, and to find ways of controlling it with medication. These have not, on the whole, been very successful (Zipf & Berntson 1987; Dech & Budow 1991; Tu *et al.* 1992; Benjamin & Buot-Smith 1993). The reason why people affected with Prader–Willi syndrome seem to experience hunger to a greater degree than the general population remains unclear. Taylor & Caldwell (1985) reported that sweet foods are often preferred and would be chosen over larger amounts of less preferred food. High-preference foods have been used successfully as positive reinforcement, to encourage activity in one sample of adults with Prader–Willi syndrome (Caldwell *et al.* 1986). Taylor (1992) cautioned that hyperphagia is not invariable in Prader–Willi syndrome and that the eating behaviour demonstrated by individuals with Prader–Willi syndrome might be similar to any other individual who is living in an environment of continuous food restriction. Obesity is usually found in association with hyperphagia and there seems to be a characteristic body fat distribution, with weight often distributed around the trunk (Cassidy 1992). Obesity can become so severe that there may be physical (and life-threatening) complications, in addi-

tion to a poor quality of life (Holland *et al.* 1995). Maintaining a reasonably low body mass index (BMI) is the key to successful management of Prader–Willi syndrome.

Other behavioural phenotypic features include skin picking, observed in up to 85% of cases (Greenswag 1987; Clarke *et al.* 1989; Cassidy 1992), temper tantrums (Cassidy 1992; Butler 1990), belligerence and stubbornness (Greenswag 1987), aggression (Taylor 1992) and poor judgement relative to measured IQ level (Sulzbacher *et al.* 1981). However, just how specific these behaviours are to Prader–Willi syndrome, rather than to moderate mental retardation, is hard to assess. Many studies lack an appropriate comparison group and have other methodological limitations. Butler (1990) suggested that some behavioural difficulties, such as temper tantrums, may begin as a consequence of the food restriction imposed upon the individual. Whitman & Greenswag (1992) noted that individuals with lower BMIs, subjected to greater restrictions on eating behaviour, were more likely to have behavioural problems. Other studies have reported no relationship between BMI and behavioural disturbance in adults (Clarke *et al.* 1989).

Children and adults with Prader–Willi syndrome are commonly described as hypoactive and lethargic. Their lack of activity may be exacerbated by co-ordination problems, resulting from hypotonia. Problems with obesity following excessive eating will be increased by inactivity (Nardella *et al.* 1983). Davies *et al.* (1992) used doubly labelled water isotopes in a study of free living children in their home environment. Children with Prader–Willi syndrome showed a significantly lower total energy expenditure than non-obese comparisons.

Sleep architecture studies have indicated that there may be a neurological basis to the reports of disruptive sleeping patterns in Prader–Willi syndrome. Helbing-Zwanenburg *et al.* (1993), using objective measures, note that 95% of their sample of Prader–Willi syndrome affected children and adults had excessive daytime sleepiness, as compared with 10% in the adult normal comparison group. During night sleep, the Prader–Willi syndrome group showed a significantly lower proportion of rapid eye movement (REM) and slow-wave sleep than the comparisons, but there was no evidence of the sleep apnoea syndrome in any Prader–Willi syndrome cases tested. Excessive daytime sleepiness is also commonly reported (Clarke *et al.* 1989) which may be exacerbated by sleep interruption during the night.

Speech difficulties occur in around 80–90% of cases (Cassidy 1992). Kleppe *et al.* (1990) found articulation problems, difficulties in terms of expressive and receptive language, including difficulties with syntax. The battery of tests in this study was extensive, with most instruments having standardized norms for the general population, but an IQ-matched control group may have been more informative in order to identify Prader–Willi syndrome-specific speech problems.

Short stature is usual. Children with Prader–Willi syndrome are usually on the 10th centile for height or below, in contrast to non-affected obese children who are usually tall for their chronological age (Donaldson *et al.* 1994). Butler (1990) noted the lack of growth spurt in adolescence results in Prader–Willi syndrome affected adults being proportionately smaller than Prader–Willi syndrome affected children. However, short stature is not invariable. There is debate whether Prader–Willi syndrome is associated with growth hormone deficiency or whether the short stature is caused by growth hormone dysregulation. Angulo et al. (1992) examined the 24-h growth hormone profile in obese and non-obese children aged 1–15 years who had Prader–Willi syndrome. They reported abnormally low levels in all the children regardless of BMI. Blichfeldt et al. (1992) found 66% with growth hormone levels below the 25th centile of the levels reported in the general population. Other studies have cast doubt on the growth hormone insufficiency theory (Ritzen et al. 1992). Other endocrine disturbances may also be associated with the condition (Muller 1997).

Genotype–phenotype relationships

Interest has been expressed in whether the form of Prader–Willi syndrome caused by uniparental disomy differs in any aspect of the cognitive or behavioural phenotype from that caused by a microdeletion of the paternally derived chromosome 15 (Cassidy et al. 1997). There do seem to be some significant differences, but they are not large. In general, those with a deletion have a lower verbal IQ (Roof et al. 2000) and there may be rather less skin-picking behaviour and fewer articulation problems among those with uniparental disomy (Cassidy et al. 1997). Genotype–phenotype correlations have also been investigated in the mouse model for the disorder, in which a variety of mutations and deletions of the PWACR have been induced. Certain of these deletions can lead to a paternally inherited pattern of severe growth retardation and hypotonia, with partial lethality (Tsai et al. 1999). Nicholls (1999) commented that in the equivalent mouse chromosome 7C region, there is a novel gene (SNURF-SNRPN) that encodes two independent proteins, and these may play a part in the phenotype. He suggested that co-localization of SNURF and SNRPN within the imprinting control region could be a critical factor, and says evolutionary arguments would suggest that this genetic locus is a prime candidate for mutations producing the failure-to-thrive phenotype of neonates with this syndrome and of corresponding mouse models.

Angelman syndrome

Angelman syndrome is phenotypically quite unlike that of Prader–Willi syndrome, despite the fact that it is also caused by anomalies in the PWACR. The mental retardation is very severe, and most individuals do not develop spoken language. There is also ataxia, seizures, hyperactivity and paroxysms of laughter. The term by which the condition used to be known ('the happy puppet syndrome') is not regarded as appropriate nowadays. The prevalence of the disorder is much the same as that of Prader–Willi syndrome, about 1 in 15 000 live births (Clayton-Smith & Pembrey 1992).

Genetic anomaly

The genetic disorder is variable (Mann & Bartolomei 1999), and comprises deletions of the PWACR, uniparental disomy for the paternally derived chromosome 15, intragenic mutations and also imprinting mutations (Nicholls et al. 1998). In stark contrast to Prader–Willi syndrome, for which no single intragenic mutation has been discovered, about 20% of cases of Angelman syndrome are associated with presumed mutations as no other abnormality in the PWACR can be discovered. Mutations in a ubiquitin protein ligase gene (ube3a) have been found in a few rare families with Angelman syndrome (Kishino et al. 1997), and it has been proposed that the ube3a gene is maternally expressed. Even if we learn that mutations in this gene are the cause of Angelman syndrome they are unlikely to tell us much about the origin of the cognitive phenotype. The gene product is part of a widely used ubiquitin-mediated protein degradation pathway, and the deletion almost certainly will have pleiotropic effects that will be 'hard if not impossible to disentangle'. Flint commented (1999): 'An immense amount of work has gone into the characterization of the small deleted region in Prader–Willi syndrome/Angelman syndrome. The basic deficit is not simply a dosage effect. However, the molecular deficit seems to be the same in both instances, but it looks increasingly unlikely that the genes act directly or specifically on the CNS.'

Genotype–phenotype relationships

It has been possible to generate a mouse model of Angelman syndrome, with disruption of the ube3a gene (Jiang et al. 1998). The deficits displayed by these mice include a context-dependent learning deficit, motor dysfunction and inducible seizures. The central part of mouse chromosome 7 is homologous to human 15q11-q13, with conservation of both gene order and imprinted features. Gabriel et al. (1999) conducted a transgene insertion into mouse chromosome 7C, which has resulted in mouse models for both Prader–Willi syndrome and Angelman syndrome dependent on the sex of the transmitting parent.

Smith–Magenis syndrome

Smith–Magenis syndrome is caused by an interstitial deletion involving 17p11.2. It is associated with some degree of mental retardation, measured IQs being in the range 40–54 (Greenberg et al. 1996) and cognitive and behavioural profiles have recently been described (Dykens et al. 1997).

Genetic anomaly

It is one of the most frequently observed human microdeletion syndromes, and seems to be caused by homologous recombination of a low-copy-number repeat region (a repeated gene cluster) flanking the junction of the deletion (Chen et al. 1997).

Cognitive and behavioural phenotype

Over half of those with the syndrome are likely to have disobedient behaviour, to be hyperactive, to be attention-seeking, with sleep disorder and toileting abnormalities including enuresis (diurnal and nocturnal) and soiling (Dykens & Smith 1998). Impulsivity, irritability and temper tantrums may also occur (Clarke & Boer 1998). Self-injurious behaviours include biting, head banging and also inserting objects into bodily orifices and pulling out finger- or toenails (Dykens & Smith 1998; Smith *et al.* 1998b). There are motor stereotypies, including inserting hands or other objects into the mouth, grinding teeth, and other repetitive behaviours, such as flipping pages of books (Dykens *et al.* 1996; Dykens & Smith 1998).

Profound sleep disturbances include reduced or absent REM sleep (Smith *et al.* 1998a,b) and Dykens & Smith (1998) claim this is a strong predictor of behaviour problems. It is not known whether it is the lack of REM sleep that leads to the associated behavioural problems, but Dykens & Smith (1998) claim that increased length of daytime napping is associated with fewer maladaptive behaviours.

Velocardiofacial syndrome

There is psychiatric interest in the velocardiofacial syndrome (VCFS) (Shprintzen *et al.* 1981) which is characterized by cardiac defects, cleft palate, learning disabilities and a characteristic facial appearance, together with a genetic anomaly on chromosome 22 at q11. The incidence is estimated to be between 1 in 3000 and 5000 live births (Papolos *et al.* 1996). Most cases are sporadic but, when inherited, it has an autosomal dominant pattern of transmission. There is an increased risk of severe behavioural problems in children with the condition, and of major psychiatric illness in adulthood including mood disorders and psychosis (Papolos *et al.* 1996). Up to 30% of adults with VCFS will develop a major psychiatric illness, with the majority fulfilling diagnostic criteria for schizophrenia (Murphy *et al.* 1999). The risk of mental health problems increases with age (Goldberg *et al.* 1993; Papolos *et al.* 1996; Carlson *et al.* 1997a). ADHD and bipolar affective disorder are the most common diagnoses in childhood, although there has yet to be published a thorough investigation of the psychiatric phenotypes at that stage of development. Much of the current literature focuses on the physical manifestations of the condition, which comprises a range of related disorders including DiGeorge syndrome (OMIM 188400). The cognitive and behavioural phenotypes of individuals with VCFS, and children in particular, have been poorly described and are largely based on clinical observation rather than systematic assessment.

Genetic anomaly

About four out of five patients with VCFS have a deletion of the VCFS critical region, with a proximal breakpoint that is similar in most cases. The distal breakpoint is variable (Morrow *et al.*

1995; Scambler 2000). The size of the deletion is usually about 3 million base pairs, so there is clearly loss of a large number of genes from the deleted chromosome. It has been proposed that a number of genes in the deleted segment are needed in two functioning copies for normal development to occur. If only one copy is present, on the intact chromosome 22, there will be insufficient gene dosage (known technically as haploinsufficiency; Fisher & Scambler 1994).

Cognitive and behavioural phenotype

The condition is associated with learning difficulties that are apparent from childhood (Goldberg *et al.* 1993; Motzkin *et al.* 1993), although up to half have an IQ within the normal range (above 70) (Swillen *et al.* 1999). There is no clinically or statistically significant verbal vs. performance IQ discrepancy (Golding-Kushner *et al.* 1985; Swillen *et al.* 1999). Some reports suggest general cognitive ability falls over time, from preschool, through middle childhood to adolescence (Golding-Kushner *et al.* 1985). Deterioration amounts to about one standard deviation on average, and is similar in verbal and non-verbal abilities. Gross and fine motor problems are frequently noted (Goldberg *et al.* 1993; Lynch *et al.* 1995) and perceptual problems may be relatively severe, although the evidence is presently lacking (Golding-Kushner *et al.* 1985; Swillen *et al.* 1999).

Children with VCFS have speech and language problems for a number of reasons. There are physical problems, secondary to the cleft palate abnormalities, with forming speech sounds and these are characteristically hypernasal (Shprintzen *et al.* 1978). Speech development is often delayed and impoverished in content (Kok & Solman 1995; Lynch *et al.* 1995; Swillen *et al.* 1999). Qualitative descriptions of poor expressive language skills include immature grammar and syntax and low utterance length (Golding-Kushner *et al.* 1985). Poor language comprehension may also occur, and language skills tend to be worse in general than would be predicted from verbal IQ measures alone (Moss *et al.* 1999). Affected children may have poor concept formation and do not develop past the concrete operations phase in problem-solving (Golding-Kushner *et al.* 1985; Motzkin *et al.* 1993; Kok & Solman 1995; Swillen *et al.* 1999). Sight-reading ability may be markedly superior to reading comprehension skills.

A relatively low level of arithmetical ability and mathematical reasoning is also suggested from anecdotal reports (Golding-Kushner *et al.* 1985; Motzkin *et al.* 1993; Kok & Solman 1995). Poor performance on this type of task requires abstract problem-solving skills and so supports the clinical observation of poor concept formation. Remedial help for mathematics is required in a high proportion of cases. However, no analysis has been made as to whether these abilities are simply commensurate with each child's general ability level.

Many children with VCFS are described as socially immature (Goldberg *et al.* 1993), with poor social skills, impulsivity or shyness (Golding-Kushner *et al.* 1985). Anecdotal reports from parents include descriptions of rigid behaviour, difficulty with changes in routine, obsessional traits and lack of emotional responsiveness. There are no systematic studies of these children's social cognition skills. It is not known to what extent the physical features of VCFS underlie the social difficulties. For example, it is important to partial out the effects on social difficulties of poor language development and articulation from primary social cognition problems. Parents report that affected children avoid using conventional instrumental gestures, such as waving goodbye. They have unresponsive facial expressions (Swillen *et al.* 1999).

None of the studies that describe the VCFS neuropsychological profile includes a comparison group with similar levels of cognitive abilities, so any conclusions drawn must be made cautiously. The most consistently reported deficits include: arithmetic and maths; poor reading comprehension in relation to decoding skills; and possible expressive and receptive language problems. Motor and perceptual problems, visual spatial deficits, abstract reasoning and attention problems are also suspected to be characteristic of the syndrome, although they may simply be aspects of generalized learning difficulties. None of the studies has controlled for IQ in analyses exploring group deficits. However, psychiatric problems are common in childhood. For instance, Carlson *et al.* (1997b) found 4 of 6 children under 10 years had ADHD, 13 of 20 older subjects had symptoms of bipolar affective disorder (10 bipolar II and 3 bipolar I), and 4 of 6 in those over 20 years had psychotic symptoms. Only 2 of 26 had no psychiatric phenotype. These findings are astonishing, even allowing for a degree of ascertainment bias.

Genotype–phenotype correlations

No correlation seems to exist between the size of the 22q11 deletion and aspects of the phenotype, including psychiatric symptoms. There have even been cases of monozygotic twins with seemingly identical deletions and different phenotypes (Vincent *et al.* 1999). This indicates that other factors act in concert with the genetic anomaly to give rise to the clinical picture. Occasionally (~5%), patients with a VCFS phenotype have no FISH-detectable deletion. In such cases there may be a point mutation in a critical gene in the 22q11 region, or at another genetic locus altogether, indicating that the same developmental processes can be disrupted by multiple genetic or non-genetic means. One or several of the 50 genes within the typically deleted region may be implicated in the syndrome. Haploinsufficiency of Tbx1, a transcription factor, has been shown accurately to mimic the cardiac phenotype in mice (Lindsay *et al.* 2001a). Whether the same gene is responsible for the cognitive and behavioural features of VCFS has yet to be determined. interestingly, it has been shown that all mice with a heterozygous deletion that includes Tbx1 show abnormal aortic arch development early in embryogenesis, but only 32% of embryos still show abnormalities at birth (Lindsay & Baldini 2001b). This indicates that some form of compensatory mechanism can ameliorate early developmental disruption to a mesenchymal structure. Whether this is also true of the neurectoderm that eventually becomes the central nervous system is not known.

Lesch–Nyhan syndrome

This devastating disorder, a recessive X-linked genetic anomaly that affects purine synthesis, was first reported over 30 years ago (Lesch & Nyhan 1964). Although the phenotype is usually caused by simple Mendelian inheritance of the recessive alleles, occasionally spontaneous mutations occur (Davidson *et al.* 1991). It is rare, occurring in no more than 1 in 10 000 live male births. Patients with the syndrome present with hyperuricaemia, choreoathetosis, dystonia and aggressive or self-injurious behaviour. The root cause of the disorder is the virtual absence of the enzyme hypoxanthine-guanine phosphoribosyltransferase (HPRT), which plays a crucial part in a pathway of purine synthesis. The effect of the disruption to purine metabolism is a serious deficit in dopaminergic functions in the brain (Ernst *et al.* 1996). The diagnosis is made by assaying fibroblast HPRT activity.

Genetic anomaly

The condition is caused by a mutation in the *HPRT* gene, which is found at Xq26-Xq27.2. Mutations may occur more frequently among males than females. Davidson *et al.* (1991) summarized the variety of known mutations, and found very many that can result in the Lesch–Nyhan syndrome. There is evidence that insertions and deletions, as well as point mutations can also be responsible for the phenotype (Renwick *et al.* 1995). There have been attempts to produce a mouse model of the disease, by means of inducing HPRT deficiency, and some success in evoking self-injurious behaviour (Wu & Melton 1993).

Cognitive and behavioural phenotype

At birth, children with the disorder (who are almost exclusively male, because of its sex-linked character) appear normal. There may be no evidence of motor or other developmental delay until the second or even the third year of life, when there is regression and often the onset of choreoathetotic movements. Affected infants are initially hypotonic; subsequently they become hypertonic and hyper-reflexic (Matthews *et al.* 1995). In middle childhood, the characteristic self-injurious behaviour is first manifested, and by the second decade nearly all children will display a range of neurological abnormalities including spasticity, choreoathetosis, opisthotonos, and facial dystonia together with pseudobulbar palsy. There has been some debate about the degree to which these clinical features are associated with mental retardation. Scherzer & Ilson (1969) took the view that intelligence was often in the normal range, and that specific impairment in expressive language could give a false impression, for receptive language skills were within the normal range; this view has been supported by more recent work (Anderson *et al.* 1992). On the other hand, Christie *et al.* (1982) found a significant range of problems on standardized IQ testing, in a moderately large sample of 19 individuals. Matthews *et al.* (1995) made a careful study of seven patients aged between 10 and 22 years. They found, on a wide range of tests carried out over several sessions, that intellectual levels varied from moderate global delay to low-average intelligence. Attention span was generally poor, as was working memory in a variety of domains. The authors suggested that although visual and verbal abilities are acquired during the first decade or so of life, there appears to be a ceiling on further development. The same team conducted a follow-up study 4 years later on the sample (Matthews *et al.* 1999), using standardized tests of verbal reasoning, abstract and verbal reasoning ability, quantitative and short-term memory skills. They confirmed their initial hypothesis that abilities did improve up until a mental age equivalent of about 13 years, but no further. This was reflected in a decline in age-standardized scores for the raw scores tended to remain constant over time. A relative strength was found in verbal reasoning ability and in vocabulary.

The self-injurious behaviour that is seen in this disorder presents a major challenge for management. Characteristically, the onset is in the preschool period, at 3 or 4 years of age. The child starts by biting lips and fingers, but in time the range of self-injurious behaviour increases and it is usually necessary to employ splints or other restraints for at least half of the time. Many children ask to be restrained. Strangely, punishment is ineffective and may even make the behaviour worse (Anderson *et al.* 1992). Anderson & Ernst (1994) reviewed the range of self-injurious behaviour found in a large sample of individuals with the syndrome. They found that there was no correlation between the degree of self-injury and age, but that it was severe and persistent in the great majority (at least 90%) of individuals with the confirmed diagnosis. Although biting of lips was one of the most common forms of self-injury it was not the only common form, and non-biting activities such as back arching and head snapping were equally prevalent. Finger biting was likely to be the first such behaviour to be observed in childhood. The majority did not show any cyclical variability in severity. Medical management may be most effectively provided with anticonvulsants, although there has not been any systematic evaluation of such treatments. Control of the excessively high purine levels by the prescription of allopurinol does not appear to have any beneficial effect on behavioural abnormalities (Christie *et al.* 1982).

Olson & Houlihan (2000) concluded that the most effective therapeutic interventions included differential reinforcement of (and especially incompatible) behaviours. The most common intervention is restraint which, interestingly, does not necessarily have to be unduly restrictive (e.g. light gloves may be as effective as splints). There is evidence that these steps can be successful, but the generalizability of techniques that are effective for single cases is open to question.

Genotype–phenotype correlations

Dopaminergic dysfunction lies at the heart of the disorder, as indicated by a variety of studies that have examined neurotransmitters and metabolites in brain tissues, blood and cerebrospinal fluid (Ernst *et al.* 1996). A mouse model for the condition has been produced (Jinnah *et al.* 1994), which shows dopamine deficiency too. Ernst *et al.* (1996) concluded that the HPRT deficiency results in the loss of dopa decarboxylase activity, and reduced dopamine storage in dopaminergic brain regions. There was a neuropathological process that affected both dopaminergic nerve terminals and cell bodies, and probably involved mesocortical, mesolimbic and nigrostriatal dopaminergic pathways. As these pathways are believed to play a part in the regulation of cognitive, emotional and motor functions the authors suggested that their dysfunction could account for the wide range of abnormalities associated with the syndrome. They hypothesized that the profound decrease in dopamine is contributory to both the cause and the mediation of the aggression shown by many such patients towards self and colleagues. However, this cannot be the only explanation and they went on to speculate that it is the maldevelopment of certain neural pathways, beginning early in infancy, which are necessary for the full clinical picture to appear.

Cri du chat syndrome (5p syndrome)

Cri du chat syndrome is a microdeletion syndrome, with the loss of chromosomal material on the short arm of chromosome 5 at 5p15 (the name 5p syndrome is now preferred). The incidence has been estimated to be no more than 1 in 50 000 live births (Niebuhr 1978). The syndrome is associated with mental and developmental retardation from birth. There are several characteristic aspects of the physical phenotype, including slow physical growth, microcephaly, hypertelorism, epicanthic folds, a high-arched palate, and microretrognathia. The hallmark of the disorder is the infant's cry, which is high-pitched and has a mewing character that is quite distinctive once heard. The full phenotypic picture seems always to be associated with the deletion of at least 1–2 Mb at the 5p15 location, and it is assumed this is a classic contiguous gene syndrome. The location of the gene whose deletion leads to the cat-like cry may be distal to the other loci that account for the physical phenotype (Church *et al.* 1995). Most cases are caused by *de novo* deletions (which may be terminal or interstitial), with 80% paternal in origin (Church *et al.* 1995), or to structural rearrangements involving unbalanced translocations. The cognitive phenotype is very variable, even among those with an apparently identical deletion, and families have been reported with multiple affected generations in whom the anomaly was detected by chance (Kushnik *et al.* 1984).

Genetic anomaly

A molecular analysis of 17 cases of 5p deletions has been made by Church *et al.* (1995) in order to identify correlations of genotype with phenotype. Because the aim of the study was to link variability in the 5p phenotype to the location and extent of the genetic anomaly, virtually all the subjects studied had partial syndromes. A number of reasons were suggested for the phenotypic heterogeneity associated with the syndrome. These potential reasons apply to a range of conditions that are associated with aneuploidy. There was the possibility that allelic variability of the normal chromosome affected the phenotype—and this was most strikingly evident from familial cases where the deletion was presumably identical in every instance. For example, recessive mutations on the equivalent part of the normal chromosome would be expressed phenotypically in regions that are hemizygous, and recombination would influence the characteristics of those regions. In order to discover just which genes contribute to the phenotype of this syndrome, it will be necessary to clone the genes lying within the critical region. These candidates could then be studied for their temporal and spatial expression; we would expect those that are associated with the cognitive and behavioural features of the disorder to be expressed early in development in the brain, for instance.

Cognitive and behavioural phenotype

The characteristic picture of profound retardation with minimal verbal abilities and severely delayed psychomotor development may partially reflect ascertainment bias (Cornish & Pigram 1996). One of the most careful evaluations of the cognitive abilities of children with 5p syndrome was conducted by Cornish et al. (1999). A group of 26 children between 6 and 15 years was studied, using standardized measures. Most were found to have both verbal and performance IQs below 50, and none was greater than 65. Both receptive and expressive language skills were retarded, the latter much more severely. Age-equivalent scores for expressive language among those who reached a baseline level ranged from 4 to 6 years, but receptive language was rarely better than a 2 year age equivalent. Articulation problems were severe, and limited the usefulness of the spoken language even among those who possessed it. In general, the results of this investigation mirrored those of previous studies (Dykens & Clarke 1997). Clearly, children with this condition should be encouraged to communicate by nonverbal means, and up to 50% are able to do so to a limited extent. Not surprisingly, the syndrome is associated with high levels of intrafamilial stress, and such stress is worse when children show high levels of maladaptive behaviours (Hodapp et al. 1997). Dykens & Clarke (1997) examined the correlates of such behaviour in a study of 146 individuals aged from 2 to 40 years. They found that the most frequent problems included excessive distractibility, restlessness and overactivity, intrusiveness, impulsivity and demanding behaviours. Many were aggressive and disobedient or unco-operative with instructions. Treatment with stimulants for hyperactivity and inattention sometimes resulted in an exacerbation of undesirable symptoms, including stereotypical behaviours and aggression to self and colleagues.

Both the physical and the cognitive/behavioural phenotype change quite markedly over time in this condition. The facial appearance changes from a round shape with hypertelorism to a longer slender face with normalization of the inner canthal distance (Niebuhr 1978). With advancing age, the hyper-

telorism becomes less marked, and the mandibular hypoplasia becomes less evident, although the microcephaly is more striking than before and the mandible becomes more prominent (Van Buggenhout et al. 2000). The outcome in early adulthood is also associated with spasticity in a minority, and with gait problems. Few adults with the condition are able to communicate verbally other than by means of very simple expressions, and it may be that frustration consequent upon the difficulty of making their needs known underlies the outbursts of aggressive and destructive behaviour that are observed from time to time.

Genotype–phenotype correlations

Dykens & Clarke (1997) found that those whose syndrome was caused by a translocation were less severely affected than those in whom it was caused by a microdeletion. In particular they were less likely to be socially withdrawn, although they were equally hyperactive, impulsive and irritable. Church et al. (1995) attempted to map the various phenotypic features of the syndrome to the location of the deleted segment of 5p15, and found the following. Speech delay was associated with distal deletions (down to the telomere) of 5p15.3. On the other hand, deletions in the more proximal band at 5p15.2 were associated with a cat-like cry, and the facial dysmorphology was probably associated with an even more proximal deletion within this same band. There have been attempts to map candidate genes within the critical region (Simmons et al. 1997). Simmons et al. (1998) suggested the human semaphorin F gene could play a part in the aetiology of the syndrome, for it seems to be involved with neuronal migration. Certainly, there is evidence for structural brain abnormalities in 5p syndrome (Kjaer & Niebuhr 1999), so this is a reasonable hypothesis. Nevertheless, we are still some way from identifying the number and identity of the genetic loci contributing to the complex range of phenotypes encountered in this rare but tragic condition.

Chromosomal aneuploides

Down syndrome

The publication in 2000 of the DNA sequence of human chromosome 21 (Hattori et al. 2000) represents an enormous scientific leap in knowledge, from the original discovery in 1959, that an extra copy of chromosome 21 causes Down syndrome (Lejeune et al. 1959). The chromosome 21 gene catalogue reflects the realization of a longtime goal for many Down syndrome researchers (Reeves 2000). It also suggests that the total number of human genes may have been overestimated: in comparison to the previous estimates of between 70 000 and 140 000 genes (Fields et al. 1994), the chromosome 21 consortium accurately predicted approximately 40 000 genes (Hattori et al. 2000).

Down syndrome is the most common identifiable cause of learning disability, which is typically moderate to severe. The estimated second trimester prevalence is currently approximately 1 in 500 (Egan *et al.* 2000), the risk increasing with maternal age. Physical features are well recognized: they include a shortening of all parts of the body; with a wide and flat face containing a small nose; abnormally shaped ears which may be low-set; and irregular teeth. The little finger is incurved, and the feet often display a wide gap between the first and second toes. Muscle tone is usually poor, and hypotonia is common. There are characteristic dermatoglyphic patterns, including the well-known single palmar crease. Down syndrome is associated with congenital heart disease, and an increased risk of specific leukaemias, immunological deficiencies and other health-related problems. Males have poorly developed genitalia, and they are invariably sterile; in females, ovarian structures are abnormal and menstruation is irregular (Mange & Mange 1990).

Genetic anomaly

The majority of individuals with Down syndrome have trisomy 21, resulting from chromosomal non-disjunction. In a small minority (1–5%) of cases the disorder results from a translocation of a portion of chromosome 21 to other chromosomes. The translocation may be inherited, whereas the most common Down syndrome genotype is non-familial. Mosaicism, with one trisomic and one normal cell line, is seen in approximately 1–2% of cases, and may be associated with a milder phenotype.

Chromosome 21 is the smallest human autosome, representing around 1–1.5% of the human genome. The sequencing of the chromosome provided evidence for 225 genetic loci: 127 known genes, 98 predicted genes and 59 pseudogenes (Hattori *et al.* 2000). The small number of untranslated genes may explain why Down syndrome is one of the only viable human autosomal trisomies (Hattori *et al.* 2000). Studies on transgenic mice suggest that dosage imbalance of only a proportion of the genes on chromosome 21 contribute to the Down syndrome phenotype (Kola & Hertzog 1997).

Cognitive and behavioural phenotype

The most notable aspect of the cognitive phenotype in Down syndrome is the marked mental retardation, with IQs typically in the 30–70 range (averaging around 50; Chapman 1999). Relatively poor expressive language and impaired verbal short-term memory are predominant aspects of the cognitive phenotype (Chapman & Hesketh 2000).

Tests of verbal short-term memory, such as digit or word span, consistently indicate impaired performance in individuals with Down syndrome, relative to mental-age-matched controls (Jarrold *et al.* 2000). In contrast, visuospatial short-term memory is relatively spared (Jarrold & Baddeley 1997; Jarrold *et al.* 1998). These findings have often been interpreted as indicating a specific deficit to the phonological loop component of Baddeley & Hitch's (1974) model of working memory in which the phonological loop component represents the system for processing verbal material, which is considered separate from the

system for processing visuospatial material (the visuospatial sketchpad). The phonological loop is fractionated into a limited capacity store and an articulatory loop. In Down syndrome, a deficit to the articulatory loop—absent or inefficient subvocal rehearsal—does not seem to explain the poor verbal short-term memory (Jarrold *et al.* 2000). This leaves a reduced capacity phonological store as a possible explanation for the poor verbal short-term memory in Down syndrome, though encoding difficulties have not been ruled out (Jarrold *et al.* 2000). As the phonological loop has a role in language development, particularly in vocabulary acquisition (Baddeley *et al.* 1998), there might be a link from the verbal short-term memory impairment to the language deficits in Down syndrome.

Infants with Down syndrome tend to reach early language milestones (first words, first two-word combinations) at an appropriate rate, given their overall retardation in cognitive development, but there are slower rates of development in expressive lexicon and syntax subsequently (Cardoso-Martins *et al.* 1985; Miller 1995; Caselli *et al.* 1998). Poor speech intelligibility, which is caused by problems with articulation (Pueschel & Hopman 1993; Kumin 1994), is common, as are associated hearing deficits (Roizen *et al.* 1993) which might play a minor part in the impaired development of speech skills (Chapman & Hesketh 2000).

Parents express rather fewer behavioural concerns about children with Down syndrome than do parents of age-matched children with mental retardation of unknown origin, or parents of children with other syndromes associated with equivalent degrees of learning difficulty, such as Prader–Willi syndrome (Chapman & Hesketh 2000). Compared to typically developing siblings, parents report more problem behaviours overall and, specifically, more attentional problems among children and adolescents with Down syndrome (Cuskelly & Dadds 1992; Stores *et al.* 1998). Adaptive behavioural skills are overall consistent with general intelligence (Chapman & Hesketh 2000).

It has been suggested that older adults with Down syndrome are subject to two stages of cognitive decline (Chapman & Hesketh 2000). The first stage, thought to correspond to the accumulation of senile plaques, involves problems in forming new long-term memories. A loss of overlearned behaviours characterizes the second stage, which is thought to result from marked neuronal cell loss.

In adulthood, Down syndrome is also associated with an increased risk of Alzheimer disease. Autopsy studies indicate the presence of brain amyloid (senile) plaques and neurofibrillary tangles that are characteristic of this disease (Wisniewski & Silverman 1998). Neuroimaging data show that dementia in older individuals with Down syndrome is associated with volume reductions in the amygdala and hippocampus, regions known to be affected in Alzheimer disease (Aylward *et al.* 1999). Despite the presence of the neuropathology of Alzheimer disease, observed in all individuals with Down syndrome over the age of 40 (Wisniewski *et al.* 1985), many of them demonstrate clinical features of dementia only when much older (Lai &

Williams 1989). Positron emission tomography data on older individuals with Down syndrome indicate abnormalities in cerebral metabolism in the parietal and temporal cortical areas (the first cortical regions typically affected in Alzhemier disease), when the functional demand on the brain is increased through audiovisual stimulation (Pietrini *et al.* 1997). These effects were observed before the onset of dementia and despite normal metabolism at rest.

Genotype–phenotype correlations

Duplication of a small region of the distal part of the long arm of chromosome 21 (21q22.1-22.3), termed the Down syndrome critical region, is associated with several of the physical features. These include the facial features, congenital heart disease and duodenal stenosis as well as some aspects of the learning difficulties. Candidate genes located within this region whose over-expression may be linked to the learning difficulties include *DRYK*, *DSCR1*, *DSCAM*, *TPRD* and *SIM2* (Chapman & Hesketh 2000). However, genes outside the Down syndrome critical region also seem to contribute to the full behavioural phenotype (Antonarakis 1998) so the picture is a complex one.

Genes that may contribute to dementia of the Alzheimer type in Down syndrome include the superoxide dismutase gene (*SOD-1*), which is associated with rapid ageing, and the beta-amyloid precursor protein gene (*APP*), which is associated with Alzheimer disease (Chapman & Hesketh 2000). Apolipopro-tein E (APOE) alleles on chromosome 19 also influence the risk for Alzheimer disease: the E2 allele offers a protective effect in both Down syndrome (Lai *et al.* 1999) and in the general popu-lation (Corder *et al.* 1994). Although the reason for the protec-tive effect of the E2 allele is not completely understood (Lai *et al.* 1999), it seems to be associated with the extent of beta-amyloid protein deposition (Polvikoski *et al.* 1995). In Down syndrome the APOE genotype seems to be linked to language ability too. Alexander *et al.* (1997) reported that language function was in-versely related to APOE genotype in a sample of non-demented Down syndrome adults. The E2 allele, relative to the E4 allele, was associated with better language skills.

Transgenic mice with three or more copies of the mouse ho-mologues of human chromosome 21 genes can serve as models for overexpression of particular genes. Segments of mouse chro-mosomes 16, 17 and 10 have homology to human chromosome 21. Mouse chromosome 16 includes the entire Down syndrome critical region. Several mouse models have been generated, which demonstrate some features similar to those observed in Down syndrome (Antonarakis 1998). Transgenic mice that overexpress individual human chromosome 21 genes have also been produced. The new techniques will enable the testing of hypotheses about the contributions of single genes, combina-tions of genes, or combinations of human chromosome 21 syn-tenic regions (Antonarakis 1998).

It is in these attempts to assess the contributions of specific genes to traits seen in Down syndrome that the chromosome 21 gene catalogue will have its greatest impact (Reeves 2000). The catalogue now enables the hypothesis-driven selection of candi-date genes, as well as a systematic search for sets of candidates without pre-existing hypotheses (Hattori *et al.* 2000).

Turner syndrome

Turner syndrome was first described by the endocrinologist Henry Turner in 1938, but it was not until 20 years later that the genetic basis of the syndrome was discovered. About 50% of clinically identified cases of Turner syndrome are associated with a single X chromosome, and subjects therefore have 45 rather than the usual 46 chromosomes (Jacobs *et al.* 1997). In the majority, there is loss of the sex chromosome donated by the father, and so the single normal X is maternal in origin. Never-theless, the diagnosis of Turner syndrome is clinical, rather than based on the result of a genetic investigation.

The most striking physical characteristics include short stature, which is not caused by growth hormone deficiency as such but is associated with the deletion of the distal portion of the short arm of the X chromosome, which contains genes that are important for normal growth in stature (Rao *et al.* 1997). There is a failure of secondary sexual characteristics to develop in most cases, and oestrogen replacement therapy is now given routinely in adolescence. The ovaries fail to develop, and the uterus and vagina are often small and immature. Other physical features are much more variable, and include a webbed neck, a wide carrying angle, and broad chest, together with a character-istic facies (Lippe 1996).

The verbal intelligence of females with Turner syndrome is usually normal (Lippe 1996). Although specific cognitive deficits may exist, especially in visuospatial skills (McCauley *et al.* 1986; Ross *et al.* 1995; Skuse *et al.* 1997), the accepted view is that there is no increased risk of moderate or severe mental retardation. The exception is relatively rare cases with a small ring X chromosome (Dennis *et al.*, 2000; Kuntsi *et al.*, 2000). On the other hand, scattered reports over the past 20 years have also suggested that Turner syndrome is associated with psychosocial difficulties (Garron *et al.* 1978; McCauley *et al.* 1986; Downey *et al.* 1989), immaturity and poor self-concept (Hier 1980; Bender *et al.* 1987; Swillen *et al.* 1993; Rovet & Ireland 1994; McCauley *et al.* 1995). Some of these social adjustment difficulties persist into adult life (Downey *et al.* 1989).

Genetic anomaly

Most investigators believe that the phenotype in Turner syn-drome is the result of a deficiency of specific genes, most of which are as yet unidentified, rather than to the consequence of a single X chromosome (45,X) *per se*. One-half of clinically identified cases possess part of a second X chromosome too, which is structurally abnormal, usually in association with some 45,X cells (Jacobs *et al.* 1997). Phenotypic features of Turner syn-drome are thought to be caused by haploid (single and insuffi-cient) dosage of these specific genes, rather than to the complete absence of gene products or the presence of abnormal products.

Monosomy (loss of one complete chromosome) in humans is normally lethal. It is thought that Turner syndrome is an exception because, in normally developing females, one X chromosome normally undergoes condensation and transcriptional silencing (X inactivation) very early in embryogenesis. Thus, only *one* X chromosome is normally active during most of development. If a single X chromosome is associated with a phenotype (Turner syndrome) this implies that in humans X inactivation is incomplete, and some essential gene products are transcribed from the 'silent' X chromosome too. A relatively large number of such genes are now known (Brown *et al.* 1997). It therefore seems likely that the genes involved in most features of Turner syndrome are X-linked and are not subject to X inactivation. They are needed in two expressed copies (diploid dosage) for normal development to take place (Zinn *et al.* 1993).

If X-linked genes are required in diploid dosage for normal development, how can we account for the situation in males who develop normally yet have only a single X chromosome? One possibility is that there are functionally equivalent genes on the Y chromosome. Rao *et al.* (1997) identified *SHOX*, a gene that contributes to the short stature associated with the syndrome, by molecularly characterizing a region at the tip of the X and Y chromosomes that is active on both sex chromosomes and contains homologous genes. They did this by studying a small series of male and female individuals with structural abnormalities and short stature, and comparing them to an equivalent series in which there was *no* height deficit.

In genomic imprinting the allele inherited from one parent is silenced, so that normal development is dependent solely on the function of the allele from the other parent. This imprint is normally erased at some time between generations. Female mammals have a maternally derived X chromosome (X^m) and a paternally derived X chromosome (X^P) in each cell, but in males the single X is invariably maternal in origin (X^m). Until very recently no imprinted gene had been described on the X chromosome in humans. However, there is now evidence suggesting imprinted X-linked genes play a part in the aetiology of some aspects of the behavioural phenotype of Turner syndrome. In 70% of monosomic (45,X) Turner syndrome the single X chromosome is maternal in origin (Jacobs *et al.* 1997); in the remainder it is paternal in origin. The single X chromosome in X monosomy is never inactivated. The strongest evidence is for an imprinted locus on the X chromosome that is preferentially expressed from the paternally inherited chromosome. If such a mechanism exists, it would lead to the preferential expression of a genetic locus in females, which was always normally silent in males (whose single X chromosome is always maternally derived). The imprinting mechanism is deceptively simple. The genetic locus is silenced when it is transmitted by a mother and is switched on when transmitted by a father. A mother passes a silent copy of the locus to both her sons and daughters, but fathers will only pass on an expressed copy to their daughters. There are various mechanisms by which an imprinted X-linked locus could result in sexual dimorphism in phenotypic characteristics. The nature of the dimorphism would depend not only

on the parental allele from which the imprinted genes were expressed. It would also depend on whether or not the alleles in question were subject to X inactivation (Lyon 1996) and whether or not there was a gene homologue (which was not imprinted) on the Y chromosome (Skuse 1999).

Cognitive and behavioural phenotype

Deficient visuospatial functioning is a reliable finding in Turner syndrome, first noted by investigators using standard IQ tests, who reported that performance IQ was impaired relative to verbal IQ, the latter being normal. Deficits in performance IQ, in copying complex designs, and in a speeded peg-moving task (a motor task with visuospatial demands) are seen in 45,X subjects. The underlying nature of the visuospatial deficit remains poorly understood (Temple & Carney 1995). 45,X subjects have substantial impairment in simple numerical tasks, including biologically based abilities to subitize and to compare number magnitudes (Alexander & Money 1966; Rovet *et al.* 1994; Temple & Marriott 1998; Butterworth *et al.* 1999). Face recognition ability is impaired, and this includes both the ability to recognize a familiar face and the detection of facial emotions (Ross *et al.* 1997). Buchanan *et al.* (1998) suggested there is a working memory deficit for visuospatial information in Turner syndrome that links impaired facial recognition to poor performance on arithmetic tasks.

Certain aspects of social behaviour are relatively less adaptive in 45,X^m compared to 45,X^P subjects on a 'social cognition' questionnaire (Skuse *et al.* 1997). Adjustment of 45,X^m females is poorer than for those with a 45,X^P karyotype in several aspects of behaviour (Skuse *et al.* 1999), as rated by parents, teachers and by the girls themselves on standardized instruments. Approximately 5% of all subjects have been found to have either childhood autism, or autistic features compatible with a broader phenotype. In all confirmed cases the normal X chromosome was maternal in origin. It is possible that there is increased vulnerability to autism in females who lack a normal paternally derived X chromosome (Creswell & Skuse 1999; Skuse 1999, 2000a; Thomas *et al.* 1999).

In an investigation contrasting the cognitive abilities of 45,X females whose single X chromosome was either paternal or maternal in origin, intriguing differences in memory dysfunction were discovered (Bishop *et al.* 2000). There was no significant impairment in immediate recall of verbally encoded information, presented in the form of a story, in either group, compared to normal females. However, those with a 45,X^m karyotype forgot the information relatively easily, whereas 45,X^P females did not differ from controls. On a non-verbal memory task, the Rey figure (Waber & Holmes 1985, 1986), the complementary pattern was seen. Both 45,X^m and 45,X^P females had visuospatial problems that affected their ability to copy the complex figure. However, those with a 45,X^P karyotype showed a disproportionate amount of forgetting when asked to redraw it from memory after a delay, whereas those with a 45,X^m karyotype did not differ from normal controls. The implication from these findings is that imprinted X-linked genes may contribute to the development of distinct cognitive brain systems, and that verbal and visuospatial memory can be genetically disassociated.

Investigations of the neuropathology of Turner syndrome are limited to a small number of autopsy studies with heterogeneous findings, including abnormalities of cerebral cortical organization and developmental deviation of structures in the posterior fossa (Reske-Nielsen *et al.* 1982; Della Giustina *et al.* 1985). Brain structure in Turner syndrome has also been investigated with imaging techniques. These have reported changes in the parieto-occipital region (Reiss *et al.* 1993), and also in subcortical structures, especially the hippocampus (Murphy *et al.* 1993; Reiss *et al.* 1995). Attempts to link the findings of structural brain imaging to deficits in cognitive functioning have not previously been fruitful. One potentially confounding variable is ovarian dysgenesis, which is almost invariable in cases of X monosomy (Lippe 1996). Exogenous oestrogen has to be provided to induce secondary sexual characteristics, and this may have independent structural and functional effects on the central nervous system (Ross *et al.* 1995). Other potential confounding variables include X chromosome mosaicism, an excessively wide age range, and sociocultural or educational heterogeneity.

When contrasts are made between individuals with Turner syndrome and normal females, it is not possible to distinguish the behavioural effects of former oestrogen deficiency from that of haploinsufficiency for X-linked genes (Zinn & Ross 1998). Ross *et al.* (1997) showed that some non-verbal tasks and motor-related skills are performed more rapidly by oestrogen-treated subjects. Structural changes consequent upon oestrogen deficiency have been demonstrated in the hippocampus of the rat (Gazzaley *et al.* 1996) and the hormone could have a broader role in gene regulation in the brain (Toran-Allerand *et al.* 1999). However, differences in brain structure and associated cognitive functions between Turner females whose single X is paternal or maternal in origin could not be caused by oestrogen, or any other endocrine deficiency. Growth hormone treatment does not influence the cognitive function of Turner females (Ross *et al.* 1997).

Genotype–phenotype relationships

Many phenotypic features of Turner syndrome are caused by haploinsufficiency for a gene, or several genes, that are expressed from both X chromosomes in normal females (and not subject to X inactivation) and which may have homologues on the Y chromosome. Using molecular methods, it is possible to map the breakpoints in structural anomalies of the X chromosome, in samples of isochromosomes (James *et al.* 1997; Dalton *et al.* 1998), partial deletions of the short arm of the X chromosome (James *et al.* 1998), and also ring chromosomes (Dennis *et al.*, 2000). More detailed information is needed on the cognitive and behavioural phenotypes of these structural anomalies, in order to correlate systematic variations with the nature and extent of chromosomal material that has been lost. This technique is known as deletion mapping, and was successfully

applied in a study of minor X-linked structural anomalies by Rao *et al.* (1997). The methods they employed for deletion-mapping an X-linked gene (*SHOX*) that influences growth in stature, is also potentially applicable to phenotypes such as cognition (Ross *et al.* 1997).

Klinefelter syndrome

Klinefelter syndrome, first described in the 1940s, is caused by an extra X chromosome in males that can be either maternal or paternal in origin. It occurs with remarkable frequency, perhaps as many as 1 in 500 male live births (Smyth & Bremner 1998). The physical phenotype is often not apparent until after puberty, and it is very variable. Tall stature is usual, with long limbs. Testis development is characteristically inadequate, and the majority of affected men are infertile. Learning difficulties may lead to identification in childhood but, if not, diagnosis is likely to be delayed until infertility raises concerns. Our own cytogenetic laboratory data suggest that very few cases are identified in childhood, with the majority probably never identified clinically at all.

Genetic anomaly

There is considerable variability in the cognitive and behavioural phenotype, but this is not caused by mosaicism. In fact, mosaicism for a normal 46,XY cell line is unusual in Klinefelter syndrome, indicating that the genetic anomaly must have occurred at an early stage of development. The great majority are thought to be a result of non-disjunction, either in the formation of gametes in mother or in father. There is no paternal age effect, but there may be a slightly increased risk of non-disjunction in older mothers.

Cognitive and behavioural phenotype

Klinefelter syndrome is not closely associated with mental retardation, although there is a tendency for cases that have been detected in childhood, other than by antenatal screening, to have learning difficulties. Bender *et al.* (1999) reported a follow-up into young adulthood of an unselected sample determined from a consecutive birth cohort. The mean full-scale IQ was 91, significantly lower than a comparison group.

Features such as 'more tender-minded, passive' (Mandoki *et al.* 1991) have been reported for some, whereas others are said to be aggressive with poor impulse control (Netley 1991). To date there have been no systematic attempts to link the phenotype to the parental origin of the additional X chromosome, which is maternal or paternal in equal proportion. A preliminary investigation by Ratcliffe *et al.* (1990) found no relationship between the parental origin of the additional X chromosome and either verbal or non-verbal abilities. Most studies of the syndrome have recruited children and adolescents, although it would be important to have follow-up information on adult outcomes.

Geschwind *et al.* (2000) reviewed the neurobehavioural phenotype. There is a tendency for verbal abilities to be lower than non-verbal abilities (Mandoki *et al.* 1991; Rovet *et al.* 1996). This provides an interesting contrast to the situation in X monosomy (45,X), in which the reverse pattern is found. Geschwind *et al.* (2000) commented that there is an association with specific impairments in language, arithmetic and frontal-executive functions—such as the tendency to make perseverative responses on the Wisconsin Card Sort test. However, others have not found this (Bender *et al.* 1995).

Longitudinal studies show fundamental language processing difficulties in up to 80% of Klinefelter males and a specific reading disability in up to one-half (Graham *et al.* 1988). Besides a general language delay, there may be more specific difficulties in articulation, verbal fluency and possibly auditory working memory. These latter problems may persist into adulthood.

The condition seems to be associated with introversion and social withdrawal (Sorensen 1992), but also with aggressive behaviour and social maladjustment (Bender *et al.* 1999). Geschwind *et al.* (2000) speculated that the more disinhibited forms of Klinefelter syndrome, which are associated with attention deficits and hyperactivity in many cases, are caused by dysfunction in frontal brain neurocognitive systems. Testosterone is used clinically to encourage sexual maturation, but the impact on behaviour or cognition is uncertain. In Bender *et al.*'s (1999) unbiased sample, there was no evidence on standard measures of maladjustment but about half had been diagnosed with mild to moderate psychiatric disorders during adolescence (Bender *et al.* 1995). The evidence on motor skills is contradictory, with some reports suggesting impairment (Salbenblatt *et al.* 1989; Geschwind *et al.* 2000), but others not (Bender *et al.* 1995).

Patwardhan *et al.* (2000) published the first detailed report on brain morphology in the condition. Inevitably the sample size was small (just 10 subjects) because they recruited an unbiased sample. In general, the Klinefelter syndrome group had a significant reduction in the grey matter of the left temporal lobe compared with 46,XY normal comparison subjects. The extent to which this reduction occurred appeared to be associated with testosterone supplementation. These findings echoed, to some extent, those of another structural MRI study conducted by Warwick *et al.* (1999), who compared 10 47,XXY males with 47,XYY and 46,XY males. They found Klinefelter males had smaller brains than normal controls, and bilaterally enlarged lateral ventricles relative to whole brain volume. There were no significant differences in right or left temporal lobe volume between all three groups. However, inspection of the data shows the mean volume of the left temporal lobe was approximately 12% less in the Klinefelter group than normal males, and the magnitude of difference was slightly greater on the right. If these findings are generalizable, it is possible that they do provide some basis for understanding the origin of the verbal deficits associated with the syndrome.

Other sex chromosome aneuploides

There have been relatively few reports on Klinefelter syndrome,

given how commonly it occurs in liveborn males, but there are even fewer on the other relatively common sex chromosome aneuplopides, 47,XXX and 47,XYY syndromes. In the classic Edinburgh-based UK study of sex chromosome anomalies 34 380 consecutive live births were screened (Ratcliffe 1994). This showed the prevalence of both XYY and XXX syndromes to be about 1 in 1000, slightly less common than Klinefelter syndrome, but far less likely to be encountered in clinical practice. Boys with an XYY karyotype are likely to be taller than average (probably caused by overexpression of the *SHOX* gene; Rao *et al.* 1997; Ogata *et al.* 2000). They may have slightly poorer motor co-ordination than control males, and are also more likely to have delayed speech development, although intelligence is virtually normal (Ratcliffe 1994). There is an increased rate of overactivity and impulsivity. It may be that a form of ADHD impairs their ability to cope with an educational curriculum, and there is evidence of a reading level significantly behind that of their peers. Remedial support, especially in reading, was required for about half the cohort identified by Ratcliffe (1994) and in a comparable study in Boston (Walzer *et al.* 1990).

Boys with an XYY karyotype are not much more aggressive or difficult to manage than other children (Ratcliffe 1994) but there is some increase in antisocial behaviour and psychiatric referral (nearly half of cases)—usually for oppositional/defiant or conduct problems. Sexual development is normal. In the only study to have examined brain structure in this condition, Warwick *et al.* (1999) report no significant differences from controls.

Females with 47,XXX syndrome are likely to be smaller than normal at birth, in terms of birth weight, length and head circumference (Ratcliffe 1994). The size of the head correlated with later IQ, and no catch-up in this variable was observed as Ratcliffe's cohort was followed into adulthood. As is the case for boys with additional sex chromosomes, stature is significantly greater than for typically developing females at the same age. In this sample, there were associated problems in fine motor co-ordination and balance.

47,XXX syndrome is associated with a degree of mental retardation which amounts to about one standard deviation below normal, in respect of verbal IQ (Bender *et al.* 1995). Performance IQ is less impaired—an interesting comparison with Klinefelter syndrome—and quite distinct from the situation in X monosomy. There is no evidence of a deterioration over time in cognitive skills. Remedial help at school was required for over two-thirds of the sample in the Ratcliffe (1994) cohort study, and that was mainly concerned with reading retardation as a consequence of the lowered IQ.

There is little objective information on the behavioural and emotional adjustment of 47,XXX females. Anecdotally, they are said to be emotionally less mature than their peers, and to have particular difficulty relating to others in group situations. They will be taller than their peers throughout childhood, and adult stature is also a little above average. Pubertal development takes place at the normal time, and the condition is not associated with infertility. It is worth bearing in mind that adults tend to use stature as a yardstick by which to judge children's age. Those children who are tall for their age, as will be the case for most 47,XXX females, will be judged older than they actually are and will be expected to behave accordingly. As it is likely that the girls in question are going to have relatively poor verbal skills in comparison with their peers, and perhaps also to be somewhat emotionally less mature, the discrepancy between expectations and behaviour could lead to conflict, and other undesirable consequences. However, there is no evidence of any specific forms of behaviour problem being associated with this syndrome, and the vast majority of cases go undetected throughout their lives.

Conclusions

The challenge in developing a truly scientific nosology of child psychopathology is to bring together expertise from multiple complementary disciplines. Such a plea has already been expressed in respect of adult psychiatric disorders, and the study of schizophrenia in particular. Andreasen (1999) argued that the phenotype of this archetypal psychiatric illness should be defined in terms of abnormalities in neural circuits and fundamental cognitive processes. Cognitive psychology has aimed to divide the adult mind into component domains, such as perception, language and executive functions, often employing evidence from lesions to determine localization by observing the absence of function after injury. It is arguable that the very plasticity and flexibility of the developing child's central nervous system makes it less susceptible to study by that approach (Karmiloff-Smith 1998). If we could identify the genetic mechanisms that guide neurobiological systems of development, we could begin to understand the origins of the cognitive dysfunction that underlies much child psychiatric disorder. In a discipline for which there are few if any clear boundaries between 'disease' and 'normal' states of mind, categorical disease (or disorder) models may not be appropriate for the investigation of these putative genetic mechanisms. We suspect the genetic predisposition to certain cognitive deficits, particularly those underlying social communicative skills, will eventually be found to underlie a wide range of neurodevelopmental disorders.

Accordingly, in the search for genes that predispose to the development of child psychiatric disorders it may make little sense to seek the genetic components of relatively amorphous diseases (still less 'comorbid' disorders). Rather, we should look for the genetic basis of cognitive processing deficits that may be common to a number of diseases or disorders. Creating a heuristic cognitive model of developmental disorders will in due course lead to the integration of disciplines, and this is already happening in child psychiatry to some extent. We need to learn how genes control neurobiological development and, in so doing, increasing use will be made of animal models (Skuse 2000a). The appropriate use of behavioural phenotypes could guide the development of such models. Studies of the genetic influences upon specific cognitive processes could reveal 'double dissociations', analogous to the procedure used by cognitive neuroscientists to contrast cognitive profiles among groups with distinct brain lesions (Young et al. 2000). In other words, we could discover, through the appropriate use of behavioural phenotypes, that certain cognitive systems are influenced by relatively independent genetic mechanisms. Were it possible to generalize this technique with the discovery of other genes for specific cognitive functions (which may in turn have neurobehavioural consequences), a more rational and scientific basis for the classification and treatment of child psychiatric disorders could be developed.

In conclusion, specific cognitive phenotypes can be found in individuals with genetic disorders, but they are not isolated deficits. They are associated with behavioural, personality and other psychological characteristics, which make the identification of features which are causally related to the genetic anomaly difficult. It is rare to find examples of such phenotypes in which the cognitive deficit is explicit, and such specificity is likely only to be found in association with a single gene mutation (such as the language disorders in the KE family, see above).

We may be sceptical about the degree to which even very well-studied disorders with a known genetic aetiology and cognitive or psychiatric phenotypes have yet told us much about the development of the brain. Flint (1999) discussed autosomal Mendelian disorders that have cognitive disabilities in their phenotype. He commented that the study of these disorders has told us nothing about how genes affect cognitive processes. Take, for instance, the neurodegenerative disorders, such as cortical and subcortical dementias. The relatively specific deterioration in memory in Alzheimer disease might suggest that genetic analysis could lead to new advances in our understanding of the biology of memory, but this has not been the case. Nor, he commented, has the cause of the cognitive decline in Huntington disease been explained, despite the fact that there is a relatively specific neuropathology, which affects the caudate nucleus, the putamen and the globus pallidus. A mouse model has been developed, which apparently shows that there is altered expression of multiple neurotransmitters in the condition which cannot be explained on the basis of the dysfunction of a particular cell type (Cha 2000). Molecular genetics, developmental neurobiology and cognitive neuroscience have not yet been integrated into a satisfactory causal model of disease in any single condition, but the potential is there.

References

Adler, L.E., Freedman, R., Ross, R.G., Olincy, A. & Waldo, M.C. (1999) Elementary phenotypes in the neurobiological and genetic study of schizophrenia. *Biological Psychiatry*, **46**, 8–18.

Alexander, D. & Money, J. (1966) Turner's syndrome and Gerstmann's syndrome: neuropsychological comparisons. *Neuropsychologia*, **4**, 265–273.

Alexander, G.E., Saunders, A.M., Szczepanik, J. *et al.* (1997) Relation of age and apolipoprotein E to cognitive function in Down syndrome adults. *Neuroreport*, **8**, 1835–1840.

Amir, R., Dahle, E.J., Toriolo, D. & Zoghbi, H.Y. (1999) Candidate gene analysis in Rett syndrome and the identification of 21 SNPs in Xq. *American Journal of Medical Genetics*, **90**, 69–71.

Anderson, L. & Ernst, M. (1994) Self-injury in Lesch–Nyhan disease. *Journal of Autism and Developmental Disorders*, **24**, 67–81.

Anderson, L., Ernst, M. & Davis, S.V. (1992) Cognitive abilities of patients with Lesch–Nyhan syndrome. *Journal of Autism and Developmental Disorders*, **22**, 189–203.

Andreasen, N.C. (1999) Understanding the causes of schizophrenia. *New England Journal of Medicine*, **340**, 645–647.

Angulo, M., Castro-Magana, M., Uy, J. & Rosenfeld, W. (1992) Growth hormone evaluation and treatment in Prader–Willi syndrome. In: *NATO Series ASI*, Vol. H 61, *Prader–Willi Syndrome* (ed. S.B. Cassidy), pp. 172–187. Springer-Verlag, Berlin.

Antonarakis, S.E. (1998) 10 years of Genomics, chromosome 21, and Down syndrome. *Genomics*, **51**, 1–16.

Ashkenas, J. (1996) Williams syndrome starts making sense. *American Journal of Human Genetics*, **59**, 756–761.

Aylward, E.H., Li, Q., Honeycutt, N.A. *et al.* (1999) MRI volumes of the hippocampus and amygdala in adults with Down's syndrome with and without dementia. *American Journal of Psychiatry*, **156**, 564–568.

Baddeley, A.D. & Hitch, G.J. (1974) Working memory. In: *The Psychology of Learning and Motivation* (ed. G. Bower), Vol. 8, pp. 47–89. Academic Press, New York.

Baddeley, A., Gathercole, S. & Papagno, C. (1998) The phonological loop as a language learning device. *Psychological Review*, **105**, 158–173.

Bailey, A., LeCouteur, A., Gottesman, I. *et al.* (1995) Autism as a strongly genetic disorder: evidence from a British twin study. *Psychological Medicine*, **25**, 63–77.

Bardoni, B., Schenck, A. & Mandel, J.L. (1999) A novel RNA-binding nuclear protein that interacts with the fragile X mental retardation (FMR1) protein. *Human Molecular Genetics*, **8**, 2557–2566.

Baumer, A., Dutly, F., Balmer, D. *et al.* (1998) High level of unequal meiotic crossovers at the origin of the 22q11.2 and 7q11.23 deletions. *Human Molecular Genetics*, **7**, 887–894.

Baumgardner, T.L., Reiss, A., Freund, L.S. & Abrams, M.T. (1995) Specification of the neurobehavioural phenotype in males with fragile X syndrome. *Pediatrics*, **95**, 744–752.

Bellugi, U., Sabo, H. & Vaid, J. (1988) Spatial deficits in children with Williams syndrome. In: *Spatial Cognition: Brain Bases and Development* (eds J. Stiles-Davis, M. Kritchevsky & U. Bellugi), pp. 273–298. Erlbaum, Hillsdale, NJ.

Bellugi, U., Lichtenberger, L., Mills, D., Galaburda, A. & Korenberg, J.R. (1999) Bridging cognition, the brain and molecular genetics: evidence from Williams syndrome. *Trends in Neuroscience*, **22**, 197–207.

Bender, B.H., Puck, M., Salbenblatt, J. & Robinson, A. (1987) Cognitive development of children with sex chromosome abnormalities. In: *Genetics and Learning Disabilities* (ed. S. Smith), pp. 175–201. College Hill Press, San Diego.

Bender, B.G., Harmon, R.J., Linden, M.G. & Robinson, A. (1995) Psychosocial adaptation of 39 adolescents with sex chromosome abnormalities. *Pediatrics*, **96**, 302–308.

Bender, B.G., Harmon, R.J., Linden, M.G., Bucher-Bartelson, B. & Robinson, A. (1999) Psychosocial competence of unselected young adults with sex chromosome abnormalities. *American Journal of Medical Genetics*, **88**, 200–206.

Benjamin, E. & Buot-Smith, T. (1993) Naltrexone and fluoxetine in Prader–Willi syndrome. *Journal of the American Academy of Child and Adolescent Psychiatry*, **32**, 870–873.

Bertrand, J., Mervis, C.B. & Eisenberg, J.D. (1997) Drawing by children with Williams syndrome: a developmental perspective. *Developmental Neuropsychology*, **13**, 41–67.

Bihrle, J.M., Bellugi, U., Delis, D. & Marks, S. (1989) Seeing either the forest or the trees: dissociation in visuospatial processing. *Brain and Cognition*, **11**, 37–49.

Bishop, D.V.M. (1999) Perspectives: cognition—an innate basis for language? *Science*, **286**, 2283–2284.

Bishop, D.V.M., Canning, E., Elgar, K., Morris, E., Jacobs, P.A. & Skuse, D.H. (2000) Genetic fractionation of perception and memory: evidence from Turner syndrome of distinct loci on the X chromosome affecting neurodevelopment. *Neuropsychologia*, **38**, 712–721.

Blichfeldt, S., Main, K., Ritzen, M. & Skakkebaek, N.E. (1992) Diminished 24-hour urinary growth hormone excretion in patients with Prader–Willi syndrome. In: *Prader–Willi Syndrome* (ed. S.B. Cassidy), pp. 175–179. Springer Verlag, New York.

Bolton, P.F. & Griffiths, P.D. (1997) Association of tuberous sclerosis of temporal lobes with autism and atypical autism. *Lancet*, **349**, 392–395.

Bresolin, N., Castelli, E., Comi, G.P. *et al.* (1994) Cognitive impairment in Duchenne muscular dystrophy. *Neuromuscular Disorders*, **4**, 359–369.

Brown, C.J., Carrel, L. & Willard, H.F. (1997) Expression of genes from the human active and inactive X chromosomes. *American Journal of Human Genetics*, **60**, 1333–1343.

Browne, C.E., Dennis, N.R., Maher, E. *et al.* (1997) Inherited interstitial duplications of proximal 15q: genotype–phenotype correlations. *American Journal of Human Genetics*, **61**, 1342–1352.

Buchanan, L., Pavlovic, J. & Rovet, J. (1998) The contribution of visuospatial working memory to impairments in face processing and arithmetic in Turner syndrome. *Brain Cognition*, **37**, 72–75.

Bundey, S., Hardy, C., Vickers, S., Kilpatric, M.W. & Corbett, J.A. (1994) Duplication of the 15q11-13 region in a patient with autism, epilepsy and ataxia. *Developmental Medicine and Child Neurology*, **36**, 736–742.

Bushby, K.M., Appleton, R., Anderson, L.V., Welch, J.L., Kelly, P. & Gardner-Medwin, D. (1995) Deletion status and intellectual impairment in Duchenne muscular dystrophy. *Developmental Medicine and Child Neurology*, **37**, 260–269.

Butler, M.G. (1990) Prader–Willi syndrome: current understanding and diagnosis. *American Journal of Medical Genetics*, **35**, 319–332.

Butterworth, B., Grana, A., Piazza, M., Girelli, L., Price, C. & Skuse, D. (1999) Language and the origins of number skills: karyotypic differences in Turner's syndrome. *Brain and Language*, **69**, 486–488.

Caldwell, M.L., Taylor, R.L. & Bloom, S.R. (1986) An investigation of the use of high- and low-preference food as a reinforcer for increased activity of individuals with Prader–Willi syndrome. *Journal of Mental Deficiency Research*, **30**, 347–354.

Cardoso-Martins, C., Mervis, C.B. & Mervis, C.A. (1985) Early vocabulary acquisition by children with Down syndrome. *American Journal of Mental Deficiency*, **90**, 177–184.

Carlson, C., Papolos, D., Pandita, R.K. *et al.* (1997a) Molecular analysis of velocardiofacial syndrome patients with psychiatric disorders. *American Journal of Human Genetics*, **60**, 851–859.

Carlson, C., Sirotkin, H., Pandita, R. *et al.* (1997b) Molecular definition of 22q11 deletions in 151 velocardiofacial syndrome patients. *American Journal of Human Genetics*, **61**, 620–629.

Caselli, M.C., Vicari, S., Longobardi, E. *et al.* (1998) Gestures and words in early development of children with Down syndrome. *Journal of Speech, Language and Hearing Research*, **41**, 1125–1135.

Cassidy, S.B. (1984) Prader–Willi syndrome. *Current Problems in Pediatrics*, **4**, 1–55.

Cassidy, S. (1992) Introduction and overview of Prader–Willi syndrome. In: *NATO ASI Series*, Vol. H 61, *Prader–Willi Syndrome* (ed. S.B. Cassidy), pp. 1–11. Springer-Verlag, Berlin.

Cassidy, S.B., Forsythe, M., Heeger, S. *et al.* (1997) Comparison of phenotype between patients with Prader–Willi syndrome due to deletion 15q and uniparental disomy 15. *American Journal of Medical Genetics*, 68, 433–440.

Cha, J.H. Transcriptional dysregulation in Huntington's disease (2000) *Trends in Neuroscience*, 23:387–392.

Chapman, R.S. (1999) Language and cognitive development in children and adolescents with Down syndrome. In: *Improving the Communication of People with Down Syndrome* (eds J.F. Miller, L.A. Leavitt & M. Leddy), pp. 41–60. Brookes, Baltimore.

Chapman, R.S. & Hesketh, L.J. (2000) Behavioral phenotype of individuals with Down syndrome. *Mental Retardation and Developmental Disabilities Research Review*, 6, 84–95.

Cheadle, J.P., Reeve, M.P., Sampson, J.R. & Kwiatkowski, D.J. (2000) Molecular genetic advances in tuberous sclerosis. *Human Genetics*, 107, 97–114.

Chen, K.S., Manian, P., Koeuth, T. *et al.* (1997) Homologous recombination of a flanking repeat gene cluster is a mechanism for a common contiguous gene deletion syndrome. *Nature Genetics*, 17, 154–163.

Chen, R.Z., Akbarian, S., Tudor, M. & Jaenisch, R. (2001) Deficiency of methyl-CpG binding protein-2 in CNS neurons results in a Rett-like phenotype in mice. *Nature Genetics*, 27, 327–331.

Christie, R., Bay, C., Kaufman, I.A., Bakay, B., Borden, M. & Nyhan, W.L. (1982) Lesch–Nyhan disease: clinical experience with nineteen patients. *Developmental Medicine and Child Neurology*, 24, 293–306.

Chu, C.E., Donaldson, M.D.C., Kelner, C.J.H. *et al.* (1994) Possible role of imprinting in the Turner phenotype. *Journal of Medical Genetics*, 31, 840–842.

Church, D.M., Bengtsson, K.V., Nielson, J.J., Wasmuth, J.J. & Niebhur, E. (1995) Molecular definition of deletions of different segments of distal 5p that result in distinct phenotypic features. *American Journal of Human Genetics*, 56, 1162–1172.

Clarke, A., Cook, P. & Osborne, J.P. (1996) Cranial computed tomographic findings in tuberous sclerosis are not affected by sex. *Developmental Medicine and Child Neurology*, 38, 139–145.

Clarke, D.J. & Boer, H. (1998) Problem behaviors associated with deletion Prader–Willi, Smith–Magenis, and cri du chat syndromes. *American Journal of Mental Retardation*, 103, 264–271.

Clarke, D.J., Waters, J. & Corbett, J.A. (1989) Adults with Prader–Willi syndrome: abnormalities of sleep and behaviour. *Royal Society of Medicine*, 82, 21–24.

Clayton-Smith, J. & Pembrey, M.E. (1992) Angelman syndrome. *Journal of Medical Genetics*, 29, 412–415.

Cook, E.H. Jr, Lindgren, V., Leventhal, B.L. *et al.* (1997) Autism or atypical autism in maternally but not paternally derived proximal 15q duplication. *American Journal of Human Genetics*, 60, 928–934.

Corder, E.H., Saunders, A.M., Risch, N.J. *et al.* (1994) Protective effect of apolipoprotein E type 2 allele for late onset Alzheimer disease. *Nature Genetics*, 7, 180–184.

Cornish, K.M. & Pigram, J. (1996) Developmental and behavioural characteristics of cri du chat syndrome. *Archives of Disease in Childhood*, 75, 448–450.

Cornish, K.M., Cross, G., Green, A., Willatt, L. & Bradshaw, J.M. (1999) A neuropsychological–genetic profile of atypical cri du chat syndrome: implications for prognosis. *Journal of Medical Genetics*, 36, 567–570.

Creswell, C.S. & Skuse, D.H. (1999) Autism in association with Turner syndrome: genetic implications for male vulnerability to pervasive developmental disorders. *Neurocase*, 5, 101–108.

Curfs, L.M., Wiegers, A.M., Sommers, J.R., Borghgraef, M. & Fryns, J.P. (1991) Strengths and weaknesses in the cognitive profile of youngsters with Prader–Willi syndrome. *Clinical Genetics*, 40, 430–434.

Cuskelly, M. & Dadds, M. (1992) Behavioural problems in children with Down's syndrome and their siblings. *Journal of Child Psychology and Psychiatry*, 33, 749–761.

Dalton, P., Coppin, B., James, R., Skuse, D. & Jacobs, P. (1998) Three patients with a 45,X/46,X,psu dic (XP) karyotype. *Journal of Medical Genetics*, 35, 519–524.

Davidson, B.L., Tarle, S.A., Van Antwerp, M. *et al.* (1991) Identification of 17 independent mutations responsible for human hypoxanthine-guanine phosphoribosyltransferase (HPRT) deficiency. *American Journal of Human Genetics*, 48, 951–958.

Davies, M., Howlin, P. & Udwin, O. (1997) Independence and adaptive behavior in adults with Williams syndrome. *American Journal of Medical Genetics*, 70, 188–195.

Davies, P.S.W., Joughin, C., Livingstone, M.B.E. & Barnes, N.D. (1992) Energy expenditure in the Prader–Willi syndrome. In: *Prader–Willi Syndrome* (ed. S.B. Cassidy), pp. 181–187. Springer-Verlag, New York.

Dech, B. & Budow, L. (1991) The use of fluoxetine in an adolescent with Prader–Willi syndrome. *Journal of the American Academy of Child and Adolescent Psychiatry*, 30, 298–302.

Della Giustina, E., Forabosco, A., Botticelli, A.R. & Pace, P. (1985) Neuropathology of the Turner syndrome. *Pediatric Medicine Chirurgie*, 7, 49–55.

Dennis, N., Coppin, B., Turner, C., Skuse, D. & Jacobs, P. (2000) A clinical, cytogenetic and molecular study of 47 females with r (X) chromosomes. *American Journal of Human Genetics*, 64, 295–305.

Deruelle, C., Mancini, J., Livet, M.O., Casse-Perrot, C. & de Schonen, S. (1999) Configural and local processing of faces in children with Williams syndrome. *Brain Cognition*, 41, 276–298.

DeVries, B.B.A., van den Ouweland, A.M.W., Mohkamsing, S. *et al.* (1997) Screening and diagnosis for the Fragile X syndrome among the mentally retarded: an epidemiological and psychological survey. *American Journal of Human Genetics*, 61, 660–667.

Dobkin, C., Rabe, A., Dumas, R., El Idrissi, A., Haubenstock, H. & Brown, T.W. (2000) Fmr1 knockout mouse has a distinctive strain-specific learning impairment. *Neuroscience*, 100, 423–429.

Donaldson, M.D.C., Chu, C.E., Cooke, A., Wilson, A., Greene, S.A. & Stephenson, J.B.P. (1994) The Prader–Willi syndrome. *Archives of Disease in Childhood*, 70, 58–63.

Downey, J., Ehrhardt, A.A., Gruen, R., Bell, J.J. & Morishima, A. (1989) Psychopathology and social functioning in women with Turner syndrome. *Journal of Nervous and Mental Disorders*, 177, 191–201.

Dykens, E.M. & Cassidy, S.B. (1995) Correlates of maladaptive behaviour in children and adults with Prader–Willi syndrome. *American Journal of Medical Genetics*, 60, 546–549.

Dykens, E.M. & Clarke, D. (1997) Correlates of maladaptive behaviour in individuals with 5p- (Cri du Chat) syndrome. *Developmental Medicine and Child Neurology*, 39, 752–756.

Dykens, E.M. & Rosner, B.A. (1999) Refining behavioral phenotypes: personality-motivation in Williams and Prader–Willi syndromes. *American Journal of Mental Retardation*, 104, 158–169.

Dykens, E.M. & Smith, A.C. (1998) Distinctiveness and correlates of maladaptive behaviour in children and adolescents with Smith–Magenis syndrome. *Journal of Intellectual Disability Research*, 42, 481–489.

Dykens, E.M. & Volkmar, F.R. (1997) Medical conditions associated with autism. In: *Handbook of Autism and Developmental Disorders* (eds D. Cohen & F. Volkmar), pp. 388–410. John Wiley and Sons, New York.

Dykens, E.M., Hodapp, R.M., Walsh, K. & Nash, L. (1992) Profiles, correlates and trajectories of intelligence in Prader–Willi syndrome. *Journal of American Academy of Child and Adolescent Psychiatry*, **31**, 1125–1130.

Dykens, E.M., Finucane, B.M. & Gayley, C. (1996) Brief report: cognitive and behavioral profiles in persons with Smith–Magenis syndrome. *Journal of Autism and Developmental Disorders*, **27**, 203–211.

Dykens, E.M., Goff, B.J., Hodapp, R.M. *et al.* (1997) Eating themselves to death: have 'personal rights' gone too far in treating people with Prader–Willi syndrome. *Mental Retardation*, **35**, 312–314.

Egan, J.F., Benn, P., Borgida, A.F., Rodis, J.F., Campbell, W.A. & Vintzileas, A.M. (2000) Efficacy of screening for fetal Down syndrome in the United States from 1974–1997. *Obstetrics and Gynaecology*, **96**, 979–985.

Ehara, H., Ohno, K. & Takeshita, K. (1993) Growth and developmental patterns in Prader–Willi syndrome. *Journal of Intellectual Disability Research*, **37**, 479–485.

Ernst, M., Zametkin, A.J., Matochik, J.A. *et al.* (1996) Presynaptic dopaminergic deficits in Lesch–Nyhan disease. *New England Journal of Medicine*, **334**, 1568–1572.

Feil, R. & Kelsey, G. (1997) Genomic imprinting: a chromatin connection. *American Journal of Human Genetics*, **61**, 1213–1219.

Fields, C., Adams, M.D., White, O. & Venter, J.C. (1994) How many genes in the human genome? *Nature Genetics*, **7**, 345–346.

Finegan, J.A. (1998) Study of behavioral phenotypes: goals and methodological considerations. *American Journal of Medical Genetics*, **81**, 148–155.

Fisher, E. & Scambler, P. (1994) Human haploinsufficiency: one for sorrow, two for joy. *Genomics*, **41**, 75–83.

Fisher, S.E., Marlow, A.J., Lamb, J. *et al.* (1999) A quantitative-trait locus on chromosome 6p influences different aspects of developmental dyslexia. *American Journal of Human Genetics*, **64**, 146–156.

Flint, J. (1996) Annotation: behavioural phenotypes—a window onto the biology of behaviour. *Journal of Child Psychology and Psychiatry*, **37**, 355–367.

Flint, J. (1999) The genetic basis of cognition. *Brain*, **122**, 2015–2032.

Flint, J. & Yule, W. (1994) Behavioural phenotypes. In: *Child and Adolescent Psychiatry: Modern Approaches* (eds M. Rutter, E. Taylor & L. Hersov), pp. 666–687. Blackwell Scientific Publications, Oxford.

Frangiskakis, J.M., Ewart, A.K., Morris, C.A. *et al.* (1996) LIM-kinase1 hemizygosity implicated in impaired visuospatial constructive cognition. *Cell*, **86**, 59–69.

Franke, P., Leboyer, M., Hardt, J. *et al.* (1999) Neuropsychological profiles of FMR-1 premutation and full-mutation carrier females. *Psychiatry Research*, **87**, 223–231.

Frankel, W.N. & Schork, N.J. (1996) Who's afraid of epistasis? *Nature Genetics*, **14**, 371–373.

Gabel, S., Tarter, R.E., Gavaler, J., Golden, W.L., Hegedus, A.M. & Maier, B. (1986) Neuropsychological capacity of Prader–Willi children: general and specific aspects of impairment. *Applied Research in Mental Retardation*, **7**, 459–466.

Gabriel, J.M., Merchant, M., Ohta, T. *et al.* (1999) A transgene insertion creating a heritable chromosome deletion mouse model of Prader–Willi and Angelman syndromes. *Proceedings of the National Academy of Sciences, USA*, **96**, 9258–9263.

Galaburda, A.M., Wang, P.P., Bellugi, U. & Rossen, M. (1994) Cytoarchitectonic anomalies in a genetically based disorder: Williams syndrome. *Neuroreport*, **5**, 753–757.

Garron, D.C., Branda, H.B. & Lindsten, J. (1978) An early behavioral description of a person with Turner syndrome. *Behavior Genetics*, **8**, 73–75.

Gayan, J., Smith, S.D., Cherny, S.S. *et al.* (1999) Quantitative-trait locus for specific language and reading deficits on chromosome 6p. *American Journal of Human Genetics*, **64**, 157–164.

Gazzaley, A.H., Weiland, N.G., McEwen, B.S. & Morrison, J.H. (1996) Differential regulation of NMDAR1 mRNA and protein by estradiol in the rat hippocampus. *Journal of Neuroscience*, **16**, 6830–6838.

Geschwind, D.H., Boone, K.B., Miller, B.L. & Swerdloff, R.S. (2000) Neurobehavioral phenotype of Klinefelter syndrome. *Mental Retardation and Developmental Disability Research Review*, **6**, 107–116.

Gibbons, R.J., Picketts, D.J., Villard, L. & Higgs, D.R. (1995) Mutations in a putative global transcriptional regulator cause X-linked mental retardation with alpha-thalassemia (ATR-X syndrome). *Cell*, **80**, 837–845.

Gillberg, C. (1994) Debate and argument: having Rett syndrome in the ICD-10 PDD category does not make sense. *Journal of Child Psychology and Psychiatry*, **35**, 377–378.

Gillberg, I.C., Gillberg, C. & Ahlsen, G. (1994) Autistic behaviour and attention deficits in tuberous sclerosis: a population-based study. *Developmental Medicine and Child Neurology*, **36**, 50–56.

Gilmour, J. & Skuse, D. (1996) Short stature: the role of intelligence in psychosocial adjustment. *Archives of Disease in Childhood*, **75**, 25–31.

Gilmour, J., Skuse, D.H. & Pembrey, M. (2001) Hyperphagic short stature and Prader–Willi syndrome: a comparison of behavioural phenotypes, genotypes and indices of stress. *British Journal of Psychiatry*, **179**, 129–137.

Goldberg, R., Motzkin, B., Marion, R., Scambler, P. & Shprintzen, R.J. (1993) Velocardiofacial syndrome: a review of 120 patients. *American Journal of Medical Genetics*, **45**, 313–319.

Golding-Kushner, K.J., Weller, G. & Shprintzen, R.J. (1985) Velocardiofacial syndrome: language and psychological profiles. *Journal of Craniofacial Genetics and Developmental Biology*, **5**, 259–266.

Gomez, M.R. (1995) History of the tuberous sclerosis complex. *Brain Development*, **17** (Suppl. 55), 57.

Gopnik, M. (1990) Genetic basis of grammar defect. *Nature*, **347**, 26.

Gosch, A. & Pankau, R. (1997) Personality characteristics and behaviour problems in individuals of different ages with Williams syndrome. *Developmental Medicine and Child Neurology*, **39**, 527–533.

Graham, J.M. Jr, Bashir, A.S., Stark, R.E., Silbert, A. & Walzer, S. (1988) Oral and written language abilities of XXY boys: implications for anticipatory guidance. *Pediatrics*, **81**, 795–806.

Gray, J.M., Young, A.W., Barker, W.A., Curtis, A. & Gibson, D. (1997) Impaired recognition of disgust in Huntington's disease carriers. *Brain*, **120**, 2029–2038.

Greenberg, F., Lewis, R.A., Potocki, L. *et al.* (1996) Multi-disciplinary clinical study of Smith–Magenis syndrome. *American Journal of Medical Genetics*, **62**, 247–254.

Greenswag, L.R. (1987) Adults with Prader–Willi Syndrome: a survey of 232 cases. *Developmental Medicine and Child Neurology*, **29**, 145–152.

Grigorenko, E.L., Wood, F.B., Meyer, M.S. *et al.* (1997) Susceptibility loci for distinct components of developmental dyslexia on chromosomes 6 and 15. *American Journal of Human Genetics*, **60**, 27–39.

Hagberg, B., ed. (1993) *Rett syndrome: clinical and biological aspects. Clinics in Developmental Medicine.* No. 127. MacKeith Press, London.

Hardelin, J.P., Levilliers, J., del Castillo, I. *et al.* (1992) X chromosome-linked Kallmann syndrome: stop mutations validate the candidate gene. *Proceedings of the National Academy of Sciences, USA*, 89, 8190–8194.

Harrison, J.E. & Bolton, P.F. (1997) Annotation: tuberous sclerosis. *Journal of Child Psychology and Psychiatry*, 38, 603–614.

Harrison, J.E., O'Callaghan, F.J., Hancock, E., Osborne, J.P. & Bolton, P.F. (1999) Cognitive deficits in normally intelligent patients with tuberous sclerosis. *American Journal of Medical Genetics*, 88, 642–646.

Hattori, M., Fujiyama, A., Taylor, T.D. *et al.* (2000) The DNA sequence of human chromosome 21. *Nature*, 405, 311–319.

Helbing-Zwanenburg, B., Kamphuisen, H.A.C. & Mourtazev, M.S. (1993) The origin of excessive daytime sleepiness in the Prader–Willi syndrome. *Journal of Intellectual Disability*, 37, 533–541.

Hermelin, B., Pring, L., Buhler, M., Wolff, S. & Heaton, P.A. (1999) Visually impaired savant artist: interacting perceptual and memory representations. *Journal of Child Psychology and Psychiatry*, 40, 1129–1139.

Hier, D.B. (1980) Learning disorders and sex chromosome aberrations. *Journal of Mental Deficiency Research*, 24, 17–26.

Higgs, D.R. (1993) The thalassaemia syndromes. *Quarterly Journal of Medicine*, 86, 559–564.

Hodapp, R.M. (1997) Direct and indirect behavioral effects of different genetic disorders of mental retardation. *American Journal of Mental Retardation*, 102, 67–79.

Hodapp, R.M., Dykens, E.M. & Masino, L.L. (1997) Families of children with Prader–Willi syndrome: stress support and relations to child characteristics. *Journal of Autism and Developmental Disorders*, 27, 11–24.

Holland, A.J., Treasure, J., Coskeran, P. & Dallow, J. (1995) Characteristics of the eating disorder in Prader–Willi syndrome: implications for treatments. *Journal of Intellectual Disability and Research*, 39, 373–381.

Holm, V.A., Butler, S.B., Hanchett, J.M., Greenberg, F. & Greenswag, L.R. (1992) Diagnostic criteria for Prader–Willi syndrome. In: *Nato ASI*, Vol. H 61 *Prader–Willi Syndrome* (ed. S.B. Cassidy), pp. 104–113. Springer-Verlag, Berlin.

Holm, V.A., Cassidy, S.B., Butler, M.G. *et al.* (1993) Prader–Willi syndrome: consensus diagnostic criteria. *Pediatrics*, 91, 398–402.

Howlin, P., Davies, M. & Udwin, O. (1998) Cognitive functioning in adults with Williams syndrome. *Journal of Child Psychology and Psychiatry*, 39, 183–189.

Hunt, A. & Shepherd, C. (1993) A prevalence study of autism in tuberous sclerosis. *Journal of Autism and Developmental Disorders*, 23, 323–339.

The Huntington's Disease Collaborative Research Group (1993) A novel gene containing trinucleotide repeat that is expanded and unstable on Huntington's disease chromosomes. *Cell*, 72, 971–983.

Inoue, S.B., Siomi, M.C. & Siomi, H. (2000) Molecular mechanism of fragile X syndrome. *Journal of Medical Investigation*, 47, 101–107.

Jacobs, P., Dalton, P., James, R. *et al.* (1997) Turner syndrome: a cytogenetic and molecular study. *Annals of Human Genetics*, 61, 471–483.

Jambaque, I., Cusmai, R., Curatolo, P., Cortesi, F., Perrot, C. & Dulac, O. (1991) Neuropsychological aspects of tuberous sclerosis in relation to epilepsy and MRI findings. *Developmental Medicine and Child Neurology*, 33, 698–705.

James, R.S., Dalton, P., Gustashaw, K. *et al.* (1997) Molecular characterisation of isochromosomes of Xq. *Annals of Human Genetics*, 61, 485–490.

James, R.S., Coppin, B., Dalton, P. *et al.* (1998) A study of females with deletions of the short arm of the X chromosome. *Human Genetics*, 102, 507–516.

Jarrold, C. & Baddeley, A.D. (1997) Short-term memory for verbal and visuospatial information in Down's syndrome. *Cognitive Neuropsychiatry*, 2, 101–122.

Jarrold, C., Baddeley, A.D. & Hewes, A.K. (1998) Verbal and nonverbal abilities in the Williams syndrome phenotype: evidence for diverging developmental trajectories. *Journal Child of Psychology and Psychiatry*, 39, 511–523.

Jarrold, C., Baddeley, A.D. & Hewes, A.K. (2000) Verbal short-term memory deficits in Down syndrome: a consequence of problems in rehearsal? *Journal of Child Psychology and Psychiatry*, 40, 233–244.

Jiang, Y.H., Armstrong, D. & Albrecht, U. *et al.* (1998) Mutation of the Angelman ubiquitin ligase in mice causes increased cytoplasmic p53 and deficits of contextual learning and long-term potentiation. *Neuron*, 21, 799–811.

Jinnah, H.A., Wojcik, B.E., Hunt, M. *et al.* (1994) Dopamine deficiency in a genetic mouse model of Lesch–Nyhan disease. *Journal of Neuroscience*, 14, 1164–1175.

Karmiloff-Smith, A. (1997) Developmental differences between developmental cognitive neuroscience and adult neuropsychology. *Developmental Neuropsychology*, 13, 513–524.

Karmiloff-Smith, A. (1998) Development itself is the key to understanding developmental disorders. *Trends in Cognitive Sciences*, 2, 389–398.

Karmiloff-Smith, A., Grant, J., Berthoud, I., Davies, M., Howlin, P. & Udwin, O. (1997) Language and Williams syndrome: how intact is 'intact'? *Child Development*, 68, 246–262.

Kirchgessner, C.U., Warren, S.T. & Willard, H.F. (1995) X inactivation of the FMR1 fragile X mental retardation gene. *Journal of Medical Genetics*, 32, 925–929.

Kishino, T., Lalande, M. & Wagstaff, J. (1997) UBE3A/E6-AP mutations cause Angelman syndrome. *Nature Genetics*, 15, 70–73.

Kjaer, I. & Niebuhr, E. (1999) Studies of the cranial base in 23 patients with cri-du-chat syndrome suggest a cranial developmental field involved in the condition. *American Journal of Medical Genetics*, 82, 6–14.

Kleppe, S.A., Katayama, K.M., Shipley, K.G. & Foushee, D.R. (1990) The speech and language characteristics of children with Prader–Willi syndrome. *Journal of Speech and Hearing Disorders*, 55, 300–309.

Kok, L.L. & Solman, R.T. (1995) Velocardiofacial syndrome: learning difficulties and intervention. *Journal of Medical Genetics*, 32, 612–618.

Kola, I. & Hertzog, P.J. (1997) Animal models in the study of the biological function of genes on human chromosome 21 and their role in the pathophysiology of Down syndrome. *Human Molecular Genetics*, 6, 1713–1728.

Krams, M., Quinton, R., Ashburner, J. *et al.* (1999) Kallmann's syndrome: mirror movements associated with bilateral corticospinal tract hypertrophy. *Neurology*, 52, 816–822.

Kumin, L. (1994) Intelligibility of speech in children with Down syndrome in natural settings: parents' perspective. *Perceptual and Motor Skills*, 78, 307–313.

Kuntsi, J., Skuse, D.H., Elgar, K., Morris, E. & Turner, C. (2000) Ring-X chromosomes: their cognitive-behavioural phenotype. *Annals of Human Genetics*, 64, 295–305.

Kushnik, T., Rao, K.W. & Lamb, A.N. (1984) Familial 5p syndrome. *Clinical Genetics*, 26, 472–476.

Lachiewicz, A.M. & Dawson, D.V. (1994) Behavior problems of young girls with fragile X syndrome: factor scores on the Conners' Parents' Questionnaire. *American Journal of Medical Genetics*, 51, 364–369.

Lachman, H.M., Papolos, D.F., Saito, T., Yu, Y.M., Szumlanski, C.L. & Weinshilboum, R.M. (1996) Human catechol-O-methyltransferase pharmacogenetics: description of a functional polymorphism and its potential application to neuropsychiatric disorders. *Pharmacogenetics*, 6, 243–250.

Lai, R., Kammann, E., Rebeck, G.W. *et al*. (1999) APOE genotype and gender effects on Alzheimer disease in 100 adults with Down syndrome. *Neurology*, 53, 331–336.

Lai, F. & Williams, R.S. (1989) A prospective study of Alzheimer's disease in Down syndrome. *Archives of Neurology*, 46, 849–853.

Lawrence, A.D., Hodges, J.R., Rosser, A.E. *et al*. (1998) Evidence for specific cognitive deficits in preclinical Huntington's disease. *Brain*, 121, 1329–1341.

LeCouteur, A., Bailey, A., Goode, S. *et al*. (1996) A broader phenotype of autism: the clinical spectrum in twins. *Journal of Child Psychology and Psychiatry*, 37, 785–801.

Lejeune, J., Gautier, M. & Turpin, R. (1959) Etude des chromosomes somatique des neufs enfants mongoliens. *CR Academie Scientifique de Paris*, 248, 1721–1722.

Lencer, R., Malchow, C.P., Krecker, K. *et al*. (1999) Smooth pursuit performance in families with multiple occurrence of schizophrenia and nonpsychotic families. *Biological Psychiatry*, 45, 694–703.

Lesch, M. & Nyhan, W.L. (1964) A familial disorder of uric acid metabolism and central nervous system function. *American Journal of Medicine*, 36, 561–570.

Lindsay, E.A., Vitelli, F., Su, H. *et al*. (2001a) Tbx1 haploinsufficiency in the DiGeorge syndrome region causes aortic arch defects in mice. *Nature*, 401, 97–101.

Lindsay, E.A. & Baldini (2001b). Recovery from arterial growth delay reduces penetrance of cardiovascular defects in mice deleted for the DiGeorge syndrome region. *Human Molecular Genetics*, 10, 997–1002.

Lippe, B.M. (1996) Turner syndrome. In: *Pediatric Endocrinology* (ed. M.A. Sperling), pp. 387–421. W.B. Saunders, Philadelphia.

Lynch, D.R., McDonald-McGinn, D.M., Zackai, E.H. *et al*. (1995) Cerebellar atrophy in a patient with velocardiofacial syndrome. *Journal of Medical Genetics*, 32, 561–563.

Lyon, M.F. (1996) X-chromosome inactivation: pinpointing the centre. *Nature*, 379, 116–117.

Maddox, L.O., Menold, M.M., Bass, M.P. *et al*. (1999) Autistic disorder and chromosome 15q11-q13: construction and analysis of a BAC/PAC contig. *Genomics*, 62, 325–331.

Mandoki, M.W., Sumner, G.S., Hoffman, R.P. & Riconda, D.L. (1991) A review of Klinefelter's syndrome in children and adolescents. *Journal of the American Academy of Child and Adolescent Psychiatry*, 30, 167–172.

Mange, E.J. & Mange, A.P. (1990) *Basic Human Genetics*. Sinauer Associates, MA.

Mann, M.R. & Bartolomei, M.S. (1999) Towards a molecular understanding of Prader–Willi and Angelman syndromes. *Human Molecular Genetics*, 8, 1867–1873.

Margolis, R.L., McInnis, M.G., Rosenblatt, A. & Ross, C.A. (1999) Trinucleotide repeat expansion and neuropsychiatric disease. *Archives of General Psychiatry*, 56, 1019–1031.

Matthews, W.S., Solan, A. & Barabas, G. (1995) Cognitive functioning in Lesch–Nyhan syndrome. *Developmental Medicine and Child Neurology*, 37, 715–722.

Matthews, W.D., Solan, A., Barabas, G. & Robey, K. (1999) Cognitive functioning in Lesch–Nyhan syndrome: a 4-year follow-up study. *Developmental Medicine and Child Neurology*, 41, 260–262.

Mazzocco, M.M., Baumgardner, T., Freund, L.S. & Reiss, A.L. (1998) Social functioning among girls with fragile X or Turner syndrome and their sisters. *Journal of Autism and Developmental Disorders*, 28, 509–517.

McCabe, E.R., de la Cruz, F. & Clapp, K. (1999) Workshop on fragile X: future research directions. *American Journal of Medical Genetics*, 85, 317–322.

McCauley, E., Ito, J. & Kay, T. (1986) Psychosocial functioning in girls with the Turner syndrome and short stature. *Journal of the American Academy of Child Psychiatry*, 25, 105–112.

McCauley, E., Ross, J.L., Kushner, H. & Cutler, G. (1995) Self-esteem and behavior in girls with Turner syndrome. *Developmental and Behavioral Pediatrics*, 16, 82–88.

McInnis, M.G. (1996) Anticipation: an old idea in new genes. *American Journal of Human Genetics*, 59, 973–979.

Mein, C.A., Esposito, L., Dunn, M.G. *et al*. (1998) A search for type 1 diabetes susceptibility genes in families from the United Kingdom. *Nature Genetics*, 19, 297–300.

Merenstein, S.A., Sobesky, W.E., Taylor, A.K., Riddle, J.E., Tran, H.X. & Hagerman, R.J. (1996) Molecular-clinical correlations in males with an expanded FMR1 mutation. *American Journal of Medical Genetics*, 64, 388–394.

Miller, J.F. (1995) Individual differences in vocabulary acquisition in children with Down syndrome. *Progress in Clinical Biological Research*, 393, 93–103.

Moizard, M.P., Billard, C., Toutain, A., Berret, F., Marmin, N. & Moraine, C. (1998) Are Dp71 and Dp140 brain dystrophin isoforms related to cognitive impairment in Duchenne muscular dystrophy? *American Journal of Medical Genetics*, 80, 32–41.

Morrow, B., Goldberg, R., Carlson, C. *et al*. (1995) Molecular definition of the 22q11 deletions in velocardiofacial syndrome. *American Journal of Human Genetics*, 56, 1391–1403.

Moss, E.H., Batshaw, M.L., Solot, C.B. *et al*. (1999) Psychoeducational profile of the 22q11.2 microdeletion: a complex pattern. *Journal of Pediatrics*, 134, 193–198.

Motzkin, B., Marion, R., Goldberg, R., Shprintzen, R. & Saenger, P. (1993) Variable phenotypes in velocardiofacial syndrome with chromosomal deletion. *Journal of Pediatrics*, 123, 406–410.

Mount, R.H., Hastings, R.P., Reilly, S., Cass, H. & Charman, T. (2001) Behavioural and emotional features in Rett syndrome. *Disability and Rehabilitation*, 23, 129–138.

Muller, J. (1997) Hypogonadism and endocrine metabolic disorders in Prader–Willi syndrome. *Acta Paediatrica Supplement*, 423, 58–59.

Murphy, D.G., DeCarli, C., Daly, E. *et al*. (1993) X-chromosome effects on female brain: a magnetic resonance imaging study of Turner's syndrome. *Lancet*, 342, 1197–1200.

Murphy, K.C., Jones, L.A. & Owen, M.J. (1999) High rates of schizophrenia in adults with velocardiofacial syndrome. *Archives of General Psychiatry*, 56, 940–945.

Nardella, M.T., Sulzbacher, S.I. & Worthington-Roberts, B.S. (1983) Activity levels of persons with Prader–Willi syndrome. *American Journal of Mental Deficiency*, 87, 498–505.

Netley, C. (1991) Personality in 47,XXY males during adolescence. *Clinical Genetics*, 39, 409–418.

Nicholls, R.D. (1999) Incriminating gene suspects, Prader–Willi style. *Nature Genetics*, 23, 132–134.

Nicholls, R.D., Saitoh, S. & Horsthemke, B. (1998) Imprinting in Prader–Willi and Angelman syndromes. *Trends in Genetics*, 14, 194–200.

Niebuhr, E. (1978) The cri du chat syndrome: epidemiology, cytogenetics, and clinical features. *Human Genetics*, 44, 227–275.

Nyhan, W.L. (1997) The recognition of Lesch–Nyhan syndrome as an inborn error of purine metabolism. *Journal of Inheritable Metabolic Disorders*, 20, 171–178.

Ogata, T., Kosho, T., Wakui, K., Fukushima, Y., Yoshimoto, M. & Miharu, N. (2000) Short stature homeobox-containing gene duplication on the der (X) chromosome in a female with 45,X/46,X, der (X), gonadal dysgenesis, and tall stature. *Journal of Clinical and Endocrinology Metabolism*, **85**, 2927–2930.

Olson, L. & Houlihan, D. (2000) A review of behavioral treatments used for Lesch–Nyhan syndrome. *Behavior Modification*, **24**, 202–222.

Osborne, J.P., Fryer, A. & Webb, D. (1991) Epidemiology of tuberous sclerosis. *Annals of the New York Academy of Science*, **615**, 125–127.

Papolos, D.F., Faedda, G.L., Veit, S. *et al.* (1996) Bipolar spectrum disorders in patients diagnosed with velocardiofacial syndrome: does a hemizygotic deletion of chromosome 22q11 result in bipolar affective disorder. *American Journal of Psychiatry*, **153**, 1541–1547.

Paterson, S.J., Brown, J.H., Gsodl, M.K., Johnson, M.H. & Karmiloff-Smith, A. (1999) Cognitive modularity and genetic disorders. *Science*, **286**, 2355–2358.

Patwardhan, A.J., Eliez, S., Bender, B., Linden, M.G. & Reiss, A.L. (2000) Brain morphology in Klinefelter syndrome: extra X chromosome and testosterone supplementation. *Neurology*, **54**, 2218–2223.

Perez Jurado, L.A., Peoples, R., Kaplan, P., Hamel, B.C. & Francke, U. (1996) Molecular definition of the chromosome 7 deletion in Williams syndrome and parent-of-origin effects on growth. *American Journal of Human Genetics*, **59**, 781–792.

Petronis, A., Gottesman, I.I., Crow, T.J. *et al.* (2000) Psychiatric epigenetics: a new focus for the new century. *Molecular Psychiatry*, **5**, 342–346.

Pickles, A., Starr, E., Kazak, S., Bolton, P. & Papanikolaou, K. (2000) A variable expression of the autism broader phenotype. *Journal of Child Psychology and Psychiatry*, **41**, 491–502.

Pietrini, P., Dani, A., Furey, M.L. *et al.* (1997) Low glucose metabolism during brain stimulation in older Down's syndrome subjects at risk for Alzheimer's disease prior to dementia. *American Journal of Psychiatry*, **154**, 1063–1069.

Pinker, S. (1994) *The Language Instinct*, pp. 52–53. Penguin, London.

Polvikoski, T., Sulkava, R., Haltia, M. *et al.* (1995) Apolipoprotein E, dementia, and cortical deposition of β-amyloid protein. *New England Journal of Medicine*, **333**, 1242–1247.

Pueschel, S. & Hopman, M. (1993) Speech and language abilities of children with Down syndrome. In: *Enhancing Children's Communication* (eds A.P. Kaiser & D.B. Gray), pp. 335–362. Brookes, Baltimore.

Quinton, R., Duke, V.M., de Zoysa, P.A. *et al.* (1996) The neuroradiology of Kallmann's syndrome: a genotypic and phenotypic analysis. *Journal of Clinical and Endocrinological Metabolism*, **81**, 3010–3017.

Rao, E., Weiss, B., Fukami, M. *et al.* (1997) Pseudoautosomal deletions encompassing a novel homeobox gene cause growth failure in idiopathic short stature and Turner syndrome. *Nature Genetics*, **16**, 54–63.

Ratcliffe, S.G. (1994) The psychological and psychiatric consequences of sex chromosome abnormalities in children, based on population studies. In: *Basic Approaches to Genetic and Molecularbiological Developmental Psychiatry* (ed. F. Poutska), pp. 99–122. Quintessenz Library of Psychiatry, Munich.

Ratcliffe, S.G., Butler, G.E. & Jones, M. (1990) Edinburgh study of growth and development of children with sex chromosome abnormalities IV. *Children and Young Adults with sex chromosome aneuploidy birth defects: Original Article Series*, 26 (eds A. Robinson, J. Evans & J. Hamerton), pp. 1–44. John Wiey & Sons, New York.

Reeves, R.H. (2000) Recounting a genetic story. *Nature* **405**, 283–284.

Reiss, A.L., Abrams, M.T., Greenlaw, R, Freund, L. & Denckla, M.B. (1995) Neurodevelopmental effects of the FMR-1 full mutation in humans. *Nature Genetics*, **1**, 159–167.

Reiss, A.L., Freund, L., Plotnick, L. *et al.* (1993) The effects of X monosomy on brain development: monozygotic twins discordant for Turner's syndrome. *Annals of Neurology*, **34**, 95–107.

Renwick, P.J., Birley, A.J., McKeown, C.M. & Hulten, M. (1995) Southern analysis reveals a large deletion at the hypoxanthin phosphoribosyltransferase locus in a patient with Lesch–Nyhan syndrome. *Clinical Genetics*, **48**, 80–84.

Reske-Nielsen, E., Christensen, A.L. & Nielsen, J. (1982) A neuropathological and neuropsychological study of Turner's syndrome. *Cortex*, **18**, 181–190.

Ritzen, E.M., Bolme, P. & Hall, K. (1992) Endocrine physiology and therapy in Prader–Willi syndrome. In: *Nato Series*, Vol. H 61 *Prader–Willi Syndrome* (ed. S.B. Cassidy), pp. 153–169. Springer-Verlag, Berlin.

Roizen, N.J., Wolters, C., Nicol, T. & Blondis, T.A. (1993) Hearing loss in children with Down syndrome. *Journal of Pediatrics*, **123**, S9–S12.

Roof, E., Stone, W., MacLean, W., Feurer, I.D., Thompson, T. & Butler, M.G. (2000) Intellectual characteristics of Prader–Willi syndrome: comparison of genetic subtypes. *Journal of Intellectual Disability Research*, **44**, 25–30.

Ross, J.L., Stefanatos, G., Roeltgen, D., Kushner, H. & Cutler, G.B. Jr (1995) Ullrich–Turner syndrome: neurodevelopmental changes from childhood through adolescence. *American Journal of Medical Genetics*, **58**, 74–82.

Ross, J.L., Kushner, H. & Zinn, A.R. (1997) Discriminant analysis of the Ullrich–Turner syndrome neurocognitive profile. *American Journal of Medical Genetics*, **72**, 275–280.

Rovet, J.F. & Ireland, L. (1994) The behavioral phenotype in children with Turner syndrome. *Pediatric Psychology*, **19**, 779–790.

Rovet, J., Szekely, C. & Hockenberry, M.-N. (1994) Specific arithmetic calculation deficits in children with Turner syndrome. *Journal of Clinical and Experimental Neuropsychology*, **16**, 820–839.

Rovet, J., Netley, C., Keenan, M. & Bailey, J. & Stewart, D. (1996) The psychoeducational profile of boys with Klinefelter syndrome. *Journal of Learning Disability*, **29**, 180–196.

Rugarli, E.I. (1999) Kallmann syndrome and the link between olfactory and reproductive development. *American Journal of Human Genetics*, **65**, 943–948.

Rutter, M. (1994a) Psychiatric genetics: research challenges and paths forward. *American Journal of Medical Genetics* (*Neuropsychiatric Genetics*), **54**, 185–198.

Rutter, M. (1994b) Debate and argument: there are connections between brain and mind and it is important that Rett syndrome be classified somewhere. *Journal of Child Psychology and Psychiatry*, **35**, 379–381.

Rutter, M., Silberg, J., O'Connor, T. & Simonoff, E. (1999) Genetics and child psychiatry. II. Empirical research findings. *Journal of Child Psychology and Psychiatry*, **40**, 19–55.

Sacks, O. (1995) *An Anthropologist on Mars*. Picador, London.

Salbenblatt, J.A., Meyers, D.C., Bender, B.G., Linden, M.G. & Robinson, A. (1989) Gross and fine motor development in 45,X and 47,XXX girls. *Pediatrics*, **84**, 678–682.

Scambler, P.J. (2000) The 22q11 deletion syndromes. *Human Molecular Genetics*, **9**, 2421–2426.

Scherzer, A.L. & Ilson, J.B. (1969) Normal intelligence in the Lesch–Nyhan syndrome. *Pediatrics*, **44**, 116–120.

Schroer, R.J., Phelan, M.C., Michaelis, R.C. *et al.* (1998) Autism and maternally derived aberrations of chromosome 15q. *American Journal of Medical Genetics*, **76**, 327–336.

Shprintzen, R.J., Goldberg, R.B., Lewin, M.L. *et al.* (1978) A new syndrome involving cleft palate, cardiac anomalies, typical facies, and learning disabilities: velocardiofacial syndrome. *Cleft Palate Journal*, **15**, 56–62.

Shprintzen, R.J., Goldberg, R.B., Young, D. & Wolford, L. (1981) The velocardiofacial syndrome: a clinical and genetic analysis. *Pediatrics*, **67**, 167–172.

Simmons, A.D., Overhauser, J. & Lovett, M. (1997) Isolation of cDNAs from the cri-du-chat critical region by directly screening of a chromosome 5-specific cDNA library. *Genome Research*, **7**, 118–127.

Simmons, A.D., Puschel, A.W., McPherson, J.D., Overhauser, J. & Lovett, M. (1998) Molecular cloning and mapping of human semaphorin F from the cri-du-chat candidate interval. *Biochemical and Biophysical Research Communications*, **242**, 685–691.

Simonoff, E., Bolton, P. & Rutter, M. (1996) Mental retardation: genetic findings, clinical implications and research. *Journal of Child Psychology and Psychiatry*, **37**, 259–280.

Sirianni, N., Naidu, S., Pereira, J., Pillotto, R.F. & Hoffman, E.P. (1998) Rett syndrome: confirmation of X-linked dominant inheritance, and localization of the gene to Xq28. *American Journal of Human Genetics*, **63**, 1552–1558.

Skuse, D.H. (1999) Genomic imprinting of the X-chromosome: a novel mechanism for the evolution of sexual dimorphism. *Journal of Laboratory and Clinical Medicine*, **133**, 23–32.

Skuse, D.H. (2000a) Behavioural neuroscience and child psychopathology: insights from model systems. *Journal of Child Psychology and Psychiatry*, **41**, 3–31.

Skuse, D.H. (2000b) Imprinting, the X chromosome and the male brain: explaining sex differences in the liability to autism. *Pediatric Research*, **47**, 1–8.

Skuse, D.H., James, R.S., Bishop, D.V.M. *et al.* (1997) Evidence from Turner's syndrome of an imprinted X-linked locus affecting cognitive function. *Nature*, **387**, 705–708.

Skuse, D., Elgar, K. & Morris, E. (1999) Quality of life in Turner syndrome is related to chromosomal constitution: implications for genetic counselling and management. *Acta Paediatrica Supplement*, **428**, 110–113.

Smalley, S.L. (1998) Autism and tuberous sclerosis. *Journal of Autism and Developmental Disorders*, **28**, 407–414.

Smith, A.C., Dykens, E. & Greenberg, F. (1998a) Sleep disturbance in Smith–Magenis syndrome (del 17 p11.2). *American Journal of Medical Genetics*, **81**, 186–191.

Smith, A.C., Dykens, E. & Greenberg, F. (1998b) Behavioral phenotype of Smith–Magenis syndrome (del 17p11.2). *American Journal of Medical Genetics*, **81**, 179–185.

Smyth, C.M. & Bremner, W.J. (1998) Klinefelter syndrome. *Archives of Internal Medicine*, **158**, 1309–1314.

Sobesky, W.E., Taylor, A.K., Pennington, B.F. *et al.* (1996) Molecular/clinical correlations in females with fragile X. *American Journal of Medical Genetics*, **64**, 340–345.

Sorensen, K. (1992) Physical and mental development of adolescent males with Klinefelter syndrome. *Hormone Research*, **37** (Suppl. 3), 55–61.

Stores, R., Stores, G., Fellows, B. *et al.* (1998) Daytime behaviour problems and maternal stress in children with Down's syndrome, their siblings, and non-intellectually disabled and other intellectually disabled peers. *Journal of Intellect Disability Research*, **42**, 228–237.

Strachan, T. & Read, A.P. (1999). *Human Molecular Genetics*, 2nd edn. Wiley-Liss, New York.

Sulzbacher, S., Wong, B., McKeen, J., Glock, J. & MacDonald, B. (1981) Long-term therapeutic effects of a three-month intensive growth group. *Journal of Clinical Psychiatry*, **42**, 148–153.

Swillen, A., Fryns, J.P., Kleczkowska, A. *et al.* (1993) Intelligence, behaviour and psychosocial development in Turner syndrome: a cross-sectional study of 50 preadolescent and adolescent girls (4–20 years). *Genetic Counselling*, **4**, 7–18.

Swillen, A., Devriendt, K., Legius, E. *et al.* (1999) The behavioural phenotype in velocardiofacial syndrome (VCFS): from infancy to adolescence. *Genetic Counselling*, **10**, 79–88.

Tassabehji, M., Metcalfe, K., Karmiloff-Smith, A. *et al.* (1999) Williams syndrome: use of chromosomal microdeletions as a tool to dissect cognitive and physical phenotypes. *American Journal of Human Genetics*, **64**, 118–125.

Tassone, F., Hagerman, R.J., Ikle, D. *et al.* (1999) FMRP expression as a potential prognostic indicator in fragile X syndrome. *American Journal of Medical Genetics*, **84**, 250–261.

Taylor, R.L. (1992) Cognitive and behavioural characteristics. In: *Prader–Willi Syndrome: Selected Research and Management Issues* (eds M.L. Caldwell & R.L. Taylor), pp. 29–42. Springer Verlag, New York.

Taylor, R.L. & Caldwell, M.L. (1985) Type and strength of food preferences of individuals with Prader–Willi syndrome. *Journal of Mental Deficiency Research*, **29**, 109–112.

Temple, C.M. & Carney, R.A. (1995) Patterns of spatial functioning in Turner's syndrome. *Cortex*, **31**, 109–118.

Temple, C.M. & Marriott, A.J. (1998) Arithmetical ability and disability in Turner's syndrome: a cognitive neuropsychological analysis. *Developmental Neuropsychology*, **14**, 47–67.

Thomas, N.S., Sharp, A.J., Browne, C.E. & Dennis, N.R. (1999) Xp deletions associated with autism in three females. *Human Genetics*, **104**, 43–48.

Thompson, N.M., Gulley, M.L., Rogeness, G.A. *et al.* (1994) Neurobehavioral characteristics of CGG amplification status in fraile X females. *American Journal of Medical Genetics*, **54**, 378–383.

Tilghman, S.M. (1999) The sins of the fathers and mothers: genomic imprinting in mammalian development. *Cell*, **96**, 185–193.

Todd, J.A. (1991) A protective role of the environment in the development of type 1 diabetes? *Diabetic Medicine*, **8**, 906–910.

Todd, J.A. (1999) From genome to aetiology in a multifactorial disease, type 1 diabetes. *Bioessays*, **21**, 164–174.

Toran-Allerand, C.D., Singh, M. & Setalo, G. Jr (1999) Novel mechanisms of estrogen action in the brain: new players in an old story. *Frontiers of Neuroendocrinology*, **20**, 97–121.

Tsai, T.F., Jiang, Y.H., Bressler, J., Armstrong, D. & Beaudet, A.L. (1999) Paternal deletion from Snrpn to Ube3a in the mouse causes hypotonia, growth retardation and partial lethality and provides evidence for a gene contributing to Prader–Willi syndrome. *Human Molecular Genetics*, **8**, 1357–1364.

Tu, J.B., Hartridge, C. & Izawa, J. (1992) Psychopharmacogenetic aspects of Prader–Willi syndrome. *Journal of the American Academy of Child and Adolescent Psychiatry*, **31**, 1137–1140.

Turk, J. & Cornish, K. (1998) Face recognition and emotion perception in boys with fragile X syndrome. *Journal of Intellectual Disability Research*, **42**, 490–499.

Turner, G., Robinson, H., Wake, S., Laing, S. & Partington, M. (1997) Case finding for the fragile X syndrome and its consequences. *British Medical Journal*, **315**, 1223–1226.

Udwin, O. & Yule, W. (1991) A cognitive and behavioral phenotype in Williams syndrome. *Journal of Clinical and Experimental Psychology*, **13**, 232–244.

Udwin, O., Yule, W. & Martin, N. (1987) Cognitive abilities and behavioural characteristics of children with idiopathic infantile hypercalcaemia. *Journal of Child Psychology and Psychiatry*, **28**, 297–309.

Van Buggenhout, G.J., Pijkels, E., Holvoet, M., Schaap, C., Hamel, B.C. & Fryns, J.P. (2000) Cri du chat syndrome: changing phenotype in older patients. *American Journal of Medical Genetics*, **90**, 203–215.

Vargha Khadem, F., Watkins, K.E., Price, C.J. *et al.* (1998) Neural basis of an inherited speech and language disorder. *Proceedings of the National Academy of Sciences, USA*, **95**, 12695–12700.

Verkerk, A.J., Pieretti, M., Sutcliffe, J.S. *et al.* (1991) Identification of a gene (FMR-1) containing a CGG repeat coincident with a breakpoint cluster region exhibiting length variation in fragile X syndrome. *Cell*, **65**, 905–914.

Vincent, M.C., Heitz, F., Tricoire, J. *et al.* (1999) 22q11 deletion in DGS/VCFS monozygotic twins with discordant phenotypes. *Genetic Counselling*, **10**, 43–49.

Waber, D.P. & Holmes, J.M. (1985) Assessing children's copy productions of the Rey–Osterrieth Complex Figure. *Journal of Clinical and Experimental Neuropsychology*, **7**, 264–280.

Waber, D.P. & Holmes, J.M. (1986) Assessing children's memory productions of the Rey–Osterrieth Complex Figure. *Journal of Clinical and Experimental Neuropsychology*, **8**, 563–580.

Walzer, S., Bashir, A. & Silbert, A. (1990) Cognitive and behavioral factors in the learning disabilities of 47,XXY and 47,XYY boys. In: *Children and Young Adults with Sex Chromosome Aneuploidy Birth Defects. Original Articles Series*, 26 (eds J.A. Evans, J.L. Hamerton & A. Robinson), pp. 45–58. John Wiley & Sons, New York.

Warwick, M.M., Doody, G.A., Lawrie, S.M., Kestelman, J.N., Best, J.J. & Johnstone, E.C. (1999) Volumetric magnetic resonance imaging study of the brain in subjects with sex chromosome aneuploidies. *Journal of Neurology, Neurosurgery and Psychiatry*, **66**, 628–632.

Weatherall, D. (1999) From genotype to phenotype: genetics and medical practice in the new millennium. *Philosophical Transactions of the Royal Society of London B, Biological Sciences*, **354**, 1995–2010.

Weatherall, D. & Clegg, J.B. (1999) Genetic disorders of hemoglobin. *Seminars in Hematology*, **36** (4 Suppl. 7), 24–37.

Webb, D.W., Fryer, A.E. & Osborne, J.P. (1996) Morbidity associated with tuberous sclerosis: a population study. *Developmental Medicine and Child Neurology*, **38**, 146–155.

Wechsler, D. (1986) *Wechsler Adult Intelligence Scales–Revised*. Psychological Corporation, New York.

Wechsler, D. (1992) *Wechsler Intelligence Scales For Children–Revised*. Psychological Corporation, New York.

Whitman, B., Y., Greenswag, L. & R. (1992) The use of psychotropic medications in persons with Prader–Willi syndrome. In: *Nato ASI Series*, Vol. H 61, *Prader–Willi Syndrome* (ed. S.B. Cassidy), pp. 223–231. Springer-Verlag, Berlin.

Wilkie, A.O., Zeitlin, H.C., Lindenbaum, R.H. *et al.* (1990a) Clinical features and molecular analysis of the alpha thalassemia/mental retardation syndromes. II. Cases without detectable abnormality of the alpha globin complex. *American Journal of Human Genetics*, **46**, 1127–1140.

Wilkie, A.O., Buckle, V.J., Harris, P.C. *et al.* (1990b) Clinical features and molecular analysis of the alpha thalassemia/mental retardation syndromes. I. Cases due to deletions involving chromosome band 16p13.3. *American Journal of Human Genetics*, **46**, 1112–1126.

Willard, H.F. & Hendrich, B.D. (1999) Breaking the silence in Rett syndrome. *Nature Genetics*, **23**, 127–128.

Wing, L. & Gould, J. (1979) Severe impairments of social interaction and associated abnormalities in children: epidemiology and classification. *Journal of Autism and Developmental Disorders*, **9**, 11–29.

Wisniewski, H.M. & Silverman, W. (1998) Aging and dementia of the Alzheimer type in persons with mental retardation. *Advances in Experimental Medical Biology*, **446**, 223–225.

Wisniewski, K.E., Wisniewski, H.M. & Wen, G.Y. (1985) Occurrence of neuropathological changes and dementia of Alzheimer disease in Down syndrome. *Annals of Neurology*, **17**, 278–282.

Wolff, D.J., Schwartz, S. & Carrel, L. (2000) Molecular determination of X inactivation pattern correlates with phenotype in women with a structurally abnormal X chromosome. *Genet Med*, **2**, 136–141.

Wu, C.L. & Melton, D.W. (1993) Production of a model for Lesch–Nyhan syndrome in hypoxanthine phosphoribosyltransferase-deficient mice. *Nature Genetics*, **3**, 235–240.

Young, M.P., Hilgetag, C.C. & Scannell, J.W. (2000) On imputing function to structure from the behavioural effects of brain lesions. *Philosophical Transactions of the Royal Society of London B, Biological Sciences*, **355**, 147–161.

Zatz, M., Vallada, H., Melo, M.S. *et al.* (1993) Cosegregation of schizophrenia with Becker muscular dystrophy: susceptibility locus for schizophrenia at Xp21 or an effect of the dystrophin gene in the brain? *Journal of Medical Genetics*, **30**, 131–134.

Zinn, A.R., Page, D.C. & Fisher, E.M.C. (1993) Turner syndrome: the case of the missing sex chromosome. *Trends in Genetics*, **9**, 90–93.

Zinn, A.R. & Ross, J.L. (1998) Turner syndrome and haploinsufficiency. *Current Opinion in Genetic Development*, **8**, 322–327.

Zipf, W.B. & Berntson, G.G. (1987) Characteristics of abnormal food-intake patterns in children with Prader–Willi syndrome and study of effects of naloxone. *American Journal of Clinical Nutrition*, **46**, 277–281.

14 Brain Disorders

Robert Goodman

Introduction

This chapter focuses on the psychiatric consequences of childhood brain disorders, including epilepsy. It offers no more than a few glimpses of the interesting but largely unexplored territory that has variously been called 'organic child psychiatry', 'paediatric behavioural neurology', and 'developmental neuropsychiatry'. Our current knowledge of the childhood links between brain and behavioural disorders is extremely sketchy, partly because of limitations in the 'parent' disciplines of child psychiatry and paediatric neurology. Readers who appreciate how little is known about the classification, aetiology, course and management of child psychiatric disorders may be surprised to learn that the situation is no better for most of the common neurological disorders of childhood. The classification of seizure disorders has changed repeatedly, and the existence and nosological status of many named syndromes (such as the Lennox–Gastaut syndrome) remains controversial. The classification of cerebral palsy is also problematic. Everyone agrees that cerebral palsy should be thought of as a group of disorders rather than a single disorder, but there is much less agreement about what to include under that rubric, or how to subclassify the varieties of cerebral palsy. In these areas, paediatric neurology has lagged at least two decades behind child psychiatry in the use of epidemiological samples and multivariate statistics to refine clinical classification. Cerebral palsy also exemplifies many of the uncertainties in paediatric neurology about aetiology, course and management. What causes cerebral palsy? What becomes of children with cerebral palsy when they grow up? Is very intensive physiotherapy more effective than less intensive alternatives? None of these questions can be answered satisfactorily at present.

This dismal account of the state of paediatric neurology is not the whole story. In some areas, much has already been learned and progress is rapid. This is true, for example, of the biochemistry and molecular genetics of many neurodegenerative and neuromuscular disorders. However, most of these disorders are rare and advances in the assessment and management of common neurological and neurosurgical problems are less impressive. In this context, it is bound to be difficult to make sense of the links between brain and behavioural problems in childhood. For example, given the crude and changing classifications of both psychiatric disorders and epilepsy, it is obviously harder to examine the psychiatric correlates of epilepsy. These difficulties are not mentioned to discourage readers, but to put them on their guard against simplistic conclusions drawn from inadequate data.

Brain damage?

This chapter is deliberately entitled 'brain disorders' rather than 'brain damage'. The term 'damage' suggests that the brain was developing normally until something happened to damage it. This is accurate in some instances: athetoid cerebral palsy following rhesus haemolytic disease; hydrocephalus following tuberculous meningitis; epilepsy following a penetrating head injury; and so on. In other instances, however, brain development may have been abnormal from the beginning, rather than proceeding normally until derailed by some insult. Brain abnormalities can be caused by inherited disorders, new mutations and chromosomal aberrations. The power of language is such that an ill-chosen term, such as 'brain damage', can seriously distort clinical and scientific reasoning. Once children with cerebral palsy or mental retardation are labelled as 'brain damaged', parents and researchers tend to assume that the cause must be some insult, such as a difficult birth, and the possible role of genetically or chromosomally determined malformations tends to be forgotten. As far as the common brain disorders in childhood are concerned, we do not even know if acquired or intrinsic aetiologies are more important.

Another disadvantage of the term 'brain damage' is that it suggests permanence to anyone who has been taught that the brain cannot regenerate lost or damaged parts. This connotation of irreversibility is potentially misleading (see also Rutter, Chapter 19). For example, children do commonly grow out of epilepsy and may even grow out of cerebral palsy (Taudorf *et al.* 1986). In some instances, reversible brain disorders may arise not from fixed abnormalities of neuronal organization but from delayed or precocious neuronal maturation. It is plausible but unproven, for instance, that transient childhood epilepsy reflects temporarily delayed development of inhibitory neurotransmitter systems, or prematurely accelerated development of excitatory systems. Once again, 'damage' is too narrow a concept to embrace all possible brain disorders.

Birth damage

The best known 'brain damage' theories are those that

emphasize birth damage. Generations of medical students have been taught that cerebral palsy, epilepsy and severe learning difficulties (mental retardation) are commonly caused by perinatal complications. This view is almost certainly false. Obstetric and neonatal complications are common but are generally innocuous. Thus, in one study based on detailed records, over half the *normal* controls had experienced one such complication (Jacobsen & Kinney 1980).

Even severe perinatal complications are usually harmless. In one prospective study, for example, children who had an Apgar score of 3 or less at 5 min after birth were roughly 30 times more likely to be neurologically normal at the age of 7 years than to have cerebral palsy (Freeman & Nelson 1988). The same study showed that only 21% of children with cerebral palsy had at least one of three markers suggestive of birth asphyxia (Nelson & Ellenberg 1986). Even among the children with cerebral palsy who did experience birth asphyxia, many had congenital malformations or microcephaly at birth, suggesting that these fetuses were already abnormal before labour began (Nelson & Ellenberg 1986). This suggestion is reinforced by Miller's (1989) study of 36 patients with ataxic cerebral palsy: 25 of these patients had multiple minor congenital anomalies, suggesting that development had already gone awry in the first half of pregnancy, and 16 of these 25 also experienced perinatal or early postnatal complications.

Because the fetus is an active participant in the delivery process, and not simply a passive passenger who is expelled when his or her time is up, it is not surprising that an abnormal fetus is particularly liable to an abnormal birth. It is possible that perinatal complications compound whatever damage has already occurred prenatally, just as labour may compound the existing damage in spina bifida (Luthy *et al.* 1991). Alternatively, perinatal complications may simply be harmless markers for an abnormal fetus. This 'harmless marker' possibility is supported by findings that cerebral palsy rates in children born at term have been fairly steady over the recent past, despite major advances in perinatal management and a dramatic fall in perinatal mortality (Paneth & Kiely 1984; Hagberg *et al.* 1996). If perinatal complications commonly converted normal or vulnerable fetuses into children with cerebral palsy, improvements in obstetrics and neonatal paediatrics should have resulted in a clear fall in the rate of cerebral palsy — and this does not seem to have occurred.

Although this account has focused on the extent to which birth complications are largely irrelevant to cerebral palsy, probably accounting for fewer than 10% of cases (Nelson & Ellenberg 1986), similar considerations may apply to severe learning difficulties (mental retardation). Thus, Rantakallio & von Wendt (1985) described a high rate of perinatal complications in children whose severe learning difficulties were genetic or chromosomal in origin. Had the prenatal origin not been established in these cases, it is easy to imagine that the perinatal complications would have been blamed for the learning difficulties. For epilepsy too, prenatal risk factors seem far more important than perinatal risk factors (Wallace 1992).

These new views on the relationship between birth complications and brain damage are clearly relevant to obstetricians, paediatricians and their lawyers. The findings also carry two important lessons for child psychiatrists. First, neurological theories about aetiology are as error-prone as psychiatric theories — psychiatrists should not be too willing to take neurological theories on trust simply because neurology is a high-status discipline. Secondly, if birth complications are not common causes of overt brain disorders, such as cerebral palsy, it is even less likely that birth complications commonly result in 'minimal brain damage' manifesting solely in behavioural or learning difficulties. Child psychiatrists who make detailed enquiries about obstetric and neonatal complications will often elicit positive histories from the parents of their patients (as they would from the parents of normal children). This information may be clinically useful, e.g. when it reveals that the father blames the mother for their child's behavioural problems because she chose to have an epidural and this made a forceps delivery necessary. It is important that child psychiatrists do not fall into the same sort of trap, pinning the blame on birth complications without scientific justification. The combination of birth complications and psychiatric problems will often occur by chance because both are common in the general population.

Is there any truth in the notion of 'minimal brain damage'? Do birth complications sometimes cause brain damage that results in psychiatric symptoms but no neurological signs? There is no reason to suppose that this sort of causal link is at all common (Goodman 1993), except in the special case of children born very prematurely. Follow-up studies of children born weighing less than 1500 g show that even when those with overt neurological disorders are excluded, there is a consistently higher rate of attention deficit hyperactivity disorder (ADHD), with less evidence for an increase in the rate of conduct or emotional disorders (Breslau 1995; Chapieski & Evankovich 1997; Wolke 1998). The increased rate of ADHD primarily reflects problems with inattention rather than with hyperactivity or associated behavioural problems (Wolke 1998). Szatmari *et al.* (1993) suggest that the excess of ADHD is entirely explained by the lower IQ of very prematurely born children; the children are no more inattentive than would be expected for their IQ. By contrast, the findings of Whitaker *et al.* (1997) suggest that the excess of ADHD is only partly explained by the link with lower IQ; after adjusting for gender and social disadvantage, very prematurely born children of normal intelligence had elevated rates of ADHD as well as tics and separation anxiety. Studies using neonatal ultrasound scans have shown that the periventricular white matter damage that particularly commonly occurs in children born before 28 weeks' gestation is strongly associated with subsequent cognitive and psychiatric problems, even when the children do not develop overt neurological disorders (Whitaker *et al.* 1996, 1997). When the white matter damage in very prematurely born children results in cerebral palsy, this is associated with an especially high risk of comorbid psychiatric problems (see below).

How to recognize a hardware defect

If a computer is not working properly, three sorts of explanation need to be considered:

1 the computer is being used inappropriately;

2 there is a 'software' problem in the way the computer has been programmed; or

3 there is a 'hardware' fault in the electronic circuits.

Although the analogy is crude, three similar sorts of explanation need to be considered, singly or in combination, for a child's psychiatric problems:

1 the child's social world is making inappropriate demands on him or her;

2 the child has learned or internalized maladaptive ways of being in the world; or

3 the child has an abnormal brain.

This is an oversimplification, of course, but it is a useful starting point. Parents and professionals have a shared interest in establishing how far a child's problems can be attributed to underlying 'hardware' defects in the child's brain. The issue is potentially relevant to further investigations, referral to a paediatrician or paediatric neurologist, prognosis and treatment—not to mention the question of blame. There are several sorts of pointers to a hardware defect. Some of these pointers are persuasive while others are best ignored. In a rough and ready sort of way, it is worth distinguishing between six sorts of pointers.

1 Brain abnormalities are most convincingly inferred from the sorts of evidence acquired in a standard neurological assessment, e.g. a clear-cut history of seizures, the signs of a spastic diplegia, an unequivocally abnormal electroencephalogram (EEG), or a focal lesion on computed tomography (CT) or magnetic resonance imaging (MRI) scanning.

2 Less weight can be placed on 'soft neurological signs' (mostly reflecting immature motor development), abnormal neuropsychological profiles, or abnormalities of derived neurophysiological measures. In each case, abnormalities add extra weight to the suspicion that something is wrong with the child, but these abnormalities do not prove that the something is the child's brain (Goodman 1993).

3 Brain abnormalities may also be inferred from a history of exposure to the sorts of insults that can damage the brain, e.g. a head injury, an encephalitic illness or high-dose cranial irradiation. There are several potential problems with this sort of inference. First, some members of a high-risk group may escape unscathed. Secondly, changes in behaviour after a potential brain insult may be mediated by maladaptive parental responses (such as overprotectiveness or inconsistent discipline) rather than by biological damage. After mild head injuries, for example, the increased rate of child psychiatric disorders seems to owe more to disrupted parenting than to acquired brain damage (Hjern & Nylander 1964). Finally, when risk factors for brain injury are associated with psychiatric problems, it may be unclear what is cause and what is effect. For example, it is equally plausible a priori that head injury leads to hyperactivity, that hy-peractivity and impulsiveness lead to head injury, or that some third factor, such as psychosocial disadvantage, independently predisposes a child to both head injury and hyperactivity.

4 There is accumulating evidence that genetic factors play an important part in at least some child psychiatric disorders (Rutter et al. 1999; see McGuffin & Rutter, Chapter 12). Although this genetic liability may be mediated by an inherited hardware fault in the child's brain, this is not necessarily the case. In a prejudiced society, for example, genes for skin pigmentation, short stature or adiposity may be risk factors for peer rejection, low self-esteem, and secondary behavioural problems that have nothing to do with brain abnormalities.

5 When a child develops psychiatric problems despite apparently favourable home and school circumstances, it is tempting to suppose that the child's problems are biological in origin. This is a very weak argument. Until relatively recently, this sort of argument led to the consequences of child sexual abuse being attributed to constitutional factors in the child. Absence of proof of psychosocial causation is not proof of absence.

6 The presence of a specific behavioural syndrome is sometimes taken as suggestive or even sufficient evidence that the child has an abnormal brain. This is rarely warranted because few behavioural syndromes are commonly associated with *independent* evidence of underlying brain abnormalities—the exceptions being progressive dementia, severe learning difficulties (mental retardation), and perhaps autism. Inferring 'minimal brain damage' or 'minimal cerebral dysfunction' from common child psychiatric problems is currently no more than an exercise in faulty reasoning. Thus, although it is true, as described later in this chapter, that neurologically impaired children are particularly prone to hyperactivity, it does not necessarily follow that all hyperactive children have brain damage. (Consider the logic of: people with strokes are prone to limp, so anyone with a limp must be suffering from a stroke or a 'minimal stroke'.)

Given the potential difficulties in deciding whether or not a child does have a hardware defect, the following sections on the links between brain and behavioural problems are based on studies of children with the best authenticated brain abnormalities, as established by the first set of criteria on the preceding list.

Brain disorders increase the risk of child psychiatric disorders

The neuropsychiatric component of the classical Isle of Wight epidemiological study showed that brain disorders are powerful risk factors for psychiatric disorders: the rates of psychiatric disorders were 44% among children with structural brain disorders and 29% among children with idiopathic epilepsy, as compared with just 12% among children with non-cerebral physical disorders and 7% among children free from physical disorders (Rutter et al. 1970). The finding that cerebral disorders carry a much higher psychiatric risk than non-cerebral disorders strongly suggests direct brain–behaviour links in addition to the risks attendant on any chronic or stigmatizing disorder. This conclusion was supported by a companion study (Seidel *et al.* 1975) that compared children who had cerebral disorders with a matched group of children disabled by other disorders (mainly musculoskeletal). The children with cerebral disorders were twice as likely to have psychiatric problems, even though children with an IQ of under 70 were excluded from both groups, and the two groups were well matched for social background and degree of physical incapacity. Many other studies have since confirmed that psychiatric problems are more likely to result from brain disorders than from other physical disorders (Breslau 1985; Howe *et al.* 1993; Austin *et al.* 1996). Different brain disorders increase psychiatric risk to different extents, e.g. the higher risk associated with structural brain disorders than with idiopathic epilepsy in the Isle of Wight study.

Although the evidence that brain abnormalities increase the risk of child psychiatric disorders is persuasive, it is important to remember not only that many children with brain disorders are free from psychiatric problems, but also that the great majority of children with psychiatric problems are free from overt brain disorders. In the Isle of Wight study, for example, 65% of the children with cerebral palsy or epilepsy had no psychiatric disorders, and fewer than 10% of the children with psychiatric disorders also had definite brain disorders (as judged by the presence of epilepsy, severe mental retardation, cerebral palsy and related disorders).

At risk for which psychiatric disorders?

There is a long-running controversy about the extent to which brain disorders are specific risk factors for particular sorts of psychiatric problems, as opposed to non-specific risk factors for all types of psychiatric problems. It is now clear that the truth lies between these two extremes: brain disorders increase the risk of most psychiatric problems, but not to the same extent. For example, hyperkinesis was particularly over-represented among children with cerebral palsy or epilepsy in the Isle of Wight study (Rutter *et al.* 1970). Thus, while the overall prevalence of psychiatric disorders was about seven times higher in children with brain disorders than in neurologically intact children, the prevalence of hyperkinesis was about 90 times higher. The conclusion that neurological factors do influence the type of psychiatric disorder is supported by numerous studies reporting associations between particular brain abnormalities and specific psychiatric disorders, e.g. between tuberous sclerosis and pervasive developmental disorders (Hunt & Dennis 1987; Hunt & Shepherd 1993), between Sydenham's chorea and obsessive-compulsive disorder (Swedo *et al.* 1989; Asbahr *et al.* 1998), between developmental abnormalities of the temporal lobe and schizophrenia (Taylor 1975; Ounsted *et al.* 1987), and between hemiplegic (but not diplegic) cerebral palsy and hyperkinesis (Ingram 1955). When the neurological disorder is genetic, as in the case of tuberous sclerosis, the associated psychiatric problems are increasingly referred to as part of the 'behavioural phenotype'

of the underlying genetic disorder (see Skuse & Kuntsi, Chapter 13)—a term that would be misleading if it was taken to refer to an invariable link rather than some degree of statistical association.

Left vs. right hemisphere syndromes?

As asymmetrical specialization of the two cerebral hemispheres is evident in early childhood and even in prenatal life (Goodman 1994), it is certainly plausible that unilateral brain disorders could have different effects on the rate and type of associated psychiatric disorder depending on which side of the brain is affected. Such laterality differences have indeed been reported, but these positive reports have typically derived from small series of children, often attending specialized clinics. Such reports may well be capitalizing on the effects of chance in small and atypical samples—a possibility that is rendered all the more plausible by the contradictory nature of these reports. Thus, while Voeller (1986) described a high rate of hyperactivity in children with right-sided lesions, Stores (1977) reported that boys (but not girls) were more likely to be hyperactive if they had left-sided epileptic foci. Similarly, while Sollee & Kindlon (1987) found an association between left hemisphere lesions and externalizing problems, Nass & Koch (1987) found an association between right hemisphere lesions and the sort of difficult temperament associated with later conduct problems.

Studies of larger or more representative samples have not generally suggested any laterality effects on child psychopathology. Thus, the rate of hyperactivity was not influenced by the laterality of lesion in several large studies of children with brain disorders (Ingram 1955, 1956; Ounsted 1955; Rutter *et al.* 1970; Uvebrant 1988). A study of 98 children with localized brain injury caused by penetrating head injuries did not find an association between laterality of lesion and liability to any type of psychopathology (Rutter *et al.* 1984). Goodman *et al.* studied an epidemiological sample of over 400 children with left- or right-sided hemiplegias, all of whom were assessed by behaviour questionnaires, and 149 of whom were assessed by detailed parent and child interviews. The rate of psychiatric problems in this group was high but did not vary significantly by laterality (Goodman & Graham 1996). Neither did laterality of lesion influence the type of psychopathology as judged by a variety of dimensional and categorical measures (Goodman & Yude 1997). Children with left- and right-sided hemiplegias did not differ on measures of affective or interpersonal problems (including autistic problems), contrary to the results of several small studies that have linked developmental lesions of the right (or non-dominant) hemisphere with persistent affective or interpersonal difficulties (Weintraub & Mesulam 1983; Voeller 1986; Sollee & Kindlon 1987). The absence of laterality effects in childhood hemiplegia is evident in the cognitive as well as the psychiatric domain. Whereas damage to the left hemisphere in adult life is specifically linked to verbal deficits, and adult-onset damage to the right hemisphere is specifically linked to visuospatial deficits, comparable unilateral damage sustained early in life does not have laterality-specific effects on memory or intelligence (Vargha-Khadem *et al.* 1992; Goodman & Yude 1996).

Is there any strong evidence that the laterality of childhood brain disorders can influence psychiatric consequences? The best evidence for such an effect comes from studies linking temporal lobe epilepsy in childhood with subsequent psychosis in adult life. Although the literature is contradictory, there is growing evidence that adults with schizophrenia have structural and functional abnormalities that are more prominent in the left cerebral hemisphere, including tissue loss in the left temporal lobe (Gur & Chin 1999; Highley *et al.* 1999; Petty 1999). In line with this, children with temporal lobe epilepsy seem more likely to develop schizophrenia in adult life if their temporal lobe lesion is on the left rather than the right (Taylor 1975; Ounsted *et al.* 1987).

In summary, early brain lesions probably can have side-specific psychiatric consequences, but these seem to be the exception rather than the rule. Further advances in this field will probably depend on studies that correlate psychopathology with detailed information from structural and functional brain scans, while avoiding the trap of extrapolating from small or unrepresentative groups of patients.

How do neurological and non-neurological risk factors interact?

As described in the rest of this volume, a multitude of psychosocial and genetic factors influence a child's liability to psychiatric disorders. How do these 'ordinary' risk factors interact with neurological risk factors? The first point to note is that children with brain disorders are not generally immune to ordinary risk factors. In the Isle of Wight study, for example, children with brain disorders were more likely to have a psychiatric problem if they also came from a 'broken home' or had an emotionally disturbed mother (Rutter *et al.* 1970). The most obvious explanation for this finding is that parental discord or distress resulted in child psychiatric problems, although a plausible alternative is that neurologically determined behavioural problems in the child had an adverse impact on the parents' marriage and mental state. The direction of causality is clearer in the prospective study of childhood head injury carried out by Rutter *et al.* (1984). Although the severity of head injury was the most powerful single predictor of whether a child would develop a psychiatric problem, ordinary risk factors were also influential. Thus, considering just children with severe head injuries, new psychiatric disorders developed in 60% of children who also experienced high levels of psychosocial adversity, but only in 14% of the children who experienced low levels of psychosocial adversity. In this instance, the child's behavioural problems could not have created the psychosocial adversity because the presence or absence of adversity predated both the head injury and the psychiatric problem.

There is one instance in which the presence of brain disorders may 'override' an ordinary risk factor for child psychiatric problems. Among prepubertal children without neurological problems, boys are at considerably greater psychiatric risk than girls (Rutter *et al.* 1975). This male vulnerability is not evident in several studies of children with brain disorders. Psychiatric disorder was equally common in the two sexes in the Isle of Wight sample of children with brain disorders (Rutter *et al.* 1970), and in a sample of children followed prospectively after a severe head injury (Rutter *et al.* 1984). Similarly, the rate of autism in tuberous sclerosis seems to be roughly equal in boys and girls (Hunt & Shepherd 1993).

If a child's liability to psychiatric problems can be increased both by brain abnormalities and by ordinary risk factors, it is important to consider whether neurological and non-neurological risk factors act independently or synergistically. For the sake of clarity, it is worth distinguishing between 'vulnerability' and 'separate paths' models, although hybrid models are certainly plausible. According to the vulnerability model, neurological abnormalities are relatively or totally innocuous on their own, but amplify the effects of any coexistent non-neurological risk factors. By contrast, the separate paths model suggests that there are independent routes into psychiatric disorder: neurological routes that are unaffected by the presence or absence of additional psychosocial or genetic adversity; and non-neurological routes that are unaffected by the presence or absence of brain abnormalities. In statistical terms, the vulnerability model predicts a significant additive interaction between neurological and non-neurological risk factors, whereas the separate paths model variables predicts separate main effects without an interaction. While there is growing evidence for the separate paths model (Breslau 1990; Whitaker *et al.* 1997), it would be premature to write off the notion that brain abnormalities sometimes act as risk multipliers rather than as risks in themselves.

Our current understanding of the interaction of neurological and ordinary risk factors suggests two lessons for clinicians. First, because children with brain disorders are not immune to ordinary risk factors, the rate of psychiatric problems in this high-risk group could be reduced by tackling coexistent risk factors, such as parental discord or inadequate supervision. Secondly, if there is any truth in the separate paths model, some children with brain disorders will develop psychiatric problems even in the most favourable of environments. Clinicians who bear this in mind will often be able to reassure parents and teachers who blame themselves for not having done enough to prevent the emergence of psychiatric problems. Families and schools who are doing a good enough job with an extremely challenging group of children deserve to feel admired rather than blamed.

What are the mediating links?

Establishing that children with brain disorders have strikingly high rates of psychiatric problems should be the beginning

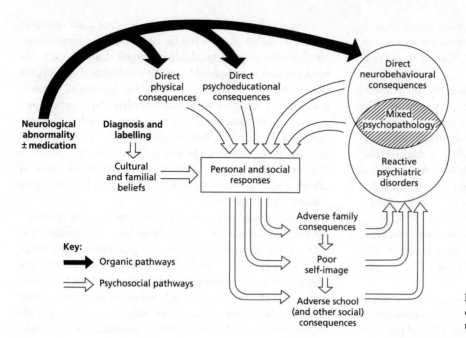

Fig. 14.1 A simplified representation of organic and psychosocial pathways from brain to behavioural abnormalities.

rather than the end of neuropsychiatric inquiry. All too often, however, neuropsychiatrists have been content to call a halt to their inquiries once they have demonstrated that brain–behaviour links exist. This is particularly unfortunate because a better understanding of the mediating mechanisms would be of great theoretical and practical interest. From a theoretical point of view, the links between brain and behavioural disorders in childhood potentially provide a unique window on the biological determinants of psychological development. From a practical point of view, we need to know much more about mediating processes if we are to prevent or treat psychiatric disorders in neurologically impaired children. Imagine, for example, that the main reason brain disorder X leads to psychiatric problems is because it results in specific learning problems that engender marked frustration with schooling, leading on to defiant and disruptive behaviour in class. Imagine also that brain disorder Y leads to psychiatric problems largely as a result of inducing parental overprotectiveness and inconsistent discipline. To be as effective as possible, preventative efforts should mainly be school-based for disorder X but home-based for disorder Y. There are multitudes of possible links between neurological and psychiatric problems, and until we know how to identify the major links for any particular child or group of children, we will misdirect much of our preventative and curative effort.

Given the current dearth of relevant studies, this account of the mediating processes has had to be based largely on clinical plausibility. Before considering the ways in which brain disorders may result in psychiatric problems, it is worth reiterating that just because a child has both neurological and psychiatric problems, it does not necessarily follow that the neurological problems caused the psychiatric problems. It is possible that the two sets of problems are a coincidence, e.g. the child's psychi-

atric problems may be attributable to school stresses that are unrelated to the child's brain disorder. Alternatively, the two sets of problems may reflect a common origin, e.g. the child's head injury and conduct disorder may both be attributable to inadequate parental supervision. Finally, the psychiatric problem may have caused the neurological problem, e.g. when a child with hyperkinesis impulsively runs into the road, gets hit by a car, and ends up with permanent brain damage as a result. With these reservations, it is now appropriate to consider those instances in which the child's brain disorder will have played some direct or indirect part in the origin of the concomitant psychiatric problems. For the sake of clarity, it is helpful to distinguish between the organic and psychosocial consequences of a brain disorder (see Fig. 14.1), acknowledging that these consequences are often intimately interrelated and that the distinction is sometimes impossible in practice.

The organic consequences of a brain disorder may be evident in the physical, psycho-educational and neurobehavioural domains. Physical disabilities, ranging from easy fatigability to lack of independent mobility, may have an indirect impact on psychological well-being, e.g. by influencing self-esteem or peer relationships. In many cases, the treatments of physical problems have their own psychological costs. Children may spend many hours each week in physiotherapy (sacrificing time when they could have been playing and occasioning 'I don't want to' battles), and some children experience repeated hospital admissions, with their attendant separations and disruptions.

Specific learning problems and below-average intelligence are common psycho-educational consequences of brain abnormalities (Rutter *et al.* 1970; Goodman & Yude 1996; Frampton *et al.* 1998). This probably reflects a direct link between brain disorders and impaired cognitive processing, although the situation is sometimes aggravated by restricted educational opportunities, lower expectations and lengthy absences from school for therapy or operations. For children with epilepsy, cognitive and scholastic skills can be disrupted not only by their clinical and subclinical seizures, but also by the effects of their antiepileptic medication (see below).

The evidence that brain disorders lead directly to some types of childhood psychopathology is largely circumstantial. First, there are adult parallels for direct brain–behaviour links (Lishman 1998), and even some animal models (Robinson 1979). Secondly, various medications have an adverse impact on children's behaviour, e.g. barbiturates on activity and attention control (Ounsted 1955). Thirdly, organic links seem to provide the best explanation for the wide variety of specific neuropsychiatric associations in childhood, such as the association between Prader–Willi syndrome and characteristic sleep and appetite problems, or the association between Lesch–Nyhan syndrome and severe self-injury (see Skuse & Kuntsi, Chapter 13).

Brain disorders can lead to a multitude of adverse psychosocial consequences. Physical disabilities can result in teasing, poor self-image and reduced opportunities for peer interaction. Repeated hospitalizations may disrupt friendships and predispose to behavioural disorders, perhaps as a result of repeated separations from family. Specific learning problems and low intelligence are associated with a much higher rate of psychiatric problems in children with brain disorders, just as they are in ordinary children (Rutter *et al.* 1970; Goodman & Graham 1996; Frampton *et al.* 1998). There are several possible reasons for this association, including the frustration engendered by school failure, and its impact on self-esteem. If brain abnormalities do have organic neurobehavioural consequences, such as hyperkinesis or an impaired ability to decipher social and emotional cues, then these organic consequences may, in turn, have adverse effects on family relationships and friendship patterns. The beliefs and attitudes of the family and the wider social world also have a major impact. Parents, teachers and peers respond to a neurologically impaired child in the light of their beliefs and prejudices about 'brain damaged' children. These beliefs influence the likelihood of overprotection, peer rejection and unrealistic expectations. Beliefs can also interfere with parents' abilities to set limits to unacceptable behaviours. This can happen, for example, if parents assume that all bad behaviour is neurologically driven and beyond the child's control, or if they fear that any reproof will trigger off an epileptic seizure and further damage the child's brain. Family relationships can be disrupted for other reasons too. Sibling rivalry, for example, can be fuelled by the resentment of disabled children who see themselves being overtaken by younger siblings, or by the resentment of non-disabled siblings who feel they are missing out on parental attention. These are only a few of the many possible psychosocial pathways from brain disorders to child psychiatric problems. Others are well described, with a wealth of case histories, in Taylor's (1989) account of the psychosocial consequences of childhood epilepsy.

It is one thing to describe a mixture of organic and psychosocial pathways from neurological abnormalities to psychiatric disorder, and it is quite another thing to establish the importance of any given pathway in practice. There are disappointingly few good studies in this area, but relevant research strategies can be summarized fairly briefly (with a more detailed account available in Goodman 1993). If we want to establish whether factor X (e.g. marital breakdown, self-esteem, friendships) is an important mediating link between neurological and psychiatric disorders in childhood, several research strategies are available. The most basic strategy, although it is sometimes overlooked, is to establish whether factor X is more common in a representative sample of children with some particular brain disorder than in the general child population. Thus, several studies suggest that the parents of children with chronic physical disorders are *not* at increased risk of marital breakdown (Sabbeth & Leventhal 1984), making it most unlikely that the high rate of psychiatric disorder in neurologically impaired children can be attributed to a high rate of marital breakdown brought on by the strains of looking after a disabled child.

If factor X *is* more common in a neurologically impaired group, the next step is to examine whether factor X predicts which neurologically impaired children will also develop a psychiatric problem. Once again, the answers may be surprising. There is no convincing evidence, for example, that a high level of physical disability increases the risk of psychiatric problems within a neurologically impaired group (Rutter *et al.* 1970; Seidel *et al.* 1975). By contrast, not only are specific reading retardation and low IQ particularly common among children with brain disorders, but these children with additional learning problems are at considerably greater psychiatric risk (Rutter *et al.* 1970; Goodman & Graham 1996; Frampton *et al.* 1998). When factor X does predict psychiatric risk, multivariate statistical techniques can be used to quantify the possible importance of X as a mediating factor (Breslau 1985). However, it is important to remember that even strong associations are not proof of causation. The presence of factor X may be a consequence rather than a cause of psychiatric disorder, or some third factor may independently increase both X and psychiatric disorder (so that X is a marker for the mediating process rather than the mediator itself).

Longitudinal studies provide a valuable research strategy for investigating the causal mechanisms underlying cross-sectional associations. For example, findings from a longitudinal study of children with hemiplegic cerebral palsy suggested that adverse family factors, including low parental warmth or marital discord, were more likely to be consequences than causes of the child's psychiatric problems (Goodman 1998). The level of adverse family factors initially did not independently predict whether that child would have improved or deteriorated at follow-up. Intervention studies could also be powerful research strategies for investigating the causal mechanisms underlying brain–behaviour links—although this potential has hardly been tapped in developmental neuropsychiatry to date.

Psychiatric consequences of specific brain disorders

Turning from the general to the particular, the following sections review a range of childhood brain disorders from a psychiatric perspective. It is obviously impossible to cover the whole of paediatric neurology and neurosurgery in a few pages; disorders have been selected on the basis of frequency, severity or particular relevance to child psychiatry. The main clinical features of each disorder are reviewed along with the psychiatric consequences. Readers who want to learn more about specific aspects of paediatric neurology are recommended to turn to Aicardi *et al.* (1998), Brett (1997) or Menkes (1995) for succinct, readable and well-referenced accounts.

Childhood dementias and other conditions involving the loss of skills

A variety of dementing disorders present in childhood with an insidious loss of skills, often accompanied by rather non-specific psychiatric problems. Child psychiatrists have a key part to play in recognizing these disorders at an early stage so that the child can be referred to a paediatric neurologist for detailed assessment. In disorders such as Wilson disease where there is a specific treatment, delayed diagnosis and treatment can result in unnecessary and irreversible damage. In most childhood dementias there is no specific treatment—but that does not mean that delayed diagnosis is trivial. Until the organic basis is recognized, the child's problems may be blamed on his or her laziness, or on parental mishandling, causing unnecessary anguish and subsequent guilt or anger. Occasionally, prompter diagnosis and genetic counselling would have averted the birth of a second affected child. Finally, once the diagnosis has been made, a child psychiatrist may be able to offer useful help to the child, the parents, and the siblings—and this help is much more likely to be accepted if the child psychiatrist referred the case on for physical investigation at an early stage.

Although desirable, prompt recognition of a dementing disorder is undoubtedly difficult. Normal development often involves some degree of 'two steps forward, one step back'; many children revert to more babyish ways when physically ill or under stress; and almost any child psychiatric disorder can interfere with concentration or application at school, leading to a falling off in classroom performance. Even when there is a marked loss of skills in several areas, the cause may be psychosocial rather than organic. For example, Brown & Perkins (1989) described child sexual abuse presenting with marked loss of skills. The presence of psychosocial or organic risk factors can sometimes be misleading in individual cases. For example, the children of prostitutes or drug addicts are clearly at psychiatric risk for psychosocial reasons, but they are also at risk of HIV infection and its associated dementia (see Havens *et al.*, Chapter 49). Conversely, because the children of patients with Huntington disease have a 50% chance of carrying the gene themselves, psychiatric problems in these children could be caused by early

onset Huntington disease—but the problems could also be caused by the abuse, neglect and disorganization that are common in affected families (Dewhurst *et al.* 1970; Folstein *et al.* 1983). In practice, an organic cause needs to be considered (and appropriate referrals or investigations initiated) when the child meets one or more of the following three criteria.

1 Progressive loss of well-established linguistic, academic or self-help skills—with performance being well below previous levels even when the child seems content, motivated and not preoccupied. Psychometric testing is sometimes helpful, particularly if repeated measures are available (Lobascher & Cavanagh 1980).

2 Emergence of other features suggestive of a brain disorder, such as seizures, evidence of visual impairment, tremor or postural disturbance.

3 Risk factors for relevant genetic or infectious diseases, e.g. father with Huntington disease, mother with AIDS.

Clinicians who make a practice of reviewing their initial diagnostic formulation at regular intervals will be less likely to miss insidiously progressive disorders that initially present with apparently straightforward psychiatric symptoms. The following are the dementing disorders that are most likely to present to child psychiatrists.

Batten disease

Batten disease (which is also known as neuronal ceroid lipofuscinosis) refers to a group of inherited neurodegenerative disorders, most of which are autosomal recessive. Child psychiatrists are most likely to encounter children with the juvenile form, which is the most common neurodegenerative disorder of childhood, affecting up to 1 in 25 000 births. Patients usually present with visual failure at age 5–7 years but disease does not generally result in obvious dementia for a further few years. If no cause is initially found for the visual failure, the child may be referred for psychiatric assessment of 'hysterical' blindness. Alternatively, if the visual impairment is attributed to a non-progressive cause, psychiatric referral may occur several years later when deteriorating schoolwork and non-specific behavioural problems (such as disruptive and aggressive behaviour) are mistakenly attributed to the psychological consequences of blindness or family stresses. Seizures may occur fairly early in the disorder, but the emergence of hard neurological signs is usually a late feature. Exceptionally, dementia and seizures may be the presenting features without any visual failure (Scully *et al.* 1978). The gene has now been located (Mole & Gardiner 1999). Blood tests can be used to diagnose the disorder and carrier status.

Wilson disease

Wilson disease is an autosomal recessive disorder of copper metabolism. As a rule of thumb, children presenting before the age of 10 years do so with progressive liver failure, whereas children presenting after the age of 10 years do so with neurological features, insidious dementia, or non-specific emotional or behavioural problems. Early neurological features include extrapyramidal and cerebellar signs. Dystonic movements and postures can be bizarre, unilateral and exacerbated by stress—so misdiagnosis as conversion hysteria is all too easy. The child's writing may change to a crabbed Parkinsonian style, or may provide evidence of involuntary jerks of the pen. Urinary copper is high, while plasma copper and caeruloplasmin are both low. Ophthalmological examination with a slit lamp may reveal the pathognomonic Kayser–Fleischer ring on the iris. Liver biopsy is necessary in doubtful cases. The disorder can be treated successfully by copper chelation, with earlier treatment resulting in a better outcome.

Huntington disease

Huntington disease is an autosomal dominant disorder that typically presents with chorea and dementia in mid-adult life. The disorder has its onset in childhood in about 5–10% of cases, with early onset cases more often having an affected father than an affected mother. Chorea may occur but a rigid Parkinsonian picture is more common. Epilepsy is an early feature in a substantial minority. The first presentation may be with disturbed or withdrawn behaviour, including loss of interest in games and lessons. These psychiatric features are particularly difficult to interpret in the context of the marked psychosocial disturbance that is common in families where one parent has Huntington disease (Dewhurst et al. 1970). The child's fear of developing the same disease may also be important. Just as a positive family history does not make the diagnosis, a negative family history does not rule out the diagnosis because the presence of affected relatives may be concealed, may be masked by misdiagnosis, or may not be apparent as a result of 'non-paternity'. CT or MRI scanning may demonstrate caudate atrophy, and positron emission tomography (PET) scans may show caudate hypometabolism. The disorder is caused by an unstable expansion of a CAG trinucleotide repeat in a gene on chomosome 4 (DiFiglia 2000). The normal number of repeats is between 6 and 34, with more than 37 resulting in a mutated protein product. More trinucleotide repeats result in earlier onset: childhood onset is associated with 55 or more repeats. A simple DNA test can now confirm the presence of the expanded repeat. Harper & Clarke (1990) have discussed some of the ethical issues involved in predictive DNA testing of children.

Adrenoleucodystrophy

Adrenoleucodystrophy is an X-linked recessive disorder. The most characteristic presentation is a combination of adrenal insufficiency, progressive dementia and neurological features. However, even within the same family the presentation can be very variable, with adrenal failure predominating in some affected boys and dementia and neurological features predominating in others. Problems with restlessness, poor coordination, disruptiveness and deteriorating school progress are often the earliest manifestations. Psychotic symptoms may also be prominent (Corbett et al. 1977). Unequivocal neurological abnormalities usually begin at 5–9 years of age, with pyramidal and extrapyramidal signs, convulsions, deafness or visual failure (sometimes caused by cortical blindness). If present, severe adrenal failure results in diarrhoea, vomiting, hypotension and pigmentation. Subtle adrenocortical insufficiency may only be evident from the results of an adrenocorticotrophic hormone (ACTH) challenge. A leucodystrophy with occipital predominance is often evident on CT scan. The combination of leucodystrophy and adrenal failure is pathognomonic. The diagnosis can be confirmed by high levels of saturated very long chain fatty acids in tissues and body fluids, and by DNA mutation analyses (Gartner et al. 1998).

Juvenile onset metachromatic leucodystrophy

Juvenile onset metachromatic leucodystrophy is an autosomal recessive disorder with an onset at 6–10 years of age. It often presents insidiously with cognitive decline, deteriorating school performance, and the emergence of oppositional, aggressive or antisocial behaviours. As the disorder progresses, the dementia worsens, Parkinsonian signs emerge, and fits may occur. Optic atrophy and visual failure are late signs. The presence of metachromatic material in the urine can be a reliable test, but the definitive diagnosis is based on markedly reduced arylsulphatase A activity in white cells or cultured fibroblasts.

Subacute sclerosing panencephalitis

Subacute sclerosing panencephalitis is a slow virus infection caused by measles virus. It is much more common after 'wild' measles (particularly if contracted during infancy) than after immunization with live attenuated measles virus. Boys are affected five times more often than girls. Onset is between 5 and 15 years, usually starting with insidious intellectual deterioration and personality change. The emergent behaviours range from irritability to withdrawal, and from defiance to inappropriate affection. Myoclonic jerks without interruption of consciousness begin several months later. Initially these jerks are infrequent and lead to occasional episodes of the child falling or staggering backwards. As the disorder progresses, the jerks become increasingly evident as shock-like movements affecting the head or the whole body, recurring every 5–20s (accompanied by characteristic periodic complexes on the EEG). These myoclonic jerks are accentuated by excitement or loud noises, and are absent in sleep. The serum and cerebrospinal fluid levels of measles antibodies are markedly elevated.

HIV encephalopathy

HIV encephalopathy may now be the most common cause of childhood dementia worldwide. Some congenitally infected children make slow developmental progress, others reach a developmental 'plateau' and fail to advance further, and yet others suffer from a true dementia, with loss of early acquired skills.

Antiretroviral therapies may halt or even reverse neurocognitive decline, although the benefits may not be sustained in the long term. The neurological and psychiatric features of congenital and acquired HIV infections are described in Brown *et al.* (2000; see also Havens *et al.*, Chapter 49).

Pervasive developmental disorders

Pervasive developmental disorders may present with loss of established skills in the domains of communication, social interaction and play—sometimes accompanied by general intellectual deterioration. Loss of skills is always present at the start of disintegrative disorder. In addition, a substantial minority of autistic children also come to medical attention after losing skills in the second year of life (Kurita 1985); such children are particularly likely to be referred to paediatric neurologists to rule out progressive neurodegenerative disorders. Clinical features supporting a pervasive developmental disorder rather than a neurodegenerative disorder include:

• the presence of subtle abnormalities in communication;
• social interaction or play *prior* to the phase when skills were lost;
• the absence of abnormalities on neurological examination and investigation; and
• a resumption of developmental progress and new learning in the months following the initial loss of skills.

The pervasive developmental disorders are described by Lord & Bailey (Chapter 38).

Rett syndrome

Rett syndrome is a progressive neurological disorder that only affects girls. After a period of normal development for the first 7–18 months, there is a phase of developmental stagnation, and then a rapid period of skill loss, commonly accompanied by screaming attacks. The disorder is described in detail in Lord & Bailey (Chapter 38).

Sanfilippo syndrome

Sanfilippo syndrome is the only mucopolysaccharidosis that commonly presents with cognitive decline and behavioural problems; the associated coarsening of the facial features is subtle and may go unnoticed because it occurs so gradually. Measuring urinary mucopolysaccharides is the simplest screening test.

Skill loss and epilepsy

As described in the following section, there are several circumstances in which epilepsy may be associated with cognitive decline. Loss of skills is prominent in some epileptic syndromes, such as the Lennox–Gastaut syndrome. In addition, potentially reversible cognitive decline can be caused by non-convulsive status epilepticus, to toxic levels of antiepileptic medication,

or to the folate deficiency induced by some antiepileptic medication.

Epilepsy

Convulsions are the most common problem encountered in paediatric neurology. Wallace (1995) provides a convenient introduction to childhood epilepsy; the three-volume textbook by Engel & Pedley (1999) provides a more detailed and densely referenced account. References are only provided in this section for topics that are not well covered in the main texts.

At least 1 child in 200 experiences repeated epileptic seizures without a detectable extracerebral cause—the usual definition of epilepsy. This definition excludes children who have hypoglycaemic seizures brought on by their diabetes, or children who have anoxic seizures as a result of faints or breath-holding attacks. The definition also excludes the 3% of preschool-age children who have one or more convulsions provoked by febrile illnesses—these febrile convulsions are generally benign, with about 98% of affected individuals *not* developing true epilepsy. Distinguishing epilepsy from other sorts of paroxysmal disorders (such as faints and parasomnias) can be surprisingly difficult, and misdiagnoses are all too common in both directions. Stores (1985) has summarized the clinical and EEG evaluation of seizures and seizure-like disorders, and has also reviewed possible confusions between sleep disorders and epilepsy (Stores 1991).

Psychiatrists may be asked to help distinguish between true seizures and pseudoseizures. This is not an easy task, particularly because most children with pseudoseizures do also suffer from true seizures, because emotional stresses can precipitate true seizures, and because many children with true epilepsy have psychiatric problems as well. Possible pointers to pseudoseizures include:

• they occur when the child is being observed but not when the child is alone;
• the onset is gradual rather than sudden;
• the paroxysm involves quivering or uncontrolled flailing rather than true clonus;
• there are theatrical semipurposive movements accompanied by loud screaming or shouting;
• painful stimuli are actively avoided during an attack and serious injury does not occur;
• the offset is sudden with an immediate return to an alert and responsive state; and
• the EEG does not show any paroxysmal discharge during an episode.

All these observations are easier to make when the child is assessed with combined EEG and video monitoring. However, none of the pointers is infallible and some sorts of true seizures (most notably frontal lobe seizures) are easily mistaken for pseudoseizures. Williams *et al.* (1978), Holmes *et al.* (1980), Goodyer (1985) and Stores (1999) have written helpful accounts of the assessment and management of pseudoseizures.

The classification of epileptic seizures and syndromes has

changed repeatedly over recent decades. In the current classification of the International League Against Epilepsy (ILAE), the most basic distinction in seizure type is between generalized and partial seizures (Commission on Classification and Terminology of the ILEA 1981, 1989). Generalized seizures are bilaterally symmetrical and the first clinical symptoms do *not* suggest a focal onset. Examples of generalized seizures include generalized tonic–clonic seizures ('grand mal'), absence seizures ('petit mal'), atypical absences, tonic seizures, atonic seizures and myoclonic seizures. In partial seizures, the first clinical symptoms *do* indicate activation of a relatively localized group of neurones, accompanied by a correspondingly localized EEG discharge. Partial seizures are further subclassified as simple or complex. In ILAE's 1969 classification (Gastaut 1970), partial seizures were described as simple when symptoms just involved elementary sensory or motor functions, and as complex when symptoms involved 'higher functions' (e.g. déjà vu, forced thinking). In ILAE's 1981 revision, however, the definition was radically changed: partial seizures were described as simple if full consciousness was retained (even if the symptoms involved 'higher functions'), and as complex if consciousness was impaired (even if the symptoms did not involve 'higher functions'). Either sort of partial seizure can evolve into generalized tonic–clonic seizures. Changes in classification make it difficult to compare studies conducted at different times. Thus studies of psychomotor epilepsy, temporal lobe epilepsy, complex partial seizures (1969 definition), and complex partial seizures (1981/1989 definition) have investigated overlapping but not identical groups of subjects, making it hard to integrate the findings of different eras.

The link between epilepsy and cognitive impairment is complex and controversial. Some of the complexities are illustrated by findings from the National Collaborative Perinatal Project (NCPP), which followed a large representative sample of children from before birth until 7 years of age (Ellenberg *et al.* 1986). When tested at 7 years, the children who had experienced one or more non-febrile seizures had an average IQ about 10 points lower than the sample average. When children with seizures were compared with siblings who had never had seizures, the difference was much less marked (4 points), and even this non-significant difference disappeared when the case–sibling comparisons were restricted to cases who appeared neurologically normal prior to the onset of seizures. When cases whose seizures began after the age of 4 years were compared with carefully matched controls, there was no evidence that the onset of seizures led to a fall in IQ by age 7. The results of this study suggest that the average IQ of children with seizures is reduced not because of the seizures themselves but because seizures are often markers either for adverse family factors, whether social or genetic, or for other neurological abnormalities. Children whose epilepsy is associated with other neurological abnormalities have a significantly lower mean IQ than children with idiopathic epilepsy (Rutter *et al.* 1970; Bourgeois *et al.* 1983). Intellectual deterioration as a direct result of the seizures themselves is probably rare, although it may sometimes

occur among the small number of children with frequent treatment-resistant seizures (Rodin 1989).

Clinical studies suggest that cognitive impairment is associated with frequent seizures, multiple seizure types, early onset and chronicity (Corbett & Trimble 1984; Farwell *et al.* 1985; Seidenberg *et al.* 1986). Two other factors are potentially relevant to cognitive impairments in children with epilepsy. First, subclinical seizure discharges in the EEG are sometimes associated with significant impairments in cognitive processing (Binnie *et al.* 1990 and Chapter 11). Secondly, antiepileptic medication may also impair cognition: phenobarbital and phenytoin are the worst offenders, while carbamazepine and sodium valproate seem less harmful, particularly when they are used singly (Cull & Trimble 1989). Folate deficiency induced by antiepileptic medication, particularly phenytoin, may also result in cognitive impairment (Corbett & Trimble 1984). Although most studies of cognition and epilepsy have focused on IQ, there is good evidence that children with seizures have a high rate of specific learning problems *after allowing for their IQ* (Rutter *et al.* 1970; Seidenberg *et al.* 1986). In the Isle of Wight study, for example, children with idiopathic epilepsy had specific reading retardation almost three times more often than children without physical disorders (Rutter *et al.* 1970).

Epilepsy in childhood is a powerful risk factor for emotional and behavioural disorders. In the Isle of Wight study (Rutter *et al.* 1970), 29% of 63 children with idiopathic epilepsy had a psychiatric disorder: four times the rate in children without physical disorders, and over twice the rate in children with physical disorders not affecting the brain. Similarly, Meltzer *et al.* (2000) reported that 37% of an epidemiological sample of schoolchildren with epilepsy had at least one psychiatric diagnosis, as compared with 10% of community controls. Although children with epilepsy have a high rate of psychiatric problems, the nature of these problems is not particularly distinctive (with a few rare exceptions, as described below). In the Isle of Wight study, over 90% of the epileptic children who had a psychiatric problem had either a conduct or an emotional disorder, or a mixture of the two (Rutter *et al.* 1970).

What factors predict which children with epilepsy develop a psychiatric disorder? One powerful predictor is the presence or absence of associated neurological abnormalities. In the Isle of Wight study, for example, psychiatric disorders were twice as common among epileptic children when there were additional neurological problems (Rutter *et al.* 1970). Similarly, in the study of temporal lobe epilepsy (TLE) carried out by Ounsted *et al.* (1966), the rate of hyperkinesis was several times more common if the TLE was secondary to a known brain insult rather than idiopathic. It is possible that many of the other predictors of psychopathology (such as frequency of seizures or presence of cognitive impairment) are primarily markers for the extensiveness of underlying brain abnormalities. The other predictors can be divided into seizure factors, medication, cognitive factors, social factors and family factors, each of which will be discussed in turn.

Possible seizure factors include type and frequency of seizures, and age of onset. As described below, TLE may be associated with a particular rate of psychiatric disorder, although the matter remains somewhat controversial. Stores (1977) reported that boys (but not girls) with TLE had more behavioural problems if the focus was in the left rather than the right hemisphere, but others have not replicated this finding (Camfield *et al.* 1984; Caplan *et al.* 1998; Schoenfeld *et al.* 1999). The existence of a link between frequent seizures and more psychopathology is also controversial, with some studies reporting such a link (Pond & Bidwell 1960; Herman *et al.* 1989; Schoenfeld *et al.* 1999) and others not (Berg *et al.* 1984; Caplan *et al.* 1998). Early onset of seizures may also be a risk factor (Pond & Bidwell 1960).

Choice of medication probably also influences psychopathology, although the evidence is surprisingly weak (Taylor 1991). Phenobarbital has been linked to a variety of behavioural problems, including aggression and hyperactivity (Ounsted 1955). Vigabatrin also seems particularly likely to result in agitation, aggression or hyperactivity—side-effects that are often reduced or abolished by lowering the dose (Luna *et al.* 1989). Polytherapy (treatment with two or more antiepileptic medications at the same time) may also increase psychiatric risk (Hermann *et al.* 1989).

Cognitive predictors of psychopathology include impaired neuropsychological functioning (Hermann 1982) and specific reading retardation (Rutter *et al.* 1970). One possible social predictor is the extent to which the child is rejected or stigmatized as a result of community prejudices about epilepsy. While there can be no doubt that such prejudices are common (Gordon & Sillanp 1997), the study of Rutter *et al.* (1970) suggests that peer rejection is more often a consequence than a cause of psychiatric problems in children with epilepsy. The link with family factors is well illustrated by Grunberg & Pond's (1957) study of children with epilepsy who did and did not have additional conduct disorders. The children with conduct disorders were much more likely to have been exposed to marital friction, disrupted care, and parental hostility or neglect, i.e. the same sorts of adverse family factors that are also associated with conduct disorders in non-epileptic children. Parental separation or divorce has also been linked to more psychopathology in children with epilepsy (Hermann *et al.* 1989). Epilepsy does not render children immune to adverse family factors, but neither does it necessarily accentuate their vulnerability to these factors. (Our current ignorance of the interaction of neurological and psychosocial risk factors is reviewed in an earlier section of this chapter.) Finally, it is worth noting that a child's epilepsy can affect the psychological well-being and coping style of other family members (Hoare 1987), and these effects potentially influence the course of the child's development.

Although child psychiatrists assess and treat children with all varieties of epilepsy, the following epileptic syndromes have behavioural correlates that are particularly relevant to psychiatrists.

Temporal lobe epilepsy

Temporal lobe epilepsy generally involves a mixture of complex partial seizures and generalized tonic–clonic seizures, combined with EEG evidence of a temporal lobe origin. The onset (aura) of seizures may involve a rising epigastric feeling or fear. Déjà vu, forced thinking, and other distortions of 'higher functions' are rare in young children. In the longitudinal clinic-based study of 100 children with TLE carried out by Ounsted *et al.* (1966, 1987), only 15% were wholly free from psychological problems in childhood, and almost half had catastrophic rage outbursts, or hyperkinesis, or both. Rutter *et al.*'s (1970) epidemiological study and Hoare's (1984) clinic-based study also found that children with TLE were at particularly high psychiatric risk (although the number of subjects in the epidemiological sample was small). By contrast, two clinic-based comparisons of children with TLE and primary generalized epilepsy suggest that the two groups may have comparable levels of psychopathology once suitable allowance had been made for confounding factors such as IQ (Whitman *et al.* 1982; Caplan *et al.* 1998). This controversy is unlikely to be resolved without a large epidemiological study.

From a psychiatric perspective, three reported features of TLE are of particular note.

1 TLE is a risk factor for a schizophrenia-like psychosis in adult life (Davison & Bagley 1969; Ounsted *et al.* 1987), perhaps particularly when the TLE arises from the left hemisphere (Taylor 1975; Perez *et al.* 1985; Ounsted *et al.* 1987). In two series of children with relatively severe TLE, 10% subsequently developed a psychosis (Ounsted *et al.* 1987; Caplan *et al.* 1998).

2 Boys whose TLE persists through puberty are more likely to be sexually indifferent during adulthood, and to remain unmarried (Taylor 1969; Ounsted *et al.* 1987).

3 Despite everything, many children with TLE and psychiatric problems grow up to be well-adjusted adults (Ounsted *et al.* 1987).

Frontal lobe epilepsy

Frontal lobe epilepsy is primarily of interest to child psychiatrists because the seizures are easily misdiagnosed as pseudoseizures or sleep disorders (Stores *et al.* 1991). Complex partial seizures arising from the frontal lobe can be very bizarre, with odd movements, postures and vocalizations. Possible features include rocking from side to side, thrashing about, making cycling movements of the legs, punching into the air, turning to one side, arching backwards, squealing, screaming, or swearing. Seizures may occur primarily or exclusively during sleep. Other clinical features that make these episodes hard to recognize as true seizures include short duration (generally under 1 min), absence of tonic–clonic movements, and abrupt termination with prompt return of responsiveness. To make matters worse, the EEG recorded between or even during seizures may be unhelpful. Combined video and EEG monitoring can be extremely useful in doubtful cases (Stores *et al.* 1991).

Infantile spasms

Infantile spasms often have psychiatric sequelae. In a typical case, runs of brief jack-knife spasms begin at about 6 months of age, accompanied by the loss of previously acquired skills and the presence of a hypsarrhythmic EEG. A cause, such as tuberous sclerosis or a major brain malformation, can be identified in most cases. Children with no identifiable cause have a better prognosis. Most affected children have severe learning difficulties (mental retardation). In a large follow-up study, Riikonen & Amnell (1981) found that serious psychiatric sequelae were common: autism was diagnosed in 12% of the sample and hyperkinesis in 23% (with considerable overlap between the two diagnoses). Using similar diagnostic criteria, Hunt *et al.* have reported considerably higher rates of autism and hyperkinesis among children whose infantile spasms were caused by tuberous sclerosis (Hunt & Dennis 1987; Hunt & Shepherd 1993). It has yet to be established how far the risk for autistic disorders stems directly from the infantile spasms themselves as opposed to specific aspects of the underlying neuropathology, e.g. presence of tubers in temporal lobes (Bolton & Griffiths 1997). Child psychiatrists should always enquire about infantile spasms when assessing children with severe learning difficulties plus autistic or hyperkinetic features. When there is a history of infantile spasms, the child should be examined particularly thoroughly for the skin signs of tuberous sclerosis—a disorder that may have important genetic implications for the family.

Lennox–Gastaut syndrome

Lennox–Gastaut syndrome accounts for about 3–10% of childhood epilepsy. There are several good paediatric reviews of the syndrome (Beaumanoir 1985a; Livingston 1988; Wheless & Constantinou 1997). Although there are continuing doubts about the nosological validity of the syndrome, both because of its heterogeneity and because typical Lennox–Gastaut syndrome grades off into a wide range of atypical variants and other syndromes, most paediatric neurologists find Lennox–Gastaut syndrome a useful diagnostic category.

The onset of Lennox–Gastaut syndrome is typically between the age of 1 and 7 years, with 'stare, jerk and fall' epilepsy, involving frequent myoclonic, tonic and atonic seizures, as well as atypical absences. Generalized tonic–clonic and partial seizures may also occur. EEG accompaniments include diffuse and irregular episodes of slow spike-waves that are more prominent in non-REM sleep (see Binnie *et al.*, Chapter 11). The great majority of affected individuals have severe learning difficulties (mental retardation). In most cases, slow development and neurological abnormalities (including infantile spasms) were evident prior to the onset of Lennox–Gastaut syndrome. In a significant minority, however, early development was normal, with marked cognitive deterioration at the onset of

Lennox–Gastaut syndrome. Incapacitating seizures often persist despite medication, and many affected children need helmets to prevent them being injured by their frequent drop attacks. Although neurological accounts mention problems with social responsiveness, attention and aggression, there have been no systematic studies of psychiatric aspects of Lennox–Gastaut syndrome. One feature of the disorder that may bring a child to psychiatric attention is a tendency to prolonged episodes of minor status. During such an episode, which may last for weeks, the child can still engage in a variety of everyday activities but may appear 'switched off', socially unresponsive, aggressive, less articulate than normal, and unusually wobbly, with minor twitching of the face and hands. If the organic basis for the episode is not recognized, the deterioration may be attributed to psychological or social factors, leading to psychiatric referral.

Landau–Kleffner syndrome

Landau–Kleffner syndrome is further discussed by Bishop (Chapter 39) and Binnie *et al.* (Chapter 11). In a typical case, a child of between 3 and 9 years of age loses receptive and expressive language skills, either suddenly or gradually. This acquired aphasia is accompanied by EEG changes, involving paroxysmal discharges that affect both hemispheres, often independently. The EEG abnormalities may be most prominent during non-REM sleep. Seizures occur in approximately 70% of cases, usually starting about the same time as the aphasia, and taking the form of generalized or simple partial seizures that are infrequent and mainly nocturnal. Seizures cease by adulthood, but the prognosis for language recovery is far more variable. It is uncertain whether the likelihood of language recovery is increased by vigorous treatment with antiepileptic medication designed to suppress EEG abnormalities. Neurosurgical treatment is potentially an option for severe and unresponsive cases. Paediatric features of Landau–Kleffner syndrome are reviewed by Beaumanoir (1985b), Gordon (1990) and Appleton (1995). Perplexity, anxiety and tantrums are common at the time of onset. In the longer term, affected children do not generally show autistic impairments in social interactions, but often show some degree of hyperactivity.

Epilepsy and CSWS

Epilepsy and continuous spike-waves during slow-wave sleep (CSWS) usually affects previously normal children, generally beginning between 2 and 9 years, and being associated with mental deterioration and behavioural disorders (Tassinari *et al.* 1985; Perez *et al.* 1993). It may be an acquired epileptic frontal lobe syndrome. Parents typically notice the behavioural deterioration before the cognitive deterioration, although it is possible that subtle neuropsychological deficits predate the emergence of psychiatric symptoms. The main psychiatric manifestations are inattention, hyperactivity, impulsiveness, aggressiveness, labile mood, disinhibition, mouthing of objects, reduced play, perseveration and lack of a sense of danger. Treatment with antiepileptic medication or corticosteroids may result in marked improvement in behaviour as well as in cognition and seizure control.

Cerebral palsy

Cerebral palsy is the single largest cause of severe physical disability in childhood. The label refers to a heterogeneous group of congenital and early acquired brain disorders that meet three criteria:

1 the disorders are chronic rather than transient;

2 the underlying brain lesions are static, although the clinical manifestations may change as the child grows up (this criterion rules out progressive neurodegenerative conditions or brain tumours); and

3 the clinical manifestations include abnormalities of motor function.

These motor defects are often accompanied by other clinical manifestations of brain abnormalities, including epilepsy, learning problems and sensory impairments.

The American term 'static encephalopathy' is roughly equivalent to cerebral palsy except that motor involvement is not obligatory. The subclassification of cerebral palsy is based on the type and distribution of motor problems, although no one scheme is entirely satisfactory. Spasticity is usually the dominant motor problem: affecting just one side of the body in spastic hemiplegia; affecting both legs to a severe extent and both arms to a mild extent in spastic diplegia; and affecting all four limbs severely in spastic quadriplegia (which is also known as tetraplegia or double hemiplegia). Less commonly, the motor problems are dominated by ataxia, or by dyskinesia (athetosis).

The aetiology of cerebral palsy is largely unknown, although there are some recognized associations: e.g. between severe rhesus disease and athetosis; between cerebrovascular accidents and hemiplegia; and between a variety of severe generalized brain insults and quadriplegia. Heredity seems particularly relevant to ataxia. Prematurity is an important risk factor for diplegia and, to a lesser extent, for other varieties of cerebral palsy too.

In the Isle of Wight study (Rutter et al. 1970), psychiatric problems were evident in almost half of the children with cerebral palsy or related disorders. The likelihood of psychiatric problems was significantly increased by two common accompaniments of cerebral palsy: low intelligence and specific reading retardation. When the child with cerebral palsy also had seizures, the rate of psychiatric disorder was higher (58 vs. 38%), although this difference fell short of statistical significance. The type of psychiatric disorder was not particularly distinctive, although there was a hint that hyperkinesis was disproportionately common. Ingram's (1955) large epidemiological study also suggested a link between cerebral palsy and hyperkinesis, with this link being most evident for hemiplegic and ataxic cerebral palsy.

Hemiplegic cerebral palsy has been the focus of a decade of psychiatric studies (Goodman 1997; Goodman & Yude 2000), making it the best-characterized type of cerebral palsy from a psychiatric perspective. Even though hemiplegia is a relatively mild physical disability and most children with hemiplegia are of normal intelligence and attend mainstream schools, around half of all children with hemiplegia have at least one psychiatric disorder (Goodman & Graham 1996). Conduct and emotional disorders each affect around one-quarter of children with hemiplegia, with hyperkinesis affecting around 10% and autistic disorders around 3%. A more detailed account of clinical presentation and management is provided in Goodman & Yude (2000). The best predictor of which children with hemiplegia develop psychiatric problems is IQ, which is itself well predicted by the degree of neurological impairment (Goodman & Graham 1996; Goodman & Yude 1996). Psychiatric problems are more common in the presence of specific learning difficulties (Frampton et al. 1998), but are not related to whether the hemiplegia is left- or right-sided (Goodman & Yude 1997). Questionnaire follow-up suggests that psychiatric problems are often very persistent, with around 70% of children with psychiatric disorders initially still having them 4 years later (Goodman 1998). Children with hemiplegia are at increased risk of peer problems, including victimization, marginalization and lack of friends, perhaps in part because of constitutional problems with social understanding and relatedness (Yude et al. 1998; Yude & Goodman 1999). Future studies will need to examine how far lessons learned from these studies of hemiplegia apply more widely to other varieties of cerebral palsy, and indeed to other chronic neurodevelopmental problems, such as hydrocephalus.

Head injury

The nature and consequences of children's head injuries are well reviewed in a chapter by Rutter et al. (1984) and in two books (Johnson et al. 1989; Broman & Michel 1995). Interested readers are advised to turn to these sources for more detailed accounts and further references.

Head injuries are major causes of hospitalization, severe disability and death in childhood. It is useful to distinguish between open head injuries, which typically involve localized brain damage caused by a penetrating injury, and closed head injuries, which typically involve widespread bilateral damage caused by acceleration–deceleration and rotation injuries secondary to a road traffic accident or a fall. Closed head injuries are more common, are much more likely to result in prolonged unconsciousness and post-traumatic amnesia, and are less likely to result in epilepsy.

The victims are not a random cross-section of children. For example, children who are male, hyperkinetic or of below-average intelligence are more likely to sustain head injuries (particularly mild head injuries), as are children who are poorly supervised because of parental illness or depression. In other words, child psychiatric problems (such as hyperkinesis) may be antecedents rather than consequences of head injury, or may reflect third factors (such as lack of parental supervision) that independently increase the risk of psychiatric disorder and head injury. This has made it particularly hard to determine if mild head injuries cause psychiatric disorders or cognitive deficits. A review of 40 recent studies of the psychological consequences of mild head injury found that those studies demonstrating no persistent impairment were both more numerous and of higher methodological quality than studies suggesting an adverse effect (Satz *et al.* 1997). However, even if mild head injury generally has no lasting effect on academic or psychosocial outcome, it is still conceivable that mild head injury does result in permanent damage to a small subgroup of susceptible children, depending on the child's age or prior risk factors.

Whatever the residual doubts about the effects of mild head injuries, there is no longer any doubt that severe head injuries often result in cognitive impairments and psychiatric problems (Rutter *et al.* 1984). Closed head injuries that result in at least 2 weeks of post-traumatic amnesia commonly result in impaired performance on a wide range of cognitive tests (affecting visuomotor and visuospatial tasks somewhat more than verbal tasks). Cognitive recovery may be partial or complete. Catch-up is fastest in the first year after injury, but may continue at a slower pace thereafter. Open head injuries also result in cognitive impairments, with performance IQ being more affected than verbal IQ, whatever the laterality or locus of injury. Damage before the age of 5 years may result in faster but less complete recovery, with persisting impairments in scholastic attainments.

The short-term psychiatric sequelae of severe head injuries are well summarized by Hill (1989). Three overlapping phases may be evident: an early phase of confusion, regression, or denial; a middle phase of demanding and arrogant behaviour or listlessness and depression; and a final phase of gradual accommodation to disability.

In the longer term, psychiatric disorders are evident in roughly half of the survivors of severe closed or open head injuries (Rutter *et al.* 1984; Lehmkuhl & Thoma 1990; Max *et al.* 1998). Within this group, the risk of psychiatric disorder is not related to age, sex, or locus of injury, is only weakly related to the severity of the injury, and is best predicted by preinjury characteristics, social adversity and parental handling. Children who had minor emotional or behavioural symptoms prior to injury are at greater psychiatric risk than children whose preinjury behaviour was normal. Coexistent psychosocial adversities (such as maternal depression, paternal criminality or overcrowding) further increase the child's psychiatric risk. This risk is probably also increased when parents respond to the injury by becoming overprotective and reluctant to discipline their child.

Although the psychiatric disorders of children with head injuries mostly involve the sorts of emotional and conduct problems that dominate ordinary child psychiatric practice, severe closed head injury can result in a distinctive syndrome of social disinhibition resembling an adult 'frontal lobe syndrome' (Rutter *et al.* 1984). These disinhibited children are unduly outspoken, ask embarrassing questions, make very personal comments and get undressed in inappropriate contexts. They may also be forgetful, overtalkative, impulsive or careless about their own cleanliness and appearance. The localization of an open head injury has little if any influence on psychiatric symptomatology; hints that depression is particularly linked with right anterior or left posterior damage have yet to be confirmed.

Prognosis of psychiatric problems in children with brain disorders

Is the prognosis of a psychiatric disorder worse if the child also has a brain disorder? Clinicians and parents often suppose so, and this pessimism may be self-fulfilling if it leads to inappropriately low expectations and therapeutic nihilism. The pessimism has more to do with theoretical expectations than empirical evidence. If a damaged brain cannot mend, it seems to follow that associated psychiatric problems cannot mend either. This is faulty reasoning. The association between brain and behavioural disorders is sometimes simply a coincidence. For example, the child's psychiatric disorder may reflect stresses at school that have nothing to do with the child's neurological problems; if the stresses at school resolve, so may the child's psychiatric disorder. Even when the psychiatric disorder is secondary to the child's brain disorder, the causal chain may be indirect and easy to interrupt. For instance, if a boy with epilepsy develops a conduct disorder, the mediating link may be the parents' fear that he will have a seizure if they discipline him in any way. Helping the parents to reinstate appropriate discipline may cure the conduct disorder. Even when psychiatric problems are direct consequences of the brain disorder, the psychiatric problems may still be temporary (just as some children with fixed brain lesions have seizures for a few months or years and then grow out of them). As noted earlier in the chapter, brain disorders do not necessarily arise from irreversible brain damage. On theoretical grounds, there is no reason to suppose that psychiatric disorders are bound to be persistent just because the child also has a brain disorder.

There is little empirical evidence on prognosis because there have been so few longitudinal neuropsychiatric studies. In the Institute of Psychiatry study of children with closed head injuries (Brown *et al.* 1981), psychiatric disorders attributable to head injury were somewhat more persistent than psychiatric disorders that were not attributable to head injury, but the difference was not statistically significant. Breslau & Marshall (1985) used a brief screening inventory to assess the stability of psychiatric problems over the course of 5 years in a group of children with a mixture of brain disorders, and in a comparison group of children with cystic fibrosis. Judging from this limited assessment, psychiatric problems were more likely to persist in the children with brain disorders—a persistence that was only partially explained by coexistent mental retardation. Follow-up of children with hemiplegic cerebral palsy also suggests that childhood psychiatric problems are often persistent (Goodman 1998). However, this evidence for persistence needs to be set against the more optimistic findings of Ounsted *et al.* (1987) who followed up 100 children with temporal lobe epilepsy for over 20 years. Although 85% of the sample had some psychological problems during childhood, the adult outcome was surprisingly good. When individuals with mental retardation were excluded, 70% of the survivors were entirely free of psychiatric disorder in adult life.

Individuals can grow into as well as out of the psychiatric consequences of childhood brain disorders. For example, a child who initially adjusts well to an acquired hemiplegia may subsequently become increasingly depressed as recovery slows down and the implications of lifelong disability sink in. Brain maturation may also be relevant. It is possible, for example, that some psychiatric consequences of head injury do not emerge until the child reaches the age when damaged late-maturing cortex normally comes 'on line' (Goodman 1989).

Prevention and treatment of psychiatric problems in children with brain disorders

Because children with brain disorders commonly develop psychiatric problems, and because combined physical and psychiatric problems impose a severe burden on parents and teachers, children with brain disorders seem an obvious target for interventions designed to prevent psychiatric problems. Unfortunately, few such studies have been conducted. Hjern & Nylander (1964) found that children with head injuries were significantly less likely to develop psychiatric problems if their parents had been counselled that the sequelae of head injury were generally transient, and that children with head injuries benefit from a graded reintroduction to all normal activities. Lewis et al. (1990, 1991) compared two educational programmes for children with epilepsy and their parents. Families were randomly allocated either to lecture sessions followed by question-and-answer periods, or to a specially devised series of parent and child groups. The group counselling approach was more likely to reduce parental anxiety and foster children's self-perceptions of social competency. Although the gains were modest, this study does demonstrate the feasibility of randomized controlled trials of preventative interventions in this area.

The psychiatric problems of children with brain disorders can be treated in just the same ways as the psychiatric problems of neurologically intact children. Biological treatments are neither more nor less useful than in ordinary child psychiatric practice. There is no empirical basis, for example, for treating a child's conduct disorder with carbamazepine rather than with behavioural therapy or parent management training simply because the child also has a brain disorder. Individual, family and school-based treatment approaches can all be helpful. As far as drug treatment is concerned, five points are worth emphasizing.

1 The indications for, and choice of, psychotropic medication differs little from standard practice (see Heyman & Santosh, Chapter 59).

2 Epilepsy is not a strong contraindication to using antipsychotics or antidepressants even though these drugs may increase seizure frequency. In practice, an increase in seizure frequency is rarely a major problem, and can often be countered by adjusting the dose of antiepileptic medication. Of the commonly used antipsychotics, risperidone, sulpiride and haloperidol are probably less likely than chlorpromazine to exacerbate seizures, while olanzapine and clozapine are better avoided if possible because they are associated with a particularly high risk of seizures.

3 Although brain disorders are often mentioned as a risk factor for antipsychotic-induced tardive dyskinesias, the evidence is decidedly weak (Kane & Smith 1982).

4 Stimulant medication can be very helpful for hyperkinetic children who also have a neurological problem, although the risk of a dysphoric reaction to stimulants may be higher than in other hyperkinetic children (Ounsted 1955; Ingram 1956). Both methylphenidate and dexamfetamine are commonly used, and although there are theoretical reasons for supposing that methylphenidate may be more likely than dexamfetamine to lower seizure threshold, methylphenidate does appear to be safe and effective for children with well-controlled seizures (Gross-Tsur et al. 1997).

5 When children with epilepsy develop behavioural problems, changing the type or dosage of antiepileptic medication can sometimes help. Behavioural problems may improve dramatically, for example, if toxic levels of phenytoin are reduced, or if phenobarbital is replaced by carbamazepine. Changes in antiepileptic medication should obviously be discussed with the child's paediatrician.

Prospects for the future

Research in developmental neuropsychiatry is gathering momentum and it is likely that studies conducted over the next 10 years will make major contributions to the field. There is still much to be done to chart the psychiatric risk profile associated with common and less common neurological disorders—clinical studies, cross-sectional epidemiological studies and longitudinal epidemiological studies all have important contributions to make. Prevention and treatment trials have the potential to be both practically and theoretically illuminating. At a practical level, they will provide the evidence base for planning neuropsychiatric services, while at a theoretical level, they will provide crucial tests of proposed causal pathways. Advances in molecular genetics and neuroimaging should provide new opportunities to examine possible explanations for the marked heterogeneity of psychiatric outcome after apparently similar brain lesions. For example, if additive 'anxiety' genes can be identified, it will be possible to test directly the hypothesis that brain disorders primarily increase an individual's risk of an anxiety disorder if that individual also has what would normally be a subthreshold dose of these genes. As functional neuroimaging can be used to localize the brain systems involved in specific cognitive processes, this approach provides a window on how brain function may be localized differently when particular areas of the brain are damaged at specific stages of development. Given several lines of evidence that neuronal reorganization can potentially impair as well as promote adaptive functioning (Goodman 1994), it is possible that the heterogeneity of psychiatric outcome in children with brain disorders will turn out to be related to different patterns of cerebral reorganization.

References

Aicardi, J., Gillberg, C., Ogier, H. & Bax, M. (1998) *Diseases of the Nervous System in Children: Clinics in Developmental Medicine*, 2nd edn. MacKeith Press, London.

Appleton, R.E. (1995) The Landau–Kleffner syndrome. *Archives of Disease in Childhood*, 72, 386–387.

Asbahr, F.R., Negrvo, A.B., Gentil, V. *et al.* (1998) Obsessive-compulsive and related symptoms in children and adolescents with rheumatic fever with and without chorea; a prospective 6-month study. *American Journal of Psychiatry*, 155, 1122–1124.

Austin, J.K., Huster, G.A., Dunn, D.W. & Risinger, M.W. (1996) Adolescents with active or inactive epilepsy or asthma: a comparison of quality of life. *Epilepsia*, 37, 1228–1138.

Beaumanoir, A. (1985a) The Lennox–Gastaut syndrome. In: *Epileptic Syndromes in Infancy, Childhood and Adolescence* (eds J. Roger, C. Dravet, M. Bureau, F.E. Dreifuss & P. Wolf), pp. 89–99. John Libbey, London.

Beaumanoir, A. (1985b) The Landau–Kleffner syndrome. In: *Epileptic Syndromes in Infancy, Childhood and Adolescence* (eds J. Roger, C. Dravet, M. Bureau, F.E. Dreifuss & P. Wolf), pp. 181–191. John Libbey, London.

Berg, R.A., Bolter, J.F., Ch'ien, L.T. & Cummins, J. (1984) A standardized assessment of emotionality in children suffering from epilepsy. *International Journal of Clinical Neuropsychology*, 4, 247–248.

Binnie, C.D., Channon, S. & Marston, D. (1990) Learning disabilities in epilepsy: neurophysiological aspects. *Epilepsia*, 31 (Suppl.4), S2–S60.

Bolton, P.F. & Griffiths, P.D. (1997) Association of tuberous sclerosis of temporal lobes with autism and atypical autism. *Lancet*, 349, 392–395.

Bourgeois, B.F.D., Prensky, A.L., Palkes, H.S., Talent, B.K. & Busch, S.G. (1983) Intelligence in epilepsy: a prospective study in children. *Annals of Neurology*, 14, 438–444.

Breslau, N. (1985) Psychiatric disorder in children with physical disabilities. *Journal of the American Academy of Child Psychiatry*, 24, 87–94.

Breslau, N. (1990) Does brain dysfunction increase children's vulnerability to environmental stress? *Archives of General Psychiatry*, 47, 15–20.

Breslau, N. (1995) Psychiatric sequelae of low birth weight. *Epidemiologic Reviews*, 17, 96–106.

Breslau, N. & Marshall, I.A. (1985) Psychological disturbance in children with physical disabilities: continuity and change in a 5-year follow-up. *Journal of Abnormal Child Psychology*, 13, 199–216.

Brett, E.M., ed. (1997) *Paediatric Neurology*, 3rd edn. Churchill Livingstone, Edinburgh.

Broman, S.H. & Michel, M.E. (1995) *Traumatic Head Injury in Children*. Oxford University Press, New York.

Brown, R.M.A. & Perkins, M.J. (1989) Child sexual abuse presenting as organic disease. *British Medical Journal*, 299, 614–615.

Brown, G., Chadwick, O., Shaffer, D., Rutter, M. & Traub, M. (1981) A prospective study of children with head injuries. III. Psychiatric sequelae. *Psychological Medicine*, 11, 63–78.

Brown, L.K., Lourie, K.J. & Pao, M. (2000) Children and adolescents living with HIV and AIDS: a review. *Journal of Child Psychology and Psychiatry*, 41, 81–96.

Camfield, P.R., Gates, R., Ronen, G., Camfield, C., Ferguson, A. & MacDonald, W. (1984) Comparison of cognitive ability, personality profile, and school success in epileptic children with pure right versus left temporal lobe EEG foci. *Annals of Neurology*, 15, 122–126.

Caplan, R., Arbelle, S., Magharious, W. *et al.* (1998) Psychopathology in pediatric complex partial and primary generalized epilepsy. *Developmental Medicine and Child Neurology*, 40, 805–811.

Chapieski, M.L. & Evankovich, K.D. (1997) Behavioral effects of prematurity. *Seminars in Perinatology*, 21, 221–239.

Commission on Classification and Terminology of the International League Against Epilepsy (1981) Proposal for revised clinical and electroencephalographic classification of epileptic seizures. *Epilepsia*, 22, 489–501.

Commission on Classification and Terminology of the International League Against Epilepsy (1989) Proposal for revised clinical and electroencephalographic classification of epileptic seizures. *Epilepsia*, 30, 389–399.

Corbett, J.A. & Trimble, M.R. (1984) Epilepsy and anticonvulsant medication. In: *Developmental Neuropsychiatry* (ed. M. Rutter), pp. 112–129. Churchill Livingstone, Edinburgh.

Corbett, J., Harris, R., Taylor, E. & Trimble, M. (1977) Progressive disintegrative psychosis of childhood. *Journal of Child Psychology and Psychiatry*, 18, 211–219.

Cull, A. & Trimble, M.R. (1989) Effects of anticonvulsant medications on cognitive functioning in children with epilepsy. In: *Childhood Epilepsies: Neuropsychological, Psychosocial and Interventions Aspects* (eds B.P. Hermann & M. Seidenberg), pp. 83–103. John Wiley, Chichester.

Davison, K. & Bagley, C.R. (1969) Schizophrenia-like psychoses associated with organic disorders of the central nervous system: a review of the literature. *British Journal of Psychiatry, Special Publication* 4, 113–184.

Dewhurst, K., Oliver, J.E. & McKnight, A.L. (1970) Socio-psychiatric consequences of Huntington's disease. *British Journal of Psychiatry*, 116, 255–258.

DiFiglia, M. (2000) Genetics of childhood disorders. X. Huntington disease. *Journal of the American Academy of Child and Adolescent Psychiatry*, 39, 120–122.

Ellenberg, J.H., Hirtz, D.G. & Nelson, D.B. (1986) Do seizures in children cause intellectual deterioration? *New England Journal of Medicine*, 314, 1085–1088.

Engel, J. & Pedley, T.A. (1999) *Epilepsy: a Comprehensive Textbook*. Lippincott, Williams & Wilkins, Philadelphia.

Farwell, J.R., Dodrill, C.B. & Batzel, L.W. (1985) Neuropsychological abilities of children with epilepsy. *Epilepsia*, 26, 395–400.

Folstein, S.E., Franz, M.L., Jensen, B.A., Chase, G.A. & Folstein, M.F. (1983) Conduct disorder and affective disorder among the offspring of patients with Huntington's disease. *Psychological Medicine*, 13, 45–52.

Frampton, I., Yude, C. & Goodman, R. (1998) The prevalence and correlates of specific learning difficulties in a representative sample of children with hemiplegia. *British Journal of Educational Psychology*, 68, 39–51.

Freeman, J.M. & Nelson, K.B. (1988) Intrapartum asphyxia and cerebral palsy. *Pediatrics*, 82, 240–249.

Gartner, J., Braun, A., Holzinger, A., Roerig, P., Lenard, H.-G. & Roscher, A.A. (1998) Clinical and genetic aspects of X-linked adrenoleukodystrophy. *Neuropediatrics*, 29, 3–13.

Gastaut, H. (1970) Clinical and electroencephalographical classification of epileptic seizures. *Epilepsia*, 11, 102–113.

Goodman, R. (1989) Limits of cerebral plasticity. In: *Children's Head Injury: Who Cares?* (eds D.A. Johnson, D. Uttley & M. Wyke), pp. 12–22. Taylor & Francis, London.

Goodman, R. (1993) Brain abnormalities and psychological development. In: *Precursors and Causes in Development and Psychopathology* (eds D.F. Hay & A. Angold), pp. 51–85. John Wiley, Chichester.

Goodman, R. (1994) Brain development. In: *Developmental Principles and Clinical Issues in Psychology and Psychiatry* (eds M.L. Rutter & D.F. Hay), pp. 49–78. Blackwell Scientific Publications, Oxford.

Goodman, R. (1997) Psychological aspects of hemiplegia. *Archives of Disease in Childhood*, 76, 177–178.

Goodman, R. (1998) The longitudinal stability of psychiatric problems in children with hemiplegia. *Journal of Child Psychology and Psychiatry*, 39, 347–354.

Goodman, R. & Graham, P. (1996) Psychiatric problems in children with hemiplegia: cross-sectional epidemiological survey. *British Medical Journal*, 312, 1065–1069.

Goodman, R. & Yude, C. (1996) IQ and its predictors in childhood hemiplegia. *Developmental Medicine and Child Neurology*, 38, 881–890.

Goodman, R. & Yude, C. (1997) Do unilateral lesions of the developing brain have side-specific psychiatric consequences in childhood? *Laterality*, 2, 103–115.

Goodman, R. & Yude, C. (2000) Emotional, behavioural and social consequences. In: *Congenital Hemiplegia, Clinics in Developmental Medicine No. 150* (eds B. Neville & R. Goodman), pp. 166–178. MacKeith Press, London.

Goodyer, I.M. (1985) Epileptic and pseudoepileptic seizures in childhood and adolescence. *Journal of the American Academy of Child Psychiatry*, 24, 3–8.

Gordon, N. (1990) Acquired aphasia in childhood: the Landau–Kleffner syndrome. *Developmental Medicine and Child Neurology*, 32, 270–274.

Gordon, N. & Sillanp, M. (1997) Epilepsy and prejudice with particular relevance to childhood. *Developmental Medicine and Child Neurology*, 39, 777–781.

Gross-Tsur, V., Manor, O., Van Der Meere, J. & Shalev, J.A. (1997) Epilepsy and attention deficit hyperactivity disorder: is methylphenidate safe and effective? *Journal of Pediatrics*, 130, 40–44.

Grunberg, F. & Pond, D.A. (1957) Conduct disorders in epileptic children. *Journal of Neurology, Neurosurgery and Psychiatry*, 20, 65–68.

Gur, R.E. & Chin, S. (1999) Laterality in functional brain imaging studies of schizophrenia. *Schizophrenia Bulletin*, 25, 141–156.

Hagberg, B., Hagberg, G. & Olow, L. (1996) The changing panorama of cerebral palsy in Sweden. VII. Prevalence and origin during the birth year period 1987–90. *Acta Paediatrica*, 85, 954–960.

Harper, P.S. & Clarke, A. (1990) Should we test children for adult genetic diseases? *Lancet*, 335, 1205–1206.

Hermann, B.P. (1982) Neuropsychological functioning and psychopathology in children with epilepsy. *Epilepsia*, 23, 545–554.

Hermann, B.P., Whitman, S. & Dell, J. (1989) Correlates of behaviour problems and social competence in children with epilepsy, aged 6–11. In: *Childhood Epilepsies: Neuropsychological, Psychosocial and Interventions Aspects* (eds B.P. Hermann & M. Seidenberg), pp. 143–157. John Wiley, Chichester.

Highley, J.R., McDonald, B., Walker, M.A., Esiri, M.M. & Crow, T.J. (1999) Schizophrenia and temporal lobe asymmetry: a post-mortem stereological study of tissue volume. *British Journal of Psychiatry*, 175, 127–134.

Hill, P. (1989) Psychiatric aspects of children's head injury. In: *Children's Head Injury: Who Cares?* (eds D.A. Johnson, D. Uttley & M. Wyke), pp. 134–146. Taylor & Francis, London.

Hjern, B. & Nylander, I. (1964) Acute head injuries in children: traumatology, therapy and prognosis. *Acta Paediatrica Scandinavica Supplement*, 152, 1–37.

Hoare, P. (1984) The development of psychiatric disorder among school children with epilepsy. *Developmental Medicine and Child Neurology*, 26, 3–13.

Hoare, P. (1987) Children with epilepsy and their families. *Journal of Child Psychology and Psychiatry*, 28, 651–655.

Holmes, G., Sackellares, J.C., McKiernan, J., Ragland, M. & Dreifuss, F.E. (1980) Evaluation of childhood pseudoseizures using EEG telemetry and video tape monitoring. *Journal of Pediatrics*, 97, 554–558.

Howe, G.W., Feinstein, C., Reiss, D., Molock, S. & Berger, K. (1993) Adolescent adjustment to chronic physical disorders. I. Comparing neurological and non-neurological conditions. *Journal of Child Psychology and Psychiatry*, 34, 1153–1171.

Hunt, A. & Dennis, J. (1987) Psychiatric disorder among children with tuberous sclerosis. *Developmental Medicine and Child Neurology*, 29, 190–198.

Hunt, A. & Shepherd, C. (1993) A prevalence study of autism in tuberous sclerosis. *Journal of Autism and Developmental Disorders*, 23, 323–339.

Ingram, T.T.S. (1955) A study of cerebral palsy in the childhood population of Edinburgh. *Archives of Disease in Childhood*, 30, 85–98.

Ingram, T.T.S. (1956) A characteristic form of overactive behaviour in brain damaged children. *Journal of Mental Science*, 102, 550–558.

Jacobsen, B. & Kinney, D.K. (1980) Perinatal complications in adopted and non-adopted schizophrenics and their controls: preliminary results. *Acta Psychiatrica Scandinavica Supplement*, 285, 337–346.

Johnson, D.A., Uttley, D. & Wyke, M.A., eds. (1989) *Children's Head Injury: Who Cares?* Taylor & Francis, London.

Kane, J.M. & Smith, J.M. (1982) Tardive dyskinesia. *Archives of General Psychiatry*, 39, 473–491.

Kurita, H. (1985) Infantile autism with speech loss before the age of thirty months. *Journal of the American Academy of Child Psychiatry*, 24, 191–196.

Lehmkuhl, M. & Thoma, W. (1990) Development in children after severe head injury. In: *Brain and Behavior in Child Psychiatry* (ed. A. Rothenberger), pp. 267–282. Springer-Verlag, Berlin.

Lewis, M.A., Salas, I., de la Sota, A., Chiofalo, N. & Leake, B. (1990) Randomized trial of a program to enhance the competencies of children with epilepsy. *Epilepsia*, 31, 101–109.

Lewis, M.A., Hatton, C.L., Salas, I., Leake, B. & Chiofalo, N. (1991) Impact of the children's epilepsy program on parents. *Epilepsia*, 32, 365–374.

Lishman, W.A. (1998) *Organic Psychiatry: the Psychological Consequences of Cerebral Disorder*, 3rd edn. Blackwell Science, Oxford.

Livingston, J.H. (1988) The Lennox–Gastaut syndrome. *Developmental Medicine and Child Neurology*, 30, 536–549.

Lobascher, M.E. & Cavanagh, N.P.C. (1980) Patterns of intellectual change in the dementing school child. *Child: Care, Health and Development*, 6, 255–265.

Luna, D., Dulac, O., Pajot, N. & Beaumont, D. (1989) Vigabatrin in the treatment of childhood epilepsies: a single-blind placebo-controlled study. *Epilepsia*, 30, 430–437.

Luthy, D.A., Wardinsky, R., Shurtleff, D.B. *et al.* (1991) Cesarean section before the onset of labor and subsequent motor function in infants with meningomyelocele diagnosed antenatally. *New England Journal of Medicine*, **324**, 662–666.

Max, J.E., Koele, S.L., Smith, W.L. Jr *et al.* (1998) Psychiatric disorders in children and adolescents after severe traumatic brain injury: a controlled study. *Journal of the American Academy of Child and Adolescent Psychiatry*, **37**, 832–840.

Meltzer, H., Gatward, R., Goodman, R. & Ford, F. (2000) *Mental Health of Children and Adolescents in Great Britain*. The Stationery Office, London.

Menkes, J.H. (1995) *Textbook of Child Neurology*, 5th edn. Lippincott, Williams & Wilkins, Philadelphia.

Miller, G. (1989) Minor congenital anomalies and ataxic cerebral palsy. *Archives of Disease in Childhood*, **64**, 557–562.

Mole, S. & Gardiner, M. (1999) Molecular genetics of the neuronal ceroid lipofuscinoses. *Epilepsia*, **40** (Suppl.3), 29–32.

Nass, R. & Koch, D. (1987) Temperament differences in toddlers with early unilateral right- and left-brain damage. *Developmental Neuropsychology*, **3**, 93–99.

Nelson, K.B. & Ellenberg, J.H. (1986) Antecedents of cerebral palsy: multivariate analysis of risk. *New England Journal of Medicine*, **315**, 81–86.

Ounsted, C. (1955) The hyperkinetic syndrome in epileptic children. *Lancet*, **ii**, 303–311.

Ounsted, C., Lindsay, J. & Norman, R. (1966) *Biological Factors in Temporal Lobe Epilepsy*. Clinics in Developmental Medicine No. 22. S.I.M.P./Heinemann, London.

Ounsted, C., Lindsay, J. & Richards, P. (1987) *Temporal Lobe Epilepsy 1948–86: a Biographical Study*. Clinics in Developmental Medicine No. 103. MacKeith Press/Blackwell Scientific Publications, Oxford.

Paneth, N. & Kiely, P. (1984) The frequency of cerebral palsy: a review of population studies in industrialized nations since 1950. In: *The Epidemiology of the Cerebral Palsies* (eds F. Stanley & E. Alberman), pp. 46–56. S.I.M.P./Blackwell Scientific Publications, Oxford.

Perez, M.M., Trimble, M.R., Murray, N.M.F. & Reider, I. (1985) Epileptic psychosis: an evaluation of PSE profiles. *British Journal of Psychiatry*, **146**, 155–163.

Perez, E.R., Davidoff, V., Despland, P.-A. & Deonna, T. (1993) Mental and behavioural deterioration of children with epilepsy and CSWS: acquired epileptic frontal syndrome. *Developmental Medicine and Child Neurology*, **35**, 661–674.

Petty, R.G. (1999) Structural asymmetries of the human brain and their disturbance in schizophrenia. *Schizophrenia Bulletin*, **25**, 121–139.

Pond, D.A. & Bidwell, B.H. (1960) A survey of epilepsy in the general practices. II. Social and psychological aspects. *Epilepsia*, **1**, 285–299.

Rantakallio, P. & von Wendt, L. (1985) Risk factors for mental retardation. *Archives of Disease in Childhood*, **60**, 946–952.

Riikonen, R. & Amnell, G. (1981) Psychiatric disorders in children with earlier infantile spasms. *Developmental Medicine and Child Neurology*, **23**, 747–760.

Robinson, R.G. (1979) Differential behavioral and biochemical effects of right and left hemispheric cerebral infarction in the rat. *Science*, **205**, 707–710.

Rodin, E. (1989) Prognosis of cognitive functions in children with epilepsy. In: *Childhood Epilepsies: Neuropsychological, Psychosocial and Interventions Aspects* (eds B.P. Hermann & M. Seidenberg), pp. 33–50. John Wiley, Chichester.

Rutter, M., Graham, P. & Yule, W. (1970) *A Neuropsychiatric Study in Childhood*. Clinics in Developmental Medicine Nos. 35/36. S.I.M.P./Heinemann, London.

Rutter, M., Cox, A., Tupling, C., Berger, M. & Yule, W. (1975) Attainment and adjustment in two geographical areas. I. The prevalence of psychiatric disorder. *British Journal of Psychiatry*, **126**, 493–509.

Rutter, M., Chadwick, O. & Shaffer, D. (1984) Head injury. In: *Developmental Neuropsychiatry* (ed. M. Rutter), pp. 83–111. Churchill Livingstone, Edinburgh.

Rutter, M., Silberg, J., O'Connor, T. & Simonoff, E. (1999) Genetics and child psychiatry. II. Empirical research findings. *Journal of Child Psychology and Psychiatry*, **40**, 19–55.

Sabbeth, B.F. & Leventhal, J.M. (1984) Marital adjustment to chronic childhood illness: a critique of the literature. *Pediatrics*, **73**, 762–768.

Satz, P., Zaucha, K., McCleary, C., Light, R., Asarnow, R. & Becker, D. (1997) Mild head injury in children and adolescents: a review of studies (1970–95). *Psychological Bulletin*, **122**, 107–131.

Schoenfeld, J., Seidenberg, M., Woodard, A. *et al.* (1999) Neuropsychological and behavioral status of children with complex partial seizures. *Developmental Medicine and Child Neurology*, **41**, 724–731.

Scully, R.E., Galdabini, J.J. & McNeely, B.U. (1978) Case records of the Massachusetts General Hospital, Case 29–1978. *New England Journal of Medicine*, **299**, 189–194.

Seidel, U.P., Chadwick, O.F.D. & Rutter, M. (1975) Psychological disorders in crippled children: a comparative study of children with and without brain damage. *Developmental Medicine and Child Neurology*, **17**, 563–573.

Seidenberg, M., Beck, N., Geisser, M. *et al.* (1986) Academic achievement of children with epilepsy. *Epilepsia*, **27**, 753–759.

Sollee, N.D. & Kindlon, D.J. (1987) Lateralized brain injury and behavior problems in children. *Journal of Abnormal Child Psychology*, **15**, 479–490.

Stores, G. (1977) Behavior disturbance and type of epilepsy in children attending ordinary school. In: *Epilepsy: the Eighth International Symposium* (ed. J.K. Penry), pp. 245–249. Raven Press, New York.

Stores, G. (1985) Clinical and EEG evaluation of seizures and seizure-like disorders. *Journal of the American Academy of Child Psychiatry*, **24**, 10–16.

Stores, G. (1991) Confusions concerning sleep disorders and the epilepsies in children and adolescents. *British Journal of Psychiatry*, **158**, 1–7.

Stores, G. (1999) Recognition of pseudoseizures in children and adolescents. *Journal of Child Psychology and Psychiatry*, **40**, 851–857.

Stores, G., Zaiwalla, A. & Bergel, N. (1991) Frontal lobe complex partial seizures in children: a form of epilepsy at particular risk of misdiagnosis. *Developmental Medicine and Child Neurology*, **33**, 998–1009.

Swedo, S.E., Rapoport, J.L., Cheslow, D.L. *et al.* (1989) High prevalence of obsessive-compulsive symptoms in patients with Sydenham's chorea. *American Journal of Psychiatry*, **146**, 246–249.

Szatmari, P., Saigal, S., Rosenbaum, P. & Campbell, D. (1993) Psychopathology and adaptive functioning among extremely low birthweight children at eight years of age. *Development and Psychopathology*, **5**, 345–357.

Tassinari, C.A., Bureau, M., Dravet, C., Dalla Bernardina, B. & Roger, J. (1985) Epilepsy with continuous spikes and waves during slow sleep. In: *Epileptic Syndromes in Infancy, Childhood and Adolescence* (eds J. Roger, C. Dravet, M. Bureau, F.E. Dreifuss & P. Wolf), pp. 194–204. John Libbey, London.

Taudorf, K., Hansen, F.J. & Melchior, J.C. (1986) Spontaneous remission of cerebral palsy. *Neuropediatrics*, **17**, 19–22.

Taylor, D.C. (1969) Sexual behaviour and temporal lobe epilepsy. *Archives of Neurology*, **21**, 510–516.

Taylor, D.C. (1975) Factors influencing the occurrence of schizophrenia-like psychosis in patients with temporal lobe epilepsy. *Psychological Medicine*, **5**, 249–254.

Taylor, D.C. (1989) Psychosocial components of childhood epilepsy. In:

Childhood Epilepsies: Neuropsychological, Psychosocial and Interventions Aspects (eds B.P. Hermann & M. Seidenberg), pp. 119–142. John Wiley, Chichester.

Taylor, E. (1991) Developmental neuropsychiatry. *Journal of Child Psychology and Psychiatry*, **32**, 3–47.

Uvebrant, P. (1988) Hemiplegic cerebral palsy aetiology and outcome. *Acta Paediatrica Scandinavica Supplement*, **345**, 1–100.

Vargha-Khadem, F., Isaacs, E., Van der Werf, S., Robb, S. & Wilson, J. (1992) Development of intelligence and memory in children with hemiplegic cerebral palsy. *Brain*, **115**, 315–329.

Voeller, K.K.S. (1986) Right-hemisphere deficit syndrome in children. *American Journal of Psychiatry*, **143**, 1004–1009.

Wallace, S.J. (1992) Prenatal and perinatal risk factors for epilepsy. In: *Recent Advances in Epilepsy, No. 5* (eds T.A. Pedley & B.S. Meldrum), pp. 91–108. Churchill Livingstone, Edinburgh.

Wallace, S. (1995) *Epilepsy in Children*. Lippincott, Williams & Wilkins, Philadelphia.

Weintraub, S. & Mesulam, M.-M. (1983) Developmental learning disabilities of the right hemisphere: emotional, interpersonal and cognitive components. *Archives of Neurology*, **40**, 463–468.

Wheless, J.W. & Constantinou, J.E.C. (1997) Lennox–Gastaut syndrome. *Pediatric Neurology*, **17**, 203–211.

Whitaker, A.H., Feldman, J.F., Van Rossem, R. *et al.* (1996) Neonatal cranial ultrasound abnormalities in low birth weight infants: relation to cognitive outcomes at six years of age. *Pediatrics*, **98**, 719–729.

Whitaker, A.H., Van Rossem, R., Feldman, J.F. *et al.* (1997) Psychiatric outcomes in low-birth-weight children at age six years: relation to neonatal cranial ultrasound abnormalities. *Archives of General Psychiatry*, **54**, 847–856.

Whitman, S., Hermann, B.P., Black, R.B. & Chhabria, S. (1982) Psychopathology and seizure type in children with epilepsy. *Psychological Medicine*, **12**, 843–853.

Williams, D.T., Spiegel, H. & Mostofsky, D.I. (1978) Neurogenic and hysterical seizures in children and adolescents: differential diagnostic and therapeutic considerations. *American Journal of Psychiatry*, **135**, 82–86.

Wolke, D. (1998) Psychological development of prematurely born children. *Archives of Disease in Childhood*, **78**, 567–570.

Yude, C. & Goodman, R. (1999) Peer problems of 9–11 year old children with hemiplegia in mainstream schools: can these be predicted? *Developmental Medicine and Child Neurology*, **41**, 4–8.

Yude, C., Goodman, R. & McConachie, H. (1998) Peer problems of children with hemiplegia in mainstream primary schools. *Journal of Child Psychology and Psychiatry*, **39**, 533–541.

15 Chronic Adversities

Ruth J. Friedman and P. Lindsay Chase-Lansdale

Introduction

Chronic adversities are environmental stressors that endure for extended periods of time. The intensity of these stressors may wax and wane, but the key characteristic that differentiates them from acute trauma is their pervasive and lasting nature. The most notable chronic adversities—poverty, parental psychopathology, parental death, interparental discord, community violence, child maltreatment, foster care, and child medical illness—are seen as creating environments of persistent stress and challenge to healthy development. The past two decades have witnessed an explosion of research examining the impact of such chronic adversities on children and youth (Garmezy & Masten 1994; Rutter 1996). In addition, a related body of work on children's resiliency has also developed, investigating the factors that promote adaptation under duress (Garmezy & Rutter 1983; Masten *et al.* 1999; Luthar *et al.* 2000).

What can we conclude about the effects of chronic adversities on child and adolescent development? What are the key processes underlying these effects? Why do some children develop healthily despite considerable, ongoing stressors in their lives? These are the questions that we address in this chapter.

We begin by briefly reviewing the empirical literature on four of the above major chronic adversities: interparental discord, poverty, parental psychopathology, and community violence. As child maltreatment, foster care, bereavement and physical illness are the topics of separate chapters in this volume, we do not include them here. Our goal in this brief literature review is to present a summary of the type, extent and severity of negative outcomes related to these chronic adversities. We then move to a discussion of two central cross-cutting themes in these literatures: the role of cumulative risk and the impact of protective factors leading to resilience.

A central goal of this chapter is to address what has largely been missing from the study of chronic adversity: a focus on the pathways leading to the negative effects on children. What are the mechanisms that explain why poor developmental outcomes occur in these problematic contexts? Conversely, what are the mechanisms that explain why some children and youth are not harmed by chronic adversity? Toward this end, we present a heuristic model that outlines the processes involved in both negative and positive outcomes for children and youth under stressful conditions. To present and critique this model, we first consider some of the normative developmental processes that are essential for healthy child development. This permits an illustration from the model of how chronic adversity interferes with these normative processes. We then evaluate the merits of the model by reviewing the existing evidence, and suggest directions for future research. Finally, we briefly discuss the implications of our review and our model for clinical practice and intervention.

Brief summary of effects of chronic adversities

Marital discord and interparental conflict

One of the most widespread adversities for children is the experience of parental discord and divorce. The annual divorce rate has been rising in the USA since the 1850s, and the rate more than doubled between 1960 and 1980, from about 9 divorces per 1000 marriages in 1960 to about 22 in 1980 (US National Center for Health Statistics 1990). Since then the divorce rate has modestly decreased and stabilized (20.9 in 1990), but the USA has the highest divorce rate of industrialized countries except the former Soviet Union. In Europe, the UK and Denmark are the next highest with rates in 1991 of 13.3 and 12.3, respectively, and Italy has the lowest rate at 2.1 (UN Demographic Yearbook 1995). Of US adults marrying in the first part of the twenty-first century, half will experience divorce over the course of their lifetimes, followed by high proportions of remarriage (75% of men and 66% of women; Cherlin 1992). Second marriages are often more problematic for children and less stable than first marriages (Hetherington *et al.* 1998). In addition, cohabitation has been on the rise in the USA, from 11% of those who married in the 1960s to 44% of those who married in the 1980s, with even higher rates for those entering remarriage (60% in the 1980s; Cherlin 1992). Cohabitation is more prevalent in parts of Europe (Kiernan 1999). Cohabiting unions in the USA dissolve more readily than do marriages, and those marriages that are preceded by cohabitation have a higher likelihood of divorce (Cherlin 1992).

It is not the focus of this review to address all of the changes in children's lives brought about by their parents' marital and partnership transitions. Rather, we address marital discord, or more broadly, interparental conflict, a difficult context for children that often predates the dissolution of marriages and cohabitations, or occurs during the dissolution or in the aftermath of separation and divorce, as well as within enduring marriages or partnerships. Of the chronic adversities reviewed in this chapter, interparental conflict is the most extensively researched.

Marital discord and interparental conflict expose children and youth to hostility, acrimony, arguments and anger. Witnessing angry adults—whether they are strangers in laboratory-based studies or parents in laboratories or at home—is emotionally disturbing and causes physiological distress in children (Cummings *et al.* 1985; El-Sheikh *et al.* 1989; Hetherington 1999). Two meta-analyses have found that marital conflict is related to child and adolescent behaviour problems, including aggression with peers, poor psychological well-being and inadequate social functioning (Reid & Crisafulli 1990; Depner *et al.* 1992). These links remain when studies are statistically controlled for gender, age, race, socioeconomic status, family structure, family psychiatric history and parenting style (Lorenz *et al.* 1995; Davies & Windle 1997).

Interparental conflict appears to be related to elevated levels of behaviour and adjustment problems for all ages of children and adolescents. In early and middle childhood, interparental conflict predicts emotional disturbance and disruptive behaviour problems (Cummings *et al.* 1994; Davies & Cummings 1998; Kerig 1998a,b; Shaw *et al.* 1999), and these same patterns are found in studies of adolescents (Lorenz *et al.* 1995). Perhaps most important, the few existing longitudinal studies show that the negative effects of interparental discord are lasting. For example, in a study of more than 400 adolescents, marital discord predicted depressive symptoms, delinquency and alcohol problems in girls 6 months later (Davies & Windle 1997). Similarly, in a prospective study of 400 nationally representative families, marital discord early in children's lives was associated with subsequent lower levels of closeness to parents, life satisfaction, happiness and self-esteem, in addition to higher levels of psychological distress and violence in adolescents' later relationships (McNeal & Amato 1998).

Interparental discord is a chronic adversity that is detrimental to the psychological health of children and youth. However, the extent of interparental conflict in the USA and in Europe is not known, and we cannot draw firm conclusions about the prevalence or severity of the poor developmental outcomes in the empirical literature.

Poverty

In 1997, 19% of children in the USA lived in families with incomes below the poverty line ($16 400 for a family of four). Poverty is an official measure of economic standing, defined by the government as the income necessary for basic support of food, clothing and shelter. The poverty line is a monetary threshold, and those falling just above the poverty line are usually not meaningfully better off than those falling just below it. One study found that 50% of all US children, at some point during childhood, live in families whose income is near the poverty line, and almost one-third of children live below the poverty line by age 15 (Duncan & Rodgers 1988).

For children growing up in poor families, poverty usually entails a much broader set of challenges than just insufficient economic resources. Children in poor families are more likely to have parents with low levels of education, to live in single-mother households, and to reside in neighbourhoods characterized by overcrowding, substandard housing conditions, high rates of unemployment, inadequate schools and higher levels of crime (Brooks-Gunn *et al.* 1997b). These correlates of economic poverty create an ecological context that may impede social, psychological and educational domains. Distinguishing the relative influences of these different dimensions of poverty has been a central challenge in the area of poverty research (Chase-Lansdale *et al.* 1995).

Poverty is related to poorer physical, cognitive and social outcomes for children and adolescents (Duncan & Brooks-Gunn 1997). Low birth weight and other health problems, such as asthma, have higher prevalence rates in low-income populations (Korenman & Miller 1997; McConnochie *et al.* 1999). Family poverty is linked to more behaviour problems and poorer cognitive functioning during early and middle childhood (Dodge *et al.* 1994; Duncan *et al.* 1994; Bolger *et al.* 1995; Chase-Lansdale *et al.* 1997; Chase-Lansdale 1999). Similarly, neighbourhood poverty is related to cognitive delay, antisocial behaviour and emotional disturbance concurrently and over time (Guerra *et al.* 1995; Chase-Lansdale & Gordon 1996; Brooks-Gunn *et al.* 1997a; Dubow *et al.* 1997; Leventhal & Brooks-Gunn 2000), controlling for gender, age and race (Dubow & Ippolito 1994). Research with adolescents finds a similar pattern, with poverty predicting school behaviour problems, poor achievement, and both emotional difficulties and disruptive behaviour problems (Conger *et al.* 1993; Hanson *et al.* 1997), although some recent work finds that poverty during children's preschool years is the most damaging (Duncan *et al.* 1998). This body of work demonstrates that low socioeconomic status is linked to behavioural, emotional and cognitive problems for children and youth.

Another point of debate in the literature involves causality. For example, Mayer (1997) contends that the major reason why children and youth in poverty fare poorly is because of selection bias. In other words, the same factors that lead an adult into poverty (low abilities, poor education, emotional problems, disabilities) can be genetically shared with offspring and can also limit poor adults' abilities to parent effectively, thus resulting in unhealthy child outcomes. We take the position that both selection bias and experience may be influential causal factors. We liken them to Rutter *et al*'s (2001) discussion of the effects of cigarette smoking on health; certain genetic and other selection biases contribute to a young person's decision to smoke, but the actual experience of smoking also brings new risks. The same logic may be true for becoming impoverished and experiencing poverty.

Parental psychopathology

Having a parent with a mental disorder is a significant risk to healthy child and adolescent development. Children with mentally ill parents are vulnerable to developmental problems because of genetic and environmental characteristics that create a situation of multiple risk. For example, parental psychopathology often co-occurs with marital difficulties, parenting problems and spousal psychopathology (Beardslee *et al.* 1998). Children are additionally at-risk because many forms of psychopathology (e.g. alcoholism, antisocial behaviour, schizophrenia and affective illness) are believed to have varying hereditary components (Rutter *et al.* 1990). A significant proportion of the population is affected by mental health problems (Kessler *et al.* 1994). Although we will discuss various types of parental psychopathology as discrete disorders, many mental disorders actually occur comorbidly and so the differential effects of specific psychopathology are often not clear (Sameroff & Seifer 1990; Garmezy & Masten 1994).

Parental alcoholism, antisocial behaviour, schizophrenia and affective illness are all associated with poorer child development. Children of alcoholics demonstrate heavier drinking (Colder *et al.* 1997), more behaviour problems (Martin *et al.* 1994), and more emotional difficulties (Roosa *et al.* 1988; for reviews see Sher 1991 and Chassin *et al.* 1997). Many of these problems continue on through adulthood (Domenico & Windle 1993). In addition, parental criminality and antisocial personality disorder predict poorer child outcomes. These forms of parental psychopathology are associated with more mental health problems and antisocial behaviour in children (Factor & Wolfe 1990; Patterson & Capaldi 1991; Guzder *et al.* 1999), including conduct problems (Loeber & Dishion 1983; Christ *et al.* 1990), attention deficit hyperactivity disorder (ADHD; Lahey *et al.* 1995), and conduct disorder (Frick *et al.* 1992). Schizophrenia, a rare but severe form of mental disorder, has a strong genetic component and relates to other mental health problems more generally (Sameroff & Seifer 1990).

A review of research in the past decade concludes that children of adults with affective illness are more vulnerable to the development of psychopathology in general and to depression specifically (Beardslee *et al.* 1998). Maternal depressive symptoms in a child's first year of life predict developmental delays at age 1 year (Field 1995) and child behaviour problems at 28 and 36 months (Leadbeater *et al.* 1996). Maternal depression is also associated longitudinally with children's social withdrawal and anxious behaviours at age 5 (Rubin *et al.* 1991), and lower child popularity and higher levels of internalizing and externalizing problems in later childhood (Goodman *et al.* 1993).

A robust literature shows that parental psychopathology poses a combination of negative psychosocial, environmental and genetic conditions that place children at-risk for numerous mental health and behaviour problems.

Violence exposure

As violent crime has become increasingly frequent in many urban low-income US communities, researchers have begun to examine the impact of violence exposure on children and adolescents. According to statistics from the Centers for Disease Control, the USA has the highest homicide rate of any industrialized country (Fingerhut *et al.* 1998), and police estimates suggest there are many more assaults than homicides (Bell & Jenkins 1993). Some violence exposure comes in the form of acute trauma, such as witnessing shootings and homicides (Pynoos & Nader 1990), but children living in high-crime US communities are often chronically exposed to violence through hearsay, as witnesses and victims, and by the ever-present threat of violence. Most research in this area does not specifically measure chronicity of exposure, but rather asks children about the frequency of exposure to specific violent events as witnesses and as victims. A survey with over 1000 children and adolescents from low-income urban communities found that 75% of boys and 70% of girls reported witnessing a shooting, stabbing, robbery or murder (Shakoor & Chalmers 1991). This work suggests many children living in low-income urban areas repeatedly experience numerous types of violence witnessing and victimization, ranging from drug use, arrests and shootings to assault (Richters & Martinez 1993).

Greater violence exposure is associated with higher rates of psychosocial problems in young children and adolescents. The level of violence exposure in young school-age children living in high crime neighbourhoods predicts higher peer-rated aggression (Attar *et al.* 1994). Frequency of violence exposure also predicts aggression and hopelessness in young children (Guerra *et al.* 1995), as well as internalizing and externalizing behaviour problems in children in early and middle childhood (Osofsky *et al.* 1993; Richters & Martinez 1993; Friedman 1999). Furthermore, older children and adolescents exposed to violence also demonstrate more behaviour problems than adolescents living in the same low-income communities but with lower levels of violence exposure (Fitzpatrick 1993; DuRant *et al.* 1995). The link between violence exposure and academic achievement is less clear. Violence exposure has been found to have no longitudinal relation to achievement over 1 year for young school-age children (Attar *et al.* 1994), but is related to poorer achievement in girls in early teenage years (Spencer *et al.* 1993).

The predominantly cross-sectional nature of this research introduces the possibility that the association between violence exposure and negative outcomes stems from adolescents with more emotional problems self-selecting into environments with greater violence. This explanation might be particularly relevant for older children and adolescents who have more autonomy to choose their peer groups and activities in the community. However, violence exposure is also related to more behaviour problems and adjustment in young children who have less ability to self-select into violent contexts, suggesting that much of the link between exposure and negative outcomes may be attributable to the experience of violence itself.

Risk and resilience

Our brief review chronicles the damaging nature of chronic adversities for children and adolescents. An important question throughout the literature is the probability of problematic outcomes for children in these contexts. Who are the most vulnerable children: who are the most likely to develop problems? The concept of cumulative risk has been developed to answer this. Conversely, who are the children least likely to develop problems: who are most likely to escape the ravages of these contexts? Resiliency may be able to provide the key. We briefly take up each of these topics.

Cumulative risk

The model of cumulative risk proposes that most children have the resources to cope with one risk without serious developmental consequences. However, the accumulation of many risk factors renders children vulnerable to psychopathology and other negative outcomes (Rutter *et al.* 1986; Sameroff *et al.* 1987, 1993; Garmezy & Masten 1994). Indeed, our brief review of the four chronic adversities—interparental discord, poverty, parental psychopathology and community violence—illustrates that multiple risk factors co-occur within each of these adverse contexts. For example, families with high levels of interparental conflict often evidence parental psychopathology. Similarly, poverty and economic hardship are linked with single parenthood, psychological distress and emotional disorders, low social support, and communities with crime and violence.

Rutter (1985) first proposed the cumulative risk model, and this approach has since been expanded and largely replicated in subsequent investigations (Sameroff *et al.* 1987, 1993; Kolvin *et al.* 1988; Liaw & Brooks-Gunn 1994; Fergusson & Lynskey 1996). The risk factors across the studies are similar, although not identical. They range in number and include such risks as:

- biological risks (physical health, low birth weight);
- socioeconomic risks (race, ethnicity, unemployment, education, income, family size);
- maternal mental health and intelligence (psychiatric disorder, verbal ability, anxiety, depressive symptoms); and
- family dynamics and support (marital discord, negativity, social support, stressful life events).

Similar findings emerge across the studies of cumulative risk: as the number of risk factors increases, the developmental status of the child decreases. The probability of negative outcomes (such as lower IQ, higher levels of behaviour problems or psychiatric disorder) increases significantly, often doubling or tripling for children with higher numbers of risk factors than those with only one risk factor. The concept of cumulative risk has also been assessed by creating an indicator of multiple risk; a construct that combines demographic, family psychosocial and neighbourhood risks. These studies also find that higher levels of the multiple risk indicator predict increased behaviour problems and poorer social competence in early (Seifer *et al.* 1996; Shaw *et al.* 1998) and middle childhood (Dumka *et al.* 1997; Greenberg *et al.* 1999).

Resilience

A rich literature identifies risk factors and demonstrates their association with poorer outcomes for children. Yet many children are able to adapt to stress and to develop adequate or competent social, emotional and cognitive functioning, despite the enormity of stressors often present within contexts of risk. Indeed, it is important to remember that most children faced with stressors and chronic adversity demonstrate competence in at least one domain of functioning, and some even thrive despite the presence of risk factors. But why do some children fare better in extreme circumstances than others? The concept of resilience has been developed to answer this question, partly to determine the best method for prevention and intervention in the lives of children in difficult contexts (Rutter 1979, 2000a).

Resilience refers to the ability to demonstrate successful development and adaptation within contexts of risk. Although there is new discourse on the definition and meaning of resiliency (Luthar *et al.* 2000), most agree that 'resilient' children are those who show adequate social and cognitive competence despite the presence of risk factors (Garmezy & Rutter 1983, 1985; Rutter *et al.* 1986; Masten & Coatsworth 1998). Three main dimensions of characteristics distinguish stress-resistant from stress-vulnerable children:

1 dispositional attributes (e.g. temperament, cognitive abilities, self-beliefs);
2 family characteristics (e.g. warmth, closeness, cohesion); and
3 the availability and use of external support systems by family members (Garmezy & Rutter 1985).

The presence of one or more of these protective factors is associated with better child and adolescent outcomes in contexts of risk (Werner & Smith 1982, 1992; Luthar & Zigler 1991; Fergusson & Lynskey 1996; Dumont & Provost 1999; Masten *et al.* 1999).

The identified dispositional characteristics are an easy temperament, at least average intelligence and self-efficacy. A close emotional tie with an adult family member or an organized family with routines and clear expectations buffer children, despite the presence of other negative family characteristics, such as parental discord. Perceived social support for parents or children from outside of the family seems to help protect children from difficult environments. These individual, family and community qualities and conditions are integral to the process of resilience and child development in the context of chronic adversity.

Heuristic model for processes underlying the impact of chronic adversities

A central goal of this chapter is to create a more process-orientated, theory-based understanding of the ways in which exposure to chronic adversities affects child and adolescent development, trajectories and outcomes. Although the field of

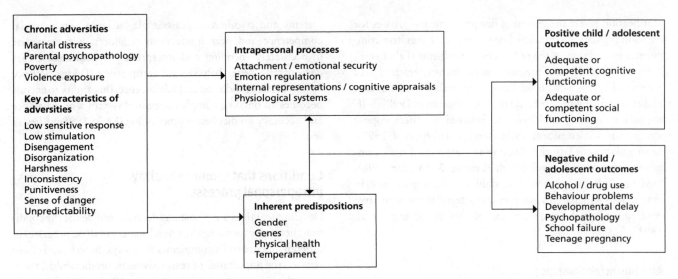

Fig. 15.1 Heuristic model for processes underlying the impact of chronic adversities.

risk and resiliency has grown substantially in the past two decades, it is still missing a unified theoretical model that attempts to explain the underlying mechanisms of resiliency in contexts of chronic risk. We are not the first to point out this gap in the field (Davies & Cummings 1994; O'Connor & Rutter 1996), nor are we the first to propose a theoretical framework for understanding children's reactions to difficult contexts (Grych & Fincham 1990; Egeland *et al.* 1993; Davies & Cummings 1994; Kumpfer 1999; Wyman *et al.* 1999). However, efforts to investigate the processes underlying the development of stress-resilient children remain scarce and disparate.

We believe that the ways in which adversities influence child trajectories cut across many risk contexts and, as such, call for an integrated approach. Therefore, in an effort to push this field forward, we have developed a heuristic model (Fig. 15.1) that proposes an integrated framework for explaining how and why chronic adversities increase the likelihood of poorer behavioural and social outcomes for children. It is our hope that this model promotes a more process-orientated approach to thinking about the meaning of chronic adversities *per se*, as well as a more process-orientated approach to investigating the impact of chronic adversities on children and families. We first turn to a discussion of normative development before presenting our model.

Intrapersonal processes and normative development

To understand the ways in which chronic adversities affect children and adolescents, we first need to consider some of the developmental processes that influence normal trajectories. We view development as a transactional process, as an interplay between the environment and the child's inherent predispositions (e.g. gender, temperament, genes; Collins *et al.* 2000). The role of genetic factors in individual development is important (see

McGuffin & Rutter, Chapter 12; Skuse & Kuntsi, Chapter 13). In recent years, genetic susceptibility for more negative developmental pathways and the interaction between genetic and environmental risk factors have become the focus of considerable research (Pike *et al.* 1996; Plomin *et al.* 1997; Rutter *et al.* 1999; Reiss *et al.* 2000; Shonkoff & Phillips 2000). For heuristic purposes, we will emphasize the role of environmental conditions as part of our framework for presenting our model. For the same reasons, we will not address the role of other biological factors (e.g. physical health and nutrition), but these factors also have a role in the transactional process. We focus on emotion regulation, attachment and emotional security, and internal representations and appraisal systems as the main processes that are fundamental to competent emotional, social and cognitive functioning. Ecological contexts can both foster and hinder the normative development of these core influential systems.

Emotion regulation

Emotion regulation refers to the process through which emotional arousal is controlled and modulated. It is central to an individual's ability to function in emotionally and physiologically arousing situations and is influenced by biological characteristics and environmental conditions (Cicchetti *et al.* 1991; Kochanska *et al.* 1997). In early childhood, caregivers help moderate and regulate arousal states by responding to infants' needs. This interaction is critical to the maintenance of physiological homeostasis and is the foundation for ongoing emotion regulation in infant development. During the first years of life, the maturation of neurological inhibitory systems, cognitive development and parental socialization all influence young children's ability to regulate and differentiate their emotions which, in the long term, influences children's adaptation to stressful situations. Demonstrating effortful control, delay of gratification and management of disappointment—proxies for emotion regulation—predicts better social and cognitive competence in addition to fewer behaviour problems (Fabes *et al.* 1999). Conversely, poor emotion regulation, often referred to as emotional reactivity, is linked to higher levels of internalizing and externalizing problems (Davies & Cummings 1998). Self-regulation in early childhood is believed to affect coping strategies in adolescence and adulthood (Eisenberg *et al.* 1997). Self-regulation in late childhood is also associated with competent psychosocial development (Lengua & Sandler 1996). Environmental responsiveness, stability and consistency in interactions with parents and peers are integral to the normative development of these systems (Sroufe 1988; Cicchetti *et al.* 1991).

Attachment relationships

The formation of secure attachment relationships is another domain of intrapersonal process with long-term implications for developmental trajectories. Attachments are individuals' representations of their relationships with significant others, usually primary caregivers. The attachment system is based upon the interaction among environmental conditions (e.g. arousing stimuli), internal child states (e.g. distress), and the behaviour and responsiveness of attachment figures (Bowlby 1969, 1982; see Cassidy 1999 for a review of attachment theory; also O'Connor, Chapter 46). Security of attachment refers to the degree to which a child has an internalized sense of significant others as trustworthy, available and loving (Bowlby 1969, 1982; Ainsworth *et al.* 1978) and, as such, can be generalized beyond relationships with parents to relationships with others. Emotional security from attachment relationships reflects a child's confidence in available and responsive attachment figures and is central to emotional well-being (Davies & Cummings 1994). Secure attachments in early childhood predict better peer relations and fewer behaviour problems in later childhood and adolescence (Shaw *et al.* 1997; Greenberg 1999) and healthier relationships and trajectories throughout life (Allen & Land 1999; Thompson 1999).

Cognitive processes

Mechanisms involved in cognitive processing, such as a child's internal representations of the world, are a third developmental domain affecting long-term adjustment and behaviour. In early childhood, children assimilate and integrate observations and appraisals of their experiences into an internalized understanding about cultural rules and expectations regarding behaviour, as well as internal representations of others and self (Zahn-Waxler & Kochanska 1988; Davies & Cummings 1994). Children use these internal working models of human interaction to evaluate and interpret the current behaviour of others and to anticipate future behaviour (Bowlby 1969, 1982; Bretherton & Munholland 1999). Consequently, these internal models, belief

systems and cognitive appraisals play a large part in social competence and peer interactions. Children with expertise in accurately encoding and interpreting environmental cues demonstrate better behavioural competency (Dodge & Price 1994). In later childhood and adolescence, this ability to encode becomes an ongoing complex appraisal system whose balance and accuracy predict better functioning (Kerig 1998a; Kliewer *et al.* 1998).

Conditions that promote healthy intrapersonal processes

Developmentalists and clinicians describe and define the conditions necessary for the healthy development of these processes in different but generally complementary ways. Investigators have stressed the importance of responsiveness, predictability, trust, warmth and sense of security (Bowlby 1969, 1982; Sroufe & Waters 1977; Sroufe 1988; Ainsworth 1990; Davies & Cummings 1994; Chase-Lansdale *et al.* 1995). These experiences are instrumental in facilitating children's emotional, behavioural and physiological abilities to cope with and adjust to stressful and arousing situations. In supportive environmental contexts, children are more likely to learn to regulate their emotions, form close attachments, and develop positive internal representations and accurate appraisal systems. Normative development of these intrapersonal processes greatly increases the likelihood that children will be able to respond to their environment with behavioural, emotional, cognitive and social competence.

We believe that the quality of early relationships is integral to future adaptation, largely through their influence upon these important intrapersonal processes. In early childhood, the family environment is often the context providing the framework for children's early experiences with others. Parent–child interactions reflect a complex bidirectional process of genetic and personality influences (Collins *et al.* 2000; Shonkoff & Phillips 2000). Children's genetically influenced tendencies (such as a sociable or difficult temperament) influence parental behaviour toward their offspring. In turn, parents can act as models of interaction, and their responsiveness, discipline and teaching techniques can directly affect children's emotional and cognitive awareness of others' behaviour and feelings (Zahn-Waxler & Radke-Yarrow 1990). During early childhood, children develop prototypical knowledge of self, others and relationships that serves as a filter for subsequent experiences (Sroufe & Fleeson 1986). The quality of early attachment relationships sets the foundation for the child's sense of effectance, curiosity about the world and, in particular, the ability to engage in intimate relationships (Sroufe 1983, 1996). Primary caregivers' emotional availability and sensitive responsiveness to the infant and growing child are critical factors in the development of secure attachment relationships, and they are important for promoting emotion regulation and providing a beneficial model of behavioural interaction (Ainsworth *et al.* 1978; Lyons-Ruth *et al.* 1989; Bretherton 1996; Eisenberg *et al.* 1997; Bretherton & Munholland 1999). Thus, responsiveness, organization, consistency, safety and warmth are all environmental qualities essential to create a context of security, caring and trust in which children can develop secure attachments, positive models for interaction and emotion regulation.

Although studied extensively in the context of parent–child interactions, relationship quality can and should also be extended to include the child's broader environment. For example, a child's interactions with and observations of interadult, peer, and other social behaviour in the home, apartment building or neighbourhood will also influence the scripts and working models they develop to make sense of their world. Furthermore, the sense of predictability and safety that a child derives in the neighbourhood can also influence emotional security and self-regulation, although more distally than from a caregiver relationship.

Later events certainly play an important part in shaping life trajectories. For instance, negative peer groups can have a deleterious effect on behaviour in middle childhood (Rutter, Giller & Hagell 1998b) and adult experiences can influence psychopathology (Brown & Harris 1989; Laub et al. 1998). However, early experience appears to have some lasting influences on development, caused in part by the internal structures that the child carries forward through each developmental stage as well as by continuity in environmental contexts (Sameroff 1994; Shonkoff & Phillips 2000). This does not mean that change is impossible at later ages (Nelson 1999), but rather that moving from an unhealthy to a healthy developmental trajectory during adolescence and young adulthood is not as easy as starting off healthily in early childhood (Chase-Lansdale et al. 1995).

Processes underlying chronic adversity

Our heuristic model proposes that chronic adversities influence developmental trajectories through the following series of mechanisms. Chronic risk creates environments characterized by disengagement, disorganization, harshness, inconsistency, insensitive responsiveness, poor stimulation, punitiveness, sense of danger and unpredictability. These qualities can exist both for proximal relationships between a child and caregiver and more distal relationships between a child and its broader community. These cross-cutting dimensions in chronic risk environments decrease a child's sense of emotional security, interrupt attachment relationships, foster emotion dysregulation, modify physiological maturation, distort internal representations and bias cognitive appraisals. The disruption in emotional security diminishes a child's ability to regulate emotional and behavioural reactions to arousing events. Modified physiological systems limit the body's ability to cope with stress. In addition, violations of trust, caring and safety negatively influence understanding of relationships and help foster biased appraisals and internal representations. The consequence of these circumstances is an increased likelihood of internalizing and externalizing behaviour problems.

The ongoing interplay between a child's inherent predisposi-

tions and the environment also serves an important role in this model. Children's inherent predispositions are conceptualized here as gender, temperament, genetics and physical health. These influence the processes between chronic adversity and child outcomes in a number of ways. First, inherent predispositions are bidirectionally related to the key characteristics of the chronic adversities. For example, certain child temperaments may facilitate greater parental disengagement or negativity. Alternatively, children of affectively ill parents are more likely to have a genetic make-up that predisposes them to poorer mental health outcomes. Secondly, these inherent qualities are bidirectionally related to intrapersonal processes. For instance, genetic predispositions and temperament can influence the development of emotion regulation (Kochanska 1997). Finally, children's inherent characteristics also have a direct relation to child outcomes. This is consistently seen in the higher rates of disruptive behaviour in males and the higher rates of emotional disorders in females (Canter 1982; Kandel & Davies 1982; Lex 1991; Huselid & Cooper 1994; Nolen-Hoeksema & Girgus 1994).

Empirical evidence

Commonalities across adverse environments

What is the evidence for psychological commonalities across adversities? Chronic interadult conflict creates a home environment in which parents are less emotionally available and where frequent and intense arguments are frightening and threatening to the child (El-Sheikh 1997; Owen & Cox 1997). Discord is related to more coercive parenting patterns (Dadds et al. 1990) and less engagement or poorer parent–child relationship quality (Harrist & Ainslie 1998). Poverty entails financial and social strains that interfere with engaged, responsive and consistent parenting (Conger et al. 1993; Klebanov et al. 1997). The frequent residential mobility and inconsistent routines that are associated with unemployment or transitory employment also can create a sense of unpredictability. Similarly, symptoms of psychopathology can be barriers to effective parenting. For example, parental depression is related to less engaged, less stimulating and less responsive parenting (Field 1995; Leadbeater et al. 1996). A chronic violent community promotes a pervasive sense of danger and disorganization as well as creating an environment that is frequently harsh and unpredictable.

The common theme across all of these chronic risk environments is that children are immersed in a context that can be threatening, disorganized, unpredictable, harsh and conflictual. This is also true of other chronic adversities, such as maltreatment, not reviewed in this chapter. Furthermore, environments in which more than one of these adversities is present are even more likely to be characterized by these psychological dimensions.

We do not contend that disorganization, for example, is the same in a household functioning under the strain of poverty as in a household with frequent interparental discord. Rather, we believe that in both cases the environmental disorganization threatens a child's need for security and predictability. We also do not mean to imply that all of these key commonalities are found in all chronically adverse environments. For instance, inconsistency, harshness and low rates of sensitive responsiveness may figure prominently in certain poverty contexts, while a sense of danger and unpredictability figure prominently in violent communities or in homes characterized by extreme parental discord. It is the pervasiveness of these characteristics, in regard to length of time and extensiveness, which makes the impact of chronic adversities so different from exposure to an acute trauma. Exposure to unpredictability, danger and insensitive responsiveness that is short or limited to one relationship is less likely to influence the developmental path of intrapersonal processes than when those conditions are persistent and pervasive. In comparison to chronic adversities, infrequent or singular acute events can be more easily assimilated as aberrations and are less likely to influence emotion regulation or necessitate the formation of new internal representations. However, chronic exposure to these contextual characteristics can be quite detrimental to these critical developmental processes.

Links to child outcomes

In the previous section, we assembled evidence from the literature for our assertion that varying chronic adversities embody similar psychological experiences for children and adolescents. In this section, we present evidence for our contention that the core features of chronic adversities in fact lead to negative child outcomes. Research across contexts of chronic risk demonstrates the links between problematic child outcomes and the key characteristics of chronic adversities in our model: harshness, inconsistency, punitiveness, unresponsiveness, unpredictability, disengagement, low stimulation and danger. Many, but not all, of these components of chronic adversities are experienced in parental behaviour. For example, parenting quality and practices (e.g. harshness of discipline, low maternal social support and low maternal warmth) explain much of the relation between socioeconomic status and psychosocial problems in children (Dodge et al. 1994; Hanson et al. 1997; Wyman et al. 1999). Maternal responsiveness, rejection and harshness also predict poorer child behaviour and academic outcomes in low-income populations (Conger et al. 1997; Myers & Taylor 1998; Shaw et al. 1998). Numerous studies also find economic stress influences children and adolescents through disruptions in parental mood and behaviour, which could be proxies for inconsistency, punitiveness and harshness (Conger et al. 1993; Duncan et al. 1994; McLoyd et al. 1994; Masten et al. 1995). Moreover, ineffective parental monitoring and discipline, which can reflect disengagement, punitiveness or inconsistency, explain the relation between socioeconomic status and delinquency in early adolescence (Larzelere & Patterson 1990), as well as the relation between parental alcohol abuse and adolescent behaviour problems (Chassin et al. 1991). In addition, lower socioeconomic status is associated with children growing up in less cognitively stimulating homes (Klebanov et al. 1997),

which in turn mediates the relation between socioeconomic status and child outcomes (Dubow & Ippolito 1994; Duncan et al. 1994).

Likewise, some of the work examining the moderating effect of protective factors supports the saliency of the key characteristics of chronic adversities. For example, the relation between maternal depression and problematic preteen outcomes is lessened when the parent–child relationship is warmer and the family demonstrates more cohesion and less conflict (Garber & Little 1999). Warmth, cohesion and low conflict reflect the absence of the key characteristics of chronic adversity we have identified, such as harshness, disorganization, inconsistency, unpredictability and punitiveness. Likewise, family cohesion is a salient buffer in contexts of parental drinking (Roosa et al. 1996) and community violence exposure (Friedman 1999). Moreover, children from high-conflict homes are less likely to demonstrate socioemotional behaviour problems if they receive authoritative parenting—a parenting style characterized by high warmth, responsiveness and monitoring (Hetherington et al. 1998). Thus, this research shows that resiliency outcomes are more likely to develop in contexts of chronic adversity when the environment is not defined by the presence of some key characteristics.

Role of intrapersonal processes in children's responses to chronic adversity

There is strong evidence that the conflictual, inconsistent and punitive characteristics of the adverse environment influence child outcomes in the context of chronic risk. However, little research examines the saliency of intrapersonal processes as a meaningful underlying mechanism. We now turn to a review of the modest existing empirical evidence for the role of intrapersonal process in children's reactions to chronic adversity.

Several theoretical models address the importance of intrapersonal process (Egeland et al. 1993; Crick & Dodge 1994; Davies & Cummings 1994, 1998; Wyman et al. 1999), but only a few studies examine this aspect of our model (Dodge et al. 1995). For the most part, research demonstrating the links between key characteristics of chronic adversities and child outcomes acknowledges the involvement and potential importance of the intrapersonal processes, but does not directly test them. The few studies examining these intermediary intrapersonal processes support their saliency as an important mechanism within the context of chronic adversity. Yet only a handful of studies addresses the four intrapersonal processes we propose: security, emotional regulation, internal representations and physiological processes. For example, maltreated children evidence internal representations that are more negative (McCrone et al. 1994). In addition, marital conflict is related to problematic attachment status in infant–parent relationships (Owen & Cox 1997), and children growing up with severely depressed mothers are more likely to have insecure attachments (Teti et al. 1995).

A relatively new area of research suggests that exposure to

chronic adversity may detrimentally affect the physiological systems designed to help humans adapt to arousing and stressful situations (see also Sandberg & Rutter, Chapter 17). The hypothalamic–pituitary–adrenal (HPA) system is one of two systems centrally involved in stress modulation. When a child or adult encounters a stressful or stimulating situation, this system is activated and helps mobilize and regulate the physiological response to stress. Chronic hyperactivity of the HPA, a possible consequence of chronic adversity, is believed to lead to dysregulated functioning of the system, which may impair stress reactivity and regulation (Hart et al. 1996). Children with a history of neglect and abuse are more likely to demonstrate altered and dysregulated HPA systems (Hart et al. 1996; Rogeness & McClure 1996; Kaufman et al. 1997). Furthermore, some children in Romanian orphanages, who have experienced severe neglect and lack of stimulation, demonstrate physiological dysregulation (Hart et al. 1996). This research suggests that immersion in a chronically stressful environment may lead to alterations in physiological stress responses, which in turn interfere with brain development and emotion regulation (Shonkoff & Phillips 2000).

Evidence for the full model

Up until now, we have tackled separate parts of the model, reviewing evidence for:

1 psychological commonalities across adversities;
2 links between these psychological commonalities and child outcomes; and
3 links between adversity commonalities and the child's intrapersonal processes.

The structure of our review reflects the status of the literature. The majority of the empirical work provides evidence for crosscutting psychological experiences of chronic adversities as well as links to child outcomes. We now highlight two programmes of research that come the closest to examining the complete process model that we propose.

The first exemplar addresses interparental discord, its effects on cognitive appraisals and links to child outcomes. The cognitive–contextual framework developed by Grych & Fincham (1990) proposes that children's understanding of conflict mediates the relation between interparental discord and child adjustment. They hypothesized that children's prior exposure to conflict leads to schemas of beliefs and expectations about what happens in conflict situations. These schemas are then used to interpret behaviour in other relationships (Grych 1998). For example, children exposed to higher levels of interparental verbal and physical aggression view conflict-orientated vignettes as more threatening and have more negative expectations about outcomes of these vignettes than children experiencing lower levels of interparental discord (Grych 1998). Similarly, children from high conflict homes perceive more anger and especially more fear during and after simulated disputes (El-Sheikh 1997). Children's perception of threat has also been associated with negative affective responses (Grych 1998).

Appraisals of conflict properties (perception of frequency, intensity and resolution), self-blame in girls and threat appraisals in boys mediate the relation between marital conflict and child outcomes, with higher levels of conflict interpretations, self-blame and threat appraisals predicting more behaviour problems (Kerig 1998b). This research supports the theory that exposure to interparental conflict distorts children's perceptions of conflict and fear, and that these biased perceptions and appraisals are used to interpret parental behaviour as well as the interactions of others. In turn, the types of appraisals children make are associated with their behavioural adjustment.

The second programme of research that provides empirical support for our heuristic model involves a social information-processing theory of social adjustment. Crick & Dodge's (1994) social information-processing model views behaviour as a function of processing environmental cues in six steps:

1 encoding of external and internal cues;
2 interpretation and mental representation of cues;
3 clarification or selection of a goal;
4 response access or construction;
5 response decision; and
6 behavioural enactment (Crick & Dodge 1994).

Crick and Dodge hypothesized that children's past experiences heavily influence these steps because memories create a general 'mental structure' (which we call internal models) that guide processing of future social cues. For example, early harsh discipline might lead to specific mental representations that would bias children toward hostile and negative interpretations of non-hostile interactions, distracting them from relevant social cues. Hypervigilance to hostile cues would lead children to assume hostile intent in others and because of this misattribution and highly accessible aggressive responses in memory, they would be more likely to behave aggressively (Dodge et al. 1997). The authors of this model also suggest that early experiences create neural paths that become activated in future interactions and that emotion is a central influence in each step of processing.

This explanatory model is empirically supported in laboratory studies using videotaped vignettes of social interactions. In school-age children, a history of physical abuse is associated with errors in all steps of information processing—attending to and encoding of relevant cues, interpretation of peers' intentions, accessing possible behavioural responses, and evaluation of consequences—controlling for socioeconomic status and temperament. Furthermore, these types of information-processing cues mediate the relation between abuse history and elevated rates of externalizing problems (Dodge et al. 1997).

In a separate longitudinal study that followed a representative sample of more than 500 pre-K children for 4 years, higher numbers of processing errors were associated with more conduct problems. The risk of later conduct problems was four times greater for children with multiple processing errors than for children with no or few processing errors (Dodge et al. 1995). In similar but less detailed research, inappropriate or inaccurate inferences about interpersonal situations have mediated the link between maltreatment and behaviour dysregulation, maltreatment and isolation by peers, and maltreatment and social effectiveness (Rogosch *et al*. 1995).

Toward understanding resilience

Timing

Our model also creates a framework for understanding risk and resiliency and why contexts of chronic adversity do not lead to poor outcomes for all children. One important aspect of this framework is the issue of timing. We believe that children who experience chronic risk later in development are more likely to demonstrate resilience. A relatively low-risk environment during infancy and early childhood would permit normative development of the identified intrapersonal processes. With normative internal representations, emotion regulation and coping systems, older children and adolescents will be more capable of adapting to chronic risks, and the likelihood of poor outcomes will decrease. In contrast, children who are born into environments of chronic adversity or who experience adverse environments early in life will be more likely to have negative prenatal influences and salient disruptions in the normative development of social, emotional and behavioural processes. A wealth of empirical evidence supports the view that healthy experiences in early childhood increase the likelihood of positive life trajectories (Shonkoff & Phillips 2000). However, very little empirical research addresses intrapersonal processes as specific components of resilience in early vs. later childhood. Evidence is accruing on the potential for recovery after abusive, neglectful or violent conditions in early childhood (Rutter *et al*. 1998a; Shonkoff & Phillips 2000), but considerably more research is needed on the reasons why this is the case.

Extent of risk

The second important issue is the degree of comprehensiveness of negative environmental dimensions. While we do not dismiss the theory of cumulative risk, we propose that it overly emphasizes the additive nature of risk, and it does not address the processes underlying multiple vs. few risks. We believe that the chance for resilience decreases with increasing aspects of the chronic adversity that limit normative intrapersonal processes. Thus, the less extensive the proximal and distal characteristics of adversities, the more likely various intrapersonal processes will develop normatively, and the more likely the child will demonstrate resilience. Are the characteristics of chronic adversities dominating the child's experience or not? For instance, a child with an affectively ill mother will be more likely to develop secure attachments, healthy emotion regulation and positive internal representations if a responsive father, free of psychopathology, is present to model healthy interactions and provide environmental organization. This scenario can indeed be understood within the model of cumulative risk: a child will fare better with two risks (maternal psychopathology,

genetic predispositions) than with three risks (maternal psychopathology, genetic predisposition, paternal psychopathology). We reframe this to focus on whether or not the commonalities across chronic adversities are widespread and pervasive vs. intermittent and restricted.

A focus on the comprehensiveness of environmental characteristics also provides a framework for understanding how the triad of protective factors might promote resilience in situations of chronic adversity. For instance, a good relationship with an adult family member acts as a protective factor for children in difficult environments (Rutter 1979; Werner & Smith 1982; Gonzales *et al*. 1996), but little research has examined the underlying process for how or why social support promotes more effective adjustment in children. Our model proposes that social support acts as a buffer by creating a meaningful attachment relationship, modelling positive social interaction, and promoting emotional security and a sense of safety. A child with social support is more likely to develop normative internal representations, cognitive appraisals and better emotion regulation, all of which promote effective coping under stressful circumstances. The protective influence of family cohesion or organization (Roosa *et al*. 1996; Friedman 1999) can be explained similarly. A child living in poverty but within a cohesive family experiences less unpredictability, less disorganization and warmer interrelationships.

The protective influence of inherent predispositions can likewise be understood. For example, children with certain temperaments seem to fare better than children with more difficult temperaments (Sanson & Prior 1999). Within the framework of this model, the underlying processes through which this occurs are specified. Children in high-risk settings who have calmer or easier temperaments may be less likely to invoke punitive parenting styles, thus facilitating healthier intrapersonal processes than would otherwise develop. Easier temperaments might also reflect a more effective inherent capacity for emotion regulation. Children with other types of inherent predispositions, such as outgoing, engaging personalities, may also elicit more positive social relationships from the environment, perhaps with a teacher, grandparent or neighbour, which foster more positive internal representations and cognitive appraisals. Thus, children are most likely to demonstrate resilience when environmental characteristics facilitate more normative development and interaction between inherent predispositions and intrapersonal processes.

Additional considerations

We would like to conclude the discussion of our model with a few caveats. It is beyond the scope of this chapter to address every nuance of this heuristic model, but some final comments are necessary. First, we believe that the model represents a dynamic transactional process, although this has not been the focus of our discussion. The model is not meant to convey a linear or one-way process. We presume that child outcome behaviours listed in the final box influence every aspect of the model.

For example, a behaviourally aggressive or disordered child likely elicits more harshness and disengagement from their environment (Ge *et al.* 1996). Similarly, an aggressive child will often self-select into more conflictual settings, and these environments will further confirm and influence negative or biased cognitive appraisal systems. Not only is the environment acting upon the child, but the child is constantly shaping the environment (Kandel & Wu 1995; Rutter *et al.* 1997; see also Rutter, Chapter 19).

Secondly, we have not fully discussed the potential influence of inherent predispositions although we believe these interact at every point in the model. The genetic contribution to both the chronic adversity and child outcome may be considerable (Pike *et al.* 1996). Parents who pass on genetic risks are also more likely to provide distal and proximal environments with increased risk (Rutter 1999; see also McGuffin & Rutter, Chapter 12). In addition, genetic factors may affect adaptation to chronic adversity by influencing individual susceptibility (Rutter 2000a). Thus, differentiating the genetic contribution from the environmental contribution is difficult. A recent report of the US National Academy of Sciences has renamed these processes 'nature through nurture' (Shonkoff & Phillips 2000), arguing that the two go hand in hand and that a focus on trying to separate them is simplistic. Nevertheless, there is a range of research strategies that may be used to test for environmental mediation of risks (Rutter *et al.*, 2001) and these have shown the importance of many of the environmental risks discussed here (Rutter 2000b).

It is beyond the scope of this chapter to review the important fields informing gene–environment correlations in development. Our uneven presentation here is not meant to imply that genetic predispositions are not relevant to the model but, rather, we have chosen to focus specifically on intrapersonal processes in this chapter and to highlight the relative lack of research on the topic. Finally, we would like to acknowledge that in many instances, parents partially select into chronically adverse environments. Exposure to chronic adversity, as an adult or child, is rarely a random event (Rutter *et al.* 1995). This is important for understanding the nature of chronic adversities because the characteristics that lead to this self-selection into adversity may also influence some portion of our model. However, our model attempts to specify what happens once a family is living in a context of chronic adversity.

Moving the field of resiliency forward

We believe that the fields of resiliency and chronic adversity will be best served by focusing on the processes underlying the developmental trajectories for children and families living within adverse circumstances. This has implications for intervention and research. From the standpoint of intervention, our model and the existing literature suggest two main pathways for effecting change. The first pathway involves the policy arena. One clear way to promote healthy development is to limit children's exposure to chronic adversities. Reducing environmental chronic adversity is no easy task, but the importance of minimizing children's exposure to chronic adversity should not be overlooked. Moreover, policymakers should recognize the difficulties inherent in trying to change developmental trajectories for children and youth. The removal of a chronic adversity after years of exposure will not produce a quick or radical behaviour change. This speaks to the importance of prevention as well as early intervention.

Secondly, our model and the empirical evidence suggest specific directions for clinicians working with children and families exposed to chronic adversities. Resilience is influenced by the child's interpersonal relationships and thus family therapy may be critical to successful intervention (Rutter 1999). For young children, the salience of intrapersonal processes means that clinical intervention at the family level should assist parents in promoting an environment that can support healthier development. This might involve helping parents understand the importance of consistent predictable parenting, and working with parents to facilitate healthier attachments, regulation and cognitions. For older children and adolescents, intervention at the family level would be similarly important. In addition, individual clinical work focused on cognitive appraisal systems, emotion regulation and coping strategies would be a helpful supplement (Sandler *et al.*, 2000; Wyman *et al.*, 2000). Finally, clinical intervention could also facilitate alternative structured activities for children and adolescents outside of the family, where they can experience consistency and positive interactions within a demanding context (Allen *et al.* 1997).

Turning to the future of empirical work on chronic adversity, we urge investigators to focus on process-orientated research. We ask that research not stop at examining *what* factors are protective, but also to determine *why* they are protective. For example, we know that IQ and cognitive functioning lead to better outcomes, but we still do not know why (Masten *et al.* 1999). Future research should seek to test competing processes. For example, which of the intrapersonal processes we propose are most important for coping? Many additional questions remain. How do inherent predispositions pull for resilience? What key characteristics of chronic adversities are potentially the most harmful? What defines chronicity and how should it be measured? In addition, the methodological difficulties associated with this area of research must continue to be addressed. Specifically, the cross-sectional nature of many studies, the bidirectionality and transactional nature of effects, and the co-occurrence of risk factors, all pose methodological challenges that researchers must continue to tackle. Our hope is that this heuristic model provides a theoretical framework for answering some of the questions remaining in the literature and for guiding the direction of future research. This will be beneficial not only for deepening our research knowledge, but also for informing clinicians and policymakers about how to best assist families living under chronically difficult circumstances.

References

Ainsworth, M.D.S. (1990) Some considerations regarding theory and assessment relevant to attachments beyond infancy. In: *Attachment in the Preschool Years* (eds M.T. Greenberg, D. Cicchetti & E.M. Cummings), pp. 463–488. University of Chicago Press, Chicago.

Ainsworth, M.D.S., Blehar, M.C., Waters, E. & Wall, S. (1978) *Patterns of Attachment: a Psychological Study of the Strange Situation.* Erlbaum, Hillsdale, NJ.

Allen, J.P. & Land, D. (1999) Attachment in adolescence. In: *Handbook of Attachment: Theory, Research, and Clinical Applications* (eds J. Cassidy & P.R. Shaver), pp. 319–335. Guilford Press, New York.

Allen, J.P., Philliber, S., Herrling, S. & Kuperminc, G.P. (1997) Preventing teen pregnancy and academic failure: experimental evaluation of a developmentally based approach. *Child Development*, 64, 729–742.

Attar, B.K., Guerra, N.G. & Tolan, P.H. (1994) Neighborhood disadvantage, stressful life events, and adjustment in urban elementary-school children. *Journal of Clinical Child Psychology*, 23, 391–400.

Beardslee, W.R., Versage, E.M. & Gladstone, T.R.G. (1998) Children of affectively ill parents: a review of the past 10 years. *Journal of the American Academy of Child and Adolescent Psychiatry*, 37, 1134–1141.

Bell, C.C. & Jenkins, E.J. (1993) Community violence and children on Chicago's southside. *Psychiatry: Interpersonal and Biological Processes*, 56, 46–54.

Bolger, K.E., Patterson, C.J., Thompson, W.W. & Kupersmidt, J.B. (1995) Psychosocial adjustment among children experiencing persistent and intermittent family economic hardship. *Child Development*, 66, 1107–1129.

Bowlby, J. (1969) *Attachment and Loss*, Vol. 1, *Attachment*. Basic Books, New York.

Bowlby, J. (1982) Attachment and loss: retrospect and prospect. *American Journal of Orthopsychiatry*, 52, 664–678.

Bretherton, I. (1996) Internal working models of attachment relationships as related to resilient coping. In: *Development and Vulnerability in Close Relationships* (eds G.G. Noam & K.W. Fischer), pp. 3–27. Erlbaum, Mahwah, New Jersey.

Bretherton, I. & Munholland, K.A. (1999) Internal working models in attachment relationships: a construct revisited. In: *Handbook of Attachment: Theory, Research, and Clinical Applications* (eds J. Cassidy & P.R. Shaver), pp. 88–111. Guilford Press, New York.

Brooks-Gunn, J., Duncan, G.J. & Aber, J.L., eds (1997a) *Neighborhood Poverty*, Vol. 1. *Context and Consequences for Children*. Russell Sage Foundation, New York.

Brooks-Gunn, J., Duncan, G.J. & Maritato, N. (1997b) Poor families, poor outcomes: the well-being of children and youth. In: *Consequences of Growing Up Poor* (eds G.J. Duncan & J. Brooks-Gunn), pp. 1–17. Russell Sage Foundation, New York.

Brown, G.W. & Harris, T.O., eds (1989) *Life Events and Illness*. Guilford Press, New York.

Canter, R.J. (1982) Sex differences in self-report delinquency. *Criminology*, 20, 373–393.

Cassidy, J. (1999) The nature of the child's ties. In: *Handbook of Attachment: Theory, Research, and Clinical Applications* (eds J. Cassidy & P.R. Shaver.), pp. 3–20. Guilford Press, New York.

Chase-Lansdale, P.L. (1999) Effects of poverty on children and families. In: *Families, Poverty, and Welfare Reform: Confronting a New Policy Era* (ed. L.B. Joseph), pp. 245–281. University of Illinois Press, Chicago.

Chase-Lansdale, P.L. & Gordon, R.A. (1996) Economic hardship and the development of five and six year olds: neighborhood and regional perspectives. *Child Development*, 67, 3338–3367.

Chase-Lansdale, P.L., Wakschlag, L.S. & Brooks-Gunn, J. (1995) A psychological perspective on the development of caring in children and youth: the role of the family. *Journal of Adolescence*, 18, 515–556.

Chase-Lansdale, P.L., Gordon, R.A., Brooks-Gunn, J. & Klebanov, P.K. (1997) Neighborhood and family influences on the intellectual and behavioral competence of preschool and early school-age children. In: *Neighborhood Poverty: Context and Consequences for Children*, Vol. 1 (eds J. Brooks-Gunn, G.J. Duncan & J.L. Aber), pp. 79–118. Russell Sage Foundation, New York.

Chassin, L., Rogosch, F. & Barrera, M. (1991) Substance use and symptomatology among adolescent children of alcoholics. *Journal of Abnormal Psychology*, 100, 449–463.

Chassin, L., Barrera, M.J. & Montgomery, H. (1997) Parental alcoholism as a risk factor. In: *Handbook of Children's Coping: Linking Theory and Intervention* (eds S.A. Wolchik & I.N. Sandler), pp. 101–129. Plenum Press, New York.

Cherlin, A.J. (1992) *Marriage, Divorce, Remarriage*. Harvard University Press, Cambridge, MA.

Christ, M.A., Lahey, B.B., Frick, J. & Russo, M.F. (1990) Serious conduct problems in the children of adolescent mothers: disentangling confounded correlations. *Journal of Consulting and Clinical Psychology*, 58, 840–844.

Cicchetti, D., Ganiban, J. & Barnett, D. (1991) Contributions from the study of high-risk populations to understanding the development of emotion regulation. In: *The Development of Emotion Regulation and Disregulation* (eds J. Garber & K.A. Dodge), pp. 15–48. Cambridge University Press, New York.

Colder, C.R., Chassin, L., Stice, E.M. & Curran, P.J. (1997) Alcohol expectancies as potential mediators of parent alcoholism effects on the development of adolescent heavy drinking. *Journal of Research on Adolescence*, 7, 349–374.

Collins, W.A., Maccoby, E.E., Steinberg, L., Hetherington, E.M. & Bornstein, M.H. (2000) Contemporary research on parenting. *American Psychologist*, 55, 1–15.

Conger, R.D., Conger, K.J., Elder, G.H. *et al.* (1993) Family economic stress and adjustment of early adolescent girls. *Developmental Psychology*, 29, 206–219.

Conger, R.D., Conger, K.J. & Elder, G.H. (1997) Family economic hardship and adolescent adjustment: mediating and moderating process. In: *Consequences of Growing Up Poor*, Vol. 1 (eds G.J. Duncan & J. Brooks-Gunn), pp. 289–310. Russell Sage Foundation, New York.

Crick, N.R. & Dodge, K.A. (1994) A review and reformulation of social information-processing mechanisms in children's social adjustment. *Psychological Bulletin*, 115, 74–101.

Cummings, E.M., Iannotti, R.J. & Zahn-Waxler, C. (1985) Influence of conflict between adults on the emotions and aggression of young children. *Developmental Psychology*, 21, 495–507.

Cummings, E.M., Davies, P.T. & Simpson, K.S. (1994) Marital conflict, gender, and children's appraisals and coping efficacy as mediators of child adjustment. *Journal of Family Psychology*, 8, 141–149.

Dadds, M.R., Sheffield, J.K. & Holbeck, J.F. (1990) An examination of the differential relationship of marital discord to parents' discipline strategies for boys and girls. *Journal of Abnormal Child Psychology*, 18, 121–129.

Davies, P.T. & Cummings, E.M. (1994) Marital conflict and child adjustment: an emotional security hypothesis. *Psychological Bulletin*, 116, 387–411.

Davies, P.T. & Cummings, E.M. (1998) Exploring children's emotional security as a mediator of the link between marital relations and child adjustment. *Child Development*, **69**, 124–139.

Davies, P.T. & Windle, M. (1997) Gender-specific pathways between maternal depressive symptoms, family discord, and adolescent adjustment. *Developmental Psychology*, **33**, 657–668.

Depner, C.E., Leino, E.V. & Chun, A. (1992) Interparental conflict and child adjustment: a decade review and meta-analysis. *Family and Conciliation Courts Review*, **30**, 323–341.

Dodge, K.A. & Price, J.M. (1994) On the relation between social information processing and socially competent behavior in early school-aged children. *Child Development*, **65**, 1385–1897.

Dodge, K.A., Pettit, G.S. & Bates, J.E. (1994) Socialization mediators of the relation between socioeconomic status and child conduct problems. *Child Development*, **65**, 649–665.

Dodge, K.A., Pettit, G.S., Bates, J.E. & Valente, E. (1995) Social information-processing patterns partially mediate the effect of early physical abuse on later conduct problems. *Journal of Abnormal Psychology*, **104** (4), 632–643.

Dodge, K.A., Pettit, G.S. & Bates, J.E. (1997) How the experience of early physical abuse leads children to become chronically aggressive. In: *Developmental Perspectives on Trauma: Theory, Research, and Intervention, Rochester Symposium on Developmental Psychology*, Vol. 8 (ed. D. Cicchetti), pp. 263–288. University of Rochester Press, Rochester, NY.

Domenico, D. & Windle, M. (1993) Intrapersonal and interpersonal functioning among middle-aged female adult children of alcoholics. *Journal of Consulting and Clinical Psychology*, **61**, 659–666.

Dubow, E.F. & Ippolito, M.F. (1994) Effects of poverty and quality of the home environment on changes in the academic and behavioral adjustment of elementary school-age children. *Journal of Clinical Child Psychology*, **23**, 401–412.

Dubow, E.F., Edwards, S. & Ippolito, M.F. (1997) Life stressors, neighborhood disadvantage and resources: a focus on inner-city children's adjustment. *Journal of Clinical Child Psychology*, **26**, 130–144.

Dumka, L.E., Roosa, M.W. & Jackson, K.M. (1997) Risk, conflict, mothers' parenting, and children's adjustment in low-income, Mexican immigrant, and Mexican American families. *Journal of Marriage and the Family*, **59**, 309–323.

Dumont, M. & Provost, M.A. (1999) Resilience in adolescents: protective role of social support, coping strategies, self-esteem, and social activities on experience of stress and depression. *Journal of Youth and Adolescence*, **28**, 343–363.

Duncan, G.J. & Brooks-Gunn, J., eds (1997) *Consequences of Growing Up Poor*. Russell Sage Foundation, New York.

Duncan, G.J. & Rodgers, W.L. (1988) Longitudinal aspects of childhood poverty. *Journal of Marriage and the Family*, **50**, 1007–1021.

Duncan, G.J., Brooks-Gunn, J. & Klebanov, P.K. (1994) Economic deprivation and early childhood development. *Child Development*, **65**, 296–318.

Duncan, G.J., Yeung, W.J., Brooks-Gunn, J. & Smith, J.R. (1998) How much does childhood poverty affect the life chances of children? *American Sociological Review*, **63**, 406–423.

DuRant, R.H., Getts, A., Cadenhead, C., Emands, S.J. & Woods, E.R. (1995) Exposure to violence and victimization and depression, hopelessness, and purpose in life among adolescents living in and around public housing. *Journal of Developmental and Behavioral Pediatrics*, **16**, 233–237.

Egeland, B.R., Carlson, E. & Sroufe, A.L. (1993) Resilience as process. *Development and Psychopathology* **5**, 517–528.

Eisenberg, N., Fabes, R.A. & Guthrie, I.K. (1997) Coping with stress: the roles of regulation and development. In: *Handbook of Children's Coping: Linking Theory and Intervention—Issues in Clinical Child Psychology* (eds S.A. Wolchik & I.N. Sandler), pp. 41–70. Plenum Press, New York.

El-Sheikh, M. (1997) Children's responses to adult–adult and mother–child arguments: the role of parental marital conflict and distress. *Journal of Family Psychology*, **11**, 165–175.

El-Sheikh, M., Cummings, E.M. & Goetsch, V.L. (1989) Coping with adults' angry behavior: behavioral, psychological, and self-reported responding in preschoolers. *Developmental Psychology*, **25**, 490–498.

Fabes, R.A., Eisenberg, N., Jones, S. *et al.* (1999) Regulation, emotionality, and preschoolers' socially competent peer interactions. *Child Development*, **70**, 432–442.

Factor, D.C. & Wolfe, D.A. (1990) Parental psychopathology and high-risk children. In: *Children at Risk: an Evaluation of Factors Contributing to Child Abuse* (eds R.T. Ammerman & M. Hersen), pp. 171–198. Plenum Press, New York.

Fergusson, D.M. & Lynskey, M.T. (1996) Adolescent resiliency to family adversity. *Journal of Child Psychology and Psychiatry*, **37**, 281–292.

Field, T. (1995) Infants of depressed mothers. *Infant Behavior and Development*, **18**, 1–13.

Fingerhut, L.A., Cox, C.S. & Warner, M. (1998) *International Comparative analysis of Injury Mortality: Findings from the ICE on Injury Statistics*. DHHS Publication No. (PHS) 98–1250. Hyattsville, MD. US Department of Health and Human Services, Public Health Service, Centers for Disease Control and Prevention, National Center for Health Statistics.

Fitzpatrick, K.M. (1993) Exposure to violence and presence of depression among low-income African American youth. *Journal of Consulting and Clinical Psychology*, **61**, 528–531.

Frick, P.J., Lahey, B.B., Loeber, R. & Stouthamer-Loeber, M. (1992) Familial risk factors to oppositional defiant disorder and conduct disorder: parental psychopathology and maternal parenting. *Journal of Consulting and Clinical Psychology*, **60**, 49–55.

Friedman, R.J. (1999) *Violence exposure and child mental health: direct effects and protective factors*. Dissertation in Clinical Psychology. Arizona State University.

Garber, J. & Little, S. (1999) Predictors of competence among offspring of depressed mothers. *Journal of Adolescent Research*, **14**, 44–71.

Garmezy, N. & Masten, A.S. (1994) Chronic adversities. In: *Child and Adolescent Psychiatry* (eds M. Rutter, E. Taylor & L. Hersov), pp. 191–208. Blackwell Scientific Publications, Boston.

Garmezy, N. & Rutter, M. (1985) Acute reactions to stress. In: *Child and Adolescent Psychiatry*, 2nd edn (eds M. Rutter & L. Hersov), pp. 152–176. Blackwell Scientific Publications, Oxford.

Garmezy, N. & Rutter, M. (1983) *Stress, Coping, and Development in Children*. McGraw-Hill, New York (later published in 1988 by John Hopkins University Press, Baltimore, MD).

Ge, X., Conger, R.D., Cadoret, R.J. *et al.* (1996) The developmental interface between nature and nurture: a mutual influence model of child antisocial behavior and parent behaviors. *Developmental Psychology*, **32**, 574–589.

Gonzales, N.A., Cauce, A.M., Friedman, R.J. & Mason, C.A. (1996) Family, peer, and neighborhood influences on academic achievement among African American adolescents: one-year prospective effects. *American Journal of Community Psychology*, **24**, 365–387.

Goodman, S.H., Brogan, D., Lynch, M.E. & Fielding, B. (1993) Social and emotional competence in children of depressed mothers. *Child Development*, **64**, 516–531.

Greenberg, M.T. (1999) Attachment and psychopathology in childhood. In: *Handbook of Attachment: Theory, Research, and Clinical*

Applications (eds J. Cassidy & Shaver, P.R.), pp. 469–496. Guilford Press, New York.

Greenberg, M.T., Lengua, L.J., Coie, J.D. *et al.* (1999) Predicting developmental outcomes at school entry using a multiple-risk model: four American communities. *Developmental Psychology*, 35, 403–417.

Grych, J.H. (1998) Children's appraisals of interparental conflict: situational and contextual influences. *Journal of Family Psychology*, 12, 437–453.

Grych, J.H. & Fincham, F.D. (1990) Marital conflict and children's adjustment: a cognitive–contextual framework. *Psychological Bulletin*, 108, 267–290.

Guerra, N.G., Huesmann, L.R., Tolan, P.H., Van Acker, R. & Eron, L.D. (1995) Stressful events and individual beliefs as correlates of economic disadvantage and aggression among urban children. *Journal of Consulting and Clinical Psychology*, 63, 518–528.

Guzder, J., Paris, J., Zelkowitz, P. & Feldman, R. (1999) Psychological risk factors for borderline pathology in school-age children. *Journal of the American Academy of Child and Adolescent Psychiatry*, 38, 206–212.

Hanson, T.L., McLanahan, S. & Thompson, E. (1997) Economic resources, parental practices and children's well-being. In: *Consequences of Growing Up Poor* (eds G.J. Duncan & J. Brooks-Gunn), pp. 191–238. Russell Sage, New York.

Harrist, A.W. & Ainslie, R.C. (1998) Marital discord and child behavior problems: parent–child relationship quality and child interpersonal awareness as mediators. *Journal of Family Issues*, 19, 140–163.

Hart, J., Gunnar, M. & Cicchetti, D. (1996) Altered neuroendocrine activity in maltreated children related to symptoms of depression. *Development and Psychopathology*, 8, 201–214.

Hetherington, E.M. (1999) Should we stay together for the sake of the children?. In: *Coping with Divorce, Single Parenting, and Remarriage: a Risk and Resiliency Perspective* (ed. E.M. Hetherington), pp. 93–116. Erlbaum, Mahwah, NJ.

Hetherington, E.M., Bridges, M. & Insabella, G.M. (1998) What matters? What does not? Five perspectives on the association between marital transitions and children's adjustment. *American Psychologist*, 53, 167–184.

Huselid, R.F. & Cooper, M.L. (1994) Gender roles as mediators of sex differences in expressions of pathology. *Journal of Abnormal Psychology*, 103, 595–603.

Kandel, D.B. & Davies, M. (1982) Epidemiology of depressive mood in adolescents. *Archives of General Psychiatry*, 39, 1205–1212.

Kandel, D.B. & Wu, P. (1995) The contributions of mothers and fathers to the intergenerational transmission of cigarette smoking in adolescence. *Journal of Research on Adolescence*, 5, 225–252.

Kaufman, J., Birmaher, B., Perel, J. *et al.* (1997) The corticotropin-releasing hormone challenge in depressed abused, depressed nonabused, and normal control children. *Biological Psychiatry*, 42, 669–679.

Kerig, P.K. (1998a) Gender and appraisals as mediators of adjustment in children exposed to interparental violence. *Journal of Family Violence*, 13, 345–363.

Kerig, P.K. (1998b) Moderators and mediators of the effects of interparental conflict on children's adjustment. *Journal of Abnormal Child Psychology*, 26, 199–212.

Kessler, R.C., McGonagle, K.A., Zhao, S. *et al.* (1994) Lifetime and 12 month prevalence of DSM-III-R psychiatric disorders in the USA: results from the National Comorbidity Survey. *Archives of General Psychiatry*, 51, 8–19.

Kiernan, K. (1999) Cohabitation in Western Europe. *Population Trends*, 96. The Stationery Office, London.

Klebanov, P., Brooks-Gunn, J., Chase-Lansdale, P.L. & Gordon, R.A. (1997) Are neighborhood effects on young children mediated by features of the home environment? In: *Neighborhood Poverty: Context and Consequences for Children*, Vol. 1 (eds J. Brooks-Gunn, G.J. Duncan & L.J. Aber), pp. 119–145. Russell Sage, New York.

Kliewer, W., Fearnow, M.D. & Walton, M.N. (1998) Dispositional, environmental, and context-specific predictors of children's threat perceptions in everyday stressful situations. *Journal of Youth and Adolescence*, 27, 83–100.

Kochanska, G. (1997) Multiple pathways to conscience for children with difficult temperaments: From toddlerhood to age 5. *Developmental Psychology*, 33, 228–240.

Kochanska, G., Murray, K. & Coy, K.C. (1997) Inhibitory control as a contributor to conscience in childhood: from toddler to early child age. *Child Development*, 68, 263–277.

Kolvin, I., Miller, F.J.W., Fleeting, M. & Kolvin, P.A. (1988) Risk/protective factors for offending with particular reference to deprivation. In: *Studies of Psychosocial Risk: the Power of Longitudinal Data* (ed. M. Rutter), pp. 77–95. Cambridge University Press, Cambridge.

Korenman, S. & Miller, J.E. (1997) Effects of long-term poverty on physical health of children in the national longitudinal survey of youth. In: *Consequences of Growing Up Poor* (eds G.J. Duncan & J. Brooks-Gunn), pp. 70–99. Russell Sage, New York.

Kumpfer, K.L. (1999) Factors and processes contributing to resilience: the resilience framework. In: *Resilience and Development: Positive Life Adaptations* (eds M.D. Glantz & J.L. Johnson), pp. 179–224. Kluwer Academic/Plenum Publishers, New York.

Lahey, B.B., Loeber, R., Hart, E.L. & Frick, P.J. (1995) Four-year longitudinal study of conduct disorder in boys: patterns and predictors of persistence. *Journal of Abnormal Psychology*, 104, 83–93.

Larzelere, R.E. & Patterson, G.R. (1990) Parental management: mediator of the effects of socioeconomic status on early delinquency. *Criminology*, 28, 301–323.

Laub, J.H., Nagin, D.S. & Sampson, R.J. (1998) Trajectories of change in criminal offending: good marriages and the desistance process. *American Sociological Review*, 63, 225–238.

Leadbeater, B.J., Bishop, S.J. & Raver, C.C. (1996) Quality of mother–toddler interactions, maternal depressive symptoms, and behavior problems in preschoolers of adolescent mothers. *Developmental Psychology*, 32, 280–288.

Lengua, L.J. & Sandler, I.N. (1996) Self-regulation as a moderator of the relation between coping and symptomatology in children of divorce. *Journal of Abnormal Child Psychology*, 24, 681–701.

Leventhal, T. & Brooks-Gunn, J. (2000) The neighborhoods they live in: the effects of neighborhood residence upon child and adolescent outcomes. *Psychological Bulletin*, 126, 309–337.

Lex, B.W. (1991) Some gender differences in alcohol and polysubstance uses. *Health Psychology*, 10, 121–132.

Liaw, R. & Brooks-Gunn, J. (1994) Cumulative familial risks and low-birthweight children's cognitive and behavioral development. *Journal of Clinical Child Psychology*, 23, 360–372.

Loeber, R. & Dishion, T. (1983) Early predictors of male delinquency: a review. *Psychological Bulletin*, 94, 68–99.

Lorenz, G., Hoven, C., Andrews, H.F. & Bird, H. (1995) Marital discord and psychiatric disorder in children and adolescents. *Journal of Child and Family Studies*, 4, 341–358.

Luthar, S.S. & Zigler, E. (1991) Vulnerability and competence: a review of research on resilience in childhood. *American Journal of Orthopsychiatry*, 61, 6–22.

Luthar, S.S., Cicchetti, D. & Becker, B. (2000) The construct of resilience: a critical evaluation and guidelines for future work. *Child Development*, 71, 543–562.

Lyons-Ruth, K., Connell, D. & Zoll, D. (1989) Patterns of maternal behavior among infants at risk for abuse: relations with infant attachment behavior and infant development at 12 months of age. In: *Child Maltreatment* (eds D. Cicchetti & V. Carlson), pp. 464–493. Cambridge University Press, Cambridge.

Martin, C.S., Earleywinde, M., Blackson, T.C. *et al.* (1994) Aggressivity, inattention, hyperactivity, and impulsivity in boys at high and low risk for substance abuse. *Journal of Abnormal Child Psychology*, **22**, 177–203.

Masten, A.S. & Coatsworth, J.D. (1998) The development of competence in favorable and unfavorable environments. *American Psychologist*, **53**, 205–220.

Masten, A.S., Coatsworth, D.J., Neemann, J. *et al.* (1995) The structure and coherence of competence from childhood through adolescence. *Child Development*, **66**, 1635–1659.

Masten, A.S., Hubbard, J.J., Gest, S.D. *et al.* (1999) Competence in the context of adversity: pathways to resilience and maladaptation from childhood to late adolescence. *Development and Psychopathology*, **11**, 143–169.

Mayer, S.E. (1997) *What Money Can't Buy: Family Income and Children's Life Chances*. Harvard University Press, Cambridge, MA.

McConnochie, K.M., Russo, M.J., McBride, J.T. *et al.* (1999) Socioeconomic variation in asthma hospitalization: excess utilization or greater need? *Pediatrics*, **103**, e75.

McCrone, E.R., Egeland, B., Kalkoske, M. & Carlson, E. (1994) Relations between early maltreatment and mental representations of relationships assessed with projective storytelling in middle childhood. *Development and Psychopathology*, **6**, 99–120.

McLoyd, V.C., Jayaratne, T.E., Ceballo, R. & Borques, J. (1994) Unemployment and work interruption among African American single mothers: effects on parenting and adolescent socioemotional functioning. *Child Development*, **65**, 562–589.

McNeal, C. & Amato, P.R. (1998) Parents' marital violence: long-term consequences for children. *Journal of Family Issues*, **19**, 123–139.

Myers, H.F. & Taylor, S. (1998) Family contributions to risk and resilience in African American children. *Journal of Comparative Family Studies*, **29**, 215–229.

Nelson, C.A. (1999) How important are the first years of life? *Applied Developmental Science*, **3**, 235–238.

Nolen-Hoeksema, S. & Girgus, J.S. (1994) The emergence of gender differences in depression during adolescence. *Psychological Bulletin*, **115**, 424–443.

O'Connor, T.G. & Rutter, M. (1996) Risk mechanisms in development: some conceptual and methodological considerations. *Developmental Psychology*, **32**, 787–795.

Osofsky, J.D., Wewers, S., Hann, D.M. & Fick, A.C. (1993) Chronic community violence: what is happening to our children? *Psychiatry of Interpersonal and Biological Processes*, **56**, 36–45.

Owen, M.T. & Cox, M.J. (1997) Marital conflict and the development of infant–parent attachment relationships. *Journal of Family Psychology*, **11**, 152–164.

Patterson, G.R. & Capaldi, D.M. (1991) Antisocial parents: unskilled and vulnerable. In: *Family Transitions* (eds P.A. Cowan & E.M. Hetherington), pp. 195–218. Advances in Family Research Series. Erlbaum, Hillsdale, NJ.

Pike, A., McGuire, S., Hetherington, E.M., Reiss, D. & Plomin, R. (1996) Family environment and adolescent depressive symptoms and antisocial behavior: a multivariate genetic analysis. *Developmental Psychology*, **32**, 590–603.

Plomin, R., Defries, G.E. & Rutter, M. (1997) *Behavioral Genetics*, 3rd edn. W.H. Freeman, New York.

Pynoos, R.S. & Nader, K. (1990) Children's exposure to violence and traumatic death. *Psychiatric Annals*, **20**, 334–344.

Reid, W.J. & Crisafulli, A. (1990) Marital discord and child behavior problems: a meta-analysis. *Journal of Abnormal Child Psychology*, **18**, 105–117.

Reiss, D., Neiderhiser, J.M., Hetherington, E.M. & Plomin, R. (2000) *The Relationship Code: Deciphering Genetic Social Influence on Adolescent Development*. Harvard University Press, Cambridge, MA.

Richters, J.E. & Martinez, P. (1993) The NIMH community violence project. I. Children as victims of and witnesses to violence. *Psychiatry of Interpersonal and Biological Processes*, **56**, 7–21.

Rogeness, G.A. & McClure, E.B. (1996) Development and neurotransmitter–environmental interactions. *Development and Psychopathology*, **8**, 183–199.

Rogosch, F.A., Cicchetti, D. & Aber, J.L. (1995) The role of child maltreatment in early deviations in cognitive and affective processing abilities and later peer relationship problems. *Development and Psychopathology*, **7**, 591–609.

Roosa, M.W., Sandler, I.N., Beals, J. & Short, J.L. (1988) Risk status of adolescent children of problem drinking parents. *American Journal of Community Psychology*, **16**, 225–239.

Roosa, M.W., Dumka, L. & Tein, J.Y. (1996) Family characteristics as mediators of the influence of problem drinking and multiple risk status on child mental health. *American Journal of Community Psychology*, **24**, 607–624.

Rubin, K.H., Both, L., Zahn-Waxler, C. *et al.* (1991) Dyadic play behaviors of children of well and depressed mothers. *Development and Psychopathology* **3**, 243–251.

Rutter, M. (1979) Maternal deprivation, 1972–78: new findings, new concepts, new approaches. *Child Development*, **50**, 283–305.

Rutter, M. (1985) Resilience in the face of adversity: protective factors and resistance to psychiatric disorder. *British Journal of Psychiatry*, **147**, 598–611.

Rutter, M. (1996) Stress research: Accomplishments and tasks ahead. In: *Stress, Risk and Resilience in Children and Adolescents: Processes, Mechanisms and Interventions* (eds R.J. Haggerty, L.R. Sherrod, N. Garmezy & M. Rutter), pp. 354–385. Cambridge University Press, New York.

Rutter, M. (1999) Resilience concepts and findings: implications for family therapy. *Journal of Family Therapy*, **21**, 119–144.

Rutter, M. (2000a) Resilience reconsidered: conceptual considerations, empirical findings, and policy implications. In: *Handbook of Early Childhood Intervention*, 2nd edn (eds J.T. Shonkoff & S.J. Meisels), pp. 651–682. Cambridge University Press, New York.

Rutter, M. (2000b) Psychosocial influences: critiques, findings and research needs. *Development and Psychopathology*, **12**, 375–405.

Rutter, M., Izard, C.E. & Read, P.B. (eds) (1986) *Depression in Young People: Developmental and Clinical Perspectives*. Guilford Press, New York.

Rutter, M., Macdonald, H., Le Couteur, A. *et al.* (1990) Genetic factors in child psychiatric disorders. II. Empirical findings. *Journal of Child Psychology, Psychiatry*, **31**, 39–83.

Rutter, M., Champion, L., Quinton, D., Maughan, B. & Pickles, A. (1995) Understanding individual differences in environmental risk exposure. In: *Examining Lives in Context: Perspectives on the Ecology of Human Development* (eds P. Moen, R.H. Elder, Jr & K. Lüscher), pp. 61–93. American Psychological Association, Washington, D.C.

Rutter, M., Dunn, J., Plomin, P. *et al.* (1997) Integrating nature and nurture: implications of person–environment correlations and interactions for developmental psychopathology. *Development and Psychopathology*, 9, 335–364.

Rutter, M. & the English and Romanian Adoptees Study Team (1998a) Developmental catch-up, and deficit, following adoption after severe global early privation. *Journal of Child Psychopathology and Psychiatry*, 39, 465–476.

Rutter, M., Giller, H. & Hagell, A. (1998b) *Antisocial Behaviour by Young People*. Cambridge University Press, London.

Rutter, M., Andersen-Wood, L., Beckett, C. *et al.* (1999) Quasi-autistic patterns following severe early global privation. *Journal of Child Psychology and Psychiatry*, 40, 537–549.

Rutter, M., Pickles, A., Murray, R. & Eaves, L. (2001) Testing hypotheses on specific environmental causal effects on behavior. *Psychological Bulletin*, 127, 291–324.

Sameroff, A. (1994) Developmental systems and family functioning. In: *Exploring Family Relationships with Other Social Contexts: Family Research Consortium—Advances in Family Research* (eds R.D. Parke & S.G. Kellam), pp. 199–214. Erlbaum, Hillsdale, NJ.

Sameroff, A.J. & Seifer, R. (1990) Early contributors to developmental risk. In: *Risk and Protective Factors in the Development of Psychopathology* (eds J.E. Rolf & A.S. Masten), pp. 52–66. Cambridge University Press, New York.

Sameroff, A.J., Seifer, R., Baldwin, A. & Baldwin, C. (1993) Stability of intelligence from preschool to adolescence: the influence of social and family risk factors. *Child Development*, 64, 80–97.

Sameroff, A.J., Seifer, R., Barocas, R., Zax, M. & Greenspan, S. (1987) Intelligence quotient scores of 4-year-old children: social environmental risk factors. *Pediatrics*, 79, 343–350.

Sandler, I.N., Tein, J.Y., Mehta, P., Wolchik, S. & Ayers, T. (2000) Coping efficacy and psychological problems of children of divorce. *Child Development*, 71, 1097–1118.

Sanson, A. & Prior, M. (1999) Temperament and behavioral precursors to oppositional defiant disorder and conduct disorder. In: *Handbook of Disruptive Behavior Disorders* (eds H.C. Quay & A.E. Hogan), pp. 397–417. Kluwer Academic/Plenum Publishers, New York.

Seifer, R., Sameroff, A.J., Dickstein, S., Keitner, G. & Miller, I. (1996) Parental psychopathology, multiple contextual risks, and one-year outcomes in children. *Journal of Clinical Child Psychology*, 25, 423–435.

Shakoor, B.H. & Chalmers, D. (1991) Co-victimization of African American children who witness violence: effects on cognitive, emotional, and behavior development. *Journal of the National Medical Association*, 83, 233–238.

Shaw, D.S., Keenan, K., Vondra, J.I., Delliquadri, E. & Giovannelli, J. (1997) Antecedents of preschool children's internalizing problems: a longitudinal study of low-income families. *Journal of the American Academy of Child and Adolescent Psychiatry*, 36, 1760–1767.

Shaw, D.S., Winslow, E.B., Owens, E.B. & Hood, N. (1998) Young children's adjustment to chronic family adversity: a longitudinal study of low-income families. *Journal of the American Academy of Child and Adolescent Psychiatry*, 37, 545–553.

Shaw, D.S., Winslow, E.B. & Flanagan, C. (1999) A prospective study of the effects of marital status and family elations on young children's adjustment among African American and European American families. *Child Development*, 70, 742–755.

Sher, K.J. (1991) *Children of Alcoholics: a Critical Appraisal of Theory and Research*. University of Chicago Press, Chicago.

Shonkoff, J.P. & Phillips, D.A. (2000) *From Neurons to Neighborhoods: the Science of Early Child Development*. National Academy Press, Washington, D.C.

Spencer, M.B., Cole, S.P., Dupree, D., Glymph, A. & Pierre, P. (1993) Self-efficacy among urban African American early adolescents: exploring issues of risk, vulnerability, and resilience. *Development and Psychopathology*, 5, 719–739.

Sroufe, L.A. (1983) Infant–caregiver attachment and patterns of adaptation in preschool: the roots of maladaptation and competence. In: *Minnesota Symposium on Child Psychology*, Vol. 16 (ed. M. Perlmutter), pp. 41–83. Erlbaum, Hillsdale, NJ.

Sroufe, L.A. (1988) The role of infant–caregiver attachment in development. In: *Clinical Implications of Attachment* (eds J. Belsky & T. Neworski), pp. 18–38. Erlbaum, Hillsdale, NJ.

Sroufe, L.A. (1996) *Emotional Development: the Organization of Emotional Life in the Early Years*. Cambridge University Press, New York.

Sroufe, L.A. & Fleeson, J. (1986) Attachment and the construction of relationships. In: *Relationships and Development* (eds W. Hartup & Z. Rubin), pp. 51–71. Erlbaum, Hillsdale, NJ.

Sroufe, L.A. & Waters, E. (1977) Attachment as an organizational construct. *Child Development*, 48, 1184–1199.

Teti, D., Gelfand, D., Messinger, D. & Isabella, R. (1995) Maternal depression and the quality of early attachment: an examination of infants, preschoolers, and their mothers. *Developmental Psychology*, 31, 364–376.

Thompson, R.A. (1999) Early attachment and later development. In: *Handbook of Attachment: Theory, Research, and Clinical Applications* (eds J. Cassidy & P.R. Shaver), pp. 265–286. Guilford Press, New York.

UN Demographic Yearbook 1995 (1997) Issue 47. Department of Economic and Social Office, United Nations.

US National Center for Health Statistics (1990) *Annual Summary of Births, Deaths, Marriages and Divorces: Monthly Vital Statistics Report*, 43 (9).

Werner, E.E. & Smith, R.S. (1982) *Vulnerable But Invincible: a Longitudinal Study*. McGraw-Hill, New York.

Werner, E.E. & Smith, R.S. (1992) *Overcoming the Odds: High Risk Children from Birth to Adulthood*. Cornell University Press, Ithaca, NY.

Wyman, P.A., Cowen, E.L., Work, W.C., Hoyt-Meyers, L., Magnus, K.B. & Fagen, D.B. (1999) Caregiving and developmental factors differentiating young at-risk urban children showing resilient versus stress-affected outcomes: a replication and extension. *Child Development*, 70, 645–659.

Wyman, P., Sandler, I., Wolchik, S. & Nelson, K. (2000) Resilience theory and interventions: cumulative developmental promotion and protection. In: *The Promotion of Wellness in Children and Adolescents* (eds D. Cicchetti, J. Rappaport, I. Sandler & R. Weissberg), pp. 133–184. CWLA Press, Washington D.C.

Zahn-Waxler, C. & Kochanska, G. (1988) The origins of guilt. In: *Nebraska Symposium on Motivation, Socioemotional Development* (ed. R. Thompson), pp. 183–258. University of Nebraska Press, Lincoln, NE.

Zahn-Waxler, C. & Radke-Yarrow, M. (1990) The origins of empathic concern. *Motivation and Emotion*, 14, 107–130.

16 Culture, Ethnicity, Society and Psychopathology

Michael Rutter and Anula Nikapota

Concepts of culture and ethnicity

Many modern industrialized societies are multicultural, multiethnic and multireligious. Indeed, almost all countries have some degree of cultural diversity. Sometimes such variation is thought of either in terms of immigration or skin colour, but both constitute a seriously misleading oversimplification. Although immigration is likely to have been responsible for the cultural or ethnic diversity in the first instance, it may go back many generations. That is obviously the case with the French and English communities in Canada, and with African-Americans and Caucasian-Americans of European origin in the USA. The fact that ethnicity may not be the defining dimension is also obvious in the clashes between Protestants and Catholics in Northern Ireland, between Hindus and Muslims in the Indian Subcontinent and between Jews and Arabs in the Middle East. In all three examples, religion is the predominant defining feature rather than ethnicity.

It may also be the case that the problems faced by subgroups within a broader community derive from features that are independent of culture or ethnicity. The evil of racial discrimination is an obvious example of this kind. It applies to very heterogeneous 'non-white' groups, many of which would see themselves as having little in common with the others (Jones 1993; Modood *et al.* 1997). A further misconception is that most people have just one culture of which they are a part. Manifestly that is not the case for many people. For example, the recent UK survey by the Policy Studies Institute (Modood *et al.* 1997) showed the very high frequency of intermarriage for people of African-Caribbean origin, although very low rates for some other ethnic groups. The children may feel part of the cultural background of either, or both, parents, but also their community of rearing may be a prime identifier. Many young people rightly regard themselves as Glaswegians or Cockneys, while at the same time identifying with being 'black'. For first-generation immigrant parents the prime identification may be with their birthplace in Jamaica or Nigeria, but for the children (who may not even have visited the country), that may not be the most important feature. It cannot be assumed that parents and children have the same cultural affiliations or values, a consideration that has service implications (see Nikapota, Chapter 69).

Group identifications extend well beyond groups as defined in this way. It may be very important for individuals that they are miners or dockers or lawyers or psychologists, and these identifications, in some circumstances, may be as important as those related to their ethnic, religious or geographical origins.

'Culture', 'ethnicity', and 'religion' all concern features that involve group characteristics that define values and styles of life. As early scholars expressed it, membership of such groups implies that individuals in them will think and act in certain ways; will conceptualize their lives in relation to group-defined goals, values and pictures of the world; and, to an important extent, behave as expected on the basis of their group membership (Berlin 1976; Shweder *et al.* 1998). However, population group characteristics may operate in several other, rather different, ways. For example, community or area influences may concern a *paucity* of group identification, values or shared goals (Sampson *et al.* 1997). The key feature may then concern *disorganization* and a *lack* of cohesion. Alternatively, the crucial element may lie in living conditions (poverty, overcrowding, absence of community resources) that derive from discriminatory value systems or from a lack of educational or employment opportunities, or from housing (or other) policies. In these cases, the subgroup is characterized by how they are treated by society, rather than by their own values. This may be important either in terms of group-based stigma or personal social circumstances that stem from societal actions. Another possibility is that the relevant group feature concerns genetic risk or protective factors that vary across ethnic groups (see below).

What we consider in this chapter is why any of these identifications or memberships of population subgroups might be important. In discussing this issue, it is essential to be aware of the multiple meanings and diverse implications of variations that are labelled 'cultural' or 'ethnic' (Rack 1982; Greenfield & Cocking 1994; Nettles & Pleck 1994; Bhugra & Bahl 1999; Masten 1999; García Coll *et al.* 2000).

Implications of group differences

Their possible importance comes in part from the evidence of marked differences among subgroups in rates of particular disorders. Within the UK, the higher rate of schizophreniform disorders in people of African-Caribbean origin has been the subject of much enquiry (Rutter *et al.*, 2001; Hollis, Chapter 37); the much higher proportion of African-Americans in prison in the USA constitutes another example (Rutter *et al.* 1998; see also Earls & Mezzacappa, Chapter 26); the lower rates of suicide among African-Americans compared with Caucasian-Americans constitutes a third example (Nettles & Pleck 1994;

see also Shaffer & Gutstein, Chapter 33). In each case, it is necessary to ask whether the differences in rates of disorder are real or whether they are a function either of biases in processing (by health services or the courts), referral patterns, or responses to psychopathology. It should be appreciated that the issue is one that is pervasive across the whole field of disorder in relation to any kind of subgroup differences. Comparable questions arise with respect to age or sex differences in disorder (see Taylor & Rutter, Chapter 1); to rates of psychopathology in seriously visually impaired or hearing-impaired children (see Hindley & van Gent, Chapter 50); or to the social class differences in some forms of behavioural disturbance (see Fombonne, Chapter 4; Verhulst & Van der Ende, Chapter 5).

Arising out of that first issue is the second question of whether population groups differ in their frequency of exposure to risk and protective factors. Such factors may be genetic or experiential. The best documented example of the former concerns the genetically determined flushing response to alcohol seen in some Asiatics (which is protective against alcoholism) and the range of single gene disorders (such as thalassaemia or the cerebral lipoidoses) that vary by ethnic group. Differences in experiential risk are obvious in the disproportionate involvement of some ethnic groups in social disadvantage. The key question is whether the associations with psychosocial functioning or disorder stem from ethnicity, from racial discrimination, from the associated social risks (e.g. unemployment, poor housing, educational disadvantage; Wilson 1987), or some complex interaction between these variables.

Cultural differences may also be important in the variations across groups in which factors provide risk or protection. An early study by Christensen (1960) showed, for example, the marked differences among cultural groups in the effects of a premarital pregnancy on subsequent marriage. More recently, the research by Stevenson *et al.* (1990) has shown the differences among countries in their response to variations in educational attainment. Studies of physical punishment suggest that both their meaning and their effects may vary by ethnicity, presumably because of different attitudes to the use of corporal punishment (Deater-Deckard & Dodge 1997). Similar issues arise with respect to people's responses to obesity and the accompanying effects in relation to eating disorders (Richards *et al.* 1990; Russell 2000).

Cultural influences may be important in people's attitudes to different indications of possible psychopathology. There has been much discussion of the diversity among cultures in the ways in which they express depression or other forms of emotional distress (Kleinman & Good 1986). In some groups, there may be a straightforward reporting of sadness, misery or hopelessness, whereas in others much the same feelings may be expressed in terms of either the somatic accompaniments or inferences or interpretations about what the negative feelings might mean. There are similar variations among groups in their attitudes to taking recreational drugs, to deliberate self-harm and suicide, and to confrontational behaviour. In many Asian cultures, confrontational behaviour in children and adolescents will be so-

cially disapproved rather than viewed as an expression of distress or frustration. Clinicians need to be aware of the variations in the ways in which different people may express what are basically the same phenomena and, similarly, they need to be aware of the variations in the values attached to such phenomena.

A related issue concerns so-called culture-bound syndromes. Despite the fact that they have been recognized for many years, there has been surprisingly little systematic research into such syndromes. At least three different possibilities need to be considered.

1 Culture-bound syndromes could arise because the main risk factors for particular disorders are largely confined to particular population subgroups.

2 Diseases or disorders that are primarily biologically based may be expressed in somewhat different ways in different groups because of variations in attitudes to the phenomena or symptomatology.

3 There may be disorders that arise primarily as a result of a particular set of beliefs within a particular subculture.

Systematic research is obviously needed to differentiate among these possibilities. In each of these instances, there are important methodological issues to be dealt with and particular research strategies needed in order to understand the mechanisms that may be involved. There are also service implications that derive out of the findings, the specific implications varying with the nature of the differences found and the nature of the mechanisms involved.

Cultural vs. cross-cultural studies

One of the major paradigm shifts in recent years has been from cross-cultural comparisons, in which a measure established and tested in one culture is used to compare two or more cultures, to cultural studies in which measures for each culture derive from the lifestyles and modes of communication in that culture (Shweder *et al.* 1998). The aim of the first approach is to study the effects of context on the universals of psychological functioning; by contrast, the second rejects the notion of universals and presupposes that there is a more intimate (and nonseparable) connection between culture and psyche such that the focus needs to be on that which is unique to each culture as expressed in its own terms.

The main rationale for the shift is that the concepts and measures as derived in any one culture cannot be assumed to cover the universe of features relevant in all cultures. For example, if the starting point was a non-literate society, the investigative tools would not include tests that could pick up the variations in reading skills in a literate society (or their consequences and correlates). Less obviously, tests of problem-solving skills are much influenced by cultural context (Ceci & Roazzi 1994; Ceci *et al.* 1994). On the whole, schooled individuals solve abstract problems better than unschooled individuals when the problems are couched in the language of schooling, whereas the reverse is the case when the same cognitive tasks are couched in the language of the workplace if the work conditions do not apply to the schooled group. The consequence is that the conclusions would be opposite according to which culture provided the starting point for the development of tests—as shown, for example, by studies involving Brazilian street vendors (Schliemann & Carraher 1994). The clear implication is that it is essential to use the context of each culture in order to conceptualize the issues and to develop appropriate measures.

However, these findings also serve to bring out the complementary points that there *are* some universals in psychological functioning and that both the differences and similarities between cultures can be assessed and understood if the comparisons are rooted in *both* the cultures to be assessed. This is evident in relation to age and gender effects on emotional disturbance and disruptive behaviour, as shown in a variety of epidemiological studies both cross-cultural comparisons and within nationalities (Bird 1996). Exactly the same point comes from comparisons among spoken languages (Maratsos 1983). Not only is the human capacity for language universal, but also there are many fundamental features that are shared across languages, as well as some that are different. The differences concern both the course of acquisition of syntax and semantics, and also some of the ways in which language is used in social discourse (Shweder *et al.* 1998). The same issues apply to psychopathology. The point that both within-group studies and between-group comparisons are needed is far from restricted to cultures. Very similar considerations arose with respect to the possibility that depression might be expressed differently in childhood from its mode of manifestation in adult life (Rutter 1986). In the event, it has turned out that the similarities outweighed the differences, although both are present (see Harrington, Chapter 29). Equally, it has been proposed that antisocial behaviour in females is expressed differently from that in males; the findings giving rise to the same conclusion (Rutter *et al.* 1998; Moffitt *et al.*, 2001). In short, the need for both within- and between-group studies applies to any situation in which either the biology or the environmental context are sufficiently different to affect the rate or expression of psychological features, irrespective of the operation of culture. The aim throughout is to use such studies to understand the range of causal factors (cultural and other) that influence the rate, form, expression and recognition of psychopathology in different groups. That requires an appreciation of how culture operates but it also requires culturally sensitive comparisons across groups (Verhulst & Achenbach 1995; Bird 1996).

Generalities vs. specificities

The extent to which psychological and psychopathological characteristics are universal across cultures is a matter to be determined by empirical enquiry. Nevertheless, some expectations may be expressed. It is very likely that all human beings experience sadness, misery, anxiety and fear because they reflect the basic biology (Izard & Shwartz 1986). It is equally probable that there will be some variations across cultures in the focus of such emotions, in their cognitive correlations, and in the ways they

are conceptualized and expressed. Equally, there is every reason to suppose that the development of selective social attachments is culture-universal (Bowlby 1969, 1980; Rajecki *et al.* 1978; see also O'Connor, Chapter 46), as a biological phenomenon that stems from humans being social animals. Moreover, the evidence suggests a substantial commonality in its correlates (van Ijzendoorn & Sagi 1999), but it would be surprising if the patterns were identical, irrespective of household composition and style of rearing.

Concepts of mental disorder

The same considerations apply to psychopathology. There are a few conditions, such as Mendelian disorders (e.g. tuberous sclerosis or Williams syndrome) that are wholly a result of some mutant gene (see McGuffin & Rutter, Chapter 12; Skuse & Kuntsi, Chapter 13), that are likely to be culture-universal provided that the genetic mutations occur in all ethnic/cultural groups. The same applies to disorders caused by chromosomal anomalies—such as Down syndrome or the fragile X anomaly. That is probably also the case with disorders that are based on neural pathology, even though they are multifactorial in origin: autism (see Lord & Bailey, Chapter 38) and schizophrenia (see Hollis, Chapter 37) possibly fit such a category. The social context may influence how these disorders are expressed and interpreted, but it may be expected that they occur in all societies; the empirical evidence (in so far as it is available) supports that expectation.

However, that cannot be expected for the broad run of common disorders involving emotional disturbance or disrupted behaviour. Of course, they reflect psychological universals and they, too, will have a biological substrate. Nevertheless, psychosocial factors are more influential and the form of the disorder is quite likely to be shaped in part by social context and cultural mores. On the other hand, the extent to which such disorders actually vary across societies will depend on the degree to which the societies differ in the sociocultural features that play the greatest part in pathogenesis and in individual response. In a later section of this chapter, we consider the empirical evidence on this matter.

Implications of cultural normality

It is sometimes assumed that if either some form of psychopathology or some psychosocial (or physical) experience is accepted as normal within a culture, it cannot be of clinical significance. A moment's thought makes it clear that that is an unsafe assumption. For many years slavery was accepted as normal and acceptable in many parts of the world but that does not mean that it had no adverse psychological consequences. Within our own lifetimes, racial segregation and discrimination (even lynching) was seen as acceptable within subcultures of the USA. Beating children was seen as normal, even beneficial, in the UK until quite recently and, even today, the law allows English parents to give permission for other caregivers to administer physical punishment to their children. Similarly, before

Bowlby's (1951) World Health Organization report, it was thought to be beneficial severely to restrict parents' visiting of their children in hospital, and residential group care was viewed quite positively. Children's emotional detachment when left in institutions used to be seen as evidence of 'contentment', whereas now we view it as psychopathology. The former may still be the view in some developing or non-industrialized countries. In addition, child labour is still a socially accepted solution to family poverty in some societies and it constitutes a large-scale problem in many developing countries, despite the emerging evidence of the damage that may result.

The reverse assumption is equally unsafe: the mere fact that some pattern of behaviour, or some type of child-rearing, is perceived as abnormal in one culture, does not automatically mean that is so in all cultures. The need in all cases is to determine the correlates and consequences within each culture. Nevertheless, there is one implication of cultural acceptability that is reasonably safe and which is clinically important. If a pattern of parental care is highly unusual and socially disapproved within a culture, it is reasonable to suppose that its occurrence may reflect personal psychopathology in the parents (although an exception to this would be those rebelling against a rigid or restrictive value system). By contrast, if the same pattern is both common and accepted as normal within a culture, it is much less likely that its occurrence will reflect psychopathology (although it may do so). In other words, the fact of cultural acceptability has fairly strong implications for the *origins* of a child-rearing practice, but much weaker implications for the *consequences* of that practice.

Measurement of disorder across societies

Tackling questions on possible differences among cultural or ethnic geographically defined groups in rates of psychopathology (either generally or confined to specific disorders) requires attention to a range of methodological issues (Hackett & Hackett 1999; López & Guarnaccia 2000). These include comparability in sampling, as well as in the assessment of disorder, paying particular attention to the need to ensure sensitivity to concepts and features that may be much more applicable in one group than others. In addition, it is essential to evaluate the possibly relevant features of each societal group in order to determine the causes of any differences found, using strategies that can pit one possible explanation (or hypothesis) against competing ones. The needs may be explicated most easily by taking several different examples from the research literature.

Rutter *et al.* (Berger *et al.* 1975; Rutter *et al.* 1975a,b; Rutter & Quinton 1977) sought to compare rates of disorder in 10-year-olds in inner London and on the Isle of Wight (an area of small towns). Rates of both emotional/behavioural disturbance and reading difficulties were found to be twice as high in London—whether measured by screening instruments or detailed individual assessments. In this case, major differences in culture were neither expected nor found and ethnic differences were bypassed by confining attention to Caucasian children. However, it was crucial to check that there was complete coverage of the population in both areas, that the differences were not an artefact of selective in- or out-migration, and that the disorders had the same meaning in the two populations. In addition, it was crucial to use the same measuring instruments in the same way. The findings showed that the differences were indeed valid. The higher rate of disorder in inner London was found to apply to earlier onset conditions more than to those beginning in adolescence, and the area difference was found to be accounted for by the higher rate of psychosocial adversity in London, together with a higher rate of school adversity. In short, in this study, the group difference seemed to reflect some aspect of the ways in which inner-city life made the good functioning of families and schools more difficult; these family and school difficulties then, in turn, had adverse effects on the children.

A rather similar study by the same research group involved a comparison, within inner London, of children of West Indian immigrants and children from non-immigrant Caucasian families (Rutter *et al.* 1974, 1975c; Yule *et al.* 1975). In this case, the findings showed important differences between the groups in the patterns of disturbance found. Teachers rated the children of West Indian immigrants as showing more disruptive behaviour but this was not found in the detailed reports of parents when interviewed personally. Also, the two groups did not differ with respect to peer relationship problems as reported by teachers, an important negative finding in view of the fact that in most studies disruptive behaviour is associated with difficulties in peer relationships. It was concluded that, although the children of West Indian immigrants showed more disruptive behaviour at school, this did not necessarily have the clinical implications of a conduct disorder that extended to other situations. There were also differences between the groups in the patterns of family functioning, which also indicated the need for caution in making cross-ethnic comparisons.

Since the early 1970s, the situation has changed markedly in several key respects. To begin with, most children today whose families derived from the West Indies were themselves born and raised in the UK. Their parents, too, face a rather different situation: their unemployment rate now is far higher; and the proportion of single-parent households has risen greatly (Modood *et al.* 1997). In the large Policy Studies Institute survey, one-third of the children in Caribbean families had single never-married mothers compared with scarcely any in South Asian families and about 5% in white families (Modood *et al.* 1997). The unemployment rate (especially the rate of long-term unemployment) was twice as high for Caribbeans as for whites. The recent Office of Statistics health survey showed that the rate of mental disorder in 'black' children was only slightly above that in 'whites', with the rate in 'Asian' children rather lower (Meltzer *et al.* 2000). However, this picture altered as the children got older, with a significantly higher rate of conduct disorder among black teenagers. The implication overall is that the psychosocial features (such as single parenthood) may not have quite the same meaning in all ethnic groups.

The third example had as its starting point an explicit focus on one particular disorder, hyperkinetic disorder, for which there were contradictory reports on whether the rate was higher or lower in Chinese children. A research team that spanned Hong Kong and the UK examined the question in a pilot study that involved observational and psychometric measures as well as questionnaire and interview data (Luk *et al.*, in press). The findings were illuminating in showing that although teachers in Hong Kong tended to rate slightly more children as hyperactive than was the case in the UK, observational data suggested that, if anything, the true difference ran in the opposite direction. The results underline the fact that most ratings of psychopathology are inherently comparative and hence are very dependent on people's views on what is 'normal'. Many diagnoses are not open to independent validation through psychometric and observational measures but hyperactivity syndromes differ in that connection. The findings serve as a warning to be careful in drawing conclusions on the basis of group differences on ratings of dimensions such as overactivity, depression or anxiety.

The fourth set of studies, by Weisz *et al.* (1997), compared childhood rates of emotional disturbance and of disruptive behaviour in Thailand and the USA using a mixture of parent and teacher questionnaires, together with observations in the classroom. Clinical vignettes were used to tap perceptions of psychopathology and clinical records were studied to examine referral practices. Despite very marked cultural differences between the two countries, the overall rates of child psychopathology were broadly similar. However, the pattern was somewhat different, with reported emotional difficulties more frequent in Thailand and disruptive behaviour more prevalent in the USA. Interestingly, this was associated in Thailand with a *lesser* tendency to make clinic referral for pure emotional problems, together with a marked tendency to regard children's problems as less serious, less worrisome and more likely to improve. It was also striking that the national differences in rates of problem behaviour on observer ratings were in the opposite direction to those on teacher ratings (the former showing higher rates in Thailand and the latter higher in the USA). The findings from this important set of studies emphasize that differences in perception and expectation have major effects on rates of reported disturbance and that the service implications of these differences may be greater that those of the (usually minor) differences in overall prevalence of psychopathology.

Somewhat similarly, Rothbaum *et al.* (2000) combined a range of quantitative and qualitative studies of parent–child and adult male relationships to investigate the development of close relationships in Japan and the USA. They concluded that the importance and strength of relationships were similar in the two countries, but their meaning and dynamics were different. Provocatively, they argued that in Japan the developmental path mainly involves symbiotic harmony, whereas in the USA it particularly comprises generative tension. They speculate about possible psychopathological implications but acknowledge the limited data on these. The report well illustrates the complementarity of different research approaches, the need to use empirical findings to derive overarching concepts, and the difficulty of drawing unambiguous answers from such endeavours.

The next example, that of ethnic variations in crime rates, concerns a set of data from numerous investigations, rather than those from one study or research programme. The starting point here is the official crime statistics that show, both in the UK and the USA, a vastly higher rate of imprisonment (for both teenagers and young adults) in blacks than in whites or South Asians (Sampson & Lauritsen 1994, 1997; Smith 1997). The differences are greatest for violent crime and for driving offences. The key questions are: whether the differences are real or reflect some sort of artefact in official records; whether, if real, they reflect ethnic variations in antisocial behaviour or in police practice or judicial processing; whether the antisocial behaviour has the same psychopathological meaning in all ethnic groups; and what causal factors might be operating (Rutter *et al.* 1998). The US data show dramatically that, at least in that country, the differences are all too real. Not only are homicide and violent crime rates higher in African-Americans than in whites, but so too are killings and the experience of physical assault. A young black male in the early 1990s was *eight* times more likely to be killed than a young white male. McCord & Freeman (1990) estimated that a male resident of rural Bangladesh had a greater chance of surviving to age 40 than a black male in Harlem. Self-report data in the UK and the USA tell a somewhat different story. In the USA, self-report findings have shown a substantially higher rate of serious offending among African-American teenagers than among whites (Robins *et al.* 1991; Farrington *et al.* 1996). By contrast, self-report data in the UK and in other European countries have shown ethnic variations that are quite minor compared with the official crime statistics (Junger-Tas *et al.* 1994; Graham & Bowling 1995).

Findings from both sides of the Atlantic have shown some differences in the ways in which offenders from different ethnic groups are dealt with by the police and the courts (these differences being rather greater in the USA). Rutter *et al.* (1998) concluded that the cumulative effects of biases in processing were probably greater than recognized by most reviewers but, nevertheless, it was implausible that they could account for the huge differences in imprisonment for serious violent crime. The evidence on possible ethnic variations in the psychopathological significance of antisocial behaviour is decidedly thin. However, it is noteworthy that the American Epidemiological Catchment Area (ECA) study found no increase among African-Americans in antisocial personality disorder, despite their substantially higher crime rate (Robins *et al.* 1991). The possibility that the meaning of crime may vary across different ethnic groups warrants more serious study than it has received so far.

The evidence on causal influences is also less conclusive than one would like. Sampson & Lauritsen (1997), in relation to the US situation, argued that it was the combination of adverse under-the-roof family circumstances and living in a ghetto neighbourhood without social cohesion or informal controls that provided the main risks. Undoubtedly, that constitutes an important part of the story. Certainly, within the USA, there are major area differences in crime rates, with socially disadvantaged blacks being much more likely than similarly disadvantaged whites to live in a ghetto, and the ethnic differences may well be much less for those not living in underclass areas (Peeples & Loeber 1994). Nevertheless, there are some puzzling anomalies. Ghettoes are much less marked in the UK and therefore less likely to be a major factor. Also, there seem to be important ethnic variations in the ways in which risk factors operate. Several studies have shown that a single-parent home is less of a risk factor for African-American young people than for whites (Peeples & Loeber 1994; Smith & Krohn 1995) and physical punishment too seems to be less of a risk factor (Deater-Deckard & Dodge 1997). There is also some suggestive evidence emerging in the UK that there may be an increase in antisocial behaviour among Asian second- and third-generation adolescents living in socially disadvantaged situations, as compared with that in their parents. We conclude that there are ethnic variations in antisocial behaviour that require explanation but the causal processes involved remain only very partially understood.

The last example is provided by schizophrenia. Numerous reports (McKenzie & Murray 1999; Bhugra 2000) have noted unusually high rates of schizophrenia in people from the Caribbean area now living in the UK (or in the Netherlands; Selten & Sijben 1994). A series of systematic studies have been undertaken both to check the validity of the observation and to test alternative hypotheses regarding the possible causes of the raised rate of schizophrenia (Rutter *et al.*, 2001). Population studies have confirmed that the rate of schizophrenia is indeed at least double that in whites; that the rate is similarly raised in relation to the rate among those of similar ethnicity living in the Caribbean (Hickling & Rodgers-Johnson 1995; Bhugra *et al.* 1996); that the high rate is not found in South Asians; that it mainly applies to schizophrenia but also includes atypical affective psychoses to some extent; and that it is not associated with an increased familial loading (and hence is unlikely to be caused by a difference in genetic risk). Rediagnosis of psychotic cases by a Caribbean psychiatrist provided no indication of diagnostic bias (Hickling *et al.* 1999) and other evidence has indicated that the explanation is unlikely to lie in an increased use of drugs or increased exposure to obstetric complications. Prenatal viral exposure remains a possibility as a contributory factor, although it seems unlikely to account for the high rate. Social adversities seem likely to have been influential, although it remains unclear why these should have had this effect in African-Caribbeans but not in South Asians. Whether or not the excess rate of schizophrenia represents 'ordinary' schizophrenia is uncertain. A 4-year follow-up study of one sample by McKenzie *et al.* (1995) showed a somewhat better clinical course than in whites but a less good social course. Thus, the African-Caribbeans were less likely to engage in suicidal behaviour but more likely to experience involuntary hospital admission and more likely to have spent some time in jail. A secondary analysis of a large sample of patients with research diagnoses, however, did not confirm the increased involuntary hospital care or prison, although it did confirm that African-Caribbeans were less likely to have a continuous illness and to receive treatment with antidepressants or psychotherapy (McKenzie *et al.* 2001). Kirov & Murray (1999) suggested that, overall, the findings suggest a socially reactive psychosis, but just what those social causal factors are remains quite unclear.

Culture-bound syndromes

The term 'culture-bound' syndromes has been applied to clusters of signs and symptoms that are largely restricted to a particular culture or group of cultures (Prince 1985). Western psychiatrists tend to think of these in terms of apparently exotic clinical pictures found in other countries—with diagnoses such as 'brain fag syndrome' or 'koro' coming to mind. However, it is important to recognize that there are culture-based syndromes much closer to home. Thus, anorexia nervosa is largely limited to Westernized or industrialized nations and is closely associated with the cultural pressures on women to be thin (Russell 2000). Similarly, dissociative identity (multiple personality) disorder is largely restricted to North America, and rates of hysterical ('conversion') disorders have varied greatly over time in keeping with cultural mores (Merskey 2000). Chronic fatigue syndrome probably has features in common with culture-based syndromes (Sharpe & Wessely 2000). The implication is not to memorize exotic clinical pictures, but rather to recognize the extent to which cultural influences and attitudes can shape the manifestations of psychopathology within our own cultures, as well as in those of other people. In each case, it is necessary to appreciate the range of mechanisms that may be involved in the cultural influences, but also to remember that their operation does not mean that individual biological factors will be unimportant.

Conclusions on differential rates of disorder

For the most part, the evidence suggest that, despite wide variations in culture, ethnicity, religion and living conditions, societies differ surprisingly little in overall rates of child and adolescent psychopathology (Bird 1996; Hackett & Hackett 1999). Moreover, there is substantial commonality in the general patterning of mental disorder (Crijnen *et al.* 1999). To some extent, this may reflect constraints imposed by the use of instruments reflecting the concepts of Western societies. Nevertheless, as illustrated by the examples given, studies that have attempted to deal sensitively with cultural variations in concept and perception have also tended to show more similarities than differences among societies.

However, that rather anodyne conclusion requires the addition of several important qualifiers and modifiers. First, there are several major exceptions to the general finding of a lack of variation. The best documented concern the relatively high rate of schizophrenia and schizoaffective psychoses in African-Caribbeans living in the UK or the Netherlands (but not in those living in the West Indies), and the relatively high rate of violent and drug-related antisocial behaviour in African-Caribbeans in the UK and USA. In both cases, the explanations are likely to involve some aspects of social adversity but quite what these are and how they operate is unknown. A possible third exception concerns the apparently higher rate of autism spectrum disorders in African-Caribbeans in the UK (Wing 1979; Akinsola & Fryers 1986; Goodman & Richards 1995), a difference usually attributed to prenatal viral infections. Although there are few systematic comparisons, the findings also suggest a slightly lower rate of overall psychopathology among South Asians in the UK despite their relatively high exposure to both social adversity and racial discrimination. Family and community cohesion may be protective but this hypothesis has yet to be put to rigorous test.

The second qualifier is that there are major group differences in rates of psychopathology within societies. These have been shown to be systematically associated with variations in exposure to social adversity. In the UK and USA, the high risks have mainly been associated with inner-city life but that has not always been the case in other societies (Quinton 1994). It is not city living as such that creates the risk but rather the accumulation of social adversities that involve social disorganization, poor job opportunities, disadvantageous housing, poor schooling, a lack of community resources, racial discrimination and social exclusion (Rutter *et al.* 1998). The specifics will vary according to whether the location is an inner city in an industrialized society or within a rural setting in a developing country. The extent to which this leads to a situation of learned helplessness and the impact on child and family needs further study. The importance of societal influences (including schooling and peer group effects) is well documented, although uncertainties remain on the precise risk and protective mechanisms involved.

Third, although there are important cultural influences on perceptions and attitudes to child psychopathology, it would be seriously misleading to conceptualize cultures as generally risky or protective in relation to mental disorder. These variations in perception are clinically important for two rather different reasons (see Nikapota, Chapter 69). Obviously, clinicians need to be aware that the ways in which families view their difficulties may not coincide with their own concepts. In addition, people's attitudes to their circumstances and to the problems they face are likely to influence their impact. The environment cannot be thought of as something objective that impinges mechanically on a passive organism. People actively *process* their experiences and *how* they do so will affect the impact of those experiences. In many instances, the *relative* nature of *experiences* may be more influential than their absolute characteristics. Thus, Hackett *et al.* (1999) in their South Indian study found that, as in Western societies, social disadvantage was associated with a higher risk for disorders involving disruptive behaviour (but not for those with emotional disturbance). However, most of the socially advantaged children would be among the poorest groups in the West; yet they did not have a high rate of disorder.

We have already drawn attention to the clinically important findings that, although many psychosocial features operate similarly across societies, some do not. The apparently lower psychopathological risks associated with a single-parent household and with physical punishment in the African-American group were given as examples. These may reflect differences in the origins of these features or in their meaning. Thus, if single parenthood is more likely to reflect social mores rather than personal psychopathology, it may involve less risk. In their study of London secondary schools, Rutter *et al.* (1979) found, for example, that although unofficial (unauthorized) physical sanctions, such as cuffing children, were associated with worse pupil outcomes, this did not apply to corporal punishment when administered to a predetermined set of rules and procedures.

Two crucially important points need to be added to the role of culture. First, although culture tends to be conceptualized as all-encompassing, there are marked individual variations within cultures. Many people feel part of several different cultures. Secondly, cultures are far from static. They represent dynamic social processes that reflect a complex changing mix of ethnic, class, gender, religious and societal influences. For example, over the last half century, there has been a huge increase in most Western societies in the proportion of young people living together while unmarried, and having children in that situation (Rutter & Smith 1995). As a consequence, the meaning of illegitimacy has changed out of all recognition, from being an index of social alienation to one of social acceptability. So far there have been few attempts to study the extent to which these changes have altered the associated psychopathological risks (but see Maughan & Lindelow 1997 for an exception dealing with teenage parenthood), and investigations of this kind are much needed. Another example of apparent attitude change within cultures concerns the current trend for women from South Asia, from relatively traditional poor backgrounds, to travel abroad for employment, particularly to the Middle East. Until relatively recently, this would have been the subject of social disapproval but now it seems to be socially sanctioned. So far, there has been a lack of study of the associated risks and benefits for either the women or the children left behind.

Both parental and professional concepts of psychopathology have varied over time, as well as across societies. For example, during the 1960s and 1970s, there were huge differences between the USA and the UK in the diagnoses of both schizophrenia (Cooper *et al.* 1972) and hyperactivity disorders (Prendergast *et al.* 1988); neither of these apply now to anything like the same extent. Similarly, childhood depressive disorders were regarded as quite rare during the same period (Rutter *et al.* 1986), whereas now they are accepted as relatively common (see Harrington, Chapter 29). Cultural studies have attempted to chart possible similar differences between societies in lay concepts of mental disorder. The studies by Weisz *et al.* (1997) were given as a high quality exemplar. There are equally telling examples in the field of scholastic attainment, as shown by the rigorous research undertaken by Stevenson *et al.* (Chen & Stevenson 1989, 1995; Stevenson *et al.* 1990, 1993; Crystal *et al.* 1994; Randel *et al.* 2000). East Asian Americans have been shown to outperform both other Americans and Europeans in mathematics and that this is associated with a higher set of expectations and different attitudes to homework.

Cultural and ethnic groups vary both in the extent to which they retain the attitudes and lifestyles of their backgrounds and the extent to which they adopt those of another culture. Some become assimilated within the host culture and others adopt cultural dualism. Mass media, consumerism and education may all be influential. On the whole, it seems that non-Western families living in the UK and USA tend to adopt Western attitudes to body size and shape. Accordingly, the apparent variations across industrialized and developing nations in rates of anorexia nervosa are not reflected within ethnic/cultural groups living in the West (see Steinhausen, Chapter 34). On the other hand, educational values of East Asian groups have tended to be maintained. Nikapota *et al.*'s (1998) study of four cultural groups in London found no differences in parents' ability to identify problems (as compared with professionals) but South Asian parents were least likely to ascribe emotional reasons for a problem and more likely than white or African-Caribbean parents to access help for educational difficulties. They were also less forthcoming in their answers to questions on problems—a reporting style that could have implications for their response to screening questionnaires.

The main messages that come out of the findings on cultural influences are that:

1 these apply as much within Western societies as in developing countries;

2 they are likely to influence both psychopathology and service utilization (see Nikapota, Chapter 69);

3 they vary greatly within societal groups and over time; and

4 the perceptions and attitudes of parents and children in the same family may not be the same—especially when the older generation was raised in a quite different culture to that in the host society.

The implication is that clinicians should not try to learn stereotypes about different cultural groups because they will not apply to all members of those groups and because the values are likely to change over the generations and as a result of changing social circumstances. Rather, the implication is that clinicians should be sensitive to the operation of cultural influences on all families that they see, not just those of ethnic minorities, and that they should be sensitive to the need to pick up cues on those cultural factors as they operate on individual families and children.

Conclusions

In this chapter we have emphasized the multiple facets of cultural, ethnic and societal variations and their implications for psychopathology. The main focus throughout has been on the conceptual and methodological issues that need to be taken into account in any study of possible social group or population differences. It cannot be assumed that measures of psychopathology or of family functioning have the same meaning in

all groups; within-group studies are necessary to explore the matter. Equally, however, systematic standardized comparisons across groups are possible, and informative, provided they are undertaken with appropriate cultural sensitivity. There are many similarities among societies but attention has been drawn to some clinically relevant differences (see also Nikapota, Chapter 69). These may operate in several contrasting ways. Rutter (1999) summarized these in terms of five broad concepts.

1 The effects of social *connotation* or meaning in changing the impact of risk or protective features or the implication of particular psychological patterns.

2 Social *comparative* effects by which the influence of a factor derives from its reflection of a person's social standing or value in relation to others.

3 A *compositional* effect in which an aggregative group characterization is used to infer some characteristic of an individual.

4 A social *contextual* effect deriving from the ethos or qualities of the broader social environment, such as a school or geographical area.

5 A social *group characteristic* effect, whereby the influence derives from the behaviour and values of a person's peer group or sociocultural group with which they identify.

References

Akinsola, H.A. & Fryers, T. (1986) A comparison of patterns of disability in severely mentally handicapped children of different ethnic origins. *Psychological Medicine*, **16**, 127–133.

Berger, M., Yule, W. & Rutter, M. (1975) Attainment and adjustment in two geographical areas. II. The prevalence of specific reading retardation. *British Journal of Psychiatry*, **126**, 510–519.

Berlin, I. (1976) *Vico and Herder*. Hogarth Press, London.

Bhugra, D. (2000) Migration and schizophrenia. *Acta Psychiatrica Scandinavica*, **102** (Suppl. 407), 68–73

Bhugra, D. & Bahl, V. (eds) (1999) *Ethnicity: an Agenda for Mental Health*. Royal College of Psychiatrists/Gaskell, London.

Bhugra, D., Hilwig, M., Hossein, T. *et al.* (1996) First-contact incidence rates of schizophrenia in Trinidad and one-year follow-up. *British Journal of Psychiatry*, **169**, 587–592.

Bird, H.R. (1996) Epidemiology of childhood disorders in a cross-cultural context. *Journal of Child Psychology and Psychiatry*, **37**, 35–49.

Bowlby, J. (1951) *Maternal Care and Mental Health*. World Health Organization, Geneva.

Bowlby, J. (1969) *Attachment and Loss*, Vol. 1, *Attachment*. Hogarth Press, London.

Bowlby, J. (1980) *Attachment and Loss*, Vol. 3. *Loss, Sadness and Depression*. Hogarth Press, London.

Ceci, S.J. & Roazzi, A. (1994) The effects of context on cognition: postcards from Brazil. In: *Mind in Context: Interactionist Perspectives on Human Intelligence* (eds R.J. Sternberg & R.K. Wagner), pp. 74–101. Cambridge University Press, New York.

Ceci, S.J., Baker-Sennett, J.G. & Bronfenbrenner, U. (1994) Psychometric and everyday intelligence: synonyms, antonyms and anonyms. In: *Development Through Life: a Handbook for Clinicians* (eds M. Rutter & D. Hay), pp. 260–283. Blackwell Scientific Publications, Oxford.

Chen, C. & Stevenson, H.W. (1989) Homework: a cross-cultural examination. *Child Development*, 60, 551–561.

Chen, C. & Stevenson, H.W. (1995) Motivation and mathematics achievement: a comparative study of Asian-American, Caucasian-American, and East Asian high school students. *Child Development*, 66, 1214–1234.

Christensen, H.T. (1960) Cultural relativism and premarital sex norms. *American Sociological Review*, 25, 31–39.

Cooper, J.E., Kendell, R.E., Gurland, B.J., Sharpe, L., Copeland, J.R.M. & Simon, R. (eds) (1972) Psychiatric Diagnosis in New York and London: a Comparative Study of Mental Hospital Admissions. *Maudsley Monograph 20*. Oxford University Press, London.

Crijnen, A.A., Achenbach, T.M. & Verhulst, F.C. (1999) Problems reported by parents of children in multiple cultures: the Child Behaviour Check List syndrome constructs. *American Journal of Psychiatry*, 156, 569–574.

Crystal, D.S., Chen, C., Fuligni, A.J. *et al.* (1994) Psychological maladjustment and academic achievement: a cross-cultural study of Japanese, Chinese, and American high school students. *Child Development*, 65, 738–753.

Deater-Deckard, K. & Dodge, K.A. (1997) Externalizing behavior problems and discipline revisited: nonlinear effects and variation by culture, context, and gender. *Psychological Inquiry*, 8, 161–175.

Farrington, D.P., Loeber, R., Stouthamer-Loeber, M., Van Kammen, W.B. & Schmidt, L. (1996) Self-reported delinquency and a combined delinquency seriousness scale based on boys, mothers, and teachers: concurrent and predictive validity for African-Americans and Caucasians. *Criminology*, 34, 501–525.

García Coll, C., Akerman, A. & Cicchetti, D. (2000) Cultural influences on developmental processes and outcomes: implications for the study of development and psychopathology. *Development and Psychopathology*, 12, 333–356.

Goodman, R. & Richards, H. (1995) Child and adolescent psychiatric presentations of second-generation Afro-Caribbeans in Britain. *British Journal of Psychiatry*, 167, 362–369.

Graham, J. & Bowling, B. (1995) Young People and Crime. *Home Office Research Study 145*. HMSO, London.

Greenfield, P.M. & Cocking, R.R., eds (1994) Cross-Cultural Roots of Minority Child Development. Erlbaum, Hillsdale, NJ.

Hackett, R. & Hackett, L. (1999) Child psychiatry across cultures. *International Review of Psychiatry*, 11, 225–235.

Hackett, R., Hackett, L., Bhakta, P. & Gowers, S. (1999) The prevalence and associations of psychiatric disorder in children in Kerala, South India. *Journal of Child Psychology and Psychiatry*, 40, 801–807.

Hickling, F.W. & Rodgers-Johnson, P. (1995) The incidence of first contact schizophrenia in Jamaica. *British Journal of Psychiatry*, 167, 193–196.

Hickling, F.W., McKenzie, K., Mullen, R. & Murray, R.M. (1999) A Jamaican psychiatrist evaluates diagnoses at a London psychiatric hospital. *British Journal of Psychiatry*, 175, 283–285.

van Ijzendoorn, M.H. & Sagi, A. (1999) Cross-cultural patterns of attachment: universal and contextual dimensions. In: *Handbook of Attachment: Theory, Research, and Clinical Applications* (eds J. Cassidy & P.R. Shaver), pp. 713–734. Guilford Press, New York.

Izard, C. & Shwartz, G.M. (1986) Patterns of emotion in depression. In: *Depression in Young People: Developmental and Clinical Perspectives* (eds M. Rutter, C.E. Izard & P. Read), pp. 33–70. Guilford Press, New York.

Jones, T. (1993) Britain's Ethnic Minorities: an Analysis of the Labour Force Survey. Policy Studies Institute, London.

Junger-Tas, J., Terlouw, G.-J. & Klein, M.W. (1994) Delinquent Behavior Among Young People in the Western World: First Results of the International Self-Report Delinquency Study. Kugler, Amsterdam.

Kirov, G. & Murray, R.M. (1999) Ethnic differences in the presentation of bipolar affective disorder. *European Psychiatry*, 14, 199–204.

Kleinman, A. & Good, B., eds (1986) Culture and depression: Studies in the Anthropology and Cross-Cultural Psychiatry of Affect and Disorder. University of California Press, Berkeley, CA.

López, S.R. & Guarnaccia, P.J.J. (2000) Cultural psychopathology: uncovering the social world of mental illness. *Annual Review of Psychology*, 51, 571–598.

Luk, E.S.L., Leung, P.W.L. & Ho, T.P. (in press) Cross-cultural/ethnical aspects of childhood hyperactivity. In: *Attention Deficit and Hyperactivity Disorders in Childhood* (ed. S. Sandberg), 2nd edn. Cambridge University Press, Cambridge.

Maratsos, M. (1983) Some current issues in the study of the acquisition of grammar. In: *Handbook of Child Psychology*, Vol. III. *Cognitive Development* (series ed. P.H. Mussen; volume eds J.H. Flavell & E.M. Markman), 4th edn, pp. 707–786. John Wiley & Sons, New York.

Masten, A.S., ed. (1999) Cultural Processes in Child Development: the Minnesota Symposia on Child Psychology, Vol. 29. Erlbaum, Mahwah, NJ.

Maughan, B. & Lindelow, M. (1997) Secular change in psychosocial risks: the case of teenage motherhood. *Psychological Medicine*, 27, 1129–1144.

McCord, C. & Freeman, H. (1990) Excess mortality in Harlem. *New England Journal of Medicine*, 322, 173–175.

McKenzie, K. & Murray, R.M. (1999) Risk factors for psychosis in the UK African-Caribbean population. In: *Ethnicity: an Agenda for Mental Health* (eds D. Bhugra & V. Bahl), pp. 48–59. Gaskell, London.

McKenzie, K., van Os, J., Fahy, T. *et al.* (1995) Psychosis with good prognosis in Afro-Caribbean people now living in the United Kingdom. *British Medical Journal*, 311, 1325–1328.

McKenzie, K., Samele, C., van Horn, E., Tattan, T., van Os, J. & Murray, R. (2001) Comparison of the outcome and treatment of psychosis in people of Caribbean origin living in the UK and British Whites. Report from the UK700 trial. *British Journal of Psychiatry*, 178, 160–165.

Meltzer, H., Gatward, R., Goodman, R. & Ford, T. (2000) The Mental Health of Children and Adolescents in Great Britain. The Stationery Office, London.

Merskey, H. (2000) Conversion and dissociation. In: *New Oxford Textbook of Psychiatry* (eds M.G. Gelder, J.J. López-Ibor & N. Andreasen), Vol. 2, pp. 1088–1098. Oxford University Press, Oxford.

Modood, T., Berthoud, R., Lakey, J. *et al.* (1997) Ethnic Minorities in Britain: Diversity and Disadvantage. Policy Studies Institute, London.

Moffitt, T.E., Caspi, A., Rutter, M. & Silva, P. (2001) Sex Differences in Antisocial Behaviour: Conduct Disorder, Deliquency and Violence in the Dunedin Longitudinal Study. Cambridge University Press, Cambridge.

Nettles, S.M. & Pleck, J.H. (1994) Risk, resilience, and development: the multiple ecologies of black adolescents in the United States. In: *Stress, Risk, and Resilience in Children and Adolescents* (eds R.J. Haggerty, L.R. Sherrod, N. Garmezy & M. Rutter), pp. 147–181. Cambridge University Press, New York.

Nikapota, A., Cox, A.D., Sylva, K. & Rai, D. (1998) Development of Culturally Appropriate Child Mental Health Services: Perceptions and Use of Services. Report, Department of Health, London.

Peeples, F. & Loeber, R. (1994) Do individual factors and neighbourhood context explain ethnic differences in juvenile delinquency? *Journal of Quantitative Criminology*, 10, 141–157.

Prendergast, M., Taylor, E., Rapoport, J.L., Bartko, J., Donnelly, M., Zametkin A., *et al.* (1988) The diagnosis of childhood hyperactivity: a US–UK cross-national study of DSM-III and ICD-9. *Journal of Child Psychology and Psychiatry*, 29, 289–300.

Prince, R. (1985) The concept of culture-bound syndromes: anorexia nervosa and brain fag. *Social Science and Medicine*, 21, 197–203.

Quinton, D. (1994) Cultural and community influences. In: *Development Through Life: a Handbook for Clinicians* (eds M. Rutter & D.F. Hay), pp. 159–184. Blackwell Scientific Publications, Oxford.

Rack, P. (1982) *Race, Culture, and Mental Disorder*. Tavistock Publications, London.

Rajecki, D.W., Lamb, M.E. & Obmascher, P. (1978) Toward a general theory of infantile attachment: a comparative review of aspects of the social bond. *Brain and Behavioral Sciences*, 1, 417–464.

Randel, B., Stevenson, H.W. & Witruk, E. (2000) Attitudes, beliefs, and mathematics achievement of German and Japanese high school students. *International Journal of Behavioral Development*, 24, 190–198.

Richards, M.H., Boxer, A.M., Petersen, A.C. & Albrecht, R. (1990) Relation of weight to body image in pubertal girls and boys from two communities. *Developmental Psychology*, 26, 313–321.

Robins, L.N., Tipp, J. & Przybeck, T. (1991) Antisocial personality. In: *Psychiatric Disorders in America: the Epidemiologic Catchment Area Study* (eds L. Robins & D.A. Regier), pp. 258–290. Free Press, New York.

Rothbaum, F., Pott, M., Azuma, H., Miyake, K. & Weisz, J. (2000) The development of close relationships in Japan and the United States: paths of symbiotic harmony and generative tension. *Child Development*, 71, 1121–1142.

Russell, G. (2000) Anorexia nervosa. In: *New Oxford Textbook of Psychiatry* Vol. 1 (eds M.G. Gelder, J.J. López-Ibor & N. Andreasen), pp. 835–855. Oxford University Press, Oxford.

Rutter, M. (1986) The developmental psychopathology of depression: issues and perspectives. In: *Depression in Young People: Developmental and Clinical Perspectives* (eds M. Rutter, C.E. Izard & P. Read), pp. 3–30. Guilford Press, New York.

Rutter, M. (1999) Social context: meanings, measures and mechanisms. *European Review*, 7, 139–149.

Rutter, M. & Quinton, D. (1977) Psychiatric disorder: ecological factors and concepts of causation. In: *Ecological Factors in Human Development* (ed. H. McGurk), pp. 173–187. North-Holland, Amsterdam.

Rutter, M. & Smith, D.J., eds (1995) *Psychosocial Disorders in Young People: Time Trends and Their Causes*. John Wiley & Sons, New York.

Rutter, M., Yule, W., Berger, M., Yule, B., Morton, J. & Bagley, C. (1974) Children of West Indian immigrants. I. Rates of behavioural deviance and of psychiatric disorder. *Journal of Child Psychology and Psychiatry*, 15, 241–262.

Rutter, M., Cox, A., Tupling, C., Berger, M. & Yule, W. (1975a) Attainment and adjustment in two geographical areas. I. The prevalence of psychiatric disorder. *British Journal of Psychiatry*, 126, 493–509.

Rutter, M., Yule, B., Quinton, D., Rowlands, O., Yule, W. & Berger, M. (1975b) Attainment and adjustment in two geographical areas. III. Some factors accounting for area differences. *British Journal of Psychiatry*, 126, 520–533.

Rutter, M., Yule, B., Morton, J. & Bagley, C. (1975c) Children of West Indian immigrants. III. Home circumstances and family patterns. *Journal of Child Psychology and Psychiatry*, 16, 105–123.

Rutter, M., Maughan, B., Mortimore, P., Ouston, J. & Smith, A. (1979) *Fifteen Thousand Hours: Secondary Schools and Their Effects on Children*. Open Books, London.

Rutter, M., Izard, C.E. & Read, P. (1986) *Depression in Young People: Developmental and Clinical Perspectives*. Guilford Press, New York.

Rutter, M., Giller, H. & Hagell, A. (1998) *Antisocial Behaviour by Young People*. Cambridge University Press, New York.

Rutter, A., Pickles, R., Murray & Eaves, L. (2001) Testing hypotheses on specific environmental causal effects on behavior. *Psychological Bulletin*, 127, 291–324.

Sampson, R.J. & Lauritsen, J.L. (1994) Violent victimization and offending: individual, situational, and community-level risk factors. In: *Understanding and Preventing Violence: Vol. 3: Social Influences* (eds A.J. Reiss & J. Roth), pp. 1–114. National Academy Press, Washington D.C.

Sampson, R.J. & Lauritsen, J.L. (1997) Racial and ethnic disparities in crime and criminal justice in the United States. In: *Crime and Justice*, Vol. 21 (ed. M. Tonry), pp. 311–374. University of Chicago Press, Chicago, IL.

Sampson, R.J., Raudenbush, S.W. & Earls, F. (1997) Neighborhoods and violent crime: a multilevel study of collective efficacy. *Science*, 277, 918–924.

Schliemann, A.D. & Carraher, D.W. (1994) Proportional reasoning in and out of school. In: *Context and Cognition: Ways of Learning and Knowing* (eds P. Light & G. Butterworth), pp. 47–73. Erlbaum, Hillsdale, NJ.

Selten, J.P. & Sijben, N. (1994) First admission rates for schizophrenia in immigrants to the Netherlands. The Dutch National Register. *Social Psychiatry and Psychiatric Epidemiology* 29, 71–77.

Sharpe, M. & Wessely, S. (2000) Chronic fatigue syndrome. In: *New Oxford Textbook of Psychiatry*, Vol. 2 (eds M.G. Gelder, J.J. López-Ibor & N. Andreasen), pp. 1112–1121. Oxford University Press, Oxford.

Shweder, R.A., Goodnow, J., Hatano, G., LeVine, R.A., Markus, H. & Miller, P. (1998) The cultural psychology of development: one mind, many mentalities. In: *Handbook of Child Psychology*, Vol. 1. *Theoretical Models of Human Development* (eds W. Damon & R.M. Lerner), pp. 865–937. John Wiley & Sons, New York.

Smith, D.J. (1997) Race, crime and criminal justice. In: *The Oxford Handbook of Criminology* (eds M. Maguire, R. Morgan & R. Reiner), pp. 703–759. Clarendon Press, Oxford.

Smith, C. & Krohn, M.D. (1995) Delinquency and family life among male adolescents: the role of ethnicity. *Journal of Youth and Adolescence*, 24, 69–93.

Stevenson, H.W., Chen, C. & Lee, S.Y. (1993) Mathematics achievement of Chinese, Japanese, and American children: ten years later. *Science*, 259, 53–58.

Stevenson, H.W., Lee, S.-Y., Chen, C., Stigler, J.W., Hsu, C.-C. & Kitamura, S. (1990) Contexts of achievement: a study of American, Chinese and Japanese children. *Monographs of the Society for Research in Child Development, Serial No 221*, 55, 1–2.

Verhulst, F.C. & Achenbach, T.M. (1995) Empirically based assessment and taxonomy of psychopathology: cross-cultural applications. *European Child and Adolescent Psychiatry*, 4, 61–76.

Weisz, J.R., McCarty, C.A., Eastman, K.L., Chaiyasit, W. & Suwanlert, S. (1997) Developmental psychopathology and culture: ten lessons from Thailand. In: *Developmental Psychopathology: Perspectives on Adjustment, Risk, and Disorder* (eds S.S. Luthar, J.A. Burack, D. Cicchetti & J.R. Wiesz), pp. 568–592. Cambridge University Press, Cambridge.

Wilson, W.J. (1987) *The Truly Disadvantaged: the Inner City, the Underclass, and Public Policy*. University of Chicago Press, Chicago, IL.

Wing, L. (1979) Mentally retarded children in Camberwell (London). In: *Estimating Needs for Mental Health Care* (ed. H. Hafner), pp. 77–91. Springer-Verlag, Berlin.

Yule, W., Berger, M., Rutter, M. & Yule, B. (1975) Children of West Indian immigrants. II. Intellectual performance and reading attainment. *Journal of Child Psychology and Psychiatry*, 16, 1–17.

The Role of Acute Life Stresses

Seija Sandberg and Michael Rutter

Introduction

Over the years, many clinical and epidemiological studies have shown associations between life events of a severely negative kind and psychiatric disorder in children and adolescents (Goodyer *et al.* 1985, 1987, 1993; Berden *et al.* 1990; Goodyer 1990; Jensen *et al.* 1991; Sandberg *et al.* 1993, 1998, 2001; Höök *et al.* 1995; Beautrais *et al.* 1997).

In this chapter we consider four broad questions.

1 What do these findings mean?

2 What mechanisms might they represent?

3 What are their implications for our understanding of the causes and course of psychiatric disorder in children and young people?

4 How should the findings affect clinical practice?

First, however, we present a brief historical background of the concept of stress in relation to illness, mental disorder, and on the measurement of stressful life events.

Historical background

It has long been generally recognized that stressful life experiences may have an adverse effect on well-being and predispose to physical and mental disorder (Riese 1969; Garmezy & Rutter 1985; Harris *et al.* 1986; Haavet & Grünfeld 1997). Physiologists focused on the relationship between bodily changes and life experiences containing an emotional component. Through experimental and clinical studies, Cannon (1914, 1929) laid the groundwork for psychophysiological research by demonstrating that external stimuli associated with emotional arousal caused changes in basic physiological processes.

Some three decades later, a bridge to psychiatry was firmly laid out. Meyer (1957), a physician and psychiatrist, argued that life events need not be catastrophic or particularly unusual to be pathogenic. He advocated the value of life charts to bring out temporal links between such happenings as change of habitat, school entrance, graduation, marriage, divorce and bereavement, and the onset of psychiatric disorder.

This proposition was further developed in the 1960s by Holmes & Rahe (1967) through their production of questionnaires to provide overall scores of degree of life change—the assumption being that it was the extent of life change that was stressful and not necessarily the unpleasant nature of the life experiences. The first generation life event measures in childhood

(Coddington 1972; Johnson & McCutcheon 1980; Johnson 1982) were based on similar questionnaire format. In parallel with these overall approaches to life events, there were numerous studies of specific life events such as family break-up or bereavement, and disasters such as floods or hijacking.

The 1970s saw a major reappraisal of psychosocial stress research through the work of Paykel (1974, 1978), who noted the importance of differentiating between desirable and undesirable life changes; of Lazarus (Lazarus & Launier 1978), who emphasized the role of cognitive appraisal of the events; and especially of Brown & Harris (1978, 1989a), who emphasized the need to differentiate between *independent* and *dependent* events (those that could and could not have been brought about by the person's own behaviour) and who developed the notion of the psychological *threat* to the individual as viewed in the light of that person's personal *social context*. The work of Goodyer *et al.* (1985, 1987, 1990a,b), of Monck & Dobbs (1985) and, subsequently, of Sandberg *et al.* (Glen *et al.* 1993; Sandberg *et al.* 1993, 1994), building on these principles, has been instrumental in extending the use of interview assessments with children and adolescents.

At first, the distinction between *independent* and *dependent* life events was mainly based on the possibility that early symptoms of the acute psychiatric disorder might have brought about the life event (Brown & Harris 1978). Thus, someone who was becoming depressed might, through their irritability and agitation, have precipitated quarrels with other people or fallen out with friends. However, it soon became apparent that it was necessary to take a broader view of this possibility (Lazarus *et al.* 1985). Acute disorders often arise against a background of personality difficulties (see Moore & Farmer, Chapter 42; J. Hill, Chapter 43) and may be associated with comorbidity that also needs to be taken into account. It came to be accepted that it was necessary to evaluate independence in relation to any aspects of a person's behaviour and not just the early symptoms of a particular mental disorder (Brown & Harris 1986; Sandberg *et al.* 1993). In keeping with this conceptual distinction Kendler *et al.* (1999), in an adult twin study, found a genetic liability underlying the reporting of dependent, but not independent, negative life events. The results of a comparable study of children and adolescents (Thapar & McGuffin 1996), however, were less conclusive.

Although the original concept of a stressful life event was based on the degree of life change, it was evident that this was not the most important dimension. The degree of unpleasantness seemed more relevant, but it became apparent that the psychological threat involved was most influential with respect to the overall psychopathological risk. Thus, although being bitten by a dog is an exceedingly frightening experience and may induce a fear of dogs, it would be quite unusual for it to precipitate a psychiatric disorder. On the other hand, being rejected by a close friend or humiliated in a public situation, although involving little objective environmental change, may be felt as very threatening because of the damage to self-esteem. Similarly, it became clear that normative life transitions that involve huge change, such as the 'internal' event of puberty or the 'external' event of moving to secondary school, may or may not carry risk, the key feature being how the person views the event in the light of their own particular life circumstance. Thus, an unwanted pregnancy in a teenager following a casual encounter may carry major threat, whereas a planned wanted pregnancy in the context of a stable harmonious committed relationship is much less likely to do so.

Investigators were sensitive to the certainty of bias if threat was judged on the basis of asking people what they thought about an event. If a person has become depressed following some negative life experience, he or she is much more likely to view the experience as having been stressful. Accordingly, it became standard practice for researchers to rate threat on the basis of an account of social context as they would judge its significance for an average person in that circumstance. Studies with both children and adults that used the degree of contextual threat to assess stressfulness of life experiences have generally found that it is only (or mainly) events carrying high long-term threat that are associated with psychiatric disorder to any substantial degree (Brown & Harris 1978; Goodyer et al. 1985; Sandberg et al. 1993). However, in practice, many such events are associated with chronic psychosocial adversities, raising the issue of the relative importance of the acute event and of the long-standing adversity (Sandberg et al. 1993).

Measurement of life events

Broadly speaking, two main approaches have been used for the assessment of life events. First, questionnaires have asked about the occurrence of specified life events during a particular time period. Good design can ensure that there is coverage of the major common events likely to carry long-term psychological threat, and it is reasonably straightforward to differentiate between probably independent and possibly dependent events on the basis of their nature. Thus, bereavement would fall in the former category and rejection by a close friend in the latter. However, with children there is the further complication that events brought about by parents, although independent of the child, could reflect genetic mediation. This would apply to events such as parental divorce, abuse or neglect (Jockin et al. 1996; O'Connor et al. 2000). The major advantage of questionnaires lies in their low cost and ease of administration to large samples, making them readily applicable for large-scale epi-

demiological enquiries (Silberg et al. 1999). However, they have the considerable disadvantage that they cannot readily deal with the personal meaning or social context of events and they are limited in their power to obtain accurate timing.

Secondly, interviews have been used to obtain detailed descriptions of events, and of their surrounding circumstances, during a defined time period. Accurate timing is facilitated by using personalized time points such as birthdays, family holidays, school terms and the like. Contextual threat, both short-term and more enduring, can be assessed according to a range of components (Goodyer et al. 1985, 1997; Sandberg et al. 1993). In the Psychosocial Assessment of Childhood Experiences (PACE; Glen et al. 1993; Sandberg et al. 1993, 1994) these include the following:

• loss of an attachment figure (such as a parent or close friend);
• loss of a valued idea (major disappointment/humiliation);
• physical jeopardy (being in physical danger because of accident, etc.);
• trauma as witness (being witness to a frightening incident involving someone else); and
• psychological challenge (taking on a new role or new responsibilities).

Origins of life events

The early literature on life events seemed to carry the implicit assumption that most arose by chance. The introduction of the concept of dependent events provided a recognition that this was often not the case, because people's own behaviour shaped their experiences to a considerable extent. That recognition highlighted the need for systematic study of the causal factors involved in individual differences in exposure to acute and chronic negative experiences as well as the psychological mechanisms reflecting psychopathology and risk (Adams & Adams 1993, 1996; Rutter et al. 1995; Williamson et al. 1995, 1998).

Longitudinal studies have shown the huge importance of a person's own behaviour. Thus, Robins' (1966) follow-up of child guidance clinic attenders into mid-adult life found that antisocial behaviour in childhood was associated with a massive increase in negative experiences many years later. These included multiple divorce, unemployment, frequent job changes, lack of friends and lack of social support. Similarly, Champion et al.'s (1995) 20-year follow-up of London school children showed that psychopathology at age 10 years (especially conduct problems but, to a lesser extent, emotional disturbance) was associated with a more than doubling in the risk of both acute and chronic life experiences in adult life that caused long-term psychological threat. Many of the events and experiences carrying psychopathological risk involve social interactions (Rutter 2000a) and it is to be expected that these will be influenced by a person's own behaviour. Shorter term longitudinal studies have given rise to the same conclusion. Thus, Daley et al. (1997), in a 2-year longitudinal study of late adolescent women, showed that those with depression that was comorbid with other problems at the outset had more stress experiences later, and that this held even after controlling for chronic adversity. They concluded that stress generation is not just a product of individual behaviour but, rather, it arises out of a person's social world, a world that has been constructed as a result of both interpersonal and intrapersonal factors.

Other studies have shown the role of parental psychopathology in generating stress experiences for children (Rutter & Quinton 1984; Compas 1987; Rutter 1989a; Jensen *et al.* 1991; Adrian & Hammen 1993; Murray & Cooper 1997; Rutter *et al.* 1997). One study showed that parental personality disorder was associated with a major increase in the rate of marital discord and of hostility to the children, as compared with community controls (Rutter & Quinton 1984). The findings raise two different issues. First, as also shown by other research (Brown & Harris 1986; Sandberg *et al.* 1993), acutely negative experiences are more common in individuals who also suffer from chronic psychosocial adversities. That finding underlines the need to determine the relative psychopathological risk associated with the acute stresses, as distinct from the associated chronic adversities. Secondly, because the parents who are providing their children with negative experiences are also passing on genes, there is the possibility that the risks from life events are, at least partially, genetically mediated. It is relevant that twin studies with both children (Thapar *et al.* 1998; Silberg *et al.* 1999) and adults (Kendler *et al.* 1993) have shown a significant genetic effect on individual differences in the experience of negative life events.

Adoption studies have similarly shown that psychopathology in the biological parents (who did not provide rearing) is associated with more negative parenting by the adoptive parents who did not transmit genes (Ge *et al.* 1996; O'Connor *et al.* 1998). This effect derives from the effects on the parents of the children's (genetically influenced) disruptive behaviour. The same research has also shown effects on the children of the parents' behaviour: the reality is a two-way interactive process. It is evident that any rigorous study of environmental risk mediation must consider the possible role of genetic mediation.

In addition to the influences on life experiences deriving from a person's own behaviour, differences in exposure to negative life events may also stem from societal influences and broad living conditions. This has been shown for family risk factors, such as family discord and disruption, through evidence that these are more common in socially disadvantaged inner-city areas than in less disadvantaged areas of small towns (Rutter & Quinton 1977). Although not focused on acute life events as such, recent area comparisons examining the effects of community social disintegration on antisocial behaviour (Brooks-Gunn *et al.* 1997; Sampson *et al.* 1997) and of the effects of housing policies on such disintegration (Power 1997) suggests that some city areas function (or, rather, dysfunction) in ways that predispose to negative life experiences. Racial discrimination and harassment, which unfortunately remain as features of most industrialized societies (Brown 1984; Madood *et al.* 1997), will do the same. In adults, life events carrying long-term threat have been found to be more common in socially disadvantaged groups (Brown & Harris 1978); in children the same applies, probably mediated by the effects of disadvantage on chronic psychosocial adversity (Sandberg *et al.* 1993, 1998, 2000). Again, the implication is that research into the risks associated with acute life events will have to take account of these broader environmental adversities.

Testing for a causal effect

The early studies of life events simply showed that individuals with psychiatric disorder tended to experience more negative life events than did general population controls. Brown & Harris (1978) recognized that, in itself, this association did not prove causation. Accordingly, they focused on independent events (to rule out reverse causation) and tested the causal hypothesis by comparing the occurrence of events in the period immediately preceding the onset of psychiatric disorder in cases with the parallel occurrence in a similar time period preceding interview in controls. The design has become the standard life events method, and findings have been consistent in showing that life events frequently precede the onset of a psychiatric disorder. That has been so in both adults (Bebbington *et al.* 1993; Brown *et al.* 1994; Frank *et al.* 1994; Kendler *et al.* 1995) and children (Goodyer *et al.* 1985, 1987, 1990a,b; Jensen *et al.* 1991; Beautrais *et al.* 1997). The findings with adults showing a depressive disorder are the most clear-cut. Thus, Brown & Harris (1978) found that the great majority of episodes was preceded by a high threat event in the preceding 9 weeks. Surtees & Wainwright (1999) found the same, with the provoking effect on onset mainly evident in the first 6 or 7 weeks. There are far fewer findings with respect to the role of stressors in provoking the onset of child psychiatric disorders, but the available data do not show the same strong timing effect (Goodyer *et al.* 1985, 1987, 1990a, 1993; Berden *et al.* 1990; Beautrais *et al.* 1997; Sandberg *et al.* 2001). Rather, it seems that the increase in negative life events applies over an extended period of time, and not just in the weeks leading up to the onset of disorder (Rowlison & Felner 1988; Allgood-Merten *et al.* 1990; Goodyer *et al.* 1990b; Garrison *et al.* 1991; Jensen *et al.* 1991; duBois *et al.* 1992; Esser *et al.* 1993; Sandberg *et al.* 1993; Olsson *et al.* 1999).

Although the standard life events method, it involves several important methodological limitations with respect to the causal inference (Rutter, 2000a,c; Sandberg *et al.* 2001). First, the case–control comparison for a specific time period will be affected by any general (non-time-specific) difference in life events as brought about by either genetic liability or other environmental factors (such as chronic adversity). A more rigorous test is provided by within-individual comparisons of the pre-onset time period with other time periods. The only study so far to use this method gave rise to weak inconclusive time effects, although showing the usual case–control difference (Sandberg *et al.* 2001). Secondly, with very few exceptions, studies with both adults and children have used the same informant for data on life events and data on the onset of disorder. The possibility of reporting bias is clear, and recent research has moved to using different informants for the two features (Silberg *et al.* 1999, 2001; Sandberg *et al.* 2001). Thirdly, the timing method presupposes that each episode of disorder has a simple unambiguous time point when it began. The available findings suggest that this is the exception rather than the rule. Some onsets are gradual, some symptoms begin before others, and often there is a different point when symptoms lead to social impairment (Rutter & Sandberg 1992; Sandberg *et al.* 2001). Moreover, interinformant and retest reliability on the timing of onsets is weak (Angold *et al.* 1996). Fourthly, most psychiatric disorders are recurrent or chronic; this is so in both childhood and adult life. Accordingly, a more basic question with respect to the causal role of life events is whether they affect liability to psychopathology over time, rather than just having a provoking role with respect to the timing of onset.

Twin studies in both childhood (Silberg *et al.* 1999, 2001) and adult life (Kendler *et al.* 1999) have tackled this question using two complementary research strategies. The first examines the effects of life events on psychopathology within monozygotic (MZ) twin pairs. As these are genetically identical, any within-pair association between life events and disorder must represent some form of environmental mediation. The second uses bivariate analysis in which life events are treated as a phenotype. Cross-twin cross-trait analyses (using both MZ and DZ pairs) enables the association to be partitioned into genetic and environmental components. Both strategies have shown clear (although not strong) environmentally mediated effects. However, it has to be recognized that, if only life events are measured, the findings could be a consequence of life events indexing a broader range of psychosocial risk factors. In short, life events have been shown to be part of those psychosocial features that involve environmentally mediated risk for psychopathology. The extent to which acute life events carry risk that is independent of chronic adversities is not known, but we consider below the limited evidence on this point.

Although the distinction between independent and dependent life events constituted an important methodological step, the fact that a person brought about a particular experience through their own behaviour does not mean that the experience cannot then influence the person's later behaviour or predispose to disorder (Rutter 1986; Rutter *et al.* 1993). Cigarette smoking constitutes an obvious example. People choose to smoke but that does not account for the environmentally mediated effect of smoking on lung cancer, heart disease and osteoporosis. In comparable fashion, appropriately analysed longitudinal data have shown that a harmonious marriage makes it less likely that antisocial behaviour will persist from childhood to adult life (Zoccolillo *et al.* 1992; Rutter *et al.* 1997; Laub *et al.* 1998). In the same way, the fact that a person behaves in a way that leads to rebuffs or rejections from peers, or predisposes to scapegoating in the family, does not mean that the rejection or scapegoating will not constitute a significant stress event for them. It is essential to use research designs and analyses that can provide a rigorous test of the postulated stress effect but it is important to

appreciate that the implication is for research strategy and not for an automatic ruling out of a stress effect. That is pertinent to the finding that children and adolescents with psychiatric disorder differ from community controls in their exposure to both independent and dependent life events, as well as chronic psychosocial adversities (Sandberg *et al.* 1993; Williamson *et al.* 1995; Olsson *et al.* 1999).

Some life events rate high on contextual threat because they cause a major alteration in the child's life circumstances (e.g. death of a parent). In other cases, the threat is primarily cognitive. Thus, there may be little actual change in the external environment but, nevertheless, a drastic alteration in the child's self-perception or self-esteem (as through a severe humiliation) or sense of security (such as stemming from a threat to abandon the child). Many events involve a combination of real life change and cognitively mediated threat (this would be so with a parental divorce or separation).

Some events carry both a negative and a positive affective valence. The contextually positive features usually refer to hedonic qualities, enhancement of self-esteem, or favourable effect on life circumstances. Thus, a father's loss of his job may mean that the child has more pleasurable interactions with him. However, there has been limited study of positive aspects, and the findings have been inconclusive (Jensen *et al.* 1991; Brown *et al.* 1992; Sandberg *et al.* 1993; Leenstra *et al.* 1995).

Many studies have shown that negative life events are frequently associated with, and may arise from, chronic psychosocial adversities ranging from poor housing and neighbourhood problems to illness and discordant relationships within the family (Brown & Harris 1978, 1989b; Goodyer *et al.* 1988, 1997; Jensen *et al.* 1991; Sandberg *et al.* 1993, 1998; Tiet *et al.* 1998). A key issue concerns the extent to which the psychopathological risk derives from some acute event or, rather, from these more long-standing adversities that precede and succeed the event. Thus, it is necessary to ask whether, for example, the main risk derives from the event of a parental divorce or separation or from the discordant conflict that brought about marital disruption (Fergusson *et al.* 1992). In that connection, it is necessary to distinguish between the possible effects on the timing of onset of disorder and the effects on an overall liability to psychopathology. We discuss that issue below, but the point to be made here is that it has been realized that the measurement of life events must be accompanied by assessment of more long-standing difficulties and adversities (Glen *et al.* 1993; Sandberg *et al.* 1993, 2000).

Effect of negative experiences

In so far as negative experiences have enduring effects, it is necessary to consider the mediating mechanisms by which the sequelae are carried forward in time (Rutter 2000a,c). In short, what do the experiences do to the organism? There are many possibilities (Rutter 1989b). Thus, persistence may come about because the initial adverse experiences led to altered patterns of interpersonal interaction that, in turn, brought about further negative experiences (Rutter *et al.* 1995, 1998). Alternatively, as suggested by the findings on experiences of physical abuse, there may be altered cognitive sets or styles of emotional and cognitive processing (Dodge *et al.* 1990, 1995). A third possibility is that the stress affects neuroendocrine structure and function, as suggested by findings in both animals (Hennessey & Levine 1979; Levine 1982; Sapolsky 1993, 1998; Liu *et al.* 1997) and humans (Hart *et al.* 1996). Interestingly, there is some indication that this may even happen with prenatal stressors (Barbazanges *et al.* 1986; Kraemer 1992; Kraemer & Clarke 1996; Schneider *et al.* 1998).

The mechanism with respect to severe and lasting early adversities, but probably not acute stressors, could also lie in the developmental programming of the brain. It has been well demonstrated through animal studies that sensory input is necessary for the normal development of the visual cortex (Blakemore 1991), and it is likely that there are parallel experience-dependent neural development effects with respect to other experiences (Greenough *et al.* 1987; Thoenen 1995; Pollak *et al.* 1997).

Animal studies of severe stress have shown that this can result in hippocampal damage (O'Brien 1997). There is also limited evidence that the neural effects of social privation may differ from those of separation stresses (Matthews *et al.* 1996; Robbins *et al.* 1996). It remains uncertain whether similar effects apply in humans but it is reasonable to suppose that they may (Bremner *et al.* 1997).

Finally, it has been shown that stress experiences have adverse effects on the body's immunological responses (Drummond & Hewson-Bower 1997; Cohen *et al.* 1999), this possibly providing the mediating factor in relation to the demonstrated effects of adverse life events in increasing people's susceptibility to infections (Turner Cobb & Steptoe 1996, 1998; Cohen *et al.* 1993, 1998). Stress has also been implicated as a provoking factor in a wide range of somatic conditions such as asthma and rheumatoid arthritis (Heisel *et al.* 1973; Jacobs & Charles 1980; Walker & Green 1987; Mrazek *et al.* 1999; Sandberg *et al.* 2000), although whether this derives from immunological effects remains unclear.

Acute life events and chronic adversities

There is abundant evidence that chronic adversities carry a substantial psychopathological risk (see Friedman & Chase-Lansdale, Chapter 15) and, as these overlap greatly with acute negative life events (Jensen *et al.* 1991; Sandberg *et al.* 1993), it is necessary to assess their relative importance. However, in spite of the obvious relevance of the issue, few studies have specifically examined this question and their results are inconsistent (Brown & Harris 1978; Goodyer *et al.* 1988, 1990b; Jensen *et al.* 1991; Tiet *et al.* 1998). Instead, most studies have reported the effects of composite measures of cumulative life stress (Johnson 1986; Berden *et al.* 1990). Such composites often com-

bine acute stressors and chronic adversity (Coddington 1972; Johnson & McCutcheon 1980), so precluding examination of the relative importance of acute and chronic experiences.

Of the studies that have examined the differential and joint effects of acute negative life events and chronic psychosocial stressors in children, one found that the risk of psychiatric disorder was largely caused by chronic adversity, with acute events adding little to that (Jensen *et al.* 1991). Another study reported almost equal risks from acute and chronic stressors which, when they co-occurred, had a multiplicative effect (Goodyer *et al.* 1990a); and two further studies found acute events and chronic adversities exerting independent effects (Goodyer *et al.* 1990b; Tiet *et al.* 1998). Thus, Jensen *et al.* (1991), in a study of clinic referred children, found that most of the case–control differences disappeared after controlling for life events connected with chronic parent-related adversity (such as parental psychopathology or divorce). Goodyer *et al.* (1988) reported independent effects of almost equal magnitude stemming from recent negative life events, and two forms of chronic adversity (maternal distress and poor maternal confiding) but, when occurring together, they had a multiplicative effect on risk of disorder. Another study by the same team (Goodyer *et al.* 1990) showed that acute events and child's friendship difficulties (as a form of chronic adversity) each exerted an independent effect; Tiet *et al.*'s (1998) findings were rather similar. Our own study (Sandberg *et al.* 1993, 1998) showed that psychiatric clinic attenders and community controls differed with respect to both acute stresses and chronic adversities. The two tended to co-occur, with the risks being greatest when this was the case. In that inner-city sample, it was uncommon for psychiatric disorder to be associated with acute events that had no connection with chronic adversity. However, the findings could be different in the case of acute onset depressive disorders, of which there were scarcely any in the sample studied.

There is a great need for research to examine the relative risks for psychopathology associated with chronic adversity and with acute events when each occurs without the other. Such risks will need to be examined separately, with respect to overall liability and in relation to the provocation of onset. It is possible that chronic adversities may prove to be more important for the former and acute events for the latter. The findings on suicide (see Shaffer & Gutstein, Chapter 33) are consistent with that possibility, but the matter has not been systematically investigated as yet.

Specificity/generality of effects

Both in children and in adults, not only have negative life events been associated with a wide range of psychopathology (Goodyer 1990; Sandberg *et al.* 1993; Gowers *et al.* 1996) but they have also been shown to precede the onset of many somatic illnesses (Heisel *et al.* 1973; Jacobs & Charles 1980; Turner Cobb & Steptoe 1998) and to relate to recurrence or chronicity (Bedell *et al.* 1977; Randolph & Fraser 1999; Sandberg *et al.*

2000). Inevitably, the generality of these effects raises questions about mechanisms. If the effects are so non-specific, can they be conceptualized as at all central to the causal processes? Perhaps it is just that negative experiences give rise to a general lowering of resistance to other factors that are more directly implicated in causation.

In adults, some findings have suggested a degree of specificity, with 'loss' events more important in the provocation of depression, and 'danger' events in the onset of anxiety disorders (Finlay-Jones & Brown 1981; Miller & Ingham 1985; Finlay-Jones 1989; Brown et al. 1996). Goodyer et al. (1990a,b) did not find this was so with children; Eley & Stevenson (2000) did. There has been so little investigation of the possibility that the question must be regarded as still open.

There may also be some specificity with respect to the occurrence of post-traumatic stress disorder (PTSD) following quite exceptional events such as floods, earthquakes, shipping disasters and being taken hostage (see Yule, Chapter 32). PTSD involves a variety of specific psychopathogical features but there is considerable comorbity with a broader range of emotional disorders (Goenjian et al. 1995; Hubbard et al. 1995; Tyano et al. 1996; Bolton et al. 2000). It may be concluded that such very severe stressors can precipitate disorders other than PTSD. On the other hand, such events constitute only a tiny minority of the life events that provoke disorder (Giaconia et al. 1995).

Bereavement may be associated with a characteristic immediate grief reaction (see Black, Chapter 18). It may also predispose to a wider range of later psychopathology, although the risks are less than those associated with parental separation or divorce (Rutter 1971). It seems that the key risk feature concerns the conflict, discord and hostility associated with break-up rather more than the event of break-up itself (Fergusson et al. 1992). Similarly, with respect to the risks for depression arising in adult life stemming from childhood loss, the evidence suggests that the key risk feature concerns poor parenting, rather than loss per se (Harris et al. 1986).

All the findings point to the need to consider individual differences in susceptibility to stress; we consider that issue next.

Individual differences in susceptibility to life events

A universal finding of research into all manner of environmental stresses and adversities has been the huge heterogeneity in response (Rutter 2000a,b,c). Even after experiencing the most severe of psychosocial hazards, some succumb to disorder but others escape. There are numerous methodological problems to be overcome before a confident inference on variations in susceptibility can be made. It could be that the heterogeneity of response lies simply in individual differences in the severity of the stressor experienced, in the presence of other risk factors, or in outcomes not measured. Nevertheless, even when experiences can be experimentally controlled, as through regulated exposure to disease-inducing bacteria or viruses (Petitto & Evans

1999), or through studies of unusual events such as parachute jumping (Cox 1978; Rose 1980), or enemy attack during warfare (Bourne et al. 1968), marked individual differences in susceptibility have been found.

Some of this variation in susceptibility is a function of genetic influences, as shown by molecular genetic research in relation to features as diverse as infections (Hill 1998a,b), head injuries (Teasdale et al. 1997), cardiovascular accidents (McCarron et al. 1998), allergens (Cookson 1999) and smoking (Talmud et al. 2000). Less is known about specific genetic factors in relation to psychosocial stressors but twin data have pointed to genetic moderation of psychopathological responses to life stressors (Kendler et al. 1995; Rutter 2000b; Silberg et al., 2001), probably through the mediation of effects on neuroticism (Kendler 1996), although that has still to be demonstrated.

Past experiences may either have a sensitizing or steeling effect (Rutter 1981). Early animal experiments showed that stress experiences, through their effects on the neuroendocrine systems, could affect resistance to later stressors (Hennessy & Levine 1979). A parallel may be drawn with protection against infections (Tyrell 1977). Protection and immunity lies not in the avoidance of infection, but rather in exposure to small doses, with the body having learned to cope successfully with the pathogen (either through immunization or natural exposure). It is likely that there is a similar sort of adaptation in relation to psychosocial stresses and adversity. There are several studies in which findings suggest that children have been strengthened by having coped successfully with life's difficulties (Stacey et al. 1970; Elder 1974). Conversely, previous stresses or adversity may make children more vulnerable if they did not cope well (Quinton & Rutter 1976). The findings on what leads to experiences having a sensitizing or steeling effect are sparse and inconclusive but probably the crucial factor is whether or not the experience resulted in successful coping and adaptation.

Early experiences may also render children unusually susceptible to later stresses if they left the individuals with impaired feelings of self-efficacy (Bandura 1997) or lacking in social problem-solving skills (see Compas et al., Chapter 55). Brown & Harris (1978), in their studies of depression in women, found that this vulnerability was particularly associated with a lack of adequate parental care in childhood (Harris et al. 1986; Brown 1993; Brown et al. 1993; Bifulco et al. 1998). The empirical findings on the role of coping in children's response to life stresses are few. However, there is some evidence that an active (rather than avoidance) style using emotion-focused (rather than action-focused) strategies may reduce the risks associated with stress experiences (Armistead et al. 1990; Eisenberg et al. 1993; Sandler et al. 1994; Lengua et al. 1999; Mazur et al. 1999). An anxious temperament, negative affectivity, low self-esteem or poor cognitive ability may do the opposite (Davies & Cummings 1995; Sheets et al. 1996).

Concurrent social support may also moderate children's responses to stress. Goodyer et al. (1988, 1989; Goodyer 1994) found that peer relationship difficulties predicted emotional disorders in childhood, and Sandberg et al. (1993) found that a lack of a confiding relationship with parents or some other close adult relative increased the psychopathological risk associated with negative life events. Silberg *et al.* (2001) found that parental anxiety or depressive disorder increased children's vulnerability to negative life events. Better family functioning and close parental monitoring have also been shown to predict resilience in young people subjected to stressful life events (Tiet *et al.* 1998).

The effects of risk experiences are also influenced by the ways in which people think and feel about what has happened to them. The same event (such as becoming team captain or school prefect) may be seen as either very positive, because it serves as a mark of prestige and accomplishment, or very negative, because it brings new challenges, new uncertainties and new people to deal with. This has been little studied in children but research with adults (Teasdale & Barnard 1993) suggests its possible importance.

In relation to long-term sequelae, how children respond to the initial negative experience may set off either negative or positive chain reactions that will bring psychological sequelae. Thus, reliance on drugs or alcohol to relieve stress, or dropping out of education, or leaping into a teenage pregnancy or impulsive marriage as a way of escaping family conflict, are all likely to increase the chances that adverse sequelae will persist. Conversely, some sorts of response may serve to elicit supportive reactions from other people and, by so doing, may predispose to positive chain reactions that foster resilience (Rutter 1999).

The topic of resilience/vulnerability in relation to stress and adversity is important, both theoretically and practically, because of the well-demonstrated individual variations in response. However, as briefly summarized here, although there are reasonable leads on some of the underlying risk and protective factors, much remains to be learned (Rutter 1999, 2000b,c; Luthar *et al.* 2000).

Clinical implications

The issues considered above give some indications for life events enquiries to be adopted as part of routine clinical practice. This applies particularly to disorders that appear to have had a sudden onset. In practice, these are most likely to involve conditions characterized by anxiety, depression or phobias. In such acute presentations, a stressful life event, even if not the main cause of the disorder, may well have triggered it off. An example may be a very unpleasant and frightening incident of a child being bullied and refusing to go to school thereafter. However, given the general run of referrals to child and adolescent mental health services, such *de novo* sudden onset cases are likely to constitute a minority. Most referrals concern youngsters with a mixture of emotional and behavioural problems that often also have evidenced a fairly lengthy existence. The psychosocial experiences usually detected in the background of these tend to consist of a mixture of chronic and acute stress exposures. Therefore, both of these should be included in the initial enquiry. Occasionally, it may still turn out that some recent stressful life event to the child

or to the parents has brought the situation to a head, and the need for professional help has become urgent. The main issue in such situations may be support to the parents in order to enable them to regain control of their lives, and to effectively cope with the child's challenging behaviour.

The questions considered above also raise issues relevant for treatment and prevention. The overrepresentation of behaviour-related negative life events among psychiatrically disturbed children and adolescents points to an important therapeutic need for interventions directed at the children themselves, to help to modify their behaviour. Moreover, the interpersonal family conflicts, commonly involving active participation of the young person, also indicate a need for therapeutic interventions for the child and the whole family. Although unlikely to cause the disorder in the first place in most cases, such behaviour-dependent negative events may well exacerbate it.

Conversely, the preventive measures should explicitly involve the parents in order to reduce the risk of the child's enduring stressful life events stemming from parental actions, often reflecting either their personal psychopathology or marital conflicts. Likewise, the need for socioeconomic interventions by the society at large is implicated by the excess of chronic psychosocial adversities, such as poverty and unemployment, as well as those stemming from parental psychopathology and criminality, all of which are more common in the socially disadvantaged. This observation therefore introduces a further significant issue; the likelihood of familial transmission, with regard to the origins of stressful life events commonly found in excess in psychiatric samples.

Looking into the future

At this stage of the chapter it is appropriate to consider what we have learned from research about the importance of stressful life events on the mental health of children and adolescents, and what are the gaps to be filled and the challenges that should be met in the future. It seems appropriate to begin such a 'forecast' with a brief statement about where the field is now. This means acknowledging that the available evidence strongly suggests that severely negative life events play a significant part in increasing the overall risk of psychiatric disorder in children and adolescents. This is especially so with regard to acutely stressful life events occurring in conjunction with high levels of chronic psychosocial adversity. Furthermore, this combination of acute and chronic life stress increasing the risk is not unique to psychiatric disorder, but appears to exert much the same influence on physical illness, such as asthma (Sandberg *et al.* 2000). The topic is therefore of undoubted importance.

Although substantial progress has been made in the development of research strategies capable of testing environmental mediation hypotheses, their utilization so far has been almost rudimentary. Compared with our knowledge about psychosocial risk indicators, relatively little is known about the actual environmental mechanisms and processes that underlie the risk mediation. Also, the knowledge concerning diagnostic specificities in relation to risk processes remains very limited. Most research has been concerned with antisocial behaviour; and therefore much more needs to be learned about the role of environmental factors in the genesis of depression and anxiety disorders in this age group.

Future research also needs to pay attention to factors determining individual differences in exposure to stressful life events. Likewise, better research is needed to differentiate environmental effects on the person, and person-effects on the environment. More detailed knowledge about individual differences in responses to psychosocial stress and adversity is also of crucial importance. Likewise, in so far as these differences relate to mechanisms of resilience, that too remains a topic requiring research (Rutter 2000b). A shift in research focus is also needed, from the precipitants of the onset of disorder to an understanding of processes operating over time—both in the initiation and course of psychiatric disorders as they remit and relapse. In addition, the need to understand indirect chain reactions and to learn about how they operate is crucial. In that connection, perhaps the least well understood of all issues is what psychosocial risks do to the organism. More than anything else, this last question requires that psychosocial research be part of biological psychiatry.

In this spirit, it is also hoped that in the future the identification of all the genes in the human genome will open up opportunities for a more thorough analysis of neurotransmitter-related and other genes involved in personality dimensions and behaviour. Given this, a fuller understanding of how individual genetic variation influences susceptibilities to environmental hazards would be possible (see also McGuffin & Rutter, Chapter 12). This should offer new insights enabling better treatments for the mental health consequences of stress in children and young people.

References

Adams, J. & Adams, M. (1993) Effects of a negative life event and negative perceived problem-solving alternatives on depression in adolescents: a prospective study. *Journal of Child Psychology and Psychiatry*, 34, 743–747.

Adams, J. & Adams, A. (1996) The association among negative life events, perceived problem solving alternatives, depression, and suicidal ideation in adolescent psychiatric patients. *Journal of Child Psychology and Psychiatry*, 37, 715–720.

Adrian, C. & Hammen, C. (1993) Stress exposure and stress generation in children of depressed mothers. *Journal of Consulting and Clinical Psychology*, 61, 354–359.

Allgood-Merten, B., Lewinsohn, P.M. & Hops, H. (1990) Sex differences in adolescent depression. *Journal of Abnormal Psychology*, 99, 55–63.

Angold, A., Erkanlis, A., Costello, E.J. & Rutter, M. (1996) Precision, reliability and accuracy in the dating of symptom onsets in child and adolescent psychopathology. *Journal of Child Psychology and Psychiatry*, 37, 657–664.

Armistead, L., McCombs, A., Forehand, R., Wierson, M., Long, N. & Fauber, R. (1990) Coping with divorce: a study of young adolescents. *Journal of Clinical Child Psychology*, 19, 79–84.

Bandura, A. (1997) *Self-Efficacy: the Exercise of Control*. Freeman, New York.

Barbazanges, A., Piazza, P.V., Le Moal, M. & Maccari, S. (1986) Maternal glucocorticoid secretion mediates long-term effects of prenatal stress. *Journal of Neuroscience*, 3943–3949.

Beautrais, A.L., Joyce, P.R. & Mulder, R.T. (1997) Precipitating factors and life events in serious suicide attempts among youths aged 13 through 24 years. *Journal of the American Academy of Child and Adolescent Psychiatry*, 36, 1543–1551.

Bebbington, P., Der, G., MacCarthy, B. *et al.* (1993) Stress incubation and the onset of affective disorders. *British Journal of Psychiatry*, 162, 358–362.

Bedell, J.L., Diordani, B., Amour, J.L., Tavormina, J. & Boll, T. (1977) Life stress and the psychological and medical adjustment of chronically ill children. *Journal of Psychosomatic Research*, 21, 237–242.

Berden, G.F.M.G., Althaus, K. & Verhulst, F.C. (1990) Major life events and changes in the behavioural functioning of children. *Journal of Child Psychology and Psychiatry*, 31, 949–959.

Bifulco, A., Brown, G.W., Moran, P., Ball, C. & Campbell, C. (1998) Predicting depression in women: the role of past and present vulnerability. *Psychological Medicine*, 28, 39–50.

Blakemore, C. (1991) Sensitive and vulnerable periods in the development of the visual system. In: *The Childhood Environment and Adult Disease. Ciba Foundation Symposium 156* (eds G.R. Bock & J. Whelan), pp. 129–146. Wiley, Chichester.

duBois, D.L., Felner, R.D., Brand, S., Adam, A.M. & Evans, F.J. (1992) A prospective study of life stress, social support, and adaptation in early adolescence. *Child Development*, 63, 542–557.

Bolton, D., O'Ryan, D., Udwin, O., Boyle, S. & Yule, W. (2000) The long-term psychological effects of a disaster experienced in adolescence. II. General psychopathology. *Journal of Child Psychology and Psychiatry*, 41, 513–523.

Bourne, P.G., Rose, R.M. & Mason, J.W. (1968) 17-OCHS levels in combat: Special Forces 'A' Team under threat of attack. *Archives of General Psychiatry*, 19, 135–140.

Bremner, J.D., Innis, R.B., Ng, C.K. *et al.* (1997) Positron emission tomography measurement of cerebral metabolic correlates of yohimbine administration in combat-related post-traumatic stress disorder. *Archives of General Psychiatry*, 54, 246–254.

Brooks-Gunn, J., Duncan, G.J. & Aber, J.L. (1997) *Neighborhood Poverty*, Vol. 1. *Context and Consequences for Children*. Russell Sage Foundation, New York.

Brown, C. (1984) *Black and White Britain: the Third PSI Survey*. Heinemann, London.

Brown, G.W. (1993) Life events and affective disorder: replications and limitations. *Psychosomatic Medicine*, 55, 248–259.

Brown, G.W. & Harris, T.O. (1978) *The Social Origins of Depression: a Study of Psychiatric Disorder in Women*. Tavistock, London.

Brown, G.W. & Harris, T.O. (1986) Establishing causal links: the Bedford College studies of depression. In: *Life Events and Psychiatric Disorders: Controversial Issues* (ed. H. Katschnig), pp. 107–187. Cambridge University Press, London.

Brown, G.W. & Harris, T.O. (1989a) *Life Events and Illness*. Guilford, New York.

Brown, G.W. & Harris, T.O. (1989b) Depression. In: *Life Events and Illness* (eds G.W. Brown & T.O. Harris), pp. 49–93. Unwin Hyman, London.

Brown, G.W., Lemyre, L. & Bifulco, A. (1992) Social factors and recovery from anxiety and depressive disorders: a test of specificity. *British Journal of Psychiatry*, 161, 44–54.

Brown, G.W., Harris, T.O. & Eales, M.J. (1993) Aetiology of anxiety and depressive disorders in an inner-city population. II. Comorbidity and adversity. *Psychological Medicine*, 23, 155–165.

Brown, G.W., Harris, T. & Hepworth, C. (1994) Life events and 'endogenous' depression: a puzzle reexamined. *Archives of General Psychiatry*, 51, 525–534.

Brown, G.W., Harris, T.O. & Eales, M.J. (1996) Social factors and comorbidity of depressive and anxiety disorders. *British Journal of Psychiatry*, 168 (Suppl.30), 50–57.

Cannon, W.B. (1914) The emergency function of the adrenal medulla in pain and the major emotions. *American Journal of Physiology*, 33, 356–372.

Cannon, W.B. (1929) *Bodily Changes in Pain, Hunger, Fear and Rage.* Appleton, New York.

Champion, L.A., Goodall, G.M. & Rutter, M. (1995) Behavioural problems in childhood and stressors in early adult life: a 20-year follow-up of London school children. *Psychological Medicine*, 25, 231–246.

Coddington, R.D. (1972) The significance of life events as aetiological factors in the diseases of children. I. A study of professionals. *Journal of Psychosomatic Research*, 16, 7–18.

Cohen, S., Tyrrell, D.A. & Smith, A.P. (1993) Life events, perceived stress, negative affect and susceptibility to the common cold. *Journal of Personality and Social Psychology*, 64, 131–140.

Cohen, S., Frank, E., Doyle, W.J., Skoner, D.P., Rabin, B.S. & Gwaltney, J.M.J. (1998) Types of stressors that increase susceptibility to the common cold in healthy adults. *Health Psychology*, 17, 214–223.

Cohen, S., Doyle, W.J. & Skoner, D.P. (1999) Psychological stress, cytokine production, and severity of upper respiratory illness. *Psychosomatic Medicine*, 61, 175–180.

Compas, B.E. (1987) Stress and life events during childhood and adolescence. *Clinical Psychology Review*, 7, 275–302.

Cookson, W. (1999) The alliance of genes and environment in asthma and allergy. *Nature*, 402, B5–B11.

Cox, T. (1978) *Stress.* Macmillan, London.

Daley, S.E., Hammen, C., Burge, D., Davila, J., Paley, B., Lindberg, N. & Herzberg, D.S. (1997) Predictors of the generation of episodic stress: A longitudinal study of late adolescent women. *Journal of Abnormal Psychology*, 106, 251–259.

Davies, P.T. & Cummings, E.M. (1995) Children's emotions as organizers of their reactions to interadult anger: a functionalist perspective. *Developmental Psychology*, 31, 677–684.

Dodge, K.A., Bates, J.E. & Pettit, G.S. (1990) Mechanisms in the cycle of violence. *Science*, 250, 1678–1683.

Dodge, K.A., Pettit, G.S., Bates, J.E. & Valente, E. (1995) Social information-processing patterns partially mediate the effects of early physical abuse on later conduct problems. *Journal of Abnormal Psychology*, 104, 632–643.

Drummond, P.D. & Hewson-Bower, B. (1997) Increased psychosocial stress and decreased mucosal immunity in children with recurrent upper respiratory tract infections. *Journal of Psychosomatic Research*, 43, 271–278.

Eisenberg, N., Fabes, R.A., Bernzweig, J., Karbon, M., Poulin, R. & Hanish, L. (1993) The relations of emotionality and regulation to preschoolers' social skills and sociometric status. *Child Development*, 64, 1418–1438.

Elder, G.H. (1974) *Children of the Great Depression.* University of Chicago Press, Chicago.

Eley, T.C. & Stevenson, J. (2000) Specific life events and chronic experiences differentially associated with depression and anxiety in young twins. *Journal of Abnormal Child Psychology*, 28, 383–394.

Esser, G., Schmidt, M.H. & Blanz, B. (1993) Influence of early and recent as well as acute and chronic stressors on the emotional development of children and adolescents: results of a prospective epidemiological study from age 8–18. *Zeitschrift für Kinder- und Jugendpsychiatrie* 21, 82–89.

Fergusson, D.M., Horwood, L.J. & Lynskey, M.T. (1992) Family change, parental discord and early offending. *Journal of Child Psychology and Psychiatry*, 33, 1059–1075.

Finlay-Jones, R. (1989) Anxiety. In: *Life Events and Illness* (eds G.W. Brown & T.O. Harris), pp. 95–112. Unwin & Hyman, London.

Finlay-Jones, R. & Brown, G.W. (1981) Types of stressful life event and the onset of anxiety and depressive disorders. *Psychological Medicine*, 11, 803–815.

Frank, E., Anderson, B., Reynolds, C.F., Ritenour, A. & Kupfer, D.J. (1994) Life events and the research diagnostic criteria endogenous sub-type: a confirmation of the distinction using the Bedford College methods. *Archives of General Psychiatry*, 51, 519–524.

Garmezy, N. & Rutter, M. (1985) Acute reactions to stress. In: *Child and Adolescent Psychiatry: Modern Approaches* (eds M. Rutter & L. Hersov), 2nd edn, pp. 152–176. Blackwell Scientific Publications, Oxford.

Garrison, C.Z., Addy, C.L., Jackson, K.L., McKeown, R.E. & Waller, J.L. (1991) A longitudinal study of suicidal ideation in young adolescents. *Journal of the American Academy of Child and Adolescent Psychiatry*, 30, 597–603.

Ge, X., Conger, R.D., Cadoret, R.J. et al. (1996) The developmental interface between nature and nurture: a mutual influence model of child antisocial behavior and parenting. *Developmental Psychology*, 32, 574–589.

Giaconia, R.M., Reinherz, H.Z., Silverman, A.B., Pakiz, B., Frost, A.K. & Cohen, E. (1995) Traumas and post-traumatic stress disorder in a community population of older adolescents. *Journal of the American Academy of Child and Adolescent Psychiatry*, 34, 1369–1380.

Glen, S., Simpson, A., Drinnan, D., McGuinness, D. & Sandberg, S. (1993) Testing the reliability of a new measure of life events and experiences in childhood: the psychosocial assessment of childhood experiences (PACE). *European Journal of Child and Adolescent Psychiatry*, 2, 98–110.

Goenjian, A.K., Pynoos, R.S., Steinberg, A.M. & Najarian, L.M. (1995) Psychiatric comorbidity in children after the 1988 earthquake in Armenia. *Journal of the American Academy of Child and Adolescent Psychiatry*, 34, 1174–1184.

Goodyer, I. (1990) *Life Experiences, Development and Childhood Psychopathology.* Wiley, Chichester.

Goodyer, I.M. (1994) Developmental psychopathology: the impact of recent life events in anxious and depressed children. *Journal of the Royal Society of Medicine*, 87, 327–329.

Goodyer, I.M., Kolvin, I. & Gatzanis, S. (1985) Recent undesirable life events and psychiatric disorder in childhood and adolescence. *British Journal of Psychiatry*, 147, 517–523.

Goodyer, I.M., Kolvin, I. & Gatzanis, S. (1987) The impact of recent undesirable life events on psychiatric disorders in childhood and adolescence. *British Journal of Psychiatry*, 151, 179–184.

Goodyer, I.M., Wright, C. & Altham, P.M.E. (1988) Maternal adversity and recent life events in anxious and depressed children. *Journal of Child Psychology and Psychiatry*, 29, 651–667.

Goodyer, I.M., Wright, C. & Altham, P.M.E. (1989) Recent friendships in anxious and depressed school age children. *Psychological Medicine*, 19, 165–174.

Goodyer, I., Wright, C. & Altham, P. (1990a) The friendships and recent life events of anxious and depressed school-age children. *British Journal of Psychiatry*, **156**, 689–698.

Goodyer, I.M., Wright, C. & Altham, P. (1990b) Recent achievements and adversities in anxious and depressed school-age children. *Journal of Child Psychology and Psychiatry*, **31**, 1063–1077.

Goodyer, I.M., Cooper, P.J., Vize, C. & Ashby, L. (1993) Depression in 11–16-year-old girls: the role of past parental psychopathology and exposure to recent life events. *Journal of Child Psychology and Psychiatry*, **34**, 1103–1115.

Goodyer, I.M., Herbert, J., Tamplin, A., Secher, S.M. & Pearson, J. (1997) Short term outcome of major depression. II. Life events, family dysfunction, and friendship difficulties as predictors of persistent disorder. *Journal of American Academy of Child and Adolescent Psychiatry*, **36**, 474–480.

Gowers, S.G., North, C.D. & Byram, V. (1996) Life event precipitants of adolescent anorexia nervosa. *Journal of Child Psychology and Psychiatry*, **37**, 469–477.

Greenough, W.T., Black, J.E. & Wallace, C.S. (1987) Experience and brain development. *Child Development*, **58**, 539–559.

Haavet, O.R. & Grünfeld, B. (1997) Are life experiences of children significant for the development of somatic disease? A literature review. *Tidsskrift för den Norske Laegeföre* **117**, 3644–3647.

Harris, T., Brown, G.W. & Bifulco, A. (1986) Loss of parent in childhood and adult psychiatric disorder: the role of lack of adequate parental care. *Psychological Medicine*, **16**, 641–659.

Hart, J., Gunnar, M. & Cicchetti, D. (1996) Altered neuroendocrine activity in maltreated children related to symptoms of depression. *Development and Psychopathology*, **8**, 201–214.

Heisel, J.S., Ream, S., Raitz, R., Rappaport, M. & Coddington, R.D. (1973) The significance of life events as contributing factors in the diseases of children. *Behavioral Pediatrics*, **83**, 119–123.

Hennessey, J.W. & Levine, S. (1979) Stress, arousal, and the pituitary–adrenal system: a psychoendocrine hypothesis. In: *Progress in Psychobiology and Physiological Psychology* (eds J.M. Sprague & A.N. Epstein), pp. 133–178. Academic Press, New York.

Hill, A.V.S. (1998a) The immunogenetics of human infectious diseases. *Annual Review of Immunology*, **16**, 593–617.

Hill, A.V.S. (1998b) Genetics and genomics of infectious disease susceptibility. *British Medical Bulletin*, **55**, 401–413.

Holmes, T.H. & Rahe, R.H. (1967) The social readjustment rating scale. *Journal of Psychosomatic Research*, **11**, 213–218.

Höök, B., Hägglöf, B. & Thernlund, G. (1995) Life events and behavioural deviances in childhood: a longitudinal study of normal population. *European Child and Adolescent Psychiatry*, **4**, 153–164.

Hubbard, J., Realmuto, G.M., Northwood, A.K. & Masten, A. (1995) Comorbidity of psychiatric diagnoses with post-traumatic stress disorder in survivors of childhood trauma. *Journal of the American Academy of Child and Adolescent Psychiatry*, **34**, 1167–1173.

Jacobs, T.J. & Charles, E. (1980) Life events and the occurrence of cancer in children. *Psychosomatic Medicine*, **42**, 11–24.

Jensen, P.S., Richters, J., Ussery, T., Bloedau, L. & Davis, H. (1991) Child psychopathology and environmental influences: discrete life events versus ongoing adversity. *Journal of the American Academy of Child and Adolescent Psychiatry*, **30**, 303–309.

Jockin, V., McGue, M. & Lykken, D.T. (1996) Personality and divorce: a genetic analysis. *Journal of Personality and Social Psychology*, **71**, 288–299.

Johnson, J.H. (1982) Life events as stressors in childhood and adolescence. In: *Advances in Clinical Child Psychology* (eds B.B. Lahey & A.E. Kazdin), pp. 219–253. Plenum Press, New York.

Johnson, J.H. (1986) Life events as stressors in childhood and adolescence: a comparison of approaches. *Life Events as Stressors in Childhood and Adolescence* (ed J.H. Johnson), pp. 31–35. Sage, Beverly Hills, CA.

Johnson, J.H. & McCutcheon, S. (1980) Assessing life stress in older children and adolescents: preliminary findings with the life events checklist. In: *Stress and Anxiety* (eds I.G. Sarason & C.D. Spielberger), pp. 111–125. Hemisphere Publishing Group, Washington D.C.

Kendler, K.S. (1996) Major depression and generalised anxiety disorder: same genes, (partly) different environments—revisited. *British Journal of Psychiatry*, **168** (Suppl. 30), 68–75.

Kendler, K.S., Neale, M., Kessler, R., Heath, A. & Eaves, L. (1993) A twin study of recent life events and difficulties. *Archives of General Psychiatry*, **50**, 789–796.

Kendler, K.S., Kessler, R.C., Walters, E.E. *et al.* (1995) Stressful life events, genetic liability, and onset of an episode of major depression in women. *American Journal of Psychiatry*, **152**, 833–842.

Kendler, K.S., Karkowski, L.M. & Prescott, C.A. (1999) Causal relationship between stressful life events and the onset of major depression. *American Journal of Psychiatry*, **156**, 837–841.

Kraemer, G.W. (1992) Psychobiological Attachment Theory (PAT) and psychopathology. *Behavioral and Brain Sciences*, **15**, 525–534.

Kraemer, G.W. & Clarke, A.S. (1996) Social attachment, brain function, and aggression. *Annals of the New York Academy of Sciences*, **794**, 121–135.

Laub, J.H., Nagin, D.S. & Sampson, R.J. (1998) Trajectories of change in criminal offending: good marriages and the desistance process. *American Sociological Review*, **63**, 225–238.

Lazarus, R.S. & Launier, R. (1978) Stress-related transactions between person and environment. In: *Perspectives in International Psychology* (eds L.A. Pervin & M. Lewis), pp. 287–327. Plenum Press, New York.

Lazarus, R.S., DeLongis, A., Folkman, S. & Gruen, R. (1985) Stress and adaptational outcomes: the problem of confounded measures. *American Psychologist*, **40**, 770–779.

Leenstra, A.S., Ormel, J. & Giel, R. (1995) Positive life change and recovery from depression and anxiety: a three-stage longitudinal study of primary care attenders. *British Journal of Psychiatry*, **166**, 333–343.

Lengua, L.J., Sandler, I.N., West, S.G., Wolchik, S.A. & Curran, P.J. (1999) Emotionality and self-regulation, threat appraisal, and coping in children of divorce. *Development and Psychopathology*, **11**, 15–37.

Levine, S. (1982) Comparative and psychobiological perspectives on development. In: *Minnesota Symposia on Child Psychology*, Vol. 15. *The Concept of Development* (ed. W.A. Collins), pp. 29–53. Lawrence Erlbaum, Hillsdale, NJ.

Liu, D., Diorio, J., Tannenbaum, B., Caldji, C. *et al.* (1997) Maternal care, hippocampal glucocorticoid receptors, and hypothalamic–pituitary–adrenal responses to stress. *Science*, **277**, 1659–1662.

Luthar, S.S., Cicchetti, D. & Becker, B. (2000) The construct of resilience: a critical evaluation and guidelines for future work. *Child Development*, **71**, 543–562.

Madood, T., Berthoud, R., Lakey, J. *et al.* (1997) *Ethnic Minorities in Britain: Diversity and Disadvantage*. Policy Studies Institute, London.

Matthews, K., Wilkinson, L.S. & Robbins, T.W. (1996) Repeated maternal separation of preweanling rats attenuates behavioral responses to primary and conditioned incentives in adulthood. *Physiology and Behavior*, **59**, 99–107.

Mazur, E., Wolchik, S.A., Virdin, L., Sandler, I.N. & West, S.G. (1999) Cognitive moderators of children's adjustment to stressful divorce events: the role of negative cognitive errors and positive illusions. *Child Development*, **70**, 231–245.

McCarron, M.O., Muir, K.W., Weir, C.J. *et al.* (1998) The apolipoprotein E e4 allele and outcome in cerebrovascular disease. *Stroke*, **29**, 1882–1887.

Meyer, A. (1957) *Psychobiology: a Science of Man.* Charles C. Thomas, Springfield, IL.

Miller, P.M. & Ingham, J.G. (1985) Dimensions of experience and symptomatology. *Journal of Psychosomatic Research*, **29**, 475–488.

Monck, E. & Dobbs, R. (1985) Measuring life events in an adolescent population: methodological issues and related findings. *Psychological Medicine*, **15**, 841–850.

Mrazek, D.A., Klinnert, M.D., Mrazek, P.J. *et al.* (1999) Prediction of early-onset asthma in genetically at risk children. *Pediatric Pulmonology*, **27**, 85–94.

Murray, L. & Cooper, P.J. (1997) *Postpartum Depression and Child Development.* Guilford Press, New York.

O'Brien, J.T. (1997) The 'glucocorticoid cascade' hypothesis in man: prolonged stress may cause permanent brain damage. *British Journal of Psychiatry*, **170**, 199–201.

O'Connor, T.G., Deater-Deckard, K., Fulker, D., Rutter, M. & Plomin, R. (1998) Genotype-environment correlations in late childhood and early adolescence: antisocial behavioral problems and coercive parenting. *Developmental Psychology*, **34**, 970–981.

O'Connor, T.G., Caspi, A., DeFries, J.C. & Plomin, R. (2000) Are associations between parental divorce and children's adjustment genetically mediated? An adoption study. *Developmental Psychology*, **36**, 429–437.

Olsson, I.G., Nordström, M.-L., Arinell, H. & Von Knorring, A.-L. (1999) Adolescent depression and stressful life events: a case–control study within diagnostic subgroups. *Nordic Journal of Psychiatry*, **53**, 339–346.

Paykel, E.S. (1974) Life stresses and psychiatric disorders. In: *Stressful Life Events: Their Nature and Effects* (eds B.S. Dohrenwend & B.P. Dohrenwend), pp. 139–149. Wiley, New York.

Paykel, E.S. (1978) Contribution of life events to causation of psychiatric illness. *Psychological Medicine*, **8**, 245–253.

Petitto, J.M. & Evans, D.L. (1999) Clinical neuroimmunology. In: *Neurobiology of Mental Illness* (eds D.S. Charney, E.J. Nestler & B.S. Bunney), pp. 162–169. Oxford University Press, New York.

Pollak, S.D., Cicchetti, D., Klorman, R. & Brumaghim, J.T. (1997) Cognitive brain event-related potentials and emotion processing in maltreated children. *Child Development*, **68**, 773–787.

Power, A. (1997) *Estates on the Edge: the Social Consequences of Mass Housing in Northern Europe.* Macmillan, London.

Quinton, D. & Rutter, M. (1976) Early hospital admissions and later disturbances of behaviour: an attempted replication of Douglas' findings. *Developmental Medicine and Child Neurology*, **18**, 447–459.

Randolph, C. & Fraser, B. (1999) Stressors and concerns in teen asthma. *Current Problems in Pediatrics*, **29**, 82–93.

Riese, W. (1969) *The Legacy of Philippe Pinel.* Springer, New York.

Robbins, T.W., Jones, G.H. & Wilkinson, L.S. (1996) Behavioural and neurochemical effects of early social deprivation in the rat. *Journal of Psychopharmacology*, **10**, 39–47.

Robins, L. (1966) *Deviant Children Grown Up: a Sociological and Psychiatric Study of Sociopathic Personality.* Williams & Wilkins, Baltimore.

Rose, R.M. (1980) Endocrine responses to stressful psychological events. *Psychiatric Clinics of North America*, **2**, 53–71.

Rowlison, R.T. & Felner, R.D. (1988) Major life events, hassles, and adaptation in adolescence: confounding in the conceptualization and measurement of life stress and adjustment revisited. *Journal of Personality and Social Psychology*, **55**, 432–444.

Rutter, M. (1971) Parent–child separation: psychological effects on the children. *Journal of Child Psychology and Psychiatry*, **12**, 233–260.

Rutter, M. (1981) Stress, coping and development: some issues and some questions. *Journal of Child Psychology and Psychiatry*, **22**, 323–356.

Rutter, M. (1986) Meyerian psychobiology, personality development and the role of life experiences. *American Journal of Psychiatry*, **143**, 1077–1087.

Rutter, M. (1989a) Psychiatric disorder in parents as a risk factor for children. In: *Prevention of mental disorders, alcohol and other drug use in children and adolescents. OSAP Prevention Monograph 2* (eds D. Shaffer, I. Philips & E.B. Enzer), pp. 157–189. Office for Substance Abuse Prevention, US Department of Health and Human Services, Rockville, Maryland.

Rutter, M. (1989b) Pathways from childhood to adult life. *Journal of Child Psychology and Psychiatry*, **30**, 23–51.

Rutter, M. (1999) Resilience concepts and findings: implications for family therapy. *Journal of Family Therapy*, **21**, 119–144.

Rutter, M. (2000a) Negative life events and family negativity: accomplishments and challenges. In: *Where Inner and Outer Worlds Meet: Psychosocial research in the tradition of George W. Brown* (ed. T. Harris), pp. 123–149. Routledge, London.

Rutter, M. (2000b) Resilience reconsidered: conceptual considerations, empirical findings, and policy implications. In: *Handbook of Early Childhood Intervention* (eds J.P. Shonkoff & S.J. Meisels), 2nd edn, pp. 651–682. Cambridge University Press, New York.

Rutter, M. (2000c) Psychosocial influences: critiques, findings, and research needs. *Development and Psychopathology*, **12**, 375–405.

Rutter, M. & Quinton, D. (1977) Psychiatric disorder: ecological factors and concepts of causation. In: *Ecological Factors in Human Development* (ed. H. McGurk), pp. 173–187. North-Holland, Amsterdam.

Rutter, M. & Quinton, D. (1984) Parental psychiatric disorder: effects on children. *Psychological Medicine*, **14**, 853–880.

Rutter, M. & Sandberg, S. (1992) Psychosocial stressors: concepts, causes and effects. *European Journal of Child and Adolescent Psychiatry*, **1**, 3–13.

Rutter, M., Silberg, J. & Simonoff, E. (1993) Whither behavioral genetics? A developmental psychopathological perspective. In: *Nature, Nurture, and Psychology* (eds R. Plomin & G.E. McClearn), pp. 433–456. APA Books, Washington, D.C.

Rutter, M., Champion, L., Quinton, D., Maughan, B. & Pickles, A. (1995) Understanding individual differences in environmental risk exposure. In: *Examining Lives in Context: Perspectives on the Ecology of Human Development* (eds P. Moen, G.H. Elder Jr & K. Lüscher), pp. 61–93. American Psychological Association, Washington D.C.

Rutter, M., Maughan, B., Meyer, J. *et al.* (1997) Heterogeneity of antisocial behavior: causes, continuities, and consequences. In: *Nebraska Symposium on Motivation*, Vol. 44. *Motivation and Delinquency* (eds R. Dienstbier & D.W. Osgood), pp. 45–118. University of Nebraska Press, Lincoln, NB.

Rutter, M., Giller, H. & Hagell, A. (1998) *Antisocial Behaviour by Young People: the Main Messages from a Major New Review of the Research.* Cambridge University Press, New York.

Sampson, R.J., Raudenbush, S.W. & Earls, F. (1997) Neighborhoods and violent crime: a multilevel study of collective efficacy. *Science*, **277**, 918–924.

Sandberg, S., Nicholls, J., Prior, V. & Hillary, C. (1994) *PACE: Life Events and Long-Term Experiences Dictionary.* University of Glasgow, Glasgow.

Sandberg, S., Rutter, M., Giles, S. *et al.* (1993) Assessment of psychosocial experiences in childhood: methodological issues and some illustrative findings. *Journal of Child Psychology and Psychiatry*, **34**, 879–897.

Sandberg, S., McGuinness, D., Hillary, C. & Rutter, M. (1998) Independence of childhood life events and chronic adversities: a comparison of two patient groups and controls. *Journal of the American Academy of Child and Adolescent Psychiatry*, **37**, 728–735.

Sandberg, S., Paton, J.Y., Ahola, S. *et al.* (2000) The role of acute and chronic stress in asthma attacks in children. *Lancet*, **356**, 982–987.

Sandberg, S., Rutter, M., Pickles, A., McGuinness, D. & Angold, A. (2001) Do high threat life events really provoke the onset of psychiatric disorder in children? *Journal of Child Psychology and Psychiatry*, **42**, 523–532.

Sandler, I.N., Tein, J.Y. & West, S.G. (1994) Coping, stress, and the psychological symptoms of children of divorce: a cross-sectional and longitudinal study. *Child Development*, **65**, 1744–1763.

Sapolsky, R.M. (1993) Endocrinology alfresco: psychoendocrine studies of wild baboons. *Recent Progress in Hormone Research*, **48**, 437–468.

Sapolsky, R.M. (1998) *Why Zebras Don't Get Ulcers: an Updated Guide to Stress, Stress-Related Diseases, and Coping.* W.H. Freeman, New York.

Schneider, M.L., Clarke, A.S., Kraemer, G.W. *et al.* (1998) Prenatal stress alters brain biogenic amine levels in primates. *Development and Psychopathology*, **10**, 427–440.

Sheets, V., Sandler, I.N. & West, S.G. (1996) Negative appraisals of stressful events by pre-adolescent children of divorce. *Child Development*, **67**, 2166–2182.

Silberg, J., Pickles, A., Rutter, M. *et al.* (1999) The influence of genetic factors and life stress on depression among adolescent girls. *Archives of General Psychiatry*, **56**, 225–232.

Silberg, J., Rutter, M., Neale, M. & Eaves, L. (2001) Genetic moderation of environmental risk for depression and anxiety in adolescent girls. *British Journal of Psychiatry*, **179**, 116–121.

Stacey, M., Dearden, R., Pill, R. & Robinson, D. (1970) *Hospitals, Children and Their Families: The Report of a Pilot Study.* Routledge & Kegan Paul, London.

Surtees, P.G. & Wainwright, N.W.J. (1999) Surviving adversity: event decay, vulnerability and the onset of anxiety and depressive disorder. *European Archives of Psychiatry and Clinical Neuroscience*, **249**, 86–95.

Talmud, P.J., Bujac, S.R., Hall, S., Miller, G.J. & Humphries, S.E. (2000) Substitution of asparagine for aspartic acid at residue 9 (D9N) of lipoprotein lipase markedly augments risk of ischaemic heart disease in male smokers. *Atherosclerosis*, **149**, 75–81.

Teasdale, J.D. & Barnard, P.J. (1993) *Affect, Cognition, and Change: Re-Modelling Depressive Thought.* Erlbaum, Hove.

Teasdale, G.M., Nicoll, J.A.R., Murray, G. & Fiddes, M. (1997) Association of apolipoprotein E polymorphism with outcome after head injury. *Lancet*, **350**, 1069–1071

Thapar, A. & McGuffin, P. (1996) Genetic influences on life events in childhood. *Psychological Medicine*, **26**, 813–820.

Thapar, A., Harold, G. & McGuffin, P. (1998) Life events and depressive symptoms in childhood: shared genes or shared adversity? A research note. *Journal of Child Psychology and Psychiatry*, **39**, 1153–1158.

Thoenen, H. (1995) Neurotrophins and neuronal plasticity. *Science*, **270**, 593–598.

Tiet, Q.Q., Bird, H.R., Davies, M. *et al.* (1998) Adverse life events and resilience. *Journal of the American Academy of Child and Adolescent Psychiatry*, **37**, 1191–1200.

Turner Cobb, J.M. & Steptoe, A. (1996) Psychosocial stress and susceptibility to upper respiratory tract illness in an adult population sample. *Psychosomatic Medicine*, **58**, 404–412.

Turner Cobb, J.M. & Steptoe, A. (1998) Psychosocial influences on upper respiratory infectious illness in children. *Journal of Psychosomatic Research*, **45**, 319–330.

Tyano, S., Iancu, I., Solomon, Z. *et al.* (1996) Seven-year follow-up of child survivors of a bus–train collison. *Journal of the American Academy of Child and Adolescent Psychiatry*, **35**, 365–373.

Tyrell, D. (1977) Aspects of infection in isolated communities. In: *Health and Diseases in Tribal Societies. Ciba Foundation Symposium 49*, pp. 137–153. Elsevier/Excerpta Medica, Amsterdam.

Walker, L.S. & Greene, J.W. (1987) Negative life events, psychosocial resources and psychophysiological symptoms in adolescents. *Journal of Clinical Child Psychology*, **16**, 29–36.

Williamson, D.E., Birmaher, B., Anderson, B., Al-Shabbout, M. & Ryan, N. (1995) Stressful life events in depressed adolescents: the role of dependent events during the depressive episode. *Journal of the American Academy of Child and Adolescent Psychiatry*, **34**, 591–598.

Williamson, D.E., Birmaher, B., Frank, E., Anderson, B.P., Matty, M.K. & Kupfer, D.J. (1998) Nature of life events and difficulties in depressed adolescents. *Journal of the American Academy of Child and Adolescent Psychiatry*, **37**, 1049–1057.

Zoccolillo, M., Pickles, A., Quinton, D. & Rutter, M. (1992) The outcome of childhood conduct disorder: implications for defining adult personality disorder and conduct disorder. *Psychological Medicine*, **22**, 971–986.

Bereavement

Dora Black

Introduction

The loss of a parent by death is one of the most significant developmental challenges a dependent child can face, one which has been implicated as a major risk factor for psychiatric disorder in childhood and later. This chapter reviews the known effects of parental bereavement on children of different ages and varying levels of cognitive development, drawing on research on humans and higher primates, sets out the principles for clinical assessment of the impact of bereavement on child and family, and discusses the selection of appropriate preventive and therapeutic interventions. The effects of bereavements other than parental are less well researched but will be touched upon. The effects of traumatic bereavement (the loss by death which is sudden, unexpected and horrific as occurs in war, civil conflict, accidents, suicide and homicide) will be considered separately. The effects of witnessing or being caught up in traumatic events which do not necessarily result in bereavement are considered in Chapter 17.

In Western countries between 1.5 and 4% of children are orphaned of at least one parent in childhood (Haskey 1993). In developing countries, and those affected by natural disasters, war and civil conflict, the figures are much higher. In Britain in 1995, 1 in 5 of all dependent children was living in a one-parent family, but only 1 in 25 lone parents is widowed (compared with 1 in 4 in 1971) (Haskey 1998). As the proportion of children reared in single-parent households increases, the death of a sole parent figure is likely to be associated with an increased incidence of morbidity in the children. As premature deaths from other infectious diseases decline, deaths of parents from AIDS presents a new scourge, leaving large numbers of doubly orphaned children in many parts of the world.

The biology of loss

The poignant description by Goodall (1996) of the suffering of the infant chimpanzee in the wild, when bereft of her mother, is echoed by the experimental laboratory work of Hinde (Hinde & McGinnis 1977), Harlow (Seay & Harlow 1965) and Suomi (1983) with monkeys, and Hofer (1996) with rats, indicating that primates, at least, react in ways similar to humans when deprived of their caregiver.

In an attempt to understand the biological aspects of loss that are central to its role as a risk factor for disease, Hofer carried out a study looking at physiological and behavioural responses of infant rats to separation from their mothers before the normal weaning time. The rats in Hofer's study displayed an initial 'distress' calling, followed more slowly by profound behavioural inhibition, said to be very similar to the sequence of 'protest' and 'despair' phases described by Bowlby in human infants (Bowlby 1969). Hofer explores the effect of the loss of 'hidden maternal regulators', such as touch and smell, on infant and later behaviour in rats. Early separation induced a susceptibility to a complex and widespread regulatory disturbance which was still manifest later in life and increased susceptibility to stress-induced pathology. However, the response was dependent to some extent on the quality of the pre-separation mother–infant relationship. He suggests that this may give a clue to understanding how regulatory interactions, such as feeding or warming, become linked in the memory with the same pattern of maternal olfactory, auditory and visual cues giving an 'internal working model' of the mother as an attachment figure. Her loss is then experienced at a deep visceral level as well as at the psychological level of sadness. He elaborates this theory to hypothesize about the way that older human children develop the ability to predict future events as a result of this internal working model and how early loss of the mother interferes with this information processing and thus shapes adult behavioural traits and future vulnerability to stress.

Recent studies on the effect of trauma on the developing brain suggest that a traumatic experience, such as the sudden and permanent loss of the main caregiver, can alter the way the brain of the infant organizes and internalizes new information, which can influence the subsequent regulation of affect and may permanently alter neurophysiological function and emotional development. The right orbito-frontal cortex, which is responsible for regulating and mediating affect, social relations and emotional balance, among other functions, may develop differentially, depending on early infantile experiences and the responsiveness or even availability of the primary caregiver in allaying fear (Schore 1994; Perry *et al.* 1995). Schore suggested that the experiences 'that fine-tune brain circuitries in critical periods of infancy are embedded in socio-emotional interchanges between an adult brain and a developing brain'. Although a good deal of caution is needed at this stage, if these findings are confirmed, they help to understand why the loss of the adult who has made such an accommodation is likely to affect the infant profoundly. Perry *et al.* (1995) found that, in the infants they studied, there were various adaptive mental and physical responses to trauma, including physiological hyper-arousal and dissociation. These acute adaptive states can become maladaptive traits. Their findings have implications for clinical assessment, intervention and prevention and can help to explain the increase in anxiety and depressive disorders in bereaved children both in childhood and adult life. Some of the findings may not be specific to loss but might be the effect of chronic or severe adversity.

Why should bereavement concern psychiatrists?

Grief is a normal response to bereavement, but it causes at least as much suffering as, say, fever, the normal response to an infection and may be as dangerous to the organism. Grief has many of the components of what would otherwise be regarded as a major depressive episode (e.g. feelings of sadness, insomnia, poor appetite, weight loss) and this is recognized by the DSM-IV definition of bereavement (V62.82). However, the normal processes of grief usually lead eventually to recovery, even though a new identity has to be assumed: widow, orphan, etc. (Parkes 1972). Symptoms such as guilt, thoughts of death, morbid preoccupation with worthlessness, marked psychomotor retardation, prolonged and marked functional impairment, and hallucinatory experiences are usually considered to be more typical of a pathological grief reaction. This definition is an adult-orientated one, but older children and adolescents may also fit this picture. It has been argued that the DSM-IV definition does not satisfy the observations made about childhood bereavement (Vida & Grizenko 1989) but it does at least acknowledge the need for recognition of the trigger to the development of symptoms. On the other hand, the ICD-10 does not recognize bereavement as having the possibility of generating *specific* psychopathology. What evidence there is favours the development of specific depressive disorders in adult life associated with bereavement, particularly when it occurs in childhood (Brown & Harris 1978) although chronic adversity following the loss of a parent may be the intervening variable (Harris *et al.* 1986). This is developed in more detail below.

The loss of a parent by death has interested theoreticians and clinicians for many years. Freud (1917) noted the effect of the death of a loved one on his adult patients and Bowlby (1969, 1972, 1980) developed the theory of attachment as a biological organizer of human behaviour, with the inevitable converse phenomenon of loss. Parkes (1972) was one of the first researchers to study widows systematically and to identify the high morbidity that occurs after the loss of a spouse, both immediately and in the longer term. Studies on the origins of depressive illness in adults have found life-events involving some kind of loss occur significantly more often in individuals suffering from these disorders than in controls (Paykel *et al.* 1969; Birtchnell 1970; Brown & Harris 1978; Berlinsky & Biller 1982; Paykel & Dowlatshahi 1988).

Rutter was one of the first researchers to establish that be-reaved children were at enhanced risk of developing psychiatric problems compared with non-bereaved controls, finding that children attending the child psychiatric department of the Maudsley Hospital were significantly more likely to have lost a parent by death, than controls attending a dental clinic (Rutter 1966). Many early studies of the effects of bereavement on children used parental reports (Black 1978; Black & Urbanowicz 1985, 1987; Elizur & Kaffman 1983; Van Eerdewegh *et al.* 1985) but more recently the children have been studied directly (Raphael 1982; Kranzler *et al.* 1990; Weller *et al.* 1991; Silverman & Worden 1992; Thompson *et al.* 1998). All these studies found that children bereaved of a parent, when compared with controls, had higher levels of psychiatric symptoms in the immediate aftermath and on follow-up 1 or 2 years later. When children are studied directly, higher levels of morbidity are found. For example, a controlled study of 38 bereaved children aged 5–12 years (from 26 families out of a potential 101 families) found that 37% of the bereaved children met DSM-III-R criteria for major depressive episode 3–12 weeks after the loss (Weller *et al.* 1991).

A prospective study of 26 recently bereaved 3–6-year-olds, using matched non-bereaved controls, showed that there were significantly more symptoms, particularly symptoms of anxiety and depression in the bereaved children than in controls. Bereaved children, especially girls, reported significantly more sadness when thinking of their parents than did controls. Depression in the surviving parent was the most powerful predictor of child disturbance (Kranzler *et al.* 1990). Multiple bereavements are likely to enhance the risk of later psychopathology (Goodyer & Altham 1991).

Young children are more likely than adults to have difficulties with the comprehension of death and the processes of grief and mourning. They are more likely to develop pathological mourning reactions because of limitations in their understanding, lack of information and changes in their lives (Bowlby & Parkes 1970; Goodyer 1990b). Symptoms in bereaved children may be delayed in onset, so that studies of recently bereaved children may underestimate the distress. This may be a response, not to the bereavement itself, but to the consequences of the death. Children who lose their mothers suffer a reduction in the quantity as well as quality of care (Weller *et al.* 1991) and the finding that adult psychopathology following childhood loss of a parent is correlated with the adequacy of care following the death (Harris *et al.* 1986) has implications for preventive intervention.

Goodyer *et al.* (1990a), on the basis of a series of population studies on school-aged children, concluded that recent undesirable life events exert a significant (about five times) adverse effect on the probability of being anxious or depressed which was independent of maternal adversities (poor confiding relations in mothers' own lives and the presence of maternal distress). Emotional disorders in the children were best predicted by the presence of all three adversities. The Christchurch longitudinal study had a similar finding (Fergusson & Lynskey 1996).

Disruption of attachment because of the death of a caregiver—usually a mother—during early childhood increases the risk to the child of developing an attachment disorder, a separation anxiety disorder, anxiety, depression or other emotional disorder during childhood and adolescence.

A literature review of the effects on children of bereavement concluded that findings were inconsistent and that there was a lack of appropriate measurement tools (Berlinsky & Biller 1982). The Harvard Bereavement Study (Silverman & Worden 1993) attempted to remedy this using multiple measures, some of which they devised. They noted that preadolescent children often did not express grief directly but there was a high incidence of somatic symptoms. They suggest that bereavement outcomes need to be conceptualized in terms that emphasize change and adaptation rather than the presence or absence of diagnostic categories.

Mental health professionals may be asked to help in the immediate aftermath of a bereavement because of dysfunction. They may also find themselves treating long-term psychopathology which is associated with an earlier bereavement. They may also be called upon to advise on or set up preventative services after a bereavement, especially a sudden, unexpected and traumatic one.

Resilience

Although bereavement enhances the risk of developing psychopathology, the majority of bereaved children do not develop psychiatric disorders either in childhood or adult life and epidemiological studies indicate that childhood bereavement in itself is not a major risk factor for later psychopathology (Harrington & Harrison 1999). Studies on the resilience of children (Rutter 1985) note that resistance to stress is relative, not absolute; the bases of the resistance are both environmental and constitutional and the degree of resistance is not a fixed entity, but varies over time and according to circumstance. For example, genetic factors (such as temperament or cognitive level) have their impact through their role in influencing individual differences in susceptibility to environmental risk, as do children's prior experiences (Rutter 1999). Later experiences are not independent of what has occurred before and vicious cycles can build up unless prevented by therapeutic intervention. Rutter makes the point that the reduction of the negative impact of an event or adversity becomes a critical issue in prevention and this forms the basis for the rationale of intervening with bereaved children and those about to be bereaved.

Children's grief reactions

Children who have reached school age are as capable as adults of comprehending death, of expressing grief and taking part in community mourning rituals. The reactions may appear different because they often take an immature form. The influences on the expression of grief and the ability to mourn by children are related to their cognitive, emotional and physical developmental levels.

Cognitive development

The child's ability to comprehend the various components of the concept of death has been well-studied and the consensus is that by 5 years most children of normal intelligence can understand that death is irreversible, universal, has a cause, involves permanent separation and that dead people differ from live people in a number of respects: they are immobile, unfeeling, cannot hear, see, smell, taste, speak and all their bodily functions cease. The concept of corporeal deterioration is more difficult for young children to comprehend and this concept is not fully formed until nearer puberty (Kane 1979; Reilly et al. 1983; Lansdown & Benjamin 1985). In a review of children's reactions to death (Cuddy-Casey & Orvaschel 1997) the concepts of irreversibility and universality were found to be understood before causality, and external events, such as moving and speaking, were believed by children to cease before internal ones, such as thinking and feeling. Children younger than 5 years generally appear unable to give a narrative account of the sequence of events around bereavement.

Other cognitive difficulties involve immaturity in searching for the dead parent, an important component of the process of mourning, and anticipating both the death and the prospect of missing the dead parent. There is a developmental progression in the ability to envisage how one might feel on future occasions. For example, it would be difficult for young children to imagine that they might miss their mother all over again when they next go on holiday. Anticipatory mourning for all the small and large events and situations at which the mother will no longer be present is therefore more difficult and, when the event comes, the child is unprepared for the emotional experience of renewed loss.

Cognition plays a part in reunion fantasies, which are concrete in early childhood:

Harry, aged 3 when his father died in hospital, said when he visited his grandmother in the same hospital, one year later: 'Good, now we can see daddy again.' His mother thought he had understood that his father's death was permanent and was surprised that he had held on to the hope of reunion for so long. It clearly was revived by the visit to the last place he had seen his father alive.

Children are rarely prepared for the death of a parent or a sibling. In adults mourning is aided by anticipation of the inevitability and proximity of death (Parkes 1972). The evidence for children is contradictory. While several studies have found that if children are prepared, the morbidity is subsequently lower (Rosenheim & Reicher 1985; Siegel et al. 1997), Saldinger et al. (1999) found, in a community study of parentally bereaved young children, that forewarning of death does not lead to better mental health outcomes than when there is a sudden death. Other studies have noted similar findings (Kranzler et al. 1990; Freeman et al. 1991; Fristad et al. 1993). It may be a function of developmental stage. Younger children cannot perform the cognitive task of anticipating and most studies do not analyse their findings according to age.

Cognitive limitations also affect the child's ability to recall memories, especially in the absence of contextual cues (Johnson & Foley 1984). These are often denied to them by protective adults who do not wish to remind them of their loss. The places they visited with their parent are avoided, so mourning for the lost parent is inhibited. Whereas adults can take themselves to the places in reality and in fantasy, it is more difficult for children to do so.

At least one study (Van Eerdewegh *et al.* 1982) found that the loss of a parent is associated with difficulties in learning and failure to maintain progress in school in the presence of a normal intelligence.

Learning disability

Children with moderate or severe learning disability have not been studied in relation to bereavement. Studies of adults with learning disability have found that they are often not told about significant deaths in the family, and are not given the support that both adults and children of normal intelligence receive. Their reactions to the death may be misunderstood, they may not be allowed to participate in family or community rituals (Cathcart 1995). Even when they experience a bereavement, their understanding of death may not have improved, although their reactions indicate that they are aware of a change in their lives and they can be helped to grieve and to relinquish their attachment to the dead person (Hollins & Esterhuyzen 1997; Bonell-Pascual *et al.* 1999).

Emotional development

Children's capacity to sustain sad affects increases gradually with age and maturity. Not only may they avoid the experience of the pain of grief but young children do not sustain affects for long periods and their apparent lack of sadness may deceive their caregivers into believing that they are unaffected by the loss.

One way in which children obtain understanding of events is through repetitive play, which may be distressing to adults because it lacks appropriate affective expression. Children need to be able to understand the reality of death in order to mourn and yet they are given less opportunity to see for themselves the physical deterioration and then the immobility and unresponsiveness of the dead parent. They may be prevented from going to the funeral and protected from the grief of the adults. Yet the evidence is that, properly supported, children who view the (unmutilated) body after death and attend the funeral, even of a parent, have lower morbidity levels than those who do not.

Weller *et al.* (1988) looked at an unselected parentally bereaved group of 6–12-year-olds. Twenty-six of 56 children of families approached entered the study which used structured and semistructured interviews with children and surviving parents. Ninety-two per cent attended the funeral—more of the

older than the younger ones. Their psychiatric state was assessed 2 months after the bereavement. Neither the type of death, nor the sex of child and parent, influenced the child's participation or reaction to funeral activities and there was no association between psychiatric state and attendance or transient 'atypical' reactions. Although the contrast group was too small to draw conclusions, it seemed that attending the funeral only had adverse consequences if the child was forced to go. There is little research on the advantages or disadvantages of children viewing the dead body; most of what we know comes from adult studies (Cathcart 1988). My clinical experience is that it helps children to a greater cognitive understanding of the differences between life and death. They need to be properly supported, by someone who is familiar with the appearance of a corpse (the GP is the ideal person), and it is not advisable to allow children to view a body which is mutilated, especially if the face is unrecognizable.

Children may be protected from reminders of the dead parent and this handicaps them in the normal process of grieving and resolving grief. Their concrete thinking and egocentric view of the world make it more likely that young children will feel guilty and responsible for the parent's disappearance. Longings for death and even suicidal ideas are common as part of reunion fantasies but are rarely acted upon (Weller *et al.* 1991) and although in adolescents, suicide can commonly be precipitated by loss of peers, it is rarely triggered by loss of a parent (Brent *et al.* 1988; Prosser & McArdle 1996).

Children can be taught to recognize and name emotions. Kranzler *et al.* (1990) found that children as young as 3 years were able to recognize sad affects in themselves, and that recognizing these grieving emotions correlated with a better outcome. This has important implications for preventive intervention and therapy.

Children may not understand the source of the emotions of grief and suffer alone without seeking elucidation from carers or other adults. The misconstruing of emotions may lead to hypochondriasis or other psychosomatic symptoms and these in turn may bind the surviving parent to the child, thus reinforcing the symptoms.

Carla was 4 when her mother died after a short illness. At 6 she was seen by a child psychiatrist because of disturbed sleep and hypochondriasis. Assessment revealed that she interpreted every delay in her father's return from work as evidence that he too had died. Her various symptoms served to keep him at home where she could keep an eye on him.

The ability to attribute anxiety, depression and other dysphoric emotions accurately develops with maturation. Bereaved children may feel ashamed of their reactions, believing themselves to be experiencing unique emotions. Education about emotional reactions can usefully be part of the school curriculum and a handbook for teachers has been published (Ward 1993).

Another aspect of emotional development is the continuing need for caregivers. Children who have lost one parent feel anxious lest the other one will also die or disappear. This leads them to monitor their surviving parent, and parental expressions of grief may be misinterpreted as illness. Children may hide their own grief in order to protect their parent and avoid upsetting them. Adolescents in the process of separating from parents may either take a step back in the process and become more involved with the family, particularly if they are the eldest or the same sex as the deceased parent (Birtchnell 1971), or they may react by rejecting the family and developing new and possibly premature procreative partnerships.

Physical development

Pre-verbal children react to loss with bodily responses. They may lose their recently acquired control over urination or defecation, lose their appetites, fail to settle to sleep or become restless. Motility or speech may be temporarily lost. The immune system may be affected so that infections and other illnesses are more common in young children following the loss of a parent (Raphael *et al.* 1980; Schleifer *et al.* 1983).

Effect of parental grief on children

Parents who lose a partner, a child or a parent will undergo a grief reaction. A normal grief reaction in adults is characterized by an acute phase which lasts for a few weeks or months, during which their normal functioning may be disrupted (Parkes 1996). It is important that relatives, friends and neighbours who may be less affected by the death rally round and, by offering respite care, relieve the children of exposure to the continuing and possibly overwhelming sorrow of the parent.

Parents who lose a child experience a fundamental change in their beliefs about their family's future security. Their grief reaction is more likely to take a pathological course. Grief may be absent, delayed, prolonged or distorted and may affect their sensitivity and ability to parent their remaining children. A review of the studies of the effect on parents of the death of a child, points out that there is surprisingly little methodologically sound research in this area but that what seems to be emerging from a very limited body of sound research is that the effect of loss of a child extends beyond psychological distress for a limited duration, to, in some studies, long-term effects on mental and physical health and even to disruption of marriages (Dijkstra & Stroebe 1998).

Other bereavements

Siblings

The death of a sibling has been less well studied than that of a parent (Newman *et al.* 1997). One study of 28 children found that 2 or 3 years after the death, a high proportion of the children were emotionally or behaviourally disturbed and had a low self-esteem. The dead sibling was idealized and school work was

suffering. If the child had been prepared for the death, had participated in the patient's care and had been able to take leave of him or her and joined in the community rituals, the outcome appeared to be better. Interestingly, there was no correlation between parental and child adaptation (Pettle Michael & Lansdown 1986).

A study of 25 unselected suicide-bereaved adolescent siblings and their parents, compared them with a demographic-matched sample of adolescents unexposed to suicide, and found that the siblings were at a sevenfold risk of developing major depression within 6 months subsequent to their sibling's death. Those who developed depression had a personal and/or family history of depression or other psychiatric disorder. Their mothers were much more likely to become depressed also (Brent *et al.* 1993). A longitudinal follow-up over the ensuing 3 years of this group (20 subjects out of the original 25 participated) found no significantly increased risk for the development of depression, post-traumatic stress disorder (PTSD) or other disorders in siblings, although they did discover prolonged high levels of grief symptomatology. This was particularly marked in younger siblings. The mothers were also more likely to show more marked and long-lasting effects, those with prebereavement histories of depression faring the worst (Brent *et al.* 1997). Although there was a correlation between mother and sibling depression at 6 months, this did not persist.

Peers

Brent *et al.* (1994) compared the friends and acquaintances of the adolescent who committed suicide with the siblings and found that their rates of depression were also high and that, in contrast to the siblings, this persisted on follow-up. The authors suggest that the siblings were more likely to have been given support and encouragement to mourn than were friends and acquaintances and that this may have aided the resolution of the depressive symptoms.

Relatives

Grandparents and other close relatives are often involved as carers for bereaved children and supports for the widowed parent. They may even take over the care completely of orphaned children. There are no studies which look at the effect on the children of the grief of grandparents or how they help their charges with their own bereavement. The death of a grandparent, particularly one who has had a major caring role, has been little studied although the effect on grandparents of the death of a grandchild has (Ponzetti & Johnson 1991).

Traumatic bereavement

While all bereavements can be traumatic to children, there are types of deaths which tend to produce more frequent, severe and longer lasting morbidity. Sudden, unexpected, violent and mutilating deaths, particularly if witnessed by the child, and which affect their lives—deaths of family members, for example—have consistently been shown to produce more serious psychological problems. Children can get caught up in war and civil conflict, and community violence, and may witness the murder of parents, siblings and other familiar people (Richman 1993; Kuterovac et al. 1994; Osofsky 1997; Saigh et al. 1998). Domestic violence can lead to the death of a parent, and in at least 50% of cases of such homicides, the children may witness it (Harris Hendriks et al. 1993). Other homicides, suicide by a parent or sibling, and accidents, may all be witnessed by the child. The effects on children of traumatic events is discussed by Sandberg & Rutter (Chapter 17). There is still uncertainty about the factors that make some children more vulnerable to developing psychiatric morbidity after traumatic events. The degree of exposure to the event is probably important, and witnessing death or injury in others, being separated from family and friends, a subjective fear of a threat to life, feelings of helplessness and guilt, and academic ability, may all affect outcome (Terr 1991; Harris Hendriks et al. 1993).

A comparative study of 10 siblings who had lost a brother or sister by accidental death with 10 who had been bereaved of a sibling by homicide (Applebaum & Burns 1991) found that all the siblings reported symptoms of PTSD with 45% meeting full criteria for the disorder. Parents were not necessarily aware of their child's distress, perhaps because they were struggling with their own symptoms. There was a correlation between the severity of PTSD symptoms in child and parent.

Of the children who experience the death of a loved one, those who witness a sudden, horrific and unexpected one and those who perceive a threat to their own life are more likely to develop PTSD (Pynoos et al. 1987a; Harris Hendriks et al. 1993). Post-traumatic stress disorder can inhibit the normal response to bereavement (Pynoos et al. 1987b) and it is sound clinical practice to treat PTSD before attempting to deal with the grief reaction (Raphael 1997).

> Yolande was 4 when her brother died from maltreatment by her parents. She had witnessed the chronic abuse of her sibling but had not been physically abused herself. She developed troubling nightmares in which a monster kept coming for her, and other symptoms of PTSD. She was not able to accept the reality of her brother's death until her PTSD symptoms had been successfully treated. She then started to grieve for her brother, and her mourning was aided by bereavement counselling, seeing the dead body and going to the funeral. Yolande had to adjust not only to her brother's death, but to the loss of her parents who were found guilty of manslaughter and given custodial sentences. She has been successfully adopted and is doing well, although at 13 she still has to negotiate adolescence.

Family survivors of homicide are among the most likely to develop dysfunctional symptoms. One large survey found that over 25% developed PTSD at some stage following the homicide (Amick-McMullan et al. 1991), and the pain, rage, guilt and revenge fantasies are likely to persist far longer than in other bereavements, both for children and adults (Masters et al. 1988).

Clinical assessment of bereaved children

Children and adolescents may reach the clinician as a result of referral from health practitioners because of psychiatric symptoms, but they may also be referred for consideration for preventive intervention and therapy, or for advice to schools, social services or the courts from sources such as social workers, teachers, lawyers, voluntary organizations working with victims of crime and the bereaved, and self-referrals. The usual clinical examination may be aided by some recently developed reliable and valid questionnaires for use in assessing PTSD: Children's PTSD Inventory (Saigh et al. 2000); Child Post-Traumatic Stress Reaction Index (Pynoos et al. 1987b; Pynoos et al. 1993), Revised Child Impact of Events Scale (Joseph et al. 1993); and Psychosocial Assessment of Childhood Experiences (PACE) (Sandberg et al. 1993). These may be particularly useful as screening instruments when there is a mass disaster and individual assessment interviews cannot be conducted with every individual (Nader 1997). Questionnaires to aid in the assessment of depression, anxiety and other symptoms are also available and the clinician may wish to develop a package of relevant and useful aids to his or her clinical examination.

Assessing children who have been bereaved, especially by a traumatic bereavement, must involve not only evaluation for the presence of psychiatric disorders, but also their attachment needs, where they should live, if it is not possible or desirable to live with the parent(s), and what contact they should have with a perpetrator parent. The children's parents and/or caregivers must be part of the assessment, which has to include an evaluation of the effect of the bereavement on their parenting functions.

While it may be helpful to spend some time with the family together, it is essential to interview each child (and adult) individually. This is of particular importance when the experience of a child may be idiosyncratic and horrific so that secondary traumatization of other children in the family is avoided where possible. Children often strive to protect their surviving carer when they have been bereft of one, and will not easily describe or play out distressing events in their presence for fear of upsetting the adult.

With young children, exploration of their understanding of the components of the concept of death, particularly concepts of permanence and irreversibility, the degree of responsibility they have assumed for the death, and their perception of changes in a surviving parent or caregiver, will aid in devising appropriate interventions. The specific assessment of post-traumatic reactions is necessary in traumatic bereavements and should probably be a feature of the assessment of all bereaved children. When there has been loss of a parent(s), assessment for attachment disorders is indicated. Feelings of responsibility for the death, guilt for sins of omission or commission, fears that others in the family might die, rage at others (including the dead parent or sibling) and fantasies of revenge should be specifically enquired for in both child and adult.

When exploring the impact of a death on a child's functioning, taking note of possible anniversary reactions in child or parent may help to answer the question, 'Why are they presenting now?' Exploring previous losses both for the child and the family, and any other vulnerabilities (traumatic separations, familial mental illness, loss of home or country, etc.) will enable the clinician to evaluate the meaning for the child and family of this loss. For example, a child reacting to the neonatal death of a sibling he or she barely knew, is probably responding to the parents' grief and his or her relative neglect by them. Support for the parent in their grieving may be more appropriate than therapy for the child in such a case (Hindmarch 1995).

If the family come from a different ethnic or religious background from the prevailing one, exploration of the way that culture views and deals with death is an essential preliminary to intervention (Parkes *et al.* 1997).

After the sudden death from heart failure of their lone parent, the three daughters, aged 6, 8 and 11 years, were cared for by a fellow member of the Jehovah's Witness church. She brought them to a family counselling service because of their profound grief at their mother's death. The carer had little time for this grief. She told them that their mother might be resurrected at any time and therefore they should be full of joy, not sorrow.

Intervention and treatment

The majority of children who are bereaved will not require psychiatric treatment, although most will benefit from contact with a concerned adult outside the family who will provide a listening ear and an opportunity to understand and come to terms with their loss. This may be provided by a school counsellor, a health visitor or counsellor attached to a GP's surgery, or volunteer bereavement counselling services. Child and adolescent mental health services can provide useful support, training and consultation to such services. Bereavement counselling is one of the few preventive interventions where sound evidence exists for it having a significant effect on community mental health (Parkes 1980; Kreitman 1989). However, this evidence is based on adult studies and the evidence of the benefits of bereavement counselling for children is nowhere near so clear-cut.

Who are the high risk groups where resources should be concentrated in an effort to prevent morbidity? Assessment of the following groups as a routine is recommended.
- Children under 10 years.
- Those with learning difficulties.
- Those who have suffered previous losses.
- Where there is a family or personal history of psychiatric disorder.
- Where the death is sudden or otherwise traumatic.

- Children caught up in witnessing violent deaths of those known to them (homicide, accident, suicide).
- Where there is a perceived threat to their own life.
- Those where there are multiple adversities.
- Those where the surviving parent(s) are failing in their care of the child.

Good quality controlled trials of interventions for bereaved children are few. Black & Urbanowicz (1985) randomly allocated unselected recently bereaved children into a family intervention group who were offered six family therapy sessions and a group who had no intervention. Follow-up at 1 year of both groups (45 families, 83 children) showed that the post-bereavement morbidity had been reduced from 40 to 20% in the intervention group. The sessions concentrated on helping the surviving parent to help the children to understand what had happened to their dead parent, supporting the parent and sharing mourning. By the second year follow-up there were no statistical differences between the groups, possibly because of the loss to follow-up of the most disturbed families (Black & Urbanowicz 1987). This study did not interview the children directly at follow-up but had almost no attrition in the intervention group.

The Family Bereavement Program of Sandler *et al.* (1992) in Arizona is a well-researched intervention programme, designed to improve the variables in the family environment which have been found to affect child mental health. The evaluation used a random assignment of families to either an intervention or control group ($N = 46$); there was a manual for the intervention and the outcome was measured with several instruments and self-evaluation. They found that use of the programme increased parental perceptions of the warmth of their relationship with their children; increased satisfaction with social support; and reduced parental reports of depression and conduct disorders in their older children. There were fewer positive reports from the children and younger children did not seem to benefit significantly.

Preventive intervention groups for bereaved children have been described (Fleming & Balmer 1991; Lohnes & Kalter 1994; Morrison Tonkins & Lambert 1996) but few have been adequately evaluated. Most did not have control groups, had small selected numbers, and relied on adult reports of the children's progress. Stokes *et al.* (1997), who run a bereavement service for children which includes children's camps, have pointed out the difficulties of providing control groups, but are attempting to develop measures to evaluate outcome.

Individual psychodynamically orientated therapy is well described by Furman (1974) but there has not been specific evaluation of such work in relation to bereavement. Various techniques are described for working with bereaved children but there are no controlled trials described (Smith & Pennells 1995).

When specific pathology has set in, treatment must be that of the condition diagnosed. There are specific issues in relation to children who have developed a psychiatric disorder resulting from bereavement which need to be addressed. Clinicians can help the carers to promote mental health by being truthful about what has happened to the parent or sibling, by involving the children in community rituals (funeral, cremation, memorial services; Weller *et al.* 1988), visiting the grave and by monitoring explanations given to the children to ensure that they do not violate the child's logic. If the child is told that 'Mummy is in heaven', he will expect her to return, as she did when she went to visit grandma in Brighton the other week. Parents may need help in distinguishing for the child what it is that went to heaven — was it the body of mother, or only the spirit? Building an inner representation of the dead parent appears to aid coping in bereaved children and can be a focus for therapeutic work (Nickman *et al.* 1998).

With traumatic bereavements, the attention must be to treating the effects of the trauma, before turning to grief work. There were hopes that PTSD might be prevented by 'de-briefing' techniques of crisis intervention. Recent evidence has not supported this hope. A follow-up of the children where one parent killed the other showed that brief intervention was not sufficient to protect the children from developing psychiatric problems (Harris-Hendriks *et al.*, 2nd edn. 2000). A controlled trial in children and adolescents of cognitive behavioural therapy for PTSD showed that in a population sample with a single traumatic incident it was effective (March *et al.* 1998). A meta-analysis of treatments for PTSD looked at 61 outcome trials and found that behaviour therapy and eye movement desensitization and reprocessing (EMDR) were the most effective (Van Etten & Taylor 1998).

Brom *et al.* (1989) conducted a controlled trial of psychodynamic psychotherapy with traumatized adults, comparing it with systematic desensitization and hypnotherapy with waiting list controls. All treatment groups had better symptoms than the controls, with psychotherapy having more effect on avoidance symptoms, while the other two achieved grater reduction in intrusive symptoms. As yet there has been no controlled comparison of treatments in children.

Children who are traumatically bereaved by the homicide of a parent or sibling require many interventions. Those responsible for their care (relatives, social services, the courts) may seek advice in regard to placement, contact with a perpetrator parent, as well as therapeutic needs. The clinician may find it helpful to see the perpetrator parent him- or herself and perhaps to conduct an initial therapeutic session with him or her and the child/children if appropriate, before making recommendations (Harris Hendriks *et al.* 1993; Black 1995).

Conclusions

Although over the last decade there has been considerable increase in interest in bereaved children, we still lack definitive large-scale studies of the effect of the death of a parent or sibling on children, both immediately and in the longer term. Common sense as well as clinical experience leads one to the conclusion that children, even more than adults, are likely to be profoundly affected by such deaths, although longitudinal studies indicate

that divorce and separation of parents pose greater risks for the mental health of children than death of a parent. Such intervention and treatment studies as we have point to a modest but significant decrease in morbidity with many modes of treatment, and much client satisfaction. In the area of traumatic bereavement we are on firmer ground and some well-conducted studies have shown us the extent of suffering endured by even very young children and given us the means to mitigate it. In our present state of knowledge and given finite resources, psychiatric resources should be restricted to treating high-risk children, such as those experiencing traumatic bereavements, and those with defined psychiatric disorders or dysfunctional symptoms, and supporting other counselling services for bereaved children by offering consultation, training and encouragement.

References

Amick-McMullan, A., Kilpatrick, D.G. & Resnick, H.S. (1991) Homicide as a risk factor for PTSD among surviving family members. *Behaviour Modification*, 15, 545–559.

Applebaum, D.R. & Burns, G.L. (1991) Unexpected childhood death: post-traumatic stress disorder in surviving siblings and parents. *Journal of Clinical Child Psychology*, 20, 114–120.

Berlinsky, E.B. & Biller, H.B. (1982) *Parental Death and Psychological Development.* Lexington Books, Lexington.

Birtchnell, J. (1970) Early parent death and mental illness. *British Journal of Psychiatry*, 116, 281–288.

Birtchnell, J. (1971) Early parent death in relation to size and constitution of sibship. *Acta Psychiatrica Scandinavica*, 47, 250–270.

Black, D. (1978) Annotation: the bereaved child. *Journal of Child Psychology and Psychiatry*, 19, 287–292.

Black, D. (1995) Parents who have killed their partner. In: *Assessment of Parenting* (eds P. Reder & C. Lucey), pp. 219–234. Routledge, London.

Black, D. & Urbanowicz, M.A. (1985) Bereaved children-family intervention. In: *Recent Research in Developmental Psychopathology* (ed. J.E. Stevenson), pp. 179–187. Pergamon, Oxford.

Black, D. & Urbanowicz, M.A. (1987) Family intervention with bereaved children. *Journal of Child Psychology and Psychiatry*, 28, 467–476.

Bonell-Pascual, E., Huline-Dickens, S., Hollins, S. *et al.* (1999) Bereavement and grief in adults with learning disabilites. *British Journal of Psychiatry*, 175, 348–350.

Bowlby, J. (1969) *Attachment and Loss*, Vol. 1, *Attachment.* Basic Books, New York.

Bowlby, J. (1972) *Attachment and Loss*, Vol. 2. Hogarth, London.

Bowlby, J. (1980) *Attachment and Loss*, Vol. 3. Hogarth, London.

Bowlby, J. & Parkes, C.M. (1970) Separation and loss within the family. In: *The Child in His Family* (eds C.J. Anthoney & C. Koupernik), pp. 180–198. J.Wiley, New York.

Brent, D.A., Perper, J.A., Goldstein, C.E. *et al.* (1988) Risk factors for adolescent suicide: a comparison of adolescent suicide victims with suicidal inpatients. *Archives of General Psychiatry*, 45, 581–588.

Brent, D.A., Perper, J.A., Moritz, G. *et al.* (1993) Psychiatric impact of the loss of an adolescent sibling to suicide. *Journal of Affective Disorders*, 28, 249–256.

Brent, D.A., Perper, J.A., Moritz, G., Liotus, L., Schweers, J. & Canobbio, R. (1994) Major depression or uncomplicated bereavement: a follow-up of youth exposed to suicide. *Journal of the American Academy of Child and Adolescent Psychiatry*, **33**, 231–239.

Brent, D.A., Moritz, G., Bridge, J. & Perper, J. (1997) The impact of adolescent suicide on siblings and parents: a longitudinal follow-up. *Suicide and Life-Threatening Behaviour*, **26**, 253–259.

Brom, D., Kleber, R.J. & Defares, P.B. (1989) Brief psychotherapy for post-traumatic stress disorders. *Journal of Consulting and Clinical Psychology*, **57**, 607–612.

Brown, G.W. & Harris, T.O. (1978) *Social Origins of Depression: a Study of Psychiatric Disorder in Women*. Unwin Hyman, London.

Cathcart, F. (1988) Seeing the body after death [Editorial]. *British Medical Journal*, **297**, 997–998.

Cathcart, F. (1995) Death and people with learning disabilities: interventions to support clients and carers. *British Journal of Clinical Psychology*, **34**, 165–175.

Cuddy-Casey, M. & Orvaschel, H. (1997) Children's understanding of death in relation to child suicidality and homicidality. *Clinical Psychology Review*, **17**, 33–45.

Dijkstra, I.C. & Stroebe, M.S. (1998) The impact of a child's death on parents: a myth (not yet) disproved? *Journal of Family Studies*, **4**, 185.

Elizur, E. & Kaffman, M. (1983) Factors influencing the severity of childhood bereavement reactions. *American Journal of Orthopsychiatry*, **53**, 668–676.

Fergusson, D.M. & Lynskey, M.T. (1996) Adolescent resiliency to family adversity. *Journal of Child Psychology and Psychiatry*, **37**, 281–292.

Fleming, S. & Balmer, L. (1991) Group intervention with bereaved children. In: *Children and Death* (eds D. Papadatou & C. Papadatos), pp. 105–124. Hemisphere, Washington.

Freeman, N.L., Perry, A. & Factor, D.C. (1991) Child behaviours as stressors: replicating and extending the use of the Cars as a measure of stress–a research note. *Journal of Child Psychology and Psychiatry*, **32**, 1025–1030.

Freud, S. (1917) *Mourning and Melancholia*. Hogarth Press, London.

Fristad, M.A., Jedel, R., Weller, R.A. & Weller, E.B. (1993) Psychological functioning in children after the death of a parent. *American Journal of Psychiatry*, **150**, 511–513.

Furman, E. (1974) *A Child's Parent Dies*. Yale University Press, New Haven.

Goodall, J. (1996) *In the Shadow of Man*. Phoenix, London.

Goodyer, I.M. (1990a) Annotation: recent life-events and psychiatric disorder in school age children. *Journal of Child Psychology and Psychiatry*, **31**, 839–848.

Goodyer, I.M. (1990b) *Life Experiences, Development and Childhood Psychopathology*. Wiley, Chichester.

Goodyer, E.M. & Altham, P.M.E. (1991) Lifetime exit events and recent social and family adversities in anxious and depressed school-age children and adolescents. I. *Journal of Affective Disorders*, **21**, 219–228.

Harrington, R. & Harrison, L. (1999) Unproven assumptions about the impact of bereavement on children. *Journal of the Royal Society of Medicine*, **92**, 230–233.

Harris Hendriks, J., Black, D. & Kaplan, T. (1993) (2nd edn, 2000) *When Father Kills Mother: Guiding Children Through Trauma and Grief*. Routledge, London.

Harris, T., Brown, G.W. & Bifulco, A. (1986) Loss of parent in childhood and adult psychiatric disorder: the role of lack of adequate parental care. *Psychological Medicine*, **16**, 641–659.

Haskey, J. (1993) Trends in the numbers of one-parent families in Great Britain. *Population Trends*, **71**, 26–33.

Haskey, J. (1998) One-parent families and their dependent children in Great Britain. *Population Trends*, **91**, 5–14.

Hinde, R.A. & McGinnis, L. (1977) Some factors influencing the effect of temporary mother–infant separation: some experiments with rhesus monkeys. *Psychological Medicine*, **7**, 192–212.

Hindmarch, C. (1995) Secondary losses for siblings. *Child Care, Health and Development*, **21**, 425–431.

Hofer, M.A. (1996) On the nature and consequences of loss. *Psychosomatic Medicine*, **58**, 570–581.

Hollins, S. & Esterhuyzen, A. (1997) Bereavement and grief in adults with learning disabilites. *British Journal of Psychiatry*, **170**, 497–501.

Johnson, M.K. & Foley, M.A. (1984) Differentiating fact from fantasy: the reliability of children's memory. *Journal of Social Issues*, **40**, 33–50.

Joseph, S., Yule, W., Williams, R. & Hodgkinson, P. (1993) The Herald of Free Enterprise disaster: measuring post-traumatic symptoms 30 months on. *British Journal of Clinical Psychology*, **32**, 327–331.

Kane, B. (1979) Children's concepts of death. *Journal of Genetic Psychology*, **134**, 141–153.

Kranzler, E.M., Shaffer, D., Wasserman, G. & Davies, M. (1990) Early childhood bereavement. *Journal of the American Academy of Child and Adolescent Psychiatry*, **29**, 513–520.

Kreitman, N. (1989) Mental health for all. *British Medical Journal*, **299**, 1292–1293.

Kuterovac, G., Dyregrov, A. & Stuvland, R. (1994) Children in war: a silent majority under stress. *British Journal of Medical Psychology*, **67**, 363–375.

Lansdown, R. & Benjamin, G. (1985) The development of the concept of death in children aged 5–9 years. *Child: Care, Health and Development*, **11**, 13–20.

Lohnes, K.L. & Kalter, N. (1994) Preventive intervention groups for parentally bereaved children. *American Journal of Orthopsychiatry*, **64**, 594–603.

March, J.S., Amaya-Jackson, L., Murray, M.C. & Schulte, A. (1998) Cognitive-behavioural psychotherapy for children and adolescents with posttraumatic stress disorder after a single-incident stressor. *Journal of the American Academy of Child and Adolescent Psychiatry*, **37**, 585–593.

Masters, R., Friedman, L.N. & Getzel, G. (1988) Helping families of homicide victims: a multidimensional approach. *Journal of Traumatic Stress*, **1**, 109–125.

Morrison Tonkins, S.A. & Lambert, M.J. (1996) A treatment outcome study of bereavement groups for children. *Child and Adolescent Social Work Journal*, **13**, 3–21.

Nader, K.O. (1997) Assessing traumatic experiences in children. In: *Assessing Psychological Trauma and PTSD* (eds J.P. Wilson & T.M. Keane), pp. 291–348. Guilford Press, London.

Newman, M., Black, D. & Harris-Hendriks, J. (1997) Victims of disaster, war, violence or homicide: psychological effects on siblings. *Child Psychology and Psychiatry Review*, **2**, 140–149.

Nickman, S.L., Silverman, P.R. & Normand, C. (1998) Children's construction of a deceased parent: the surviving parent's contribution. *American Journal of Orthopsychiatry*, **68**, 126–134.

Osofsky, J.D. (1997) *Children in a Violent Society*. Guilford Press, New York.

Parkes, C.M. (1972) *Bereavement: Studies of Grief in Adult Life*. Tavistock, London.

Parkes, C.M. (1980) Bereavement counselling: does it work? *British Medical Journal*, **281**, 3–6.

Parkes, C.M. (1996) *Bereavement: Studies of Grief in Adult Life*, 3rd edn. Routledge, London.

Parkes, C.M., Laungani, P. & Young, B., eds (1997) *Death and Bereavement Across Cultures*. Routledge, London.

Paykel, E.S. & Dowlatshahi, D. (1988) Life events and mental disorder.

In: *Handbook of Life Stress, Cognition and Health* (eds S. Fisher & J. Reason), pp. 241–263. John Wiley, Chichester.

Paykel, E.S., Myers, J., Dienelt, M., Klerman, G., Lindethal, J. & Pepper, P. (1969) Life events and depression. *Archives of General Psychiatry*, 5, 340–347.

Perry, B.D., Pollard, R.A., Blakley, T.L., Baker, W.L. & Vigilante, D. (1995) Childhood trauma, the neurobiology of adaptation and 'use-dependent' development of the brain: how 'states' become 'traits'. *Infant Mental Health Journal*, 16, 271–291.

Pettle Michael, S.A. & Lansdown, R.G. (1986) Adjustment to the death of a sibling. *Archives of Disease in Childhood*, 61, 278–283.

Ponzetti, J.J. & Johnson, M.A. (1991) The forgotten grievers: grandparents' reactions to the death of grandchildren. *Death Studies*, 15, 157–167.

Prosser, J. & McArdle, P. (1996) The changing mental health of children and adolescents. *Psychological Medicine*, 26, 715–725.

Pynoos, R.S., Frederick, C., Nader, K. *et al.* (1987a) Life threat and post-traumatic stress in school-age children. *Archives of General Psychiatry*, 44, 1057–1063.

Pynoos, R.S., Nader, K., Frederick, C. *et al.* (1987b) Grief reactions in school-age children following a sniper attack at school. Special issue: grief and bereavement. *Israel Journal of Psychiatry and Related Sciences*, 24, 53–63.

Pynoos, R.S., Goenjian, A., Tashjian, M. *et al.* (1993) Post-traumatic stress reactions in children after the 1988 Armenian earthquake. *British Journal of Psychiatry*, 163, 239–247.

Raphael, B. (1982) The young child and the death of a parent. In: *The Place of Attachment in Human Behaviour* (eds C.M. Parkes & J. Stevenson-Hinde), pp. 131–150. Tavistock, London.

Raphael, B. (1997) The interaction of trauma and grief. In: *Psychological Trauma: a Developmental Approach* (eds D. Black, J. Harris Hendriks, M. Newman & G. Mezey), pp. 31–43. Gaskell, London.

Raphael, B., Field, J. & Kvelde, H. (1980) Childhood bereavement: a prospective study as a possible prelude to future preventive intervention. In: *The Child in his Family, Vol. 6. Preventive Psychiatry in an Age of Transition* (eds E.J. Anthony & C. Chiland), pp. 507–519. Wiley, New York.

Reilly, T.P., Hasazi, J.E. & Bond, L.A. (1983) Children's conceptions of death and personal mortality. *Journal of Pediatric Psychology*, 8, 21–31.

Richman, N. (1993) Children in situations of political violence. *Journal of Child Psychology and Psychiatry*, 34, 1286–1302.

Rosenheim, E. & Reicher, R. (1985) Informing children about a parent's terminal illness. *Journal of Child Psychology and Psychiatry*, 26, 995–998.

Rutter, M. (1966) *Children of Sick Parents*. Oxford University Press, Oxford.

Rutter, M. (1985) Resilience in the face of adversity: protective factors and resistance to psychiatric disorder. *British Journal of Psychiatry*, 147, 598–611.

Rutter, M. (1999) Resilience concepts and findings: implications for family therapy. *Journal of Family Therapy*, 21, 119–145.

Saigh, P.A., Fairbank, J.A. & Yasik, A.E. (1998) War-related post-traumatic stress disorder among children and adolescents. In: *Children of Trauma: Stressful Life Events and Their Effects on Children* (ed. T.W. Miller), pp. 119–140. International Universities Press, Madison, CT.

Saigh, P.A., Yasik, A.E., Oberfield, R.A. *et al.* (2000) The Children's PTSD Inventory: development and reliability. *Journal of Traumatic Stress*, 13, 369–380.

Saldinger, A., Cain, A., Kalter, N. & Lohnes, K. (1999) Anticipating parental death in families with young children. *American Journal of Orthopsychiatry*, 69, 39–48.

Sandberg, S., Rutter, M., Giles, S. *et al.* (1993) Assessment of psychosocial experiences in childhood: methodological issues and some illustrative findings. *Journal of Child Psychology and Psychiatry*, 34, 879–898.

Sandler, I.N., West, S.G., Baca, L. *et al.* (1992) Linking empirically based theory and evaluation: the family bereavement program. *American Journal of Community Psychology*, 20, 491–521.

Schleifer, S.J., Keller, S.E., Camerino, M., Thornton, J.C. & Stein, M. (1983) Suppression of lymphocyte stimulation following bereavement. *Journal of the American Medical Association*, 250, 374–377.

Schore, A.N. (1994) *Affect Regulation and the Origin of the Self*. Lawrence Erlbaum Associates, Hove.

Seay, B.M. & Harlow, H.F. (1965) Maternal separation in the rhesus monkey. *Journal of Nervous and Mental Disorders*, 140, 434–441.

Siegel, K., Karus, D. & Raveis, V.H. (1997) Adjustment of children facing the death of a parent due to cancer. *Journal of the American Academy of Child and Adolescent Psychiatry*, 35, 442–450.

Silverman, P.R. & Worden, J.W. (1992) Children's reactions in the early months after the death of a parent. *American Journal of Orthopsychiatry*, 62, 104.

Silverman, P. & Worden, J.W. (1993) Children's reaction to the death of a parent. In: *Handbook of Bereavement, Theory, Research and Intervention* (eds M. Stroebe, W. Stroebe & R. Hansson), pp. 300–316. Cambridge University Press, New York.

Smith, S.C. & Pennells, M. (1995) *Interventions with Bereaved Children*. Jessica Kingsley, London.

Stokes, J., Wyer, S. & Crossley, D. (1997) The challenge of evaluating a child bereavement programme. *Palliative Medicine*, 11, 179–190.

Suomi, S. (1983) Models of depression in primates. *Psychological Medicine*, 13, 465–468.

Terr, L. (1991) Childhood traumas: an outline and overview. *American Journal of Psychiatry*, 148, 10–20.

Thompson, M.P., Kaslow, N.J., Kingree, J.B., King, M., Bryant, L. Jr & Rey, M. (1998) Psychological symptomatology following parental death in a predominantly minority sample of children and adolescents. *Journal of Clinical Child Psychology*, 27, 434–441.

Van Eerdewegh, M.M., Bieri, M.D., Parrilla, R.H. & Clayton, P.J. (1982) The bereaved child. *British Journal of Psychiatry*, 140, 23–29.

Van Eerdewegh, M.M., Clayton, P.J. & Van Eerdewegh, P. (1985) The bereaved child: variables influencing early psychopathology. *British Journal of Psychiatry*, 147, 188–194.

Van Etten, M.L. & Taylor, S. (1998) Comparative efficacy of treatments for PTSD: a meta-analysis. *Clinical Psychology and Psychotherapy*, 5, 126–144.

Vida, S. & Grizenko, N. (1989) DSM-III-R and the phenomenology of childhood bereavement: a review. *Canadian Journal of Psychiatry*, 34, 148–155.

Ward, B. (1993) *Good Grief 1*, 2nd edn. Jessica Kingsley, London.

Weller, E.B., Weller, R.A., Fristad, M.A., Cain, S.E. & Bowes, J.M. (1988) Should children attend their parent's funeral? *Journal of the American Academy of Child and Adolescent Psychiatry*, 27, 559–562.

Weller, R.A., Weller, E.B., Fristad, M.A. & Bowes, J.M. (1991) Depression in recently bereaved prepubertal children. *American Journal of Psychiatry*, 148, 1536–1540.

19 Development and Psychopathology
Michael Rutter

Introduction

One of the major changes that has taken place in psychiatry over recent decades has been the growing appreciation of the need to take into account developmental considerations. This has led to the concept of developmental psychopathology (Sroufe & Rutter 1984; Cicchetti 1989; Cicchetti & Toth 1995; Rutter 1996a; Cummings *et al.* 2000; Rutter *et al.* 2000). At one time, many people would have assumed that a developmental perspective meant a focus on the role of very early life experiences in creating a risk for later mental disorders. It is now appreciated that this constitutes much too narrow a view of development. It has to include the biology of brain development as well as the psychology of the development of the mind and the various ways in which developmental level influences people's response to their experiences. This chapter reviews some of the key findings on these three facets of development and considers the clinical implications that flow from them.

Biology of development

The biology of development is genetically programmed to follow a particular course. The genes that regulate development are non-segregating genes that have come to be present in all humans as a result of evolution (Bock *et al.* 2000). Genes determine the fact that everyone is born with a potential to develop communicative language, to walk in an upright position and to develop selective social attachments. These non-segregating genes, present in everyone, differ in their effects from the segregating genes considered in the chapters by McGuffin & Rutter (Chapter 12), Skuse & Kuntsi (Chapter 13) and Simonoff (Chapter 66). Of course, at a basic level, both sorts of genes are directly comparable, and there is no sharp demarcation between the two. Thus, for example, although there are non-segregating genes that determine the universal capacity for language, there are also segregating genes that underlie individual differences in people's language skills.

A key feature of the genetically programmed biology of development is that it is probabilistic in the way that it works (Finch & Kirkwood 2000); there are inbuilt self-correcting mechanisms to ensure that development proceeds appropriately. For example, in brain development there is an initial overproduction of neurones, accompanied by their migration from one part of the brain to another, followed by selective pruning

(Greenough *et al.* 1987; Greenough & Black 1992; Nelson & Bloom 1997; Bateson & Martin 1999; Bruer 1999; see also Goodman, Chapter 14). Genes determine that this always happens, but genes do not determine precisely what happens with each individual neurone. The process of neuronal migration and functional differentiation, as well as the selective pruning, is influenced by cell–cell interactions that are, in turn, influenced in part by experiential input. This has given rise to simplified aphorisms such as, 'Cells that fire together wire together' and 'Use it or lose it'. The general notion is that, just as brain structure influences brain function, so function shapes brain development.

This general style of development applies just as much to other parts of the body as it does to the brain. Parallel considerations apply to the development of the neuroendocrine system. The general plan and course of neuroendocrine development is the same in all humans but development is also shaped by experiences—as shown, for example, by the effects on structure and function of the neuroendocrine system of severe stressful experiences in early life (Hennessey & Levine 1979; Levine 1982). Segregating genes and experiences both influence the timing of puberty, as do exercise and body weight (Pickles *et al.* 1994; Graber *et al.* 1995).

There has been a tendency in the writings of some behaviour geneticists to assume that everything is determined by either genetic or environmental factors or some form of interplay between the two. There is a recognition that there is need to break down each into further components, such as the differentiation between additive genetic effects and epistatic or synergistic genetic effects and that between shared and non-shared environmental effects (see McGuffin & Rutter, Chapter 12). However, on its own, this view constitutes an oversimplification, for two rather different reasons. First, it ignores the need to consider the universals of biological development with respect to the interplay between genes and environment. Secondly, the partitioning of population variance into genetic and environmental effects ignores the fact that chance variation also plays a part (Goodman 1991; Jensen 1997; Finch & Kirkwood 2000). Thus, all females are born with two X chromosomes, and it is invariable that one of the X chromosomes is inactivated. On the other hand, it seems to be largely a chance matter which of the X chromosomes is inactivated.

Role of chance in determining individual differences

Molenaar *et al.* (1993) have written about chance as something that constitutes a 'third force' in the determination of individual differences. At first sight, that might seem nothing more than recourse to an unmeasurable variable to account for that which is currently beyond our understanding. However, it is rather more than that. For example, most people exhibit minor imperfections of physical development (Waldrop & Halverson 1971; Vogel & Motulsky 1997; Tarrant & Jones 2000). These may be evident in features such as an extra rudimentary nipple, extra teeth, missing muscles, and other oddities (the great majority of which are without serious functional significance). Often, people are unaware that they have these imperfections but they are readily detectable by systematic examination. It is known that such minor congenital anomalies tend to be more common in children born to older mothers, and they are also more common in monozygotic twins than dizygotic twins (monozygotic twinning itself being a variety of congenital anomaly). With respect to these general risk factors, it is clear that the occurrence of developmental anomalies is open to influences on groups of individuals that are potentially understandable and measurable, but the details of their presence in any one individual are essentially unpredictable. A higher than usual number of congenital anomalies have been found to be associated with an increased risk for various different forms of psychopathology, including autism, schizophrenia, and attention deficit hyperactivity disorder (ADHD; Marenco & Weinberger 2000). The mechanisms involved in these pleiotropic risk mechanisms are unknown. It is unlikely that the anomalies themselves mediate risk; it is more probable that they index some form of perturbation in the developmental process as it has occurred at an early intrauterine phase.

Apart from the presence of congenital anomalies, which could have arisen through a variety of mechanisms, there have been other attempts to assess whether or not individuals have been subjected to unusual developmental perturbation. Asymmetry in dermatoglyphic patterns has been one suggested way forward (Tarrant & Jones 2000). At the moment, there are few hard findings on the role of chance variation in developmental processes but the possibility of their importance needs to be taken seriously.

Developmental programming

The concept of developmental programming is that particular experiences influence the structural and functional development of the organism in a lasting way. In the context of brain development, the role of visual input shaping the structure and function of the visual cortex is much the best known and best demonstrated example. This was first demonstrated by the Nobel Prize winning research of Hubel, Wiesel and their colleagues (Hubel & Wiesel 1965) and has been amply confirmed since (Blakemore 1991). One practical consequence is that, if a child's strabismus is not corrected in the first few years of life, it is highly likely that binocular vision will not be possible later. There is a possible parallel in the field of language development. In the early months of life, all babies show roughly the same skills in phonological discrimination but, as they become more exposed to the language input, their phonological discriminations come to be adapted to the language to which they are exposed (Kuhl 1994; Kuhl *et al.* 1997). At a later age, individuals find very difficult phonological discriminations that are not part of the language with which they grew up. A somewhat similar pattern of development arises with grammatical constructions. Older second-language learners have no difficulty in acquiring the vocabulary of a second or third language, but both their phonology and their grammar tend to betray the origins of their first language. Functional imaging findings (Kim *et al.* 1997) also suggest that the neural basis of later second-language learning differs from that which underlies normal first-language learning. With respect to brain development, Greenough *et al.* (1987) conceptualized the process of experiential influences on brain growth in terms of experience-expectant development. In other words, biological development is programmed on the basis of an expectation that a particular range (albeit a very wide range) of expectable experiences occur.

What has proved much more controversial is the question as to how far this concept may be extrapolated to the effects on brain development of variations in experiential input within the normal range. Extrapolation has seemed to be encouraged by the findings from animal research that brain development differs between caged animals given extra experiences and ordinary laboratory caged animals. The implication has seemed to be that environmental enrichment has somatic effects that are both lasting and of functional importance. The research is of high quality but the problem is that it is doubtful whether the so-called enriched environment is in fact superior to the environment that the animals would have experienced in the wild. Rather, the researchers in this field have concluded that additional experiences have done something to counteract the severe deprivation that is ordinarily the state of affairs with caged laboratory animals. The evidence suggests that the biology of normal brain development requires experiential input but that the range of experiences providing it is very wide. Clearly, this makes evolutionary sense in that development needs to be able to occur in a wide variety of environmental conditions. Gross departures from the average expectable environment may be damaging in their developmental consequences, but the extent of environmental variation that is consistent with normal brain development is very wide. Accordingly, the notion that particularly high-quality experiences in early life will make for 'better' brain development does not have empirical support. It may well be advantageous for children to have particularly rich, varied and emotionally supportive experiences in early life but this does not mean that such experiences programme brain development. Of course, all learning has neural consequences (how else could learning occur?) but that is not quite the same thing as effects on the programming of the structure of brain development.

We may conclude that it is likely that rather extreme and extensive restriction of experiences are likely to be important for this type of developmental programming to occur. The one well-documented recent human experience that provides just such a restriction is that obtained in Romanian orphanages, prior to the fall of the Ceaușescu regime, of severe institutional privation (see O'Connor, Chapter 46). The findings are provocative with respect to developmental programming notions (Rutter, in press; Rutter, O'Connor & the English and Romanian Adoptees Research Team, submitted). The implication for developmental programming is that serious effects should persist despite radical changes of a beneficial kind in the environment. In so far as that suggests that recovery cannot take place if the change of environment does not occur until after the age of 2 or 3 years, the findings clearly contradict the expectation. To the contrary, dramatic developmental gains across all domains were apparent (Rutter *et al.* 1998c; O'Connor *et al.* 2000a). On the other hand, the findings were equally striking in showing a higher frequency of substantial deficits in the children whose depriving institutional care extended after the age of 2 years, as compared with those who left the institutions under the age of 6 months. The two groups differed with respect to their general cognitive index at age 6 years by 24 points — a very large difference indeed (O'Connor *et al.* 2000a). The findings with respect to sociobehavioural deficits were of the same magnitude (Rutter *et al.*, 2000a).

Several queries need to be raised before making assumptions of developmental programming. To begin with, the children were severely malnourished as well as psychologically deprived. However, the deficit findings according to age of leaving the institution were similarly apparent in the subgroup of children who did not show significant malnourishment (Rutter, O'Connor & the English and Romanian Adoptees Research Team, submitted). Accordingly, the persistence of effects cannot be wholly attributed to malnutrition, although the deficits were greater in those who were severely malnourished. Also, it was necessary to check that the findings were not a consequence of the duration of time in the adoptive home, rather than the period in the institution (the one ordinarily leading directly to the other). Longitudinal data showed that (after a period of some 2.5 years in the adoptive home) it was the length of time in the institution that was the decisive factor (Rutter *et al.* 2000b). The gains between age 4 and age 6 were quite minor, and neither the outcome at age 6 nor the gains between 4 and 6 were systematically related to variations in the qualities of the adoptive family, although these were generally of high quality and therefore exhibited a narrow range of variation. In short, evidence suggested that there were substantial cognitive and social sequelae that persisted for some years (findings from the currently ongoing follow-up at age 11 years will be needed to determine how long), despite a radical change of environment.

The question is what basic process mediates these persistent effects and whether that process can reasonably be conceptualized as some type of developmental programming. A further question is how far the findings on this very extremely deprived group have implications for more ordinary variations and circumstances in the industrialized world. Yet another question has to be posed about the nature of the experiential restriction that led to these effects. On the face of it, it would seem unlikely that the same type of restriction led to the cognitive impairment as that which led to the social deficits (e.g. quasi-autistic patterns, impaired selective social attachment, inattention/overactivity). There were modest intercorrelations between these different outcomes but the correlations were not high. Perhaps it was the general restriction of conversation and play that had the major role in the cognitive impairment (the children were generally confined to cribs without toys, without experiences outside the crib, and without much talk — most of the children being entirely without language at the time they left the institution). Conversely, perhaps the lack of interchanges with people, together with a lack of personalized caregiving, played a greater part with respect to the social sequelae. What is relevant is that studies of children reared in much better functioning institutions in the UK have shown somewhat comparable (albeit much milder) social sequelae that have occurred in the absence of cognitive impairment (Hodges & Tizard 1989a,b; Roy *et al.* 2000; Rutter *et al.*, in press).

The first concept of developmental programming is based on the need of the organism to have certain experiences (within a broad range) if somatic development is to proceed normally. A somewhat different programming concept has been put forward by Barker *et al.* (Barker 1991, 1997; O'Brien *et al.* 1999) to describe the ways in which early somatic development adapts to the prevailing environmental circumstances. One of the stimuli for this notion was the empirical association that was observed between low birth weight and an increased risk of cardiovascular disease. The finding was of developmental interest because, although undernutrition in early life is a risk factor for cardiovascular disease, it is overnutrition that is the risk factor later on. The hypothesis is that the organism is programmed to deal with subnutrition and that, as a consequence, this means that it is wrongly programmed to cope with overnutrition, if that is what happens in later life. This second concept is crucially different from the first in three crucial respects.

1 It is concerned with the effects of variations in experiences within (as well as outside) the normal range.

2 It is concerned with organismic *adaptation* to particular environmental circumstances (rather than normal growth that is dependent only on a type of environmental input that would be present in any ordinary circumstances).

3 The developmental effects of the early experiences do not concern either optimal functioning or even generally normal functioning. Rather, they prepare the organism to be in the best state to cope with *continuation* of the same environmental circumstances. If the environment changes, the consequence may be malfunction because the organism was adapted to be responsive to the needs provided by a different set of circumstances.

In the metabolic domain, the implication is the important, but counterintuitive, implication that compensatory feeding in middle childhood to make up for subnutrition in the womb or infancy may actually be damaging. In the psychological arena, there are possible parallels in the effects of institutional deprivation on the development of social relationships (O'Connor *et al.* 1999, 2000b; Rutter *et al.*, 2000a). Perhaps the brain becomes adapted to coping with an extremely barren environment that is largely lacking in interpersonal play or communication, and is thereby maladapted to dealing with a normal social post-adoption environment. The 'programming' notion is possibly relevant because it suggests that developmental effects become relatively fixed after a particular sensitive period of openness to environmental influences, and that the effects involve adaptation to a particular environment.

There may even be a third type of programming effects. Early experimental studies of stress on the development of the neuroendocrine system in rodents (Hennessey & Levine 1979) showed that the usual effect was enhancement of structure and function. In other words, the effects of early exposure to a noxious environment provided a degree of resistance later to similar noxious experiences—a so-called 'steeling' effect (Rutter 1981b). However, clinical experience suggests that the reverse may also occur—a 'sensitization' effect. Experimental studies are now beginning to confirm the reality of such effects in which early stresses *increase* vulnerability to later stresses (Heim *et al.* 2000; Ruda *et al.* 2000). What remains unclear is what determines which occurs (steeling or sensitization), and what biological processes mediate each type of effect.

Brain plasticity re-responses to physical injury

At one time, it used to be thought that the effects of early brain injury were much less than those of later brain injury (the so-called 'Kennard principle'). It is now known that that is a misleading oversimplification, although there are indeed major effects of age on responses to brain injury (Rutter 1993; Goodman 1994; see also Goodman, Chapter 14). The key finding is that unilateral brain lesions in infancy do not lead to either lasting language impairment or distinctive patterns of differences in verbal and visuospatial skills, regardless of which hemisphere is injured. On the other hand, early injuries do lead to general cognitive impairment. It is also striking that the degree of cognitive impairment seems to be influenced at least as much by active epileptic activity, suggesting that the impairments come from abnormal brain discharges as much as from lack of brain function (Vargha-Khadem *et al.* 1992). The implication is that, in early life, the brain has the plasticity required for either hemisphere to take up responsibility for specialized functions, such as language. The precise neural processes that provide this plasticity are as yet not well understood but their importance is clear.

It is important not to overgeneralize these findings on interhemispheric plasticity because it is quite clear that early brain impairments can lead to severe lasting deficits in specialized skills. The findings with respect to both developmental language

disorders (see Bishop, Chapter 39) and autism (see Lord & Bailey, Chapter 38) clearly make that point. The implication, however, is that such specialized deficits are likely to stem from systems failures or bilateral lesions, rather than from any focal lesion, however severe, on just one side of the brain.

Implications of cognitive processing and memory

It has long been known that there are major developmental changes in the ways in which children process their experiences. Even very young babies think about what happens to them and, moreover, they conceptualize and draw conclusions about their experiences. This is evident, for example, in the ways in which young children understand and respond to what is said to them, conceptualizing the meaning of what they have heard and so initially both undergeneralizing and overgeneralizing as they 'play with' the language concepts and their meaning (Rutter 1987). It is evident too, in the ways in which babies' initial somewhat indiscriminate response to other people's social overtures changes in the middle of the first year of life to a high degree of specificity (see O'Connor, Chapter 46; Rutter 1981a). It has also been found that it is only towards the end of the second year of life that toddlers develop a well-articulated set of standards that they apply both to themselves and to the world around them (Kagan 1982).

The concept of so-called 'infantile amnesia' is also well-established (Rutter *et al.* 1998a). It is not that children forget all that they have learned during the first two years of life or that their experiences during that age period do not register; it is obvious that language learning in those early years persists into adult life, as does all sorts of other learning. The key distinction is between implicit and explicit memories (Tulving 1983; Baddeley 1990). Children maintain the skills and knowledge that they have learned in early life but what is largely lost is recall of particular events and experiences during that early period. Few people have much in the way of memories of discrete happenings during their first 2 or 3 years. Although the precise reasons for this amnesia are not well understood, it does seem related to the process of recall rather than registration of the original learning. Perhaps this is a consequence of the fact that the concepts and ways of thinking, at the time of attempted recall in later life, are so different from those operating in the infancy period. The implication is that, although early experiences may well have enduring effects, they are unlikely to operate through the triggering of particular discrete memories of events or happenings.

Once more, questions have to be asked about the neural substrate for these different forms of learning, memory and recall. The Zero to Three movement has sought to extrapolate from neuroscientific findings, to argue that major experiences have to operate in the first three years if they are to have enduring effects. That is a misleading assumption, for at least three rather different reasons. First, as already noted, explicit memories of an enduring kind are not usually present until after the age of 2 or 3 years. Children's ability to conceptualize about their experiences also increases greatly with age. It was on these grounds that Kagan (1980) argued that, completely contrary to the views of the Zero to Three group, it is only *after* infancy that experiences are likely to have enduring effects. That is because it is only after the infancy years that children develop more complex conceptualizations of what has happened to them.

The second reason that the extrapolation is unwarranted is that neuroscientific findings have shown that brain development is far from complete by the end of the second or third year. Many important developments take place during childhood and adolescence, even extending into adult life (Krasnegor *et al.* 1997). It is true that brain growth is at its most rapid and extensive during early life but it goes on much longer. Furthermore, although the new growth of neurones is predominantly a feature of early brain development, recent research has shown that, at least in some parts of the brain and in some circumstances, there can be neuronal proliferation even in adult life (Eriksson *et al.* 1998; Gould *et al.* 1999; Scharff *et al.* 2000).

Thirdly, although it may be that new learning is supported by the acquisition of new synapses (Greenough & Black 1992), the initial proliferation of synapses does not seem to be environmentally driven. Learning probably results in a loss of some connections and a strengthening of others as a result of competitive interactions among populations of neurones (Goldman-Rakic *et al.* 1997). In so far as that is the case, that suggests that brain plasticity is likely to extend through the period of synaptic loss extending into early adult life (Huttenlocher 1979, 1994).

Much remains to be learned about the interconnections between brain functioning and the workings of the mind, and between both of these and the input of experiences. Tentatively, it may be concluded that, although developmental programming effects (by which brain growth is sculpted by experiences) are most evident in the first few years of life, even then the effects are not necessarily permanent and irreversible. Also, the sculpting effects of experiences on brain development probably mainly applies to rather gross variations in pervasive experiences, rather than to variations in experiences within the normal range. However, later experiences may also have effects on brain structure. Because cognitive and affective processing is so important in response to experiences, it is also the case that in some ways later experiences may make more of an impact. They, too, will bring about changes in the neural structure, albeit ones that differ from developmental programming effects.

It should be added that it is highly unlikely that the concept of developmental programming reflects a single process. The notion of brain sculpting as a result of universally expectable experiences suggests that variations within the normal range of experiences will not have structural effects. By contrast, the rather different programming concept as applied to the effects of nutrition on metabolic functioning or of infections on immunity is thought to apply to experiences within the normal range. It is not known whether, or how, that concept might operate in relation to brain development.

'Switching on' of genes

Although all genes are present at birth, they may not exert their effects until much later in life. Most obviously, that is the case with genetic influences on the timing of the menarche or menopause. It is also apparent in the case of Mendelian disorders of late onset, such as Huntington disease. It is necessary to consider whether similar 'switching on' effects apply with respect to genetically influenced psychiatric disorders that do not usually begin until late adolescence or early adult life — such as schizophrenia or bipolar affective disorder. The processes may well differ among these various later onset disorders. For example, although the psychotic features of schizophrenia are not usually present until the late teens, non-psychotic cognitive, social and behavioural abnormalities are frequently present from the early childhood years onwards (Weinberger 1987; McGrath & Murray 1995; Marenco & Weinberger 2000; McDonald *et al.* 2000; see also Hollis, Chapter 37). In other words, it has become increasingly apparent that it is necessary to conceptualize many cases of schizophrenia as neurodevelopmental in origin, rather than as adult-onset psychoses. That leaves open the question as to what are the factors that underlie the transition from the behavioural precursors of childhood to the overt psychotic features of adult life. Do they rely, for example, on the changes in brain development that take place in the adolescent period? To what extent does the schizophrenia that involves childhood precursors differ from schizophrenia where these are apparently absent? It has become very apparent that a more developmental approach to the understanding of schizophrenia is going to be required.

The situation with respect to bipolar affective disorder may not be quite the same (see Harrington, Chapter 29). Although there is some association between early neurodevelopmental delays and bipolar disorder, the effects are very much weaker than they are with schizophrenia (McDonald *et al.* 2000). Although Biederman *et al.* (Biederman *et al.* 1996; Faraone *et al.* 1997) have argued that it is relatively common for ADHD to lead on to mania in adult life, this has not been evident in other follow-up studies of children with ADHD (see Schachar & Tannock, Chapter 25). It seems more likely that the apparent connection derives from a surface similarity between particular behaviours, rather than progression from one form of psychopathology to another. Large-scale systematic follow-up studies of children and adolescents with major depressive disorders (Weissman *et al.* 1999a,b; Fombonne *et al.*, 2001a,b) have also shown the infrequency with which early depressive conditions develop into bipolar disorders in early adult life. Although bipolar disorders can, and sometimes do, begin in childhood, it is much more frequent for them to begin in later adolescence or early adult life. It is possible, although not as yet demonstrated, that this is a function of genes whose effects usually 'switch on' during this age period.

The situation with respect to unipolar depression may be different again. To begin with, it is striking that the sex ratio changes during adolescence (Rutter *et al.* 1986; Weissman *et al.*

1999a,b; Fombonne *et al.*, 2001a,b). In childhood, depression is more common in boys whereas, from adolescence onwards, it is substantially more common in girls. Genetic liability for depression increases substantially from childhood to adolescence/adult life but this increase is mainly evident in the case of females (Thapar & McGuffin 1994; Silberg *et al.* 1999). This rise in genetic effect is accompanied by substantial gene–environment correlations and, also, interactions (Silberg *et al.*, in press); and it is possible that, to an important extent, the genetic effect is operating as a result of its influence on the interplay with the environment. It is not clear at the moment why that should mainly apply to females rather than males.

Age-related variations in responses to psychosocial experiences

To an important extent, people's responses to psychosocial experiences vary according to their age at the time. However, it is necessary to exercise caution in drawing conclusions about the reasons for these age-related variations. That is because, in a real sense, age is an ambiguous variable because it indexes biological maturity, because different elements of biological maturation do not proceed together; and because age also reflects past experiences and current social situations (Rutter 1989a). Before drawing conclusions about the underlying causal mechanisms, it is important to determine which of these various aspects of age are responsible for the association.

Hospital admission, and other forms of stressful separation, may be taken as an example (Rutter 1979). The evidence suggests that adverse psychological effects are infrequent in the case of separations during the early infancy period; are maximal during the toddler period; and less evident, again, in the case of separations during the school-age years. It is probable that these changes reflect the role of selective social attachments. The effects are less likely in infancy because infants have yet to develop such attachments and therefore do not have well-developed selective relationships that can be disrupted by separation. Conversely, older children have developed such relationships but, with increasing cognitive capacity, have learned that it is possible to maintain relationships during the course of a separation. Accordingly, although they may be upset at the time, the sequelae are less marked and less prolonged. In short, in this case the age-related effects seem to be a function of both what is taking place developmentally in relation to the establishment of selective social relationships and also what is occurring in the parallel development of cognitive understanding.

Somewhat similarly, it seems that the relative failure to develop intense selective social relationships, the so-called disinhibited attachment disorder, is a consequence of institutional rearing in the first few years of life; whereas (although not well documented) apparently it is not found with respect to the occurrence of institutional care in older children (see O'Connor, Chapter 46). The effects on a function that has still to develop and on one that is already well established are likely to be different.

A possibly rather different age trend is apparent in the case of marked grief reactions (Dowdney 2000; see also Black, Chapter 18). Although young children may well be greatly distressed by a bereavement, they are less likely to exhibit the severe grief reaction at the time that is characteristic in adults. This may be because they think about the loss in ways that involve less preoccupation with its meaning and less projections forwards and backwards in time. Of course, that does not mean that the effect of early loss are less than those of later loss. Indeed, the converse may be the case, because, although the loss itself may not have direct long-lasting stress effects, if it leads to impaired patterns of parental care (as is sometimes the case), that will carry with it important vulnerabilities (Harris *et al.* 1986). Poor parental care in the absence of parental loss is a major risk factor for psychopathology, whereas loss that is accompanied by good parenting is not. As is the case with brain injury, the issue is not the age at which effects are most marked but, rather, that the effects differ in type according to children's age at the time.

Hormonal effects

The effects of hormones need to be considered in relation to two main age periods: just before birth and puberty. It is well established from animal studies that androgens have a programming effect on early brain development such that there are subtle, but important, differences between males and females (Greenough *et al.* 1987; Gorski 1996; Goy 1996). These effects have some implications for later sex-typical behaviours of various kinds. It seems likely that something comparable takes place with respect to human development (Collaer & Hines 1995; Ruble & Martin 1998). There is some supporting evidence deriving from studies of individuals with physical anomalies of one kind or another but it is not at all clear whether or not these play any significant part in relation to sexual disorders (see Zucker, Chapter 44).

The massive hormonal changes, and the extent to which they differ between males and females, during adolescence are well known and have physical effects that are obvious and striking. What is much less clear are their psychopathological implications. These need to be considered in relation to four types of disturbance: antisocial behaviour, depression, eating disorders, and drug and alcohol use and abuse.

Antisocial behaviour

It is well established that androgens have a major effect in both sexes in relation to sex drive and patterns of dominance (Rubinow & Schmidt 1996). There is a rise in the production of androgens in both males and females, although it is much greater in the former (where the testes have a major role), the rise in females deriving from the adrenals. At first sight, it might seem obvious that the much greater rise in androgens that occurs in males is likely to account for the male preponderance in antisocial behaviour, and especially in violence and sex crimes. However, the empirical research findings raise doubts about this explanation. To begin with, contrary to what one might expect, the sex difference in antisocial behaviour is least evident in adolescence, rather than most evident as the hormonal explanation would lead one to suppose (Rutter *et al.* 1998b; Moffitt *et al.*, 2001). The male preponderance is more marked, both before puberty and in adult life. Also, variations in androgen levels within males are not particularly strongly associated with variations in aggression, although they are more strongly linked with variations in dominance (Tremblay *et al.* 1997). It would be foolish to suppose that hormones have no role in relation to the sex differences in antisocial behaviour but, equally, it would be quite wrong to suppose that they provide the main explanation (Rutter *et al.* 1998b; Moffitt *et al.*, 2001). The main difference between males and females lies in early onset antisocial behaviour that is associated with hyperactivity, and that continues into adult life. Some sort of mechanism that involves neurodevelopmental function seems more likely than one that resides in hormonal effects.

A distinction needs to be drawn, however, between the effects of puberty as such, and the effects of reaching puberty at a much earlier (or later) age than usual. Stattin & Magnusson (1990), in Sweden, found that girls who had an unusually early menarche were more likely than other girls to become involved in socially disapproved behaviour. Caspi *et al.* (1993), in New Zealand, found the same. Both studies, however, found that although the stimulus was biological, the mediating mechanism was social. The effect was found only in early maturing girls who became part of an older peer group that provided antisocial models. Risk mechanisms need to be considered in terms of causal claims in which the influences on the origin of a risk factor may not be the same as the mode of risk mediation with respect to the pathological outcome (Rutter *et al.* 1993).

Depression

Note has already been made of the marked rise in depression in females during adolescence, and similar questions need to be asked about the possible role of hormones. An early study of a clinical sample suggested that the main association was with chronological age rather than puberty as such (Angold & Rutter 1992) but a more recent general population study suggested the reverse (Angold *et al.* 1999). The latter found evidence of stronger associations with hormonal levels than with the physical manifestations of puberty. It seems rather unlikely that there is direct effect of hormones on depressive disorder because of the lack of consistent associations with either hormonal changes associated with the menstrual cycle or with the menopause. On the other hand, the female preponderance in depression does seem less marked in old age than it is in mid-adult life (Bebbington 1996, 1998). The causal processes involved have yet to be established, but two possibilities seem most likely. First, although the hormonal changes do not directly cause depression, it may be that the changes associated with puberty in females in some way serve as a longer lasting predisposing vulnerability factor that makes women more susceptible to depression. Alternative-

ly, it may be that the hormonal changes are not themselves the most important feature; instead, it may be that they index other features of biological development that are more directly responsible for the risk of depression.

Eating disorders

Eating disorders constitute the third group showing a dramatic rise in frequency that occurs roughly around puberty (see Steinhausen, Chapter 34). The question is what it means, and what causes it. One possibility is that a key stimulus is provided by the marked increase in deposition of fat that is characteristic of puberty in females but less so in males. The hypothesis, then, is that it is the dissatisfaction with weight gain that leads to dieting, and that the dieting in turn leads on to anorexia nervosa. The story seems likely to be valid with respect to the very frequent dieting behaviour that is so characteristic of female adolescents in Western society (Attie & Brooks-Gunn 1989). However, although dissatisfaction with weight gain in adolescence may provoke the onset of dieting, it seems that depression and disturbed family relationships may play a greater part in the persistance of disturbed eating patterns (Attie & Brooks-Gunn 1989; Patton *et al.* 1997).

Although dissatisfaction with weight gain may be the key factor provoking the beginning of dieting, it is much more doubtful whether it accounts for the rise in anorexia nervosa in adolescence. If it was critical, it might be supposed that the severe dieting that is characteristic of both ballet dancers and some athletes should frequently lead on to anorexia nervosa; however, the evidence suggests that that is surprisingly unusual (Szmukler *et al.* 1985; Patton *et al.* 1990). It might also be supposed that the less frequent occurrence of anorexia nervosa in boys should be found particularly often in those with an unusual deposition of fat. The evidence on this point is fragmentary but that does not seem to be the case. Although it seems likely that the changes associated with puberty do indeed play a part in the genesis of anorexia nervosa, queries remain on the mechanisms involved. The mere association between eating disorders and puberty does not, in itself, provide a causal explanation. The same applies to the sex difference. It is important to appreciate that age-related differences in rates of psychopathology provide crucially important leads for questions to be tackled but they do not, in themselves, provide an answer.

Substance use/abuse

The fourth type of psychopathology showing a marked rise during adolescence concerns use and abuse of alcohol and other drugs (see Weinberg *et al.*, Chapter 27). The cause of the rise in drug use in the teenage years is not obvious. It is possible that part of the explanation may lie in age-related psychological responses to the physical substance. For example, it seems that most children do not experience the euphoric response to stimulants that is characteristic in adults (see Heyman & Santosh, Chapter 59). However, whether this applies more generally to other drugs is doubtful. It could be that drug use stems in part from the rise in risk-taking behaviour that is evident during adolescence. That might explain why drug-taking is more likely, and tends to begin earlier, in individuals showing antisocial behaviour that includes risk-taking features (Robins & McEvoy 1990). In some cases it may be that there is recourse to drugs as a way of dealing with negative mood (see Weinberg *et al.*, Chapter 27). Longitudinal studies of depressed youths, however, provide little support for this possibility; the effects of depression seem much weaker than those of antisocial behaviour with respect to the predisposition to drug-taking (see Rutter, Chapter 28). Alternatively, it may be that part of the explanation lies in the role of social groups. Much consumption of alcohol and taking of drugs takes place in social settings, and these come to occupy a much greater part of young people's social lives during adolescence. Still, that leaves the question as to why the taking of drugs and alcohol should be such prominent features of these social groups. Does that derive from cultural features, biological features, or some interplay between the two?

An unusually early menarche is associated with an increase in smoking and drinking of alcohol in girls (Stattin & Magnusson 1990), as well as the already mentioned increase in socially disapproved behaviour. A Finnish twin study (Dick *et al.* 2000) showed that the effect was confined to girls in urban (rather than rural) settings. It also found that the effect was not caused by any shared genetic liability between early puberty and drinking/smoking. The effect of early puberty on drinking does not persist into adult life to any marked extent. As the social context alters, so the meaning and impact of early puberty changes. The initial effect did not bring about lasting personality change. Rather, the early puberty made a difference because it altered the peer group and extent of parental supervision, but (as with other influences) if the person's social circumstances change, the environmental effects may well prove to be evanescent (Clarke & Clarke 1976, 2000).

Response to physical substances

Over the last few decades, there has been a growing awareness of the ways in which substances ingested by the mother during pregnancy may have adverse effects on the fetus. The thalidomide tragedy, with its devastating effects in causing limb deformities, is the most dramatic example of this kind. However, from a psychopathological perspective, infection, alcohol and recreational drugs occupy a greater importance. The evidence on the role of maternal infections is greatest in the case of influenza as a contributory predisposing factor to schizophrenia (McGrath & Murray 1995; see also Hollis, Chapter 37). There is circumstantial evidence that influenza, when it occurs during the second trimester, is associated with an approximate doubling of the risk of schizophrenia (but see Westergaard *et al.* 1999 for contrary evidence). Maternal rubella has well-established devastating effects on fetal development, leading to mental retardation, blindness and deafness. This is associated with an increase in

autistic-like patterns, although they differ in course from those seen with 'ordinary' autism (Chess *et al.* 1971; Chess 1977).

Heavy consumption of alcohol in the first trimester is known to be associated with physical consequences to fetal development (the so-called 'fetal alcohol' syndrome) and indeed has important psychological consequences, particularly in relation to patterns of inattention/overactivity (Streissguth & Kanter 1997). It also seems that there are likely to be adverse effects at levels of alcohol consumption that are very high but yet do not lead to the identifiable physical anomalies. The evidence is inconclusive as to whether even moderate levels of alcohol consumption carry psychological risks, but the available evidence suggests that with modest levels of consumption the risks are minimal, even though it may be prudent to avoid taking alcohol at all during the early months of pregnancy (Stratton *et al.* 1996; Streissguth & Kanter 1997). The animal evidence (Schneider *et al.* 1997, 1999) is provocative in its suggestion that stress experiences in pregnancy increase the fetus' vulnerability to maternal alcohol and that these effects are most marked in early gestation.

Although there is abundant evidence that the occurrence of depression in young people is associated with a much increased rate of recurrence of major disorder in adult life (see Harrington, Chapter 29), it appears that the response to tricyclic medication is not the same. All the major well-controlled trials of tricyclic medication in young people have failed to show substantial benefits (Hazell *et al.* 1995), whereas almost all such trials in adults have shown significant effects. Even in adults, there are marked individual differences in response, and in childhood too there are occasional individuals who seem to show beneficial responses. Nevertheless, considered as a whole, there seem to be marked age differences in the likelihood of a person having a beneficial response to tricyclic medication. The reasons for this age difference remain unknown. It is not, apparently, that there is a general insensitivity to antidepressant medication because response to selective serotonin re-uptake inhibitors (SSRIs) has been more positive (Emslie *et al.* 1997, 1999).

Neural substrate of continuities and discontinuities in psychopathology

The need to consider a possible neural substrate for changes in psychopathology as people grow older arises with respect to several different mental disorders. Mention has already been made of the transition in schizophrenia from the neurodevelopmental delays, attention difficulties, social deficits and behavioural problems that are characteristic of childhood manifestations, to the more florid negative symptoms in adult life, together with thought disorder, delusions and hallucinations. It is necessary to ask whether this change is a function of progression in the disease process itself or, rather, whether it reflects the effects on psychopathological manifestations that derive from normal changes in brain development that, as it were, 'unmask' a psychotic vulnerability (McDonald *et al.* 2000). Attempts are being made to tackle this question by determining whether imaging studies can show progressive changes in the period leading up to the onset of psychotic manifestations. The same basic strategy has also been applied with respect to the cognitive impairment that is associated with schizophrenia (Cosway *et al.* 2000). As discussed by Marenco and Weinberger (2000), there is some preliminary evidence of brain changes during this prodromal period, although uncertainty remains on the neural processes that they reflect.

Somewhat similar questions arise with respect to the frequent development of epileptic attacks during late adolescence and early adult life in individuals with autism (Rutter 1970; Howlin, S. Goode & M. Rutter, in preparation). In this case, the issue is not a change in psychopathology as such but rather the development of epileptic activity. Although it has been claimed that this is often associated with psychopathological deterioration (Gillberg & Steffenburg 1987), that has not been found in other studies (Hutton, S. Goode & M. Rutter, in preparation). Although epileptic attacks can begin at any age in autistic individuals, onset in late adolescence/early adult life is peculiarly characteristic, and it is rather different from the predominance of onset in early childhood that is usually found in both mentally retarded individuals and in general population samples (Cooper 1965; Richardson & Koller 1996). Once more, the question is whether this reflects changes in the disease process of autism, or whether normal brain development during this age period is unmasking an epileptic liability.

A further phenomenon of neural substrate concerns the feature that has come to be called 'kindling' (Post 1992). It has been observed that the experience of a major depressive disorder has effects that seem to create a self-perpetuating tendency to an increased liability to recurrence, despite a decreased susceptibility to the effects of negative life events (Brown *et al.* 1994; Frank *et al.* 1994). Kendler *et al.* have used a twin design to test for the reality of this effect, with confirmatory findings (Kendler *et al.* 2000, in press). Curiously, however, the data also seemed to show that the kindling effect was greatest in individuals inferred to be at low genetic risk (Kendler *et al.*, 2001). Much has still to be learned about this phenomenon but its existence seems to be confirmed, and it serves as a reminder that the experience of a major mental disorder may have effects on the organism that carry implications for the likelihood of a recurrence.

Personality development

Over the years, there have been major changes in concepts of what is involved in personality development (Rutter & Rutter 1993; Caspi 1998; Rutter *et al.* 1998b). Four features warrant particular emphasis. First, although it is the case that, as with other psychological attributes, consistency in temperamental features increases over the years of childhood, measures at ages as early as 3 years do predict later psychopathological functioning to a significant (but only moderate) degree.

Secondly, temperamental characteristics should not be conceptualized as representing the genetic basis of personality. They are subject to genetic influences but not to any greater extent than other behaviours. Temperament evolves over the course of development through the combined effect of genetic and environmental influences.

Thirdly, nature and nurture are not independent of one another (see also McGuffin & Rutter, Chapter 12). Genetic effects operate in part through their role in bringing about differences in environmental risk exposure—as a result of influences on behaviours that serve to shape and select environments—and in susceptibility to risk environments.

Finally, from infancy onwards, personality involves not only biologically influenced behavioural propensities, such as activity level or autonomic reactivity, but also thinking and feeling patterns (Rutter 1987). Children develop ideas about standards and values (Kagan 1982), and they gain a self-concept of what sort of person they are (Harter 1998). This includes a view of their value (self-esteem) and their ability to cope with different life challenges and situations (self-efficacy; Bandura 1995, 1997). It also involves an internal model of their past experiences and their expectations of how other people are likely to respond to them. Their concept of the world being a loving or hostile environment will, in turn, influence how they behave in their interactions and relationships with other people (Dodge *et al.* 1990, 1995; Thompson 1998).

Psychological substrate of continuities and discontinuities

These personality features, together with other characteristics, contribute to psychological mechanisms in continuities and discontinuities in psychopathology. It is not that these mechanisms do not have a neural substrate; they do (all learning and thinking has to involve brain processes), but the brain changes are of a type that can adapt to, and incorporate, new learning and new concepts.

At least three rather different features need to be considered with respect to continuities and discontinuities. First, there is the most fundamental question of what it is that environmental experiences do to the organism that leads to the carrying forward of effects that persist beyond the time span of the negative experience itself (Rutter 2000a). Numerous possibilities exist (Rutter 1989a). Mention has already been made of developmental programming effects, although it is likely that these apply to only a minority of rather severe experiences. There are also effects on neuroendocrine function. Animal studies have, on the whole, suggested that negative experiences lead to an enhancement of neuroendocrine structure and function that is protective against later stresses (Hennessey & Levine 1979; Levine 1982), whereas human evidence suggests rather the reverse (see Sandberg & Rutter, Chapter 17). The reasons for this disparity remain ill-understood at the moment. In addition, there are the effects on thought processes. Attachment theorists have placed great weight on the likelihood that the experience of negative relationships in early childhood leads children to develop negative internal working models of both themselves and of the relationships that they may expect with others. The supposition is that it is these negative cognitive sets that provide the mechanisms that are the carrying forward of psychological sequelae. There is no doubt that children do, indeed, think about their experiences and do develop concepts and ideas about their meaning with respect to themselves and to the world about them. It is plausible that such cognitive and affective models influence the persistence, or non-persistence, of adverse effects of negative experiences, but the empirical research to test this proposition is largely a task for the future. Dodge *et al.* (1990, 1995) have asked similar questions in relation to the mechanisms by which adverse experiences, such as physical abuse, become transformed into an increased liability for antisocial behaviour. They hypothesize that the process might involve effects on cognitive processing of experiences leading to an increase in the tendency to make hostile attributions. Their findings provided modest support for the hypothesis but the cognitive measures accounted for a relatively small proportion of the variance in the outcome measure. It is unclear whether this means that other mechanisms were involved or, rather, that there were measurement problems with respect to such cognitions in early childhood. The findings so far may not provide a solid answer, but there is no doubt that this is the type of question that needs to be asked.

A second, somewhat related, issue concerns the effects of psychopathology on cognitive processing. It was once thought that negative cognitive attributions constituted a key risk factor for depressive disorder. That may be the case to some extent but, at least with adults, the available evidence casts doubt on the role of negative cognitions as an independent risk factor for depression. On the other hand, the same evidence does suggest that the experience of depression leads to negative cognitions that, in turn, do play a substantial part in the continuation of the depressive features (Teasdale & Barnard 1993). It is observations of this kind that have played a major part in the development of cognitive behavioural approaches in the treatment of emotional disorders (see Brent, Chapter 54).

The third issue concerns the role of major life experiences in bringing about continuities or discontinuities in behaviour. It was once thought that the 'norm' or 'ordinary expectation' was that, once a behaviour was present, it would continue indefinitely unless something happened to change it. It is now clear that that is a wholly mistaken and misleading assumption (Rutter 1994). The expectation cannot be simply of unchanging continuity. Rather, both continuity and discontinuity have to be accounted for, and the role of life experiences needs to be part of those considerations. Caspi & Moffitt (1991) have made the important point that when there were continuities between life experiences (which is usually the case), stresses and adversities will usually operate to enhance pre-existing behavioural tendencies, rather than change them. It is only when experiences are of a kind that show discontinuity with the past that turning point effects may be found (Rutter 1996b). For individuals who have shown antisocial behaviour in childhood, a supportive harmonious marriage makes a big difference in leading to a much reduced

likelihood that antisocial behaviour will continue, and to an increased likelihood of adaptive social functioning (Zoccolillo *et al.* 1992; Sampson & Laub 1993; Rutter *et al.* 1997; Laub *et al.* 1998). Of course, it is only a minority of antisocial individuals who make such a supportive marriage, and it is important to consider the possibility that the apparent protective effect is an artefact of the pre-existing behaviour or pre-existing psychosocial risk factors associated with individuals who are fortunate enough to land up in that situation. Nevertheless, detailed and careful statistical analyses have shown that the protective effect is, indeed, a real one. The likelihood of making a marriage to a supportive partner is strongly predicted by prior behaviour and prior circumstances (Quinton *et al.* 1993) but the positive adult life experience clearly makes a difference. Amongst other things, the findings point to the fact that the experiences that people bring about themselves can, nevertheless, have important effects on their own behaviour (Rutter *et al.* 1993).

Risk and resilience

One of the central concepts in modern medicine is that of risk factors and vulnerability. Very few disorders have a single main cause; rather they arise through an interplay among risk factors, each of which involves an increase in vulnerability or susceptibility, but none of which causes disorder directly. The likelihood of developing coronary artery disease is increased by low birth weight, high cholesterol levels, smoking, an increased clotting tendency, lack of exercise, and by a high waist:hips ratio—a rather diverse range of risk features. Similarly, osteoporosis in women is more likely if the person smokes, takes little exercise, lacked an adequate calcium intake in early life, and has low sex hormone levels. Much the same applies with psychiatric disorders in childhood and adult life. The greatest psychopathological risk arises from the cumulative effect of multiple environmental and genetic risk factors (Rutter 1999, 2000a,b). From a developmental perspective, the key questions are *how* these come together and *which* mediating mechanisms are implicated. Do they concern an increased reactivity to later psychosocial hazards, a negative mental set, a lack of self-efficacy, or a propensity to behave in ways that tend to engender stress situations—to mention just a few possibilities (Rutter 1989b)?

With all kinds of environmental risks (physical and psychosocial), there is huge individual variability in response (Rutter 2000a,b). The term resilience is applied when there is relatively normal functioning despite the experience of major risk factors. The evidence suggests that multiple factors play a part in this important phenomenon (Luthar *et al.* 2000; Rutter 2000b): including temperamental and other genetically influenced features; prior experiences; the impact of the risk experience at the time; the ways in which the individual conceptualized and thought about the experience; compensatory protective features that counteract the risk; and subsequent circumstances and happenings. A consideration of how these might be operative in the individual case will be relevant in planning therapeutic interventions (Rutter 1999; see also Rutter & Taylor, Chapter 2).

Psychopathological progressions

There are several examples in the field of mental disorders where it is necessary to account for apparent progressions in psychopathology: drug dependency; antisocial personality disorder; suicide; progression from anxiety disorders to depression; and the progression from dieting to anorexia or bulimia nervosa.

In order to become dependent upon drugs or alcohol, it is necessary to make the first transition from no use of drugs to taking the substances at all; to move on to take them regularly at a high level; to become psychologically and/or physically dependent on the substances; and ultimately, to develop physical and social damage from the substance abuse (see Weinberg *et al.*, Chapter 27). In addition, there is likely to be a progression from taking just one drug to being reliant on multiple drugs. The features that provide maximum risks are by no means necessarily the same at all stages in this progression, as shown for example by Robins's (1993) research with heroin dependence in Vietnam veterans. African-Americans from the inner cities were the group most likely to take heroin but, on the return from Vietnam, it was rural whites who were more likely to continue to be dependent on the drug.

Genetically influenced specific responses to individual substances may be important in some circumstances. The unpleasant flushing response to alcohol that is present in some orientals constitutes a good example of a pharmacological response that is protective because of its unpleasantness (Vanyukov & Tarter 2000). There are other parallels, too, with respect to physiological responses that increase or decrease the risks of heavy use of substances. In addition, there may be genetically influenced or environmentally influenced features that have a role in the use of drugs, but not necessarily in the transition to dependence (Kendler *et al.* 1999). For example, longitudinal studies as well as retrospective cross-sectional studies have made clear the high frequency with which antisocial behaviour predisposes both to drug-taking in general and, especially, to the early use of drugs (Robins & McEvoy 1990). In other circumstances, dysthymic mood may constitute a predisposing factor, albeit a weaker one, to the use of drugs to relieve negative emotional states (Rao *et al.* 1999). However, findings also show that effects are bidirectional. Alcohol intoxication, possibly through its disinhibiting effects, makes violent crime more likely; and dependence on 'hard' drugs predisposes to thefts, probably because of the money needed to support the drug habit (Rutter *et al.* 1998b).

Although there is some evidence that the causal factors operate in somewhat different ways at different points in this progression, it is also necessary to consider the possibility that the different features all represent varied manifestations of the same underlying liability. The genetic evidence suggests that, to some extent, that is probably the case although that does not represent the whole of the story. The causal pathways for these progressions in psychopathology are not at all well worked out, and there is a considerable need to try to investigate the causal mechanisms for each of the various phases and transitions.

Somewhat similar issues arise with respect to the transitions from hyperkinetic behaviour in early childhood to oppositional/defiant disturbance during middle childhood, to conduct problems in later childhood and adolescence, and then on to antisocial personality disorder (and other forms of personality disorder) in adult life. Although, according to traditional systems of classification, these are all considered different mental disorders, the genetic findings suggest that, to a considerable extent, they reflect the same underlying genetic liability (Rutter *et al.* 1998b). Thus, oppositional/defiant problems and conduct disorders share the majority of their genetic liability (Nadder *et al.* in press; Eaves *et al.*, 2000); and the same applies to the associations between both of those and prior ADHD. What is different here, however, is that the available genetic findings so far (much more needs to be done in order to sort out the mechanisms) suggest that the co-occurrence of hyperactivity indexes a different form of antisocial behaviour that involves a stronger genetic liability (Silberg *et al.* 1996). It is nevertheless the case that by no means all children with hyperactivity go on to develop antisocial behaviour, and also the transition is largely in the direction of earlier hyperactivity to later antisocial behaviour (with the reverse pattern distinctly uncommon); and this raises the possibility that either the transition requires an interplay of environmental risk factors (for which there is some evidence; see Moffitt 1990) or that the phenotype of hyperactivity creates an increased likelihood of negative family interactions that themselves predispose to the transition. Again, a developmental perspective requires that the causal mechanisms be viewed in terms of possible indirect chain effects as well as in terms of direct causes.

Mention has already been made of the need to examine continuities and discontinuities between the severe dieting and dissatisfaction with body shape that is so common in females during adolescence and the much rarer clinical syndrome of anorexia or bulimia nervosa. Is there a transition from the one to the other, perhaps requiring a different set of risk factors, or are the apparent similarities just surface parallels without there being a common underlying liability? Clearly, dieting predicts eating disorders (at least at a partial syndrome level) but is that because dieting represents the early phase of the disorder or is it because dieting itself serves as a risk factor (Patton *et al.* 1999)?

The situation with respect to anxiety and depression is rather different in that it is clear that there is a strong association at the individual level, and that both involve the shared liability factor of neuroticism or emotional liability (see Rutter & Taylor, Chapter 2). However, there is the additional consideration that longitudinal studies suggest that the usual course is for anxiety in childhood to lead on to depression in adolescence or early adult life, with the reverse pattern being much less common. Does this mean that age-related factors influence which manifestations are most striking at different ages, or are there mechanisms of one kind or another that are implicated in the transition from anxiety to depression?

A further example is provided by the risk factors for suicide. Longitudinal studies suggest that depressive disorder and anti-social behaviour both constitute risks but, presumably, the former does so through the effects of severe depression of mood leading to feelings of hopelessness and despondency about the future, whereas the latter operates through the role of risk-taking behaviour and use of drugs (Harrington *et al.* 1994). Again, the question that needs to be asked is whether these are two parallel risk factors that operate in additive fashion or whether the developmental findings imply that there are two different developmental chains operating differently and yet which both increase the risk of suicide.

So far, most of the research that has been undertaken has focused on statistical associations in order to identify risk and protective factors, and much less attention has been paid to the possibility that the causal processes may differ at different points in the causal chain. We need to investigate that possibility. That is perhaps one of the main features to derive from the developmental perspective.

Sex differences

Throughout this chapter, there has been frequent reference to the presence of major sex differences in psychopathology. The reasons for that remain largely unexplained; nevertheless, the patterns are somewhat consistent. There is a male preponderance in almost all of the early onset disorders that seem to involve some form of neurodevelopmental impairment: autism (see Lord & Bailey, Chapter 38); developmental language disorders (see Bishop, Chapter 39); and hyperactivity (see Schachar & Tannock, Chapter 25). At first sight, antisocial behaviour might seem an exception to this trend but careful analysis of the evidence indicates that the main male preponderance applies to early onset antisocial behaviour that is associated with hyperactivity (Moffit *et al.*, 2001) and, hence, even that may be attributable to some form of neurodevelopmental feature. Of course, that leaves entirely open the question why these neurodevelopmental impairments are more common in males, but it narrows the question in so far as it focuses on the neurodevelopmental features rather than on a diverse range of psychopathology.

The other pattern is exemplified by the female preponderance that arises in adolescence, especially with respect to eating disorders and depression. It seems most unlikely that that sex difference is related to neurodevelopmental impairment; a rather different set of mechanisms need to be implicated. Genetic factors seem likely to play a part but such evidence as is available in the case of depression suggests that they may operate through their impact on nature–nurture interplay, rather than directly on disorder as such (Silberg *et al.* 1999, in press).

There are other disorders where the situation is more complex. For example, with schizophrenia it is not so much that there is an overall sex difference but that in males onset tends to be earlier than it is in females (Castle *et al.* 1998; Tarrant & Jones 2000). It is not yet known why that is so. Similarly, with respect to the use and abuse of substances, it is not so much that there is an overall sex difference but that the particular pattern of sex difference varies with each substance. Again, we lack a good explanation.

Much of the research into sex differences up to now has been based on the sociological feminist perspective, focusing on the role of women in society. Those considerations may well be important with respect to some sex differences, but the strong likelihood is that a range of different explanations may need to be invoked, and that some of these will be largely biologically, rather than socially, influenced. This remains a high priority for future research.

Conclusions

Developmental considerations arise at all points in chapters throughout this volume. In this chapter, we have simply sought to pull together some of the different considerations and topics that must be investigated. Developmental approaches to psychopathology have brought some important advances but, even more than that, they have raised a rather different set of research questions that have still to be addressed. The purpose of this chapter has been to indicate what some of these might be.

References

Angold, A. & Rutter, M. (1992) Effects of age and pubertal status on depression in a large clinical sample. *Development and Psychopathology*, 4, 5–28.

Angold, A., Costello, E.J., Erkanli, A. & Worthman, C.H. (1999) Pubertal changes in hormone levels and depression in girls. *Psychological Medicine*, 29, 1043–1053.

Attie, I. & Brooks-Gunn, J. (1989) Development of eating problems in adolescent girls: a longitudinal study. *Developmental Psychology*, 25, 70–79.

Baddeley, A.D. (1990) *Human Memory: Theory and Practice*. Lawrence Erlbaum Associates, Hove & London; Allyn & Bacon, Needham Heights MA.

Bandura, A., ed. (1995) *Self-Efficacy in Changing Societies*. Cambridge University Press, New York.

Bandura, A. (1997) *Self-Efficacy: the Exercise of Control*. Freeman, New York.

Barker, D.J.P. (1991) The intrauterine environment and adult cardiovascular disease. In: *The Childhood Environment and Adult Disease*, Ciba Foundation Symposium 156 (eds G.R. Bock & J. Whelan), pp. 3–10. John Wiley & Sons, Chichester.

Barker, D.J. (1997) Fetal nutrition and cardiovascular disease in later life. *British Medical Bulletin*, 53, 96–108.

Bateson, P. & Martin, P. (1999) *Design for a Life: How Behaviour Develops*. Jonathan Cape, London.

Bebbington, P. (1996) The origins of sex differences in depressive disorder: bridging the gap. *International Review of Psychiatry*, 8, 295–332.

Bebbington, P.E. (1998) Sex and depression [Editorial]. *Psychological Medicine*, 28, 1–8.

Biederman, J., Faraone, S., Mick, E. *et al.* (1996) Attention deficit hyperactivity disorder and juvenile mania: an overlooked cormorbidity? *Journal of the American Academy of Child and Adolescent Psychiatry*, **35**, 997–1008.

Blakemore, C. (1991) Sensitive and vulnerable periods in the development of the visual system. In: *The Childhood Environment and Adult Disease, Ciba Foundation Symposium 156* (eds G.R. Bock & J. Whelan), pp. 129–147. John Wiley & Sons, Chichester.

Bock, G., Goode, J. & Webb, K. (2000) *The Nature of Intelligence, Novartis Foundation Symposium 233*. John Wiley & Sons, Chichester.

Brown, G.W., Harris, T.O. & Hepworth, C. (1994) Life events and endogenous depression: a puzzle reexamined. *Archives of General Psychiatry*, **51**, 525–534.

Bruer, J.T. (1999) *The Myth of the First Three Years*. The Free Press, New York.

Caspi, A. (1998) Personality development across the life course. In: *Handbook of Child Psychology*, Vol. 3, *Social, Emotional, and Personality Development* (eds W. Damon, series ed & N. Eisenberg, volum ed), 5th edn, pp. 311–388. John Wiley & Sons, New York.

Caspi, A. & Moffitt, T.E. (1991) Individual differences are accentuated during periods of social change: the sample case of girls at puberty. *Journal of Personality and Social Psychology*, **61**, 157–168.

Caspi, A., Lynam, D., Moffitt, T.E. & Silva, P.A. (1993) Unraveling girls' delinquency: biological, dispositional, and contextual contributions to adolescent misbehavior. *Developmental Psychology*, **29**, 19–30.

Castle, D.J., Wessely, S., Van Os, J. & Murray, R.M. (1998) The effect of gender in age at onset of psychosis. In: *Psychosis in the Inner City: the Camberwell First Episode Study, Maudsley Monograph No 40*, pp. 27–36. Psychology Press, Hove.

Chess, S. (1977) Follow-up report on autism in congenital rubella. *Journal of Autism and Childhood Schizophrenia*, **7**, 69–81.

Chess, S., Kern, S.J. & Fernandez, P.B. (1971) *Psychiatric Disorders of Children with Congenital Rubella*. Brunner/Mazel, New York.

Cicchetti, D. (1989) Developmental psychopathology: past, present, and future. In: *The Emergence of a Discipline: Rochester Symposium on Developmental Psychopathology*, Vol. 1 (ed. D. Cicchetti), pp. 1–12. Erlbaum, Hillsdale, NJ.

Cicchetti, D. & Toth, S. (1995) Developmental psychology and disorders of affect. In: *Developmental Psychopathology*, Vol. 2 (eds D. Cicchetti & D. Cohen), pp. 369–420. Wiley, New York.

Clarke, A.M. & Clarke, A.D.B. (eds) (1976) *Early Experience: Myth and Evidence*. Open Books, London.

Clarke, A.M. & Clarke, A.D.B. (2000) *Early Experience and the Life Path*. Jessica Kingsley, London.

Collaer, M.L. & Hines, M. (1995) Human behavioral sex differences: a role of gonadal hormones during early development? *Psychological Bulletin*, **118**, 55–107.

Cooper, J.E. (1965) Epilepsy in a longitudinal survey of 5000 children. *British Medical Journal*, **1**, 1020–1022.

Cosway, R., Byrne, M., Clafferty, R. *et al.* (2000) Neuropsychological change in young people at high risk for schizophrenia: results from the first two neuropsychological assessments of the Edinburgh High Risk Study. *Psychological Medicine*, **30**, 1111–1121.

Cummings, E.M., Davies, P.T. & Campbell, S.B. (2000) *Developmental Psychopathology and Family Process: Theory, Research, and Clinical Implications*. Guilford Press, New York.

Dick, D.M., Rose, R.J., Viken, R.J. & Kaprio, J. (2000) Pubertal timing and substance use: associations between and within families across late adolescence. *Developmental Psychology*, **36**, 180–189.

Dodge, K.A., Bates, J.E. & Pettit, G.S. (1990) Mechanisms in the cycle of violence. *Science*, **250**, 1678–1683.

Dodge, K.A., Pettit, G.S., Bates, J.E. & Valente, E. (1995) Social information-processing patterns partially mediate the effect of early physical abuse on later conduct problems. *Journal of Abnormal Psychology*, **104**, 632–643.

Dowdney, L. (2000) Childhood bereavement following parental death. *Journal of Child Psychology and Psychiatry*, **41**, 819–830.

Eaves, L.J., Rutter, M., Silberg, J.L., Shillady, L., Maes, H. & Pickles, A. (2000) Genetic and environmental causes of covariation in interview assessments of disruptive behavior in child and adolescent twins. *Behavior Genetics*, **30**, 321–334.

Emslie, G.J., Rush, A.J., Weinberg, W.A. *et al.* (1997) A double-blind, randomized, placebo-controlled trial of fluoxetine in children and adolescents with depression. *Archives of General Psychiatry*, **54**, 1031–1037.

Emslie, G.J., Walkup, J.T., Pliszka, S.R. & Ernst, M. (1999) Nontricyclic antidepressants: current trends in children and adolescents. *Journal of the American Academy of Child and Adolescent Psychiatry*, **38**, 517–528.

Eriksson, P.S., Perfilieva, E., Björk-Eriksson, T. *et al.* (1998) Neurogenesis in the adult human hippocampus. *Nature Medicine*, **4**, 1313–1317.

Faraone, S.V., Biederman, J., Wozniak, J., Mundy, E., Mennin, D. & O'Donnell, D. (1997) Is comorbidity with ADHD a marker for juvenile-onset mania? *Journal of the American Academy of Child and Adolescent Psychiatry*, **36**, 1046–1055.

Finch, C.E. & Kirkwood, T. (2000) *Chance, Development, and Aging*. Oxford University Press, Oxford.

Fombonne, E., Wostear, G., Cooper, V., Harrington, R. & Rutter, M. (2001a) The Maudsley long-term follow-up of child and adolescent depression. I. Psychiatric outcomes in adulthood. *British Journal of Psychiatry*, **179**, 210–217.

Fombonne, E., Wostear, G., Cooper, V., Harrington, R. & Rutter, M. (2001b) The Maudsley long-term follow-up of child and adolescent depression. II. Suicidality, criminality and social dysfunction in adulthood. *British Journal of Psychiatry*, **179**, 218–223.

Frank, E., Anderson, B., Reynolds, C.F., Ritenour, A. & Kupfer, D.J. (1994) Life events and the research diagnostic criteria endogenous subtype: a confirmation of the distinction using the Bedford College methods. *Archives of General Psychiatry*, **51**, 519–524.

Gillberg, C. & Steffenburg, S. (1987) Outcome and prognostic factors in infantile autism and similar conditions: a population-based study of 46 cases followed through puberty. *Journal of Autism and Developmental Disorders*, **17**, 273–287.

Goldman-Rakic, P.S., Bourgeois, J.-P. & Rakic, P. (1997) Synaptic substrate of cognitive development: life-span analysis of synaptogenesis in the prefrontal cortex of the nonhuman primate. In: *Development of the Prefrontal Cortex: Evolution, Neurobiology, and Behavior* (eds N.A. Krasnegor, G.R. Lyon & P.S. Goldman-Rakic), pp. 27–47. Paul H. Brookes, Baltimore.

Goodman, R. (1991) Growing together and growing apart: the non-genetic forces on children in the same family. In: *The New Genetics of Mental Illness* (eds P. McGuffin & R. Murray), pp. 212–224. Heinemann Medical, Oxford.

Goodman, R. (1994) Brain development. In: *Development Through Life: a Handbook for Clinicians* (eds M. Rutter & D.F. Hay), pp. 49–78. Blackwell Scientific Publications, Oxford.

Gorski, R.A. (1996) Gonadal hormones and the organization of brain structure and function. In: *The Lifespan Development of Individuals: Behavioral, Neurobiological, and Psychosocial Perspectives* (ed. D. Magnusson), pp. 315–340. Cambridge University Press, Cambridge.

Gould, E., Reeves, A.J., Graziano, M.S.A. & Gross, C.G. (1999)

Neurogenesis in the neocortex of adult primates. *Science*, **286**, 548–552.

Goy, R.W. (1996) Patterns of juvenile behavior following early hormonal interventions. In: *The Lifespan Development of Individuals: Behavioral, Neurobiological and Psychosocial Perspectives* (ed. D. Magnusson), pp. 296–314. Cambridge University Press, Cambridge.

Graber, J.A., Brooks-Gunn, J. & Warren, M.P. (1995) The antecedents of menarcheal age: heredity, family environment, and stressful life events. *Child Development*, **66**, 346–359.

Greenough, W.T. & Black, J.E. (1992) Induction of brain structure by experience: substrates for cognitive development. In: *Developmental Behavior Neuroscience*, Vol. 24 (eds M. R. Gunnar & C. A. Nelson), pp. 155–200. Erlbaum, Hillsdale, NJ.

Greenough, W.T., Black, J.E. & Wallace, C.S. (1987) Experience and brain development. *Child Development*, **58**, 539–559.

Harrington, R., Bredenkamp, D., Groothues, C., Rutter, M., Fudge, H. & Pickles, A. (1994) Adult outcomes of childhood and adolescent depression. III. Links with suicidal behaviours. *Journal of Child Psychology and Psychiatry*, **35**, 1309–1319.

Harris, T., Brown, G.W. & Bifulco, A. (1986) Loss of parent in childhood and adult psychiatric disorder: the role of lack of adequate parental care. *Psychological Medicine*, **16**, 641–659.

Harter, S. (1998) The development of self-representations. In: *Handbook of Child Psychology*, Vol. 3: *Social, Emotional, and Personality Development* (eds W. Damon & N. Eisenberg), 5th edn, pp. 553–617. John Wiley & Sons, New York.

Hazell, P., O'Connell, D., Heathcote, D., Robertson, J. & Henry, D. (1995) Efficacy of tricyclic drugs in treating child and adolescent depression: a meta-analysis. *British Medical Journal*, **310**, 897–901.

Heim, C., Newport, J., Heit, S. *et al.* (2000) Pituitary–adrenal and autonomic responses to stress in women after sexual and physical abuse in childhood. *Journal of the American Medical Association*, **284**, 592–597.

Hennessey, J.W. & Levine, S. (1979) Stress, arousal, and the pituitary–adrenal system: a psychoendocrine hypothesis. In: *Progress in Psychobiology and Physiological Psychology* (eds J.M. Sprague & A.N. Epstein), pp. 133–178. Academic Press, New York.

Hodges, J. & Tizard, B. (1989a) IQ and behavioural adjustment of ex-institutional adolescents. *Journal of Child Psychology and Psychiatry*, **30**, 53–75.

Hodges, J. & Tizard, B. (1989b) Social and family relationships of ex-institutional adolescents. *Journal of Child Psychology and Psychiatry*, **30**, 77–97.

Hubel, D.H. & Wiesel, T.N. (1965) Binocular interaction in striate cortex of kittens reared with artificial squint. *Journal of Neurophysiology*, **28**, 1041–1059.

Huttenlocher, P.R. (1979) Synaptic density in human frontal cortex: developmental changes and effects of aging. *Brain Research*, **163**, 195–205.

Huttenlocher, P.R. (1994) Synaptogenesis, synapse elimination, and neural plasticity in human cerebral cortex. In: *Threats to Optimal Development: Integrating, Biological, Psychological, and Social Risk Factors* (ed. C.A. Nelson) *Minnesota Symposia on Child Psychology*, Vol. 27, pp. 35–54. Lawrence Erlbaum Associates, Hillsdale, NJ.

Jensen, A.R. (1997) The puzzle of nongenetic variance. In: *Intelligence, Heredity, and Environment* (eds R.J. Sternberg & E.L. Grigorenko), pp. 42–88. Cambridge University Press, Cambridge.

Kagan, J. (1980) Perspectives on continuity. In: *Constancy and Change in Human Development* (eds O.G. Brim & J. Kagan), pp. 26–74. Harvard University Press, Cambridge, MA.

Kagan, J. (1982) The emergence of self. *Journal of Child Psychology and Psychiatry*, **23**, 363–381.

Kendler, K.S., Karkowski, L.M., Corey, L.A., Prescott, C.A. & Neale, M.C. (1999) Genetic and environmental risk factors in the aetiology of illicit drug initiation and subsequent misuse in women. *British Journal of Psychiatry*, **175**, 351–356.

Kendler, K.S., Thornton, L.M. & Gardner, C.O. (2000) Stressful life events and previous episodes in the etiology of major depression in women: an evaluation of the 'kindling' hypothesis. *American Journal of Psychiatry*, **157**, 1243–1251.

Kendler, K.S., Thornton, L.M. & Gardner, C.O. (2001) Genetic risk, number of previous depressive episodes and stressful life events in predicting onset of major depression. *American Journal of Psychiatry*, **158**, 582–586.

Kim, K.H.S., Relkin, N.R., Lee, K.-M. & Hirsch, J. (1997) Distinct cortical areas associated with native and second languages. *Nature*, **388**, 171–174.

Krasnegor, N.A., Lyon, G.R. & Goldman-Rakic, P.S., eds (1997). *Development of the Prefrontal Cortex: Evolution, Neurobiology, and Behavior*. Paul H. Brookes, Baltimore.

Kuhl, P.K. (1994) Learning and representation in speech and language. *Current Opinion in Neurobiology*, **4**, 812–822.

Kuhl, P.K., Andruski, J.E., Chistovich, I.A. *et al.* (1997) Cross-language analysis of phonetic units in language addressed to infants. *Science*, **277**, 684–686.

Laub, J.H., Nagin, D.S. & Sampson, R.J. (1998) Trajectories of change in criminal offending: good marriages and the desistance process. *American Sociological Review*, **63**, 225–238.

Levine, S. (1982) Comparative and psychobiological perspectives on development. In: *The Minnesota Symposia on Child Psychology*, Vol. 15, *The Concept of Development* (ed. W.A. Collins), pp. 29–53. Lawrence Erlbaum Associates, Hillsdale, NJ.

Luthar, S.S., Cicchetti, D. & Becker, B. (2000) The construct of resilience: a critical evaluation and guidelines for future work. *Child Development*, **71**, 543–562.

Marenco, S. & Weinberger, D.R. (2000) The neurodevelopmental hypothesis of schizophrenia: following a trail of evidence from cradle to grave. *Development and Psychopathology*, **12**, 501–527.

McDonald, C., Fearon, P. & Murray, R. (2000) Neurodevelopmental hypothesis of schizophrenia 12 years on: data and doubts. In: *Childhood Onset of 'Adult' Psychopathology: Clinical and Research Advances* (ed. J.L. Rapoport), pp. 193–220. American Psychiatric Press, Washington D.C.

McGrath, J. & Murray, R.M. (1995) Risk factors for schizophrenia: from conception to birth. In: *Schizophrenia* (eds S. Hirsch & D. Weinberger), pp. 187–205. Blackwell, Oxford.

Moffitt, T.E. (1990) Juvenile delinquency and Attention Deficit Disorder: boys' developmental trajectories from age 3 to age 15. *Child Development*, **61**, 893–910.

Moffitt, T.E., Caspi, A., Rutter, M. & Silva, P. (2001) Sex differences in antisocial behaviour: conduct disorder, delinquency, and violence in the Dunedin Longitudinal Study. Cambridge University Press, Cambridge.

Molenaar, P.C.M., Boomsma, D.I. & Dolan, C.V. (1993) A third source of developmental differences. *Behavior Genetics*, **23**, 519–524.

Nadder, T.S., Silberg, J.L., Maes, H.H., Rutter, M. & Eaves, L.J. (in press) Genetic effects on the variation and covariation of ADHD and ODD/CD symptomatologies across informant and occasion of measurement. *Psychological Medicine*.

Nelson, C.A. & Bloom, F.E. (1997) Child development and neuroscience. *Child Development*, **68**, 970–987.

O'Brien, P.M.S., Wheeler, T. & Barker, D.J.P. (eds) (1999) *Fetal Programming: Influences on Development and Disease in Later Life*. Royal College of Obstetricians and Gynaecologists Press, London.

O'Connor, T.G., Bredenkamp, D., Rutter, M. & the English and Romanian Adoptees (ERA) Study Team (1999) Attachment disturbances and disorders in children exposed to early severe deprivation. *Infant Mental Health Journal*, 20, 10–29.

O'Connor, T., Rutter, M., Beckett, C., Keaveney, L., Kreppner, J.M. & the English and Romanian Adoptees (ERA) Study Team (2000a) The effects of global severe privation on cognitive competence: extension and longitudinal follow-up. *Child Development*, 71, 376–390.

O'Connor, T., Rutter, M. & the English and Romanian Adoptees Study Team (2000b) Attachment disorder behavior following early severe deprivation: extension and longitudinal follow-up. *Journal of the American Academy of Child and Adolescent Psychiatry*, 39, 703–712.

Patton, G.C., Johnson-Sabine, E., Wood, K., Mann, A.H. & Wakeling, A. (1990) Abnormal eating attitudes in London schoolgirls: a prospective epidemiological study: outcome at twelve month follow-up. *Psychological Medicine*, 20, 383–394.

Patton, G.C., Carlin, J.B., Shao, Q. *et al.* (1997) Adolescent dieting: healthy weight control or borderline eating disorders? *Journal of Child Psychology and Psychiatry*, 38, 299–306.

Patton, G.C., Selzer, R., Coffey, C., Carlin, J.B. & Wolfe, R. (1999) Onset of adolescent eating disorders: population based cohort study over 3 years. *British Medical Journal*, 318, 765–768.

Pickles, A., Crouchley, R., Simonoff, E. *et al.* (1994) Survival models for developmental genetic data: age of onset of puberty and antisocial behavior in twins. *Genetic Epidemiology*, 11, 155–170.

Post, R.M. (1992) Transduction of psychosocial stress into the neurobiology of recurrent affective disorder. *American Journal of Psychiatry*, 149, 999–1010.

Quinton, D., Pickles, A., Maughan, B. & Rutter, M. (1993) Partners, peers, and pathways: assortative pairing and continuities in conduct disorder. *Development and Psychopathology*, 5, 763–783.

Rao, U., Ryan, N.D., Dahl, R.E. *et al.* (1999) Factors associated with the development of substance use disorder in depressed adolescents. *Journal of the American Academy of Child and Adolescent Psychiatry*, 38, 1109–1117.

Richardson, S.A. & Koller, H. (1996) *Twenty-Two Years: Causes and Consequences of Mental Retardation*. Harvard University Press, Cambridge, MA.

Robins, L.N. (1993) The sixth Thomas James Okey Memorial Lecture. Vietnam veterans' rapid recovery from heroin addiction: a fluke or normal expectation? *Addiction*, 88, 1041–1054.

Robins, L.N. & McEvoy, L. (1990) Conduct problems as predictors of substance abuse. In: *Straight and Devious Pathways from Childhood to Adulthood* (eds L. Robins & M. Rutter), pp. 182–204. Cambridge University Press, Cambridge.

Roy, P., Rutter, M. & Pickles, A. (2000) Institutional care: risk from family background or pattern of rearing? *Journal of Child Psychology and Psychiatry*, 41, 139–149.

Rubinow, D.R. & Schmidt, P.J. (1996) Androgens, brain, and behavior. *American Journal of Psychiatry*, 153, 974–984.

Ruble, D.N. & Martin, C.L. (1998) Gender development. In: *Handbook of Child Psychology*, Vol. 3, *Social, Emotional, and Personality Development* (eds W. Damon & N. Eisenberg), 5th edn, pp. 933–1016. John Wiley & Sons, New York.

Ruda, M.A., Ling, Q.-D., Hohmann, A.G., Peng, Y.B. & Tachibana, T. (2000) Altered nociceptive neuronal circuits after neonatal peripheral inflammation. *Science*, 289, 628–631.

Rutter, M. (1970) Autistic children: infancy to adulthood. *Seminars in Psychiatry*, 2, 435–450.

Rutter, M. (1979) Separation experiences: a new look at an old topic. *Journal of Pediatrics*, 95, 147–154.

Rutter, M. (1981a) *Maternal Deprivation Reassessed*, 2nd edn. Penguin, Harmondsworth.

Rutter, M. (1981b) Stress, coping and development: some issues and some questions. *Journal of Child Psychology and Psychiatry*, 22, 323–356.

Rutter, M. (1987) The 'what' and 'how' of language development: a note on some outstanding issues and questions. In: *Language Development and Disorders* (eds W. Yule & M. Rutter), pp. 159–170. MacKeith Press, London.

Rutter, M. (1989a) Pathways from childhood to adult life. *Journal of Child Psychology and Psychiatry*, 30, 23–51.

Rutter, M. (1989b) Age as an ambiguous variable in developmental research: some epidemiological considerations from developmental psychopathology. *International Journal of Behavioral Development*, 12, 1–34.

Rutter, M. (1993) An overview of developmental neuropsychiatry. *Educational and Child Psychology*, 10, 4–11.

Rutter, M. (1994) Continuities, transitions and turning points in development. In: *Development Through Life: a Handbook for Clinicians* (eds M. Rutter & D.F. Hay), pp. 1–25. Blackwell Scientific Publications, Oxford.

Rutter, M. (1996a) Developmental psychopathology: concepts and prospects. In: *Frontiers of Developmental Psychopathology* (eds M.F. Lenzenweger & J.J. Haugaard), pp. 209–237. Oxford University Press, New York.

Rutter, M. (1996b) Transitions and turning points in developmental psychopathology: as applied to the age span between childhood and mid-adulthood. *International Journal of Behavioral Development*, 19, 603–626.

Rutter, M. (1999) Resilience concepts and findings: implications for family therapy. *Journal of Family Therapy*, 21, 119–144.

Rutter, M. (2000a) Psychosocial influences: critiques, findings, and research needs. *Development and Psychopathology*, 12, 375–405.

Rutter, M. (2000b) Resilience reconsidered: conceptual considerations, empirical findings, and policy implications. In: *Handbook of Early Childhood Intervention* (eds J.P. Shonkoff & S.J. Meisels), pp. 651–682. Cambridge University Press, New York.

Rutter, M. (in press) Nature, nurture and development: From evangelism through science towards policy and practice, *Child Development*.

Rutter, M. & Rutter, M. (1993) *Developing Minds: Challenge and Continuity Across the Lifespan*. Penguin, Harmondsworth/Basic Books, New York.

Rutter, M. & Sroufe, L.A. (2000) Developmental psychopathology: concepts and challenges. *Development and Psychopathology*, 12, 265–296.

Rutter, M., Izard, C.E. & Read, P.B., eds (1986) *Depression in Young People: Developmental and Clinical Perspectives*. Guilford Press, New York.

Rutter, M., Silberg, J. & Simonoff, E. (1993) Whither behavioral genetics? A developmental psychopathological perspective. In: *Nature, Nurture, and Psychology* (eds R. Plomin & G.E. McClearn), pp. 433–456. APA Books, Washington D.C.

Rutter, M., Maughan, B., Meyer, J. *et al.* (1997) Heterogeneity of antisocial behavior: causes, continuities, and consequences. In: *Nebraska Symposium on Motivation*, Vol. 44, *Motivation and Delinquency* (eds R. Dienstbier & D.W. Osgood), pp. 45–118. University of Nebraska Press, Lincoln, NB.

Rutter, M., Maughan, B., Pickles, A. & Simonoff, E. (1998a) Retrospective recall recalled. In: *Methods and Models for Studying the Individual Essays in Honor of Marian Radke-Yarrow* (eds R.B. Cairns, L.R. Bergman & J. Kagan), pp. 219–242. Sage Publications, Thousand Oaks, CA.

Rutter, M., Giller, H. & Hagell, A. (1998b) *Antisocial Behavior by Young People*. Cambridge University Press, New York.

Rutter, M. & the English and Romanian Adoptees (ERA) Study Team (1998c) Developmental catch-up, and deficit, following adoption after severe global early privation. *Journal of Child Psychology and Psychiatry*, **39**, 465–476.

Rutter, M., O'Connor, T., Beckett, C. *et al.* (2000b) Recovery and deficit following profound early deprivation. In: *Intercountry Adoption: Developments, Trends and Perspectives* (ed. P. Selman), pp. 107–125. British Association for Adoption and Fostering, London.

Rutter, M., Kreppner, J., O'Connor, T. & the English and Romanian Adoptees (ERA) Study Team (2000a) Risk and resilience following profound early global privation. *British Journal of Psychiatry Special Issue*,

Rutter, M., O'Connor, T., & the English and Romanian Adoptees Research Team (submitted). Are there biological programming effects for psychological development? Findings from a study of Romanian adoptees.

Rutter, M., Roy, P. & Kreppner, J. (in press) Institutional care as a risk factor for inattention/overactivity. In: *Hyperactivity and Attention Deficits in childhood* (ed. S. Sandberg), 2nd edn. Cambridge University Press, Cambridge.

Sampson, R.J. & Laub, J.H. (1993) *Crime in the Making: Pathways and Turning Points Through Life*. Harvard University Press, Cambridge, MA.

Scharff, C., Kirn, J.R., Grossman, M., Macklis, J.D. & Nottebohm, F. (2000) Targeted neuronal death affects neuronal replacement and vocal behavior in adult songbirds. *Neuron*, **25**, 481–492.

Schneider, M.L., Roughton, E.C. & Lubach, G.R. (1997) Moderate alcohol consumption and psychological stress during pregnancy induce attention and neuromotor impairments in primate infants. *Child Development*, **68**, 747–759.

Schneider, M.L., Roughton, E.C., Koehler, A.J. & Lubach, G.R. (1999) Growth and development following prenatal stress exposure in primates: an examination of ontogenetic vulnerability. *Child Development*, **70**, 263–274.

Silberg, J., Meyer, J., Pickles, A. *et al.* (1996) Heterogeneity among juvenile antisocial behaviours: findings from the Virginia Twin Study of Adolescent Behavioural Development. In: *Genetics of Criminal and Antisocial Behaviour, Ciba Foundation Symposium 194* (eds G.R. Bock & J.A. Goode), pp. 76–86. John Wiley & Sons, Chichester.

Silberg, J., Pickles, A., Rutter, M. *et al.* (1999) The influence of genetic factors and life stress on depression among adolescent girls. *Archives of General Psychiatry*, **56**, 225–232.

Silberg, J., Rutter, M., Neale, M. & Eaves, L. (2001) Genetic moderation of environmental risk for depression and anxiety in adolescent girls. *British Journal of Psychiatry*, **179**, 116–121.

Sroufe, L.A. & Rutter, M. (1984) The domain of developmental psychopathology. *Child Development*, **55**, 17–29.

Stattin, H. & Magnusson, D. (1990) *Pubertal Maturation in Female Development*. Erlbaum, Hillsdale, NJ.

Stratton, K., Howe, C. & Battaglia, F. (1996) *Fetal Alcohol Syndrome: Diagnosis, Epidemiology, Prevention, and Treatment*. National Academy Press, Washington D.C.

Streissguth, A.P. & Kanter, J. (1997) *The Challenge of Fetal Alcohol Syndrome: Overcoming Secondary Disabilities*. University of Washington Press, Seattle.

Szmukler, G.I., Eisler, I., Gillies, C. & Hayward, M.E. (1985) The implications of anorexia nervosa in a ballet school. *Journal of Psychiatric Research*, **19**, 177–181.

Tarrant, C.J. & Jones, P.B. (2000) Biological markers as precursors to schizophrenia: specificity, predictive ability, and etiological significance. In: *Childhood Onset of 'Adult' Psychopathology: Clinical and Research Advances* (ed. J.L. Rapoport), pp. 65–102. American Psychiatric Press, Washington D.C.

Teasdale, J.D. & Barnard, P.J. (1993) *Affect, Cognition, and Change: Re-Modelling Depressive Thought*. Erlbaum, Hove.

Thapar, A. & McGuffin, P. (1994) A twin study of depressive symptoms in childhood. *British Journal of Psychiatry*, **165**, 259–265.

Thompson, R.A. (1998) Early sociopersonality development. In: *Handbook of Child Psychology*, Vol. 3, *Social, Emotional, and Personality Development* (eds W. Damon & N. Eisenberg), 5th edn, pp. 25–104. John Wiley & Sons, New York.

Tremblay, R.E., Schaal, B., Boulerice, B. & Pérusse, D. (1997) Male physical aggression, social dominance and testosterone levels at puberty: a developmental perspective. In: *Unlocking Crime: the Biosocial Key* (eds A. Raine, P. Brennan, D.P. Farrington & S.A. Mednick), pp. 271–292. Plenum, New York.

Tulving, E. (1983) *Elements of Episodic Memory*. Oxford University Press, New York.

Vanyukov, M.M. & Tarter, R.E. (2000) Genetic studies of substance abuse. *Drug and Alcohol Dependence*, **59**, 101–123.

Vargha-Khadem, F., Isaacs, E., van der Werf, S., Robb, S. & Wilson, J. (1992) Development of intelligence and memory in children with hemiplegic cerebral palsy: the deleterious consequences of early seizures. *Brain*, **115**, 315–329.

Vogel, F. & Motulsky, A.G. (1997) *Human Genetics: Problems and Approaches*, 3rd edn. Springer-Verlag. Berlin.

Waldrop, M.F. & Halverson, C.F. Jr (1971) Minor physical anomalies and hyperactive behavior in young children. In: *Exceptional Infant*, Vol. 2, *Studies in Abnormalities* (ed. J. Hellmuth), pp. 343–380. Brunner/Mazel, New York.

Weinberger, D.R. (1987) Implications of normal brain development for the pathogenesis of schizophrenia. *Archives of General Psychiatry*, **44**, 660–669.

Weissman, M.M., Wolk, S., Wickramaratne, P. *et al.* (1999a) Children with prepubertal-onset major depressive disorder and anxiety grown up. *Archives of General Psychiatry*, **56**, 794–801.

Weissman, M.M., Wolk, S., Goldstein, R.B. *et al.* (1999b) Depressed adolescents grown up. *Journal of the American Medical Association*, **281**, 1707–1713.

Westergaard, T., Mortensen, P.B., Pedersen, C.B., Wohlfahrt, J. & Melbye, M. (1999) Exposure to prenatal and childhood infections and the risk of schizophrenia: suggestions from a study of sibship characteristics and influenza prevalence. *Archives of General Psychiatry*, **56**, 993–998.

Zoccolillo, M., Pickles, A., Quinton, D. & Rutter, M. (1992) The outcome of childhood conduct disorder: implications for defining adult personality disorder and conduct disorder. *Psychological Medicine*, **22**, 971–986.

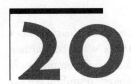

20 Child Abuse

Robert E. Emery and Lisa Laumann-Billings

Introduction

In this chapter, we discuss physical child abuse, neglect and psychological abuse, although for the sake of brevity, we frequently use the term 'abuse' to refer collectively to these three subtypes. We also distinguish between *child violence* (abuse that causes serious harm to a child) and *child maltreatment* (abuse that causes little or no serious harm). Child sexual abuse is covered by Glaser (Chapter 21).

Child abuse is a distressingly prevalent problem. The abuse of children has been ignored historically, and instances of abuse continue to be overlooked, minimized or wrongly perceived as minor, both in individual cases and in entire countries. The minimization of child abuse can lead to tragic results for individual children and for groups of children growing up in harmful and hurtful societal circumstances. Thus, the overriding goal of this chapter is to address the most important empirical, clinical and policy concerns in relation to the unacceptably high prevalence of child abuse and its adverse consequences for children. Shockingly, much of the world has yet to accept that child abuse is a widespread problem, and legal policies in many countries and social practices in many cultures continue to tolerate extreme acts of physical injury and/or neglect of children.

We also raise some cautions about the potential for overreaching in research and practice in regard to the emotionally and politically charged topic of child abuse, particularly in the USA. As we have detailed elsewhere (Emery & Laumann-Billings 1998), many estimates of the prevalence or incidence of abuse use broad definitions that include identified cases that depart widely from the everyday connotations of the term 'abuse'. In addition, evidence on aetiology highlights the contributions of life stress to the risk for abuse, while research on the consequences of abuse underscores the importance of considering the influence of third variables, such as troubled parenting. These empirical findings lead us to suggest that, especially in the USA, well-intentioned efforts have come to focus too much on physical abuse *per se*, and not enough on the correlates of abuse, such as social isolation, poverty, parenting problems and family adversity. Finally, and most importantly, we suggest that a balanced perspective on the problem of child abuse can lead to improved intervention. In the USA, law, policy and many treatment efforts have come to focus on policing abusive families to the exclusion of efforts to support these families under stress. Evidence on child abuse leads us to conclude that, whereas some families do require policing, many would benefit from a more supportive stance in direct intervention and in broader policies, as has been the practice in the UK and much of Western Europe.

Because of problems at the extremes of ignoring abuse, and of overinclusive definitions, we have proposed that abuse should be divided into two levels of seriousness: child maltreatment and child violence (Emery & Laumann-Billings 1998). *Child maltreatment* involves intentional acts or omissions on the part of a caregiver that lead to minimal physical or psychological harm or endangerment of the child, whereas *child violence* involves intentional acts or omissions on the part of a caregiver that result in serious physical injury or profound psychological trauma (Emery & Laumann-Billings 1998). We recognize that numerous problems arise in defining the boundary between these two categories of abuse, and we only briefly address that thorny issue here. Nevertheless, as we review in this chapter, the distinction is supported by epidemiological studies, research on the causes and consequences of child abuse, and by the radically different intervention practices associated with the contrasting philosophies of whether abusive individuals and families should be policed or supported.

Definitions of child abuse

There are no universal legal or scientific definitions of child physical abuse, neglect or psychological abuse (Korbin 1997), but a useful starting point is to consider a general definition of each problem. The legal definition of physical child abuse in our home state of Virginia (USA) is:

> A physical injury, threat of injury or creation of a real and significant danger of substantial risk of death, disfigurement or impairment of bodily functions. Such injury or threat of injury, regardless of intent, is inflicted or allowed to be inflicted by non-accidental means.

The state of Virginia actually defines six separate types of child neglect/psychological abuse: physical neglect; medical neglect; failure to thrive; mental abuse/neglect; educational neglect; and bizarre discipline. Physical neglect is defined as 'the failure to provide food, clothing, shelter or supervision for a child to the extent that the child's health or safety is endangered.' The state of Virginia defines mental abuse/neglect as 'a pattern of acts or omissions by the caregiver which result in harm to a child's psychological or emotional health or development.'

These definitions of abuse are typical of law in the USA (which can differ from state to state), and the definitions clearly include many acts of violence. However, the definitions of physical abuse, neglect and mental abuse also are very broad, and problems of overinclusiveness become apparent when we consider them more closely. A literal interpretation might define spanking as an act of physical abuse, while the existence of a behaviour problem in a child could be interpreted to be sufficient to consider the child as psychologically abused.

Given the very broad nature of such definitions, it is hardly surprising that operational definitions of child abuse for research and practice are the source of much scientific, legal and cultural controversy (Straus & Gelles 1990; Wald 1991; Finkelhor 1995). In the USA, statutory definitions differ from state to state (Wang & Harding 1999), and broad differences in the definition of abuse and neglect are found across the world. For example, in Sweden, Finland and Norway (but not Denmark), the corporal punishment of children by teachers and parents is illegal (Roberts 2000). At the other extreme, China has no government programmes to identify or prevent child abuse, no legal mechanisms for removing children from abusive homes and, in fact, even cases of infanticide can be overlooked under the 'one couple, one child' regime (Littlewood 1997; Fitzgibbon 1998).

Intermediate examples include Japan, where corporal punishment by parents and teachers remains common, and recent governmental efforts to address child abuse have been impeded by a strong tradition of family privacy (Kozu 1999; WuDunn 1999). In 1994, for example, only 1961 cases of abuse were officially reported in Japan, and only one case resulted in the loss of custody rights (Kozu 1999). In England, child abuse is defined similarly as in the USA, but the social service system tends to focus more on the provision of services than on the identification of abuse. For example, home visiting programmes are universal in England but scattered in the USA and, in contrast to the USA, the reporting of suspected cases of abuse is not mandatory in England (although failure to report may lead to disciplinary actions; Berridge 1997).

Such observations make it clear that definitions of child abuse are based on social judgements, not immutable objective standards (Emery 1989). It is also true that definitions of abuse can vary depending upon their purpose. For instance, demographers often employ broad definitions when assessing the prevalence of maltreatment in the general population, whereas child protection workers more typically apply a stringent definition when recommending coercive interventions for abusive parents. Such differences are understandable but, at least for research purposes, there is a need for a consensual *operational* definition of different categories of child abuse in order to facilitate communication and avoid misunderstanding (National Research Council 1993). The importance of such a definition becomes evident in examining evidence on the epidemiology of child abuse.

Epidemiology of child abuse

Child abuse is disturbingly common, even given the most stringent definition: an estimated 1200–1500 children (0.018 per 1000 children) are killed in the USA each year by their parent or parent figure (Sedlak & Broadhurst 1996; Wang & Harding 1999). However, extreme instances of child abuse comprise only a minority of identified cases in epidemiological studies. For example, consider the National Incidence Studies (NIS) that are based on official reports of child abuse and surveys of a nationally representative US sample of community professionals who come in contact with maltreated children (e.g. teachers, paediatricians). These studies are widely regarded as among the best estimates of child abuse incidence. The third survey (NIS-3; Sedlak & Broadhurst 1996) estimated that between 1.5 and 2.8 million children (23–42 per 1000) in the USA were abused in 1993. The lower figure is obtained when abuse is defined as acts or omissions that result in demonstrable harm to a child, whereas the higher figure includes all of these children, plus children who were in danger of being harmed according to the views of community professionals and Child Protection Services (CPS) agencies.

The more serious (demonstrable harm) cases in NIS-3 were divided into serious, moderate and inferred categories. Serious injury was defined as 'a life-threatening condition or long-term impairment of physical, mental, or emotional capacities, or requiring professional treatment aimed at preventing such long-term impairment.' Moderate injury was defined as an injury that 'persisted in observable form (including pain or impairment) for at least 48 h (e.g. bruises, depression, or emotional distress not serious enough to require professional treatment).' Inferred harm was defined as 'the nature of the maltreatment itself gave reasonable cause to assume the injury or impairment probably occurred' (Sedlak & Broadhurst 1996, chapter 3, pp. 13–14).

Figure 20.1 illustrates how the NIS-3 estimates break down in terms of the number of cases in different categories of abuse, and the figure also includes a rating of the seriousness of abuse within each category. Consideration of this figure indicates, to the present authors at least, a pattern that seems inconsistent with everyday assumptions about the prevalence of child abuse.

First, consider the general categories of abuse (pie chart). Emotional abuse and educational neglect are the most common forms of abuse, whereas physical abuse comprises about one-quarter of all cases. Regular school attendance is obviously essential to children, but we are dubious about the benefits of terming educational neglect as 'abuse'. Secondly, consider further that only about 15% of cases of physical abuse were designated serious (bar chart). In 85% of the cases, a parent's punishment left the child with an observable bruise, pain or emotional distress that lasted at least 48 h, but professional treatment was not required (Sedlak & Broadhurst 1996). We do not condone, for example, a hard spanking that leaves a temporary mark, but such acts seem to differ from the popular conception of child abuse. In both the academic literature and the popular media, it is common, for example, to cite a statistic indicating a very high prevalence of child abuse followed by a case example of physical abuse involving torture. Such a pairing is misleading, and we believe that distorted popular ideas about

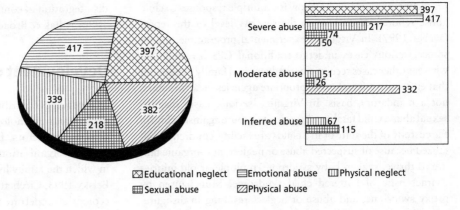

Fig. 20.1 A close look at subtypes of abuse (pie chart) and severity ratings within each type (bar chart) indicates that the category 'child abuse' is a broad one that includes many actions outside of the usual connotations of the term. Data are based on the Third National Incidence Study of Child Abuse and Neglect (Sedlak & Broadhurst 1996), a leading epidemiological study of child abuse in the United States conducted in 1993. Number of cases are presented in 1000s; all cases of educational and emotional abuse were severe by definition.

the severity of the more typical cases of child abuse can handcuff intervention efforts by generating only public wrath and no compassion for maltreating parents under stress (discussed below). We are not arguing that we should only be concerned with the 50 000 (0.74 per 1000 children) cases of severe physical abuse. However, we are arguing that commonly touted prevalence figures are misleading unless abuse is defined with great care.

The same sort of analysis can be applied to official reports of abuse in the USA. For example, the National Center on Child Abuse Prevention Research (NCCAPR) 50 State Survey found approximately 3 million cases (45 per 1000 children) of *reported* child abuse in the USA in 1998, but only one-third (1 009 000 or 15 per 1000 children) were *substantiated*, that is, determined by a case worker to have sufficient probability of abuse (Wang & Harding 1999). Moreover, the majority of the substantiated cases involved neglect (54%), the form of maltreatment most clearly associated with poverty (Pelton 1992). About one-fifth of the substantiated cases were of physical abuse, 10% were primarily sexual abuse, 3% were emotional maltreatment, and 14% did not clearly fall into any of these categories (Wang & Harding 1999).

Variations in reported cases across countries also reflect differences in definitions. Gilbert (1997) compiled child abuse reporting for various Western European and North American countries. Reporting rates ranged from a high of 43 per 1000 children in the USA to a low of 2.9 per 1000 children in Belgium. Rates in the province of Ontario, Germany, England (estimated), and the Netherlands were 21, 15, 13.6, and 4.9 per 1000 children, respectively. Cross-national comparisons are complicated not only by different definitions of abuse, but also by reporting laws (or the absence of reporting laws), the method of data collection and more general cultural factors. Nevertheless, the variations again call attention to the fact that the term 'abuse' is ill-defined, and in the USA at least, applied broadly at the reporting phase.

Reporting differences indicate large variations in definitions of child abuse, but they do not indicate with precision where a line is drawn between abuse and acceptable (if perhaps inadequate or problematic) parenting. One of the clearest sources

of evidence in the USA about specific acts that may be deemed abusive comes from a Gallup poll of a random, representative sample of 1000 families. The poll concluded that approximately 5% of children had been physically abused in the previous year. However, different rates can be computed for different operational definitions because the poll identified very specific acts. For instance, for those who consider spanking to be abusive (Finkelhor & Dziuba-Leatherman 1994), an estimated two-thirds of children in the USA are victims. When violence is defined as hitting with an object other than on the bottom (the definition used in the Gallup poll), the rate drops to 5%. The rate drops to about one-tenth of that level if one were to use a definition of serious physical abuse that included hitting with a fist, kicking hard, or beating up a child (Gallup *et al.* 1995).

Distinguishing levels of abuse

We do not encourage spanking or condone parental acts that hurt a child physically or emotionally. We do suggest, however, that the term 'abuse' connotes serious physical or psychological harm, yet mild to moderate acts account for most cases of abuse in most epidemiological surveys. Furthermore, most parents currently labelled as abusive are under a great deal of stress, and they are not endangering their children's long-term physical health and safety. Such families are more likely to benefit from interventions designed to support them through the challenges of parenting, not from interventions that first label them as abusive. Distinguishing between what we have termed child maltreatment vs. child violence could be an important step on the path to providing supportive interventions to those who might benefit from support, while pursuing forceful coercive interventions in the most serious cases.

In arguing for this distinction, we realize that there is not a 'bright line' between maltreatment and violence and that any specific definitions immediately create controversy. For these reasons, we offer no preferred definitions here. Instead, we note that a handful of states in the USA, including Virginia, Missouri, Florida, Iowa, North Dakota, South Dakota and Kentucky, are experimenting with fundamentally altering their child protection programmes to allow for multiple responses to child abuse reports, depending on the severity level of the report (Weber 1997). In Virginia's experimental programme, for instance, serious cases undergo traditional CPS investigation, whereas other cases receive a non-adversarial family assessment that ends with referrals to appropriate agencies on a voluntary, not a mandatory, basis. In Virginia, 'serious' cases include: sexual abuse, child fatality, allegations of abuse against a child in the custody of the state or in a child care facility, children hospitalized because of suspected abuse or neglect, non-organic failure to thrive, shaken baby syndrome, multiple or old injuries characteristic of battered child syndrome, Münchausen by proxy syndrome, and abuse or neglect resulting in disfigurement, fracture, severe burn or laceration, mutilation, maiming, forced ingestion of a dangerous substance, or life-threatening internal injuries. All other cases—the majority of CPS referrals—are offered assessment, and referral to other community agencies for supportive services (Community Partnerships for Protecting Children 1996).

Is family violence increasing?

In 1976, 669 000 cases of child abuse were reported to social service agencies in the USA (Besharov & Laumann 1996) but that number grew steadily to 3 154 000 reports in 1998 (Wang & Harding 1999). Similar increases in reports of child abuse were noted in the UK and other European countries during this time (Hess 1995). Much of the increased reporting was a result of increased recognition of child abuse, and this represents an important social achievement in these countries—one that needs to be repeated elsewhere in the world. In the USA, however, dramatic increases in child abuse reporting have created a new problem as they have solved an old one. Social service agencies are so overwhelmed with investigating reports of abuse, most of which go unsubstantiated, that they are left with few resources to offer supportive interventions (US Advisory Board on Child Abuse and Neglect 1993). In fact, as policing families for abuse has increasingly dominated social service agencies since the 1970s, the philosophy of offering support to families in need has been lost (Besharov & Laumann 1997). Thus, another reason to differentiate maltreatment from violence is the potential to reduce the resources devoted to adversary investigation and redirect efforts into supportive family interventions.

Although increased reporting largely reflects greater public concern with child abuse, there may have been some real increase in child abuse in recent years. The number of cases of moderate child abuse remained stable between 1986 and 1993 in the NIS, but the number of *serious* cases quadrupled from 142 000 to 565 000 (Sedlak & Broadhurst 1996). The number of cases of 'grave concern' also increased in the UK in the late 1980s (Hess 1995). If the increase was solely caused by 'definitional creep' (Besharov 1996), one would expect increases across all levels of severity. Researchers who believe that serious abuse is rising attribute the growing problem to increased use of illegal drugs, greater poverty, increased overall violence and the disintegration of communities (Garbarino 1995; Lung & Daro 1996; Sedlak & Broadhurst 1996).

Development of child abuse

Many factors contribute to the development of physical abuse, neglect and psychological maltreatment, including individual personality factors, family interaction patterns, poverty and social disorganization, acute stressors, and the cultural context in which the family lives (Bronfenbrenner 1979; Vondra 1990; Belsky 1993; Cicchetti & Toth 1995). Bronfenbrenner's (1979) ecological model often has been used to integrate research on the multiple risks at four levels of analysis:

1 individual characteristics;
2 the immediate social context;
3 the broader ecological context; and
4 the societal/cultural context.

We briefly review research on each of these broad topics in the following sections. For the most part, the risk factors we review apply to physical abuse, neglect and psychological abuse, although we occasionally note exceptions.

Individual characteristics

Personality factors, such as low self-esteem, poor impulse control, external locus of control, negative affectivity and heightened response to stress, all increase the likelihood of child abuse (Pianta *et al.* 1989). Alcohol and/or drug dependence also play a part as both a background risk factor for all forms of child abuse and as an immediate precipitant of physical abuse (Kantor & Straus 1990). Although evidence is less consistent, some research has also suggested that child abuse *victims* share some common characteristics, including poor physical or mental health, behavioural deviancies and difficult temperament or personality features (Belsky 1993). The child's age also seems to have a crucial role. Children are at greatest risk for physical abuse and neglect between the ages of 3 months and 3 years, with a second peak in physical and psychological abuse during adolescence (Azar & Wolfe 1998). The increased risk for these age groups may be related to the developmentally related oppositional behaviour that both age groups display. This is supported by findings that physical and psychological abuse is commonly associated with child disciplinary situations that involve aversive child behaviours (e.g. non-compliance, aggressive behaviour, uncontrollable crying; Herrenkohl *et al.* 1983).

Related to this, there is evidence to suggest that child abusers may differ from non-abusers in how they perceive their children, being more prone to cognitive distortions and deficits concerning their children's behaviour. Specifically, studies have found that abusive parents tend to ascribe greater negative intentionality to their children's behaviour than do normal parents, even when the behaviour is within developmental norms (Larrance & Twentyman 1983; Plotkin 1983). Similarly, other studies have found that abusive parents have more unrealistic expectations of what is developmentally appropriate behaviour in their children (e.g. 3-month-olds can stop crying on demand; Azar *et al.* 1984; Azar & Rohrbeck 1986). Abusive parents also tend to find their child's behaviour more stressful than parents who are not abusive (Frodi & Lamb 1980; Susman *et al.* 1985).

Substance abuse has been found to have a role in both the onset as well as the continuation of both child physical abuse and neglect (Kelleher *et al.* 1994; Harrington *et al.* 1995; Chaffin *et al.* 1996). In her review of the literature, Widom (1992) found alcoholism rates ranging from 18 to 45% in child-maltreating parents, which are much higher than matched controls. Substance abuse has also been shown to be a common outcome of the effects of early maltreatment in adulthood (Duncan *et al.* 1996). The association between alcohol abuse and family violence is complicated, involving the interplay of a number of other variables including personality style, the nature of the relationship, the type of alcohol problem and the degree of family conflict (Widom 1992; Murphy & O'Farrell 1994). An important question for further study is whether heavy alcohol use disinhibits aggression, interacting with personality type to predict violence (Murphy & O'Farrell 1994), or whether aggressive personality-types act violently whether or not they are drinking (Pernanen 1991).

Research also indicates that children who are victims of abuse are at an increased risk for becoming violent themselves as adults (Widom 1989). It is important to note that only a minority of physically abused or neglected children (perhaps one-third) go on to become violent in their own families (Kaufman & Zigler 1987; Widom 1989; Malinosky-Rummel & Hansen 1993). Furthermore, some (or much) of the familiality of family violence may be accounted for by genetic rather than environmental risk (DiLalla & Gottesman 1991).

Immediate context

Characteristics of the immediate social context, especially the family, have important implications for the aetiology or perpetuation of child abuse (Emery 1989). Studies have examined a host of contributing factors, including family structure and size, acute stressors (e.g. the loss of a job or death in the family) and characteristic styles of resolving conflicts or parenting.

Research on family stress illustrates this area of investigation. In one of the few prospective studies of child abuse, Egeland *et al.* (1981) found that the number of stressful life events distinguished families who were reported for child abuse. However, most stressed families did not abuse their children; thus it was essential to distinguish stressed families who abused from those who did not. Holding life stress constant, abusers were found to be more aggressive, anxious and defensive, and less succorant, than their non-maltreating counterparts. Similar findings were found in later work (Egeland *et al.* 1988). Thus, it seems clear that coping style, as well as stress, contributes to the development of family violence.

High levels of marital conflict and aggression are also associated with child abuse (Straus & Gelles 1990; Cummings 1997).

A recent study found that in 30–60% of families where wife-battering is occurring, physical child abuse also occurred (Edelson 1999). This may be because the escalation of emotional arousal that often accompanies adult conflict carries over to interactions with the child. This is not surprising as marital conflicts most often arise over disagreements over child-rearing, discipline, and each parent's responsibilities in child care (Edleson *et al.* 1991). Children may be caught in the conflict between parents, or they may precipitate parental arguments by misbehaving (Jaffe *et al.* 1990).

Broader ecological context

Physical child abuse, and especially neglect and psychological maltreatment, are related to qualities of the community in which the family is embedded, such as poverty, absence of family services, social isolation and the lack of social cohesion in the community. As Garbarino & Kostelny (1992, p. 463) have noted, child abuse is 'a social as well as a psychological indicator'. The relation between poverty, social isolation and child abuse has now been well established across all categories of abuse (Garbarino 1977; Garbarino & Sherman 1980; Pelton 1981; Polansky *et al.* 1985; Zuravin 1989; Garbarino & Kostelny 1992; Gelles 1992; Pan *et al.* 1994). High levels of unemployment, inadequate housing, daily stresses and community violence also contribute to an increased risk.

Most poor parents do not abuse their children (Garbarino 1977; Bronfenbrenner 1979), so this relation is not simple or direct. Garbarino *et al.* have consistently shown that the principal difference between poor families who do and do not abuse their children lies in the degree of social cohesion and mutual caring found in their communities (Garbarino & Crouter 1978; Garbarino & Kostelny 1992; Coulton *et al.* 1995). For example, neighbourhoods with high concentrations of child abuse or neglect reports tend to suffer from severe social disorganization and lack of community identity. They also have higher rates of juvenile delinquency, drug trafficking and violent crime (Coulton *et al.* 1995).

Social isolation is one of the most commonly noted features of maltreating families (Gabarino & Kostelny 1992). Maltreating parents often lack social connections to others in their extended family, the neighbourhood, the community, and the social agencies most likely to provide needed assistance (Furstenburg 1993; Korbin 1994). Neglectful families are especially prone to isolation and insularity (Wolfe 1999). Some contend that individual personality factors cause this sense of social isolation and that selection factors contribute to these individuals living in more chaotic neighbourhoods (Polansky *et al.* 1985), but others argue that the causal arrow points in the opposite direction (Vondra 1990; Garbarino & Kostelny 1992; Cicchetti & Lynch 1993).

Societal or cultural context

A number of commentators contend that family violence is perpetuated by the broad cultural beliefs and values (e.g. the use of physical punishment, extremes in family privacy, and violence) in the popular media (Garbarino 1977; Vondra 1990; Finkelhor & Dziuba-Leatherman 1994). As discussed earlier, some of these differences are reflected in the differing cross-national rates of reports of child abuse and in countries' different approaches to intervening in the problem and supporting families under stress. Societal policies may not *cause* family violence, but some practices appear to condone it. Unfortunately, there is little sound empirical evidence on how broad social policies and cultural practices affect the incidence of abuse.

Biological factors

Although they are often overlooked, biological factors clearly contribute to the aetiology of child abuse, both in terms of normative human propensities and individual differences in behaviour (Daly & Wilson 1980, 1988, 1995; Burgess et al. 1983; Burgess & Draper 1989; Malkin & Lamb 1994). In regard to normative increases in child abuse, evolutionary psychologists have pointed to the role of biological relatedness as one key risk (or protective) factor. As a dramatic example, Daly & Wilson (1988) reported that step-parents were responsible for a drastically higher rate of homicide of children in comparison to biological parents. Differences in risk were truly astronomical (a 10 000% or even greater increase; Daly & Wilson 1988, see fig. 1, p. 520) for infants and preschool-age children, who in general are at much greater risk of homicide than are older children. Even as we point to the fact that step-parents are over-represented among abusive parents, we also want to underscore that, while step-parenting poses many normative struggles, the majority of step-parents have good relationships with their stepchildren (Booth & Dunn 1994; Hetherington et al. 1998).

The evolutionary psychology approach offers an innovative framework for conceptualizing other contributing causes of child abuse (Daly & Wilson 1982, 1985, 1996b; Burgess et al. 1983). For example, the evolutionary perspective offers a thought-provoking twist on the well-documented link between poverty and child neglect (Pelton 1981, 1989; Straus & Gelles 1990). When resources are insufficient to meet basic needs, parents may differentially allocate their investment in and resources to their offspring. Evidence supporting this theorizing is inconsistent (Belsky 1993), but it is true that stepchildren, unplanned children, and children in larger families all are at greater risk for child abuse (Daly & Wilson 1988; Zuravin 1989).

Research on aversively stimulated aggression offers strong evidence on another normative biologically based propensity toward aggression. A variety of studies indicate that humans and other animals are prone to respond to a variety of unpleasant stimuli, including stressful family interactions, with aggression (Berkowitz 1983). Like evolutionary psychology, the aversively stimulated aggression perspective offers new conceptualizations for some conditions of child abuse. For example, it helps to explain why physical abuse is more likely in circumstances where child-rearing places added demands on parents, such as in the care of infants, temperamentally difficult children or children with disabilities.

Finally, it should be noted that biological factors contribute to individual differences as well as normative tendencies in the risk for child abuse. The familiality (or intergenerational transmission) of child abuse is consistent with biological as well as environmental models of causation, because families obviously share genes as well as environments (DiLalla & Gottesman 1991). Although we know of no behaviour genetic studies of the risk for child abuse, it is likely that at least some intergenerational risk is accounted for by genetic influences on personality (e.g. antisocial characteristics) and/or psychopathology (e.g. substance abuse).

Environmental implications of biological aetiologies

Strong objections have been raised about various aspects of biological theorizing in regard to the development of child abuse. Here, we wish to respond to only one aspect of these objections: that evidence on biological contributions to child abuse is irrelevant to the pressing task of intervention. In fact, just the opposite is true. Evidence on biological contributions suggests important new components to intervention.

Consider two direct implications of the evidence that step-parenting is linked with an increased risk for child abuse. First, step-parents (and biological parents) might benefit from recognizing that the bond with children can be different for step- and biological parents. If some problems are normative, then there is less reason for guilt, disappointment and recrimination in negotiating parenting roles in step-families. In fact, a recognition of normative struggles would seem to be an appropriate starting point for improving step-parenting through education or intervention. Secondly, recognizing the difference in step-parent–child relationships, single biological parents may want to alter their 'marital search strategies' so as to select potential mates based, in part, on qualities reflecting the individual's likely investment in children (e.g. patience, empathy).

An important practical implication stemming from the aversively stimulated aggression perspective is that frustration and anger are normal, not abnormal, parts of parenting. In raising our own children (without physical abuse or corporal punishment), we have come to recognize that the frustrations that sometimes end in physical child abuse are more familiar than foreign. For example, the demands of infants, especially when they cannot be soothed, can be extremely frustrating, particularly under conditions of stress (e.g. no sleep, multiple competing demands). Perhaps normalizing some of these feelings of frustration would prove helpful in preventing abusive acts. More generally, the framework that parents need to learn to recognize emotions and control normative impulses may help to improve intervention and public education. Research and intervention on child abuse have overwhelmingly emphasized the social learning of violence, but the focus needs to be expanded to include learning to inhibit or otherwise express the natural frustrations of parenting.

Multiple pathways: typologies of abusers

As a final point regarding aetiology, it is important to highlight that theorists increasingly recognize the importance of *multiple pathways*, as well as multiple risk factors, in the development of family maltreatment and violence. Early research on the aetiology of child abuse attempted to capture the 'pathological' personality of the perpetrator (Steele & Pollock 1968; Melnick & Hurley 1969), whereas later reviewers abandoned the psychopathological model (Parke & Collmer 1975; Emery 1989; Belsky 1993). More recent efforts have sought to identify the different typologies of abusers (so far focusing only on abusive men who batter their wives), some of whom suffer from psychological disorders and many of whom do not (Francis *et al.* 1992; Saunders 1992; Murphy *et al.* 1993, 1994; Gottman *et al.* 1995; Heyman *et al.* 1995; Jacobson *et al.* 1995).

No consistent typology has yet emerged, but the approach is promising and needs to be extended more into the area of child abuse. In their review of the literature, Holtzworth-Munroe & Stuart (1994) identified three primary types of spouse batterers.

Type 1: generally violent, antisocial. Type 1 batterers tend to be violent across situations and potential victims. They also are more likely to abuse alcohol, be more belligerent and contemptuous, and have antisocial personality traits.

Type 2: family only. Type 2 makes up the majority of spouse abusers, who tend to abuse only in the family, commit less severe acts, be less aggressive in general, suppress angry emotions and feel remorseful. Type 2 abusers often are dependent and jealous and are unlikely to have personality or other disorders.

Type 3: dysphoric, borderline (emotionally volatile) batterers. Type 3 batterers also tend to be violent only within their family. However, they are more socially isolated and socially incompetent than other batterers and often are depressed, feel inadequate and are emotionally volatile. Type 3 abusers are more likely to have schizoid or borderline personalities.

Some initial research supports the value of dividing abusive men into these three categories (Waltz *et al.* 2000). Although this and other typologies are best viewed as tentative and have focused only on the issue of spouse abuse, they do imply that all child abusers—and all acts of abuse—are not the same. Increasing recognition of alternative pathways to child abuse is critically important to future research and intervention, and is broadly consistent with our suggestion of distinguishing child maltreatment and violence.

Consequences of child abuse

Child abuse can cause a wide range of adverse consequences, including serious physical injury, immediate and delayed psychological distress and/or disorder, and a variety of practical upheavals (e.g. placement in foster care). The consequences for children are a function of at least five broad classes of variables:

1 the nature of the abusive act, as well as its frequency, intensity and duration;

2 individual characteristics of the victim;

3 the nature of the relationship between the child and the abuser;

4 the response of others to the abuse; and

5 factors correlated with abuse which may exacerbate its effects or, in fact, may account for some of the putative consequences of abuse.

The number of variables involved, as well as methodological limitations (Kendall-Tackett *et al.* 1993; Malinosky-Rummell & Hansen 1993; National Research Council 1993), prevent us from reaching unambiguous conclusions about the consequences of child abuse, let alone for differences between physical abuse, neglect and psychological abuse. However, we are able to point to some general patterns concerning physical, emotional and practical outcomes.

Physical harm

Physical harm is a clear consequence of many instances of physical child abuse and neglect, but information on the prevalence of specific physical consequences of child abuse is surprisingly incomplete. As noted earlier, an estimated 1200–1500 children, most of whom are under the age of 5 years, die each year as a result of either physical abuse (52%), neglect (42%), or both (5%) by a parent or parent figure (Wang & Harding 1999). However, official data may somewhat underestimate actual deaths caused by child abuse because of misclassification of causes of death (McClain *et al.* 1993).

Information on non-lethal injuries is much more sketchy. According to NIS-3, nearly 50 000 children were victims of 'serious' physical abuse in 1993; that is, they suffered from life-threatening injuries, long-term physical impairment or required professional treatment to prevent long-term physical impairment (Sedlak & Broadhurst 1996). It has also been estimated that over 18 000 children become severely disabled each year as a result of severe physical child abuse (Baladerian 1991). We could not locate epidemiological data on more specific physical outcomes, such as the rate of non-organic failure to thrive (weight loss and psychomotor delays resulting from gross neglect) among infants or specific injuries such as broken bones. Clearly, we need more information on the specific physical consequences of child abuse (see Feldman 1997 for review of identifying signs of physical abuse vs. accidental injury during a physician's examination).

Münchausen by proxy syndrome

Münchausen by proxy syndrome (MBPS) is a unique rare, but potentially very harmful, form of physical child abuse that merits special consideration. In MBPS a parent (98% of whom are female) feigns, exaggerates or induces illness in a child, often resulting in unneeded diagnostic tests, medication trials, hospitalizations and even surgery. In most cases, MBPS involves a parent and young child. In the more benign cases, the parent simply fabricates the child's illness; in more serious cases, the parent actually induces illness. No prevalence data exist on MBPS, although since it was first diagnosed in the late 1970s, there have been hundreds of case reports. The most common fabrications or modes of symptom inducements in MBPS involve seizures, apnoea, failure to thrive, vomiting and diarrhoea, asthma and allergies, and infections.

A study in England used covert video surveillance to monitor parents bringing their children to the hospital with suspicions of induced illness (Southall *et al.* 1997). The results were alarming. Of the 39 children in the experimental group, video recording in the hospital captured 30 parents attempting to intentionally suffocate, one mother break her child's arm, and another mother attempt to poison her child with disinfectant. Alarmingly, of the 41 siblings of the target children, 12 had previously died suddenly and unexpectedly. After being confronted, four of the parents admitted to having suffocated these siblings. These results clearly illustrate that MBPS can be a severe and ultimately deadly form of child abuse.

Psychological consequences

Physical abuse, neglect and psychological abuse have considerable psychological importance, because these experiences happen as part of ongoing relationships that are expected to be protective and nurturing. Thus, the child is often faced with an emotionally wrenching dilemma: the child wants to be protected from physical and emotional harm but, at the same time, the child also has strong emotional ties to the parent. Another dilemma is that the parent may often oscillate between perpetrating physical violence or emotional abuse at one time and offering the child warmth and attention at other times.

A number of recent books and papers have reviewed the large body of research on the psychological adjustment of abused children (National Research Council 1993; Cicchetti & Toth 1995; Wolfe 1999). We can draw two global conclusions from this broad and sometimes conflicting literature. First, although some have found child neglect to be more psychologically harmful than physical abuse (Erickson & Egeland 1996), victims of child abuse are at an increased risk for a variety of psychological problems. Secondly, there may be a modest relation between the types of abusive acts and specific psychological outcomes; for example, physical abuse and aggression among victims (Widom 1989; Malinosky-Rummell & Hansen 1993). However, the more prominent finding is that child abuse is linked with diverse psychological problems ranging from aggression and anxiety to depression. Evidence on more specific psychological outcomes may be clouded by the need to consider:

1 risk factors correlated with family violence;
2 clusters of symptoms (e.g. post-traumatic stress disorder, PTSD) in addition to specific symptoms;
3 subtle psychological consequences that are difficult to document empirically, particularly among children; and
4 psychological processes (not just psychological outcomes)

set into motion or disrupted by the experience of family violence.

Correlated risk factors

Child abuse is associated with a number of factors known to place children at risk for psychological problems: poverty (Pelton 1992); troubled family environments (Egeland 1997); and genetic liability (DiLalla & Gottesman 1991). These risk factors may account for the apparent relation between child abuse and psychological problems, or their effects may interact with the consequences of abuse. Thus, research comparing abused and non-abused children may actually reflect the psychological effects of anxious attachments, social isolation or general family stress rather than the consequences of violence *per se* (National Research Council 1993; Cicchetti & Toth 1995; Egeland 1997). If so, interventions might appropriately focus on these risk factors in addition to, or even instead, of the abuse, particularly in cases where abuse is relatively mild.

Acute and post-traumatic stress disorders

Assessment at the level of psychological disorders, not just psychological symptoms, should also further understanding of the psychological consequences of child abuse. Recent research on PTSD illustrates the promise of such broader assessments. Several investigators have now documented PTSD among between one-quarter and one-half (or more) of child victims of physical abuse (Kiser *et al.* 1991; Famulro *et al.* 1992, 1994; Livingston *et al.* 1993). Moreover, the risk for PTSD increases when physical abuse is more severe and long lasting (Kiser *et al.* 1991). The PTSD diagnosis suggests new possibilities for psychological intervention, especially given recent research on the successful treatment of PTSD (Frueh *et al.* 1995; Rothbaum & Foa 1996; see also Yule, Chapter 32). However, the difficulties involved in diagnosing PTSD in children, as well as the need to develop sound measures of acute stress disorder, pose basic challenges to researchers and clinicians.

Subtle psychological effects on victims

The diagnoses of PTSD and acute stress disorder include symptoms such as re-experiencing and dissociation, and thus offer further impetus for studying some of the more subtle psychological consequences of child abuse (Friedrich *et al.* 1992; Wolfe *et al.* 1989). We also urge more attention to such reactions as guilt and self-blame in response to being a victim of abuse (Wolfe *et al.* 1994).

The vehement controversy over 'recovered memories' of abuse provides another rationale for research on more subtle psychological reactions (Loftus 1994; Koss 1995). A review of the recovered memories controversy is beyond the scope of this chapter, but we do note that there is now widespread agreement that many false memories have been implanted by recovered memory therapists; that there is no way to discern if a memory is recovered or implanted in the absence of independent corroborative evidence; and that many professional organizations explicitly recommend against the use of techniques to recover memories (Kihlstrom 1998). At the same time, we recognize that one longitudinal study found that documented sexual abuse among girls aged 10 months to 12 years was not reported by nearly 40% of the victims when they were asked about their history as young adults (Williams 1994a). Our present concern is not whether this study documents dissociation or simple forgetting (Loftus 1994; Williams 1994b), but the need to increase our understanding of children's cognitive and emotional processing of abusive experiences over long periods of time.

We similarly are intrigued by the psychological mechanisms that may underlie other long-term outcomes, particularly the intergenerational transmission of abuse. Our main question in the present context is how a propensity toward violence might be carried forward in the child's psyche across the years from childhood to adult life. Because fear is children's most immediate response to abuse, we believe that processes more subtle than direct imitation must account for this continuity (Margolin 1998).

Process of adaptation

Most research focuses on the outcomes of child abuse, but the psychological consequences are best described as a process that unfolds over time. We need more adequate models describing this process. For example, Cicchetti & Toth (1995) have articulated how physical abuse and neglect may disrupt the normal tasks of child development, such as the formation of attachments, affect regulation, the self system and peer relationships.

Practical consequences

Finally, we must underscore the fact that child abuse—and interventions with abusive families—can have tremendously adverse practical consequences for children and families. For example, 254 000 children were placed in foster care in the USA in 1994, most as a result of abuse or neglect (Tatara 1996). Foster care placements are often less than ideal in many ways, but even excellent foster care causes considerable upheaval for children. In focusing on children's psychological concerns, mental health professionals must not overlook the practical consequences of well-intended interventions. When intervening with abusive families, it must be clear that a better alternative can be offered. When mental health or social service professionals can offer better alternatives, we suggest that supportive rather than adversarial intervention should be more effective—except in cases of serious abuse.

Prevention and intervention

In much of the world, the physical abuse, neglect and psychological maltreatment of children continues to be ignored, as it was until relatively recent times in the USA and Western Europe. As has happened in the West over the last several decades, the task in preventing and intervening with child abuse in countries such as China must begin with public recognition of the problem, making acts of child abuse illegal, and offering publicly supported interventions that break some traditions of family privacy and autonomy in order to protect children. Obviously, these are difficult but extremely important goals, particularly because non-Western countries encompass the great majority of the world's population. Nevertheless, in drawing some implications for prevention and practice, we focus not on the need for increased recognition of the problem of child abuse in most of the world, but on the need for a moderation of the extreme adversarial legalistic approaches that have developed in some Western countries, particularly the USA.

In the West, attempts to prevent or stop child abuse, or treat victims or perpetrators, involve a huge array of interventions involving mental health, social service and legal professionals, as well as other professionals who have regular contact with children and families (e.g. teachers, family physicians). Unfortunately, the creation and implementation of new interventions has far outstripped research on their effectiveness, as previous reviewers have noted (National Research Council 1993; Becker et al. 1995; Melton et al. 1995; Wolfe et al. 1995). Especially in the USA, the child protection system has come to be dominated by identifying, reporting and investigating abuse with the expectation that something can and will be done to help children. Unfortunately, research does not point clearly to interventions that work, and the ever-growing investigative approach to child abuse has consumed so many resources that little is left for attempts to help abused children and families under stress.

Thus, while increased recognition of child abuse is the task for most of the world, it seems time for moderation in the USA. Specifically, we offer three recommendations, all of which relate to distinguishing levels of abuse and, more generally, to moderating the legalistic approach.

1 We urge clarification and revision of child abuse reporting laws.
2 We encourage the rediscovery of the helping model of social services for less serious cases of abuse and for families under stress.
3 We advocate for more forceful legal intervention in cases of serious family violence.

At the outset, we should note that the first two goals would bring policy in the USA closer to that of the UK, where reporting is not mandatory but is encouraged by the possibility of professional sanctions, and where, despite some problems with overreporting, the goal of supporting families under stress has remained in the provision of social services (Duquette 1992; Berridge 1997).

Child abuse reporting

By all accounts, child protective services in the USA are driven by—and overwhelmed with—the investigation of child abuse reports (Kamerman & Kahn 1990). As we have noted, over three million reports are made every year in the USA, but less than one-third are substantiated. Moreover, social service workers are so swamped with reports and investigations that about 40% of *substantiated* cases receive no services at all (McCurdy & Daro 1993). Finally, only a small proportion of substantiated cases (<20%) involve any type of formal court action, with child protective workers encouraging the great majority of substantiated cases to enter treatment voluntarily (Melton *et al.* 1995).

Mental health professionals are in a rather ironic position in regard to reporting child abuse. Most cases involve only suspected or mild abuse, families are stressed and parents have indicated at least some interest in receiving help by virtue of their contact with the mental health professional. Yet, under existing law, mental health professionals are required to report these cases, while knowing that the likely outcomes are failure to substantiate, no provision of services, no legal action and, eventually, encouraging the family to seek treatment—exactly where they began the long expensive and intrusive process. Not surprisingly, mental health professionals commonly report that they have little faith in the reporting system and believe that it undermines therapeutic relationships (Zellman 1990; Levine *et al.* 1991). Indeed, one prominent group of commentators termed the resultant failure to report cases among American mental health professionals an action of 'civil disobedience' (Melton *et al.* 1995, p. 52).

Given this circuitous chain of events, a simple but not necessarily minor change, in the USA and other countries with similar requirements, would be to alter reporting requirements for mental health professionals in order to reduce investigations and improve services. Specifically, we would exempt mental health professionals from reporting less serious cases of abuse, whether known or suspected, when a family is actively engaged in treatment. We do not attempt to define these cases here, but we do note the need to define less serious cases (what we have called maltreatment) clearly in the law, as has been done in some experimental programmes. Such a change would be a first step toward the broader goal of refocusing the child protection system to supporting rather than policing more families under stress, while simultaneously pursuing more vigorous coercive intervention with cases of serious family violence.

Supportive interventions

A number of supportive interventions have been developed in an attempt to reduce child abuse, including individual and group therapies for both victims and perpetrators, parent-training and family therapy, and home visiting programmes for the prevention of child abuse. In general, the more serious and chronic the nature of the abuse, the less successful these programmes are in changing behaviours (Cohn & Daro 1987; Barth 1991; National Research Council 1993; Guterman 1999). However, with problems of mild to moderate abuse, multilevel programmes, which combine behavioural methods, stress manage-

ment, and parent–child relationship skills, lower stress in families and may reduce the likelihood of continued aggression in child abuse cases (Lutzker & Rice 1984; National Research Council 1993; Murphy 1994).

Until 30 years ago, treatment for maltreating families focused on intrapsychic approaches, guided by the belief that maltreating parents had deviant personalities that needed to be changed (Steele & Pollock 1968). It is now clear that only a small minority of abusive parents are significantly psychiatrically disturbed and, furthermore, that these approaches to treatment are too narrow and ineffective (Azar & Wolfe 1998). Behavioural approaches that focus on parent–child interaction patterns and take into account the family's larger ecological context (e.g. nature of family life, environmental stressors affecting family, other parental problems and sociodemographic factors) have proven to be the most promising alternative (Wolfe & Wekerle 1994; Schellenbach 1998). Additionally, behavioural approaches tend to be less threatening to child abuse perpetrators, as they are more concrete and problem-focused.

Comprehensive family assessment is crucial in working with maltreating families, as this is a heterogeneous population and many of these families have additional issues that need to be addressed concomitantly (e.g. parental substance abuse, marital problems) for successful treatment outcomes. In assessing maltreating families, Azar & Wolfe (1998) suggested that clinicians need to consider at least four areas, in order of importance:

1 determination of danger to the child;
2 identification of general strengths and problem areas of the family system;
3 identification of specific parental needs vis-à-vis child-rearing demands; and
4 identification of child needs.

A number of behavioural strategies have been used with abusive parents, either alone or in combination. Such strategies include:

1 modelling and behavioural rehearsal, in which parents practice more appropriate responses to children's aversive behaviour;
2 cognitive restructuring of distorted interpretations of child behaviour;
3 anger control management and relaxation training; and
4 skills-training which teaches parents contingency management principles (Azar & Wolfe 1998).

Some studies have found support for combining group parenting sessions with home visitation to promote generalization of new behaviours to the home environment (Azar *et al.* 1984). Treatment services that focus on maltreated children are much less common than parent-orientated interventions. Part of the reason is the age of the child, with the majority being preschool-age or younger. Another part is that parental behaviour is often the primary concern. Nevertheless, recent efforts have been made to address maltreated children's developmental needs and reduce long-term impairments (Jones 1997; Kempe 1997). For example, improvements in social behaviour and cognitive development were found in one preschool-aged programme which matched maltreated children who tended to be withdrawn with resilient peers (Davis & Fantuzzo 1989; Fantuzzo *et al.* 1996). Therapeutic preschools also show promising results (Kempe 1997). With older children, non-compliance and aggression is often addressed through parent training.

It is important for clinicians working with maltreating parents to recognize some of the characteristics of these families that may impede treatment. First, many maltreating families live very chaotic lives, affecting treatment in several ways, including missing appointments and failing to comply with treatment. Secondly, abusive parents typically do not identify themselves as having a problem, thus making the establishment of a therapeutic relationship especially challenging. Specific factors that lower the likelihood of successful treatment outcomes include:

1 parental personality disorder;
2 substance abuse;
3 lack of empathy for the child;
4 disordered attachment;
5 severe abuse/neglect;
6 Münchausen by proxy syndrome;
7 premeditated abuse;
8 child with developmental delay and/or special needs;
9 family with pervasive diverse family violence; and
10 extreme social isolation (Jones 1997).

Project 12-Ways, an intervention programme for maltreating families that has been operating in rural Illinois since 1979, addresses many of the above principles and has been shown to lower recidivism rates in families reported for child abuse and neglect (Lutzker & Rice 1984; Lutzker *et al.* 1998). With most of the services delivered in the home, this programme conducts a comprehensive family assessment and then provides a multitude of supportive services based on each family's needs. The services include: parent–child training; stress reduction; basic skills training for children; money management training; social support; home safety training; multiple setting behaviour management; health and nutrition; marital counseling; problem-solving; alcohol/substance abuse referral; and single mother services.

Some interventions show promise, but the need for early intervention and especially prevention is underscored by the difficulty of changing child abuse and the stressful life circumstances that promote it (Garbarino & Kostelny 1992; Pelton 1992). Home visitor programmes for new parents living in difficult circumstances are one especially promising form of prevention. Home visitor programmes simultaneously assist with material needs (e.g. cribs, child care, transportation), psychological needs (e.g. parenting education and support), and educational needs (e.g. job skills), and may both improve general family well-being and reduce child maltreatment (MacMillan *et al.* 1994). One controversy about home visitor programmes is whether they should be universal or targeted to families at greater psychosocial risk. Although the targeted strategy is more economical, greater reductions in abuse have been found for the universal programme, perhaps because targeted families are less likely to benefit from home visiting (Guterman 1999).

An outstanding example of home visiting is the Prenatal and Infancy Home Visitors' Program which targeted low-income teen and single-parent mothers who were pregnant with their first child. Based on evaluations conducted during the programme (Olds, Henderson, Chamberlin, Tatelbaum 1986), 1–2 years following termination (Olds *et al.* 1994, 1995) and 15 years later (Olds *et al.* 1999), home visited mothers had fewer and less serious CPS reports, fewer subsequent births, spent fewer months on welfare, had fewer arrests and were less likely to abuse substances in comparison to control families. In large part due to such benefits, in 1992 the National Committee to Prevent Child Abuse launched a national initiative of home visitor programmes, Healthy Families America, in over 300 communities. Some programme evaluations completed to date suggest that Healthy Families America may be reducing reports of abuse and neglect. However, three randomized trials have failed to find differences between Healthy Families America participants and controls, although the null findings may be a result of relatively small samples and low statistical power (Daro & Harding 1999).

Coercive intervention

Although this has not been the main focus of this chapter, we should note that distinguishing between levels of abuse may also help to improve intervention in cases of serious and extreme child abuse. One benefit would be to free investigators and police to focus on the most serious cases. Shockingly, between 35 and 50% of all fatalities brought about by child abuse/neglect in the USA occur in cases already brought to the attention of law enforcement and child protection agencies (Wang & Harding 1999). Another benefit might be to help to clarify when coercive legal intervention is and is not appropriate. For example, many commentators have questioned the overriding goal of family reunification following child abuse, especially in cases of serious physical and sexual abuse. In extreme cases like these, the termination of parental rights and early adoption may be the appropriate intervention, especially given the many problems with the overwhelmed foster case system (Tatara 1996).

Distinguishing between levels of abuse should help to resolve controversy and thereby clarify the appropriate use of coercive legal intervention. The idea of termination of parental rights is far more threatening when our definitions of abuse include relatively minor acts, as they currently do. Clearly, it is difficult to draw a line between cases that should or should not lead to termination of parental rights (Azar *et al.* 1995), but the challenge of distinguishing between levels of abuse should not deter us from the task. What we have called maltreatment may be on a continuum with what we have termed violence, and both acts of abuse may differ from normal family aggression only by a matter of degree. However, drawing distinctions between levels of abuse seems consistent with the state of our knowledge about the prevalence of abuse, its development, consequences and appropriate intervention.

Levels of abuse, present clinical practice and future research

As a final note, we highlight that our focus on distinguishing levels of abuse holds implications for present clinical practice and future research. Child abuse can be horrific but, in many cases, clinicians can understand and even empathize with the behaviour of parents who, to a mild or moderate degree, physically hurt, neglect or psychologically maltreat their children. Such families are more likely to benefit from a supportive rather than an adversarial stance in the clinical setting, in the provision of social services and in legal interventions. Child abuse should never be tolerated, but mildly or moderately abusive parents may benefit from disclosure, discussion, education and practical support with their children and with managing their own work and family lives.

In cases of serious abuse, clinical treatment of perpetrators may simply be inappropriate. Although parents who seriously abuse their children may have mental health treatment needs, family reunification seems to be an inappropriate and unattainable goal, at least in the more extreme cases. Distinguishing levels of abuse, accompanied by better triage of cases, should allow mental health and social services to concentrate resources and efforts on those cases most appropriate for supportive intervention, while the legal system focuses on those cases most appropriate for policing, termination of parental rights and prosecution.

Future research could help practitioners by working to develop a better typology of child abuse and of abusive parents. We recognize that the distinction that we argue for here is only a very crude initial grouping. We look forward to the development of far more refined categories of abuse.

References

Azar, S.T. & Rohrbeck, C.A. (1986) Child abuse and unrealistic expectations: Further validation of the Parent Opinion Questionnaire. *Journal of Consulting & Clinical Psychology*, **54**, 867–868.

Azar, S.T. & Wolfe, D. (1998) Child physical abuse and neglect. In: *Treatment of Childhood Disorders*, 2nd edn (eds E.J. Mash & R.A. Barkley), pp. 251–268. American Psychological Association, Washington D.C.

Azar, S.T., Robinson, D.R., Hekimian, E. & Twentyman, C.T. (1984) Unrealistic expectations and problem-solving ability in maltreating and comparison mothers. *Journal of Consulting and Clinical Psychology*, **52**, 687–691.

Azar, S.T., Benjet, C.L., Fuhrmann, G.S. & Cavallero, L. (1995) Child maltreatment and the termination of parental rights: can behavioral research help Soloman? *Behavior Therapy*, **26**, 599–623.

Baladerian, N.J. (1991) Abuse causes disabilities. In: *Disability and the Family*, p. 35. Spectrum, Culver City, CA.

Barth, R.P. (1991) An experimental evaluation of in-home child abuse prevention services. *Child Abuse and Neglect*, **15**, 363–375.

Becker, J.V., Alpert, J.L., BigFoot, D.S. et al. (1995) *Journal of Clinical Child Psychology*, **24** (Suppl.), 23–47.

Belsky, J. (1993) Etiology of child maltreatment: a developmental–ecological analysis. *Psychological Bulletin*, **114**, 413–434.

Berkowitz, L. (1983) Aversively stimulated aggression: some parallels and differences in research with animals and humans. *American Psychologist*, **38**, 1135–1144.

Berridge, D. (1997) England: child abuse reports, responses, and reforms. In: *Combating Child Abuse: International Perspectives and Trends* (ed. N. Gilbert), pp. 72–101. Oxford University Press, New York.

Besharov, D.J. (1996) Child abuse: threat or menace? How common is it really? *Slate*, **9**, 1–5.

Besharov, D.J. & Laumann-Billings, L. (1996) Child abuse reporting. In: *Social Policies for Children* (eds I. Garfinkel, J. Hochschild & S. McLanahan), pp. 257–274. Brookings Institute Press, Washington D.C.

Besharov, D. & Laumann (Billings), L. (1997) Don't call it child abuse if it's really poverty. *Journal of Children and Poverty*, **3**, 5–36.

Booth, A. & Dunn, J., eds. (1994) *Stepfamilies: Who benefits? Who does not?* Lawrence Erlbaum, Hillsdale, NJ.

Bronfenbrenner, U. (1979) *The Ecology of Human Behavior*. Harvard University Press, Cambridge, MA.

Brunk, M., Henggeler, S.W. & Whelan, J.P. (1987) Comparison of multisystemic therapy and parent training in the brief treatment of child abuse and neglect. *Journal of Consulting and Clinical Psychology*, **55**, 171–178.

Burgess, A. & Draper, P. (1989) The explanation of family violence: the role of biological, behavioral, and cultural selection. In: *Family Violence* (eds L. Ohlin & M. Tonry), pp. 59–116. University of Chicago Press, Chicago.

Burgess, R.L., Garbarino, J. & Gilstrap, B. (1983) Violence to the family. In: *Lifespan developmental psychology: Non-normative life events* (eds E.J. Callahan & K. McCluskey). Academic Press, San Diego, CA.

Chaffin, M., Kelleher, K. & Hollenberg, J. (1996) Onset of physical abuse and neglect: Psychiatric, substance abuse, and social risk factors from prospective community samples. *Child Abuse & Neglect*, **20**, 191–203.

Cicchetti, D. & Lynch, M. (1993) Toward an ecological/transactional model of community violence and child maltreatment: consequences for children's development. *Psychiatry*, **56**, 96–118.

Cicchetti, D. & Toth, S.L. (1995) A developmental psychopathology perspective on child abuse and neglect. *Journal of the American Academy of Child and Adolescent Psychiatry*, **34**, 541–565.

Cohn, A.H. & Daro, D. (1987) Is treatment too late: what ten years of evaluative research tell us. *Child Abuse and Neglect*, **11**, 433–442.

Community Partnerships for Protecting Children (1996, Winter) *Newsletter*, 1.

Coulton, C.J., Korbin, J.E., Su, M. & Chow, J. (1995) Community level factors and child maltreatment rates. *Child Development*, **66**, 1162–1176.

Cummings, E.M. (1997) Marital conflict, abuse, and adversity in the family and child adjustment: A developmental psychopathology perspective. In: *Child abuse: New directions in prevention and treatment across the lifespan* (eds D.A. Wolfe, R.J. McMahon & R. Joseph), pp. 3–26. Sage Publications: Thousand Oaks, CA.

Daly, M. & Wilson, M. (1980) Discriminative parental solicitude: a biological perspective. *Journal of Marriage and the Family*, **42**, 277–288.

Daly, M. & Wilson, M. (1982) Male sexual jealousy. *Ethology and Sociobiology*, **3**, 11–27.

Daly, M. & Wilson, M. (1985) Child abuse and other risk factors of not living with both parents. *Ethology & Sociobiology*, **6**, 197–210.

Daly, M. & Wilson, M. (1988) Evolutionary social psychology and family homicide. *Science*, **242**, 519–524.

Daly, M. & Wilson, M.I. (1996) Violence against stepchildren. *Current Directions in Psychological Science*, **5**, 77–81.

Daro, D.A. & Harding, K.A. (1999) Healthy Families America: using research to enhance practice. *Future of Children*, **9**, 152–176.

Davis, S.P. & Fantuzzo, J.W. (1989) The effects of adult and peer social initiations on the social behavior of withdrawn and aggressive maltreated preschool children. *Journal of Family Violence*, **4**, 227–248.

DiLalla, L.F. & Gottesman, I.I. (1991) Biological and genetic contributors to violence: Widom's untold tale. *Psychological Bulletin*, **109**, 125–129.

Duncan, R.D., Saunders, B.E., Kilpatrick, D.G., Hanson, R.F. & Resnick, H.S. (1996) Childhood physical assault as a risk factor for PTSD, depression, and substance abuse: Findings from a national survey. *American Journal of Orthopsychiatry*, **66**, 437–448.

Duquette, D.N. (1992) Child protection legal process: comparing the USA and Great Britain. *University of Pittsburgh Law Review*, **54**, 239–287.

Edleson, J.L. (1999) The overlap between women battering and child maltreatment. *Violence Against Women*, **5**, 134–154.

Edleson, J.L., Eisikovits, Z.C., Guttmann, E. & Sela-Amit, M. (1991) Cognitive and interpersonal factors in woman abuse. *Journal of Family Violence*, **6**, 167–182.

Egeland, B., Jacobovitz, D. & Sroufe, A. (1988) Breaking the cycle of abuse. *Child Development*, **59**, 1080–1088.

Emery, R.E. (1989) Family violence. *American Psychologist*, **44**, 321–328.

Emery, R.E. & Laumann-Billings, L. (1998) An overview of the nature, causes, and consequences of abusive family relationships: Toward differentiating maltreatment and violence. *American Psychologist*, **53**, 121–135.

Erickson, M.F. & Egeland, B.J. (1996) Child neglect. In: *The APSAC Handbook on Child Maltreatment* (eds J. Briere, L. Berliner, J. Bulkley, C. Jenny & T. Reid), pp. 4–20. Sage, Thousand Oaks, CA.

Famulro, R., Fenton, T. & Kinscherff, R. (1992) Psychiatric diagnoses of maltreated children: preliminary findings. *Journal of the American Academy of Child and Adolescent Psychiatry*, **31**, 863–867.

Famulro, R., Fenton, T., Kinscherff, R., Ayoub, C. & Barnum, R. (1994) Maternal and child posttraumatic disorder in cases of child maltreatment. *Child Abuse and Neglect*, **18**, 27–36.

Fantuzzo, J., Sutton-Smith, B. & Atkins, M. *et al.* (1996) Community-based resilient peer treatment of withdrawn maltreated preschool children. *Journal of Consulting & Clinical Psychology*, **64**, 1377–1386.

Feldman, K.W. (1997) Evaluation of physical abuse. In: *The Battered Child*, 5th edn (eds M.E. Helfer, R.S. Kempe & R.D. Krugman), pp. 175–220. University of Chicago Press, Chicago.

Finkelhor, D. (1995) The victimization of children: A developmental perspective. *American Journal of Orthopsychiatry*, **65**, 177–193.

Finkelhor, D. & Dziuba-Leatherman, J. (1994) Victimization of children. *American Psychologist*, **49**, 173–183.

Fitzgibbon, T.J. (1998) The United Nations Convention on the rights of the child: Are children really protected? A case study of China's implementation. *Loyola International Law Journal*, **20**, 325–363.

Francis, C.R., Hughes, H.M. & Hitz, L. (1992) Physically abusive parents and the 16-PF: a preliminary psychological typology. *Child Abuse and Neglect*, **16**, 673–691.

Friedrich, W.N., Grambsch, P., Damon, L., Hewitt, S.K., Koverola, S. & Wolfe, V. (1992) Child Sexual Behavior Inventory: Normative and clinical comparisons. *Psychological Assessment*, **4**, 303–311.

Frodi, A.M. & Lamb, M.E. (1980) Infants at risk for child abuse. *Infant Mental Health Journal*, **1**, 240–247.

Frueh, B.C., Turner, S. & Beidel, D. (1995) Exposure-therapy for combat-related PTSD: A critical review. *Clinical Psychology Review*, **15**, 799–817.

Furstenburg, F.F. (1993) How families manage risk and opportunity in dangerous neighborhoods. In: *Sociology and the Public Agenda* (ed. W.J. Wilson), pp. 231–258. Sage, Newbury Park, CA.

Gallup, G.H., Moore, D.W. & Schussel, R. (1995) *Disciplining children in America: A Gallup Poll Report*. The Gallup Organization, Princeton, NJ.

Garbarino, J. (1977) The human ecology of child maltreatment: a conceptual model for research. *Journal of Marriage and Family*, **39**, 721–735.

Garbarino, J. (1995) Growing up in a socially toxic environment: Life for children and families in the 1990s. In: *The individual, the family, and social good: Personal fulfillment in times of change. Nebraska Symposium on Motivation* (ed G. Melton), pp. 1–20. University of Nebraska Press, Lincoln, NE.

Garbarino, J. & Crouter, A. (1978) Defining the community context of parent–child relations: the correlates of child maltreatment. *Child Development*, **49**, 604–612.

Garbarino, J. & Kostelny, K. (1992) Child maltreatment as a community problem. *Child Abuse and Neglect*, **16**, 455–467.

Garbarino, J. & Sherman, D. (1980) High-risk neighborhoods and high-risk families: the human ecology of child maltreatment. *Child Development*, **51**, 188–198.

Gelles, R.J. (1992) Poverty and violence toward children. *American Behavioral Scientist*, **35**, 258–274.

Gilbert, N. (1997) Conclusion: a comparative perspective. In: *Combating Child Abuse: International Perspective and Trends*. (ed. N. Gilbert), pp. 232–240. Oxford University Press, New York.

Gottman, J.M., Jacobson, N.S., Rushe, R.H. *et al.* (1995) The relationship between heart rate reactivity, emotionally aggressive behavior, and general violence in batterers. *Journal of Family Psychology*, **9**, 227–248.

Guterman, N.B. (1999) Enrollment strategies in early home visitation to prevent physical child abuse and neglect and the 'universal versus targeted' debate: a meta-analysis of population-based and screening-based programs. *Child Abuse and Neglect*, **23**, 863–890.

Harrington, D., Dubowitz, H., Black, M.M., & Binder, A. (1995) Maternal substance use and neglectful parenting: Relations with children's development. *Journal of Clinical Child Psychology*, **24**, 258–263.

Herrenkohl, R.C., Herrenkohl, E.C. & Egolf, B.P. (1983) Circumstances surrounding the occurrence of child maltreatment. *Journal of Consulting and Clinical Psychology*, **51**, 424–431.

Hess, L.E. (1995) Changing family patterns in Western Europe: opportunity and risk factors for adolescent development. In: *Psychosocial Disorders in Young People: Time Trends and Their Causes* (eds M. Rutter & D.J. Smith), pp. 150–178. Wiley, New York.

Hetherington, E.M., Bridges, M.B. & Insabella, G.M. (1998) What matters? What does not? Five perspectives on the association between marital transitions and children's adjustment. *American Psychologist*, **53**, 167–184.

Heyman, R., O'Leary, D. & Jouriles, E. (1995) Alcohol and aggressive personality styles: potentiators of serious physical aggression against wives? *Journal of Family Psychology*, 9, 44–57.

Holtzworth-Munroe, A. & Stuart, G.L. (1994) Typologies of male batterers: three subtypes and the differences among them. *Psychological Bulletin*, 116, 476–497.

Jacobson, N.S., Gottman, J.M. & Shortt, J.W. (1995) The distinction between Type 1 and Type 2 batterers: further considerations—reply to Ordnuff *et al.* (1995), Margolin *et al.* (1995), and Walker (1995). *Journal of Family Psychology*, 9, 272–279.

Jaffe, P.G., Wolfe, D.A. & Wilson, S.K. (1990) *Children of Battered Women*. Sage, Newbury Park, CA.

Jones, D.P. (1997) Treatment of the child and the family where child abuse or neglect has occurred. In: *The Battered Child*, (eds M.E. Helfer, R.S. Kempe & R.D. Krugman), 5th edn, pp. 521–543. University of Chicago Press, Chicago.

Kamerman, S.B. & Kahn, A.J. (1990) The problems facing social services for children, youth, and families. *Children and Youth Services Review*, 12, 7–20.

Kantor, G.K. & Straus, M.A. (1990) The 'drunken bum' theory of wife beating. In: *Physical Violence in American Families* (eds M.A. Straus & R.J. Gelles), pp. 203–224. Transaction, New Brunswick, NJ.

Kaufman, J. & Zigler, E. (1987) Do abused children become abusive parents? *American Journal of Orthopsychiatry*, 57, 186–192.

Kelleher, K., Chaffin, M., Hollenberg, J. & Fischer, E. (1994) Alcohol and drug disorders among physically abusive and neglectful parents in a community-based sample. *American Journal of Public Health*, 84, 1586–1590.

Kempe, R.S. (1997) A developmental approach to the treatment of abused children. In: *The Battered Child* (eds M.E. Helfer, R.S. Kempe & R.D. Krugman), 5th edn, pp. 543–566. University of Chicago Press, Chicago.

Kendall-Tackett, K.A., Williams, L.M. & Finkelhor, D. (1993) Impact of sexual abuse on children: a review and synthesis of recent empirical studies. *Psychological Bulletin*, 113, 164–180.

Kihlstrom, J.F. (1998) Exhumed memory. In: *Truth in Memory* (eds S.J. Lynn & K.M. McConkey), pp. 3–31. Guilford, New York.

Kiser, L.J., Heston, J., Millsap, P.A. & Pruitt, D.B. (1991) Physical and sexual abuse in childhood: relationship with post-traumatic stress disorder. *Journal of the American Academy of Child and Adolescent Psychiatry*, 30, 776–783.

Korbin, J.E. (1994) Sociocultural perspective in child maltreatment. In: *Protecting children from abuse and neglect: Foundations for a new strategy* (eds G.B. Melton & F.D. Barry), pp. 182–223. The Guilford Press: New York.

Korbin, J.E. (1997) Culture and child maltreatment. In: *The Battered Child* (eds M.E. Helfer, R.S. Kempe & R.D. Krugman), pp. 29–48. University of Chicago Press, Chicago.

Koss, M.P., Tromp, S. & Tharan, M. (1995) Traumatic memories: Empirical foundations, forensic, and clinical implications. *Clinical Psychology: Science and Practice*, 2, 111–132.

Kozu, J. (1999) Domestic violence in Japan. *American Psychologist*, 54, 50–54.

Larrance, D.T. & Twentyman, C.T. (1983) Maternal attributions and child abuse. *Journal of Abnormal Psychology*, 92, 449–457.

Levine, M. (1990) The need for a special relationship doctrine in the child protection context. *Brooklyn Law Review*, 56, 329–376.

Littlewood, P.C. (1997) Domestic child abuse under the U.N. Convention on the rights of the child: Implications for children's rights in four Asian countries. *Pacific Rim Law and Policy Journal*, 6, 411–446.

Livingston, R., Lawson, L. & Jones, J.G. (1993) Predictors of self-reported psychopathology in children abused repeatedly by a parent. *Journal of the American Academy of Child and Adolescent Psychiatry*, 32, 948–953.

Loftus, E. (1994) The repressed memory controversy. *American Psychologist*, 49, 443–445.

Loftus, E.F., Garry, M. & Feldman, J. (1994) Forgetting sexual trauma: What does it mean when 38% forget? *Journal of Consulting and Clinical Psychology*, 62, 1177–1181.

Lung, C.T. & Daro, D. (1996) *Current trends in child abuse reporting and fatalities: the results of the 1995 annual fifty state survey.* National Committee to Prevent Child Abuse, Chicago.

Lutzker, J. & Rice, J.M. (1984) Project 12-Ways: measuring outcome of a large in home-service for the treatment and prevention of child abuse and neglect. *Child Abuse and Neglect*, 8, 519–524.

Lutzker, J.R., Bigelow, K.M., Doctor, R.M., Gershater, R.M. & Greene, B.F. (1998) An ecobehavioral model for the prevention and treatment of child abuse and neglect: history and applications. In: *Handbook of Child Abuse Research and Treatment: Issues in Clinical Child Psychology* (ed. J.R. Lutzker), pp. 239–266. Plenum Press, New York.

MacMillan, H.L., MacMillan, J.H., Offord, D.R., Griffith, L. & MacMillan, A. (1994) Primary prevention of child abuse and neglect: a critical review. Part I. *Journal of Child Psychology, Psychiatry*, 35, 835–856.

Malinosky-Rummell, R. & Hansen, D.J. (1993) Long-term consequences of child abuse and neglect. *Psychological Bulletin*, 114, 68–79.

Malkin, C.M. & Lamb, M.E. (1994) Child maltreatment: a test of sociobiological theory. *Journal of Comparative Family Studies*, 25, 121–133.

McCurdy, K. & Daro, D. (1993) *Current trends in child abuse reporting and fatalities: the results of the 1992 annual fifty state survey.* National Center on Child Abuse Prevention Research, Chicago.

Melnick, B. & Hurley, J.R. (1969) Distinctive personality of child-abusing mothers. *Journal of Consulting and Clinical Psychology*, 33, 746–749.

Murphy, C.M. & O'Farrell, T.J. (1994) Factors associated with marital aggression in male alcoholics. *Journal of Family Psychology*, 8, 321–335.

Murphy, C.M., Meyer, S.L. & O'Leary, K.D. (1993) Family of origin and MCMI-II psychopathology among partner-assaultive men. *Violence and Victims*, 8, 165–176.

Murphy, C.M., Meyer, S.L. & O'Leary, K.D. (1994) Dependency characteristics of partner-assaultive men. *Journal of Abnormal Psychology*, 103, 729–735.

National Research Council (1993) *Understanding Child Abuse and Neglect.* National Academy Press, Washington D.C.

Olds, D.L., Henderson, C.R. & Kitzman, H. (1994) Does prenatal and infancy home visitation have enduring effects on qualities of parental caregiving and child health at 25–50 months of life? *Pediatrics*, 93, 89–98.

Olds, D.L., Henderson, C.R., Kitzman, H. & Cole, R. (1995) Effects of prenatal and infancy nurse home visitation on surveillance of child maltreatment. *Pediatrics*, 95, 365–372.

Olds, D.L., Henderson, C.R., Kitzman, H.J., Eckenrode, J.J., Cole, R.E. & Tatelbaum, R.C. (1999) Prenatal and infancy home visitation by nurses: recent findings. *Future of Children*, 9, 44–65.

Pan, H.S., Neidig, P.H. & O'Leary, K.D. (1994) Predicting mild and severe husband to wife physical aggression. *Journal of Consulting and Clinical Psychology*, 62, 975–981.

Parke, R.D. & Collmer, C.W. (1975) Child abuse: an interdiscplinary analysis. In: *Review of Child Development Research*, Vol. 5 (ed. E.M. Hetherington), pp. 509–590. University of Chicago Press, Chicago.

Pelton, L.H. (1981) *The Social Context of Child Abuse and Neglect.* Human Services Press, New York.

Pelton, L.H. (1989) *For Reasons of Poverty.* Praeger Press, New York.

Pelton, L.H. (1992) *The role of material factors in child abuse and neglect.* Paper prepared for the US Advisory Board on Child Abuse and Neglect.

Pernanen, K. (1991) *Alcohol in Human Violence.* Guilford Press, New York.

Pianta, R.B., Egeland, B. & Erickson, M.F. (1989) The antecedents of maltreatment: results of the Mother–Child Interaction Research Project. In: *Child Maltreatment: Theory and Research on the Causes and Consequences of Child Abuse and Neglect* (eds D. Cicchetti & V. Carlson), pp. 203–253. Cambridge University Press, New York.

Plotkin, R.C. (1983) Cognitive mediation in disciplinary action among mothers who have abused or neglected their children: Dispositional and environmental factors. *Dissertation Abstracts International,* **45,** 684.

Polansky, N.A., Gaudin, J.M., Ammons, P.W. & Davis, K.B. (1985) The psychological ecology of the neglectful mother. *Child Abuse and Neglect,* **9,** 265–275.

Roberts, J.V. (2000) Changing public attitudes towards corporal punishment: the effects of statutory reform in Sweden. *Child Abuse and Neglect,* **24,** 1027–1103.

Rothbaum, B.O. & Foa, E.B. (1996) Cognitive-behavioral therapy for posttraumatic stress disorder. In: *Traumatic stress: The effects of overwhelming experience on mind, body, and society* (eds B.A. Van der Kolk, A.C. MacFarlane & L. Weisaeth), pp. 491–509. Guilford Press: New York.

Saunders, D.G. (1992) A typology of men who batter: three types derived from cluster analysis. *American Journal of Orthopsychiatry,* **62,** 264–275.

Schellenbach, C.J. (1998) Child maltreatment: a critical review of research on treatment for physically abusive parents. In: *Violence Against Children in the Family and the Community* (eds P. Trickett & C.J. Schellenbach), pp. 251–268. American Psychological Association, Washington D.C.

Sedlak, A.J. & Broadhurst, D.D. (1996) *Third National Incidence Study on Child Abuse and Neglect.* Department of Health and Human Services, Washington D.C.

Southall, D.P., Plunkett, M.C., Banks, M.W., Falkov, A.F. & Samuels, M.P. (1997) Covert video recordings of life-threatening child abuse: lessons for child protection. *Pediatrics,* **100,** 735–774.

Steele, B.F. & Pollock, C.B. (1968) A psychiatric study of parents who abuse their infants and small children. In: *The Battered Child* (eds R.E. Helfer & C.H. Kempe), pp. 89–133. University of Chicago Press, Chicago.

Straus, M.A. & Gelles, R.J. (1990) *Physical Violence in American Families.* Transaction Press, New Brunswick, NJ.

Tatara, T. (1996) *US child substitute care flow data for FY 1994 and trends in the state child substitute care populations: technical report.* American Public Welfare Association, Washington D.C.

Thompson, R.A. (1994) Social support and the prevention of child maltreatment. In: *Protecting Children From Abuse and Neglect: Founda-*tions for a new strategy (eds. G.B. Melton & F.D. Barry), pp. 40–130. Guilford Press, New York.

Trickett, P.K. & Susman, E.J. (1988) Parental perceptions of child-rearing practices in abusive and nonabusive families. *Developmental Psychology,* **24,** 270–276.

US Advisory Board on Child Abuse & Neglect (1993) *Neighbors Helping Neighbors: a New National Strategy for the Protection of Children (Fourth Report).* US Government Printing Office, Washington D.C.

Vondra, J.I. (1990) The community context of child abuse. *Marriage and Family Review,* **15,** 19–38.

Wald, M.S. (1991) Defining psychological maltreatment: The relationship between questions and answers. *Developmental Psychopathology,* **3,** 111–118.

Waltz, J., Babcock, J.C., Jacobson, N.S. & Gottman, J.M. (2000) Testing a typology of batterers. *Journal of Consulting and Clinical Psychology,* **68,** 658–669.

Wang, C.T. & Harding, K. (1999) *Current trends in child abuse reporting and fatalities: The results of the 1998 Annual Fifty State Survey.* National Center on Child Abuse Prevention Research, Chicago.

Weber, M.W. (1997) Assessment of child abuse. In: *The Battered Child* (eds M.E. Helfer, R.S. Kempe & R.D. Krugman), 5th edn, pp. 120–149. University of Chicago Press, Chicago.

Widom, C.S. (1989) The cycle of violence. *Science,* **244,** 160–166.

Widom, C.S. (1992) Child abuse and alcohol use and abuse. In: *Alcohol and Interpersonal Violence: Fostering Interdisciplinary Research (National Institute on Alcohol Abuse and Alcoholism (NIAAA) Research Monograph No. 24, NIH Publication No. 93–3496,* (ed. S.E. Martin), pp. 291–314. National Institutes of Health, Rockville, MD.

Willliams, L.M. (1994a) Recall of childhood trauma: A prospective study of women's memories of childhood sexual abuse. *Journal of Consulting and Clinical Psychology,* **62,** 1167–1176.

Williams, L.M. (1994b) What does it mean to forget childhood sexual abuse? A reply to Loftus, Garry, and Feldman. *Journal of Consulting and Clinical Psychology,* **62,** 1182–1186.

Wolfe, D.A. (1999) *Child Abuse: Implications for Child Development and Psychopathology,* 2nd edn. Sage, Thousand Oaks, CA.

Wolfe, V.V., Gentile, C. & Wolfe, D.A. (1989) The impact of sexual abuse on children: a PTSD formulation. *Behavior Therapy,* **20,** 215–228.

Wolfe, D.A., Sas, L. & Wekerle, C. (1994) Factors associated with the development of post-traumatic stress disorder among child victims of sexual abuse. *Child Abuse and Neglect,* **18,** 37–50.

Wolfe, D.A., Reppucci, N.D. & Hart, S. (1995) Child abuse prevention: knowledge and priorities. *Journal of Clinical Child Psychology,* **24,** 5–23.

WuDunn, S. (1999) Child abuse has Japan rethinking family autonomy. *New York Times,* August 15, pp. A1, A8.

Zellman, G. (1990) Report decision-making patterns among mandated child abuse reporters. *Child Abuse and Neglect,* **14,** 325–336.

Zuravin, S.J. (1989) The ecology of child abuse and neglect: review of the literature and presentation of data. *Violence and Victims,* **4,** 101–120.

21 Child Sexual Abuse
Danya Glaser

Introduction

Sexual abuse is a physical act but its deleterious consequences are primarily psychological. It is a significant risk factor for the development of psychopathology in childhood, adolescence and adulthood. Familiarity with the phenomenon (including its presentation and treatment) is therefore of particular importance to the practice of child and adolescent psychiatry.

The hallmarks of child sexual abuse are its secret nature and the very frequent denial of the abuse by the abuser, once it is alleged to have happened. These two factors play a central part in the process of the abuse and in its aftermath. Sexual abuse includes a far wider spectrum than incest, occurs both within the family and outside it but, in either circumstance, the abuser is frequently already known to the child. Indeed, this acquaintance may be based on a deliberate befriending or 'grooming' of the child by the abuser for the purposes of preplanned abuse. Because it involves sexuality, this form of abuse is particularly emotive.

Child sexual abuse is not a new phenomenon. The incest taboo has been in existence for over 4000 years, first records being in the Babylonian code of Hammurabi (≈ 2150 BC) which referred to 'a man be known to his daughter' (Handcock 1932) where 'known' has been translated as 'to conceive a child' (ten Bensel *et al.* 1997). The laws of Moses (*c.* 3000 BC) describe incest as a sin (Leviticus 18:6). General Booth, founder of the Salvation Army, wrote in 1890: 'I understand that the Society for the Protection of Children prosecuted last year a fabulous number of fathers for unnatural sins with their children' (Booth 1890). Despite sporadic earlier pronouncements, child sexual abuse only began to be noted as a significant form of child abuse in the 1970s. Increasing recognition came with the development of the women's movement, reports by adult women survivors of their childhood abuse and a greater openness regarding sexuality. This pattern of increasing recognition has swept through successive countries, with reports appearing in the scientific press, in particular in *Child Abuse and Neglect, the International Journal* (Sariola & Uutela 1996; Luo 1998; Rhind *et al.* 1999).

The universal disapproval of child sexual abuse is exemplified in the UN Convention on the Rights of the Child. Nationally, this disapproval is expressed by the legal prohibition of incest and sexual contact between an adult and a child, and its inclusion as various offences under criminal law. However, some of the harmful effects of child sexual abuse, such as the denial of the abuse by the abuser, and guilt and self-blame by the victim, are largely consequent on this expressed disapproval by society. Moreover, the fact that child sexual abuse is a relatively common experience for children and young persons implies a lack of protection and care for these vulnerable members of society. Despite the now repeated findings of very high reported rates of child sexual abuse (see below), most suspicions of sexual abuse continue to be met with caution, and disclosures are often regarded with suspicion. The fact that an apparently common phenomenon is so often doubted or disbelieved is probably explained by the social taboo surrounding adult sexual contact with children and by at least two further factors. First, the absence of non-involved witnesses to this (secret) activity helps to support the frequent denial of the abuse by the alleged abuser. Secondly, the potentially serious consequences for the alleged abuser if found guilty, govern the attitude to investigation. Alongside the high rate of reports of sexual abuse of children and adolescents, the rates of prosecution and conviction are low. In an English sample of 188 cases of contact abuse, the rate of prosecution was 36% with 17% convictions. A further 5% received a caution (Prior *et al.* 1997). Two independent studies from the USA found that less than one in five cases of alleged abuse reached the stage of prosecution (Tjaden & Thoennes 1992; Martone *et al.* 1996). The stringent test of the evidence in criminal law, 'beyond reasonable doubt', which is higher than 'on balance of probabilities' required in civil law, may help to explain this low rate. Many children who have been abused find difficulty in comprehending the lack of more frequent criminal convictions, especially when they have been prepared to testify in court.

Definitions

The most influential and time-honoured definition of child sexual abuse is by Schechter & Roberge (1976): 'Sexual abuse is defined as the involvement of dependent, developmentally immature children and adolescents in sexual activities they do not truly comprehend, to which they are unable to give informed consent, or that violate the social taboos of family roles.' Inherent, although not specifically stated in this definition, is the notion of coercion or a power differential between the abuser and the child. It is also important to note that the abuser's intentions or motivations are not considered necessary to be included in many definitions. Despite the wide applicability of this definition, a myriad of definitions for legal, research and other purposes continue to be developed and used.

Cultural practices

The above definition refers to social norms. In our multicultural societies, the question of what is a culture-specific practice needs to be considered. This is particularly relevant where ethnic minority groups are living in a majority host culture whose norms differ. Cultural practices are expected to alter with time and context, and the dominant culture tends to set prevailing child-rearing standards (Korbin 1997). However, Ahn & Gilbert (1992), for example, found that among Koreans living in the USA, a grandfather touching the genitalia of his preschool-age grandson was seen as an expression of pride in the fact that this child would continue the family line. Cultural practices may not be benign and culturally sanctioned normative practices may affect adversely the well-being of children (McKee 1984). A particular case is the issue of female genital mutilation (Davis 1998; Eke & Nkanginieme 1999). There is also individual deviation in child care and other practices within cultures (Korbin 1981). Whereas it is important to avoid misidentifying culture as abuse and vice versa (Abney & Gunn 1993), this can be quite difficult in practice. An admittedly small sample (33) of Filipino, Asian and Pacific Island persons working in human services in the USA showed a divergence of opinion about the acceptability, for example, of fathers checking a girl's vaginal area for medical reasons; and for family members to kiss and fondle a baby boy's genitals as an expression of joy about his gender (Okamura *et al.* 1995).

Legal considerations

Under English civil law, child sexual abuse is recognized in the Children Act (1989) as a form of Significant Harm. For child protection purposes, a working definition employed in England is that:

> 'Sexual abuse involves forcing or enticing a child or young person to take part in sexual activities, whether or not the child is aware of what is happening. The activities may involve physical contact, including penetrative . . . or non-penetrative acts . . . ' and 'non-contact activities, such as involving children in looking at, or in the production of, pornographic material or watching sexual activities, or encouraging children to behave in sexually inappropriate ways.' (Department of Health *et al.* 1999)

In criminal law, child sexual abuse is subsumed under a number of different offences. These include incest, which applies to vaginal intercourse between a male and a female whom the offender knows to be his (legal) daughter, granddaughter, sister or mother. Incest is thus not necessarily child sexual abuse. Other offences include indecent exposure, sexual assault, indecent assault, gross indecency, buggery, unlawful sexual intercourse (where one of participants is under 16 years) and rape. Rape requires proof of lack of consent.

In some jurisdictions, such as in England and the USA, civil and criminal proceedings can continue in parallel and independently of each other. This means that, in theory although not always in practice, a child may be protected from an abuser by being moved from his care under civil law, when there has been no criminal trial and potentially even if a criminal trial failed to convict the alleged abuser. In other jurisdictions, child protective procedures will only be undertaken following the criminal conviction of the abuser. This confers considerably less protection on children, especially as the rate of convictions worldwide is relatively low compared with the number of allegations.

Epidemiology

From the perspective of mental health care planning, sufficient provision needs to be made for the treatment of the consequences of a common problem. Planning and resource issues also affect other related agencies, including social services, the police and the courts. However, the published figures for incidence and prevalence of child sexual abuse vary considerably according to the definition used, the source of data and the population studied (Finkelhor 1994). Whereas broad definitions point to the extent of the problem, they are less helpful in indicating severity and the kind of therapeutic services required.

Although annual reports of child sexual abuse could, in theory, indicate incidence, such figures are inaccurate underestimates. Many occurrences of child sexual abuse are not reported at the time of the abuse (Finkelhor *et al.* 1990) and some are not reported at all. Rates of reporting have increased over the past 30 years, both in the UK (Markowe 1988) and in the USA (Finkelhor 1991). More recently, the number of reports of child sexual abuse has decreased (Jones *et al.* 2001). Despite these reported variations, there is little evidence to suggest that the actual incidence has changed significantly (Feldman *et al.* 1991).

The most accurate prevalence figures are from population studies. Even here, responses to interviews or questionnaires may be underestimates, because there may be reluctance or a feeling of shame in describing previous abuse. For instance, Williams (1994) found that 38% of 129 women aged 18–31 years who were interviewed by her, did not mention their previous sexual abuse, which had been documented some 17 years earlier. Whether this represented lack of recall in every case, or some reluctance to talk is still debated. It has been suggested that interviews, which tend to yield higher rates of reported abuse, may be more specific in their questions and more likely to prompt recall of abuse (Wyatt & Peters 1986).

Prevalence of child sexual abuse

Nature of the abuse

Within the spectrum of sexual abuse, the first distinction that needs to be made is between non-contact and contact abuse (Peters *et al.* 1986).

Non-contact abuse

This includes deliberate exposure of children to adult genitalia or sexual activity, either live or depicted in photographs or film. It also includes intrusive looking at the young person's body, inducing children to interact sexually with each other and the taking of photographs for pornographic purposes. There has been debate about the point at which the threshold for Significant Harm or actual abuse is reached when the concerns are about non-contact sexual interaction. When considering the question of harm, it is important to ascertain whether the interaction was deliberate and the extent of coercion used, with greater coercion increasing the harm. Although the most serious effects of sexual abuse are associated with contact, and especially penetrative abuse, many young persons report the experience of being intrusively observed as humiliating and intimidating.

Population studies of adults that have included contact and non-contact abuse by age 18 have yielded rates of between 54% (Russell 1983) and 62% (Wyatt 1985) for women in the USA. In an English interview study of both men and women aged over 15, Baker & Duncan (1985) found 10% positive responses for experiences before the age of 16, whereas Kelly et al. (1991) found rates of 43% for women and 18% for men for at least one unwanted/abusive experience before the age of 16.

Contact abuse

Broadly, in Western societies including specifically the UK and the USA, any physical contact between the breasts and genitalia of a child or adult and a part of the other's body, with the exception of isolated accidental touch (e.g. in the bath or in bed), and for developmentally and age-appropriate cleaning or for applying medication or ointment, is considered to be sexual abuse. Abusive contact includes fondling, masturbation, oral–genital contact or penetration, attempted or actual digital and penal penetration, and the insertion of objects into the vagina or anus. Active abuse is often preceded by an insidious process of 'grooming' in which the abuser, having identified a particular child or children, finds ways of befriending the child or increasing the opportunities for being with the child unobserved. Given the addictive nature of much child sexual abuse, it is in the abuser's interest to be able to continue to abuse a child. There is therefore typically a gradual progression from touching to more penetrative abuse (Berliner & Conte 1990), so as to avoid causing initial pain or injury which would be more likely to lead the child to complain about or report the abuse. Anal abuse is understandably more common in boys, although younger girls are not infrequently anally abused (Hobbs & Wynne 1989). In a small proportion of cases, actual physical violence is used, either as a way of intimidating or coercing the child, or as an integral aspect of the abuse (30% in the study reported by Gomes-Schwartz et al. 1990).

In population studies of women, as opposed to victim samples, non-penetrative contact abuse is the form most commonly described (Haugaard & Reppucci 1988). Russell (1983), in her urban community study of 930 women found that 38% had suffered contact abuse under the age of 18 years, and very serious sexual abuse (forced vaginal or anal intercourse and oral–genital abuse) in 27% of intrafamilial cases. In a British study of female and male students (Kelly et al. 1991), 27 and 11% of respondents, respectively, reported contact abuse. Four per cent of female, and 2% of male respondents, respectively, reported serious, penetrative or coercive abuse, with an age difference between abuser and victim of more than 5 years. Finkelhor (1979), in his questionnaire study of 796 college students, found that 4% had experienced abuse with full intercourse. By contrast, the rate for these serious forms of abuse in clinical samples rises to over 65% (Cupoli & Sewell 1988; Gomes-Schwartz et al. 1990).

Frequency and duration

Whereas population studies have shown a majority for whom sexual abuse is a single episode, in clinical samples the majority of children have been abused more than once by the same abuser. It appears that single episodes of abuse are less likely to be reported and subsequently referred to helping agencies. There is evidence that a child who has been sexually abused is vulnerable to further abuse by others: 14% in the Baker & Duncan (1985) study. This is likely to be a result of a combination of the original vulnerability of the child and the added vulnerability conferred by the experience of having been abused. A distinction needs to be made between repeat victimization by the same abuser and revictimization by different abusers (Hamilton & Browne 1999). Children subjected to organized abuse are often multiply abused. Repeated abuse often continues for several years (Gomes-Schwartz et al. 1990). Duration, frequency and severity, including penetration, are thus linked factors.

Age of victims

Children may be abused from infancy onwards. Children who experience intercourse tend to be older, with an average age of 11.4 years in the Gomes-Schwartz et al. (1990) study, compared with 9.1 years for other forms of significant contact abuse.

Gender of victims

Girl victims are about four times as common as boy victims (Adams-Tucker 1984; Badgley et al. 1984). There is a tendency for sexual abuse of boys to be underreported, in part because of shame and the fear of homosexuality. Adolescent boys are increasingly reluctant to talk about their abuse, even in therapy (Nasjleti 1980). This may explain some reports that boys are abused at a younger mean age than girls (Singer 1989). Younger boys are not infrequently abused alongside their sisters rather than in isolation (Vander Mey 1988). Extrafamilial abuse more commonly involves boys although there is no agreement about whether boys are more commonly abused by strangers (Watkins & Bentovim 1992).

Disability

National statistics on child abuse do not contain data on abused children's disabilities (Kelly 1992). However, in studies of children with disabilities the rate of sexual abuse is two or three times that in 'normal' children (Crosse *et al.* 1993; Sullivan & Knutson 2000). The reasons for this greater prevalence include: the children's' difficulties in communicating abuse (Morris 1999); their dependency on intimate physical care; social isolation in institutional care (Utting *et al.* 1997); and care by staff rather than parents (Westcott & Jones 1999).

Abusers

The majority of abusers (85–95%) are male. Whereas male abusers who abuse prepubertal children may well target both boys and girls, there is some gender specificity in relation to adolescent girl victims. By the time a sexual abuser is identified, his pattern of abusing has often been well established. A small proportion of child sexual abuse is carried out by female abusers (Saradjian 1996), often in conjunction with a man. Women abusers on their own are more likely to abuse boys (Faller 1989).

Sexual abuse by adolescents, mostly boys, has become widely recognized (Abel *et al.* 1987) and is no longer considered an acceptable variant of adolescent sexual development. Many adult abusers report the onset of their abusive activities in adolescence and abuse by an adolescent cannot be considered safely to 'burn out' in adulthood (Vizard *et al.* 1995). A significant proportion of adolescent abusers are of low intellectual ability. Age is no bar to sexually abusive interactions and older men may well continue to abuse children.

There has been much debate about a possible psychological profile of abusers or about a commonality of childhood experiences that might have led them to abuse children. Whereas many will have experienced disruption and physical abuse in their formative years (Seghorn *et al.* 1987), their own sexual abuse is one predisposing, but not a prerequisite, factor for sexually abusing children (summarized in Watkins & Bentovim 1992). A study sought differences between the previous experiences of four comparison samples, each consisting of 15 boys aged 11–15 years who had, respectively,

1 been sexually abused;
2 abused other children;
3 been abused as well as abused other children; and
4 suffered from a conduct disorder (Skuse *et al.* 1998).

Factors predating the sexually abusive activity by the boys included discontinuity of care, exposure to or experience of physical violence and emotional abuse. Such findings help to explain why, in practice, sexual abusers constitute a heterogeneous group in terms of personal, social and demographic factors.

Abuser–child relationship

The majority of children knew their abuser before commencement of the abuse. This acquaintance may have been deliber-ately fostered by the abuser as part of a grooming process, or the abuser and child may be part of the same family or social network. In community studies, the most common relationship is stepfather–stepdaughter (Finkelhor 1984). The same abuser may abuse children both within and outside the family, and include biological as well as stepchildren. Risk to other children in the family and in contact with the abuser is therefore difficult to predict and an assumption must be made that the proven capacity to actually abuse children renders all children in contact with that abuser at risk.

Organized abuse

Many abusers abuse in isolation. However, there are also organized forms of abuse involving more than one abuser and multiple children, some of whom are recruited in sex rings (Wild & Wynne 1986). Organized abuse may include formalized rituals (Frude 1996); debate continues about the extent to which sexual abuse is a part of sadistic or satanic practices. There are, in these cases, questions about the reliability, verifiability and credibility of the reports (Young *et al.* 1991). Organized abuse also includes the use of children and young persons for prostitution, and for the production of child pornography. Children in residential settings in particular may be subject to sexual abuse. These children, who are already vulnerable, are dependent on staff and often isolated from confiding contact with adults outside the residential setting (Utting *et al.* 1997).

Ethnicity, culture and socioeconomic status

Both in the UK and the USA, population-based studies have shown no ethnic differences in the rates of child sexual abuse (Korbin 1997). In the UK, Kelly *et al.* (1991) found no differences between white and black respondents. In the USA, studies have included African-American college students (Priest 1992); Latino, Asian, African-American and European-American women in Russell's (1986) study in San Francisco; and Wyatt's (1985) study which specifically sought equal representation of African- and European-American women respondents. Child sexual abuse has also been described in Filipino, Pacific Island, Cambodian and Asian communities living in the USA by Okamura *et al.* (1995), Rao *et al.* (1992) and Scully *et al.* (1995). However, data on the incidence of child sexual abuse in these communities are lacking, partly because of decisions on data collection criteria which do not classify racial/ethnic background sufficiently finely, and partly because shame and denial about sexual abuse within some cultures conspire against reporting (Okamura *et al.* 1995), particularly when the group has a minority status within a larger host culture. Accurate data on incidence within a particular ethnic group may reflect effects of that group's recent traumatic migration and experiences, rather than aspects of the particular culture, as exemplified by Cambodians living in the USA (Scully *et al.* 1995). Lastly, some societies continue to find difficulty in facilitating open acknowledgement of the existence of child abuse in general, and sexual abuse in particular, within their countries (personal information).

Socioeconomic status is unrelated to the incidence of child sexual abuse in population studies (Berliner & Elliott 1996) but there is an overrepresentation of lower socioeconomic groups in clinic samples (Bentovim *et al.* 1987; Haugaard & Reppucci 1988). This may be because these groups are more likely to come to the attention of child protective agencies than middle class families who may find ways of hiding the abuse or avoiding its reporting (Gomes-Schwartz *et al.* 1990). Different forms of child abuse and neglect are not infrequently found in the same family and the same child (Mullen *et al.* 1994; Ney *et al.* 1994), especially among the socially disadvantaged. Child sexual abuse is associated with troubled family life including family disruption (Russell 1986), reconstituted families, intra-familial violence (Bifulco *et al.* 1991) and parents who are perceived as emotionally distant and uncaring (Alexander & Lupfer 1987).

Theories of risk and causation, and maintaining factors for child sexual abuse

There is no unitary theory of causation to explain child sexual abuse (Glaser & Frosh 1993). In 1896, Freud in his essay entitled 'The Aetiology of Hysteria' postulated that hysterical symptoms found in his patients were attributable to actual sexual experiences in early childhood. Later he changed his views and suggested instead that his patients' difficulties were based not on actual abuse but, rather, on incestuous fantasies or wishes for sexual contact and on young children's seductive capacities. The possible reasons for this change, which was to have a major influence on some later theories of child development, are discussed by Masson (1984). They include the consequent social isolation and pressure that Freud experienced, and the fact that by attributing experiential origins to his patients' difficulties, he was rejecting the prevalent explanations of mental illness in terms of heredity.

The current understanding of sexual abuse is that although, by definition, it is an interaction between the abuser and the child, or the perpetrator and the victim, intention and responsibility rest with the abuser. The abuser's wish for power and sexual gratification are the two main aspects. Sexual arousal to prepubertal children or paedophilia is likely to be a motivating force for abusers of prepubertal children.

Finkelhor (1984) has brought together several factors in a systemic model of four preconditions which, he postulates, are necessary for child sexual abuse to occur. They include both the necessary presence of motivating factors and the absence of inhibiting factors. They are:

1 motivation to sexually abuse children;
2 absence of internal inhibitors;
3 absence of external inhibitors; and
4 absence of child's resistance (or a child's vulnerability).

Preconditions for potential abusers

Motivations refer to the abuser's sexuality and sexual development and include paedophilia, fear/avoidance of peer sexual relationships and sadism. They also address interpersonal motivators, such as a need to overpower or gain mastery over more vulnerable persons, arising as a result of one's own past abuse and low self-esteem. It is noteworthy that in a survey of male undergraduates, 5–9% expressed sexual interest in children (Briere & Runtz 1989). This suggests that the predisposition to sexual abuse is far more common than the action, supporting the postulated need for other factors to exist before abuse will actually occur. Some of the motivations for women abusers are discussed by Welldon (1988) who described incestuous mothers as simultaneously attacking and emotionally engulfing or possessing their children.

Absence of internal inhibitors includes the effects of alcohol and stress. It also refers particularly to the cognitive distortions or rationalizations that abusers employ in continuing to perpetrate abuse and which have been studied by those treating sexual abusers. These cognitive distortions include minimization of the harmful effect of the abuse on the child; conceptualizing the abuse as 'love' or 'education'; and placing responsibility on the child or adolescent who is described as inviting or requesting the abuse.

Child risk factors

External inhibitors of sexual abuse include protective family structures and relationships surrounding the child, in particular a secure attachment to primary caregiver(s), good monitoring of the child's whereabouts and the existence of confiding relationships for the child. Their lack provides a risk for sexual abuse.

The child's vulnerability by virtue of age, disability, neglect or social isolation, all increase the likelihood of sexual abuse. Indeed, abusers recognize these factors as rendering a child suitable for abuse (Budin & Johnson 1989; Conte *et al.* 1989).

This explanatory schema does not remove the abuser's responsibility for the abuse, whatever the nature of contributory risk factors.

Maintaining factors

Summit (1983, 1992) hypothesized a child sexual abuse accommodation syndrome or pattern to explain how children progressively adjust to sexual abuse by a trusted person, by accommodating psychologically to the inherent contradictions, confusions and enforced secrecy accompanying the experience, and which also explains the way in which many children come to disclose sexual abuse. He postulated five stages:

1 secrecy;
2 helplessness;
3 entrapment and accommodation;
4 delayed, unconvincing disclosure; and
5 retraction.

This accommodation pattern enables some children to remain asymptomatic during the abuse, helping to maintain the secrecy and leaving the abuse undiscovered. The abuser's own pattern of denial of the abuse through cognitive distortions lessens his potential discomfort and enables him to continue the abuse. By the time sexual abuse is discovered in childhood, it has usually occurred many times.

Effects of child sexual abuse

The majority of children who have suffered sexual abuse experience a variety of problems (Beitchman *et al.* 1991; Kendall-Tackett *et al.* 1993), some of which extend into adulthood (Wyatt & Powell 1988); there is no specific post child sexual abuse syndrome (Kendall-Tackett *et al.* 1993). Some effects are direct consequences of the sexual experience, such as age-inappropriate sexualized behaviour. Others develop as a response to the abusive nature of what happened. The actual effects are shaped by the child's gender, age, family circumstances (Chaffin *et al.* 1997), ethnicity and social class. In non-clinical samples, adolescents report higher levels of depression and anxiety than younger children (Gidycz & Koss 1989), suggesting that with increasing maturity the adolescent more fully comprehends the implications of having been abused sexually. This is also supported by the finding that distress following child sexual abuse is greater in girls with higher cognitive functioning (Shapiro *et al.* 1992). This is despite the fact that, in general, higher innate ability and the capacity to understand are considered to be protective factors in overcoming adverse life experiences.

Effects in childhood

Sexual abuse may lead to unwanted pregnancy or sexually transmitted disease. Rarely, it may cause genital injuries. However, less than 50% of children with documented sexual abuse have physical findings (Muram 1989). Deleterious psychological effects constitute the starting points for suspecting sexual abuse but often they are only recognized retrospectively, because many are non-specific. About 1 in 3 young people show no outward indicators (Kendall-Tackett *et al.* 1993), allowing abuse to be undetected over prolonged periods. This is particularly likely with children as compared with adolescents (McLeer *et al.* 1998). Although most findings derive from clinical samples, studies of non-clinical adolescents also show raised rates of emotional/behavioural difficulties (Hibbard *et al.* 1990; McLeer *et al.* 1998).

Sexualized behaviour

Most children include in their activity and play some aspects of exploration of their body and its functions, including genitalia, pregnancy, 'mummies and daddies' and 'doctors and nurses'. Friedrich *et al.* (1991) developed the Child Sexual Behaviour Inventory (CSBI) based on parent report. Observations of preschool-age children have also shown that masturbation in preschool-age children is a part of normal development; many preschool-age children touch women's breasts, look at or touch each other's genitalia and some simulate sexual intercourse while remaining fully clothed (Lindblad *et al.* 1995). A significant proportion add genitalia to their figure drawings at some point in their early years (Marjorie Smith, personal communication, 1998).

Age-inappropriate sexualized behaviour is found significantly more commonly in, although not in most, sexually abused children (Friedrich *et al.* 1992; Friedrich 1993; Cosentino *et al.* 1995) and is an important outcome of child sexual abuse (Gale *et al.* 1988). It refers to rarely seen behaviour and talk about genitalia and sexual activity, often involving another child, a doll or, sometimes, an adult. These inappropriate behaviours include inserting fingers, objects or a penis into the vagina or anus, and oral–genital contact (Lloyd Davies *et al.* 2000). It also includes more commonly seen genitally orientated behaviours, such as looking at, touching or drawing genitalia or simulating sexual intercourse fully clothed, when these are repeated, become a preoccupation for the child, or are accompanied by coercion of another child in the activity. This troubling behaviour is particularly likely to follow abuse at an early age (McClellan *et al.* 1996). In boys, it may be regarded as a way of reasserting their masculinity (Rogers & Terry 1984). It may also be a form of reexperiencing the abuse as part of a post-traumatic response (Kiser *et al.* 1988). It is often intractable, a challenge to treatment (see below) and leads to serious difficulties in finding alternative placements for these children, who are considered to pose a risk to other children and who may become socially excluded as a result (Hall *et al.* 1998). In some children, this behaviour comes to be regarded as actual sexual abuse of another child.

Unplanned pregnancy

In adolescence, there is an association between early pregnancy and a history of sexual abuse (Mullen *et al.* 1994). This reflects the sexual vulnerability of these girls to sexual abuse which is expressed in a number of ways including: low self-esteem which leads to a lowered threshold to, or welcoming of, sexual approaches; a confusion between affectionate approaches and sexual attention towards the girls; and actual behaviour which is perceived by others as inviting sexual approaches. A history of child sexual abuse is also frequently found in both boy and girl child prostitutes.

Guilt and self-blame

Clinical experience suggests that many children blame themselves for having been abused, for not stopping the abuse or for not disclosing it earlier. Interestingly, empirical studies do not support this impression (Hunter *et al.* 1992). Tremblay *et al.* (1999) found that a majority of 7–12-year-old children who had been sexually abused maintained a relatively high sense of global worth, and Cohen & Mannarino (1998) made similar findings. By contrast, Mannarino *et al.* (1994) found that sexually abused children more commonly blame themselves for other negative events in their lives.

Post-traumatic stress disorder and dissociation

Post-traumatic stress disorder (PTSD) has been found as a sequel of child sexual abuse, the frequency varying from 44% in an abused group being evaluated for psychiatric disorders and treatment needs (McLeer *et al.* 1992) to 71% in a clinical symptomatic sample (Trowell *et al.* 1999). Moreover, many sexually abused children who do not meet the full diagnostic criteria of PTSD show symptoms of re-experiencing behaviours (McLeer *et al.* 1992), fear, anxiety and difficulty in sustaining concentration (Conte & Schuerman 1988).

Emotional problems

Depression is found more commonly among sexually abused than non-abused children (Wozencraft *et al.* 1991). Whereas depression is found in all age groups, suicidal ideation and self-injurious behaviour is mainly confined to adolescence (Lanktree *et al.* 1991). Low self-esteem (Wozencraft *et al.* 1991) is associated with a history of sexual abuse, and the association holds when family dysfunction is controlled for (Hotte & Rafman 1992). This continues into adolescence (Cavaiola & Schiff 1989). Anxiety is encountered in both sexually abused boys and girls, and in both clinical and non-clinically referred children post abuse. In children, these difficulties may become apparent only on direct questioning or when using specific measures that seek psychopathology (Berliner & Elliott 1996). However, adolescents more readily report higher levels of depression and anxiety than younger children (Gidycz & Koss 1989).

Disorders of behaviour

Aggression and disruptive behaviour may also follow sexual abuse (Kendall-Tackett *et al.* 1993). However, reporting also reflects parental difficulties (Everson *et al.* 1989) and behavioural problems are therefore more severe in clinical populations (Tong *et al.* 1986). Running away, substance abuse and vulnerability to HIV infection both through illicit drug usage and unprotected sex is found in both boy and girl adolescents following sexual abuse (Rotheram-Borus *et al.* 1996).

Peer relationship and school difficulties

Difficulties with peer relationships may arise because of sexualized behaviour, low self-esteem, shame and lack of trust (Mannarino *et al.* 1994). Educational underachievement is commonly encountered and can be explained by a combination of factors leading to poor attention. These include preoccupation with the abuse, fear of the abuser and post-traumatic phenomena. In addition, there is often considerable anxiety and disruption to daily life following the discovery of the abuse and because of the events and responses that ensue. These include uncertainty about the child's future placement and nature of contact with the child's family, and possible change of school and disruption of friendships.

Patterns and continuities

Charting the 'natural history' of sexual abuse-related symptomatology is difficult, because prognosis depends not only on the child's coping and adaptation (Friedrich *et al.* 1988) but also on the nature of the response that the child encounters. This includes treatment which, if successful, will modify outcomes. Moreover, some difficulties are related to age and developmental stage so that new difficulties may arise with maturation. Some children become more symptomatic than when initially seen (Bentovim *et al.* 1987; Gomes-Schwartz *et al.* 1990; Kendall-Tackett *et al.* 1993). Some symptoms resolve more rapidly than others; dissociation, post-traumatic phenomena and sexualized behaviour all attenuate only slowly (Beitchman *et al.* 1991), even with treatment (Lanktree & Briere 1995). Improvement in family functioning, particularly in the domain of problem-solving, correlates with improvement in children's behaviour while maternal coping through avoidance strategies correlates with deterioration in behaviour (Oates *et al.* 1994). Family functioning post abuse is related to the closeness between the abuser, the child and the remaining family. If the abuser is a close family member, and especially if he is denying the fact of the abuse, the family will be more troubled. Whereas there is an overall trend towards improvement in children's functioning, the path is neither smooth nor is its direction straight or entirely predictable.

Effects in adulthood

Studies of male and female adult survivors of child sexual abuse show a clear pattern of interpersonal and intrapsychic difficulties, although this does not constitute a syndrome (Stein *et al.* 1988; Fontes 1995). Interestingly, in their community study from New Zealand, Mullen *et al.* (1996) found that sexually abused women tended not to attribute their mental health problems to their (serious) childhood sexual abuse.

The most commonly reported symptom is depression; deliberate self-harm is significantly higher in women abused in childhood than in non-abused women (e.g. 16 vs. 6%), even in community samples (Saunders *et al.* 1992). Anxiety is also reported but less commonly. Drug and alcohol abuse are important long-term sequelae (Mullen *et al.* 1993), found more commonly in male survivors (Stein *et al.* 1988).

Mullen *et al.* (1994) also found difficulties in the sexual functioning and intimate interpersonal relationships, and distrust of men in women who had been abused, and all the deleterious effects were exacerbated by abuse that had included intercourse. Less disturbance of sexual functioning has been found in men survivors (Stein *et al.* 1988). Only a minority of homosexual men had been sexually abused in childhood, and they have no greater sexual interest in children than heterosexual men.

One study that tested the validity of Finkelhor and Browne's traumagenic model (see below) in a sample of 192 adult women survivors, found that stigma and self-blame, but not betrayal and powerlessness, mediated the effects of sexual abuse on adult psychological functioning (Coffey *et al.* 1996). Some of these difficulties, including low self-esteem, impact on the parenting functions of adult survivors and contribute to the explanation of intergenerational continuities of child abuse. Continuing low self-esteem is also reflected in higher rates of unskilled or semiskilled work among women sexually abused in childhood (Mullen *et al.* 1994).

Eating disorders have been reported as occurring more commonly in women survivors of childhood sexual abuse (Mullen *et al.* 1993).

Neurobiological responses to sexual abuse

There is accumulating evidence of neurobiological effects of child abuse and neglect, including sexual abuse, in both children and adults (Glaser 2000). They include the hypothalamic–pituitary–adrenal (HPA) axis and catecholamine responses, as well as changes in cerebral volume. In children, dysregulation of the HPA axis with blunting of the adenocorticotrophic hormone (ACTH) response to ovine corticotrophin-releasing hormone, but without increased cortisol secretion, has been found in sexually abused girls at a mean of 5 years after the abuse, suggesting downregulation of the HPA axis following the stress of the abuse (De Bellis *et al.* 1994a). De Bellis *et al.* (1999a) found increased 24-h urinary cortisol secretion in children still suffering from PTSD following serious abuse including sexual abuse. Similarly, Kaufman *et al.* (1997) found an elevated ACTH response in children who had been abused and who were still living in adversity, experiencing active emotional abuse. Raised secretion of catecholamines has been found in sexually abused girls (De Bellis *et al.* 1994b). Finally, magnetic resonance imaging (MRI) brain scans of children suffering from PTSD following serious abuse (De Bellis *et al.* 1999b) showed 7% smaller cerebral volume and increased cortical cerebrospinal fluid volume in comparison to non-abused children. Unlike adults, the abused children did not show decreased hippocampal volume.

Golier & Yehuda's (1998) review suggested that some years after sexual abuse, lower cortisol levels are found, in conjunction with a possibly enhanced negative feedback in the HPA axis. Deficits in verbal, but not visual, short-term memory have been found in men and women who had experienced severe childhood physical, sexual and/or emotional abuse, often of early onset (Bremner *et al.* 1995). The severity of the verbal memory deficits correlated positively with the severity of the abuse, as measured on a specially developed instrument relying on past recall, the Early Trauma Inventory. The short-term verbal memory impairment shown in this study is not to be confused with memory for the past abuse which, as the methodology assumes, must be intact. It is suggested (Sapolsky 1996) that

excess cortisol secretion brought on by the stress of the abuse leads to hippocampal damage.

Factors contributing to the effects of sexual abuse

Tremblay *et al.* (1999) found that abuse variables, parental support and the child's coping strategies contributed independently to the psychological outcome for a group of 50 7–12-year-old children. Pre-abuse circumstances, child characteristics and post-abuse responses were also relevant.

Abuse variables

Abuse variables include the nature, duration, and severity of the abuse, and the relationship between the abuser and the child. Abuse factors that are associated with more severe psychological sequelae include prolonged duration and greater frequency of abuse (Caffaro-Rouget *et al.* 1989), penetration of mouth, anus or vagina and abuse accompanied by threats or force (Gomes-Schwartz *et al.* 1990).

Closeness in the relationship between the abuser and the child adversely affects prognosis. Clinical impression suggests a worse prognosis when there have been several abusers, although empirical findings are equivocal on this point (Kendall-Tackett *et al.* 1993). Abuse by mothers of their boy neonates, e.g. by sucking their penises, has shown a powerful sexualizing effect on the boys at a very young age (Chasnoff *et al.* 1986). There are few available data about the specific effects on girls of abuse by women.

Child variables

There is no consistent difference in the magnitude or severity of response between boys and girls. Contrary to expectations, there is no conclusive empirical evidence indicating that boys who have been sexually abused show more externalizing disorders than girls. However, boys experience more anxiety about becoming homosexual or about latent homosexuality within them that, they sometimes believe, had been detected by the abuser (Watkins & Bentovim 1992). The evidence on effects of age at onset of abuse is inconclusive when studied independently of duration of abuse. However, many studies indicate that older children are more symptomatic at the time of presentation. Early sexual abuse, before the age of 7 years, appears to be a risk factor for later inappropriate sexualized behaviour (Mian *et al.* 1996).

Interestingly, the child's coping strategies and cognitive evaluation of the abusive experiences have been shown to contribute less to the child's later functioning than severity of the abuse and the support of the non-abusing carer (Spaccarelli & Kim 1995).

Pre-abuse and family circumstances

The child's family and the nature of caregiving experienced by the child influence the outcome for the child (Waterman *et al.* 1993). Pre-existing adverse family relationships and circumstances may have increased the child's prior vulnerability to abuse as well as contributing to the adverse impact of the abuse on the child (Conte & Schuerman 1988). This includes neglect of supervision; lack of provision for basic needs which renders the child more vulnerable to predatory abusers; the formation of insecure attachments by the child which lessens the likelihood of the child talking about worrying experiences, such as sexual abuse; and social isolation. In some cases, sexual abuse can be regarded as a marker for other detrimental factors in the family which in themselves contribute significantly to later psychopathology (Mullen *et al.* 1993, 1996).

Post-abuse response

The post-abuse response includes the investigation, the response of the non-abusing caregiver(s) and the abuser, as well as protective steps taken to ensure the child's future safety. Denial of the allegation by the alleged abuser naturally leads to a stringent testing and even discrediting of the child's verbal descriptions (Summit 1992). Child protective steps, which may include removing the child from the home, are often necessary because of the denial of the abuse by the abuser (Glaser 1991).

Many mothers remain supportive of their child following discovery of sexual abuse (Sirles & Franke 1989). The non-abusing carer's belief, support and active protection of the child are significant determinants of a good outcome for the child, regardless of the nature of the sexual abuse (Everson *et al.* 1989; Runyan *et al.* 1992). Conversely, the mother's emotional distress adversely affects outcome for the child (Cohen & Mannarino 1998). This points to the need to ensure that at the time of discovery of sexual abuse, help and support are directed at the non-abusing caregiver(s) who are often faced with a conflict of interests, between the abuser and the child. The closer the relationship between the abuser and the non-abusing caregiver, the less supported will the child be by her family (Berliner & Elliott 1996) and the worse the adjustment of the child (Spaccarelli & Kim 1995). Abuse by a stepfather or a mother's current boyfriend is a particularly risky circumstance, compromising support of the child by the mother (Elliott & Briere 1994).

Belief in the child's account of abuse is the first step towards support for the child. It is not, however, synonymous with consistent protection of the child; this requires the primary carer(s) to distance themselves and the child from the abuser, both emotionally and physically. This is particularly difficult when the abuser is the mother's partner (Heriot 1996).

Model for the effects of child sexual abuse

Finkelhor & Browne (1985) developed a model to explain the effects of child sexual abuse. This eclectic and comprehensive model reflects the complexity, and consequently the heterogeneous nature of the effects of child sexual abuse. It comprises the following: traumatic sexualization, betrayal, stigmatization and powerlessness.

Traumatic sexualization refers to the abuse experience and combines the trauma and the developmentally inappropriate sexual aspects of the abuse. Finkelhor (1988) postulated that the process of the abuse fetishises children's genitalia in a developmentally inappropriate way, rewards children for, and confuses children about the meaning and involvement of their sexual behaviour, and leads to an association of sexuality with trauma. These aspects are considered to be unique to child sexual abuse.

A *sense of betrayal* refers to aspects of the child–abuser and child–caregiver relationships. It reflects the fact that abusers have usually been trusted by the child, either inherently by the nature of the relationship, or by the relationship that has been created by the abuser, sometimes deliberately, prior to the abuse. The sense of betrayal also extends to the experience of not being believed by their non-abusing caregivers, especially mothers (Herman 1981). Young children, who believe in the power of their parents to protect them from harm, lose this sense of safety and protection when they become abused.

Stigmatization concerns the child's emotional response and self-view. It includes the sense of shame, blame/guilt and worthlessness which are both communicated to the child in the process of the abuse and by the way sexual abuse is regarded. Children often seek to 'explain' why they were targeted and ascribe self-denigrating meanings. Boys sometimes believe that they must have been recognized as homosexual in order to have been 'chosen'. Many girls express feelings of having become 'spoilt goods' (Rogers & Terry 1984).

Powerlessness refers to the child's experience of threat or overwhelming fear sometimes associated with sexual abuse and the origin of post-traumatic stress responses. Less traumatically, it also encompasses the child's experience of being overruled and their body invaded and spoiled.

Shapiro (1989) discussed a reciprocal relationship between self-blame and helplessness or powerlessness in sexually abused children. If the child's perception of helplessness is confined to the abuse situation, this may mitigate against self-blame for the abuse. Conversely, if the child blames herself, this may help to overcome her perception of herself as powerless.

Role of child and adolescent mental health services in child sexual abuse

Child sexual abuse is sometimes part of the referral presentations and sometimes its occurrence is discovered incidentally during assessment or treatment. Also, some troubled parents will have been sexually abused in childhood. The possibility of abuse in family members therefore always needs to be considered; familiarity with its effects as well as with its investigation, and with protection and legal aspects, is important. Sexual abuse needs to be considered especially in children showing age-inappropriate sexualized behaviour and in depressed or suicidal adolescents. At times, an unsolicited disclosure is made by a child during therapeutic work. Child psychologists, psychiatrists and psychotherapists may contribute to investigations of child sexual abuse, particularly in assessment interviews of young or very traumatized children, or in children with communication difficulties. Consultation to social services in case management and to carers of children who have been sexually abused is often requested. A particular role is the provision of individually appropriate treatment for abused children and their families.

Child sexual abuse may also call for forensic work. This includes assessments for Children Act 1989 proceedings, providing expert reports and oral evidence (Wall 2000). Comments are usually requested on the presence or absence of Significant Harm and on the nature of the Care Plan, which includes the future care and residence of the child, contact with family members including the abuser, and the child's and family's therapeutic needs. Risk assessments on adolescent abusers may also be required. Children who have been sexually abused are eligible for Criminal Injury Compensation Authority awards, and child mental health professionals may be requested to provide reports about the nature and extent of the harm to the child and their treatment needs.

Initial professional encounters with child sexual abuse

Principles

Whenever sexual abuse is suspected or presented explicitly to a professional, including child mental health practitioners, multidisciplinary professional involvement follows inevitably. Its broad aims are to ascertain what, if anything, has happened to the child and to gain an understanding of the child's development and family context and needs. If the child has been abused, the child's needs will include the following.
1 The immediate and long-term protection of the child from sexual abuse.
2 The amelioration of the effects of the abuse including:
   • reduction of distress and the resolution of internal conflicts for the child;
   • resolution of interpersonal conflicts surrounding the child; and
   • treating physical consequences of the abuse.
3 Ensuring optimal development for the child following cessation of abuse.

Although these aims are clear, their achievement in practice is fraught with difficulties. Suspicions need to be verified and a child's account tested, because protection comes at a cost and therapy can only follow protection. As there are rarely witnesses to the abuse, establishing whether it has occurred will rest heavily on the child's verbal description, which may be retracted even if it was true. Discovery of abuse is often accompanied by

denial by the alleged abuser, and some doubt or disbelief, and usually constitutes a crisis for the family and a challenge to the professional system. The child's ultimate well-being will, to a significant extent, be determined by the support given by the family. The nature of the early intervention by professionals and their consideration of the position and needs of the mother or non-abusing caregivers, will have long-lasting effects on the child's and the family's subsequent expectations and attitudes towards professionals with whom they may need to continue to work (Sharland et al. 1996).

In some countries, including the UK, the responsibility for child protection rests with social services to whom suspicions or actual abuse are reported. The subsequent multidisciplinary and multiagency process involves, in addition, the police, health and education and the courts. In other countries, the responsibility for child protection remains with the courts. A number of well-established steps in the process have been identified (Jones 1997; Department of Health et al. 1999), each step depending on the outcome of the previous one.
1 Suspicion or recognition leading to referral to (child protection) social services.
2 Establishing whether there is a need for immediate protection.
3 Planning the investigation including:
   • interagency discussion;
   • interviewing the child;
   • medical examination of the child; and
   • initial assessment of the family.
4 Validation and initial child protection meeting (conference).
5 Protection plan and a more comprehensive assessment.
6 Implementation of plans and review.
7 Prosecution.
8 Therapy.
Different combinations of agencies are involved in the many stages.

Suspicion, recognition and disclosure

Suspicion is based on one or more indicators, both specific and non-specific (Glaser & Frosh 1993). Specific indicators include: inappropriate sexualized behaviour (see above); genital physical signs (Hobbs & Wynne 1989) including sexually transmitted diseases and pregnancy in a young girl or when the identity of the father is unclear; running away and deliberate self-harm in adolescence; sexual abuse of other children in the family; and known contact with a sexual abuser. Non-specific indicators include a variety of behavioural, emotional and educational difficulties. Sexual abuse needs to be considered especially when there is a sudden onset of difficulties in a previously untroubled child and when no other obvious explanations are available. These difficulties include inability to sustain attention, deterioration in educational progress, social isolation or aggressiveness, indicators of low self-esteem, marked unhappiness or depression, disturbed sleep and nightmares, fearfulness and separation anxiety, and eating disorders.

In child and adolescent psychiatric practice, it is important to consider the possibility of sexual abuse as one explanation for those difficulties that are recognized as effects of sexual abuse. Rather than an initial direct enquiry about sexual abuse, it is preferable to enquire about upsetting and unwanted experiences and previous contact with social services. With adolescents, a direct enquiry could be made, especially following deliberate self-harm. Careful notes should be made of such assessment interviews (Jones *et al.* 1993) and it is always advisable to discuss one's concerns and suspicions with a colleague. It is also possible to request an 'anonymous consultation' with a social worker, in which the child's identity is not divulged. As a result of such assessments, sexual abuse may come to light which may or may not already be known about by child protection agencies. If it is a new disclosure, the child needs to be listened to, avoiding interruptions and questions, and the conversation needs to be carefully recorded in writing.

Although in the UK, unlike in the USA, there is no *mandatory* reporting of seriously suspected or actual sexual abuse, it is considered to be good professional practice to report serious suspicions or disclosures to child protective agencies or social services (Department of Health *et al.* 1999). This overrides the usual rules of confidentiality. A child may not wish for their disclosure to be divulged to another agency. When it is not possible to accede to the child's wishes, the child's misgivings need to be explored, the reasons given for the need to report the abuse, and the child needs to be involved in the process of notifying social services. Referral is usually made with the knowledge of the family, unless there are indicators that this will place the child at increased risk, including pressure on the child to retract an allegation.

Abuse more usually comes to light when a child talks about it to a relative, friend or teacher (Bradley & Wood 1996). Children who spontaneously describe sexual abuse and who make an intentional disclosure are likely to be accurate in their account.

The need for immediate protection is a decision of social services in consultation with other professionals and agencies and might require an emergency protection order in respect of the child (Children Act 1989).

Investigation and formal interview

The next step in the investigative and protection process is a professional (or strategy) meeting, which is convened by the statutory agencies — police and social services. It will also include any professionals with immediate relevant knowledge about the concerns and about the child and the family, including a professional to whom an allegation or disclosure has been made. This could therefore be a child psychiatrist or other mental health professional.

The purpose of the strategy discussion is to plan the investigation, the approach to the family, the formal interview with the child and the medical examination (Heger & Emans 2000). Children will be interviewed formally if there are clear suspicions of abuse or if the child has already disclosed the abuse informally. Both clinical experience and empirical evidence (Keary & Fitzpatrick 1994) show that children (especially younger ones) will not usually describe sexual abuse during a formal interview, unless they have previously spoken about it. (The converse is not, however, true.) Consideration therefore needs to be given to the relative merits of enabling a child to talk informally, with the attendant risk of this being later construed as suggestive, against submitting a child who is not ready to talk to a formal interview which may not yield a description of abuse which had, nevertheless, occurred.

Talking about an event either at the time or afterwards, enables a child to organize the experience in a more coherent way and enhances the laying down of a more coherent account and memory of the experience (Haden *et al.* 1997). Although the fact of a conversation will distort the memory to some extent, talking continues to improve the capacity to recall an experience as well as to make sense of it, especially when the experience is stressful or traumatic (Goodman & Quas 1997).

The formal interview is video recorded and may be used both as prosecution evidence in a subsequent criminal trial, and in civil child protection legal proceedings. It is therefore carried out by police and social services according to strictly specified guidelines. Rarely, children are encountered whose distressed or traumatized mental state, or whose difficulties in communication indicate the need for interviewing skills of a child mental health professional. Some people have used facilitated communication with autistic children who are suspected of having been abused, but systematic studies have made it clear that what is communicated usually does *not* derive from the child (see Rutter & Yule, Chapter 7). This is an unsafe procedure.

Ceci *et al.* (Chapter 8) discuss what is known about children's memory and their reliability as witnesses. Among many other factors not associated with memory but which may, nevertheless, be misinterpreted as poor recall, is the extent to which the child is motivated to talk about past events. The child may well continue to be cared for, or be in close contact with an abuser, and may therefore consider disclosure of the abuse to be a betrayal of the abuser. Silence may be one way of dealing with this dilemma (Freyd 1996). Children who are interviewed some time after the abuse, and who may be suffering from PTSD, may find difficulty in talking about the abuse.

The child's responses are by no means related only to the strength of memories or the power of recall. As well as challenging the child's capacity to recall, the child's truthfulness, clarity of thought as opposed to confusion, and the child's capacity to withstand misleading suggestions, are all often questioned. There is now much research evidence to show that the circumstances in which the child's account is sought and obtained, and the power differential in the relationship between the interviewer and the child, have a significant bearing on the child's 'performance' (for a review see Lamb *et al.* 1997). Interviewing styles and forms of questioning are capable of significantly distorting children's accounts which do not then reflect what the child had previously recalled. For instance, when the rapport-building stage of the interview consists of open questions, children's response to the first open question regarding a past experience yields 2.5 more details and words than following a closed question. Moreover, this initial pattern continues in response to open questions throughout the interview. Repeated occasions *per se*, in which the child is simply invited to describe past experiences, without pressure or suggestion, do not compromise accuracy of recall (Fivush & Schwarzmueller 1995). By contrast, closed questions requiring a forced choice, yes/no answers (and not infrequently used by advocates in court) yield far less accurate information. However, in order to obtain optimal information and verify certain facts, closed questions can be alternated with open ones.

There has been much debate about the use of anatomically correct dolls in the interviewing of children. There is little evidence that young non-abused children proceed beyond exploration of the dolls' genitalia to enact sexualized behaviour (Glaser & Collins 1989). Nevertheless, the dolls should not be used as a screening tool (Boat & Everson 1994) or cue (Everson & Boat 1994), but rather to enable young children to illustrate what they have conveyed verbally.

Validation

Validation of child sexual abuse requires assessment of the evolution of suspicions, and the circumstances as well as the content of the child's first description or disclosure of abuse. The outcome of a formal interview and the findings in a medical examination receive obvious scrutiny, particularly in legal proceedings, both civil and criminal. Other factors include family circumstances; the child's relationship with the alleged abuser; the responses to the allegation by the mother or the non-abusing caregivers, and by the alleged abuser. In a retrospective review of 551 case notes of reported concerns about possible child sexual abuse, 43% were substantiated, 21% were inconclusive, and 34% were not considered to be abuse cases. Only 2.5% were erroneous concerns emanating from children, and included only eight (1.5%) of false allegations originating from the child, and three made in collusion with a parent (Oates *et al.* 2000). In other studies, false allegations were most commonly made under the influence of a parent in the context of disputed contact or residence disputes between warring parents.

The nature of protection

A child who is believed to have been abused is deemed to be protected providing all contact with the alleged abuser is either fully supervised or stopped. A child can only be protected in a context in which there is belief in the child's allegations, without explicit blame of the child, and where there is a commitment by the child's non-abusing caregiver to protect the child. Children abused by persons outside the family tend to be excluded from child protective services on the, sometimes erroneous (Tebbutt *et al.* 1997), assumption that they will be protected by their families. If protection is achieved, and if no legal proceedings ensue,

there may never be a formal record of the validated fact of the abuse.

Child protection conference and planning

A multidisciplinary child protection conference is convened if there is a reasonable likelihood that a child has been abused and remains unprotected. The purpose of a conference is to determine, on the basis of information gathered, whether the child continues to be at risk of Significant Harm and, if so, the nature of the protection plan which will ensure the child's safety. This plan will include a comprehensive assessment of the child and the family's needs and commencement of therapeutic work, to both of which child mental health services are often required to contribute.

Legal proceedings

There are both civil and criminal proceedings in which the question of child sexual abuse is at issue. Civil proceedings concern the future safety of the child. In England under the Children Act (1989) the child's welfare is paramount. The child does not attend court or give evidence; hearsay and expert evidence are allowed. Civil proceedings include the following.

1 Public law care proceedings in which Significant Harm is determined and a finding may be made about sexual abuse having occurred. The court may grant an order (care or supervision) to ensure the child's well-being and a care plan is required, for which the local authority is responsible.

2 Private law family proceedings in which residence and contact disputes between parents are sometimes based on allegations of sexual abuse of the child while in the care of one of the parents.

In criminal proceedings, the child is an accessory to the court process, whose interest is the determination of the guilt or innocence of the alleged abuser. Unless the alleged abuser pleads guilty, both the child's account of the abuse (which may have previously been video-recorded) and cross-examination of the child, are required. Expert evidence and opinion regarding the child's credibility is not permitted in English courts, that being an issue for the jury and the judge to decide.

Therapeutic work

A systemic treatment approach to the effects of child sexual abuse requires consideration of the child's needs, both individually and in the context of the family. Just as there is no post abuse syndrome, so is the application of a programmatic universal treatment not appropriate. It is more useful to consider in each case which likely issues might require treatment. A starting point is consideration of the individual needs, and relationships between the three participants in the 'abuse triangle': the abuser, the child and the non-abusive caregiver (Glaser 1991).

The fulfilment of the child's and family members' needs often requires social work support as well as more formal psychological therapy and psychiatric treatment. An integrated multi-disciplinary and multiagency approach is required (Furniss 1991) in which therapy both deals with needs as they arise and according to their severity, and is offered at appropriate points in the post-abuse process (Jones 1996). For instance, it is not appropriate for a child to receive group or individual therapy for the effects of the abuse while the child remains unprotected; children in transition from one family to a new permanent home are often more preoccupied with their impermanence and their family's response than with the sexual abuse. It may be inadvisable for a child to join a therapeutic group before testifying in impending criminal proceedings; therapy might need to await outcome of criminal proceedings if a child has retracted allegations or the alleged abuser denies the abuse (Home Office *et al.* 2001). Furthermore, work with the child is most beneficial when undertaken in parallel with work with the parent(s) or carers and family (Monck *et al.* 1996). Some of the child's needs can only be addressed by work with the non-abusing carers alone or with the child and mother/parents together (Celano *et al.* 1996). For other difficulties, it is appropriate to work with the child alone or in a peer-group setting.

Children's therapeutic needs

Not all children who have been sexually abused require prolonged or even systematic therapy. However, as a minimum requirement it is important to ascertain that the child is able to talk about their experiences to a parent or other identified person, who believes the child and is able to listen to the child supportively and uncritically. Children who have been sexually abused also require age-appropriate education about sexuality and the nature and risks of sexual abuse. As stated earlier, many children are symptomatic and therefore require treatment. Whereas some symptoms, such as sexualized behaviour, are readily apparent, others, such as PTSD or depression, may need to be actively sought. Specific instruments, such as the Children's Impact of Traumatic Events Scale–Revised (CITES-R) (Wolfe *et al.* 1991), the Trauma Symptom Checklist for Children (Brierea 2001) and measures of depression such as the Childhood Depression Inventory (Kovacs 1983) are of particular help. It is important to include children who have been abused by strangers or by someone outside the family (Van Scoyk *et al.* 1988; Grosz *et al.* 2000), whose therapeutic needs may be overlooked when protection from re-abuse is not considered to be an issue (Sharland *et al.* 1996).

Overall, treatments that are directed at specific difficulties have been shown to be more effective than no treatment (Finkelhor & Berliner 1995) or the mere passage of time (Deblinger *et al.* 1996) and length of treatment has been found to be predictive of outcome for depression (Lanktree & Briere 1995). There are some findings of no effect (Oates *et al.* 1994; Tebbutt *et al.* 1997) or some deterioration for a minority of children during therapy (Jones & Ramchandani 1999). It is not clear what the relative contribution of intercurrent developments in the child's life or the therapy itself made to the reported deterioration. In the light of the mostly positive outcome for therapy, it would not be appropriate to withhold treatment from symptomatic children. However, these findings point to the importance of monitoring the child's psychological state during treatment and a preparedness to halt therapy if necessary.

There are several ways by which treatment approaches for children can be categorized. Children may be treated individually or in groups; treatment may be directed at specific symptoms; and specific therapeutic approaches, such as psychodynamic or cognitive behavioural therapy (Cohen & Mannarino 1993; Deblinger & Heflin 1996), may be selected.

Group and individual therapy

The shared membership of a group offers an alternative to the secretiveness, isolation and shame experienced by most sexually abused children; this may explain findings from a small sample of children who expressed a preference for group over individual therapy (Prior *et al.* 1994). The group setting is appropriate for learning about sexuality and for developing a socially appropriate 'story' about one's own abuse. The observation of children in groups enables professionals to assess children's further therapeutic needs, which may include longer term individual psychotherapy.

It is preferable for a group to have more than one child with a particular attribute, such as minority ethnicity, abuse by a stranger or living away from home. Groups for children aged over 7 years are more appropriately offered separately for boys and girls and broadly age-banded (Nelki & Watters 1989). Groups require two therapists, of whom one should be a woman. Groups for pre-adolescent children are usually activity-based and follow a programme which addresses issues commonly encountered by children who have been abused. These include a range of distressing feelings, such as shame, guilt, anger and low self-esteem; sexuality; confiding and secrets (Berliner 1997). Adolescents are able to use groups for a more reflective exploration of their feelings (Furniss *et al.* 1988).

Children's attendance in therapy, whether group or individual, is dependent on their parents' psychological and physical support. The provision of support or therapy for the accompanying parent or carer in conjunction with the child's therapy is therefore useful in addressing both emotional and practical issues of the parents (Damon & Waterman 1986). This can be offered individually or in a group. It also enables the parents to remain involved in, and informed about relevant aspects of the child's therapy, in order to support that process (Rushton & Miles 2000).

Whereas groups are widely used and their process well documented (Berman 1990), a recent review of published outcome studies of therapy for sexually abused children (Jones & Ramchandani 1999) found overall little difference in effect between group and individual treatments in improving children's symptoms. In one of the studies reviewed (Trowell *et al.* 1995), the outcome for very troubled girls randomly assigned to individual psychodynamic psychotherapy or group therapy showed significant improvement of a comparable extent at 1- and 2-year follow-up after both forms of therapy. The only significant difference was a greater decrease in PTSD re-experiencing of trauma, and persistent avoidance of stimuli dimensions, for girls receiving individual therapy.

Specific symptoms and therapeutic modalities

Sexualized behaviour (Trowell *et al.* 1999) and PTSD have been found to be particularly difficult to alleviate. However, cognitive behavioural therapy directed at particular difficulties has been shown to be significantly more efficacious than non-directive supportive therapy in improving outcome for young sexually abused children, including a significant decrease in sexualized behaviour (Cohen & Mannarino 1997). Interestingly, both psychodynamic therapy (see above) and cognitive behavioural therapy which was directed specifically at symptoms of PTSD (Deblinger *et al.* 1996) have been shown to be effective in reducing PTSD.

Therapeutic work with caregivers and family

Mothers and non-abusing caregivers

The mental health of the non-abusing mother or caregiver, as well as her belief in and support of the child are important factors determining the outcome for a sexually abused child. In the absence of parental support, children may not remain living with their biological family, because of both blame and lack of protection. There are many obstacles to maternal or parental support following discovery of abuse, which are amenable to change through specific therapeutic work, either individually or in a group. The obstacles include the nature of the relationship between the carer and the abuser, and the need for an imposed distance or termination of that relationship; the mother or carer's guilt about not protecting the child; anger towards the child; and memories of some mothers' own abuse. The discovery of sexual abuse and its aftermath also offer opportunities for helping parents with parenting issues (Celano *et al.* 1996).

Siblings and the family

Siblings are sometimes the silent witnesses of abuse and their needs and feelings may be overlooked in the process of attending to the sexually abused child and the mother. Meetings with the whole family can redress this balance, also enabling the family to talk openly about the fact of the abuse, whose mention is often avoided despite the fact that family members are acutely aware of it. However, family meetings would not include the abuser unless he has taken responsibility for the abuse and is receiving treatment. Family work is important when there are indications of blaming or scapegoating of the

abused child. Other dysfunctional aspects of family interactions that are associated with child sexual abuse include, in particular, inappropriate intergenerational boundaries, disorganization, parental neglect and unavailability (Madonna *et al.* 1991; Bentovim 1992). They require more formal family therapy (Elton 1988).

Work with abusers

Adolescent abusers

The treatment of adolescent abusers is important in order to prevent progression of abuse into adulthood. The prognosis may be more encouraging than with adult abusers because the adolescent may be less defensive and at a developmental stage when he is emotionally vulnerable and responsive to change. Moreover, the child protective and youth justice systems can be instrumental in encouraging attendance at therapy. A particularly important factor is the support, by the young abuser's parents, for the adolescent to own up to the abuse. Without this, it is difficult to offer therapy. A dual approach is required, which encompasses both the young abuser's responsibility for the abuse and his likely past emotional, physical or sexual victimization. Therapy may be offered individually (Woods 1997) or in groups (Smets & Cebula 1987). Using activities as well as words, a group can offer the following:

- peer support;
- challenging denial and minimization of the abuse and responsibility for it;
- sex education;
- development of social skills;
- victim awareness;
- recognition of cognitive distortions concerning the abuse; and
- mapping the abuse cycle (Hawkes 1999) and learning to halt its progression.

Adult abusers

The issue of treatment for adult abusers is important for those children who are closely related to their abuser and who wish to resume a meaningful relationship with him. Central to treatment, often carried out in group settings, is reduction of denial by the abuser (Salter 1988). Initial denial of their involvement is encountered in the majority of abusers. There is commonly also denial of the extent of the abuse, responsibility for the abuse, the harm caused to the child or the inappropriate nature of the sexual contact. Therapy needs to recognize the emotional comfort which denial offers and to acknowledge the cost of assuming responsibility. The issues described above in adolescent abuser groups also apply to adult abusers. Common to both is the recognition that the risk for returning to child sexual abuse remains a possibility.

Conclusions

Child sexual abuse is a discrete, definable and often repeated event that is embedded in a complex web of contextual factors, both historical and relational. Its antecedents and consequences are manifold and not necessarily specific. For these reasons, specific prevention is particularly difficult and alertness to the possibility and early recognition offer the best hope for damage limitation. Children cannot be relied upon to protect themselves. Secrecy, denial and disbelief are integrally related to sexual abuse and exert a very significant influence on the professional response and outcome for the children and their families.

References

Abel, G., Becker, J., Mittelman, M., Cunningham-Rathier, J., Rouleau, J. & Murphy, W. (1987) Self reported sex crimes in nonincarcerated paraphiliacs. *Journal of Interpersonal Violence*, 2, 3–25.

Abney, V. & Gunn, K. (1993) Culture: a rationale for cultural competency. *APSAC Advisor*, 6, 19–22.

Adams-Tucker, C. (1984) The unmet psychiatric needs of sexually abused youths: referrals form a child protection agency and clinical evaluations. *Journal of the American Academy of Child and Adolescent Psychiatry*, 23, 659–667.

Ahn, H. & Gilbert, N. (1992) Cultural diversity and sexual abuse prevention. *Social Service Review*, 66, 410–427.

Alexander, P. & Lupfer, S. (1987) Family characteristics and long-term consequences associated with sexual abuse. *Archives of Sexual Behaviour*, 16, 235–245.

Badgley, R., Allard, H., McCormich, N. *et al.* (1984) *Sexual Offences Against Children*. Canadian Government Publishing Centre, Ottawa.

Baker, A. & Duncan, S. (1985) Child sexual abuse: a study of prevalence in Great Britain. *Child Abuse and Neglect*, 9, 457–467.

Beitchman, J., Zucker, K., Hood, J., da Costa, G. & Akman, D. (1991) A review of the short-term effects of child sexual abuse. *Child Abuse and Neglect*, 15, 537–556.

ten Bensel, R., Rheinberger, M. & Radbill, S. (1997) Children in a world of violence: the roots of child maltreatment. In: *The Battered Child* (eds M. Helfer, R. Kempe & R. Krugman), pp. 3–28. University of Chicago Press, Chicago.

Bentovim, A. (1992) *Trauma Organised Systems: Physical and Sexual Abuse in Families*. Karnac, London.

Bentovim, A., Boston, P. & van Elburg, A. (1987) Child sexual abuse: children and families referred to a treatment project and the effects of intervention. *British Medical Journal*, 295, 1453–1457.

Berliner, L. (1997) Intervention with children who experienced trauma. In: *Developmental Perspectives on Trauma: Theory, Research and Intervention* (eds D. Cicchetti & S. Toth), pp. 491–514. University of Rochester Press, Rochester, NY.

Berliner, L. & Conte, J. (1990) The process of victimization: the victim's perspective. *Child Abuse and Neglect*, 14, 29–40.

Berliner, L. & Elliott, D. (1996) Sexual abuse of children. In: *APSAC Handbook on Child Maltreatment* (eds J. Briere, L. Berliner, J. Bulkley, C. Jenny & T. Reid), pp. 51–71. Sage, London.

Berman, P. (1990) Group therapy techniques for sexually abused preteen girls. *Child Welfare*, 69, 239–252.

Bifulco, A., Brown, G. & Adler, Z. (1991) Early sexual abuse and clinical depression in adult life. *British Journal of Psychiatry*, 159, 115–122.

Boat, B. & Everson, M. (1994) Exploration of anatomical dolls by non-referred pre-school aged children: Comparisons by age, gender, race and socio-economic status. *Child Abuse and Neglect*, 18, 139–153.

Booth, W. (1890) A preventive home for unfallen girls when in danger. In: *In Darkest England and the Way Out*, pp. 192–193. International Headquarters of the Salvation Army, London.

Bradley, A. & Wood, J. (1996) How do children tell? The disclosure process in child sexual abuse. *Child Abuse and Neglect*, 20, 881–891.

Bremner, J., Randall, P., Scott, T. *et al.* (1995) Deficits in short-term memory in adult survivors of childhood abuse. *Psychiatry Research*, 59, 97–107.

Briere, J., Johnson, K., Blissada, A. *et al.* (2001) The Trauma Symptom Checklist for Young Children (TSCYC): reliability and association with abuse exposure in multi-site study. *Child Abuse and Neglect*, 25, 1001–1014.

Briere, J. & Runtz, M. (1989) University males' sexual interest in children predicting potential indices of 'paedophilia' in a non-forensic sample. *Child Abuse and Neglect*, 13, 65–75.

Budin, L. & Johnson, C. (1989) Sex abuse prevention programmes: offenders' attitudes about their efficacy. *Child Abuse and Neglect*, 13, 77–87.

Caffaro-Rouget, A., Lang, R. & van Santen, V. (1989) The impact of child sexual abuse. *Annals of Sex Research*, 2, 29–47.

Cavaiola, A. & Schiff, M. (1989) Self esteem in abused chemically dependent adolescents. *Child Abuse and Neglect*, 13, 327–334.

Celano, M., Hazard, A., Webb, C. & McCall, C. (1996) Treatment of traumagenic beliefs among sexually abused girls and their mothers: an evaluation study. *Journal of Abnormal Child Psychology*, 24, 1–17.

Chaffin, M., Wherry, J. & Dykman, R. (1997) School aged children's coping with sexual abuse: abuse stresses and symptoms associated with four coping strategies. *Child Abuse and Neglect*, 21, 227–240.

Chasnoff, M., Burns, W., Schnoll, S., Burns, K., Chisum, G. & Kyle-Spore, L. (1986) Maternal–neonatal incest. *American Journal of Orthopsychiatry*, 56, 577–580.

Coffey, P., Leitenberg, H., Henning, K., Turner, T. & Bennett, R. (1996) Mediators of the long-term impact of child sexual abuse: perceived stigma, betrayal, powerlessness, and self-blame. *Child Abuse and Neglect*, 20, 447–455.

Cohen, J. & Mannarino, A. (1993) A treatment model for sexually abused pre-schoolers. *Journal of Interpersonal Violence*, 8, 115–131.

Cohen, J. & Mannarino, A. (1997) A treatment outcome study for sexually abused preschool children: outcome during a one year follow-up. *Journal of the American Academy of Child and Adolescent Psychiatry*, 36, 1228–1335.

Cohen, J. & Mannarino, A. (1998) Factors that mediate treatment outcome of sexually abused preschool children: six and 12 month follow-up. *Journal of the American Academy of Child and Adolescent Psychiatry*, 37, 44–51.

Conte, J. & Schuerman, J. (1988) The effects of sexual abuse on children: a multidimensional view. In: *The Lasting Effects of Child Sexual Abuse* (eds G. Wyatt & G. Powell), pp. 157–170. Sage, CA.

Conte, J., Wolfe, S. & Smith, T. (1989) What sexual offenders tell us about prevention strategies. *Child Abuse and Neglect*, 13, 293–302.

Cosentino, S., Meyer-Bahlburg, H., Alpert, J., Weinberg, S. & Gaines, R. (1995) Sexual behavior problems and psychopathology symptoms in sexually abused girls. *Journal of the American Academy of Child and Adolescent Psychiatry*, 34, 1033–1042.

Crosse, S., Kaye, E. & Ratnofsky, A. (1993) *A report on the maltreat-*

ment of children with disabilities. National Center on Child Abuse and Neglect, Washington D.C.

Cupoli, J. & Sewell, P. (1988) 1059 children with a chief complaint of sexual abuse. *Child Abuse and Neglect*, **12**, 151–162.

Damon, L. & Waterman, J. (1986) Parallel group treatment of children and their mothers. In: *Sexual Abuse of Young Children* (eds K. MacFarlane & J. Waterman), pp. 244–298. Guilford, New York.

Davis, A. (1998) Female genital mutilation. *Medicine and Law*, **17**, 143–148.

De Bellis, M., Chrousos, G., Dorn, L. *et al.* (1994a) Hypothalamic–pituitary–adrenal axis disregulation in sexually abused girls. *Journal of Clinical Endocrinology and Metabolism*, **7**, 249–255.

De Bellis, M., Lefter, L., Trickett, P. & Putnam, F. (1994b) Urinary catecholamine excretion in sexually abused girls. *Journal of the American Academy of Child and Adolescent Psychiatry*, **33**, 320–327.

De Bellis, M., Baum, A., Birmaher, B. *et al.* (1999a) Developmental traumatology. I. Biological stress systems. *Biological Psychiatry*, **45**, 1259–1270.

De Bellis, M., Keshavan, M., Clark, D. *et al.* (1999b) Developmental traumatology. II. Brain development. *Biological Psychiatry*, **45**, 1271–1284.

Deblinger, E. & Heflin, A. (1996) *Treating Sexually Abused Children and Their Non-Offending Parents: a Cognitive Behavioural Approach*. Sage, London.

Deblinger, E., Lippman, J. & Steer, R. (1996) Sexually abused children suffering post-traumatic stress symptoms: initial treatment outcome findings. *Child Maltreatment*, **1**, 310–321.

Department of Health, Home Office & Department for Education and Employment (1999) *Working Together to Safeguard Children*. The Stationery Office, London.

Eke, N. & Nkanginieme, K. (1999) Female genital mutilation: a global bug that should not cross the millennium bridge. *World Journal of Surgery*, **23**, 1082–1086.

Elliott, D. & Briere, J. (1994) Forensic sexual abuse evaluations: disclosures and symptomatology. *Behavioural Sciences and the Law*, **12**, 261–277.

Elton, A. (1988) Working with substitute carers. In: *Child Sexual Abuse Within the Family: Assessment and Treatment* (eds A. Bentovim, A. Elton, J. Hildebrand, M. Tranter & E. Vizard), pp. 238–251. John Wright, London.

Everson, M. & Boat, B. (1994) Putting the anatomical doll controversy in perspective: An examination of major uses of the dolls in child sexual abuse evaluations. *Child Abuse and Neglect*, **18**, 113–129.

Everson, M., Hunter, W., Runyan, D., Edelsohn, G. & Coulter, M. (1989) Maternal support following disclosure of incest. *American Journal of Orthopsychiatry*, **59**, 198–207.

Faller, K. (1989) Characteristics of a clinical sample of sexually abused children: how boy and girl victims differ. *Child Abuse and Neglect*, **13**, 281–291.

Feldman, W., Feldman, E., Goodman, J. *et al.* (1991) Is child sexual abuse really increasing in prevalence? Analysis of the evidence. *Pediatrics*, **88**, 29–33.

Finkelhor, D. (1979) *Sexually Victimised Children*. Free Press, New York.

Finkelhor, D. (1984) *Child Sexual Abuse*. Free Press, New York.

Finkelhor, D. (1988) The trauma of child sexual abuse. In: *The Lasting Effects of Child Sexual Abuse* (eds G. Wyatt & G. Powell), pp. 61–82. Sage, CA.

Finkelhor, D. (1991) The scope of the problem. In: *Intervening in Child Sexual Abuse* (eds K. Murray & D. Gough), pp. 9–17. Scottish Academic Press, Glasgow.

Finkelhor, D. (1994) Current information on the scope and nature of child sexual abuse. *Future of Children*, **4**, 31–53.

Finkelhor, D. & Berliner, L. (1995) Research on the treatment of sexually abused children: a review and recommendations. *Journal of the American Academy of Child and Adolescent Psychiatry*, **34**, 1408–1423.

Finkelhor, D. & Browne, A. (1985) The traumatic impact of child sexual abuse: a conceptualization. *American Journal of Orthopsychiatry*, **55**, 530–541.

Finkelhor, D., Hotaling, G., Lewis, L. & Smith, C. (1990) Sexual abuse in a national survey of adult men and women: prevalence, characteristics and risk factors. *Child Abuse and Neglect*, **14**, 19–28.

Fivush, R. & Schwarzmueller, A. (1995) Say it once again: effects of repeated questions on children's event recall. *Journal of Traumatic Stress*, **8**, 555–580.

Fontes, L., ed. (1995) *Sexual Abuse in Nine North American Cultures*. Sage, CA.

Freyd, J. (1996) *Betrayal Trauma: the Logic of Forgetting Childhood Abuse*. Harvard University Press, Cambridge, MA.

Friedrich, W. (1993) Sexual victimization and sexual behavior in children: a review of recent literature. *Child Abuse and Neglect*, **17**, 59–66.

Friedrich, W., Beilke, R. & Urquiza, A. (1988) Behavior problems in young sexually abused boys: a comparison study. *Journal of Interpersonal Violence*, **3**, 21–28.

Friedrich, W., Grambach, P., Broughton, D., Kuiper, J. & Beilke, R. (1991) Normative sexual behavior in children. *Pediatrics*, **88**, 456–464.

Friedrich, W., Grambach, P., Damon, L. *et al.* (1992) Child sexual behavior inventory: normative and clinical comparison. *Psychological Assessment*, **4**, 303–311.

Frude, N. (1996) Ritual abuse: conceptions and reality. *Clinical Child Psychology and Psychiatry*, **1**, 59–77.

Furniss, T. (1991) *The Multiprofessional Handbook of Child Sexual Abuse*. Routledge, London.

Furniss, T., Bingley-Miller, I. & Van Elburg, A. (1988) Goal-oriented group treatment for sexually abused adolescent girls. *British Journal of Psychiatry*, **152**, 97–106.

Gale, J., Thompson, R., Moran, T. & Sack, W. (1988) Sexual abuse in young children: its clinical presentation and characteristic patterns. *Child Abuse and Neglect*, **12**, 163–170.

Gidycz, C. & Koss, M. (1989) The impact of adolescent sexual victimization: standardized measures of anxiety, depression and behavioral deviancy. *Violence and Victims*, **4**, 139–149.

Glaser, D. (1991) Treatment issues in child sexual abuse. *British Journal of Psychiatry*, **159**, 769–782.

Glaser, D. (2000) Child abuse and neglect and the brain: a review. *Journal of Child Psychology and Psychiatry*, **41**, 97–116.

Glaser, D. & Collins, C. (1989) The response of young non-sexually abused children to anatomically correct dolls. *Journal of Child Psychology and Psychiatry*, **30**, 547–560.

Glaser, D. & Frosh, S. (1993) *Child Sexual Abuse*. Macmillan, London.

Golier, J. & Yehuda, R. (1998) Neuroendocrine activity and memory-related impairments in posttraumatic stress disorder. *Development and Psychopathology*, **10**, 857–869.

Gomes-Schwartz, B., Horowitz, J. & Cardarelli, A. (1990) *Child Sexual Abuse: the Initial Effects*. Sage, CA.

Goodman, G. & Quas, J. (1997) Trauma and memory: individual differences in children's recounting of a stressful experience. In: *Memory for Everyday and Emotional Events* (eds L. Stein, P. Ornstein, B. Tversky & C. Brainerd), pp. 267–294. Lawrence Erlbaum, Mahwah, NJ.

Grosz, C., Kempe, R. & Kelly, M. (2000) Extrafamilial sexual abuse: treatment for child victims and their families. *Child Abuse and Neglect*, 24, 9–23.

Haden, C., Haine, R. & Fivush, R. (1997) Developing narrative structure in parent–child conversations about the past. *Developmental Psychology*, 33, 295–307.

Hall, D., Matthews, F. & Pearce, J. (1998) Factors associated with sexual behavior problems in young sexually abused children. *Child Abuse and Neglect*, 22, 1045–1063.

Hamilton, C. & Browne, K. (1999) Recurrent maltreatment during childhood: a survey of referrals to police child protection units in England. *Child Maltreatment*, 4, 275–286.

Handcock, P., ed. (1932) *The Code of Hammurabi*. Macmillan, New York.

Haugaard, J. & Reppucci, N. (1988) *The Sexual Abuse of Children*. Jossey-Bass, San Francisco.

Hawkes, C. (1999) Linking thoughts to actions: using the integrated abuse cycle. In: *Good Practice in Working with Violence* (eds H. Kemshall & J. Pritchard), pp. 149–167. Jessica Kingsley, London.

Heger, A. & Emans, J. (2000) *Evaluation of the Sexually Abused Child*, 2nd edn. Oxford University Press, Oxford.

Heriot, J. (1996) Maternal protectiveness following the disclosure of intrafamilial child sexual abuse. *Journal of Interpersonal Violence*, 11, 181–194.

Herman, J. (1981) *Father–Daughter Incest*. Harvard University Press, Cambridge, MA.

Hibbard, R., Ingersoll, G. & Orr, D. (1990) Behavior risk, emotional risk and child abuse among adolescents in a non-clinical setting. *Pediatrics*, 86, 896–901.

Hobbs, C. & Wynne, J. (1989) Sexual abuse of English boys and girls: the importance of anal examination. *Child Abuse and Neglect*, 13, 195–210.

Home Office, Crown Prosecution Service, Department of Health (2001) *Provision of Therapy for Child Witnesses Prior to a Criminal Trial*. The Stationery Office, London.

Hotte, J. & Rafman, S. (1992) The specific effects of incest on prepubertal girls from dysfunctional families. *Child Abuse and Neglect*, 16, 273–283.

Hunter, J., Goodwin, D. & Wilson, R. (1992) Attributions of blame in child sexual abuse victims: an analysis of age and gender influences. *Journal of Child Sexual Abuse*, 1, 75–90.

Jones, D.P.H. (1996) Management of the sexually abused child. *Advances in Psychiatric Treatment*, 2, 39–45.

Jones, D.P.H. (1997) Assessment of suspected child sexual abuse. In: *The Battered Child* (eds M. Helfer, R. Kempe & R. Krugman), pp. 296–312. University of Chicago Press, Chicago.

Jones, D.P.H. & Ramchandani, P. (1999) *Child Sexual Abuse: Informing Practice from Research*. Radcliffe Medical Press, Abingdon.

Jones, D.P.H., Hopkins, C., Godfrey, M. & Glaser, D. (1993) The investigative process. In: *Investigative Interviewing with Children* (eds W. Stainton-Rogers & M. Worrel), pp. 12–18. Open University Press, Milton Keynes.

Jones, L., Finkelhor, D. & Kopiec, K. (2001) Why is sexual abuse declining? A survey of state child protection administration. *Child Abuse and Neglect*, 25, 1139–1158.

Kaufman, J., Birmaher, B., Perel, J. *et al.* (1997) The corticotropin-releasing hormone challenge in depressed abused, depressed non-abused, and normal control children. *Biological Psychiatry*, 42, 669–679.

Keary, K. & Fitzpatrick, C. (1994) Children's disclosure of sexual abuse during formal investigations. *Child Abuse and Neglect*, 18, 543–548.

Kelly, L. (1992) The connections between disability and child abuse: a review of the research evidence. *Child Abuse Review*, 1, 157–167.

Kelly, L., Regan, L. & Burton, S. (1991) *An Exploratory Study of the Prevalence of Sexual Abuse in a Sample of 16–21-Year-Olds*. Polytechnic of North London, London.

Kendall-Tackett, K., Williams, L. & Finkelhor, D. (1993) Impact of sexual abuse on children: a review and synthesis of recent empirical studies. *Psychological Bulletin*, 113, 164–180.

Kiser, L., Ackerman, B., Brown, E. *et al.* (1988) Post-traumatic stress disorder in young children: a reaction to purported sexual abuse. *Journal of the American Academy of Child and Adolescent Psychiatry*, 27, 258–264.

Korbin, J. (1997) Culture and child maltreatment. In: *The Battered Child* (eds M. Helfer, R. Kempe & R. Krugman), pp. 29–48. University of Chicago Press, Chicago.

Korbin, J., ed. (1981) *Child Abuse and Neglect: Cross-Cultural Perspectives*. University of California Press, Berkeley and Los Angeles.

Kovacs, M. (1983) *The Children's Depression Inventory: A Self-rated Depression Scale for School-aged Youngsters*. University of Pittsburgh School of Medicine, Pittsburgh, PA.

Lamb, M., Sternberg, J., Esplin, P., Hershkowitz, I. & Orbach, Y. (1997) Assessing the credibility of children's allegations of sexual abuse: a survey of recent research. *Learning and Individual Differences*, 9, 175–194.

Lanktree, C. & Briere, J. (1995) Outcome of therapy for sexually abused children: a repeated measures study. *Child Abuse and Neglect*, 19, 1145–1156.

Lanktree, C., Briere, J. & Zaidi, L. (1991) Incidence and impact of sexual abuse in a child outpatient sample: the role of direct inquiry. *Child Abuse and Neglect*, 15, 447–453.

Lindblad, F., Gustafsson, P., Larson, I. & Lundig, B. (1995) Preschoolers' sexual behavior at day care centers: an epidemiological study. *Child Abuse and Neglect*, 19, 569–577.

Lloyd Davies, S., Glaser, D. & Kossoff, R. (2000) Children's sexual play and behavior in pre-school settings: staff's perceptions, reports, and responses. *Child Abuse and Neglect*, 24, 1329–1343.

Luo, T. (1998) Sexual abuse trauma among Chinese survivors. *Child Abuse and Neglect*, 22, 1013–1026.

Madonna, P., Van Scoyk, S. & Jones, D.P.H. (1991) Family interactions within incest and non-incest families. *American Journal of Psychiatry*, 148, 46–49.

Mannarino, A., Cohen, J. & Berman, S. (1994) The Children's Attributions and Perceptions Scale: a new measure of sexual abuse-related factors. *Journal of Clinical Child Psychology*, 23, 204–211.

Markowe, H. (1988) The frequency of child sexual abuse in the UK. *Health Trends*, 20, 2–6.

Martone, M., Jaudes, P. & Cavins, M. (1996) Criminal prosecution of child sexual abuse cases. *Child Abuse and Neglect*, 20, 457–464.

Masson, J. (1984) *Freud: the Assault on Truth*. Faber and Faber, London.

McClellan, J., McCurry, C., Ronnei, M., Adams, J., Eisner, A. & Storck, M. (1996) Age of onset of sexual abuse: relationship to sexually inappropriate behaviours. *Journal of the American Academy of Child and Adolescent Psychiatry*, 35, 1375–1383.

McKee, L. (1984) Sex differentials in survivorship and customary treatment of infants and children. *Medical Anthropology*, 8, 91–108.

McLeer, S., Deblinger, E., Henry, D. & Orvaschel, H. (1992) Sexually abused children at high risk for post-traumatic stress disorder. *Journal of the American Academy of Child and Adolescent Psychiatry*, 31, 875–879.

McLeer, S., Dixon, J., Henry, D. *et al.* (1998) Psychopathology in non-clinically referred sexually abused children. *Journal of the American Academy of Child and Adolescent Psychiatry*, 37, 1326–1333.

Mian, M., Marton, P. & LeBaron, D. (1996) The effects of sexual abuse on 3–5-year old girls. *Child Abuse and Neglect*, 20, 731–745.

Monck, E., Bentovim, A., Goodall, G. et al. (1996) *Child Sexual Abuse: a Descriptive and Treatment Study*. HMSO, London.

Morris, J. (1999) Disabled children, child protection systems and the Children Act 1989. *Child Abuse Review*, 8, 91–108.

Mullen, P., Martin, J. & Anderson, J. (1993) Childhood sexual abuse and mental health in adult life. *British Journal of Psychiatry*, 163, 721–732.

Mullen, P., Martin, J., Anderson, J., Romans, S. & Herbison, G. (1994) The effect of child sexual abuse on social, interpersonal and sexual function in adult life. *British Journal of Psychiatry*, 165, 35–47.

Mullen, P., Martin, J., Anderson, J., Romans, S. & Herbison, G. (1996) The long-term impact of the physical, emotional, and sexual abuse of children: a community study. *Child Abuse and Neglect*, 20, 7–21.

Muram, D. (1989) Child sexual abuse: relationship between sexual acts and genital findings. *Child Abuse and Neglect*, 13, 211–216.

Nasjleti, M. (1980) Suffering in silence: the male incest victim. *Child Welfare*, 59, 269–275.

Nelki, J. & Watters, J. (1989) A group for sexually abused young children: unravelling the web. *Child Abuse and Neglect*, 13, 369–377.

Ney, P., Fung, T. & Wickett, A. (1994) The worst combinations of child abuse and neglect. *Child Abuse and Neglect*, 18, 705–714.

Oates, R., O'Toole, B., Lynch, D., Stern, A. & Cooney, G. (1994) Stability and change in outcomes for sexually abused children. *Journal of the American Academy of Child and Adolescent Psychiatry*, 33, 945–953.

Oates, R., Jones, D.P.H., Denson, D., Sirotnak, A., Gary, N. & Krugman, R. (2000) Erroneous concerns about child sexual abuse. *Child Abuse and Neglect*, 24, 149–157.

Okamura, A., Heras, P. & Wong-Kerberg, L. (1995) Asian, Pacific Island, and Filipino Americans and sexual child abuse. In: *Sexual Abuse in Nine North American Cultures* (ed. L. Fontes), pp. 67–96. Sage, CA.

Peters, S., Wyatt, G. & Finkelhor, D. (1986) Prevalence. In: *A Sourcebook of Child Sexual Abuse* (ed. D. Finkelhor), pp. 15–59. Sage, CA.

Priest, R. (1992) A preliminary examination of child sexual victimization in college African-American populations. *American Journal of Orthopsychiatry*, 63, 367–371.

Prior, V., Lynch, M.A. & Glaser, D. (1994) *Messages from Children: Children's Evaluations of the Professional Response to Child Sexual Abuse*. NCH Action For Children, London.

Prior, V., Glaser, D. & Lynch, M.A. (1997) Responding to child sexual abuse: the criminal justice system. *Child Abuse Review*, 6, 128–140.

Rao, K., Di Clemente, R. & Pontion, L. (1992) Child sexual abuse of Asians compared with other populations. *Journal of the American Academy of Child and Adolescent Psychiatry*, 31, 880–886.

Rhind, N., Leung, T. & Choi, F. (1999) Child sexual abuse in Hong Kong: double victimization? *Child Abuse and Neglect*, 23, 511–517.

Rogers, C. & Terry, T. (1984) Clinical interventions with boy victims of sexual abuse. In: *Victims of Sexual Aggression: Treatment of Children, Women and Men* (eds I. Stuart & J. Greer), pp. 91–104. Van Nostrand Reinhold, New York.

Rotheram-Borus, M., Mahler, K., Koopman, C. & Langabeer, K. (1996) Sexual abuse history and associated multiple risk behavior in adolescent runaways. *American Journal of Orthopsychiatry*, 66, 390–400.

Runyan, D., Hunter, W. & Everson, M. (1992) *Maternal support for child victims of sexual abuse: determinants and implications*. National Center on Child Abuse and Neglect, Washington D.C.

Rushton, A. & Miles, G. (2000) A study of a support service for the current carers of sexually abused girls. *Clinical Child Psychology and Psychiatry*, 5, 1359–1045.

Russell, D. (1983) The incidence and prevalence of intrafamilial and extrafamilial sexual abuse of female children. *Child Abuse and Neglect*, 7, 133–146.

Russel, D. (1986) *The Secret Trauma: Incest in the Lives of Girls and Women*. Basic Books, New York.

Salter, A. (1988) *Treating Child Sex Offenders and Victims*. Sage, CA.

Sapolsky, R. (1996) Why stress is bad for your brain. *Science*, 273, 749–750.

Saradjian, J. (1996) *Women Who Sexually Abuse Children*. Wiley, Chichester.

Sariola, H. & Uutela, A. (1996) The prevalence and context of incest abuse in Finland. *Child Abuse and Neglect*, 20, 843–850.

Saunders, B., Villeponeaux, L., Lipovsky, J. & Kilpatrick, D. (1992) Child sexual assault as a risk factor for mental disorder among women: a community survey. *Journal of Interpersonal Violence*, 7, 189–204.

Schechter, M. & Roberge, L. (1976) Child sexual abuse. In: *Child Abuse and Neglect: the Family and the Community* (eds R. Helfer & C. Kempe), pp. 127–142. Ballinger, Cambridge, MA.

Scully, M., Kuoch, T. & Miller, R. (1995) Cambodians and sexual child abuse. In: *Sexual Abuse in Nine North American Cultures* (ed. L. Fontes), pp. 97–127. Sage, CA.

Seghorn, T., Prensky, R. & Boucher, R. (1987) Childhood sexual abuse in the lives of sexually aggressive offenders. *Journal of the American Academy of Child and Adolescent Psychiatry*, 26, 262–267.

Shapiro, J. (1989) Self-blame versus helplessness in sexually abused children: an attributional analysis with treatment recommendations. *Journal of Social and Clinical Psychology*, 8, 442–455.

Shapiro, J., Leifer, M., Martone, M. & Kassem, L. (1992) Cognitive functioning and social competence as predictors of maladjustment in sexually abused girls. *Journal of Interpersonal Violence*, 7, 156–164.

Sharland, E., Seal, H., Croucher, M., Aldgate, J. & Jones, D.P.H. (1996) *Professional Intervention in Child Sexual Abuse*. HMSO, London.

Singer, K. (1989) Group work with men who experienced incest in childhood. *American Journal of Orthopsychiatry*, 59, 468–472.

Sirles, E. & Franke, P. (1989) Factors influencing mothers' reactions to intrafamilial sexual abuse. *Child Abuse and Neglect*, 13, 131–139.

Skuse, D., Bentovim, A., Hodges, J. et al. (1998) Risk factors for the development of sexually abusive behaviour in sexually victimised adolescent males: cross-sectional study. *British Medical Journal*, 317, 175–179.

Smets, A. & Cebula, C. (1987) A group treatment program for adolescent sex offenders: five steps towards resolution. *Child Abuse and Neglect*, 11, 247–254.

Spaccarelli, S. & Kim, S. (1995) Resilience criteria and factors associated with resilience in sexually abused girls. *Child Abuse and Neglect*, 19, 1171–1182.

Stein, J., Golding, J., Siegel, J., Burnam, M. & Sorensen, S. (1988) Long-term psychological sequelae of child sexual abuse. *Journal of the American Academy of Child and Adolescent Psychiatry*, 27, 650–654.

Sullivan, P. & Knutson, J. (2000) Maltreatment and disabilities: a population-based epidemiological study. *Child Abuse and Neglect*, 10, 1257–1273.

Summit, R. (1983) The child sexual abuse accommodation syndrome. *Child Abuse and Neglect*, 7, 177–193.

Summit, R. (1992) Abuse of the child sexual accommodation syndrome. *Journal of Child Sexual Abuse*, 1, 153–163.

Tebbutt, J., Swanston, H., Oates, R. & O'Toole, B. (1997) Five years after child sexual abuse: persisting dysfunction and problems of prediction. *Journal of the American Academy of Child and Adolescent Psychiatry*, 36, 330–339.

Tjaden, P. & Thoennes, N. (1992) Predictors of legal intervention in child maltreatment cases. *Child Abuse and Neglect*, **16**, 807–821.

Tong, L., Oates, K. & McDowell, M. (1986) Personality development following sexual abuse. *Child Abuse and Neglect*, **11**, 371–383.

Tremblay, C., Herbert, M. & Piche, C. (1999) Coping strategies and social support as mediators of consequences in child sexual abuse victims. *Child Abuse and Neglect*, **23**, 929–945.

Trowell, J., Berelowitz, M. & Kolvin, I. (1995) Design and methodological issues in setting up a psychotherapy outcome study with girls who have been sexually abused. In: *Research Foundations for Psychotherapy Practice* (eds M. Aveline & D. Shapiro), pp. 247–262. Wiley, London.

Trowell, J., Ugarte, B., Kolvin, I., Berelowitz, M., Sadowski, J. & Le Couteur, A. (1999) Behavioural psychopathology of child sexual abuse in schoolgirls referred to a tertiary centre: a North London study. *European Journal of Child and Adolescent Psychiatry*, **8**, 107–116.

Utting, W., Baines, C., Stuart, M., Rolands, J. & Vialva, R. (1997) *People Like Us: The Report of the Review of the Safeguards for Children Living Away from Home*. The Stationery Office, London.

Van Scoyk, S., Gray, J. & Jones, D.P.H. (1988) A theoretical framework for evaluation and treatment of the victims of child sexual assault by a non-family member. *Family Process*, **27**, 105–113.

Vander Mey, B. (1988) Sexual victimisation of male children: a review of previous research. *Child Abuse and Neglect*, **12**, 61–72.

Vizard, E., Monck, E. & Misch, P. (1995) Child and adolescent sex abuse perpetrators: a review of the research literature. *Journal of Child Psychology and Psychiatry*, **36**, 731–756.

Wall, N. (2000) *Handbook for Expert Witnesses in Children Act Cases*. Family Law, Bristol.

Waterman, J., Kelly, R., McCord, J. & Oliveri, M. (1993) *Behind the Playground Walls: Sexual Abuse in Preschools*. Guilford Press, New York.

Watkins, B. & Bentovim, A. (1992) The sexual abuse of male children and adolescents: a review of current research. *Journal of Child Psychology and Psychiatry*, **33**, 197–248.

Welldon, E. (1988) *Mother, Madonna, Whore*. Free Association Books, London.

Westcott, H. & Jones, D.P.H. (1999) The abuse of disabled children. *Journal of Child Psychology and Psychiatry*, **40**, 497–506.

Wild, N. & Wynne, J. (1986) Child sex rings. *British Medical Journal*, **293**, 183–185.

Williams, L. (1994) Recall of childhood trauma: a prospective study of women's memories of child sexual abuse. *Journal of Consulting Clinical Psychology*, **62**, 1167–1176.

Wolfe, V., Gentile, C., Michienzi, T., Sas, L. & Wolfe, D. (1991) The children's impact of traumatic events scale: a measure of post-sexual abuse PTSD symptoms. *Behavioral Assessment*, **13**, 359–383.

Woods, J. (1997) Breaking the cycle of abuse and abusing: individual psychotherapy for juvenile sex offenders. *Clinical Child Psychology and Psychiatry*, **2**, 379–392.

Wozencraft, T., Wagner, W. & Pellegrin, A. (1991) Depression and suicidal ideation in sexually abused children. *Child Abuse and Neglect*, **15**, 505–510.

Wyatt, G. (1985) The sexual abuse of Afro-American and white-American women in childhood. *Child Abuse and Neglect*, **9**, 507–519.

Wyatt, G. & Peters, S. (1986) Methodological considerations in research on the prevalence of child sexual abuse. *Child Abuse and Neglect*, **10**, 241–251.

Wyatt, G. & Powell, G. (1988) Identifying the lasting effects of child sexual abuse. In: *The Lasting Effects of Child Sexual Abuse* (eds G. Wyatt & G. Powell), pp. 11–17. Sage, CA.

Young, W., Sachs, R., Braun, B. & Watkins, R. (1991) Patients reporting ritual abuse in childhood: a clinical syndrome. *Child Abuse and Neglect*, **15**, 181–189.

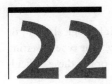

Residential and Foster Family Care

Alan Rushton and Helen Minnis

Introduction

'In the home for abandoned children, they are sad and sometimes die of sadness.' From the Diary of a Spanish Bishop, 1725 (Spitz 1945)

It has been known for centuries that a loving reciprocal early relationship is essential for healthy development. Most families provide this. However, when birth parents have psychological or health problems, learning or physical disability, and/or live under adverse conditions, such as poverty or overcrowding, parenting capacity may be compromised and the child may become vulnerable. Short-term substitute care to deal with a crisis will sometimes follow, or the family may be investigated by the child protection services and the child removed. Some children may not return home because they remain at risk or because the parents have rejected them.

We are concerned, in this chapter, with children placed in foster family or residential care and with factors related to this placement including: the children's emotional and behavioural functioning; the characteristics of the care environments; abuse in care; children's relationships within and outside the setting; the perspectives of the children; the longer term outcomes and treatment interventions. The approach we have taken is to make direct comparisons between the effects of two environments—foster family care (mostly longer term) and residential care—on the children placed there. The chapter will not address forms of residential care such as inpatient psychiatric units (see Green, Chapter 61), hospital wards, young offender institutions (see S. Bailey, Chapter 60) or, the largest group of all, boarding schools in the independent sector. However, some of the issues discussed will be equally relevant to these groups. Nor will we attempt to deal with the specialized problems of children with significant learning or physical disabilities in residential care (see Bernard, Chapter 67).

The placement of healthy infants in adoptive homes seems to be achievable with no worse long-term outcome than for children never separated from their birth families (Maughan & Pickles 1990; Bohman 1997). A more pertinent question for the current child welfare system is whether children who have had a history of broken attachments, abuse, neglect and other adversities make adequate developmental recoveries in a new environment and, where appropriate, form sufficiently strong psychological ties to their new carers. A crucial question is whether the substitute care provided is of sufficient quality and stability to avoid further harm and serves a remedial purpose (Rutter 2000).

Nearly 50 children in every 10 000 are being 'looked after' by the local authority in England and Wales (Department of Health 1999), but these rates vary widely across the world (e.g. 75 in 10 000 in the USA). In the UK, after a steady fall, the proportion of children under 18 'in care' may have been rising again (from 80 in 10 000 in 1987, to 45 in 1995 and to 49 in 1999). Of the two major placement categories, most children (65%) are looked after in foster placements and 12% in children's homes. The remaining children include those placed under supervision with birth parents and those placed for adoption. The number of children in residential care in England and Wales fell by almost 80% from the late 1970s to the 1990s, but for the past 5 years the foster:residential care ratio has been constant. In Europe, Australasia and North America, a general trend exists towards reducing numbers and lengths of stay in residential care. However, this has not been evident in other parts of the world (Hill 2000).

The move towards briefer stays in residential care is not wholly positive; some children experience both foster and residential care and, with greater emphasis on family preservation, it is not unusual for children to spend short periods in foster or residential placements interspersed with periods in a less than optimal family environment. This is a particularly difficult area to research, but it is important to track the effects of numerous changes of environment and of such complex care careers. Current knowledge of the likely consequences of maltreatment has recently been summarized (Cicchetti & Toth 1995; Glaser 2000) and the stresses involved in living in adverse preplacement environments put children at risk for health, developmental and academic problems.

Historical background

The social arrangement called family foster care has had a longer history than residential placement, in the sense that the care of children in need has always been provided by other families (Werner 1984). Fortunately, humans are sometimes driven by acts of generosity and community spirit and parentless children can be successfully brought up by others. In the modern more formally organized fostering system, alternative care is provided by unrelated families who are recruited, assessed, regulated and paid for their services.

The history of residential care in the UK can be traced to the first Poor Law of 1531 when there was a need to take over the functions of the dissolved monasteries. However, the growth of institution building three centuries later, which saw the arrival of the orphanage and the workhouse, has had the most powerful influence on its character. Attempts to document and analyse the history of residential care (Parker 1990; Frost *et al.* 1999) have considered the ill effects of industrialization and urbanization on family life on the one hand and the part played by religion and philanthropy in 'rescuing' children from poverty and crime on the other.

Fostering and residential care have run in parallel as alternative arrangements for children since the nineteenth century, often competing for status and resources. The introduction, in 1857, by the Foundling Hospital in London of a new system in which children were boarded out with families may have been the origin of rivalry between residential and foster care (Frost *et al.* 1999).

Theoretical developments have contributed to the preference for family rather than institutional care, including Bowlby's (1951) emphasis on preserving attachment with an adult caregiver, Goffman's (1961) critique of institutions in general and Maluccio *et al.*'s (1986) theories on the importance of 'permanence'. Influenced by these ideas, a hierarchy of out-of-home placement choices is now often advocated with adoption first, foster family care second and residential care as the least desirable option.

International comparisons

It is instructive when exploring evidence on placement alternatives to embrace international comparisons of fostering and residential care. Although now absent from the Western world, horrifying examples of poor child care in large insanitary institutions with inadequate nutrition and lack of personal warmth are still to be found (Chisholm *et al.* 1995). Within Europe wide variations exist in the total number of children in public care, the proportion living in children's homes, opportunities for training for carers and levels of remuneration (Gottesman 1991; Madge 1994; Sellick 1998). Colton & Hellinkx (1994) identified a number of common developments across Europe, such as the reduction in the size of homes, the professionalization of carers and a preference for placements that are inclusive rather than exclusive of the family and community. Although we are aware of important practice advances in various parts of the world (e.g. Australasia and Scandinavia), little has reached the academic literature other than work from the UK and the USA. We hope that a more genuinely international perspective will emerge in the near future.

What characterizes the foster family and residential care environment?

Child and adolescent mental health professionals may be asked for opinions about appropriate placements for children in diffi-

culty who need to be placed away from their biological family or they may be providing a therapeutic service. The type of setting will have an important impact on whether or not these difficulties are resolved.

Since the 1940s, researchers have observed the effects of institutions on children. Spitz (1945) concluded that adequate stimulation and presence of the child's mother were crucial in preventing physical and intellectual delay. This and later research, demonstrating that the effects of institutionalization on children's behaviour include the 'indiscriminate' giving of affection and a tendency to go easily to strangers, has transformed social care (Goldfarb 1945; Dennis & Najarian 1957; Tizard & Hodges 1978; Chisholm *et al.* 1995; Vorria *et al.* 1998). In the developed world, many of the remaining residential institutions attempt to address these findings by providing smaller units with better family and community links.

Systematic research on fostering has developed since the 1960s with attempts to investigate the stability of foster family placements and to establish predictors of successful outcome (Trasler 1960; Parker 1966; George 1970; Fanshel & Shinn 1978; Berridge & Cleaver 1987). Despite attempts to reduce the extent of serial placements, fostering can still be an unstable arrangement for many children.

Foster care clearly differs in many ways from residential care and there may be different expectations about what each environment can offer a child. Fresh attachments may be more likely to develop where the caregiver is available most of the time, as in foster family care, as opposed to various carers operating on a shift basis as in residential care. In addition, relationships between children and their foster carers, who tend to be older than parents of similar aged children in the general population (Triseliotis *et al.* 2000), will undoubtedly differ from relationships that residential care staff, who may be only a few years older, have with the teenagers they look after. This has important implications for limit setting and for the maintenance of emotional and sexual boundaries. In a small but influential study, Colton (1988) gathered both qualitative and quantitative data from 12 foster carers and the senior member of staff of 12 children's homes in England. Data from structured interviews suggested that foster placements were more child-orientated, had better physical amenities and children had more community contacts than those in residential care. Direct observation of care practices showed that foster carers used fewer ineffective and inappropriate techniques of control and used warmer, more approving, informative (as opposed to controlling) speech than residential care staff. Children received more adult attention in foster homes and their perceptions of their environments compared favourably with those in residential care. Berridge & Brodie (1998) confirmed these findings and also found that, in the residential homes they visited, virtually no specialist educational input or professional help was available to enable the young people to deal with psychological problems.

However, Sinclair & Gibbs (1998) found that children who had experienced painful foster care breakdowns sometimes preferred the residential environment and that child outcomes can be improved where a set of coherent goals promotes a healthy staff culture (Brown *et al.* 1998). A significant proportion of foster placements 'break down'; that is, the child has to leave the placement, in a manner that is not in accord with the plans of the social work department. Rates of breakdown as high as 35% have been quoted for what were planned as long-term placements (Strathclyde Regional Council Social Work Department 1991) and 10% for short-term placements (Berridge & Cleaver 1987). Many see this high rate of breakdown as one of the major flaws of foster care. For all concerned, a precipitous placement ending is traumatic, not least for the child who is left with an uncertain future. When a child has experienced a series of placement breakdowns, residential care may be seen as the 'end of the road' or, alternatively, as a relief from the pain of forming relationships that may fail again.

Table 22.1 sets out some of the similarities and differences between foster family and residential care in the UK, although it offers only broad comparisons. The information has been taken from UK studies and national statistics (Colton 1988; Knapp 1997; Sinclair & Gibbs 1998; Triseliotis *et al.* 2000).

Some evidence exists of important differences between the population of children in residential care and that in foster care (see Table 22.1; Sinclair & Gibbs 1998; Triseliotis *et al.* 2000). While children of all ages are in foster care, residential care accommodates mainly teenagers. The length of stay in foster care ranges from a few days to a whole childhood, whereas in residential care the length of stay is now much reduced to an average of 6 months. In the UK, the collection of data on ethnicity for children in local authority care is now mandatory, but accurate statistics do not yet exist. UK research suggests that between 8 and 22% of looked-after children are 'black' (Barn 1993; Mehra 1996), but differences in definitions of ethnic groups make interpretation difficult and the ethnic mix in different care environments is as yet unknown.

Abuse in care

The experience of children in public care cannot now be discussed without reference to scandals over extensive physical and sexual abuse by residential workers which have resulted in highly publicized inquiries in the UK. For example, a study of Welsh children's homes described extensive abuse of residents by staff (Welsh Office 2000). The protection of children who have been sexually abused may be inadequate in both foster and residential care, with vulnerable children sharing rooms with children with a known abuse history (Farmer & Pollock 1998). Residential care has been so much vilified that many have questioned whether there remains a place for such provision at all. Scandals sometimes alert public attention dramatically and can trigger reform, better training, more inspection, stricter quality control and quality assurance. Foster care has also been criticized, although the discussion of these forms of alternative care is best undertaken in comparison with the outcome for children who had not been removed from home.

Table 22.1 A comparison between foster family care and residential care in the UK

Foster family care	Residential care
Carers live in own home	Carers live away from setting
Paid an allowance	Paid a wage
On average 1.7 children present	On average 7 children present
4 out of 10 children over 10 years old	9 out of 10 children over 10 years old
Age range 0–18	Age range usually 5–18
Roughly equal sex ratio	6 out of 10 boys
Individualized care	Group care by a sequence of carers
More child orientated, e.g. child generally has access to all areas of the family home	More institution orientated, e.g. child usually excluded from the office
Better physical amenities (e.g. higher ratio of baths/locking toilets to residents, more personal effects such as photos, posters, etc., in bedrooms)	Poorer physical amenities
Emphasis on good family and community contacts	Traditionally more isolated from family and community, but improving in this respect
Long-term placement common	Long-term placement now rare
Direct costs low	Direct costs high (staff and building)
Indirect costs high (social work support, carer recruitment and training)	Indirect costs low
Pre-placement training almost universal but variable in quality. Qualifications rare	In-service training common, but variable in quality. 1 in 5 staff have a residential social work qualification
Composition of the family group generally more consistent	Permanent peer group unlikely
Balance of care and control	Frequently more control than care
Often more children than adults	More staff than residents

A British study (Hobbs *et al.* 1999) has compared reported abuse in foster and residential care with that in a general urban population. Children in foster care were 7–8 times, and children in residential care were 6 times more likely to be reported as physically or sexually abused compared with children in the general population. The study points out that in addition to abuse by carers, abuse could be perpetrated by, amongst others, birth family during contact or by other looked-after children. This highlights the risks of placing vulnerable children together in the same home, where victims may become perpetrators. A Scottish study found that 91% of residential placements caring for children who had sexually abused others also cared for children who had been sexually abused (Lindsay 1999). Farmer & Pollock (1998) found that one in five sexually abused children in care had sexually abused other residents in children's homes, or foster homes. Little therapeutic help was being directed specifically at the abusing behaviour and carers had great uncertainty about managing the sexually indiscriminate behaviour of adolescent girls.

Does the reported increase in abuse in foster family care reflect the real prevalence? Foster families in Baltimore had over a threefold increase in the frequency of maltreatment reports, particularly physical abuse, as compared to non-foster families, although a smaller proportion were substantiated. There are various possible reasons for this finding. First, increased vigilance over children in foster care may increase *reports* of abuse. For example, in Baltimore, no corporal punishment at all is allowed by foster carers, whereas some of the local schools still allow corporal punishment, so a lower threshold for reports undoubtedly exists for foster families (Benedict *et al.* 1994). Secondly, children in foster care tend to have more of the risk factors for child abuse, such as physical and learning disabilities and behavioural problems. A study comparing 78 children who had been abused or neglected while in foster care with 229 who had not, showed that those abused while in foster care were significantly more likely to have mental health and development problems (Benedict *et al.* 1996a). Thirdly, some biological families may make reports of abuse in foster care in the hope of making a return home more likely (Benedict *et al.* 1994). It is possible that foster carers may be more likely to abuse children who are not biologically their own, but this is unproven.

There has been increasing recognition that certain adults may actively seek out opportunities to abuse vulnerable children. This, plus the past experiences of looked-after children and those children with whom they are placed, put this group at heightened risk of abuse in the very settings designed to protect and care for them (Gallagher 1999).

What is known about the emotional and behavioural functioning in each environment during childhood?

Knowledge of the clinical status of children and young people in the care system has often relied upon research enquiries conducted in specific child welfare organizations or in selected areas of the country without the benefit of not-in-care controls. Until information in child care agencies is routinely collected, processed and analysed—a promise held out by the Looking After Children materials promoted by the UK Department of Health (Parker *et al.* 1991; Ward 1996)—the following findings are the best information on children in care. Studies have consistently shown elevated rates of problems compared with children never in public care. The range of findings suggest real variations in the prevalence of mental health problems in foster care because of location, placement length and characteristics of children, but no decrease in prevalence with time.

Early studies (Parker 1966; Lambert *et al.* 1977) showed between one-third and one-half of children to have problems of clinical significance. The study by Rowe *et al.* (1984) on long-term foster care was one of the first in the UK to use an established measure: the Rutter A Scale. The study concluded that 29% of children in long-term foster care between the ages of 5 and 15 years scored at or above the cut-off for disturbance. Common problems were temper tantrums and lack of concentration. Although this rate was many times higher than found in general population data, it was not as high as other studies of similar populations. This may have been because the children were a fairly stable group. Thorpe (1980), in contrast, found that 39% of her sample were disturbed.

St. Claire & Osborn (1987) found that children in foster care, and more so in residential care, had substantial cognitive deficits and problem behaviour even after allowing for possible confounding variables. Although those who had spent time in residential care showed more antisocial behaviour, it is possible that behaviour problems were present before admission to the residential placement. Problems were thought to be caused by pre-care experiences and pre-existing behavioural difficulties rather than aspects of the current placement environment.

More recent studies have also shown a high rate of mental health problems. Quinton *et al.* (1998) found high levels in a neglected and abused sample immediately after being placed from care into new intended permanent family placement: 54% of boys and 58% of girls were beyond the cut-off for psychopathology. That the mean scores for the group did not differ significantly across the first year of placement shows this was not a momentary phenomenon as a result of the transition to a new family. A two-stage cross-sectional study of all adolescents in care in Oxfordshire, with a comparison group matched for age and sex, used the Achenbach Child Behaviour Checklist (CBCL) as a screening instrument, then interviewed high-scorers using the semistructured Kiddie Schedule for Affective Disorders and Schizophrenia (K-SADS; Chambers *et al.* 1985). The prevalence of psychiatric disorder was 67%: 57% for adolescents in foster care and 98% in residential care. This contrasted with only 15% in the comparison group (McCann *et al.* 1996). A replication of the McCann study, based in a small local authority in Scotland (A. Addo, A. Blower, L. Lamington & K. Towlson, personal communication 2000), has found lower rates (54%) of psychopathology in looked-after children.

Dumaret *et al.* (1997) have examined psychological problems in fostered children of below-average IQ. A cross-sectional case note review was made of all children with IQs of 60–90 who were in foster care (*n* = 127) in seven areas in France. All were adopted from foster care after the age of 4 years and had had a full assessment in the year before adoption. At the pre-adoption assessment, nearly half had emotional/psychological problems—nearly four times the French average. Factors associated with mental health status included maternal learning disability, late age at first adoption and a history of abuse and neglect.

Few studies have focused solely on residential care, but a UK study examined the psychological status of the residents (Sinclair & Gibbs 1998) using an interview-based well-being measure (Angold *et al.* 1987) on their sample (*n* = 216) and found the following problems were present for more than half the group: 'worried', 'unhappy', 'nervous', 'easily upset' and 'poor self-opinion'. Forty per cent had thought about killing themselves. This was clearly a very troubled population.

Prevalence studies such as these beg the question 'to what extent were these problems present prior to entering local authority care?' A case–control study compared 50 children who were in foster care as a result of abuse or neglect for at least 3 months with 50 children eligible for Medicaid (from low-income families). Mean CBCL scores were higher for the foster care sample, but differences were no longer significant when controlled for family structure and stability, suggesting that the experience of foster care itself was not contributing to the children's problems (Hulsey & White 1989). At entry to an episode of care, children appear to have approximately twice the prevalence of emotional and behavioural problems expected in the general population (Dimigen *et al.* 1999).

Although not definitive, the research suggests that residential care is detrimental to children's mental health, whereas foster care may improve it. A Finnish longitudinal study of 53 children in residential care found that emotional and behavioural problems worsened over 2.5 years, while a UK study of 141 children in 48 children's homes reported little change in mood or adjustment over 6–9 months follow-up (Gibbs & Sinclair 1998). In contrast, prospective studies of children in permanent family placements have shown that emotional and behavioural problems are improved or unchanged 9 months–1 year into placement (Rushton *et al.* 1995; Quinton *et al.* 1998; Minnis 1999).

One of the most direct pieces of evidence that foster care can, of itself, be therapeutic compared to other forms of care, comes from Iraqi Kurdistan. Fifty-four orphans (24 in orphanages and 30 in foster families) were assessed using the CBCL and a checklist for post-traumatic stress disorder (PTSD). Total problems on the CBCL increased in the orphanage group while significantly decreasing in the fostered group. The orphanage sample reported a higher incidence of PTSD than the fostered group (Ahmad & Mohamad 1996). This suggests that mental health may improve in foster care and deteriorate in residential care, but the story is unlikely to be that simple. Children may be placed in residential care because their problems are considered too severe for a family to deal with, therefore these children may be a more disturbed group when first accommodated. A paper reporting on a study carried out in the 1970s has helped to tease out the effects of prior problems from the effects of the care environment by studying children from similar social environments who experienced either residential or family foster care. Both groups were compared with classroom controls and although both were more prone to hyperactivity/inattention, such a problem was substantially more marked in the group who had experienced residential care (Roy *et al.* 2000).

Several points need to be made about the higher levels of problems frequently found in residential care samples.

1 These differences are likely to be most evident when the placement environments are very distinctly dissimilar, for example, when comparing lack of individualized care in a children's home

with stable life in a foster family. However, if the comparison were to be drawn between similar children, one group in a small stable children's home with a family atmosphere and the other in a large foster family, the differences might reduce or disappear.
2 The differences could result from the fact that populations entering these environments are different, particularly in age, background and abuse histories, and comparisons can be misleading without employing matched controls.
3 The means of assessment may have a biasing effect. Interviews with children may detect emotional problems better than child self-reports and biases may be inherent in using the carer as the informant. For example, it is possible that foster carers and residential workers may underrate problems, as they are used to living with children with a high rate of difficulty and so minimize the difference from the general population.

Perspectives of the children

Information about in-care populations has tended to be gathered via carers, social workers and teachers. A recent research development has been to elicit information from the children more directly. This has so far produced softer data, but developments in appropriate techniques for conducting research interviews with children may add an important dimension to knowledge about substitute care. Several investigations have asked the children themselves about their experiences as foster children or children's home residents. In a study by Kufeldt *et al.* (1995), 40 foster children were asked to complete a structured assessment both on their own family and on their foster family. They regarded their foster family as significantly more 'healthy' than their birth family. McAuley's (1996) small-scale study used semistructured questionnaires to elicit responses from foster children about their lives, feelings and wishes. Sinclair & Gibbs (1998) used structured interviews with over 200 children, asking especially about their experience of the children's home and its 'social climate', their families and their social workers. Not surprisingly, the young people wanted a good physical environment and friendly staff. They found their sense of subjective well-being was strongly related to the extent of current bullying and harassment by other residents. These direct interviews may help to bring out features of the children's world to which adult assessors may be less attuned. For example, one boy described to Biehal & Wade (1996) his feeling of alienation from family life:

'It were just a family I saw in the park once. Christmas day. So I went out for a ride on me bike, sat on a park bench watching these kids play. They were flying a kite so I went up to them and says 'what's it like having Christmas with your family?'

Physical health

This chapter is concerned mostly with psychological problems but we briefly mention physical health because of the obvious links between the two areas. It is not unusual for physical health problems to fall through the net, often because of difficulties with tracking medical notes and poor communication between services. A US study of children in kinship care, showed that approximately half the children had not clearly received all their immunizations and the level of undetected health problems suggested inadequate primary care (Dubowitz *et al.* 1994). In the UK, all children entering an episode of care are meant to have a routine medical, but Polnay *et al.* (1996) have concluded that the system of assessment and treatment of physical and mental health problems of children in residential care is often unsuccessful because the routine medical examination is frequently avoided by young people. They recommend the use of self-completion health questionnaires and improved training of residential care staff in health promotion to further the goal of optimum health.

Education

Education is known to protect the mental health of high-risk children (Rutter 1985), yet many looked-after adolescents attend school only intermittently and are at considerably higher risk of exclusion than others (Blyth & Milner 1996; Fletcher-Campbell 1997). In England and Wales, over 75% of care leavers have no educational qualifications at all and only 3% attain five GCSEs compared with 60% in the general population. Educational expectations have been found to be low and academic success limited in both residential and foster care (Jackson 1989; Cheung & Heath 1994; Heath *et al.* 1994) and school absence of children in residential care is particularly high (Sinclair & Gibbs 1998).

A study comparing ex-care adults who had been particularly successful in educational terms with their less successful peers has emphasized the importance of school for children in care. Educational success was associated with better mental health and greater life satisfaction, whereas children who had not achieved educationally were many times more likely to be unemployed, single parents or homeless. Factors associated with educational success in care included experiencing at least one stable placement, having a parent or carer who valued education, having out-of-care friends and interests, learning to read early and attending school regularly. High educational achievers were no more likely to have had educated birth parents. Residential care seemed to be a particularly discouraging environment. Ex-residents described a lack of interest in school by staff and poor facilities for homework. In contrast, carers who read to children and encourage the use of books and libraries may be providing them with some of the most important protective factors for their psychosocial development (Jackson & Martin 1998).

Relationships within and outside the placement

Relationships in any family are complex, but children looked after in foster or residential care are expected to negotiate a network of relationships of a different order of magnitude. Children in foster care may have attachments with foster carers, the carers' biological children, their own siblings (either in the same placement, living in a different placement or with the birth family), other foster children from different birth families, and with their own biological parents. Children in residential care may have attachments to a range of residential social workers, with their own biological family and with other children in the residential placement.

Attachment relationships assume great importance for children in foster or residential care who have inevitably suffered separation and loss and are likely to have had insecure attachments with primary caregivers. Insecure attachment is known to be an important risk factor for later psychosocial functioning (Crowell & Feldman 1988; Goldberg 1991; Lyons-Ruth 1996; Warren *et al.* 1997), and there is limited evidence that relationship styles with birth parents may predict the formation of fresh attachments with foster carers. A US study measured internal representations of self and primary attachment figures in 32 children entering foster care for the first time from a birth family in which they had suffered abuse. These representations significantly predicted children's subsequent views of their relationships with their foster mothers and their behaviour in the new placement (Milan & Pinderhughes 2000). Stovall & Dozier (2000) investigated the development of attachment between young children and foster carers by asking carers to complete a daily diary of attachment behaviours over the first 2 months, and by using more traditional methods to measure carer–child attachment and the foster mother's state of mind regarding attachment with her own parents. For infants placed below 12 months of age, the attachment style with the carer tended to reflect that of the foster mother with her own parents. However, those placed after 12 months tended to have persistently insecure attachment styles with the foster carer.

The question of whether or not a 'blood bond' is important for the formation of secure attachment is obviously pertinent to foster family and residential care, but most of the evidence in this area relates to adoption. The attachment styles of adoptive mother–infant pairs and controls appear to be similar (Singer *et al.* 1985) and no differences are found in middle childhood between the adjustment of biological children and those children adopted in infancy. This suggests that a blood bond is not fundamental for secure attachment. Late adopted children have more problems (Triseliotis *et al.* 1995). Emotional and behavioural problems themselves do not appear to be associated with placement breakdown but, when attachment problems are also present, the balance may be tipped towards placement instability (Rushton *et al.* 2000). Satisfying relationships do develop within the first few years of placement, even with older children placed with the intention of permanence (Rushton & Mayes 1997). Whether 'permanency' in terms of adoption helps attachment with new caregivers remains controversial, although a review of the literature on permanency planning and its effects on foster children found no difference in the psychosocial adjustment of children where permanency planning had taken place and those where it had not (Seltzer & Bloksberg 1987).

Contact with the birth family

Which relationships are most important for looked-after children? Interviews with children in residential care on the subject of contact have given perhaps surprising results. Around half wanted more contact with siblings, one-third more contact with their mother and a significant minority wanted more contact with former foster carers. However, 25% of the children wanted *less* contact with their mother (Sinclair & Gibbs 1998). Qualitative research with foster families suggests that, within the foster family itself, children feel most able to confide in the foster mother. However, they tend to love and to think that they are loved by their birth families 'most in the world', despite usually being admitted to care because of abuse or neglect by the birth family. One year into placement, they still think and dream about birth parents frequently (McAuley 1996), but tend to rate their emotional involvement with both birth parents and carers as low (Kufeldt *et al.* 1995). These studies paint a picture of children lacking in warm trusting reciprocal relationships whose yearnings for closeness and support from their birth parents are unfulfilled.

Where the plan for a child in a family placement is not to return home, the degree of contact with birth parents that is beneficial remains controversial (Quinton *et al.* 1997). It has been found that the less contact a child has with the birth mother, the less secure they feel in the foster home (Fanshel *et al.* 1990) and that children who visit their birth parents more frequently are more likely to rate their parents as healthy/normal (Kufeldt *et al.* 1995). This has been seen as evidence that contact with birth parents is good. However, children coming from better functioning birth families may be more able to maintain relationships in general—both with the birth and the foster family. Also, better functioning birth parents may be more able to maintain contact with their children. It may be unwise therefore to assume that relationships with birth parents should be maintained regardless of the nature of that relationship. Where co-operative working between foster and birth families can be maintained, however, there is evidence that contact may benefit the child. Foster placements appear to be more stable where birth parents have prepared children for placement (Palmer 1996) and foster carers' anxiety about young children's contact with birth parents is associated with poorer child adjustment (Gean *et al.* 1985).

A child's entry to care can be traumatic for all the family, and parents are often left confused about their rights and obligations, making visiting difficult (Millham *et al.* 1986). Around one-third of children in UK residential care see one or more of their birth parents more than once a week compared with around two-fifths of children in medium to long-term foster care, while around one-fifth of children in both settings have no contact with parents (Sinclair & Gibbs 1998; Minnis 1999). A Scottish survey of 835 foster carers found that, while the majority of foster carers were well disposed towards birth parents, negative reactions were also common. Most carers preferred contact to take place outside their home. Just over half had experienced difficulties with contact, including verbal and physical attacks, seeing children being let down by parents who keep inconsistent contact and having the family routine disrupted by parents coming late or staying too long. Such difficult relationships between adults who have significant roles in a child's life are likely to place additional stresses on children (Triseliotis *et al.* 2000). Until recently, children in residential care have tended to be relatively isolated in institutions, and there has been little focus on building relationships with their families, whose relationship difficulties may often be very entrenched. The nature of institutions may prove more of a barrier for visiting for some families, while others may find it more difficult to enter another family home, but practitioners are being urged to remove barriers and to work more in partnership with families (Hill 2000).

For the majority of children, placement in foster or residential care leads to separation from siblings, and looked-after children may have siblings living in a variety of situations, both in and out of the care system (Kosonen 1996a). Siblings can provide much care and support for each other (Cicirelli 1995; Kosonen 1996b) and the inclusion of siblings in planning for looked-after children has been a relatively neglected area of research and practice.

A new initiative of 'concurrent planning' (Katz 1999) is an attempt 'to work towards family reunification while, at the same time, developing an alternative permanent placement'. Foster carers recruited to these schemes are expected to work towards family reunification, but to accept the child on a permanent basis if this is not successful. This will clearly require a different attitude on the part of biological parents and foster carers towards one another, plus a great deal of training and resources for it to be a success. The effect on the mental health of children in care of having to negotiate new relationships, separations and losses is an area requiring research. Whether or not concurrent planning can make these transitions easier for children remains to be seen. Until this information is available, practitioners must continue to work with individual cases while attempting to balance the full complexity of the child's situation.

How does kinship foster care compare with traditional foster care?

Kinship foster care can be defined as the placement of children in public care into the homes of extended family members who have been formally approved in a similar way to traditional foster parents. This relatively new development is the fastest growing placement practice in the USA, particularly for African-American families, and is more developed than in Europe. A major aim is to reduce dislocation for children placed in care and to retain them in the extended families and communities familiar to them, thereby maintaining their cultural and ethnic identity. Many questions remain as to whether this practice genuinely benefits the children and the focus here will be on findings from outcome research.

A comprehensive review of research reports (Scannapieco 1999) has compared findings and concluded that kinship foster care research is still in its infancy, being frequently compromised by small samples and problems with representativeness, lack of equivalence in the samples and differing outcome measures. Berrick *et al.* (1994) and Iglehart (1994) have reported that children in kinship care have fewer developmental and behavioural problems than those in foster care, but it is possible that children with more serious maltreatment histories are generally placed away from their relatives. Maternal grandmothers are the most frequent carers and kinship carers in general are likely to be older, less educated, have lower incomes and be in poorer health than foster carers (Dubowitz *et al.* 1994). This suggests that although the children remain in a familiar environment, it is also a materially poor environment, similar to that of the birth families. Research on the intergenerational transmission of attachment styles (Fonagy *et al.* 1991) implies caution in placing children with grandparents. Parents who provided inadequate parenting may have themselves been brought up by parents who did not provide adequate care.

The Benedict *et al.* (1996b) study has produced some of the most valuable follow-up data. Former foster children were between 25 and 35 years old when interviewed to assess their adult functioning. Comparisons were made between the total sample of former foster children (*n* = 71), comprising kinship foster care children (*n* = 31) and non-relative foster children (*n* = 40) and groups of children matched age, gender and ethnicity who were never separated from their birth families. Both fostered groups fared less well than never-placed comparisons. Differences in social support, behavioural adjustment and mental health status were not very pronounced, but those placed in non-relative foster homes were more likely to have experienced homelessness, to have been unemployed and to have a lower standard of living. This reinforces the argument for helping foster children leaving care to find and maintain adequate accommodation and to enhance their educational achievements. However, it is not possible to establish from research based on a cross-sectional follow-up whether the differences the researchers found resulted from the types of placement in themselves or from other mediating variables, such as preplacement experiences.

What is the longer term outcome for foster family and residential care?

Considering the levels of emotional and behavioural problems noted in childhood, studies of ex-foster care adults, as a whole, give a surprisingly positive picture. However, inherent difficulties exist in evaluating longitudinal studies of this group. The type of care provided in various settings may have changed radically in the years since the subjects were in foster care, so the

findings may have limited relevance for today's practice. It is also hard to compare residential with foster care on these outcomes as the populations entering different kinds of care may differ. Notwithstanding these differences various studies are worthy of comment. Buchanan (1999), in a recent analysis of the National Child Development Study data, showed that children who had been in care (types of placement cannot be distinguished in this cohort) were less satisfied with their lives at age 16 and significantly more at risk of depression at age 33. Despite this, three-quarters of 16-year-olds and four-fifths of 33-year-olds did not have psychological problems. Life satisfaction was associated with qualifications, jobs and partners.

Fanshel *et al.* (1990), in a retrospective cohort study of 'special needs' children in foster care, showed that 66% of respondents were wage-earners, with only 10% receiving public assistance. Thirteen per cent had serious drug problems, with one-third having had such problems in the past. One-quarter had had alcohol problems, 13% currently. In a later cross-sectional survey of 'alumni' of the same programme, most saw their experiences in foster care as positive and only 6% were unemployed, although there was no control group with which to compare (Wedeven *et al.* 1997).

A French retrospective cohort study of 63 adults reared in long-term foster care (for at least 5 years) found that the social class spread was similar to France as a whole and similar proportions of 'alumni' to the French national averages were married, were home owners and were employed. More were divorced (9 vs. 3.9%) and had no high school diploma (67 vs. 21.8%), one-third had used drugs, one-quarter had had charges or arrests for criminal activity and 13% described themselves as having health problems. Participants had better educational achievement the longer they had been in foster care and a poor educational outcome was associated with learning difficulties *before* going into care. Poor adult outcome was associated with social or psychiatric disorder in the birth parents and with problems such as abuse before going into care (Dumaret *et al.* 1997). A retrospective cohort study from the USA of adults who had been in long-term foster care gave a less rosy picture. Forty-two per cent had not completed high school, 31% were unemployed, 27% had been homeless, 54% had used drugs, 20% had been arrested, 45% had been violent to their partner and 35% had been victims of their partner's violence (Benedict *et al.* 1996b). The reasons for these geographical differences in outcomes are unknown, but they may indicate different levels of difficulty in children being fostered, different fostering environments, or different levels of psychosocial problems in the base populations in the USA as opposed to France. Little is known about outcomes for adults who spent a shorter time in foster care.

Studies of adult outcome from residential care are probably even more difficult to relate to the present day as the nature of residential care, and the kinds of children placed there, have changed a great deal in recent decades. One notable prospective study examined the long-term consequences for a sample of boys and girls raised in group homes in the 1960s (Quinton & Rutter 1984; Rutter *et al.* 1990). The adult follow-up of this ex-care sample showed different outcomes for men and women. Outcomes for women, when compared with controls, showed an increased rate of psychiatric disorder and parenting problems. One-third were faring poorly at follow-up and predictors of poor outcome were found to be disrupted early years and having multiple caregivers. Predictors of positive outcome were good school experiences, the capacity to plan ahead, avoidance of relationships with men with problems and not having babies in adolescence. For both men and women, adult outcomes were, to some extent, dependent on the quality of relationships made after leaving care.

Almost all children in residential and foster family care in the UK eventually return to their families. For a young person still to be in care or enter care in late adolescence tends to indicate particularly poor family relationships. A UK study showed that only 8% of 16–18-year-olds leaving care returned to live with a parent, suggesting that those still in care in their late teens are those for whom a return home has not been negotiable. Only a minority of this age group had positive supportive relationships with a parent, although contact with extended family or older siblings could provide important sources of support for a significant minority. This was also true of foster families. However, many young people did not receive ongoing support from foster carers and voiced a great sense of loss after leaving care. Almost one-quarter of the young women had their own children on discharge from care (compared with only 5% of women of the same age in the general population; Biehal & Wade 1996).

Young people who leave care at 16–18 years may, in fact, have spent most of their lives with birth families, having been placed in adolescence. The successful placement of adolescents in foster family care is generally hard to achieve because of the difficulties recruiting families, the fact that these young people may have been exposed to adversity for longer and because of the severity of their emotional and behavioural problems. Residential care is therefore a common placement option (Department of Health 1999) but may fail to contain their difficult behaviour (Berridge & Brodie 1998). Specialist foster care has been considered as an alternative, but the rate of breakdown can be as high as 40% (Fratter *et al.* 1991; Strathclyde Regional Council Social Work Department 1991). An evaluation of one specialist fostering scheme for adolescents has identified possible predictors of placement breakdown (Fenyo *et al.* 2000). This confirmed the findings of placement research on younger children: the presence of a teenager near in age to a child in the foster home is a strong predictor of breakdown, as is previous placement breakdown and behavioural difficulties, specifically delinquency and truancy. Teenage fostering schemes are being subjected to local audit, but a prospective study which controls for preplacement adversities and which compares foster with residential care outcomes is still lacking.

To what extent does the environment a young person enters upon leaving care have an impact upon their later functioning? The years immediately after leaving the care system are likely to be crucial for adult adjustment. A UK study surveyed 75% of the Leaving Care Projects in England and Wales in 1996 and compared the results with a similar study from 1992. Only 11% of care leavers between the ages of 16 and 21 were in full-time employment in 1996 while over half were unemployed, with a decline since 1992 in benefits and in financial assistance for further education and training. No doubt the economic and social climate into which a young person is 'discharged' from care will have an impact on his or her psychosocial adjustment. The study points out that 65% of 19-year-olds in the UK still live at home yet young people leaving care, who as a group have considerably greater difficulties than the general population, receive substantially less support in the crucial years of early adult life (Broad 1998). Young people from the general population go through a number of transitions in their late teens to early twenties, including leaving school, leaving home, setting up a home of their own and perhaps becoming a parent. For young people leaving care, these transitions are accelerated.

Young people leaving residential care may be doubly disadvantaged in their transition to independence compared to those leaving foster care. First, because of the greater likelihood of psychosocial problems in the birth family, residential care leavers may be less able to re-establish family links than those leaving foster care. Secondly, it is almost certainly harder to maintain relationships with members of a rotating staff group than with a foster carer. These young people may leave care with no one to confide in or who can offer them support. A large proportion of homeless youth and prison inmates have been in local authority care, evidencing a common transition from care into social exclusion (Jackson & Martin 1998). More research is urgently needed on this most vulnerable of groups.

Research on risk and protective factors helps explain why some children do well after local authority care while others do not. Earlier admission to long-term foster care and later discharge are associated with better outcomes for children, as is the absence of conduct problems. Recent policies emphasizing short-term placements may have allowed children to go in and out of care and caused delays in settling children who would benefit from long-term placements. The possibility exists of behavioural improvement for children placed under the age of 10, but this is much less likely for those exposed to longer periods of neglect and/or abuse (Minty 1999). Studies in the general population have shown that the most important predictor for good long-term outcome is a child's ability to form one good relationship, not necessarily with a parent or relative (Rosenfeld *et al.* 1997). Helping a child form and maintain that one crucial relationship within the complexity of a life in care would be a useful 'gold standard' towards which services could aim.

Treatment in residential and foster care

Delivering treatment to children in the care system is notoriously difficult: partly because of the problem of continuity for children who may move placement (Bondy *et al.* 1990) and partly because of lack of recognition of children's problems. A notable proportion of those diagnosed as suffering from major mental illness in McCann *et al.*'s (1996) study had hitherto unrecognized problems and this was particularly true of major depression. Those who work exclusively with looked-after children may have particular difficulty in recognizing problems warranting referral because they have become accustomed to working with disturbed children. This suggests that more systematic screening for looked-after children is essential and the new Looking After Children materials may go some way towards achieving this in the UK (Polnay & Ward 2000).

Undertreatment may not be the rule in all countries. A US study of medication use by looked-after children suggested that children in foster care were prescribed medication three times more frequently than similar children from the general population, while being approximately twice as likely to have a diagnosis of attention deficit hyperactivity disorder (ADHD) or major depression (Zima *et al.* 1999). There was no mention, in this study, of psychological treatments, and prescribing in isolation from other therapies would be a cause for concern.

Accounts of treatment of children in foster care are rare and evaluation unsatisfactory (Bondy *et al.* 1990; Barrows 1996), but received wisdom states that psychotherapists are often reluctant to begin treatment because of the difficulties that arise when children, who may have made an attachment to carers, peers and a therapist, have to move placement, school and clinic, breaking all of these bonds at once (Bondy *et al.* 1990). Research on treatment in residential care has been equally sparse. Some residential placements, particularly in the USA, are seen as treatment *per se* but studies of residential treatment have rarely been randomized. Comparisons of different residential treatment modalities (e.g. behaviour therapy vs. transactional analysis) suggest that, regardless of the content of the programme, a proportion of children show behavioural improvement while in the placement, but these improvements tend not to be sustained on leaving care, depending on the family and social circumstances into which the child is discharged. Carefully selected children, however, may respond well to a period of residential treatment within a continuum of care which includes family placement (Curry 1991).

One innovative US model for improving the emotional and behavioural functioning of children in foster care was the Fostering Individualized Assistance Programme (FIAP) in which children aged 7–15, deemed 'at risk' of behaviour problems after screening, were assigned a specialist caseworker who coordinated and/or delivered such services as individual and family therapy, advocacy, educational assistance and financial help. This was assessed by randomized single-blind controlled trial and showed that, after 18 months, the FIAP group were doing better as measured by the CBCL than controls and there were fewer runaways in this group (Clark *et al.* 1994). Presumably a children's social worker could perform this task, but success would require ease of access to, and good ongoing communication with, a range of services.

Whatever specific mental health problems a child in foster or residential care displays, children in this group are united in having suffered separation and loss. The vast majority probably also had grossly distorted attachment relationships prior to coming into care. The social and relationship difficulties displayed by children who have either been maltreated or have never had the opportunity to form selective attachments are well documented (Tizard & Hodges 1978; Gaensbauer & Sands 1979; George & Main 1979; Chisholm *et al.* 1995) and include indiscriminate friendliness, restless inattentive behaviour, aggression and unpredictable social responses. These problems may not precipitate referral to mental health services, yet may make it difficult for new relationships to develop between foster carers or residential workers and the children they look after. Rushton *et al.* (1998) have shown that children with restless inattentive behaviour may not benefit even from concerted attempts to help them settle into new placements.

The development of methods for treating children with serious attachment difficulties is one of the major challenges to child psychiatry. A large body of research has demonstrated the association between reciprocal communication between parent and infant in early childhood and the quality of attachment (Ainsworth 1979; Denham 1994; Freitag *et al.* 1996; Klann-Delius & Hofmeister 1997; Reddy *et al.* 1997). Interventions that help carers to communicate sensitively with children and to understand behaviour as communication—a basic tenet of parental behaviour management training programmes (Webster-Stratten & Herbert 1994)—may prove to be beneficial for looked-after children. A randomized trial using a communication training programme for foster carers showed trends towards improvement in general mental health and attachment disorders in children (Minnis 1999). The training was based on 'Communicating with Children: Helping Children in Distress' (Richman 1993) and was delivered by a social worker using an adult education model (Minnis *et al.* 1999). The implementation of such programmes on a larger scale could perhaps be achieved by effective joint working between health and social services.

How can child and adolescent psychiatry best serve this group within the current structure of services? An English study of health provision showed that child and adolescent psychiatry provided patchy provision for children in care across the country (Kurtz *et al.* 1994). The needs of this group are now being recognized more widely, but service evaluations are still rare. Arcelus *et al.* (1999), in an account of a mental health service for children in care, found that more than two-thirds of referrals were for children with aggressive behaviour, but there was a striking absence of adult carers and informants present in the assessment. This presents a major treatment challenge because the therapies indicated for such difficulties usually involve parents or families. Where children engaged in treatment, and when there was enough stability in the child's life for treatment to be supported, both psychodynamic and cognitive–behavioural therapeutic techniques appeared to enhance children's coping skills. Family therapy in foster care is an area that appears to have been neglected by research. Newer treatments based on 'holding therapy' designed for children with attachment difficulties are being used in some centres (Hughes 1997), but no formal trials have been carried out and such intervention remains controversial.

The only interventions with demonstrated effectiveness in reducing the emotional and behavioural problems of looked-after children are those delivered either in close liaison with foster carers, or directly through foster carers. A randomized controlled trial of a specialized fostering programme in the USA has shown benefits to children's mental health for those with the most severe emotional and behavioural problems. This scheme offered, on a weekly basis, 2-h group sessions for foster carers, 3–5 h of face-to-face plus frequent telephone contact with staff each week, therapy for child and family where appropriate and a significantly improved fostering allowance. While such interventions are clearly expensive, this trial also demonstrated cost effectiveness with an estimated $10 000 reduction in hospitalization costs per child (Chamberlain & Weinrott 1990).

If such benefits can emerge using highly trained and supported foster carers, could similar results be achieved in residential care? Residential staff may have little contact with child and adolescent mental health services and lack support in dealing with difficult emotional and behavioural problems (Hatfield *et al.* 1996), therefore interventions designed to support staff in dealing with such problems would be expected to benefit residents. However, Gibbs & Sinclair (1998) have pointed out that virtually all the therapies possible in residential care (including group and individual work) are also possible in foster care, without the same dangers of bullying and sexual harassment from other residents, or involvement in a delinquent culture. If lack of secure attachment is a fundamental difficulty for many looked-after children, placement with expertly supported foster carers who can provide this may be the most therapeutic option. Many child and adolescent mental health services in the UK provide one-off consultation for social workers or foster carers working with looked-after children with emotional and behavioural problems. While this model has merit in that it assumes foster families to be the main agents of change in children they look after, there is no evidence for its effectiveness. Ongoing partnership between mental health professionals and foster carers has, however, been shown to be successful. The work of the Clark and Chamberlain groups suggest that even children and young people with the most severe emotional and behavioural problems can be contained and successfully treated in foster care if the carers are well trained, supported and remunerated (Chamberlain & Weinrott 1990; Clark *et al.* 1994).

Conclusions

We now have good epidemiological data on the emotional and behavioural problems of looked-after children, but information is still lacking on the efficacy of interventions with these children and their carers. The rare attempts that have been made to conduct experimental trials of such interventions require replication and expansion. The extant literature shows a very high prevalence of emotional and behavioural problems both in children going into residential or foster care, and in children already being looked after. The prevalence of problems is particularly high among children in residential care, and while some studies suggest that problems may diminish in foster care and worsen in residential care, a direct comparison is difficult because the types of child entering the two environments are probably very different. The concept of an adoption–foster care–residential care hierarchy becomes even more pronounced in the context of revelations of appalling abuse by child care staff. This argues for a smaller number of high-quality safe residential places for those who need and prefer them. A complementary need would then be recruitment and support of foster families and/or more emphasis on family preservation. Foster care appears to be more child-centred and has not suffered from the blanket adverse publicity directed at residential care. On the other hand, placement breakdown and indeterminate placements remains a problem in foster care. At the policy level, every country must scrutinize potential carers, maintain high standards of staff conduct, strengthen children's rights, listen to children's allegations and provide them with advocates. Recruitment of foster carers must be maintained in order to provide a pool of high-quality placements.

Improved channels of referral to existing Child and Adolescent Mental Health Services (CAMHS) would be one model for tackling the children's problems. However, the historical origins and culture of the child mental health and social services differ and it will be a major challenge to achieve genuinely joint working between these agencies. It may be that the structure of CAMHS, in which diagnosis depends in part on adult informants who know the child well, may not be entirely appropriate for delivering treatment to children in care. An alternative model of service provision is specialist CAMHS services for looked-after children and some of these are currently being evaluated. Specialist foster care, in which carers receive significantly improved stipends and training plus close and ongoing liaison with CAMHS, aims to help the child gain a secure base from which development and treatment can take place. This third model is the only one which has been shown to be cost-effective. Excellent 'joined-up working' between social services, health and education will be essential in achieving such a service and a positive change in this direction will take research, money and political will.

References

Ahmad, A. & Mohamad, K. (1996) The socioemotional development of orphans in orphanages and traditional foster care in Iraqi Kurdistan. *Child Abuse and Neglect*, 20, 1161–1173.

Ainsworth, M.D. (1979) Infant–mother attachment. *American Psychologist*, 34, 932–937.

Angold, A., Costello, E., Messer, S.C. & Pickles, A. (1985) The development of a short questionnaire for use in epidemiological studies of depression in children and adolescents. *International Journal of Methods in Psychiatric Research*, 5, 237–249.

Arcelus, J., Bellerby T. & Vostanis P. (1999) A mental health service for young people in the care of the local authority. *Clinical Child Psychology and Psychiatry*, 4, 233–245.

Barn, R. (1993) *Black Children in the Public Care System*. British Agencies for Adoption and Fostering/Batsford, London.

Barrows, P. (1996) Individual psychotherapy for children in foster care: possibilities and limitations. *Clinical Child Psychology and Psychiatry*, 1, 385–397.

Benedict, M.I., Zuravin, S., Brandt, D. & Abbey, H. (1994) Types and frequency of child maltreatment by family foster care providers in an urban population. *Child Abuse and Neglect*, 18, 577–585.

Benedict, M.I., Zuravin, S., Somerfield, M. & Brandt, D. (1996a) The reported health and functioning of children maltreated while in family foster care. *Child Abuse and Neglect*, 20, 561–571.

Benedict, M.I., Zuravin, S. & Stallings, R.Y. (1996b) Adult functioning of children who lived in kin versus non-relative family foster homes. *Child Welfare*, 75, 529–549.

Berrick, J.D. & Barth R.P. (1994) Research on kinship foster care: What do we know? Where do we go from here? *Children and Youth Services Review*, 16, 1–5.

Berridge, D. & Brodie, I. (1998) *Children's Homes Revisited*. Jessica Kingsley, London.

Berridge, D. & Cleaver, H. (1987) *Foster Home Breakdown*, 2nd edn. Blackwell, Oxford.

Biehal, N. & Wade, J. (1996) Looking back, looking forward: care leavers, families and change. *Children and Youth Services Review*, 18, 425–445.

Blyth, E. & Milner, J. (1996) *Exclusion from School*. Routledge, London.

Bohman, M. (1997) Nature and nurture: lessons from Swedish adoption surveys. *Adoption and Fostering*, 21, 19–27.

Bondy, D., Davis, D., Hagen, S., Spiritos, A. & Winnick, A. (1990) Mental health services for children in foster care. *Children Today*, 19, 28–32.

Bowlby, J. (1951) *Maternal Care and Mental Health*. World Health Organization, Geneva.

Broad, B. (1998) *Young People Leaving Care: Life After the 1989 Children Act*. Jessica Kingsley, London.

Brown, E., Bullock, R., Hobson, C. & Little, M. (1998) *Making Residential Care Work: Structure and Culture in Children's Homes*. Ashgate, Aldershot.

Buchanan, A. (1999) Are care leavers significantly dissatisfied and depressed in adult life? *Adoption and Fostering*, 23, 35–40.

Chamberlain, P. & Weinrott, M. (1990) Specialized foster care: treating seriously emotionally disturbed children. *Children Today*, 19, 24–27.

Chambers, W., Puig-Antich, J., Hirsh, M. *et al.* (1985) The assessment of affective disorders in children and adolescents by semi-structured interview: test–retest reliability of the K-SADS-P. *Archives of General Psychiatry*, 42, 702.

Cheung, Y. & Heath, A. (1994) After care: the education and occupation of children who have been in care. *Oxford Review of Education*, 20, 361–374.

Chisholm, K., Carter, M.C., Ames, E.W. & Morison, S.J. (1995) Attachment security and indiscriminately friendly behaviour in children adopted from Romanian orphanages. *Development and Psychopathology*, 7, 283–294.

Cicchetti, D. & Toth, S.L. (1995) A developmental psychopathology perspective on child abuse and neglect. *Journal of the American Academy of Child and Adolescent Psychiatry*, 34, 541–565.

Cicirelli, V.G. (1995) *Sibling Relationships Across the Life Span*. Plenum, New York.

Clark, H.B., Prange, M.E., Lee, B., Boyd, L.A., McDonald, B.A. &

Stewart, E.S. (1994) Improving adjustment outcomes for foster children with emotional and behavioral disorders: early findings from a controlled study on individualized services. *Journal of Emotional and Behavioral Disorders*, 2, 207–218.

Colton, M. (1988) *Dimensions of Substitute Child Care*, 1st edn. Avebury, Aldershot.

Colton, M. & Hellinkx, W. (1994) Residential and foster care in the European Community: current trends in policy and practice. *British Journal of Social Work*, 24, 559–576.

Crowell, J. & Feldman, S. (1988) Mother's internal models of relationships and children's behavioural and developmental status: a study of mother–child interaction. *Child Development*, 59, 1273–1285.

Curry, J.F. (1991) Outcome research on residential treatment: implications and suggested directions. *American Journal of Orthopsychiatry*, 61, 348–357.

Denham, S.A. (1994) Mother–child emotional communication and preschoolers' security of attachment and dependency. *Journal of Genetic Psychology*, 155, 119–121.

Dennis, W. & Najarian, P. (1957) Infant development under environmental handicap. *Psychological Monographs*, 71, 1–13.

Department of Health (1999) *The Government's Objectives for Children's Social Services*. Department of Health, London.

Dimigen, G., Del Priore, C., Butler, S., Evans, S., Ferguson, L. & Swan, M. (1999) The need for a mental health service for children at commencement of being looked after and accommodated by the local authority: questionnaire survey. *British Medical Journal*, 319, 675–675.

Dubowitz, H., Feigelman, S., Harrington, D., Starr, R., Jr., Zuravin, S. & Sawyer, R. (1994) Children in kinship care: how do they fare? *Children and Youth Services Review*, 16, 85–106.

Dumaret, A.-C., Coppel-Batsch, M. & Couraud, S. (1997) Adult outcome of children reared for long-term periods in foster families. *Child Abuse and Neglect*, 21, 911–927.

Dumaret, A.C., Duyme, M. & Tomkiewicz, S. (1997) Foster children: risk factors and development at a preschool age. *Early Child Development and Care*, 134, 23–42.

Fanshel, D., Finch, S.J. & Grundy, J.F. (1990) *Foster Children in a Life Course Perspective*. Columbia University Press, New York.

Fanshel, D. & Shinn, E.B. (1978) *Children in Foster Care: a Longitudinal Investigation*. Columbia University Press, New York.

Farmer, E. & Pollock, S. (1998) *Sexually Abused and Abusing Children in Substitute Care*. John Wiley & Sons, Chichester.

Fenyo, A., Knapp, M. & Baines, B. (2000) Foster care breakdown: a study of a special teenager fostering scheme. In: *The State as Parent: International Research Perspectives on Interventions with Young Persons* (eds J. Hudson & B. Galaway), pp. 315–329. Kluwer Academic Publishers, Dordrecht.

Fletcher-Campbell, F. (1997) *The Education of Children Who Are Looked-After*. National Foundation for Educational Research, Slough.

Fonagy, P., Steel, H. & Steele, M. (1991) Maternal representations of attachment during pregnancy predict the organization of infant–mother attachment at one year of age. *Child Development*, 62, 891–905.

Fratter, J., Rowe, J., Sapsford, D. & Thoburn, J. (1991) *Permanent Family Placement: a Decade of Experience*. British Agencies for Adoption and Fostering, London.

Freitag, M.K., Belsky, J., Grossmann, K., Grossman, K.E. & Scheurer-Englisch, H. (1996) Continuity in parent–child relationships from infancy to middle childhood and relations with friendship competence. *Child Development*, 67, 1437–1454.

Frost, N., Mills, M. & Stein, M. (1999) *Understanding Residential Child Care*. Ashgate Publishing, Aldershot.

Gaensbauer, T. & Sands, K. (1979) Distorted affective communication in abused/neglected infants and their caretakers. *Journal of the American Academy of Child and Adolescent Psychiatry*, **18**, 236–250.

Gallagher, B. (1999) The abuse of children in public care. *Child Abuse Review*, **8**, 357–365.

Gean, M.P., Gillmore, J.L. & Dowler, J.K. (1985) Infants and toddlers in supervised custody: a pilot study of visitation. *Journal of the American Academy of Child Psychiatry*, **24**, 608–612.

George, V. (1970) *Foster Care: Theory and Practice*. Routledge, London.

George, C. & Main, M. (1979) Social interactions of young abused children: approach, avoidance and aggression. *Child Development*, **50**, 318.

Gibbs, I. & Sinclair, I. (1998) Treatment outcomes in children's homes. *Child and Family Social Work*, **4**, 1–8.

Glaser, D. (2000) Child abuse and neglect and the brain: a review. *Journal of Child Psychology and Psychiatry*, **41**, 97–116.

Goffman, E. (1961) *Asylums*. Penguin, Harmondsworth.

Goldberg, S. (1991) Recent developments in attachment theory and research. *Canadian Journal of Psychiatry*, **36**, 393–400.

Goldfarb, W. (1945) Effects of psychological deprivation in infancy and subsequent stimulation. *American Journal of Psychiatry*, **102**, 18–33.

Gottesman, M. (1991) *Residential Care: an International Reader*. Whiting and Birch, London.

Hatfield, B., Harrington, R. & Mohamad, H. (1996) Staff looking after children in local authority residential units: the interface with child mental-health professionals. *Journal of Adolescence*, **19**, 127–139.

Heath, A.F., Colton, M.J. & Aldgate, J. (1994) Failure to escape: a longitudinal study of foster children's educational attainment. *British Journal of Social Work*, **24**, 241–260.

Hill, M. (2000) The residential childcare context. In: *Residential Child Care: International Perspectives on Links with Families and Peers* (eds M. Chakrabarti & M. Hill), pp. 9–29. Jessica Kingsley, London.

Hobbs, G., Hobbs, C. & Wynne, J. (1999) Abuse of children in foster and residential care. *Child Abuse and Neglect*, **23**, 1239–1252.

Hughes, D. (1997) *Facilitating Developmental Attachment*. Jason Aronson, New Jersey.

Hulsey, T.C. & White, R. (1989) Family characteristics and measures of behavior in foster and non-foster children. *American Journal of Orthopsychiatry*, **59**, 502–509.

Iglehart, A.P. (1994) Kinship foster care: Placement, service and outcome issues. *Children and Youth Services Review*, **16**, 107–122.

Jackson, S. (1989) Residential care and education. *Children and Society*, **4**, 335–350.

Jackson, S. & Martin, P.Y. (1998) Surviving the care system: education and resilience. *Journal of Adolescence*, **21**, 569–583.

Katz, L. (1999) Concurrent planning: benefits and pitfalls. *Child Welfare*, **78**, 71–87.

Klann-Delius, G. & Hofmeister, C. (1997) The development of communicative competence of securely and insecurely attached children in interactions with their mothers. *Journal of Psycholinguistic Research*, **26**, 69–88.

Knapp, M. (1997) Economic evaluations and interventions for children and adolescents with mental health problems. *Journal of Child Psychology and Psychiatry*, **38**, 3–25.

Kosonen, M. (1996a) Maintaining sibling relationships-neglected dimension in child care practice. *British Journal of Social Work*, **26**, 809–822.

Kosonen, M. (1996b) Siblings as providers of support and care during

middle childhood: children's perceptions. *Children and Society*, **10**, 267–279.

Kufeldt, K., Armstrong, J. & Dorosh, M. (1995) How children in care view their own and their foster families: a research study. *Child Welfare*, **74**, 695–715.

Kurtz, Z., Thornes, R. & Wolkind, S. (1994) *Services for the Mental-Health of Children and Young People in England: a National Review*. Department of Public Health, London.

Lambert, L., Essen, J. & Head, J. (1977) Variations in behaviour ratings of children who have been in care. *Journal of Child Psychology and Psychiatry*, **18**, 335–346.

Lindsay, M. (1999) The neglected priority: sexual abuse in the context of residential child care. *Child Abuse Review*, **8**, 418.

Lyons-Ruth, K. (1996) Attachment patterns among children with aggressive behaviour problems: the role of disorganized early attachment patterns. *Journal of Consulting and Clinical Psychology*, **64**, 64–73.

Madge, N. (1994) *Children in Residential Care in Europe*. National Children's Homes, London.

Maluccio, N., Fein, E. & Olmstead, A. (1986) *Permanency Planning for Children: Concepts and Methods*. Tavistock Publications, London.

Maughan, B. & Pickles, A. (1990) Adopted and illegitimate children growing up. In: *Straight and Devious Pathways from Childhood to Adulthood* (eds L.N. Robins & M. Rutter), pp. 36–61. Cambridge University Press, Cambridge.

McAuley, C. (1996) *Children in Long-Term Foster Care*. Avebury, Aldershot.

McCann, J.B., James, A., Wilson, S. & Dunn, G. (1996) Prevalence of psychiatric disorders in young people in the care system. *British Medical Journal*, **313**, 1529–1530.

Mehra, H. (1996) *Residential Care for Ethnic Minorities Children: Meeting the Needs of Ethnic Minority Children*. Jessica Kingsley, London.

Milan, S.E. & Pinderhughes, E.E. (2000) Factors influencing maltreated children's early adjustment in foster care. *Development and Psychopathology*, **12**, 63–81.

Millham, S., Bullock, R., Hosie, K. & Haak, M. (1986) *Lost in Care: The Problems of Maintaining Links Between Children in Care and Their Families*. Gower, Aldershot.

Minnis, H. (1999) *Evaluation of a training programme for foster carers*. PhD thesis, University of London.

Minnis, H., Devine, C. & Pelosi, A. (1999) Foster carers speak about training. *Adoption and Fostering*, **23**, 42–47.

Minty, B. (1999) Outcomes for long-term foster family care. *Journal of Child Psychology and Psychiatry*, **40**, 991–999.

Palmer, S. (1996) Placement stability and inclusive practice in foster care: an empirical study. *Children and Youth Services Review*, **18**, 589–601.

Parker, R.A. (1966) *Decision in Child Care: a Study of Prediction in Fostering*. George Allen & Unwin, London.

Parker, R. (1990) *Away from Home: a History of Child Care*. Barnardos, Ilford.

Parker, R., Ward, H., Jackson, S., Aldgate, J. & Wedge, P. (1991) *Looking After Children: Assessing Outcomes in Child Care*. HMSO, London.

Polnay, L. & Ward, H. (2000) Promoting the health of looked after children. *British Medical Journal*, **320**, 661–662.

Polnay, L., Glaser, A. & Rao, V. (1996) Better health for children in resident care. *Archives of Disease in Childhood*, **75**, 263–265.

Quinton, D. & Rutter, M. (1984) Parents with children in care: current circumstances and parenting skills. *Journal of Child Psychology and Psychiatry*, 25, 231–250.

Quinton, D., Rushton, A., Dance, C. & Mayes, D. (1997) Contact between children placed away from home and their birth parents: research issues and evidence. *Clinical Child Psychology and Psychiatry*, 2, 393–413.

Quinton, D., Rushton, A., Dance, C. & Mayes, D. (1998) *Joining New Families: a Study of Adoption and Fostering in Middle Childhood.* Wiley, Chichester.

Reddy, V., Hay, D., Murray, L. & Trevarthen, C. (1997) Communication in infancy: mutual regulation of affect and attention. In: *Infant Development: Recent Advances* (eds G. Bremner & A. Slater), pp. 247–273. Psychology Press/Erlbaum, Hove.

Richman, N. (1993) *Communicating with Children: Helping Children in Distress.* Save the Children, London.

Rosenfeld, A.A., Pilowsky, D.J., Fine, P. *et al.* (1997) Foster care: an update. *Journal of the American Academy of Child and Adolescent Psychiatry*, 36, 448–457.

Rowe, J., Caine, M., Hundleby, M. & Keane, A. (1984) *Long-Term Foster Care.* Batsford, London.

Roy, P., Rutter, M. & Pickles, A. (2000) Institutional care: risk from family background or pattern of rearing? *Journal of Child Psychology and Psychiatry*, 41, 139–149.

Rushton, A. & Mayes, D. (1997) Forming fresh attachments in childhood: a research update. *Child and Family Social Work*, 2, 121–127.

Rushton, A., Treseder, J. & Quinton, D. (1995) An eight-year prospective study of older boys placed in permanent substitute families: a research note. *Journal of Child Psychology and Psychiatry*, 36, 687–695.

Rushton, A., Quinton, D., Dance, C. & Mayes, D. (1998) Preparation for permanent placement: evaluating direct work with older children. *Adoption and Fostering*, 21, 41–48.

Rushton, A., Dance, C. & Quinton, D. (2000) Findings from a UK based study into late permanent placements. *Adoption Quarterly*, 2, 5–17.

Rutter, M. (1985) Resilience in the face of adversity: protective factors and resistance to psychiatric disorder. *British Journal of Psychiatry*, 147, 589–611.

Rutter, M. (2000) Children in substitute care: some conceptual considerations and research implications. *Children and Youth Services Review*, 22, 658–703.

Rutter, M., Quinton, D. & Hill, J. (1990) Adult outcomes of institution reared children: males and females compared. In: *Straight and Devious Pathways from Childhood to Adulthood* (eds L.N. Robins & M. Rutter), pp. 135–157. Cambridge University Press, Cambridge.

Scannapieco, M. (1999) Kinship care in the public welfare system: a systematic review of research. In: *Kinship Foster Care* (eds R. Hegar & M. Scannapieco), pp. 141–154. Oxford University Press, Oxford.

Sellick, C. (1998) The use of institutional care for children across Europe. *European Journal of Social Work*, 1, 301–310.

Seltzer, M.M. & Bloksberg, L.M. (1987) Permanency planning and its effects on foster children: a review of the literature. *Social Work*, 32, 65–68.

Sinclair, I. & Gibbs, I. (1998) *Children's Homes: a Study in Diversity.* Wiley, Chichester.

Singer, L.M., Brodzinsky, D.M., Ramsay, D., Steir, M. & Waters, E. (1985) Mother–infant attachment in adoptive families. *Child Development*, 56, 1543–1552.

Spitz, R.R. (1945) Hospitalism: an inquiry into the genesis of psychiatric conditions in early childhood. *Psychoanalytic Study of the Child*, 1, 54–74.

St. Claire, L. & Osborne A.F. (1987) The ability and behaviour of children who have been 'in care' or separated from their parents. *Early Development and Care*, 28, Special Issue.

Stovall, K.C. & Dozier, M. (2000) The development of attachment in new relationships: single subject analysis for 10 foster infants. *Development and Psychopathology*, 12, 133–156.

Strathclyde Regional Council Social Work Department (1991) Fostering and adoption disruption research in Strathclyde region: the permanent placements. In: *Adoption and Fostering: the Outcome of Permanent Family Placements in Two Scottish Local Authorities*, pp. 47–123. Scottish Office, Edinburgh.

Thorpe, M. (1980) The experience of children and parents living apart. In: *New Developments in Foster Care and Adoption* (ed. J. Triseliotis), pp. 85–100. Routledge & Kegan Paul, London.

Tizard, B. & Hodges, J. (1978) The effect of early institutional rearing on the development of eight year old children. *Journal of Child Psychology and Psychiatry*, 19, 99–118.

Trasler, G. (1960) *In Place of Parents.* Routledge & Kegan Paul, London.

Triseliotis, J., Sellick, C. & Short, R. (1995) *Foster Care: Theory and Practice.* Batsford, London.

Triseliotis, J., Borland, M. & Hill, M. (2000) *Delivering Foster Care.* British Agencies for Adoption and Fostering, London.

Vorria, P., Rutter, M., Pickles, A., Wolkind, S. & Hobsbaum, A. (1998) A comparative study of Greek children in long-term residential group care and in two-parent families. I. Social, emotional, and behavioural differences. *Journal of Child Psychology and Psychiatry*, 39, 225–236.

Ward, H. (1996) Constructing and implementing measures to assess the outcomes of looking after children away from home. In: *Child Welfare Services: Developments in Law, Policy, Practice and Research* (eds M. Hill & J. Aldgate), pp. 240–254. Jessica Kingsley, London.

Warren, S., Huston, L., Egeland, B. & Sroufe, A. (1997) Child and adolescent anxiety disorders and early attachment. *Journal of the American Academy of Child and Adolescent Psychiatry*, 36, 637–644.

Webster-Stratten, C. & Herbert, M. (1994) *Troubled Families: Problem Children.* Wiley, New York.

Wedeven, T., Pecora, P.J., Hurwitz, M., Howell, R. & Newell, D. (1997) Examining the perceptions of alumni of long-term family foster care: a follow-up study. *Community Alternatives: International Journal of Family Care*, 9, 88–106.

Welsh Office (2000) *Lost in Care.* Stationery Office, Cardiff.

Werner, E.E. (1984) *Child Care: Kith, Kin and Hired Hands.* University Park Press, Baltimore.

Zima, B.T., Bussing, R., Crecelius, G.M., Kaufman, A. & Belin, T. (1999) Psychotropic medication use among children in foster care: relationship to severe psychiatric disorder. *American Journal of Public Health*, 89, 1732–1735.

23 Adoption

Nancy J. Cohen

Contemporary trends in adoption policy and practice

Creating a family through adoption has changed considerably over the past four decades. Historically, adoption was a service for childless couples. Selection was based on finding a match between children, most typically healthy white infants, and prospective parents. Over time, adoption has become focused on the needs of children and on adoptive parents' actual aptitude for parenting. Further, the number of infants available for adoption has declined because of increases in effective contraception, available abortion and social acceptability for young single women keeping their babies. As a consequence, the criteria for adoption in Western countries have changed. Ethnic origins, age, and the physical and emotional health of the child, once limiting factors when the goal was to match infant and parents, are now less of an issue. Adoption of children who are older and have other special needs as well as interracial and intercountry adoptions are more common. In the last two decades the definition of parents' suitability to adopt also has changed to embrace single parents, gay and lesbian parents, older individuals, and families who are less economically advantaged. Finally, there is greater concern for all members of the adoption triad with some form of open adoption and the option to search for a birth child or birth parent becoming more common.

Drawing on an international literature base, this chapter reviews the outcomes of multiple forms of adoption and considers related conceptual, clinical and social issues. Risks for socioemotional disturbance are examined in the light of developmental tasks and transitions for adopted children and their families. Implications of research findings are discussed in relation to mental health and prevention service needs of adopted children and their families.

Best interests of children in care

Children need a sensitive, caring and secure environment and individualized care. These needs provide the basis for serving the best interests of children when removal from their birth families is inevitable. When one considers the socioemotional or educational outcomes of children in care, adoption is preferable to being raised in foster care or in a residential setting (Bohman & Sigvardsson 1990; Maughan & Pickles 1990). Long-term foster care is the second best option in so far as it pro-

vides continuous individual caregiving (Minty 1999; Roy *et al.* 2000) and, in that sense, mirrors the situation for adopted children. This is also an important option because older children may refuse adoption, choosing returning to birth parents as their long-term goal. As is the case for adoption, older children placed in foster or residential care are more likely to have special needs and this affects the choice for placement (see Rushton & Minnis, Chapter 22).

While change is possible at many developmental points, the potential for change may be constrained by prior adaptations, highlighting the need for early decisions (Rutter 1999). Although delays should be avoided in deciding whether a child in care should be released for adoption or returned to their birth family, there is no consensus regarding the point at which delay becomes deleterious to child adjustment. Much is dependent on the child's age, experiences and, for older children, readiness for adoption. Unfortunately, decisions regarding children in care are often made in an adversarial environment where one camp is working toward removal of the child and the other toward maintaining the integrity of the birth family. To terminate parental rights, it must be proven that birth parents, usually the mother, has not acted responsibly in caring for and protecting her child, is erratic or errant in visiting and showing interest in her child's activities and well-being, and does not co-operate with child welfare and mental health systems to demonstrate convincingly that rehabilitation or life style change is likely. Birth mothers often love their children but cannot care for them. Removal of the child is another blow to their self-esteem, salvaged only by winning back the child or getting pregnant again. In some instances the adversarial process may be averted by including the birth mother and other family members in the planning process with arrangements made simultaneously for the birth mother and the child (Triseliotis *et al.* 1997). Providing empathy, options and resources (e.g. education, therapy or support), and access to some ongoing information about the child may facilitate a mutually beneficial decision. This approach may also increase opportunities for obtaining information about the birth family's biological and psychosocial history which is important for both adopted children and their adoptive families.

Delay may be caused in placement because keeping a sibling group together is the preferred option. The benefit of this remains controversial and results tend to be mixed (Triseliotis *et al.* 1997). On the positive side, harmonious sibling groups provide continuity and support for one another and an effort should be made to keep such groups together (Barth & Berry 1988). However, limitations in adoptive family financial and personal resources may reduce the feasibility of this option.

Outcomes of adoption

Studies of community samples show a heightened risk for learning difficulties (Brodzinsky & Steiger 1991) and adjustment problems, particularly disruptive behaviour, in middle childhood and early adolescence (Wierzbicki 1993). This pattern applies to children adopted as infants as well as to those adopted later (Smyer et al. 1998). Recent criticisms of research methodology—related to use of convenience samples, lack of adequate comparison groups, small sample size, retrospective methods and subjective measurement—have renewed debate over whether or not adopted children exhibit more psychopathology (Haugaard 1998; Brand & Brinich 1999; Peters et al. 1999). Results of controlled epidemiological and longitudinal studies (Lipman et al. 1992) conclude that only a small subset of adopted children have socioemotional problems; thus, most adopted children adjust well. It is also notable that, with rare exceptions (Smith & Brodzinsky 1994; Sobol et al. 1994), children's perceptions of their own problems have not been solicited.

Conclusions regarding adjustment apply to heterogeneous samples. In the next sections, the risks for different forms of adoptions will be considered.

Children with special needs

Adoption policy supports a commitment to finding homes for all children, including children with special needs. The term 'special needs' applies to children who are adopted later (usually over the age of 5), are members of a sibling group, have medical conditions, physical and developmental disabilities, or mental health problems. Despite concerns to the contrary, most of these placements are successful (Barth & Needell 1995). Characteristics of adoptive mothers predicting positive adjustment at 5-year follow-up include having fewer initial reservations, more experience, strong religious beliefs and not being depressed (Glidden 1994). Low maternal education, child functioning and family income are unrelated to outcome. Vulnerability to adjustment problems and disruption is greatest in late adopted children, particularly when there has been an accumulation of adverse experiences (e.g. abuse, privation and rejection) and serious behaviour problems prior to adoption (Verhulst et al. 1992; Rushton et al. 1995; Howe 1998).

Interracial adoption

Discussions of interracial adoption focus on within-country adoption of non-white minority status children, typically adoption of black children by white parents in the USA (McRoy et al. 1997) and African-Caribbean children in the UK (Rushton & Minnis 1997). Some members of the black community maintain that this trend reflects a bias against black families because of lower income status. Historically, black families have had more difficulty being approved for adoption. While there have been more assertive attempts to enlist black adoptive families, there is still a disproportionate number of black children in care (McRoy et al. 1997). Political issues aside, the outcomes for interracial adoptions have been positive and similar to that of intraracial adoptions (Rushton & Minnis 1997).

Interracial adoption also concerns native North American children. The history of adoption of native Indian children is rooted in violation of native rights and culture in the nineteenth and twentieth century when children were forcibly taken from parents and community and taught to depreciate their ethnic roots. Adoption into non-native families also violated the native practice of caring for children within the extended family. Moreover, the cultural distinctiveness, limited assimilation of native peoples, and paucity of models within the larger society may make it more difficult for native than for black children (Griffith & Duby 1991). In addition, native children have experienced poor relationships with adoptive parents and low self-esteem (Bagley 1990). As a result, adoption of native Indian children has decreased markedly.

Although society has moved toward greater acceptance of interracial adoption, the fact that the social context remains racist suggests that, when given an option, children should be placed in ethnically matched households (Rushton & Minnis 1997). When children are placed interracially, careful attention should be given to ensuring that adoptive parents have the understanding and sensitivity to support their children's ethnic identity.

Intercountry adoption

Intercountry adoption originated with efforts to rescue children victimized by war, epidemics and other calamities, or abandoned because of poverty and population control policies. Along with these humanitarian concerns, in some cases, intercountry adoption is motivated by preference of white parents for adopting infants and children who are not observably racially different or have special needs. Reports from a number of countries attest to the success of this form of adoption from parents' perspectives (Hoksbergen 1997; Cederblad et al. 1999). Moreover, children fare well with respect to ethnic identity and self-esteem (Cohen & Westhues 1995).

Intercountry adoptions do include children with special needs. Some children are in poor health, have neurological and developmental disabilities that are initially unknown or undisclosed (Johnson et al. 1992; Miller & Hendrie 2000), and have been exposed to prolonged privation. Such was the case for children adopted from Romania in the early 1990s, who have been the most comprehensively studied international adoptees. Although length of institutionalization of these children was related to cognitive deficits, even those exposed to extreme privation made medical, physical and cognitive gains, functioning within normal limits within 2 years on average (Marcovitch et al. 1997; Rutter et al. 2000). Moreover, cognitive gains were retained when followed at 4 and 6 years of age (Castle *et al.* 1999; O'Connor *et al.* 2000b). Nevertheless, late adopted children continued to exhibit significantly lower cognitive test scores relative to earlier adopted Romanian and within-country adopted children.

Socioemotional outcomes are less positive. High rates of insecure and unusual attachment patterns, behaviour problems, inattention/hyperactivity (O'Connor *et al.* 1999, 2000a), and autistic symptoms (Rutter *et al.* 1999a) have been observed, particularly among late adopted children (Chisholm *et al.* 1995; Fisher *et al.* 1997; Marcovitch *et al.* 1997; O'Connor *et al.* 1999). Although some of these symptoms abate, insecure attachments were stable over at least 3 years (Chisholm 1998; O'Connor *et al.* 2000a). Relationship problems with peers also persisted even when family attachments were formed (Fisher *et al.* 1997; O'Connor *et al.* 1999). It must be recognized that indices of attachment developed from normative Western samples may not have the same meaning. For instance, behaviour such as indiscriminate approach was associated with being a favourite in the institution, an adaptive behaviour in an environment with limited caregiving resources (Chisholm 1998). It must also be recognized that although parents were not concerned at first, family relations and stress may worsen if time proves that children's initial interpersonal problems do not abate (Chisholm 1998).

Adoption by non-traditional families

Past prejudices against single-parent adoption have given way to acceptance with good result (Glidden 1994). When followed into adolescence, children adopted by single parents continue to do well (Groze & Rosenthal 1991). Single parents are usually older non-white and lower income women willing to adopt children with special needs. Although it would appear that the most difficult children are placed with those with the fewest resources, children in single-parent homes experience fewer emotional and behavioural problems than children in two-parent adoptive homes (Rosenthal & Groze 1991). There are some strengths in single parenthood, including commitment to both the child and adoption, capacity to handle crises, relatively simple family structure, independence, self-confidence, and ability to develop and use supportive networks (Shireman 1995). However, encouraging single parents to adopt means that financial subsidies, counselling, education concerning child development, and help with planning for the child's future are critical.

Adoption by gay and lesbian parents has also increased (Hersov 1994). Systematic studies of outcome are not available. There are probably more adoptions by gay and lesbian couples than is known to adoption agencies, as some single-parent adoptions fall into this category. Supports are provided within the gay and lesbian community but fuller acceptance would open access to a broader service system.

Open adoption

Traditionally, members of the adoption triad were protected from the perceived stigma of adoption by confidentiality, with the intention of creating a situation in which all members of the adoption triad could get on with their lives. The reality was otherwise. In the 1970s, concerns with human rights and freedom of information coalesced with the human need to know and open adoption increased, as has search for birth parents by adopted children and adopted children by birth parents (Grotevant & McRoy 1997).

The term 'open adoption' refers to a continuum of arrangements ranging from confidential adoption, time-limited meetings with information relayed by the caseworker, ongoing information sharing mediated by the caseworker, to fully open adoption with direct meetings. The findings to date have applied to same-race infant private or independent adoptions. Grotevant and McRoy (1997) found that for 4–11-year-old children, outcomes of openness could be beneficial. Moreover, adoptive parents felt satisfied and birth mothers with ongoing contact showed better grief resolution than those without (Christian *et al.* 1997). It is also apparent that initial choices are not always permanent. Although most birth parents were interested in having information about their child, many did not want to interfere with their child's life or make the long-term commitment to a contact agreement (Hughes 1995). Contacts have been shown to decrease or stop after 5 years (Berry *et al.* 1998). Further, adoptive parents who chose open adoption for fear that they would not be able to adopt otherwise, tended to reduce frequency of contact over time. At this point it appears that adoptive and birth parents must negotiate arrangements regarding openness to fit their unique situations. Of prime importance is the impact of contact on the child and whether reduction in contact is perceived as a loss. Many issues regarding openness remain, such as how to deal with differing access to birth families for multiple children within a family and the fact that for some children contact is impossible.

With older children, the terminology is 'adoption with contact'. Triseliotis (1991) made a strong case for this, drawing a parallel with literature indicating that children's adjustment following divorce is related to consistent ongoing relationships with both parents. Opposing arguments claim that continuing contact will interfere with the children's bonding to their new family. Contact is adversely affected when the birth family opposes adoption (Parker 1999). However, lack of contact can also interfere if children continue to worry about their birth families and this can precede adoption disruption (Cohen & Duvall 1996). Some benefit accrues when a foster family, who have a relationship with the birth parent, are the adoptive family (Howe 1998). Clearly, empirical studies are required to show the conditions under which contact does or does not ease adjustment to the adoptive home.

Search for birth parents and birth children

The majority of adopted adults think about obtaining information or reuniting with birth relatives (Howe & Feast 2000).

Adoptees who search are usually female and relatively young. Although those who search are more likely to be ambivalent or dissatisfied about their adoption, this is not the sole reason for searching. Concerns regarding identity and understanding reasons for relinquishment are primary and a relationship with the birth parent only secondary (Howe & Feast 2000). Various types of relationships evolve following reunion, and early contact usually diminishes over time with approximately half of reunited individuals continuing to have contact after 5 years (Howe & Feast 2000). While feelings of emotional closeness are important, outcome is also mediated by geography, perceived response of birth relatives, or adoptive family members, sexual attraction, and expectations each party had of the other.

There are few social guidelines for how these family members should behave towards one another and clinicians may be able to help in negotiating the relationship. Consequently, they need to become knowledgeable about the search process (Gladstone & Westhues 1998). For instance, it may be necessary for the adoptee to deal with feelings regarding disloyalty towards their adoptive family. In addition, aspects of the reunion experience may underlie other issues that an adopted person presents within therapy. Also, help may be needed to resolve conflicts associated with expectations, inappropriate behaviour, role ambiguity, and differences in attitudes or values. Finally, help may be sought in dealing with the reality of post-reunion relationships and their outcomes.

Determinants of adjustment

Determinants of adjustment go beyond a specific type of adoption arrangement and entail an interdependent transaction between child characteristics, experiences prior to adoption and adoptive family characteristics.

There is now strong evidence of the importance that genetically determined traits bring to relationships. Evidence is strongest for a genetic basis for cognitive outcomes. Although adopted children's IQ scores correlate significantly with those of birth parents, children raised in adoptive homes score higher than those who remain with birth parents in disadvantaged social environments (Dumaret 1985). With respect to socioemotional characteristics, certain conditions—e.g. bipolar disorder, attention deficit hyperactivity syndrome (ADHD) and autism—appear to be more heritable than others (Rutter et al. 1999b). However, inheritance of other traits—e.g. temperament, criminality, other mental illnesses and substance abuse—is not so clear. Children born to parents with psychiatric disorder and antisocial behaviour are at higher risk for those problems but the risks are greater when the problems are also present in the adoptive family (Peters et al. 1999). The way genetics influences socioemotional functioning is probably indirect. There is a bidirectional transactional process between genetic and environmental influences, such that genetic factors contribute to children's experiences, making them susceptible to or protecting them from environmental influence and shaping the way that others act toward them (Ge et al. 1996; Rutter 2000). For instance, adopted children at genetic risk for antisocial behaviour have been shown to receive more negative control from parents than children who were not at risk (O'Connor et al. 1998).

As well as genetic risks, clinical samples often include children adopted late who have been exposed to adverse experiences including abuse and neglect, multiple moves into care, early hospitalizations, admission to care after the age of 2 years, prolonged institutional experiences, lack of satisfactory parenting and birth parent rejection. Outcomes for children with adverse early histories are improved by being placed in cohesive families who are flexible decision-makers (Groze 1994), can tolerate differences in the child in relation to other family members, have realistic expectations (Barth & Berry 1988), and where fathers are actively involved in parenting (Westhues & Cohen 1990).

Developmental issues in adoptive family adjustment

Changes in family structure and relationships created by having a child bring stresses to all families. Becoming an adoptive family, however, involves additional features. Common to all adoptions, parents are required to go through an intrusive investigation for suitability to parent and readiness to adopt, and live with the uncertainties of the timing of placement and legal finalization of the adoption. Once placed, the child must be integrated into the immediate and extended family and social network.

For families adopting infants, the transition process is relatively non-stressful (Levy-Shiff et al. 1990) and the mother–infant attachment relationship is as likely to be secure as in non-adoptive samples (Juffer & Rosenboom 1997). Adjustment problems, if they occur, emerge in middle childhood and early adolescence when children have the cognitive maturity to understand that to be adopted necessarily means that they were relinquished by another family. Some adopted children subsequently become ambivalent about their adoption, experience feelings of loss and grief, and emotional or behavioural problems ensue. Another developmental milestone occurs when adopted adolescents grapple with the unknowns in their biological and personal histories which complicates normal developmental preoccupations. Although adjustment problems peak in middle childhood and early adolescence, they tend to dissipate in later adolescence and adulthood (Bohman & Sigvardsson 1990; Sobol et al. 1994). Therefore, it would appear that long-term adjustment for infant adoptees is related to normal developmental processes (Brodzinsky 1987) and individual coping styles (Smith & Brodzinsky 1994).

The transition to adoptive family life in older and other special needs children is more complex and the adjustment period lengthier. Not surprisingly, children who have experienced inadequate caregiving have difficulty putting trust in adults for love and protection and may be less adaptive in a new setting. While adoptive parents can usually understand the implications of trauma, abuse and rejection that their adopted child experienced in the past, actually making accommodations can be difficult. Following placement, symptoms such as lying, stealing, challenges to family rules and lack of empathy may appear in adopted children (Pinderhughes 1996). When an adoption disrupts it is frequently attributed to children's attachment problems reflected in these symptoms. When at their most disruptive, adopted children may actually be testing the security of the placement, but these are not the signs of attachment formation that parents expect (Cohen & Duvall 1996). Restabilizing as a new family involves tasks for both adults and children, such as forming attachments and establishing rituals and rules. For adoptive parents, providing a secure environment while managing and setting limits on child behavioural problems without rejection by the child can be a challenge (Reitz & Watson 1992; Rushton *et al.* 2000). The restabilization process depends on family resources, supports and coping strategies (Groze 1994). Factors that interfere with this process include adoptive parents' inflexibility and difficulties in dealing with the adopted child's emotional needs, unresolved grief associated with infertility, unrealistic expectations and perceiving the child as incompatible with the family (Grotevant & Kohler 1999). Problems also arise when a child is placed in a family with a birth infant or child close to his or her age (Beckett *et al.* 1998). Step-parents who adopt older children may have difficulties in the transition process in tolerating their child's attachment to the absent birth parent. This is an important issue because step-parent adoption comprises the largest proportion of older child adoptions.

Although successful restabilization is the norm, ambivalence about the adoption may ensue and the child be returned to care during the probation period (Festinger 1990). All of this suggests that for families adopting older children and children who have experienced early severe adversity, selection and preparation of families and post-adoption services and supports have special importance.

Selection and preparation of children and families for adoption

Child welfare services and private adoption agencies are responsible for determining eligibility, evaluating tolerance for the risks of older and other special needs adoptions, and supporting and assisting parents in the adoption process (Triseliotis *et al.* 1997). Available information on children's genetic, medical and psychosocial history is described to parents and the implications for physical, cognitive and socioemotional functioning are discussed. For parents adopting children with special needs, meetings with experienced adoptive parents are arranged where they can talk about challenges and rewards of adopting these children. Adopting parents also are helped to reflect on the individual and family strengths and weaknesses they bring to adoption (Parker 1999). Despite these efforts, prospective parents have reported that there is insufficient discussion of the impact of adoption on birth children, inadequate targeted information for

subgroups of adopting parents (e.g. single parents), and that challenging behaviour is not always accurately presented. The need for both adopted and birth children's involvement in the adoption process has also been emphasized (Parker 1999).

Because it is not possible to know how parents will actually respond to their adopted child's emotional needs and behavioural characteristics, post-placement services should become a routine part of the adoption process for families adopting children with special needs. These must be health focused and aimed at helping adopted children and their families negotiate an important transition period. Such services could also permit timely intervention if difficulties arise. In fact, behavioural problems sometimes can be capitalized upon during the post-placement period to promote secure attachment; secure attachment is not threatened by children's emotional pain but how it is handled. Post-placement programmes can also help parents and adopted children when a return to care seems inevitable. These tasks cannot be accomplished by post-adoption support groups organized by the adoption agencies or by parent-run organizations. Such groups are important but cannot address struggles of individual families in developing relationships and usually do not involve children directly.

Some programmes have been developed specifically for use with adoptive families in the post-placement transition period. The Family Attachment Programme applies principles from both attachment theory and brief interactional family therapy in a series of exercises with the whole family (Cohen & Duvall 1996). The goal is to assist parents to understand and empathize with their child's pre-adoption experiences, explore losses the child and family have had and move into the future by punctuating new family roles, rituals and rules, establishing realistic expectations, facilitating effective communication, and encouraging risk-taking in self-disclosure in the service of building trusting relationships. To help children to situate themselves in terms of time, place and relationships with important people in their histories, tools such as the Life Story Book, Life Story Map, and genealogical diagrams are used. These help children express feelings, put confusing events into order, and create a more coherent narrative of the child's life that can be shared with their new family (Cohen & Duvall 1996; Triseliotis *et al.* 1997). Creation of a coherent narrative is recognized as an especially important component of an integrative sense of identity throughout the life cycle of adopted children (Grotevant 1997). Including all family members is critical in the post-placement period, when the primary task is family formation. Therefore, family focused programmes should take precedence over individual therapy for the child.

For infants, toddlers and preschool-age children, less verbally based services are most appropriate. With healthy international infant adoptees, Juffer *et al.* (1997) found a positive effect on attachment security, maternal sensitivity and infant exploration using a brief intervention involving a book concerning sensitive parenting coupled with an intervenor commenting on videotaped mother–infant interactions that illustrated sensitive responses. This was more effective than giving parents the book alone. Infant-led approaches (Muir *et al.* 1999) also have been used in the post-placement period although systematic studies have not been carried out on adoptive families specifically (Cohen *et al.* 1999).

Post-adoption services should not be provided by the adoption worker responsible for placement whom parents may perceive as having the power to remove the child if problems emerge in the transitional probationary period. An arms's length arrangement whereby the family is seen by a mental health practitioner who maintains contact with the adoption agency is likely to facilitate a positive outcome.

Adopted children and their families in the clinic

Adopted children and adolescents have been shown to be over-represented in both outpatient and inpatient services, especially for disruptive behaviour problems such as conduct disorder and ADHD (Wierzbicki 1993; Moore & Fombonne 1999). In one study, although parents of adopted adolescents were more likely to make a mental health referral than parents of non-adopted adolescents with problems of similar severity, for children with more severe problems the referral rates did not differ (Warren 1992). Potential reasons for the increased mental health referrals of children with moderate problems include adoptive parents' greater comfort accessing services, hypervigilance about difficulties coupled with perception of their children as more susceptible to adjustment problems, and the fragility and consequent reactivity of adoptive families to even low level problems (Warren 1992).

Most families who seek clinical service receive the same service as non-adoptive families and often feel their problems are overly pathologized (Cohen *et al.* 1993). Mental health professionals typically do not have specialized training and may not understand the adoption process, characteristics of adoptive parents, the issues with which adopted children and their families struggle, the fact that the child's problems preceded adoption (Nickman & Lewis 1994), and that some difficulties arise as part of normative developmental transitions and crises in the adopted child or adoptive family life cycle (Brodzinsky 1987). In fact, it has been shown that adoptive families in treatment have greater psychosocial resources and better familial and marital functioning than non-adoptive families in treatment (Cohen *et al.* 1993). This suggests that strengths of adoptive parents can be utilized to bring about rapid changes. Treatment of non-adoptive families may be lengthier and more complex because marital and family problems contribute to and maintain child problems. Practitioners also may erroneously believe that some issues are specific to adoption and this could colour intervention. For instance, descriptive reports have indicated that adoptive families may not feel entitled to be parents and, as a consequence, have difficulty setting limits on child behaviour for fear of being rejected (Reitz & Watson 1992). However, when adoptive and non-adoptive families who were and were not re-ceiving mental health services were studied, these traits were found to apply to families seeking service regardless of adoption status (Cohen *et al.* 1996). As suggested above, the difference may be that, given adoptive families strengths, they have greater potential for change. Finally, clinicians are not always aware of the patterns of recovery for children exposed to adverse pre-adoption experiences when placed in a positive family environment so that accurate information can be given (Rutter *et al.* 2000).

Unfortunately, the research literature has not examined outcomes of interventions with adoptive families. As discussed above, research findings suggest that adoptive families do well with less complicated brief interventions that help them to provide structure and limits for their child's behaviour (Schaffer & Lindstrom 1990; Cohen *et al.* 1993). For children who exhibit attachment disorders, interventions with a relational focus appear to be helpful (Jernberg 1989; Juffer *et al.* 1997; Muir *et al.* 1999). Children also may benefit from environmental manipulations, such as gradual exposure to stimulation, directing selective social approach and display of affection, and facilitating social pragmatic skills (Rutter *et al.* 2000). Cline (1990) has suggested a more extreme measure, holding therapy, which has gained attention from parents desperate for help with their severely attachment disordered children. However, the reputation of holding therapy is based on its extreme methods and extravagant claims and not on empirical evidence. There is an urgent need to test empirically all of these possible avenues of treatment.

An alternate solution to treatment of severe child behaviour problems is to remove the child from the adoptive family. Cohen *et al.* (1993) found that among adoptive families presenting for clinical service 5 or more years after adoption, 25% considered removal of the child whose behaviour they perceived as unmanageable as a solution to problems and 9% ultimately did so. Although in most cases removal could be averted with treatment, therapists must be sensitive to clues that removal of the child is the preferred solution so that this can be addressed directly. In other situations, a different kind of living arrangement that involves living away while maintaining contact can be an option. The intimacy of family life may be too threatening for children with significant attachment problems, although they do not want to sever connection. Unfortunately, in some cases a child has been removed from the adoptive home when the family only wanted respite care. It is important that clinicians have the flexibility to weigh a range of possible solutions.

Conclusions and future challenges

This chapter has reviewed advances in understanding the various forms of adoption. In the last decade, many of the prejudices and dire predictions of the past have given way either to acceptance or to serious systematic consideration. Although more is known about the process of adoption and its outcomes, challenges remain for both researchers and practitioners. Specifically, the literature consistently supports the strengths of adoptive parenthood and the resilience of children, even those who have experienced adversity. There is a subgroup of children with special needs, however, who pose challenges to their families and to practitioners. Some of the challenges to practitioners arise because of lack of specialized training regarding adoption. It must be acknowledged that training can only go so far because we are lacking essential empirical information on the treatment of adoptive families. The need for information extends beyond special needs adoption and encompasses understanding the many forms of open adoption and adoption with contact, the critical time frame for making placement decisions and the exact criteria on which they should be based, and the long-term consequences of opening adoption records. Challenges also remain regarding intercountry adoption in terms of regulation of adoption procedures and working collaboratively with countries offering children for adoption to ensure that pre-placement care serves children's best interests. There does not appear to be evidence of the kind of political heat with respect to intercountry interracial adoption that is associated with within-country interracial adoption. Nevertheless, given the increase of intercountry adoptions, some of which are also interracial, it is important to track the experiences of the children with attention paid to issues of racism and identity.

Clearly, complex questions remain in the field of adoption for which there are no easy answers. They must continue to be explored systematically in order to create policies and practices that will protect children while being flexible enough to accommodate a variety of arrangements.

References

Bagley, C. (1990) Adoption of Native children in Canada. In: *Intercountry Adoption: a Multinational Perspective* (eds H. Altstein & R. Simon), pp. 55–79. Praeger, New York.

Barth, R.P. & Berry, M. (1988) *Adoption and Disruption: Rates, Risks, and Responses.* Aldine De Gruyter, New York.

Barth, R.P. & Needell, B. (1995) Outcomes for drug-exposed children four years post-adoption. *Children and Youth Services Review*, **18**, 37–56.

Beckett, C., Groothues, C. & O'Connor, T. (1998) Adopting from Romania: the role of siblings in adjustment. *Adoption and Fostering*, **22**, 25–34.

Berry, M., Dylla, D.J., Barth, R.P. & Needell, B. (1998) The role of open adoption in the adjustment of adopted children and their families. *Children and Youth Services Review*, **20**, 151–168.

Bohman, J. & Sigvardsson, S. (1990) Outcome in adoption: lessons from longitudinal studies. In: *The Psychology of Adoption* (eds D.M. Brodzinsky & M.D. Schechter), pp. 93–107. Oxford University Press, New York.

Brand, A.E. & Brinich, P. (1999) Behavior problems and mental health contacts in adopted, foster, and nonadopted children. *Journal of Child Psychology and Psychiatry*, **40**, 1221–1230.

Brodzinsky, D.M. (1987) Adjustment to adoption: a psychosocial perspective. *Clinical Psychology Review*, **7**, 25–47.

Brodzinsky, D.M. & Steiger, C. (1991) Prevalence of adoptees among special education populations. *Journal of Learning Disabilities*, **24**, 484–489.

Castle, J., Groothues, C., Bredenkamp, D. *et al.* (1999) Effects of qualities of early institutional care on cognitive attainment. *American Journal of Orthopsychiatry*, **69**, 424–437.

Cederblad, M., Höök, B., Irhammar, M. & Mercke, A.M. (1999) Mental health in international adoptees as teenagers and young adults: an epidemiological study. *Journal of Child Psychology and Psychiatry*, **40**, 1239–1248.

Chisholm, K. (1998) A three year follow-up of attachment and indiscriminate friendliness in children adopted from Romanian orphanages. *Child Development*, **69**, 1092–1106.

Chisholm, K., Carter, M., Ames, E.W. & Morison, S.J. (1995) Attachment security and indiscriminately friendly behavior in children adopted from Romanian orphanages. *Development and Psychopathology*, **7**, 283–294.

Christian, C.L., McRoy, R.G., Grotevant, H.D. & Bryant, C.M. (1997) Grief resolution of birth mothers in confidential, time-limited mediated, ongoing mediated, and fully disclosed adoptions. *Adoption Quarterly*, **1**, 35–58.

Cline, F. (1990) Understanding and treating the severely disturbed child. In: *Adoption Resources for Mental Health Professionals* (ed. P.V. Grabe), pp. 137–150. Transaction Publishers, London.

Cohen, N.J. & Duvall, J.D. (1996) *Manual for The Family Attachment Program: An Innovative Program for Working with Families Adopting Older Children.* Hincks-Dellcrest Institute, Toronto.

Cohen, J.S. & Westhues, A. (1995) A comparison of self-esteem, school achievement, and friends between intercountry adoptees and their siblings. *Early Child Development and Care*, **106**, 205–224.

Cohen, N.J., Coyne, J. & Duvall, J. (1993) Adopted and biological children in the clinic: family, parental and child characteristics. *Journal of Child Psychology and Psychiatry*, **34**, 55–562.

Cohen, N.J., Coyne, J.C. & Duvall, J.D. (1996) Parents' sense of 'entitlement' in adoptive and nonadoptive families. *Family Process*, **35**, 441–456.

Cohen, N.J., Muir, E., Lojkasek, M. *et al.* (1999) Watch, Wait, and Wonder: testing the effectiveness of a new approach to mother–infant psychotherapy. *Infant Mental Health Journal*, **20**, 429–451.

Dumaret, A. (1985) IQ, scholastic performance and behaviour of sibs raised in contrasting environments. *Journal of Child Psychology and Psychiatry*, **26**, 553–580.

Festinger, T. (1990) Adoption disruption: rates and correlates. In: *The Psychology of Adoption* (eds D.M. Brodzinsky & M.D. Schechter), pp. 201–220. Oxford University Press, New York.

Fisher, L., Ames, E.W., Chisholm, K. & Savoie, L. (1997) Problems reported by parents of Romanian orphans adopted to British Columbia. *International Journal of Behavioral Development*, **20**, 67–82.

Ge, X., Conger, R.D., Cadoret, R.J. *et al.* (1996) The developmental interface between nature and nurture: a mutual influence model of child antisocial behavior and parenting. *Developmental Psychology*, **32**, 574–589.

Gladstone, J. & Westhues, A. (1998) Adopted reunions: a new side to intergenerational family relationships—family relations. *Interdisciplinary Journal of Applied Family Studies* **47**, 177–184.

Glidden, L. (1994) Not under my heart, but in it: families by adoption. In: *When There's No Place Like Home: Options for Children Living Apart from Their Natural Families* (ed. J. Blacher), pp. 181–209. Paul H. Brookes, Baltimore.

Griffith, E.E. & Duby, J.L. (1991) Recent developments in the transracial adoption debate. *Bulletin of the American Academy of Psychiatry and Law*, **19**, 339–350.

Grotevant, H.D. (1997) Coming to terms with adoption: the construction of identity from adolescence into adulthood. *Adoption Quarterly*, **1**, 3–27.

Grotevant, H.D. & Kohler, J.K. (1999) Adoptive families. In: *Parenting and Child Development In 'Nontraditional' Families* (ed. M.E. Lamb), pp. 161–190. Erlbaum, Mahwah, NJ.

Grotevant, H.D. & McRoy, R.G. (1997) The Minnesota/Texas adoption research project: implications of openness in adoption for development and relationships. *Applied Developmental Science*, **1**, 168–186.

Groze, V. (1994) Clinical and nonclinical adoptive families of special-needs children. *Families in Society*, **75**, 90–104.

Groze, V. & Rosenthal, J. (1991) Single parents and their adopted children: a psychosocial analysis. *Families in Society*, **72**, 67–77.

Haugaard, J.J. (1998) Is adoption a risk factor for the development of adjustment problems? *Clinical Psychology Review*, **18**, 47–69.

Hersov, L. (1994) Adoption. In: *Child and Adolescent Psychiatry: Modern Approaches* (eds M. Rutter & L. Hersov), 3rd edn, pp. 267–282. Blackwell, London.

Hoksbergen, R.A.C. (1997) Turmoil for adoptees during their adolescence? *International Journal of Behavioral Development*, **20**, 33–46.

Howe, D. (1998) *Patterns of Adoption*. Blackwell, London.

Howe, D. & Feast, J. (2000) *Adoption, Search and Reunion: The Long Term Experience of Adopted Adults*. The Children's Society, London.

Hughes, B. (1995) Openness and contact in adoption: a child centered perspective. *British Journal of Social Work*, **25**, 729–747.

Jernberg, A.M. (1989) Training parents of failure to attach children. In: *Handbook of Parent Training Parents as Co-Therapists for Children's Behavior Problems* (eds J.E. Schaeffer & J.E. Briesmester), pp. 392–413. Wiley, New York.

Johnson, A., Miller, L., Iverson., S. *et al.* (1992) The health of children adopted from Romania. *Journal of the American Medical Association*, **268**, 3446–3451.

Juffer, F. & Rosenboom, L.G. (1997) Infant–mother attachment of internationally adopted children in the Netherlands. *International Journal of Behavioral Development*, **20**, 93–107.

Juffer, F., Hoksbergen, R.A.C., Riksen-Walraven, J.M. & Kohnstamm, G.A. (1997) Early intervention in adoptive families: supporting maternal sensitive responsiveness, infant–mother attachment and infant competence. *Journal of Child Psychology and Psychiatry*, **38**, 1039–1050.

Levy-Shiff, R., Goldshmidt, I. & Har-Even, B. (1990) Transition to parenthood in adoptive families. *Developmental Psychology*, **27**, 131–140.

Lipman, E.L., Offord, D.R., Racine, Y.A. & Boyle, M.H. (1992) Psychiatric disorders in adopted children: a profile from the Ontario Child Health Study. *Canadian Journal of Psychiatry*, **37**, 627–633.

Marcovitch, S., Goldberg, S., Gold, A. *et al.* (1997) Determinants of behavioural problems in Romanian children adopted in Ontario. *International Journal of Behavioral Development*, **20**, 17–31.

Maughan, B. & Pickles, A. (1990) Adopted and illegitimate children grown up. In: *Straight and Deviant Pathways from Childhood to Adulthood* (eds L. Robins & M. Rutter), pp. 36–61. Cambridge University Press, New York.

McRoy, R.G., Oglesby, Z. & Grape, H. (1997) Achieving same-race adoptive placements for African-American children: culturally sensitive practice approaches. *Child Welfare*, **76**, 85–104.

Miller, C. & Hendrie, N.W. (2000) Health of children adopted from China. *Pediatrics*, **105**, 76–82.

Minty, B. (1999) Annotation: outcomes in long-term foster family care. *Journal of Child Psychology and Psychiatry*, **40**, 991–999.

Moore, J. & Fombonne, E. (1999) Psychopathology in adopted and nonadopted children: a clinical sample. *American Journal of Orthopsychiatry*, **69**, 403–409.

Muir, E., Lojkasek, M. & Cohen, N.J. (1999) *Watch, Wait, and Wonder: A Manual Describing an Infant-Led Approach to Problems in Infancy and Early Childhood*. Hincks-Dellcrest Institute, Toronto.

Nickman, S.L. & Lewis, R.G. (1994) Adoptive families and professionals: when the experts make things worse. *Journal of the American Academy of Child and Adolescent Psychiatry*, **33**, 753–755.

O'Connor, T.G., Deater-Deckard, K., Fulker, D., Rutter, M. & Plomin, R. (1998) Genotype–environment correlations in late childhood and early adolescence: antisocial behavior problems and coercive parenting. *Developmental Psychology*, **34**, 970–981.

O'Connor, T.G., Bredenkamp, D., Rutter, M. *et al.* (1999) Attachment disturbances and disorders in children exposed to early severe deprivation. *Infant Mental Health Journal*, **20**, 10–29.

O'Connor, T.G. & Rutter, M. & the English and Romanian Adoptees Study Team (2000a) Attachment disorder behavior following early deprivation: extension and longitudinal follow-up. *Journal of the American Academy of Child and Adolescent Psychiatry*, **39**, 703–712.

O'Connor, T.G., Rutter, M., Beckett, C. *et al.* (2000b) The effects of global severe privation on cognitive competence: extension and longitudinal follow-up. *Child Development*, **71**, 376–390.

Parker, R. (1999) *Adoption Now*. Wiley, West Sussex.

Peters, B.R., Atkins, M.S. & McKernan McKay, M. (1999) Adopted children's behavior problems: a review of five explanatory models. *Clinical Psychology Review*, **19**, 297–328.

Pinderhughes, E.E. (1996) Toward understanding family readjustment following older child adoptions: the interplay between theory generation and empirical research. *Children and Youth Services Review*, **18**, 115–138.

Reitz, M. & Watson, K.W. (1992) *Adoption and the Family System*. Academic Press, Orlando, FL.

Rosenthal, J.A. & Groze, V. (1991) Behavioral problems of special needs adopted children. *Children and Youth Services Review*, **13**, 343–361.

Roy, P., Rutter, M. & Pickles, A. (2000) Institutional care: risk from family background or pattern of rearing. *Journal of Child Psychology and Psychiatry*, **41**, 139–150.

Rushton, A. & Minnis, H. (1997) Transracial family placements. *Journal of Child Psychology and Psychiatry*, **38**, 147–160.

Rushton, A., Treseder, J. & Quinton, D. (1995) An eight-year prospective study of older boys placed in permanent substitute families: a research note. *Journal of Psychology and Psychiatry*, **36**, 687–695.

Rushton, A., Dance, C. & Quinton, D. (2000) Findings from a UK based study of late permanent placements. *Adoption Quarterly*, **3**, 51–71.

Rutter, M. (1999) Resilience concepts and findings: implications for family therapy. *Journal of Family Therapy*, **21**, 119–144.

Rutter, M. (2000) Children in substitute care: some conceptual considerations and research implications. *Children and Youth Services Review*, **22**, 685–702.

Rutter, M., Anderson-Wood, L., Beckett, C. *et al.* (1999a) Quasi-autistic patterns following severe early global privation. *Journal of Child Psychology and Psychiatry*, **40**, 537–555.

Rutter, M., Silberg, T., O'Connor, T. & Simonoff, E. (1999b) Genetics and child psychiatry. I. Advances in quantitative and molecular genetics. *Journal of Child Psychology and Psychiatry*, **40**, 3–18.

Rutter, M., O'Connor, T., Beckett, C. *et al.* (2000) Recovery and deficit following profound early deprivation. In: *Intercountry Adoption: Developments, Trends and Perspectives* (ed. P. Selman), pp. 107–125. British Association for Adoption and Fostering, London.

Schaffer, J. & Lindstrom, C. (1990) Brief solution-focused therapy with adoptive families. In: *The Psychology of Adoption* (eds D. Brodzinsky & M. Schechter), pp. 240–252. Oxford University Press, New York.

Shireman, J.F. (1995) Single parent adoptive homes. *Children and Youth Services Review*, **18**, 23–36.

Smith, D.W. & Brodzinsky, D.M. (1994) Stress and coping in adopted children: a developmental study. *Journal of Clinical Child Psychology*, **23**, 91–99.

Smyer, M.A., Gatz, M., Simi, N.L. & Peterson, N.L. (1998) Childhood adoption: long term effects in adulthood. *Psychiatry*, **61**, 191–205.

Sobol, M.P., Delaney, S. & Earn, B.M. (1994) Adoptees' portrayal of the development of family structure. *Journal of Youth and Adolescence*, **3**, 385–401.

Triseliotis, J. (1991) Maintaining the links in adoption. *British Journal of Social Work*, **21**, 401–414.

Triseliotis, J., Shireman, J. & Hundleby, M. (1997) *Adoption: Theory, Policy, and Practice*. Cassell, London.

Verhulst, F.C., Althaus, M. & Versluis-Den Bieman, H.J.M. (1992) Damaging backgrounds: later adjustment of international adoptees. *Journal of the American Academy of Child and Adolescent Psychiatry*, **31**, 518–524.

Warren, S.B. (1992) Lower threshold referral for psychiatric treatment for adopted adolescents. *Journal of the American Academy of Child and Adolescent Psychiatry*, **31**, 512–517.

Westhues, A. & Cohen, J.S. (1990) *How to Reduce the Risk: Healthy Functioning Families for Adoptive and Foster Children*. Report No. 2, The research report. University of Toronto Press, Toronto.

Wierzbicki, M. (1993) Psychological adjustment of adoptees: a meta-analysis. *Journal of Clinical Child Psychology*, **22**, 447–454.

24 History of Child and Adolescent Psychiatry

Michael Neve and Trevor Turner

Introduction

The importance of a historical account of the development of child and adolescent psychiatry is threefold. First, the history displayed is one that illustrates change, disagreement and innovation in attitudes to childhood (Stone 1979) and then within the specialism itself, showing how nothing is constant through time and very few apparent truths are independent of historical circumstance and limitation. Even definitions of what constitutes a child and when adulthood begins remain in constant flux.

Secondly, history makes abundantly clear how psychiatry is fashioned within social and familial ideas of childhood and adolescence (Walvin 1984; Parry-Jones 1989, 1992). A world where children were put to work changed, in the late nineteenth century, into a world where children were sent to school. There they were inspected and tested and urged to embody social and legal values which had serious implications for their futures and for their mental and physical health. No longer hidden in the mines and back alleys, they generated a diverse psychoeducational enterprise, part of which was the child psychiatrist and the child psychotherapist.

Thirdly, history is the story of progress and assists in the task of estimating the future. More importantly, it seeks to avoid simple ideas of progress or prophecy and, instead, to show how all medical practices have their rationality and their purpose, even when seeming outdated to the modern mind. The most modern of therapies and the most sophisticated of disease entities will share in that fate, and history can both teach the need for modesty as well as describing how modern psychiatry came into being (Jones 1972) and helped fashion the present state of affairs (Collingwood 1946; Carr 1961; Evans 1997). This perspective also has the advantage of summoning a world where interest in children and adolescents as psychiatric subjects was at a minimum.

'Until about a generation ago most psychiatrists knew little about children from first-hand experience', wrote Leo Kanner (1935) in his seminal textbook. The history of the asylum and the growth of the psychiatric profession in the nineteenth and early twentieth centuries is paralleled by a history of marginality for the investigating of insanity in children. Unusual or difficult behaviour was enmeshed in conventional, often Christian, accounts of early social life, family experience and innate dispositions to evil doing. The language of morality and good conduct dominated both parents and children, and medicalized accounts of the life of the child made small—if any—inroads into that

established vocabulary (Pollock 1983; Steedman 1995). Some clinicians (Clouston 1880, 1891) attempted a psychiatry of adolescence, seeing it as the developmental stage wherein semiadult notions of will and responsibility might be invoked. In this enterprise they hoped to display how genuine forms of mental illness might be separable from whole clusters of moral judgements and moral accusations (Kett 1977). A true childhood psychology was also a late starter within the often contested growth of psychiatry as a whole and, in the twentieth century, had to face challenges from related but essentially adult-centred practices such as psychoanalysis (Walk 1964; Bynum *et al.* 1985/1988; Von Gontard 1988; Scull 1993; Shorter 1997). Even the specific developmental theories of the modern era, the psychosexual (Freud 1905), the social/generational (Erikson 1959), or the cognitive (Piaget 1926), can be seen to be overarching, to lack empirical evidence and to ignore key biological details.

There is also the historical need to distinguish childhood insanity from mental deficiency. The entry under 'insanity in children' in Daniel Hack Tuke's (1892) *Dictionary of Psychological Medicine* sets a useful historical precedent, stating that insanity in prepubescent, non-imbecilic children was a subject of importance '*but not commonly observed*'. They might be managed at home and avoid the asylum, would not go to idiot schools and thereby would escape notice. The child, as imagined by the author of the entry, T. Clifford Allbutt, Regius Professor of Physic at Cambridge, lived in a world of fantasy and simplicity and imitation—suicide in children was for example an 'imitative act'. The child's internal world of simple and primary forms indicated a lack of reflection and yet was full of affect. Insanity in children was apparently almost always hereditary, although it might be brought on by bad upbringing and excessive study and was the 'vestibule of the insanity of adults'. Allbutt even affirmed that: 'There is as it were a veil between the mind of earlier and the mind of later life' (Allbutt 1892), and his approach gives a sense of the late Victorian dilemma in dealing with the reality of 'childhood insanity', a dilemma matched only in its uncertainty by the elusive nature of the condition itself.

Early accounts

Early accounts of the development of child psychiatry (Walk 1964; Stone 1973; Brandon 1986; Von Gontard 1988) tended to focus on clinical anecdotes beginning in late Enlightenment

England. Walk began with one of the cases most repeated in the subsequent literature, that of a child born 'raving mad' and mentioned by Alexander Crichton in his *Inquiry into the Nature and Origin of Mental Derangement* (1798). When 4 days old it took four women to hold the child down, and he was also prone to uncontrollable fits of laughter. Walk also described a case in William Perfect's *Annals of Insanity* (1787) and three in John Haslam's *Observations on Madness* (1809). A notable aspect of the latter was his somewhat dismissive telling of stories about patients for whom nothing could be done, and one case being a 'convincing description of simple schizophrenia' in a boy of 10 (Walk 1964). The distinguished ethnologist and doctor, J. C. Prichard (1835), also used a case of moral insanity in a girl of 7 to illustrate the proximity of a psychiatric diagnosis to common Christian notions of foul and immoral behaviour.

Other important contributions can be found in the work of W.A.F. Browne (1805–1885) and his son James Crichton-Browne (1840–1938), and in the phrenological writings of Andrew Combe (1797–1847), all of whom admired the French psychiatrists J.E.D. Esquirol (1772–1840) and Felix Voisin (1794–1872). Esquirol actually wrote that infancy is 'secure from insanity', while then going on to discuss a manic child aged 8, another aged 9 and a melancholic aged 11. He stated that mental alienation can only begin at puberty, and that it is only 'dementia' that is sometimes observed among the young. Suicide could appear in schoolchildren but usually after a 'vicious' education. None the less, for those believing in the notion of infantile insanity, Esquirol was the champion. He gave enough authoritative, although exceptional, examples for later writers to highlight and amplify: a 3-year-old girl behaving obscenely in church was mentioned by Henry Maudsley (1867), for example.

Charles West and the origins of Great Ormond Street can at first sight seem important but the strict concern for insanity in children was not highly developed in his early writings (West 1848), and the hospital made no initial provision for mentally ill children. West wrote of hypochondriasis and night terrors but had little to say on brain disorders (West 1854). However, his work from the 1860s increasingly concentrated on moral insanity and mental illness, acting as an index of the growth of a paediatric specialism from the mid-nineteenth century (West 1860, 1871). The British situation was wholly altered in the 1860s by James Crichton-Browne who, among other things, stated a full case for the 'psychical diseases of early life' (Neve & Turner 1995).

A number of philosophical obstacles to the concept of childhood madness were strong in the early nineteenth century. Children were seen to reside in the world of *unreason* and were thus exempted from disorders of *reason*. The exceptions to this were monstrous, aberrant or occurring at an age close to precocious adulthood and always rare. Private madhouses did not generally admit children, for financial reasons, and very few children were admitted to public institutions—about 0.15% of asylum admissions in the first half of the century were in the 0–10 age group. Between 1796 and 1840 at the York Retreat, the percent-age of patients aged between 0 and 10 admitted was 0.96 compared to 12.77 in the age group 10–20 (Bucknill & Tuke 1858). Between 1815 and 1899, some 1000 children and adolescents were admitted to Bethlem (Wilkins 1993), while only two or three children under 14 years were likely to be admitted annually to other lunatic asylums. Textbooks from the 1870s onwards, in both Europe and the USA, found room, however, for sophisticated discussion separating juvenile insanity from idiocy, epilepsy and neurological disorders and concentrating on adolescence as the developmental moment where both hereditary legacies and future dangers were made manifest (Clouston 1892, 1898; Maudsley 1895; Kraepelin 1919; Bleuler 1950).

There is an important relationship between this growing medicalization of childhood diseases and the wider context of family life and family fortunes. Examining a wide range of evidence, especially letters and diaries, Pollock (1983) contested the claim that good mothering is a modern invention, or that children were seen as evil or unimportant, or even went unmourned, prior to some eighteenth century discovery of 'sentiment' or notions of 'primitive innocence'. She looked at the case for construing ideas of childhood via the history of child labour or the rise of various educational systems—and schooling was a key influence in generating a demand for a child psychiatry—but stressed that, if there is one thing that might have taught a cruel lesson before the late nineteenth century, it would be the high infant mortality rate. However, despite this general uniformity in the parent–child relationship between 1500 and 1900, Pollock did admit that in the early nineteenth century there was evidence for a growth in expressions of both ambivalence and nostalgia for the world of childhood, suggesting that punishment was on the increase especially in schools, and that both home and school were crueller. Pollock's work is historically significant in that, at the same time as psychiatry was becoming professionally organized (Scull 1993), there was a social and moral conservatism at work. The difficulty of advancing psychiatric views of behaviour—famously in criminal insanity cases—might equally have applied to the early life of children, an ascendant moral language insisting on goodness and badness rather than trying to formulate imprecise notions of mental illness.

A Haslam case history

John Haslam (1764–1844) was apothecary to Bethlem between 1795 and 1816, and in his *Observations on Madness and Melancholy* (1809) he included three cases of insane children. In 1803 he was asked to see a 10-year-old 'young gentleman', whose history had been well established by another 'learned and respectable' physician. Despite having parents of sound mind, at the age of 2 this child had been sent away from home to an aunt's house because he had become so 'mischievous and uncontrollable'. At his parents' request he was indulged in every wish, becoming thereby 'the creature of volition and the terror of the family'. Subsequent attempts at limiting his behaviour failed, hence the referral to Haslam.

Although of healthy appearance, the boy's countenance was

'decidedly maniacal'. There was some 'deficiency of the skin's sensibility' (he did not complain at the painful removal of a dressing for a boil), and he showed normal physical functions, apart from seeming to sleep more than usual. Haslam also described his memory as 'very retentive', but noted that he had a limited attention span, being only attracted 'by fits and starts'. 'He had been several times to school and was the hopeless pupil of many masters, distinguished for their patience and rigid discipline . . . it may therefore be concluded that . . . he had derived all the benefits which could result from privations to his stomach, and from the application of the rod to the more delicate parts of his skin.'

At the physician's first interview, this boy managed to 'break a window and tear the frill of my shirt'. He was gratified regularly by other destructive acts (china, windows, tearing lace), and he tended to abuse cats and dogs, throwing them on the fire or tearing out their whiskers. When spoken to, apparently he usually said, 'I do not choose to answer.' He formed no friendships with other children and 'would as readily kick or bite a girl as a boy'. Although attached to the keeper who looked after him, the keeper himself was of a different opinion, being persuaded that the boy would 'destroy him, whenever he found the means and opportunity' when he grew older. The boy also showed some insight, suggesting that 'God had not made him like other children', and regularly threatened suicide. Haslam's final comments are informative:

> 'During the time he [the boy] remained here, I conducted him to the hospital, and pointed out to him several patients who were chained in their cells; he discovered no fear or alarm; and when I showed him a mischievous maniac who was more strictly confined that the rest, he said, with great exultation "this would be the right place for me". Considering the duration of his insanity, and being ignorant of any means by which he was likely to recover, he returned to his friends.'

In other words, for Haslam he was not a suitable case for treatment. Theoretical diagnoses were not even mentioned (although hinted at in the term 'maniacal') but the modern child psychiatrist may find many parallels to the clinical dilemmas of today. The combination of parental and educational despair, the troubling prognosis, the uncertain diagnostic framework and the therapeutic impotence are not artefacts of history. Troubled twenty-first century children may be better delineated in terms of developmental psychology and family systems but reviewing these historical stories is a useful antidote to complacency. A number of them can be found in the work of Burrows (1828), Morison (1828, 1848), Combe (1831, 1835, 1841), Browne (1837) and Conolly (1862), as well as the standard continental authors.

The nineteenth century

In *Psychical Diseases of Early Life*, read before the Royal Medical Society of Edinburgh in the winter of 1859, James Crichton-Browne (1860) insisted that insanity did occur *in utero*, in infancy and in childhood, other writings notwithstanding. Esquirol was quoted approvingly on the power of hereditary taint. Those parents who had violated natural laws through self-abuse, lust and intemperance could expect punishment. The transmission of syphilis, measles and smallpox could occur *in utero*; idiocy could result from a blow to the abdomen. The results of fear were there—Browne quoted the famous case of the effect of a mother's fear of Spanish invasion on the birth of that philosopher of fear, Thomas Hobbes. Illegitimate children carried the marks of their mother's anxiety, although some natural children were the product of 'ardent passion' and thus close to genius. Dementia was a fact in early life, although not the same thing as idiocy, because in dementia 'the mind has existed but is veiled and diseased'. 'Acute dementia is frequently met with in this country between 10 and 16', and (in Scottish fashion) Crichton-Browne deemed it curable, in many cases, by generous diet. Drawing on cases from the Crichton Royal Hospital at Dumfries and other sources (including that of Samuel Taylor Coleridge's son, Hartley), he also cited theomania, demonomania, kleptomania, pyromania and cases of night terrors from Charles West. He also discussed suicidal impulse and choreamania, and the need to attend to early training, mental culture and physical education, but the point of his paper was expressed in a sentence near the end: 'Those influences that are productive of psychical disease are coextensive with existence.'

This founding text in British child psychiatry made a developmental, phrenological and ambitious claim for the rectitude of breaking ranks from the standard authorities who declared infantile insanity impossible. The importance of this for Crichton-Browne's own career was that it became part of a sustained ideal of the crucial importance of early experience, of early nurturing of the brain, so as to lower the rate of admissions to lunatic asylums (Neve & Turner 1995). He called for practical paediatrics based on social and moral hygiene because his own clinical experience had taught him that, for too many patients, the arrival in the asylum was too late. The psychical diseases of early life had to become objects of concern for parents and for teachers because it was then that the damage would be done. Children's sleep, children's breakfasts, children's avoidance from destructive examinations at primary school ('over-pressure') and morally upright parents whose brains were healthily matched, these were the 'weapons'—as he called them in 1859—with which to resist the advance of mental disease. His later time as an influential Lord Chancellor's Visitor in lunacy and society doctor continued this crusade, with a re-emphasis of all these themes.

Crichton-Browne's various concerns can also be felt in the work of the Yorkshireman Henry Maudsley (motherless from the age of 7) and the Scotsman Thomas Clouston (1840–1915). The most useful works of Maudsley's are *The Physiology and Pathology of Mind* (1867) and his revised third edition published as *The Pathology of Mind* (1895), the latter having two sections on 'The insanities of children' (22 pages), and 'Pubescent or adolescent insanities' (also 22 pages). Between these two editions was passed (in Great Britain) the ground-breaking Education Act of 1870 (children had to go to school), and in about 1875 the birth rate started to decline. Thus, in 1870, some 40% of 10-year-olds (and 2% of 14-year-olds) were in full-time education, but by 1902 this was officially 100% (Marsh 1958).

Contributions from T. Clifford Allbutt (1892), Fletcher Beach (1898) and William Ireland (1898) on psychological problems in children were published in the last decade of the century, the latter suggesting that children experienced an 'involuntary analysis of sensations'. Maudsley, however, while his hereditarian approach represented the degenerationist fears of the time, saw his key purpose in outlining the insanities of early life as being to confirm 'the principles of the study of the development of mind'. Thus, a child cannot have an hallucination until it has acquired 'a definite sensation', because 'children like brutes live in the present'. He acknowledged the eidetic imagination of children and discussed the 'phantasms' that are visible representations of their thoughts. In other words, 'what they think they actually see'. Such precocious imagination he regarded as something not to be fostered 'as a wonderful evidence of talent' (he cited William Blake as a warning), but preferred that 'the child should be solicited to regular intercourse with the realities of nature'. Damping down playful fantasizing was essential (Maudsley 1867). The child-led elaborations and creative play (Klein 1950; Winnicott 1958, 1971) encouraged by the twentieth century child guidance clinic would have been anathema to Maudsley and his contemporaries. Their concern was for diagnostic dilemmas, such as moral insanity, its causes, course and treatment, and the dawning awareness that as often as not such conditions were recognizable in childhood, as seen in the new schools, the courts and in their own private 'nervous clinics'.

Moral insanity

Illustrative of a late-nineteenth century trend towards considering moral defects in children as a disorder of brain function was the work of George Still, assistant physician for diseases of children at King's College Hospital and at Great Ormond Street. In three Goulstonian Lectures, entitled 'Some abnormal psychical conditions in children', Still (1902) discussed 'an abnormal defect of moral control', defined as 'control of action in conformity with the idea of the good of all'. He was dealing with an issue that he felt had a 'far-reaching' importance 'for the welfare of these unfortunate children and for the good of society'. In particular he stressed the problem of education, the method of providing supervision, how far one should resort to 'confinement in special institutions', and how far 'these children are to be held responsible for their misdoings'.

In Still's analysis, moral control required, as an essential factor, normal intellectual capacity. Impaired intellect was often the basis for moral defect, and many examples were given in the lectures. He also suggested that there could still be a primary failure to develop moral control, or there could be a morbid loss (permanent or temporary) of an already acquired moral control,

brought about by physical illness. While such conditions accounted for most cases, Still accepted that there was a residual group of children who suffered from 'a defect of moral consciousness which cannot be accounted for by a fault of environment'. He asserted that this had an evolutionary basis, quoting Darwin's phrase, 'so-called moral sense is aboriginally derived from the social instincts'. In a reflection of the psychophysiology of Henry Maudsley, he felt that this 'psychical defect' not only represented a 'perversion of function in the higher nervous centres' but was 'an actual physical abnormality underlying the moral defect'. Some cases might be temporary, some could be improved by careful training, but all should be *protected*, and all should be seen as a potential danger.

Elaborating on this socioneurological approach, Still also suggested that this defect could be caused by the same conditions as those that created idiocy or imbecility in other children. He listed family histories, degenerative stigmata and 'associated mental and nervous disorders' as being especially prevalent in his case sample (some 20 cases). Although acknowledging that 'a moral sense' was difficult to define, he could still conceive of it as the most recent and therefore most unstable product of mental evolution. His version can be seen as a contemporary, and perhaps logical, extension of that put forward by James Crichton-Browne, as a newer neurological account of phenomena once seen as immoral, while still using the older language of morality (e.g. 'vicious', 'depraved') to describe abnormal psychological function.

This version of disorderly children was an understandable attempt to discover order in the fitful debate around 'moral insanity' in the latter part of the nineteenth century. The influential co-editors of the *Journal of Mental Science*, Daniel Hack Tuke (1885) and George Savage (1891), published significant contributions and the topic was also raised by Robert Steen (1913). There was a general unanimity on typical cases and potential causes, with childhood onset accepted as a key principle. Savage felt that no one was 'capable of being intellectually complete and yet morally defective' and high moral control equated to high intellectual control, and often moral insanity was a stage of a progressing mental disease. He stressed the health of the parents and wrote of 'children saturated with insanity while still in the womb'. He defined most cases as coming on between the ages of 5 and 10 years, with behaviours such as lying, stealing, disruption in school, and non-response to punishment as indicative of the limited therapeutic options. These were the results apparently of 'badly built minds', and he coined the phrase 'a kind of partial moral dementia'.

Tuke, who also provided the entry for 'moral insanity' in the *Dictionary of Psychological Medicine* (1892) wrote of 'moral or emotional insanity', collected case material and even suggested that such individuals might be 'a reversion to an old savage type . . . born by accident in the wrong century'. While agreeing that moral influences might modify such tendencies, he quoted a Dr Kerlin who would have had these pupils banned from the school room to 'lifelong detention', because 'early detection' was not difficult. However, Tuke had to admit that diagnosis required individual case assessment, because there was no absolute rule to distinguishing moral insanity from moral depravity.

The most interesting aspect of Steen's paper (1913) was its acknowledged purpose, to persuade parliament to include moral insanity in the Mental Deficiency Bill then being considered. Steen gave figures of 3.5 in 1000 private cases, and 1 in 1000 pauper cases, to indicate the relative rarity of the condition and its likely congenital origin, but recognized the similarity with Kraepelin's 'psychopathic personality' concept. He concluded that the term 'moral insanity' had come to him through 'many different types of cases'; that moral defectives were a distinct class within the broader category; and that confinement in an asylum could be beneficial. Any 'display of temper' could be 'met with a few days rest in bed', and 'after a few weeks they adapt themselves to the institutional routine and have an excellent time, as they are usually proficient in games and amusements'. While this therapeutic approach, based on social structure and control, may seem somewhat amateur, it is striking that these brief comments remain one of the few articulated treatment outlines within the moral insanity literature. It is also striking that Steen stressed early recognition, based on the history rather than the 'present state', emphasizing the central role of the moral insanity question within the wider understanding of the elusive nature of 'childhood insanity'.

Maudsley's contribution to this complex debate is noteworthy because, although his language is full of apparent Victorian disgust (e.g. 'vice', 'defect', 'perverted'), even describing children as having a 'hideous and uncontrollable propensity to acts of cruelty', his explicit object was to provide a scientific basis to morality. Children, to him, were of necessity 'extremely selfish' because they operated by the two basic instincts of self-conservation and propagation. He described a boy being 'the most vicious of all wild beasts', yet insisted on the 'purity and innocence of a child's mind', testifying to 'an absence of mind'. He asserted forcefully the reality of child sexuality, with 'frequent manifestations of its existence throughout early life', thus, 'whosoever avers otherwise . . . must be strangely or hypocritically oblivious of the events of his own early life.' Nevertheless, children were 'little more than an organic machine automatically impelled by disordered nerve centres'. It has been suggested that in some sense Maudsley hated children, with the insane child as the original Morelian degenerate, but he could still look for love 'or a congenial pursuit' to 'divert self devastating feelings to channels of outward activity'. This apparently worked 'by increasing and strengthening their relations, with the outside world of not-self, and therewith its hold on them'.

The work of Thomas Clouston introduced the notion of adolescent insanity to British psychiatry. It should be stressed that Clouston's version of adolescence is a discovery (just as hebephrenia, first described by Kahlbaum, is also a late asylum invention) and aimed at describing the age between 18 and 25 years (Clouston 1880, 1891, 1892). He emphasized the distinction, pointing out that: 'The boy enjoys Ballantyne and Captain Marryat; at puberty the adolescent takes to Scott and Dickens and only the man enjoys and understands Shakespeare, George Eliot and Thackeray.' Thus, 'the adolescent feels instinctively that he has now entered a new country, the face of which he does not know.' He also noted that the period between 21 and 25 years of age showed the highest incidence of uncomplicated insanity, to him the most hereditary of all forms of mental disease, although curable in terms of discharge. He felt that 'psychologically and physiologically they emerged from the attack as men and women'.

In other words, Clouston was partaking in a physiological analysis of 'growing-up'. Eschewing quotes from the old cases, he outlined a highly structured version of normal developmental psychology; in particular, its dangerous sexuality. Careful education (not 'over-pressure'), mental hygiene, diet and exercise were central to his therapeutic regime, nurturing the brain (and soul—he was a committed Christian) through the stormy currents of puberty and adolescence, and breaking down the neurological fixations (or deviations) that might develop. His work represented the apogee of the established belief outlined by Crichton-Browne (1860), and elaborated by Froebel (1893), Maudsley (1895), Beach (1898), Keay (1888) and Allbutt (1892), that 'early training, mental culture, and physical education act, not merely in modelling disposition and laying the foundation of character, but in the rearing up of barriers opposed to the incursion of disease' (Clouston 1892).

Clouston also contributed to a new specialism within British and Continental psychiatry—the study of child suicide (Bartmann 1994). A number of authors included cases of young people killing themselves, discussing whether such acts were voluntary or partly imitative and whether new pressures in modern life—especially schooling and examination—were contributing to the statistical increase in such behaviour (Morselli 1881; Westcott 1885; Strahan 1893). The socially well-connected novelist, Thomas Hardy, who knew both Crichton-Browne and Allbutt, tapped into the anxieties of the age by portraying a child suicide (who first murders two infants as an act of compassion) in his 1895 novel, *Jude the Obscure*. The scandal the novel caused should not detract from the way that Hardy reflected growing concerns about the range and early appearance of psychiatric illness in children.

Conclusions

The collective view of the psychiatry of the child before the twentieth century—as summarized by Allbutt (1892)—agreed the following 'scientific' facts. Insane children were not defective enough to be sent to idiot schools and could be managed at home. The insanity of children was 'the vestibule' of insanity in adults, signifying an 'unstable nervous system'. The child's insanity was the insanity of the senses, of simpler impressions and of the instincts, of the lower and earlier organized centres. Suicide or homicide in children was imitative and unreflective, thus 'the child hangs himself or drowns himself to escape a lesson for which he is not prepared'. 'If man lives in a vain show, far more so does the child', and the normal child's mind was deemed 'fantastic', with 'daydreams as the only realities'.

Disturbances therefore occurred in the world of the affective and the imitative rather than in the world of thought. Insanity in the baby presented as kicking and biting. Insanity in children was often hereditary, or a gift from syphilitic parents. Prognosis was variable but melancholy, timidity and mild mania could be dealt with over 2–3 years under 'judicious management' and by following hygienic modes of life. However, such management was very difficult to obtain because the number of properly trained governesses was low, and Allbutt 'earnestly hoped that the number of ladies having the mental and moral endowments necessary for such difficult duties . . . will increase' (Allbutt 1892). He feared that otherwise adolescence would be reached in a state of greater or less imbecility and concluded by reporting several recent cases of 'degenerative cerebral disease', with his core references being Moreau de Tours (1888), Maudsley (1879) and Down (1887).

The patchwork nineteenth century psychiatric construction of the reality of childhood insanity, e.g. Wilmarth (1894) generated an unsystematic variety of medical accounts, but all placed great importance on family, school and society. In the next century, this conjunction of the medical, the educational, the legal and the social, e.g. Hall (1904) would receive formal recognition in the development of specialist units, psychological theories (Claparède 1911), juvenile courts and dedicated child therapists and social workers. Fuelled by advances in nutrition, public health acts (e.g. against child labour), world wars and education for all (Dwork 1987; Hendrick 1994, 1997), the bringing up of children in both Europe and the USA became a matter of municipal and, to some extent, state responsibility (Burke & Miller 1929; Cooter 1992). By 1914, Mott, a leading psychiatrist, wrote (in a monograph on *Nature and Nurture in Mental Development*) that the 'medical inspection of school children and health visiting' was of essential importance in 'the development of body and mind'. He even allowed a chapter of his book to be specially written by a lady sanitary inspector and school nurse (Mott 1914).

History of child psychiatry in the twentieth century

'When the twentieth century made its appearance, there was not—and there could not be—anything that might in any sense be regarded as child psychiatry. It took a series of definite steps in the development of cultural attitudes to make possible the inclusion of children in the domain of psychiatry.' (Kanner 1935)

Any review of the developments in child psychiatry over the last 100 years has to acknowledge the range of studies already available. These include broader surveys such as by Lowrey (1944), Nissen (1974, 1991), Howells & Osborn (1981), Wardle (1991a,b), Rydelius (1995), Stone (1997) and Geissman & Geissman (1998). Further reviews by Heywood (1959), Eisenberg (1969), Horn (1984), Clarke & Clarke (1986), Hersov (1986), Cless (1988) and Duché (1990) are more specific, but there is also

a large secondary literature (Staples 1995; Kern 1973; Donaldson 1996, Levy 1968) dealing especially with developments in the field of child psychoanalysis. According to Parry-Jones (1994), Kanner (1960) attributed the origin of the term 'child psychiatry' to its use at a Swiss psychiatric society meeting in 1933. In essence, the difference from the nineteenth century and its anecdotal accounts of 'insane' offspring and their bad behaviour, lies in the emergence of near-universal schooling. Once most children came under the eye of institutions and professionals, their more subtle forms of disturbance could be noted. Instead of idiots, epileptics and grossly disordered psychotics (requiring asylum care), society felt the need to deal with 'troubled' or 'delinquent' children (Sullivan 1915), Healy 1917), and to formulate a range of social and clinical terms so as to comprehend them.

Although the rise of eugenics and child-rearing concerns (Beers 1908), the development of child guidance units (Crutcher 1943; Wardle 1991a), the influence of Freudian psychoanalysis (Freud 1905, 1953–74), and the advances in educational psychology (Binet & Simon 1905; Burt 1925; Gesell 1925; Piaget 1926) are seen as the essential strands, in the preceding century there was already a considerable specialist literature (Emminghaus 1887; Hurd 1895; Harms 1960). Hysteria was of particular importance (Kern 1973), with school pressures, concerns about child labour, heredity (e.g. the mother transmitting her dispositions to the child), and poverty in general, providing possible explanations for disturbed childhood behaviour. In 1896, there appeared a yearly periodical devoted to the study of character disorders in children (*Die Kinderfehler*), and in 1905 Sigmund Freud took on Little Hans. In fact Freud himself never saw a child in his consulting room (using parents as go-betweens instead) but the work of his daughter, Anna, in considerable and notorious competition with Melanie Klein, became a landmark cultural debate in the psychoanalytic, educational and child guidance worlds (Zaretsky 1999), a debate linked to the increasing acceptance of a welfare state and the professionalization of child care procedures.

Influence of Leo Kanner

Kanner's textbook, *Child Psychiatry*, was first published in 1935 with the second edition appearing in 1948. The preface to the former was by Adolf Meyer who considered that 'the personality of the child' had been given 'vital status', and that child psychiatry was now 'more and more on a safe and broad middle of the road course between the extremes of reluctance and of excessive zeal'. An additional preface insisted on the paediatrician understanding also 'parents, teachers, and all those surrounding the child'. The second edition (1948) recalled the 'somewhat strident notes of conflicting and doctrinaire claims agitating this field in the 1930s' and suggested they have now been largely 'quieted by sobering responsible work'. The author suggested that there had been advances in projective methods, somatic approaches and an understanding of attitudes and relationships in early childhood deriving from experience during the Second World War.

To Kanner, the important factors giving impetus to 'the century of the child' included the introduction of psychometry (Binet & Simon 1905, 1914), the element of dynamic psychiatry (looking for the origins of mental problems in one's upbringing), the setting up of juvenile courts (the first in 1895 in South Australia and then in 1899 in Illinois and Colorado), and the mental hygiene movement (Beers 1908). The discovery that 'any amount of tutoring, drilling, admonitions, punitive measures, promises or bribes' did not actually work, and that magistrates and judges wanted to know just why children were misbehaving, led to changes of some significance before 1920. This included the 'environmental cushioning of the decidedly delinquent, the noticeably retarded, the woefully neglected and mistreated, foster home placements, special education, removal from parental mismanagement or gang associations', and the preference for 'wholesome recreational facilities'. Kanner was particularly impressed by the Heilpädagogik movement in Europe and the subsequent development in the 1920s and 1930s of dealing with 'the everyday problems of the everyday child'.

He defined the Boston Habit Clinic of 1921 as the first child guidance clinic, and by 1930 some 500 clinics had opened when the first International Congress of Mental Hygiene was held in Washington D.C. Other work (Wickman 1928) called for a shift towards 'the psychology of the social development of children', whereas August Aichhorn (1878–1949) in his 1925 book *Wayward Youth* outlined an approach to caring for delinquent children.

The 1930s and 1940s led to developments in working psychologically with children (e.g. play therapy as outlined by Anna Freud), and liaison paediatric/psychiatric clinics, but the paediatric perception of childhood conditions remained doggedly organic. Kanner quoted a popular 1928 textbook giving eight possible causes of enuresis, only one of which was 'neurotic', and which baldly stated that children with 'unstable nervous equilibrium from chorea, epilepsy and similar conditions are prone to incontinence of urine'. Under 'psychical influences, especially in dreams, the child imagines a convenient place for urination and the reflexes act'. That was the full section. By contrast, Kanner saw the work of Cameron (1919) as exceptional, including as it did a detailed section that began with a thoughtful recognition of 'the apprehensions of the grown-up people who have charge of the (enuretic) children' and their 'unwise suggestions'.

Kanner's textbook continues to have a modern feel. It is divided into four parts: 'history of child psychiatry'; 'basic orientation'; 'clinical considerations'; and 'phenomenology', the latter being divided into three sections: 'personality problems arising from physical illness'; 'psychosomatic problems'; and 'problems with behaviour'. The clinical section deals with the symptom 'as an admission ticket, or signal, or safety valve, or as a means of solving problems, or as a nuisance'. It includes practical details of dealing with the initial contact, the case history, projective methods in psychotherapy, and prevention. Physical aspects concentrate on brain disease, epilepsies and endocrinopathies, while psychosomatic problems are dealt with under the various orders and groups (e.g. digestive system).

By far the longest section, some 300 pages, deals with behavioural presentations, such as eating, sleeping, speech and language, scholastic performance or even anger. Treatment approaches are based on psychotherapy, particularly using rapport, transference and the relationship. With regard to rapport, Kanner advises the child, 'I'll tell you what it is all about and what I want you to do.' In terms of transference, he suggests that one should say something like, 'I'll tell you what has been going on in your unconscious. See for yourself what you can do with it.' As for the relationship, the line is 'You go ahead and be yourself. Thereby you tell yourself and me about the way you feel about yourself and your status in the world. Let us see together what you can do with your resources.' Warning about parents and jealousies between parent and child, Kanner advises the use of a referee in arguments, the dangers of being invited to dinner ('noodle soup psychiatry'), and the usefulness of minor psychotherapy by general paediatricians. Social factors, in terms of casework and looking at what was going on in the classroom, are never forgotten or minimized.

Service developments

Sources generally agree that the pioneering child-focused clinic set up by Witmer in 1896, in Pennsylvania, was a core model of service development. In 1909, Healy founded the Chicago Juvenile Psychopathic Institute (aimed essentially at delinquency treatment), and in 1922 a number of demonstration clinics were set up (e.g. Klopp 1932; Witmer 1940) in the USA via the Commonwealth Fund (Stevenson & Smith 1934). The subsequent developments in England (Wardle 1991a) included interested visitors to the USA (e.g. Mrs Strachey, a London magistrate, whose husband was the editor of the *Spectator*), and the sending of some social workers to train in child guidance methods. In 1927, Emanuel Miller set up the East London Child Guidance Clinic; in 1929, the London Child Guidance Clinic, in Canonbury, was established using US methods. By 1930, in the USA there were some 500 clinics (Kanner 1935), while in England there were some 95 clinics by 1944 (Howells 1965), and 367 by 1970 (Wardle 1991a). According to Parry-Jones (1984), 'an entirely new model of interdisciplinary collaboration by psychologist, psychiatric social workers and psychiatrists was created which shaped child psychiatrists' working relationships and service delivery patterns for half a century'. Such developments occurred together with outpatient clinics in hospital departments, the increasing employment of child psychiatrists (in the UK 68 consultants in 1953, 365 in 1986), academic and professorial posts, and the increasing expansion of the speciality in terms of training places and speciality status (Kanner 1959; Wardle 1991a). Unfortunately, services became distant from asylum psychiatry, a particular problem for the more difficult adolescents, such units only being established in Britain in the 1950s and 1960s, although earlier in the USA (Curran 1939). Formal research into the impact and effectiveness of these child guidance centres and inpatient units tended to lag behind, not least because of the difficulties in establishing an agreed diagnostic classification system (Rutter *et al.* 1975).

A useful summary of developments can be found in Warren's historical survey of the Maudsley Hospital Child Psychiatry Unit ('Child psychiatry and the Maudsley Hospital: an historical survey', unpublished Third Kenneth Cameron Memorial Lecture, Institute of Psychiatry Library, 1974). Harking back to the establishment of the Child Guidance Council (set up in 1926), Warren acknowledged the role of 'aments' (those with learning disabilities) in providing the first child patients. By the late 1920s there were three psychiatric clinics looking after child patients, but in 1930 a playgroup was set up (to look after bored children within an indefinite appointment system), and possibilities for observation were developed. By 1930, there were weekly conferences on child problems, and eventually a full children's department was established in 1939, with formal treatment. The inpatient unit had to wait until after the war (1947); however, its design was still more appropriate to physically sick children than those with psychological problems. In 1947, a full-time occupational therapist was appointed, a teacher and a school were set up in 1950 and by the late 1940s most trainee psychiatrists were spending some time rotating through the children's departments (Cameron 1949). The actual publishing and development of research was limited until the appointment of the first senior lecturer in child psychiatry (James Anthony) in 1952.

Reviewing child psychiatry in general in 1968, Rutter was moved to state that 'the history of research in child psychiatry is a short one'. The most important insights came from Kanner (1943) in his description of infantile autism, and Levy (1941) in his study of maternal overprotection. Further studies during the 1950s on encopresis, psychosis in childhood, sleep disturbances and manic depressive psychosis began to establish clearer diagnostic entities and developmental and behavioural norms. A focus of work at the Maudsley Hospital related to links between disorders in childhood and adult life, in particular the diagnostic development of those suffering from neurosis in childhood. Such patients were demonstrated to have continuing problems of depression, anxiety or other neurotic disorders, although a number showed problems with immature/inadequate personalities. Delinquent children tended to move towards antisocial disorders, while children with conduct disorders had milder disorders of personality (Rutter 1968). In essence, the core studies of the post-war period, between about 1950 and 1975, were aimed at establishing the epidemiology, diagnostic boundaries, specificities and relationship factors (particularly within the family) germane to child psychiatric problems. This very much reflected the dominant epidemiological and social bias of the Maudsley Hospital under the influence of Aubrey Lewis and Michael Shepherd.

Mid-century developments

In a more general sense, and variably attached to the highly influential child psychoanalytic movement (see below), routine child psychiatry in the 1940s and 1950s could not avoid the impact of the Second World War. The most outstanding document deriving from this, *Maternal Care and Mental Health* (Bowlby 1951), has probably been the most influential piece of writing of the century. Later expanded into *Child Care and the Growth of Love* (1953), this widely read and neopopulist piece of work combined a psychoanalytic perspective with a careful clinical approach. Bowlby's most striking contribution was an understanding of maternal deprivation which has continued to inform services, education, populist understanding and political approaches (Van Dijken 1998).

By the 1970s further research had shown the need for 'a more precise delineation of the different aspects of "badness" . . . and the reasons why children differ in their responses' (Rutter 1972b) to bad care in early life, but the stimulus to research has been immense. Thus, Bowlby's opening statement can be considered as true today as it was then: 'The quality of the parental care which a child receives in his earliest years is of vital importance for his future mental health.' His conclusion remains equally accepted: 'The proper care of children deprived of a normal home life can now be seen to be not really an act of common humanity, but to be essential for the mental and social welfare of a community.' His expressed hope, that 'all over the world men and women in public life will recognize the relation of mental health to maternal care, and will seize their opportunities for promoting courageous and far-reaching reforms', remains to be put into practice. In fact, the increasing recognition of child physical and sexual abuse (e.g. the National Family Violence survey in the USA, in 1973), the rise of the single-parent family and the continued widespread impoverishment of children globally, all represent a significant failure of the influence of the psychiatric establishment.

Yet it is not as if there has been a lack of other texts popularizing the importance of the process of childhood development. Eric Erikson's *Childhood and Society* (1951) and Donald Winnicott's *The Child, the Family and the Outside World* (1964) are just two among many. The link between childhood misbehaviour and broken homes had been well understood earlier in the century. A study of head injuries (Fabian & Bender 1947) showed that 83% of children attending with significant head injuries had 'mental abnormality more than their parents', and that the 'home atmosphere in these cases was one of hate, rejection and violence'. The problem of 'identification with a sadistic father was marked in boys', and the healthy influence of police officers and the youth club movement, in a 1947 report of the Commissioner of Metropolitan Police (Scott 1947), showed a marked drop in juvenile crime when such projects were developed. A survey from the Cambridge Child Guidance Clinic (Banister & Ravden 1944) correlated nervous symptoms with broken homes and commented on well-adjusted children having more strongly developed interest in hobbies and 'much less frequent attendance at cinemas'. The Chief Clerk to the London Juvenile Courts (Giles 1946) considered that problem parents much exceeded problem children.

In the 1950s, apart from the insights of John Bowlby, with respect to maternal deprivation, the influence of the films made by James and Joyce Robertson (1971) about children's admission to hospital, and a residential nursery, cannot be exaggerated (Freud A. 1953). This led to a completely altered attitude towards mothers visiting their children in hospital, allowing virtually open access in an attempt to combat the problems of separation. Equally influential were the large-scale studies of Spitz (1951) on 'pathological mothering', and Lewis (1954) on deprived children who reviewed 500 cases, with over 100 being followed-up directly. The traumatizing effects of separation before the age of 5 were established, but the circumstances, the quality of mothering and the subsequent care were seen as determining an outcome.

The problems of adolescents, in the increasing economic well-being of the 1950s, also came to the fore (Underwood 1955). As with the original developments in child psychiatry, social influences were the Education Act of 1944 and the National Health Act of 1948 (in the UK), placing specific responsibilities on child psychiatric services. Particular confusions developed around the notions of childhood and/or adolescent psychosis, and there was considerable debate as to its reality, causation and key symptoms. Cameron outlined these confusions, suggesting that the psychopathological concepts deriving from Kleinian psychoanalysis did not really fit with the manifest clinical syndromes, and that at times it was difficult to be clear as to whether 'a manifest clinical entity or a psychopathological postulate was under consideration'. Cameron's (1956) article 'Past and present trends in child psychiatry' summarized a number of these issues.

However, perhaps most important in practical terms were the continuing 'developments' in the range of treatments used. Essentially, from the 1950s, family and group approaches were offered, with a flourishing of family therapy in the 1960s and 1970s. Alongside this, the work of a number of behavioural psychologists (Bandura 1969; Yule 1984) has shown effectiveness in relevant diagnostic cases but, as Wardle (1991a) pointed out, there has been a tendency for different approaches to denigrate each other. Likewise, the difficulties of co-ordinating multidisciplinary teams have been lambasted (e.g. the 1987 Butler-Sloss Inquiry into child abuse in Cleveland, UK), and the persisting interdisciplinary rivals within the broad child care movement (education, psychiatry, psychoanalysis, social work, home support, educational psychology) have never been fully resolved. Certain practical advances, in terms of causation, development, psychopathology and treatment, do have a general importance in illustrating post-war trends. Dyslexia, once an intrapsychic conflict of 'streptosymbolia' (Rosen 1947) is now an established neurological disorder, while studies of the offspring of psychotic parents have demonstrated the genetic and biological bases of conditions such as schizophrenia (Mednick et al. 1984; Stone 1997). The pharmacological treatment of hyperactivity, using methylphenidate or similar stimulants (Gittelman-Klein & Klein 1976), the recognition and classification of depression in childhood (Rutter et al. 1986; Carlson &

Cantwell 1979), and the clear separation between infantile autism and early onset schizophrenia in childhood (Rutter 1972a) are other significant clarifications. Not only have these findings demonstrated an increasingly biological perspective, they have also enabled a more realistic understanding of developmental psychopathology and reflect the improved nutrition and infant mortality figures of the period. Nevertheless, compared with adults, the use of medication has been significantly inhibited by ethical issues, differential age responses and the limited reliability of diagnoses.

Psychoanalytic approaches

To many lay observers, child psychiatry has been seen to be coterminous with child psychoanalysis. The influence of Freudian theory, psychotherapeutically orientated child guidance clinics (Freud 1946), and the Tavistock Institute (in the UK) have led to some marginalization of the routine services. These include multidisciplinary teams, inpatient units, medication approaches (e.g. the use of stimulants for ADHD or antidepressants for significant depressive illnesses) or the practicalities of educational psychology in schools. Childhood loss (real or imagined), play therapy, systems theory in the context of family dynamics, and the clear diagnostic differences between childhood disorders and those of adulthood have enhanced a predominantly psychotherapeutic culture within the speciality. In terms of journals, for example, *The Psychoanalytic Study of the Child* was first published in 1945, and *The Journal of Child Psychotherapy* in December 1963. More eclectic journals, such as *The Journal of Child Psychology and Psychiatry* (first published in 1960) or *The Journal of the American Academy of Child and Adolescent Psychiatry* (first published in 1961) also include considerable amounts of psychoanalytic and psychotherapeutic material. In a review of *The Psychoanalytic Study of the Child* (between 1945 and 1975), it was seen as providing the 'major repository of the science of psychoanalysis, centred on the child', and as 'a scholarly forum in which psychoanalysis as a developmental psychology in general theory could be systematically reviewed and elaborated'. Some 500 papers of both US and European origin were published in that 30-year period, with three leading editors (Anna Freud, Henry Hartmann and Ernst Kris) contributing significantly, especially the first.

In terms of the celebrated debate during the late 1920s and early 1930s between Anna Freud (1895–1982) and Melanie Klein (1882–1960), detailed biographies of the two protagonists provide fascinating background material on their core influences on child psychoanalysis (Peters 1985; Grosskurth 1986). A more recent review (Donaldson 1996) has concluded that Anna Freud focused on theory and the strength of the ego, following in her father's footsteps, whereas Klein's observations challenged the traditional psychoanalytic account, resulting thereby in the development of object-relations theory. It is of note, however, that both Anna Freud and Melanie Klein were lay psychoanalysts, the former being a qualified school teacher who derived her initial guidance from a retired teacher and lecturer in child education in Vienna, Hermine Hug-Hellmuth. In fact, Hug-Hellmuth was murdered in 1924, at the age of 53, by her 18-year-old nephew, apparently a young man brought up on liberal and psychoanalytic principles by his mother and aunt. This inauspicious start reflected a number of difficulties in the early history of child psychoanalysis, necessitating, for example, Ernest Jones' removing to Toronto from the UK, and other accusations of abuse (Kern 1973) directed by children at male analysts in particular. The influence of Maria Montessori, for example, in her popular work *The Montessori Method* (1919), derived from a popular series of lecture tours. She emphasized the importance of children freely choosing their own activities merely guided by teachers or parents.

Anna Freud's early work propagated the view that it was possible to carry out a proper Freudian psychoanalysis even on difficult patients such as children. The difficulties included minimum insight, a maximum of resistance and no possible transference apart from through the parents. She combined therapeutic and educational approaches, using drawing, knitting and play, and felt that a special theory was not needed. Her later *The Ego and the Mechanisms of Defence* (1936) extended her views into the adult world.

By contrast, Melanie Klein, whose first analysis was carried out on her own sons, tended to be aggressive in symbolically interpreting every act and suggested that it was possible to analyse children at a much younger age. Moving to the UK in 1926, and treating among her first patients Ernest Jones' children, her first written piece was *The family novel in status nascendi* (see Donaldson 1996). More detailed discussions of her technique occurred in her 1932 book, including over 570 sessions on one 6-year-old child with a compulsive neurosis. The first overt clash arose in 1927 when the proceedings of a symposium on child analysis were published in the *International Journal of Psychoanalysis* (editor Ernest Jones). This was, in fact, a response to Anna Freud's criticism of Klein's technique published in a monograph entitled 'Introduction to the technique of child analysis' (seee Donaldson 1996), and in September 1927 Sigmund Freud wrote to Ernest Jones accusing him of organizing a 'regular campaign' against his daughter. The technical difficulties in this debate are not relevant to a broad survey but are central to understanding the differing strands of child psychotherapeutic practice. The modern use of studying children's play, drawings and non-verbal expressions, for example in paediatric assessments of possible sexual abuse, have developed a considerable sophistication. Klein felt that all children should be psychoanalysed as a prophylactic measure, whereas Anna Freud felt that all school teachers should be psychoanalytically trained to deal with young pupils within the educational system. The most important effect, the development of Bowlby's investigations into the effects of maternal deprivation, initially on behalf of the World Health Organization (Bowlby 1951), has been the central influence in the day-to-day routine of the modern child guidance unit.

The practical outcome of these issues can be seen in a contribution by Winnicott (1964) on the training for child psychiatry. Winnicott felt that 'the basis of much of the work of the child psychiatrist is the psycho-therapeutic interview with the child', while acknowledging that the child psychiatrist is also engaged in working with the parents, and work that is 'essentially practical' in that 'in respect of each case we meet a challenge'. However, Winnicott felt that 'paediatrics has failed as a parental figure for child psychiatry, and so has psychiatry', and thus he insisted on autonomy for the child psychiatric profession. He felt that the only solution was for 'child psychiatry to become a thing in its own right and to devise its own training' as, in his view, 'the really necessary preparation for child psychiatry is in the psychoanalytic training'. Apart from the emotional development of children, he considered that 'the interferences with maturational processes that come from the environment and from conflict within the child' were the essence of the problem, and in that sense child psychiatry was akin to paediatrics (Phillips 1988).

Conclusions

To Leo Kanner, the twentieth century was 'the century of the child', and the richness of both 'vitalist' and 'mechanist' research into the normal and disordered child may represent one facet of this understanding. Whether or not the range of insights (e.g. Kahr 1991) and treatment approaches has served to improve the quality of childhood, in itself a much more prolonged process in the twentieth century, remains a moot point. The development of child psychiatry as a speciality at first concentrating on the mentally retarded, then moving into areas of education and delinquency, incorporating sociological and psychological disciplines, and growing into the widespread child guidance clinic established throughout much of the world after the Second World War, was a paradigm of the increasing acceptance of psychiatry as part of the history of ideas. Paradoxically, the work in the USA—Eric Erikson, Margaret Mahler, Moritz Tramer, Beata Rank and Rene Spitz, among many others—reflected a strongly psychotherapeutic tradition, yet medication and the use of inpatient care, especially for adolescents, have been prominent in treatment. The more clinical, epidemiological and neuropsychological approach of the English school (as represented at the Maudsley Hospital) generated more practical insights, yet a less medicalized therapeutics.

For example, the celebrated study of the children of the Isle of Wight (Rutter *et al.* 1970) provided the reassuring news that most adolescents actually like their parents. The importance of the family, the effects of parental mental illness on children, the influence of subtle learning or emotional difficulties (e.g. ADHD, dyspraxia, dyslexia) on subsequent 'difficult' or antisocial behaviour, and the establishment of robust treatment approaches can all be seen as advances. As Wardle (1991a) has pointed out, 'Studies of social and family factors underlying childhood disorder have helped clinicians to build more accurate models of the interaction of causes, enabling them to focus on attainable therapeutic aims and to look for positive and protective factors to work with in the child's environment and family.' The same author lamented the unfortunate role of fashion in terms of the public's view of child psychiatric services. From autism in the 1950s and 1960s, to anorexia and hyperactivity in the 1970s, and sexual or even satanic abuse in the 1990s, the speciality has been peculiarly prone to political, media and populist interference (e.g. Wolff 1989). The establishment of a robust classification (Rutter *et al.* 1975) brought some order to an often obscure descriptive system but future developments must take a grasp of the strange eventful history that has already preceded them.

If, as Bowlby has emphasized, 'the proper care of children deprived of a normal home' (whatever 'normal' may mean) remains of the essence, perhaps the iconic heart of twentieth century child psychiatry lies in the experience of the child in wartime. Whether it be Anna Freud's monthly reports of children's reactions to sleeping in underground stations, and bombings, etc., or Wicks' (1988) memories of children in his collection of personal records entitled *No Time to Wave Goodbye*, the simple requests of the children cannot be ignored. Their song from Lionel Bart's musical 'Blitz' echoes the metaphor of their journey.

'We're going to the country, we're going to see the cows,
We are going to have a real good time, in a country house,
It's called evacuation
They take you to the station,
They put you on a train,
Let's hope it doesn't rain,
We are going to the country.'

References

Aichhorn, A. (1925) English translation 1936, *Wayward Youth*. Putnam, London.

Allbutt, T.C. (1892) Insanity in children. In: *A Dictionary of Psychological Medicine* (ed. D. Hack Tuke). J.A. & A. Churchill, London.

Arnold, T. (1782/1786) *Observations on the Nature, Kinds, Causes, and Prevention of Insanity, Lunacy or Madness*, Vol. 1. Containing Observations on the Nature, and Various Kinds of Insanity; Vol. 2. Containing Observations on the Causes and Prevention of Insanity. G. Robinson, Leicester.

Bartmann, H. (1994) Child suicide and harsh punishment in Germany at the turn of the last century. *Paediatric History*, 30, 849–864.

Bandura, A. (1969) *Principles of Behavior Modification*. Holt Rhinehart Winston, New York.

Banister, H. & Ravden, M. (1944) The Problem Child and his Environment. *British Journal of Psychology*, 34, 60–65.

Beach, F. (1898) Insanity in children. *Journal of Mental Science*, 44, 459–474.

Beers, C. (1908) *A Mind That Found Itself*. Longmans Green, New York.

Binet, A. & Simon, T. (1905) Application des méthodes nouvelles au diagnostic du niveau intellectuel chez les enfants normaux et anormaux d'hospice et d'école primaire. *L'Année Psychologique*, 11, 245–366.

Binet, A. & Simon, T. (1914) *Mentally Defective Children* (trans. W.B. Drummond). E. Arnold, London.

Bleuler, E. (1950) *Dementia Praecox or the Group of Schizophrenias* (trans. J. Zinkin). International Universities Press, New York.

Bowlby, J. (1951) *Maternal Care and Mental Health*. World Health Organization, Geneva.

Bowlby, J. (1953) *Child Care and the Growth of Love*. Penguin Books, Harmondsworth.

Brandon, S. (1986) The early history of psychiatric care of children. In: *Child Care Through the Centuries* (eds T. Turner & J. Cule), pp. 61–78. STS Publishing, Cardiff.

Browne, W.A.F. (1837) *What Asylums Were, Are and Ought to Be*. Black, Edinburgh.

Bucknill, J.C. & Tuke, D.H. (1858) *A Manual of Psychological Medicine*. Blanchard & Lea, Philadelphia.

Burke, N.H.M. & Miller, E. (1929) Child mental hygiene: its history, methods and problems. I. The history of the movements towards child mental hygiene. *British Journal of Medical Psychology*, 9, 218–242.

Burrows, G.M. (1828) *Commentaries on the Causes, Forms, Symptoms, and Treatment, Moral and Medical of Insanity*. Underwood, London.

Burt, C. (1925) *The Young Delinquent*. University of London Press, London.

Bynum, W.F., Porter, R. & Shepherd, M. (1985/1988) *The Anatomy of Madness*, Vols I–III. Routledge, London.

Cameron, H.C. (1919) *The Nervous Child at School*. Oxford University Press, London.

Cameron, K.L. (1949) A psychiatric inpatient department for children. *Journal of Mental Science*, 95, 560–566.

Cameron, K. (1956) Past and present trends in child psychiatry. *Journal of Mental Science*, 102, 599–603.

Carlson, G.A. & Cantwell, D.P. (1979) A survey of depressive symptoms in a child and adolescent psychiatric population. *Journal of the American Academy of Child Psychiatry*, 18, 587–599.

Carr, E.H. (1961) *What Is History?* Penguin, London.

Chess, S. (1988) Child and adolescent psychiatry come of age: a 50 year perspective. *Journal of the American Academy of Child and Adolescent Psychiatry*, 27, 1–7.

Claparède, E. (1911) *Experimental Pedagogy and the Psychology of the Child* (trans. M. Louch & H. Holman). E. Arnold, London.

Clarke, A.M. & Clarke, A.D.B. (1986) Thirty years of child psychology: a selective review. *Journal of Child Psychology and Psychiatry*, 27, 719–759.

Clouston, T.S. (1880) *Puberty and Adolescence Medico-Psychologically Considered*. Oliver & Boyd, Edinburgh.

Clouston, T.S. (1891) *The Neuroses of Development: the Morison Lectures for 1890*. Oliver & Boyd, Edinburgh.

Clouston, T.S. (1892) Development insanities and psychoses. In: *A Dictionary of Psychological Medicine* (ed. D.H. Tuke), 1, pp. 357–371. Churchill, London.

Clouston, T.S. (1898) *Clinical Lectures on Mental Disorders*, 5th edn. J. & A. Churchill, London.

Collingwood, R.G. (1946) *The Idea of History*. Oxford University Press, Oxford.

Combe, A. (1831) *Observations on Mental Derangement*. J. Anderson, Edinburgh.

Combe, A. (1835) *The Principles of Physiology Applied to the Preservation of Health and to the Improvement of Physical and Mental Education*, 3rd edn. Maclachlan & Stewart, Edinburgh.

Combe, A. (1841) *A Treatise on the Physiological and Moral Management of Infancy*, 2nd edn. Maclachlan & Stewart, Edinburgh.

Conolly, J. (1862) Recollections of the varieties of insanity. II. Cases and consultations. Nos. I–V Juvenile insanity. *Medical Times and Gazette*, i, 27–29; 130–132; 234–236; 372–374: ii, 2–4.

Cooter, R. (ed) (1992) *In the name of the child: health and welfare 1880–1940*. Routledge, London.

Crichton, A. (1798) *An Inquiry Into the Nature and Origin of Mental Derangement*. T. Cadell & W. Davies, London.

Crichton-Browne, J. (1860) Psychical diseases of early life. *Journal of Mental Science*, 6, 284–320.

Crutcher, R. (1943) Child psychiatry: a history of its development. *Psychiatry*, 6, 191–201.

Curran, F.J. (1939) Organisation of a ward for adolescents in Bellevue Psychiatric Hospital. *American Journal of Psychiatry*, 95, 1365–1388.

Donaldson, G. (1996) Between practice and theory: Melanie Klein, Anna Freud and the development of child analysis. *Journal of the History of the Behavioural Sciences*, 32, 160–176.

Down, J.L. (1887) *On Some of the Mental Affections of Childhood and Youth: the Lettsomian Lectures delivered to the Medical Society of London in 1887*. J. & A. Churchill, London.

Duché, D.-J. (1990) *Histoire de la Psychiatrie*. Presses Universitaires de France, Paris.

Dwork, D. (1987) *War Is Good for Babies and Other Young Children*. Tavistock, London.

Eisenberg, L. (1969) Child psychiatry: the past quarter century. *American Journal of Orthopsychiatry*, 39, 389–401.

Emminghaus, H. (1887) *Die Psychischen Störungen Des Kindesalters*. Laupp, Tubingen.

Erikson, E.H. (1951) *Childhood and Society*. Imago, New York.

Erikson, E. (1959) *Identity and the Life Cycle*. W.W. Norton, New York.

Evans, R.J. (1997) *In Defence of History*. Granta Books, London.

Fabian, A.L. & Bender, L. (1947) An inquiry into predisposing factors in children with head injury. *American Journal of Orthopsychiatry*, 17, 68–85.

Freud, A. (1936) *The Ego and the Mechanisms of Defence*. International Universities Press, New York.

Freud, A. (1946) *The Psychoanalytic Treatment of Children*. Imago, London.

Freud, A. (1953) Film Review—A two-year-old goes to hospital (scientific film by James Robertson). *International Journal of Psychoanalysis* 34, 284–287.

Freud, S. (1905) *Drei abhandlungen zur sexualtheorie*. Deuticke, Leipzig/Vienna.

Freud, S. (1953–74) *The Standard Edition of the Complete Works of Sigmund Freud* (eds J. Strachey, A. Freud, A. Strachey & A. Tyson). Hogarth Press/Institute of Psychoanalysis, London.

Froebel, F.W.A. (1893) *The Education of Man*. D. Appleton, New York.

Geissman, C. & Geissman, P. (1998) *A History of Child Psychoanalysis*. Routledge, London.

Gesell, A. (1925) *Mental Growth in the Preschool Child*. Macmillan, New York.

Giles, F.T. (1946) *The Juvenile Courts: Their Work and Problems*. Allen & Unwin, London.

Gittelman-Klein, R. & Klein, D. (1976) Comparative effects of methylphenidate and thioridazine in hyperactive children. I. Clinical results. *Archives of General Psychiatry*, 33, 1217–1231.

Grosskurth, P. (1986) *Melanie Klein, her world and her work*. Hodder and Stoughton, London.

Hall, G.S. (1904) *Adolescence: Its Psychology and its Relations to Physiology, Anthropology, Sociology, Sex, Crime, Religion and Education*. D. Appleton, New York.

Harms, E. (1960) At the cradle of child psychiatry. Hermann Emminghaus' Psychische Stoerungen des Kindesalters (1887). *American Journal of Orthopsychiatry*, 30, 186–190.

Haslam, J. (1809) *Observations on Madness and Melancholy including Practical Remarks on these Diseases together with Cases*. J. Callow, London.

Healy, W. (1917) *The Individual Delinquent*. Little, Brown, Boston.

Hendrick, H. (1994) *Child Welfare: England 1872–1989*. Routledge, London.

Hendrick, H. (1997) *Children, Childhood and English Society 1880–1990*. Cambridge University Press, Cambridge.

Hersov, L. (1986) Child psychiatry in Britain: the last 30 years. *Journal of Child Psychology and Psychiatry*, 27, 781–801.

Heywood, J.S. (1959) *Children in Care The Development of the Service for the Deprived Child*. Routledge & Kegan Paul, London.

Horn, M. (1984) The moral message of child guidance 1925–45. *Journal of Social History*, 18, 25–36.

Howells, J.G. (1965) Organization of child psychiatric services. In: *Modern Perspectives in Child Psychiatry* (ed. J.G.Howells), pp. 251–284. Oliver & Boyd, Edinburgh.

Howells, J.G. & Osborn, M.L. (1981) The history of child psychiatry in the United Kingdom. *Acta Paedopsychiatrica (Basel)*, 46, 193–202.

Hurd, H.M. (1895) *Some Mental Disorders of Childhood and Youth*. Friedenwald, Baltimore, MD.

Ireland, W.W. (1898) *The Mental Affections of Children, Idiocy, Imbecility and Insanity*. J. & A. Churchill, London.

Jones, K. (1972) *A History of the Mental Health Services*. Routledge & Kegan Paul, London.

Kahr, B. (1991) The sexual molestation of children: historical perspectives. *Journal of Psychology*, 19, 191–214.

Kanner, L. (1935) *Child Psychiatry*. Charles C. Thomas, Springfield, IL.

Kanner, L. (1943) Autistic disturbances of affective contact. *Nervous Child*, 2, 217–250.

Kanner, L. (1959) The thirty-third Maudsley Lecture: trends in child psychiatry. *Journal of Mental Science*, 105, 581–593.

Kanner, L. (1960) Child psychiatry: retrospect and prospect. *American Journal of Psychiatry*, 117, 15–22.

Keay, J. (1888) A case of insanity of adolescence. *Journal of Mental Science*, 34, 69–72.

Kern, S. (1973) Freud and the birth of child psychiatry. *Journal of the History of the Behavioural Sciences*, 9, 360–368.

Kett, J.F. (1977) *Rites of Passage: Adolescence in America 1790 to the Present*. Basic Books, New York.

Klein, M. (1932) *The psycho-analysis of children*. Hogarth Press, London.

Klein, M. (1950) *The Psychoanalysis of Children*, 4th edn. Hogarth Press, London.

Klopp, H.I. (1932) The children's institute of the Allentown state hospital. *American Journal of Psychiatry*, 88, 1108–1118.

Kraepelin, E. (1919) *Dementia Praecox and Paraphrenia* (trans. R.M. Barclay). E. & S. Livingstone, Edinburgh.

Levy, D. (1941) Maternal overprotection. *Psychiatry*, 4, 393–438.

Levy, D. (1968) Beginnings of the child guidance movement. *American Journal of Orthopsychiatry*, 38, 799–804.

Lewis, H. (1954) *Deprived Children*. Oxford University Press, Oxford.

Lowrey, L.G. (1944) Psychiatry for children: a brief history of developments. *American Journal of Psychiatry*, 101, 375–388.

Marsh, D.C. (1958) *The Changing Social Structure of England and Wales 1871–1961*. Routledge & Kegan Paul, London.

Maudsley, H. (1867) *The Physiology and Pathology of the Mind*. Macmillan, London.

Maudsley, H. (1879) *The Pathology of Mind*. Macmillan, London.

Maudsley, H. (1895) *The Pathology of Mind A Study of its Distempers, Deformities, and Disorders*. Macmillan, London.

Mednick, S.A., Cudeck, R., Griffith, J.J., Talovic, S.A. & Schulsinger, F. (1984) The Danish high risk project: recent methods and findings. In: *Children at High Risk for Schizophrenia* (eds N.F. Watts, E.J.

Anthony, L.C. Wynne & J.E. Rolf), pp. 21–78. Cambridge University Press, Cambridge.

Montessori, M. (1919) English translation. *The Montessori Method.* William Heinemann, London.

Moreau de Tours, P. (1888) *La Folie Chez les Enfants.* Baillière, Paris.

Morison, A. (1828) *Cases of Mental Disease, with Practical Observations on the Medical Treatment: For the Use of Students.* Longman/S. Highley, London.

Morison, T.C. (1848) Case of mania occurring in a child 6 years old. *Journal of Psychological Medicine and Mental Pathology,* 1, 317–318.

Morselli, H. (1881) *Suicide: an Essay on Comparative Moral Statistics.* Kegan Paul, London.

Mott, F.W. (1914) *Nature and Nurture in Mental Development.* John Murray, London.

Neve, M. & Turner. T. (1995) What the doctor thought and did: Sir James Crichton-Browne (1840–1938). *Medical History,* 39, 399–432.

Nissen, G. (1974) History of child psychiatry in Germany. *Medical Bulletin of the US Army, Europe,* 31, 228–234.

Nissen, G. (1991) The history of child and adolescent psychiatry. In: *The European Handbook of Psychiatry and Mental Health* (ed. A. Seva), Vol. 2, pp. 1459–1467. Editorial Anthropos, Barcelona.

Parry-Jones, W. Ll. (1984) Adolescent psychiatry in Britain: a personal view of its development and present position. *Bulletin of the Royal College of Psychiatry,* 8, 230–233.

Parry-Jones, W. Ll. (1989) The history of child and adolescent psychiatry: its present day relevance. *Journal of Child Psychology and Psychiatry,* 30, 3–11.

Parry-Jones, W. Ll. (1992) Historical research in child and adolescent psychiatry: scope, methods and application. *Journal of Child Psychology and Psychiatry,* 33, 803–811.

Parry-Jones, W. L. (1994) History of child and adolescent psychiatry. In: *Child and Adolescent Psychiatry: Modern Approaches* (eds M. Rutter, E. Taylor & L. Hersov), 3rd edn, pp. 794–812. Blackwell Scientific, Oxford.

Perfect, W. (1787) *Select Cases in the Different Species of Insanity, Lunacy or Madness, with the Modes of Practice as adopted in the Treatment of Each.* Gillman, Rochester, UK.

Peters, U.H. (1985) *Anna Freud. A life dedicated to children.* Weidenfeld and Nicholson, London.

Phillips, A. (1988) *Winnicott.* Fontana, London.

Piaget, J. (1926) *The Language and Thought of the Child* (trans. M. Gabain). Routledge & Kegan Paul, London.

Pollock, L.A. (1983) *Forgotten Children: Parent–Child Relationships 1500–1900.* Cambridge University Press, Cambridge.

Prichard, J.C. (1835) *A Treatise on Insanity and Other Disorders Affecting the Mind.* Sherwood, Gilbert & Piper, London.

Robertson, J. & Robertson, J. (1971) Young children in brief separation: a fresh look. *Psychoanalytic Study of the Child,* 26, 264–315.

Rosen, V. (1947) Streptosymbolia: an intra-systemic disturbance of the synthetic function of the ego. *Psychoanalytic Study of the Child,* 10, 83–99.

Rutter, M. (1968) Child Psychiatry. In: *Studies in Psychiatry* (eds M. Shepherd & D.L. Davies), pp. 147–167. Oxford University Press, London.

Rutter, M. (1972a) Childhood schizophrenia reconsidered. *Journal of Autism and Childhood Schizophrenia,* 2, 315–338.

Rutter, M. (1972b) *Maternal Deprivation Reassessed.* Penguin, Harmondsworth.

Rutter, M., Schaffer, D. & Shepherd, M. (1975) *A Multiaxial Classification of Child Psychiatric Disorders,* World Health Organization, Geneva.

Rutter, M., Tizard, J. & Whitmore, K. (eds) (1970) *Education, Health and Behaviour.* Longmans, London.

Rutter, M., Izard, C. & Read, P. (1986) *Depression in Young People: Developmental and Clinical Perspectives.* Guilford Press, London.

Rydelius, P.A. (1995) History of Swedish child and adolescent psychiatry (1900–95). *Acta Paedopsychiatrica (Basel)*, 84, 703–704.

Savage, G.H. (1891) Moral insanity. *Journal of Mental Science,* 27, 147–155.

Scott, H. (1947) *Report of Commissioner of Metropolitan Police.* HMSO, London.

Scull, A. (1993) *The Most Solitary of Afflictions: Madness Society in Britain, 1700–1900.* Yale University Press, New Haven & London.

Shorter, E. (1997) *A History of Psychiatry: from the Era of the Asylum to the Age of Prozac.* John Wiley, New York.

Spitz, R. (1951) The psychological diseases of infancy: an attempt at their etiologic classification. *Psychoanalytic Study of the Child,* 6, 255–278.

Staples, H.D. (1995) Reflections on the history of adolescent psychiatry (1900–95). *Adolescent Psychiatry,* 20, 39–49.

Steedman, C. (1995) *Strange dislocations: Childhood and the idea of human interiority 1780–1930.* Virago, London.

Steen, R.H. (1913) Moral insanity. *Journal of Mental Science,* 59, 478–486.

Stevenson, G.S. & Smith, G. (1934) *Child Guidance Clinics: A Quarter Century of Development.* The Commonwealth Fund, New York.

Still, G.F. (1902) The Goulstonian Lectures. *Lancet,* April 12, 1008–1012; April 19, 1077–1082; April 26, 1163–1168.

Stone, L. (1979) *The Family, Sex and Marriage In England 1500–1800.* Penguin Books, Harmondsworth.

Stone, M.H. (1973) Child psychiatry before the 20th century. *International Journal of Child Psychotherapy,* 2, 264–308.

Stone, M.H. (1997) *Healing the Mind: A History of Psychiatry from Antiquity to the Present.* W.W. Norton & Co, New York & London.

Strahan, S.A.K. (1893) *Suicide and Insanity: A Physiological Sociological Study.* Swan Sonnenschein, London.

Sullivan, W.C. (1915) Criminal children. In: *Defective Children* (ed. T.N. Kelynack), pp. 81–97. J. Bale & Danielsson, London.

Tuke, D.H. (1885) Moral or educational insanity. *Journal of Mental Science,* 31, 174–190.

Tuke, D.H. (1892) *A Dictionary of Psychological Medicine.* J & A Churchill, London.

Underwood, J.A.E. (1955) *Report of the Committee on Maladjusted Children.* HMSO, London.

Van Dijken, S. (1998) *John Bowlby: his early life.* Free Association Books, London.

Von Gontard, A. (1988) The development of child psychiatry in 19th century Britain. *Journal of Child Psychology and Psychiatry,* 29, 569–588.

Walk, A. (1964) The pre-history of child psychiatry. *British Journal of Psychiatry,* 110, 754–767.

Walvin, J. (1984) *A Child's World: A Social History of English Childhood 1800–1914.* Penguin, Harmondsworth.

Wardle, C.J. (1991a) Twentieth-century influences on the development in Britain of services for child and adolescent psychiatry. *British Journal of Psychiatry,* 159, 53–68.

Wardle, C.J. (1991b) Historical influences on services for children and adolescents before 1900. In: *150 Years of British Psychiatry 1841–1991* (eds G.E. Berrios & H. Freeman), pp. 279–293. Gaskell, London.

Warren, W. (1974) *Child Psychiatry and the Maudsley Hospital: An Historical Survey*. Unpublished Third Kenneth Cameron Memorial Lecture, Institute of Psychiatry Library.

West, C. (1848) *Lectures on the Diseases of Infancy and Childhood*, 1st edn, pp. 128–131 Longman, Brown, Green & Longmans, London.

West, C. (1854) *Lectures on the Diseases of Infancy and Childhood*, 3rd edn, pp. 185–206 Longman, Brown, Green & Longmans, London.

West, C. (1860) On the mental peculiarities and mental disorders of childhood. *Medical Times and Gazette*, **1**, 133–137.

West, C. (1871) *On Some Disorders of the Nervous System in Childhood: the Lumleian Lectures Delivered . . . in March 1871*. Longmans, Green, London.

Westcott, W.W. (1885) *Suicide: its History, Literature, Jurisprudence, Causation and Prevention*. H.K. Lewis, London.

Wickman, E.K. (1928) *Teachers and Behavior Problems*. Commonwealth Fund, New York.

Wicks, B. (1988) *No Time to Wave Goodbye*. Bloomsbury, London.

Wilkins, R. (1993) Delusions in children and teenagers admitted to Bethlem Royal Hospital in the 19th century. *British Journal of Psychiatry*, **162**, 487–492.

Wilmarth, A.W. (1894) Causation and early treatment of mental disease in children. *Journal of American Medical Association*, **23**, 271–274.

Winnicott, D.W. (1958) *Collected Papers: Through Paediatrics to Psychoanalysis*. Tavistock Publications, London.

Winnicott, D.W. (1964) *The Child, the Family and the Outside World*. Penguin Books, Harmondsworth.

Winnicott, D.W. (1971) *Therapeutic Consultations in Child Psychiatry*. Hogarth Press, London.

Witmer, H.L. (1940) *Psychiatric Clinics for Children, with Special Reference to State Programs*. Commonwealth Fund, New York.

Wolff, S. (1989) Fact and fashion: changing perspectives in child psychiatry. *Journal of the Royal Society of Medicine*, **82**, 324–328.

Yule, W. (1984) Child behaviour therapy in Britain: 1962–82. *Newsletter of the Association of Child Psychology and Psychiatry*, **6**, 15–20.

Zaretsky, E. (1999) One large secure solid background: Melanie Klein and the origins of the British welfare state. *Psychoanalysis and History*, **1**, 136–154.

PART THREE

Clinical Syndromes

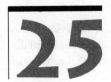

25 Syndromes of Hyperactivity and Attention Deficit

Russell Schachar and Rosemary Tannock

Introduction

Restlessness, inattention and impulsiveness are common behavioural problems during the preschool- and school-age years. Adolescents and adults also exhibit these traits but usually to a lesser extent. In the extreme, these characteristics are impairing to the affected individuals and disturbing to those around them. Consequently, they are thought to be symptoms of a mental disorder. Persons affected by this disorder in childhood are at risk for learning, conduct and social problems, and are more likely to develop serious impairment in adolescence and adulthood. As a result, this disorder places substantial demands on the health care, educational and legal resources of the community and is of considerable importance from a public health perspective.

The purpose of this chapter is to review the current understanding of the aetiology, nosology and treatment of this disorder. We begin by describing the clinical features and by tracing the evolution of our understanding of the syndrome.

As a result of enduring controversy about nosology, we adopt the convention suggested by Taylor (1998) of using the term 'hyperactivity' to refer to the cardinal symptoms (overactivity, inattention, impulsiveness) that define the syndrome and of using specific diagnostic terms, such as hyperkinetic disorder (HD) or attention deficit hyperactivity disorder (ADHD) when addressing a particular diagnostic entity and set of criteria. We will use the acronym AD-HKD when referring to characteristics that are shared by ADHD and HD. In referring to the syndrome as 'hyperactivity' we do not intend to convey the impression that gross motor activity is either the defining symptom of the disorder or its essential deficit. In fact, motor activity is only one of the important manifestations of the disorder and may not be as important as others such as inattention and cognitive deficit. Hyperactivity is used in a purely descriptive manner as a proxy for all the other labels that have been used. A wide range of terms have been used to describe this syndrome and each has taken on a specific meaning. Any choice of label such as ADHD or HD would convey the impression that the chapter pertains to children defined by one set of diagnostic criteria only.

Even though clinicians, scientists and authors find 'ADHD' or 'hyperactive children' a convenient shorthand, diagnoses actually describe disorders not individuals. People change as do labels. In this chapter, all references to hyperactive individuals should be understood as statements about disorders not people.

Clinical features

The cardinal features of children with AD-HKD are excessive motor activity, inattention and impulsiveness. Compared with their peers, these children are restless, fidgety and boisterous when required to be still and quiet. This is true both in structured situations, such as the classroom, and in unstructured situations, such as the playground. They have difficulty attending to instructions in academic and social situations. They tend to look away when spoken to, require frequent repetition of directions or appear unable to comprehend the nuances of an instruction. At school, their work is characterized by careless errors, poor organization and forgetfulness. They lose things such as books, notes and assignments that are crucial to school work but they also lose possessions that are of obvious personal value. They are typically the last to start a designated activity (often because they cannot find the necessary materials, forget to gather them together or have been daydreaming) and last to finish (because of staring off into space, failing to concentrate and being distracted). They shout out their replies, interrupt others and are reckless and accident-prone. On the other hand, they may not speak when they are supposed to (Zentall 1988). They seem to have trouble interrupting their course of action, and appear unable to adjust an incorrect or maladaptive response. They make careless errors in their school work and in other activities.

The characteristics of AD-HKD are variable both within and among individual children. It is rare to find a person who exhibits every characteristic of hyperactivity to a comparable extent. Some children are particularly restless and impulsive but are quite attentive (Goldstein 1987). Others are primarily inattentive and relatively inactive or even hypoactive (McGee et al. 1992). The behaviour of hyperactive children is context-dependent; a child may be highly distractible and inattentive in the classroom setting but restless and impulsive around the home. Moreover, the extent of behavioural excess varies with the demands of the situation. A child who is markedly symptomatic at school may be described as quite average in behaviour by their parents, or a child who is highly distractible while performing a structured task in the classroom may be described as perfectly average when playing a computer game, interacting with peers or while engaged in an unstructured activity. Parents frequently comment that it is the marked variability day-to-day, hour-by-hour and minute-by-minute that is the most salient feature of these children.

The manifestations of this syndrome change with development. In preschool-age children, overactivity is most obvious and possibly most impairing. Inattention becomes more salient once a child confronts the demands of the classroom. As children reach adolescence and adulthood, the motor overactivity seems to diminish and inattention and impulsiveness become most impairing and are particularly noticeable in social situations.

Some authorities point to the variability described above and question the objectivity of the symptoms of hyperactivity and therefore the validity of the syndrome. To others, this variability is not surprising given the complexity of human behaviour and psychopathology. Ample research demonstrates that hyperactivity is more than the subjective impression of adults. There is sufficient convergence between ratings of hyperactive, inattentive and impulsive symptoms and direct measures of the same behaviours to support the validity of the core symptoms of the syndrome (see Sandberg et al. 1996 for review). For example, when observed in a playroom, hyperactive children are more often off-task and persist less on a particular activity than their non-hyperactive peers (Milich & Fitzgerald 1985). Hyperactive children are demonstrably more active throughout the day (Porrino et al. 1983) and are less attentive in a range of laboratory situations (Sergeant 2000). However, the extent to which agreement between subjective ratings of hyperactive symptoms and objective measures of the same behaviours is only modest suggests that we do not fully understand the exact nature of these behaviours, the role of context or the factors that influence observer judgement (Sandberg et al. 1996).

There are many reasons for these modest levels of agreement among informants.

1 Informants may not share a common definition of each behaviour. An observer might consider failure to persist in a task to be evidence of defiance, lack of interest, low motivation, boredom or learning disability rather than inattention.

2 Children's behaviour is a function of the demands of the setting. Parents may have fewer opportunities than teachers to observe their child in situations that demand attention. Inattention might be particularly impairing in school and therefore salient to a teacher's judgement of psychopathology, whereas restlessness might be more conspicuous at home (Hewitt et al. 1997). By contrast, parents and teachers are more likely to agree about which children are impaired than they are to agree about the presence of particular symptoms (Mota & Schachar 2000).

3 The informant's mental state or cultural expectations may influence perceptions of child behaviour (Boyle & Pickles 1997). Age-appropriate levels of activity may seem more aversive for a depressed socially isolated mother, for those with high expectations for academic attainment or for a teacher of a class that does not include other children with special needs.

4 Cultures may differ in their sensitivity to hyperactive behaviours. Leung et al. (1996) reported that parents in Hong Kong rated their children as highly hyperactive even though objective measures did not distinguish them. Informants seem to have difficulty discriminating among various dimensions of disturbance. This inability to discriminate among behaviours may result in a halo effect whereby the presence of defiance and disobedience is taken as evidence of hyperactivity (Schachar et al. 1986; Abikoff et al. 1991).

5 Parents have a tendency to exaggerate the differences among their children when making behavioural judgements (Eaves et al. 1997).

It is also true that many of these features describe all children to some extent at some times, such as when a child is tired or unwell. However, in hyperactive children, these behaviours are more frequent, severe and persistent and interfere with a child's peer and parental relationships, impede their academic performance and undermine their psychological well-being. The problem is how much of which behaviours in what settings assessed in what way by whom is sufficient to constitute a discrete disorder. We return to this issue in the discussion of nomenclature and assessment.

Associated impairment

Children with AD-HKD experience serious social, academic and psychological impairment at every stage of development. They are rejected by peers and adults and are treated in a controlling and negative fashion by them (Barkley et al. 1985; Hinshaw & James 1991). Their parents experience considerable stress and feelings of incompetence. Child management problems can increase social isolation and marital discord. Hyperactivity in a child may even be a risk factor for parental alcohol consumption (Pelham et al. 1998). The economic burden of having a hyperactive child is considerable but currently unspecified. Children with AD-HKD are more likely than their unaffected peers to live in families that are disrupted by poverty, characterized by marital discord and parental psychopathology and to have siblings who are at risk for the development of psychopathology (Faraone et al. 1996a; Hechtman 1996; Woodward et al. 1998).

Compared with their normally developing peers, children with AD-HKD get lower marks, fail more grades at school, and are more likely to have a diagnosis of a learning disability (Weiss & Hechtman 1993; Zentall et al. 1994; Mannuzza et al. 1998). Failure at school results in demoralization, low self-esteem, peer rejection and feelings of anxiety and depression. In turn, these responses result in premature school drop-out, increased exposure to delinquent peer groups and consequent risk of delinquency and substance abuse.

Hyperactive adolescents and adults show many of the same features as their younger counterparts, although earlier overt restlessness may be replaced by a sense of inner restlessness. Affected adolescents are more likely to drop out of school with lower marks and to have lower paid and lower status occupations than their non-hyperactive peers and siblings. Their self-esteem may suffer, although sometimes one observes what appears to be a defensively inflated sense of self-esteem (Slomkowski et al. 1995). Poor driving habits, accidental injuries or death are more common among hyperactive individuals as are suicide attempts and substance abuse disorder (Barkley *et al.* 1996; Nada-Raja *et al.* 1997). Hyperactive adults are more likely than others to have a discordant marriage and to have hyperactive children (Weiss & Hechtman 1993; Biederman *et al.* 1995).

Comorbidity

Many children with ADH-HKD meet the criteria for another psychiatric disorder—a phenomenon known as comorbidity (see Taylor & Rutter, Chapter 1). Estimates of comorbidity depend on the criteria used to define hyperactivity, the criteria used to define the comorbid disorder and the sample under study. In general, oppositional/defiant disorder is observed in 35–50% of cases, conduct disorder in 25%, depressive disorder in 15% and anxiety disorder in 25% (Jensen *et al.* 1997; Kuhne *et al.* 1997). In fact, over 50% of children with AD-HKD meet criteria for two comorbid conditions (Szatmari *et al.* 1989a). Learning disability occurs in 15–40% of children, particularly among those with inattentive symptoms, and language impairment in about 15–75% of children (Cohen *et al.* 2000; Tannock 2000).

Several factors may contribute to the rate high rate of comorbidity but none accounts for it completely (Caron & Rutter 1991).

1 The rate of comorbidity is affected by referral bias (individuals with more than one disorder get preferentially referred for services), overlapping diagnostic criteria (e.g. inattention counts as a symptom of AD-HKD and of depression), or the inability of informants and clinicians to draw precise distinctions among disorders (e.g. an aggressive child may appear restless).

2 AD-HKD may increase the risk of a second disorder. For example, school failure associated with hyperactivity may result in gravitation toward delinquent peer groups or in demoralization that develops into depression.

3 AD-HKD and a comorbid disorder, such as reading disability, may occur together because they are alternate manifestations of a shared underlying cause.

4 AD-HKD in the presence of a comorbid disorder may be a distinct condition.

5 The comorbid condition could represent a phenocopy of one of the 'pure' disorders (e.g. conduct disorder children are restless, impulsive, etc. but their AD-HKD symptoms do not carry the same implications as does AD-HKD in the absence of conduct disorder (Schachar & Tannock 1995).

There are several ways to test the validity of these competing hypotheses. One way is to compare AD-HKD with and without the comorbid disorder with individuals affected only by the pure comorbid disorder on a range of important correlates such as impairment, aetiological indicator, associated pathology, natural history and the like. Secondly, one can treat each of the two conditions and examine the impact on the other. Thirdly, one can use family genetic strategies to determine the risk in family members of each of the separate disorders.

Although these strategies have been applied widely, none of the common comorbidities has as yet been fully explained. For example, AD-HKD with comorbid conduct disorder differs from 'pure' AD-HKD on a wide range of cognitive, prognostic and family measures suggesting that it may be a distinct entity (MacDonald & Achenbach 1996; Jensen *et al.* 1997; Faraone *et al.* 1998a). Conversely, the hybrid hypothesis for AD-HKD and conduct disorder gains support from the considerable clinical and neuropsychological research showing that the comorbid group shares the characteristics of both AD-HKD and conduct disorder (Szatmari *et al.* 1989b); from twin studies that point to a shared genetic risk for conduct disorder and AD-HKD (Silberg *et al.* 1996; Faraone *et al.* 1997a); and from studies that show improvement in symptoms of conduct disorder following the reduction in hyperactivity that occurs with methylphenidate (Klein *et al.* 1997).

Similarly, there is evidence for each of the mechanisms of comorbidity acting in comorbid AD-HKD and reading disability. Neuropsychological and family history studies demonstrate that AD-HKD and reading disability are distinct conditions with separate correlates and causes, but that they frequently co-occur as a true hybrid (Douglas & Benezra 1990; Faraone *et al.* 1993; Shaywitz *et al.* 1995). Twin studies indicate that AD-HKD and reading disability have shared genetic influences suggesting that they may be heterogeneous manifestations of a single genetic diathesis (Gillis *et al.* 1992; Stevenson *et al.* 1993). Others argue that the combined condition may be a phenocopy of AD-HKD and that comorbid AD-HKD and reading disorder is a variant of reading disorder not AD-HKD (Pennington *et al.* 1993).

In summary, existing research does not clarify which mechanism is responsible for comorbidity of AD-HKD with other conditions. It is possible that each of the mechanisms for comorbidity described above accounts for some of these comorbid cases.

Development of the concept

Excessively hyperactive, inattentive and impulsive children have been described in the medical literature since the late-nineteenth century (for reviews see Schachar 1986; Sandberg & Barton 1996). In fact, early descriptions and aetiological theories of hyperactivity were, in many ways, strikingly similar to current descriptions of the syndrome (Still 1902; Tredgold 1908). The syndrome was characterized by morbid inability to sustain attention, a lack of will or self-control (insufficiency of inhibitory volition), restlessness and impulsiveness (exaggeration of excitability) together with soft neurological signs such as clumsiness and minor congenital anomalies or stigmata (Tredgold 1908). Befitting prevailing Darwinist and evolutionary views of society and psychopathology, these early concepts focused on a lack of sustained 'will' as the cardinal manifestation of the disorder and labelled the disorder a syndrome of 'moral dyscontrol'. The prevailing notions of 'will' and 'morality' were rather like theories of executive control and self-regulation that play such an important part in current neuropsychological theories of AD-HKD.

Will, morality, sustained effort and the like were held to be the highest and latest achievements of evolution and were localized in the most recently evolved parts of the brain (Tredgold 1908). As a result, these processes were especially vulnerable to loss as a result of relatively minor pre- or postnatal brain injury, infection, malnutrition or exposure to toxins, especially in individuals with a hereditary predisposition. Moral dyscontrol was not thought to be a result of adverse social circumstances that were common at the time but rather was thought to be a biological affliction. This perspective reflected the prevailing philosophical and sociological inclination of the late-nineteenth century that attributed extremes of behaviour, as well as poverty and its correlates (e.g. medical illness, alcoholism and immorality), to physiological rather than to psychological or social causes (Tredgold 1908). Defined in this way, moral dyscontrol provided a neurobiological formulation for many of the childhood problems of the times.

In many respects, essential theories of AD-HKD changed little over the decades. However, with detailed study of the behaviour of hyperactive children and accumulating knowledge of brain function during the century, concepts of the fundamental behavioural and neuropathological deficit of AD-HKD changed dramatically. By the middle of the nineteenth century, the manifestations and impairment associated with AD-HKD were attributed to restlessness arising from abnormal arousal mechanisms in the reticular activating system. More recently, the fundamental deficit in AD-HKD was believed to be deficient sustained attention (Douglas 1972, 1988), a central impairment in self-regulation, and impairments in executive processes (Barkley 1998). Current theory favours the fundamental role of deficient inhibition—the future-orientated, delaying mechanism involved in the timing, initiation and interruption of action and of neuropathology in the frontal and related regions of the brain (Barkley et al. 1992a). Competing models have also been proposed, which attribute poor performance in ADHD to the impact of state moderators (e.g. arousal, activation, effort, motivation), or to differential sensitivity to reward, rather than to fundamental cognitive deficits (Laufer et al. 1957; Chess 1960; Wender 1971; Glow & Glow 1979; Haenlein & Caul 1987).

Evolution in nomenclature

Many different diagnostic terms have been used to label the hyperactive child over the years. When the syndrome first appeared in the modern North American diagnostic classifications of mental disorders, *Diagnostic and Statistical Manual of the American Psychiatric Association*, it was known as hyperkinetic reaction of childhood (DSM-II; American Psychiatric Association 1968). This term stressed overactivity as the cardinal feature of the syndrome rather than notions of minimal brain damage or dysfunction that had been current until that time (Clements 1966). The name of the disorder was changed to attention deficit disorder (ADD) in 1980 (DSM-III; American Psychiatric Association 1980) to reflect the opinion emerging, particularly in North America, that inattention and impulsive-

ness rather than motor overactivity *per se* was the cardinal behavioural manifestation of the disorder and possibly the central deficit (Douglas 1972).

DSM-IV (American Psychiatric Association 1994) differs from DSM-III-R (American Psychiatric Association 1987) and DSM-III in that it separates inattention criteria from those of hyperactivity and impulsiveness but does not distinguish the later two aspects of the syndrome. The shifts in diagnostic criteria complicate research efforts because it is not possible to extrapolate from studies using earlier criteria to those based on DSM-IV criteria.

Over the last half century, diagnostic traditions of North America and Europe diverged. In Europe, two parallel notions of hyperactivity evolved. The average hyperactive child was thought to have a behaviour disorder arising from the effects of social or familial adversity. These children were typically diagnosed with conduct or behaviour disorder rather than hyperactivity. The few children with severe persistent and pervasive symptoms and with documented neuropathology, such as a history of head injury or seizure disorder (Ounsted 1955; Bax & McKeith 1963), were diagnosed with hyperkinetic disorder (International Classification of Diseases, ICD; World Health Organization 1978).

Current approaches to categorization

The most recent editions of the DSM and ICD classifications reflect an effort to bring the definitions of ADHD and HD closer together. DSM-IV and ICD-10 (World Health Organization 1994) have adopted almost identical criteria for the identification of inattentive, hyperactive and impulsive symptoms. However, significant differences between the European and North American approaches are still evident in their diagnostic algorithms (the number of criteria in each domain required for a diagnosis), the role of inattention, the definition of pervasiveness and the handling of comorbidity.

According to DSM-IV, the diagnosis of ADHD requires the presence of six inattentive or six hyperactive–impulsive symptoms, or both. Three different subtypes of ADHD are therefore permitted:

1 predominantly inattentive—the presence of six or more symptoms of disordered attention and fewer than six symptoms of hyperactivity–impulsivity;
2 predominantly hyperactive–impulsive—the presence of six or more symptoms of hyperactivity–impulsivity and fewer than six symptoms of inattention; and
3 combined—the presence of six or more inattentive and six or more hyperactive–impulsive symptoms.
To establish a diagnosis of HD based on ICD-10, at least six inattentive, three hyperactive, and one impulsive symptom must be present. The diagnosis cannot be made in the absence of each type of symptom so no symptomatic subtypes are permitted. The relative weight given to inattention in ICD criteria is ironic given the name but accurately reflects current emphasis on inattention as the cardinal and most impairing symptom.

ICD-10 is also more demanding about cross-situational pervasiveness, requiring that all necessary criteria be present, both at home and at school (or other situations such as in the clinic). DSM-IV is more lenient: it demands that criteria be met in at least one situation and that impairment arising from ADHD symptoms be present in another. The definition of impairment, the number of symptoms that must be present or the severity of the symptoms in this second situation are not stipulated. Nevertheless, DSM-IV is an advance over DSM-III-R, which instructed clinicians to give priority to the judgement of teachers over that of parents.

Perhaps the most salient difference between the DSM-IV and ICD-10 classifications is the approach to the diagnosis when more than one disorder coexists with AD-HKD. DSM-IV recognizes all diagnoses that are present, except for schizophrenia, autism and pervasive developmental disorder. In contrast, ICD-10, in general, discourages multiple diagnoses. In the presence of internalizing disorders, such as anxiety or mood disorders, ICD-10 does not recommend the HD diagnosis. The only exception occurs when both HD and conduct disorder coexist. ICD-10 labels this combination hyperkinetic conduct disorder. This new subcategory is intended to deal with the tendency of clinicians in Europe to prefer the diagnosis of conduct disorder to HD when both disorders are evident (Prendergast *et al.* 1988).

Considerable evidence supports the validity of both ADHD and HD. Children with ADHD diagnosed according to DSM criteria or HD diagnosed according to ICD can be distinguished reliably from children with other disorders, such as conduct disorder, and differ in important ways from normally developing children on a wide range of laboratory measures of attention, social interaction and outcome (Barkley 1995). For example, conduct disorder is associated with hostile attributional bias, greater exposure to psychosocial adversity and higher prevalence of delinquency in adolescence. By contrast, ADHD and HD are associated with cognitive deficit of various kinds (Schachar 1991; Tannock 1998a) and with later antisocial behaviour above and beyond the risk associated with early conduct disorder (Taylor *et al.* 1996).

There have been few direct comparisons of non-overlapping groups of ADHD and HD children (Tripp & Luk 1997). Based on available evidence, ADHD that is not severe enough to fulfil criteria for HD is common in the general population. In many cases, these children are not particularly impaired (Taylor *et al.* 1991). Nevertheless, ADHD of this degree of severity may identify a group of children at high risk for the development of disturbance. HD (as defined by ICD-10) constitutes the most severe 20% of those with ADHD (as defined by DSM-IV) as judged by an increased rate of important clinical correlates, such as neurodevelopmental delay, risk of comorbidity, psychosocial impairment, poor academic and cognitive function and comorbid psychopathology. HD may also be more responsive to methylphenidate (Taylor *et al.* 1987, 1991).

Northern European clinicians continue to stress the centrality of delay in motor development to the diagnosis (Bax & McKeith 1963; Kalverboer 1975; Nichols & Chen 1981). Accordingly,

disorder of attention, motor control and perception (DAMP) came to refer to the coincidence of these deficits (Gillberg & Gillberg 1988, 1989). DAMP overlaps with but is not coincident with ADHD or HD. Approximately half of children with ADHD meet criteria for DAMP (Landgren *et al.* 1996). DAMP plus ADHD delineates a subset of children with more marked classroom dysfunction and poorer academic test scores than either ADHD or DAMP alone. By contrast, the majority of those with HD meet criteria for DAMP (Taylor *et al.* 1991). The validity of the concept of DAMP has been questioned because the association of neurodevelopmental abnormality and hyperactivity does not appear to be specific to hyperactivity nor is there a uniform behaviour consequence of brain injury (Rutter 1982; Rutter *et al.* 1983; Shaffer *et al.* 1985; Rydelius 2000).

Subtypes

Various subtypes of AD-HKD have been distinguished, based on phenomenology, pervasiveness of symptoms and patterns of comorbidity. Subgrouping based on the children's response to treatment is less well established, but is suggested by the existence of differences between children who do and do not respond favourably to methylphenidate (Buitelaar *et al.* 1995; Taylor *et al.* 1987). Subgroups based on the presence or absence of genetic risk factors involved in the dopaminergic and noradrenergic systems remains speculative (Swanson *et al.* 2000).

DSM-IV makes a distinction between hyperactive–impulsive, inattentive and combined hyperactive–impulsive and inattentive subtypes, although the true significance of this distinction is unknown. The inattentive and combined subtypes are about equally prevalent among school-age children and are more common than the hyperactive–impulsive subtype (Morgan *et al.* 1996; Faraone *et al.* 1998b). The hyperactive–impulsive subtype is more common in very young children but decreases in prevalence with age. Many children with the hyperactive–impulsive subtype have combined subtype on follow-up (Cantwell & Baker 1988), suggesting that subtypes may represent developmental stages rather than distinct entities.

Hyperactive and impulsive behaviour tends to be predictive of delinquent and aggressive behaviour (Taylor *et al.* 1996; Eiraldi *et al.* 1997; Babinski *et al.* 1999). Inattentive behaviour predicts lower IQ, more abnormalities in cognition and delayed language development. Inattentive children are also less impulsive, aggressive, distractible and socially disinhibited (Lahey & Carlson 1991; Cantwell & Baker 1992; McBurnett *et al.* 1999; Warner-Rogers *et al.* 2000). Taylor *et al.* (1991) found that the majority of attention deficits associated with the inattentive subtype (DSM-III ADD without hyperactivity) were artefacts of lower IQ: differences in attention between ADD and normal children disappeared once IQ was controlled.

Quantitative and categorical approaches to diagnosis

Arguments about the relative validity of criteria for ADHD, HD and DAMP are all conducted from a categorical perspective on diagnosis. This approach assumes that individuals who meet specific criteria and those who do not differ in kind rather than in degree. There is another broad perspective on classification of AD-HKD: the dimensional approach. According to this approach, the constituent behaviours of AD-HKD vary widely in the general population and so individuals are more or less affected and impaired (Fergusson *et al.* 1991; Meehl 1995). Accordingly, AD-HKD is best viewed as the extreme of some continuously distributed but unobservable or latent trait, rather than as a discrete entity: affected persons are quantitatively but not qualitatively distinct from unaffected persons. Which approach is correct is not easily resolved. It is likely that certain aspects of the syndrome are captured best by the categorical approach, while others are better characterized by the dimensional, or quantitative, perspective.

The quantitative approach is supported by the observation that no bimodal distribution of scores is observed in behavioural data and that there does not seem to be an obvious discontinuity between a group of individuals with high hyperactivity and a group with low hyperactivity. A bimodal distribution, if present, would indicate that there is both temperamental variation and the presence of a discrete 'hyperactive' group (Meehl 1995). In addition, one typically observes a continuous and generally linear dose–response function relating symptom severity and outcome risk (substance abuse behaviour, juvenile offending, heritability and school drop-out at age 16; Fergusson & Horwood 1995; Levy *et al.* 1997). Dimensionally scored variables are often better predictors of outcome than are measures based on a diagnostic classification (extreme scores; Fergusson & Horwood 1995).

Course and prognosis

Hyperactive preschool-age children are referred for clinical assessment. However, most individuals are referred after they start school. In most but not all cases, the history reveals AD-HKD symptoms from an early age.

Originally, AD-HKD was thought to be a transient phenomenon because of the tendency for symptoms, especially restlessness, to diminish as children reached adolescence. Inattention and impulsiveness are more persistent manifestations (Hart *et al.* 1995). It is now clear that the disorder persists into adolescence in half or more of affected persons, and into adulthood in half or more of adolescent cases (Klein & Mannuzza 1991; Weiss & Hechtman 1993; Mannuzza *et al.* 1998).

Compared with their non-AD-HKD peers, previously affected persons are at approximately five times greater risk for substance abuse (tobacco, alcohol, illicit drugs), antisocial behaviour (aggression, trouble with the law, admission to juvenile facilities), and other psychiatric disorders, such as depression and anxiety (Levin & Kleber 1995; McArdle *et al.* 1997). Academic and educational problems persist into adolescence; by the time they are adults, hyperactive children have completed

significantly less schooling and hold lower status jobs than their non-hyperactive peers (Fergusson *et al.* 1997; Mannuzza *et al.* 1997). Even those who no longer meet the criteria for AD-HKD in adolescence are at increased risk for substance abuse and antisocial disorders, suggesting the persistence of some residual or latent deficit (Mannuzza *et al.* 1993).

Poor outcome in adolescence and young adulthood is more likely when the affected child experiences stressful life circumstances, such as those that are commonly associated with poverty, overcrowding, negative expressed emotion in the parent–child relationship, and parental psychopathology (Barkley *et al.* 1990a; Farrington *et al.* 1990; Fischer *et al.* 1993; Taylor *et al.* 1996). Prognosis is also worse when the AD-HKD symptoms are severe, and predominantly hyperactive–impulsive in nature and when the child exhibits early conduct, language or learning disorder (Moffitt 1990; Lynskey & Fergusson 1995; Babinski *et al.* 1999; Merrell & Tymms 2001). Nevertheless, the poor outcome of children with AD-HKD is not simply a function of these early associated impairments; AD-HKD increases the risk of a poor outcome, even when due allowance is made for the associated risk factors (Babinski *et al.* 1999; Farrington *et al.* 1990; Taylor *et al.* 1996).

Epidemiology

The prevalence of AD-HKD depends, to a great extent, on the diagnostic measures used (e.g. questionnaires or interviews), diagnostic criteria (ICD-10, DSM-IV), sampling method, number of informants used (parents only, teachers only or both), handling of comorbidity (exclusion of cases with comorbid diagnosis), age of population, country, and the nature of the population studied (e.g. inner city or rural; Boyle *et al.* 1996). Screening with behavioural questionnaires identifies 10–20% of the population as affected (Wolraich *et al.* 1998). Studies that use definitions based on DSM, requiring some degree of pervasiveness and impairment and include comorbid cases, report prevalence rates in the 5–10% range (Offord *et al.* 1987; Fergusson *et al.* 1993; Newman *et al.* 1996). When the more stringent ICD-based criteria are used and the diagnosis is restricted to the presence of the full syndrome without comorbid conditions, 1–2% prevalence rates are found (for review see Danckaerts & Taylor 1995; Swanson *et al.* 1998a). The prevalence of combined ADHD and DAMP is about 6% (Kadesjo & Gillberg 1998). In clinical samples, fewer than half of children meeting criteria for ADHD also meet criteria for HD (Tripp *et al.* 1999).

Prevalence of the diagnosis of AD-HKD varies by culture although there is little difference among cultures in rates of hyperactive behaviour as assessed by questionnaire rating (Leung *et al.* 1996). The diagnosis of AD-HKD is only recently becoming more common in Mediterranean countries.

The ratio of males : females with the diagnosis in community samples is approximately 3 : 1 (Szatmari *et al.* 1989c). The prevalence of AD-HKD is highest among school-aged boys and lower among adolescents. In contrast, its prevalence among females is lower, but is more stable across ages. AD-HKD is more common in urban than rural communities (Szatmari *et al.* 1989c).

There has been a lot of speculation about the apparent increase in prevalence of the disorder over the last half century. The rapid increase in prevalence of the diagnosis was largely a North American phenomenon (Danckaerts & Taylor 1995). One reason for increased prevalence lies with the broadening of diagnostic criteria resulting from changes in DSM. However, rates may be increasing in Europe of late as clinicians shift from emphasizing only the social and psychological factors in hyperactivity to appreciating the role of neurobiological influences. Some have emphasized the potential impact that the marked changes in the *pace* or *speed* of everyday life could have on neural development. Others attribute the increasing use of the diagnosis to the discovery by Charles Bradley (1937) that dexamphetamine was a safe and effective treatment. Changes in educational practice, societal expectations and allocation of health care resources have also played a part.

Aetiology

AD-HKD is an aetiologically heterogeneous disorder that can be caused by a range of biological, psychological and social conditions that act individually or together to increase the risk of AD-HKD. Although we now know a good deal about the individual genetic, neurochemical, neuropathological and cognitive mechanisms involved in AD-HKD, we do not understand fully how these influences interact to cause AD-HKD, what part is played by environmental factors or whether there are distinct subgroups caused by particular factors or combinations of factors.

Much of the available evidence points to the importance of abnormal higher order cognitive functions caused by dysfunction in catecholamine metabolism and neurotransmission in the prefrontal cortex and associated subcortical structures. Primate lesion studies as well as human imaging, electrophysiological and neuropathological studies (Pardo *et al.* 1990; Corbetta *et al.* 1993; Posner & Raichle 1998) indicate that executive functions, self-regulation, arousal and motivation involve a distributed neural system that includes the orbital prefrontal, anterior cingulate cortex and related subcortical structures (basal ganglia) (Goldman-Rakic 1996, 1987; Posner *et al.* 1997). These higher order functions are the delaying, future-orientated and intentional control processes of the cognitive system that guide action and behaviour (Denckla 1996). They have a role in maintenance of alertness, sustaining of attention and effort, inhibition of inappropriate actions, and adjustment of response strategies when errors are made or circumstances change. Deficits in these processes are common among children with AD-HKD and are thought to be the proximal cause of their poorly regulated everyday behaviour and impaired performance on laboratory tasks (Pennington & Ozonoff 1996; Barkley 1997).

The neurones in the regions of the brain implicated in executive control are particularly rich in catecholamines (dopamine, adrenaline and noradrenaline), as well as other neurotransmitters. These neurotransmitters have multiple functions and vary in their distribution but are involved in motivation, action and attention. Other neurotransmitters, such as serotonin, may have a role in modulating dopamine transmission and in the expression of AD-HKD (Swanson *et al.* 1998b; Zametkin & Liotta 1998; Gainetdinov *et al.* 1999; Quist *et al.* 2000).

At low doses, stimulants reduce locomotion in both humans and animals. These drugs raise the resting extracellular levels of dopamine primarily by blocking the dopamine transporter that is involved in re-uptake of dopamine at presynaptic neurones thereby preventing re-entry of dopamine into the neurone. Dexamphetamine also directly releases dopamine from presynaptic neurones. The result is a resting increase in the availability of dopamine at the synaptic cleft and at dopamine receptor sites. During a normal nerve impulse, there is a transient rise in extracellular dopamine. The net effect of the rise in resting dopamine level with low-dose drug treatment is a reduction in the relative rise in dopamine that is triggered by an impulse (Seeman & Madras 1998).

Neuroimaging studies confirm structural and functional abnormalities in those regions of the brain that are implicated in executive function (for a review see Casey *et al.* 1997; Tannock 1998b). These studies report significantly smaller less symmetrical prefrontal and basal ganglia structures, particularly on the right side, in children with AD-HKD than in matched controls (Giedd *et al.* 1996; Casey *et al.* 1997; Filipek *et al.* 1997).

Family, twin, adoption and molecular studies offer strong evidence of genetic susceptibility to AD-HKD. Relatives of individuals with AD-HKD have an increased risk for AD-HKD (Schachar & Wachsmuth 1990; Szatmari *et al.* 1993; Faraone *et al.* 1996b). For example, siblings of children with AD-HKD have a 2–3 times greater risk of AD-HKD than siblings of normal controls (Faraone & Biederman 1994). Twin studies find a markedly higher concordance of AD-HKD for monozygotic (79%) than dizygotic (32%) twins that is consistent with high heritability of AD-HKD. Heritability estimates range from 0.7 to 0.9 (Goodman & Stevenson 1989; Gilger *et al.* 1992; Edelbrock *et al.* 1995; Eaves *et al.* 1997; Levy *et al.* 1997). Adoption studies (van den Oord *et al.* 1994) provide further evidence of a genetic component to AD-HKD; biological parents of AD-HKD individuals are more likely to exhibit AD-HKD or related disorders than are adoptive parents.

The strong evidence of genetic effects, the effect of stimulant medication on children with AD-HKD, and the concentration of neurones rich in dopamine and norepinephrine in the neural areas involved in executive function led to investigation of the role of candidate genes involved in the noradrenergic and dopaminergic systems (McCracken 1991; Castellanos 1997). To date, AD-HKD has been associated with the dopamine transporter gene (*DAT1*) (Cook *et al.* 1995; Gill *et al.* 1997; Barr *et al.*

2000) and the dopamine D4 receptor gene (LaHoste *et al.* 1996; Smalley *et al.* 1998).

Presumably, these polymorphisms or mutations in the respective genes may give rise to the AD-HKD phenotype by altering the function of the proteins involved in the transcription of the various receptors in these pathways. For example, signal transmission is blunted when dopamine binds to the 7-repeat allele receptor compared to the 2- or 4-repeat alleles. The association between specific alleles and AD-HKD could be caused by a direct pathophysiological effect or the observed polymorphism could be a marker for a nearby DNA site that influences risk for AD-HKD.

Although the evidence for a genetic mechanism involving the neurochemical and structural substrate of executive control is strongly supported by these lines of research, there is ample evidence that other mechanisms also have an important role. For example, twin studies show a small but important shared and non-shared environmental effect for AD-HKD (Eaves *et al.* 1997). Gene–environment interactions may be more important than currently believed and may be inflating estimates of the genetic component of AD-HKD in twin studies. Moreover, the magnitude of genetic influence in AD-HKD may be inflated in family, adoption and twin studies by methodological eventualities, such as parental rater bias, contributing to sibling contrast effects (Simonoff *et al.* 1998) and bias in selection of adoptive parents.

A range of psychosocial factors are associated with AD-HKD, including maternal stress during pregnancy and poor quality or disrupted early caregiving as may be seen in children in institutions or foster care (Jacobvitz & Sroufe 1987; Roy *et al.* 2000). Neurobiological risk factors, especially those acting during the period of rapid brain growth during fetal development and early life, could have a direct adverse impact on cognitive development or an indirect effect through increasing risk for neurobiological hazards. These factors include fetal exposure resulting from the mother's use of alcohol, drugs or cigarettes, and the adverse effects of perinatal obstetrical complications or prematurity (Streissguth *et al.* 1994; Breslau *et al.* 1996; Milberger *et al.* 1998). AD-HKD occurs after traumatic brain injury in 25% of cases (Max *et al.* 1997; Gerring *et al.* 1998) or after exposure to environmental toxins such as zinc or lead (Toren *et al.* 1996). The brain region involved in executive control may be particularly sensitive to perinatal hypoxia or toxins because of the terminal nature of the arterial supply to the anterior forebrain. These environmental risks probably interact among themselves and with genetic risks, making the specific role of any single factor difficult to assess accurately.

Treatment

Currently, the accepted approach to treatment involves long-term multimodal intervention in which various pharmacological and psychological treatments and combinations of treatment are used together with a supportive management strategy. Family, school and other agencies have a major role in intervention. The mainstay of treatment is stimulant medication (Miller 1999). Psychological therapy involving family, group or behaviour therapy or those involving special education are thought to be effective but have received relatively less empirical support. Special diets, dietary supplements, megavitamins, antimotion-sickness medication, and electroencephalographic biofeedback are also used but are not proven therapies (Goldstein & Ingersoll 1992; Richters *et al.* 1995; Jadad *et al.* 1998).

Current estimates place the number of US children receiving special education provisions for AD-HKD at 1 million although they are typically labelled as learning disabled, emotionally disordered or as having 'other health impairments'. The costs associated with these provisions are estimated to be in the order of 3 billion dollars annually above what is typically spent on children with a learning disability. Yet, two-thirds of children with AD-HKD receive no services: females, members of minority groups, the poor, those living in rural areas and those in health maintenance organizations are less likely to be served. AD-HKD is associated with a high family burden arising from the cost of psychological testing, tutoring, medication and other out-of-pocket expenses.

Methylphenidate (Ritalin) and, to a much lesser extent, dexamphetamine are the most frequently prescribed treatments for AD-HKD in North America (Rappley *et al.* 1995; Safer *et al.* 1996). Tricyclic antidepressants and α_2-noradrenergic agonists, such as clonidine and guanfacine, are second-line drug treatments for children who have an inadequate response to stimulants (Greenhill *et al.* 1996; Cantwell 1998).

The number of prescriptions of medication for children with AD-HKD has more than doubled over the last two decades to 5 million in the USA: about 3% of persons aged 5–18 years (1.5 million children) are taking medication for AD-HKD (Safer *et al.* 1996). The prevalence of the use of medication is lower in Canada, Europe and Australasia (about 1%) than in the USA, but is beginning to rise (Miller 1999). Community physicians rely heavily on medication for the treatment of AD-HKD: as many as 88% of diagnosed children receive drug treatment at some point in time (Wolraich & Baumgaertel 1997).

The steady growth in the use of medication is driven by the more frequent identification of affected persons, in particular, those with inattention only; the growth in rate of identification and treatment of girls, preschool-age children, adolescents and adults; and the increased length of the treatment for each individual. The rising prevalence of the use of medication may also be linked to a lack of affordable and feasible non-drug treatment; greater familiarity with and acceptance of medication; and an absence of convincing evidence that non-pharmacological interventions are as effective as those involving medication.

Therapeutic effects of stimulants

Heyman & Santosh (Chapter 59) deal with the main efficacy

and pharmacokinetic issues for these medications. Numerous placebo-controlled randomized control trials (for meta-analyses see Jadad *et al.* 1998; Miller 1999) confirm the substantial short-term benefits of stimulants. Stimulants markedly and rapidly reduce the overt clinical manifestations of AD-HKD, such as restlessness, inattentiveness and impulsiveness, improve the quality of social interactions, decrease aggression and increase compliance (Cunningham *et al.* 1991; Hinshaw & James 1991; Whalen & Henker 1991). By comparison, the effect on laboratory measures of attention is evident but less robust. Stimulants increase accuracy, facilitate error detection, improve the ability to focus on the most relevant aspects of a stimulus array and decrease impulsive responses without causing undue narrowing of attention or rigidity of thought in most cases (Douglas *et al.* 1995; Tannock *et al.* 1995; Brumaghim & Klorman 1998). Moreover, stimulants increase persistence, effort and frustration tolerance (Milich *et al.* 1991). Improvement is evident on a range of demanding divergent thinking tasks, not just on boring, simple or repetitive tasks (Nigg *et al.* 1997) and stimulants also improve academic productivity (Tannock *et al.* 1989; Rapport *et al.* 1994). However, stimulants have far less of a beneficial effect on school work. There is no evidence that the information learned while a child is receiving medication is recalled less easily later when the child is not medicated (this is known as state-dependent learning; Becker-Mattes *et al.* 1985).

In a substantial proportion of children mood, self-esteem and anxiety improve (Buhrmester *et al.* 1992; Ahmann *et al.* 1993; Pelham *et al.* 1997) although in some there is a decrease in social interaction (Whalen *et al.* 1989). Medication does not seem to engender attribution of success to external factors rather than to personal effort (Pelham *et al.* 1997). Even prolonged treatment with stimulants does not appear to increase the risk of drug use or abuse and may even prevent them (Hechtman & Weiss 1986; Biederman *et al.* 1999). No adverse events or reduction in height or weight have been demonstrated over long periods of treatment (Schertz *et al.* 1996; Spencer *et al.* 1998).

Preschool-age children and those with low intelligence respond favourably to stimulants (Firestone *et al.* 1998) but are somewhat less responsive to stimulants than are school-aged children of average intelligence and somewhat more prone to develop side-effects (Pisterman *et al.* 1989; Handen *et al.* 1991; Mayes *et al.* 1994). Stimulants are effective among adolescents (Klorman *et al.* 1990), adults (Spencer *et al.* 1996) and children with neurodevelopmental delay (Handen *et al.* 1991), aggression (Klorman *et al.* 1994; Klein *et al.* 1997) or comorbid tics (Gadow *et al.* 1995). A greater severity of AD-HKD symptoms, younger age and, possibly, absence of symptoms of anxiety predict a better clinical response to stimulants (Taylor *et al.* 1987; DuPaul *et al.* 1994; Pliszka *et al.* 1994; Buitelaar 1995; Diamond *et al.* 1999). Tolerance to methylphenidate can develop in some children over months or years of continuous therapy (Sleator *et al.* 1974; Kupietz *et al.* 1988; Swanson *et al.* 1999). About one-third of these children may require increased dosage (Safer & Allen 1989).

Limitations of stimulant medication

Although stimulants have proved effective, they have their limitations. They are thought by many to be prescribed too frequently and inappropriately and to be a public health risk in their own right because of their potential for undetected long-term adverse events, for abuse and for the way that they can distract from 'genuine' treatments.

Medication is not an acceptable treatment option for many children and families. Many families believe that their child's problems reside in the context of key relationships or in the child's school. Others are more concerned about comorbid learning, behaviour or emotional disorders and less interested in treatment of hyperactivity *per se*. Other families are concerned about the biological or ethical implications of treating young children with drugs or about the potential for unknown long-term risks of treatment.

Lack of adherence limits the effectiveness of medication, as it does with all medical treatments. Adherence is lower among adolescents because of their increased autonomy, their determination to make important decisions for themselves and their dislike of being 'different' from their friends. A substantial number of individuals are able to manage quite well after discontinuing medication but many choose to restart medication following a medication-free period because of deteriorating behaviour or school performance.

Typically, children take immediate-release stimulant medication twice daily or a sustained-release preparation once daily. Medication has a limited duration of action and difficulties may arise during medication-free periods (Schachar *et al.* 1997). Administration of medication three times daily can have advantages when tolerated but can be associated with an increase in side-effects in some children (Kent *et al.* 1995; Greenhill *et al.* 1996; Corkum *et al.* 1998).

Even though a beneficial impact of behaviour, as rated by their teachers, may occur in about 70% of treated children (Spencer *et al.* 1996), treatment normalizes the behaviour of only about half of children (Rapport *et al.* 1994) and many disabilities remain. Stimulants have only a limited impact on school grades (Rapport *et al.* 1994). One-quarter of children with AD-HKD who are aggressive before treatment show no increase in prosocial behaviour or improvement in processing of social information (Hinshaw *et al.* 1989). Stimulant medication may increase socially inhibited behaviour, social withdrawal and dysphoria. Consequently, the child may be perceived as socially unresponsive, with the result the child may be less liked by peers or adults (Buhrmester *et al.* 1992; Granger *et al.* 1993a,b).

Children with AD-HKD and comorbid anxiety may have a somewhat less robust behavioural response to stimulants and possibly a greater incidence of side-effects than children with AD-HKD without comorbid anxiety (DuPaul *et al.* 1994). However, a differential treatment response has not been detected with long-term treatment (Diamond *et al.* 1999) and many children with AD-HKD and comorbid anxiety may show a reduction in anxiety as their hyperactivity abates.

Although generally safe, stimulant medication does have side-effects in a significant proportion of recipients that, in some cases, result in the termination of treatment. Loss of appetite, weight loss, insomnia, headaches and stomach aches are the most frequent side-effects although many children with AD-HKD have these complaints before starting treatment (Barkley *et al.* 1990b; Ahmann *et al.* 1993). Stimulant-related disruption of sleep is not uncommon (e.g. delayed sleep onset; Corkum *et al.* 1998; Tirosh *et al.* 1993; Kent *et al.* 1995). Initial physiological side-effects tend to persist, whereas other side-effects, such as irritability and moodiness, tend to have delayed onset (Schachar *et al.* 1997).

One of the most significant limitations of stimulant medication is the lack of evidence of its efficacy over prolonged periods of treatment. Available evidence indicates that extended treatment with stimulants improves core behavioural symptoms for as long as it is taken, although few subjects become indistinguishable from their normal peers (Conrad *et al.* 1971; Abikoff & Gittelman 1985). On cessation of the medication, benefits dissipate rapidly (Brown *et al.* 1986; Gillberg *et al.* 1997). Even with prolonged administration, stimulants may not reliably improve academic attainment, reduce the risk of developing antisocial behaviour, facilitate peer relationships or enhance self-esteem (Barkley *et al.* 1990a; Fischer *et al.* 1993).

Health care costs are an important measure of effectiveness. However, no evidence is available about how well stimulant medication reduces the overall health care costs associated with AD-HKD.

Psychological treatments

Various psychological therapies have been used for AD-HKD, either as an alternative to medication or as a method of augmenting the effects of medication. Behaviour parent training is the most commonly prescribed psychological intervention for AD-HKD. Parent training is predicated on the observation that parents of children with AD-HKD use overly controlling and inefficient parenting strategies (Mash & Johnston 1990) and that adversity in the parent–child relationship is predictive of poor outcome (Taylor *et al.* 1996). Parent-training programmes are based on social learning theory. They use direct instruction, modelling and role-playing to teach parents to reinforce positive behaviour, decrease the use of punitive strategies, and manage defiant, stubborn and inappropriate behaviour effectively (Cunningham *et al.* 1993).

Parent-training programmes improve the parents' child-management skills, enhance their self-confidence, reduce family stress and mitigate oppositional behaviour (Barkley *et al.* 1992b; Pisterman *et al.* 1992; Anastopoulos *et al.* 1993; Webster-Stratton & Hammond 1997). The important advantages of parent training are its relatively low cost, its ability to be delivered in the community rather than in clinics, thereby reducing barriers to participation, and its ability to be adapted to the needs of specific ethnic or cultural groups (Cunningham *et al.* 1995). However, parent training does not reduce the core symp-

toms of AD-HKD as effectively as does stimulant medication, nor does it appear to enhance the effectiveness of stimulants (Firestone *et al.* 1986; Horn *et al.* 1991; Jadad *et al.* 1998). Benefits tend not to persist beyond the period of treatment.

Behavioural therapy involves trained therapists, parents or teachers who reinforce positive behaviour and academic accomplishment, and who use response–cost procedures (withholding rewards when inappropriate behaviour occurs) to reduce disruptive behaviour (Abramowitz *et al.* 1992). Cognitive-behaviour therapy attempts to enhance self-control by teaching children self-instructional strategies. Social skills training targets the child's problems with peers and adults, typically in a group setting. These therapies may yield short-term improvement when administered on their own (Abikoff 1991; Carlson *et al.* 1992; Frankel *et al.* 1997; Pfiffner & McBurnett 1997), but there is little evidence that they are as potent as medication or routinely add to the effects of medication (MTA Cooperative Group 1999a,b).

Multimodal treatment

Families most frequently choose combined treatments, although the additional benefits accruing from treatment combinations are unclear (Jadad *et al.* 1998, 1999). A large multisite study in the USA recently tested the relative effectiveness of various treatment strategies delivered individually and in combination in 576 school-aged children with AD-HKD (MTA Cooperative Group 1999a,b). Four treatment strategies were compared:
1 drug treatment (mostly methylphenidate);
2 drug treatment combined with an intensive psychosocial intervention strategy (family therapy, social skills training, an intensive summer camp programme and classroom management);
3 psychosocial intervention alone; and
4 a typical community-based intervention.
All subjects received the same assessment, but those in the community-based intervention were referred to facilities in the community and their family physicians for treatment. The other treatments were administered by research personnel.

The implications of this study are currently being debated. Psychosocial treatment, when administered without medication, was generally equivalent to that of community-based treatment even though community treatment involved medication in two-thirds of cases. Combined intervention was minimally superior to medication administered alone across the entire group of participants. The additional benefit was most evident among the small subgroup of children who had more emotional symptoms and poorer home life. Combined treatment achieved equivalent improvement to medication alone but with lower doses of medication. Many children in the community-based intervention received medication, but they did not seem to progress as well as those who received medication from study physicians. This was particularly true for children with AD-HKD who also had prominent anxiety symptoms. This finding suggests that medication management that is intensive and coupled with supportive counselling and that is responsive to the presence of anxiety may be superior to the medication treatment most children receive in the community.

In summary, psychological interventions are an important treatment option, particularly for families who do not wish to use medication. On their own, they are less effective than well-delivered medication but as effective as medication administered in the community. The primary benefit of combined parent training and medication may be reduction of secondary impairments, such as the conflict between parents and children in subgroups of AD-HKD cases with emotional symptoms or poor parent–child relationships (MTA Cooperative Group 1999a,b). However, both the medication management protocol and the intensive psychosocial interventions used in this study are not typically available in the community. There are many unanswered questions about timing, intensity, duration, availability and cost of psychological interventions (Boyle & Pickles 1997; Cunningham 1999; Pelham 1999).

Management

Diagnosis and assessment

The preceding description of the range of AD-HKD manifestations, situational variability, comorbidity and associated impairment points to the complexity of the assessment and treatment of the disorder (Dulcan & Benson 1997; Goldman *et al.* 1998). Reports of hyperactive behaviour are quite subjective and there is considerable variability across settings. Consequently, the diagnostician would be wise to employ converging measures of behaviour derived from more than a single informant. Typically, the assessor will obtain information from the child's parents, the child and the child's classroom teacher. The diagnostician should elicit descriptions of child behaviour because global impressions of AD-HKD symptoms can be very misleading and subject to bias or halo effect arising from the informant's mental state or beliefs about the nature of AD-HKD. Behaviour rating scales provide a valuable, simple and inexpensive means to collect descriptions of child behaviour from various informants but they are subject to the same bias and error as other measures.

During the assessment, the physician must investigate the presence of a concurrent disorder and the relationship of the symptoms of a comorbid disorder and AD-HKD. For example, are the restlessness and inattention of a child limited to a period of anxiety or depression? Are the AD-HKD symptoms part of a conduct disorder, substance abuse disorder, or Tourette syndrome?

Children with AD-HKD are able to suppress their inattention, restlessness and impulsiveness to a great extent in novel and highly structured situations, such as those afforded by the typical visit to the physician's office. Direct examination of the younger child may be limited by the child's apparent lack of insight into his or her behaviour or an inability to communicate

as a result of learning or language impairment. Nevertheless, the interview with the child may be useful for identifying comorbid disorders, assessing the relationship of symptoms to anxiety or academic demands, monitoring treatment, and establishing the rapport that is required to sustain a prolonged intervention.

Because many children meet AD-HKD criteria almost exclusively on the basis of behavioural difficulties within the school context, it is essential to assess the presence of learning difficulties, the nature of the educational experience and the quality of the child's relationships with peers and teachers. Consultation from an educational psychologist and speech pathologist is very important in assessing the nature of the academic difficulties and the potential contribution of speech and language delay to deviant child behaviour.

Assessment of adolescents and adults

The diagnostic process in adolescents and adults is complicated in several ways. The manifestations of the disorder change with age. Gross motor activity decreases and an inner sense of restlessness, fidgeting and inattention emerges as the primary expression of disorder. It becomes more difficult to obtain an accurate description of the adolescent's behaviour, especially in the school and work settings, because of the absence of a consistent informant. These considerations place increased importance on the interview of the adolescent concerning their own social, scholastic and behavioural problems.

It is generally accepted that an adult diagnosis of AD-HKD requires a childhood history of AD-HKD (Shaffer & Greenhill 1979). In many cases, there is no informant who knew the person as a child and there may be no possibility of obtaining reliable school records. Despite these obvious difficulties, the diagnosis of AD-HKD in adults based on self-report seems to be reliable (Spencer *et al.* 1994; Faraone *et al.* 1997b).

The diagnostic process among adolescents and adults is also complicated by high rates of anxiety, mood disorder, personality disorder and substance abuse, for which they may have received extensive treatment. AD-HKD uncomplicated by comorbid psychopathology is rare in this age group, in part because of the consequences of lifetime AD-HKD. Distinguishing 'primary' hyperactivity that has led to secondary psychopathology from hyperactivity that arises as a secondary manifestation of another disorder can be challenging.

Differential diagnosis

There are several conditions that can mimic AD-HKD but which require very different treatment. These conditions include the effects of prescription medication (phenobarbital, antihistamines, theophylline, sympathomimetics or steroids), substance abuse, metabolic disorders (hyperthyroidism), toxic conditions (lead poisoning), anxiety and mood disorder. In its early stages, Tourette syndrome may be evident in symptoms of hyperactivity. Despite robust evidence for cognitive, neuropsychological, neurophysiological and biochemical deficits in children with AD-HKD, there are no known laboratory tests that have sufficient diagnostic sensitivity and specificity to distinguish children with AD-HKD from unaffected children or from those with other disorders. Specific laboratory tests may be necessary to exclude suspected problems, such as poor hearing or vision, metabolic disease, drug abuse or exposure to toxins. Although there is an increased prevalence of AD-HKD among persons with a generalized resistance to the thyroid hormone, thyroid abnormalities are rare among individuals with AD-HKD and routine screening for thyroid abnormality is not indicated (Hauser *et al.* 1997; Woodward *et al.* 1989).

Not infrequently, children with AD-HKD also present with severe emotional and behavioural dysregulation, high irritability, extremely low frustration tolerance and episodes of aggression. Although these individuals show subtle rather than clear evidence of mania, euphoria or grandiosity, some believe that a diagnosis of bipolar disorder is warranted and a trial of mood-stabilizing medication appropriate. This subgroup of AD-HKD individuals is more likely than others to have a family member affected by bipolar disorder (Wozniak *et al.* 1995a,b). It is not yet clear whether the disturbance of these individuals is best understood as a variant of mood disorder or as a particularly extreme form of AD-HKD.

Other conditions may be identified at the time of assessment, such as fetal alcohol syndrome or the consequences of traumatic brain injury. For the most part, hyperactivity associated with these disorders leads to the same treatment as for primary AD-HKD although the evidence to support this practice is largely lacking.

Management strategies

AD-HKD is a chronic condition that affects many aspects of a child's life over a prolonged period of time. Consequently, it requires a comprehensive management strategy that targets all facets of the disorder. The persistent nature of the disorder dictates the need for consistent long-term case management. Treatment must be flexible, both in kind and in intensity, to reflect the social, physiological and cognitive developments and variations in the life of each child and his or her family. Medication is unlikely to be the only course of action. Drug and psychological interventions need to be layered according to the needs of the child and family. There are families who are not ready for or capable of undertaking treatments other than those involving medication. For many of these families, a period of symptomatic improvement resulting from successful drug therapy may provide the impetus for entry into other essential non-pharmacological components of therapy. Some families may not consider non-pharmacological interventions until they observe that an immediate increase in academic productivity does not necessarily translate into better grades at the end of the year and that teachers' report of improved behaviour at school does not ensure improved family and peer relationships. Other families may be too chaotic to use medications appropriately and may first need to try psychological interventions under close supervision. Some

components of behavioural intervention, such as time out or punishment tactics, can be used in a punitive manner and are not necessarily more benign than medication. Some families are more content with the decision to use medication if it follows a period of counselling or behavioural intervention (Slimmer & Brown 1985).

It is often recommended that pharmacological treatment commence with a systematic double-blind trial of immediate-release methylphenidate or dexamphetamine. Many parents are reassured by the rigor of a systematic trial (Johnston & Fine 1993). Systematic trials are not particularly complicated and can be organized in typical clinical practice. On the other hand, systematic trials seem to have little advantage over open trials. There is little evidence of a sustained placebo effect, and doses determined by a systematic trial tend to be similar to those determined by open titration. Consequently, the extra cost of a double-blind trial may not be justified (Pliszka *et al.* 2000).

Education is an important part of treatment because it helps parents and the affected child to develop an understanding of the nature of the disorder. Moreover, increased knowledge may result in more realistic expectations of and better adherence to treatment. Regular contact with the child's teacher is useful to monitor behavioural improvement and side-effects in the school setting. Behavioural response and side-effects must be monitored regularly (MTA Cooperative Group 1999a,b).

Comparison of physicians' actual clinical practice with the results of recommendations of authorities for the medical management of AD-HKD show that management may be suboptimal in about one-third of cases (Miller 1999). Diagnosis often fails to include consideration of behaviour in multiple settings, presence of comorbid psychopathology, and associated impairments. Medication may not be monitored closely enough and non-pharmacological components of care are not implemented. Although stimulant medication may be relatively easy to prescribe because of its favourable effects and low risk of adverse effects, there is ample evidence that the quality of medical management has an impact on treatment outcome (MTA Cooperative Group 1999a,b).

Prevention

Primary prevention of AD-HKD, like that of other mental illnesses, requires intervention to alter identified population health risks. Apparently, hyperactivity has a multifactorial aetiology and each factor accounts for only a small portion of the variance in the incidence of the disorder or outcome. Unless we can identify subgroups in which specific causes have a large impact, it will be very difficult to effect a public health intervention.

The validity of HD, the most narrowly defined syndrome, is most easily supported by current research. Consequently, this may be the optimal subgroup for research purposes. However, the most narrowly defined syndrome might not be optimal from a public health perspective because it may be more effective to reduce the overall burden of suffering in the population by diminishing impairment across the severity spectrum.

Several groups of hyperactive children seem to be at particularly great risk and targeted intervention seems appropriate for these groups. For example, preschool-age children with the triad of AD-HKD, aggression and impairment of language and learning are at particularly high risk for persistent AD-HKD and for significant impairment in later life (Moffitt 1990). Children at any age who have marked learning problems, pervasive hyperactivity and conduct disturbance are also at high risk. Early detection and intervention for targeted groups of children with AD-HKD may reduce impairment for the affected child and the burden of suffering for the families and communities. Given the high prevalence of AD-HKD, it is not reasonable to assume that traditional clinic-based services will be able to meet this considerable mental health need. Nevertheless, there is a clear need for a multidimensional, multidisciplinary and comprehensive clinical assessment to establish the initial diagnosis, plan treatment and support the long-term management of affected persons.

Conclusions

AD-HKD is likely to remain a controversial disorder among professionals and lay individuals. This is not surprising given questions about the measurement of individual symptoms and differences in diagnostic practice among professionals. Moreover, the widespread use of stimulant medication will rightly remain a contentious social and scientific issue. The same social factors that aided the development in the nineteenth century of the concept of hyperactivity as a medical condition may be operating today. A clearer understanding of these social factors can benefit our understanding of this entity, enhance our ability to prevent disorder and assist affected individuals.

We have learned much about the biological, psychological and social causes of this particular constellation of behaviours. There is little doubt that hereditary and acquired biological factors have a role in the genesis of hyperactivity, although no single genetic or biological risk factor seems adequate to account for AD-HKD in most cases. Psychosocial factors also increase the risk of hyperactivity. There is clear evidence that cognitive factors are involved in AD-HKD and may serve to span the gap between brain and behaviour. Despite frequent changes in nosology, hyperactivity has aided communication among professionals, facilitated our understanding of the relationship between brain and behaviour and stimulated the development of intervention programmes and research.

Much remains to be learned about the effective management of hyperactivity. Despite our growing understanding of the role of the cognitive, genetic and neuropathological substrate of AD-HKD, our clinical and therapeutic concepts of the disorder remain primarily at a descriptive level, emphasizing and treating the observable behavioural deficits and associated impairments rather than the fundamental abnormality of the disorder. Med-

ication is effective for many children and can provide respite from the symptoms of AD-HKD during which time other essential aspects of therapy can be implemented. Nevertheless, several of the worst outcomes of AD-HKD are seen in adolescence and adulthood. The risk for these adverse outcomes must be reduced. To date, no intervention in childhood is demonstrably effective for this purpose. The development of acceptable, cost-effective and widely available non-pharmacological therapies for AD-HKD remains a priority for the field, as is the development of further pharmacological options for those children who do not benefit from stimulants or other currently available medications. In the short term, there is much to be done to improve the quality of care provided to affected children and their families even given our current limited understanding of the disorder and its treatment.

References

Abikoff, H. (1991) Cognitive training in ADHD children: less to it than meets the eye. *Journal of Learning Disabilities*, 24, 205–209.

Abikoff, H. & Gittelman, R. (1985) The normalizing effects of methylphenidate on the classroom behavior of ADDH children. *Journal of Abnormal Psychology*, 13, 33–44.

Abikoff, H., Courtney, M. & Koplewicz, H. (1991) Halo effects and teachers' ratings of children's classroom behavior. *38th Annual Meeting of the American Academy of Child and Adolescent Psychiatry*, San Francisco.

Abramowitz, A.J., Eckstrand, D., O'Leary, S.G. & Dulcan, M.K. (1992) ADHD children's responses to stimulant medication and two intensities of a behavioral intervention. *Behavior Modification*, 16, 193–203.

Ahmann, P.A., Waltonen, S.J., Olson, K.A., Theye, F.W., Van Erem, A.J. & LaPlant, R.J. (1993) Placebo-controlled evaluation of Ritalin side effects. *Pediatrics*, 91, 1101–1106.

American Psychiatric Association (1968) *Diagnostic and Statistical Manual of Mental Disorders: DSM-II*, 2nd edn. Washington D.C.

American Psychiatric Association (1980) *Diagnostic and Statistical Manual of Mental Disorders: DSM-III*, 3rd edn. Washington D.C.

American Psychiatric Association (1987) *Diagnostic and Statistical Manual of Mental Disorders–Revised: DSM-III-R*, 3rd edn. Washington D.C.

American Psychiatric Association (1994) *Diagnostic and Statistical Manual of Mental Disorders: DSM-IV*, 4th edn. Washington D.C.

Anastopoulos, A.D., Shelton, T.L., DuPaul, G.J. & Guevremont, D.C. (1993) Parent training for attention-deficit hyperactivity disorder: its impact on parent functioning. *Journal of Abnormal Child Psychology*, 21, 581–596.

Babinski, L.M., Hartsough, C.S. & Lambert, N.M. (1999) Childhood conduct problems, hyperactivity–impulsivity, and inattention as predictors of adult criminal activity. *Journal of Child Psychology and Psychiatry*, 40, 347–355.

Barkley, R. (1995) Is there an attention deficit in ADHD? *ADHD Report*, 3, 1–4.

Barkley, R.A. (1997) Behavioral inhibition, sustained attention, and executive functions: constructing a unifying theory of ADHD. *Psychological Bulletin*, 121, 65–94.

Barkley, R.A. (1998) Attention-deficit hyperactivity disorder. *Scientific American*, 279, 66–71.

Barkley, R.A., Karlsson, J., Pollard, S. & Murphy, J.V. (1985) Developmental changes in the mother–child interactions of hyperactive boys: effects of two dose levels of Ritalin. *Journal of Child Psychology and Psychiatry*, 26, 705–715.

Barkley, R.A., Fischer, M., Edelbrock, C.S. & Smallish, L. (1990a) The adolescent outcome of hyperactive children diagnosed by research criteria. I. An 8-year prospective follow-up study. *Journal of the American Academy of Child and Adolescent Psychiatry*, 29, 546–557.

Barkley, R.A., McMurray, M.B., Edelbrock, C.S. & Robbins, K. (1990b) Side effects of methylphenidate in children with attention deficit hyperactivity disorder: a systemic, placebo-controlled evaluation. *Pediatrics*, 86, 184–192.

Barkley, R.A., Grodzinsky, G. & DuPaul, G.J. (1992a) Frontal lobe functions in attention deficit disorder with and without hyperactivity: a review and research report. *Journal of Abnormal Child Psychology*, 20, 163–188.

Barkley, R.A., Guevremont, D.C., Anastopoulos, A.D. & Fletcher, K.E. (1992b) A comparison of three family therapy programs for treating family conflicts in adolescents with attention-deficit hyperactivity disorder. *Journal of Consulting and Clinical Psychology*, 60, 450–462.

Barkley, R.A., Murphy, K.R. & Kwasnik, D. (1996) Motor vehicle driving competencies and risks in teens and young adults with attention deficit hyperactivity disorder. *Pediatrics*, 98, 1089–1095.

Barr, C.L., Wigg, K.G., Bloom, S. *et al.* (2000) Further evidence from haplotype analysis for linkage of the dopamine D4 receptor gene and attention-deficit hyperactivity disorder. *American Journal of Medical Genetics*, 96, 262–267.

Bax, M. & McKeith, R. (1963) *Minimal Cerebral Dysfunction*. NSS-MEIU/Heineman.

Becker-Mattes, A., Mattes, J.A., Abikoff, H. & Brandt, L. (1985) State-dependent learning in hyperactive children receiving methylphenidate. *American Journal of Psychiatry*, 142, 455–459.

Biederman, J., Faraone, S.V., Mick, E. *et al.* (1995) High risk for attention deficit hyperactivity disorder among children of parents with childhood onset of the disorder: a pilot study. *American Journal of Psychiatry*, 152, 431–435.

Biederman, J., Wilens, T., Mick, E., Spencer, T. & Faraone, S.V. (1999) Pharmacotherapy of attention-deficit/hyperactivity disorder reduces risk for substance use disorder. *Pediatrics*, 104, e20.

Boyle, M.H. & Pickles, A.R. (1997) Influence of maternal depressive symptoms on ratings of childhood behavior. *Journal of Abnormal Child Psychology*, 25, 399–412.

Boyle, M.H., Offord, D.R., Racine, Y., Szatmari, P., Fleming, J.E. & Sanford, M. (1996) Identifying thresholds for classifying childhood psychiatric disorder: issues and prospects. *Journal of the American Academy of Child and Adolescent Psychiatry*, 35, 1440–1448.

Bradley, C. (1937) The behavior of children receiving benzedrine. *American Journal of Psychiatry*, 94, 577–585.

Breslau, N., Brown, G.G., DelDotto, J.E. *et al.* (1996) Psychiatric sequelae of low birth weight at 6 years of age. *Journal of Abnormal Child Psychology*, 24, 385–400.

Brown, R.T., Borden, K.A., Wynne, M.E., Schleser, R. & Clingerman, S.R. (1986) Methylphenidate and cognitive therapy with ADD children: a methodological reconsideration. *Journal of Abnormal Child Psychology*, 14, 481–497.

Brumaghim, J.T. & Klorman, R. (1998) Methylphenidate's effects on paired-associate learning and event-related potentials of young adults. *Psychophysiology*, 35, 73–85.

Buhrmester, D., Whalen, C.K., Henker, B., MacDonald, V. & Hinshaw, S.P. (1992) Prosocial behavior in hyperactive boys: effects of stimulant medication and comparison with normal boys. *Journal of Abnormal Child Psychology*, 20, 103–121.

Buitelaar, J.K., Van der Gaag, R.J., Swaab-Barneveld, H. & Kuiper, M. (1995) Prediction of clinical response to methylphenidate in children with attention-deficit hyperactivity disorder. *Journal of the American Academy of Child and Adolescent Psychiatry*, 34, 1025–1032.

Cantwell, D.P. (1998) ADHD through the life span: the role of bupropion in treatment. *Journal of Clinical Psychiatry*, 59, 92–94.

Cantwell, D.P. & Baker, L. (1988) Issues in the classification of child and adolescent psychopathology. *Journal of the American Academy of Child and Adolescent Psychiatry*, 27, 521–533.

Cantwell, D.P. & Baker, L. (1992) Attention deficit disorder with and without hyperactivity: a review and comparison of matched groups. *Journal of the American Academy of Child and Adolescent Psychiatry*, 31, 432–438.

Carlson, C.L., Pelham, W.E. Jr, Milich, R. & Dixon, J. (1992) Single and combined effects of methylphenidate and behavior therapy on the classroom performance of children with attention-deficit hyperactivity disorder. *Journal of Abnormal Child Psychology*, 20, 213–232.

Caron, C. & Rutter, M. (1991) Comorbidity in child psychopathology: concepts, issues and research strategies. *Journal of Child Psychology and Psychiatry*, 32, 1063–1080.

Casey, B.J., Castellanos, F.X., Giedd, J.N. *et al.* (1997) Implication of right frontostriatal circuitry in response inhibition and attention-deficit/hyperactivity disorder. *Journal of the American Academy of Child and Adolescent Psychiatry*, 36, 374–383.

Castellanos, F.X. (1997) Toward a pathophysiology of attention-deficit/hyperactivity disorder. *Clinical Pediatrics*, 36, 381–393.

Chess, S. (1960) Diagnosis and treatment of the hyperactive child. *New York State Journal of Medicine*, 60, 2379–2385.

Clements, S.D. (1966) *Minimal Brain Dysfunction in Children: Terminology and Identification—Phase one of a three-phase project*. US Department of Health, Education and Welfare, Washington D.C.

Cohen, N.J., Vallance, D.D., Barwick, M. *et al.* (2000) The interface between ADHD and language impairment: an examination of language, achievement, and cognitive processing. *Journal of Child Psychology and Psychiatry*, 41, 353–362.

Conrad, W.G., Dworkin, E.S., Shai, A. & Tobiessen, J.E. (1971) Effects of amphetamine therapy and prescriptive tutoring on the behavior and achievement of lower class hyperactive children. *Journal of Learning Disabilities*, 4, 45–53.

Cook, E.H. Jr, Stein, M.A., Krasowski, M.D. *et al.* (1995) Association of attention-deficit disorder and the dopamine transporter gene. *American Journal of Human Genetics*, 56, 993–998.

Corbetta, M., Miezin, F.M., Shulman, G.L. & Petersen, S.E. (1993) A PET study of visuospatial attention. *Journal of Neuroscience*, 13, 1202–1226.

Corkum, P., Tannock, R. & Moldofsky, H. (1998) Sleep disturbances in children with attention-deficit/hyperactivity disorder. *Journal of the American Academy of Child and Adolescent Psychiatry*, 37, 637–646.

Cunningham, C.E. (1999) In the wake of the MTA: charting a new course for the study and treatment of children with attention-deficit hyperactivity disorder. *Canadian Journal of Psychiatry*, 44, 999–1006.

Cunningham, C.E., Siegel, L.S. & Offord, D.R. (1991) A dose–response analysis of the effects of methylphenidate on the peer interactions and simulated classroom performance of ADD children with and without conduct problems. *Journal of Child Psychology and Psychiatry*, 32, 439–452.

Cunningham, C.E., Davis, J.R., Bremner, R., Dunn, K.W. & Rzasa, T. (1993) Coping modeling problem solving versus mastery modeling: effects on adherence, in-session process, and skill acquisition in a residential parent-training program. *Journal of Consulting and Clinical Psychology*, 61, 871–877.

Cunningham, C.E., Bremner, R. & Boyle, M. (1995) Large group community-based parenting programs for families of preschoolers at risk for disruptive behaviour disorders: utilization, cost effectiveness, and outcome. *Journal of Child Psychology and Psychiatry*, **36**, 1141–1159.

Danckaerts, M. & Taylor, E. (1995) The epidemiology of childhood hyperactivity. In: *The Epidemiology of Child and Adolescent Psychopathology* (eds F.C. Verhulst & H.M. Koot), pp. 178–209. Oxford University Press, Oxford.

Denckla, M.B. (1996) Research on executive function in a neurodevelopmental context: application of clinical measures. *Developmental Neuropsychology*, **12**, 5–15.

Diamond, I.R., Tannock, R. & Schachar, R.J. (1999) Response to methylphenidate in children with ADHD and comorbid anxiety. *Journal of the American Academy of Child and Adolescent Psychiatry*, **38**, 402–409.

Douglas, V.I. (1972) Stop, look and listen: the problem of sustained attention and impulse control in hyperactive and normal children. *Canadian Journal of Behavioral Science*, **4**, 259–282.

Douglas, V.I. (1988) Attention deficit disorder: criteria, cognition, intervention. In: *Cognitive Deficits in Children with Attention Deficit Disorder with Hyperactivity* (eds L.M. Bloomingdale & J. Sergeant), pp. 65–82. Pergamon, New York.

Douglas, V.I. & Benezra, E. (1990) Supraspan verbal memory in attention deficit disorder with hyperactivity normal and reading-disabled boys. *Journal of Abnormal Child Psychology*, **18**, 617–638.

Douglas, V.I., Barr, R.G., Desilets, J. & Sherman, E. (1995) Do high doses of stimulants impair flexible thinking in attention-deficit hyperactivity disorder? *Journal of the American Academy of Child and Adolescent Psychiatry*, **34**, 877–885.

Dulcan, M.K. & Benson, R.S. (1997) AACAP Official Action: summary of the practice parameters for the assessment and treatment of children, adolescents, and adults with ADHD. *Journal of the American Academy of Child and Adolescent Psychiatry*, **36**, 1311–1317.

DuPaul, G.J., Barkley, R.A. & McMurray, M.B. (1994) Response of children with ADHD to methylphenidate: interaction with internalizing symptoms. *Journal of the American Academy of Child and Adolescent Psychiatry*, **33**, 894–903.

Eaves, L.J., Silberg, J.L., Meyer, J.M. *et al.* (1997) Genetics and developmental psychopathology. II. The main effects of genes and environment on behavioral problems in the Virginia Twin Study of Adolescent Behavioral Development. *Journal of Child Psychology and Psychiatry*, **38**, 965–980.

Edelbrock, C., Rende, R., Plomin, R. & Thompson, L.A. (1995) A twin study of competence and problem behavior in childhood and early adolescence. *Journal of Child Psychology and Psychiatry*, **36**, 775–785.

Eiraldi, R.B., Power, T.J. & Nezu, C.M. (1997) Patterns of comorbidity associated with subtypes of attention-deficit/hyperactivity disorder among 6- to 12-year-old children. *Journal of the American Academy of Child and Adolescent Psychiatry*, **36**, 503–514.

Faraone, S.V. & Biederman, J. (1994) Is attention deficit hyperactivity disorder familial? *Harvard Review of Psychiatry*, **1**, 271–287.

Faraone, S.V., Biederman, J., Lehman, B.K. *et al.* (1993) Evidence for the independent familial transmission of attention deficit hyperactivity disorder and learning disabilities: results from a family genetic study. *American Journal of Psychiatry*, **150**, 891–895.

Faraone, S.V., Biederman, J., Mennin, D., Gershon, J. & Tsuang, M.T. (1996a) A prospective four-year follow-up study of children at risk for ADHD: psychiatric, neuropsychological, and psychosocial outcome. *Journal of the American Academy of Child and Adolescent Psychiatry*, **35**, 1449–1459.

Faraone, S.V., Biederman, J., Mick, E. *et al.* (1996b) Attention deficit hyperactivity disorder in a multigenerational pedigree. *Biological Psychiatry*, **39**, 906–908.

Faraone, S.V., Biederman, J., Jetton, J.G. & Tsuang, M.T. (1997a) Attention deficit disorder and conduct disorder: longitudinal evidence for a familial subtype. *Psychological Medicine*, **27**, 291–300.

Faraone, S.V., Biederman, J. & Mick, E. (1997b) Symptom reports by adults with attention deficit hyperactivity disorder: are they influenced by attention deficit hyperactivity disorder in their children? *Journal of Nervous and Mental Disease*, **185**, 583–584.

Faraone, S.V., Biederman, J., Mennin, D., Russell, R. & Tsuang, M.T. (1998a) Familial subtypes of attention deficit hyperactivity disorder: a 4-year follow-up study of children from antisocial-ADHD families. *Journal of Child Psychology and Psychiatry*, **39**, 1045–1053.

Faraone, S.V., Biederman, J., Weber, W. & Russell, R.L. (1998b) Psychiatric, neuropsychological, and psychosocial features of DSM-IV subtypes of attention-deficit/hyperactivity disorder: results from a clinically referred sample. *Journal of the American Academy of Child and Adolescent Psychiatry*, **37**, 185–193.

Farrington, D.P., Loeber, R. & van Kammen, W.B. (1990) Long-term criminal outcomes of hyperactivity-impulsivity-attention deficit and conduct problems in childhood. In: *Straight and Devious Pathways from Childhood to Adulthood* (eds L. Robins & M. Rutter), pp. 62–81. Cambridge University Press, Cambridge.

Fergusson, D.M. & Horwood. L.J. (1995) Predictive validity of categorically and dimensionally scored measures of disruptive childhood behaviors. *Journal of the American Academy of Child and Adolescent Psychiatry*, **34**, 477–485.

Fergusson, D.M., Horwood. L.J. & Lloyd, M. (1991) Confirmatory factor models of attention deficit and conduct disorder. *Journal of Child Psychology and Psychiatry*, **32**, 257–274.

Fergusson, D.M., Horwood. L.J. & Lynskey, M.T. (1993) Prevalence and comorbidity of DSM-III-R diagnoses in a birth cohort of 15-year-olds. *Journal of the American Academy of Child and Adolescent Psychiatry*, **32**, 1127–1134.

Fergusson, D.M., Lynskey, M.T. & Horwood. L.J. (1997) Attentional difficulties in middle childhood and psychosocial outcomes in young adulthood. *Journal of Child Psychology and Psychiatry*, **38**, 633–644.

Filipek, P.A., Semrud-Clikeman, M., Steingard, R.J., Renshaw, P.F., Kennedy, D.N. & Biederman, J. (1997) Volumetric MRI analysis comparing subjects having attention-deficit hyperactivity disorder with normal controls. *Neurology*, **48**, 589–601.

Firestone, P., Crowe, D., Goodman, J.T. & McGrath, P. (1986) Vicissitudes of follow-up studies: differential effects of parent training and stimulant medication with hyperactives. *American Journal of Orthopsychiatry*, **56**, 184–194.

Firestone, P., Musten, L.M., Pisterman, S., Mercer, J. & Bennett, S. (1998) Short-term side effects of stimulant medication are increased in preschool children with attention-deficit/hyperactivity disorder: a double-blind placebo-controlled study. *Journal of Child and Adolescent Psychopharmacology*, **8**, 13–25.

Fischer, M., Barkley, R.A., Fletcher, K.E. & Smallish, L. (1993) The adolescent outcome of hyperactive children: predictors of psychiatric, academic, social, and emotional adjustment. *Journal of the American Academy of Child and Adolescent Psychiatry*, **32**, 324–332.

Frankel, F., Myatt, R., Cantwell, D.P. & Feinberg, D.T. (1997) Parent-assisted transfer of children's social skills training: effects on children with and without attention-deficit hyperactivity disorder. *Journal of the American Academy of Child and Adolescent Psychiatry*, **36**, 1056–1064.

Gadow, K.D., Sverd, J., Sprafkin, J., Nolan, E.E. & Ezor, S.N. (1995) Efficacy of methylphenidate for attention-deficit hyperactivity disorder in children with tic disorder. *Archives of General Psychiatry*, **52**, 444–455.

Gainetdinov, R.R., Wetsel, W.C., Jones, S.R., Levin, E.D., Jaber, M. & Caron, M.G. (1999) Role of serotonin in the paradoxical calming effect of psychostimulants on hyperactivity. *Science*, **283**, 397–401.

Gerring, J.P., Brady, K.D., Chen, A. *et al.* (1998) Premorbid prevalence of ADHD and development of secondary ADHD after closed head injury. *Journal of the American Academy of Child and Adolescent Psychiatry*, **37**, 647–654.

Giedd, F.N., Snell, J.W., Lange, N. *et al.* (1996) Quantitative magnetic resonance imaging of human brain development: ages 4–18. *Cerebral Cortex*, **6**, 551–560.

Gilger, J.W., Pennington, B.F. & DeFries, J.C. (1992) A twin study of the etiology of comorbidity: attention-deficit hyperactivity disorder and dyslexia. *Journal of the American Academy of Child and Adolescent Psychiatry*, **31**, 343–348.

Gill, M., Daly, G., Heron, S., Hawi, Z. & Fitzgerald, M. (1997) Confirmation of association between attention deficit hyperactivity disorder and a dopamine transporter polymorphism. *Molecular Psychiatry*, **2**, 311–313.

Gillberg, I.C. & Gillberg, C. (1988) Children with deficits in attention, motor control and perception (DAMP): need for specialist treatment. *Acta Paediatrica Scandinavica*, **77**, 450–451.

Gillberg, I.C. & Gillberg, C. (1989) Children with preschool minor neurodevelopmental disorders. IV. Behaviour and school achievement at age 13. *Developmental Medicine and Child Neurology*, **31**, 3–13.

Gillberg, C., Melander, H., von Knorring, A.L. *et al.* (1997) Long-term stimulant treatment of children with attention-deficit hyperactivity disorder symptoms: a randomized, double-blind, placebo-controlled trial. *Archives of General Psychiatry*, **54**, 857–864.

Gillis, J.J., Gilger, J.W., Pennington, B.F. & DeFries, J.C. (1992) Attention deficit disorder in reading-disabled twins: evidence for a genetic etiology. *Journal of Abnormal Child Psychology*, **20**, 303–315.

Glow, P.H. & Glow, R.A. (1979) Hyperkinetic impulse disorder: a developmental defect of motivation. *Genetic Psychology Monographs*, **100**, 159–231.

Goldman, L.S., Genel, M., Bezman, R.J. & Slanetz, P.J. (1998) Diagnosis and treatment of attention-deficit/hyperactivity disorder in children and adolescents. Council on Scientific Affairs, American Medical Association. *Journal of the American Medical Association*, **279**, 1100–1107.

Goldman-Rakic, P.S. (1987) Development of cortical circuitry and cognitive function. *Child Development*, **58**, 601–622.

Goldman-Rakic, P.S. (1996) Regional and cellular fractionation of working memory. *Proceedings of the National Academy of Sciences, USA*, **93**, 13473–13480.

Goldstein, H.S. (1987) Cognitive development in low attentive, hyperactive and aggressive 6 through 11 year old children. *Journal of the American Academy of Child and Adolescent Psychiatry*, **26**, 214–218.

Goldstein, S. & Ingersoll, B. (1992) Controversial treatments for children with attention deficit hyperactivity disorder. *Chadder*, Fall/Winter, 1–4.

Goodman, R. & Stevenson, J. (1989) A twin study of hyperactivity. I. An examination of hyperactivity scores and categories derived from Rutter teacher and parent questionnaires. *Journal of Child Psychology and Psychiatry*, **30**, 671–689.

Granger, D.A., Whalen, C.K. & Henker, B. (1993a) Malleability of social impressions of hyperactive children. *Journal of Abnormal Child Psychology*, **21**, 631–647.

Granger, D.A., Whalen, C.K. & Henker, B. (1993b) Perceptions of methylphenidate effects on hyperactive children's peer interactions. *Journal of Abnormal Child Psychology*, **21**, 535–549.

Greenhill, L.L., Abikoff, H.B., Arnold, L.E. *et al.* (1996) Medication treatment strategies in the MTA Study: relevance to clinicians and researchers. *Journal of the American Academy of Child and Adolescent Psychiatry*, **35**, 1304–1313.

Haenlein, M. & Caul, W.F. (1987) Attention deficit disorder with hyperactivity: a specific hypothesis of reward dysfunction. *Journal of the American Academy of Child and Adolescent Psychiatry*, **26**, 356–362.

Handen, B.L., Feldman, H., Gosling, A., Breaux, A.M. & McAuliffe, S. (1991) Adverse side effects of methylphenidate among mentally retarded children with ADHD. *Journal of the American Academy of Child and Adolescent Psychiatry*, **30**, 241–245.

Hart, E.L., Lahey, B.B., Loeber, R., Applegate, B. & Frick, P.J. (1995) Developmental change in attention-deficit hyperactivity disorder in boys: a four-year longitudinal study. *Journal of Abnormal Child Psychology*, **23**, 729–749.

Hauser, P., Soler, R., Brucker-Davis, F. & Weintraub, B.D. (1997) Thyroid hormones correlate with symptoms of hyperactivity but not inattention in attention deficit hyperactivity disorder. *Psychoneuroendocrinology*, **22**, 107–114.

Hechtman, L. (1996) Families of children with attention deficit hyperactivity disorder: a review. *Canadian Journal of Psychiatry*, **41**, 350–360.

Hechtman, L. & Weiss, G. (1986) Controlled prospective fifteen year follow-up of hyperactives as adults: non-medical drug and alcohol use and anti-social behaviour. *Canadian Journal of Psychiatry*, **31**, 557–567.

Hewitt, J.K., Silberg, J.L., Rutter, M. *et al.* (1997) Genetics and developmental psychopathology. I. Phenotypic assessment in the Virginia Twin Study of Adolescent Behavioral Development. *Journal of Child Psychology and Psychiatry*, **38**, 943–963.

Hinshaw, S. & McHale, J. (1991) Stimulant medication and the social interactions of hyperactive children. In: *Personality, Social Skills and Psychopathology: an Individual Difference Approach* (eds G.G. David & C.J. James), pp. 229–253. Plenum Press, New York.

Hinshaw, S.P., Henker, B., Whalen, C.K., Erhardt, D. & Dunnington, R.E. Jr (1989) Aggressive, prosocial, and nonsocial behavior in hyperactive boys: dose effects of methylphenidate in naturalistic settings. *Journal of Consulting and Clinical Psychology*, **57**, 636–643.

Horn, W.F., Ialongo, N.S., Pascoe, J.M. *et al.* (1991) Additive effects of psychostimulants, parent training, and self-control therapy with ADHD children. *Journal of the American Academy of Child and Adolescent Psychiatry*, **30**, 233–240.

Jacobvitz, D. & Sroufe, L.A. (1987) The early caregiver–child relationship and attention-deficit disorder with hyperactivity in kindergarten: a prospective study. *Child Development*, **58**, 1496–1504.

Jadad, A.R., Booker, L., Gauld, M. *et al.* (1999) The treatment of attention-deficit hyperactivity disorder: an annotated bibliography and critical appraisal of published systematic reviews and meta-analyses. *Canadian Journal of Psychiatry*, **44**, 1025–1035.

Jadad, A.R., Boyle, M., Cunningham, C., Kim, M. & Schachar, R. (1998) *The treatment of attention-deficit/hyperactivity disorder: a evidence report*. Agency for Healthcare Research and Quality, US Department of Health and Human Services, Rockville, MD.

Jensen, P.S., Martin, D. & Cantwell, D.P. (1997) Comorbidity in ADHD: implications for research, practice, and DSM-V. *Journal of the American Academy of Child and Adolescent Psychiatry*, **36**, 1065–1079.

Johnston, C. & Fine, S. (1993) Methods of evaluating methylphenidate in children with attention deficit hyperactivity disorder: acceptability, satisfaction, and compliance. *Journal of Pediatric Psychology*, **18**, 717–730.

Kadesjo, B. & Gillberg, C. (1998) Attention deficits and clumsiness in Swedish 7-year-old children. *Developmental Medicine and Child Neurology*, **40**, 796–804.

Kalverboer, A.F. (1975) *A Neurobehavioural Study in Preschool Children*. Lippincott, Philadelphia.

Kent, J.D., Blader, J.C., Koplewicz, H.S., Abikoff, H. & Foley, C.A. (1995) Effects of late-afternoon methylphenidate administration on behavior and sleep in attention-deficit hyperactivity disorder. *Pediatrics*, **96**, 320–325.

Klein, R.G. & Mannuzza, S. (1991) Long-term outcome of hyperactive children: a review. *Journal of the American Academy of Child and Adolescent Psychiatry*, **30**, 383–387.

Klein, R.G., Abikoff, H., Klass, E., Ganeles, D., Seese, L.M. & Pollack, S. (1997) Clinical efficacy of methylphenidate in conduct disorder with and without attention deficit hyperactivity disorder. *Archives of General Psychiatry*, **54**, 1073–1080.

Klorman, R., Brumaghim, J.T., Fitzpatrick, P.A. & Borgstedt, A.D. (1990) Clinical effects of a controlled trial of methylphenidate on adolescents with attention deficit disorder. *Journal of the American Academy of Child and Adolescent Psychiatry*, **29**, 702–709.

Klorman, R., Brumaghim, J.T., Fitzpatrick, P.A., Borgstedt, A.D. & Strauss, J. (1994) Clinical and cognitive effects of methylphenidate on children with attention deficit disorder as a function of aggression/oppositionality and age. *Journal of Abnormal Psychology*, **103**, 206–221.

Kuhne, M., Schachar, R. & Tannock, R. (1997) Impact of comorbid oppositional or conduct problems on attention-deficit hyperactivity disorder. *Journal of the American Academy of Child and Adolescent Psychiatry*, **36**, 1715–1725.

Kupietz, S.S., Winsberg, B.G., Richardson, E., Maitinsky, S. & Mendell, N. (1988) Effects of methylphenidate dosage in hyperactive reading-disabled children. I. Behavior and cognitive performance effects. *Journal of the American Academy of Child and Adolescent Psychiatry*, **27**, 70–77.

Lahey, B.B. & Carlson, C.L. (1991) Validity of the diagnostic category of attention deficit disorder without hyperactivity: a review of the literature. *Journal of Learning Disabilities*, **24**, 110–120.

LaHoste, G.J., Swanson, J.M., Wigal, S.B. *et al.* (1996) Dopamine D4 receptor gene polymorphism is associated with attention deficit hyperactivity disorder. *Molecular Psychiatry*, **1**, 121–124.

Landgren, M., Pettersson, R., Kjellman, B. & Gillberg, C. (1996) ADHD, DAMP and other neurodevelopmental/psychiatric disorders in 6-year-old children: epidemiology and co-morbidity. *Developmental Medicine and Child Neurology*, **38**, 891–906.

Laufer, M.W., Denhoff, E. & Solomons, G. (1957) Hyperkinetic impulse disorder in children's behavior problems. *Psychosomatic Medicine*, **19**, 38–49.

Leung, P.W., Luk, S.L., Ho, T.P., Taylor, E., Mak, F.L. & Bacon-Shone, J. (1996) The diagnosis and prevalence of hyperactivity in Chinese schoolboys. *British Journal of Psychiatry*, **168**, 486–496.

Levin, F.R. & Kleber, H.D. (1995) Attention-deficit hyperactivity disorder and substance abuse: relationships and implications for treatment. *Harvard Review of Psychiatry*, **2**, 246–258.

Levy, F., Hay, D.A., McStephen, M., Wood, C. & Waldman, I. (1997) Attention-deficit hyperactivity disorder: a category or a continuum? Genetic analysis of a large-scale twin study. *Journal of the American Academy of Child and Adolescent Psychiatry*, **36**, 737–744.

Lynskey, M.T. & Fergusson, D.M. (1995) Childhood conduct problems, attention deficit behaviors, and adolescent alcohol, tobacco, and illicit drug use. *Journal of Abnormal Child Psychology*, **23**, 281–302.

MacDonald, V.M. & Achenbach, T.M. (1996) Attention problems versus conduct problems as six-year predictors of problem scores in a national sample. *Journal of the American Academy of Child and Adolescent Psychiatry*, **35**, 1237–1246.

Mannuzza, S., Klein, R.G., Bessler, A., Malloy, P. & LaPadula, M. (1993) Adult outcome of hyperactive boys: educational achievement, occupational rank, and psychiatric status. *Archives of General Psychiatry*, **50**, 565–576.

Mannuzza, S., Klein, R.G., Bessler, A., Malloy, P. & Hynes, M.E. (1997) Educational and occupational outcome of hyperactive boys grown up. *Journal of the American Academy of Child and Adolescent Psychiatry*, **36**, 1222–1227.

Mannuzza, S., Klein, R.G., Bessler, A., Malloy, P. & LaPadula, M. (1998) Adult psychiatric status of hyperactive boys grown up. *American Journal of Psychiatry*, **155**, 493–498.

Mash, E.J. & Johnston, C. (1990) Determinants of parenting stress: illustration from families of hyperactive children and families of physically abused children. *Journal of Clinical Psychology*, **19**, 313–328.

Max, J.E., Robin, D.A., Lindgren, S.D. *et al.* (1997) Traumatic brain injury in children and adolescents: psychiatric disorders at two years. *Journal of the American Academy of Child and Adolescent Psychiatry*, **36**, 1278–1285.

Mayes, S.D., Crites, D.L., Bixler, E.O., Humphrey, F.J. II, & Mattison, R.E. (1994) Methylphenidate and ADHD: influence of age, IQ and neurodevelopmental status. *Developmental Medicine and Child Neurology*, **36**, 1099–1107.

McArdle, P., O'Brien, G. & Kolvin, I. (1997) Is there a comorbid relationship between hyperactivity and emotional psychopathology? *European Child and Adolescent Psychiatry*, **6**, 142–150.

McBurnett, K., Pfiffner, L.J., Willcutt, E. *et al.* (1999) Experimental cross-validation of DSM-IV types of attention-deficit/hyperactivity disorder. *Journal of the American Academy of Child and Adolescent Psychiatry*, **38**, 17–24.

McCracken, J.T. (1991) A two-part model of stimulant action on attention-deficit hyperactivity disorder in children. *Journal of Neuropsychiatry and Clinical Neurosciences*, **3**, 201–209.

McGee, R., Williams, S. & Feehan, M. (1992) Attention deficit disorder and age of onset of problem behaviors. *Journal of Abnormal Child Psychology*, **20**, 487–502.

Meehl, P.E. (1995) Bootstraps taxometrics: solving the classification problem in psychopathology. *American Psychologist*, **50**, 266–275.

Merrell, C. & Tymms, P.B. (2001) Inattention, hyperactivity and impulsiveness: their impact on academic achievement and progress. *British Journal of Educational Psychology*, **71**, 43–56.

Milberger, S., Biederman, J., Faraone, S.V. & Jones, J. (1998) Further evidence of an association between maternal smoking during pregnancy and attention deficit hyperactivity disorder: findings from a high-risk sample of siblings. *Journal of Clinical Child Psychology*, **27**, 352–358.

Milich, R. & Fitzgerald, G. (1985) Validation of inattention/overactivity and aggression ratings with classroom observations. *Journal of Consulting and Clinical Psychology*, **53**, 139–140.

Milich, R., Carlson, C.L., Pelham, W.E. Jr & Licht, B.G. (1991) Effects of methylphenidate on the persistence of ADHD boys following failure experiences. *Journal of Abnormal Child Psychology*, **19**, 519–536.

Miller, A. (1999) Appropriateness of psychostimulant prescription to children: theoretical and empirical perspectives. *Canadian Journal of Psychiatry*, **44**, 1017–1024.

Moffitt, T.E. (1990) Juvenile delinquency and attention deficit disorder: boys' developmental trajectories from age 3 to age 15. *Child Development*, **61**, 893–910.

Morgan, A.E., Hynd, G.W., Riccio, C.A. & Hall, J. (1996) Validity of DSM-IV ADHD predominantly inattentive and combined types:

relationship to previous DSM diagnoses/subtype differences. *Journal of the American Academy of Child and Adolescent Psychiatry*, 35, 325–333.

Mota, V.L. & Schachar, R. (2000) Reformulating attention deficit hyperactivity disorder according to sensitivity and specificity: could DSM be wrong? *Journal of the American Academy of Child and Adolescent Psychiatry*, 39, 1144–1151.

MTA Cooperative Group (1999a) A 14-month randomized clinical trial of treatment strategies for attention-deficit/hyperactivity disorder. *Archives of General Psychiatry*, 56, 1073–1086.

MTA Cooperative Group (1999b) Moderators and mediators of treatment response for children with attention-deficit/hyperactivity disorder. *Archives of General Psychiatry*, 56, 1088–1096.

Nada-Raja, S., Langley, J.D., McGee, R., Williams, S.M., Begg, D.J. & Reeder, A.I. (1997) Inattentive and hyperactive behaviors and driving offenses in adolescence. *Journal of the American Academy of Child and Adolescent Psychiatry*, 36, 515–522.

Newman, D.L., Moffitt, T.E., Caspi, A., Magdol, L., Silva, P.A. & Stanton, W.R. (1996) Psychiatric disorder in a birth cohort of young adults: prevalence, comorbidity, clinical significance, and new case incidence from ages 11–21. *Journal of Consulting and Clinical Psychology*, 64, 552–562.

Nichols, P.L. & Chen, T.-C. (1981) *Minimal Brain Dysfunction: A Prospective Study*. Erlbaum, Hillsdale, NJ.

Nigg, J.T., Swanson, J.M. & Hinshaw, S.P. (1997) Covert visual spatial attention in boys with attention deficit hyperactivity disorder: lateral effects, methylphenidate response and results for parents. *Neuropsychologia*, 35, 165–176.

Offord, D.R., Boyle, M.H., Szatmari, P. *et al.* (1987) Ontario Child Health Study. II. Six-month prevalence of disorder and rates of service utilization. *Archives of General Psychiatry*, 44, 832–836.

van den Oord, E.J., Boomsma, D.I. & Verhulst, F.C. (1994) A study of problem behaviors in 10- to 15-year-old biologically related and unrelated international adoptees. *Behavior Genetics*, 24, 193–205.

Ounsted, C. (1955) The hyperkinetic syndrome in epileptic children. *Lancet*, 2, 303–311.

Pardo, J.V., Pardo, P.J., Janer, K.W. & Raichle, M.E. (1990) The anterior cingulate cortex mediates processing selection in the Stroop attentional conflict paradigm. *Proceedings of the National Academy of Sciences, USA*, 87, 256–259.

Pelham, W.E.J. (1999) The NIMH multimodal treatment study for attention-deficit hyperactivity disorder: just say yes to drugs alone? *Canadian Journal of Psychiatry*, 44, 981–990.

Pelham, W.E., Hoza, B., Kipp, H.L., Gnagy, E.M. & Trane, S.T. (1997) Effects of methylphenidate and expectancy of ADHD children's performance, self-evaluations, persistence, and attributions on a cognitive task. *Experimental and Clinical Psychopharmacology*, 5, 3–13.

Pelham, W.E. Jr, Lang, A.R., Atkeson, B. *et al.* (1998) Effects of deviant child behavior on parental alcohol consumption: stress-induced drinking in parents of ADHD children. *American Journal on Addictions*, 7, 103–114.

Pennington, B.F. & Ozonoff, S. (1996) Executive functions and developmental psychopathology. *Journal of Child Psychology and Psychiatry*, 37, 51–87.

Pennington, B.F., Grossier, D. & Welsh, M.C. (1993) Contrasting cognitive deficits in attention deficit hyperactivity disorder versus reading disability. *Developmental Psychology*, 29, 511–523.

Pfiffner, L.J. & McBurnett, K. (1997) Social skills training with parent generalization: treatment effects for children with attention deficit disorder. *Journal of Consulting and Clinical Psychology*, 65, 749–757.

Pisterman, S., McGrath, P., Firestone, P., Goodman, J.T., Webster, I.

& Mallory, R. (1989) Outcome of parent-mediated treatment of preschoolers with attention deficit disorder with hyperactivity. *Journal of Consulting and Clinical Psychology*, 57, 628–635.

Pisterman, S., Firestone, P., McGrath, P. *et al.* (1992) The role of parent training in treatment of preschoolers with ADHDDH. *American Journal of Orthopsychiatry*, 62, 397–408.

Pliszka, S.R., Maas, J.W., Javors, M.A., Rogeness, G.A. & Baker, J. (1994) Urinary catecholamines in attention-deficit hyperactivity disorder with and without comorbid anxiety. *Journal of the American Academy of Child and Adolescent Psychiatry*, 33, 1165–1173.

Pliszka, S.R., Greenhill, L.L., Crismon, M.L. *et al.* (2000) The Texas Children's Medication Algorithm Project: report of the Texas Consensus Conference Panel on mediation and treatment of childhood attention-deficit/hyperactivity disorder. Part I. Attention-deficit/hyperactivity disorder. *Journal of the American Academy of Child and Adolescent Psychiatry*, 39, 908–919.

Porrino, L.J., Rapoport, J.L., Behar, D., Sceery, W., Ismond, D.R. & Bunney, W.E. Jr (1983) A naturalistic assessment of the motor activity of hyperactive boys. I. Comparison with normal controls. *Archives of General Psychiatry*, 40, 681–687.

Posner, M.I. & Raichle, M.E. (1998) The neuroimaging of human brain function. *Proceedings of the National Academy of Sciences, USA*, 95, 763–764.

Posner, M.I., DiGirolamo, G.J. & Fernandez-Duque, D. (1997) Brain mechanisms of cognitive skills. *Consciousness and Cognition*, 6, 267–290.

Prendergast, M., Taylor, E., Rapoport, J.L. *et al.* (1988) The diagnosis of childhood hyperactivity: a US–UK cross-national study of DSM-III and ICD-9. *Journal of Child Psychology and Psychiatry*, 29, 289–300.

Quist, J.F., Barr, C.L., Schachar, R. *et al.* (2000) Evidence for the serotonoin HTR2A gene as a susceptibility factor in attention deficit hyperactivity disorder (ADHD). *Molecular Psychiatry*, 5, 537–541.

Rappley, M.D., Gardiner, J.C., Jetton, J.R. & Houang, R.T. (1995) The use of methylphenidate in Michigan. *Archives of Pediatrics and Adolescent Medicine*, 149, 675–679.

Rapport, M.D., Denney, C., DuPaul, G.J. & Gardner, M.J. (1994) Attention deficit disorder and methylphenidate: normalization rates, clinical effectiveness, and response prediction in 76 children. *Journal of the American Academy of Child and Adolescent Psychiatry*, 33, 882–893.

Richters, J.E., Arnold, L.E., Jensen, P.S. *et al.* (1995) NIMH collaborative multisite multimodal treatment study of children with ADHD. I. Background and rationale. *Journal of the American Academy of Child and Adolescent Psychiatry*, 34, 987–1000.

Roy, P., Rutter, M. & Pickles, A. (2000) Institutional care: risk from family background or pattern of rearing? *Journal of Child Psychology and Psychiatry*, 41, 139–149.

Rutter, M. (1982) Syndromes attributed to minimal brain dysfunction in childhood. *American Journal of Psychiatry*, 139, 21–33.

Rutter, M., Chadwick, O. & Schachar, R. (1983) Hyperactivity and minimal brain dysfunction: epidemiological perspectives on questions of cause and classification. In: *The Child at Psychiatric Risk* (ed. R.E. Tarter), pp. 80–107. Oxford University Press, New York.

Rydelius, P.-A. (2000) Commentary: DAMP and MBD versus AD/HD and hyperkinetic disorders. *Acta Paediatrica*, 89, 266–268.

Safer, D.J. & Allen, R.P. (1989) Absence of tolerance to the behavioral effects of methylphenidate in hyperactive and inattentive children. *Journal of Pediatrics*, 115, 1003–1008.

Safer, D.J., Zito, J.M. & Fine, E.M. (1996) Increased methylphenidate usage for attention deficit disorder in the 1990s. *Pediatrics*, 98, 1084–1088.

Sandberg, S. & Barton, J. (1996) Historical development. In: *Hyperactivity Disorders of Childhood* (ed. S. Sandberg), pp. 1–25. Cambridge University Press, Cambridge.

Sandberg, S., Day, R. & Trott, G.E. (1996) Clinical aspects. In: *Hyperactivity Disorders of Childhood* (ed. S. Sandberg), pp. 69–110. Cambridge University Press, Cambridge.

Schachar, R.J. (1986) The history of the hyperkinetic syndrome. In: *The Overactive Child* (ed. E. Taylor), pp. 19–40. Spastics International Medical, London.

Schachar, R. (1991) Childhood hyperactivity. *Journal of Child Psychology and Psychiatry*, 32, 155–191.

Schachar, R. & Tannock, R. (1995) Test of four hypotheses for the comorbidity of attention-deficit hyperactivity disorder and conduct disorder. *Journal of the American Academy of Child and Adolescent Psychiatry*, 34, 639–648.

Schachar, R. & Wachsmuth, R. (1990) Hyperactivity and parental psychopathology. *Journal of Child Psychology and Psychiatry*, 31, 381–392.

Schachar, R., Sandberg, S. & Rutter, M. (1986) Agreement between teachers' ratings and observations of hyperactivity, inattentiveness, and defiance. *Journal of Abnormal Child Psychology*, 14, 331–345.

Schachar, R.J., Tannock, R., Cunningham, C. & Corkum, P.V. (1997) Behavioral, situational, and temporal effects of treatment of ADHD with methylphenidate. *Journal of the American Academy of Child and Adolescent Psychiatry*, 36, 754–763.

Schertz, M., Adesman, A.R., Alfieri, N.E. & Bienkowski, R.S. (1996) Predictors of weight loss in children with attention deficit hyperactivity disorder treated with stimulant medication. *Pediatrics*, 98, 763–769.

Seeman, P. & Madras, B.K. (1998) Anti-hyperactivity medication: methylphenidate and amphetamine. *Molecular Psychiatry*, 3, 386–396.

Sergeant, J. (2000) The cognitive–energetic model: an empirical approach to attention-deficit hyperactivity disorder. *Neuroscience and Biobehavioral Reviews*, 24, 7–12.

Shaffer, D. & Greenhill, L. (1979) A critical note on the predictive validity of 'the hyperkinetic syndrome'. *Journal of Child Psychology and Psychiatry*, 20, 61–72.

Shaffer, D., Schonfeld, I., O'Connor, P.A. *et al.* (1985) Neurological soft signs: their relationship to psychiatric disorder and intelligence in childhood and adolescence. *Archives of General Psychiatry*, 42, 342–351.

Shaywitz, B.A., Fletcher, J.M. & Shaywitz, S.E. (1995) Defining and classifying learning disabilities and attention-deficit/hyperactivity disorder. *Journal of Child Neurology*, 10, S50–S57.

Silberg, J., Rutter, M., Meyer, J. *et al.* (1996) Genetic and environmental influences on the covariation between hyperactivity and conduct disturbance in juvenile twins. *Journal of Child Psychology and Psychiatry*, 37, 803–816.

Simonoff, E., Pickles, A., Hervas, A., Silberg, J.L., Rutter, M. & Eaves, L. (1998) Genetic influences on childhood hyperactivity: contrast effects imply parental rating bias, not sibling interaction. *Psychological Medicine*, 28, 825–837.

Sleator, E.K., Von Neumann, A. & Sprague, R.L. (1974) Hyperactive children: a continuous long-term placebo-controlled follow-up. *Journal of the American Medical Association*, 229, 316–317.

Slimmer, L.W. & Brown, R.T. (1985) Parents' decision-making process in medication administration for control of hyperactivity. *Journal of School Health*, 55, 221–225.

Slomkowski, C., Klein, R.G. & Mannuzza, S. (1995) Is self-esteem an important outcome in hyperactive children? *Journal of Abnormal Child Psychology*, 23, 303–315.

Smalley, S.L., Bailey, J.G., Palmer, C.G. *et al.* (1998) Evidence that the dopamine D4 receptor is a susceptibility gene in attention deficit hyperactivity disorder. *Molecular Psychiatry*, 3, 427–430.

Spencer, T., Biederman, J. & Wilens, T. (1998) Growth deficits in children with attention deficit hyperactivity disorder. *Pediatrics*, 102, 501–506.

Spencer, T., Biederman, J., Wilens, T. & Faraone, S.V. (1994) Is attention-deficit hyperactivity disorder in adults a valid disorder? *Harvard Review of Psychiatry*, 1, 326–335.

Spencer, T., Biederman, J., Wilens, T., Harding, M., O'Donnell, D. & Griffin, S. (1996) Pharmacotherapy of attention-deficit hyperactivity disorder across the life cycle. *Journal of the American Academy of Child and Adolescent Psychiatry*, 35, 409–432.

Stevenson, J., Pennington, B.F., Gilger, J.W., DeFries, J.C. & Gillis, J.J. (1993) Hyperactivity and spelling disability: testing for shared genetic aetiology. *Journal of Child Psychology and Psychiatry*, 34, 1137–1152.

Still, G.F. (1902) The Coulstonian Lectures on some abnormal psychical conditions in children. *Lancet*, 1, 1008–1012; 1077–1082; 1163–1168.

Streissguth, A.P., Barr, H.M., Sampson, P.D. & Bookstein, F.L. (1994) Prenatal alcohol and offspring development: the first fourteen years. *Drug and Alcohol Dependence*, 36, 89–99.

Swanson, J.M., Sergeant, J.A., Taylor, E., Sonuga-Barke, E.J., Jensen, P.S. & Cantwell, D.P. (1998a) Attention-deficit hyperactivity disorder and hyperkinetic disorder. *Lancet*, 351, 429–433.

Swanson, J., Castellanos, F.X., Murias, M., LaHoste, G. & Kennedy, J. (1998b) Cognitive neuroscience of attention deficit hyperactivity disorder and hyperkinetic disorder. *Current Opinion in Neurobiology*, 8, 263–271.

Swanson, J., Gupta, S., Guinta, D. *et al.* (1999) Acute tolerance to methylphenidate in the treatment of attention deficit hyperactivity disorder in children. *Clinical Pharmacology and Therapeutics*, 66, 295–305.

Swanson, J., Oosterlaan, J., Murias, M. *et al.* (2000) Attention deficit-hyperactivity disorder children with a 7-repeat allele of the dopamine receptor D4 gene have extreme behavior but normal performance on critical neuropsychological tests of attention. *Proceedings of the National Academy of Sciences, USA*, 97, 4754–4759.

Szatmari, P., Boyle, M.H. & Offord, D.R. (1993) Familial aggregation of emotional and behavioral problems of childhood in the general population. *American Journal of Psychiatry*, 150, 1398–1403.

Szatmari, P., Offord, D.R. & Boyle, M.H. (1989a) Correlates, associated impairments and patterns of service utilization of children with attention deficit disorder: findings from the Ontario Child Health Study. *Journal of Child Psychology and Psychiatry*, 30, 205–217.

Szatmari, P., Boyle, M. & Offord, D.R. (1989b) ADHD and conduct disorder: degree of diagnostic overlap and differences among correlates. *Journal of the American Academy of Child and Adolescent Psychiatry*, 28, 865–872.

Szatmari, P., Offord, D.R. & Boyle, M.H. (1989c) Ontario Child Health Study: prevalence of attention deficit disorder with hyperactivity. *Journal of Child Psychology and Psychiatry*, 30, 219–230.

Tannock, R. (1998) Attention deficit hyperactivity disorder: advances in cognitive, neurobiological, and genetic research. *Journal of Child Psychology and Psychiatry*, 39, 65–99.

Tannock, R. (2000) Attention deficit disorders with learning disorders. In: *Attention Deficit Disorder and Comorbidities in Children, Adolescents and Adults* (ed. T.E. Brown), pp. 231–295. American Psychiatric Press, Washington D.C.

Tannock, R., Schachar, R.J., Carr, R.P. & Logan, G.D. (1989) Dose-response effects of methylphenidate on academic performance and overt behavior in hyperactive children. *Pediatrics*, **84**, 648–657.

Tannock, R., Schachar, R. & Logan, G. (1995) Methylphenidate and cognitive flexibility: dissociated dose effects in hyperactive children. *Journal of Abnormal Psychology*, **23**, 235–266.

Taylor, E. (1998) Clinical foundations of hyperactivity research. *Behavioural Brain Research*, **94**, 11–24.

Taylor, E., Schachar, R., Thorley, G., Wieselberg, H.M., Everitt, B. & Rutter, M. (1987) Which boys respond to stimulant medication? A controlled trial of methylphenidate in boys with disruptive behaviour. *Psychological Medicine*, **17**, 121–143.

Taylor, E.A., Sandberg, S., Thorley, G. & Giles, S. (1991) *The Epidemiology of Childhood Hyperactivity*. Oxford University Press, London.

Taylor, E., Chadwick, O., Heptinstall, E. & Danckaerts, M. (1996) Hyperactivity and conduct problems as risk factors for adolescent development. *Journal of the American Academy of Child and Adolescent Psychiatry*, **35**, 1213–1226.

Tirosh, E., Sadeh, A., Munvez, R. & Lavie, P. (1993) Effects of methylphenidate on sleep in children with attention-deficient hyperactivity disorder: an activity monitor study. *American Journal of Diseases of Children*, **147**, 1313–1315.

Toren, P., Eldar, S., Sela, B.A. *et al.* (1996) Zinc deficiency in attention-deficit hyperactivity disorder. *Biological Psychiatry*, **40**, 1308–1310.

Tredgold, A.F. (1908) *Mental Deficiency (Amentia)*. W. Wood, New York.

Tripp, G. & Luk, S.L. (1997) The identification of pervasive hyperactivity: is clinic observation necessary? *Journal of Child Psychology and Psychiatry*, **38**, 219–234.

Tripp, G., Luk, S.L., Schaughency, E.A. & Singh, R. (1999) DSM-IV and ICD-10: a comparison of the correlates of ADHD and hyperkinetic disorder. *Journal of the American Academy of Child and Adolescent Psychiatry*, **38**, 156–164.

Warner-Rogers, J., Taylor, A., Taylor, E. & Sandberg, S. (2000) Inattentive behavior in childhood: epidemiology and implications for development. *Disabilities*, **33**, 520–536.

Webster-Stratton, C. & Hammond, M. (1997) Treating children with early-onset conduct problems: a comparison of child and parent training interventions. *Journal of Consulting and Clinical Psychology*, **65**, 93–109.

Weiss, G. & Hechtman, L.T. (1993) *Hyperactive Children Grown Up*. Guilford Press, New York.

Wender, P.H. (1971) *Minimal Brain Dysfunction in Children*. Wiley, New York.

Whalen, C.K. & Henker, B. (1991) Social impact of stimulant treatment for hyperactive children. *Journal of Learning Disabilities*, **24**, 231–241.

Whalen, C.K., Henker, B., Buhrmester, D., Hinshaw, S.P., Huber, A. & Laski, K. (1989) Does stimulant medication improve the peer status of hyperactive children? *Journal of Consulting and Clinical Psychology*, **57**, 545–549.

Wolraich, M.L. & Baumgaertel, A. (1997) The practical aspects of diagnosing and managing children with attention deficit hyperactivity disorder. *Clinical Pediatrics*, **36**, 497–504.

Wolraich, M.L., Hannah, J.N., Baumgaertel, A. & Feurer, I.D. (1998) Examination of DSM-IV criteria for attention deficit/hyperactivity disorder in a county-wide sample. *Journal of Developmental and Behavioral Pediatrics*, **19**, 162–168.

Woodward, L., Taylor, E. & Dowdney, L. (1998) The parenting and family functioning of children with hyperactivity. *Journal of Child Psychology and Psychiatry*, **39**, 161–169.

Woodward, C.A., Thomas, H.B., Boyle, M.H., Links, P.S. & Offord, D.R. (1989) Methodologic note for child epidemiological surveys: the effects of instructions on estimates of behavior prevalence. *Journal of Child Psychology and Psychiatry*, **30**, 919–924.

World Health Organization (1978) *Mental Disorders: Glossary and Guide to their Classification in Accordance with the Ninth Revision of the International Classification of Diseases*. World Health Organization, Geneva.

World Health Organization (1994) *ICD-10: Classification of Mental and Behavioural Disorders*. World Health Organization, Geneva.

Wozniak, J., Biederman, J., Kiely, K., Ablon, J.S., Faraone, S.V., Mundy, E. & Mennin, D. (1995a) Mania-like symptoms suggestive of childhood-onset bipolar disorder in clinically referred children. *Journal of the American Academy of Child and Adolescent Psychiatry*, **34**, 867–876.

Wozniak, J., Biederman, J., Mundy, E., Mennin, D. & Faraone, S.V. (1995b) A pilot family study of childhood-onset mania. *Journal of the American Academy of Child and Adolescent Psychiatry*, **34**, 1577–1583.

Zametkin, A.J. & Liotta, W. (1998) The neurobiology of attention-deficit/hyperactivity disorder. *Journal of Clinical Psychiatry*, **59**, 17–23.

Zentall, S.S. (1988) Production deficiencies in elicited language but not in the spontaneous verbalizations of hyperactive children. *Journal of Abnormal Child Psychology*, **16**, 657–673.

Zentall, S.S., Smith, Y.N., Lee, Y.B. & Wieczorek, C. (1994) Mathematical outcomes of attention-deficit hyperactivity disorder. *Journal of Learning Disabilities*, **27**, 510–519.

Conduct and Oppositional Disorders

Felton Earls and Enrico Mezzacappa

Introduction

Conduct disorder constitutes a constellation of antisocial and aggressive behaviours that may become prominent in early childhood and persist through adolescence, even into adulthood. Sufficient understanding of the risk factors and early presentation of this disorder holds the promise of not only reducing the prevalence of a common childhood dysfunction, but also preventing much negligent, abusive and criminal behaviour. Oppositional disorder shares the negative and conflictual attributes of conduct disorder, but presents in a more limited fashion.

In this chapter these two disorders are examined from historical and theoretical perspectives prior to reviewing knowledge about their prevalence, course, causes, treatment and prevention. Two principal concepts are emphasized throughout. First, conduct disorder frequently develops in social and family contexts that are marked by conflict and adversity. This finding raises the question of the extent to which the specific symptoms of the disorder represent deviations from normal behaviour and emotions that are precipitated and sustained by pathogenic situations and relationships. The primacy given the social setting and interpersonal relationships does not mean that individual differences are unimportant. Even when children are exposed to high-risk conditions, many do not develop the disorder. Secondly, the dysfunctional nature of conduct and oppositional disorders can be conceptualized either in terms of a categorical diagnostic category or as a dimension of behaviour that everyone shows to a greater or lesser degree. A categorical approach is necessary for clinical decision-making but a dimensional one may better reflect the quantitative way that many causal processes, involving risk and protective factors, operate. In practice, both orientations can operate simultaneously in a complementary fashion.

Historical background

A historical excursion into efforts to understand and treat conduct disorder is warranted because it marks one of the earliest organized activities that defined the discipline of child psychiatry. With the establishment of clinics attached to juvenile courts and the ascendancy of the mental hygiene movement, a systematic and therapeutic approach to delinquent and antisocial youths began (Levy 1952). William Healy, an obstetrician and founder of the first juvenile court clinics in Chicago and Boston,

interpreted the presence of both physical and mental defects in patients as supporting hereditary origins of delinquent behaviour. Cyril Burt (1925), the English psychologist, also recognized this combination of factors, but stopped short of placing primary emphasis on either hereditary or social factors.

As psychoanalytic ideas gained prominence, the concept of a poorly developed superego became a popular approach that attracted a great deal of speculation and some interesting therapeutic approaches (Aichorn 1935; Johnson & Szurek 1952). Because these approaches were seldom systematically evaluated, there is little evidence to support their success in the literature.

Cleckley's monograph, *The Mask of Sanity* (1941), provided an influential summary of clinical experience with adults over the first half of the twentieth century. His detailed case descriptions were based on an assessment of prevailing constitutional and psychodynamic theories of psychopathy. The review of his own patients, many of whom were outwardly successful in their occupations, led him to devise an inventory of cardinal features that still remains useful:

1 an absent sense of responsibility;
2 refusal to accept blame for wrongdoing;
3 an absent sense of shame, humiliation, regret;
4 lying and cheating;
5 a failure to learn from experience;
6 a marked self-centredness that interferes with the capacity to love;
7 poverty of affect;
8 a lack of insight;
9 alcoholic indulgences;
10 sexual peculiarities; and
11 lack of goal directedness, resulting in a chaotic life style.

Cleckley was careful to claim that not all cases exhibited these behaviours at young ages and that some psychopaths came from undeniably 'good stock.' He did, however, postulate that the basic defect was a deep-seated one, justifying use of the term 'emotional dementia' to describe the apparent absence of personal insight and responsibility in the lives of the patients he treated.

While this work in adults was becoming influential, clinicians working with children were endeavouring to understand the origins of behavioural syndromes that were conceivably linked to adult psychopathy. John Bowlby carried out some of the most influential work in this vein. In his early studies, the developmental histories of delinquent boys were systematically reconstructed (Bowlby 1944). In acknowledging the need to classify these cases as a first step towards studying their origins, Bowlby devised a system consisting of six types, the most common of which were the affectionless character, the hyperthymic character and the depressive character. As will be seen in a later section of this chapter, this subtyping is similar to the major classes of conduct disorder currently adopted in the International Classification of Diseases (ICD-10; World Health Organization 1987). Bowlby was particularly drawn to the affectionless character as the prototype of the psychopath:

'It is my hope that the Affectionless Characters will be studied in great detail in the future, for I believe that they form the real hard core of the problem of recidivism. There can be no doubt that they are essentially delinquent characters, which is not true of the other characters discussed in this paper. The Depressed, Circular, Hyperthymic and Schizoid all had counterparts among the controls. We can get a Depressive who does not steal as well as one who does; we can find a law-abiding Hyperthymic as well as his antisocial brother. I am doubtful, however, whether the law-abiding Affectionless Character exists.' (Bowlby 1944, p. 39)

Making this diagnostic distinction led him to characterize the early histories of such children as marked by 'prolonged separations from their mothers and foster-mothers'. His intense interest in the early development of this subgroup became the inspiration for his subsequent work on attachment and has had a major influence on the field of developmental psychology (Bowlby 1969; Ainsworth *et al.* 1978; see also O'Connor, Chapter 46).

Although the multiple determinants of delinquency and psychopathy have not led to the isolation of specific causal factors, the work of Robins (1966) provided a grasp of its natural history. This work ranks as one the most important empirical studies in psychiatry of its era. By tracing the adult outcomes of children who were initially seen in a St. Louis child guidance clinic, a convincing link was established between childhood conduct problems and adult psychopathology. The most common outcome was antisocial personality disorder, a constellation of problems that was similar to the descriptions provided by Cleckley. This important study has been replicated in several different samples and the findings remain some of the most secure in modern psychiatry (Robins 1978). Recognition of this fact has been of enormous value in underscoring both the seriousness and chronicity of antisocial disorders (Loeber & LeBlanc 1990).

Classification

The effort to classify conduct and oppositional disorders has been informed by both theory and empirical research. The work of Hewitt & Jenkins (1946) was of fundamental importance in demonstrating that there were two distinct organizing features of conduct disorder: a socialization dimension and an aggressive behaviour dimension. Building on this work, the major contemporary classification systems used in psychiatry, the Diagnostic and Statistical Manual (DSM) of the American Psychiatric Association (APA) (1994) and the International Classification of Diseases (ICD) of the World Health Organization (WHO) (1992), capture these two cardinal features, but in somewhat different ways.

Compared to previous renditions of this system (DSM-II and DSM-III), the criteria in the current edition of DSM (DSM-IV) for making the diagnosis of conduct disorder have been made more stringent, with greater emphasis placed on objectively defined behavioural symptoms rather than on the moral or socialization elements of this disorder. The diagnosis is subclassified according to age of onset, broadly reflecting Moffitt's (1993b) distinction between 'adolescence-limited' and 'life-course-persistent' antisocial behaviour, the latter typically being first manifest in early childhood. Although important questions remain on these categories there is now a substantial body of empirical evidence supporting the validity of the distinction (Rutter *et al.* 1998).

ICD-10 includes socialized and unsocialized types of conduct disorder. In this system the concept of 'socialized' has been widened to include those who are integrated into either deviant or non-deviant peer networks. Both classification systems have specified symptom thresholds and duration criteria. Similar to the changes brought about in the revisions of DSM, the revisions of ICD have raised the threshold of clinical severity by including more seriously harmful and negligent behaviours to the list of possible symptoms.

However, important distinctions between these two systems remain. In contrast to DSM, which appears to have diminished the centrality of the quality of the child's social relations as a diagnostic feature, ICD places a higher priority on the quality of socialization than on the 'severity of the offence'. It has been pointed out that the latter feature may be most important in determining the prognosis of the disorder, especially as it is in keeping with the personality characteristics that are of fundamental importance to the definition of the adult syndrome (Rutter 1989; Christian *et al.* 1997).

The relationship between oppositional and conduct disorders is also handled somewhat differently in the two systems. In DSM the rules specify that oppositional disorder is to be excluded if conduct disorder is present. This reflects the inclination to view oppositional disorder as a milder form of conduct disorder, one that may represent a developmental precursor of conduct disorder (Schachar & Wachsmuth 1990; Frick *et al.* 1991a; Loeber *et al.* 1991a). ICD views the symptoms of oppositional/defiant disorder as a subcategory of conduct disorder, a position that is consistent with the classic work of Levy (1952) who described persistent patterns of resistant and negativistic behaviour as follows:

'Negativism has been contrasted with aggression and referred to as a more primitive and also safer expression of antagonism. In the form of open defiance it is difficult and probably unnecessary to differentiate it from aggression. As in the case of aggression, numerous modifications of the extreme act are seen . . . The mixtures or patterns of both forms of behaviour depend on the situation and on the available aggression in the personality.' (Levy 1952, p. 225)

The distinction between normative and deviant forms of negativism is especially important in pointing how a feature of one's temperament may be shaped into a maladaptive syndrome (Lahey *et al.* 1999). In a study that independently examined symptoms of children with oppositional and conduct disorders, it was found that fighting and lying were present in both groups (Loeber *et al.* 1991a). The suggestion was made that these two symptoms could effectively be eliminated from the definition of conduct disorder and placed on an expanded list of symptoms associated with oppositional disorder. The effect of such a change would be to make oppositional disorder a more serious problem, thereby enhancing the rationale to consider it a psychiatric disorder. Consistent with this proposal is some evidence that oppositional disorder in young children is more likely to predict mood disorders than conduct disorder on follow-up to middle childhood (Speltz *et al.* 1999). Whichever choice represents the more valid case, the separation of the two disorders splits the more interpersonal symptoms of oppositionality from the violations of social norms that characterize the prevailing definition of conduct disorder.

Another difference between the two systems is reflected in the distinction between 'splitters and lumpers'. The DSM system has a penchant for subdividing diagnostic groups into smaller categories, as illustrated by its separation of oppositional and conduct disorder. An important consequence of this convention is to encourage the tendency to diagnose multiple disorders in the same child. On the other hand, a preference is shown for maintaining larger domains of symptoms in ICD. For example, the broad category 'mixed disorder of conduct and emotions' includes three subtypes:

1 depressive conduct disorder;
2 other mixed disorders of conduct and emotions (implying anxiety symptoms); and
3 unspecified mixed disorders of conduct and emotions.

Another example of this type of convergent definition is the ICD-10 category of hyperactive conduct disorder.

The observation that antisocial behaviour can exist transiently or in relative isolation from other conduct problems is reflected in the categories, Adjustment Disorder with Disturbance of Conduct and Adjustment Disorder with Disturbance of Conduct and Emotion. In this instance, symptoms are observed to be triggered by acute stressful events, such as birth of a sibling, death of a relative or exposure to a catastrophic event. DSM makes it explicit that these symptoms should not last for more than 3 months. DSM-IIIR also includes a V code diagnosis, Childhood or Adolescent Antisocial Behaviour. This is to be used in cases of an isolated behaviour which is not associated with a recognizable stressful event.

Another approach to definition and classification in child psychiatry has been to assume that these disorders represent statistical departures from normal behaviour. If the categorical approach is fuelled by assumptions about the nature of a disorder, the statistical or dimensional approach rests on a tradition that avoids such assumptions. Many instruments have been devised for this purpose over the years (see Verhulst & Van der Ende, Chapter 5). Two of the most widely used in current research are the Child Behaviour Checklist (CBCL) (Achenbach *et al.* 1989) and the Revised Behaviour Problem Checklist (RBPC) (Quay & Peterson 1987). The two methods include nearly the same number of conduct disorder related items (38 and 39), but the CBCL makes none of the distinctions (socialized, unsocialized, oppositional) discussed so far in its single factor termed 'aggressive'. The RBPC, on the other hand, lists two separate factors: conduct disorder and socialized aggression.

The statistical approach is based on empirically derived behavioural items that can be shown to distinguish clinically referred from non-referred children, while the categorical approach relies on inductive process derived from consensual observations and clinical experience. Despite their conceptual differences, considerable overlap exists between these two approaches in practice (Edelbrock & Costello 1988; Jensen *et al.* 1996). In relation to conduct disorder, the issue concerns the nature of the disorder. Is it more like a deviation from normal, or a category with boundaries that separate it from normal behaviour as well as other types of disorders (Hill & Maughan 2001)? It is important to note that scale scores that include aggressive behaviour frequently capture other types of behaviour, while by concentrating on boundaries between disorders, the categorical approach excludes this possibility (Jensen *et al.* 1993).

Prevalence

Epidemiological studies over a 20-year period provide a developmental profile on the prevalence of conduct and oppositional disorders and specific antisocial behaviours (Costello 1989). From the preschool period to middle childhood there is an overall decrease in the frequency of temper tantrums, management problems, bullying and destructiveness, behaviours relating more to oppositional disorder than conduct disorder (Olweus 1979). Nevertheless, about half of those found to display early aggressive behaviour as preschool-age children develop persistent problems (Richman *et al.* 1982; Fischer *et al.* 1984). Any trend towards reduction of aggression in the first decade of life would appear to be offset by the increase in more serious antisocial behaviour during early to middle adolescence. In late adolescence the reduction in antisocial behaviour appears nearly as marked as the increase did in early adolescence. However, this picture is the sum of several cross-sectional and short-term longitudinal studies (Earls 1989). What is less clear is how often the same individuals might receive the diagnosis of conduct disorder at different points in time.

One of the first investigations to estimate the prevalence of conduct disorder in the general population was the Isle of Wight study (Rutter *et al.* 1970). Given an overall rate of 4.2% among 10–11-year-olds, the rate in boys was four times higher than the rate in girls: 6.2% compared to 1.6%. Conduct disorder was found to be by far the most common disorder in males, accounting for about three-quarters of all disorders in this group. When similar methods were used in a relatively poor area of London, the rate of conduct disorder doubled (Rutter *et al.* 1975).

The Ontario Child Health Survey provides a comprehensive picture of conduct disorder in the general population (Offord *et al.* 1987, 1991). In this study of children ranging in age from 4 to 16 and sampled throughout the province of Ontario, a diagnostic method was produced that conformed to criteria established in DSM-III. For younger children (4–11 years), scales were used to rate both parent- and teacher-reported symptoms, while for adolescents (12–16 years) parent and self-report data were collected (teacher data were found not to be reliable). Care was taken to measure the accuracy of the scales prior to launching the project.

The overall rate of conduct disorder, 5.5%, is similar to the rate reported 25 years earlier in the Isle of Wight study. The male : female ratio was also similar, 8.2% for males and 2.8% for females. However, geographical area differences were not found, the urban rate being just slightly higher than the rural rate: 5.6% compared to 5.2%. There was an unexpected reversal in relationship of area differences to age. For both sexes younger children in urban areas had a higher rate, but rural adolescents had higher rates than urban adolescents. The investigators interpret these findings as showing the importance of socioeconomic factors. The effect of geographical area was diminished when the degree of poverty in the different contexts was taken into account.

The prevalence of individual symptoms varied in a number of ways. As expected, the frequency of symptoms of lesser seriousness declined with age while those of a more serious nature increased with age. Predictably, males exceeded females in prevalence for most symptoms. For all 15 symptoms surveyed, adolescents reported more symptoms than did their parents. This was especially true for the more serious symptoms, such as vandalism, threats to hurt someone and cruelty to animals. For younger children, parents and teachers varied considerably in their reporting patterns.

The amount of agreement between any pair of informants was so slight as not to exceed that expected by chance alone. Thus, less than 10% of males had a pervasively defined disorder and not a single case of pervasive conduct disorder was found in young females. The proportion of cases defined by both parents and adolescents increased slightly at the older age level, but it still left over 80% of males and 90% of females with a disorder defined by only one informant. An interesting and perhaps unanticipated result was the large number of cases of conduct disorder found among the younger children, which were defined only by teachers (80%). Offord *et al.* (1991) suggest that this finding reflects the fact that conduct disorder is highly conditioned by school settings. This reasoning, however, may not extend to the findings with the older group, because self-reported symptoms cannot be regarded as suggesting situation specificity.

Further confirmation that the prevalence rate for conduct disorder is in the range of 3–5% is reported in a study of a predominantly rural population of children between the ages of 9 and 13 in the state of North Carolina in the USA (Costello *et al.* 1996). The overall rate of conduct disorder was 3.3%, males experiencing a fourfold higher rate than females (5.4% compared to 1.3%). The prevalence of oppositional disorder was 2.7% with a lower sex ratio still favouring males (3.2% compared to 2.3%). As in the Ontario study, but not in keeping with the London study of several decades ago, these results show that exposure to urban life does not increase the rate of conduct disorder appreciably. Family income, on the other hand, is strongly and inversely correlated with prevalence of conduct disorder. This picture of the prevalence and demographic correlates of conduct disorder is nearly paralleled by findings of antisocial personality in adults (Kessler *et al.* 1994).

In contrast to the consistent replications of estimates of the prevalence and correlates of conduct disorder in developed countries, much less information exists from studies in developing countries. There is reason to believe that conduct disorder may vary as a function of cultural differences in the strength of family preservation and child-rearing methods (Weisz *et al.* 1988). A relatively low prevalence of conduct disorder was reported by Bird *et al.* (1988) in Puerto Rico, suggesting that local cultural factors were at play. Bird (1996) discussed some of the challenges surrounding cross-cultural and cross-national research in child psychiatric epidemiology.

Risk factors and correlates

Many characteristics of children and their environments have been studied in relation to conduct disorders of childhood and adolescence. However, few have been examined in such a way as to establish causal relationships to conduct disorders. Understanding temporal relationships is critical to the process of identifying causal relationships between any set of relevant indices (Kraemer *et al.* 1997). Causal risk factors precede the onset of the disorder and to the extent that they can be manipulated, such factors should then alter its course.

Identification of risk factors is an important step in eventually identifying the causal mechanisms of morbidity. For example, child abuse is an identified causal risk factor for conduct disorder. Child abuse, in turn, has been associated with concurrent alterations in a variety of cognitive, emotional, neurohumoral and neuroendocrinological regulatory processes. Variations in each of these dimensions have also been associated with conduct disorder, and may contribute directly or indirectly to its symptoms and course. More detailed investigation of temporal–developmental relations between child abuse and these underlying regulatory processes is likely to lead to a better understanding of the pathogenesis of behavioural disturbances resulting from child abuse.

Some causal risk factors are important throughout the course of development, and merely change form according to the developmental level of the child (e.g. caregiver involvement and disciplinary practices). Other factors appear to be more crucial during particular developmental stages (e.g. peer influences during pre-adolescence and the acceptance/rejection of a child into deviant or adaptive social groups, and the biases present in social information processing that influence how an individual responds in ambiguous social situations).

Environmental causal risk factors loom large in the onset and evolution of conduct disorder. These factors begin in the intrauterine environment. Maternal smoking has been one of the more extensively studied prenatal risk factors for later psychopathology in children, adolescents and adults. Maternal smoking during pregnancy has been associated in a number of prospective longitudinal studies with an increased risk of conduct disorder in children and adolescents, and antisocial personality disorder in adults (Wakschlag *et al.* 1997; Fergusson *et al.* 1998; Brennan *et al.* 1999; Rasanen *et al.* 1999; Weissman *et al.* 1999). The preponderance of these studies examined only males. Where gender effects were studied, maternal smoking was markedly stronger for males than for females. In most of these studies, the effect of maternal smoking during pregnancy was either specific to, or more strongly predictive of violent criminality, than non-violent criminality. It also seems that maternal smoking predisposes to more persistent forms of conduct disorder, rather than transient forms. In all instances, the effects of maternal smoking were noted above and beyond those effects caused by a host of other postnatal environmental factors.

To date, the most compelling evidence for causal elements in the onset and course of conduct disorder is the familial aggregation of disturbances of conduct and antisocial behaviour in those children identified with early onset aggressive conduct disorder. Such familial aggregation of disturbances of conduct and antisocial behaviours reflects multiple interacting genetic and environmental determinants. The factors repeatedly identified in this body of literature include parental psychopathology, particularly antisocial behaviour, and parent child-rearing practices. The latter cover a range of behaviours from supervision, attentiveness–responsiveness, validation, and conflict resolution and disciplinary tactics.

The genetic component(s) of such familial aggregation of conduct and antisocial disorders have been difficult to study and quantify for a variety of reasons, even in the case of carefully conducted twin studies. Foremost among these is the dependence of the statistical estimates of genetic and environmental contributions to conduct disorder on the methods used to ascertain conduct disorder, and on the informant providing the data upon which the ascertainment of conduct disorder is based. Estimates vary depending on whether children or adults provide relevant information, and on whether questionnaires or structured interviews are used to ascertain conduct disorder. Secondly, it is not clear if inherited aspects apply broadly to all or many forms and symptoms of conduct disorders, or if inheritance patterns are more specific to certain symptoms or types of conduct disorder, such as the overt or covert subtypes of conduct disorder.

Reliable estimation of the shared and unique environments of children is critical to obtaining valid estimates of the genetic contributions to conduct disorders. Such reliable estimation of environmental contributions is often difficult to obtain. In the Virginia Twin Study of Adolescent Behavioural Development (Eaves *et al.* 1997; Simonoff *et al.* 1998), child ratings of twin differences in conduct disorder suggested stronger unique environmental influences, and a genetic contribution that was common to both aggression and property violations, as well as overt destructive forms of conduct disorder behaviours. Maternal ratings, on the other hand, not surprisingly suggested the importance of the shared environment as well, when compared with child ratings of differences between twins in conduct disorder outcomes. Mothers' ratings gave some, but less importance to unique environmental factors, and little or no support to a common genetic factor, but some support for specific genetic factors contributing to aggression, to property violations and to oppositional behaviours.

Finally, despite all indications that a genetic component is present, what is very unclear in the case of conduct disorders is exactly what is inherited. The syndrome of conduct disorder itself, with all its attendant complex behavioural patterns, is unlikely to be inherited *in toto*. In this regard, some of the correlates of conduct disorder identified below, such as autonomic underarousal, insensitivity to punishment, deficiencies in neurohumoral regulation and deficits of executive controls, have been put forth in a speculative fashion by various investigators as those heritable traits that may predispose an individual singly or in concert to develop conduct disorder. These trait predispositions would presumably lead to conduct disorder when the environment also presents with factors that act to increase risk for conduct disorder by modelling the sorts of complex social behaviours that are characteristic of the syndrome, and through the absence of other behaviours considered essential to healthy and adaptive development.

The risk factors for conduct disorder reported in the Ontario Child Health Survey (Offord *et al.* 1987) are similar to those noted in many other studies. The three most significant risk factors exerting independent effects on conduct disorder were:
1 family dysfunction (relative odds 3.1);
2 parental mental illness (relative odds 2.2); and
3 low income. Low income had its effect on children aged 4–11 (relative odds 3.7), but not on adolescents.
These factors resemble the six described by Rutter (1978) as gereral indicators of psychosocial adversity: low socioeconomic status; criminality of the father; overcrowding; maternal neurosis; chronic marital discord; and institutional care.

Throughout the age range covered, those children with conduct disorder were more likely to have impairments as reflected in school underachievement and interpersonal problems. At the younger age level, 62% were thought to be in need of intervention compared to 8% without conduct disorder; in adolescence 74% of those with conduct disorder were in need of treatment compared to 44% of those wthout this disorder. These findings provide a source of external validity for the method of selecting children with conduct disorder.

In terms of peers and social relations outside the home, causal risk has been identified for peer rejection/acceptance, and for the part played by social information processing biases. Aggressive individuals often exhibit biases in interpreting the intent of others, whereby hostile attributions are more likely to be generated over more benign interpretations of the ambiguous social–interpersonal behaviours of others (Dodge *et al.* 1995).

Risk factors that may be causal factors

In studies comparing children with conduct disturbances to those with emotional disturbances and those without disturbances, those with conduct disorder have consistently shown lower levels of electrodermal activity (EDA), lower mean resting heart rate (HR), lower heart rate reactivity (HRR), and lower heart rate variability (HRV). These characteristics are most marked in individuals whose behavioural disturbances and impairments are earlier in onset, and involve predatory aggression and poor socialization. This has led to theories suggesting that autonomic underarousal is a fundamental characteristic of individuals manifesting such forms of conduct disorder. Many of these findings are closely linked conceptually and physiologically to sympathetic modulation, which in turn is known to be associated with anxiety and arousal mechanisms subserving the inhibition of behaviours associated with negative consequences.

Of all the physiological indices examined in relation to conduct disorder, HR is by far the most extensively studied. Taking the body of literature on HR indices together, the fact that similar relationships between HR regulatory indices and behaviour have been reported in samples of different ages, from infancy and preschool through adolescence and adulthood, suggests several things.

1 HR indices are, at the very least, important time-varying correlates of behaviour throughout the life span, from infancy to adolescence and beyond. Individual differences in HR regulation appear to be present from very early on in life, in both genders (Raine *et al.* 1990, 1995, 1997; Porges *et al.* 1996; Mezzacappa *et al.* 1997; Pine *et al.* 1998).

2 The direction of reported effects appears to be consistent across studies, and over the life span. Where difficult, disruptive, aggressive or antisocial behaviours are concerned, it is lower HR or lower HR variability that are consistently associated with these behavioural patterns (Raine *et al.* 1990, 1995, 1997; Mezzacappa *et al.* 1997; Pine *et al.* 1998).

3 The status of a risk factor for onset or for persistence of conduct disorder has been established for HR and HRV. HR indices have been noted to predict later onset of aggression in childhood (lower HR; lower vagal tone) (Porges *et al.* 1996; Raine *et al.* 1997), and the desistence of antisocial behaviour in young adulthood (higher HR) (Raine *et al.* 1995).

Correlates and concomitants of conduct disorder

These indices have been found to co-occur in time with manifestations of conduct disorder. In many instances, temporal relations have simply not been studied (correlates). Therefore some of these may very well turn out to be risk or causal risk factors, or they may simply be concomitants of conduct disorder.

Associations of conduct disturbances with alterations in the regulation of neuroendocrinological and neurohumoral indices—such as plasma or salivary cortisol and testosterone levels; activity of platelet monoamine oxidase (MAO); and plasma, cerebrospinal fluid or urinary levels of the monoamines dopamine, norepinephrine, serotonin and their respective metabolites—have been less consistent than those found with the autonomic indices (McBurnett *et al.* 1991; Rogeness *et al.* 1992; Scerbo & Kolko 1994; Coccaro & Kavoussi 1996; Schaal *et al.* 1996; Stoff & Vitello 1996; Pine *et al.* 1997). None the less, when individuals with disturbances of conduct are subcategorized, and those with earlier onset, persistent aggression are identified, then findings of diminished levels of salivary cortisol and elevated levels of salivary testosterone have been replicated in some studies.

Another finding that has been replicated in both animal and human studies, including those involving children and adolescents, has been the deficiency of serotonergic (5-hydroxytryptamine; 5-HT) activity in subjects displaying patterns of aggressive behaviour (Coccaro & Kavoussi 1996; Stoff & Vitello 1996; Pine *et al.* 1997). Individuals with histories of earlier onset and persistently high levels of impulsive aggressive behaviours were those whose serotonergic activity was found to be the most deficient.

Three principal neuropsychological deficits have been reported in relation to conduct disorder (Moffitt 1993a): differences in IQ, language deficits and impaired executive control functions (ECF). The presence of conduct disorder has been associated with lower IQ scores, even after controlling for socioeconomic and demographic factors. On specific tests of language function, conduct disorder is associated with deficits even when IQ and demographic variables are controlled. Performance IQ (PIQ)–verbal IQ (VIQ) differences, where PIQ is noticeably higher than VIQ, are among these findings.

Executive control functions (e.g. planning or delay of actions, anticipation of outcome, inhibiting or changing responses, maintaining purposeful effort and self-monitoring of behaviour) have been noted to be impaired in children and adolescents affected with conduct disorder. These deficits, when present, can add characteristics to the conduct disturbances such as impulsivity, and may also influence the course of disorder through factors such as academic underachievement.

Recent studies (Seguin *et al.* 1995, 1999; Toupin *et al.* 2000) of both population-based and clinical samples, using well-specified models and methods for assessing ECF, improved classification of subjects, and inclusion of relevant confounds such as IQ and socioeconomic status, indicate that ECF and disturbances of conduct are related, even in the absence of attention deficit hyperactivity disorder (ADHD). Children with more persistent pervasive conduct disorder with aggression seem more likely to demonstrate such ECF deficits. The relationship of ECF indices to behavioural problems also appears to be relatively independent of IQ and non-executive cognitive functions such as memory (Seguin *et al.* 1995, 1999; Oosterlaan & Sergeant 1996; Oosterlaan *et al.* 1998).

A study of adults by Raine *et al.* (2000) lends further support to the notion that ECF may be important to the understanding of conduct disorder and its course. Using magnetic resonance imaging and autonomic indices, these investigators studied adult males with antisocial personality, and compared them to matched controls with other psychiatric disorders and no disorder. They found volumetric reductions in prefrontal cortical regions in the antisocial group only, which are believed to subserve ECF.

Challenges to ECF with strong motivational influences have been utilized to identify individuals with difficulties in the monitoring and modification of behaviour resulting from a lack of concern over the consequences of behaviour. Tasks of passive avoidance learning, which require withholding responses to avoid negative consequences, have been used to demonstrate deficits in this capacity in children with undersocialized aggressive forms of conduct disorder (UACD). In the opinion of some investigators, it is the children with UACD who are at greatest risk for persistent disorder and adult antisocial personality disorder (ASP) (Daugherty & Quay 1991; Quay 1993). These authors ascribe the course and persistence of disorder to this lack of concern for the consequences and outcomes of behaviour.

Course and persistence

In the classic study by Robins (1966), 45% of those with conduct disorders went on to develop ASP, highlighting the potential lifelong course of these disturbances. The progression of conduct disorders through childhood and adolescence and into adulthood has since received considerable attention, and a number of conceptually useful, overlapping pathway models have emerged.

Some models focus on the timing of onset, and the accrual and persistence of disturbances of conduct over time (Farrington 1995). Here primary distinctions have been made between earlier and later onset disturbances, and the timing of desistence of disturbances. In an effort to integrate knowledge in the existing empirical literature, Moffitt (1993b) proposed that multiple pathways could lead to the same constellation of antisocial behaviours. She outlined in some detail two developmental trajectories: one termed 'early onset, life-course-persistent', and the other termed 'adolescent limited'. The early onset variety was postulated to include children with neuropsychological and temperamental profiles that represented enduring traits placing them at high and continuing risk for antisocial behaviour. The adolescent onset type includes persons who are particularly susceptible to the influence of deviant peers.

The type and severity of the symptomatology, and the progression to include more symptom types over time, is also a useful manner of conceptualizing the course of disturbances in conduct (Loeber *et al.* 1993). Here distinctions are made between prevalence of symptoms related to conflicts with authority (e.g. truancy and disobeying curfew), symptoms related to covert delinquent behaviours (e.g. theft, deceit and destruction of property) and symptoms related to overt disturbances of conduct (e.g. cruelty and predatory aggression towards persons or animals).

Applying and integrating these two approaches to the course of conduct disorder, early onset disturbances of conduct are more frequently persistent and more often associated with symptoms involving conflictual, covert and overt delinquent behaviours. Individuals whose course begins with conflictual behaviours later in the course of development rather than earlier, are much less likely to progress on to covert and overt delinquent acts, or to have persistent disorder into adulthood (Loeber *et al.* 1993; Moffitt 1993b). Those individuals who manifest disturbances of conduct earlier in life, not only tend to display more symptoms of greater severity, they commit more severe criminal offences, and account for a disproportionately large number of the total offences in their respective age groups. In some reports, the most problematic 10% of individuals account for more than half the criminal offences committed (Farrington 1995).

An important qualifier in the matter of life-course symptoms and patterns of comorbidity of conduct disorder is the influence of gender (Cohen *et al.* 1993; Zahn-Waxler 1993; Zoccolillo 1993; Loeber & Keenan 1994). While reports of the overall prevalence of conduct disorder tend to highlight the male preponderance for this syndrome, sex-related differences in prevalence vary with age, being least in mid-adolescence (Moffitt *et al.*, 2001). The sex difference is most marked with respect to life-course-persistent antisocial behaviour, which is decidedly uncommon in females. This means that both early onset conduct problems (often accompanied by hyperactivity) and crime in adult life are much more frequent in males.

Despite the strong relationships repeatedly identified between early onset, aggressive variants of conduct disorder, and persistent problems throughout childhood and adolescence often leading to adult antisocial behaviours, not all children displaying this more severe form of conduct disorder become antisocial adults. The work of Magnusson & Bergman (1988) is especially instructive in this regard, highlighting the complex multifactorial relationships involved with the features and course of conduct disorders. Taking a developmental, person-orientated approach to the study of aggressive conduct disorder, these investigators noted that highly aggressive children who were impaired in other ways, including poor peer relations, low school motivation and academic underachievement, frequently progressed on to adult antisocial behaviour. Children with comparable levels of aggression without such impairments did not persist and progress on to adult antisocial behaviours nearly as often.

An additional distinction useful in understanding the course of conduct disorders is whether or not deviant behaviours occur in the company of a peer group (Reiss & Farrington 1991). It appears that the majority of delinquent offences committed by adolescents occur in the company of small groups of two or more persons, highlighting the impact of social networks on behaviour in this age category (Cairns *et al.* 1988). It also seems that those children and adolescents whose symptoms of conduct disorder involve aggression, and who carry out their deviant behaviours in isolation of others, sometimes referred to as UACD (Quay 1993), are at increased risk for more persistent and impairing disorder.

Perhaps the most useful way of conceptualizing the evolution of disturbances of conduct is to apply a developmental model to the transactional processes occurring between the characteristics of the individual, and the multiple levels of environment (home, school, neighbourhood, and the larger community and culture) to which he or she is continuously exposed. In such transactional models one may construct a number of plausible pathways leading to serious and persistent disturbances of conduct, and serious impairment in the life of the child (Nagin & Tremblay 1999).

Central to reconstructing the evolution of the symptomatology of conduct disorders is the matter of time-variance. Rarely do all the manifestations and complications of these disorders present simultaneously, nor do they manifest at maximum levels of severity at all times. Risk factors for conduct disorder are generally also time-varying in nature. The time-variance of symptoms and the relations of symptomatic behaviours to time-varying risk factors within the child and in the environment are an extremely important perspective for understanding the developmental psychopathology of conduct disorders. Three examples are considered here.

1 Children of difficult temperament raised by caregivers who themselves have difficulty with impulse control, may become involved in transactions around behavioural control and coercion that involve increasingly severe forms of discipline aimed at controlling problematic behaviour. The 'slippery slope' to child maltreatment is not difficult to imagine in such instances, and may be more likely to occur during times when caregivers themselves are under greater stress from extraneous factors. Child maltreatment is known to be a particularly virulent risk factor for subsequent persistent conduct disorders.

2 Children with language deficits, or problems with executive control, such that the requirements of planning and maintenance of effortful work will often find them at odds with the demands of the classroom. This process culminates in both disciplinary problems and academic underachievement. The consequences of this may fuel frustration, loss of self-esteem and a gravitation towards increasingly disruptive behaviours, disenchantment with school, and gravitation towards more deviant peers.

3 Children whose frustration tolerance is lower, and whose responses to frustration tend to be more aggressive or disruptive in nature, often find themselves excluded from peer groups and later in the course of development find social affiliations only with more deviant individuals in their peer cohort. The nature in which individuals are accepted or rejected by networks of peers operates as an important conduit into either socially conforming or deviant behaviour (Cairns *et al.* 1988). For example, a child who behaves aggressively in elementary school in response to exposure to domestic violence, may by virtue of these experiences have acquired a bias in social information processing whereby he or she is inclined to attribute hostile intentions to others in ambiguous situations, and to reactively behave in an aggressive fashion towards them (Dodge *et al.* 1995). This may lead to increasing alienation, anger and more maladaptive behaviours on the part of the isolated individual, and eventually to association with other (deviant) peers. This group of deviant peers may enhance the repertoire of maladaptive behaviours of the individual, often at the expense of the acquisition of age-appropriate adaptive social skills. The increasingly maladaptive behaviours and relative lack of age appropriate skills then reinforce the cycle of rejection by more functional peers, and the more stable socialization of the individual into a deviant peer group, thereby contributing to the evolution of conduct disorder into a more intractable variant.

Diagnostic assessment

The point was raised previously that changes in the number and type of symptoms, thresholds and boundaries between closely related disorders have changed frequently over the past few decades. Cognisant of these distinctions, the process of making a diagnosis represents a means of putting a classification system to work. However, it is important to realize that the diagnosis should be viewed as only one component of an overall process of assessment.

The reliability and validity of diagnostic groupings are important metrics used to establish the utility of classification systems. A number of considerations are involved in these determinations, including identifying the informant (parent, teacher, child), determining the situation or setting in which the symptoms are manifest (home, school), estimating the degree of impairment associated with the symptom load, and selecting an instrument to conduct the assessment. In general, the results of studies using highly structured interviews indicate that conduct disorder is among the most reliable and valid disorders in children (Jensen *et al.* 1995; Schwab-Stone *et al.* 1996). Despite this, there remain sufficient levels of inconsistency between parent, teacher and child reports to leave open the question of situational specificity in the expression of symptoms in a majority of cases. Unlike the assessment of attentional and oppositional disorders, child reports are at least as reliable and valid as are parent reports (Jensen *et al.* 1995).

Because the nature of conduct disturbances is such that they are more likely to be of concern to others than to the patient, such children are prone to view themselves as victims of adult authority. Indeed, the clinic contact may all too readily be perceived as punishment for the conflict generated at home or school. To counteract this tendency, it is wise to establish direct contact with the child.

Evaluation of a child's personality and peer relations is of great importance in terms of understanding the nature of the child's disturbance. Research has shown peer unpopularity to be an unstable feature among aggressive children (Cairns & Cairns 1991), thus personality traits weigh in heavily along with peer acceptance and the number of friends. The types of activities engaged in with peers and their apparent behavioural norms is important because these factors may represent important indicators of the potential for escalation (Elliot *et al*. 1985).

Keeping in mind the issues of different classification systems as discussed in an earlier section, the pattern of symptoms becomes especially significant when evaluating the presence of problems that fall outside the realm of narrowly defined conduct disturbance. As demonstrated in several studies, children with symptoms of ADHD and conduct disorder are at greater risk for poor outcomes than children with ADHD or conduct disorder alone (Stewart *et al*. 1981; McGee *et al*. 1984; Gittelman *et al*. 1985; Moffitt 1990; Mannuzza *et al*. 1991). Moreover, the combination of cognitive impairment and antisocial behaviour may act synergistically (Loeber *et al*. 1990a; Frick *et al*. 1991a). Children with conduct and anxiety symptoms, on the other hand, are less likely to have police contacts or to be perceived by their peers as bullies than conduct disordered children without anxiety symptoms (Walker *et al*. 1991). The assumption is that the presence of anxiety acts as a 'braking system' on the seriousness of antisocial behaviour.

Conduct disorder appears to be more closely related to substance abuse than to other psychiatric disorders. The association covers alcohol and several types of drugs, including stimulants, depressants, inhalants, opiates and cocaine (Kandel *et al*. 1978; Elliot *et al*. 1989; Greenbaum *et al*. 1991; Milin *et al*. 1991). In a large group of seriously delinquent youths, Weisz *et al*. (1991) found that substance abuse predicted the escalation of violent behaviour.

The assorted nature of antisocial symptoms makes it essential to obtain the reports of teachers as well as parents. While children and parents agree to a fair extent on symptoms of conduct disorder, greater degrees of disagreement are found when inquiring about attentional, impulse control and oppositional symptoms. On analysing these patterns of agreement and disagreement, Loeber *et al*. (1990b, 1991b) found that parents and teachers report more symptoms of ADHD and oppositional behaviour than did children. Information from parents was found to be more useful in predicting police contacts than the two other sources. Both parents and teachers predicted placement in special classes better than children. However, the three informants were about equally good in predicting school suspensions.

Because the pattern of symptoms in conduct disorder follows a developmental trend to become more heterogeneous over time, it is essential to establish a history of antisocial behaviour at the time the clinical assessment is made. A number of studies have shown that symptoms may become prominent in the preschool period, creating a noticeable pressure on parental authority and control (Campbell & Ewing 1990; White *et al*. 1990; Tremblay *et al*. 1991). Early onset may be an indicator of persistence simply because it reflects a degree of skill and control acquired by the child in adapting to his or her environment. As Patterson *et al*. (1989) adroitly stated, '. . . the child can become both victim and architect of a maladaptive lifestyle in which investment in aggressive behaviour is paramount'.

The evaluation should include a search for diagnosable and possibly treatable diseases of the central nervous system. In addition to a neurological examination, the history should include a detailed review of head injuries, especially those associated with a loss of consciousness, infectious diseases involving the brain, and seizures. It is essential to inquire specifically about exposure to sources of lead contamination. Often young children will have had lead levels determined in the past and, if so, a record of the actual level should be ascertained. The neuropsychiatric status of a child may be particularly important in the case of more severe offences. A study of adolescent youths incarcerated for homicide revealed a disproportionately high incidence of head injuries and other insults to the central nervous system in the medical histories of the inmates (Lewis 1990; Lewis *et al*. 1988). The authors speculated that compromise to cognitive functions and impulse control as a direct result of the central nervous system insult may have been a contributing factor to the commission of such serious crimes.

A psychological assessment is a critically important component to the overall evaluation. Measures of intellectual capacity, language development, reading and arithmetic skills should be included to evaluate school performance and intelligence and the extent to which one predicts the other. It is worth emphasizing that careful attention to performance in these areas is important at all ages, including adolescence. The presence of above average intellectual functioning and achievement should be considered as a good prognostic sign (White *et al*. 1989). Under circumstances where detailed psychometric assessment is impractical or not obtainable, a careful review of academic performance from school records may be substituted and still be very helpful for identifying areas of weakness or underachievement. Addressing these areas will not only improve competence and self-esteem, but will also likely improve long-term prognosis where conduct disorder is concerned.

School records are a valuable source of information beyond their contribution to the evaluation of academic performance. Information on behaviour problems, absenteeism, truancy, reasons for parent conferences and extracurricular activities may all be helpful in completing a comprehensive picture of the child's functioning. Review of such records prior to contacting the school may also assist in preparing for an efficient use of time with school personnel.

Once these multiple sources of information are at hand, a differential diagnosis can be entertained. Other disorders may be of primary or secondary importance relative to symptoms of oppositional and conduct disorders. Among the diagnoses to consider are psychoses, seizure disorders, mental retardation, specific developmental disorders, attention deficit disorders, substance abuse, post-traumatic stress disorder as well as other anxiety disorders and major depressive disorder.

Conduct disorder is routinely associated with impairments in the areas of family and peer relations, and school and job performance. These should be carefully assessed because they may have implications for the types of treatment recommended. In judging the seriousness of behavioural disturbance, attention must also be given to patterns of risk-taking. Frequency of fighting and the types of injuries sustained in such conflicts, the possession and use of weapons, patterns of offending and co-offending, gang membership, use of drugs, and the use of coercion in sexual encounters are the areas of inquiry that will help determine severity.

As a final step in determining prognosis, two other considerations should be added to knowledge about the severity of the symptom pattern. These are the degree to which the individual manifests a restricted range of reasoning about interpersonal relationships and conflict negotiation, and the degree of support provided by immediate family members. The inability to view social encounters as events that require thinking about the feelings and rights of others and the consequences of one's actions in these regards, may well represent the most profound problem associated with conduct disorder (Joffe *et al.* 1990). The child's lack of sensitivity to other family members may make parents feel futile in knowing how to help the child. This, in turn, may serve to justify their withdrawal of support and care. Of course, these problems exist in a nexus, which is usually impossible to disentangle during a clinical evaluation. More important than understanding the dynamics of such predicaments, is the need to acknowledge their presence as a complicating factor towards recovery.

Another way to evaluate the family in this regard is in relation to the resources available to them that might be mobilized to support the well-being or rehabilitation of an antisocial child. Much has been made of the role of family conflict and harsh rearing conditions as risk factors in the development of conduct disorder. If these conditions are present, the treatment plan must undoubtedly address efforts to reduce the level of disharmony in the home or the child's exposure to it but, at the same time, the presence of a caring adult within the family or in the community should not be missed (Jenkins & Smith 1990).

Treatment

General considerations

Given the multiplicity of factors identified as risk, causal or perpetuating forces in the onset and evolution of conduct disorder, it is fundamentally inconceivable to envision interventions for this condition that do not comprehensively address all these facets. In assessing conduct disorder, it is essential to obtain information from multiple informants who know the child in a variety of contexts. This is important in order to place disturbances of conduct in a perspective that allows one to address not only individual symptoms, but possible risk and causal factors as well, in a fashion that is developmentally appropriate. Self-reports of behaviour are essential to uncovering covert behaviours that have been successfully kept from the awareness of adults.

A comprehensive diagnostic assessment and history-gathering from multiple informants will have helped to identify the presence of conduct disorder and any coexisting conditions and problem areas that must be addressed in order for the healthy development of adaptive functioning to be restored over time. The most common coexisting clinical conditions found with conduct disorder are ADHD, mood and anxiety disorders, and substance use disorders. Furthermore, it is common to encounter academic underachievement and outright school failure, even in the absence of any learning disorders. Social isolation and arrest of development of age-appropriate social skills often result.

Once a child or adolescent has been identified as exhibiting conduct disorder, the clinician must be thinking along multiple, intersecting dimensions as he or she plans the approaches to the treatment of the patient. These dimensions include the developmental level and gender of the child, the presence of any coexisting problems and conditions, the planning and provision of interventions that will be carried out by the clinician in the clinical setting itself, the planning and co-ordination of interventions that will evolve outside the clinical setting, the involvement of caregivers and educators, and the possible recruitment of other agencies and providers, particularly those representing community resources, including the courts and juvenile justice system. For the extremely resistant child or adolescent, it may be necessary to involve the juvenile court to implement and supervise assessments and treatments.

Many of the interventions that evolve outside the clinical setting are similar both in principle and implementation to those interventions designed to prevent the onset of conduct disorder discussed elsewhere in this chapter. The clinician is unlikely to be a direct agent of change in these types of interventions. However, it is important for the clinician to be aware of the existing community resources, such as after-school programmes, and to recommend and assist if necessary the enrolment of the patient in such programmes. This may be especially indicated in situations where adult-supervised activities are deemed appropriate to either prevent association with deviant peers, or to enhance the acquisition of adaptive social skills. Advocating that the child receive supplementary academic services when indicated, is another crucial role of the child clinician, and will serve to enhance developmental competence in academic skills.

The literature concerning the clinical treatment of conduct disorders acknowledges the multifactorial causality of this group of disturbances, and their chronicity. Hence, once conduct disorder has been identified, it is not surprising that multimodal approaches, and extended time periods for the treatments are recommended and carried out. These multimodal approaches address not only the symptomatology of the conduct problems, but the fact that many children so affected require remediation in the areas of academic and social skills. Few studies have examined the long-term outcomes of programmes providing such complex interventions. The work of Grizenko *et al.* (1993; Grizenko 1997), suggests that such multimodal treatment approaches can lead to sustained benefits long after termination of the interventions, particularly when there is good parental participation during the intervention.

Specific psychosocial interventions

To a large extent, interventions that have been shown to be effective in randomized clinical trials follow closely from those factors that have been clearly identified as causal risk factors or risk factors of conduct disorder. In the case of conduct disorder, the most compelling evidence has been accrued around the causal role of caregiver practices. As a result, interventions targeted at this level are essential and most likely to lead to positive behavioural change, particularly when combined with strategies supporting the role of parents in the community and school. Some of the intervention strategies to address parenting behaviours may serve both as therapeutic and as preventive efforts.

Interventions will follow according to the developmental level of the child. For preschool- and elementary school-aged children, interventions will focus heavily on the training of primary caregivers and educators. The training will involve how these adults should alter and structure the environment of the child, how to prevent maladaptive behaviours, how to respond to the child when such behaviours do occur, how to teach the child to assume responsibility and control for his or her own behaviours, and how to impart adaptive skills and behaviours to the child. These techniques all draw heavily from operant–behavioural and cognitive–behavioural approaches to behavioural change (see Herbert, Chapter 53).

For adolescents, considerations involving the training of adults remain valid. Here, however, the need to provide interventions that impact the socialization process is critical. It is not that younger children would not benefit from socially based interventions, but adolescents are considerably more mobile than younger children, and can access peer groups far beyond those of their homes, immediate neighbourhoods, and their schools. Therefore it is important to devise interventions that can instill the inherent desire to associate with more functional peers, and the skills to engage successfully in such peer interactions.

For the interventions that are provided in the clinical setting itself by clinicians, those involving parent management training (PMT) have been the most successful and promising for altering the course of conduct disorder (Offord & Bennett 1994; Kazdin 1997; Brestan & Eyberg 1998). A number of studies involving randomized assignment to treatment or control conditions have been conducted, attesting to the efficacy of this general approach. Among the most widely studied of these approaches is the method developed by Patterson & Guillon (1968). This method stresses an operant–behavioural approach to behaviour management. This involves parental monitoring, ignoring or punishing deviant behaviours, and rewarding appropriate and incompatible (with problems) behaviours.

Various methods of imparting PMT are employed. For example, Webster-Stratton (1994; Webster-Stratton & Hammond 1997) have successfully conducted PMT with groups of parents using video tapes and group leaders, to model effective parenting behaviours. This modality of treatment delivery renders a technique of known efficacy and even more cost-effective intervention. These same investigators have also highlighted the importance of identifying and addressing how parents resolve marital conflicts, as a means of reducing behavioural problems in children (Webster-Stratton 1994; Webster-Stratton & Hammond 1999).

Home-based family therapy, such as the Family Project Approach (Verwaaijen *et al.* 1993a,b; Van Acker & de Kemp 1997), provides a means of working intensively with severely disturbed children and adolescents. By providing in-home training and support to primary caregivers in their parenting roles, such interventions may avert the need for institutional care of symptomatic children and adolescents. Furthermore, in vulnerable families, such interventions may reduce the risk of escalation of conflicts to the point where caregivers become overwhelmed and child maltreatment results.

Other therapeutic techniques aimed at individuals, that have shown clear promise in treating conduct disorders but are lacking in the type of evidence accrued for the various forms of PMT, include anger management and assertiveness training techniques, problem-solving skills training, and interventions designed to address biases in social cognition and information processing (Offord & Bennett 1994; Kazdin 1997; Brestan & Eyberg 1998). Each of these approaches is targeted to a specific factor thought to have a potential role in the onset or the evolution of conduct disorder. Symptomatic children may receive interventions to improve anger and aggression management, to learn appropriate means of asserting themselves in non-aggressive ways, to recognize and address biases in social cognition, and to improve problem-solving skills, so that during conflicts more adaptive solutions may be generated that can avoid outcomes such as aggressive confrontations.

A conceptual–empirical approach that is gaining increasing attention for the understanding and treatment of conduct disorders is attachment theory. Interventions for conduct disorder based on attachment theory begin with the premise that the children who display persistent disturbances of conduct are first and foremost 'disconnected' from the individuals and the norms of the society within which they live. Therefore, it is insufficient to focus on the identification and management of maladaptive behaviours. First, a meaningful connection must be established with the child, and with key individuals in the child's life (Moretti *et al.* 1994; Moore *et al.* 1998). Interventions informed by this theory have been extended to caregiving adults too. Studies indicate that mothers of children with conduct disorders report histories of problematic attachment to caregivers in their own childhood (Routh *et al*. 1995). Reparations in adult attachment behaviours towards their children is seen as central to influencing both child attachment behaviours and the symptoms of conduct disorder.

Psychopharmacological interventions

The psychopharmacological management of symptoms of conduct disorder *per se* has been a relatively neglected area of child psychiatric treatment. In fact, the longstanding clinical wisdom has been such that coexisting conditions, such as ADHD and mood disorders, are routinely treated medically. However, there has been widespread belief that symptoms specific to conduct disorder are not responsive to medications. This belief has been understandably sustained by the clear salience of environmental contributions to the causation of conduct disorder. However, this stance has recently been placed in question by the growing evidence of biological correlates of conduct disorder (Rogeness *et al*. 1992; Coccaro & Kavoussi 1996; Stoff & Vitiello 1996) and by a few well-designed and conducted medication trials involving randomized double-blind conditions, with assessment of change in some of the defining features of conduct disorder.

Once again, one would not consider medications in the absence of other interventions, nor would one expect that the complexity of a syndrome such as conduct disorder would respond *in toto* to medications. However, judicious targeting of certain conduct disorder-specific symptoms may be indicated where there is considerable severity and impairment resulting from such symptoms. Among the symptoms most commonly targeted with medical interventions are those involving the overt behaviours of explosive temper, interpersonal aggression and destruction of property. In two randomized double-blind placebo-controlled trials involving psychiatric inpatients, Campbell *et al*. (1995) and Malone *et al*. (2000) found that lithium carbonate reduced target symptoms of aggression and temper outbursts significantly more than placebo, independent of other mood effects of lithium. In an open-label study Kafantaris *et al*. (1992) found carbamazepine to be useful in reducing aggressive and explosive behaviours in hospitalized children diagnosed with conduct disorder. A follow-up study of inpatients by these investigators using double-blind placebo-controlled conditions and randomized assignment (Cueva *et al*. 1996), however, did not find carbamazepine to be superior to placebo in reducing these same target symptoms. It is important to recognize in the case of these studies, that inpatients were targeted for medication intervention. These results may not apply equally to outpatients, who might presumably display less severe forms of the same symptoms.

The use of psychostimulants has generally been reserved for the management of symptoms of ADHD. Klein *et al*. (1997) recently explored the efficacy of methylphenidate in reducing conduct disorder-specific symptoms in a randomized double-blind placebo-controlled trial of outpatients. They found that independent of pretreatment levels of comorbid symptoms of ADHD, methylphenidate significantly reduced levels of some conduct disorder-specific symptomatology, including verbal and physical aggression, stealing and cruelty.

There have been a number of other open-label studies involving the use of a variety of psychotropic medications to treat conduct disorder, including stimulants, beta-blockers, alpha-2 adrenergic agonists, antidepressants, mood stabilizers and neuroleptics (Lavin & Rifkin 1993). These studies suffer not only from the limitations inherent in the open-label design — including the lack of blinding of patients and raters, and the absence of randomized assignment to treatment conditions — but they often also suffer from the absence of a differentiated focus on symptoms of conduct disorder and on other comorbid conditions. Therefore it is difficult to ascertain in many of these trials if improvement was a direct result of treatment effects on conduct disorder-specific symptoms, or an indirect effect on behaviour caused by improvement in comorbid symptoms such as mood or hyperactivity.

Given the rapidly expanding field of paediatric psychopharmacology, and the increasing pressures and indications for biological therapies in multimodal approaches to conduct disorders, it will be necessary for more well-conducted clinical trials to be carried out involving blinded conditions and randomized assignment of patients, together with the use of well-validated assessment tools, to evaluate the efficacy of the wide range of medications that could plausibly be utilized to ameliorate specific target symptoms of conduct disorder.

Prevention

The high prevalence and chronicity of conduct disorder, combined with its refractoriness to treatment and high costs to society, make it a prime candidate for primary prevention (see Offord & Bennett, Chapter 52). It is far from obvious, however, what to emphasize in a programme of prevention, because the risk factors represent such a complex configuration of environmental and personal factors (Price *et al*. 1989; Walter *et al*. 1991).

Public health approaches to prevention generally work in one of two ways: either the environment harbouring the risk conditions is improved; or the personal resources and competence of children to deal with such conditions are strengthened. Offord (1987, 1989) has supplied a balanced account of prevention efforts in this area, and provided a rationale for the design of experiments based on the analysis of risk factors from the Ontario Child Health Study (Boyle & Offord 1989). While considerable effort has been directed towards community- and school-based efforts to reduce prevalence, it is important to contrast these with those that target high-risk groups of families or children. The decision to design programmes that can be universally applied, in contrast to interventions that target high-risk groups, is a major source of uncertainty in the prevention of conduct disorder.

An informative community-based experiment conducted in a

public housing area in Canada reported limited but important results (Offord & Jones 1983; Jones & Offord 1989). A comprehensive programme of non-academic skill development was established in one of two comparable areas for boys between 5 and 15 years. In the area receiving the intervention, the number of police and fire calls was reduced, as was the frequency of vandalism over a 3-year period. At the same time evidence was amassed to show that the children actually achieved new levels of athletic and physical skills. A cost analysis demonstrated that the money saved by government agencies far exceeded the programme's expenditures. These results are in keeping with the findings of studies that have examined the contribution of lack of adult supervision to and monitoring to disruptive behaviour in adolescents (Pettit *et al.* 1999). A caveat of this experiment is that the benefits were limited to non-academic areas. There was little evidence that the results generalized to areas of school performance or social skills.

School-based interventions have been popular for a number of years but have produced varying degrees of success in prevention (Gottfredson 1987). Recently, Hawkins *et al.* (1991) combined parent and teacher training programmes to promote social skill development in children aged 6 to 8 years old. The intervention, carried out over the first 2 years of primary school, significantly reduced the level of aggressive behaviour for white students, but did not have a significant impact on African-American children. While the possibility of biased teacher ratings cannot be discounted, it is conceivable that the level of risk in African-American children was beyond the level reachable by this experiment. These results are broadly similar to the Newcastle experiment in which group therapy and behaviour modification produced improvements in behavioural outcomes in children in primary school (Kolvin *et al.* 1981).

As the execution of well-designed school level intervention experiments have improved, the problems that complicate programme effectiveness have been better documented. Two examples will suffice. The Tri-Ministry study in Canada compared academic and social skills components separately and in combination, and followed children over a sufficiently long interval to document both transient and more lasting benefits (Hundert *et al.* 1999). The findings were sporadic and inconsistent in showing the expected increases in prosocial and decreases in antisocial behaviour. Among the several limitations discussed by the authors of this report, a particularly sobering one concerns the heavy reliance placed on outside experts in the design of the intervention. They suggest that a more collaborative approach from the beginning of conceptualizing such a programme may be fundamental to maximizing programme effectiveness. A similar prevention trial designed for children in the elementary school years and conducted in a US public school system demonstrated the formidable problems of random classroom and teacher allocation. The system's bias to cluster aggressive children in the same classroom worked to undermine interventions to reduce aggressive behaviour (Kellam *et al.* 1998).

The nationwide effort to reduce the level of interpersonal violence among school children in Norway is unique in its scope (Olweus 1991). The intervention was initiated by the Ministry of Education in the wake of an outbreak of suicides among boys who had apparently been victimized by peers. The endeavour involved mobilizing all the resources of the school system to educate teachers, administrators, parents and students in understanding the nature and seriousness of the aggressor–victim relationship. The programme was designed as a quasi-experiment in which results were assessed in a time-lagged fashion, permitting an estimate to be made about the size of the intervention effect in the absence of a control group. Judged by this standard, the effort was not only remarkably successful in reducing the level of violence, but also in diminishing antisocial behaviour in the school environment.

Prevention experiments that target preschool-aged children should conceivably have a more powerful impact than those that start later (McGuire & Earls 1991). Some evidence that this approach might work to reduce the prevalence of conduct disorder was provided by the Perry preschool intervention. Although this effort was designed as an educational enrichment programme for poor children, one follow-up study indicated that reduction in officially recorded delinquency was achieved in the experimental group (Schweinhart & Weikart 1997). To date, preschool experiments explicitly designed to reduce the rate of conduct problems have not been conducted, but the evidence derived from studies such as these must be regarded as promising.

Experiments designed to judge the long-term benefits of home-based parent training interventions beginning in the prenatal period and extending through the first few years of postnatal life have been closely watched. Although many of the same problems confronting school-based experiments have strained these types of efforts, the results represent a somewhat more optimistic picture. The work of Olds *et al.* (1998) is noteworthy in showing a long-term reduction of antisocial behaviour through adolescence. The positive effects of this intervention were restricted to the children at the highest risk in the sample. Such results argue for targeting resources to selective subgroups in contrast to interventions designed for universal application (Earls 1998).

The Montreal Prevention Experiment is a prime example of a high-risk design (Tremblay *et al.* 1992). In this study of kindergarten boys, all from low-income families, positive screening for oppositional and aggressive behaviour was performed prior to randomly assigning the subjects to one of three groups: experimental, control and placebo (these subjects were observed frequently but did not receive an intervention). The 2-year programme of intervention included PMT, social skill development for children, and a television viewing training curriculum for both parents and children. Follow-up at 3 years post-intervention demonstrated higher levels of grade retention, less fighting and delinquent behaviour in the experimental group. The study is now tracking subjects into their adolescent years to observe if these promising results endure (Vitaro *et al.* 1999).

Conclusions

As this chapter reveals, a considerable body of knowledge and experience exist about conduct problems, yet it would be an overstatement to say that this understanding is any where near being sufficient to address the disruptive and potentially dangerous consequences that are associated with this disorder. The control of this problem remains a challenge for child psychiatry and its associated disciplines and services. A necessity for meeting this challenge requires professionals to be closely attuned to the ways in which modern societies are changing in responding to the unvarying needs for nurture and guidance that all children require.

This is far from a straightforward task. Efforts to isolate the causes of conduct disorder have been complicated by a variety of contributing factors. The heterogeneity of factors exist at different levels of organization rendering a reductionistic approach inadvisable (see HTTP://phdcn.harvard.ed for description of a research programme that is designed to capture such multiple levels of influence in a single design). Yet, treatment plans and prevention efforts must have a target. Maintaining a balance between a comprehensive approach towards assessment and a focused intervention is one of the most demanding aspects of caring for children with this disorder.

References

Achenbach, T.M., Conners, C.K., Quay, H.C., Verhulst, F.C. & Howell, C.T. (1989) Replication of empirically derived syndromes as a basis for taxonomy of child/adolescent psychopathology. *Journal of Abnormal Child Psychology*, 17, 299–323.

Aichorn, A. (1935) *Wayward Youth*. Viking Press. New York.

Ainsworth, M.D.S., Blehar, M.C., Waters, E. & Wall, S. (1978) *Patterns of Attachment, A Psychological Study of the Strange Situation*. Lawrence Erlbaum, Hillsdale, NJ.

American Psychiatric Association (1994) *Diagnostic and Statistical Manual of Mental Disorders (DSM-IV)*, 4th ed. American Psychiatric Association, Washington D.C.

Bird, H. (1996) The epidemiology of childhood disorders in cross-cultural context. *Journal of Child Psychology and Psychiatry*, 37, 35–39.

Bird, H., Canino, G. & Rubio-Stipec, M. (1988) Estimates of the prevalence of childhood maladjustment in a community survey in Puerto Rico: the use of combined measures. *Archives of General Psychiatry*, 45, 1120–1126.

Bowlby, J. (1944) Forty-four juvenile thieves: their characters and home-life. *International Journal of Psychoanalysis*, 25, 1–57.

Bowlby, J. (1969) *Attachment*. Basic Books, New York.

Boyle, M.H. & Offord, D.R. (1989) Primary prevention of conduct disorder: issues and prospects. *Journal of the American Academy of Child and Adolescent Psychiatry*, 29, 227–233.

Brennan, P., Grekin, E.R. & Mednick, S.A. (1999) Maternal smoking during pregnancy and adult male criminal outcomes. *Archives of General Psychiatry*, 56, 215–222.

Brestan, E.V. & Eyberg, S.M. (1998) Effective psychosocial treatments of conduct-disordered children and adolescents: 29 years, 82 studies, and 5272 kids. *Journal of Clinical Child Psychology*, 27, 180–189.

Burt, C. (1925) *The Young Delinquent*. D. Appleton, New York.

Cairns, R.B. & Cairns, B.D. (1991) Social cognition and social networks: a developmental perspective. In: *The Development and Treatment of Childhood Aggression* (eds D.J. Pepler & K.H. Rubin), pp. 249–278. Lawrence Erlbaum, Hillsdale, NJ.

Cairns, R.B., Cairns, B.D., Neckerman, H.J. *et al.* (1988) Social networks and aggressive behavior: peer support or peer rejection? *Developmental Psychology*, 24, 815–823.

Campbell, S.B. & Ewing, L.J. (1990) Follow-up of hard-to-manage preschoolers: adjustment at age 9 and predictors of continuing symptoms. *Journal of Child Psychology and Psychiatry*, 31, 871–889.

Campbell, M., Adams, P.B., Small, A.M. *et al.* (1995) Lithium in hospitalized aggressive children with conduct disorder: a double-blind and placebo-controlled study. *Journal of the American Academy of Child and Adolescent Psychiatry*, 34, 445–453.

Christian, R.E., Frick, P.J., Hill, N.L. *et al.* (1997) Psychopathy and conduct problems in children. II. Implications for subtyping children with conduct problems. *Journal of the American Academy of Child and Adolescent Psychiatry*, 36, 233–241.

Cleckley, H. (1941) *The Mask of Sanity*. C.V. Mosby, St. Louis.

Coccaro, E.F. & Kavoussi, R.J. (1996) Neurotransmitter correlates of impulsive aggression. In: *Aggression and Violence: Genetic, Neurobiological and Biosocial Perspectives* (eds D.M. Stoff & R.B. Cairns), pp. 66–86. Lawrence Erlbaum, Mahwah, NJ.

Cohen, P., Cohen, J., Kasen, S. *et al.* (1993) An epidemiological study of disorders in late childhood and adolescence. I. Age- and gender-specific prevalence. *Journal of Child Psychology and Psychiatry*, 34, 851–867.

Costello, E. (1989) Developments in child psychiatric epidemiology. *Journal of the American Academy of Child and Adolescent Psychiatry*, 28, 836–841.

Costello, E.J., Angold, A., Burns, B.J. *et al.* (1996) The Great Smoky Mountains Study of Youth. *Archives of General Psychiatry*, 53, 1129–1136.

Cueva, J.E., Overall, J.E., Small, A.M. *et al.* (1996) Carbamazepine in aggressive children with conduct disorder: a double-blind and placebo-controlled study. *Journal of the American Academy of Child and Adolescent Psychiatry*, 35, 480–490.

Daugherty, T. & Quay, H.C. (1991) Response perseveration and delayed responding in childhood behavior disorders. *Journal of Child Psychology and Psychiatry*, 32, 453–461.

Dodge, K.A., Pettit, G.S., Bates, J.E. & Valente, E. (1995) Social information processing patterns partially mediate the effect of early physical abuse on later conduct problems. *Journal of Abnormal Psychology*, 104, 632–643.

Earls, F. (1989) Epidemiology and child psychiatry: entering the second phase. *American Journal of Orthopsychiatry*, 59, 279–283.

Earls, F. (1998) Positive effects of prenatal and early childhood interventions. *Journal of the American Medical Association*, 280, 1271–1273.

Eaves, L.J., Silberg, J.L., Meyer, J.M. *et al.* (1997) Genetics and developmental psychopathology. II. The main effects of genes and environment on behavioral problems in the Virginia Twin Study of Adolescent Behavioral Development. *Journal of Child Psychology and Psychiatry*, 38, 965–980.

Edelbrock, C. & Costello, A.J. (1988) Convergence between statistically derived behavior problem syndromes and child psychiatric diagnoses. *Journal of Abnormal Child Psychology*, 16, 219–232.

Elliot, D.S., Huizinga, D. & Ageton, S.S. (1985) *Explaining Delinquency and Drug Use*. Sage, Newbury Park, CA.

Elliot, D.S., Huizinga, D. & Menard, S. (1989) *Multiple Problem Youth:*

Delinquency, Substance Use and Mental Health Problems. Springer-Verlag, New York.

Farrington, D.P. (1995) The development of offending and antisocial behavior from childhood: key findings from the Cambridge Study in Delinquent Development. *Journal of Child Psychology and Psychiatry*, **36**, 929–964.

Fergusson, D.M., Woodward, L.J. & Horwood, L.J. (1998) Maternal smoking during pregnancy and psychiatric adjustment in late adolescence. *Archives of General Psychiatry*, **55**, 721–728.

Fischer, M., Rolf, J.E., Hasazi, J.E. & Cummings, L. (1984) Follow-up of a preschool epidemiological sample: cross-age continuities and predictions of later adjustment with internalizing and externalizing dimensions of behavior. *Child Development*, **55**, 137–150.

Frick, P.J., Lahey, B.B., Loeber, R. *et al.* (1991) Oppositional defiant disorder and conduct disorder in boys: patterns of behavioral covariation. *Journal of Clinical Child Psychology*, **20**, 202–208.

Gittelman, R., Mannuzza, S., Shenker, R. & Bonagura, N. (1985) Hyperactive boys almost grown up. I. Psychiatric status. *Archives of General Psychiatry*, **42**, 937–947.

Gottfredson, D.C. (1987) An empirical test of school-based environmental and individual interventions to reduce the risk of delinquent behavior. *Criminology*, **24**, 705–731.

Greenbaum, P.E., Prange, M.E., Friedman, R.M. & Silver, S.E. (1991) Substance abuse prevalence and comorbidity with other psychiatric disorders among adolescents with severe emotional disturbances. *Journal of the American Academy of Child and Adolescent Psychiatry*, **30**, 575–583.

Grizenko, N. (1997) Outcome of multimodal day treatment for children with severe behavior problems: a five-year follow-up. *Journal of the American Academy of Child and Adolescent Psychiatry*, **36**, 989–997.

Grizenko, N., Papineau, D. & Sayegh, L. (1993) Effectiveness of a multimodal day treatment program for children with disruptive behavior problems. *Journal of the American Academy of Child and Adolescent Psychiatry*, **32**, 127–134.

Hawkins, J.D., Von Cleve, E. & Catalano, R.F. (1991) Reducing early childhood aggression: results of a primary prevention program. *Journal of the American Academy of Child and Adolescent Psychiatry*, **30**, 208–217.

Hewitt, L.E. & Jenkins, R.L. (1946) *Fundamental Patterns of Maladjustment: the Dynamics of Their Origins.* State of Illinois, Springfield, IL.

Hill, J. & Maughan, B. (2001) *Conduct Disorders in Childhood and Adolescence.* Cambridge University Press, Cambridge.

Hundert, J., Boyle, M.H., Cunningham, C.E. *et al.* (1999) Helping children adjust: a Tri-Ministry study. II. Program effects. *Journal of Child Psychology and Psychiatry*, **40**, 1061–1073.

Jenkins, J.M. & Smith, M.A. (1990) Factors protecting children in disharmonious homes. *American Academy of Child and Adolescent Psychiatry*, **29**, 60–69.

Jensen, P.S., Salzberg, A.D., Richters, J.E. & Watanabe, H.K. (1993) Scales, diagnoses, and child psychopathology. I. CBCL and DISC relationships. *Journal of the American Academy of Child and Adolescent Psychiatry*, **32**, 397–406.

Jensen, P.S., Roper, M., Fisher, P. *et al.* (1995) Test–retest reliability of the Diagnostic Interview Schedule for Children (DISC 2.1). *Archives of General Psychiatry*, **52**, 61–71.

Jensen, P.S., Watanabe, H.K., Richters, J.E. *et al.* (1996) Scales, diagnoses, and child psychopathology. II. Comparing the CBCL and the DISC against external validators. *Journal of Abnormal Child Psychology*, **24**, 151–168.

Joffe, R.D., Dobson, K.S., Fine, S., Marriage, K. & Haley, G. (1990) Social problem-solving in depressed, conduct-disordered and normal adolescents. *Journal of Abnormal Child Psychology*, **18**, 565–575.

Johnson, A.M. & Szurek, S.A. (1952) The genesis of antisocial acting-out in children and adolescents. *Psychoanalytic Quarterly*, **21**, 323–343.

Jones, M.B. & Offord, D.R. (1989) Reduction of antisocial behavior in poor children by nonschool skill-development. *Journal of Child Psychology and Psychiatry*, **30**, 737–750.

Kafantaris, V., Campbell, M., Padron-Gayol, M.V. *et al.* (1992) Carbamazepine in hospitalized aggressive conduct disorder children: an open pilot study. *Psychopharmacology Bulletin*, **28**, 193–199.

Kandel, D., Kessler, R.C. & Margulies, R.Z. (1978) Antecedents of adolescent initiation into stages of drug use: a developmental analysis. In: *Longitudinal Research and Drug Use: Empirical Findings and Methodological Issues* (ed. D.B. Kandel), pp. 73–98. Hemisphere, Washington D.C.

Kazdin, A.E. (1997) Practitioner review: psychosocial treatments for conduct disorder in children. *Journal of Child Psychology and Psychiatry*, **38**, 161–178.

Kellam, S.G., Ling, X., Mersica, R., Brown, C.H. & Ialongo, N. (1998) The effect of the level of aggression in the first grade classroom on the course and malleability of aggressive behavior into middle school. *Development and Psychopathology*, **10**, 165–185.

Kessler, R.C., McGonagle, K.A., Zhao, S. *et al.* (1994) Lifetime and 12-month prevalence of DSM-III-R psychiatric disorders in the United States. *Archives of General Psychiatry*, **51**, 8–19.

Klein, R.G., Abikoff, H., Klass, E. *et al.* (1997) Clinical efficacy of methylphenidate in conduct disorder with and without attention deficit hyperactivity disorder. *Archives of General Psychiatry*, **54**, 1073–1080.

Kolvin, I., Garside, R.F., Nicol, A.R., MacMillen, A., Wolstenhome, F. & Leitch, I.M. (1981) *Help Starts Here: the Maladjusted Child in the Ordinary School.* Tavistock Publications, New York.

Kraemer, H.C., Kazdin, A.E., Offord, D.R. *et al.* (1997) Coming to terms with the terms of risk. *Archives of General Psychiatry*, **54**, 337–343.

Lahey, B.B., Waldman, I.D. & McBurnett, K. (1999) The development of antisocial behavior: an integrative causal model. *Journal of Child Psychology and Psychiatry*, **40**, 669–682.

Lavin, M.R. & Rifkin, A. (1993) Diagnosis and pharmacotherapy of conduct disorder. *Progress in Neuro-Psychopharmacology and Biological Psychiatry*, **17**, 875–885.

Levy, D.M. (1952) Oppositional syndromes and oppositional behavior. In: *Psychopathology of Childhood* (eds P.H. Hach & J. Zubin), pp. 204–226. Grune and Stratton, New York.

Lewis, D.O. (1990) Neuropsychology and experiential correlates of violent juvenile delinquency. *Neuropsychology Review*, **1** (2), 125–136.

Lewis, D.O., Lovely, R., Yeager, C., Ferguson, G. & Friedman, M. (1988) *Journal of the American Academy of Child and Adolescent Psychiatry*, **27**, 582–587.

Loeber, R. & Keenan, K. (1994) Interaction between conduct disorder and its comorbid conditions: effects of gender and age. *Clinical Psychology Review*, **14**, 497–523.

Loeber, R. & Le Blanc, M. (1990) Toward a developmental criminology. In: *Crime and Justice: a Review of Research* (eds M. Tonry & N. Morris), pp. 375–473. University of Chicago Press, Chicago, IL.

Loeber, R., Brinthaupt, V.P. & Green, S.M. (1990a) Attention deficits, impulsivity, and hyperactivity with or without conduct problems: relationships to delinquency and unique contextual factors. In: *Behavior Disorders of Adolescence. Research, Intervention and Policy in Clinical and School Settings* (eds R.J. McMahon & R.DeV. Peters), pp. 39–61. Plenum Press, New York.

Loeber, R., Green, S.M. & Lahey, B.B. (1990b) Mental health professionals' perception of the utility of children, mothers, and teachers as informants on childhood psychopathology. *Journal of Clinical Child Psychology*, **19**, 136–143.

Loeber, R., Green, S.M., Lahey, B.B. & Stouthamer-Loeber, M. (1991a) Differences and similarities between children, mothers, and teachers as informants on disruptive child behavior. *Journal of Abnormal Child Psychology*, **19**, 75–95.

Loeber, R., Lahey, B.B. & Thomas, C. (1991b) Diagnostic conundrum of oppositional defiant disorder and conduct disorder. *Journal of Abnormal Psychology*, **100**, 379–390.

Loeber, R., Wung, P., Keenan, K. *et al.* (1993) Developmental pathways in disruptive child behavior. *Development and Psychopathology*, **5**, 103–134.

Magnusson, D. & Bergman, L. (1988) Individual and variable-based approaches to longitudinal research on early risk factors. In: *Studies of Psychosocial Risk: the Power of Longitudinal Data* (ed. M. Rutter), pp. 45–61. Cambridge University Press, Cambridge.

Malone, R.P., Delaney, M.A., Luebbert, J.F., Cater, J. & Campbell, M. (2000) A double-blind placebo-controlled study of lithium in hospitalized aggressive children and adolescents with conduct disorder. *Archives of General Psychiatry*, **57**, 649–658.

Mannuzza, S., Klein, R.G., Bonagura, N., Malloy, P., Giampino, T.L. & Addalli, K.A. (1991) Hyperactive boys almost grown up. V. Replication of psychiatric status. *Archives of General Psychiatry*, **48**, 77–83.

McBurnett, K., Lahey, B.B., Frick, P.J. *et al.* (1991) Anxiety, inhibition, and conduct disorder in children. II. Relation to salivary cortisol. *Journal of the American Academy of Child and Adolescent Psychiatry*, **30**, 192–196.

McGee, R., Williams, S. & Silva, P.A. (1984) Behavioral and developmental characteristics of aggressive, hyperactive, and aggressive-hyperactive boys. *Journal of the American Academy of Child Psychiatry*, **23**, 270–279.

McGuire, J. & Earls, F. (1991) Prevention of psychiatric disorders in early childhood. *Journal of Child Psychology and Psychiatry*, **32**, 129–154.

Mezzacappa, E., Tremblay, R.E., Kindlon, D. *et al.* (1997) Anxiety, antisocial behavior and heart rate regulation in adolescent males. *Journal of Child Psychology and Psychiatry*, **38**, 457–470.

Milin, R., Halikas, J.A., Meller, J.E. & Morse, C. (1991) Psychopathology among substance abusing juvenile offenders. *Journal of the American Academy of Child and Adolescent Psychiatry*, **30**, 569–574.

Moffitt, T.E. (1990) Juvenile delinquency and attention deficit disorder: boys' developmental trajectories from age 3 to age 15. *Child Development*, **61**, 893–910.

Moffitt, T. (1993a) The neuropsychology of conduct disorder. *Development and Psychopathology*, **5**, 135–152.

Moffitt, T.E. (1993b) Adolescence-limited and life-course-persistent antisocial behavior: a developmental taxonomy. *Psychological Review*, **100**, 674–701.

Moffitt, T.E., Caspi, A., Rutter, M. & Silva, P. (2001) *Sorting Out Sex Differences in Antisocial Behaviour: Conduct disorder, delinquency and violence in the Dunedin Longitudinal Study.* Cambridge University Press, Cambridge.

Moore, K., Moretti, M.M. & Holland, R. (1998) A new perspective on youth care programs: using attachment theory to guide interventions for troubled youth. *Residential Treatment of Children and Youth*, **15**, 1–24.

Moretti, M.M., Holland, R. & Peterson, S. (1994) Long term outcome of an attachment-based program for conduct disorder. *Canadian Journal of Psychiatry*, **39**, 360–370.

Nagin, D. & Tremblay, R.E. (1999) Trajectories of boys' physical aggression, opposition, and hyperactivity on the path to physically violent and nonviolent juvenile delinquency. *Child Development*, **70**, 1181–1196.

Offord, D.R. (1987) Prevention of behavioral and emotional disorders in children. *Journal of Child Psychology and Psychiatry*, **28**, 9–19.

Offord, D.R. (1989) Conduct disorders: risk factors and prevention. In: *Prevention of Mental Disorders, Alcohol and Other Drug Use in Children and Adolescents* (eds D. Shaffer, I. Philips, N.B. Enzer & M.M. Silverman), pp. 273–307. OSAP Prevention Monograph 2, US Department of Health and Human Services, Rockville, MD.

Offord, D.R. & Bennett, K.J. (1994) Conduct disorder: long-term outcomes and intervention effectiveness. *Journal of the American Academy of Child and Adolescent Psychiatry*, **33**, 1069–1078.

Offord, D.R. & Jones, M.B. (1983) Skill development: a community intervention program for the prevention of antisocial behavior. In: *Childhood Psychopathology and Development* (eds S.B. Guze, F. Earls & J.E. Barrett), pp. 165–188. Raven Press, New York.

Offord, D.R., Boyle, M.H., Szatmari, P. *et al.* (1987) Ontario Child Health Study. I. Six-month prevalence of disorder and service utilization. *Archives of General Psychiatry*, **44**, 832–836.

Offord, D.R., Boyle, M.C. & Racine, Y.A. (1991) The epidemiology of antisocial behavior in childhood and adolescence. In: *The Development and Treatment of Childhood Aggression* (eds D.J. Pepler & K.H. Rubin), pp. 31–54. Lawrence Erlbaum, Hillsdale, NJ.

Olds, D., Henderson, C.R. & Cole, R. (1998) Long-term efffects of nurse home visitation on children's criminal and antisocial behavior: 15-year follow-up of a randomized controlled trial. *Journal of the American Medical Association*, **280**, 1238–1244.

Olweus, D. (1979) Stability of aggressive reaction patterns in males: a review. *Psychological Bulletin*, **86**, 852–875.

Olweus, D. (1991) Bully/victim problems among schoolchildren: basic facts and effects of a school based intervention program. In: *The Development and Treatment of Childhood Aggression* (eds D.J. Pepler & K.H. Rubin), pp. 411–448. Lawrence Erlbaum, Hillsdale, NJ.

Oosterlaan, J. & Sergeant, J.A. (1996) Inhibition in ADHD, aggressive and anxious children: a biologically based model of child psychopathology. *Journal of Abnormal Child Psychology*, **24**, 19–36.

Oosterlaan, J., Logan, G. & Sergeant, J.A. (1998) Response inhibition in AD/HD, CD, comorbid AD/HD + CD, anxious and control children: a meta-analysis of studies with the stop task. *Journal of Child Psychology and Psychiatry*, **39**, 411–425.

Patterson, G.R. & Guillon, M.E. (1968) *Living With Children: New Methods for Parents and Teachers.* Research Press, Champaign, IL.

Patterson, G.R., DeBarysh, B.D. & Ramsey, E. (1989) A developmental perspective on antisocial behavior. *American Psychologist*, **44**, 329–335.

Pettit, G.S., Bates, J.E., Dodge, K.A. & Meece, D.W. (1999) The impact of after-school peer contact on early adolescent externalizing problems is moderated by parental monitoring, perceived neighborhood safety, and prior adjustment. *Child Development*, **70**, 768–778.

Pine, D.S., Coplan, J.D., Wasserman, G.A. *et al.* (1997) Neuroendocrine response to fenfluramine challenge in boys: associations with aggressive behavior and adverse rearing. *Archives of General Psychiatry*, **54**, 839–846.

Pine, D.S., Wasserman, G.A., Miller, L. *et al.* (1998) Heart period variability and psychopathology in boys at risk for delinquency. *Psychophysiology*, **35**, 521–529.

Porges, S.W. & Doussard-Roosevelt, J.A., Portales, A.L., & Greenspan, S. (1996) Infant regulation of the vagal 'brake' predicts child behavior problems: a psychobiological model of social behavior. *Developmental Psychobiology*, **29**, 697–712.

Price, R.H., Cowen, E.L., Lorion, R.P. & Ramos-McKay, J. (1989) The search for effective prevention programs: what we learned along the way. *American Journal of Orthopsychiatry*, **59**, 49–58.

Quay, H.C. (1993) The psychobiology of undersocialized aggressive conduct disorder: a theoretical perspective. *Development and Psychopathology*, **5**, 165–180.

Quay, H.C. & Peterson, D.R. (1987) *Manual for the Revised Behavior Problem Checklist*. University of Miami, Coral Gables, FL.

Raine, A., Venables, P.H. & Williams, M. (1990) Relationships between central and autonomic measures of arousal at age 15 years and criminality at age 24 years. *Archives of General Psychiatry*, **47**, 1003–1007.

Raine, A., Venables, P.H. & Williams, M. (1995) High autonomic arousal and electrodermal orienting at age 15 years as protective factors against criminal behavior at age 29 years. *American Journal of Psychiatry*, **152**, 1595–1600.

Raine, A., Venables, P.H. & Mednick, S.A. (1997) Low resting heart rate at age 3 years predisposes to aggression at age 11 years: evidence from the Mauritius Child Health Project. *Journal of the American Academy of Child and Adolescent Psychiatry*, **36**, 1457–1464.

Raine, A., Lencz, T., Bihrle, S., LaCasse, L. & Colletti, P. (2000) Reduced prefrontal gray matter and reduced autonomic activity in antisocial personality disorder. *Archives of General Psychiatry*, **57**, 119–127.

Rasanen, P., Hakko, H., Isohanni, M., Hodgins, S., Jarvelin, M.R. & Tiihonen, J. (1999) Maternal smoking during pregnancy and risk of criminal behavior among adult male offspring in the Northern Finland 1966 birth cohort. *American Journal of Psychiatry*, **156**, 857–862.

Reiss, A.J. & Farrington, D.P. (1991) Advancing knowledge about co-offending: results from a prospective longitudinal survey of London Males. *Journal of Criminal Law and Criminology*, **82**, 360–395.

Richman, N., Stevenson, J. & Graham, P.J. (1982) *Pre-school to School: a Behavioural Study*. Academic Press, London.

Robins, L.N. (1966) *Deviant Children Grown Up*. Williams & Wilkins, Baltimore.

Robins, L.N. (1978) Sturdy childhood predictors of adult antisocial behavior: replications from longitudinal studies. *Psychological Medicine*, **8**, 611–622.

Rogeness, G.A., Javors, M.A. & Pliszka, S.R. (1992) Neurochemistry and child and adolescent psychiatry. *Journal of the American Academy of Child and Adolescent Psychiatry*, **31**, 765–781.

Routh, C.P., Hill, J.W., Steele, H. *et al.* (1995) Maternal attachment status, psychosocial stressors and problem behavior: follow-up after parent training courses for conduct disorder. *Journal of Child Psychology and Psychiatry*, **36**, 1179–1198.

Rutter, M. (1978) Family, area, and school influences in the genesis of conduct disorders. In: *Aggression and Anti-Social Behavior in Childhood and Adolescence* (eds L.A. Hersov & M. Berger), pp. 95–114. Pergamon, London.

Rutter, M. (1989) Annotation: child psychiatric disorders in ICD-10. *Journal of Child Psychology and Psychiatry*, **30**, 499–513.

Rutter, M., Tizard, J. & Whitmore, K. (1970) *Education, Health and Behavior*. Longman, London.

Rutter, M., Cox, A., Tupling, C., Berger, M. & Yule, W. (1975) Attainment and adjustment in two geographical areas. I. Prevalence of psychiatric disorder. *British Journal of Psychiatry*, **126**, 493–509.

Rutter, M., Giller, H. & Hagell, A. (1998) *Antisocial Behavior by Young People*. Cambridge University Press, New York.

Scerbo, A.S. & Kolko, D.J. (1994) Salivary testosterone and cortisol in disruptive children: relationship to aggressive, hyperactive, and internalizing disorders. *Journal of the American Academy of Child and Adolescent Psychiatry*, **33**, 1174–1184.

Schaal, B., Tremblay, R.E., Soussignan, R. & Susman, E.J. (1996) Male testosterone linked to high social dominance but low physical aggres-

sion in early adolescence. *Journal of the American Academy of Child and Adolescent Psychiatry*, **35**, 1322–1330.

Schachar, R. & Wachsmuth, R. (1990) Oppositional disorder in children: a validation study comparing conduct disorder, oppositional disorder and normal control children. *Journal of Child Psychology and Psychiatry*, **31**, 1089–1102.

Schwab-Stone, M., Shaffer, D., Dulcan, M.K. *et al.* (1996) Criterion validity of the NIMH Diagnostic Interview Schedule for Children, Version 2.3 (DISC-2.3). *Journal of the American Academy of Child and Adolescent Psychiatry*, **35**, 878–888.

Schweinhart, L.J. & Weikart, D.P. (1997) The High/Scope Preschool Curriculum Comparison study through age 23. *Early Childhood Research Quarterly*, **12**, 117–143.

Seguin, J.R., Pihl, R.O., Harden, P.W. *et al.* (1995) Cognitive and neuropsychological characteristics of physically aggressive boys. *Journal of Abnormal Psychology*, **104**, 614–624.

Seguin, J.R., Boulerice, B., Harden, P.W. *et al.* (1999) Executive functions and physical aggression after controlling for attention deficit hyperactivity disorder, general memory, and IQ. *Journal of Child Psychology and Psychiatry*, **40**, 1197–1208.

Simonoff, E., Pickles, A., Meyer, J., Silberg, J. & Maes, H. (1998) Genetic and environmental influences on subtypes of conduct disorder behavior in boys. *Journal of Abnormal Child Psychology*, **26**, 495–509.

Speltz, M.L., McClellan, J., DeKlyen, M. & Jones, K. (1999) Preschool boys with oppositional defiant disorder: clinical presentation and diagnostic change. *Journal of the American Academy of Child and Adolescent Psychiatry*, **38**, 838–845.

Stewart, M.A., Cummings, C., Singer, S. & DeBlois, C.S. (1981) The overlap between hyperactive and unsocialized aggressive children. *Journal of Child Psychology and Psychiatry*, **22**, 35–45.

Stoff, D.M. & Vitiello, B. (1996) Role of serotonin in aggression of children and adolescents: biochemical and pharmacologic studies. In: *Aggression and Violence: Genetic, Neurobiological and Biosocial Perspectives* (eds D.M. Stoff & R.B. Cairns), pp. 101–124. Lawrence Erlbaum, Mahwah, NJ.

Toupin, J., Dery, M., Pauze, R., Mercier, H. & Fortin, L. (2000) Cognitive and familial contributions to conduct disorder in children. *Journal of Child Psychology and Psychiatry*, **41**, 333–344.

Tremblay, R.E., Vitaro, F., Bertrand, L., *et al.* (1992) Parent and child training to prevent early onset of delinquency: The Montreal Longitudinal-Experimental Study. In: *Parenting Antisocial Behaviour: Interventions from Birth Through Adolescence* (eds. J. McCord, R.E. Tremblay), pp. 151–236. Guilford, New York.

Tremblay, R.E., Loeber, R., Gagnon, C., Charlebois, P., Larivee, S. & LeBlanc, M. (1991a) Disruptive boys with stable and unstable high fighting behavior patterns during junior elementary school. *Journal of Abnormal Child Psychology*, **19**, 285–299.

Tremblay, R.E., McCord, J., Boileau, H. *et al.* (1991b) Can disruptive boys be helped to become competent? *Psychiatry*, **54**, 148–161.

Van Acker, J.C. & de Kemp, R.A.T. (1997) The Family Project Approach. *Journal of Adolescence*, **20**, 419–430.

Verwaaijen, A.A. & Van Acker, J.C. (1993a) Family treatment for adolescents at risk of placement. I. Theory and treatment process. *Family Therapy, Special Issue*, **20**, 73–102.

Verwaaijen, A.A. & Van Acker, J.C. (1993b) Family treatment for adolescents at risk of placement. II. Treatment process and outcome. *Family Therapy, Special Issue*, **20**, 103–132.

Vitaro, F., Brendgen, M. & Tremblay, R.E. (1999) Prevention of school dropout through reduction of disruptive behaviors and school failure in elementary school. *Journal of School Psychology*, **37**, 205–226.

Wakschlag, L.S., Lahey, B.B., Loeber, R., Green, S.M., Gordon, R.A. & Leventhal, B.L. (1997) Maternal smoking during pregnancy and the risk of conduct disorder in boys. *Archives of General Psychiatry*, 54, 670–676.

Walker, L.J., Lahey, B.B., Russo, M.F. *et al.* (1991) Anxiety, inhibition, and conduct disorder in children. I. Relations to social impairment. *Journal of the American Academy of Child and Adolescent Psychiatry*, 30, 187–191.

Walter, H.J., Vaughn, R.D. & Cohall, A.T. (1991) Risk factors for substance use among high school students: implications for prevention. *Journal of the American Academy of Child and Adolescent Psychiatry*, 30, 556–562.

Webster-Stratton, C. (1994) Advancing videotape parent training: a comparison study. *Journal of Consulting and Clinical Psychology*, 62, 583–593.

Webster-Stratton, C. & Hammond, M. (1997) Treating children with early onset conduct problems: a comparison of child and parent training interventions. *Journal of Consulting and Clinical Psychology*, 65, 93–109.

Webster-Stratton, C. & Hammond, M. (1999) Marital conflict management skills, parenting style and early onset conduct problems: processes and pathways. *Journal of Child Psychology and Psychiatry*, 40, 917–927.

Weissman, M.M., Warner, V., Wickramaratne, P.J. & Kandel, D.B. (1999) Maternal smoking during pregnancy and psychopathology in offspring followed to adulthood. *Journal of the American Academy of Child and Adolescent Psychiatry*, 38, 892–899.

Weisz, J.R., Suwanert, S., Chaiyasit, W., Weiss, B., Walter, B.R. & Anderson, W.W. (1988) Thai and American perspectives on over- and undercontrolled behavior problems: exploring the threshold model among parents, teachers, psychologists. *Journal of Consulting and Clinical Psychology*, 56, 601–609.

Weisz, J.R., Martin, S.L., Walter, B.R. & Fernandez, G.A. (1991) Differential prediction of young adult arrests for property and personal crimes: findings of a cohort follow-up study of violent boys from North Carolina's Willie M. Program. *Journal of Child Psychology and Psychiatry*, 32, 783–792.

White, J.L., Moffitt, E. & Silva, P.A. (1989) A prospective replication of the protective effects of IQ in subjects at high risk for juvenile delinquency. *Journal of Clinical and Consulting Psychology*, 57, 719–724.

White, J.L., Moffitt, T.E., Earls, F., Robins, L. & Silva, P.A. (1990) How early can we tell? Predictors of childhood conduct disorder and adolescent delinquency. *Criminology*, 28, 507–533.

World Health Organization (1992) *The ICD-10 Classification of Mental and Behavioural Disorders: Clinical Descriptions and Diagnositic Guidelines*. World Health Organization, Geneva, Switzerland.

Zahn-Waxler, C. (1993) Warriors and worriers: gender and psychopathology. *Development and Psychopathology*, 5, 79–90.

Zoccolillo, M. (1993) Gender and the development of conduct disorder. *Development and Psychopathology*, 5, 65–78.

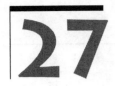

27 Substance Use and Abuse: Epidemiology, Pharmacological Considerations, Identification and Suggestions Towards Management

Warren A. Weinberg, Caryn R. Harper and Roger A. Brumback

Introduction

One of the major problems confronting society at the beginning of the twenty-first century is the increasing substance use and abuse by young people. Despite many studies of this problem, there is still little understanding of the causes, appropriate treatment and, most importantly, successful approaches to prevention. Farrell & Taylor (1994) and Bukstein & Tarter (1998) reviewed much of the relevant literature. An excellent review of adolescent substance abuse and dual disorders was published in 1996 in *Child and Adolescent Psychiatric Clinics of North America* with S.L. Jaffe as guest editor. Rather than duplicating those efforts, this chapter highlights important older studies, introduces some newer information, and then emphasizes an approach to identifying and studying those underlying conditions that may predispose children and adolescents to substance use and abuse.

Definitions

One of the stumbling blocks to understanding substance use and abuse has been the confusion over terminology and definitions. People query whether nicotine and alcohol are 'drugs', whether the abuse of medically prescribed drugs (e.g. benzodiazepines) is comparable with the abuse of illicit drugs (e.g. heroin), whether drug use is synonymous with abuse, and whether abuse and dependence are different. There has also been a reluctance to label young people as having substance abuse problems because of the wide-spread pejorative lay usage of terms such as 'junkie' or 'addict' to describe adults with these problems.

There are many prescribed and illegal substances that can be used recreationally and which can result in abuse (see Table 27.1). They share the quality of having mental effects that are considered desirable, and most can give rise to some form of intoxication, but they vary in the extent to which there is pharmacological dependence, and some do not result in withdrawal symptoms. There are also performance-enhancing illicit drugs that involve substantial health risks but they are not considered here, other than in terms of a note on pharmacology, because the problems with which they are associated are rather different.

For medical purposes, substance use, abuse, misuse, dependence and withdrawal must all be differentiated (Farrell & Taylor 1994). The problem drug-taker may be defined as: 'Any person who experiences social, psychological, physical or legal problems related to intoxication and/or regular excessive consumption and/or dependence as a consequence of his own use of drugs or other chemical substances' (Advisory Council on the Misuse of Drugs 1982). The World Health Organization (1992, 1996) in their ICD-10 defined *acute intoxication* as psychoactive substance use resulting in disturbed 'level of conscience, cognition, perception, affect or behaviour, or other psychophysiological functions and responses ... directly related to the acute pharmacological effects of the substance and resolve with time, with complete recovery, except where tissue damage or other complications have arisen'. *Harmful use* was defined as 'a pattern of psychoactive substance use that is causing damage to health ... physical ... or mental.' *Dependence* was defined as 'a cluster of behavioural, cognitive, and physiological phenomena that develop after repeated substance use and that typically include a strong desire to take the drugs, difficulties in controlling its use, persisting in its use despite harmful consequences, a higher priority given to drug use than to other activities and obligations, increased tolerance, and sometimes a physical withdrawal state ... chronic alcoholism ... drug addiction'. *Withdrawal state* was defined as 'a group of symptoms of variable clustering and severity occurring on absolute or relative withdrawal of a substance after persistent use of that substance.'

The Diagnostic and Statistical Manual of Mental Disorders, fourth edition (DSM-IV; American Psychiatric Association 1994) distinguishes between *substance use disorders* (substance dependence and substance abuse) and the *substance-induced disorders* (e.g. intoxication, withdrawal or delirium). *Tolerance* is the 'need for greatly increased amounts of the substance to achieve intoxication (or the desired effect) or a markedly diminished effect with continued use of the same amount of the substance.' *Withdrawal* is defined as 'a maladaptive behavioural change, with physiological and cognitive concomitants, that occurs when blood or tissue concentrations of substance decline in an individual who had maintained prolonged heavy use of the substance. After developing unpleasant withdrawal symptoms the person is likely to take the substance to relieve or to avoid

Table 27.1 Substances of abuse. After Halikas (1990).

Alcohol
- Ingested through drinking.
- Manifestation of intoxication—slurred speech; staggering gait; slowed reflexes; and personality change, including argumentativeness, belligerence, melancholia, irritability, euphoria, social disinhibition, and a variety of other significant personality changes. Memory blackouts, related to the rapidity of the rise in blood alcohol level, which in turn is related to the rapidity of ingestion coupled with the lack of other food contents in the stomach, are the most common medical consequence. Overdose, especially in this non-tolerant population, can result in death.
- Treatment—a youngster who is non-arousable and believed to have ingested significant quantities of alcohol (or any other drug) should be considered a medical emergency and hospitalized for close management. There, appropriate intervention including support, gastric lavage and dialysis, if necessary, can be instituted.

Amphetamines (stimulants)
- Generally taken orally, although occasionally injectable amfetamine preparations are still used.
- Manifestation of intoxication—acute effects are generally those of stimulation, with increased energy, euphoria, grandiosity, increased irritability, increased physical activity and decreased sleep. Acute toxicity generally includes paranoid symptoms and panic and can easily include spontaneous violence. Hypertension leading to cerebral haemorrhage and cardiac failure, hyperthermia and seizures may occur.
- Treatment—caution should be exercised in dealing with adolescents intoxicated with amphetamines. Any rapid movement or any movement in the direction of the patient may be misinterpreted as an aggressive act, and the patient may become violent. Use of injections may be seen as particularly threatening. Intervention must include a great deal of supportive talk and calming agents such as benzodiazepines. Chronic amphetamine use generally requires hospitalization for withdrawal because of the withdrawal depression that occurs uniformly.

Cannabis (marijuana, hashish)
- Generally smoked but occasionally ingested.
- Manifestation of intoxication—generally sedating with a euphoriant quality. It has a relatively rapid onset of action by inhalation and the intoxication lasts 15–30 min unless renewed. Time is slowed down, the senses seem heightened, the person is happy, and everyone is 'mellow'. The most consistent physiological concomitant is hunger, and snacking is common. Occasionally, novice users develop symptoms of a panic anxiety attack because of tachycardia or sensory effects. Sensory effects that are generally perceived as pleasurable, but can be seen as frightening, include visual distortion with trails or streaks of light following movement of objects (e.g. shimmering of walls or waving of light or air). These misperceptions can become frightening and reach the proportion of hallucinations in the panicked user. A marijuana toxic delirium exists but is rarely seen.
- Treatment—in the face of a marijuana-induced panic attack, benzodiazepine might be used to provide some sedation. In the face of a toxic delirious state, brief hospitalization and supportive care would be appropriate, because the active constituents of marijuana, the cannabinoids, are fat soluble and can have impact over several days.

Cocaine
- Generally snorted or smoked, although injectable forms are also occasionally used.
- Manifestation of intoxication—similar to the amphetamines but subtler and more reinforcing. Apparently there are fewer adverse acute effects. This drug has a rapid onset of action by the routes used. Cardiac failure and seizures can be lethal.
- Treatment—this is probably the hardest single drug in which to achieve abstinence and stable remission. The relapse rate is almost universal. Withdrawal cannot hope to be achieved on an outpatient basis. Inpatient withdrawal could include therapy with amantadine and desipramine. There is some recent interest in carbamazepine as an adjunct to control cravings. Many drugs are being tried in the management of this resistant addiction. The acute intoxication requires hospitalization and appropriate treatment of the medical symptoms.

Hallucinogens (phencyclidine [PCP], LSD, mescaline, and 'designer drugs')
- Ingested orally.
- Manifestation of intoxication—will vary from mild stimulation, euphoria, sensory enhancement and increased energy to delirious states with hallucinations, fluctuating sensorium and disorientation.
- Treatment—acute intoxication with hallucinogens that result in a 'bad trip' can be managed generally with verbal supportive care and the use of calming agents such as the benzodiazepines. However, PCP is an extremely troublesome drug. Toxic psychotic states associated with its use seem to occur among chronic users, while the acute delirious toxic state occurs among more irregular or novice users. This chronic toxic state requires long-term inpatient management and has been known to last several months: it clears very slowly. Hallucinations and delusions, confusion and bewilderment, and an overall decrease in mental functioning are hallmarks of this chronic state. It is often misdiagnosed as a schizophrenic condition when seen in adolescents. Treatment of the acute intoxication includes acidification of the urine with ammonium chloride in an effort to accelerate the excretion of the substance from the body. Management of the long-term condition generally includes major neuroleptics, which unfortunately are not very useful but are commonly used for behaviour control.

Opiates including heroin (narcotics)
- Oral narcotics are occasionally used with regularity and are frequently at least tried among multiple-drug users in this group. Intravenous use is also prominent.
- Manifestation of intoxication—the opiate overdose is often acute and life-threatening with the patient found in semicomatose condition with evidence of a recent intravenous injection. Physical signs will often show decreased respirations, cyanosis, pinpoint pupils and, if life-threatening, evidence of pulmonary oedema, cardiac dysrhythmias and/or convulsions progressing to cerebral oedema (Schuckit 1979).

Continued

Table 27.1 *continued*

- Treatment—narcotic overdose is a medical emergency requiring aggressive management. Any adolescent brought to an emergency department in a comatose state should receive an intravenous narcotic antagonist, naloxone hydrochloride, because of the possibility of a narcotic overdose. Should the patient be roused by this medication, it would indicate that at least one of the drugs that this person has overdosed with was a narcotic. Multiple drugs are generally involved so that the management is not just for narcotics. Also, illegal availability of the long-acting narcotic methadone in large cities means that some youngsters will overdose with that substance. While they will be aroused by naloxone, left to themselves they will soon become unconscious again. They should therefore be watched closely for at least 24 h. Cardiac dysrhythmias and pulmonary oedema, if present, will require appropriate medical management.

Inhalants (hydrocarbons, glue-sniffing, toluene-sniffing)
- The sniffing of any of the volatile hydrocarbons, whether directly from cans of gasoline, from glue, or from other substances placed into plastic bags, is a habit or behaviour that is likely to occur at ages 10–14 years. It is the most common type of adolescent drug abuse, after alcohol, in developing countries. In recent years, for example, the sniffing of typewriter-correcting chemicals became popular among 10–12 year-old children.
- Manifestation of intoxication—these young people are only brought to the attention of the medical community in an acute state when toxic and delirious. At that time they have all of the usual signs and symptoms of an acute delirium.
- Treatment—hospitalization is usually required. Supportive care, close observation and close protection are necessary. Aggressive treatment for the long-term problem is crucial. It would appear that the volatile hydrocarbons have the worst long-term impact on the user. A chronic organic state can result that will include decreased cognitive functions, hallucinations, irritability and aggressiveness, and a persistent drive for an altered euphoric mental state. Because of their youth, this drive and their aggressiveness, these patients often require chronic hospitalization and generally are mislabelled as 'young chronic schizophrenics'.

Nicotine
- Inhaled or 'chewed' as in snuff and chewing tobacco.
- Manifestation of intoxication—similar to stimulants, including improved alertness, memory and decreased appetite.
- Treatment—transdermal patch (slowly tapering the dose) with adjunctive psychological support.

Sedative and tranquillizers (barbiturates, methaqualone, sleeping pills, benzodiazepines)
- Ingested orally in pill or capsule form.
- Manifestation of intoxication—includes sedation, somnolence or sleep. The state sought and achieved, while awake, is that of 'mellow' oblivious neutrality. These drugs are sometimes used in conjunction with one of the stimulants to counteract agitation or other adverse psychological effects.
- Treatment—overdose with these drugs is a medical emergency. The barbiturates and barbiturate-like compounds can cause severe respiratory depression. The benzodiazepines, when combined with alcohol, can be especially lethal from respiratory depression. Unresponsive patients should be hospitalized and medically treated. Withdrawal from the benzodiazepines can last up to 2 weeks because of their fat solubility. Therefore, it is not surprising that patients addicted to these substances become irritable and paranoid and demand discharge at day 10–14 of hospitalization. Withdrawal from these drugs should proceed at about a 10% reduction per day after changing the patient to a seconal or diazepam withdrawal schedule.

those symptoms.' *Compulsive substance use* refers to taking a substance in larger amounts or over a longer period than was originally intended, often accompanied by a persistent desire to cut down or discontinue usage. Typically, the individual spends a great deal of time obtaining the substance, using it or recovering from its effects. Despite recognizing the contributing role of the substance to a psychological or physical problem, the person continues to use the substance.

The American Academy of Pediatrics (1996) used broadly similar definitions. *Substance intoxication* was applied to the 'development of a reversible substance-specific syndrome due to recent ingestion of (or exposure to) a substance resulting in clinically significant maladaptive behavioural and psychological changes'.

Substance use starts with the experimental initiation of occasional drug-taking, progresses to regular usage to achieve the pleasurable effects, the development of tolerance and increasing 'dosage' to obtain the same effects, the development of associated psychosocial impairment or other harmful consequences,

and finally dependence or compulsive usage (Chaltos 1996; see Fig. 27.1). The risk factors that have been identified are many and various (American Academy of Pediatrics Committee on Substance Abuse 1998; Bukstein & Tarter 1998; Reinherz *et al.* 2000; Table 27.2).

Epidemiology

Over the last 20 years, there have been several large-scale epidemiological studies of drug use and abuse in young people, in both North America and Europe (Silbereisen *et al.* 1995; Kandel & Davies 1996; McKeganey *et al.* 1996; Miller & Plant 1996; Reid 1996; American Academy of Pediatrics Committee on Substance Abuse 1998, 1999; Bukstein & Tarter 1998; Maxwell & Liu 1999; Silberg *et al.*, unpublished data; Weinberg N.Z. *et al.* 1998). The precise rates vary somewhat across investigations, according to methods of assessment, definition and population studied. However, there is broad agreement on most key findings.

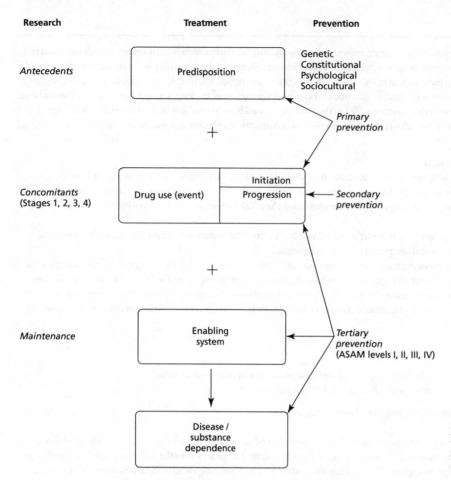

Fig. 27.1 Developmental biopsychosocial disease model. With permission from Chatlos, J.C. (1996).

- Alcohol and nicotine are the most frequently used substances, followed closely by marijuana, with inhalants (e.g. glue-sniffing), 'uppers' (e.g. stimulants such as amphetamines), 'downers' (e.g. sleeping pills) and hallucinogens next in frequency, and cocaine or opiates somewhat less frequent.
- About one-half to three-quarters of older adolescents have taken an illicit drug at some time.
- A substantial minority (20–40%) of those who have used drugs have tried multiple drugs.
- Only about 1 in 12 who have taken drugs are heavy users.
- Drug use is uncommon in children under the age of 12 years but becomes much more frequent during the teenage years, with the exception of inhalants which are more used by younger age groups.
- Drug use, overall, is about as common in girls as boys but there are marked gender differences in types of drug used, with alcohol abuse much more common in males.
- Although secular trends vary according to type of drug, overall drug usage in young people tended to increase during the 1990s.
- Associations with social background vary considerably, according to type of drug.
- Drug use is more frequent among young people with poor scholastic achievement.

Longitudinal course

General population studies have been consistent in showing that the younger people are when they first use drugs, the more likely they are to progress from experimental usage to dependence or abuse (Robins & McEvoy 1990; Tubman *et al.* 1990; Anthony & Petronis 1995; Fergusson & Horwood 1997; Maxwell & Liu 1999). This finding has been used to argue for the value of prevention programmes to delay drug use, on the grounds that this should reduce major drug problems (Robins & McEvoy 1990). However, although that might be so, it seems equally likely that the late onset is itself a reflection of a lower liability (in which case, any success in delaying first drug usage might have little or no effect).

Longitudinal studies of drug abusers have all shown the very considerable psychopathological and physical risks, especially with respect to suicide and accidental deaths, delinquency, depression and psychosocial malfunction (Crumley 1990; Deykin & Buka 1994; Kandel & Davies 1996; Kandel *et al.* 1997; Brook *et al.* 1998; Borowsky *et al.* 1999). Oyefeso *et al.* (1999) found a teenage-specific mortality excess of 11 times the general population rate in males, and 21 times in females. Conversely, studies of suicide have shown the high frequency with which it was preceded by substance abuse (Fowler *et al.* 1986). There is also a substantially increased risk of HIV and of hepatitis C among drug users who inject, because of transmission of infection by contaminated needles (Gilvarry 2000; see also Havens *et al.*, Chapter 49).

Neuropharmacology of substances

The substances used can be grouped according to chemical or pharmacological similarities. We highlight the major points adapted from the following exhaustive reviews: Schuckit (1979), Cooper *et al.* (1991, 1996), Karch (1996), Stahl (1996), Carvey (1998) and Siegel *et al.* (1999). Sites and pharmacological actions of common drugs of abuse are shown in Table 27.3. All these substances produce dysemotionality symptomatic of depression, mania, or a rapid cycling between these affective states. Affective symptoms can be acutely induced and chronically promoted by the continued substance use. Sedation, lethargy and the impairment in diligence and volition are also common, both in acute and chronic substance use.

Alcohol (Carvey 1998)

One of the most ubiquitous substances used and abused is 'alcohol' (ethyl alcohol), which is a product of the fermentation of a variety of sugars. It is consumed orally ('drinking'). It is rapidly and almost completely absorbed from the gastrointestinal tract (primarily the duodenum) and is quickly distributed throughout the body. Because of its partial lipid solubility, alcohol easily penetrates tissues but is preferentially distributed in the brain, which has a particularly high lipid content. Alcohol is metabolized primarily through the alcohol dehydrogenase system in the liver where it is converted to acetaldehyde and then acetate. It interacts with membranes, reducing function of embedded proteins (e.g. interfering with the sodium–potassium adenosine triphosphatase pump in the cell membrane and interfering with the electron transport chain in the mitochondrial membrane). Alcohol has numerous and variable effects on neuronal function, including:
- potentiating the gamma-aminobutyric acid (GABA) (A) receptor (inhibitory ligand-gated chloride channel);
- decreasing excitability of the N-methyl-D-aspartate (NMDA) glutamate receptor (excitatory ligand-gated calcium channel);
- facilitating the release of dopamine, norepinephrine, serotonin and endogenous opioids;
- inhibiting the release of acetylcholine;
- binding to the delta opioid receptors; and
- reacting (as acetaldehyde) with catecholamines (dopamine and norepinephrine) to form tetrahydroisoquinolines and salsolinol (which possess opiate-like properties).

The interaction with GABA (A) receptors explains the additive and perhaps synergistic effects that occur when ethanol and benzodiazepines are used together (Carvey 1998). The

Table 27.2 Risk factors for adolescent substance use disorders. Adapted from American Academy of Pediatrics Committee on Substance Abuse (1998) and Bukstein & Tarter (1998).

Individual risk factors
Early childhood characteristics
    Early conduct problems, aggression
    Poor academic performance/school failure
Early onset of substance use
Adolescent's attitudes and beliefs about substance use
Risk-taking behaviours or antisocial behaviours
Rebelliousness and alienation
Low self-esteem
Psychopathology, particularly affective disorders (depression, bipolar disorders) and conduct disorders
Negative character traits (e.g. lying, lack of empathy)
Previous dependence on substances (tobacco, alcohol, drugs)
Early sexual activity

Peer-related risk factors
Peer substance use
Peer attitudes about substance use
Greater orientation (attachment) to peers
Perception(s) of peer substance use/attitudes
Disorganization in the community

Parent/family risk factors
Parent, sibling or other family member with history of substance use
Parental beliefs/attitudes about substance use
Parental tolerance of substance use/deviant behaviour
Lack of closeness/attachment with parents
Lack of parental involvement in youth's life
Lack of appropriate supervision/discipline
Family history of antisocial behaviour
Child abuse and neglect

acute opiate-like actions contribute to analgesic, euphorigenic and sedative-hypnotic properties of alcohol (Carvey 1998). Effects on peripheral and central biogenic amines are competitive on cardiovascular function but eventually produce an overall depressant effect on cardiac output. The inhibition of acetylcholine release in the brainstem reticular formation probably contributes to the acute sedating properties of alcohol. Effects on the hypothalamus include an alteration in temperature homeostasis (usually resulting in a reduction in body temperature) and an inhibition of the antidiuretic hormone release (resulting in increased urine production).

Considerable interest relates to the proposed teratogenic effects of alcohol on the developing fetus in women who abuse alcohol during pregnancy. It is not clear whether the reported alterations in body development and facial features and changes in head size and brain function are actually an effect of alcohol or the result of other genetic and environmental factors that may have predisposed the mother to alcohol abuse as well as nutritional factors during the pregnancy.

Alcohol is not only a sedative, but also induces dysphoric states of agitation, anxiety and depression. Symptomatic of in-

Table 27.3 Sites and pharmacological actions of common drugs of abuse. Used with permission from Bukstein & Tarter (1998).

Substance	Proposed action	Brain site
Alcohol	Facilitation	GABA receptors
	Inhibition	NMDA (glutamate receptors)
Cannabis/marijuana	Agonist	Cannabinoid receptors
Hallucinogens (e.g. LSD)	Partial agonist	5-HT2 receptors
Opiates	Agonist	Opioid receptors
Cocaine	Inhibition	Monoamine reuptake systems (dopamine, norepinephrine, serotonin)
Nicotine	Agonist	Nicotinic acetylcholine receptors

GABA, gamma-aminobutyric acid; 5-HT2, 5-hydroxytryptamine (serotonin); LSD, lysergic acid diethylamide; NMDA, N-methyl-D-aspartate.

toxication is impaired alertness, decreased cognitive functioning and motor impairment (including ataxia) that may progress to coma and even death.

Nicotine (Stahl 1996; Carvey 1998; Siegel 1999)

Nicotine is the major psychoactive substance in tobacco. It can be released by burning tobacco leaves (cigarettes) and then inhaled in the cigarette smoke, or it can be released by saliva digestion of tobacco leaves (snuff and chewing tobacco). It is a tertiary amine that readily crosses membranes of the lungs and mouth to enter the bloodstream, where it can be quickly metabolized to cotinine; it is also rapidly distributed in the brain (Carvey 1998). Nicotine is a direct-acting nicotinic cholinergic receptor agonist (Carvey 1998; Siegel et al. 1999). It acts on the autonomic nervous system ganglia to increase both sympathetic and parasympathetic activity, and it stimulates the nicotinic acetylcholine receptors at the neuromuscular junction (Carvey 1998; Siegel et al. 1999). In the central nervous system it stimulates nicotinic cholinergic receptors (Siegel et al. 1999). Its action on the brainstem reticular activating system probably has some relationship to its alerting effects, and its action on emotion and memory areas of the temporal lobe limbic system structures has some relationship to the behavioural patterning associated with individual use of the substance. Its enhancement of release of biogenic amines (e.g. dopamine and norepinephrine) probably contributes to its euphorigenic properties. Overall, the effects of nicotine and its metabolites are similar to those of stimulants, including improved alertness and memory and decreased appetite (Carvey 1998).

Marijuana (Carvey 1998)

Marijuana is the dried female flower of the *Cannabis sativa* plant of the hemp family. The major psychoactive chemicals in marijuana are a class of substances called cannabinoids of which delta-9 tetrahydrocannabinol (THC) is the chemical thought to be most responsible for the mental effects, but other cannabinoids, such as delta-8-tetrahydrocannabinol, connabidiol and cannabinol, have not been systematically evaluated (Carvey 1998). Burning marijuana releases about 20% of the cannabinoids in the smoke which when inhaled allows the lipid-soluble cannabinoids to rapidly pass into the bloodstream. In contrast, only about 6% of cannabinoids are released by oral ingestion of marijuana (Carvey 1998). Soaking the flower buds of the *Cannabis sativa* plant in resin concentrates the cannabinoids in a material called hashish.

Cannabinoids are metabolized almost exclusively in the liver and excreted in the bile but do not induce the P-450 system. THC is an exceptionally lipophilic substance that quickly distributes throughout the body but it is only slowly cleared and remains detectable for months. THC readily dissolves in membranes, disrupting functioning in a manner similar to alcohol. THC enters membranes of specific receptors that are widely distributed in the brain with highest density in the basal ganglia, cerebellum, hippocampus, and layers I and VI of the cerebral cortex (Carvey 1998). These THC binding sites interact with G-proteins and other secondary messenger systems serving as neuromodulators effecting the action of various neurotransmitters (except THC receptor sites seem to have little effect on dopaminergic systems). One effect is to inhibit the voltage regulated N-channel for calcium that regulates neurotransmitter release (Carvey 1998).

In various situations THC can have effects ranging from stimulant/euphoric, to depressive/sedative, to marked anxiety and panic/toxic delirium (Carvey 1998). Acute effects include: euphoria, relaxation and disinhibition; impaired problem-solving skills and difficulty organizing thoughts and conversing; and significantly lowered cognitive function (such as reaction time). Chronic use in adolescents and young adults is associated with decreased diligence and volition—the 'amotivational syndrome' (Musty & Kaback 1995; Carvey 1998). However, this may not be the direct result of the marijuana use, but rather the result of genetic and environmental factors that produce such behaviour and also predispose the individual to chronic marijuana abuse. Depression can be induced or promoted by the ongoing use of marijuana; marijuana appears to be a 'gateway' illicit drug towards the use of other drugs (American Academy of Pediatrics Committee on Substance Abuse 1999). It is our experience that acute marijuana use induces depression in genetically susceptible adolescents, and chronic use of marijuana promotes deepening depression and the maladaptation associated with a chronically depressed state (Musty & Kaback 1995).

Inhalants (Schuckit 1979; Karch 1996; Carvey 1998)

Inhalants are a diverse set of volatile organic compounds found in aerosols, glues, cleaning fluids, marking pens, lighter fluid, fingernail polish, typewriter correction fluid, paint and paint removers, room deodorizers, engine fuels and gasoline, and gaseous anaesthetic agents. These agents are inhaled by 'sniffing' through the nose or 'huffing' through the mouth either directly from the container or from bags into which the substance has been placed (Carvey 1998). The effects of the inhalants generally last approximately 30 min or less but can be sustained by repeated usage (Carvey 1998). Because the inhalants are strongly lipophilic chemicals, they readily pass through mucous membranes of the upper respiratory tract and lungs to enter the bloodstream (Karch 1996). They are also rapidly distributed throughout the body and easily pass into the brain (Karch 1996). Despite their structural diversity, the major effect is to dissolve in membrane lipids and disrupt membrane function in a manner similar to alcohol (Carvey 1998). Depending upon the compound, metabolism varies from excretion unchanged through the lungs, catabolism though the liver P-450 system with excretion in the bile, or excretion in the urine. The act of inhaling the vapours in a closed environment can result in hypoxaemia with consequent central nervous system neuronal injury. Disruption of mitochondrial membranes in cells of both the central and peripheral nervous systems can also produce cell injury or cell death. Damage to organ systems, other than the brain, such as the kidneys, liver or bone marrow, which occurs with use of benzene or halogenated hydrocarbons, can produce metabolic derangements that secondarily disrupt brain functioning (Carvey 1998). Contaminants, such as lead in gasoline, can also damage the nervous system. Death is rare but can occur from cardiac dysrhythmias with the halogenated hydrocarbons (Carvey 1998). Inhalants are used as illicit drugs by younger age groups (children and adolescents). Chronic inhalant users have been found to have a high rate of depression (Zur & Yule 1990).

Cocaine (Karch 1996; Carvey 1998)

Cocaine is derived from the leaf of the coca plant. In powder form it can be inhaled and after dissolving in mucous membranes it is rapidly transported into the blood. 'Crack' cocaine is a more powerful concentrated form of cocaine produced by extracting the free base into an organic solvent, such as ether, and smoking it (Carvey 1998). Crack smokers have blood levels twice as high as those who snort cocaine. It is quickly distributed to the brain. Half-life of cocaine is only 20–45 min. Cocaine plus alcohol produces cocaethylene, a psychoactive chemical that has a much longer half-life and is more likely to cause cardiac conduction abnormalities than either cocaine or alcohol alone. Cocaine increases biogenic amines by acting as an inhibitor of the reuptake mechanisms. In particular, cocaine binds to the dopamine transporter and induces a structural change that reduces the capacity to bind neurotransmitters (Leshner 1996). Cocaine can also act as a competitive inhibitor of dopamine. Unlike amfetamines, the large cocaine molecule cannot be transported across the neuronal membrane and biogenic amine release does not occur (Carvey 1998). Acute central nervous system effects of cocaine include anxiety, paranoia, hallucinations, emotional lability, irritability, stereotypic behaviour, tremor and seizures. Cocaine increases alertness and attention. In those individuals with a genetic susceptibility to affective illness, cocaine use can result in a state of mania.

There are several external markers of intense and repeated cocaine abuse and the presence of these external markers is a strong confirmatory sign of cocaine abuse. These markers include: perforated nasal septum, cocaine 'tracks' (salmon-coloured bruises that turn blue and yellow over time), 'crack keratitis' (damage to the cornea where the abuser has rubbed his or her anaesthetized eyes too roughly), enamel erosion of the teeth, calloused thumb from lighters, superficial burns and blackened, hyperkeratotic lesions on the palmar aspect of the hand (from handling crack pipes) and, in some cases, bite marks on the lips and tongue from seizure activity (Karch 1996).

Mittleman et al. (1999) analysed data from 3946 patients who were interviewed an average of 4 days after myocardial infarction (MI), of whom 38 reported using cocaine in the year preceding their myocardial infarction. Of these 38, nine reported using cocaine within 1 h of onset of MI symptoms; another two had used it within 1–3 h. Cocaine users were younger than non-users and were more likely to be males, current smokers or members of minority groups. Analysis showed that the risk for MI increased more than 20-fold within 1 h of using cocaine but the risk declined to levels that were not statistically significant after 1 h. Death from cardiovascular causes is more common with crack.

Cocaine abuse during pregnancy may cause vascular injury to the fetus. This effect seems to be related to the level of prenatal cocaine exposure (Frank et al. 1999). This has led certain states in the USA to regard cocaine during pregnancy as a criminal act. Cocaine smoke, just like cigarette smoke, can be passively absorbed and can lead to positive urine, blood and hair tests in those who have been in the environment while cocaine is being smoked.

In young adult homosexual males, cocaine abuse has been reported to be a significant independent predictor of the failure to

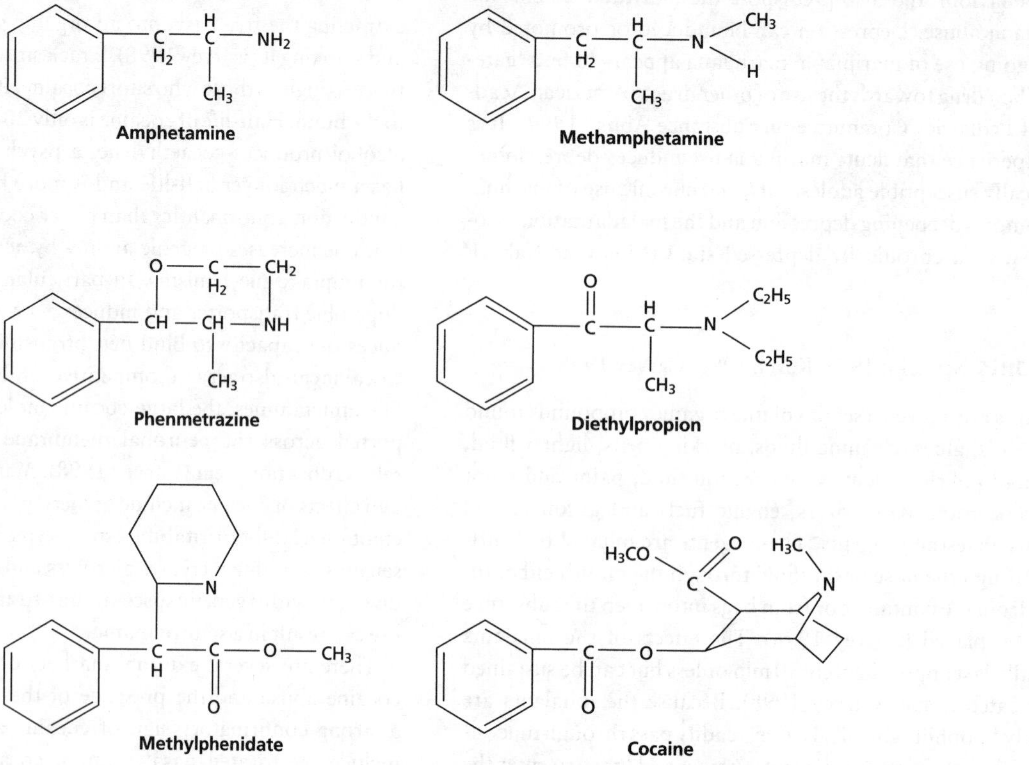

Fig. 27.2 The chemical structures of common psychostimulants. Used with permission from: Carvey, P.M. (1998) *Drug Action in the Central Nervous System*, p. 325. Oxford University Press.

use condoms during anal intercourse. Why this group (rather than those abusing amfetamines and other substances) chooses not to practice 'safe sex' remains unknown (McNall & Remafedi 1999).

Stimulants (Karch 1996; Carvey 1998; Siegel *et al.* 1999)

The psychostimulants are a structurally diverse group of drugs (Fig. 27.2). The most commonly used psychostimulants are dexamphetamine, methamphetamine, 3,4-methylene-dioxymethamphetamine (MDMA or 'ecstasy'), phenmetrazine and diethylpropion (Carvey 1998). When amphetamine or methamphetamine is injected intravenously it is called 'speed'. Methamphetamine is called 'ice' when its free base is extracted into an organic solvent, such as ether, and smoked (Carvey 1998), similar to the technique of producing crack cocaine. The stimulants are indirect-acting agonists of catecholamines (dopamine and norepinephrine), and competitively inhibit the biogenic amine transporters (reuptake pump) for dopamine, norepinephrine and serotonin, cause calcium-independent release (release independent of nerve terminal depolarization) of the biogenic amines from nerve terminals in the brain, and competitively inhibit monoamine oxidase (Carvey 1998). Half-life is 8–12 h and these drugs are mostly excreted unchanged in the

urine (Karch 1996). Effects on biogenic amines also occur in the peripheral nervous system, resulting in hypertension, cardiac dysrhythmias, vasculitis, arterial thrombosis and cardiac failure (Schuckit 1979). High-dose abuse can also produce severe vasoconstrictive effects, resulting in intracranial ischaemia or haemorrhage, myoglobinuria and renal failure. Chronic use promotes—particularly in those with a genetic susceptibility to affective illness—agitation, irritability and homicidal ideation.

Downers (Stahl 1996; Carvey 1998)

Downers include sleeping pills, barbiturates, other sedatives and minor tranquillizers such as the benzodiazepines: diazepam and chlordiazepoxide. The prototype sedative-hypnotic are the barbiturates (phenobarbital, secobarbital) and the prototype tranquillizers are diazepam (Valium) and chlordiazepoxide (Librium). These central nervous system depressants reduce the electrical activity of the brain, facilitate sleep, promote muscle relaxation, treat seizures, produce anaesthesia and reduce anxiety. The liver metabolizes many of these drugs but some are excreted unchanged in the urine. Half-lives vary from hours to days (Cooper *et al.* 1991, 1996; Stahl 1996; Carvey 1998).

The barbiturates increase chloride conductance by binding to one of the GABA (A) receptor subunits, increasing the amount of time that the chloride channel remains open (Cooper *et al.* 1996; Stahl 1996). The increase in chloride conductance occurs even in the absence of GABA (Stahl 1996; Carvey 1998). Barbiturates depress respiration in a dose-dependent fashion, inducing coma and fatal respiratory depression at high doses (Carvey 1998). Death caused by a barbiturate overdose can be the result of drug autonomism rather than an intentional act (Carvey 1998). Drug autonomism is a behavioural pattern in which the patient takes drugs unnecessarily because the drugs have interfered with the individual's ability to determine if doses are really needed (Stahl 1996; Carvey 1998). Because barbiturates continue to open the chloride channel in the absence of GABA, a ceiling effect will not occur and can lead to fatal respiratory depression (Carvey 1998). Both pharmacokinetic and physiological tolerances develop during the use of barbiturates. Barbiturates (especially the longer acting agents, such as phenobarbital) induce the P-450 system, making increased doses necessary to maintain steady state plasma levels. Continued use results in dependence, especially if used for euphoria or sleep.

Benzodiazepines bind to a specific receptor site (or benzodiazepine receptor site) on the GABA (A) receptor (Carvey 1998). In the presence of benzodiazepine receptor binding, GABA more frequently activates the chloride channel, thus producing a greater degree of GABA-mediated inhibition (Stahl 1996; Carvey 1998). Because GABA (A) receptors are widely distributed in the brain, the benzodiazepines produce an overall reduction in brain electrical activity (Carvey 1998). Benzodiazepines also inhibit the reuptake of adenosine, promoting vasodilatation (including coronary artery dilation) and reducing acetylcholine release from the terminals of certain reticular formation neurones, thereby lowering the state of arousal. Some of the benzodiazepines (e.g. oxazepam and loriazepam) are conjugated extrahepatically (Carvey 1998). The degree of lipid solubility of the benzodiazepines varies > 50-fold and accounts in great part for the differences in rates of absorption, onset of action and redistribution (Carvey 1998). The benzodiazepines are generally completely absorbed following oral administration. Chlorazepate is decarboxylated in gastric juice to the active agent N-desmethyldiazepam, while the other benzodiazepines are biotransformed into active metabolites by the liver (Carvey 1998). The benzodiazepines are classified as short- (triazolam), intermediate- (lorazepam), or long-acting (diazepam, chlordiazepoxide) based upon the method of biotransformation, the lipid solubility and the half-lives (Schuckit 1979; Carvey 1998). Enterohepatic recirculation of conjugated benzodiazepine metabolites also increases their duration of action, and deposition in muscle and fat with subsequent delayed release over a long period of time produces some of the 'hangover effects' (Carvey 1998). Tolerance results in part from receptor alterations that decrease the amount of enhanced chloride conductance (Yu *et al.* 1988).

Although withdrawal symptoms occur, compulsive drug-seeking behaviour (addiction) to downers is considered unlikely (Carvey 1998). In our experience, these drugs may lower anxiety at the expense of inducing or promoting dysphoria symptomatic of depression in those vulnerable to depression.

Hallucinogens (Carvey 1998)

The hallucinogenic (or psychedelic) drugs produce hallucinations without delirium in the presence of intact cognitive functioning and intact orientation to the environment (Carvey 1998). Hallucinations are perceptions that result from disruption of brain systems responsible for the recognition and interpretation of external events and may be visual, auditory, tactile, olfactory, gustatory or kinetic. The hallucinogens can also produce pleasurable moods or frightening experiences with sympathetic arousal. It has been suggested that nearly 8% of the population over age 12 years has used these drugs at least once (Carvey 1998).

The hallucinogens fall into three major classes: lysergic acid diethylamide (LSD), phenylalkylamines (mescaline) and indolealkylamines (psilocybin). In addition to these chemical groups, designer drugs (substituted amphetamines or phenylethylamine derivatives) with hallucinogen-like effects have been developed (Table 27.4; Carvey 1998). The hallucinogens generally act on 5-hydroxytryptamine (5-HT or serotonin) receptors but also act as dopamine agonists, although dopamine antagonists do not block hallucinations induced by these drugs (Carvey 1998).

LSD-induced hallucinations often occur in a temporal sequence as unformed bursts of light, then as geometric forms and finally as complex images which involve faces, scenes and movement within those scenes. This suggests that the hallucinogenic drugs reduce the threshold for activation of neurones along sequential sensory pathways, and once these thresholds have been reduced, neurones fire in response to background activity in the absence of an external event, thereby producing the hallucination. LSD is one of the most potent drugs known, with 50 μg being the threshold dose. LSD is a powder ingested orally either with sugar cubes or dissolved in a liquid, but it is unstable to heating which prevents inhalation in smoke (Carvey 1998).

The psilocybins and mescaline-like drugs are much less potent than LSD (Carvey 1998). The psilocybins are found in 'magic mushrooms' indigenous to Mexico, Texas, Florida, Hawaii and the Pacific Northwest USA. They are eaten raw or dry, brewed in tea or eaten in a stew (Carvey 1998). Mescaline, the least potent hallucinogenic, comes from the peyote cactus found in North and South America. The sun-dried crowns of these cacti are consumed either dry or in various recipes (Karch 1996; Carvey 1998). Mescaline is associated with nausea and vomiting and the hallucinogenic experience reflects its potent dopamine agonist properties (Carvey 1998).

LSD, mescaline and psilocybins are absorbed by oral ingestion with the hallucination beginning within 1 h and persisting for 6–12 h. Tolerance to these compounds is rapid and develops within 24 h, making dependence unlikely (Carvey 1998). These

Table 27.4 Designer drugs. From Carvey (1998).

Drug	Distinguishing characteristics
2,4,5-Trimethoxyamphetamine (TMA)	Structurally resembles both mescaline and amphetamine Effects are similar to those of mescaline
4-Methyl-2,5-dimethoxyamphetamine (DOM)	Also known as Serenity, Tranquillity and Peace (STP) Hallucinations occur with significant sympathetic autonomic nervous system activation
Paramethoxyamphetamine (PMA)	Very potent hallucinogen associated with excessive sympathetic autonomic nervous system stimulation and fatalities Most frequently used as a contaminant to enhance psychic effects of other drugs
Brom-DOM	The most potent phenylethylamine compound, distributed in a microdot formulation Effects last for 10 h Overdose is rarely fatal
3.4-Methylenedioxyamphetamine (MDA)	Mild intoxication without hallucination Produces feelings of empathy and euphoria Higher doses produce hallucinations with delirium
3–4-Methylenedioxymethamphetamine (MDMA)	Also known as 'ecstasy', Adam, and M&M Initially synthesized as an appetite suppressant Used in conjunction with group therapy because of its ability to produce empathy Known to have induced several deaths secondary to cardiac dysrhythmias
3–4-Methylenedioxyethamphetamine (MDEA)	Also known as Eve, with effects similar to those of MDMA

drugs are excreted rapidly in the urine, are not lipophilic, and thus not stored in muscle and fat. Serious medical consequences are unusual and most often secondary to some type of trauma occurring while experiencing the hallucinations (Carvey 1998). Cardiovascular or other serious medical problems also can result from combined use of another substance, such as phencyclidine (PCP) or a designer drug.

Designer drugs are substituted amphetamines or phenylethylamine. These drugs do not produce clear-cut psychostimulant effects or true hallucinations, but they do deplete serotonin, dopamine and norepinephrine (Carvey 1998). These drugs enhance self-esteem that leads to increased use (Carvey 1998). The designer drugs have much lower therapeutic indices than LSD with resultant overdose associated with morbidity and even mortality (Carvey 1998). They produce more sympathomimetic effects, which complicates emergency treatment of overdose (Carvey 1998). Signs and symptoms of sympathetic activation represent states of toxicity requiring immediate treatment, similar to amfetamine toxicity (Karch 1996).

Anabolic steroids (Karch 1996; Carvey 1998)

The anabolic steroids are all derivatives of the androgenic hormone testosterone: cypionate, nandrolone decanoate, methandrostenolone and boldenone undecylenate (Carvey 1998). These chemical modifications increase oral absorption and prolong the half-life. Their effects are to alter nitrogen balance and muscle growth and they are used with the goals of in-

creasing lean body mass, increasing strength, reducing recovery time between athletic activities and increasing aggressiveness. Anabolic steroid use was introduced during the Second World War to improve healing and speed recoveries in wounded soldiers and improve symptoms of depression (Karch 1996). Anabolic steroids can be taken orally or injected intramuscularly. Use occurs as 'stacking' (use of several different preparations at once) which maximizes the 'anabolic effect' while minimizing any 'androgenic effect'; 'cycling' (using combinations in alternating 6–12-week cycles) which reduces tolerance; and 'pyramiding' (initial use of low doses progressing to large doses for several weeks, followed by tapering before an athletic contest) which reduces the chance of detection by drug-screening programmes (Karch 1996; Carvey 1998).

The anabolic steroids are metabolized in the liver and excreted in the bile (Karch 1996). Half-life and onset of action is minutes to days (Karch 1996). Muscle hypertrophy and increased strength following anabolic steroid use is the result of massive increase in the size of type 2 (fast twitch, anaerobic) muscle fibres. However, collagen in tendons and ligaments is altered and weakened, resulting in a mismatch such that the hypertrophic muscle fibres cause tears and other injuries (sprains and strains). Adverse effects of anabolic steroids on the liver include peliosis hepatis, cholestatic jaundice and hepatic neoplasms. Myocardial fibrosis and cardiomyopathy have also been reported. Other systemic symptoms include testicular atrophy, hyperpigmentation of the skin, acne on the extremities and hirsutism. Metabolic conversion of anabolic steroids to estradiols may be responsible for the gynaecomastia and reduced sperm production. Anabolic steroids bind with the sigma opiate receptors in the brain (Karch 1996).

Widespread use of anabolic steroids by athletes has been associated with euphoria, aggression, depression, irritability, hallucinations, paranoid ideation, manic symptoms and violent crime (Pope & Katz 1988, 1990; Conacher & Workman 1989; Oliva & Middleton 1990; Cooper & Noakes 1994). One report described a 16-year-old boy with school and social phobia, increasing symptoms of depression as he reached puberty, and a passive temperament, who began using anabolic steroids when he started weight-lifting. He then became increasingly aggressive and violent and in a rage murdered his girlfriend. He was diagnosed with depression and treated successfully with medication while awaiting trial for murder (Pope *et al.* 1996). Evaluation of 133 male convicts in the same facility (mean age 30.7 ± 7.6 years) uncovered two other cases of apparent anabolic steroid-induced crimes, suggesting the induction of manic-type (homicidal) anger (Pope *et al.* 1996).

Opiates/heroin (Schuckit 1979; Karch 1996; Carvey 1998)

Opiates are among the oldest substances used for psychoactive effects, with ancient Greek literature referring to the use of poppies for sleep and pain relief. The Greek word for the poppy seed 'opion' is derived from 'opos' for juice. The smoking of opium developed in China during the sixteenth century and was abetted by the colonial powers. Also in the sixteenth century, the famous physician Paracelsus (Philippus Aureolus Theophrastus Bombast von Hohenheim) popularized opium-containing formulations as the treatment of choice for all diseases. His 'laudanum' consisted of 25% opium and was the most popular formulation for disease treatment. Sydenham shared this enthusiasm for opium as a panacea and influenced Thomas Dover to create a powdered opium formula known as 'Dover's Powder' as a home remedy for all types of ills and its use continued well into the twentieth century. In the 1850s, the Scottish physician Alexander Wood popularized the injection of opium preparations for pain. The US Civil War further popularized the injection of opiate formulations for war injuries or other painful conditions and many of these people became addicted. Sigmund Freud suggested that chewing cocaine antagonized the sedative effects of opiates and was a treatment for opium addiction, but instead this resulted in simultaneous addiction to both opiates and cocaine. In 1874, Wright first synthesized heroin from morphine, and in 1898 Strube showed its effectiveness in relieving severe tubercular coughs. The Bayer Company then began commercial production of heroin, thinking this to be a safe and effective cough suppressant. Thus, widespread opiate abuse, particularly in the middle class population (and mostly in women), developed in Europe and the USA in the early 1900s as the result of purchases of legally produced opiate formulations containing morphine, heroin, codeine and other compounds. This led to the banning of some manufacture and the non-prescription dispensing of opiate analogues in the 1920s. Also in the 1920s, the practice of intravenous injection of heroin (and other opiates) to maintain addiction developed among addicts. Legal bans did result in a decline in opiate use until the 1960s and the Vietnam War (Karch 1996).

Currently, a wide variety of chemical substances used and abused fall into the category of opiates. This category includes the natural substance opium (the raw material derived from poppy seeds) and its purified derivatives such as morphine and codeine. It also includes semisynthetic agents produced by minor chemical alterations of the basic poppy-derived substances, e.g. heroin, hydromorphone (Dilaudid), oxymorphone (Numorphan), hydrocodone (Tussend), oxycodone (Percodan) and methadone (Dolophine). There are also purely synthetic opiates, e.g. propoxyphene (Darvon), fentanyl (Actiq), meperidine (Demerol), pentazocine (Talwin) and diphenoxylate (Lomotil) (Schuckit 1979).

Opiates are well absorbed from all routes of administration including intravenously, subcutaneously, orally, rectally, intranasally (snorting), inhalation (smoking) and transcutaneously (patch) (Schuckit 1979). Once in the bloodstream, opiates are rapidly distributed throughout the body (Karch 1996). Various opiates undergo metabolism, although some are excreted with only minimal changes (Karch 1996). Morphine is quickly conjugated in the liver to morphine-3-glucuronide and morphine-6-glucuronide. The half-life of these glucuronides is 3–4 h and they are excreted in the urine in 24–48 h. There is also some enterohepatic recirculation of the glucuronides excreted in the bile with deconjugation by gut bacteria followed by reabsorption, prolonging the half-life. Within 10–15 min heroin is rapidly converted to morphine in the body. Over 80% of codeine is conjugated to codeine-6-glucuronide which, unlike the morphine conjugates, is an inactive metabolite, but codeine is converted by demethylation to active metabolites morphine and norcodeine. N-demethylation is the most common route of metabolism for the other opiates (Karch 1996).

The opiate agents are all lipid soluble, rapidly distributing throughout the body and crossing the blood–brain barrier. In the brain, opiates interact with membrane receptors on neurones. The opiate receptors are G-protein-coupled receptors (GPCRs) that have a variety of actions. The major receptor is the mu opiate receptor but there also are kappa and sigma opiate receptors, which are normally neurotransmitter receptors for the endogenous endorphin, enkephalin and dynorphin peptides. The behavioural effects of opiates appear to be mediated mainly by the mu opiate receptor, which on various neuronal populations produces alterations in potassium channels, calcium channels and adenylyl cyclase. The effect on adenylyl cyclase is upregulation of the cyclic adenosine monophosphate (cAMP) pathways (Karch 1996). The acute effect of mu opiate receptor stimulation and upregulation of cAMP in locus caeruleus neurones is inhibition of neuronal firing, but with chronic use the neuronal firing returns to normal (resulting in tolerance). After chronic stimulation, acute cessation (withdrawal) of mu opiate receptor stimulation causes a 7–10-fold increase above normal in neuronal firing. Such changes in neurones explain some of the physiological and behavioural symptoms experienced by individuals using and abusing opiates (Busquets *et al.* 1995; Karch 1996; Carvey 1998).

Opiates increase the pain threshold, and produce sedation and motor inco-ordination. In adolescents with genetic suscep-tibility for affective illness, opiates can induce manic symptoms (euphoria, giddiness, racing thoughts) or depression (dyspho-ria, irritability). A variety of systemic effects are evident with opiate use. Some of these are specific to the route of administra-tion, e.g. skin puncture wounds, scarring, abscesses, fasciitis and lymphoedema occur with administration by injection. Peri-pheral thrombophlebitis often follows intravenous administra-tion. Pulmonary oedema is a common consequence of intravenous opiate administration. It is unclear whether this is a direct result of the opiates, a reaction to the various substances mixed with the agents, or a combination. Damage to the heart valves (particularly the tricuspid valve) from both drug contam-inates (especially particulate) in the injected solution and any pulmonary oedema predispose to subsequent endocarditis (most commonly staphylococcal endocarditis). Acute opiate overdose produces coma with decreased respiration, cyanosis and pinpoint pupils, and can progress to pulmonary oedema, cardiac dysrhythmias and/or convulsions, with death resulting from a combination of respiratory depression and pulmonary and cerebral oedema (Schuckit 1979).

Use of other substances adds to the potential of a fatal outcome. Granulomas from embolized particulate materials (adulterants such as talc, cotton, starch or cellulose) in the intravenously injected opiates are common in the lungs and result in a progressive thromboembolic microarteriopathy with resulting pulmonary hypertension. Almost all individuals who have used intravenous opiates have at least some pathologic ev-idence of this microarteriopathy. Infections transmitted through contamination of needles, syringes or opiate mixtures are very common and can be bacterial or viral (particularly prominent are hepatitis B and C, and human immunodeficiency virus). Renal damage (focal segmental glomerulosclerosis) following chronic intravenous opiate use may be the result of immunolog-ical changes and can result in renal failure (Schuckit 1979; Karch 1996; Carvey 1998).

As a consequence of pulmonary problems and/or cardiac dis-ease, strokes can be observed in opiate abusers. Transverse myelitis has also been observed in patients abusing opiates and this is thought to relate to either thromboembolism or toxicity from contaminants. One contaminant of amateur synthesis of meperidine-like opiates is 1-methyl-4-phenyl-1,2,3,6-tetrahydropyridine (MPTP) that destroys pigmented neurones in the zona compacta of the substantia nigra, resulting in the acute onset of severe parkinsonism (Karch 1996).

Because an addict purchasing drugs 'on the street' has no way of determining its purity or potency, a less potent drug (less than 3% purity) often results in withdrawal symptoms, while a more potent than usual sample can produce fatal respiratory depres-sion, and a sample containing different contaminates may result in hypersensitivity reaction, toxicity from another component, or emboli to the lungs and retina (Karch 1996). There are certain

individuals who have abused heroin in the past but are no longer addicted and have an apparently stable lifestyle, yet, presumably when under stress, these individuals will use opiates. This has been termed 'chipping' and does not impair social functioning (Zinberg *et al.* 1975; Zinberg & Jacobson 1976; Zinberg *et al.* 1978; Schuckit 1979; Harding 1983–84; Harding *et al.* 1980; Harding & Zinberg 1984). In these individuals, variability in potency and purity can be lethal.

The withdrawal syndrome of the 'street abuser' is a com-bination of emotional, behavioural and physical symptoms (Schuckit 1979). The benign nature relates to the variability in the potency of heroin obtained on the street that ranges from 8 to 75%, mostly around 36% (Karch 1996). The psychological state includes a strong 'craving' with irritability and agitation (Schuckit 1979). The physical signs and symptoms of withdraw-al can be generalized as follows (Schuckit 1979, pp. 91–92).

a Within 12 hours of the last dose, physical discomfort begins with tearing of the eyes, a runny nose, sweating, and yawning, followed by a restless sleep (a 'yen') which continues for 24–48 hours. Over the same time period, other symptoms include dilated pupils, loss of appetite, gooseflesh (hence, the term 'cold turkey'), back pain, and a tremor.

b Subsequently the individual develops insomnia, incessant yawning, a flu-like syndrome (consisting of weakness, gastroin-testinal upset and chills fusing), muscle spasms, ejaculation (males), and abdominal pain.

c The symptoms then slowly decrease in intensity by the fifth day, and completely disappear by 7–10 days.

The acute withdrawal phase can be followed by a more pro-tracted abstinence of two subtypes: during weeks 4–10, a mild increase in blood pressure, temperature, respiration and dilated pupils; then a later phase, lasting 30 weeks or more, character-ized by a mild decrease in all of the above measures and a de-crease in the respiratory centre response to carbon dioxide (Schuckit 1979).

Heroin overdose, both accidentally and intentionally, is not uncommon. In a recent study of 438 heroin-users recruited in non-clinical settings, mean age of first heroin use was 21 years, 98 (23%) reported at least one overdose (unconsciousness), mean number of overdoses being 3.6, and mean age of first hero-in overdose was 24 years. Fifteen (16%) reported more than one overdose. Ninety-six of the 98 overdoses were by injected heroin, with 31% of the injectors of heroin reporting overdose, compared to 2% of the non-injectors. Users who had overdosed were more severely dependent upon heroin, older, and more likely to have been treated for a drug problem. Overdose was not related to gender or reported frequency or quantity of heroin use. In this study group both the overdose and non-overdose groups were using heroin 3–4 times per week with the average daily doses being about 0.5 g of illegal street heroin. Reasons for overdose included a higher than usual dose; stronger than usual quality of the heroin; alcohol use at the same time; and heroin use after abstinence. Up to 16% reported having taken overdose 'deliberately'. Interestingly, 48% had been present when some-one else overdosed (Gossop *et al.* 1996).

Concerns have been raised that the use of opiate analgesics (morphine, fentanyl, oxycodone, hydromorphone and, less so, meperidine) to control, prevent and relieve patients of pain may promote opiate addiction and opiate abuse. A recent study negates this concern by showing that increasing medical use of opiate analgesics to treat pain 'does not appear' to be contributing to opiate analgesic abuse (Joranson *et al.* 2000).

Acute withdrawal symptoms occur in up to 90% of the newborns of heroin-dependent mothers and this carries a mortality of up to 30%. There is usually a low birth weight, and on the second day post-delivery withdrawal symptoms begin with irritability, crying, tremor, hyperreflexia, tachypnoea, diarrhoea, hyperactivity, vomiting and sneezing/hiccups. Treatment of the withdrawal syndrome in neonates involves the use of paregoric, methadone, phenobarbital or diazepam. Medication is given for 10–20 days, with tapering doses during days 14–20 (Schuckit 1979). A prospective study of such infants remains unavailable; however, a recent prospective study (5–6 years) of prematurely born children who received morphine as neonates to facilitate mechanical ventilation showed no adverse effects on intelligence, motor function or behaviour (MacGregor *et al.* 1998).

Self-medication

The high rate of affective disturbance in opiate addicts attending a treatment programme was noted by Rounsaville *et al.* (1982), and similar associations have been found with the use/abuse of other substances (Deykin *et al.* 1987, 1992; Bukstein *et al.* 1989; Greenbaum *et al.* 1991; Swadi 1992a,b; Hovens *et al.* 1994; Clark *et al.* 1995; Young *et al.* 1995). This could reflect factors leading to clinical referral (and, doubtless, to some extent it does) but epidemiological studies of the general population have also shown a substantial association between drug use/abuse and depression (see Rutter, Chapter 28). This association has also been noted among delinquent youths manifesting conduct disorder (Riggs *et al.* 1995). Accordingly, it has been suggested that individuals start using substances in an attempt to treat themselves (Deykin *et al.* 1987; Milin *et al.* 1991; Riggs *et al.* 1995).

The selection of the substance used for self-treatment of affective illness is not random but seems to be directed towards specific moods and feelings. Certain substances seem to be used to induce a state of euphoria (amfetamines, cocaine, alcohol) while other illicit drugs are used in a more relaxing, sedative, calming manner (marijuana, heroin, alcohol). The opiates appear to dampen feelings of rage and aggression and cocaine benefits the rapid cycling moods of depression and mania (Khantzian 1985). Some substances are used to promote impulsive primitive behaviours and others to dull unpleasant feelings/moods.

The limbic system (which includes, among others, the ventral tegmental area, nucleus accumbens, hypothalamus, cingulate cortex, prefrontal cortex, hippocampus and amygdala) is a circuitry prominent in fear, hunger, sexual desire and the emotions associated with impulsivity and memories, and seemingly plays a prominent part in addiction and dependency. The primary neurotransmitter of the limbic system is dopamine but other neurotransmitters (serotonin, norepinephrine, acetylcholine, GABA) are also involved. Laboratory animal models for dependency have focused on the effects on the dopaminergic system (Gardner 1992; Bukstein & Kaminer 1993; Bukstein & Tarter 1998). A possible molecular mechanism of cocaine addiction involves changes in the dopamine-reuptake transporter to which cocaine binds strongly (Giros *et al.* 1996; Leshner 1996).

It has long been proposed that alcoholics, and especially binge drinkers, are trying to 'drown their blues'. Problem alcohol use to cope with depressive affect has been reported to be a significant risk factor in the development of alcohol dependence (Carpenter & Hasin 1999). Poor psychological well-being (poor self-esteem, anxiety, somatic symptoms, and eating concerns, most likely representing depression) in adolescents (mean age 17 years) is a significant risk factor for the development of later problem alcohol use at 22 years of age (Pitkanen 1999).

The relationship between affective disorders and problematic substance use can be explained as the interaction between genetic susceptibility for affective disorders and environmental factors, specifically exposure to the experimental use of substances as a developmental variant (American Academy of Pediatrics, Committee on Substance Abuse 1996). The families in which problematic substance use occurs tend to show a loading for a broad range of psychopathology (including sociopathy and alcohol and drug abuse) as well as affective disorder. Children and adolescents with this mixed family pattern often present early in life with multiple developmental behavioural and psychiatric symptoms (Weinberg & Emslie 1991; Weinberg & Brumback 1992). Nevertheless, if the underlying affective disorder is not recognized and appropriately managed, progression to substance dependence/abuse will often occur (Famularo *et al.* 1985; Geller *et al.* 1998; Weinberg & Glantz 1999). Winokur *et al.* (1998), studying a large cohort of adults with affective disorders and substance abuse, noted that the drug-abusing bipolar patients were significantly younger at entrance and had a higher incidence of family histories of mania or schizoaffective mania compared to the non-abusing bipolar patients. They suggested that drug abuse might precipitate an earlier onset of bipolar disorder in those who have a familial predisposition for mania.

Identification of substance use/abuse

The standard method for identifying alcohol use and abuse has long been the demonstration of ethanol in various body fluids (saliva, urine, blood) but has recently been expanded to include the demonstration of a number of oxidative and non-oxidative enzymes metabolizing ethanol to acetate (oxidative pathway) and to phosphatidylethanolamine (non-oxidative pathway). These are called ethanol 'state markers' and are possibly more quantitatively specific in gauging the severity of chronic use rather than acute toxicity (Laposata 1999).

The QED saliva test is a cost-effective method of screening for alcohol exposure in public health settings where intoxication is a common cause of a clinic visit (Bendtsen *et al.* 1999). Currently, the gold standard for identifying drug use in the previous 48 h is chemical analysis of a urine sample. Urine tests performed before an interview have been shown to be 93% accurate, but this accuracy decreased to 58% when urine testing was performed after the interview (Hamid *et al.* 1999). However, urine testing vastly underestimates the problem. The overwhelming majority of substance-using children and adolescents are unrecognized and do not seek the care of health professionals for substance use. One popular method for identifying substance use is the mandatory drug screening of children and adolescents involved in sports. Screening in other school settings is also taking place with the belief that such drug screening will lower substance use and its complications. Unfortunately, there are no data to confirm that such screening reduces the incidence of substance use, and it is possible that such screening actually increases the likelihood of school drop-out or lack of participation in activities.

A better tool for identifying substance use is the careful and detailed history-taking and examination of the child or adolescent (Weinberg W.A. *et al.* 1998). History should be obtained from a competent informed guardian (preferably the biological or adoptive mother). The physician should use a closed-end semistructured interview format to obtain information from the guardian (the child/adolescent should be present and can contribute additional information) about the present illness (concerns), developmental history (course): behaviour *in utero* (fetal hyperactivity), neonatal period and infancy (colic, irritable, little need for sleep, incessant crying or pleasant, good-natured), toddler years (hyperactive and could not be taken to the supermarket ['supermarket toddler']), 2–5 years of age (hyperactive, moody, irritable, provocative, sad, clingy, unable to separate), and each school year from kindergarten to present grade (adaptation, performance, behaviour and concerns) at school and outside of school, including home. It is particularly important to enquire about the dysphoric and vegetative symptoms of depression, hypomanic/manic behaviours, antisocial activities, bothersome compulsions and/or anxieties, sleep disturbance, diligence, volition (abiding by rules and regulations), the ability to cope with discomfort, the enjoyment of affection, development of verbal communication skills, reading ability, arithmetic skills, writing and non-verbal communication (including social interaction, competency, enjoyment) (Weinberg *et al.* 1995, 1998). A detailed three-generation family history must also be obtained. The child is often excused prior to discussing the family history but the adolescent is encouraged to remain if the parent/guardian agrees in order to learn of his or her family background. Information should be sought about affective illness, thought disorder (schizophrenia), Briquet syndrome, alcoholism (and drug and substance abuse) and sociopathy. Dynamic issues including separation, divorce (and reasons why), and problematic difficulties of finance, violence and abuse are discussed.

The examination of the child/adolescent should be conducted in a non-threatening manner using a detailed semistructured closed-end interview format, assessing moods and feelings, behaviour, substance use (including reasons for use, substances used and the sequence and frequency). The guardian may or may not be present during this examination depending upon the wishes of the child or adolescent. We have found young people to be reliable historians when not in a manic (euphoric/denial) state. Their reliability of reporting of their serious and sensitive feelings has been documented by others (Robbins & Alessi 1985). In substance-abusing adolescents, their reporting of depressive symptomatology may be more reliable than their guardians (Hovens *et al.* 1994). Information must also be obtained about physical abuse, sexual activity, attitudes towards the present problems and the desire to feel and do better. The examination must also include a detailed evaluation of higher brain functions (the Symbol Language and Communication Battery, SLCB; Weinberg W.A. *et al.* 1998) and neurological function including the evaluation of subtle motor findings (Emslie *et al.* 1998).

In most cases, substance use can be identified through this careful history-taking and examination, making routine urine drug screening unnecessary because it promotes distrust of the physician. However, there are some illicit drug abusing adolescents who find urine screening helpful towards promoting abstinence and it should be provided for that individual.

Course and treatment

The treatment of substance use/abuse disorders begins with prevention (Brook *et al.* 1999), and prevention begins with eliminating exposure and other risk factors in the environments (home, school, playground). Limiting factors are the recognition and prompt treatment of guardians manifesting affective illness with or without secondary substance use disorders. It is often the unrecognized affective illness of the caregiver that is promoting an unstable home environment with violence, physical abuse or neglect. An equally limiting variable is schools not recognizing, or meeting the needs of children and adolescents with learning disabilities. Equally significant is the recognition of affective illness in children and adolescents, thus preventing the progression to substance abuse in young people with a mixed-type family history (Weinberg *et al.* 1973; Brumback & Weinberg 1976, 1977).

Childhood or adolescent onset of problematic alcohol use seems to be persistent to late fifth decade of life. Individuals from the upper socioeconomic classes (with family and financial resources and adequate dietary intake) have a more favourable prognosis than individuals from a lower socioeconomic class who often have complications of neurological damage, family violence associated with a mood disorder, social failure and antisocial behaviour. Crack cocaine and heroin use are significantly more problematic with greater maladjustment in social/work functioning and more frequent fatality. Tobacco smoking, alcohol and/or marijuana use often precede the use of cocaine and heroin, and thus prevention of serious drug problems may not require preventing all substance use but just preventing progression during adolescence (Robins 1984) or until a predisposing affective illness is brought under control (Deykin *et al.* 1987; Clark & Neighbors 1996; Geller *et al.* 1998). The hallucinogens (psychedelic drugs) and amfetamines are generally not used regularly but are often associated with other illicit drugs in a select group of poly-substance abusing adolescents. It does appear that with cessation of substance abuse there can be remarkably improved functioning during the fourth decade of life, if the individual survives to that age. Initiation of substance abuse is uncommon in the later part of the third decade of life and problematic substance use seems to start in early rather than late adolescence (Robins 1984).

To date there are no well-controlled treatment studies in children or adolescents. Individual psychotherapy, family therapy and group education/supportive programmes including Narcotics Anonymous and Alcoholics Anonymous have anecdotal successes. A recent study of the treatment of adults with cocaine dependence, using a randomly assigned method, demonstrated benefit from intensive drug counselling plus group drug counselling as compared to two methods of professional psychotherapy (Crits-Christoph *et al.* 1999). Another study in adults with cocaine dependence noted the important variable being a longer stay in the drug treatment facility (Simpson *et al.* 1999). However, in methadone-treated opiate addicts, depression seemed to be the prominent variable in promoting the escalation to cocaine abuse (Kosten *et al.* 1987).

A variety of pharmacological treatments have been employed in adult substance abuse: drugs (disulfiram and multiple other agents) are used in treating alcoholism (Swift 1999); opiate analogues (methadone) have been used for heroin abuse; D1–D5 antagonists (ecopipam) have been tried in a small sample of cocaine-dependent abusers (Romach *et al.* 1999); opiate-dependent cocaine abusing adults maintained on buprenorphine and methadone have been successfully treated with desipramine (a norepinephrine tricyclic agonist) to facilitate opiate and cocaine abstinence (Oliveto *et al.* 1999); and lithium has been successful in treating cyclothymic (bipolar disorder) cocaine abusers (Gawin & Kleber 1984). Interestingly, opium addicts with depression who were successfully treated with methadone continued to use cocaine. More recently, one older adolescent and one young adult female with affective illness reported that their use of a synthetic amphetamine ('ecstasy'; MDMA) no longer produced euphoria when under the influence of either citalopram or paroxetine (both selective serotonin reuptake inhibitors; SSRIs) (Stein & Rink 1999). Many non-controlled and anecdotal reports have shown the usefulness of psychotropic medications in treating substance abuse.

In our experience, the most important part of management of the child or adolescent with problematic substance use is freedom from availability of illicit drugs, continued education about the social, economic and physical effects of illicit drugs ('social influence model') (Kleber 1994), and the proper diagnosis and successful treatment of predisposing underlying affective disorder, when it is present. Once recognized, the affective illness must be vigorously treated using a multimodal approach of individual and family cognitive therapy (Wilkes *et al.* 1994) and appropriate pharmacotherapy with antidepressant medications, often in conjunction with lithium (Geller *et al.* 1998; Weinberg *et al.* 1998; Winokur *et al.* 1998).

It is also important to identify any specific learning disorder that may be contributing to school failure and social exclusion that are known to be high-risk variables for substance use (school drop-outs, gangs, etc). If a specific learning disorder is identified, the child or adolescent should be provided with multimedia for learning and performance, preferably in regular mainstream classes with ordinary peers as colleagues, avoiding excessive remediation, time on the skill-area deficit, grade retention or daily failure (Weinberg *et al.* 1971; Weinberg & McLean 1986; Levy *et al.* 1992; Weinberg *et al.* 1998).

Conclusions

Increasing substance use and abuse by young people is one of the major problems to be confronted by society in the twenty-first century. Depending on their sociocultural circumstances and the availability of drugs, up to half (or even more) use substances at some time. In some societies, experimental substance use might be said to be a normal developmental variant. Why and how some of these children and adolescents go on to become chronic users/abusers of substances is a key question. Careful assessment of these chronic substance using/abusing children and adolescents suggests that some of them have evidence of affective illness, sometimes before the onset of the chronic substance use/abuse. A family loading for psychopathology suggests a genetic liability in many which, coupled with availability of substances in the environment, and family adversity, results in the substance use problem. Multimodal intervention, which includes treatment of affective illness, may be the most effective way of preventing or controlling the substance use problem.

Acknowledgements

This work was funded by contributions from Mr and Mrs Woody Hunt and the Cimarron Foundation; Caleb C. and Julia W. Dula Education and Charitable Foundations; Mr Abraham Azoulay and Mr Morton Meyerson.

References

Advisory Council on the Misuse of Drugs (1982) *Treatment and Rehabilitation Report*. Department of Health and Social Security, London.
American Academy of Pediatrics (1996) *The Classification of Child and Adolescent Mental Diagnoses in Primary Care: Diagnostics and*

Statistical Manual for Primary Care (DSM-PC) Child and Adolescent Version. American Academy of Pediatrics, Elk Grove Village, IL.

American Academy of Pediatrics Committee on Substance Abuse (1996) Testing for drugs of abuse in children and adolescents. *Pediatrics,* **98,** 305–307.

American Academy of Pediatrics Committee on Substance Abuse (1998) Tobacco, alcohol, and other drugs: the role of the pediatrician in prevention and management of substance use. *Pediatrics,* **101** (1), 125–128.

American Academy of Pediatrics Committee on Substance Abuse (1999) Marijuana: a continuing concern for pediatricians. *Pediatrics,* **104** (4), 982–985.

American Psychiatric Association (1994) *Diagnostic and Statistical Manual of Mental Disorders, (DSM-IV),* 4th edn. American Psychiatric Association, Washington D.C.

Anthony, J.C. & Petronis, K.R. (1995) Early-onset drug use and risk of later drug problems. *Drug and Alcohol Dependence,* **40,** 9–15.

Bendtsen, P., Hultberg, J., Carlsson, M. & Jones, A.W. (1999) Monitoring ethanol exposure in a clinical setting by analysis of blood, breath, saliva, and urine. *Alcoholism, Clinical and Experimental Research,* **23** (9), 1446–1451.

Borowsky, I.W., Resnick, M.D., Ireland, M. & Blum, R.W. (1999) Suicide attempts among American Indian and Alaska native youth. *Archives of Pediatrics and Adolescent Medicine,* **153,** 573–580.

Brook, J.S., Cohen, P. & Brook, D.W. (1998) Longitudinal study of co-occurring psychiatric disorders and substance use. *Journal of the American Academy of Child and Adolescent Psychiatry,* **37,** 322–330.

Brook, J.S., Balka, E.B. & Whiteman, M. (1999) The risks for late adolescence of early adolescent marijuana use. *American Journal of Public Health,* **89** (10), 1549–1554.

Brumback, R.A. & Weinberg, W.A. (1976) Mania in childhood: case studies and literature review. *American Journal of Diseases of Children,* **130,** 380–385.

Brumback, R.A. & Weinberg, W.A. (1977) Childhood depression: an explanation of a behavior disorder of children. *Perceptual and Motor Skills,* **44,** 911–916.

Bukstein, O.G. & Kaminer, Y. (1993) The nosology of adolescent substance abuse. *American Journal of Addictions,* **3,** 1–13.

Bukstein, O.G. & Tarter, R.E. (1998) Substance use disorders. In: *Textbook of Pediatric Neuropsychiatry* (eds C.E. Coffey & R.A. Brumback), pp. 595–616. American Psychiatric Press, Washington D.C.

Bukstein, O.G., Brent, D.A. & Kaminer, Y. (1989) Comorbidity of substance abuse and other psychiatric disorders in adolescents. *American Journal of Psychiatry,* **146,** 1131–1141.

Busquets, X., Escriba, P., Sastre, M. & Garcia-Sevilla, J.A. (1995) Loss of protein kinase C-alpha beta in brain of heroin addicts and morphine-dependent rats. *Journal of Neurochemistry,* **64,** 247–252.

Carpenter, K.M. & Hasin, D.S. (1999) Drinking to cope with negative affect and DSM-IV alcohol use disorders: a test of three alternative explanations. *Journal of Studies on Alcohol,* **60** (5), 694–704.

Carvey, P.M. (1998) *Drug Action in the Central Nervous System.* Oxford University Press, New York.

Chaltos, J.C. (1996) Recent trends and a developmental approach to substance abuse in adolescents. *Child and Adolescent Psychiatric Clinics of North America,* **5** (1), 1–27.

Clark, D.B. & Neighbors, B. (1996) Adolescent substance abuse and internalizing disorders. In: *Adolescent Substance Abuse and Dual Disorders: Child and Adolescent Psychiatric Clinics of North America* (ed. S.L. Jaffe), **5,** 45–57.

Clark, D.B., Bukstein, O.G., Smith, M.G., Kaczynski, N.A., Mezzich, A.C. & Donovan, J.E. (1995) Identifying anxiety disorders in adoles-

cents hospitalized for alcohol abuse or dependence. *Psychiatric Services,* **46,** 618–620.

Conacher, G.N. & Workman, D.G. (1989) Violent crime possibly associated with anabolic steroid use. *American Journal of Psychiatry,* **146,** 679.

Cooper, C.J. & Noakes, T.D. (1994) Psychiatric disturbances in users of anabolic steroids. *South African Medical Journal,* **84,** 509–512.

Cooper, J.R., Bloom, F.E. & Roth, R.H. (1991) *The Biochemical Basis of Neuropharmacology,* 6th edn. Oxford University Press, New York.

Cooper, J.R., Bloom, F.E. & Roth, R.H. (1996) *The Biochemical Basis of Neuropharmacology,* 7th edn. Oxford University Press, New York.

Crits-Christoph, P., Siqueland, L., Blaine, J. *et al.* (1999) Psychosocial treatments of cocaine dependence: National Institute on Drug Abuse collaborative cocaine treatment study. *Archives of General Psychiatry,* **56,** 493–502.

Crumley, F.E. (1990) Substance abuse and adolescent suicidal behavior. *Journal of the American Medical Association,* **263,** 3051–3056.

Deykin, E.Y. & Buka, S.L. (1994) Suicidal ideation and attempts among chemically dependent adolescents. *American Journal of Public Health,* **84** (4), 634–639.

Deykin, E.Y., Levy, J. & Wells, V. (1987) Adolescent depression, alcohol, and drug abuse. *American Journal of Public Health,* **77** (2), 178–182.

Deykin, E.Y., Buka, S.L. & Zeena, T.H. (1992) Depressive illness among chemically dependent adolescents. *American Journal of Psychiatry,* **149,** 1341–1347.

Emslie, G.J., Weinberg, W.A. & Kowatch, R.A. (1998) Mood disorders. In: *Textbook of Pediatric Neuropsychiatry* (eds C.E. Coffey & R.A. Brumback), pp. 359–391. American Psychiatric Press, Washington D.C.

Famularo, R., Stone, K. & Popper, C. (1985) Preadolescent alcohol abuse and dependence. *American Journal of Psychiatry,* **142,** 1187–1189.

Farrell, M. & Taylor, E. (1994) Drug and alcohol use and misuse. In: *Child and Adolescent Psychiatry* (eds M. Rutter, E. Taylor & L. Hersov). Blackwell Scientific Publications, Oxford.

Fergusson, D.M. & Horwood, L.J. (1997) Early onset cannabis use and psychosocial adjustment in young adults. *Addiction,* **92,** 279–296.

Fowler, R.C., Rich, C.L. & Young, D. (1986) San Diego suicide study. II. Substance abuse in young cases. *Archives of General Psychiatry,* **43,** 281–284.

Frank, D.A., McCarten, K.M., Robson, C.D. *et al.* (1999) Level of *in utero* cocaine exposure and neonatal ultrasound findings. *Pediatrics,* **104,** 1101–1105.

Gardner, E.L. (1992) Brain reward mechanisms. In: *Substance Abuse: a Comprehensive Text Book* (eds J.H. Lowinson, P. Ruiz & R.B. Millman), pp. 70–99. Williams & Wilkins, Baltimore, MD.

Gawin, F.H. & Kleber, H.D. (1984) Cocaine abuse treatment: open pilot trial with desipramine and lithium carbonate. *Archives of General Psychiatry,* **41,** 903–909.

Geller, B., Cooper, T.B., Sun, K. *et al.* (1998) Double-blind and placebo-controlled study of lithium for adolescent bipolar disorders with secondary substance dependency. *Journal of the American Academy of Child and Adolescent Psychiatry,* **37,** 171–178.

Gilvarry, E. (2000) Substance abuse in young people. *Journal of Child Psychology, Psychiatry,* **41,** 55–80.

Giros, B., Jaber, M., Jones, S.R., Wightman, R.M. & Caron, M.G. (1996) Hyperlocomotion and indifference to cocaine and amphetamine in mice lacking the dopamine transporter. *Nature,* **379,** 606–612.

Gossop, M., Griffiths, P., Powis, B., Williamson, S. & Strang, J. (1996) Frequency of non-fatal heroin overdose: survey of heroin users recruited in non-clinical settings. *British Medical Journal*, 313, 402.

Greenbaum, P.E., Prange, M.E., Friedman, R.M. & Silver, S.E. (1991) Substance abuse prevalence and comorbidity with other psychiatric disorders among adolescents with severe emotional disturbances. *Journal of the American Academy of Child and Adolescent Psychiatry*, 30, 575–583.

Halikas, J. (1990) Substance abuse in children and adolescents. In: *Psychiatric Disorders in Children and Adolescents* (eds B.D. Garfinkel, G.A. Carlson & E.B. Weller), pp. 210–234. W.B. Saunders, Philadelphia, PA.

Hamid, R., Deren, S., Beardsley, M. & Tortu, S. (1999) Agreement between urinalysis and self-reported drug use. *Substance Use and Misuse*, 34 (11), 1585–1592.

Harding, W.M. (1983–84) Controlled opiate use: fact or artifact? *Advances in Alcohological and Substance Abuse*, 3, 105–118.

Harding, W.M. & Zinberg, N.E. (1984) Controlling intoxicant use. *Journal of Psychoactive Drugs*, 16, 101–106.

Harding, W.M., Zinberg, N.E., Stelmack, S.M. & Barry, M. (1980) Formerly-addicted-now-controlled-opiate users. *International Journal of Addiction*, 15, 47–60.

Hovens, J.G.F.M., Cantwell, D.P. & Kiriakos, R. (1994) Psychiatric comorbidity in hospitalized adolescent substance abusers. *Journal of the American Academy of Child and Adolescent Psychiatry*, 33, 476–483.

Jaffe, S.L., ed. (1996) *Adolescent Substance Abuse and Dual Disorders*. Child and Adolescent Psychiatric Clinics of North America, 5, (1).

Joranson, D.E., Ryan, K.M., Gilson, A.M. & Dahl, J.L. (2000) Trends in medical use and abuse of opioid analgesics. *Journal of the American Medical Association*, 283, 1710–1714.

Kandel, D.B. & Davies, M. (1996) High school students who use crack and other drugs. *Archives of General Psychiatry*, 53, 71–80.

Kandel, D.B., Johnson, J.G., Bird, H.R. *et al.* (1997) Psychiatric disorders associated with substance use among children and adolescents. findings from the Methods for the Epidemiology of Child and Adolescent Mental Disorders (MECA) study. *Journal of Abnormal Child Psychology*, 25 (2), 121–132.

Karch, S.B. (1996) *The Pathology of Drug Abuse*, 2nd edn. CRC Press, Boca Raton.

Khantzian, E.J. (1985) The self-medication hypothesis of addictive disorders: focus on heroin and cocaine dependence. *American Journal of Psychiatry*, 142 (11), 1259–1264.

Kleber, H.D. (1994) Our current approach to drug abuse: progress, problems, proposals. *New England Journal of Medicine*, 330, 361–365.

Kosten, T.R., Rounsaville, B.J. & Kleber, H.D. (1987) A 2.5-year follow-up of cocaine use among treated opioid addicts: have our treatments helped? *Archives of General Psychiatry*, 44, 281–284.

Laposata, M. (1999) Assessment of ethanol intake: current tests and new assays on the horizon. *American Journal of Clinical Pathology*, 112 (4), 443–450.

Leshner, A.I. (1996) Molecular mechanisms of cocaine addiction. *New England Journal of Medicine*, 335 (2), 128–129.

Levy, H.B., Harper, C.R. & Weinberg, W.A. (1992) A practical approach to children failing in school. *Pediatric Clinics of North America*, 39, 895–928.

MacGregor, R., Evans, D., Sugden, D., Gaussen, T. & Levene, M. (1998) Outcome of 5–6 years of prematurely born children who received morphine as neonates. *Archives of Diseases in Children, Fetal and Neonatal Edition*, 79, F40–F43.

Maxwell, J.C. & Liu, L.Y. (1999) *1998 Texas School Survey of Substance Use Among Students: Grades 7–12*. Texas Commission on Alcohol and Drug Abuse, Austin, TX.

McKeganey, N., Forsyth, A., Barnard, M. & Hay, G. (1996) Designer drinks and drunkenness amongst a sample of Scottish schoolchildren. *British Medical Journal*, 313, 401.

McNall, M. & Remafedi, G. (1999) Relationship of amphetamine and other substance use to unprotected intercourse among young men who have sex with men. *Archives of Pediatrics and Adolescent Medicine*, 153, 1130–1135.

Milin, R., Halikas, J., Meller, J. & Morse, C. (1991) Psychopathology among substance abusing juvenile offenders. *Journal of the American Academy of Child and Adolescent Psychiatry*, 30, 569–574.

Miller, P.McC. & Plant, M. (1996) Drinking, smoking, and illicit drug use among 15 and 16-year-olds in the United Kingdom. *British Medical Journal*, 313, 394–397.

Mittleman, M.A., Mintzer, D., Maclure, M., Tofler, G.H., Sherwood, J.B. & Muller, J.E. (1999) Triggering of myocardial infarction by cocaine. *Circulation*, 99, 2737–2741.

Musty, R.E. & Kaback, L. (1995) Relationships between motivation and depression in chronic marijuana users. *Life Sciences*, 56, 2151–2158.

Oliva, C.C. & Middleton, R.K. (1990) Anabolic steroid-induced psychiatric reactions. *Drug Intelligence and Clinical Pharmacy*, 24, 388.

Oliveto, A.H., Feingold, A., Schottenfeld, R., Jatlow, P. & Kosten, T.R. (1999) Desipramine in opioid-dependent cocaine abusers maintained on buprenorphine vs. methadone. *Archives of General Psychiatry*, 56, 812–820.

Oyefeso, A., Ghodse, H., Clancy, C., Corkery, J. & Goldfinch, R. (1999) Drug abuse-related mortality: a study of teenage addicts over a 20-year period. *Social Psychiatry and Psychiatric Epidemiology*, 34 (8), 437–441.

Pitkanen, T. (1999) Problem drinking and psychological well-being: a five-year follow-up study from adolescence to young adulthood. *Scandinavian Journal of Psychology*, 40 (3), 197–207.

Pope, H.G. Jr & Katz, D.L. (1988) Affective and psychotic symptoms associated with anabolic steroid use. *American Journal of Psychiatry*, 145, 487–490.

Pope, H.G. Jr & Katz, D.L. (1990) Homicide and near-homicide by anabolic steroid users. *Journal of Clinical Psychiatry*, 51, 28–31.

Pope, H.G. Jr, Kouri, E.M., Powell, K.F., Campbell, C. & Katz, D.L. (1996) Anabolic–androgenic steroid use among 133 prisoners. *Comprehensive Psychiatry*, 37, 322–327.

Reid, D. (1996) Teenage drug use. *British Medical Journal*, 313, 375.

Reinherz, H.Z., Giaconia, R.M., Hauf, A.M., Wasserman, M.S. & Paradis, A.D. (2000) General and specific childhood risk factors for depression and drug disorders by early adulthood. *Journal of the American Academy of Child and Adolescent Psychiatry*, 39 (2), 223–231.

Riggs, P.D., Baker, S., Mikulich, S.K., Young, S.E. & Crowley, T.J. (1995) Depression in substance-dependent delinquents. *Journal of the American Academy of Child and Adolescent Psychiatry*, 34 (6), 764–771.

Robbins, D.R. & Alessi, N.E. (1985) Depressive symptoms and suicidal behavior in adolescents. *American Journal of Psychiatry*, 142, 588–592.

Robins, L.N. (1984) The natural history of adolescent drug use. *American Journal of Public Health*, 74, 656–657.

Robins, L.N. & McEvoy, L. (1990) Conduct problems as predictors of substance abuse. In: *Straight and Devious Pathways from Childhood to Adulthood* (eds L. Robins & M. Rutter), pp. 182–204. Cambridge University Press, Cambridge.

Romach, M.K., Glue, P., Kampman, K. *et al.* (1999) Attenuation of the euphoric effects of cocaine by the dopamine D1/D5 antagonist ecopipam (SCH39166). *Archives of General Psychiatry*, **56**, 1101–1106.

Rounsaville, B.J., Weissman, M.M., Crits-Christoph, K., Wilber, C. & Kleber, H. (1982) Diagnosis and symptoms of depression in opiate addicts: course and relationship to treatment outcome. *Archives of General Psychiatry*, **39**, 151–156.

Schuckit, M.A. (1979) *Drug and Alcohol Abuse: A Clinical Guide to Diagnosis and Treatment*. Plenum, New York.

Siegel, G.J., Agranoff, B.W., Albers, R.W., Fisher, S.K. & Uhler, M.D. (1999) *Basic Neurochemistry: Molecular, Cellular, and Medical Aspects*, 6th edn. Lippincott Williams & Wilkins, Philadelphia.

Simpson, D.D., Joe, G.W., Fletcher, B.W., Hubbard, R.L. & Anglin, M.D. (1999) A national evaluation of treatment outcomes for cocaine dependence. *Archives of General Psychiatry*, **56**, 507–514.

Stahl, S.M. (1996) *Essential Psychopharmacology: Neuroscientific Basis and Practical Applications*. Cambridge University Press, Cambridge.

Stein, D.J. & Rink, J. (1999) Effects of 'ecstasy' blocked by serotonin reuptake inhibitors. *Journal of Clinical Psychiatry*, **60**, 485.

Swadi, H. (1992a) Relative risk factors in detecting adolescent drug abuse. *Drug and Alcohol Dependence*, **29**, 253–254.

Swadi, H. (1992b) Psychiatric symptoms in drug abusing adolescents. *Drug and Alcohol Dependence*, **31**, 77–83.

Swift, R.M. (1999) Drug therapy for alcohol dependence. *New England Journal of Medicine*, **340** (19), 1482–1490.

Tubman, T.G., Vicary, J.R., von Eye, A. & Lerner, J.V. (1990) Longitudinal substance use and adult adjustment. *Journal of Substance Abuse*, **2**, 317–334.

Weinberg, N.Z. & Glantz, M.D. (1999) Child psychopathology risk factors for drug abuse: overview. *Journal of Clinical Child Psychology*, **28**, 290–297.

Weinberg, N.Z., Rahdert, E., Colliver, J.D. & Glantz, M.D. (1998) Adolescent substance abuse: a review of the past 10 years. *Journal of the American Academy of Child and Adolescent Psychiatry*, **37**, 252–261.

Weinberg, W.A. & Brumback, R.A. (1992) The myth of attention deficit-hyperactivity disorder: symptoms resulting from multiple causes. *Journal of Child Neurology*, **7**, 431–445; discussion 446–461.

Weinberg, W.A. & Emslie, G.J. (1991) Attention deficit hyperactivity disorder: the differential diagnosis. *Journal of Child Neurology*, **6** (Suppl.), S23–S36.

Weinberg, W.A. & McLean, A. (1986) A diagnostic approach to developmental specific learning disorders. *Journal of Child Neurology*, **1**, 158–172.

Weinberg, W.A., Penick, E.C., Hammerman, M. & Jackoway, M. (1971) An evaluation of a summer remedial reading program. *American Journal of Diseases of Children*, **122**, 494–498.

Weinberg, W.A., Rutman, J., Sullivan, L., Penick, E.C. & Dietz, S.G. (1973) Depression in children referred to an educational diagnostic center: diagnosis and treatment—preliminary report. *Journal of Pediatrics*, **83** (6), 1065–1072.

Weinberg, W.A., Harper, C.R. & Brumback, R.A. (1995) Neuroanatomic substrate of developmental specific learning disabilities and select behavioral syndromes. *Journal of Child Neurology*, **10** (Suppl.), S78–S80.

Weinberg, W.A., Harper, C.R. & Brumback, R.A. (1998) Clinical evaluation of cognitive/behavioral functions in children and adolescents: use of the Symbol Language and Communication Battery in the physician's office for assessment of higher brain functions. In: *Textbook of Pediatric Neuropsychiatry* (eds C.E. Coffey & R.A. Brumback), pp. 171–220. American Psychiatric Press, Washington D.C.

Wilkes, T.C.R., Belsher, G., Rush, A.J. & Frank, E. (1994) *Cognitive Therapy for Depressed Adolescents*. Guilford Press, New York.

Winokur, G., Turvey, C., Akiskal, H. *et al.* (1998) Alcoholism and drug abuse in three groups: bipolar I, unipolars, and their acquaintances. *Journal of Affective Disorders*, **50**, 81–89.

World Health Organization (1992) *The ICD-10 Classification of Mental and Behavioural Disorders: Clinical Descriptions and Diagnostic Guidelines*. World Heath Organization, Geneva.

World Health Organization (1996) *Multiaxial Classification of Child and Adolescent Psychiatric Disorders. The ICD-10 Classification of Mental and Behavioural Disorders in Children and Adolescents*. Introduction by Professor Sir Michael Rutter, pp. 55–56. Cambridge University Press, Cambridge.

Young, S.E., Mikulich, S.K., Goodwin, M.B. *et al.* (1995) Treated delinquent boys' substance use: onset, pattern, relationship to conduct and mood disorders. *Drug and Alcohol Dependence*, **37**, 149–162.

Yu, O., Chiu, T.H. & Rosenburg, H.C. (1988) Modulation of GABA-gated chloride ion flux in rat brain by acute and chronic benzodiazepine administration. *Journal of Pharmacological and Experimental Therapy*, **246**, 107–113.

Zinberg, N.E. & Jacobson, R.C. (1976) The natural history of 'chipping'. *American Journal of Psychiatry*, **133**, 37–40.

Zinberg, N.E., Jacobson, R.C. & Harding, W.M. (1975) Social sanctions and rituals as a basis for drug abuse prevention. *American Journal of Drug and Alcohol Abuse*, **2** (2), 165–182.

Zinberg, N.E., Harding, W.M., Stelmack, S.M. & Marblestone, R.A. (1978) Patterns of heroin use. *Annals of the New York Academy of Sciences*, **311**, 10–24.

Zur, J. & Yule, W. (1990) Chronic solvent abuse. II. Relationship with depression. *Child Care and Health Development*, **16**, 21–34.

28 Substance Use and Abuse: Causal Pathways Considerations

Michael Rutter

Introduction

One of the crucial features of substance use and abuse is the very high frequency of occasional recreational use of drugs and the relative infrequency of drug abuse and dependency. Thus, in the Christchurch longitudinal study, nearly 70% of the study had used cannabis at some time but less than 7% showed substance abuse or dependence (Fergusson & Horwood 2000a). It is necessary to ask whether these represent opposite ends of the same continuum or whether the factors leading to one are somewhat different from those leading to the other. For example, in her study of Vietnam veterans, Robins (1993) found that prior heroin use was most frequent in inner city African-Americans but, of those using heroin in Vietnam, the likelihood of becoming and remaining dependent after return to the USA was greatest in rural whites. The question is by no means specific to drug abuse. Very comparable questions arise with respect to the possible connections between dieting in adolescent girls, which is exceedingly common, and anorexia nervosa, which is quite uncommon (see Steinhausen, Chapter 34), or between occasional delinquent acts in males, which are virtually normative, and life-course-persistent antisocial behaviour, which is both uncommon and handicapping (see Earls & Mezzacappa, Chapter 26), or between isolated brief episodes of depression and bipolar affective disorders (see Harrington, Chapter 29). In this chapter, possible causal influences are considered, mainly with reference to the findings of longitudinal studies, and with a particular focus on the meaning of associations between substance use/abuse and other forms of psychopathology or social malfunction.

Risk factors

A diverse range of risk factors for substance use and abuse have been identified through epidemiological studies, time series analyses, case–control comparisons and longitudinal studies (Hawkins *et al.* 1995; Silbereisen *et al.* 1995; Weinberg *et al.* 1998; Gilvarry 2000). They are likely to operate maximally at different stages in the progression from experimental recreational usage to dependence and abuse; they reflect a variety of possible risk mechanisms; and they vary in the degree to which the risks apply specifically to drug use and abuse. The last consideration is crucial because of the very high frequency with which drug users also show other forms of psychopathology.

Societal influences

The second half of the twentieth century saw a massive increase in both recreational illicit substance usage and alcoholism in most Western countries (Silbereisen *et al.* 1995; Rutter 1979; Gilvarry 2000). Time series analyses have shown a quite close connection between overall levels of population usage and rates of abuse disorders—for example, between alcohol consumption and deaths from cirrhosis or rates of very heavy drinking. It has also been found that time trends in both reflect accessibility and costs, as shown by the effects of changes in licensing, taxation, purchasing power and drug controls. Increased affluence tends to increase alcohol consumption, a severe sudden rise in taxation reduces consumption, and making usage illegal (as by raising the age for legal drinking) also has effects. Prohibitions on smoking have been similarly associated with changed public attitudes and a fall in the proportion of the population who smoke but, strikingly, much less so among young people than in older age groups. Effects are crucially dependent on social context. Thus, Mooney *et al.* (1992) found that the higher minimum age for drinking in North Carolina as compared to Louisiana was associated with a lower alcohol consumption by college students in controlled situations, but a *higher* rate in uncontrolled situations. Government actions to restrict importing, distribution and sales of amphetamines was followed by a marked decrease in their use (De Alarcon 1972; Wilson 1972). To be effective such steps need to have community approval and need to be accompanied by equally effective prevention of illegal production and distribution. The parallels with situational prevention of crime (Rutter *et al.* 1998) are close. Although it is evident that societal influences do affect substance use and abuse, it has not proved at all easy to use that knowledge to prevent substance abuse disorders.

Genetic influences

The evidence from both twin and adoptee studies indicates that there is a moderate genetic influence on the overall liability to substance use and abuse (van den Bree *et al.* 1998a–c; Kendler *et al.* 1999a, 2000; Vanyukov & Tarter 2000). In itself, that finding is not very informative because it applies to almost all forms of psychopathology (see McGuffin & Rutter, Chapter 12). What is more important is the light thrown on possible causal processes. Several pointers warrant emphasis. Genetic influences are much weaker on individual differences in initial experimental recreational use of drugs than on established abuse or dependency, which has a quite strong heritability. Although there is substantial overlap between the two, the genetic influences on initiation are to some extent different from those on dependence (Kendler *et al.* 1999b). On the whole, the heritability of substance abuse is somewhat stronger in males than females, although this may reflect little more than gender differences in the severity/persistence of substance abuse problems.

The liabilities to use and abuse of different categories of drugs, alcohol and tobacco share over half their genetic variance—implying that most of the genetic influences are not drug-specific. This shared genetic variance includes that between nicotine and alcohol (True *et al.* 1999). Nevertheless, there are genetic influences on individual differences in sensitivity/tolerance to specific substances and these may well have a role in vulnerability to problems with specific substances. The best demonstrated example concerns the flushing reaction to alcohol seen in about half of Orientals, because of a deficiency in one of the key enzymes involved in alcohol oxidation. This unpleasant reaction to alcohol is quite a powerful protector against alcoholism. The genetic polymorphism does not occur in Caucasian and black populations, however, and therefore cannot account for individual differences in liability to alcoholism in these groups. On the other hand, there could be comparable genetic mechanisms that do so (Schuckit 1985; Comings *et al.* 1997; Koob & Le Moal 1997). Thus, Heath *et al.* (1999) found that, in males but not females, high sensitivity to alcohol was associated with a reduced risk of alcohol dependence.

There is a paucity of evidence on the role of genetic factors in the comorbidity between substance abuse and either antisocial behaviour or depression. A longitudinal twin study of adolescents, therefore dealing with initiation more than dependence, found that there was shared genetic liability for both types of comorbidity (Silberg, Rutter, D'Onofrio & Eaves, submitted). Family and adoptee studies are somewhat inconsistent (van den Bree *et al.* 1998b). Twin and adoptee studies have confirmed the environmentally mediated risk associated with early experiences such as parental loss or sexual abuse (Kendler *et al.* 1996, 2000), adverse rearing influences (Cadoret *et al.* 1986) and contemporaneous experiences such as unusually early puberty (Dick *et al.* 2000). There is also some indication that genetic liability operates both directly as a risk factor and indirectly in relation to susceptibility to environmental hazards (Cadoret *et al.* 1995). The second route implies that environmental risks may operate only or mainly on individuals who are genetically vulnerable.

Molecular genetic findings provide valuable leads but, so far, no solid findings (Vanyukov & Tarter 2000). The early reports that allelic variations in the dopamine D2 receptor gene were associated with alcoholism were probably largely a result of stratification biases (see McGuffin & Rutter, Chapter 12 for explanation). Currently, the main attention is being focused on genes that may have a role in temperamental features (such as novelty-seeking) implicated in the risk for substance abuse, but it remains to be seen whether this will pay off.

Individual characteristics

There is abundant evidence that antisocial behaviour in middle childhood and later, and its correlates, is strongly associated with an increased risk for substance abuse (see below) but little is known about other individual characteristics that carry risk (Weinberg *et al.* 1998; Gilvarry 2000). Attention deficit disorder with hyperactivity (ADHD) is associated with an increased risk for substance abuse but it seems that this risk is largely carried by its association with antisocial behaviour (Biederman *et al.* 1997; Mannuzza *et al.* 1991; Disney *et al.* 1999). ADHD in the absence of conduct problems probably does not increase the risk of substance abuse. It has been suggested that impaired behavioural regulation and self-monitoring, and lack of foresight/planning, are associated with an increased risk for both disruptive behaviour and substance abuse (Giancola *et al.* 1996). The same applies to sensation-seeking and difficulties with affect regulation (Pandina *et al.* 1992). There is growing evidence of the associations between temperamental measures of lack of control and impulsivity in the postinfancy, preschool years and later disruptive and antisocial behaviour (Caspi 1997; Rutter *et al.* 1998). The risks are likely to include substance abuse but whether there is any increase in risk that is independent of antisocial behaviour is quite uncertain. The same applies to poor scholastic attainment. Both risk-taking behaviour and a lack of commitment to social institutions and their values may be expected to predispose to taking illicit drugs, but the strength of their effects is not known.

In view of the evidence that substance abuse is associated with drug and alcohol problems in the parents, it is also necessary to consider the possibility that some risk may derive from fetal exposure to maternal alcohol and drugs (see Marks *et al.*, Chapter 51). In that such exposure has behavioural consequences, it could be implicated in the risk processes but evidence is lacking on whether that actually is the case.

Psychosocial risk factors

There is an abundance of evidence that young people attending clinic facilities for treatment of their substance abuse problems have a much increased rate of family adversity, but this may say as much about referral factors as the causes of substance abuse. Nevertheless, longitudinal studies of non-clinic samples suggest that the associations have some validity. Four key issues have only just begun to be addressed. First, there is the query of the extent to which the risks are environmentally, rather than genetically, mediated. The possibility needs to be taken seriously because so many of the psychosocial risks involve parental psychopathology. Nevertheless, as already noted, genetically sensitive designs have shown the reality of the psychosocial risks associated with parental loss as a result of family breakdown (Kendler *et al.* 1996), with sexual abuse (Kendler *et al.* 2000) and adverse rearing (Cadoret *et al.* 1986). The nature of these risk factors suggests that they are operating on psychological functioning in childhood before there has been any involvement with either alcohol or illicit drugs. In short, the effects are likely to be on the overall liability rather than on substance use as such.

The second query is the extent to which the risks apply to the initial experimentation with drugs and how far to the progression from drug use to abuse and dependency. Surprisingly, this issue has received little attention up to now.

Thirdly, there is the question of the extent to which the risks apply specifically to substance use and abuse as distinct from socially disapproved behaviour and psychopathology more generally. It is obvious that the psychosocial risk factors closely parallel those for antisocial behaviour (see Earls & Mezzacappa, Chapter 26) and little is known about possible specificities. Lewinsohn et al. (1995) sought to differentiate shared and specific risk factors as they applied to depression and substance abuse. Both shared and specific risks were found.

The fourth query concerns the extent to which the psychosocial risks stem from the children's qualities as distinct from environmental features over which they have no control. Thus, Brook et al. (1999) found that a close parent–child identification was protective and involvement with a deviant peer group carried risk. Both are likely to have been influenced by the young people's own behaviour in shaping and selecting environments and by influencing their own personal interactions with other people. Situations brought about by the individuals themselves can undoubtedly influence the person's later behaviour—as shown, for example, by the effects of a harmonious marriage in making desistance from antisocial behaviour more likely (Zoccolillo et al. 1992; Laub et al. 1998). Nevertheless, in conceptualizing risk processes, it is necessary to consider the various ways in which persons interact with their environments.

Perhaps this applies especially to the possible influence of deviant peer groups. Fergusson & Horwood (1996, 2000a) showed that these did make an impact that was still evident after appropriate statistical control for other personal and experiential factors. Urberg et al. (1997) and Brook et al. (1999) found the same. However, few studies have used designs that could truly test the causal role of peer group influences (Rutter et al. 1998). Those that have done so have shown that the transitions into smoking and into alcohol use are significantly affected by the peer group's use of those substances.

Depression, antisocial behaviour and substance use/abuse

Although substance use/abuse can be associated with diverse forms of psychopathology (including schizophrenia), the most frequent comorbidity patterns involve either depression or antisocial behaviour or both. The key question is which leads to which? Does the co-occurrence reflect a shared liability, deriving from either genetic or environmental risks? Do conduct problems predispose to drug-taking—perhaps because they reflect risk-taking and novelty-seeking behaviour—or does drug-taking lead people into delinquent activities? Similarly, does depression cause a propensity to drug-taking—perhaps as a form of self-medication to reduce the pain of negative emotions—or does the taking of drugs with effects on the brain lead to depression?

These questions have been tackled using several different research strategies. Thus, cross-sectional data from the epidemiological catchment area (ECA) were used by Robins & McEvoy (1990) to derive pathways over time. They found that conduct disturbance in childhood was a powerful predictor of drug use/abuse in adolescence and adult life, the effect being found to follow a dose–response relationship; the effects were *not* dependent on the conduct problems being above a clinical threshold. Longitudinal methods provide a stronger test of predictive power because they can deal with the possible role of comorbidity in childhood. Harrington et al. (1990), in a long-term follow-up into adult life of a clinical sample, found that depression in childhood/adolescence caused a substantial increase in the risk for recurrence of depression in adult life but no increase in other forms of psychopathology (including drug abuse) in adult life compared with the risks associated with non-depressive psychiatric disorders in childhood. The rates of any form of substance abuse were 15% in the depressed group and 21% in the non-depressed psychopathology comparison group. Fombonne et al. (2001, a,b), in a comparable long-term 20-year follow-up of another clinic sample from the same hospital, focused more explicitly on the effects of early comorbidity. They contrasted the adult outcome for 96 children/adolescents with non-comorbid major depressive disorders and 53 whose major depression was accompanied by a conduct disorder. There was a dramatic difference between these two groups in the rate of substance abuse disorders (excluding alcoholism): 1% in the 'pure' depression group vs. 28% in the comorbid group. The between-group difference for alcoholism followed the same pattern but the difference was much less: 28% vs. 40%. The implication is that the main risks for substance abuse come from conduct problems rather than depression. The apparent risk from depression stemmed from a prior comorbidity with conduct problems.

Weissman et al. (1999a), somewhat similarly, undertook a 10–15-year follow-up of 73 adolescents with a major depressive disorder who attended a US clinical centre and 37 volunteers without psychiatric disorders in adolescence. The two groups differed little with respect to alcohol dependence (27 vs. 22%) or drug abuse (12 vs. 11%) or drug dependence (18 vs. 8%, a nonsignificant difference). A comparable follow-up study of 83 prepubertal children with major depression contrasted their outcome with that of prepubertal children with an anxiety disorder and a randomly selected sample of 91 controls living in the same neighbourhood (Weissman et al. 1999b). Both the clinical groups had a raised rate of substance abuse/dependence in adult life (45 and 39%, respectively, vs. 18%). The number of depressed children with comorbid conduct disorder was small ($n=13$) but they did not account for the increased rate of drug problems.

Yet another strategy has been to use longitudinal data to examine the temporal sequence of patterns of comorbidity. Brook et al. (1995a,b, 1996, 1998, 1999) have pioneered this approach using a longitudinal study of a general population sample followed from age 5–10 years to adolescence and then on to early adult life. They found that both childhood aggression (incorporating anger and impulsivity) and intrapsychic distress predicted adolescent illicit drug use. However, overt depression in adolescence did not predict either the initiation or continuation of drug usage in the early twenties. A multivariate analysis of marijuana initiation showed that although unconventionality (rebelliousness, deviance and sensation-seeking) was significantly predictive after taking account of other variables, emotional distress was not predictive.

Rao *et al.* (2000) examined the temporal association between depressive disorder and substance use disorder in a longitudinal study of 155 young women (aged 17–19 years). Depression had no significant risk effect on substance abuse but the effect of substance abuse in increasing the risk for further depression was substantial (an odds ratio of 2.95) and long-lasting. The findings are informative in indicating how the impression that depression predisposes to substance abuse comes about. Women with substance abuse had a rate of major depression that was nearly threefold that in women without substance abuse. This resulted in just over half of women with substance abuse (53%) having a comorbid major depressive disorder. Nevertheless, whereas substance abuse predicted the development of a major depressive disorder during the subsequent 5 years, the reverse did not occur.

Silberg, Rutter, D'Onofrio & Eaves (submitted) in a longitudinal study of a general population twin sample found that the predictive correlation over time (a cross-lagged correlation) from early conduct symptoms to later drug usage was greater than the reverse, but that the opposite was the case for depressive symptoms. That is, although early drug usage predicted later depressive symptomatology, early depression had little effect on later drug usage. However, the genetic analyses also showed that an important reason for both types of comorbidity was a shared genetic liability rather than the effect of one type of psychopathology in increasing the risk for the other.

Other investigators have tackled the issue through a focus on the extent to which comorbidity occurs as a result of shared risk factors, but again using longitudinal data (Newcomb & Bentler 1990; Henry *et al.* 1993; Fergusson *et al.* 1996a,b, 2000; Lynskey *et al.* 1998; Fergusson & Woodward 2000). The findings have been consistent in showing the importance of shared risk with respect to both the associations among the usages of different substances and the associations among depression, conduct problems and substance use and abuse. Newcomb & Bentler's (1990) findings, however, suggested that there might be some direct effects that varied across the course of development, Thus, whereas early drug usage reduced negative emotions, later drug usage increased the risk of depressive mood. Henry *et al.* (1993), using data from the Dunedin Longitudinal Study, found that neither depression nor conduct problems at 11 years predicted alcohol use at 15 years; depression at 11 years predicted multiple substance use at 15 years in males but not in females.

Much the strongest association, however, was found between contemporaneous conduct problems and multiple drug use in both sexes at age 15. Both conduct problems and depression at 15 years were associated with self-medication at the same age. However, the lack of association between depression and drug usage in females suggests that the influences on self-medication may not be the same as those on recreational drug usage. Fergusson & Horwood (2000b) found that there was evidence that alcohol abuse predisposed to crime, even after account was taken of the shared liability.

Achenbach *et al.* (1998) examined the predictive power of Child Behaviour Checklist (CBCL) scores in adolescence on alcohol and drug use at age 19–22 years in a general population sample. Delinquent subscale scores proved to be predictive in both sexes after taking account of other variables whereas 'anxious/depressive' scores were not predictive. Fergusson *et al.* (2000), in their New Zealand study, found that conduct problems at age 8 years predicted substance use at 16 years in both males and females.

Putting the findings together, it may be concluded that the predictive associations from early conduct problems to later substance use/abuse are substantially stronger than those from early depression. In childhood, it may well be that dysphoric mood predisposes to drug-taking in some individuals, but during adolescence and adult life the effects of substance usage in leading to depression are greater. However, the strongest influence on comorbidity is a shared liability that derives from both genetic and environmental influences. In considering the clinical implications of these findings, the following features warrant emphasis.

1 Conduct problems in middle childhood are common and have an early onset; therefore they could account for a substantial portion of the risk for substance use/abuse in adolescence and adult life.

2 Depressive disorders in childhood are uncommon, with a peak onset only in late adolescence; therefore it is unlikely that they could account for much of the risk for substance use/abuse.

3 The main role of dysphoric affect seems to be in childhood/early adolescence. Accordingly, although not tested systematically, presumably the main effects are on initial experimentation and self-medication, rather than on the later stages of the causal pathway concerned with abuse and dependence.

4 Substance abuse in adolescence has an important effect in increasing the risk for major depressive disorders in early adult life.

5 Much of the association between both conduct problems and depression, and later substance use/abuse, reflects a shared liability rather than a causal effect of one form of psychopathology on the other.

6 Although there is a very strong contemporaneous comorbidity between substance abuse and depression, this does not necessarily mean that one causes the other.

Drugs, alcohol and crime

Numerous studies have shown associations between drug/

alcohol use/abuse and crime (Rutter *et al.* 1998). To a substantial extent, that is bound to be because they share the same set of risk factors (Robins & Wish 1977; Jessor *et al.* 1991; Catalano & Hawkins 1997). On the other hand, that is unlikely to be the complete story if only because there is such a marked variation among crimes in the likelihood that they would be committed under the influence of alcohol (Kerner *et al.* 1997)—being lowest for fraud (2%) and simple theft (5%) and greatest for violent crimes (32%). You need to have a clear head to commit fraud successfully and it is a good idea not to be drunk as a cat burglar! The association with violence probably arises in large part because of disinhibition; experimental studies have shown that intoxication leads to aggression in the presence of frustration (Ito *et al.* 1996). However, the issue is not mainly one of the role of intoxication (by alcohol or other substances) in predisposing to a criminal act, but rather whether substance use/abuse makes crime more likely through non-situational mechanisms and, conversely, whether antisocial behaviour predisposes to the use or abuse of alcohol or illicit drugs. Longitudinal studies have been reasonably consistent in showing predictive dose–response relationships in both directions (Robins & McEvoy 1990; Hawkins *et al.* 1992; Brook *et al.* 1996; Dobkin *et al.* 1997). Fergusson & Horwood (2000b), using the Christchurch Longitudinal Study data, showed that alcohol abuse in late adolescence increased the involvement in crime (especially violent crime) and that this effect held up after control for both observed and non-observed risk factors. Brook *et al.* (1996) suggested that non-alcohol drug use predisposed to crime by reducing inhibitions, creating a need for money to purchase drugs, causing difficulty in family relationships, interfering with the development of social coping skills and establishing a peer group that supports both further drug use and antisocial activities.

'Gateway' effects

It is clear from numerous studies that young people tend to start with using just one substance and then progress to polysubstance usage, this progression being accompanied by increasing associated psychosocial problems and becoming dependent on drugs. This observation has led to various stage theories (Kandel & Faust 1975; Ellickson *et al.* 1992; Stenbacka *et al.* 1993), most of which make the assumption that the usage of one substance (the main focus has been on cannabis as a substance that is used particularly widely) has a causal effect in making it more likely that the person will go on to take other illicit, and potentially more harmful, drugs. This could come about through several rather different mechanisms. For example, the discovery that the use of cannabis may be pleasurable and seemingly without major perceived harmful effects might lead users to experiment with other drugs to see if they had similar properties (Fergusson *et al.* 1993). Alternatively, it could be that the use of cannabis brings young people into increased contact with substance-using peers and drug sellers, so that both enhanced access and a fostering social context predispose to further substance usage (Kandel 1985; Newcomb & Bentler 1989). However, the apparent gateway effect could simply reflect a general liability and process of transition from non-deviant to deviant behaviours (Osgood *et al.* 1998). According to this concept, the many young people who use cannabis but do not progress to polysubstance usage and dependence simply have a lesser liability than those who do progress.

In order to test this last possibility, several investigators have used multivariate analyses of longitudinal data to determine if cannabis use predisposes to other illicit drug use, once adequate account has been taken of other risk factors (Yamaguchi & Kandel 1984; Fergusson & Horwood 2000a). The Christchurch study well illustrates the pattern of findings (Fergusson & Horwood 2000a). Virtually all (99%) users of other illicit drugs had used cannabis first, but nearly two-thirds of cannabis users did not progress to other drugs. There was a very strong dose–response relationship between extent of cannabis usage and progression, with the likelihood of progression being over 140 times as high in young people who used cannabis on at least 50 occasions in the year compared to non-users of cannabis; the risk was 12 times higher in those using cannabis 3–11 times, and 41 times in those using cannabis on 12–49 occasions. To an important extent, this progression was a consequence of an accumulation of personal and experiential risk factors but, even after account of those had been taken, the risk for very heavy users of cannabis was still 59 times higher than for non-users (with the same linear dose–response relationship). It is possible that this risk was a function of unmeasured genetic liability, which could not be assessed in the study, but the findings supported the view that cannabis could act as a gateway drug that encouraged other forms of illicit drug use.

Implications for prevention and treatment

The first implication of causal pathways considerations is that prevention policies should begin with steps to constrain access to substances that carry major risks of abuse or dependence. That presupposes agreement on which substances carry such risks. Controversy mainly focuses on cannabis. Certainly, it is no more dangerous than alcohol, but whether it is desirable to add another drug to those legally available, given that some risks are involved (Ashton 2001; Hall & Solowij 1998; Johns 2001; see also Weinberg *et al.*, Chapter 27) and that it seems to serve a gateway function to other more harmful drugs (see above) is the question. Proponents of legalization argue that it is the very fact that cannabis is illicit that makes it have a gateway function. It is to be hoped that if it is decriminalized, the effects of the legal change will be monitored systematically, so that we may learn from the experience. With respect to alcohol, it is evident that, although taxation, laws on the drinking age and the introduction of breathalysers and blood alcohol laws (to reduce drunken driving) can all have effects, their benefits are crucially dependent on people's acceptance of the constraints. Nevertheless, attitudes can be changed by imposing rules, as evident by antismoking legislation. However, there are powerful commercial misinformation campaigns, as instanced by the actions of tobacco companies (Glantz *et al.* 1996; Ong & Glantz 2000).

A rather different prevention approach is to focus on the secondary effects of drug abuse in predisposing to crime. The controlled prescribing of methadone for heroin addicts was introduced as an attempt to avoid criminalizing the problem. It has had some success in that connection (Farrell & Taylor 1994; Ward *et al.* 1998) although concerns have been expressed regarding its appropriateness in adolescence (O'Brien 1996). In terms of predisposing factors in childhood, it is evident that the main focus needs to be on the prevention and alleviation of disruptive behaviour and conduct problems, as these constitute the strongest risk factor for substance use/abuse. What can be achieved is discussed by Offord & Bennett (Chapter 52) and by Earls & Mezzacappa (Chapter 26). In addition there have been various school-based programmes specifically targeted at drug abuse prevention (Gilvarry 2000). Some successes have been reported (Botvin *et al.* 1995a,b) but there are few systematic evaluations and firm conclusions on the approaches that are effective are not possible (White & Pitts 1998), except that experiential programmes seem more effective than educationally didactic ones (Tobler & Stratton 1997).

Adequate evaluations of the efficacy of individual targeted interventions are similarly few. Family therapies seem promising (Stanton & Shadish 1997) and comprehensive approaches, such as multisystemic therapy (Henggeler *et al.* 1998) that combine family and community methods, are particularly so. Those who are most in need of treatment are often the hardest to engage and retain; this is perhaps especially the case with street youths (Smart & Ogborne 1994; Kipke *et al.* 1997).

In some respects, decisions on how to deal with the very frequent comorbidity with both antisocial behaviour and depressive disorders are some of the most difficult. That is especially the case in view of the evidence that some of these are secondary to the substance abuse, rather than the other way round. Nevertheless, in most cases causal effects are likely to be bidirectional and good clinical care requires attention to the whole pattern of psychopathology.

A final point is that the high frequency of substance use and abuse means that, if referred, most children and adolescents with these problems will be seen in general clinics rather than specialized services for children with substance use disorders. The implication is that routine diagnostic assessment should include enquiry about substance usage and general child and adolescent psychiatrists should be aware of the issues concerned with the diagnosis and treatment of drug problems.

There have been important gains in the development of prevention and intervention programmes over the last decade (Weinberg *et al.* 1998; Gilvarry 2000) but much remains to be done. Most of all, there is a need for a better integration of the findings from epidemiological/longitudinal studies tackling causal questions, experimental investigations of basic mechanisms, and prevention/intervention initiatives leading on to randomized controlled trials designed to determine, not just whether something 'works', but also what are the crucial mediating mechanisms of success, and why the intervention works with this individual but not with that one (Rutter 1982; Rutter *et al.*, 2001).

References

Achenbach, T.M., Howell, C.T., McConaughy, S.H. & Stanger, C. (1998) Six-year predictors of problems in a national sample. IV. Young adult signs of disturbance. *Journal of the American Academy of Child and Adolescent Psychiatry*, 37, 718–727.

Ashton, C.H. (2001) Pharmacology and effects of cannabis: a brief review. *British Journal of Psychiatry*, 178, 101–106.

Biederman, J., Wilens, T., Mick, E. & Faraone, S.V. (1997) Is ADHD a risk factor for psychoactive substance use disorders? Findings from a four-year prospective follow-up study. *Journal of the American Academy of Child and Adolescent Psychiatry*, 36, 21–29.

Botvin, G., Baker, E., Dusenbury, L., Botvin, E. & Diaz, T. (1995a) Long-term follow-up results of a randomized drug abuse prevention trial in a white middle-class population. *Journal of the American Medical Association*, 273, 1106–1112.

Botvin, G.J., Schinke, S.P., Epstein, J.A., Diaz, T. & Botvin, E.M. (1995b) Effectiveness of culturally focused and generic skills training approaches to alcohol and drug abuse prevention among minority adolescents: two-year follow-up results. *Psychology of Addictive Behaviors*, 9, 183–194.

van den Bree, M.B.M., Johnson, E.O., Neale, M.C. & Pickens, R.W. (1998a) Genetic and environmental influences on drug use and abuse/dependence in male and female twins. *Drug and Alcohol Dependence*, 52, 231–241.

van den Bree, M.B.M., Svikis, D.S. & Pickens, R.W. (1998b) Genetic influences in antisocial personality and drug use disorders. *Drug and Alcohol Dependence*, 49, 177–187.

van den Bree, M.B.M., Johnson, E.O., Neale, M.C., Svikis, D.S., McGue, M. & Pickens, R.W. (1998c) Genetic analysis of diagnostic systems of alcoholism in males. *Biological Psychiatry*, 43, 139–145.

Brook, J.S., Whiteman, M., Cohen, P., Shapiro, J. & Balka, E. (1995a) Longitudinally predicting late adolescent and young adult drug use: childhood and adolescent precursors. *Journal of the American Academy of Child and Adolescent Psychiatry*, 34, 1230–1238.

Brook, J.S., Whiteman, M., Finch, S. & Cohen, P. (1995b) Aggression, intrapsychic distress, and drug use: antecedent and intervening processes. *Journal of the American Academy of Child and Adolescent Psychiatry*, 34, 1076–1084.

Brook, J.S., Whiteman, M., Finch, S.J. & Cohen, P. (1996) Young adult drug use and delinquency: childhood antecedents and adolescent mediators. *Journal of the American Academy of Child and Adolescent Psychiatry*, 35, 1584–1592.

Brook, J.S., Cohen, P. & Brook, D.W. (1998) Longitudinal study of co-occurring psychiatric disorders and substance use. *Journal of the American Academy of Child and Adolescent Psychiatry*, 37, 322–330.

Brook, J.S., Kessler, R.C. & Cohen, P. (1999) The onset of marijuana use from preadolescence and early adolescence to young adulthood. *Development and Psychopathology*, 11, 901–914.

Cadoret, R.J., Troughton, E., O'Gorman, T.W. & Heywood, E. (1986) An adoption study of genetic and environmental factors in drug abuse. *Archives of General Psychiatry*, 43, 1131–1136.

Cadoret, R.J., Yates, W.R., Troughton, E., Woodworth, G. & Stewart,

M.A. (1995) Adoption study demonstrating two genetic pathways to drug abuse. *Archives of General Psychiatry*, **52**, 42–52.

Caspi, A. (1997) Personality development across the life course. *Handbook of Child Psychology*, Vol. 3 (series ed. W. Damon; volume ed. N. Eisenberg), 5th edn, pp. 311–388. Wiley, New York.

Catalano, R.F. & Hawkins, J.D. (1997) The social developmental model: a theory of antisocial behavior. In: *Delinquency and Crime: Current Theories* (ed. J.D. Hawkins), pp. 149–177. Cambridge University Press, New York.

Comings, D.E., Gade, R., Wu, S. *et al.* (1997) Studies of the potential role of the dopamine D1 receptor gene in addictive behaviors. *Molecular Psychiatry*, **2**, 44–56.

De Alarcon, R. (1972) An epidemiological evaluation of a public health measure aimed at reducing the availability of methylamphetamine. *Psychological Medicine*, **2**, 293–300.

Dick, D.M., Rose, R.J., Viken, R.J. & Kaprio, J. (2000) Pubertal timing and substance use: associations between and within families across late adolescence. *Developmental Psychology*, **36**, 180–189.

Disney, E.R., Elkins, I.J., McGue, M. & Iacono, W.G. (1999) Effects of ADHD, conduct disorder, and gender on substance use and abuse in adolescence. *American Journal of Psychiatry*, **156**, 1515–1521.

Dobkin, P.L., Tremblay, R.E. & Sacchitelle, C. (1997) Predicting boy's early-onset substance abuse from father's alcoholism, son's disruptiveness, and mother's parenting behavior. *Journal of Consulting and Clinical Psychology*, **65**, 86–92.

Ellickson, P.L., Hays, R.D. & Bell, R.M. (1992) Stepping through the drug use sequence: longitudinal scalogram analysis of initiation and regular use. *Journal of Abnormal Psychology*, **101**, 441–451.

Farrell, M. & Taylor, E. (1994) Drug and alcohol use and misuse. In: *Child and Adolescent Psychiatry* (eds M. Rutter, E. Taylor & L. Hersov), 3rd ed, pp. 529–545. Blackwell Scientific Publications, Oxford.

Fergusson, D.M. & Horwood, L.J. (1996) The role of adolescent peer affiliations in the continuity between childhood behavioural adjustment and juvenile offending. *Journal of Abnormal Child Psychology*, **24**, 205–221.

Fergusson, D.M. & Horwood, L.J. (2000a) Does cannabis use encourage other forms of illicit drug use? *Addiction*, **95**, 505–520.

Fergusson, D.M. & Horwood, L.J. (2000b) Alcohol abuse and crime: a fixed-effects regression analysis. *Addiction*, **95**, 1525–1536.

Fergusson, D.M. & Woodward, L.J. (2000) Educational, psychosocial, and sexual outcomes of girls with conduct problems in early adolescence. *Journal of Child Psychology and Psychiatry*, **41**, 779–792.

Fergusson, D.M., Horwood, L.J. & Lynskey, M.T. (1993) The effects of conduct disorder and attention deficit in middle childhood on offending and scholastic ability at age 13. *Journal of Child Psychology and Psychiatry*, **34**, 899–916.

Fergusson, D.M., Lynskey, M.T. & Horwood, L.J. (1996a) Origins of comorbidity between conduct and affective disorders. *Journal of the American Academy of Child and Adolescent Psychiatry*, **35**, 451–460.

Fergusson, D.M., Lynskey, M.T. & Horwood, L.J. (1996b) The short-term consequences of early-onset cannabis use. *Journal of Abnormal Child Psychology*, **24**, 499–512.

Fergusson, D.M., Woodward, L.J. & Horwood, L.J. (2000) Gender differences in the relationship between early conduct problems and later criminality and substance abuse. *International Journal of Methods in Psychiatric Research*, **8**, 179–191.

Fombonne, E., Wostear, G., Cooper, V., Harrington, R. & Rutter, M. (2001a) The Maudsley long-term follow-up of child and adolescent depression. I. Psychiatric outcomes in adulthood. *British Journal of Psychiatry*, **179**, 210–217.

Fombonne, E., Wostear, G., Cooper, V., Harrington, R. & Rutter, M. (2001b) The Maudsley long-term follow-up of child and adolescent depression. II. Suicidality, criminality and social dysfunction in adulthood. *British Journal of Psychiatry*, **179**, 218–223.

Giancola, P.R., Martin, C.S., Tarter, R.E., Pelham, W.E. & Moss, H.B. (1996) Executive cognitive functioning and aggressive behavior in preadolescent boys at high risk for substance abuse/dependence. *Journal of Studies on Alcohol*, **57**, 352–359.

Gilvarry, E. (2000) Substance abuse in young people. *Journal of Child Psychology and Psychiatry*, **41**, 55–80.

Glantz, S.A., Slade, J., Bero, L.A., Hanauer, P. & Barnes, D.E. (1996) *The Cigarette Papers*. University of California Press, Berkeley, CA.

Hall, W. & Solowij, N. (1998) Adverse effects of cannabis. *Lancet*, **352**, 1611–1616.

Harrington, R., Fudge, H., Rutter, M., Pickles, A. & Hill, J. (1990) Adult outcome of childhood and adolescent depression. I. Psychiatric status. *Archives of General Psychiatry*, **47**, 465–473.

Hawkins, J.D., Catalano, R.F. & Miller, J.Y. (1992) Risk and protective factors for alcohol and other drug problems in adolescence and early adulthood: implications for substance abuse prevention. *Psychological Bulletin*, **112**, 64–105.

Hawkins, J.D., Arthur, M.W. & Catalano, R.F. (1995) Preventing substance abuse. In: *Building a Safer Society: Strategic Approaches to Crime Prevention* (eds M. Tonry & D.P. Farrington), pp. 343–428. University of Chicago Press, Chicago.

Heath, A.C., Madden, P.A.F., Bucholz, K.K. *et al.* (1999) Genetic differences in alcohol sensitivity and the inheritance of alcoholism risk. *Psychological Medicine*, **29**, 1069–1081.

Henggeler, S., Schoenwald, S., Borduin, C., Rowland, M.D. & Cunningham, P.B. (1998) *Multisystemic Treatment of Antisocial Behaviour in Children and Adolescents*. Guilford Press, New York.

Henry, B., Feehan, M., McGee, R., Stanton, W., Moffitt, T.E. & Silva, P. (1993) The importance of conduct problems and depressive symptoms in predicting adolescent substance use. *Journal of Abnormal Child Psychology*, **21**, 469–480.

Ito, T., Miller, N. & Pollock, V.E. (1996) Alcohol and aggression: a meta-analysis on the moderating effects of inhibitory cues, triggering events, and self-focused attention. *Psychological Bulletin*, **120**, 60–82.

Jessor, R., Donovan, J.E. & Costa, F.M. (1991) *Beyond Adolescence: Problem Behavior and Young Adult Development*. Cambridge University Press, Cambridge.

Johns, A. (2001) Psychiatric effects of cannabis. *British Journal of Psychiatry*, **178**, 116–122.

Kandel, D.B. (1985) On processes of peer influences in adolescent drug use: a developmental perspective. *Advances in Alcohol and Substance Abuse*, **4**, 139–163.

Kandel, D. & Faust, R. (1975) Sequence and stages in patterns of adolescent drug use. *Archives of General Psychiatry*, **32**, 923–932.

Kendler, K.S., Neale, M.C., Prescott, C.A. *et al.* (1996) Childhood parental loss and alcoholism in women: a causal analysis using a twin-family design. *Psychological Medicine*, **26**, 79–95.

Kendler, K.S., Karkowski, L.M. & Prescott, C.A. (1999a) Hallucinogen, opiate, sedative and stimulant use and abuse in a population-based sample of female twins. *Acta Psychiatrica Scandinavica*, **99**, 368–376.

Kendler, K.S., Neale, M.C., Sullivan, P., Corey, L.A., Gardner, C.O. & Prescott, C.A. (1999b) A population-based twin study in women of smoking initiation and nicotine dependence. *Psychological Medicine*, **29**, 299–308.

Kendler, K.S., Karkowski, L.M., Neale, M.C. & Prescott, C.A. (2000) Illicit psychoactive substance use, heavy use, abuse, and dependence in a US population-based sample of male twins. *Archives of General Psychiatry*, **57**, 261–269.

Kerner, H.-J., Weitekamp, E.G.M., Stelly, W. & Thomas, J. (1997) Patterns of criminality and alcohol abuse: results of the Tübingen criminal behaviour development study. *Criminal Behaviour and Mental Health*, 7, 401–420.

Kipke, M.D., Montgomery, S.B., Simon, T.R. & Iverson, E.F. (1997) 'Substance abuse' disorders among runaway and homeless youths. *Substance Use and Misuse*, 32, 969–986.

Koob, G.F. & Le Moal, M. (1997) Drug abuse: hedonic homeostatic dysregulation. *Science*, 278, 52–58.

Laub, J.H., Nagin, D.S. & Sampson, R.J. (1998) Trajectories of change in criminal offending: good marriages and the desistance process. *American Sociological Review*, 63, 225–238.

Lewinsohn, P.M., Gotlib, I.H. & Seeley, J.R. (1995) Adolescent psychopathology. IV. Specificity of psychosocial risk factors for depression and substance abuse in older adolescents. *Journal of the American Academy of Child and Adolescent Psychiatry*, 34, 1221–1229.

Lynskey, M.T., Fergusson, D.M. & Horwood, L.J. (1998) The origins of the correlations between tobacco, alcohol, and cannabis use during adolescence. *Journal of Child Psychology and Psychiatry*, 39, 995–1005.

Mannuzza, S., Klein, R.G., Bonagura, N., Malloy, P., Giampino, T. & Addali, K. (1991) Hyperactive boys almost grown up. V. Replication of psychiatric status. *Archives of General Psychiatry*, 48, 77–83.

Mooney, L.A., Gramling, R. & Forsyth, C. (1992) Legal drinking age and alcohol consumption. *Deviant Behavior: an Interdisciplinary Journal*, 13, 59–71.

Newcomb, M.D. & Bentler, P.M. (1989) Substance use and abuse among children and teenagers. *American Psychologist*, 44, 242–248.

Newcomb, M.D. & Bentler, P.M. (1990) Antecedents and consequences of cocaine use: an eight-year study from early adolescence to young adulthood. In: *Straight and Devious Pathways from Childhood to Adulthood* (eds L. Robins & M. Rutter), pp. 158–181. Cambridge University Press, Cambridge.

O'Brien, C.P. (1996) Recent developments in the pharmacotherapy of substance abuse. *Journal of Consulting and Clinical Psychology*, 64, 677–686.

Ong, E.K. & Glantz, S.A. (2000) Tobacco industry efforts subverting International Agency for Research on Cancer's second-hand smoke study. *Lancet*, 355, 1253–1259.

Osgood, D.W., Johnston, L.D., O'Malley, P.M. & Bachman, J.G. (1988) The generality of deviance in late adolescence and early adulthood. *American Sociological Review*, 53, 81–93.

Pandina, R.J., Johnson, V. & Labouvie, E.W. (1992) Affectivity: a central mechanism in the development of drug dependence. In: *Vulnerability to Drug Abuse* (eds M.D. Glantz & R.W. Pickens), pp. 179–210. American Psychological Association, Washington D.C.

Rao, U., Daley, S.E. & Hammen, C. (2000) Relationship between depression and substance use disorders in adolescent women during the transition to adulthood. *Journal of the American Academy of Child and Adolescent Psychiatry*, 39, 215–222.

Robins, L. (1993) The sixth Thomas James Okey Memorial Lecture. Vietnam veterans' rapid recovery from heroin addiction: a fluke or normal expectation? *Addiction*, 88, 1041–1054.

Robins, L.N. & McEvoy, L. (1990) Conduct problems as predictors of substance abuse. In: *Straight and Devious Pathways from Childhood to Adolescence* (eds L.N. Robins & M. Rutter), pp. 182–204. Cambridge University Press, Cambridge.

Robins, L.N. & Wish, E. (1977) Child deviance as a developmental process: a study of 223 urban black men from birth to 18. *Social Forces*, 56, 448–473.

Rutter, M. (1979) *Changing youth in a changing society: patterns of adolescent development and disorder*. Nuffield Provincial Hospitals Trust, London/Harvard University Press, Cambridge, MA.

Rutter, M. (1982) Psychological therapies in child psychiatry: issues and prospects. *Psychological Medicine*, 12, 723–740.

Rutter, M., Giller, H. & Hagell, A. (1998) *Antisocial Behaviour by Young People*. Cambridge University Press, Cambridge.

Rutter, M., Pickles, A., Murray, R. & Eaves, L. (2001) Testing hypotheses on specific environmental causal effects on behavior. *Psychological Bulletin*, 127, 291–324.

Schuckit, M. (1985) Studies of populations at high risk for alcoholism. *Psychiatric Development*, 3, 31–63.

Silbereisen, R.K., Robins, L. & Rutter, M. (1995) Secular trends in substance use: concepts and data on the impact of social changes on alcohol and drug abuse. In: *Psychosocial Disorders in Young People; Time Trends and Their Causes* (eds M. Rutter & D.J. Smith), pp. 490–543. John Wiley & Sons, Chichester.

Silberg, J., Rutter, M., D'Onofrio, B. & Eaves, L. (submitted) *Genetic and environmental risk factors in adolescent substance use*.

Smart, R.G. & Ogborne, A.C. (1994) Street youth in substance abuse treatment: characteristics and treatment compliance. *Adolescence*, 29, 733–745.

Stanton, M.D. & Shadish, W.R. (1997) Outcome, attrition, and family-couples treatment for drug abuse: a meta-analysis and review of the controlled, comparative studies. *Psychological Bulletin*, 122, 170–191.

Stenbacka, M., Allebeck, P. & Romelsjo, A. (1993) Initiation into drug use: the pathway from being offered drugs to trying cannabis and progression to intravenous drug abuse. *Scandinavian Journal of Social Medicine*, 21, 31–39.

Tobler, N.S. & Stratton, H.H. (1997) Effectiveness of school-based drug-prevention programs: a meta-analysis of the research. *Journal of Primary Prevention*, 18, 71–128.

True, W.R., Xian, H., Scherrer, J.F. *et al.* (1999) Common genetic vulnerability for nicotine and alcohol dependence in men. *Archives of General Psychiatry*, 56, 655–661.

Urberg, K.A., Degirmencioglu, S.M. & Pilgrim, C. (1997) Close friend and group influence on adolescent cigarette smoking and alcohol use. *Developmental Psychology*, 33, 834–844.

Vanyukov, M.M. & Tarter, R.E. (2000) Genetic studies of substance abuse. *Drug and Alcohol Dependence*, 59, 101–123.

Ward, J., Mattick, R. & Hall, W. (eds) (1998) *Methadone Maintenance Treatment and Other Opioid Replacement Therapies*. Harwood Academic Publishers, Amsterdam.

Weinberg, N.Z., Rahdert, E., Colliver, J.D. & Glantz, M.D. (1998) Adolescent substance abuse: a review of the past 10 years. *Journal of the American Academy of Child and Adolescent Psychiatry*, 37, 252–261.

Weissman, M.M., Wolk, S., Goldstein, R.B. *et al.* (1999a) Depressed adolescents grown up. *Journal of the American Medical Association*, 281, 1707–1713.

Weissman, M.M., Wolk, S., Wickramaratne, P. *et al.* (1999b) Children with prepubertal-onset major depressive disorder and anxiety grown up. *Archives of General Psychiatry*, 56, 794–801.

White, D. & Pitts, M. (1998) Educating young people about drugs: a systematic review. *Addiction*, 93, 1475–1487.

Wilson, C.W.M. (1972) Amphetamine abuse and government legislation. *British Journal of Addiction to Alcohol and Other Drugs*, 67, 107–112.

Yamaguchi, K. & Kandel, D.B. (1984) Patterns of drug use from adolescence to young adulthood. II. Sequences of progression. *American Journal of Public Health*, 74, 668–672.

Zoccolillo, M., Pickles, A., Quinton, D. & Rutter, M. (1992) The outcome of childhood conduct disorder: implications for defining adult personality disorder and conduct disorder. *Psychological Medicine*, 22, 971–986.

29 Affective Disorders

Richard Harrington

Depressive disorders

History

The concept of a depressive syndrome that is distinct from the broad class of childhood onset emotional disorders has a relatively short history. Until the 1970s it was believed that depressive disorders resembling adult depression were uncommon among the young. Pre-adolescent children were thought incapable of experiencing depression. Depression in adolescents was often seen as a normal feature of development, so-called 'adolescent turmoil'. However, in the 1970s and early 1980s several investigators began to diagnose depression in children using adult criteria (Weinberg *et al.* 1973; Pearce 1978; Puig-Antich 1982). These studies showed that conditions resembling adult depression could occur in even young children. As a result, the features of depressive disorder were deemed the same for children, adolescents and adults (American Psychiatric Association 1980).

The next 15 years saw intensive research into the adult-like depressive conditions that were being diagnosed with increasing frequency among the young. These investigations have led to a reappraisal of the concept of childhood depression. It is apparent that a variety of different problems have been subsumed within the concept. Moreover, there seem to be important differences between child and adolescent depressions. In comparison with adolescent depression, pre-adolescent depression is less likely to lead to adult depression (Harrington *et al.* 1990; Weissman *et al.* 1999a,b), has more overlap with other disorders (Alpert *et al.* 1999), is less prevalent (Angold *et al.* 1998), shows a male preponderance (Angold *et al.* 1998), and is more strongly associated with family dysfunction (Harrington *et al.* 1997). Pre-adolescent depression may therefore be a different diagnostic entity (Harrington 2000). This chapter is concerned mainly with depressive disorders in adolescents but, when relevant, also deals with depressive problems that arise in younger age groups.

Concepts of depression

Depression can be conceptualized both as a dimension and as a category. Epidemiological studies suggest that juvenile depression is a continuum that is associated with problems at most levels of severity (Pickles *et al.*, in press). Indeed, it seems that there is no 'good' level of depression; it is better for an adolescent to have no symptoms of depression at all than to be averagely depressed (Harrington & Clark 1998). Thus, in the Oregon Adolescent Depression Project the level of psychosocial impairment increased as a direct function of the number of depressive symptoms (Lewinsohn *et al.* 1998). Moreover, in line with studies of adults (Angst *et al.* 1997), much of the morbidity associated with depression occurred in the 'milder' but more numerous cases of minor depression. Even mild forms of adolescent depression are a risk factor for depression in early adulthood (Pine *et al.* 1999). The implication is that from the public health perspective of lowering the total burden of morbidity associated with depression, it might be better to regard depression as a continuum.

In clinical practice, however, depression is viewed not only as a dimension but also as a category. This is partly because many clinical decisions are dichotomous. For example, if a patient has a depressive disorder then a course of treatment is initiated; if not then the patient is reassured that all is well. Clinicians do not generally prescribe a little bit of antidepressant for a little bit of depression. To clinicians, then, depression usually means a diagnosis: something that a patient either does or does not have.

Nowadays most clinicians use one of the major schemes for diagnosis: ICD-10 (World Health Organization 1992) or DSM-IV (American Psychiatric Association 1994). The schemes differ in many ways, but at the core of both is the concept of an episodic disorder of varying degrees of severity that is characterized by depressed mood or loss of enjoyment that persists for several weeks. The individual must also experience other symptoms during the episode. These include *depressive thinking*, such as pessimism about the future or suicidal ideas, and *biological symptoms*, such as early waking, reduced appetite and weight loss. DSM-IV states that in children irritable mood may substitute for depressed mood, and that dysthymia (see below) need only last for 1 year (2 years in adults). It also notes that certain symptoms, such as somatic complaints and social withdrawal, are particularly common in children, while other symptoms, such as delusions, are rare. ICD-10 does not mention age differences.

Subcategories of depressive disorder

Subcategorizing depressive disorder by severity is widely accepted. Both DSM-IV and ICD-10 distinguish between mild, moderate and severe episodes of depression but differ in their definitions of severity. In ICD-10, severity is defined by symptoms, whereas in DSM-IV severity is defined in terms of symptoms and functional impairment. We shall see later that in clinical practice impairment is a useful guide both to choice of treatment and to prognosis. For example, adolescents with severe depression, defined as complete disability in one or more domains of social functioning (e.g. unable to go to school, does not see friends at all), are much less likely to respond to psychological treatment than those with mild or moderate depression (Jayson *et al.* 1998). Nevertheless, it can be difficult to link impairment to specific symptoms, and there are many cases whose impairment seems out of proportion to their symptoms (Angold *et al.* 1999c).

Both ICD-10 and DSM-IV distinguish between psychotic and non-psychotic episodes of depression. Psychotic depression is very uncommon before mid-adolescence, but the concept is useful in adults to the extent that it predicts a worse prognosis (Lee & Murray 1988). Psychotic symptoms also presage worse outcomes in adolescent depression (Strober *et al.* 1993).

Other subtypes are less well established. DSM-IV and ICD-10 have a category for chronic mild depression lasting 1 or more years—dysthymia. However, longitudinal studies have shown that in children there is much overlap of major depression and dysthymia (Kovacs *et al.* 1994) and it is likely that they are often part and parcel of the same problem.

Differential diagnosis

A problem with categorical approaches to diagnosis lies in differentiation from 'normality'. As described earlier, there is no obvious point of inflection in the dimension of depressive symptoms. It is therefore not surprising to find that diagnostic systems that are based on numbers of symptoms only (such as DSM-III-R; American Psychiatric Association 1987) give implausibly high rates of so-called depressive disorder. Depressive disorder should therefore only be diagnosed when there is impairment of social role functioning, when symptoms of unequivocal psychopathological significance are present (such as severe suicidality), or when symptoms lead to significant suffering.

A further problem arises from the fact that all epidemiological studies conducted up to now have found that depressive disorder very commonly occurs in conjunction with other psychiatric problems (see below). Indeed, one of the best discriminators in community studies between children with any form of psychiatric disorder and children with no psychiatric disorder is the symptom of depression (Rutter *et al.* 1970). Moreover, some of the symptoms that are part of the depressive constellation may arise as a symptom of other disorders. Thus, restlessness is seen in agitated depression, hypomania and hyperkinetic syndrome. As a general rule, the double diagnosis should be made only when symptoms that are not simply part of another disorder clearly indicate the separate presence of a depressive disorder.

Depression can sometimes be the result of physical disorders. For example, Lewinsohn *et al.* (1998) found that adolescents who reported that they had had a physical illness causing functional impairment (e.g. glandular fever) were at increased risk of subsequent depression. The diagnostic assessment should therefore establish whether a physical disorder may have caused the depression.

Rating scales and interviews

Many questionnaire measures are available to assess depression in children and adolescents (Costello & Angold 1988; Harrington & Shariff 1992). These can be divided into:
1 scales that were specifically designed for studies of juvenile depression, such as the Mood and Feelings Questionnaire (Angold *et al.* 1995a) and the Children's Depression Inventory (Kovacs 1981);
2 scales that were originally devised for studies of depressed adults, but which have often been used in studies of adolescents, such as the Beck Depression Inventory (Beck 1967); and
3 general scales for assessing psychopathology in children that contain some depressive items, such as the Strengths and Difficulties Questionnaire (Goodman 1997).

The choice of scale depends on the purpose to which it will be put. As a general rule, depression specific scales tend to be better measures of change in depression than general scales. However, they are often lengthy and do not provide information about comorbid symptoms, such as anxiety or behavioural problems. Questionnaire measures are also used to screen for depressive disorder in community or high-risk samples (Roberts *et al.* 1991). It should be borne in mind, however, that at the cutpoints that are often used on depression screening questionnaires, specificity and sensitivity seldom exceed 80%. This means that with a low prevalence problem, such as major depression in adolescence, it is a mathematical certainty that most cases with a 'high' score on a questionnaire will not have depressive disorder. Child mental health professionals are often unaware of this problem, assuming that a high score on a screening questionnaire means that the young person is very likely to have a depressive disorder (Clark & Harrington 1999).

Although pencil-and-paper questionnaires will often generate important information for the clinical assessment, an interview with the young person supplemented by an interview with the primary caregiver is usually considered the 'gold standard' for the diagnosis of depressive disorder. This is because careful interviewing is the only way of ensuring that the respondent is describing what the investigator is interested in. A number of standardized interviews of known reliability, such as the Child and Adolescent Psychiatric Assessment (Angold & Costello 1995; Angold *et al.* 1995b) have been developed (Hodges 1993). These are now widely used in research settings but they have some limitations: reliability is low in younger age groups; interviews can last for several hours; there is often a marked discrepancy between different sources of information; and outside of academic centres it can be difficult to obtain training.

The low reliability of the standardized interview as a means of measuring psychopathology in children aged less than 10 years has led to the development of several alternative methods of assessment in this age group (see Angold, Chapter 3). These methods include a structured pictorial questionnaire based on the DSM (Valla *et al.* 1994) and puppet interviews. Early results from the use of puppet interviews with 4–8-year-old-children have been encouraging (Ablow *et al.* 1999).

Comorbidity

Most children and adolescents who are referred for treatment of depressive disorder meet the criteria for at least one other psychiatric diagnosis. Even in community samples, there is much overlap of depression and other forms of psychopathology. In a systematic review of around 20 epidemiological studies based on DSM, Angold *et al.* (1999a) found that the most common comorbid disorders were conduct disorder (occurring, on average, in 40% of depressed cases) and anxiety disorders (34%).

ICD-10 and DSM-IV take different approaches to comorbidity (see Taylor & Rutter, Chapter 1). In ICD-10 it is assumed that a mixed clinical picture is more likely to be the result of a single disorder with different manifestations than of two or more disorders that happen to occur in the same individual at the same time. ICD-10 therefore has a category for mixed disorders, Mixed Disorders of Conduct and Emotions (F92), which includes the subcategory Depressive Conduct Disorder (F92.0). DSM-IV, by contrast, usually allows the investigator to diagnose several supposedly separate disorders, with the result that in surveys based on DSM it is quite common to find individuals with three or more diagnoses (Caron & Rutter 1991).

Conduct disorders

There are several explanations for comorbidity of depression and conduct disorder. Comorbidity might be an artefact of methodology, measurement or current diagnostic systems. However, most reviewers have concluded that this is unlikely to be the case (Caron & Rutter 1991; Angold *et al.* 1999a). Another possibility is that depression is simply an integral part of conduct disorder. Zoccolillo (1992) suggested that conduct disorder is a problem of multiple dysfunction, with depression a dysfunction of affect regulation and conduct disorder a dysfunction of social regulation. Alternatively, it may be that conduct disorder causes depression. Children with conduct disorder sometimes behave in ways that increase their risk of the kinds of adverse events that cause depression, such as inconsistent parenting (O'Connor *et al.* 1998a). However, in an elegant analysis of longitudinal data from the Christchurch Health and Development Study, Fergusson *et al.* (1996) reported that direct causal pathways between depression and conduct disorder were weak. Much of the correlation between the two could be explained by shared risk factors, such as family dysfunction. Similarly, O'Connor *et al.* (1998b) found that nearly 50% of the association between depression and conduct disorder could be explained by a common genetic liability.

Comorbidity between depression and conduct disorder has implications for assessment and management. It is easy to miss depression when the clinical picture is dominated by problems such as aggression. Comorbidity may also influence prognosis. The adult adjustment of children with depression and conduct disorder is as poor as that of children with conduct disorder alone (Harrington *et al.* 1991) and there may be an increased risk of suicide (Fombonne *et al.*, 2001b).

Anxiety disorders

Longitudinal and epidemiological studies suggest that anxiety tends to precede depression in both children (Kovacs *et al.* 1989) and adults (Merikangas *et al.* 1996), raising the possibility that depression is in some sense secondary to anxiety. It may be that they share a common temperamental basis, such as emotionality. Genetic studies suggest the possibility of a common genetic diathesis (Eley & Stevenson 1999).

Epidemiology

Prevalence

Rates of depressive disorder vary between studies. This is partly because of differences in definition and measurement (Roberts *et al.* 1998), and partly because of differences in the time period over which the rate of depression is calculated. For example, some studies report 3-month prevalence (Simonoff *et al.* 1997), others 6-month prevalence (Breton *et al.* 1999) and yet others cumulative incidence (Oldehinkel *et al.* 1999).

A review of early studies found prevalences among adolescents ranging from <1% to 6% (Fleming *et al.* 1989). Recent studies have produced similar findings, with a 1-year (or less) prevalence of major depressive disorder associated with impairment ranging from around 1% (Simonoff *et al.* 1997), through 3% (Cohen *et al.* 1993a; Lewinsohn *et al.* 1998) to 6% (Olsson & von Knorring 1999). When all kinds of depressive disorder are included, then the prevalence can be as high as 10% (Angold *et al.* 1998). The cumulative probability of having a depressive disorder by late adolescence seems to be between 10 and 20% (Lewinsohn *et al.* 1998; Oldehinkel *et al.* 1999; Olsson & von Knorring 1999). Depressive disorder is not, then, an uncommon problem in adolescence.

Developmental trends and gender differences

Almost all recent epidemiological research has found that depressive disorder is much less common among pre-adolescent children than among adolescents (Simonoff *et al.* 1997; Angold *et al.* 1998; Lewinsohn *et al.* 1998; Oldehinkel *et al.* 1999; Olsson & von Knorring 1999; Meltzer *et al.* 2000). For instance, in a large national survey in the UK the odds of having a depressive disorder for 11–15-year-olds compared to 5–10-year-olds was 8.5 (Meltzer *et al.* 2000). The origins of these reliable developmental differences are not well understood, but there are several pointers about possible causes. Age trends in depression are stronger in girls than in boys. Most studies have found that in prepubertal children there is either no gender difference in the prevalence of depression or there is a small male preponderance. In contrast, by late adolescence the female preponderance found in adult depression is well established. However, there is some uncertainty about when the gender difference emerges. The New York and Greater Smoky Mountain studies (Cohen *et al.* 1993a; Angold *et al.* 1998) found that the difference was present by around the age of 13 years, but another study has reported that it emerges later (Hankin *et al.* 1998).

The finding that the gender difference seems to be linked more to some aspect of puberty itself than age (Angold *et al.* 1998) raises important questions about the mechanisms involved. It is possible that there is some direct vulnerability arising from changes in hormone levels, such as androgens (Angold *et al.* 1999b). However, puberty is accompanied by many other changes, such as in cognition and in stressful events. Moreover, even in large samples it can be very difficult to tease apart the effects of age and puberty. Probably there are several reasons for the greater vulnerability of girls. Before adolescence, girls are more likely than boys to have risk factors for depression, such as certain personality features (Nolen-Hoeksema & Girgus 1994; see below). However, these risk factors are not sufficient to cause depression until the person experiences the biological and social challenges of adolescence (Nolen-Hoeksema & Girgus 1994; Cyranowski *et al.* 2000).

Time trends

The prevalence of depressive disorders may be increasing among young people. Evidence of a secular trend comes mainly from retrospective reports of age at onset of depression in family and community studies of depressed adults. These studies have found that people in more recent birth cohorts report higher rates and an earlier onset of depressive disorder than those born earlier in the last century (Fombonne 1999). The results of these studies may have been biased by memory artefacts (Giuffra & Risch 1994). However, repeated cross-sectional surveys have also found an increase in levels of depression. It is likely, then, that there has been a real, though probably small, increase in depression.

Changes in the biological, familial and social context of adolescence provide clues about possible candidate mechanisms that could explain these time trends (Fombonne 1995). Adolescents enter puberty much earlier nowadays than they did 100 years ago. They may also be exposed to higher levels of family conflict. It is likely that combinations of these risk factors are particularly important. For example, earlier puberty probably means that adolescents experience the stresses of making and breaking intimate relationships at an earlier age.

Course

Short-term

Studies of clinical samples have reported that young people with a depressive disorder have a high risk of recurrence or persis-

tence (Emslie *et al.* 1997b; Goodyer *et al.* 1997a). Kovacs *et al.* (1984a) undertook a follow-up of child patients with a major depressive disorder, a dysthymic disorder, an adjustment disorder with depressed mood, and some other psychiatric disorder. The development of subsequent episodes of depression was virtually confined to children with major depressive disorders and dysthymic disorders. Surveys of community samples have generally also found that depressive disorders among young people tend to be recurrent (Fleming *et al.* 1993; Lewinsohn *et al.* 1993, 1994a; Garrison *et al.* 1997). Lewinsohn *et al.* (1993, 1994a) found that the 1-year relapse rate for unipolar depression (18.4%) was much higher than the relapse rate found in most other disorders.

Long-term

Adolescent depressive disorder shows significant continuity into adult life. Harrington *et al.* (1990) followed up 63 depressed children and adolescents on average 18 years after their initial contact. The depressed group had a substantially greater risk of depression after the age of 17 years than a control group who had been matched on a large number of variables. Other groups, too, have found high rates of recurrence of major depression in clinical samples of depressed adolescents who have been followed up into adulthood (Rao *et al.* 1995; Weissman *et al.* 1999a; Fombonne *et al.* 2001a).

Continuity from childhood into adult life has also been found in community surveys, such as the Dunedin Multidisciplinary Health and Development Study (DMHDS). Follow-back longitudinal analyses found that subjects with a mood disorder at age 21 years were much more likely to have a history of previous mood disorder than of non-depressive disorders earlier in life (Newman *et al.* 1996). Similarly, prospective longitudinal analyses from the Oregon Adolescent Depression Project (Lewinsohn *et al.* 1999) found significant continuity from late adolescence (age 17 years) into early adult life (age 24 years). About 45% of depressed adolescents developed a new episode of depression between the ages of 19 and 24. In the New York study (Cohen *et al.* 1993a,b), anxiety or depression in adolescence predicted anxiety or depression in early adult life (Pine *et al.* 1998). The British birth cohort follow-up of individuals born in 1946 found that evidence of affective disturbance at ages 13 and 15 years was a strong predictor of major affective disorder in middle life (Os *et al.* 1997).

Other outcomes

Early studies reported that depression can lead to subsequent problems in social adjustment, such as marital problems (Puig-Antich *et al.* 1985a,b; Kandel & Davies 1986; Garber *et al.* 1988). However, none of these studies excluded the effects that childhood conduct problems, which we saw earlier are commonly associated with adolescent depression, could have on these outcomes. Harrington *et al.* (1991) found that juvenile depression seemed to have little direct impact on social functioning in adulthood once the association with conduct problems was controlled. Similar findings were reported by Renouf et al. (1997) who found that social dysfunction associated with comorbid depression and conduct disorder seemed to be mainly related to the effects of conduct disorder. The implication is that it is important to differentiate the course of depressive disorder from the course of other comorbid disorders.

Depressed young people very commonly have suicidal thoughts and some of them make suicidal attempts (Andrews & Lewinsohn 1992). Lewinsohn et al. (1994c) reported that depression was one of the strongest predictors of a subsequent suicidal attempt, even when the association with other risk factors was controlled. Conversely, it seems that suicidal children are at increased risk of depression. For example, Pfeffer et al. (1991) found that young people who had attempted suicide were 10 times more likely to have a mood disorder during the 6–8-year follow-up period than young people who had not made an attempt.

Three studies have reported increased rates of completed suicide in adolescent patients followed up into adulthood, with a cumulative risk of around 2–4% (Harrington et al. 1990; Rao et al. 1993; Weissman et al. 1999a; Fombonne et al. 2001b). This is around six times higher than in the general population of this age. Several psychological autopsy studies of suicide in young people have found high rates of affective disorders (Brent et al. 1988; Marttunen et al. 1991; Shaffer et al. 1996; Groholt et al. 1998; see also Shaffer & Gutstein, Chapter 33). The association between suicide and depression seems to be particularly strong in females (Marttunen et al. 1995). It is, however, important to note that other problems are also relevant in suicide. Marttunen et al. (1991) found that nearly one-fifth of suicides aged between 13 and 19 years had a conduct disorder, and that one-quarter abused alcohol or drugs.

Recovery

Although follow-up studies suggest that depressive disorders tend to recur, it should be borne in mind that the prospects of recovery from the episode are high. Indeed, the available data suggest that the majority of young people with major depression will recover within 2 years. Kovacs et al. (1984b) reported that the cumulative probability of recovery from major depression by 1 year after onset was 74% and by 2 years was 92%. The median time to recovery was about 28 weeks. This study included many subjects who had previous mental problems and some form of treatment. However, very similar results were reported by Keller et al. (1988) in a retrospective study of recovery from first episode of major depression in young people who had mostly not received treatment, and by Warner et al. (1992) in a study of the children of depressed parents. In a community survey, Garrison et al. (1997) found that only one-fifth of those with major depression at baseline continued to have it at 1 year. Recovery can be quite rapid. Harrington et al. (1998b) found that most cases of major depression following deliberate self-poisoning remitted within 6 weeks.

Patterns of relapse and remission

In summary, adolescent depression is a relapsing and remitting condition. Most adolescents will recover from major depression within a year, but a significant proportion will relapse. Persistence of depression is more likely if symptoms are severe (Pickles et al., 2001) or if the young person experiences persisting adversity (Goodyer et al. 1997b), such as family problems (Birmaher et al. 2000). Depressed adolescents are at risk of a variety of other problems later in life, including poor social functioning and suicide. However, their risk of these outcomes stems at least in part from the conditions that are often associated with depression, such as behavioural problems and drug abuse.

Aetiology

The aetiology of depressive disorders among young people is not understood completely, but the available evidence suggests that the cause is a combination of: (i) predisposing constitutional factors arising from genetic endowment or earlier experience; and (ii) precipitating stressful events. These aetiological factors act through biochemical and psychological processes to produce the depressive syndrome. Once established, the syndrome is often prolonged by maintaining factors.

Predisposing factors

Genetic factors

The offspring of depressed parents are at increased risk of depression, especially in childhood and early adult life (Wickramaratne & Weissman 1998). Many other forms of psychopathology are increased among these children (Wickramaratne & Weissman 1998) and they are also at increased risk of medical problems (Kramer et al. 1998). Prospective longitudinal studies have suggested that these increased risks extend for many years (Hammen 1991; Beardslee et al. 1993a; Weissman et al. 1997). For example, Weissman et al. (1997) evaluated the effects of parental depression on offspring over a 10-year period. High rates of depression, panic disorder and alcoholism were found among the children.

There is evidence that affective disorders in adults have a genetic component. Genetic influences seem strongest for bipolar disorders (McGuffin & Katz 1986), but unipolar major depressions also show significant heritability (Kendler et al. 1995). There have thus far been no large systematic twin or adoption studies of depressive disorder in young people. However, family studies find increased rates of depression among relatives of young probands with depressive disorder (Harrington et al. 1993). Moreover, twin studies suggest modest genetic influences on depressive symptoms in adolescence (Thapar & McGuffin 1994; Eaves et al. 1997), although this has not been replicated in adoption studies (Eley et al. 1998). Twin studies also report that some of the stability in depressive symptoms arises from genetic factors (O'Connor et al. 1998c). The mode of inheritance is uncertain, but genetic effects are likely to act through multiple mechanisms, many of which are indirect (Silberg *et al.* 1999). In some cases it seems that genetic factors act by increasing vulnerability to adverse life events (Silberg *et al.* 2001): an example of gene–environment interaction. In others, genes appear to increase the liability to experience depressing life events, such as falling out with friends, an example of active gene–environment correlation (Silberg *et al.* 1999).

Family environment

It is likely that family environment also plays an important part in predisposing to depression, although the relationship is likely to be bidirectional—children with problems may act as a stressor to the parents (Rutter 1997). Hammen *et al.* (1991) found a close temporal relationship between episodes of depression in children and episodes of depression in the mother. Fergusson *et al.* (1995) reported that maternal depression was only associated with depressive symptoms in adolescent offspring in so far as it was associated with social disadvantage or family adversity. Depression in parents is associated with many problems that could lead to depression in offspring, including impaired child management practices, personality problems, poor marital functioning and hostility towards the child (Goodman & Gotlib 1999). It is possible that the early relationship between the mother and the child partly mediates this association (Murray *et al.* 1999).

Temperament and personality

Genetic influences and family environment may also predispose to depression through the effects they have on the child's temperament and personality. Vulnerability to depression may start early in life (Sigurdsson *et al.* 1999); some temperamental features are associated with depression, particularly emotionality (Goodyer *et al.* 1993a). The child's cognitive or behavioural style, such as a tendency to blame oneself rather than other people, may also increase the risk of depression. Some of these behavioural styles are more common in girls from an early age, and may partly explain why girls are more likely to develop depression than boys (Nolen-Hoeksema & Girgus 1994). A longitudinal study in a community sample of adolescents showed that personality features predicted later development of depressive disorder (Daley *et al.* 1999).

Precipitating factors

Depressive disorders in young people often follow stressful life events (Goodyer *et al.* 1993b), such as parental discord, bullying, and physical, sexual or emotional abuse (Boney-McCoy & Finkelhor 1996; Kaplan *et al.* 1998). However, there is great variation in young people's responses to acute adversity. Most young people who experience such events do not develop mental disorder (Goodyer 1990; Silberg *et al.* 2001). Conversely, a significant minority of depressed young people show no obvious acute precipitant for their episode (Goodyer *et al.* 1993b). Moreover, many stressors are chronic (Rutter, 2000). The adolescent's experiences of adversity over time may therefore be just as important as the precipitants of a single episode (Rueter *et al.* 1999). Indeed, isolated events, such as death of a parent, seem to carry little increased risk of subsequent depression (Harrington & Harrison 1999). Much depends on the context of the event, its meaning for the young person, on what happens before it and, perhaps most importantly, on what happens after it.

Biochemical and psychological processes

Monoamine neurotransmitters

The amine hypothesis proposes that depression arises from hypoactivity in monoamine reward systems. Research has concentrated on two monoamine neurotransmitters: 5-hydroxytryptamine (5-HT) and norepinephrine. The findings have not been very robust, but two lines of evidence support an abnormality of 5-HT in juvenile depression:
1 reduced 5-HT transporter protein in platelets from the blood of children and adolescents with major depression (Salee *et al.* 1998); and
2 the positive response of some young depressed patients to the serotonin-specific reuptake inhibitor, fluoxetine (Emslie *et al.* 1997a).

It will be appreciated, however, that 5-HT metabolism in the blood may be very different from in the brain. Moreover, other drugs that enhance the functioning of 5-HT pathways, such as the tricyclic antidepressants and sertraline, do not seem to be effective antidepressants in young people (Hazell *et al.* 1995; Mandoki *et al.* 1997). Thus, while it is likely that the amine hypothesis will continue to influence biological research, in this age group it is far from proven.

Endocrine abnormalities

Many investigations have examined the links between juvenile depression and endocrine abnormalities that are not associated with obvious endocrine disease. Possible candidate hormones include melatonin (Shafii *et al.* 1996), thyroid hormone (Kutcher *et al.* 1991; Dorn *et al.* 1996), prolactin (Hardan *et al.* 1999), growth hormone (Ryan *et al.* 1994) and cortisol. Interest has focused on cortisol. Several studies have shown that in comparison with non-depressed patients, depressed young people are less likely to show suppression of cortisol secretion when the exogenous corticosteroid dexamethasone is administered (Casat & Powell 1988). There is also evidence that cortisol levels predict the course of juvenile depression. Goodyer *et al.* (1998) found that higher cortisol levels at night predicted persistence of major depression. Susman *et al.* (1997) reported that adolescents who showed increased cortisol levels in a challenging situation had higher levels of depressive symptoms a year later than adolescents whose cortisol did not change or decreased. It could be, then, that cortisol mediates the links between adversity and depression, perhaps through direct effects on some parts of the brain. However, abnormalities of cortisol metabolism are not specific. They are seen in other child psychiatric disorders (Tyrer *et al.* 1991), as well as in stressful situations such as admission to hospital. Their role as an important mechanism in juvenile depression remains to be conclusively demonstrated and the cortisol findings have not as yet had many therapeutic implications.

Cognitive processes

In cognitive theory, depression is not simply triggered by adversity but rather by the perception and processing of adverse events. Research has shown that depressed young people have a variety of cognitive deficits and distortions. They often have low self-esteem and cognitive distortions, such as selectively attending to negative features of an event (McCauley *et al.* 1988; Kendall *et al.* 1990; Hammen 1991). In addition, depressed youngsters are more likely than their non-depressed peers to develop negative attributions. For instance, they tend to attribute the cause of positive events to unstable external causes rather than to their own endeavours (Cole & Turner 1993). Depressed young people also have low perceived academic and social competence (Cole 1990) and this sense of competency predicts subsequent depression (Cole *et al.* 1997).

Although many studies have documented an association between childhood depression and various cognitive distortions, there are many unresolved questions. In particular, it is unclear whether these negative cognitions are a cause or consequence of depression (Harrington *et al.* 1998d). Dalgleish *et al.* (1998) reported that performance on information-processing tasks returned to normal when depression remitted. It is also uncertain whether some cognitive processes are more important than others. Nevertheless, research on cognitive processes in depressed children has provided a useful theoretical basis for planning treatment strategies.

Maintaining factors

Direct persistence of disorder

At first sight, the finding that most cases of major depression remit within a few months (see above) would seem to suggest that direct persistence is uncommon. However, a detailed 12-year prospective study of adults who had presented with major depression found that while only 15% had major depressive disorder during the follow-up, 43% had subthreshold depression (Judd *et al.* 1998). The same may apply to depression in young people; major depression and dysthymia often overlap and one can lead to the other (Kovacs *et al.* 1994). The symptomatic course of depression seems to be malleable, and symptoms of major depression, dysthymia and minor depression alternate over time in the same patients. Direct persistence of subthreshold symptoms is probably quite common.

Scarring or sensitization

Another potential mechanism of continuity is that individuals are changed by their first episode in such a way that they become more likely to have subsequent episodes. This notion, sometimes referred to as 'scarring' has attracted much attention from investigators of the neurobiological (Post & Weiss 1998) and psychological (Rohde *et al.* 1990) processes that may be involved in the relapsing and remitting course of depression in adults. Post *et al.* (Post 1992; Post & Weiss 1998) have suggested that the first depressive episode may sensitize people to further episodes. They hypothesized that such sensitization may help to explain three characteristics of depression in adults: the tendency to recur, the decreasing length of interval between episodes and the greater role of psychosocial stress at the first episode. The idea is that the first episode of depression, which can often be linked to a psychosocial stressor, is associated with long-lasting changes in biology and responsivity to stressors. There may be biochemical and microstructural changes in the central nervous system (such as electrophysiological kindling) that puts the individual at risk of further episodes (Post *et al.* 1996).

The idea of scarring may also be relevant to depression in young people. Lewinsohn *et al.* (1994b) found in cross-sectional comparisons that formerly depressed individuals shared many psychosocial characteristics with depressed individuals. A subsequent prospective study by the same research group identified 45 adolescents who experienced and recovered from a first episode of depression between two assessment points (Rohde *et al.* 1994). Psychosocial scars (characteristics evident after but not before the episode) included excessive emotional reliance on others and subsyndromal depressive symptoms.

Persistence of biological or cognitive vulnerability

Scarring should be distinguished from the concept of vulnerability, in which the predisposition to depression both precedes and follows the acute episode. As noted above, there are many personality, temperamental, biological and cognitive features that could act to increase vulnerability to subsequent episodes. However, the available data suggest that some of these features, such as depressive cognitions (see above), return to normal following apparent recovery from depression.

Persisting adversity

Depressive disorders are also maintained by continuing stressors. Asarnow *et al.* (1993) reported that relapse of depression after discharge from a psychiatric inpatient sample was virtually confined to children who returned to a home environment characterized by high expressed emotion and hostility. Goodyer *et al.* (1997b) found that family dysfunction and lack of a confiding relationship with the mother predicted persistent psychiatric disorder in a sample with major depression. Poor peer relationships are also associated with persistence of depression (Goodyer *et al.* 1997b).

Comorbidity

Several studies have reported that comorbidity with non-depressive disorders predicts a worse outcome for juvenile depressive disorder (Sandford *et al.* 1995; Goodyer *et al.* 1997a; Kovacs *et al.* 1997). Kovacs *et al.* (1997) found that comorbid externalizing disorder predicted a much more protracted recovery from dysthymic disorder. Goodyer *et al.* (1997a) reported that comorbid obsessive-compulsive disorder was associated with persistence of major depression at 36 weeks follow-up.

Multifactorial aetiology

It seems, then, that the onset and persistence of depression are associated with many factors. It is likely that it is the combination of several of these factors that poses the greatest risk. Beardslee *et al.* (1996a) examined risk factors for affective disorder within a random sample of 139 adolescents. Single risk factors, such as parental major depression, parental non-affective diagnosis or a previous child psychiatric diagnosis, increased the risk of subsequent affective disorder from 7 to 18%. However, when all three risk factors were present the risk jumped to 50%.

In some instances, risk factors simply 'add up' to increase the risk of depression; but more often there is some kind of interaction between them. Two common patterns are found. In the first, the one risk factor causes another; Daley *et al.* (1998) found that personality disorder features seemed to generate chronic interpersonal stress, which increased vulnerability to depression. In the second, one risk factor increases vulnerability to another, as when acute life events only lead to depression when the child is made vulnerable by pre-existing relationship problems (Goodyer 1990).

Management of the acute episode

Initial management

The initial management of depressed young people depends greatly on the nature of the problems identified during the assessment procedure. The assessment may indicate that the reaction of the child is appropriate for the situation. In such a case, and if the depression is mild, an early approach can consist of a few sympathetic discussions with the child and the parents, simple measures to reduce stress, and encouraging support. Around one-third of mild or moderately depressed adolescents will remit following this kind of brief non-specific intervention (Harrington *et al.* 1998a).

Cases that persist will require more specific and lengthy forms of treatment. However, the clinician should initially consider a number of issues. The first is whether the depression is severe enough to warrant admission to hospital. Indications for admission of depressed young people include severe suicidality, psy-

chotic symptoms or refusal to eat or drink. A related question is whether the child should remain at school. When the disorder is mild, school can be a valuable distraction from depressive thinking. When the disorder is more severe, symptoms such as poor concentration and motor retardation may add to feelings of hopelessness. It is quite common to find in such cases that ensuring that the child obtains tuition in the home, or perhaps in a sheltered school, improves mood considerably.

The second issue is whether the depression is complicated by other disorders, such as behavioural problems. If it is, then measures to deal with these other problems must be included in the treatment programme. In some cases it is best to try to deal with comorbid problems before embarking on therapy for depression. For instance, it is difficult to conduct psychological therapies for depression when a patient is very underweight because of comorbid anorexia nervosa. In other cases it may be possible to treat the comorbid problem at the same time as the depression.

Managing the social context of depression

The third issue concerns the management of the stresses that are associated with many cases of major depression (Hammen *et al.* 1999). It is sometimes possible to alleviate these stresses. For example, bullying at school may be reduced by a discreet phone-call to the head teacher or other intervention with the school (Olweus 1994). Maternal depression may resolve following treatment with an antidepressant. However, in many cases acute stressors are just one of a number of causes of the adolescent's depression. Moreover, such stressors commonly arise out of chronic difficulties, such as family discord, and may therefore be very hard to remedy. Symptomatic treatments for depression can therefore be helpful even when it is obvious that the depression occurs in the context of chronic adversity that is likely to persist.

Evidence base for psychosocial interventions

Depression is a problem with such pervasive features that one can find abnormalities in almost any domain (e.g. cognitive, interpersonal, familial, psychodynamic) to justify virtually any psychosocial intervention. The interventions reviewed here all have three features in common.

1 They are based on testable theories about the mechanisms of disorder and about how treatment reduces dysfunction.

2 They have been evaluated in randomized trials.

3 They are all relatively brief and therefore capable of implementation in clinical practice.

Table 29.1 summarizes the evidence base for the three psychosocial interventions that meet these criteria.

Cognitive-behaviour therapy

The best studied of the psychological interventions is cognitive-behaviour therapy (see Brent, Chapter 54). Cognitive-

Table 29.1 Psychosocial treatments for adolescent major depression.

Intervention	Strength of recommendation	Quality of evidence	Comments
Cognitive-behaviour therapy	✓✓	B+	Moderate MDD
Interpersonal psychotherapy	✓	B−	
Family therapy	✗✗	B	

Recommendation: ✓✓✓ (good supporting evidence) through ✓✗ (uncertain evidence) to ✗✗✗ (good evidence to reject).
Quality: A (five independent systematic randomized trials with consistent results) through C (systematic open studies) to E (opinion of respected authority).

behavioural treatment (CBT) programmes were developed to address the cognitive distortions and deficits identified in depressed children (see above). Many varieties of CBT exist for childhood depression, but they all have the following common characteristics.

1 The child is the focus of treatment (although most CBT programmes involve parents).
2 The child and therapist collaborate to solve problems.
3 The therapist teaches the child to monitor and keep a record of thoughts and behaviour. There is therefore emphasis on diary-keeping and on homework assignments.
4 Treatment usually combines several different procedures, including behavioural techniques (such as activity scheduling) and cognitive strategies (such as cognitive restructuring).

CBT has been used in both school and clinical settings. There have been at least six randomized controlled studies of CBT in samples of children with depressive symptoms recruited through schools (Reynolds & Coats 1986; Stark *et al.* 1987; Kahn *et al.* 1990; Liddle & Spence 1990; Marcotte & Baron 1993; Weisz *et al.* 1997). The design has usually been to screen for depression with a questionnaire and then to invite those with a high score to a group CBT intervention. In three of the trials CBT was significantly superior to no treatment. Although these results are promising, they may not necessarily apply to cases with depressive disorder. However, a meta-analysis (Harrington *et al.* 1998a) of six randomized trials with clinically diagnosed cases of depressive disorder (Lewinsohn *et al.* 1990; Reed 1994; Vostanis *et al.* 1996b; Wood *et al.* 1996; Brent *et al.* 1997; Clarke *et al.* 1999) found that CBT was significantly superior to comparison conditions, such as remaining on a waiting list or having relaxation training (pooled odds ratio of 2.2).

Interpersonal psychotherapy

Two other psychological treatments have been evaluated in randomized trials with clinically depressed adolescents. Interpersonal psychotherapy (IPT) is based on the premise that depression occurs in the context of interpersonal relationships (Klerman & Weissman 1992). The empirical basis for treating adolescent depression with IPT comes from research showing a strong association between depression and problems with relationships (Goodyer *et al.* 1997b). Like CBT, IPT is a brief time-

limited therapy. The two main goals are to identify and treat, first, depressive symptoms and, secondly, the problems associated with the onset of depression (Moreau *et al.* 1991; Mufson *et al.* 1993). A randomized trial in a very disadvantaged sample has shown significant benefits over non-specific counselling (Mufson *et al.* 1999).

Family interventions

Family interventions are based on the reliable observation that adolescent depression often occurs in the context of family dysfunction (see above). There are widely differing definitions of family therapy, but most therapies have the following features in common (Gorell Barnes 1994).

1 They typically involve face-to-face work with more than one family member.
2 Therapeutic work focuses on altering the interactions among family members.
3 Practitioners think of improvement at two levels: that of the presenting problem and that of the relationship patterns associated with the problem.

Two kinds of work have been undertaken with the families of depressed children. The first, exemplified by the research of Lewinsohn *et al.* (1990) and Clarke *et al.* (1999), consists of parental attendance at a course run in parallel with the child's individual psychological treatment (Lewinsohn *et al.* 1996). The aim of the parents' course is to help them promote the adolescent's learning of new skills. Parents also learn problem-solving and communication skills and adolescents and parents rehearse these skills in joint sessions. The second approach involves conjoint family work. In this approach the primary focus is usually within the treatment sessions, which aim directly to change family communication patterns and methods of solving problems. The therapist may also help the family to see depression from the relational function it could have within the family.

There have been at least four randomized controlled trials of family therapy in adolescent depressive disorder. Two involved a family intervention only (Brent *et al.* 1997; Harrington *et al.* 1998b) and two examined the value of parental sessions given in parallel with individual CBT (Lewinsohn *et al.* 1990; Clarke *et al.* 1999). None has found a significant benefit of the family

Table 29.2 Biological treatments for adolescent major depression.

Intervention	Strength of recommendation	Quality of evidence	Comments
Serotonin-specific reuptake inhibitors	✓	B	Three randomized controlled trials thus far
Tricyclic antidepressants	✗✗	A–	Second line in older adolescents
Venlafaxine	✗✓	B–	One randomized controlled trial to date
Electroconvulsive therapy	✗✓	D	Very severe cases

Recommendation: ✓✓✓ (good supporting evidence) through ✓✗ (uncertain evidence) to ✗✗✗ (good evidence to reject).
Quality: A (five independent, systematic randomized trials with consistent results) through C (systematic open studies) to E (opinion of respected authority).

treatment. However, it would be premature to conclude that family interventions have no place in managing juvenile depression. The association between juvenile depression and family dysfunction is so strong that further studies of family interventions are indicated. None the less, the failure of the early family therapy studies suggests that future research will need to reconsider the target of the intervention. For example, because juvenile depression is often associated with family negativity (Harrington *et al.* 1997), trials of therapies that seek to reduce this negativity are needed. Until there is a firmer empirical basis for family therapy, however, other interventions will be the treatment of choice.

Limitations of psychosocial treatments

Individual focused 'here-and-now' psychological interventions, such as CBT and IPT, are promising treatments for adolescent depression but they have the following limitations.
1 Adolescents with severe depressive disorders respond less well than those with mild or moderately severe conditions (Clarke *et al.* 1992; Brent *et al.* 1998; Jayson *et al.* 1998; Brent *et al.* 1999).
2 Although proponents of psychosocial treatments often claim long-term benefits for the adolescent's psychological development, this has yet to be conclusively demonstrated. Few trials have provided follow-up data for more than a few months, and those that do have not generally found long-term effects (Vostanis *et al.* 1996a; Wood *et al.* 1996; Birmaher *et al.* 2000).
3 It is unclear what psychological processes correlate with a better outcome. The therapeutic basis for change is therefore uncertain.
4 Although both CBT and IPT have been described in detailed manuals (Clarke *et al.* 1990; Mufson *et al.* 1993), few centres offer training for therapists wishing to work with this age group.

Evidence base for biological treatments

Table 29.2 summarizes the evidence base for biological treatments. Most of the research on pharmacotherapy has been with the tricyclic antidepressants (TCAs), especially imipramine and

nortryptyline. The results from early open trials were encouraging. However, with the exception of Preskorn *et al.* (1987), the randomized controlled double-blind trials have found no significant differences between oral tricyclics and placebo (Kramer & Feiguine 1981; Petti & Law 1982; Kashani *et al.* 1984; Puig-Antich *et al.* 1987; Geller *et al.* 1989, 1990; Hughes *et al.* 1990; Kutcher *et al.* 1994; Kye *et al.* 1996; Birmaher *et al.* 1998). A meta-analysis of the tricyclic trials (Hazell *et al.* 1995) found that the pooled response rate was around one-third, less than that generally found when tricyclics are given to depressed adults.

There is evidence that TCAs are an effective treatment for adult depression (Boyce & Judd 1999), raising the question as to the possible explanations of the failure of clinical trials among the young. The first possibility is that the failure is more apparent than real, and stems from some of the methodological issues involved in conducting trials in this age group. Consent must in practice be obtained from two people, and many parents are reluctant to allow their children into a study in which one of the treatments is medication. This may be especially difficult in studies involving TCAs, where regular monitoring of cardiac function is required. The result may have been that particularly severe, and perhaps less responsive, cases of depression have been admitted to the tricyclic trials. There have also been technical problems with some of the trials (Hazell *et al.* 1995), of which perhaps the most striking is their relatively small sample sizes. Significant drug effects within subgroups could easily have been missed. In addition, some trials have had very high response rates in the group given placebo (Puig-Antich *et al.* 1987), making it even more difficult to detect an effect of active drug.

The second set of explanations concern that possibility that juvenile depressions differ from adult depression in ways that make it less likely they will respond to TCAs. There are important differences between pre-adolescent and adult depression in respect of comorbidity and epidemiology (see above). It has also been suggested that young people differ from adults both in the relative balance of the cerebral neurotransmitters on which TCAs are thought to act (Strober *et al.* 1999) and in the hormonal milieu of the brain (Ryan *et al.* 1986). Finally, it could be that it is harder to get drug dosage right in children than it is in adults. There may be developmental variations in the metabolism of TCAs, such as their rate of elimination from the body (Geller 1991).

Two randomized trials have found that SSRIs may be of benefit in children and adolescents with major depression (Emslie *et al.* 1997b; Keller *et al.* 2001). It is too early to say whether this finding is robust—a small trial with fluoxetine produced a negative result (Simeon *et al.* 1990). Nevertheless, it clearly raises the possibility that young people may be more responsive to antidepressants than previously thought, perhaps especially to drugs that act more on serotonergic rather than noradrenergic systems (Ryan & Varma 1998). Negative results have been reported in a trial with the mixed serotonergic/noradrenergic antidepressant venlafaxine (Mandoki *et al.* 1997).

Electroconvulsive therapy (ECT) is very seldom used with adolescents, and then only for the most severe life-threatening depressions that have failed to respond to other treatments. It is usually best to obtain a second opinion from another psychiatrist before ECT is considered (for a review see Walter *et al.* 1999).

Limitations of biological treatments

The main limitation is side-effects. These are potentially severe with the TCAs (see Heyman & Santosh, Chapter 59), which can be cardiotoxic in overdose and which have been linked to sudden cardiac death even in therapeutic doses (Geller *et al.* 1999). SSRIs seem to have fewer side-effects (Ambrosini *et al.* 1999; Strober *et al.* 1999) and, unlike the TCAs, do not usually require specific cardiovascular monitoring (Gutgesell *et al.* 1999). However, symptoms such as dry mouth and gastrointestinal upset can be a problem (Emslie *et al.* 1999) and there has been concern about the so-called 'serotonin syndrome'. This 'syndrome', which is probably better regarded as the extreme end of the continuum of toxicity, is characterized by alterations in cognition, behaviour, autonomic and central nervous system function as a result of increased post-synaptic serotonin receptor agonism (Gillman 1999). Abrupt discontinuation of SSRIs can lead to symptoms such as dizziness, nausea and lethargy (Drug and Therapeutics Bulletin 1999), which may raise parental concerns about 'addiction'.

Another important limitation is that, as with psychosocial treatments, a significant minority fail to respond. It is unclear who is most likely to respond to drugs such as fluoxetine (Kowatch *et al.* 1999). Drug levels are unlikely to be helpful as there is tremendous interindividual variability in the metabolism of SSRIs (Findling *et al.* 1999), as there is with the TCAs.

An evidence-based treatment algorithm for moderate depression

Although the evidence base is not yet as comprehensive as one would wish, it is now possible to construct simple evidence-based algorithms for the management of juvenile depression (Fig. 29.1).

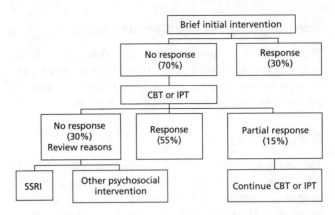

Fig. 29.1 Management of moderately severe depression.

Steps 1 and 2. Moderately severe depression of just a few months' duration remits after a brief intervention in around one-third of cases. This suggests that a sensible initial approach can consist of a thorough assessment, encouraging support and efforts to alleviate any obvious precipitating stressors (see above).

Step 3. The best treatment for persistent major depression in adolescence is not yet firmly established. SSRIs are probably cheaper than psychosocial treatments but their benefits have not yet been established in more than two published trials. This suggests that, if available, either CBT or IPT is probably the first choice treatment for moderate depression (Renaud *et al.* 1999).

Step 4. A meta-analysis (Harrington *et al.* 1998a) of CBT studies found that around one-third of clinically depressed adolescents had not improved by the end of the CBT course. Therefore, patients should be re-assessed after about 6–8 weeks to determine whether there has been a response or not. By this stage, there are likely to be two groups who still need help: those who have failed to respond or are getting worse and those who have partially improved but are still symptomatic. If an adolescent is resistant to the effects of CBT then the reasons for this should be reviewed. It may be that other problems besides depression are present. Review may also indicate some specific reasons for the failure of CBT. For example, CBT is less effective when given by an inexperienced therapist who tells the adolescent what to do (Scott 1998).

Step 5. If the review does not show a simple way of improving the adolescent's mental state, then a different line in treatment should be pursued. In some instances, this means starting an antidepressant, such as an SSRI. In other cases it may be necessary to provide treatments such as family therapy.

Less is known about the management of severe depression. Clinical experience suggests that combination of medication and individual treatment is often necessary. Antidepressants may be augmented with lithium in cases who fail to respond.

Promoting remission and preventing relapse

Young people with depressive disorders are likely to have another episode and so it is important to consider the need for prophylactic treatments. Research with depressed adults distinguishes between continuation and maintenance treatments.

Continuation treatments

The idea behind continuation treatments is that although treatment may suppress the acute symptoms of depression, the treatment should continue until the hypothesized underlying episode has finished. There have been no randomized trials of continuation treatments for juvenile depressive disorders. However, data from a non-randomized trial with depressed adolescents suggest that continuing psychological treatment for 6 months after remission is feasible and may be effective in preventing relapse (Kroll *et al.* 1996). The treatment given during the acute episode of adolescent depression should therefore be continued until the patient has been free of depression for around 6 months.

Maintenance treatments

Maintenance treatments have a different objective, which is to prevent the development of a new episode of depression. Research with adult patients suggests that both pharmacotherapy and psychotherapy may reduce the risk of relapse if maintained for several years after the index depressive episode (Frank *et al.* 1992; Kupfer 1992). Clearly, such treatments will be very time-consuming and expensive. They cannot therefore be contemplated for more than a small minority of patients. Clinical experience suggests that indications for maintenance treatment in depressed young people include a history of highly recurrent depressive disorder, severely handicapping episodes of depression and chronic major depression (for a review of maintenance treatments with adults see Keller (1999)).

Possibilities of primary prevention

The case for primary prevention

There is a strong case, at least in theory, for preventing depression in young people (Harrington & Clark 1998). Although the evidence reviewed earlier suggests that some effective psychological treatments are available, many patients fail to respond. Moreover, only a minority of depressed youngsters ever come to clinical services (Oldehinkel *et al.* 1999), possibly because parents perceive greater need for mental health services for children with disruptive disorders than for those with depression (Wu *et al.* 1999).

Strategies for primary prevention

There has been a great deal of work on general strategies for preventing child psychiatric disorders (Durlak & Wells 1997) and some of these strategies could be effective in preventing depression (e.g. reducing bullying in classrooms, improving access to special education, and maternal befriending). As many of these interventions are discussed in other parts of this book, the present section only deals with strategies in which reducing depression in young people is an important potential outcome.

It is customary to distinguish between two types of primary preventive strategy. *Universal programmes* involve all individuals in a population regardless of their level of risk. Typically, such programmes involve either attempts to change levels of depression directly (Clarke *et al.* 1993) or efforts to develop strengths that might protect against depression (King & Kirschenbaum 1990). The latter have usually consisted of educational sessions and cognitive-behavioural techniques, particularly techniques to develop social skills.

Targeted programmes aim to prevent depression in a population known to be at risk. The best-established risk factors for depressive disorder in young people are earlier depressive symptoms or a family history of depression (Harrington & Vostanis 1995). Treatments for depressive symptoms are described above. The rationale behind family interventions is that improving problems such as parenting difficulties or maternal depression should reduce the risk of depression among offspring. Preventive family interventions have been devised both for the depressed mothers of young infants (Cooper & Murray 1997) and for the families of older children in which at least one parent has an affective disorder (Beardslee *et al.* 1993b). Interventions for depressed mothers have targeted maternal depression alone (Cooper & Murray 1997), toddler–parent attachment (Cicchetti *et al.* 2000), deficits in maternal social support (Brugha *et al.* 1999) and mother–infant interactions (Field 1997).

Effectiveness of universal prevention programmes

Clarke *et al.* (1993) have conducted two randomized trials of universal interventions designed to reduce depressive symptoms in the general population of children, regardless of their levels of depression. Neither has shown significant benefits.

Effectiveness of targeting young people with high levels of depression

Interventions that target individuals with high levels of depressive symptoms have produced more promising results. King & Kirschenbaum (1990) studied primary school children with a high score on a screening questionnaire. They found that a programme of social skills training and consultation with parents and teachers was significantly better than consultation alone in reducing depressive symptoms. Clarke *et al.* (1995) randomly allocated schoolchildren with a high score on a depression questionnaire to CBT or to no treatment. The CBT group had a significantly reduced risk of depressive disorder during the following year.

Effectiveness of targeting family risk factors

There is evidence from randomized trials that some (Wickberg & Hwang 1996; Cooper & Murray 1997), but not all (Brugha *et al.* 1999), forms of brief psychological treatment are effective in reducing depression in postpartum women. Antidepressant medication also appears to be beneficial (Appelby *et al.* 1997). Nevertheless, it seems that treatment of maternal depression does not necessarily improve the infant's outcome. Cooper & Murray (1997) found no significant benefits for the parent–infant relationship, even though maternal depression had improved considerably. Similar findings were reported by Gelfand *et al.* (1996) in a non-randomized design. However, intensive interventions that help depressed mothers to parent more effectively may lead to better infant outcomes (Field 1997; Cicchetti *et al.* 2000). It remains to be seen whether these interventions will prevent depression in these infants as they grow up.

Several randomized studies have examined the efficacy of intervening with the families of older children at risk for depression. In a study of bereaved families, Sandler *et al.* (1992) found that a programme of help for the whole family reduced depressive symptoms in the child. Beardslee *et al.* (1993b, 1996b) conducted a randomized trial with families in which at least one parent had an affective disorder. They compared a clinician-facilitated educational preventive programme with a lecture group. No data are yet available on rates of depressive disorders in the offspring but early findings indicate that there are useful changes in the family's knowledge about depression and in intrafamilial communication.

Conclusions on effectiveness of prevention strategies

In summary, the preliminary evidence suggests that universal programmes that aim to reduce depression across the whole population may not be effective. Universal programmes have a number of advantages over targeted interventions (Graham 1994) but it may be better for such programmes to concentrate on increasing factors that could protect against depression (Clarke *et al.* 1993).

Targeted interventions seem more promising, particularly those that focus on youngsters with high levels of depressive symptoms. A strength of these studies is that preventive programmes have huge potential to reduce the burden of suffering arising from depression. A challenge for targeted approaches is to increase the proportion of individuals who are willing to take part. The uptake of psychological treatments offered to individuals identified as at risk has often been low (Harrington *et al.* 1998c). Future studies must also pay greater attention to the possible harmful effects that might result from targeting at risk children or their parents for treatment (Harrington & Clark 1998).

Other affective disorders

Bipolar disorder

Classification and clinical features

Bipolar disorder is characterized by the combination of depressive disorder and distinct episodes of manic disorder. By convention, all patients with mania are classified in the bipolar group, whether or not they have had depression. The central features of mania are elation or irritability, increased activity and self-important ideas. When mania is *severe* there may be grandiose delusions, hallucinations and frenzied overactivity. When mania is moderate there is sustained overactivity and pressure of speech, euphoric mood and inflated self-esteem. In mild forms of mania (*hypomania*) there is some elevated mood, increased sociability and excessive involvement in pleasurable activities.

Diagnostic uncertainties

The concept of bipolar disorder in adult life has received substantial validation, but the same cannot be said for the concept of bipolar disorder among the young. There has been particular concern about the validity of the concept of mania in pre-adolescent children.

Until relatively recently, typical 'adult-like' manic states were widely regarded as extremely uncommon among prepubertal children. However, several investigations have identified substantial numbers of children with symptoms similar to mania. Wozniak *et al.* (1995) found 43 children aged 12 years or younger who met DSM criteria for mania. Geller *et al.* (1994) found that bipolarity developed in 25 of 79 children with major depression, the majority of whom were prepubertal.

Attempts to validate these mania-like states are necessarily at an early stage, but there are at least five reasons for doubting the links between prepubertal 'mania' and mania in adulthood.

1 Although the diagnosis of mania in young people should be based on the same criteria as adults (American Academy of Child and Adolescent Psychiatry 1997), some studies seem to have applied the criteria differently (Klein *et al.* 1998). For instance, mania in adults is usually a relapsing and remitting condition, yet studies of prepubertal mania find that it is often chronic without distinct manic episodes (Geller & Luby 1997).

2 There is huge overlap between the criteria for mania and those for attention deficit disorder. Core symptoms of both conditions include reduced attention, racing thoughts, distractibility, motor overactivity and impulsive behaviour. Both are also strongly associated with irritability. Indeed, around one-half of adolescents diagnosed with bipolar disorder also meet the criteria for attention deficit hyperactivity disorder (West *et al.* 1995). There must be concern that the two are being confused.

3 All epidemiological studies find that mania is very rare or non-existent in pre-adolescent children. For example, in the Smoky Mountain study in the USA (Costello *et al.* 1996) and in the Office of National Statistics survey in the UK (Meltzer *et al.* 2000) no cases of mania were found.

4 In contrast to the study of Geller *et al.* (1994), most other longitudinal studies find that among children the rate of conversion from major depression to mania is very low (Harrington *et al.* 1990; Weissman *et al.* 1999b; Fombonne *et al.* 2001a). Conversely, studies of children diagnosed with attention deficit disorder do not generally find increased risks of bipolar disorder in adult life.

5 Studies of the school-aged children of parents with bipolar disorder (Hammen *et al.* 1990; Radke-Yarrow *et al.* 1992) do not report cases of mania.

Differential diagnosis

Mild forms of mania are easily confused with problems such as conduct disorder and attention deficit disorder (Kovacs & Pollock 1995). Severe psychotic manic states can be difficult to distinguish from schizophrenia (Carlson *et al.* 1994). Manic symptoms can also occur when susceptible subjects have been prescribed antidepressants (Briscoe *et al.* 1995).

Epidemiology and aetiology

Severe 'typical' bipolar disorder appears to be uncommon in adolescence. In the first two waves of the Oregon study only 2 of the 1500 adolescents who were evaluated met full diagnostic criteria for bipolar disorder (Lewinsohn & Klein 1995). Nevertheless, bipolar disorder may be on the increase. Possible explanations include the genetic process of anticipation, more sensitive diagnostic methods and substance or alcohol abuse (Goodwin & Ghaemi 1998).

Little is known about the aetiology of juvenile bipolar disorder. There have been no large genetically informative studies of bipolar disorders in young people. However, there is no reason for thinking that juvenile bipolar disorder is any less genetic than it seems to be in adults. Adolescent bipolar disorder is familial (Strober *et al.* 1988) and shows a distribution of affective illness in relatives that is compatible with genetic factors (Todd *et al.* 1996).

Course

Bipolar disorders that occur in adolescence tend to follow the remitting and relapsing course of adult cases. Strober *et al.* (1995) followed up 54 consecutive admissions of adolescents with bipolar illness to a university inpatient service. At the time of admission, 20 were manic and the remainder depressed or in mixed states. Nearly 50% of the sample had a relapse during the 5-year follow-up. However, the prognosis of early onset bipolar disorder is probably better than of early onset schizophrenia (Werry *et al.* 1991). A small proportion of adolescent patients who present with depression will go on to develop mania. Strober *et al.* (1993) found that 5 out of 58 adolescents with major depression developed manic or hypomanic episodes during the 24-month follow-up period. Many of these cases had psychotic features during their depressive episode. Other predictors of outcome include premorbid personality (Werry & McClellan 1992) and family history. Milder forms of bipolar disorder in adolescents also show moderate short-term stability (Lewinsohn & Klein 1995) and may be a manifestation of a temperamental vulnerability to typical manic depression (Akiskal 1995).

Treatment

In adults, lithium has been shown to be effective for both the prevention of manic and depressive episodes and the treatment of the acute episode of depression or mania. Much less is known about its use in children or adolescents but there is some evidence it is effective (Geller *et al.* 1998). As in adults, the lithium range for the acute phase should range from 0.6 to 1.2 mEq/L, with somewhat lower levels for effective prophylaxis (American Academy of Child and Adolescent Psychiatry 1997). Lithium has some significant side-effects, including hypothyroidism and neurological symptoms. Anticonvulsants may also be used in the treatment and prophylaxis of bipolar disorder among the young, perhaps especially when it is rapid cycling (Ryan *et al.* 1999).

Seasonal affective disorder

Retrospective studies suggest that adolescents report high rates of seasonal variation in affective symptoms such as energy level and mood (Sourander *et al.* 1999). Seasonal affective disorder (SAD) is characterized by depressions that occur at certain times of the year. Most often, the episodes begin in autumn or winter and remit in spring. Prominent symptoms include loss of energy, sleep disturbance and craving for carbohydrates. Carskadon & Acebo (1993) estimated a 3–5% prevalence for seasonal depression among children. Giedd *et al.* (1998) followed up six children (aged from 6 to 17 years) with a diagnosis of SAD. Subjects were followed for 7 years and outcomes were assessed using standardized methods. All subjects had persistent seasonal symptoms, which remained relatively severe. However, in most light therapy was of some benefit.

Future challenges

The past decade has seen important advances in research into the epidemiology, aetiology and treatment of depressive disorders among the young. We are beginning to understand how risk factors combine to precipitate and maintain depression. Progress has also been made in the development of effective treatments. This concluding section will consider some of the challenges that remain.

Methods

There are several outstanding methodological issues. First, better measures are needed of psychosocial risk factors for depression. Up to now, most of the research on juvenile depressive disorder has focused on acute life events. However, it is becoming clear that many cases of depression are recurrent and so we need to know how psychosocial factors contribute to long-term liability. This will mean developing measures that are better able to assess long-term psychosocial problems. Secondly, there is a need for greater use of intensive longitudinal designs that measure depression and its risk factors over several time-points. Much of what is currently known about the course of juvenile depression comes from studies with just a single follow-up. This makes it difficult to study covariation of depression and its risk factors over time.

How do genes and environment combine to produce depression?

Although many important predisposing factors for adolescent depressive disorder are familial (see above), it is still not clear how far this association is a reflection of genes, environment or both. At first sight, then, it seems obvious that the next step should be large genetically informative studies of samples with depressive disorder. Such studies could be useful. However, the data from studies carried out thus far indicate that genetic effects on depression are often indirect; they seem to operate more by making it likely that young people will experience risk environments, or be susceptible to such environments, than by direct effects on depression itself (Silberg *et al.* 1999). The implication is that further genetic studies should be concerned as much with factors that predispose to depression, such as personality dimensions, as with depression *per se*.

How can depression be prevented?

Identification of the complex gene–environment pathways leading to juvenile depression also has implications for preventive programmes. Much of the psychopathological risk to the children of depressed mothers seems to stem from factors other than maternal depression, such as chronic parenting problems. Future preventive studies probably need to target these factors at least as much as they do parental depression.

How should established depression be treated?

For the foreseeable future, however, it will not be possible to prevent more than a small number of cases of juvenile depression. Many challenges remain in the development of effective treatments for established depressive disorders, of which four stand out.

1 Although several promising treatments have been developed for the acute episode, we know very little about their relative demerits and merits. A key question for future research is how individual psychological treatments compare with the SSRIs.

2 There needs to be greater appreciation of the limitations of current designs for clinical practice. Much extant research has been based on selected samples of cases with only moderately severe depression and without the comorbid problems that often complicate the cases that are seen in everyday practice. 'Pragmatic' studies (Hotopf *et al.* 1999) with large samples of the kinds of patients who present in routine clinical practice are also required. In particular, information is needed on the efficacy of treatments within severely impaired samples.

3 There needs to be a continuation of efforts to develop and test the kinds of clinical algorithms described earlier. Treatment researchers have, up to now, tended to conceptualize an intervention as just one treatment modality given for a short time. This strategy has been a necessary first step in the development of coherent theory-driven interventions. The complexity of factors that precipitate and maintain juvenile depression suggests, however, that it is unlikely that any single treatment will be effective in all cases. 'Treatment' in research studies needs to be conceptualized more often as a programme of interventions used singly or in combination that will often follow one after the other, depending on the likely causes of the young person's problems and response to treatment.

4 There has been little attention so far to ways of preventing relapse or other complications, such as suicidal behaviour. Perhaps the most daunting challenge for the future will be to develop better ways of identifying and helping the significant minority of depressed young people in whom their first episode of depression presages further serious psychopathology.

References

Ablow, J.C., Measelle, J.R., Kraemer, H.C. *et al.* (1999) The MacArthur three city outcome study: evaluating multi-informant measures of young children's symptomatology. *Journal of the American Academy of Child and Adolescent Psychiatry*, 38, 1580–1590.

Akiskal, H.S. (1995) Developmental pathways to bipolarity: are juvenile-onset depression pre-bipolar? *Journal of the American Academy of Child and Adolescent Psychiatry*, 34, 754–763.

Alpert, J.E., Fava, M., Uebelacker, L.A. *et al.* (1999) Patterns of axis I comorbidity in early-onset versus late-onset major depressive disorder. *Biological Psychiatry*, 46, 202–211.

Ambrosini, P.J., Wagner, K.D., Biederman, J. *et al.* (1999) Multicenter open-label sertraline study in adolescent outpatients with major depression. *Journal of the American Academy of Child and Adolescent Psychiatry*, 38, 566–572.

American Academy of Child and Adolescent Psychiatry (1997) Practice parameters for the assessment and treatment of children and adolescents with bipolar disorder. *Journal of the American Academy of Child and Adolescent Psychiatry*, 36, 138–157.

American Psychiatric Association (1980) *Diagnostic and Statistical Manual of Mental Disorders (DSM-III)*, 3rd edn. American Psychiatric Association, Washington D.C.

American Psychiatric Association (1987) *Diagnostic and Statistical Manual of Mental Disorders (DSM-III-R)*, revised 3rd edn. American Psychiatric Association, Washington D.C.

American Psychiatric Association (1994) *Diagnostic and Statistical Manual of Mental Disorders (DSM-IV)*, 4th edn. American Psychiatric Association, Washington D.C.

Andrews, J.A. & Lewinsohn, P.M. (1992) Suicidal attempts among older adolescents: prevalence and co-occurrence with psychiatric disorders. *Journal of the American Academy of Child and Adolescent Psychiatry*, 31, 655–662.

Angold, A. & Costello, E.J. (1995) A test–retest reliability study of child-reported psychiatric symptoms and diagnoses using the Child and Adolescent Psychiatric Assessment (CAPA-C). *Psychological Medicine*, 25, 755–762.

Angold, A., Costello, E.J., Messer, S.C., Pickles, A., Winder, F. & Silver, D. (1995a) The development of a short questionnaire for use in epidemiological studies of depression in children and adolescents. *International Journal of Methods in Psychiatric Research*, 5, 237–249.

Angold, A., Prendergast, M., Cox, A., Rutter, M. & Harrington, R. (1995b) The Child and Adolescent Psychiatric Assessment (CAPA). *Psychological Medicine*, 25, 739–753.

Angold, A., Costello, E.J. & Worthman, C.M. (1998) Puberty and depression: the roles of age, pubertal status and pubertal timing. *Psychological Medicine*, 28, 51–61.

Angold, A., Costello, E.J. & Erkanli, A. (1999a) Comorbidity. *Journal of Child Psychology and Psychiatry*, 40, 57–87.

Angold, A., Costello, E.J., Erkanli, A. & Worthman, C.M. (1999b) Pubertal changes in hormone levels and depression in girls. *Psychological Medicine*, 29, 1043–1053.

Angold, A., Costello, E.J., Farmer, E.M.Z., Burns, B.J. & Erkanli, A. (1999c) Impaired but undiagnosed. *Journal of the American Academy of Child and Adolescent Psychiatry*, 38, 129–137.

Angst, J., Merikangas, K.R. & Preisig, M. (1997) Subthreshold syndromes of depression and anxiety in the community. *Journal of Clinical Psychiatry*, 58, 6–10.

Appleby, L., Warner, R., Whitton, A. & Faragher, B. (1997) A controlled study of fluoxetine and cognitive-behavioural counselling in the treatment of postnatal depression. *British Medical Journal*, 31, 932–936.

Asarnow, J.R., Goldstein, M.J., Tompson, M. & Guthrie, D. (1993) One-year outcomes of depressive disorders in child psychiatric inpatients: evaluation of the prognostic power of a brief measure of expressed emotion. *Journal of Child Psychology and Psychiatry*, 34, 129–137.

Beardslee, W.R., Keller, M.B., Lavori, P.W., Staley, J. & Sacks, N. (1993a) The impact of parental affective disorder on depression in offspring: a longitudinal follow-up in a nonreferred sample. *Journal of the American Academy of Child and Adolescent Psychiatry*, 32, 723–730.

Beardslee, W.R., Salt, P., Porterfield, K. *et al.* (1993b) Comparison of preventive interventions for families with parental affective disorder. *Journal of the American Academy of Child and Adolescent Psychiatry*, 32, 254–263.

Beardslee, W.R., Keller, M.B., Seifer, R. *et al.* (1996a) Prediction of adolescent affective disorder: effects of prior parental affective disorders and child psychopathology. *Journal of the American Academy of Child and Adolescent Psychiatry*, 35, 279–288.

Beardslee, W.R., Wright, E., Rothberg, P.C., Salt, P. & Versage, E. (1996b) Response of families to two preventive intervention strategies: long-term differences in behavior and attitude change. *Journal of the American Academy of Child and Adolescent Psychiatry*, 35, 774–782.

Beck, A.T. (1967) *Depression: Clinical, Experimental and Theoretical Aspects*. Harper & Row, New York.

Birmaher, B., Waterman, G.S., Ryan, N.D. *et al.* (1998) Randomized, controlled trial of amitriptyline vs. placebo for adolescents with 'treatment resistant' major depression. *Journal of the American Academy of Child and Adolescent Psychiatry*, 37, 527–535.

Birmaher, B., Brent, D., Kolko, D. *et al.* (2000) Clinical outcome after short-term psychotherapy for adolescents with major depressive disorder. *Archives of General Psychiatry*, 57, 29–36.

Boney-McCoy, S. & Finkelhor, D. (1996) Is youth victimization related to trauma symptoms and depression after controlling for prior symptoms and family relationships? A longitudinal, prospective study. *Journal of Consulting and Clinical Psychology*, 64, 1406–1416.

Boyce, P. & Judd, F. (1999) The place for the tricyclic antidepressants in the treatment of depression. *Australian and New Zealand Journal of Psychiatry*, 33, 323–327.

Brent, D.A., Perper, J.A., Goldstein, C.E. *et al.* (1988) Risk factors for adolescent suicide: a comparison of adolescent suicide victims with suicidal inpatients. *Archives of General Psychiatry*, 45, 581–588.

Brent, D., Holder, D., Kolko, D. *et al.* (1997) A clinical psychotherapy trial for adolescent depression comparing cognitive, family, and supportive treatments. *Archives of General Psychiatry*, 54, 877–885.

Brent, D.A., Kolko, D.J., Birmaher, B. *et al.* (1998) Predictors of treatment efficacy in a clinical trial of three psychosocial treatments for adolescent depression. *Journal of the American Academy of Child and Adolescent Psychiatry*, 37, 906–914.

Brent, D.A., Kolko, D.J., Birmaher, B., Baugher, M. & Bridge, J. (1999) A clinical trial for adolescent depression: predictors of additional treatment in the acute and follow-up phases of the trial. *Journal of the American Academy of Child and Adolescent Psychiatry*, 38, 263–270.

Breton, J.J., Bergeron, L., Valla, J.P. *et al.* (1999) Quebec child mental health survey: prevalence of DSM-III-R mental health. *Journal of Child Psychology and Psychiatry*, 40, 375–384.

Briscoe, J.J.D., Harrington, R.C. & Prendergast, M. (1995) Development of mania in close association with tricyclic antidepressant administration in children: a report of two cases. *European Child and Adolescent Psychiatry*, 4, 280–283.

Brugha, T., Wheatley, S.L., Shapiro, D. *et al.* (1999) *One year mental health outcomes of a randomised trial of antenatal preventative psychosocial intervention. Final report to the NHS Executive.* Department of Psychiatry, University of Leicester, Leicester.

Carlson, G.A., Fennig, S. & Bromet, E.J. (1994) The confusion between bipolar disorder and schizophrenia in youth: where does it stand in the 1990s? *Journal of the American Academy of Child and Adolescent Psychiatry*, 33, 453–460.

Caron, C. & Rutter, M. (1991) Comorbidity in child psychopathology: concepts, issues and research strategies. *Journal of Child Psychology and Psychiatry*, 32, 1063–1080.

Carskadon, M.A. & Acebo, C. (1993) Parental reports of seasonal mood and behavior changes in children. *Journal of the American Academy of Child and Adolescent Psychiatry*, 32, 264–269.

Casat, C.D. & Powell, K. (1988) The dexamethasone suppression test in children and adolescents with major depressive disorder: a review. *Journal of Clinical Psychiatry*, 49, 390–393.

Cicchetti, D., Rogosch, F.A. & Toth, S.L. (2000) The efficacy of toddler–parent psychotherapy for fostering cognitive development in offspring of depressed mothers. *Journal of Abnormal Child Psychology*, 28, 135–148.

Clark, A. & Harrington, R.C. (1999) On diagnosing rare disorders rarely: appropriate use of screening instruments. *Journal of Child Psychology and Psychiatry*, 40, 287–290.

Clarke, G., Lewinsohn, P. & Hops, H. (1990) *Leaders Manual for Adolescent Groups: Adolescent Coping with Depression Course.* Castalia, Eugene, OR.

Clarke, G.N., Hops, H., Lewinsohn, P.M., Andrews, J.A., Seeley, J.R. & Williams, J.A. (1992) Cognitive-behavioral group treatment of adolescent depression: prediction of outcome. *Behavior Therapy*, **23**, 341–354.

Clarke, G.N., Hawkins, W., Murphy, M. & Sheeber, L. (1993) School-based primary prevention of depressive symptomatology in adolescents: findings from two studies. *Journal of Adolescent Research*, **8**, 183–204.

Clarke, G.N., Hawkins, W., Murphy, M., Sheeber, L.B., Lewinsohn, P.M. & Seeley, J.R. (1995) Targeted prevention of unipolar depressive disorder in an at-risk sample of high school adolescents: a randomized trial of a group cognitive intervention. *Journal of the American Academy of Child and Adolescent Psychiatry*, **34**, 312–321.

Clarke, G.N., Rohde, P., Lewinsohn, P.M., Hops, H. & Seeley, J.R. (1999) Cognitive-behavioural treatment of adolescent depression: efficacy of acute group treatment and booster sessions. *Journal of the American Academy of Child and Adolescent Psychiatry*, **38**, 272–279.

Cohen, P., Cohen, J., Kasen, S. *et al.* (1993a) An epidemiological study of disorders in late childhood and adolescence. I. Age- and gender-specific prevalence. *Journal of Child Psychology and Psychiatry*, **34**, 851–867.

Cohen, P., Cohen, J. & Brook, J. (1993b) An epidemiological study of disorders in late childhood and adolescence. II. Persistence of disorders. *Journal of Child Psychology and Psychiatry*, **34**, 869–877.

Cole, D.A. (1990) Relation of social and academic competence to depressive symptoms in childhood. *Journal of Abnormal Psychology*, **99**, 422–429.

Cole, D.A. & Turner, J.E. (1993) Models of cognitive mediation and moderation in child depression. *Journal of Abnormal Psychology*, **102**, 271–281.

Cole, D.A., Martin, J.M. & Powers, B. (1997) A competency-based model of child depression: a longitudinal study of peer, parent, teacher, and self-evaluations. *Journal of Child Psychology and Psychiatry*, **38**, 505–514.

Cooper, P.J. & Murray, L. (1997) The impact of psychological treatments of postpartum depression on maternal mood and infant development. In: *Postpartum Depression and Child Development* (eds L. Murray & P.J. Copper), pp. 201–220. Guilford, New York.

Costello, E.J. & Angold, A. (1988) Scales to assess child and adolescent depression: checklists, screens and nets. *Journal of the American Academy of Child and Adolescent Psychiatry*, **27**, 726–737.

Costello, E.J., Angold, A., Burns, B.J. *et al.* (1996) The Great Smoky Mountains Study of Youth: goals, design, methods, and the prevalence of DSM-III-R disorders. *Archives of General Psychiatry*, **53**, 1129–1136.

Cyranowski, J.M., Frank, E., Young, E. & Shear, K. (2000) Adolescent onset of the gender difference in lifetime rates of major depression. *Archives of General Psychiatry*, **57**, 21–27.

Daley, S.E., Hammen, C., Davila, J. & Burge, D. (1998) Axis II symptomatology, depression, and life stress during the transition from adolescence to adulthood. *Journal of Consulting and Clinical Psychology*, **66**, 595–603.

Daley, S.E., Hammen, C., Burge, D. *et al.* (1999) Depression and axis II symptomatology in an adolescent community sample: concurrent and longitudinal associations. *Journal of Personality Disorders*, **13**, 47–59.

Dalgleish, T., Neshat-Doost, H., Taghavi, R. *et al.* (1998) Information processing in recovered depressed children and adolescents. *Journal of Child Psychology and Psychiatry*, **39**, 1031–1035.

Dorn, L.D., Burgess, E.S., Dichek, H.L., Putnam, F.W., Chrousos, G.P. & Gold, P.W. (1996) Thyroid hormone concentrations in depressed and nondepressed adolescent: group differences and behavioral relations. *Journal of the American Academy of Child and Adolescent Psychiatry*, **35**, 299–306.

Drug and Therapeutics Bulletin (1999) Withdrawing patients from antidepressants. *Drug and Therapeutics Bulletin*, **37**, 49–52.

Durlak, J.A. & Wells, A.M. (1997) Primary prevention mental health programs for children and adolescents: a meta-analytic review. *American Journal of Community Psychology*, **25**, 115–152.

Eaves, L.J., Silberg, J.L., Meyer, J.M. *et al.* (1997) Genetics and developmental psychopathology. II. The main effects of genes and environment on behavioral problems in the Virginia Twin Study of adolescent behavioral development. *Journal of Child Psychology and Psychiatry*, **38**, 965–980.

Eley, T.C. & Stevenson, J. (1999) Exploring the covariation between anxiety and depression symptoms: a genetic analysis of the effects of age and sex. *Journal of Child Psychology and Psychiatry*, **40**, 1273–1282.

Eley, T.C., Deater-Deckard, K., Fombonne, E., Fulker, D.W. & Plomin, R. (1998) An adoption study of depressive symptoms in middle childhood. *Journal of Child Psychology and Psychiatry*, **39**, 337–345.

Emslie, G., Rush, A., Weinberg, W. *et al.* (1997a) A double-blind, randomized placebo-controlled trial of fluoxetine in depressed children and adolescents. *Archives of General Psychiatry*, **54**, 1031–1037.

Emslie, G.J., Rush, J.A., Weinberg, W.A., Gullion, C.M., Rintelmann, J. & Hughes, C.W. (1997b) Recurrence of major depressive disorder in hospitalized children and adolescents. *Journal of the American Academy of Child and Adolescent Psychiatry*, **36**, 785–792.

Emslie, G.J., Walkup, J.T., Pliszka, S.R. & Ernst, M. (1999) Nontricyclic antidepressants: current trends in children and adolescents. *Journal of the American Academy of Child and Adolescent Psychiatry*, **38**, 517–528.

Fergusson, D.M., Horwood, L.J. & Lynskey, M.T. (1995) Maternal depressive symptoms and depressive symptoms in adolescents. *Journal of Child Psychology and Psychiatry*, **36**, 1161–1178.

Fergusson, D.M., Lynskey, M.T. & Horwood, L.J. (1996) Origins of comorbidity between conduct and affective disorders. *Journal of the American Academy of Child and Adolescent Psychiatry*, **35**, 451–460.

Field, T. (1997) The treatment of depressed mothers and their infants. In: *Postpartum Depression and Child Development* (eds L. Murray & P.J. Cooper), pp. 221–236. Guilford, New York.

Findling, R.L., Reed, M.D., Myers, C. *et al.* (1999) Paroxetine pharmacokinetics in depressed children and adolescents. *Journal of the American Academy of Child and Adolescent Psychiatry*, **38**, 952–959.

Fleming, J.E., Offord, D.R. & Boyle, M.H. (1989) Prevalence of childhood and adolescent depression in the community: Ontario Child Health Study. *British Journal of Psychiatry*, **155**, 647–654.

Fleming, J.E., Boyle, M.H. & Offord, D.R. (1993) The outcome of adolescent depression in the Ontario Child Health Study. *Journal of the American Academy of Child and Adolescent Psychiatry*, **32**, 28–33.

Fombonne, E. (1995) Depressive disorders: time trends and putative explanatory mechanisms. In: *Psychosocial Disorders in Young People: Time Trends and Their Causes* (eds M. Rutter & D. Smith), pp. 544–615. Wiley, Chichester.

Fombonne, E. (1999) Time trends in affective disorders. In: *Historical and Geographical Influences on Psychopathology* (eds P. Cohen, C. Slomkoski & L.N. Robins), pp. 115–139. Lawrence Erlbaum, NJ.

Fombonne, E., Wostear, G., Cooper, V., Harrington, R. & Rutter, M. (2001a) The Maudesly long-term follow-up of child and adolescent depression: I. Psychiatric outcomes in adulthood. *British Journal of Psychiatry*, **179**, 210–217.

Fombonne E., Wostear G., Cooper V., Harrington R. & Rutter M. (2001b) The Maudsley long-term follow-up of child and adolescent depression: II. Suicidality, criminality and social dysfunction in adulthood. *British Journal of Psychiatry*, **179**, 218–223.

Frank, E., Kupfer, D.J., Hamer, T., Grochocinski, V.J. & McEachran, A.B. (1992) Maintenance treatment and psychobiologic correlates of endogenous subtypes. *Journal of Affective Disorders*, 25, 181–190.

Garber, J., Kriss, M.R., Koch, M. & Lindholm, L. (1988) Recurrent depression in adolescents: a follow-up study. *Journal of the American Academy of Child and Adolescent Psychiatry*, 27, 49–54.

Garrison, C.Z., Waller, J.L., Cuffe, S.P., McKeown, R.E., Addy, C.L. & Jackson, K.L. (1997) Incidence of major depressive disorder and dysthymia in young adolescents. *Journal of the American Academy of Child and Adolescent Psychiatry*, 36, 458–465.

Gelfand, D.M., Teti, D.M., Seiner, S.A. & Jameson, P.B. (1996) Helping mothers fight depression: evaluation of a home-based intervention program for depressed mothers and their infants. *Journal of Clinical Psychology*, 25, 406–422.

Geller, B. (1991) Psychopharmacology of children and adolescents: pharmacokinetics and relationships of plasma/serum levels to response. *Psychopharmacology Bulletin*, 27, 401–409.

Geller, B. & Luby, J. (1997) Child and adolescent bipolar disorder: a review of the past 10 years. *Journal of the American Academy of Child and Adolescent Psychiatry*, 36, 1168–1176.

Geller, B., Cooper, T., McCombs, H., Graham, D. & Wells, J. (1989) Double-blind placebo-controlled study of nortriptyline in depressed children using a 'fixed plasma level' design. *Psychopharmacology Bulletin*, 25, 101–108.

Geller, B., Cooper, T.B., Graham, D.L., Marsteller, F.A. & Bryant, D.M. (1990) Double-blind placebo-controlled study of nortriptyline in depressed adolescents using a 'fixed plasma level' design. *Psychopharmacology Bulletin*, 26, 85–90.

Geller, B., Fox, L.W. & Clark, K.A. (1994) Rate and predictors of prepubertal bipolarity during follow-up of 6- to 12-year-old depressed children. *Journal of the American Academy of Child and Adolescent Psychiatry*, 33, 461–468.

Geller, B., Cooper, T.B., Sun, K. *et al.* (1998) Double-blind and placebo-controlled study of lithium for adolescent bipolar disorders with secondary substance dependency. *Journal of the American Academy of Child and Adolescent Psychiatry*, 37, 171–178.

Geller, B., Reising, D., Leonard, H.L., Riddle, M.A. & Walsh, B.T. (1999) Critical review of tricyclic antidepressant use in children and adolescents. *Journal of the American Academy of Child and Adolescent Psychiatry*, 38, 513–516.

Giedd, J.N., Swedo, S.E., Lowe, C.H. & Rosenthal, N.E. (1998) Case series: pediatric seasonal affective disorder—a follow-up report. *Journal of the American Academy of Child and Adolescent Psychiatry*, 37, 218–220.

Gillman, P.K. (1999) The serotonin syndrome and its treatment. *Journal of Psychopharmacology*, 13, 100–109.

Giuffra, L. & Risch, N. (1994) Diminished recall and the cohort effect of major depression: a simulation study. *Psychological Medicine*, 24, 375–383.

Goodman, R. (1997) The strengths and difficulties questionnaire: a research note. *Journal of Child Psychology and Psychiatry*, 38, 581–586.

Goodman, S.H. & Gotlib, I.H. (1999) Risk for psychopathology in the children of depressed mothers: a developmental model for understanding mechanisms of transmission. *Psychological Review*, 106, 458–490.

Goodwin, F.K. & Ghaemi, S.N. (1998) Commentary: understanding manic-depressive illness. *Archives of General Psychiatry*, 55, 23–25.

Goodyer, I.M. (1990) *Life Experiences, Development and Childhood Psychopathology*. John Wiley, Chichester.

Goodyer, I.M., Ashby, L., Altham, P.M.E., Vize, C. & Cooper, P.J. (1993a) Temperament and major depression in 11–16-year-olds. *Journal of Child Psychology and Psychiatry*, 34, 1409–1423.

Goodyer, I.M., Cooper, P.J., Vize, C. & Ashby, L. (1993b) Depression in 11–16-year-old girls: the role of past parental psychopathology and exposure to recent life events. *Journal of Child Psychology and Psychiatry*, 34, 1103–1115.

Goodyer, I.M., Herbert, J., Secher, S.M. & Pearson, J. (1997a) Short-term outcome of major depression. I. Comorbidity and severity at presentation as predictors of persistent disorder. *Journal of the American Academy of Child and Adolescent Psychiatry*, 36, 179–187.

Goodyer, I.M., Herbert, J., Tamplin, A., Secher, S.M. & Pearson, J. (1997b) Short-term outcome of major depression. II. Life events, family dysfunction, and friendship difficulties as predictors of persistent disorder. *Journal of the American Academy of Child and Adolescent Psychiatry*, 36, 474–480.

Goodyer, I.M., Herbert, J. & Altham, P.M. (1998) Adrenal steroid secretion and major depression in 8- to 16-year-olds. III. Influence of cortisol:DHEA ratio at presentation on subsequent rates of disappointing life events and persistent major depression. *Psychological Medicine*, 28, 265–273.

Gorell Barnes, G. (1994) Family therapy. In: *Child and Adolescent Psychiatry: Modern Approaches* (eds M. Rutter, E. Taylor & L. Hersov), 3rd edn, pp. 946–965. Blackwell Scientific Publications, Oxford.

Graham, P. (1994) Prevention. In: *Child and Adolescent Psychiatry: Modern Approaches* (eds M. Rutter, E. Taylor & L. Hersov), 3rd edn, pp. 815–828. Blackwell Scientific, Oxford.

Groholt, B., Ekeberg, O., Wichstrom, L. & Haldorsen, T. (1998) Suicide among children and younger and older adolescents in Norway: a comparative study. *Journal of the American Academy of Child and Adolescent Psychiatry*, 37, 473–481.

Gutgesell, H., Atkins, D., Barst, R. *et al.* (1999) AHA scientific statement: cardiovascular monitoring of children and adolescents receiving psychotropic drugs. *Journal of the American Academy of Child and Adolescent Psychiatry*, 38, 1047–1050.

Hammen, C. (1991) Depression runs in families. *The Social Context of Risk and Resilience in Children of Depressed Mothers*. Springer-Verlag, New York.

Hammen, C., Burge, D., Burney, E. & Adrian, C. (1990) Longitudinal study of diagnoses in children of women with unipolar and bipolar affective disorder. *Archives of General Psychiatry*, 47, 1112–1117.

Hammen, C., Burge, D. & Adrian, C. (1991) Timing of mother and child depression in a longitudinal study of children at risk. *Journal of Consulting and Clinical Psychology*, 59, 341–345.

Hammen, C., Rudolph, K., Weisz, J., Rao, U. & Burge, D. (1999) The context of depression in clinic-referred youth: neglected areas in treatment. *Journal of the American Academy of Child and Adolescent Psychiatry*, 38, 64–71.

Hankin, B.L., Abramson, L.Y., Silva, P.A., McGee, R. & Angell, K.E. (1998) Development of depression from preadolescence to young adulthood: emerging gender differences in a 10-year longitudinal study. *Journal of Abnormal Psychology*, 107, 128–140.

Hardan, A., Birmaher, B., Williamson, D.E. *et al.* (1999) Prolactin secretion in depressed children. *Biological Psychiatry* 46, 506–511.

Harrington, R.C. (2000) Childhood depression: is it the same disorder?. In: *Childhood Onset of 'Adult' Psychiatric Disorder: Clinical and Research Advances* (ed. J. Rapoport), pp. 223–244. American Psychiatric Press, Washington.

Harrington, R.C. & Clark, A. (1998) Prevention and early intervention for depression in adolescence and early adult life. *European Archives of Psychiatry and Clinical Neuroscience*, 248, 32–45.

Harrington, R.C. & Harrison, L. (1999) Unproven assumptions about the impact of bereavement on children. *Journal of the Royal Society of Medicine*, 92, 230–233.

Harrington, R.C. & Shariff, A. (1992) Choosing an instrument to assess depression in young people. *Newsletter of the Association of Child Psychology and Psychiatry*, **14**, 279–282.

Harrington, R.C. & Vostanis, P. (1995) Longitudinal perspectives and affective disorder in children and adolescents. In: *The Depressed Child and Adolescent: Developmental and Clinical Perspectives* (ed. I.M. Goodyer), pp. 311–341. Cambridge University Press, Cambridge.

Harrington, R.C., Fudge, H., Rutter, M., Pickles, A. & Hill, J. (1990) Adult outcomes of childhood and adolescent depression. I. Psychiatric status. *Archives of General Psychiatry*, **47**, 465–473.

Harrington, R.C., Fudge, H., Rutter, M., Pickles, A. & Hill, J. (1991) Adult outcomes of childhood and adolescent depression. II. Risk for antisocial disorders. *Journal of the American Academy of Child and Adolescent Psychiatry*, **30**, 434–439.

Harrington, R.C., Fudge, H., Rutter, M., Bredenkamp, D., Groothues, C. & Pridham, J. (1993) Child and adult depression: a test of continuities with data from a family study. *British Journal of Psychiatry*, **162**, 627–633.

Harrington, R.C., Rutter, M., Weissman, M. *et al.* (1997) Psychiatric disorders in the relatives of depressed probands. I. Comparison of prepubertal, adolescent and early adult onset forms. *Journal of Affective Disorders*, **42**, 9–22.

Harrington, R., Whittaker, J., Shoebridge, P. & Campbell, F. (1998a) Systematic review of efficacy of cognitive behaviour therapies in child and adolescent depressive disorder. *British Medical Journal*, **316**, 1559–1563.

Harrington, R.C., Kerfoot, M., Dyer, E. *et al.* (1998b) Randomized trial of a home based family intervention for children who have deliberately poisoned themselves. *Journal of the American Academy of Child and Adolescent Psychiatry*, **37**, 512–518.

Harrington, R.C., Whittaker, J. & Shoebridge, P. (1998c) Psychological treatment of depression in children and adolescents: a review of treatment research. *British Journal of Psychiatry*, **173**, 291–298.

Harrington, R.C., Wood, A. & Verduyn, C. (1998d) Clinically depressed adolescents. In: *Cognitive Behaviour Therapy for Children and Families* (ed. P. Graham), pp. 156–193. Cambridge University Press, Cambridge.

Hazell, P., O'Connell, D., Heathcote, D., Robertson, J. & Henry, D. (1995) Efficacy of tricyclic drugs in treating child and adolescent depression: a meta-analysis. *British Medical Journal*, **310**, 897–901.

Hodges, K. (1993) Structured interviews for assessing children. *Journal of Child Psychology and Psychiatry*, **34**, 49–67.

Hotopf, M., Churchill, R. & Lewis, G. (1999) Pragmatic randomized controlled trials in psychiatry. *British Journal of Psychiatry*, **175**, 217–223.

Hughes, C.W., Preskorn, S.H., Weller, E., Weller, R., Hassanein, R. & Tucker, S. (1990) The effect of concomitant disorders in childhood depression on predicting clinical response. *Psychopharmacology Bulletin*, **26**, 235–238.

Jayson, D., Wood, A.J., Kroll, L., Fraser, J. & Harrington, R.C. (1998) Which depressed patients respond to cognitive-behavioral treatment? *Journal of the American Academy of Child and Adolescent Psychiatry*, **37**, 35–39.

Judd, L.L., Akiskal, H.S., Maser, J.L. *et al.* (1998) A prospective 12-year study of subsyndromal and syndromal depressive symptoms in unipolar major depressive disorders. *Archives of General Psychiatry*, **55**, 694–700.

Kahn, J.S., Kehle, T.J., Jenson, W.R. & Clark, E. (1990) Comparison of cognitive-behavioral, relaxation, and self-modeling interventions for depression among middle-school students. *School Psychology Review*, **2**, 196–211.

Kandel, D.B. & Davies, M. (1986) Adult sequelae of adolescent depressive symptoms. *Archives of General Psychiatry*, **43**, 255–262.

Kaplan, S.J., Pelcovitz, D., Salzinger, S. *et al.* (1998) Adolescent physical abuse: risk for adolescent psychiatric disorders. *American Journal of Psychiatry*, **155**, 954–959.

Kashani, J.H., Shekim, W.O. & Reid, J.C. (1984) Amitriptyline in children with major depressive disorder: a double-blind crossover pilot study. *Journal of the American Academy of Child Psychiatry*, **23**, 348–351.

Keller, M.B. (1999) The long-term treatment of depression. *Journal of Clinical Psychiatry*, **60** (Suppl. 17), 41–45.

Keller, M.B., Beardslee, W., Lavori, P.W., Wunder, J., Drs, D.L. & Samuelson, H. (1988) Course of major depression in non-referred adolescents: a retrospective study. *Journal of Affective Disorders*, **15**, 235–243.

Keller M.B., Ryan N.D. & Strober M. *et al.* (2001) Efficacy of paroxetine in the treatment of adolescent major depression: a randomized, controlled trial. *Journal of the American Academy of Child and Adolescent Psychiatry*, **40**, 762–772.

Kendall, P.C., Stark, K.D. & Adam, T. (1990) Cognitive deficit or cognitive distortion in childhood depression. *Journal of Abnormal Child Psychology*, **18**, 255–270.

Kendler, K.S., Kessler, R.C., Walters, E.E. *et al.* (1995) Stressful life events, genetic liability, and onset of an episode of major depression in women. *American Journal of Psychiatry*, **152**, 833–842.

King, C.A. & Kirschenbaum, D.S. (1990) An experimental evaluation of a school-based program for children at risk: Wisconsin early intervention. *Journal of Community Psychology*, **18**, 167–177.

Klein, R., Pine, D.S. & Klein, D.F. (1998) Resolved: mania is mistaken for ADHD in prepubertal children—negative. *Journal of the American Academy of Child and Adolescent Psychiatry*, **37**, 1093–1096.

Klerman, G.L. & Weissman, M.M. (1992) Interpersonal psychotherapy. In: *Handbook of Affective Disorders* (ed. E.S. Paykel), 2nd edn, pp. 501–510. Churchill Livingstone, Edinburgh.

Kovacs, M. (1981) Rating scales to assess depression in school-aged children. *Acta Paedopsychiatrica*, **46**, 305–315.

Kovacs, M. & Pollock, M. (1995) Bipolar disorder and comorbid conduct disorder in childhood and adolescence. *Journal of the American Academy of Child and Adolescent Psychiatry*, **34**, 715–723.

Kovacs, M., Feinberg, T.L., Crouse-Novak, M., Paulauskas, S.L., Pollock, M. & Finkelstein, R. (1984a) Depressive disorders in childhood. II. A longitudinal study of the risk for a subsequent major depression. *Archives General Psychiatry*, **41**, 643–649.

Kovacs, M., Feinberg, T.L., Crouse-Novak, M.A., Paulauskas, S.L. & Finkelstein, R. (1984b) Depressive disorders in childhood. I. A longitudinal prospective study of characteristics and recovery. *Archives of General Psychiatry*, **41**, 229–237.

Kovacs, M., Gatsonis, C., Paulauskas, S. & Richards, C. (1989) Depressive disorders in childhood. IV. A longitudinal study of comorbidity with and risk for anxiety disorders. *Archives of General Psychiatry*, **46**, 776–782.

Kovacs, M., Akiskal, H.S., Gatsonis, C. & Parrone, P.L. (1994) Childhood-onset dysthymic disorder: clinical features and prospective naturalistic outcome. *Archives of General Psychiatry*, **51**, 365–374.

Kovacs, M., Obrosky, S., Gatsonis, C. & Richards, C. (1997) First-episode major depressive and dysthymic disorder in childhood: clinical and sociodemographic factors in recovery. *Journal of the American Academy of Child and Adolescent Psychiatry*, **36**, 777–784.

Kowatch, R.A., Carmody, T.J., Emslie, G.J., Rintelmann, J.W., Hughes, C.W. & Rush, A.J. (1999) Prediction of response to fluoxetine and placebo in children and adolescents with major depression: a hypothesis generating study. *Journal of Affective Disorders*, **54**, 269–276.

Kramer, A.D. & Feiguine, R.J. (1981) Clinical effects of amitriptyline in adolescent depression. *Journal of the American Academy of Child and Adolescent Psychiatry*, 20, 636–644.

Kramer, R.A., Warner, V., Olfson, M., Ebanks, C.M., Chaput, F. & Weissman, M.M. (1998) General medical problems among the offspring of depressed parents: a 10-year follow-up. *Journal of the American Academy of Child and Adolescent Psychiatry*, 37, 602–611.

Kroll, L., Harrington, R.C., Gowers, S., Frazer, J. & Jayson, D. (1996) Continuation of cognitive-behavioural treatment in adolescent patients who have remitted from major depression: feasibility and comparison with historical controls. *Journal of the American Academy of Child and Adolescent Psychiatry*, 35, 1156–1161.

Kupfer, D. (1992) Maintenance treatment in recurrent depression: current and future directions. *British Journal of Psychiatry*, 161, 309–316.

Kutcher, S., Malkin, D., Silverberg, J. *et al.* (1991) Nocturnal cortisol, thyroid stimulating hormone, and growth hormone secretory profiles in depressed adolescents. *Journal of the American Academy of Child and Adolescent Psychiatry*, 30, 407–414.

Kutcher, S., Boulos, C., Ward, B. *et al.* (1994) Response to desipramine treatment in adolescent depression: a fixed-dose, placebo-controlled trial. *Journal of the American Academy of Child and Adolescent Psychiatry*, 33, 686–694.

Kye, C.H., Waterman, G.S., Ryan, N.D. *et al.* (1996) A randomized, controlled trial of amitriptyline in the acute treatment of adolescent major depression. *Journal of the American Academy of Child and Adolescent Psychiatry*, 35, 1139–1144.

Lee, A.S. & Murray, R.M. (1988) The long-term outcome of Maudsley depressives. *British Journal of Psychiatry*, 153, 741–751.

Lewinsohn, P.M. & Klein, D.N. (1995) Bipolar disorders in a community sample of older adolescents: prevalence, phenomenology, comorbidity, and course. *Journal of the American Academy of Child and Adolescent Psychiatry*, 34, 454–463.

Lewinsohn, P.M., Clarke, G.N., Hops, H. & Andrews, J. (1990) Cognitive-behavioural treatment for depressed adolescents. *Behavior Therapy*, 21, 385–401.

Lewinsohn, P.M., Hops, H., Roberts, R.E., Seeley, J.R. & Andrews, J.A. (1993) Adolescent psychopathology. I. Prevalence and incidence of depression and other DSM-III-R disorders in high school students. *Journal of Abnormal Psychology*, 33, 133–144.

Lewinsohn, P.M., Clarke, G.N., Seeley, J.R. & Rohde, P. (1994a) Major depression in community adolescents: age at onset, episode duration, and time to recurrence. *Journal of the American Academy of Child and Adolescent Psychiatry*, 33, 809–818.

Lewinsohn, P.M., Roberts, R.E., Seeley, J.R., Rohde, P., Gotlib, I.H. & Hops, H. (1994b) Adolescent psychopathology. II. Psychosocial risk factors for depression. *Journal of Abnormal Psychology*, 103, 302–315.

Lewinsohn, P.M., Rohde, P. & Seeley, J.R. (1994c) Psychosocial risk factors for future adolescent suicide attempts. *Journal of Consulting and Clinical Psychology*, 62, 297–305.

Lewinsohn, P.M., Clarke, G.N., Rohde, P., Hops, H. & Seeley, J.R. (1996) A course in coping: a cognitive-behavioral approach to the treatment of adolescent depression. In: *Psychosocial Treatments for Child and Adolescent Disorders: Empirically Based Strategies for Clinical Practice* (eds E. Hibbs & P.S. Jensen), pp. 109–135. American Psychological Association, Washington D.C.

Lewinsohn, P.M., Rohde, P. & Seeley, J.R. (1998) Major depressive disorder in older adolescents: prevalence, risk factors, and clinical implications. *Clinical Psychology Review*, 18, 765–794.

Lewinsohn, P.M., Rohde, P., Klein, D.N. & Seeley, J.R. (1999) Natural course of adolescent major depressive disorder. I. Continuity into young adulthood. *Journal of the American Academy of Child and Adolescent Psychiatry*, 38, 56–63.

Liddle, B. & Spence, S.H. (1990) Cognitive-behaviour therapy with depressed primary school children: a cautionary note. *Behavioural Psychotherapy*, 18, 85–102.

Mandoki, M.W., Tapia, M.R., Sumner, G.S. & Parker, J.L. (1997) Venlafaxine in the treatment of children and adolescents with major depression. *Psychopharmacology Bulletin*, 33, 149–154.

Marcotte, D. & Baron, P. (1993) L'efficacite d'une strategie d'intervention emotivo-rationnelle aupres d'adolescents depressifs du milieu scolaire. *Canadian Journal of Counselling*, 27, 77–92.

Marttunen, M.J., Aro, H.M., Henriksson, M.M. & Lonnqvist, J.K. (1991) Mental disorders in adolescent suicide: DSM-III-R axes I and II diagnoses in suicides among 13- to 19-year-olds in Finland. *Archives of General Psychiatry*, 48, 834–839.

Marttunen, M.J., Henriksson, M.M., Aro, H.M., Heikkinen, M.E., Isometsa, E.T. & Lonnqvist, J.K. (1995) Suicide among female adolescents: characteristics and comparison with males in the age group 13–22 years. *Journal of the American Academy of Child and Adolescent Psychiatry*, 34, 1297–1307.

McCauley, E., Mitchell, J.R., Burke, P. & Moss, S. (1988) Cognitive attributes of depression in children and adolescents. *Journal of Consulting and Clinical Psychology*, 56, 903–908.

McGuffin, P. & Katz, R. (1986) Nature, nurture and affective disorder. In: *The Biology of Depression* (ed. J.F.W. Deakin), pp. 26–52. Royal College of Psychiatrists, London.

Meltzer, H., Gatward, R., Goodman, R. & Ford, T. (2000) *Mental Health of Children and Adolescents in Great Britain*. The Stationery Office, London.

Merikangas, K.R., Angst, J., Eaton, W. *et al.* (1996) Comorbidity and boundaries of affective disorders with anxiety disorders and substance misuse: results of an international task force. *British Journal of Psychiatry*, 30 (Suppl.), 58–67.

Moreau, D., Mufson, L., Weissman, M.M. & Klerman, G.L. (1991) Interpersonal psychotherapy for adolescent depression: description of modification and preliminary application. *Journal of the American Academy of Child and Adolescent Psychiatry*, 30, 642–651.

Mufson, L., Moreau, D., Weissman, M.M. & Klerman, G.L. (1993). *Interpersonal Psychotherapy for Depressed Adolescents*. Guilford Press, New York.

Mufson, L., Weissman, M.M., Moreau, D. & Garfinkel, R. (1999) Efficacy of interpersonal psychotherapy for depressed adolescents. *Archives of General Psychiatry*, 56, 573–579.

Murray, L., Sinclair, D., Cooper, P., Ducournau, P., Turner, P. & Stein, A. (1999) The socioemotional development of 5-year-old children of postnatally depressed mothers. *Journal of Child Psychology and Psychiatry*, 40, 1259–1271.

Newman, D.L., Moffitt, T.E., Caspi, A., Magdol, L., Silva, P.A. & Stanton, W.R. (1996) Psychiatric disorder in a birth cohort of young adults: prevalence, comorbidity, clinical significance, and new case incidence from ages 11–21. *Journal of Consulting and Clinical Psychology*, 64, 552–562.

Nolen-Hoeksema, S. & Girgus, J.S. (1994) The emergence of gender differences in depression during adolescence. *Psychological Bulletin*, 115, 424–443.

O'Connor, T.G., Deater-Deckard, K., Fulker, D., Rutter, M. & Plomin, R. (1998a) Genotype-environment correlations in late childhood and early adolescence: antisocial behavioral problems and coercive parenting. *Developmental Psychology*, 34, 970–981.

O'Connor, T.G., McGuire, S., Reiss, D., Hetherington, E.M. & Plomin, R. (1998b) Co-occurrence of depressive symptoms and antisocial behavior in adolescence: a common genetic liability. *Journal of Abnormal Psychology*, **107**, 27–37.

O'Connor, T.G., Neiderhiser, J.M., Reiss, D., Hetherington, E.M. & Plomin, R. (1998c) Genetic contributions to continuity, change, and co-occurrence of antisocial and depressive symptoms in adolescence. *Journal of Child Psychology and Psychiatry*, **39**, 323–336.

Oldehinkel, A.J., Wittchen, H.U. & Schuster, P. (1999) Prevalence, 20-month incidence and outcome of unipolar depressive disorders in a community sample of adolescents. *Psychological Medicine*, **29**, 655–658.

Olsson, G.I. & von Knorring, A.L. (1999) Adolescent depression: prevalence in Swedish high-school students. *Acta Psychiatrica Scandinavica*, **99**, 324–331.

Olweus, D. (1994) Annotation: bullying at school: basic facts and effects of a school based intervention program. *Journal of Child Psychology and Psychiatry*, **35**, 1171–1190.

Os, J.V., Jones, P., Lewis, G., Wadsworth, M. & Murray, R. (1997) Developmental precursors of affective illness in a general population birth cohort. *Archives of General Psychiatry*, **54**, 625–631.

Pearce, J.B. (1978) The recognition of depressive disorder in children. *Journal of the Royal Society of Medicine*, **71**, 494–500.

Petti, T.A. & Law, W. (1982) Imipramine treatment of depressed children: a double-blind pilot study. *Journal of Clinical Psychopharmacology*, **2**, 107–110.

Pfeffer, C., Klerman, G.L., Hunt, S.W., Lesser, M., Peskin, J.R. & Siefker, C.A. (1991) Suicidal children grown up: demographic and clinical risk factors for adolescent suicidal attempts. *Journal of the American Academy of Child Psychiatry*, **30**, 609–616.

Pickles, A., Rowe, R., Simonoff, E., Foley, D., Rutter, M. & Silberg, J. (2001) Child psychiatric symptoms and psychosocial impairment: relationship and prognostic significance. *British Journal of Psychiatry*, **179**, 230–235.

Pine, D.S., Cohen, E., Cohen, P. & Brook, J. (1999) Adolescent depressive symptoms as predictors of adult depression: moodiness or mood disorder? *American Journal of Psychiatry*, **156**, 133–135.

Pine, D.S., Cohen, P., Gurley, D., Brook, J. & Ma, Y. (1998) The risk for early-adulthood anxiety and depressive disorders in adolescents with anxiety and depressive disorders. *Archives of General Psychiatry*, **55**, 56–64.

Post, R.M. (1992) Transduction of psychosocial stress into the neurobiology of recurrent affective disorder. *American Journal of Psychiatry*, **149**, 999–1010.

Post, R.M. & Weiss, S.R. (1998) Sensitization and kindling phenomena in mood, anxiety, and obsessive-compulsive disorders: the role of serotonergic mechanisms in illness progression. *Biological Psychiatry*, **44**, 193–206.

Post, R.M., Weiss, S.R.B., Leverich, G.S., George, M.S., Frye, M. & Ketter, T.A. (1996) Developmental psychobiology of cyclic affective illness: implications for early therapeutic intervention. *Development and Psychopathology*, **8**, 273–305.

Preskorn, S.H., Weller, E.B., Hughes, C.W., Weller, R.A. & Bolte, K. (1987) Depression in prepubertal children: dexamethasone non-supression predicts differential response to imipramine vs. placebo. *Psychopharmacology Bulletin*, **23**, 128–133.

Puig-Antich, J. (1982) Major depression and conduct disorder in prepuberty. *Journal of the American Academy of Child Adolescent Psychiatry*, **21**, 118–128.

Puig-Antich, J., Lukens, E., Davies, M., Goetz, D., Brennan-Quattrock, J. & Todak, G. (1985a) Psychosocial functioning in prepubertal major depressive disorders. II. Interpersonal relationships after sustained recovery from affective episode. *Archives of General Psychiatry*, **42**, 511–517.

Puig-Antich, J., Lukens, E., Davies, M., Goetz, D., Brennan-Quattrock, J. & Todak, G. (1985b) Psychosocial functioning in prepubertal major depressive disorders. I. Interpersonal relationships during the depressive episode. *Archives of General Psychiatry*, **42**, 500–507.

Puig-Antich, J., Perel, J.M., Lupatkin, W. *et al.* (1987) Imipramine in prepubertal major depressive disorders. *Archives of General Psychiatry*, **44**, 81–89.

Radke-Yarrow, M., Nottelmann, E., Martinez, P., Fox, M.B. & Belmont, B. (1992) Young children of affectively ill parents: a longitudinal study of psychosocial development. *Journal of the American Academy of Child and Adolescent Psychiatry*, **31**, 68–77.

Rao, U., Weissman, M.M., Martin, J.A. & Hammond, R.W. (1993) Childhood depression and risk of suicide: preliminary report of a longitudinal study. *Journal of the American Academy of Child and Adolescent Psychiatry*, **32**, 21–27.

Rao, U., Ryan, N.D., Birmaher, B. *et al.* (1995) Unipolar depression in adolescence: clinical outcome in adulthood. *Journal of the American Academy of Child and Adolescent Psychiatry*, **34**, 566–578.

Reed, M.K. (1994) Social skills training to reduce depression in adolescents. *Adolescence*, **29**, 293–302.

Renaud, J., Axelson, D. & Birmaher, B. (1999) A risk–benefit assessment of pharmacotherapies for clinical depression in children and adolescents. *Drug Safety*, **20**, 59–75.

Renouf, A.G., Kovacs, M. & Mukerji, P. (1997) Relationship of depressive, conduct, and comorbid disorders and social functioning in childhood. *Journal of the American Academy of Child and Adolescent Psychiatry*, **36**, 998–1004.

Reynolds, W.M. & Coats, K.I. (1986) A comparison of cognitive-behavioural therapy and relaxation training for the treatment of depression in adolescents. *Journal of Consulting and Clinical Psychology*, **54**, 653–660.

Roberts, R.E., Attkisson, C. & Rosenblatt, A. (1998) Prevalence of psychopathology among children and adolescents. *American Journal of Psychiatry*, **155**, 715–725.

Roberts, R.E., Lewinsohn, P.M. & Seeley, J.R. (1991) Screening for adolescent depression: a comparison of depression scales. *Journal of the American Academy of Child and Adolescent Psychiatry*, **30**, 58–66.

Rohde, P., Lewinsohn, P.M. & Seeley, J.R. (1990) Are people changed by the experience of having an episode of depression? A further test of the scar hypothesis. *Journal of Abnormal Psychology*, **99**, 264–271.

Rohde, P., Lewinsohn, P.M. & Seeley, J.R. (1994) Are adolescents changed by an episode of major depression? *Journal of the American Academy of Child and Adolescent Psychiatry*, **33**, 1289–1298.

Rueter, M.A., Scaramella, L., Wallace, L.E. & Conger, R.D. (1999) First onset of depressive or anxiety disorders predicted by the longitudinal course of internalizing symptoms and parent–adolescent disagreements. *Archives of General Psychiatry*, **56**, 726–732.

Rutter, M. (1997) Afterword. Maternal depression and infant development: cause and consequences; sensitivity and specificity. In: *Postpartum Depression and Child Development* (eds L. Murray & P. Cooper), pp. 295–315. Guilford, New York.

Rutter, M. (2000) Negative life events and family negativity: accomplishments and challenges. In: *Where Inner and Outer Worlds Meet: Essays in Honour of George W. Brown* (ed T. Harris), pp. 25–40. Taylor & Francis, London.

Rutter, M., Tizard, J. & Whitmore, K., eds. (1970) *Education, Health and Behaviour*. Longman, London.

Ryan, N.D. & Varma, D. (1998) Child and adolescent mood disorders: experience with serotonin-based therapies. *Biological Psychiatry*, **44**, 336–340.

Ryan, N.D., Puig-Antich, J., Cooper, T. *et al.* (1986) Imipramine in adolescent major depression: plasma level and clinical response. *Acta Psychiatrica Scandinavica*, 73, 275–288.

Ryan, N.D., Dahl, R.E., Birmaher, B. *et al.* (1994) Stimulatory tests of growth hormone secretion in prepubertal major depression: depressed versus normal children. *Journal of the American Academy of Child and Adolescent Psychiatry*, 33, 824–833.

Ryan, N.D., Bhatara, V.S. & Perel, J.M. (1999) Mood stabilizers in children and adolescents. *Journal of the American Academy of Child and Adolescent Psychiatry*, 38, 529–536.

Salee, F.R., Hilal, R., Dougherty, D., Beach, K. & Nesbitt, L. (1998) Platelet serotonin transporter in depressed children and adolescents: H-paroxetine platelet binding before and after sertraline. *Journal of the American Academy of Child and Adolescent Psychiatry*, 37, 777–784.

Sandford, M., Szatmari, P., Spinner, M. *et al.* (1995) Predicting the one-year course of adolescent major depression. *Journal of the American Academy of Child and Adolescent Psychiatry*, 34, 1618–1628.

Sandler, I.N., West, S.G., Baca, L. *et al.* (1992) Linking empirically based theory and evaluation: the family bereavement program. *American Journal of Community Psychology*, 20, 491–521.

Scott, J.M.S. (1998) Cognitive therapy training for psychiatrists. *Advances in Psychiatric Treatment*, 4, 3–9.

Shaffer, D., Gould, M., Fisher, P. *et al.* (1996) Psychiatric diagnosis in child and adolescent suicide. *Archives of General Psychiatry*, 53, 339–348.

Shafii, M., MacMillan, D.R., Key, M.P., Derrick, A.M., Kaufman, N. & Nahinsky, I.D. (1996) Nocturnal serum melatonin profile in major depression in children and adolescents. *Archives of General Psychiatry*, 53, 1009–1013.

Sigurdsson, G., Fombonne, E., Sayal, K. & Checkley, S. (1999) Neurodevelopmental antecedents of early-onset bipolar affective disorder. *British Journal of Psychiatry*, 174, 121–127.

Silberg, J., Pickles, A., Rutter, M. *et al.* (1999) The influence of genetic factors and life stress on depression among adolescent girls. *Archives of General Psychiatry*, 56, 225–232.

Silberg, J., Rutter, M., Neale, M. & Eaves, L. (2001) Genetic moderation of environmental risk for depression and anxiety in adolescent girls. *British Journal of Psychiatry*, 179, 116–121.

Simeon, J.G., Dinicola, V.F., Ferguson, H.B. & Copping, W. (1990) Adolescent depression: a placebo-controlled fluoxetine treatment study and follow-up. *Progress in Neuro-Psychopharmacology and Biological Psychiatry*, 14, 791–795.

Simonoff, E., Pickles, A., Meyer, J.M. *et al.* (1997) The Virginia Twin Study of adolescent behavioral development: influences of age, sex, and impairment on rates of disorder. *Archives of General Psychiatry*, 54, 801–808.

Sourander, A., Koskelainen, M. & Helenius, H. (1999) Mood, latitude, and seasonality among adolescents. *Journal of the American Academy of Child and Adolescent Psychiatry*, 38, 1271–1276.

Stark, K.D., Reynolds, W.M. & Kaslow, N. (1987) A comparison of the relative efficacy of self-control therapy and a behavioral problem-solving therapy for depression in children. *Journal of Abnormal Child Psychology*, 15, 91–113.

Strober, M., Morrell, W., Burroughs, J., Lampert, C., Danforth, H. & Freeman, R. (1988) A family study of bipolar I disorder in adolescence: early onset of symptoms linked to increased familial loading and lithium resistance. *Journal of Affective Disorders*, 15, 255–268.

Strober, M., Lampert, C., Schmidt, S. & Morrell, W. (1993) The course of major depressive disorder in adolescents. I. Recovery and risk of manic switching in a 24-month prospective, naturalistic follow-up of psychotic and nonpsychotic subtypes. *Journal of the American Academy of Child and Adolescent Psychiatry*, 32, 34–42.

Strober, M., Schmidt-Lackner, S., Freeman, R., Bower, S., Lampert, C. &

DeAntonio, M. (1995) Recovery and relapse in adolescents with bipolar affective illness: a five-year naturalistic, prospective follow-up. *Journal of the American Academy of Child and Adolescent Psychiatry*, 34, 724–731.

Strober, M., DeAntonio, M., Schmidt-Lackner, S. *et al.* (1999) The pharmacotherapy of depressive illness in adolescents: an open-label comparison of fluoxetine with imipramine-treated historical controls. *Journal of Clinical Psychiatry*, 60, 164–169.

Susman, E., Dorn, L.D., Inoff-Germain, G., Nottelmann, E.D. & Chrousos, G.P. (1997) Cortisol reactivity, distress behavior, and behavioral and psychological problems in young adolescents: a longitudinal perspective. *Journal of Research on Adolescence*, 7, 81–105.

Thapar, A. & McGuffin, P. (1994) A twin study of depressive symptoms in childhood. *British Journal of Psychiatry*, 165, 259–265.

Todd, R.D., Reich, W., Petti, T.A. *et al.* (1996) Psychiatric diagnoses in the child and adolescent members of extended families identified through adult bipolar affective disorder probands. *Journal of the American Academy of Child and Adolescent Psychiatry*, 35, 664–671.

Tyrer, S.P., Barrett, M.L., Berney, T.P. *et al.* (1991) The dexamethasone suppression test in children: lack of an association with diagnosis. *British Journal of Psychiatry*, 159 (Suppl. 11), 41–48.

Valla, J., Bergeron, L., Berube, H., Gaudet, N. & St-Georges, M. (1994) A structured pictorial quesionnaire to assess DSM-III-R-based diagnoses in children (6–11 years): development, validity, and reliability. *Journal of Abnormal Child Psychology*, 22, 403–423.

Vostanis, P., Feehan, C., Grattan, E. & Bickerton, W. (1996a) A randomized controlled out-patient trial of cognitive-behavioural treatment for children and adolescents with depression: 9-month follow-up. *Journal of Affective Disorders*, 40, 105–116.

Vostanis, P., Feehan, C., Grattan, E. & Bickerton, W. (1996b) Treatment for children and adolescents with depression: lessons from a controlled trial. *Clinical Child Psychology and Psychiatry*, 1, 199–212.

Walter, G., Rey, J.M. & Mitchell, P.B. (1999) Practitioner review: electroconvulsive therapy in adolescents. *Journal of Child Psychology and Psychiatry*, 40, 325–334.

Warner, V., Weissman, M.M., Fendrich, M., Wickramaratne, P. & Moreau, D. (1992) The course of major depression in the offspring of depressed parents: incidence, recurrence, and recovery. *Archives of General Psychiatry*, 49, 795–801.

Weinberg, W.A., Rutman, J., Sullivan, L., Penick, E.C. & Dietz, S.G. (1973) Depression in children referred to an educational diagnostic centre: diagnosis and treatment. *Journal of Paediatrics*, 83, 1065–1072.

Weissman, M.M., Warner, V., Wickramaratne, P., Moreau, D. & Olfson, M. (1997) Offspring of depressed parents: 10 years later. *Archives of General Psychiatry*, 54, 932–940.

Weissman, M.M., Wolk, S., Goldstein, R.B. *et al.* (1999a) Depressed adolescents grown up. *Journal of the American Medical Association*, 281, 1707–1713.

Weissman, M.M., Wolk, S., Wickramaratne, P. *et al.* (1999b) Children with prepubertal-onset major depressive disorder and anxiety grown up. *Archives of General Psychiatry*, 56, 794–801.

Weisz, J.R., Thurber, C.A., Sweeney, L., Proffitt, V.D. & LeGagnoux, G.L. (1997) Brief treatment of mild-to-moderate child depression using primary and secondary control enhancement training. *Journal of Consulting and Clinical Psychology*, 65, 703–707.

Werry, J.S. & McClellan, J.M. (1992) Predicting outcome in child and adolescent (early onset) schizophrenia and bipolar disorder. *Journal of the American Academy of Child and Adolescent Psychiatry*, 31, 147–150.

Werry, J.S., McClellan, J.M. & Chard, L. (1991) Childhood and adolescent schizophrenic, bipolar, and schizoaffective disorders: a clinical and outcome study. *Journal of the American Academy of Child and Adolescent Psychiatry*, 30, 457–465.

West, S.A., McElroy, S.L., Strakowski, S.M., Keck, P.E. & McConville, B.J. (1995) Attention deficit hyperactivity disorder in adolescent mania. *American Journal of Psychiatry*, 152, 271–273.

Wickberg, B. & Hwang, C.P. (1996) Counselling of postnatal depression: a controlled study on a population based Swedish sample. *Journal of Affective Disorders*, 39, 209–216.

Wickramaratne, P.J. & Weissman, M.M. (1998) Onset of psychopathology in offspring by developmental phase and parental depression. *Journal of the American Academy of Child and Adolescent Psychiatry*, 37, 933–942.

Wood, A.J., Harrington, R.C. & Moore, A. (1996) Controlled trial of a brief cognitive-behavioural intervention in adolescent patients with depressive disorders. *Journal of Child Psychology and Psychiatry*, 37, 737–746.

World Health Organization (1992) *The ICD-10 Classification of Mental and Behavioural Disorders: Clinical Descriptions and Diagnostic Guidelines*. World Health Organization, Geneva.

Wozniak, J., Biederman, J., Kiely, K. *et al.* (1995) Mania-like symptoms suggestive of childhood-onset bipolar disorder in clinically referred children. *Journal of the American Academy of Child and Adolescent Psychiatry*, 34, 867–876.

Wu, P., Hoven, C.W., Bird, H.R. *et al.* (1999) Depressive and disruptive disorders and mental health service utilization in children and adolescents. *Journal of the American Academy of Child and Adolescent Psychiatry* 38, 1081–1090.

Zoccolillo, M. (1992) Co-occurrence of conduct disorder and its adult outcomes with depressive and anxiety disorders: a review. *Journal of the American Academy of Child and Adolescent Psychiatry*, 31, 547–556.

30 Anxiety Disorders

Rachel G. Klein and Daniel S. Pine

Diagnosis of anxiety disorders in children

Distinction between normal and pathological childhood anxiety

Defining the boundaries between extremes of normal behaviour and psychopathology is a dilemma that pervades all psychiatry. In the very extreme, diagnostic decisions are straightforward (as in mental retardation, for example), but with milder forms, the defining point for caseness is often ambiguous. A few symptoms escape this definitional conundrum by virtue of being deviant no matter what their severity, such as delusional beliefs or hallucinations. Even in these cases, some childlike fantasies may resemble these symptoms. It is especially problematic to establish the limits between normal behaviour and pathology in the case of anxiety because many childhood anxieties are not only common but also have an adaptive role in human development, signalling that self-protective action is required to ensure safety. Because anxiety can be rated on a continuum, it is often believed that the extremes represent only a severe expression of the trait, rather than a distinct or pathological state. However, distributions may be comprised of distinct entities (Alpert *et al.* 1994), and the mere fact that anxiety falls on a continuum of severity does not preclude the presence of qualitatively distinct disorders at any point in the distribution.

Anxiety may become symptomatic at any age when it prevents or limits developmentally appropriate adaptive behaviour. A useful rule of thumb for determining diagnostic threshold is the child's ability to recover from anxiety and to remain anxiety-free when the provoking situation is absent. For example, it is not necessarily deviant for a young child to respond with distress to the parent's departure. However, such reactions reach clinical levels when the child is unable to recover after the separation is effected (assuming proper care is available), when the child cannot function normally during normal separation experiences, and when the child also develops concerns about future separations and vigilance, or even avoidance of activities that require separation. Therefore, the child's lack of flexibility in affective adaptation is an important pathological indicator. In addition, the degree of distress and dysfunction influences diagnostic decisions, which vary with the child's age, as well as with cultural and familial standards. When anxiety symptoms are developmentally inappropriate, subjective distress is relatively more informative. In brief, three clinical features impinge on the definition of pathological anxiety. Two of these, distress and dysfunction, vary in importance as a function of developmental stage. The third, symptomatic inflexibility, is diagnostically relevant regardless of age (Klein 1978).

As long as signs and symptoms are the exclusive basis for establishing the presence of psychiatric disorders, it is unlikely that we will reach completely satisfactory criteria for diagnosis. Longitudinal research can provide answers by identifying specific symptom patterns and thresholds that have long-term significance. Such evidence is informative, but rarely conclusive. Even if recovery were a common ultimate outcome, it would not follow that the syndrome in question did not represent a discrete disorder or a pathological state.

Diagnosis of childhood anxiety disorders

The past two decades have witnessed great expansion in the study of childhood anxiety disorders. Until recently, determination of children's fears and anxiety largely relied on rating scales, or interviews that inquired about a multitude of unrelated fears and worries which generated a count without clear clinical meaning (Lapouse & Monk 1958). These approaches have virtually vanished as the sole strategies for documenting and quantifying childhood anxiety. The emphasis has shifted to the study of diagnostic groups that reflect explicit clinical criteria. This strategy makes sense for several reasons. The number of childhood fears is potentially very large. It is cumbersome to assess them all for their occurrence and impact on children's well-being, and the task of determining their clinical relevance would be a daunting endeavour. Generating syndromes provides a more parsimonious estimate of pathological anxiety than scales with a plethora of items. Besides their practical advantages, clinical diagnoses are intended to represent distinct forms of pathological anxiety and foster the hope that they provide a more accurate reflection of pathology than scale measures. Scale ratings can be grouped to generate overall scores of anxiety, or what has come to be called 'internalizing' symptoms, such as in the widely used Child Behaviour Checklist (CBCL; Achenbach 1991) but, as the evidence shows, these scale ratings correspond poorly to clinical entities. Except for the section concerning assessment of childhood anxiety, where the role of anxiety scales in children is discussed, we restrict this chapter to reports that have formulated diagnoses of anxiety disorders, based on interviews with children and/or parents.

ICD-10 and DSM-IV

The two nomenclatures have similar diagnoses for childhood anxiety disorders. The major difference is that the ICD-10 provides a single diagnosis for cases who have both anxiety and behaviour disorders, whereas the DSM-IV (American Psychiatric Association 1994) requires the use of several diagnoses for such children. In addition, obsessive-compulsive disorder and post-traumatic stress disorder are under the rubric of the anxiety disorders in the DSM-IV, but not in ICD-10. Longitudinal and family studies report a weak relationship between these disorders and other anxiety disorders; therefore, their coverage elsewhere is justified. The most important anxiety disorders, and the most studied, consist of phobic disorder (specific phobia in DSM-IV), separation anxiety disorder, social phobia, generalized anxiety disorder and panic disorder. This ranking approximates their modal developmental sequence. It may be that, as knowledge is accumulated, some or all anxiety disorders will be shown to have specific biological features or causes, and will warrant their own examination.

Some differences exist in the definitions of childhood anxiety disorders between ICD-10 and DSM-IV (Klein 1994); however, this summary focuses on common clinical features.

Phobic disorder

The diagnosis of phobic disorder is defined as marked unreasonable fear of a specific object (e.g. animals) or situation (e.g. heights), that is invariable (it occurs whenever the person encounters the feared object). In addition, the phobia must be of such severity that it impairs the person's well-being by causing clinically significant distress or affects normal activities through avoidance of the feared situations. Although phobic disorders may begin at any age, their typical onset is in early childhood, but it is not restricted to it.

Although there are multiple sources of phobias, the majority of children with phobic disorders share a limited number of feared situations. Attempts to differentiate among various phobias in adults have not yielded clearly differentiating features (Fyer 1998). An exception is blood phobia which has a distinct physiological profile, consisting of a sudden drop in blood pressure and heart rate, and possibly fainting (Rachman 1990). These somatic symptoms do not characterize phobic reactions to other specific stimuli.

Separation anxiety disorder

This anxiety diagnosis is the only one that must begin before adulthood (age 18). The onset is frequently in late childhood, before adolescence. As the name connotes, it reflects anxiety at separation from home or caregivers that is beyond reason and to the point of interfering with the person's well-being or age-appropriate function. It is often accompanied by resisting activities that require separation from caregivers, such as play dates in friends' home but not in their own home. In younger children, what is referred to as school phobia is usually avoidant behaviour secondary to separation anxiety. (The diagnostic underpinning of school phobia in adolescence is more varied, because social phobia may also lead to school refusal.) There is no logical content to the specific situations children with separation anxiety disorder avoid; for example, a child may have no difficulty going to school, but be very uncomfortable during play dates in thoroughly familiar settings.

Social phobia

This condition is sometimes referred to as social anxiety disorder because its key clinical feature is anxiety in social situations because of fear of scrutiny, ridicule, humiliation or embarrassment. Some children may not articulate the latter concerns, but feel self-conscious and uncomfortable in social settings. Children must experience discomfort with peers, not only with adults, and anxiety cannot be caused by impaired capacity for socialization, as evidenced by the fact that the children relate well in social interactions with those who are familiar to them.

Individuals with social anxiety disorder avoid situations which require social interactions. In severe instances, there may be avoidance even of familiar people. The diagnostic qualifier, generalized social phobia, denotes whether social anxiety occurs in most social settings. Unfortunately, no definition of the non-generalized form is provided, and it has been interpreted in divergent ways. Some apply it to individuals who experience social anxiety in only one or two situations, such as parties; others use the diagnosis of non-generalized social phobia for patients who experience performance anxiety, such as public speaking or performance, eating in front of people, as well as test anxiety, but who do not have anxiety during social interactions.

Epidemiological evidence supports the notion that the two forms of social phobia are distinct, because the generalized form has been reported to have an earlier onset, more chronicity and comorbidity, and more psychopathology in relatives (Wittchen *et al.* 1999). This work exemplifies how epidemiological studies can inform diagnostic validity.

Generalized anxiety disorder

This diagnosis encompasses multiple worries about a variety of life circumstances, such as school work, appearance, money problems, the future, etc., to the point of interference with the person's comfort and functioning. The age of onset of this disorder is poorly understood, but typically is not in early childhood. Relative to other anxiety disorders, generalized anxiety disorder, unlike other anxieties, is more likely to occur with other psychopathology, and is not typically found on its own. Also, because the symptoms consist mostly of worries, the disorder is not usually characterized by avoidant behaviour, although there are exceptions. For example, children with extreme worries about academic performance may be absent from school on testing days.

Panic disorder

The essential clinical feature of panic disorder is the repeated experience of unprovoked spontaneous panic attacks, which may lead to limited independent travel or agoraphobia. The panic attacks are characterized by intense fear of impending doom or danger, accompanied by physical symptoms, such as rapid heartbeat, shortness of breath, choking sensation, sweating, depersonalization or derealization. The onset is usually in late adolescence and early adulthood.

Young children may display panic reactions, but whether they experience spontaneous unprovoked panic attacks—the hallmark of panic disorder—is controversial. Case reports have described panic disorder in pre-adolescents (Herskowitz 1986; Biederman 1987; Alessi & Magen 1988; Ballenger et al. 1989; Last & Strauss 1989; Black & Robbins 1990; Klein et al. 1992), but several are based on retrospective reports (Herskowitz 1986; Last & Strauss 1989; Black & Robbins 1990; Klein et al. 1992). These are certainly suggestive, but they fall short of being conclusive as they may be subject to retrospective distortions. Further, it is not easy to establish spontaneity of panic attacks retrospectively, or to distinguish other forms of severe anxiety-related panic attacks. A child psychiatry clinic series of 12 cases with panic disorder included only one pre-adolescent, who had the additional diagnosis of separation anxiety disorder (Renaud et al. 1999). Whether panic disorder occurs at all in pre-adolescents is still an unresolved issue but, if it does, it must be very rare. This makes it difficult to study the condition systematically. It has been suggested that, in keeping with the cognitive model of anxiety, children may lack the cognitive resources for misinterpreting somatic experiences in a catastrophic fashion and therefore do not have panic attacks (Nelles & Barlow 1988). This conjecture seems unlikely, because panic reactions associated with terror occur in children. It is the sudden unprovoked aspect of panic that seems to be missing in childhood, not the catastrophic reaction. At the same time, it is possible that true panic attacks have age-related clinical variants.

Comorbidity of childhood anxiety disorders

Comorbidity is an important clinical feature because it has been shown repeatedly to entail relatively greater dysfunction (Newman et al. 1998). Two forms of diagnostic overlap are considered: comorbidity of anxiety disorders with each other; and comorbidity of anxiety disorders with other diagnoses.

Studies of children referred for treatment report very high comorbidity among the anxiety disorders. In the largest treatment study to date of children and adolescents with anxiety disorders, social phobia, separation anxiety and generalized anxiety disorder were each diagnosed in about 60% of the children (RUPP Anxiety Study Group 2001). Comorbidity was particularly elevated in children with generalized anxiety disorder who, in 90% of the cases, also had another anxiety disorder, a finding consistent with clinical studies that also have noted the greatest comorbidity for overanxious disorder (reclassified as generalized anxiety disorder).

In epidemiological studies, comorbidity across anxiety disorders has been a highly consistent finding (Anderson et al. 1987; Bird et al. 1988; McGee et al. 1990; Fergusson et al. 1993; Costello et al. 1996; Simonoff et al. 1997; Verhulst et al. 1997; Essau et al. 1999; Wittchen et al. 1999). An examination of Table 30.1 provides a broad estimate of comorbidity, as the total prevalence of anxiety disorders exceeds the number of children with any anxiety disorder. It also indicates that comorbidity occurs in all geographical sites, and is not a variable phenomenon.

As to comorbidity between anxiety and other types of psychopathology, there is unanimous agreement that major depression is highly comorbid with anxiety disorders. As depression is much less frequent than anxiety disorders, especially in pre-adolescents, it follows that among those with anxiety disorders the overlap with depression is not as striking as when one selects those with diagnoses of depression, and that comorbidity increases with age. Although some clinical reports have indicated marked comorbidity between anxiety and attention deficit hyperactivity disorder, this relationship has not been confirmed in population studies, whereas there is some evidence of comorbidity between anxiety disorders and substance abuse and conduct disorder. At the same time, as noted in the section on long-term outcome, children with conduct and anxiety disorders may represent a distinct subgroup of conduct disorder because their longitudinal course seems relatively favourable (Pine et al. 2000a).

Historical developments

ICD-10 and DSM-IV implemented some changes in the diagnosis of anxiety disorders in children. As the literature mostly derives from the DSM-III-R classification (American Psychiatric Association 1987), these revisions are noted. The first and obvious proviso of a nomenclature is that clinical diagnoses should reflect distinct phenomenology. This elementary desideratum was felt to be lacking in the case of avoidant and overanxious disorders in the DSM-III (American Psychiatric Association 1980) and DSM-III-R, because their symptomatic content overlapped with several other anxiety disorders, especially with social phobia. This peculiar situation was not too surprising for overanxious disorder because it was introduced in the diagnostic manual in spite of there being no literature whatever on such a clinical syndrome, much less study, and it was essentially fabricated (Klein 1994). In view of these limitations, the DSM-IV does not include overanxious disorder. Avoidant disorder has a different history (Klein 1994)—it was felt that it was encompassed adequately by the diagnosis of social phobia.

Differentiated syndromes of anxiety facilitate communication among professionals, which is not a trivial goal, but it represents a very minimum requirement as a standard for the nomenclature. The DSM-IV and ICD-10 have met the minimal goal of providing anxiety diagnoses with distinct if not unique

Table 30.1 Prevalence (%) of anxiety disorders in children and adolescents.

Location	Authors	N	Age in years	Interview	Time frame	Rates (%)					
						Any	Simple phobia	SAD	OAD	Social phobia	PD
New Zealand											
Dunedin	Anderson et al. 1987[a]	785	11	DISC-C[b]	12 mos[c]	1.8–7.5	0–2.4	0.06–3.5	0.05–2.9	0–0.9	—
					12 mos[d]	3.6[x]	1.7	1.9	2.5	0.4	—
	McGee et al. 1990[a]	943	15	DISC-C	12 mos[e]	10.7[x]	3.6	2.0	5.9	1.1	—
Christchurch	Fergusson et al. 1993	986	15	DISC-P	12 mos[e]	3.9	1.3	0.1	0.6	0.7	—
		965		DISC-C	12 mos[e]	10.8	5.1	0.5	2.1	1.7	—
Germany											
Manheim	Esser et al. 1990	191	13	Graham/Rutter P/C[f,g,m]	6 mos	5.8	—	—	—	—	—
Munich	Reed and Wittchen 1998[a]	3021	14–24	M-CIDI[h,i]	12 mos	—	—	—	—	—	0.6
					Lifetime	—	—	—	—	—	0.8
	Wittchen et al. 1999[a]	925	14–17	M-CIDI[h,i]	12 mos	—	—	—	—	3.0	—
					Lifetime	—	—	—	—	4.0	—
Bremen	Essau et al. 1999	1035	12–17	M-CIDI[h,i]	Lifetime	—	—	—	—	1.6	—
UK											
London ‡	Kramer et al. 1998	131	13–17	K-SADS[i,j]	12 mos	5.3	—	—	3.1	1.5	0.8
Holland	Verhulst et al. 1997	312/780[k]	13–18	DISC-C	6 mos	10.5	4.5	1.4	1.8	3.7	0.2
				DISC-P		16.5	9.2	0.6	1.5	6.3	0.3
				DISC[l]		23.5	12.7	1.8	3.1	9.2	0.4
				DISC[m]		5.3					
						4.4					
Puerto Rico	Bird et al. 1988	386/777[h]	4–16	DISC[m]	6 mos	7.0	2.6	4.7	—	—	—
							1.3	2.1		—	—
USA											
Missouri	Kashani et al. 1987	150	14–16	DICA[i,n]	12 mos	8.7	—	—	—	—	—
Pennsylvania	Costello et al. 1988[a]	300/789[k]	7–11	DISC-C	12 mos	10.5	6.7	4.1	2.0	1.0	—
		300/789[k]		DISC-P	12 mos	6.5	3.0	0.4	2.8	0	—
	Benjamin et al. 1990[a]	300/789[k]	7–11	DISC[e]	12 mos	15.4	9.1	4.1	4.6	1.0	—

Continued

Table 30.1 continued

Location	Authors	N	Age in Years	Interview	Time Frame	Rates (%)					
						Any	Simple Phobia	SAD	OAD	Social Phobia	PD
New York State	Velez et al. 1989	320	9–12	DISC[e]	12 mos	—	—	25.6	19.1	—	—
		456	13–18	DISC[e]		—	—	6.8	12.7	—	—
	Velez et al. 1989 (repeat evaluations)	320	11–14	DISC[e]		—	—	15.3	9.7	—	—
		456	15–20	DISC[e]		—	—	4.4	8.6	—	—
New Jersey	Whittaker et al. 1990	356/5596[k]	13–18	Study interview[j]	Lifetime	—	—	—	3.7	—	0.6
Nationwide	Magee et al. 1996	1765	15–24	CIDI[i,o]	Lifetime	—	10.8	—	—	14.9	—
North Carolina	Costello et al. 1996	1015	9, 11, 13	CAPA[i,p]	3 mos	5.7	0.3	3.5	1.4	0.6	0.03
Georgia	Shaffer et al. 1996	1285	9–17	DISC-P[q,r]	6 mos	21.0	11.7	2.5	4.3	7.9	—
New Haven				DISC-C[r]		23.7	11.2	3.1	5.4	8.5	—
New York				DISC[m]		18.5	9.5	4.1	8.0	8.2	—
Puerto Rico						13.9	6.8	3.5	6.5	6.6	—
				DISC[s]		20.5	3.3	5.8	7.7	7.6	—
Virginia	Simonoff et al. 1997	2762 (twins)	8–16	CAPA[p,t]	3 mos	—	21.2	7.2	10.8	8.4	—
							4.4	1.5	4.4	2.5	—

Note: Rates calculated from papers.

SAD = Separation Anxiety Disorder, OAD = Overanxious Disorder, PD = Panic Disorder.

‡ Adolescents in primary care clinics.

a Same cohort within site.

b DISC-C and DISC-P, Diagnostic Interview Schedule for Children, Child and Parent Version (Costello et al. 1984).

c Rates vary depending on diagnostic criteria based on DISC-C, and parent and teacher ratings, e.g. diagnostic criteria met (1) by two of three sources or by one source and symptoms confirmed by at least one other source; (2) by one source but no other source confirms symptoms; (3) by combining symptoms from all three sources.

d Percent meeting diagnostic criteria applying same standards as at age 15 in McGee et al. (1992).

e Percent meeting criteria based on DISC-C plus parent ratings.

f Interview by Graham & Rutter (1968).

g Includes anxiety and mood disorders.

h M-CIDI, Munich modification of CIDI (Wittchen et al. 1998).

i Diagnosis based on interview with adolescent.

j K-SADS, Kiddie Schedule for Affective Disorders and Schizophrenia (Ambrosini et al. 1989).

k Two stage study: N in stage 2/N in Stage 1.

l Percent meeting diagnostic criteria based on interview with parent OR child.

m Top line: percent meeting diagnostic criteria on parent OR child interview and had a C-GAS<61 (Shaffer et al. 1983). Bottom line: percent meeting diagnostic criteria on parent OR child interview and had a C-GAS between 61 and 70.

n DICA, Diagnostic Interview for Children and Adolescents (Herjanic and Reich 1982).

o CIDI, Composite International Diagnostic Interview (WHO 1990).

p CAPA, Child and Adolescent Psychiatric Assessment (Angold and Costello 1995).

q DISC Version 2.3 (Shaffer et al. 1996).

r Percent meeting diagnostic criteria only for symptom number, age of onset and duration.

s Percent meeting diagnostic criteria and impairment linked to the specific disorder.

t Top line: percent meeting diagnostic criteria. Bottom line: percent meeting diagnostic criteria and impairment criteria.

clinical content. However, do specific anxiety disorders reflect valid distinct conditions, as defined by different natural histories, different correlates and risk factors, whether environmental, genetic or biological (Robins & Guze 1970), and different treatment responses? As far as possible, we examine research findings in this light to assess whether they support the validity of the current classification of anxiety disorders in children and adolescents.

Conclusions

The specific anxiety disorders in ICD-10 and DSM-IV, separation anxiety disorder, specific phobia, social phobia, panic disorder and generalized anxiety disorder, contain sufficiently distinguishing clinical features to assure their discreteness at the descriptive level. Comorbidity among anxiety disorders is well documented. Comorbidity of anxiety disorders with other disorders has also been demonstrated, but is not universally supported, except for the association with depressive disorders.

Assessment of childhood anxiety

There has been a proliferation of instruments to quantify levels of anxiety or determine the presence of anxiety disorders in children. Assessments include paper-and-pencil scales for children, parents and teachers, as well as child and parent interviews specifically designed to assess anxiety symptoms. Several reviews have appeared of self, parent and teacher rated anxiety scales for children (Klein 1994; March & Albano 1998; Silverman & Rabian 1999). Therefore an overview is provided, rather than a detailed report.

Rating scales

Rating scales serve diverse purposes. They may be useful for screening large groups to identify children likely to have anxiety at a symptomatic level, in order to provide economical means of targeting these individuals. At times, this strategy is used in prevention programmes (Dadds et al. 1997), or in epidemiological studies, to maximize efficacy of costly treatment or interview procedures. Rating scales have also been used in very large studies to examine the relative contribution of genetics and environment on dimensions of anxiety (Topolski et al. 1997, 1999). In clinical studies, scales may serve as indices of severity and as outcome measures of treatment efficacy.

Rating scales that anteceded the nosology of anxiety disorders introduced in the DSM-III (American Psychiatric Association 1980) and ICD-10 were not designed to reflect anxiety syndromes but, rather, consisted of factors such as worry, physiological anxiety, fear of bodily harm, etc. These scales include the Revised Children's Manifest Anxiety Scale (RCMA; Reynolds & Richmond 1985), the State Trait Anxiety Inventory for Children (STAIC; Spielberger 1973) and the Revised Fear Survey

Schedule for Children (FSSC-R; Scherer & Nakamura 1968; Ollendick 1983). In addition, the CBCL (Achenbach 1991) generates a non-specific factor of emotional disturbance, called 'internalizing' factor.

A major clinical challenge is to differentiate between anxiety and depression, and there would be great value to instruments capable of doing so. However, anxiety scales do not distinguish adequately between children with anxiety disorders and those with other diagnoses (Klein 1994). The Negative Affect Self-Statement Questionnaire (Ronan et al. 1994) has been reported to discriminate anxious from depressed affect (Lerner et al. 1999), but scale factors reflecting these two affects are highly correlated (Hodges 1990; Brady & Kendall 1992; DiBartolo et al. 1998; Lerner et al. 1999). The meaning of self-ratings of anxiety is further complicated by the finding that they do not correlate with symptoms of anxiety obtained from clinical interviews. Anxiety scales may provide overall estimates of anxiety levels, but they cannot be viewed as contributing to the diagnosis of anxiety disorders, and clinicians would be unwise to rely on them for differential diagnostic decisions.

A discussion of psychometric requirements for enabling usage of scales for diagnostic purposes is beyond the purview of this chapter. Nevertheless, it is useful to recall that if a measure differentiates statistically between two groups, such as depressed vs. anxious children, the difference is not an indicator of the utility of the measure as a clinical or diagnostic tool. Many other conditions must be met before assessments can contribute to diagnostic assignment.

The limitations of the older anxiety rating scales, and renewed interest in the study of childhood anxiety disorders, have spurred the development of more sensitive and diagnostically relevant measures of childhood anxiety. Recent efforts reflect the shift in the classification of anxiety disorders, and there has been a move toward specificity of content, with relevance to diagnostic groupings. In this vein, several scales have been devised, such as the Social Anxiety Scale for Children (La Greca et al. 1988; La Greca & Stone 1993) and for adolescents (La Greca & Lopez 1998), the Multidimensional Anxiety Scale for Children (MASC; March et al. 1997; March & Albano 1998) and the Screen for Child Anxiety Related Emotional Disorders (SCARED), which has a parent version (Birmaher et al. 1997; Monga et al. 2000). The MASC and SCARED stand out as promising for clinical purposes, because they were sensitive to the effects of fluvoxamine, a serotonin-specific reuptake inhibitor (SSRI), in a placebo controlled trial in children and adolescents with anxiety disorders (Research Units on Paediatric Psychopharmacology Anxiety Group, in press).

The Hamilton Anxiety Scale (HAS; Hamilton 1959, 1969), a clinician-based assessment, was developed for use in adults. It has had limited application in younger populations (Clark & Donovan 1994), maybe because it is weighted heavily with somatic symptoms, which are not believed to be clinically relevant to young patients. Unlike other scales in the RUPP Anxiety Study Group (2001), the HAS score was not significantly affected by fluvoxamine relative to placebo at all sites, suggesting limited utility for the measure.

Diagnostic interviews

There are several systematic diagnostic interviews for children, and for parents as informants about their child (Shaffer *et al.* 1999). They have been devised to meet different purposes, and vary accordingly. The Diagnostic Interview Schedule for Children (DISC; Shaffer *et al.* 1996) was developed for use in epidemiological studies, to be administered by individuals without clinical training. It is therefore highly structured, and the interviewer has the sole function of reading the interview content. The DISC provides a computer-administered version that eliminates the interviewer. As one study reported fair agreement among clinic patients, between standard DISC diagnoses and clinicians who administered the DISC, as well as a clinical interview, it has been claimed that the interview has a role in clinical settings (Schwab-Stone *et al.* 1996). That non-clinicians can provide valid clinical diagnoses in referred groups requires better documentation, especially because diagnostic rates are relatively elevated in epidemiological studies that have relied on the DISC (see Table 30.1).

The Child and Adolescent Psychiatric Assessment (CAPA; Angold & Costello 1995), also devised for epidemiological studies, is less structured than the DISC, requires some appreciation of clinical syndromes, and allows for clarification of questions by the interviewer. As a result, it entails extensive training for proper implementation. The CAPA resembles more closely usual clinical interview procedures than other diagnostic instruments by inquiring about areas of function, such as school, social relationships, etc., as well as specific symptoms, whereas most other instruments focus on symptoms exclusively.

The Kiddie Schedule for Affective Disorder and Schizophrenia (K-SADS) was developed for use by clinicians and allows full latitude of inquiry (Chambers *et al.* 1985). Multiple versions exist (Kaufman *et al.* 1997), including a highly structured version administered by lay interviewers (Orvaschel *et al.* 1982).

The Diagnostic Interview for Children and Adolescents (DICA) (Herjanic & Reich 1982; Reich *et al.* 1991) is also highly structured, but at times has been used in semistructured format.

The Anxiety Disorders Interview Schedule for Children (ADIS) was designed originally to provide detailed information on child and adolescent anxiety disorders obtained in flexible clinical fashion (Silverman & Albano 1996). It has been expanded to provide diagnoses for other major disorders.

There is little to guide the selection of one instrument over another, in terms of better reliability or validity. All have demonstrated modest to adequate test–retest reliability, with the anxiety disorders faring no better or worse than most other diagnoses. The DISC, developed under contract from the National Institute of Mental Health (NIMH) for use in epidemiological research, has provided more information on its psychometric properties than any other interview. It is the most widely used worldwide, perhaps because of its source, which has resulted in major dissemination efforts. It has been used in large multisite clinical studies developed under the aegis of the NIMH (MTA Cooperative Group 1999). The few direct comparisons between diagnostic interviews do not support the expectation that they yield similar rates of anxiety disorders, and therefore are interchangeable (Carlson *et al.* 1987; Cohen *et al.* 1987). The finding that method variance affects rates of psychiatric disorders complicates straightforward interpretation of the disparate rates of anxiety disorders across studies.

Although conceived for research purposes, diagnostic interviews may be useful to clinicians because they provide comprehensive coverage of symptomatic status. Also, they are excellent teaching tools for training in clinical diagnosis by providing a systematic means of ensuring that no important symptom domain has been overlooked.

The key issue is whether anxiety disorders generated by structured interviews are valid. Evidence points to the validity of diagnoses of social phobia, through consistent demonstration of onsets in adolescence, and the specificity of its longitudinal course (Pine *et al.* 1998a), which is discussed below. Inconsistent findings concerning the predictive significance of childhood anxiety disorders in girls and boys (McGee *et al.* 1992; Pine *et al.* 1998a; Costello *et al.* 1999) raise questions about the validity of diagnoses in childhood. If the findings from Pine *et al.* (1998a) are replicated, showing that overanxious disorder (now generalized anxiety disorder) has no specific longitudinal course, the syndromal distinctness and significance of the disorder will be questionable. Rather, overanxious disorder might be a marker of severity in a range of pathology. It is difficult to estimate the validity of anxiety disorders based on results from any one study, because interviews are not interchangeable and findings may be specific to the measure used. As a result, each interview schedule has to have demonstrated diagnostic validity—a costly enterprise.

Conclusions

Rating scales of anxiety have not been shown to distinguish between: various anxiety disorders; anxiety disorders and other child psychiatric disorders; or anxiety and depression symptoms. As such, they have not reached a sufficient level of precision for diagnostic classification. Two scales have been found to reflect treatment effects, and can contribute to the assessment of therapeutic efficacy in children with anxiety disorders. Several diagnostic interviews have been developed, with reliability estimates for anxiety disorders that do not differ from the reliability of most other diagnoses. There is evidence of validity for social phobia diagnoses derived from systematic interviews.

Epidemiology of anxiety disorders of childhood

Across several continents, well-executed epidemiological studies have informed on the prevalence, comorbidity, possible risk factors and, to a limited extent, course of anxiety disorders. These studies have the great advantage of avoiding the confounds of self-selection and other features that bias the information obtained from clinical studies.

Prevalence of childhood anxiety disorders

Population studies that report on anxiety disorders are presented in Table 30.1. As noted, focus is on investigations that have obtained direct information from children and/or parents. Epidemiological studies that antedate such practices have been reviewed previously (Links 1983).

Problematically, an overview of the prevalence of anxiety disorders is complicated by shifts in diagnostic convention. For example, avoidant and overanxious disorders that were in the DSM-III and DSM-III-R were removed from the classification with the advent of the DSM-IV. Social phobia now encompasses what was previously avoidant disorder, and generalized anxiety disorder substitutes for overanxious disorder. These disorders are not completely equivalent; especially in the case of overanxious disorder for which it is unclear whether it is captured by generalized anxiety disorder. One study (Pine et al. 1998a) formulated diagnoses of generalized anxiety and overanxious disorder in the same cases, and either or both disorders could be given. Modest concordance between the two diagnoses was found, suggesting that they do not reflect the same syndrome. Ongoing epidemiological studies are obtaining DSM-IV and ICD-10 diagnoses, but the published literature antedates them. However, the diagnoses of separation anxiety disorder, and simple as well as social phobia, have remained virtually unchanged in the DSM-IV, so that previous studies are relevant to the current nomenclature.

Table 30.1 is limited to prevalence of anxiety diagnoses; other syndromes are discussed in other chapters. Most epidemiological studies have found that anxiety disorders are the most common mental disorders in children and adolescents. Similar results have been obtained in adults (Christie et al. 1988). Epidemiological studies do not report on panic disorder in preadolescents. The few population-based studies that have reported the disorder's frequency in adolescents have found low rates, below 1% for lifetime (Whittaker et al. 1990; Pine et al. 1998a; Reed & Wittchen 1998), and lower frequencies for the past 6 or 12 months (Verhulst et al. 1997; Reed & Wittchen 1998). In preadolescents (below age 13), separation anxiety disorder is more prevalent than overanxious disorder (Anderson et al. 1987; Costello et al. 1988, 1996; Velez et al. 1989; Gurley et al. 1996). This ranking is reversed in adolescents in some reports (McGee et al. 1990; Fergusson et al. 1993; Verhulst et al. 1997), but not all (Velez et al. 1989). In DSM-III-R, the diagnosis of overanxious disorder was heavily weighted by symptoms of social anxiety; therefore, the pattern of relative frequency of separation anxiety and overanxious disorders in childhood and adolescence fits well the developmental literature on vulnerabilities to various types of anxiety disorders at different ages.

Rates of any anxiety disorder in children or adolescents within the past 6 or 12 months, range from 1.8% in New Zealand (Anderson et al. 1987) to 23.5% in Holland (Verhulst et al. 1997). It follows that there are also large differences in the prevalence of individual anxiety disorders. These striking discrepancies point to factors that may be important in affecting the diagnosis of anxiety disorders in children.

For one, age is a key issue. The modal age of onset of anxiety disorders varies. A consistent finding of epidemiological studies is that social phobia is relatively more common in adolescence. This finding gives indirect support to the validity of the assessments of social phobia in non-clinical populations. Longitudinal epidemiological studies would be informative, but they are scarce. Exceptions, such as the New York Study (Pine et al. 1998a) and the Dunedin studies (Anderson et al. 1987; McGee et al. 1990), indicate an increase in social phobia from childhood to adolescence in the same children, confirming that the disorder occurs more frequently in adolescence than childhood.

At the same time, there is marked variation in prevalence among similar aged groups across different studies. Some of this variation may reflect true differences because it has been argued that there may be geographical discrepancies in rates of anxiety disorders, at least in adults. However, disparate rates emerge even when site differences seem minimal. Two well-executed studies of adolescents, using similar interviews and both conducted in urban sites in Germany—Bremen (Essau et al. 1999) and Munich (Wittchen et al. 1999)—report lifetime rates for social phobia of 1.6 and 4%, respectively. A greater than twofold difference in prevalence is not inconsiderable. The 1.6% prevalence for social phobia in Bremen is for 12–17-year-olds, whereas the 4% rate in Munich is for 14–17-year-olds. This age difference could be key to the divergent rates, but it is not. The Bremen study indeed found that 12–14-year-olds had a significantly lower rate of social phobia than 14–17-year-olds (0.5 vs. 2.0%) (Essau et al. 1999). However, the 14–17-year-olds in the Bremen study had half as much social phobia as a similar aged group in the Munich study (Wittchen et al. 1999). As evident in Table 30.1, another case in point are the New Zealand studies from Dunedin (McGee et al. 1990) and Christchurch (Fergusson et al. 1993) which, in spite of applying similar assessments in similar aged cohorts, report a fourfold difference in rates of separation anxiety disorder (2.0 and 0.5%, respectively). No anxiety disorder is spared discrepancies in prevalence even when diagnostic definitions are identical and sites appear indistinguishable.

Thus, in spite of applying a uniform definitional standard for diagnoses, in the hope of limiting inconsistencies because of variable means of assessment, there is considerable divergence across rates of anxiety disorders. Variability in prevalence occurs in all child psychiatric disorders, but different factors may be at play in various conditions. In determining the presence of anxiety disorders, one relies on children's and parents' judgements, often lacking corroboration through objective observations by the informant. Given the highly subjective nature of informant judgements, it is likely that the method used for eliciting anxiety symptoms affects reporting.

In addition, there is no consensus about diagnostic thresholds and what rules diagnoses in or out, so that rates vary greatly depending on the convention applied. For example, rates are relatively high if diagnoses of anxiety disorders do not require that symptoms impact function. Some ignore the issue of impairment; others require it. Yet others use an overall index of impairment which is interpreted as documenting the diagnostic importance of all symptoms reported. Table 30.1 illustrates clearly that diagnostic rates are reduced sharply if diagnoses are made only when impairment is present. Problematically, an overall index of impairment, such as that obtained from the Children's Global Assessment Scale (C-GAS; Shaffer et al. 1983), a commonly used impairment scale, may not be reflect impairment caused by a specific diagnosis. Also, when several disorders exist, each may not incur the same impairment. The use of a single global judgement of impairment is likely to exaggerate the frequency of comorbidity, because no distinction can be made among diagnosed disorders as to their respective contribution to impairment. Only one study has compared prevalence rates as a function of diagnostic definitions (Shaffer et al. 1996). The overall rate of anxiety disorders was considerably lower when diagnosis-specific rather than global impairment measures were applied (13.9 vs. 20.5%). A key problem for judging impairment is the lack of any standard definition. How much or little is enough? Moreover, because global impairment measures are not designed for dysfunctions characteristic of specific disorders, they are amenable to local interpretation, and hardly represent thermometers of functional status in children. Divergent rates may reflect, in part, different local concepts of impairment. This problem is much less likely to occur in interviews that provide specific impairment definitions for each class of symptoms (e.g. the CAPA; Angold & Costello 1995). At the same time, serious overall impairment has been found to contribute to the stability of some anxiety disorders in children (Cohen et al. 1993; Costello et al. 1999). Although requiring impairment for diagnosis has a great deal of clinical and common sense appeal, and now has empirical support, it is not known whether the standard is appropriate in all cases. For example, adolescents with social fears (Essau et al. 1999), and with panic attacks (Reed & Wittchen 1998), who did not qualify for a diagnosis of social phobia or panic disorder, had high comorbidity with other disorders. It may be that impairment is relatively more critical to diagnostic validity in younger children, whose conditions are likely to be of relatively recent origin and transient. Impairment can be especially difficult to determine for the anxiety disorders in cases where the environment accommodates the child's anxious concerns. Some families, at times without deliberate planning, eliminate activities that cause distress to the child, and avoid making demands on the child. When this pattern occurs, impairment may be masked and not obviously apparent.

Not all studies are conducted during the same time period. Could it be that there are secular changes that affect rates of anxiety disorders? This possibility cannot be ruled out, but does not seem to account for discrepancies across studies, because results do not suggest time-dependent rates of anxiety disorders in young people (see Table 30.1).

Another problem for consistent diagnosis of anxiety disorders is that informant agreement is poor. It is commonplace to interview parents about their children. Depending on their age, children also contribute valuable information about themselves, especially about internal states, such as worries and fears. Studies that specify rates of anxiety disorders reported by children and parents, separately as well as jointly, reveal very different rates for each source, with little overlap between the two sources (see Table 30.1). Whether the same discrepancies occur to a similar extent in clinical cases is not known, but seems unlikely. At the very least, there is no dilemma about the issue of impairment in children brought for treatment because children with trivial dysfunction rarely come to clinical attention. How should multiple sources be used or combined? Some consider symptoms present when endorsed either by the child or parent. Others identify an optimal informant and disregard the others. These two strategies are essentially what clinicians do, depending on the individual case, based on their opinion of each informant's ability to provide accurate information. A more sophisticated approach has been to derive a statistical estimate of the diagnosis or latent class (Fergusson et al. 1993). This strategy has generated rates that closely parallel those generated by the 'optimal informant' method, but it has not been compared to the 'either parent or child' approach to diagnosis.

It is generally agreed that the answer regarding optimal approach to diagnosis will come from studies that examine the relative accuracy of diagnostic conventions in predicting course, as well as other features such as genetics and biological markers. There is some evidence that childhood anxiety disorders without impairment are not predictive of difficulties in adolescence, whereas the same is not true for disorders with impairment (Costello et al. 1999). At the same time, it is possible for impairment to occur in syndromes that are subthreshold for diagnosis (Reed & Wittchen 1998).

Conclusions

Based on the weight of the evidence in children, a fair estimate of current prevalence for any anxiety disorder accompanied by impairment appears to be between 5 and 10% (Anderson et al. 1987; Costello et al. 1996). Results suggest that similar rates apply to adolescents (Kashani et al. 1987; McGee et al. 1990; Fergusson et al. 1993; Kramer & Garralda 1998), with some exceptions in which rates exceed 20% (Shaffer et al. 1996; Verhulst et al. 1997). Additionally, epidemiological studies have been important in confirming that child (Benjamin et al. 1990) and adolescent disorders (Wittchen et al. 1999) are associated with significant impairment in multiple functional domains.

Risk factors for childhood anxiety disorders

Epidemiological studies are potentially the most enlightening means of identifying factors associated with illness. The most consistent finding has been that, at all ages, girls are overrepresented among individuals with anxiety disorders of all ages. This sex difference is virtually universal across studies. The twofold preponderance of girls among children with anxiety disorders has been claimed to occur as early as age 6 (Lewinsohn *et al.* 1998). Sex may also influence the stability of anxiety disorders because childhood anxiety disorders have been reported to have greater predictive impact for later anxiety in girls than boys (McGee *et al.* 1992; Costello *et al.* 1999), but findings are not unanimous (Pine *et al.* 1998a). In addition, some have reported headaches to be associated with anxiety disorders in girls but not boys (Egger *et al.* 1998), but others have not (Pine *et al.* 1996).

The documentation of a sex difference in childhood anxiety has influenced theories of psychopathology. It has been conjectured that vulnerability to depression in women may be partly caused by the greater prevalence of early anxiety disorders in women (Breslau *et al.* 2000). Indeed, in a prospective epidemiological study, Breslau *et al.* (2000) found, as expected, that women were twice as likely as men to have had an anxiety disorder and to become depressed in adulthood. However, men and women with histories of anxiety were equally vulnerable to the development of depression, and early anxiety disorders accounted to a large degree for the sex difference in adult depression. Problematically, studies of adults rely on retrospective reports of anxiety whose accuracy may differ by sex. Moreover, the role of early anxiety as a risk factor for adult depression needs to be reconciled with the fact that rates of depression escalate markedly after puberty (Angold *et al.* 1998), but rates of anxiety, in general, do not. However, as noted further on in the review of the course of childhood anxiety disorders, there is support for the expectation that anxiety disorders in childhood are risk factors for depressive disorders in adulthood.

Although relationships between smoking and anxiety had been observed in cross-sectional and restrospective studies, it was not possible to disentangle their causal relationship. A recent prospective epidemiological survey of adults found that smoking predicted the onset of panic attacks, but not vice versa (Breslau & Klein 1999). A subsequent prospective epidemiological study of adolescents also found that daily smoking was a significant predictor of anxiety disorders in adulthood, including agoraphobia and panic disorder, but not social phobia (Johnson *et al.* 2000). Importantly, anxiety disorders in non-smoking adolescents did not predict smoking in adulthood. It has been suggested that it is through its dysregulation of respiratory function that smoking places individuals at risk for some forms of anxiety.

There is little consensus regarding other risk factors for anxiety disorders in children (Costello & Angold 1995). A variety of environmental and family features, including economic disadvantage, school failure, stressful life events, family dysfunction, single-parent households, parental emotional problems, and low parental education have been related either to separation anxiety or overanxious disorder. However, unlike risk factors for conduct disorders, no consistent pattern has emerged.

In the Dunedin longitudinal study, risk factors were found for behaviour disorders, but no pattern emerged for anxiety disorders (McGee *et al.* 1992). Although epidemiological studies offer unique opportunities for assessing risk factors, they also have inherent limitations. Although anxiety disorders are common in the general population, each specific anxiety disorder is relatively scarce. Consequently, the number of affected children is small. As an example, among the 1035 adolescents studied by Essau *et al.* (1999), only 17 had social phobia. The Dunedin study examined risk factors for 'internalizing disorders' by combining all cases of anxiety and depressive disorders. In spite of its large sample of over 700 children, only 23 were identified with internalizing disorder (Williams *et al.* 1990). When addressing important questions, such as distinctions between girls and boys or between ages of onset, sample sizes become vanishingly small. The challenge will be to develop strong hypotheses that can be refuted without requiring large samples of affected individuals, as well as to identify the mechanisms that account for the contribution of anxiety disorders to young people's vulnerability for later depression. So far, epidemiological studies of risk factors have been fishing expeditions. The most heuristic observation is that disparate risk factors may be associated with different anxiety disorders. On the other hand, this suggestion is difficult to reconcile with claims of high overlap across anxiety disorders.

Conclusions

The lack of uniform standards for diagnosing anxiety disorders complicates estimates of prevalence in children and adolescents. There is inconsistency in sources of information, and in the requirement for impairment in symptomatic individuals. In spite of these methodological dilemmas, the evidence from epidemiological studies, with regard to anxiety disorders, provides support for:

1 relatively elevated rates, estimated to be between 5 and 10%;

2 their causing clinically significant impairment;

3 the significant longitudinal contribution of impairment in childhood to dysfunction into adolescence;

4 an approximate twofold preponderance of girls; and

5 the possibility that childhood anxiety disorders have different longitudinal consequences in girls and boys.

Recently, smoking has been identified as a risk factor for the development of anxiety. The identification of risk factors in childhood anxiety disorders has been hampered by a lack of cogent hypotheses.

Longitudinal course

The long-term consequences of childhood anxiety disorders take on special importance given the high proportion of affected children. Although a considerable literature exists, interpretations of studies on the outcome of childhood anxiety disorders are complicated by methodological issues, such as the nature of the samples, procedures implemented to evaluate children, and definitions of outcome, including psychiatric diagnosis and indices of overall function.

Often, one cannot assume that the assessment of anxiety disorders has been established reliably. While recent approaches have fared relatively better, the longest follow-up studies necessarily relied on older measures, with questionable reliability. As reliability places an upper limit on associations, outcome findings may represent lower-bound estimates of the impact of anxiety disorders on later adjustment. Moreover, the information on outcome relies mostly on studies of clinical cases. As children with uncomplicated or pure anxiety disorders are less likely to present for treatment than those with comorbid psychopathology (Cohen *et al.* 1987; Costello *et al.* 1999), studies of children in clinical settings may not capture the broad course of childhood anxiety. Usually, no matter what the disorder, children in treatment centres experience a more sustained and impairing course than children ascertained in the community. Another strategy has been to examine children at high risk (Weissman *et al.* 1997). These studies follow the children of parents with anxiety disorders, for whom it is expected that comorbidity and outcome patterns are less influenced by referral biases than is the case in clinical patients. However, high-risk studies must grapple with referral biases among parents, and the effects of parental psychopathology on reports of psychopathology in their children (Breslau *et al.* 1988).

Some of the initial epidemiological data on outcome relied on retrospective reports from adults. Because of the influence of current emotional state on recall, it may be that adults with ongoing mood or anxiety disorders selectively report negative childhood experiences, thus exaggerating the contribution of early anxiety on later adjustment.

Two major sources of data have addressed the developmental progression of childhood anxiety disorders: studies of the relationships between early life temperament, especially behavioural inhibition, and later anxiety; and studies of the outcome of specific anxiety disorders.

Inhibited temperament and psychopathology

Kagan *et al.* (1988, 1995), in Boston, first called attention to the relationship between childhood temperament and later anxiety disorders. Kagan noted that a subset of young children react with apprehension in novel situations. These children are defined as highly reactive during infancy and as behaviourally inhibited during toddlerhood. Inhibited children are slow to speak and smile in social settings. Criteria for inhibited temperament have been set to identify approximately 15% of toddlers. Relying on different approaches but using similar criteria, at least five other groups have studied temperamentally inhibited or uninhibited children. Rubin (1993) and Calkins *et al.* (1996) used

observational methods similar to those of Kagan *et al.* (1988); Caspi *et al.* (1996) used psychologists' observations during testing of preschool-age children; Kerr *et al.* (1997) and Hayward *et al.* (1998) used rating scales in older children. Altogether, associations between inhibition and psychopathology have been examined in thousands of children. In all centres, results suggest an association between behavioural inhibition and later anxiety (Kagan *et al.* 1995), with distinct associations at different developmental periods. During school-age years, Kagan's inhibited toddlers were found to have elevated rates of various anxiety disorders, including separation anxiety disorder and various phobias (Biederman *et al.* 1995). Similarly, Rubin (1993) reported associations with a range of symptoms on anxiety rating scales in young children. Caspi *et al.* (1996) found that inhibition at age 3 was associated with measures of anxiety and depression at age 21. Across these cohorts, associations with anxiety vary in strength, but none approach the magnitude of stability found for conduct problems across similar ages. Correlations between inhibition and anxiety ratings over time fall in the 0.20–0.40 range. However, there appears to be a specific link between early behavioural inhibition and social phobia in adolescence (Hayward *et al.* 1998; Schwartz *et al.* 1999), with odds ratios in the 2.0–4.0 range.

In addition to its association with anxiety, behavioural inhibition has been reported to influence the development of later behaviour problems (Kagan *et al.* 1995). Results from the Boston group (Schwartz *et al.* 1999), and from Kerr *et al.* (1997) in Canada, indicate lower rates of behaviour disorders in inhibited compared to uninhibited children. However, it is unclear whether this difference reflects relatively low rates of behaviour problems in inhibited children or high rates in those who were uninhibited (Raine *et al.* 1998).

An Australian longitudinal study recently reported that shyness in early childhood was significantly associated with parent and self-rated anxiety in early adolescence (ages 13–14), with odds ratios around 2.0 (Prior *et al.* 2000). In addition, the *persistence* of shyness through development was a predictor of later anxiety. Among the adolescents, 11.7% of those with little or no childhood shyness were considered anxious, vs. 41.5% of those with consistent childhood shyness. However, most shy children did not have high anxiety levels later on, and most adolescents with anxiety had not been shy children. Yet, the relationships observed are impressive in so far as they relied on rating scales of shyness and of anxiety. These are likely to underestimate the extent of longitudinal relationships.

Stability of anxiety disorders

The study of diagnostic stability of anxiety disorders has been examined among community cases, high-risk children and clinical patients, using retrospective and prospective designs.

Despite limitations of retrospective studies, they may provide leads for further study. The ease with which retrospective data can be collected is a major advantage (Robins 1978). Retrospective studies of adult anxiety disorders have called attention to the possible role of childhood anxiety disorders over time. Two large epidemiological studies in the USA, the Epidemiological Catchment Area (ECA) study, and the National Comorbidity Survey (NCS) found that the majority of adults with specific and social phobia reported childhood onsets (Robins & Regier 1995; Curtis *et al.* 1998). In contrast, adults with panic disorder and generalized anxiety disorder reported onsets in early adulthood, although some anxiety symptoms during adolescence were common (Eaton *et al.* 1991; Robins & Regier 1995; Wittchen *et al.* 1998). Also, self-reports of childhood generalized anxiety disorder in the NCS were associated with major depression in adulthood (Kessler & Walters 1998). These large community-based observations are generally consistent with retrospective clinical studies of adults, which have found that a large proportion of adults with panic disorder report childhood anxiety (Alpert *et al.* 1994; Labbate *et al.* 1994; Otto & Whittal 1995; Manfro *et al.* 1996).

Five community-based studies have examined the course of specific anxiety disorders. Although the first, from Dunedin (Anderson *et al.* 1987), did not specify outcome for individual anxiety disorders, some conclusions may be inferred (McGee *et al.* 1992; Feehan *et al.* 1993; Newman *et al.* 1998). In the initial follow-up, from age 11–15, a composite index of any mood or anxiety disorder predicted later anxiety for girls, but not boys (McGee *et al.* 1992). Comparable sex differences were obtained in prospective studies (Costello *et al.* 1999; Rueter *et al.* 1999). The latter also found that internalizing symptoms predicted a diagnosis of major depression.

These studies suggest that early broad indicators of anxiety disorders at one age predict risk for mood or anxiety disorders at a later age. However, they provide limited information on the course of specific anxiety disorders. Using a school-based cohort, Hayward *et al.* (1998) reported some degree of specificity in the course of social phobia across adolescence, but they did not find an association between self-ratings of past separation anxiety disorder and later panic disorder in adolescents. Lewinsohn *et al.* (1998) found that early adolescents with an anxiety disorder faced a threefold risk for anxiety disorders in late adolescence. Consistent with other family data (Wickramaratne & Weissman 1998), Lewinsohn *et al.* (1997) also noted that adolescents with both anxiety and depression were especially likely to have poor outcomes. This study did not find significant specificity in the short-term course of individual anxiety disorders.

Another longitudinal community-based study examined the outcome of specific anxiety disorders (Cohen *et al.* 1993; Pine *et al.* 1998a). There was relatively poor stability for overanxious disorder from early to late adolescence (kappa = 0.29) (Cohen *et al.* 1993). A different longitudinal pattern characterized the course of anxiety disorders into early adulthood (Pine *et al.* 1998a). Specific phobia during childhood or adolescence predicted specific phobia exclusively in adulthood. Similarly, previous social phobia was predictive of social phobia in adult-

hood, and no other adult disorder. The two disorders yielded odd ratios in the 2.0–5.0 range. Separation anxiety disorder predicted no specific disorder, but tended to predict panic attacks, whereas overanxious disorder was associated with an array of adult disorders including any anxiety disorder and major depression.

Beyond these community-based studies, two prospective high-risk studies have followed children of parents with either major depression or panic disorder. Anxiety disorders early in life, particularly phobia and overanxious disorder, incurred a two- to fourfold increase of major depression at follow-up (Wickramaratne & Weissman 1998). Similarly, children ascertained through a family study of anxiety and substance use disorders had elevated rates of anxiety and depressive disorders (Merikangas *et al.* 1999).

The course of childhood anxiety disorders has also been reported for clinic samples. Two studies ascertained children with school refusal and prominent anxiety symptoms prior to the nosological standardization introduced in the early 1980s (Berg & Jackson 1985; Flakierska-Praquin *et al.* 1997). The majority of children experienced relatively benign clinical courses into adulthood. Two other studies (Klein 1995; Last *et al.* 1996) confirm the generally good outcome of children with anxiety disorders referred to a child psychiatric clinic. In the study by Klein (1995), separation anxiety disorder coupled with school phobia predicted panic disorder, as well as major depression, though panic disorder was uncommon.

Conclusions

Data from longitudinal studies lead to several conclusions. Childhood anxiety disorders show considerable stability, but most children with anxiety disorders do not have anxiety disorders in adulthood. However, most adults with anxiety as well as mood disorders are very likely to have suffered from a childhood anxiety disorder. Furthermore, anxiety disorders in childhood increase the risk for later depressive disorders. Specificity of course into adulthood has been found for specific phobias and social phobia and, to some extent, for separation anxiety disorder but not for overanxious disorder.

Family genetics of childhood anxiety

The sequencing of the human genome has stimulated great interest in the familial aggregation of psychiatric disorders, including childhood anxiety disorders. During the past 25 years, more than 20 studies have reported an association between various forms of parental psychopathology and childhood anxiety. A series of studies document an association between child anxiety disorders and various parental psychiatric disorders. These studies include so-called 'top-down' studies which evaluate the children of parents with anxiety disorders, as well as a handful of so-called 'bottom-up' studies, which ascertain the parents of

Table 30.2 Anxiety in children as a function of parental psychopathology.

		Odds ratio between parental psychopathology and anxiety disorders in offspring vs. normal controls
Top-down studies	*Parental diagnosis (number of offspring)*	
Weissman *et al.* (1984)	MDD and PD (19) (mothers)	10.4*
	MDD (23) (mothers)	2.3
Turner *et al.* (1987)	OCD or AGO (16)	7.2*
	Dysthymia (14)	5.5*
Rende *et al.* (1995)	MDD (164)	2.2 T1*; 2.9 T2*
	No MDD (68)	0.92 T1; 0.92 T2
Warner *et al.* (1995)	MDD (32)	2.5*
	MDD & PD (60)	1.1
	PD (17)	2.3*
Capps *et al.* (1996)	AGO (16)	3.9*
Beidel & Turner (1997)	AD (28)	5.4*
	MDD (24)	5.7*
	AD & MDD (29)	5.4*
Merikangas *et al.* (1998)	AD, AGO & OAD (36)	2.5
Bottom-up study	*Children's diagnosis (number of mothers)*	
Last *et al.* (1991)	SAD (19)	1.4
	OAD (22)	4.2*
	OAD and SAD (17)	10.7*

* 95% Confidence interval of odds ratio excludes 1.0 (statistically significant at $P < 0.05$).
Parental diagnoses: AGO, agoraphobia; MDD, major depressive disorder; OCD, obsessive-compulsive disorder; PD, panic disorder.
Offspring diagnoses: AD, anxiety disorder including PD, OCD or social phobia; GAD, generalized anxiety disorder; OAD, overanxious disorder; SAD, separation anxiety disorder.
T1, time one; T2, 2-year follow-up.

children with anxiety disorders. In light of consistent cross-generational transmission, attempts have been made to decompose the familial transmission into environmental and genetic components, and some have attempted to delineate the process by which anxiety is transmitted from parent to child. This effort has involved studies of parent–child relationships, as well as studies of temperamental or biological profiles of children born to parents with anxiety disorders.

Anxiety and parental psychopathology

Multiple studies report higher rates of anxiety disorders in children of parents with anxiety disorders, relative to children of non-ill parents. As shown in Table 30.2, they include 'top-down' and 'bottom-up' studies. Two studies of adults also suggest that a childhood-onset anxiety disorder may identify a particularly heritable form of psychopathology. Specifically, Goldstein *et al.* (1994) found higher familial aggregation of panic disorder in relatives of adult patients with early onsets compared to families in which the patients had onsets in adulthood. Similarly, Battaglia *et al.* (1995) found higher loading for panic disorder in families where patients reported a history of childhood separation anxiety disorder.

Among adults, there is a growing literature on familial and genetic aspects of conditions related to the anxiety disorders. In general, this literature parallels the literature on childhood disorders; there is evidence of specificity in familial transmission in some instances but not in others. Kendler *et al.*'s (1996, 1997) twin studies support strong associations in the genetic factors implicated in generalized anxiety disorder and major depressive disorder. These two conditions are thought to share an underlying genetic substrate, differing largely in contributions from non-shared environmental factors. In contrast, other anxiety disorders show more evidence of distinct genetic risk. For example, genetic risk for panic disorder appears distinct from the risk for phobias, for generalized anxiety disorder, as well as major depression (Kendler, 1997; Kendler *et al.*, 1999). Findings from twin studies and family studies are consistent (Goldstein *et al.* 1994). Family studies have found that 'pure' cases of panic disorder and major depression tend to 'breed true'; in other words, panic disorder in the absence of depression is not associated with major depression in relatives. Similarly, data from twin studies implicate distinct genetic factors in the phobias. These data are also consistent with family studies where phobias confer relatively specific risks among family members (Fyer *et al.* 1993; Fyer 1998). Nevertheless, firm conclusions do not readily emerge from these data on familial genetic aspects of adult anxiety disorders. The strongest evidence of specificity in family studies derives from research on 'pure' cases (those with limited if any comorbidity). In cases with comorbidity, such as in adults with panic disorder and social phobia, evidence of non-specificity emerges (Horwath *et al.* 1995). Similarly, twin studies performed in the community may be less likely than clinic-based family studies to select cases with high rates of co-morbidity, which may account for some evidence of specificity in family genetic risk. Moreover, not all twin studies support the view of specificity in genetic risk (Andrews 1990).

Ongoing twin studies are delineating the degree to which fa-milial associations may result from genetic, and shared or un-shared environmental factors. Only tentative conclusions can be drawn because twin studies have reported divergent estimates of heritability for rating scale scores of childhood anxiety (Topols-ki *et al.* 1997; Topolski 1998) and of interview-based symptom scale ratings (Silberg *et al.* 1999). As with data from adult twin studies, the twin data in children are consistent in suggesting a modest genetic component to most forms of childhood anxiety, with heritabilities generally less than 40–50%. These relatively low heritabilities across the age range have led to the suggestion that genes confer a broad diathesis towards anxiety as opposed to a predilection for one or another specific disorder. Consistent with this possibility, heritabilities for temperamental factors, such as behavioural inhibition, have been somewhat higher than those for specific anxiety symptoms or disorders. Non-shared environmental factors account for much of the remaining vari-ance in child-based twin studies of anxiety symptoms, much as they do in adults. Nevertheless, the data in children show con-siderable variability across samples in genetic and environmen-tal contributions to anxiety. Such variability may reflect distinct genetic and environmental effects across age, sex and specific forms of anxiety.

A key question arising from family and twin studies concerns the degree to which connections between parent and child anxi-ety represent specific diagnostic associations. Most studies re-port associations between parental panic disorder and a range of childhood anxiety disorders. However, several studies suggest a particular relationship between parental panic disorder and childhood separation anxiety disorder (Warner *et al.* 1995; Capps *et al.* 1996). Conversely, family studies of adults, as well as two family studies of children, suggest specificity in the trans-mission of social phobia (Fyer *et al.* 1993; Merikangas *et al.* 1998). However, the limited number of children and parents with 'pure' forms of specific anxiety disorders limits firm con-clusions with respect to the diagnostic specificity of risk con-ferred to children by parental anxiety disorders.

Other questions related to diagnostic specificity concern the degree of overlap in risk for anxiety and depression. 'Top-down' studies document a strong association between parental major depression and childhood anxiety disorders, particularly speci-fic phobia and overanxious disorder or generalized anxiety dis-order (Warner *et al.* 1995; Beidel & Turner 1997; Weissman *et al.* 1997). These findings are consistent with twin and family studies of adults, in whom common genetic factors may predis-pose to depression and generalized anxiety disorder (Kendler 1996; Kendall & Flannery-Schroeder 1998). Based on these findings, Wickramaratne & Weissman (1998) suggest that childhood anxiety signals a particularly familial form of mood disorder.

A range of factors, including environmental, temperamental and psychophysiological, have been examined in efforts to iden-tify mechanisms related to the tie between parental and child anxiety disorders. As in the area of twin research, the paucity of available data precludes conclusions in this area.

Conclusions

Findings from family studies clearly establish the cross-genera-tional transmission of anxiety from parents to children. These data have stimulated the pursuit of key questions, one of which concerns the degree of specificity in familial associations among anxiety disorders. A second question concerns the mechanisms of intergenerational transmission.

Behavioural genetic studies in child and adolescents are extending work carried out in adult anxiety disorders. Twin studies, which are highly informative, suggest that there are moderate genetic components to anxiety in adults, and a rela-tively large contribution from non-shared environmental effects (Kendler 1996). Conclusions from twin studies in children have yet to emerge, given the ambiguities in the determination of childhood anxiety. For example, heritability estimates may vary for self as opposed to parent reports. Variability in heritability may also emerge as a function of gender or developmental level (Topolski *et al.* 1999). Despite these complications, efforts to re-solve these issues may eventually clarify aetiological factors in childhood anxiety. For example, twin studies may identify mechanisms that influence comorbidity (Simonoff 2000), espe-cially because studies in adults demonstrate the utility of twin designs in this regard.

Familial features of childhood anxiety disorders

Various aspects of parent–child interactions have been sug-gested as contributing to child anxiety disorders. Parental behaviours include:

1 modelling of avoidant or anxiety promoting behaviour through parental overprotectiveness;

2 direct production of anxiety through harsh rearing practices; and

3 facilitation of anxiety through failures to soothe children.

These aspects of the parent–child relationship are generally viewed from a transactional perspective, with possible contribu-tions from parent behaviour, child behaviour, and their interac-tion. Based on these models, treatment approaches have been designed to alter parent–child interactions patterns and child anxiety (Barrett 1998).

Behavioural inhibition is thought to constrain variability in later behaviour and interact with parental behaviour ultimately to produce anxiety in the child. For example, behaviourally inhibited children raised by parents showing high levels of emotional expressivity may be particularly vulnerable to high levels of anxiety later on (Hirshfeld *et al.* 1997).

Other transactional relationships between parent and child behaviour focus on attachment and reactions to separation. Bowlby originally hypothesized that attachment behaviours reflect interactions between evolutionarily derived genetic factors and environmental influences. Warren *et al.* (1997) found that toddlers who exhibited abnormal behaviours during separation faced an elevated risk for anxiety, particularly separation anxiety disorder, during adolescence. While these findings are consistent with prior data linking childhood separation anxiety disorder to later-life panic disorder, follow-up of children's responses to separation experiences and later anxiety have yielded inconsistent results (Rutter 1997).

Psychobiological features of childhood anxiety disorders

Based on the study of the brain substrates for anxiety in lower mammals (Davis 1998), children at risk for anxiety are hypothesized to have abnormalities in physiological systems implicated in adult anxiety disorders and animal models of anxiety. Animal models of anxiety have been facilitated by a high degree of cross-species conservation in brain circuitry among mammals as well as extensive cross-species data on the pharmacology of fear. Distinct forms of fear are regulated by interrelated brain systems involving various components of the limbic system. Learned fears can be modelled by fear conditioning experiments, where an aversive stimulus, such as a shock or air-puff, is paired with a neutral stimulus, such as a light or tone. Following such pairings, an organism exhibits fear-related behaviours towards the formerly neutral stimulus. Such forms of learned fear, known as 'fear conditioning', depend upon a neural circuit involving the central nucleus of the amygdala, located within the medial temporal lobes.

Other forms of fear develop without prior experience and are regulated by distinct but related neural circuits. For example, nocturnal organisms, such as rodents, display fearful behaviour in a well-lit environment. Unlike learned fears, this fear does not habituate and actually may increase in intensity with repeated exposure. The fear involves the basolateral as opposed to the central nucleus of the amygdala; the two circuits are regulated by distinct neurochemical systems (Davis 1998). For example, infusions with corticotrophin-releasing factor may potentiate light-enhanced fear but not conditioned fear. Innate fears of other stimuli may show similar distinctions from learned fears on pharmacological and anatomical grounds.

Functional aspects of brain circuits that regulate learned and innate fears can be quantified reliably in lower mammals as well as humans by examining changes in the startle reflex following presentations of mildly stressful stimuli. Adults with various forms of anxiety exhibit startle abnormalities. A study of asymptomatic children of parents with anxiety disorders provides evidence that risk for anxiety is associated with abnormalities in startle regulation (Merikangas *et al.* 1999). However, the precise conditions under which startle is most discriminatory of family history of anxiety are incompletely understood. Kagan *et al.* (1995) suggest that behavioural inhibition, a behavioural marker of risk for anxiety, also results from abnormalities in the same brain circuits. This view is based on peripheral physiological profiles in inhibited children, using physiological indices that are influenced by components of circuits that regulate fear in mammals. Data in children implicate the same abnormalities in brain circuits that regulate fear in lower mammals. Consistent with this view, behavioural and physiological signs of behavioural inhibition have been found in children of parents with panic disorder (Biederman *et al.* 1990). However, the finding is not specific to anxiety because similar relationships characterized the offspring of depressed parents.

While these data provide scientific leads, there are crucial pharmacological inconsistencies among humans and animal models in the regulation of fear conditioning and clinical signs of anxiety. For example, medications effective in panic disorder do not affect fear conditioning (Cassella & Davis 1985), though they appear to affect certain forms of unlearned fear (Blanchard *et al.* 1997). Accordingly, risk for anxiety disorders has been hypothesized to relate more closely to inherited tendency to respond to innate unlearned fearful stimuli than to the fear conditioning circuit. The most developed line of research examines the association between respiratory dysregulation and panic disorder (Klein 1993). Much like a well-lit room for a rodent, respiratory stimulants represent unlearned fear-inducing stimuli for air-breathing organisms, including humans. A wealth of studies suggests that sensitivity to respiratory stimulants identifies individuals with a diathesis for types of anxiety closely related to spontaneous panic attacks. For example, adults with panic disorder have enhanced responses to respiratory stimulants, such as CO_2, sodium lactate, cholocystokinin-cholecystokinin or doxapram (Klein 1993). Sensitivity to CO_2 has also been found in children with anxiety disorders compared to controls (Pine *et al.* 1998b), specifically among children with separation anxiety disorder (Pine *et al.* 2000b). Syndromes, such as subclinical panic disorder, that have strong familial associations with panic disorder are also characterized by enhanced responses to respiratory stimulants. Moreover, signs of respiratory abnormalities, such as sensitivity to CO_2, occur especially among panic patients with highly familial forms of panic (Perna *et al.* 1995; Horwath *et al.* 1998). In addition, healthy first-degree relatives of panic patients also exhibit enhanced responses to respiratory stimuli (Perna *et al.* 1995; Coryell 1997). These data suggest that children at risk for panic disorder may also be sensitive to respiratory stimulation.

In brief, abnormalities in underlying fear circuitry, as assessed using startle, may quantify a child's risk for later anxiety. However, learned fear, as assessed via fear-potentiated startle, has inconsistent relation to clinical anxiety disorders in adults, as well as to risk for anxiety disorders in children (Merikangas *et al.*

1999). There also is some evidence that startle under circumstances of innate threat may index risk for anxiety, based on temperamental or familial factors. However, as with work on fear-potentiated startle, there are inconsistencies across studies, sex and age groups. The level of basic science knowledge in this area is likely to foster research in the relationships between startle regulation and childhood anxiety.

Another area of research delineates the effects of fear on cognitive processes. Fear-relevant stimuli are processed more readily than neutral stimuli; this effect can be quantified using lesions or neurophysiological recordings in animals (Gallagher & Holland 1994), and using reaction time in humans (McNally 1996). In animals, the effect of fear on cognitive processes is thought to result from changes in amygdala-based circuits. Two procedures have been used in humans to probe changes in cognitive processes. One procedure, the so-called emotional Stroop test, increases the latency required to name colours during the presentation of coloured 'threat' words as opposed to 'neutral' words. Adults with various forms of anxiety show relatively prolonged latency to name colour words that are threat cues, such as 'panic', presumably because of enhanced vigilance to the meaning of 'threat' words (Williams *et al.* 1996). In another procedure, the so-called dot-probe test, reaction time to a spatial probe is quantified based on variations in the proximity of the probe to 'threat' words or pictures. Adults with anxiety show faster reaction times to probes appearing proximal to threatening stimuli, an effect that is also attributed to enhanced vigilance. For both tasks, there are relatively subtle but consistent effects of anxiety in adults' reaction times during the presentation of threats (Williams *et al.* 1996). There is some evidence suggesting similar effects in childhood anxiety disorders (Vasey *et al.* 1995).

Two central questions emerge from work on cognitive bias. First, the cognitive bias for threat has been conceived as a risk factor for anxiety. However, among adults, enhanced cognitive bias for threat cues is related primarily to ongoing symptoms, and disappears with treatment. Similarly, asymptomatic children with behavioural inhibition do not show enhanced bias for threat cues on the emotional Stroop test. Although these negative results have been attributed to methodological factors, they raise questions about the degree to which cognitive biases are central to anxiety or represent epiphenomena. Questions also arise about the diagnostic specificity of cognitive biases, because they have been found in most forms of adult anxiety, as well as in adult depressive disorders.

Preliminary data from the only available child-based study of anxiety disorders found an enlarged amygdala volume among children with generalized anxiety disorder, as compared to healthy comparisons (De Bellis *et al.* 2000).

Clinical implications

There is evidence for non-shared environmental influences in the development of anxiety in children. However, their nature is poorly understood, and the findings do not lend themselves to clinical applications. There have been attempts to identify parental features that may affect either the development or the maintenance of anxiety in children. This is a problematical task because it is difficult to identify the direction of the relationship. Do parents behave differently because their children are anxious, or has the parental behaviour led to anxiety in the child? Furthermore, the exact nature of parental behaviour is difficult to establish. For example, in a study of parental behaviour among adolescents with social phobia, parents of socially phobic children did not differ from parents of non-socially phobic children in their ratings of their child-rearing styles and the family environment (Caster *et al.* 1999). In contrast, the anxious adolescents, compared to the non-anxious adolescents, rated their parents worse on multiple measures relating to social phobia (concern about others' opinion, etc.). The identification of parental influences on childhood anxiety will likely require a longitudinal approach among children at high risk for anxiety.

Although the evidence is hardly in, it is generally accepted, based on clinical lore (at times it may be accurate) that it is best not to accommodate the child's fears, but rather to help the child experience anxiety-provoking situations to enable the development of mastery. Such parental behaviour may be quite relevant to preventing the maintenance of anxiety in children; it is less compelling that it prevents the onset of anxiety disorders.

Conclusions

The research summarized lays the groundwork for studying psychobiological bases of childhood anxiety. Data on cognitive biases and fear conditioning suggest a need for systematic brain imaging research on the structure and functioning of human limbic brain regions linked to animal models of anxiety. Research in other areas of medicine illustrate the strategic advantages afforded by genetic studies through the identification of physiological markers indicative of an endophenotype. Work on the associations among childhood anxiety, adult panic disorder, and respiratory dysfunction holds the hope of providing similar knowledge on the genetics of anxiety disorders across the life span.

Treatment of childhood anxiety disorders

The evidence that childhood anxiety disorders cause suffering and impairment, and findings that they may entail long-term liability, highlight the need for effective treatments. Some interventions, such as cognitive-behaviour therapy (CBT), are based on a theoretical model of anxiety; others, such as medications (e.g. SSRIs), follow from demonstrated efficacy in adult anxiety disorders.

The literature is replete with case studies reporting efficacy for treatments. Were there no systematic controlled trials, it would be sensible to consider them. However, because controlled studies have been conducted, clinical reports are not contributory.

Psychotherapy

The most well-studied intervention is CBT (see Brent, Chapter 54), which is based on the notion that distorted cognitions about the dangerousness of the environment are the underlying mechanism for anxiety symptoms at all ages. Therefore, treatment focuses on the child's thought processes, aiming to replace negative beliefs with more realistic neutral cognitions. This theory implicates only the child, and some forms of CBT focus exclusively on the child (Kendall & Ronan 1990; Albano et al. 1995). Others systematically recruit the family's active involvement (Barrett et al. 1996; Barrett 1998). The contribution that parents can make to their child's progress in treatment is likely to vary as a function of the child's disorder and age. It is difficult to appreciate how a child with severe separation anxiety could receive optimal assistance without parental involvement. Also, if such a child resisted school attendance, why would one not involve the school? At times, theoretical allegiances may lead to practices that seem out of step with children's problems.

A major positive feature of CBT is the availability of treatment manuals that allow comparisons across studies. All the studies reported have used treatment manuals. The controlled studies of CBT can be classified as those that used a no-treatment waiting list control, and those that compared CBT to a non-specific control intervention. While often used in early psychotherapy trials, the use of waiting list controls is methodologically problematic when applied to clinic patients. This clinical disposition confirms to patients that they require treatment, but withholds it. Moreover, there is concern that, in some instances, waiting list controls may have a deleterious impact. Another limitation is that this control does not reveal the specific usefulness of an intervention, because there is no way of determining whether treatment was effective because of its particular nature, or because of non-specific treatment features, such as therapist's interest and concern, or the family mobilizing itself to bring the child for treatment.

The most informative studies are those that have relied on a comparison treatment that is reasonable and credible for the particular disorder. Even when a control psychotherapy is used, methodological problems remain. The treatments should be equivalently appreciated by the recipients, so that treatment effects are not a function of differences in treatment credibility. Finally, in studies of psychotherapy, it is essential that treatment outcome be evaluated by individuals who are not aware of the treatment delivered, rather than by the therapist. In this fashion, one ensures that biases introduced by treatment allegiances do not influence estimates of outcome. Thus, self-reports of patients who received psychotherapy compared to waiting list controls are not revealing of specific treatment efficacy and may reflect the wishes of the patient rather than actual improvement. These design features are very infrequently met in current studies of psychotherapy in anxiety disorders. However, most studies have the merit of examining both the immediate and long-term effects of treatment. Long-term advantages of therapies are important, because there would be little point in investing costly efforts for transient clinical advantages.

CBT was examined in two systematic studies by Kendall (Kendall 1994; Kendall et al. 1997) in which anxious children were randomized to receive CBT for 16 weeks, or be on a waiting list for 8 weeks. In both trials, relative to the waiting list group, the group that received CBT was significantly improved after treatment, as well as 1 year, and 2–5 years later (Kendall & Southam-Gerow 1996). The treatment studies are weakened by the fact that there was a twofold difference in time between the two conditions. Controlled treatment studies are meant to control for time, especially when disorders are not regularly chronic, as is the case with anxiety disorders. (Understandably, there were concerns about the ethics of keeping patients on a waiting list for 4 months.) The sustained effect of CBT over several years is impressive, but it is difficult to understand because the children in the waiting list control received CBT after the 8-week wait, if they required it. Why should their status be different from children whose treatment was not delayed? Is this an example of the psychotoxic effects of waiting list controls in clinic patients? Waiting list controls have been used in other studies of CBT; as a result, their contribution to an estimate of efficacy is difficult to establish (King et al. 1998; Silverman et al. 1999).

Three studies have used 'attention' controls. Last (1998) treated a diagnostically mixed group of school phobic children with CBT or an established manualized control treatment. This is the only study that ensured that the two treatments had equivalent credibility to children as well as parents. No difference in efficacy was obtained between the two treatment conditions.

A study by Silverman et al. (1999) examined the specific effect of a cognitive treatment component by comparing an exposure-based behavioural contingency treatment with an exposure-based cognitive programme, and a family group intervention. No outcome differences were found across the three treatments.

A well-designed study compared a behavioural approach to a control intervention in children with social phobia (Beidel et al. 2000). This study is unique in restricting patients to a single anxiety disorder. Based on independent assessors, children in the behavioural intervention were significantly more improved than their peers in the control group. Unfortunately, the credibility of the treatments was not assessed.

Other studies have examined variations in treatment, such as parental involvement and group format. A study of parent involvement compared treatment of the child only, parent only, and parent with child treatment, in children with a variety of anxiety disorders (Mendlowitz et al. 1999). The parents who received treatment with their child reported greater improvement. In the absence of independent assessment, it is difficult to draw clear conclusions. Another controlled study found that there was significant advantage to having families participate in CBT, as assessed by independent evaluators and that the advantages of family involvement were maintained over a 1-year follow-up (Barrett *et al.* 1996).

On the basis of a systematic trial of group CBT, group family CBT, and waiting list control, Barrett (1998) concluded that CBT could be implemented in a group format, but the children who received CBT were not better than the controls.

Pharmacotherapy

SSRIs have been studied extensively in adults with anxiety disorders, and have documented safety and efficacy in generalized anxiety disorder, obsessive-compulsive disorder, post-traumatic stress disorder, social phobia and panic disorder (Roy-Byrne & Cowley 1998). Although open clinical trials of SSRIs in children have appeared, only one placebo controlled study has been conducted to date RUPP Anxiety Group, 2001). A large multisite 8-week study found that fluvoxamine was significantly superior to placebo in children with mixed anxiety disorders (social phobia, separation anxiety and generalized anxiety disorders), but without major depression. The advantage of the active compound was sizeable: 79% of children on the medication improved, compared to 28% on placebo. The superiority of the medication was detectable after 3 weeks of treatment, reached its peak after 6 weeks, and was maintained over the ensuing 2 weeks.

A previous literature review (Klein 1994) indicated that there was inconsistent support for the efficacy of tricyclic antidepressants in children with separation anxiety. A recent study found that imipramine was superior to placebo in adolescents with school refusal and anxiety disorders (Bernstein *et al.* 2000). Problematically, the patients also had major depression and therefore differed from previous samples. In spite of the fact that tricyclic antidepressants have not established efficacy in adolescent major depression (Klein *et al.* 1998), the possibility remains that the disorder contributed to the treatment results.

Although there have been some reports on the use of benzodiazepines in anxious children (Klein 1994), the safety profile of the SSRIs and recent evidence of their usefulness weaken consideration of benzodiazepines.

Conclusions

Although therapeutic research in anxiety disorders has progressed considerably, few studies of psychotherapy meet adequate methodological standards. Two of the three studies that have used a psychotherapy control condition failed to find an advantage for CBT in school phobic (Last *et al.* 1998) and phobic children (Silverman *et al.* 1999). Only one study, that focused on social phobia, found superiority for a behavioural intervention over a control treatment (Beidel *et al.* 2000). There is evidence supporting the merit of parental involvement in the child's treatment.

One large placebo controlled study obtained significant clinical superiority for an SSRI in children with anxiety disorders.

No investigations of the utility of combined treatments has been conducted.

Summary

A multiplicity of findings have contributed to a growing awareness of the possible importance of childhood anxiety disorders. These include findings of the common occurrence of child and adolescent anxiety disorders; the associated functional limitations they may incur; the fact that they put children at risk for later depression; and their moderate but significant continuity with anxiety disorders in adulthood.

Epidemiological studies of childhood anxiety disorders have generated divergent rates of current anxiety disorders. The overall evidence suggests a 5–10% prevalence in the general population, with girls being overrepresented. Gender also may influence course, in that some have found greater stability of anxiety in girls. Long-term stability has been found for social phobia, but less so for other specific childhood anxiety disorders. Childhood anxiety disorders have not been found to predict adult psychopathology other than anxiety and depression.

Identification of antecedants of childhood anxiety disorders would enable the identification of children at risk, and the development of appropriate treatment. Few antecedents have been established. Early temperament, specifically inhibited temperament, is weakly related to later anxiety, especially social phobia. A modest influence for genetic transmission has been found, with non-shared environmental factors playing a greater part in the occurrence of childhood anxiety disorders. Unfortunately, the nature of non-genetic factors in childhood anxiety disorders are poorly understood. As a result, they make little contribution to the clinical management of children with anxiety disorders.

Models of brain circuits that regulate fear in animals, and that have been studied in adults, are currently being applied to investigations of anxiety in children. Early studies suggest that children show the same abnormalities in underlying fear circuitry, as measured by startle responses to non-conditioned fear stimuli, and information processing of fear-related stimuli. However, it is difficult to determine which is cause and which is effect in the relationships between startle sensitivity and anxiety disorders. Neuroimaging studies of children are under way, focusing on the hypothesis that amygdala volume is positively related to anxiety disorders in children. At this time, the most well-documented biological feature of childhood anxiety is respiratory dysregulation, as indexed by hypersensitivity to CO_2 exposure, in children with anxiety disorders, especially those with separation anxiety disorder.

Treatment of anxiety disorders encompasses psychotherapeutic and psychopharmacological interventions. Treatment studies of anxious children, with one exception, have included a mixture of anxiety disorders, and have not distinguished among various anxiety disorders. Most psychotherapy studies have methodological limitations, but there is evidence of sustained improvement over time. Comparisons of different therapeutic approaches do not demonstrate superior efficacy of any one psychotherapeutic approach over others. Fluvoxamine, an SSRI, has been found effective in reducing anxiety in a placebo controlled study of a diagnostically mixed group of anxiety disordered children and adolescents. There now are treatments based on empirical evidence that can be offered to children with anxiety disorders.

References

Achenbach, T.M. (1991) *Manual for the Child Behavior Checklist and 1991 Child Behavior Profile*. Department of Psychiatry, University of Vermont, Burlington, VT.

Albano, A.M., Marten, P.A., Holt, C.S., Heimberg, R.G. & Barlow, D.H. (1995) Cognitive-behavioral group treatment for social phobia in adolescents: a preliminary study. *Journal of Nervous and Mental Disease*, 183, 649–656.

Alessi, N.E. & Magen, J. (1988) Panic disorder in psychiatrically hospitalized children. *American Journal of Psychiatry*, 145, 1450–1452.

Alpert, J.E., Maddocks, A., Rosenbaum, J.F. & Fava, M. (1994) Childhood psychopathology retrospectively assessed among adults with early onset major depression. *Journal of Affective Disorders*, 31, 165–171.

Ambrosini, P.J., Metz, C., Prabucki, K. & Lee, J. (1989) Videotape reliability of the third revised edition of the K-SADS. *Journal of the American Academy of Child and Adolescent Psychiatry*, 28, 723–728.

American Psychiatric Association (1980) *Diagnostic and Statistical Manual of Mental Disorders*, 3rd edn. American Psychiatric Association, Washington D.C.

American Psychiatric Association (1987) *Diagnostic and Statistical Manual of Mental Disorders–Revised*, 3rd edn. American Psychiatric Association, Washington D.C.

American Psychiatric Association (1994) *Diagnostic and Statistical Manual of Mental Disorders*, 4th edn. American Psychiatric Association, Washington D.C.

Anderson, J.C., Williams, S., McGee, R. & Silva, P.A. (1987) DSM-III disorders in preadolescent children: prevalence in a large sample from the general population. *Archives of General Psychiatry*, 44, 69–76.

Andrews, G. (1990) Evidence for a general neurotic syndrome. *British Journal of Psychiatry*, 157, 6–12.

Angold, A. & Costello, E.J. (1995) A test–retest reliability study of child-reported psychiatric symptoms and diagnoses using the child and adolescent psychiatric assessment (CAPA-C). *Psychological Medicine*, 25, 755–762.

Angold, A., Costello, E.J. & Worthman, C.M. (1998) Puberty and depression: the roles of age, pubertal status and pubertal timing. *Psychological Medicine*, 28, 51–61.

Ballenger, J.C., Carek, D.J., Steele, J.J. & Cornish-McTiche, D. (1989) Three cases of panic disorder with agoraphobia in children. *American Journal of Psychiatry*, 146, 922–924.

Barrett, P.M. (1998) Evaluation of cognitive-behavioral group treatments for childhood anxiety disorders. *Journal of Clinical Child Psychology*, 27, 459–468.

Barrett, P.M., Dadds, M.R. & Rapee, R.M. (1996) Family treatment of childhood anxiety: a controlled trial. *Journal of Consulting and Clinical Psychology*, 64, 333–342.

Battaglia, M., Bertella, S., Politi, E. *et al.* (1995) Age at onset of panic disorder: influence of familial liability to the disease and of childhood

separation anxiety disorder. *American Journal of Psychiatry*, 152, 1362–1364.

Beidel, D.C. & Turner, S.M. (1997) At risk for anxiety. I. Psychopathology in the offspring of anxious parents. *Journal of the American Academy of Child and Adolescent Psychiatry*, 36, 918–924.

Beidel, D.C., Turner, S.M. & Morris, T.L. (2000) Behavioral treatment of childhood social phobia. *Journal of Consulting and Clinical Psychology*, 68, 1072–1080.

Benjamin, R.S., Costello, E.J. & Warren, M. (1990) Anxiety disorders in a pediatric sample. *Journal of Anxiety Disorders*, 4, 293–316.

Berg, I. & Jackson, A. (1985) Teenage school refusers grow up: a follow-up study of 168 subjects, ten years on average after in-patient treatment. *British Journal of Psychiatry*, 147, 366–370.

Bernstein, G.A., Borchardt, C.M., Perwien, A.R. *et al.* (2000) Imipramine plus cognitive-behavioral therapy in the treatment of school refusal. *Journal of the American Academy of Child and Adolescent Psychiatry*, 39, 276–283.

Biederman, J. (1987) Clonazepam in the treatment of prepubertal children with panic-like symptoms. *Journal of Clinical Psychiatry*, 48, 38–41.

Biederman, J., Rosenbaum, J.F., Chaloff, J. & Kagan, J. (1995) Behavioral inhibition as a risk factor for anxiety disorders. In: *Anxiety Disorders in Children and Adolescents* (ed. J. March), pp. 61–81. Guilford Press, New York, NY.

Biederman, J., Rosenbaum, J.F. & Hirshfeld, D.R. (1990) Psychiatric correlates of behavioral inhibition in young children of parents with and without psychiatric disorders. *Archives of General Psychiatry*, 47, 21–26.

Bird, H.R., Canino, G., Rubio-Stipec, M. *et al.* (1988) Estimates of the prevalence of childhood maladjustment in a community survey in Puerto Rico. *Archives of General Psychiatry*, 29, 796–803.

Birmaher, B., Khetarpal, S., Brent, D. & Cully, M. (1997) The screen for child anxiety related emotional disorders (SCARED): scale construction and psychometric characteristics. *Journal of the American Academy of Child and Adolescent Psychiatry*, 36, 545–553.

Black, B. & Robbins, D.R. (1990) Panic disorder in children and adolescents. *Journal of the American Academy of Child and Adolescent Psychiatry*, 29, 36–44.

Blanchard, R.J., Griebel, G., Henrie, J.A. & Blanchard, D.C. (1997) Differentiation of anxiolytic and panicolytic drugs by effects on rat and mouse defense test batteries. *Neuroscience and Biobehavioral Reviews*, 21, 783–789.

Brady, E.U. & Kendall, P.C. (1992) Comorbidity of anxiety and depression in children and adolescents. *Psychological Bulletin*, 111, 244–255.

Breslau, N. & Klein, D.F. (1999) Smoking and panic attacks: an epidemiologic investigation. *Archives of General Psychiatry*, 56, 1141–1147.

Breslau, N., Davis, G.C. & Prabucki, K. (1988) Depressed mothers as informants in family history research—are they accurate? *Psychiatry Research*, 24, 345–359.

Breslau, N., Chilcoat, H.D., Kessler, R.C. & Davis, G.C. (1999) Previous exposure to trauma and PTSD effects of subsequent trauma: results from the Detroit Area Survey of Trauma. *American Journal of Psychiatry*, 156, 902–907.

Breslau, N., Chilcoat, H., Peterson, E. & Schultz, L. (2000) Gender differences in major depression: the role of anxiety. In: *Gender and its Effects on Psychopathology* (ed. E. Frank), pp. 132–149. American Psychiatric Press, Washington D.C.

Calkins, S.D., Fox, N.A. & Marshall, T.R. (1996) Behavioral and psychological antecedents of inhibited and uninhibited behavior. *Child Development*, 67, 523–540.

Capps, L., Sigman, M., Sena, R., Henker, B. & Whalen, C. (1996) Fear, anxiety and perceived control in children of agoraphobic parents. *Journal of Child Psychology and Psychiatry*, 37, 445–452.

Carlson, C., Lahey, B.B., Frame, C.L., Walker, J. & Hynd, G.W. (1987) Sociometric status of clinic-referred children with attention deficit disorders with and without hyperactivity. *Journal of Abnormal Child Psychology*, 15, 537–547.

Caspi, A., Moffitt, T.E., Newman, D.L. & Silva, P.A. (1996) Behavioral observations at age 3 years predict adult psychiatric disorders: longitudinal evidence from a birth cohort. *Archives of General Psychiatry*, 53, 1033–1039.

Cassella, J.V. & Davis, M. (1985) Fear-enhanced acoustic startle is not attenuated by acute or chronic imipramine. *Psychopharmacology*, 87, 278–282.

Caster, J.B., Inderbitzen, H.M. & Hope, D. (1999) Relationship between youth and parent perceptions of family environment and social anxiety. *Journal of Anxiety Disorders*, 13, 237–251.

Chambers, W.J., Puig-Antich, J., Hirsch, M. et al. (1985) The assessment of affective disorders in children and adolescents by semi-structured interview: test–retest reliability of the Schedule for Affective Disorders and Schizophrenia for School-Age Children, Present Episode Version. *Archives of General Psychiatry*, 42, 696–702.

Christie, K.A., Burke, J.D. Jr, Regier, D.A., Rae, D.S., Boyd, J.H. & Locke, B.Z. (1988) Epidemiologic evidence for early onset of mental disorders and higher risk of drug abuse in young adults. *American Journal of Psychiatry*, 145, 971–975.

Clark, D.B. & Donovan, J.E. (1994) Reliability and validity of the Hamilton Anxiety Rating Scale in an adolescent sample. *Journal of the American Academy of Child and Adolescent Psychiatry*, 33, 354–360.

Cohen, P., O'Connor, P., Lewis, S., Velez, N. & Malachowski, B. (1987) Comparison of DISC and K-SADS-P interviews of an epidemiological sample of children. *Journal of the American Academy of Child and Adolescent Psychiatry*, 26, 662–667.

Cohen, P., Cohen, J., Kasen, S. et al. (1993) An epidemiological study of disorders in late childhood and adolescence. I. Age- and gender-specific prevalence. *Journal of Child Psychology and Psychiatry*, 34, 851–867.

Coryell, W. (1997) Hypersensitivity to carbon dioxide as a disease specific trait marker. *Biological Psychiatry*, 41, 259–263.

Costello, E.J. & Angold, A. (1995) Epidemiology. In: *Anxiety Disorders in Children and Adolescents* (ed. J.S. March), pp. 109–124. Guilford Press, New York.

Costello, A.J., Edelbrock, C.S., Dulcan, M.K., Kalas, R. & Klaric, S.H. (1984) *Development and testing of the NIMH diagnostic interview schedule for children in a clinical population. Final report (Contract No RFD-DB-81-0027)*, Center for Epidemiological Studies, NIMH, Rockville, MD.

Costello, E.J., Costello, A.J., Edelbrock, C. et al. (1988) Psychiatric disorders in pediatric primary care. *Archives of General Psychiatry*, 45, 1107–1116.

Costello, E.J., Angold, A., Burns, B.J. et al. (1996) The Great Smoky Mountains study of youth. *Archives of General Psychiatry*, 53, 1129–1136.

Costello, E.J., Angold, A. & Keeler, G. (1999) Adolescent outcomes of childhood disorders: the consequences of severity and impairment. *Journal of the American Academy of Child and Adolescent Psychiatry*, 38, 121–128.

Curtis, G.C., Magee, W.J., Eaton, W.E., Wittchen, H.U. & Kessler, R.C. (1998) Specific fears and phobias: epidemiology and classification. *British Journal of Psychiatry*, 173, 212–217.

Dadds, M.R., Spence, S.H., Holland, D.E., Barrett, P.M. & Laurens, K.R. (1997) Prevention and early intervention for anxiety disorders: a controlled trial. *Journal of Consulting and Clinical Psychology*, 65, 627–635.

Davis, M. (1998) Are different parts of amygdala involved in fear versus anxiety? *Biological Psychiatry*, 44, 1239–1247.

De Bellis, M.D., Casey, B.J., Dahl, R.E. et al. (2000) A pilot study of amygdala volumes in pediatric generalized anxiety disorder. *Biological Psychiatry*, 48, 51–57.

DiBartolo, P.M., Albano, A.M., Barlow, D.H. & Heimberg, R.G. (1998) Cross-informant agreement in the assessment of social phobia in youth. *Journal of Abnormal Child Psychology*, 26, 213–220.

Eaton, W.W., Dryman, A. & Weissman, M.M. (1991) Panic and phobia. In: *Psychiatric Disorders in America: the Epidemiological Catchment Area Study* (eds L.N. Robins & D.A. Regier), pp. 155–179. Free Press, New York, NY.

Eaves, L.J., Silberg, J.L., Meyer, J.M. & Maes, H.H. (1997) Genetics and developmental psychopathology. II. The main effects of genes and environment on behavioral problems in the Virginia Twin Study of adolescent behavorial development. *Journal of Child Psychology and Psychiatry*, 38, 965–980.

Egger, H.L., Angold, A. & Costello, E.J. (1998) Headaches and psychopathology in children and adolescents. *Journal of the American Academy of Child and Adolescent Psychiatry*, 37, 951–958.

Essau, C.A., Conradt, J. & Petermann, F. (1999) Frequency and comorbidity of social phobia and social fears in adolescents. *Behaviour Research and Therapy*, 37, 831–843.

Feehan, M., McGee, R., Williams, S.M. & Anderson, J. (1993) Mental health disorders from age 15 to age 18 years. *Journal of the American Academy of Child and Adolescent Psychiatry*, 32, 1118–1126.

Fergusson, D.M., Horwood. L.J. & Lynskey, M.T. (1993) Prevalence and comorbidity of DSM-III-R diagnoses in a birth cohort of 15 year olds. *Journal of the American Academy of Child and Adolescent Psychiatry*, 32, 1127–1134.

Flakierska-Praquin, N., Lindstroem, M. & Gillberg, C. (1997) School phobia with separation anxiety disorder: a comparative 20- to 29-year follow-up study of 35 school refusers. *Comprehensive Psychiatry*, 38, 17–22.

Fyer, A.J. (1998) Current approaches to etiology and pathophysiology of specific phobia. *Biological Psychiatry*, 44, 1295–1304.

Fyer, A.J., Mannuzza, S., Chapman, T.F. et al. (1993) A direct interview family study of social phobia. *Archives of General Psychiatry*, 50, 286–293.

Gallagher, M. & Holland, P.C. (1994) The amygdala complex: multiple roles in associative learning and attention. *Proceedings of the National Academy of Science, USA*, 91, 11771–11776.

Goldstein, R.B., Weissman, M.M., Adams, P.B. & Horwath, E. (1994) Psychiatric disorders in relatives of probands with panic disorder and/or major depression. *Archives of General Psychiatry*, 51, 383–394.

Graham, P. & Rutter, M. (1968) The reliability and validity of the psychiatric assessment of the child. II. Interview with the parents. *British Journal of Psychiatry*, 114, 581–592.

Gurley, D., Cohen, P., Pine, D.S. & Brook, J. (1996) Discriminating depression and anxiety in youth: a role for diagnostic criteria. *Journal of Affective Disorders*, 39, 191–200.

Hamilton, M. (1959) The assessment of anxiety states by rating. *British Journal of Medical Psychology*, 3, 76–79.

Hamilton, M. (1969) Diagnosis and rating of anxiety. *British Journal of Psychiatry. Special Publication*, 3, 76–79.

Hayward, C., Killen, J.D., Kraemer, H.C. & Taylor, C.B. (1998) Linking self reported childhood behavioral inhibition to adolescent social phobia. *Journal of the American Academy of Child and Adolescent Psychiatry*, 38, 1308–1316.

Herjanic, B. & Reich, W. (1982) Development of a structured psychiatric interview for children: agreement between child and parent on individual symptoms. *Journal of Abnormal Child Psychology*, 10, 307–324.

Herskowitz, J. (1986) Neurologic presentations of panic disorder in childhood and adolescence. *Developmental Medicine and Child Neurology*, 28, 617–623.

Hirshfeld, D.R., Biederman, J., Brody, L., Faraone, S.V. & Rosenbaum, J.F. (1997) Expressed emotion toward children with behavioral inhibition: associations with maternal anxiety disorder. *Journal of the American Academy of Child and Adolescent Psychiatry*, 36, 910–917.

Hodges, K. (1990) Depression and anxiety in children: a comparison of self-report questionnaires to clinical interview. *Psychological Assessment*, 2, 376–381.

Horwath, E., Wolk, S.I., Goldstein, R.B. *et al.* (1995) Is the comorbidity between social phobia and panic disorder due to familial cotransmission or other factors? *Archives of General Psychiatry*, 52, 574–582.

Horwath, E., Wagner, V., Wickramaratne, P., Pine, D.S. & Weissman, M.M. (1998) Panic disorder and smothering symptoms: evidence for increased risk in first degree relatives. *Depression and Anxiety*, 6, 147–153.

Johnson, J.G., Cohen, P., Pine, D.S., Klein, D.F., Kasen, S. & Brooks, J.S. (2000) Association between cigarette smoking and anxiety disorders during adolescence and early adulthood. *Journal of the American Medical Association*, 284, 2348–2351.

Kagan, J., Reznick, J.S. & Snidman, N. (1988) Biological bases of childhood shyness. *Science*, 240, 167–171.

Kagan, J., Snidman, N. & Arcus, D. (1995) The role of temperament in social development. In: *Stress: Basic Mechanisms and Clinical Implications. Annals of the New York Academy of Sciences* (eds G.P. Chrousos & R. McCarty), pp. 485–490. New York Academy of Sciences, New York, NY.

Kashani, J.H., Beck, N.C., Hoeper, E.W. *et al.* (1987) Psychiatric disorders in a community sample of adolescents. *American Journal of Psychiatry*, 144, 584–589.

Kaufman, J., Birmaher, B., Brent, D. *et al.* (1997) Schedule for affective reliability and validity data. *Journal of the American Academy of Child and Adolescent Psychiatry*, 36, 980–988.

Kendall, P.C. (1994) Treating anxiety disorders in children: results of a randomized clinical trial. *Journal of Consulting and Clinical Psychology*, 62, 100–110.

Kendall, P.C. & Flannery-Schroeder, E.C. (1998) Methodological issues in treatment research for anxiety disorders in youth. *Journal of Abnormal Child Psychology*, 26, 27–38.

Kendall, P.C. & Ronan, K. (1990) Assessment of children's anxieties, fears and phobias: cognitive-behavioral models and methods. In: *Handbook of Psychological and Educational Assessment of Children: Personality, Behavior and Context* (eds C. Reynolds & R. Kamphaus), pp. 223–244. Guilford Press, New York.

Kendall, P.C. & Southam-Gerow, M.A. (1996) Long-term follow-up of a cognitive-behavioral therapy for anxiety-disordered youth. *Journal of Consulting and Clinical Psychology*, 64, 724–730.

Kendall, P.C., Flannery-Schroeder, E., Panichelli-Mindel, M. *et al.* (1997) Therapy for youths with anxiety disorders: a second randomized clinical trial. *Journal of Consulting and Clinical Psychology*, 65, 366–380.

Kendler, K.S. (1996) Major depression and generalised anxiety disorder. Same genes, (partly) different environments—revisited. *British Journal of Psychiatry* (Suppl.), 30, 68–75.

Kendler, K.S. (1997) The genetic epidemiology of psychiatric disorders: a current perspective. *Social Psychiatry and Psychiatric Epidemiology*, 32, 5–11.

Kendler, K.S., Karkowski, L.M. & Prescott, C.A. (1999) Fears and phobias: reliability and heritability. *Psychological Medicine*, 29, 539–553.

Kerr, M., Tremblay, R.E., Pagani, L. & Vitaro, F. (1997) Boy's behavioral inhibition and the risk of later delinquency. *Archives of General Psychiatry*, 54, 809–816.

Kessler, R.C. & Walters, E.E. (1998) Epidemiology of DSM-III-R major depression and minor depression among adolescents and young adults in the national comorbidity survey. *Depression and Anxiety*, 7, 3–14.

King, N., Tonge, B., Heyne, D. *et al.* (1998) Cognitive-behavioral treatment of school-refusing children: a controlled evaluation. *Journal of the American Academy of Child and Adolescent Psychiatry*, 37, 395–403.

Klein, D.F. (1978) A proposed definition of mental illness. In: *Critical Issues in Psychiatric Diagnosis* (eds R.L. Spitzer & D.F. Klein), pp. 41–71. Raven Press, New York.

Klein, D.F. (1993) False suffocation alarms, spontaneous panics, and related conditions: an integrative hypothesis. *Archives of General Psychiatry*, 50, 306–317.

Klein, R.G. (1994) Anxiety disorders. In: *Child and Adolescent Psychiatry: Modern Approaches* (eds M. Rutter, L. Hersov & E. Taylor), pp. 351–373. Blackwell Scientific Publications, Oxford.

Klein, R.G. (1995) Is panic disorder associated with childhood separation anxiety disorder? *Clinical Neuropharmacology*, 18, S7–S14.

Klein, D.F., Mannuzza, S., Chapman, T. & Fyer, A.J. (1992) Child panic revisited. *Journal of the American Academy of Child and Adolescent Psychiatry*, 31, 112–116.

Klein, R.G., Mannuzza, S., Koplewicz, H.S. *et al.* (1998) Adolescent depression: controlled desipramine treatment and atypical features. *Depression*, 7, 15–31.

Kramer, T. & Garralda, E. (1998) Psychiatric disorders in adolescents in primary care. *British Journal of Psychiatry*, 173, 508–513.

La Greca, A.M. & Lopez, N. (1998) Social anxiety among adolescents: linkages with peer relations and friendships. *Journal of Abnormal Child Psychology*, 26, 83–94.

La Greca, A.M. & Stone, W.L. (1993) Social anxiety scale for children-revised: factor structure and concurrent validity. *Journal of Clinical Child Psychology*, 22, 17–27.

La Greca, A.M., Dandes, S.K., Wick, P., Shaw, K. & Stone, W.L. (1988) Development of the social anxiety scale for children: reliability and concurrent validity. *Journal of Clinical Child Psychology*, 17, 84–91.

Labbate, L.A., Pollack, M.H., Otto, M.W. & Langenauer, S. (1994) Sleep panic attacks: an association with childhood anxiety and adult psychopathology. *Biological Psychiatry*, 36, 57–60.

Lapouse, R. & Monk, M.A. (1958) An epidemiologic study of behavior characteristics in children. *American Journal of Public Health*, 48, 1134–1144.

Last, C. (1998) Cognitive-behavioral treatment of school phobia. *Journal of the American Academy of Child and Adolescent Psychiatry*, 37, 404–411.

Last, C.G. & Strauss, C.C. (1989) Panic disorder in children and adolescents. *Journal of Anxiety Disorders*, 3, 87–95.

Last, C.G., Hersen, M., Kazdin, A., Orvaschel, H. & Perrin, S. (1991) Anxiety disorders in children and their families. *Archives of General Psychiatry*, 48, 928–934.

Last, C.G., Perrin, S., Hersen, M. & Kazdin, A.E. (1996) A prospective study of childhood anxiety disorders. *Journal of the American Academy of Child and Adolescent Psychiatry*, 35, 1502–1510.

Last, C., Hansen, C. & Franco, N. (1998) Cognitive-behavioral treatment of school phobia. *Journal of the American Academy of Child and Adolescent Psychiatry*, 37, 404–411.

Lerner, J., Safren, S.A., Henin, A. *et al.* (1999) Differentiating anxious and depressive self-statements in youth: factor structure of the negative affect self-statement questionnaire among youth referred to an anxiety disorders clinic. *Journal of Clinical Child Psychology*, 28, 82–93.

Lewinsohn, P.M., Seeley, J.R. & Gotlib, I.H. (1997) Depression-related psychosocial variables: are they specific to depression in adolescents? *Journal of Abnormal Psychology*, 106, 365–375.

Lewinsohn, P.M., Gotlib, I.H., Lewinsohn, M., Seeley, J.R. & Allen, N.B. (1998) Gender differences in anxiety disorders and anxiety symptoms in adolescents. *Journal of Abnormal Psychology*, 107, 109–117.

Links, P.S. (1983) Community surveys of the prevalence of childhood psychiatric disorders: a review. *Child Development*, 54, 531–548.

Magee, W.J., Eaton, W.W., Wittchen, H.-U., McGonagle, K.A. & Kessler, R.C. (1996) Agoraphobia, simple phobia, and social phobia in the National Comorbidity Survey. *Archives of General Psychiatry*, 53, 159–168.

Manfro, G.G., Otto, M.W., McArdle, E.T. *et al.* (1996) Relationship of antecedent stressful life events to childhood and family history of anxiety and the course of panic disorder. *Journal of Affective Disorders*, 41, 135–139.

March, J.S. & Albano, A.M. (1998) New developments in assessing pediatric anxiety disorders. In: *Advances in Clinical Child Psychology* (eds T.H. Ollendick & R.J. Prinz), pp. 213–241. Plenum Press, New York.

March, J.S., Parker, J.D.A., Sullivan, K. & Stallings, P. (1997) The multidimensional anxiety scale for children (MASC): factor structure, reliability, and validity. *Journal of the American Academy of Child and Adolescent Psychiatry*, 36, 554–565.

McGee, R., Feehan, M., Williams, S. *et al.* (1990) DSM-III disorders in a large sample of adolescents. *Journal of the American Academy of Child and Adolescent Psychiatry*, 29, 161–169.

McGee, R., Feehan, M., Williams, S. & Anderson, J. (1992) DSM-III disorders from age 11 to age 15 years. *Journal of the American Academy of Child and Adolescent Psychiatry*, 31, 50–59.

McNally, R.J. (1996) Cognitive bias in the anxiety disorder. *Nebraska Symposium on Motivation*, 43, 211–250.

Mendlowitz, S.L., Manassis, K., Bradley, S. *et al.* (1999) Cognitive-behavioral group treatment in childhood anxiety disorders: the role of parent involvement. *Journal of the American Academy of Child and Adolescent Psychiatry*, 38, 1223–1229.

Merikangas, K.R., Dierker, L.C. & Szamari, P. (1998) Psychopathology among offspring of parents with substance abuse and/or anxiety disorders: a high risk study. *Journal of Child Psychology and Psychiatry*, 39, 711–720.

Merikangas, K.R., Avenevoli, S., Dierker, L. & Grillon, C. (1999) Vulnerability factors among children at risk for anxiety. *Biological Psychiatry*, 46, 1523–1535.

Monga, S., Birmaher, B., Chiappetta, L. *et al.* (2000) Screen for Child Anxiety-Related Emotional Disorders (SCARED): convergent and divergent validity. *Depression and Anxiety*, 12, 85–91.

MTA Cooperative Group (1999) A 14-month randomized clinical trial of treatment strategies for attention-deficit/hyperactivity disorder. *Archives of General Psychiatry*, 56, 1073–1086.

Nelles, W.B. & Barlow, D.H. (1988) Do children panic? *Clinical Psychological Review*, 8, 359–372.

Newman, D.L., Moffitt, T.E., Capsi, A. & Silva, P.A. (1998) Comorbid mental disorders: implications for treatment and sample selection. *Journal of Abnormal Psychology*, 107, 305–311.

Ollendick, T.H. (1983) Reliability and validity of the revised Fear Survey Schedule for Children (FSSC-R). *Behaviour Research and Therapy*, 21, 685–692.

Orvaschel, H., Puig-Antich, J., Chambers, W., Tabrizi, M.A. & Johnson, R. (1982) Retrospective assessment of prepubertal major depression with the Kiddie-SADS-E. *Journal of the American Academy of Child and Adolescent Psychiatry*, 21, 392–397.

Otto, M.W. & Whittal, M.L. (1995) Cognitive-behavior therapy and the longitudinal course of panic disorder. *Psychiatric Clinics of North America*, 18, 803–820.

Perna, G., Cocchi, S., Bertani, A., Arancio, C. & Bellodi, L. (1995) Sensitivity to 35% CO_2 in healthy first-degree relatives of patients with panic disorder. *American Journal of Psychiatry*, 152, 623–625.

Pine, D.S., Cohen, P. & Brook, J. (1996) The association between major depression and headaches: results of a longitudinal epidemiological study in youth. *Journal of Child and Adolescent Psychopharmacology*, 6, 153–164.

Pine, D.S., Cohen, P., Gurley, D., Brook, J. & Ma, Y. (1998a) The risk for early-adulthood anxiety and depressive disorders in adolescents with anxiety and depressive disorders. *Archives of General Psychiatry*, 55, 56–64.

Pine, D.S., Coplan, J.D., Papp, L.A. *et al.* (1998b) Ventilatory physiology of children and adolescents with anxiety disorders. *Archives of General Psychiatry*, 55, 123–129.

Pine, D.S., Cohen, E., Cohen, P. & Brook, J.S. (2000a) Social phobia and the persistence of conduct problems. *Journal of Child Psychology and Psychiatry*, 41, 657–665.

Pine, D.S., Klein, R.G., Coplan, J.D. *et al.* (2000b) Differential CO_2 sensitivity in childhood anxiety disorders and non-ill comparisons. *Archives of General Psychiatry*, 57, 960–967.

Prior, M., Smart, D., Sanson, A. & Oberklaid, F. (2000) Does shy-inhibited temperament in childhood lead to anxiety problems in adolescence? *Journal of the American Academy of Child and Adolescent Psychiatry*, 39, 461–468.

Rachman, S.J. (1990) *Fear and Courage*. Freeman, New York.

Raine, A., Reynolds, C., Venables, P.H., Mednick, S.A. & Farrington, D.P. (1998) Fearlessness, stimulation-seeking, and large body size at age 3 years as early predisposition to childhood aggression at age 11 years. *Archives of General Psychiatry*, 56, 283–284.

Reed, V. & Wittchen, H.U. (1998) DSM-IV panic attacks and panic disorder in a community sample of adolescents and young adults: how specific are panic attacks? *Journal of Psychiatric Research*, 32, 335–345.

Reich, W., Shayka, J.J. & Taibleson, C. (1991) *Diagnostic Interview for Children and Adolescents (DICA-R-C)*, Division of Child Psychiatry, Washington University, St. Louis.

Renaud, J., Birmaher, B., Wassick, S.C. & Bridge, J. (1999) Use of selective serotonin reuptake inhibitors for the treatment of childhood panic disorder: a pilot study. *Journal of Child and Adolescent Psychopharmacology*, 9, 73–83.

Rende, R., Wickramaratne, P., Warner, V. & Weissman, M.M. (1995) Sibling resemblance for psychiatric disorders in offspring at high and low risk for depression. *Journal of Child Psychology and Psychiatry*, 36, 1353–1363.

Reynolds, C.R. & Richmond, B.O. (1985) *Revised children's Manifest Anxiety Scale: Manual*. Western Psychological Services, Los Angeles, CA.

Robins, L.N. (1978) Sturdy childhood predictors of adult antisocial behavior: replications from longitudinal studies. *Psychological Medicine*, 8, 611–622.

Robins, E.N. & Guze, S. (1970) Establishment of diagnostic validity in psychiatric illness: its application to schizophrenia. *American Journal of Psychiatry*, **126**, 983–987.

Robins, L.N. & Regier, D.A., eds. (1995) *Psychiatric Disorders in America: the Epidemiological Catchment Area Study*. Free Press, New York, NY.

Ronan, K.R., Kendall, P.C. & Rowe, M. (1994) Negative affectivity in children: development and validation of a self-statement questionnaire. *Cognitive Therapy and Research*, **18**, 509–528.

Roy-Byrne, P.P. & Cowley, D.S. (1998) Pharmacological treatment of panic, generalized anxiety, and phobic disorders. In: *Treatments That Work* (eds P.E. Nathan & J.M. Gorman), pp. 319–338. Oxford Press, New York.

Rubin, R.K. (1993) The Waterloo longitudinal project: correlates and consequences of social withdrawal from childhood to adolescence. In: *Social Withdrawal, Inhibition, and Shyness in Childhood* (eds K.H. Rubin & J.B. Asendorpf), pp. 291–314. Lawrence Erlbaum, Hillsdale, NJ.

Rueter, M.A., Scaramella, L., Wallace, L.E. & Conger, R.D. (1999) First onset of depressive or anxiety disorders predicted by the longitudinal course of internalizing symptoms and parent–adolescent disagreements. *Archives of General Psychiatry*, **56**, 726–732.

RUPP Anxiety Study Group (The Research Units on Pediatric Psychopharmacology) (2001) Fluvoxamine treatment of anxiety disorders in children and adolescents. *New England Journal of Medicine*, **344**, 1279–1285.

Rutter, M. (1997) Clinical implications of attachment concepts: retrospect and prospect. In: *Attachment and Psychopathology* (eds L. Atkinson & K.J. Zucker), pp. 17–46. Guilford Press, New York, NY.

Scherer, M.W. & Nakamura, C.Y. (1968) A Fear Survey Schedule for Children (FSS-FC): a factor analytic comparison with manifest anxiety (CMAS). *Behavior Research and Therapy*, **6**, 173–182.

Schwab-Stone, M.E., Shaffer, D., Dulcan, M.K. & Jensen, P.S. (1996) Criterion validity of the NIMH Diagnostic Interview Schedule for Children, Version 2.3 (DISC-2.3). *Journal of the American Academy of Child and Adolescent Psychiatry*, **35**, 878–888.

Schwartz, C.E., Snidman, N. & Kagan, J. (1999) Adolescent social anxiety as an outcome of inhibited temperament in childhood. *Journal of the American Academy of Child and Adolescent Psychiatry*, **38**, 1008–1015.

Shaffer, D., Fisher, P., Dulcan, M.K. *et al.* (1996) The NIMH Diagnostic Interview Schedule for Children, Version 2.3 (DISC 2.3): description, acceptability, prevalence rates, and performance in the MECA study. *Psychiatric Clinics of North America*, **35**, 865–877.

Shaffer, D., Gould, M.S., Brasic, J. *et al.* (1983) A children's global assessment scale (CGAS). *Archives of General Psychiatry*, **20**, 1228–1231.

Shaffer, D., Lucas, C.P. & Richters, J.E. (1999) *Diagnostic Assessment in Child and Adolescent Psychopathology*. Guilford Press, New York, NY.

Silverman, W. & Albano, A.M. (1996) *Anxiety Disorders Interview Schedule for Children (ADIS-C)*. Graywind Publications, State University of New York, Albany.

Silverman, W.K. & Rabian, B. (1999) Rating scales for anxiety and mood disorders. In: *Diagnostic Assessment in Child and Adolescent Psychopathology* (eds D. Shaffer & C. Lucas), pp. 127–166. Guilford Press, New York, NY.

Silverman, W.K., Kurtines, W.M., Ginsburg, G.S. *et al.* (1999) Contingency management, self-control, and education support in the treatment of childhood phobic disorders: a randomized clinical trial. *Journal of Consulting and Clinical Psychology*, **67**, 675–687.

Simonoff, E. (2000) Extracting meaning from comorbidity: genetic analyses that make sense. *Journal of Child Psychology and Psychiatry*, **41**, 667–674.

Simonoff, E., Pickles, A., Meyer, J.M. *et al.* (1997) The Virginia Twin Study of adolescent behavioral development. *Archives of General Psychiatry*, **54**, 801–808.

Spielberger, C.D. (1973) *State-Trait Anxiety Inventory for Children*. Consulting Psychologists Press, Palo Alto, CA.

Topolski, T.D. (1998) A twin study of genetic and environmental influences on anxiety during childhood and adolescence. *Dissertation Abstracts International: Section B: the Sciences and Engineering*, **58**, 3936.

Topolski, T.D., Hewitt, J.K., Eaves, L.J. *et al.* (1997) Genetic and environmental influences on child reports of manifest anxiety and symptoms of separation anxiety and overanxious disorders: a community-based twin study. *Behavior Genetics*, **27**, 15–28.

Topolski, T.D., Hewitt, J.K., Evans, L. *et al.* (1999) Genetic and environmental influences on ratings of manifest anxiety by parents and children. *Journal of Anxiety Disorders*, **13**, 371–397.

Turner, S.M., Beidel, D.C. & Costello, A. (1987) Psychopathology in the offspring of anxiety disorder patients. *Journal of Consulting and Clinical Psychology*, **55**, 229–235.

Vasey, M.W., Daleiden, E.L., Williams, L.L. & Brown, L.M. (1995) Biased attention in childhood anxiety disorders: a preliminary study. *Journal of Abnormal Child Psychology*, **23**, 267–278.

Velez, C.N., Johnson, J. & Cohen, P. (1989) A longitudinal analysis of selected risk factors for childhood psychopathology. *Psychiatric Clinics of North America*, **28**, 861–864.

Verhulst, F.C., van der Ende, J., Ferdinand, R.F. & Kasius, M.C. (1997) The prevalence of DSM-III-R diagnoses in a national sample of Dutch adolescents. *Archives of General Psychiatry*, **54**, 329–336.

Warner, V., Mufson, L. & Weissman, M.M. (1995) Offspring at high and low risk for depression and anxiety: mechanisms of psychiatric disorder. *Journal of the American Academy of Child and Adolescent Psychiatry*, **34**, 786–797.

Warren, S.L., Huston, L., Egeland, B. & Sroufe, L.A. (1997) Child and adolescent anxiety disorders and early attachment. *Journal of the American Academy of Child and Adolescent Psychiatry*, **36**, 637–644.

Weissman, M.M., Leckman, J.F., Merikangas, K.R., Gammon, G.D. & Prusoff, B.A. (1984) Depression and anxiety disorders in parents and children: results from the Yale family study. *Archives of General Psychiatry*, **41**, 845–852.

Weissman, M.M., Bland, R.C., Canino, G.J. *et al.* (1997) The cross-national epidemiology of panic disorder. *Archives of General Psychiatry*, **54**, 305–309.

Whittaker, A., Johnson, J., Shaffer, D. *et al.* (1990) Uncommon troubles in young people: prevalence estimates of selected psychiatric disorders in a non-referred adolescent population. *Archives of General Psychiatry*, **47**, 487–496.

WHO (World Health Organization) (1990) *Composite International Diagnostic Interview (Version 1.0)*. Geneva, Switzerland.

Wickramaratne, P.J. & Weissman, M.M. (1998) Onset of psychopathology in offspring by developmental phase and parental depression. *Journal of the American Academy of Child and Adolescent Psychiatry*, **37**, 933–942.

Williams, S., Anderson, J., McGee, R. & Silva, P. (1990) Risk factors for behavioral and emotional disorder in preadolescent children. *Journal of the American Academy of Child and Adolescent Psychiatry*, **29**, 413–419.

Williams, J.M.G., Mathews, A. & MacLeod, C. (1996) The emotional stroop task and psychopathology. *Psychological Bulletin*, **120**, 3–24.

Wittchen, H.-U., Lachner, G., Wunderllich, U. & Pfister, H. (1998) Test–retest reliability of the computerized DSM-IV version of the Munich Composite International Diagnostic Interview (M-CIDI). *Social Psychiatry and Psychiatric Epidemiology*, 33, 568–578.

Wittchen, H.U., Stein, M.B. & Kessler, R.C. (1999) Social fears and social phobia in a community sample of adolescents and young adults: prevalence, risk factors and co-morbidity. *Psychological Medicine*, 29, 309–323.

31 Adjustment Disorders

Peter Hill

Introduction

Adjustment disorder has the curious distinction of being the only condition in the major classification schemes for psychiatric disorders, ICD-10 (World Health Organization 1992) and DSM-IV (American Psychiatric Association 1994) that has no characteristic psychopathological picture. Its nature is essentially defined by the exclusion of a major category axis I disorder, its relationship to a putative stressor, and its duration. It might, with reason, be regarded as a historical anachronism. Indeed, the history of the concept of adjustment reaction or disorder reflects the history of Western thought about childhood psychiatric disorder for most of the last century. In DSM-I (American Psychiatric Association 1952) it was one of only two categories of childhood psychiatric disorder listed, the other being childhood schizophrenia.

Early definitions and papers reviewing the concept reveal the extent to which earlier clinicians conceptualized childhood and adolescent psychiatric disorder as a reaction to both external stressors and to internal mental developmental processes. This approach appears to have been coupled with a prejudice against using psychiatric disorder categories when children were considered and an apparent assumption that psychiatric disorders in the young were transient and not serious (Weiner & Del Gaudio 1976). Certainly adjustment reaction or disorder were commonly used labels. In the USA, 'adjustment reaction' and 'transient situational disturbance' were the most common diagnoses in child and adolescent psychiatric practice in the early 1960s (Rosen *et al.* 1964). Originally these concepts seem to have been remarkably vague, as well as all-encompassing, and were criticized accordingly (Fard *et al.* 1978). This led to a tightening of criteria in subsequent editions of ICD and DSM, restricting the concept to a relatively brief abnormal psychological reaction (not amounting to a major psychiatric disorder) to an acute external event. Even so, criticism of the concept continued (Newcorn & Strain 1992; Hill 1994), albeit with recognition that some classificatory mechanism was required to accommodate abnormal psychological reactions to external adversity that did not amount to major psychiatric disorder.

Adjustment disorder is a popular term with many psychiatrists. Setterburg *et al.* (1991) surveyed US child psychiatrists and reported that the diagnosis was more frequently used by those who were psychodynamically trained, older, and in office rather than hospital practice. Some 55% of those surveyed stated that they employed the diagnosis specifically in order to avoid stigmatization of the patient. The authors also commented that the diagnosis retained its popularity because of the way in which its non-specific wording maintained a degree of confidentiality as to the exact nature of the psychopathology and did not prejudice subsequent life insurance application. Reviewing the published literature with this in mind, it is interesting how prevalent the term is in studies of adolescent psychiatric inpatient populations (e.g. 34% of the adolescents in Greenberg *et al.* 1995) given its supposed mildness and brevity. Its popularity is not entirely American, however; figures from Pelkonen *et al.*'s (2000) study indicate a prevalence of 29% among outpatients in a Finnish clinic.

The current approach taken in ICD-10 recognizes three main categories of reaction to acute stress, irrespective of age: acute stress reaction, post-traumatic stress disorder (PTSD) and adjustment disorder. The latter is divided further into six main subcategories defined symptomatically (with respect to presence of depression, other emotional disturbance or conduct problems) and an 'other' category.

For the core diagnosis of adjustment disorder, 'subjective distress and emotional disturbance, usually interfering with social functioning and performance' needs to have arisen 'in the period of adaptation to a significant life change or to the consequences of a stressful life event'. 'None of the symptoms is of sufficient severity or prominence in its own right to justify a more specific diagnosis.' Stressors should be more than minor, and the onset of the disorder is said to be 'usually' within 1 month of the occurrence of the stressful event, 'significant life change leading to continued unpleasant life circumstances', or life crisis. A period of more than 3 months between stressor and symptom onset indicates that the disorder should be classified differently. For most reactions, the duration of symptoms will not normally exceed 6 months, although brief and prolonged depressive reactions have maximum limits of 1 month and 2 years, respectively, and, if it does, the diagnosis should be changed to a more specific category. The identified stressful event or situation can be coded with a separate Z code or, for children and adolescents, listed in axis V (associated abnormal psychosocial situations) of the multiaxial version of ICD-10. Subsection 6 of axis 5 (acute life events) is most likely to be invoked. For an experience to be included it must be 'significantly abnormal in the context of the child's level of development, past experiences and prevailing sociocultural circumstances'.

Although adjustment disorder is intended to be a category

that can be applied to all age groups, some comments in the diagnostic guidelines apply specifically to children. The subcategory 'with predominant disturbance of other emotions' 'should also be used for reactions in children in which regressive behaviour, such as bed-wetting or thumb-sucking, are also present'. Later in the guidelines an adolescent grief reaction resulting in aggressive or dissocial behaviour is given as an instance of the subcategory 'with predominant disturbance of conduct'. Separation anxiety disorder, which must have an onset in the preschool years, is specifically excluded, but 'hospitalism' in children is included.

The definition of adjustment disorder provided in DSM-IV is very similar: marked disproportionate distress coupled with significant impairment of social, occupational or academic functioning arising within 3 months of exposure to an identifiable stressor and lasting no more than 6 months after the stressor has ceased. The stressor can be of any severity, not necessarily extreme. Bereavement is excluded unless the reaction is excessive or protracted. Severity is mild: 'the stress-related disturbance does not meet the criteria for another specific axis I disorder'. There is provision for subtyping, very much as in ICD-10. A chronic variant can be invoked if the psychological disturbance lasts more than 6 months in response to 'a stressor that has enduring consequences'.

An original notion that there is a specific type of psychological distress or disturbed behaviour that is the result of a stressor, external or internal, and which can be recognized as a disorder has thus been modified. This is in response to a mounting volume of evidence that various adversities, acute and chronic, can contribute to the causation or maintenance of psychiatric disorder in the young (see Friedman & Chase-Lansdale, Chapter 15; Sandberg & Rutter, Chapter 17; Yule, Chapter 32). The impact of adverse circumstances is now recognized to be relevant to a number of other psychiatric conditions and the concept of adjustment disorder has shrunk to indicating a mild, short-lived and non-specific reaction to an adversity that is itself circumscribed in duration.

In the ICD-10 clinical description, the points are made that there is commonly a plurality of emotional symptoms and that there needs to be a careful evaluation of relationships among form, content and severity, previous personality and the stressor. This is the kernel of the concept, which in both classification schemes has four or possibly five components.

1 Distress or disturbance of functioning that is beyond the normal expected range or is maladaptive.

2 Psychopathology less severe than a major category diagnosis would require.

3 An identifiable stressor that is an event or onset of change in circumstances occurring within a maximum of 3 months prior to onset of the disorder. This must be of significant but not overwhelming severity, and it is a necessary condition for the disorder to be diagnosed.

4 Relatively short duration (usually a maximum of 6 months).

5 Not an exacerbation of previously identified psychopathology.

From this, some critical issues emerge that have to do with caseness and normality.

Threshold issues

To qualify as a disorder, a pattern of symptoms or signs has to be associated with clinically significant distress or impairment in social, occupational or other important areas of functioning. In DSM-IV and the Diagnostic Criteria for Research edition of ICD-10 (World Health Organization 1993) a minimum number of clinical features must be present for caseness. By definition, adjustment disorder can only be diagnosed when criteria for a major category disorder are not met. The impairment criteria specified in ICD-10 are vague: '*usually* interfering with social functioning and performance'; '*some* degree of disability in the performance of daily routine'. The duration of an adjustment disorder is brief, by definition.

There is not always a predictable correlation between the number of symptoms and the degree of impairment, yet the major classification schemes determine caseness by symptom counts. This can be criticized. Harrington's group (quoted in Harrington & Clark 1998) have demonstrated that one or two severe symptoms of adolescent depression can be associated with very substantial impairment yet be an insufficient number to qualify as a major category disorder. From data accumulated in the Great Smoky Mountains epidemiological study, Angold *et al.* (1999) were able to make a similar point. If caseness is restricted to those children whose psychopathology contains a given minimum number of symptoms or signs specified in a major category psychiatric disorder, some instances of what would otherwise be considered as illness or disorder and that represent a health care need will be missed.

Impairment appears to be a fundamental variable in determining prognosis, trumping symptom counts. Costello *et al.* (1999) examined the psychiatric status of adolescents 5–7 years after first assessment in childhood. Children with 'threshold' status (symptom count satisfying DSM criteria but of insufficient severity for clinical caseness) were subdivided into those with and without impairment. Threshold status might be thought comparable with the degree of clinical severity indicated by a diagnosis of adjustment disorder. Threshold children without impairment had the same long-tem outlook as healthy children. The presence of impairment in conjunction with threshold status provided an intermediate prognosis compared with clinical-level impaired cases.

Nevertheless, functional impairment is not an all-or-none feature; it can fluctuate and be measured in its own right. Scales of personal functioning, such as the Children's Global Assessment Scale (C-GAS; Shaffer *et al.* 1983) or the Functional Impairment Scale for Children and Adolescents (FISCA; Frank & Paul 1995; Frank *et al.* 2000) do not indicate a clear cut-off for impairment, although a consensus as to the level below which *most* cases of agreed disorder fall can be established. In the Puerto Rican general population study (Bird *et al.* 1988), the prevalence of adjustment disorder in children varied from 7.6% when a C-GAS cut-off score of 70 or less was employed, to 4.2% at the inferior level of functioning of 60 or below.

The situation with respect to caseness is thus less than clearcut. The usefulness of an adjustment disorder concept is that it can accommodate some cases in which there is a clinical need but a major category disorder cannot be said to be present. It describes a subthreshold, or subsyndromal condition, something of potential importance in primary care practice. Clear assessment of associated impairment seems important, yet the time constraints on duration and the temporal relation with a stressor still limit its applicability in this respect. In the previous edition, this chapter was critical of the concept of adjustment disorder and suggested it be recast as a V code. In the same vein, Pincus et al. (1999) have suggested it be abolished and a subthreshold category created in each of the major disorder sections. This would free matters from the time constraints. A condition would be subthreshold if either the symptom count or impairment criterion were not met.

Establishing an aetiological link with the stressor

Reactions to acute stressors are already subclassified in the major classification systems. In an acute stress reaction, a state of mute disorientated bewilderment lasting only a few hours or days is typical and quite commonly seen in children subject to severe life-threatening experiences, such as road traffic accidents. Astute observation reveals them commonly to be highly aroused in autonomic terms. Clinically, it seems more likely to be evident when a child has no access to attachment figures, although their presence does not necessarily prevent its occurrence.

Post-traumatic stress disorder is a classic example of a pattern of more protracted symptoms that have a defined relationship to an extremely stressful event (see Yule, Chapter 32). It is well recognized that other psychological and psychiatric symptom patterns can follow such stress. Moreover, the classic pattern of formal PTSD is not absolute; rather, it is at the severe end of a spectrum of post-traumatic reactions displaying the same component symptoms.

Adjustment disorder is conceptualized as arising as a result of a less catastrophic but acute experience. This acute experience may not be as potent an aetiological factor as it seems. Indeed, Rutter & Sandberg (1992; see Sandberg & Rutter, Chapter 17) point out that an acute adverse experience occurring in isolation is usually not pathogenic and the interaction with chronic stressors is critical. In a particular case, the aetiological contribution of previously existing chronic stressors may be proportionally greater but masked by a recent dramatic acute event serving as the straw on the camel's back. Yet it is this event that forms the base from which are drawn the time limits specified in the diagnostic rules. Furthermore, the definition of adjustment disorder refers to a linear model of causation that does not square easily with what is known about the impact of adversities on children's

minds. For instance, the extent to which an individual's behaviour contributes to the likelihood of future adversity, even apparently independent life events, needs consideration (see Sandberg & Rutter, Chapter 17).

The association between apparent stressor and reaction will necessarily be based on post hoc reasoning. It will rest upon a clinical judgement as to how closely the stressor relates to the behaviour or emotional disorder in terms of form and content or in temporal proximity. Effectively, a verstehende concept applies in that the type of stressor and the extent and content of the psychopathology must be understood by the observer to be semantically related. However, when an attempt is made to link disorder with life events in childhood, it is apparent that the association between type of event and type of disorder is generally weak (Goodyer et al. 1985) and even extreme stressors do not consistently produce predictable types of reactions such as PTSD.

Timing

In the definition of adjustment disorder, the time elapsing between the putative stressor and the onset of the adjustment disorder is set at a maximum of 3 months. From the study of Kovacs et al. (1995) on children in whom the stressor was a first diagnosis of diabetes, this would seem appropriate. Thirty-one patients had developed an adjustment disorder in that period; extending the time frame to 6 months only identified another two.

Although not a study of adjustment disorder, it is interesting that Goodyer et al. (2000) found that when undesirable life events are considered in relation to major depression, only events in the preceding month before onset were relevant. However, only 53% of episodes of major depression were preceded by such an event. The other cases may have responded to the impact of daily hassles. Indeed, some reviewers have suggested that these are more likely to predict psychopathology than are major events (Leadbeater et al. 1995; see Sandberg & Rutter, Chapter 17). Timing obviously becomes more difficult when daily stressors rather than discrete events are considered.

Both classificatory schemes specify a 6-month maximum duration after which reclassification is required, although it is not explained why such a time was selected. Clearly, this constraint is often neglected, as admitted by the majority of those psychiatrists surveyed by Setterburg et al. (1991). Furthermore, there is the issue, not just of what the time course of understandable reactive distress might be, but whether this can be related to a definition of disorder. If one takes bereavement as the paradigm for a stressor that can lead to an adjustment reaction, then it is instructive to note that in Fristad et al.'s (1993) study, one-third of children were at their most distressed 6 months after the death, although by 13 months matters had subsided somewhat. However, duration of disorder may vary with stressor. Kovacs et al. (1995) found that the average episode length for adjustment disorder following an initial diagnosis of diabetes was 3 months. However, in that study 5 of 33 children had episodes lasting longer than 6 months, although all had recovered by 9 months. In the same group's related study of children with adjustment disorder in a psychiatric clinic, the mean duration of disorder was 9 months (range 3–24 months). In contrast to the notion of prolonged depressive reaction in ICD-10 (the only subtype to allow a 2-year duration), there was either no difference in duration between subtypes (Kovacs *et al.* 1995) or a trend for depressive subtypes to recover faster (Kovacs *et al.* 1995).

A key complicating issue is that children's response to a stressor is not just their own distress at the experience but mediated through the reactions of their carers, often exposed to the same stressor. For instance, Van Eerdewegh *et al.* (1985) and Dowdney *et al.* (1999) demonstrated a relationship between the amount of parental psychopathology and the child's emotional and behavioural status following parental bereavement. With this in mind, it is probable that the time limitations set for adults might not be appropriate for children dependent on carers who are also affected by similar life stresses.

Abnormality

There is an implicit assumption in the concept of an adjustment disorder that normal patterns of adjustment to stressors are sufficiently well defined for a normality to be identifiable by referring to:

• quality of response—a deviation from normal reaction patterns to the stressor in question;

• quantitative issues, such as number of symptoms or excessive duration; and

• adaptive vs. maladaptive response.

However, there is often no clear indication of what the limits of normality are. For instance, with respect to qualitative abnormalities in bereavement reactions (the example cited in ICD-10), Kranzler (1990) demonstrated that better studies of grief in children reveal that aspects of the bereavement response previously considered pathological may be seen in most bereaved children. This can result in normal bereavement being seen as abnormal and lead to unnecessary interventions (Harrington & Harrison 1999).

Frequency and intensity of symptoms, or chronicity would be a better indicator of abnormality rather than presence or absence of particular features. However, estimating the normal intensity or duration of responses to adverse events is not straightforward and may indeed be difficult for many psychiatrists (Malt 1986). Accurate judgement would involve an extensive knowledge of how the stressor impinges upon the individual child in terms of the child's attributions or previous sensitization, as well as being able to assess the contribution of associated chronic adversity. A more general appeal to empirical data may help but little because of the influence of development and context. With respect to children's reactions to divorce as an event, for instance, responses are known to alter by age and sex, according to the quality of previous family relationships, and to

continuing features of relationships between the parents and between parents and children (Kelly 2000).

It is also necessary to determine that the child's reaction is maladaptive, placing him or her at risk or at an avoidable disadvantage, as in repeated acts of deliberate self-harm. Clinicians seem especially likely to diagnose an adjustment reaction when an adolescent, for instance, takes an overdose (Martunnen *et al.* 1994; Greenberg *et al.* 1995; Nasser & Overholser 1999), yet such an action, although at first sight clearly maladaptive, may ultimately prove beneficial if it recruits help in resolving the child's predicament. There is a difficulty in moving beyond the descriptive to evaluating the cost to the child because this may alter according to whether short- or long-term benefits are considered. There may be potential in identifying deviation from normal patterns of coping and this is now considered further.

Coping strategies

The very term 'adjustment disorder' implies that the process of satisfactory adjustment to or coping with a stressor is awry or insufficient. The affected young person either uses a method of coping that is counterproductive and thus maladaptive, or their mind is overwhelmed and symptoms result which are not those of acute stress reaction or classical PTSD. In order to make a judgement about this, a knowledge of normal coping and normal responses to stress is necessary, but this field is young and much of what is known is provisional and culture-bound.

A major difficulty is that prediction of coping method depends upon several factors. Frydenberg (1997, p. 5), doubtless with tongue in cheek, suggested the quasi-mathematical formula:

$$C = f(P + S + pS),$$

where C is coping, P is the individual person, S the situational determinant, and pS the perceived situation).

It is possible to make some generalizations. The language and the conceptual models used in coping research are becoming useful for clinical approaches. Thus, in one model (Rice *et al.* 1993) stressors may be:

• *normative* or generic, experienced by all children during development (e.g. separation from parents in order to attend school, public examinations);

• *non-normative*, which is peculiar to the individual and may be subdivided into acute (e.g. bereavement) and chronic (e.g. bullying, parental discord) (Compas *et al.* 1993); and

• daily hassles, relatively minor but cumulative.

These become more or less stressful according to their *number*, *timing* and *synchronicity*.

A very similar position but using different terms was taken by Graber & Brooks-Gunn (1996) who suggested an interplay among *transitions* (universal experiences in development), *turning points* (unique experiences), and the ways in which the number, synchronicity and timing of these (e.g. in relation to age) govern their impact and the manner of coping. The idea that dif-

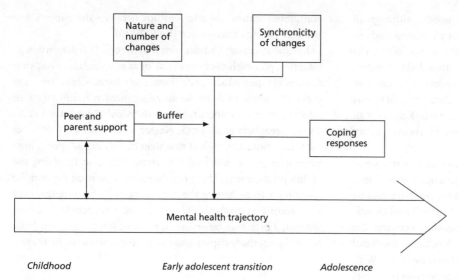

Fig. 31.1 Model of development transition in early adolescence.

ferent issues and challenges present at different ages and stages of development and are dealt with serially is not at all new and has data to support it, as in Coleman's (1974) focal theory of adolescent psychological development. There is converging agreement that the impact of experiences is a function of the above variables. Rice *et al.* suggest a diagram for their model (Fig. 31.1) (Coleman & Hendry 1999).

In determining whether a particular experience or event will be stressful, additional so-called *event parameters* are referred to. To such variables as number, synchronicity and timing, one can add unpredictability (Seiffge-Kranke 1995) so that there is no opportunity for anticipatory coping. As far as individual characteristics of the child are concerned, age, previous exposure (both sensitizing and steeling), gender, social support (family and peers) and culture will modify the perception of the stressor and thus the subjective significance of it (*event appraisal*) as well as the coping style used. With respect to event appraisal, lack of control (Lazarus & Folkman 1991) with respect to the individual's perception of the event or process seems particularly important.

Coping strategies have usually been conceptualized according to three main dichotomies:

1 emotion-focused strategies (Lazarus 1966);

2 engagement (approach) vs. disengagement (avoidance); and

3 problem-solving (primary control) vs. cognitive reframing (secondary control) (Compas 1995; Seiffge-Kranke 1995; Compas *et al.*, 2001).

Wishful thinking is also quite often included as an avoidant strategy. The type of stressor itself, considered objectively, is a weak determinant of which coping strategies are selected. Which strategies are actually used depends on a number of factors and some preliminary generalizations can be made on the basis of empirical studies.

Age and gender

Younger children are more likely to use family resources, with a particular focus on attachment relationships and figures for emotion-focused coping, and instrumentally dependent relationships for problem-solving coping; adolescents increasingly employ friends or adults outside the family. Emotion-focused coping on one's own increases with age (Compas 1995). By the teenage years, most adolescents have acquired a good range of coping strategies, mostly functional (active problem-solving, such as seeking information or advice, discovering social support and accepting it, reflecting upon a choice between possible courses of action). This stands in contrast to dysfunctional coping (social withdrawal, avoidance of confrontation, wishful thinking). Across a range of cultures, those teenagers who employ functional coping strategies outnumber those who do not by 4 : 1 (Seiffge-Kranke 1995). Generally speaking, the repertoire of coping strategies increases with age and stabilizes at around 15 (Seiffge-Kranke 1995, 2000). Boys use more problem-solving than girls who use more in the way of social supports (Schonert-Reichl & Muller 1996). This means that girls are doubly disadvantaged by avoidant strategies which deprive them of a coping resource. A child is more likely to use problem-solving approaches if the stressor is appraised as being controllable.

Family background

The type of parenting employed in a family (authoritative, authoritarian, permissive, neglectful) exerts an influence, probably by inducing control beliefs to varying degrees. Children who have confidence in their ability to control events or processes are more likely to use problem-solving strategies and come from families in which there is authoritative parenting (McIntyre & Dusek 1995). Put slightly differently, children and adolescents from families that encourage independence and the open expression of feeling are more likely to use family and social resources actively rather than withdraw (Shulman 1993).

It may be reasonable to conclude that although a framework

for beginning to understand coping and adaptation is developing, it is premature to indicate what deviant coping would be. We still must have recourse to a crude notion of maladaptation in the sense of a cost to the individual's well-being or function.

Empirical information about adjustment disorder

There is remarkably little published about adjustment disorder and there is an impression that the term is less used than previously. Some findings may be gleaned from a sparse literature.

What form does adjustment disorder predominantly take?

Clearly, any clinical account can be affected by ascertainment bias. Kovacs et al. (1994, 1995) found considerable consistency of type in two studies of adjustment disorder in children presenting either to a psychiatric clinic or following the onset of diabetes. Diagnoses were made by structured processes and formal criteria and were independent of clinicians' diagnoses. Depressive subtype predominated in both settings, followed by mixed anxiety and depression. These two subtypes accounted for 24 of 30 of the psychiatric clinic patients and 30 of 33 of the new diabetics. Other subtypes with predominantly anxiety or conduct disturbance were unusual. The same was found in the very large-scale field trial undertaken for DSM-IV (Strain et al. 1998). These findings contrast with observations deriving from older studies, such as the influential work by Andreason & Wasek (1980) which has informed a number of textbook accounts.

With respect to suicidal phenomena, just over half (58%) of the depressive subtype in the psychiatric clinic and 53% of the diabetic group had suicidal ideation. The papers cited do not mention self-harm but no children seem to have killed themselves during 7–8 years of follow-up. A related study (Kovacs et al. 1993) found lower rates of suicidal behaviour in adjustment disorder compared with dysthymic and major depressive disorder and on the basis of their own studies stated that suicide attempts occur only 'rarely in the context of adjustment disorder' (Kovacs et al. 1994). Nevertheless, that there is some risk is demonstrated by Martunnen et al. (1994) who were able to find 11 cases of adjustment disorder among all the Finnish teenagers and young adults who killed themselves in 1987–78.

How prevalent is adjustment disorder?

Because of the shift in diagnostic criteria, only recent studies can be used to determine the answer. However, recent whole population studies mainly used categories that did not include adjustment disorder. An exception is the general population study of 4–16-year-olds in Puerto Rico using DSM-III criteria which gave a prevalence rate for definite adjustment disorder of 4.2% within a total prevalence rate for psychiatric morbidity of 17.8%, i.e. about one-quarter of all cases (Bird et al. 1989). Curiously, ad-

justment disorders in this population showed no relationship with the number of life events or family dysfunction, nor with age or sex as variables. A similar figure of 3.4% was found in a total birth cohort study of 8–9-year-olds in Finland (Almqvist et al. 1999).

Within clinic populations, just under twice this rate is suggested for the prevalence of adjustment disorder by relatively recent criteria. For instance, Doan & Petti (1989) found a rate of 7% among nearly 800 patients attending day-units in Western Pennsylvania. In Steinhausen & Erdin's (1991a) study 5.9% were diagnosed as having adjustment disorder. These figures stand in contrast to the higher figures found in inpatient population studies (see above) and it seems likely that other forces are guiding the diagnostic behaviour of psychiatrists in such settings.

Viewing the questions somewhat differently, Kovacs et al. (1995) found that systematically diagnosed adjustment disorder occurred in 36% of 92 children following the onset of diabetes. It was by far the most common psychiatric diagnosis to follow this well-defined stressor and was twice as likely to occur among those children whose parents also had marital problems, suggesting that the contribution of background chronic adversity is significant. Similarly, the DSM-IV field trial (based on referrals in the 1980s) found that the diagnosis was made in about one-third of cases (Strain et al. 1998).

How reliably is the diagnosis made?

Traditionally, adjustment disorder and similar categories have had poor interrater reliability (Newcorn & Strain 1992). The development of more structured criteria have apparently improved matters somewhat but perhaps not greatly. Rey et al. (1989) calculated a mean value for Cohen's kappa of 0.41 across studies using DSM-III, the lowest for any axis I diagnosis apart from attention deficit disorder without hyperactivity. According to ICD criteria, Steinhausen & Erdin (1991b) found a high interrater agreement of 82% for the diagnosis using ICD-10 criteria applied to a written vignette. In view of the small number of vignettes (5) used in the latter study, this may be an unrepresentative finding.

Validity of the diagnosis

From examination of the literature, two sources of empirical information as to the validity of the concept emerge. One is the predictive power of the diagnosis with respect to health compared with other diagnoses as revealed on follow-up. The other is whether follow-up studies suggest that symptomatology breeds true to type.

Older work was pessimistic as to validity. Andreason & Hoenk (1982), following up a group of 50 adolescent patients with a diagnosis of adjustment reaction made 5 years earlier by clinicians in a very reputable centre, commented that with respect to diagnostic practice, 'the disorder was not transient, the reaction not acute and the stress not overwhelming'. This figure was comparable to the high rates of serious pathology of various kinds found on follow-up in studies on undiagnosable disorder in adolescence (Fard *et al.* 1979) and transient situational disturbance (Looney & Gunderson 1978).

One might dismiss such findings as merely reflecting confused diagnostic practice. Logically, the diagnostic criteria for adjustment disorder require that when psychopathology is persistent beyond 6 months, the condition be redefined diagnostically so that adjustment disorder cannot breed true by definition. Nevertheless, the conditions found at longer follow-up were often severe. Compared with the older studies, the use of somewhat more recent and tighter diagnostic criteria yields a picture less different from that which one might predict. Cantwell & Baker (1989) carried out a 4-year follow-up of children seen at a speech and language clinic with a psychiatric disorder rate of about 50%. The diagnosis of DSM-III adjustment disorder made in 19 children was the least stable (0%) of all diagnoses made, presumably an artefact of the criteria, but the overall recovery rate was remarkably low at 26%. There was no correspondence between the type of symptoms exhibited initially and those on follow-up. On the other hand, Lewinsohn *et al.* (1999) found that adolescents diagnosed with adjustment disorder with depressed mood had the same rate of major depressive disorder 5 years later in early adult life as those initially diagnosed as major depressive disorder; in other words the condition appeared to breed true in the instance of affective disorder as well as having as poor a prognosis as the major category disorder.

Kovacs *et al.* (1994, 1995) were able to follow up the cases they detected systematically for 5 years or more. The children with adjustment disorder first seen in a psychiatric clinic at an average age of 10 years were equally likely to develop a new psychiatric disorder over the next 5 years compared with a carefully matched control group. Matching had taken account of comorbid psychiatric disorder at initial diagnosis, and the lack of difference at follow-up was thought to be accounted for by the common (60%) existence of these comorbid conditions. In other words, the lack of difference was a function of sample and matching. A clearer result is found in the follow-up of children with diabetes who developed adjustment disorders; 27% had a new psychiatric disorder on follow-up, adjustment disorder increasing the risk of developing subsequent disorder by a factor of 3.4. Among those affected, depressive disorder was the most common type (36%), reflecting the predominance of this subtype at the outset; 24% had conduct disorder; and 20% an anxiety disorder. There is not enough detail in the papers to determine whether disorder bred true to type for each individual, but probably enough to indicate that adjustment disorder increases the risk for future psychiatric disorder.

The stressful experiences identified

Stressful experiences are probably no different in adjustment disorder to the types of acute stress that might be implicated in the precipitation of non-neurodevelopmental psychiatric disorder generally (Al-Ansari & Matar-Ali 1993). In the one recent study that has made the comparison, the number of adverse life-events preceding adjustment disorder in a year did not exceed that found preceding major category disorder (Kovacs *et al.* 1994), something which raises a question about the whole concept of adjustment disorder. The DSM-IV field trial finding that the rate of stressors did not differ across diagnostic groups and, in particular, was not higher in the adjustment disorder cases, raises doubts about the validity of tying the diagnosis to the association with a stress experience (Strain *et al.* 1998).

Assessment

A conventional child psychiatric assessment is as necessary for the diagnosis of an adjustment disorder as for any other psychiatric condition. It would seem particularly important to interview the child to obtain quantification of the impact of supposed adversity for the following reasons.

1 Parents may be unaware of experiences, such as bullying, which characteristically is kept secret by its victims.
2 The parents may conceal an adversity that implicates them, sexual abuse being a case in point.
3 An apparently moderate stressor may be severe for the child in question because of idiosyncratic personal elements, such as previous sensitization.
4 Skilled interviewers who know what questions to ask may reveal symptoms that would otherwise remain undisclosed.

In related vein, it may be only the child who can reveal the timing of onset of private symptoms. This should not mean that only the child can provide information; life events interviews have shown how the best data are derived from combining parental and child accounts (see Sandberg & Rutter, Chapter 17). Certainly, parental mental state must be assessed, given the evidence that this may be the maintaining factor in responses to a number of stressors (see above).

Careful formulation of the mechanisms involved in the genesis and maintenance of disorder must include specification as to how the child has attempted to cope with the stressor or new life circumstances as well as to what extent his or her efforts have contributed to exacerbating their impact. There would seem to be some advantage in documenting how previous stresses and life transitions have been successfully managed because this may indicate a logical approach to treatment (see below).

There is a potential risk in jumping to an assumption that an apparently adverse event is aetiological. In Dunn & Kendrick's (1982) work on the impact of the birth of a sibling, rather more than half of the elder siblings showed some signs of being more 'grown-up' in areas such as independence in self-care or language, suggesting that the birth of a sibling is by no means necessarily entirely adverse and can, like divorce may for some adolescents (Wallerstein & Kelly 1980), act as a developmental stimulus. To make an inferential leap in judging a psychological disturbance to be a consequence of an event may be misleading unless the content of the child's disturbance supports such a link; there may be different reasons.

If DSM-IV guidelines are followed, a reassessment at 6 months is mandatory to examine whether redesignation to a major category diagnosis is required.

Prevention

Although there are no solid data on prevention of adjustment disorders as such, the evidence that preparation by discussion, explanation, visiting and provision of mitigating circumstances will minimize the distress of young children admitted to hospital with minimal contact with their parents (Wolfer & Visintainer 1975) suggests that other predictable changes in life circumstances can be constructively prepared for along similar lines. Otherwise, the recommendations for prevention are rather diffuse: reducing the number of stressors (such as divorce) through mental health education or social support systems; building self-esteem; and educating children about how to cope with predictable stressors, such as examinations. These are untested and, in current formulation, probably too diffuse to be testable.

Treatment

There are no substantial data on treatment choice or effectiveness for adjustment disorders as currently defined. At first glance, an approach combining environmental manipulation with individual or family counselling that hinged upon removing or minimizing the stressful situation while supporting the child and family in constructive adaptation would seem appropriate.

If it were possible to identify how children's coping strategies related to immunity from stress-related psychiatric disorder then this would provide a basis on which to use a more educational model that could build coping mechanisms. However, most of the work on invulnerability documents personality characteristics rather than coping skills. Nevertheless, there are early indications as to how matters might develop. In a 3-year longitudinal study of stressors and coping styles, Seiffge-Kranke (2000) identified only withdrawal (avoidant coping) as associated with the development of psychopathology. The same study also indicated that avoidant coping in the face of major and daily stressors did not only lead to psychopathology but also maintained it; psychopathology in adolescents leading to deficits in coping skills. It may also be the case that the more extensive use of social support by girls (Seiffge-Kranke 1995) means that social withdrawal associated with depressive symptomatology deprives them of a coping resource which is less important for boys. With this in mind, tutoring in more active coping and social engagement ought to prove beneficial, yet attempts to explore the deployment of coping skills and vulnerability to disorder have not yet yielded sufficient positive results on which to build treatments (see Jenkins et al. 1989 for a well-executed but ultimately disappointing instance).

As far as secondary level care is concerned, there is evidence that cognitive therapies assist children with a mild depressive reaction (Harrington et al. 1998) and it seems plausible that this would apply to anxiety too. However, the chances of a child being detected as likely to have an adjustment disorder, accepted into a treatment programme, assessed and treated to completion within a maximum period of 6 months are not high enough to make many treatment outcome studies feasible in the future. It may be more relevant to concentrate on prevention research, particularly with a view to reducing the risk of future major category psychiatric disorder. On the other hand, most cases of adjustment disorder would be seen in primary care and counselling/social support approach would be viable. There is just a possibility that less orthodox approaches, such as relaxation/massage, might be applicable for those with anxious subtype, given some evidence for effectiveness (Field et al. 1992). Nevertheless, a generally optimistic prognosis could mask apparent effect and lead to wasted treatment resources.

Conclusions

Refining diagnostic criteria has led to a more satisfactory position with respect to the nosological validity of adjustment disorder compared with 10 years ago. It is popular, probably because of its non-pejorative status, and what is described according to diagnostic criteria seems broadly valid. However, logic leads to a reconceptualization of subthreshold minor disorder category with nearly the same time constraints as currently apply; a 9-month duration would seem more valid. Tying such minor disorder categories to a perceived adverse event to create a concept of a type of psychiatric disorder different from the way other major episodic category disorders are precipitated by adversity seems unnecessary, both from early empirical findings and given the existence of Z codes.

References

Al-Ansari, A. & Matar-Ali, M. (1993) Recent stressful life events among Bahraini adolescents with adjustment disorder. *Adolescence*, 28, 339–346.

Almqvist, F., Puura, K., Kumpulainen, K. *et al.* (1999) Psychiatric disorders in 8–9-year-old children based on a diagnostic interview with the parents. *European Child and Adolescent Psychiatry*, 8 (Suppl.4), 17–28.

American Psychiatric Association (1952) *Diagnostic and Statistical Manual of Mental Disorders*, 1st edn. American Psychiatric Press. Washington D.C.

American Psychiatric Association (1994) *Diagnostic and Statistical Manual of Mental Disorders*, 4th edn. American Psychiatric Press. Washington D.C.

Andreason, N.C. & Hoenk, P.P. (1982) The predictive value of adjustment disorders: a follow-up study. *American Journal of Psychiatry*, 139, 584–590.

Andreason, N.C. & Wasek, P. (1980) Adjustment disorders in adolescents and adults. *Archives of General Psychiatry*, 37, 1166–1170.

Angold, A., Costello, E.J., Farmer, E.M.Z., Burns, B.J. & Erkanli, A. (1999) Impaired but undiagnosed. *Journal of the American Academy of Child and Adolescent Psychiatry*, 38, 129–137.

Bird, H.R., Canino, G., Rubio-Stipec, M. *et al.* (1988) Estimates of the prevalence of childhood maladjustment in a community survey in Puerto Rico: the use of combined measures. *Archives of General Psychiatry*, 45, 1120–1126.

Bird, H.R., Gould, M.S., Yager, T., Staghezza, M.P.H. & Canino, G. (1989) Risk factors for maladjustment in Puerto Rican children. *Journal of the American Academy of Child and Adolescent Psychiatry*, 28, 847–850.

Cantwell, D.P. & Baker, L. (1989) Stability and natural history of DSM-III diagnoses. *Journal of the American Academy of Child and Adolescent Psychiatry*, 28, 691–700.

Coleman, J. (1974) *Relationships in Adolescence*. Routledge & Kegan Paul, London.

Coleman, J.C. & Hendry, L.B. (1999) *The Nature of Adolescence*, 3rd edn. Routledge, London.

Compas, B.E. (1995) Promoting successful coping during adolescence. In: *Psychosocial Disturbances in Young People* (ed. M. Rutter), pp. 247–273. Cambridge University Press, Cambridge.

Compas, B.E., Oroson, P.G. & Grant, K.E. (1993) Adolescent stress and coping: implications for psychopathology during adolescence. *Journal of Adolescence*, 16, 331–349.

Compas, B.E., Connor-Smith, J.K., Satzman, H., Thomsen, A.H. & Wadsworth, M.E. (2001) Coping with stress during childhood and adolescence: problems, progress, and potential in theory and research. *Psychological Bulletin*, 127, 87–127.

Costello, E.J., Angold, A. & Keeler, G.P. (1999) Adolescent outcomes of childhood disorders. *Journal of the American Academy of Child and Adolescent Psychiatry*, 38, 121–128.

Doan, R.J. & Petti, T.A. (1989) Clinical and demographic characteristics of child and adolescent partial hospital patients. *Journal of the American Academy of Child and Adolescent Psychiatry*, 28, 66–69.

Dowdney, L., Wilson, R., Maughan, B., Allerton, P., Schofield, P. & Skuse, D. (1999) Psychological disturbance and service provision in parentally bereaved children: prospective case–control study. *British Medical Journal*, 319, 354–357.

Dunn, J. & Kendrick, C. (1982) *Siblings: Love, Envy and Understanding*. Cambridge University Press, Cambridge.

Fard, F., Hudgens, R.W. & Welner, A. (1978) Undiagnosed psychiatric illness in adolescents: a prospective study and seven-year follow-up. *Archives of General Psychiatry*, 35, 279–282.

Field, T., Morrow, C., Valdeon, C., Larson, S., Kuhn, C. & Schanberg, S. (1992) Massage reduces anxiety in child and adolescent patients. *Journal of the American Academy of Child and Adolescent Psychiatry*, 31, 125–131.

Frank, S.J. & Paul, J.S. (1995) *The Functional Impairment Scale for Children and Adolescents*. Department of Psychology, Michigan State University.

Frank, S.J., Paul, J.S., Marks, M. & Van Egeren, L.A. (2000) Initial validation of the functional impairment scale for children and adolescents. *Journal of the American Academy of Child and Adolescent Psychiatry*, 39, 1300–1308.

Fristad, M.A., Jedel, R., Weller, R.A. & Weller, B. (1993) Psychosocial functioning in children after the death of a parent. *American Journal of Psychiatry*, 150, 511–513.

Frydenberg, E. (1997) *Adolescent Coping: Theoretical and Research Perspectives*. Routledge, London.

Goodyer, I., Kolvin, I. & Gatzanis, S. (1985) Recent undesirable life events and psychiatric disorders of childhood and adolescence. *British Journal of Psychiatry*, 147, 517–523.

Goodyer, I., Herbert, J., Tamplin, A. & Altham, P. (2000) Recent life events, cortisol, dehydroepiandrosterone and the onset of major depression in high-risk adolescents. *British Journal of Psychiatry*, 177, 499–504.

Graber, J. & Brooks-Gunn, J. (1996) Transitions and turning points: navigating the passage from childhood through adolescence. *Developmental Psychology*, 32, 768–776.

Greenberg, W.M., Rosenfeld, D.N. & Ortega, E.A. (1995) Adjustment disorder as an admission diagnosis. *American Journal of Psychiatry*, 152, 459–461.

Harrington, R. & Clark, A. (1998) Prevention and early intervention for depression in adolescence and early adult life. *European Archives of Psychiatry and Clinical Neuroscience*, 248, 32–45.

Harrington, R. & Harrison, L. (1999) Unproven assumptions about the impact of bereavement on children. *Journal of the Royal Society of Medicine*, 92, 230–233.

Harrington, R., Whittaker, J., Shoebridge, P. & Campbell, F. (1998) Systematic review of efficacy of cognitive behaviour therapies in child and adolescent depressive disorder. *British Medical Journal*, 316, 1559–1563.

Hill, P. (1994) Adjustment disorder. In: *Child and Adolescent Psychiatry: A Modern Approach* (eds M. Rutter, E. Taylor & L. Hersov). Blackwell Scientific Publications, Oxford.

Jenkins, J.M., Smith, M.A. & Graham, P.J. (1989) Coping with parental quarrels. *Journal of the American Academy of Child and Adolescent Psychiatry*, 28, 182–189.

Kelly, J.B. (2000) Children's adjustment in conflicted marriage and divorce: a decade review of research. *Journal of the American Academy of Child and Adolescent Psychiatry*, 39, 963–973.

Kovacs, M., Goldston, D. & Gatsonis, C. (1993) Suicidal behaviors and childhood-onset depressive disorders: a longitudinal investigation. *Journal of the American Academy of Child and Adolescent Psychiatry*, 32, 8–20.

Kovacs, M., Gatsonis, C., Pollock, M. & Parrone, P.L. (1994) A controlled prospective study of DSM-III adjustment disorder in childhood: short-term prognosis and long-term predictive validity. *Archives of General Psychiatry*, 51, 535–541.

Kovacs, M., Ho, V. & Pollock, M.H. (1995) Criterion and predictive validity of the diagnosis of adjustment disorder: a prospective study of youths with new-onset insulin-dependent diabetes mellitus. *American Journal of Psychiatry*, 152, 523–528.

Kranzler, E. (1990) Parental death in childhood. In: *Childhood Stress* (ed. L.E. Arnold), pp. 405–421. Wiley Interscience, New York.

Lazarus, R.S. (1966) *Psychological Stress and the Coping Process*. McGraw-Hill, New York.

Lazarus, R.S. & Folkman, S. (1991) *Stress, Appraisal and Coping*. Springer, New York.

Leadbeater, B.J., Blatt, S.J. & Quinlan, D.M. (1995) Gender-linked vulnerabilities to depressive symptoms, stress and problem behaviors in adolescents. *Journal of Research on Adolescence*, 5, 1–29.

Lewinshon, P.M., Rhode, P., Klein, D.N. & Seeley, J.R. (1999) Natural course of adolescent major depressive disorder: I. Continuity into young adulthood. *Journal of the American Academy of Child and Adolescent Psychiatry*, 38, 56–63.

Looney, J.G. & Gunderson, E. (1978) Transient situational disturbance: course and outcome. *American Journal of Psychiatry*, 135, 660–663.

Malt, U.F. (1986) Five years of experience with the DSM-III system in clinical work and research: some concluding remarks. *Acta Psychiatrica Scandinavica*, 73 (Suppl. 328), 76–84.

Martunnen, M.J., Aro, H.M., Henriksson, M.M. & Loennqvist, J.K. (1994) Adolescent suicides with adjustment disorders or no psychiatric diagnosis. *European Journal of Child and Adolescent Psychiatry*, 3, 101–110.

McIntyre, J. & Dusek, J. (1995) Perceived parental rearing practices and styles of coping. *Journal of Youth and Adolescence*, **24**, 499–509.

Nasser, E.H. & Overholser, J.C. (1999) Assessing varying degrees of lethality in depressed adolescent suicide attempters. *Acta Psychiatrica Scandinavica*, **6**, 397–398.

Newcorn, J.H. & Strain, J. (1992) Adjustment disorder in children and adolescents. *Journal of the American Academy of Child and Adolescent Psychiatry*, **31**, 318–327.

Pelkonen, M., Marttunen, M., Laippala, P. & Lonnqvist, J. (2000) Factors associated with early dropout from adolescent psychiatric outpatient treatment. *Journal of the American Academy of Child and Adolescent Psychiatry*, **39**, 329–336.

Pincus, H.A., Davis, W.W. & McQueen, L.E. (1999) 'Subthreshold' mental disorders. *British Journal of Psychiatry*, **174**, 288–296.

Rey, J.M., Plapp, J.M. & Stewart, G.W. (1989) Reliability of psychiatric diagnosis in referred adolescents. *Journal of Child Psychology and Psychiatry*, **30**, 879–888.

Rice, K.G., Herman, M.A. & Petersen, A.C. (1993) Coping with challenge in adolescence: a conceptual model and psycho-educational intervention. *Journal of Adolescence*, **16**, 235–251.

Rosen, B.M., Bahn, A.K. & Kramer, M. (1964) Demographic and diagnostic characteristics of psychiatric clinic out-patients in the USA, 1961. *American Journal of Orthopsychiatry*, **34**, 122–136.

Rutter, M. & Sandberg, S. (1992) Psychosocial stressors: concepts, causes and effects. *European Journal of Child and Adolescent Psychiatry*, **1**, 3–13.

Schonert-Reichl, K. & Muller, J. (1996) Correlates of help-seeking in adolescence. *Journal of Youth and Adolescence*, **25**, 705–732.

Seiffge-Kranke, I. (1995) *Stress, Coping and Relationships in Adolescence*. Lawrence Erlbaum Associates, Hove, UK.

Seiffge-Kranke, I. (2000) Causal links between stressful events, coping style, and adolescent symptomatology. *Journal of Adolescence*, **23**, 675–691.

Setterburg, S.R., Ernst, M., Rao, U. *et al.* (1991) Child psychiatrists,

views of DSM-III-R: a survey of usage and opinions. *Journal of the American Academy of Child and Adolescent Psychiatry*, **30**, 652–658.

Shaffer, D., Gould, M.S., Brasic, J. *et al.* (1983) A Children's Global Assessment Scale (CGAS). *Archives of General Psychiatry*, **40**, 1228–1231.

Shulman, S. (1993) Close relationships and coping in adolescence. *Journal of Adolescence*, **16**, 267–284.

Steinhausen, H.-C. & Erdin, A. (1991a) A comparison of ICD-9 and ICD-10 diagnoses of child and adolescent psychiatric disorders. *Journal of Child Psychology and Psychiatry*, **32**, 909–920.

Steinhausen, H.-C. & Erdin, A. (1991b) The inter-rater reliability of child and adolescent psychiatric disorders in the ICD-10. *Journal of Child Psychology and Psychiatry*, **32**, 921–928.

Strain, J.J., Newcorn, J., Mezzich, J. & Kirisci, L. (1998) Adjustment disorder: the MacArthur reanalysis. In: *DSM-IV Source Book*, Vol. 4 (eds T.A. Widiger, A.J. Francis, H.A. Pincus *et al.*), pp. 403–424. American Psychiatric Association, Washington D.C.

Van Eerdewegh, M.M., Clayton, P.J. & Van Eerdewegh, P. (1985) The bereaved child: factors influencing early psychopathology. *British Journal of Psychiatry*, **147**, 188–194.

Wallerstein, J. & Kelly, J. (1980) *Surviving the Breakup: How Children and Parents Cope with a Divorce*. Grant McIntyre, London.

Weiner, I.B. & Del Gaudio, A.C. (1976) Psychopathology in adolescence: an epidemiological study. *Archives of General Psychiatry*, **33**, 187–193.

Wolfer, J.A. & Visintainer, M.A. (1975) Pre-hospital psychological preparation for tonsillectomy patients: effects on children's and parents' adjustment. *Pediatrics*, **64**, 646–655.

World Health Organization (1992) *The ICD-10 Classification of Mental and Behavoural Disorders: Clinical Descriptions and Diagnostic Guidelines*. World Health Organization, Geneva.

World Health Organization (1992) *The ICD-10 Classification of Mental and Behavoural Disorders: Diagnostic Criteria for Research*. World Health Organization, Geneva.

32 Post-Traumatic Stress Disorders
William Yule

Introduction

Both ICD-10 (World Health Organization 1987, 1988, 1991) and DSM-IV (American Psychiatric Association 1994) diagnostic systems now acknowledge that major stressors can cause serious morbidity and that children may suffer from post-traumatic stress disorder (PTSD). The past 15 years has seen a great increase in studies of the effects of major stresses, as encountered in disasters, war and other life-threatening experiences. However, the question for child psychiatry remains whether severe acute stresses, as opposed to chronic ones linked to social adversity (see Friedman & Chase-Lansdale, Chapter 15), or more ordinary acute stresses (see Sandberg & Rutter, Chapter 17), carry a substantial increased risk of psychiatric sequelae. If so, what sort of stressors carry such increased risk? What are the most common psychological sequelae? Do these vary according to stressor, or according to developmental level? What is the role of the family in moderating the reactions? Are there other known risk and protective factors? Indeed, is PTSD truly a separate disorder or is it merely a variant of other well-recognized disorders, such as anxiety, phobias or depression? Finally, what is currently known about intervention?

The concept of post-traumatic stress disorder

The diagnosis of PTSD was first conceptualized in response to observations of Vietnam war veterans presenting with what came to be recognized as a particular pattern of symptoms in three clusters:

1 intrusive thoughts about a traumatic event;

2 emotional numbing and avoidance of reminders of that event; and

3 physiological hyperarousal (American Psychiatric Association 1980).

In retrospect, similar patterns were noted as reactions in earlier wars and, in prospect, the criteria were adapted, partly operationalized and applied to adult civilians. Next, the diagnosis was applied to children who had experienced an 'event outside the range of usual human experience . . . that would be markedly distressing to almost anyone' (DSM-III-R, American Psychiatric Association 1987).

Thus, it was argued that there were certain types of stressful experiences that were very severe and/or unusual and that there was a distinctive form of stress reaction to these. PTSD was classified as an anxiety disorder, but many argued that it should be included as a dissociative disorder. It was increasingly described as 'a normal reaction to an abnormal situation' and so, logically, it was queried whether it should be regarded as a psychiatric disorder at all (O'Donohue & Eliot 1992). Even if it were regarded as a normal reaction, as will be shown below, it causes substantial impairment in sufficient cases to be regarded as a disorder.

Results from studies of adults have reasonably established that PTSD, while being predominantly an anxiety disorder, differs from other anxiety disorders in important ways. Foa *et al.* (1989) showed that the trauma suffered violated more of the patients' safety assumptions than did events giving rise to other forms of anxiety. There was a much greater generalization of fear responses in the PTSD groups and, unlike other anxious patients, they reported far more frequent re-experiencing of the traumatic event. Indeed, it is this internal subjective experience that seems most to mark out PTSD from other disorders (Jones & Barlow 1992). In adults, the argument is increasingly made that PTSD is an 'abnormal reaction to an abnormal event' that involves a complex interaction of biological, psychological and social causes (Yehuda & McFarlane 1995).

Recently, Ehlers & Clark (2000) have pointed out that, unlike most anxiety disorders, PTSD involves reactions to memories of past events rather than anticipation of any impending threat. They put forward an integrative cognitive model which helps to account for previously puzzling findings and which has been useful in developing effective treatment approaches for adult patients. As yet, the model has not been applied to children and adolescents.

There is still considerable debate in the adult literature as to whether there needs to be specification of 'Criterion A', the inadequately operationalized description of the unusual traumatic event. There are cases where patients meet the criteria for the presence of all three clusters of reactions, but have either no known exposure or only a trivial exposure to a stressor. This is important because, if true, then a diagnosis of PTSD does not automatically mean that the patient has suffered a trauma. Concern has been expressed that the diagnosis is being made too liberally, without due attention being paid to the impact on social functioning. Equally, concern has been expressed that there are other forms of stress reactions to chronic stress as experienced in repeated physical or sexual abuse (see Glaser, Chapter 21). Terr (1991), for example, drew a distinction between Type I and Type II traumas, roughly the distinction between acute and chronic. While these are important debates that will alter the views taken on PTSD, here we will concentrate on acute conditions as manifested in children and adolescents.

With its roots in studies of adult psychopathology, the concept has been uneasily extended to apply to stress reactions in children and adolescents. The major difficulty from the outset has been that some of the symptoms are developmentally inappropriate for younger people. Indeed, the younger the child, the less appropriate the criteria.

Many writers agree that it is very difficult to elicit evidence of emotional numbing in children (Frederick 1985). Some children do show loss of interest in activities and hobbies that previously gave them pleasure. Preschool-age children show much more regressive behaviour as well as more antisocial, aggressive and destructive behaviour. There are many anecdotal accounts of preschool-age children showing repetitive drawing and play involving themes about the trauma they experienced.

Although parents and teachers initially report that young children do not easily talk about the trauma, recent experience has been that many young children easily give very graphic accounts of their experiences and are also able to report how distressing the re-experiencing in thoughts and images was (Sullivan *et al.* 1991; Misch *et al.* 1993). All clinicians and researchers need to have a good understanding of children's development to be able to assist them to express their inner distress.

Scheeringa *et al.* (1995) examined the phenomenology reported in published cases of trauma in infants and young children and evolved an alternative set of criteria for diagnosing PTSD in very young children. Re-experiencing is seen as being manifested in:

- post-traumatic play;
- re-enactment of the trauma;
- recurrent recollection of the traumatic event;
- nightmares; and
- flashbacks or distress at exposure to reminders of the event.

Only one positive item is needed.

Numbing is present if one of the following is manifested:

- constriction of play;
- socially more withdrawn;
- restricted range of affect; or
- loss of previously acquired developmental skill.

Increased arousal is noted if one of the following is present:

- night terrors;
- difficulty getting off to sleep;
- night waking;
- decreased concentration;
- hypervigilance; or
- exaggerated startle response.

A new subset of new fears and aggression was suggested and is said to be present if one of the following is recorded:

- new aggression;
- new separation anxiety;
- fear of toileting alone;
- fear of the dark; or
- any other unrelated new fear.

To date, these altered criteria have not been tested against the traditional ones. Almqvist & Brandell-Forsberg (1997) provided evidence on how a standard set of play materials can be used to obtain objective data on traumatic stress reactions from preschool-age children. Thus, one can anticipate a refining of criteria and methods of assessment of PTSD in preschool-age children in the next few years.

Manifestations of stress reactions in children and adolescents

Immediately following a very frightening experience, children are likely to be very distressed, tearful, frightened and in shock. They need protection and safety and to be reunited with their families wherever possible. Clinical experience, surveys and clinical descriptive studies quoted below show that the main manifestations of stress reactions are as follows.

Starting almost immediately, most children are troubled by *repetitive, intrusive thoughts* about the accident. Such thoughts can occur at any time, but particularly when the children are otherwise quiet, as when they are trying to drop off to sleep. At other times, the thoughts and vivid recollections are triggered off by reminders in their environment. Vivid dissociative *flashbacks* are uncommon. In a flashback, the child reports that he or she is re-experiencing the event, as if it were happening all over again. It is almost a dissociated experience. *Sleep disturbances* are very common, particularly in the first few weeks. *Fears* of the dark and bad dreams, *nightmares*, and waking through the night are widespread, and often manifest outside the developmental age range in which they normally occur.

Separation difficulties are frequent, even among teenagers. For the first few days, children may not want to let their parents out of their sight, even reverting to sleeping in the parental bed. Many children become much more *irritable and angry* than previously, both with parents and peers.

Although child survivors experience a *pressure to talk* about their experiences, paradoxically they also find it very *difficult to talk with their parents and peers*. Often they do not want to upset the adults, and so parents may not be aware of the full extent of their children's suffering. Peers may hold back from asking what happened in case they upset the child further; the survivor often feels this as a rejection.

Children report a number of *cognitive changes*. Many experience *difficulties in concentration*, especially in school work. Others report *memory problems*, both in mastering new material and in remembering old skills, such as reading music. They become very *alert to danger* in their environment, being adversely affected by reports of other disasters.

Survivors have learned that life is very fragile. This can lead to a loss of faith in the future or a *sense of foreshortened future*. Their priorities change. Some feel they should live each day to the full and not plan far ahead; others realize they have been overconcerned with materialistic or petty matters and resolve to rethink their values. Their 'assumptive world' has been challenged (Janoff-Bulman 1985). Not surprisingly, many develop *fears* associated with specific aspects of their experiences. They avoid situations they associate with the disaster. Many experience '*survivor guilt*'—about surviving when others died; about thinking they should have done more to help others; about what they themselves did to survive.

Adolescent survivors report significantly high rates of *depression*, some becoming clinically depressed, having suicidal thoughts and taking overdoses in the year after a disaster. A significant number become very *anxious* after accidents, although the appearance of *panic attacks* is sometimes considerably delayed. When children have been *bereaved*, they may need bereavement counselling.

In summary, children and adolescents surviving a life-threatening disaster show a wide range of symptoms that tend to cluster around signs of re-experiencing the traumatic event, trying to avoid dealing with the emotions that this gives rise to, and a range of signs of increased physiological arousal. There may be considerable overlap of symptoms with depression, generalized anxiety or pathological grief reactions although whether this indicates the presence of mixed disorders or comorbidity of separate disorders remains to be clarified.

However, this has implications for assessment. It is not sufficient to inquire solely about symptoms of PTSD. Symptoms of anxiety, depression and grief need also to be formally investigated. Nor are self-completed questionnaires measuring these aspects sufficient to make a diagnosis. They have an important role, but sensitive clinical interviews with the child and separately with the parents remain the cornerstone of good assessment.

Incidence and prevalence of post-traumatic stress disorder in children

Following initial scepticism that children develop PTSD, many studies of survivors of specific disasters appeared (see reviews in Vogel & Vernberg 1993; Shannon *et al.* 1994; Pfefferbaum 1997; Yule *et al.* 1999). These indicated that where reasonably standard assessment had been undertaken, then the incidence of PTSD in survivors was often in the range of 30–60%. More recently, studies of child survivors of road traffic accidents, again using standardized methods, report that around 25–30% develop PTSD (Yule 2000a). Thus, a substantial minority develops PTSD. At the same time, a substantial minority and often a majority are resilient and do not develop PTSD. Thus, the experience of a traumatic event is necessary but not sufficient to cause PTSD.

In community studies in adults, the Epidemiological Catchment Area (ECA) Survey found a lifetime rate of PTSD of 1% (Helzer *et al.* 1987) while the National Comorbidity Survey reported a much higher rate of 7.8% (Kessler *et al.* 1995). Breslau *et al.* (1991) reported a rate of 9.2% in younger adults while Giaconia *et al.* (1995) reported a rate of 6.3% in older adolescents.

One of the largest studies of adolescents following a disaster has been the study of survivors of the sinking of the cruise ship *Jupiter* in 1988. Out of nearly 400 children on board, 200 were traced and systematically assessed some 5–8 years later (Yule *et al.* 2000). Fifty-two per cent were found to have developed PTSD, mainly in the first few weeks after the sinking. In keeping with Meichenbaum's (1994) view, there were very few cases of late-onset PTSD. About one-third recovered within a year of onset, but one-quarter still suffered from the disorder for over 5 years, with 34% still meeting criteria 5–8 years after the sinking. Thus, not only did the survivors of this disaster develop higher rates of PTSD than had previously been recorded, the problems remained over many years in a substantial minority of cases.

The follow-up study of *Jupiter* survivors established that the adolescents also developed a wide range of other positive psychiatric disorders (Bolton *et al.* 2000). They showed considerably raised rates of anxiety and affective disorders compared with controls. Rates of diagnosis were higher in females than males. The disorders were especially raised among those children who had also developed PTSD.

Dose–response relationship

One of the key concepts in PTSD is that anyone can develop the disorder, irrespective of prior vulnerabilities, provided the stressor is sufficiently great. There is therefore considerable interest in whether there is any evidence for a dose–response relationship between stressor and pathology. A number of studies bear on this point in relation to children.

In the California School Sniper study, Pynoos *et al.* (Pynoos & Eth 1986; Pynoos *et al.* 1987; Pynoos & Nader 1988) reported that approximately 1 month after the event, nearly 40% of the children had moderate to severe PTSD on their Post-Traumatic Stress Reaction Index. There was a very strong relationship between exposure and later effects in that those children who were trapped in the playground scored much higher than those who had left the vicinity of the school before the attack or were not in school that day.

At 14-month follow-up, Nader *et al.* (1990) found that 74% of the most severely exposed children in the playground still reported moderate to severe levels of PTSD, contrasted with 81% of the unexposed children reporting no PTSD. Earlier PTSD Reaction Index scores were strongly related to those obtained at follow-up. Only among the less-exposed children did greater knowledge of the victim increase the strength of the emotional reaction to the trauma (Nader *et al.* 1990). In other words, the level of exposure to the life-threatening trauma was more important than other factors, such as knowledge of the victim. In this study, the moderating effects of families reactions was not reported, but the strength of the associations noted challenges McFarlane's (1987) claim that most effects are mediated by parental reaction.

There was a clear exposure–effect relationship among children affected by the Armenian earthquake of 1988, with the most exposed children at the epicentre reporting highest scores (Goenjian *et al.* 1995). In a systematic study of nearly 3000 9–14-year-old children following the Bosnian war in Mostar, a very strong relationship between exposure to war trauma and self-reported psychopathology was found (Smith *et al.* 2001). In a 1 in 10 sample, mothers' mental health was also assessed but, although this did account for a small but significant proportion of the variance in the children's adjustment scores, direct exposure to the war trauma remained the single most important predictor (Smith *et al.* 2001).

Further evidence linking severity to outcome comes from studies which used similar measures following different levels of disaster. The Revised Children's Manifest Anxiety Scale was used in both the study of children who survived the sinking of the cruise ship *Jupiter* (Yule *et al.* 1990b; Yule 1992), and those who experienced Hurricane Hugo in South Carolina on 21 September 1989 (Lonigan *et al.* 1991). In the hurricane study, degree of exposure was significantly associated with increased scores on both anxiety and stress reaction. However, the average anxiety scores for the hurricane survivors were much lower than those obtained from the 334 survivors of the *Jupiter* sinking (Yule 1992), suggesting that the hurricane was less of a direct threat to the children.

The findings from these studies strongly suggest that, within a single disaster, there is a strong relationship between degree of exposure to the stressor and subsequent adjustment. However, subjective factors also have a role. Studies of adult survivors find that high levels of pathology are related to the belief that the survivors were going to die during the incident, as well as to the experience of seeing dead and mutilated bodies (Williams *et al.* 1993). Similar findings are emerging from the study of the most severely affected children assessed individually after the sinking of the *Jupiter* (Yule *et al.* 1992).

Physiological reactions

Reactions to major stress have both physiological and psychological components. Any major life-threatening experience may activate primitive flight/fight/freeze mechanisms which are regarded as less adaptive in young children (Perry *et al.* 1995). In some individuals following some threats, these reactions seem to get stuck. The trauma is then relived at all levels: behavioural, emotional, physiological and neuroendocrinological. The reactions involve many systems, including the release of norepinephrine from the locus caeruleus and endogenous opiates in the septohippocampal system (van der Kolk *et al.* 1985; Goodyer 1990). Some fear that large increases in neurotransmitter activity following trauma may place children at risk of developmental disorders (Perry 1994). The main point to emphasize here is that massive threat can lead to major changes in brain function that may remain over many years, as demonstrated by Ornitz & Pynoos (1989) in their study of persisting startle reaction in a child with PTSD. Goenjian *et al.* (1996) still found a relationship

between intrusion symptoms and baseline cortisol levels 5 years after the Armenian earthquake.

Treatment of post-traumatic stress disorder

While there have been a number of single case reports of treatment of children suffering PTSD, as yet there are few accounts of randomized controlled studies. For the most part, treatment approaches are predominantly cognitive-behavioural and appear to consist of adaptations of approaches used with adults (Yule 1991). Practice guidelines have recently been issued by the American Academy of Child and Adolescent Psychiatry (Cohen 1998), the International Society for Traumatic Stress Studies (ISTSS; Foa *et al.* 2000) and the American Psychological Association (Vernberg & Vogel 1993). They show good agreement in their appraisal of the evidence on which current practice is based.

Critical incident stress debriefing

Critical incident stress debriefing techniques have been adapted for use with groups of children following a variety of traumas (Dyregrov 1991). These involve group leaders structuring discussion with a group of children in such a way that both knowledge and feelings aroused during a traumatic incident are shared and start to be processed. Such a structured crisis intervention approach was used with some children following the *Jupiter* sinking, with good effects on lowering the levels of intrusion and of fears (Yule & Udwin 1991). Stallard & Law (1993) used two debriefing sessions to reduce distress in girls who survived a school bus crash.

Currently, the role of crisis intervention with adults is being called into question with some evidence being cited to the effect that early intervention may cause more rather than less PTSD (Canterbury & Yule 1999). Following the arguments of Rachman (1980) and of Saigh (1986), there is a clear danger that inappropriate exposure sessions that are too short and leave the child in an aroused state may sensitize them rather than help the anxiety habituate. Moreover, the wide range of individual differences to experience have already been emphasized. Even as apparently simple an intervention as giving out a leaflet to survivors has been found to be helpful to the majority but distressing to a significant minority (Yule *et al.* 1990a). Thus, one must entertain the notion that any crisis intervention might have untoward effects in at least some children. The onus is on therapists to monitor which children are helped and which are not by any of the crisis intervention techniques.

There are now a number of leaflets available for distribution to children and their parents alerting them to possible emotional sequelae of accidents and other life-threatening experiences. Among these are the age-specific leaflets prepared by the Child Accident Prevention Trust (Troyna 1998).

Group treatments

Group treatments are obviously to be preferred as a first line of intervention when large numbers are involved. Gillis (1993) suggests that groups of 6–8 are optimum, and advises that separate groups should be run for boys and girls. However, different types of incident surely require different responses from professionals (Galante & Foa 1986; Yule & Williams 1990) and it is too soon to pontificate on what should be a standard approach.

As with debriefing, the aims of such therapeutic groups will be to share experiences and feelings, to boost children's sense of mastery and control, and to share ways of solving common problems. Pynoos & Nader (1993) point out that it is not sufficient for groups to provide a forum for the expression of feelings: this may only renew feelings of anxiety unless a constructive, therapeutic approach is taken.

School-based classroom interventions are particularly recommended when there is a widespread disruption of services and community life as in earthquakes or war. Returning some semblance of normality and predictability into children's lives is widely favoured, and helping them within the context of familiar groups is seen as advantageous. Klingman (1987) and Eth (1992) suggested that mental health professionals run the psychoeducational meetings, with the class teachers in attendance. Smith et al. (1999a) described a flexible, yet structured, intervention designed to be delivered by teachers or primary health care workers with minimal training but adequate support from mental health workers. The manual is currently being field tested with survivors of the Turkish and Greek earthquakes of 1999.

March et al. (1998) reported a single case group design in which 17 children who had witnessed a fire were treated in two small groups, with the treatment being staggered. Overall, symptom counts dropped only as treatment was started. Impressively, 8 of the 17 (57%) no longer met criteria for PTSD after the 18 weekly sessions and 12 out of 14 (86%) were free of PTSD at 6-month follow-up. The treatment was both psychoeducational and active cognitive-behavioural.

While the group treatment approaches reported above are well described and appear promising, there are no controlled studies providing evidence for the efficacy of such groups. There is a consensus that group interventions will be effective for some, but not all, children. However, one function of therapeutic groups is to screen for high-risk children who may need individual therapy. More generally, children whose problems persist despite group help should be treated individually.

Individual treatment

Individual treatment centres mainly on cognitive-behavioural therapies that aim both to help the survivor make sense of what happened and to master their feelings of anxiety and helplessness (Perrin et al. 2000; Smith et al. 1996). Drug treatments have little place at present. Asking children to draw their experiences can be useful in helping them recall both the event and the emotions associated with it (Newman 1976; Blom 1986; Galante & Foa 1986; Pynoos & Eth 1986) but merely drawing the trauma is not a sufficient therapy. A recent study from former Yugoslavia where great emphasis was placed on getting children to express their emotions through drawing found that 6 months after having had very structured sessions on drawing and other expressive techniques, there was no measurable change in children's adjustment on a whole range of self-report measures of stress reactions (Bunjevac & Kuterovac 1994).

Saigh (1986) was one of the first to provide clinical evidence that, as Rachman (1980) had predicted, there were dangers in using standard systematic desensitization approaches as the length of exposure sessions may be too short to permit adequate habituation of anxiety. It should also be remembered that where children are frightened by the vividness of their memories then relaxation may only serve to intensify the vividness. The theoretical aspects of exposure therapy in treating PTSD in children are discussed elsewhere (Saigh et al. 1996).

Given the nature of traumatic events, children are not infrequently bereaved as a consequence. Pynoos & Nader (1988) emphasize the need to help children to distinguish their trauma-related responses from those related to grief, and suggest that where several children are bereaved, small groups can be beneficial in the initial stages. Dyregrov's (1993) account of the distinguishing features of traumatic bereavement implies that the traumatic nature of the death and post-trauma reactions need to be addressed before grieving can begin. Black (1993) uses a wide variety of techniques including the use of drawings and play in her work with children who have been bereaved as a consequence of one parent killing another. Importantly, she also describes how family work—including that with new carers—is necessary in cases where a child has lost a parent.

Pynoos's (1994) developmental framework for understanding trauma reactions has a number of implications for therapeutic intervention. The model suggests that the interaction over time of many critical factors (including the complexity of the traumatic experience and the interactions of traumatic reminders, secondary stress, post-traumatic distress, and development) have a role in the progression from traumatic exposure to psychopathology. Each of these factors can be seen as a potential focus for intervention. Similarly, James (1989) describes the use of early intervention with subsequent 'pulsed intervention' over time using multifaceted treatment approaches.

Eye movement desensitization and reprocessing

There is considerable interest and scepticism in eye movement desensitization and reprocessing (EMDR) treatment (Shapiro 1991). In this technique, children are asked to conjure up an image of the traumatic event while simultaneously moving their eyes to follow the therapist's hand. The therapist makes few, if any, verbal interventions or interpretations. In some children, the images spontaneously alter and lose their ability to generate anxious feelings. To date there are no published accounts of controlled trials with children and adolescents. Tinker & Wilson (1999) described many successfully treated cases but no comparison data were provided. C. Chemtob, J. Nakashima, R. Hamada & J. Carlson (unpublished data, 1998) used 3–6 sessions of EMDR with adolescents traumatized following a hurricane and report good results, but again with no control data. As with all techniques that have no clear rationale, caution has to be exercised. However, if symptomatic relief can really be attained in a few brief sessions, then the approach needs to be carefully evaluated. As there does seem to be a different quality to the memories of a trauma that appear at the same time to be locked in, vivid, and unchangeable merely by talking about them, then any technique that will allow emotional processing to proceed must be examined.

Contingency planning

When trauma affects a large number of children at once, as in an accident at school, then a public health approach to dealing with the emergency is required (Pynoos *et al.* 1995). Schools need to plan ahead not only to deal with large-scale disasters, but also to respond to the needs of children after threatening incidents that affect only a few of them. Thus, there are now a number of texts written especially for schools to help them develop contingency plans to deal with the effects of a disaster (Johnson 1993; Klingman 1993; Yule & Gold 1993).

Most developed countries have well-established plans to deal with major civil emergencies. Increasingly, these include a psychosocial or mental health component and it is advisable for child and adolescent mental health services to be involved in the planning (Canterbury & Yule 1999). UN agencies are increasingly prepared to meet the mental health needs of children after war and major disasters (Report of the UN Secretary General on the Impact of Armed Conflict on Children 1966), and again mental health services need to collaborate with other agencies to meet such needs.

Overview of treatment

In formulating their recommendations for practice, the ISTSS task force (Foa *et al.* 2000) used very stringent criteria when judging the evidence for treatment efficacy. The strongest evidence was viewed as deriving from randomized well-controlled clinical trials (Level A) while the poorest evidence (Level F) encompassed anecdotal evidence from recently developed approaches that had not been tested empirically. They rated cognitive-behaviour therapy as being at Level A; EMDR as being at Level B–C; dynamic psychotherapy as being at Level D; and other forms of intervention such as debriefing, family psychotherapy, group psychotherapy and art therapy as all being at Level E.

Cognitive processing

Rachman (1980) conceptualized what was to be labelled as PTSD as a failure to process emotions that arose following exposure to a traumatic event. Since then, there has been a great deal of work examining emotional and cognitive processing in adult PTSD patients (Dalgleish 1999; Thrasher & Dalgleish 1999). More recently, the paradigms developed to study these processes in adults have been adapted to study PTSD in children. Thus, in a series of related studies of children presenting with general anxiety disorder, depression and PTSD, Dalgleish, Yule and colleagues have shown that on measures of attention and memory, the three groups of children not only differ but do so in the same way as adults; both groups of anxious children respond more quickly to threat words on the Stroop task, especially threat words directly related to the trauma in the case of children with PTSD (Dalgleish *et al.* 1998; Moradi *et al.* 1999a–c; Neshat-Doost *et al.* 1998, 2000; Taghavi *et al.* 1999).

Conclusions

Since its formulation in 1980, the diagnosis of PTSD has become widely used in child mental health practice. Using standard criteria and measures, significant minorities of children and adolescents have been diagnosed with PTSD following a variety of major stressors from transport accidents, natural disasters such as hurricanes, and war. These reactions have now been shown to be both long-lasting and disabling in many cases. Moreover, the few studies of psychophysiology and biochemistry confirm that there are underlying changes that may be difficult to reverse.

While it is comforting to children who develop PTSD following a life-threatening experience to be told that their frightening symptoms are 'normal', not all children do react this way and so greater emphasis is needed to discover why some children are more vulnerable than others. It seems clear that there is a dose–response relationship between severity of exposure and severity of symptoms, both within and between different types of incident.

There is considerable overlap in disorders that present after a major traumatic event (Pfefferbaum 1997; Bolton *et al.* 2000); however, there seems more than heuristic value in regarding PTSD to be both separate from other anxiety disorders and separate from depression. For example, following their intervention after the Armenian earthquake, Goenjian *et al.* (1996) found that in the group who had treatment first, PTSD scores reduced while depression scores remained stable. By contrast, in the waiting list control group, the PTSD did not resolve but the depression increased. In other words, the two disorders react differently to intervention.

One can also argue that these disorders are indeed different in so far as the content of the intrusive thoughts is so specific to the particular event and so characteristic of the disorder in a way that is not found in depression or other anxiety disorders. This needs to be explored more systematically. Indeed, studying PTSD has proved a remarkably fertile ground for studying child psychopathology and so one hopes that there will be more investigations of the nature of traumatic stress reactions in younger children as well as better intervention studies. In the mean time, PTSD is a diagnostic category that helps focus mental health professionals on the needs of the children—always providing that they ask the children themselves about their inner experiences and reactions.

References

Almqvist, K. & Brandell-Forsberg, M. (1997) Refugee children in Sweden: post-traumatic stress disorder in Iranian preschool children exposed to organized violence. *Child Abuse and Neglect*, 21, 351–366.

American Psychiatric Association (1980) *Diagnostic and Statistical Manual of Mental Disorders*, 3rd edn. American Psychiatric Association, Washington D.C.

American Psychiatric Association (1987) *Diagnostic and Statistical Manual of Mental Disorders*, Revised 3rd edn. American Psychiatric Association, Washington D.C.

American Psychiatric Association (1994) *Diagnostic and Statistical Manual of Mental Disorders*, 4th edn. American Psychiatric Association, Washington D.C.

Black, D. (1993) When father kills mother. In: *ACPP Occasional Papers 8* (ed. G. Forrest), pp. 19–25. ACPP, London.

Blom, G.E. (1986) A school disaster: intervention and research aspects. *Journal of the American Academy of Child Psychiatry*, 25, 336–345.

Bolton, D., O'Ryan, D., Udwin, O., Boyle, S. & Yule, W. (2000) The long-term psychological effects of a disaster experienced in adolescence. II. General psychopathology. *Journal of Child Psychology and Psychiatry*, 41, 513–523.

Breslau, N., Davis, G.C., Andreski, P. & Peterson, E. (1991) Traumatic events and post-traumatic stress disorder in an urban population of young adults. *Archives of General Psychiatry*, 48, 216–222.

Bunjevac, T. & Kuterovac, G. (1994) Report on the results of psychological evaluation of the art therapy program in schools in Hercegovina. UNICEF, Zagreb.

Canterbury, R. & Yule, W. (1999) Debriefing and crisis intervention. In: *Post Traumatic Stress Disorder* (ed. W. Yule), pp. 221–238. Wiley, Chichester.

Cohen, J.A. (1998) Practice parameters for the assessment and treatment of children and adolescents with post-traumatic stress disorder. *Journal of the American Academy of Child and Adolescent Psychiatry*, 37 (Suppl. 10), 4–26.

Dalgleish, T. (1999) Cognitive theories of post-traumatic stress disorder. In: *Post Traumatic Stress Disorder* (ed. W. Yule), pp. 193–220. Wiley, Chichester.

Dalgleish, T., Neshat-Doost, H., Taghavi, R. et al. (1998) Information processing in recovered depressed children and adolescents. *Journal of Child Psychology and Psychiatry*, 39, 1031–1035.

Dyregrov, A. (1991) *Grief in Children: a Handbook for Adults*. Jessica Kingsley, London.

Dyregrov, A. (1993) The interplay of trauma and grief. In: *ACPP Occasional Papers 8* (ed. G. Forrest), pp. 2–10. ACPP, London.

Ehlers, A. & Clark, D.M. (2000) A cognitive model of post traumatic stress disorder. *Behaviour Research and Therapy*, 38, 319–345.

Eth, S. (1992) Clinical response to traumatized children. In: *Responding to Disaster: a Guide for Mental Health Professionals*. (ed. L.S. Austin), pp. 101–123. American Psychiatric Press, Washington D.C.

Foa, E.B., Steketee, G. & Olasov-Rothbaum, B. (1989) Behavioral/cognitive conceptualizations of post-traumatic stress disorder. *Behavior Therapy*, 20, 155–176.

Foa, E.B., Keane, T.M. & Friedman, M.J., eds (2000) *Effective Treatments for PTSD: Guidelines from the International Society for Traumatic Stress Studies*. Guilford, New York.

Frederick, C.J. (1985) Children traumatized by catastrophic situations. In: *Post-Traumatic Stress Disorder in Children* (eds S. Eth & R. Pynoos), pp. 73–99. American Psychiatric Press, Washington D.C.

Galante, R. & Foa, D. (1986) An epidemiological study of psychic trauma and treatment effectiveness after a natural disaster. *Journal of the American Academy of Child Psychiatry*, 25, 357–363.

Giaconia, R.M., Reinherz, H.Z., Silverman, A.B., Pakiz, B., Frost, A.K. & Cohen, E. (1995) Traumas and post-traumatic stress disorder in a community population of older adolescents. *Journal of the American Academy of Child and Adolescent Psychiatry*, 34, 1369–1380.

Gillis, H.M. (1993) Individual and small-group psychotherapy for children involved in trauma and disaster. In: *Children and Disasters* (ed. C.F. Saylor), pp. 165–186. Plenum, New York.

Goenjian, A.K., Pynoos, R.S., Steinberg, A.M. et al. (1995) Psychiatric comorbidity in children after the 1988 earthquake in Armenia. *Journal of the American Academy of Child and Adolescent Psychiatry*, 34, 1174–1184.

Goenjian, A.K., Yehuda, R., Pynoos, R.S. et al. (1996) Basal cortisol, dexamethasone suppression of cortisol, and MHPG in adolescents after the 1988 earthquake in Armenia. *American Journal of Psychiatry*, 153, 929–934.

Goodyer, I.M. (1990) *Life Experiences, Development and Childhood Psychopathology*. Wiley, Chichester.

Helzer, J.E., Robins, L.N. & McEvoy, L. (1987) Post-traumatic stress disorder in the general population: findings of the Epidemiological Catchment Area Survey. *New England Journal of Medicine*, 317, 1630–1634.

James, B. (1989) *Treating Traumatized Children: New Insights and Creative Interventions*. Lexington Books, MA.

Janoff-Bulman, R. (1985) The aftermath of victimization: rebuilding shattered assumptions. In: *Trauma and its Wake* (ed. C.R. Figley), pp. 15–35. Brunner/Mazel, New York.

Johnson, K. (1993) *School Crisis Management: A Team Training Guide*. Hunter House, Alameda, CA.

Jones, J.C. & Barlow, D.H. (1992) A new model of post-traumatic stress disorder. In: *Post-Traumatic Stress Disorder: a Behavioral Approach to Assessment and Treatment* (ed. P.A. Saigh), pp. 147–165. Macmillan, New York.

Kessler, R.C., Sonnega, A., Bromet, E., Hughes, M. & Nelson, C.B. (1995) Post-traumatic stress disorder in the National Comorbidity Survey. *Archives of General Psychiatry*, 52, 1048–1060.

Klingman, A. (1987) A school-based emergency crisis intervention in a mass school disaster. *Professional Psychology: Research and Practice*, 18, 604–612.

Klingman, A. (1993) School-based intervention following a disaster. In: *Children and Disasters* (ed. C.F. Saylor), pp. 187–210. Plenum, New York.

van der Kolk, B., Greenberg, M., Boyd, H. et al. (1985) Inescapable shock, neurotransmitters, and addiction to trauma: toward a psychobiology of post-traumatic stress disorder. *Biological Psychiatry*, 20, 314–325.

Lonigan, C.J., Shannon, M.P., Finch, A.J., Daugherty, T.K. & Saylor, C.M. (1991) Children's reactions to a natural disaster: symptom severity and degree of exposure. *Advances in Behaviour Research and Therapy*, 13, 135–154.

March, J.S., Amaya-Jackson, L., Murray, M.C. & Schulte, A. (1998) Cognitive-behavioral psychotherapy for children and adolescents with post-traumatic stress disorders after a single incident stressor.

Journal of the American Academy of Child and Adolescent Psychiatry, 37, 585–593.

McFarlane, A.C. (1987) Family functioning and overprotection following a natural disaster: the longitudinal effects of post-traumatic morbidity. *Australia and New Zealand Journal of Psychiatry*, 21, 210–218.

Meichenbaum, D. (1994) *A Clinical Handbook/ Practical Therapist Manual for Assessing and Treating Adults with Post-Traumatic Stress Disorder (PTSD)*. Institute Press, Ontario.

Misch, P., Phillips, M., Evans, P. & Berelowitz, M. (1993) Trauma in pre-school children: a clinical account. In: *Trauma and Crisis Management* (ed. G. Forrest), pp. 11–18. ACPP Occasional Papers 8.

Moradi, A.R., Neshat-Doost, H.T., Taghavi, R., Yule, W. & Dalgleish, T. (1999a) Performance of children and adolescents with PTSD on the Stroop colour-naming task. *Psychological Medicine*, 29, 415–419.

Moradi, A.R., Neshat-Doost, H.T., Taghavi, R., Yule, W. & Dalgleish, T. (1999b) Everyday memory deficit in children and adolescents with post-traumatic stress disorder: performance on the Rivermead Behavioural Memory Test. *Journal of Child Psychology and Psychiatry*, 40, 357–361.

Moradi, A.R., Neshat-Doost, H.T., Taghavi, M.R., Yule, W. & Dalgleish, T. (1999c) Performance of children of adults with PTSD on the Stroop colour-naming task: a preliminary study. *Journal of Traumatic Stress*, 12, 663–672.

Nader, K., Pynoos, R., Fairbanks, L. & Frederick, C. (1990) Children's PTSD reactions one year after a sniper attack at their school. *American Journal of Psychiatry*, 147, 1526–1530.

Neshat-Doost, H.T., Taghavi, M.R., Moradi, A.R., Yule, W. & Dalgleish, T. (1998) Memory for emotional trait-adjectives in clinically depressed youth. *Journal of Abnormal Psychology*, 107, 642–650.

Neshat-Doost, H., Moradi, A., Taghavi, R., Yule, W. & Dalgleish, T. (2000) Lack of attentional bias for emotional information in clinically depressed children and adolescents on the dot probe task. *Journal of Child Psychology and Psychiatry*, 41, 363–368.

Newman, C.J. (1976) Children of disaster: clinical observation at Buffalo Creek. *American Journal of Psychiatry*, 133, 306–312.

O'Donohue, W. & Eliot, A. (1992) The current status of post-traumatic stress disorder as a diagnostic category: problems and proposals. *Journal of Traumatic Stress*, 5, 421–439.

Ornitz, E.M. & Pynoos, R.S. (1989) Startle modulation in children with post-traumatic stress disorder. *American Journal of Psychiatry*, 146, 866–870.

Perrin, S., Smith, P. & Yule, W. (2000) The assessment and treatment of post-traumatic stress disorder in children and adolescents. *Journal of Child Psychology and Psychiatry*, 41, 277–289.

Perry, B.D. (1994) Neurobiological sequelae of childhood trauma: post-traumatic stress disorder in children. In: *Catecholamine Function in Post-Traumatic Stress Disorder: Emerging Concepts* (ed. M.M. Murburg), pp. 233–255. American Psychiatric Press, Washington D.C.

Perry, B.D., Pollard, R.A., Blakley, T.L., Baker, W.L. & Vigilante, D. (1995) Childhood trauma, the neurobiology of adaptation, and 'use-dependent' development of the brain: how 'states' become 'traits'. *Infant Mental Health Journal*, 16, 271–291.

Pfefferbaum, B. (1997) Post-traumatic stress disorder in children: a review of the past 10 years. *Journal of the American Academy of Child and Adolescent Psychiatry*, 36, 1503–1511.

Pynoos, R.S. (1994) Traumatic stress and developmental psychopathology in children and adolescents. In: *Post-Traumatic Stress Disorder: a Clinical Review* (ed. R.S. Pynoos), pp. 65–98. Sidran Press, Lutherville, MD.

Pynoos, R.S. & Eth, S. (1986) Witness to violence: the child interview. *Journal of the American Academy of Child Psychiatry*, 25, 306–319.

Pynoos, R.S. & Nader, K. (1988) Psychological first aid and treatment approach for children exposed to community violence: research implications. *Journal of Traumatic Stress*, 1, 243–267.

Pynoos, R.S. & Nader, K. (1993) Issues in the treatment of post-traumatic stress in children and adolescents. In: *International Handbook of Traumatic Stress Syndromes* (eds J. Wilson & B. Raphael), pp. 535–549. Plenum Press, New York.

Pynoos, R.S., Frederick, C., Nader, K. *et al.* (1987) Life threat and post-traumatic stress in school-age children. *Archives of General Psychiatry*, 44, 1057–1063.

Pynoos, R.S., Goenjian, A. & Steinberg, A.M. (1995) Strategies of disaster interventions for children and adolescents. In: *Extreme Stress and Communities: Impact and Intervention* (eds S.E. Hobfoll & M. deVries), pp. 445–471. Kluwer, Dordrecht.

Rachman, S. (1980) Emotional processing. *Behaviour Research and Therapy*, 18, 51–60.

Saigh, P.A. (1986) *In vitro* flooding in the treatment of a 6-yr-old boy's post-traumatic stress disorder. *Behaviour Research and Therapy*, 24, 685–688.

Saigh, P.A., Yule, W. & Inamdar, S.C. (1996) Imaginal flooding of traumatized children and adolescents. *Journal of School Psychology*, 34, 163–183.

Scheeringa, M.S., Zeanah, C.H., Drell, M.J. & Larrieu, J.A. (1995) Two approaches to the diagnosis of post-traumatic stress disorder in infancy and early childhood. *Journal of the American Academy of Child and Adolescent Psychiatry*, 34, 191–200.

Shannon, M.P., Lonigan, C.J., Finch, A.J. *et al.* (1994) Children exposed to disaster. I. Epidemiology of post-traumatic symptoms and symptom profiles. *Journal of the American Academy of Child and Adolescent Psychiatry*, 33, 80–93.

Shapiro, F. (1991) Eye movement desensitization and reprocessing procedure: from EMD to EMD/R—a new treatment model for anxiety and related traumas. *Behavior Therapist*, 14, 133–135.

Smith, P., Dyregrov, A., Yule, W., Perrin, S., Gupta. L. & Gjestad, R. (1999a) *A Manual for Teaching Survival Techniques to Child Survivors of Wars and Major Disasters*. Foundation for Children and War, Bergen, Norway.

Smith, P., Perrin, S. & Yule, W. (1999b) Cognitive behaviour therapy for post traumatic stress disorder. *Child Psychology and Psychiatry Review*, 4, 177–182.

Smith, P., Perrin, S., Yule, W. & Rabe-Hesketh, S. (2001) War exposure and maternal reactions in the psychological adjustment of children from Bosnia-Hercegovina. *Journal of Child Psychology and Psychiatry*, 42, 395–404.

Smith, P., Perrin, S., Yule, W., Hacam, B. & Stuvland, R. (in press) War exposure and children from Bosnia-Hercegovina: psychological adjustment in a community sample.

Stallard, P. & Law, F. (1993) Screening and psychological debriefing of adolescent survivors of life-threatening events. *British Journal of Psychiatry*, 163, 660–665.

Sullivan, M.A., Saylor, C.F. & Foster, K.Y. (1991) Post-hurricane adjustment of preschoolers and their families. *Advances in Behaviour Research and Therapy*, 13, 163–171.

Taghavi, M.R., Neshat-Doost, H.T., Moradi, A.R., Yule, W. & Dalgleish, T. (1999) Biases in visual attention in children and adolescents with clinical anxiety and mixed depression–anxiety disorder. *Journal of Abnormal Child Psychology*, 27, 215–223.

Terr, L.C. (1991) Childhood traumas: an outline and overview. *American Journal of Psychiatry*, 148, 10–20.

Thrasher, S. & Dalgleish, T. (1999) The use of information-processing paradigms to investigate post-traumatic stress disorder: a review. In: *Post Traumatic Stress Disorder* (ed. W. Yule), pp. 176–192. Wiley, Chichester.

Tinker, R.H. & Wilson, S.A. (1999) *Through the eyes of a child: EMDR with children*. Norton, New York.

Troyna, A. (1998) *Guidelines for Professionals*. Child Accident Prevention Trust, London.

United Nations (1996) Report of the UN Secretary General on the impact of armed conflict on children (The Machel Report). United Nations, New York.

Vernberg, E.M. & Vogel, J.M. (1993) Task Force Report. II. Interventions with children after disasters. *Journal of Clinical Child Psychology*, 22, 485–498.

Vogel, J.M. & Vernberg, E.M. (1993) Task Force Report. I. Children's psychological responses to disasters. *Journal of Clinical Child Psychology*, 22, 464–484.

Williams, R., Joseph, S. & Yule, W. (1993) Disaster and mental health. In: *Principles of Social Psychiatry* (eds J. Leff & D. Bhugra), pp. 450–469. Blackwell Scientific Publications, Oxford.

World Health Organization (1987/1988/1991) *International Classification of Diseases (ICD-10)*, 10th edn. World Health Organization, Geneva.

Yehuda, R. & McFarlane, A.C. (1995) Conflict between current knowledge about post-traumatic stress disorder and its original conceptual basis. *American Journal of Psychiatry*, 152, 1705–1713.

Yule, W. (1991) Work with children following disasters. In: *Clinical Child Psychology: Social Learning, Development and Behaviour* (ed. M. Herbert), pp. 349–363. John Wiley, Chichester.

Yule, W. (1992) Post traumatic stress disorder in child survivors of shipping disasters: the sinking of the *Jupiter*. *Psychotherapy and Psychosomatics*, 57, 200–205.

Yule, W. (2000a) Treatment of PTSD in children following RTAs. In: *Road Accidents and the Mind* (eds E. Blanchard & E. Hickling), pp. 375–387. Elsevier, London.

Yule, W. (2000b) From 'pogroms' to 'ethnic cleansing': meeting the needs of war affected children. The Emmanuel Miller Lecture. *Journal of Child Psychology and Psychiatry*, 41, 695–702.

Yule, W. & Gold, A. (1993) *Wise Before the Event: Coping with Crises in Schools*. Calouste Gulbenkian Foundation, London.

Yule, W. & Udwin, O. (1991) Screening child survivors for post-traumatic stress disorders: experiences from the *Jupiter* sinking. *British Journal of Clinical Psychology*, 30, 131–138.

Yule, W. & Williams, R. (1990) Post traumatic stress reactions in children. *Journal of Traumatic Stress*, 3, 279–295.

Yule, W., Hodgkinson, P., Joseph, S. & Williams, R. (1990a) *Preliminary follow-up of adult survivors of the* Herald of Free Enterprise. Paper presented to Second European Conference on Traumatic Stress, Netherlands, September 1990.

Yule, W., Udwin, O. & Murdoch, K. (1990b) The *Jupiter* sinking: effects on children's fears, depression and anxiety. *Journal of Child Psychology and Psychiatry*, 31, 1051–1061.

Yule, W., Bolton, D. & Udwin, O. (1992) *Objective and subjective predictors of PTSD in adolescents*. Paper presented at World Conference of International Society for Traumatic Stress Studies, 'Trauma and Tragedy', Amsterdam. 21–26 June, 1992.

Yule, W., Perrin, S. & Smith, P. (1999) Post-traumatic stress disorders in children and adolescents. In: *Post Traumatic Stress Disorder* (ed. W. Yule), pp. 25–50. Wiley, Chichester.

Yule, W., Bolton, D., Udwin, O., Boyle, S., O'Ryan, D. & Nurrish, J. (2000) The long-term psychological effects of a disaster experienced in adolescence. I. The incidence and course of post traumatic stress disorder. *Journal of Child Psychology and Psychiatry*, 41, 503–511.

33 Suicide and Attempted Suicide

David Shaffer and Jennifer Gutstein

Introduction

Suicide and attempted suicide are two closely related phenomena but they differ in important ways. Suicide is a relatively unusual event. In the USA, about 1 in 10 000 15–19-year-olds commit suicide each year. Attempted suicide, on the other hand, is extremely common. All suicidal features are more common in females but suicide ideation is extremely common in both sexes, being present in 14% of boys and 25% of girls (Centers for Disease Control 2000). Further, most ideators also make a plan. If we assume a male attempt rate of 2.1% and a male death rate of 14.6 per 100 000, the ratio of serious attempts to completed suicides in males is about 140 : 1, compared with approximately 1000 : 1 in females.

Completed suicide

Incidence

Suicide in prepubertal children is rare in all countries (Table 33.1). Among 10–14-year-olds, most suicides occur in those who are oldest. The incidence of suicide then increases steadily through the teenage years, reaching a peak in the early or mid-twenties (see Fig. 33.1). In all developed countries (except the USA, where homicide is the second leading cause), suicides are the second leading cause of death, exceeded only by accidents. In the USA—a country with a relatively low suicide rate—the number of suicides outnumbers the number of deaths from all other natural causes combined (National Center for Health Statistics, Centers for Disease Control and Prevention 2000).

Rate changes over time

In recent years, the rate of suicide among teenagers has shown marked and sustained changes (Fig. 33.2): US male teenage suicides increased more than threefold in the 20-year period from the mid-1960s until the mid-1980s (National Center for Health Statistics, Centers for Disease Control and Prevention 2000), and similar increases were reported in many other countries (UNICEF 1996; Lynskey *et al.* 2000; McClure 2000; World Health Organization 1997–1999). However, between 1990 and 1998, in the USA as well as in other countries, the rate declined by around 20% in *both* males and females.

A number of reasons have been proposed to explain the ear-

lier increase and the more recent decrease in teenage suicide deaths. Reasons that were once proposed for the *increase* include broad social changes, such as high divorce rates and the increasing proportion of mothers in the workplace; and cultural influences, such as rock music lyrics, the broad acceptance of assisted suicide, and the increasing availability of firearms. However, empirical research suggests that a lack of family cohesion is not a powerful risk factor (Gould *et al.* 1998a), nor is there evidence for any noxious consequences of songs and lyrics that dwell on morbid subjects. A more convincing explanation is that the period of increasing rates was a period of increasing drug and alcohol use, a known risk factor for suicide (Robins *et al.* 1959; Murphy & Robins 1967; Murphy & Wetzel 1990; Shaffer *et al.* 1996a; Renaud *et al.* 1999). Furthermore, the relationship between suicide and substance and alcohol abuse is stronger in males (Shaffer *et al.* 1996a) and occurs mainly in older teenagers, the gender and age group most affected by the rate increase.

The more recent *fall* in the suicide rate does not seem to be caused by a reduction in alcohol exposure because, at least in the USA and the UK, drug and alcohol usage rates have remained steady during the period of declining suicide incidence (Centers for Disease Control 2000; UK Office for National Statistics 2000). A widely accepted explanation is that the reduction is a result of the much more frequent prescribing and acceptance of the newer antidepressants for teenagers (Isacsson *et al.* 1997; Safer 1997a; Ohberg *et al.* 1998; Olfson *et al.* 1998; C. Blanco & M. Olfson, personal communication 2000).

Gender

In adolescence, suicidal ideation and suicide attempts are more common in females (Safer 1997b; Centers for Disease Control 2000), whereas completed suicides are more common in males. In a small number of developing countries in South Asia and Latin America, the male and female suicide rates are similar or are even higher among girls (World Health Organization 1997–1999; Yip *et al.* 2000). The reasons for these gender differences are not known, but in all probability reside in gender differences in psychopathology and in method preference.

Psychopathology

Teenagers who commit suicide can be grouped into:

1 a large, predominantly male, group with a history of

Table 33.1 Youth suicide rates per 100 000, latest year available, in selected countries (World Health Organization 1997–1999).

Country	Year	Ages 5–14		Ages 15–25	
		Male	Female	Male	Female
Australia	1995	0.3	—	23.1	6.1
Belgium	1994	1.6	0.2	22.7	3.7
Canada	1997	1.9	0.6	22.4	4.5
France	1996	0.5	0.1	12.8	4.2
Germany	1997	0.6	0.2	12.9	3.2
Ireland	1996	1.3	—	25.4	4.5
Italy	1995	0.5	0.0	7.3	1.6
Japan	1997	0.5	0.03	11.3	5.5
Netherlands	1997	1.1	—	11.3	4.4
New Zealand	1996	1.0	1.5	37.8	13.9
Russian Federation	1997	3.0	0.7	53.2	9.0
UK	1997	0.1	0.1	11.1	2.3
England & Wales	1997	0.1	0.1	9.9	1.9
Northern Ireland	1997	0.7	0.8	18.6	4.4
Scotland	1997	—	—	19.5	5.3
USA	1998	1.2	0.4	18.5	3.3

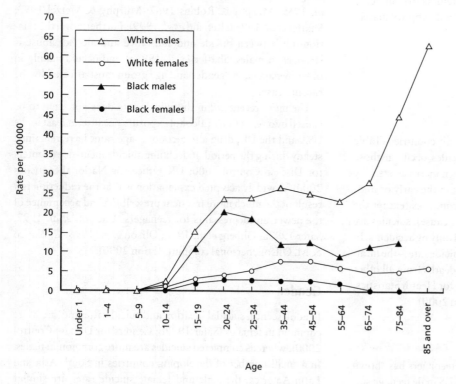

Fig. 33.1 Suicide rates at different ages (US, 1998) (NCHS, 2000).

aggressive behaviour and impulsive and intense responses to stress and comorbid substance and alcohol abuse; and

2 a much smaller group of males and females with anxious or depressive symptoms without associated antisocial behaviour (Shaffer *et al.* 1996a; Brent *et al.* 1999).

It is likely that the predominance of males in the first group accounts, in large measure, for the male excess in completed suicides.

Choice of method

Most female suicide attempts and many female suicides involve an overdose, but in most countries this is not an effective method. In some countries, the supply of rapidly lethal ingestants, such as barbiturates, is restricted and, in most developed countries, treatment resources for intentional ingestions are well developed. In countries with high female suicide rates, the

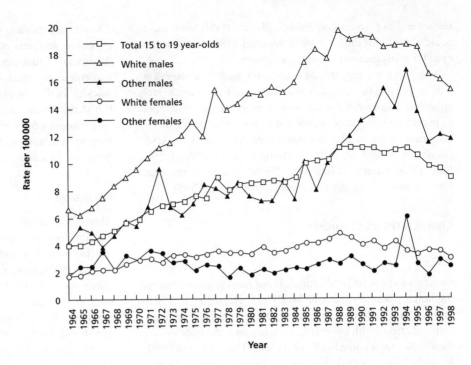

Fig. 33.2 Adolescent suicide rates (15–19-year-olds) (US, 1964–1998) (NCHS, 2000).

type of self-poisoning used cannot be treated—e.g. paraquat and organophosphate ingestion in Southeast Asia and the South Pacific (Haynes 1987; Jeyaratnam 1990; Eddleston *et al.* 1998)—and good medical services are not readily available.

Age

Completed suicide is exceedingly rare before age 12 and is, on average, less common in teenagers than in adults. The incidence increases each year until the mid-twenties when in most, but not all, countries, it increases more gradually until late middle age. This incidence pattern makes it unlikely that teenage suicide results from specifically adolescent psychological 'tasks' or stresses. If that were the case, the incidence of suicide would have a peak incidence in the mid-teenage years with a subsequent decline. The rarity of suicide before puberty has been attributed to more difficulty in accessing lethal methods and poorly developed planning skills. A youngster who intends to hang himself needs to find an appropriate and private site or a degree of technical sophistication. This is not an entirely plausible explanation, because a degree of privacy is available to most 12–15-year-olds who, nevertheless, have a very low suicide rate. Further, many suicide threats in young children involve a threat to jump from a height or into traffic—potentially effective methods that are readily accessible to most children and can be executed without much planning. It seems more likely that the incidence gradient across the teenage years is also influenced by the appearance of new risk factors in later adolescence. The two leading risk factors for suicide in adolescence—affective illness and alcohol abuse (Brent *et al.* 1989, 1993a; Gould *et al.* 1990; Shaffer *et al.* 1996a)—are uncommon before the mid-teens

(Kashani & Simonds 1979), but are increasingly prevalent after that.

Ethnicity

Cultural differences in prevalence are conveniently studied in a multiethnic country, such as the USA or the UK, where recording and reporting procedures are similar for different groups. In the USA, suicide is more common in whites than in non-whites in all age groups (see Fig. 33.1). In the UK, the suicide rate is much higher among the Scots and the Welsh than among the English (World Health Organization 1997–1999).

The reasons for these cultural differences are not known. In the USA, American Indian and Native Alaskan youth have more than twice the national rate of suicide (Indian Health Service 1996). Historically, African-Americans, both adolescents and adults, have had lower suicide rates than Caucasians. However, in the mid-1980s the African-American suicide rate in teenagers began to climb precipitously, levelling off in the mid-1990s. The current difference between African-American and Caucasian adolescent suicide rates, although still significant, is not as great. The African-American : Caucasian 15–19-year-old USA suicide rate ratio went from 1 : 2 in 1979, to 2 : 5 in 1986, to 2 : 3 in 1998. In the USA, black–white differences have been variously attributed to religiosity (Neeleman *et al.* 1998) and/or more effective social support systems (Gibbs & Martin 1964; Bush 1976; May 1987; Neeleman & Wessely 1999) or to reporting biases (Monk & Warshauer 1978). However, it is possible that variations in the suicide rates in different groups and countries are only indirectly related to culture, and that the mechanisms for the differences lie in imitation and contagion (see below) that operate *within* and not across cultural boundaries. If this were so, it could account for the quite stable regional differences that can exist for many generations within a country.

Although there appear to be cultural or regional differences in vulnerability to suicide, there is little evidence that the characteristics of suicide differ in different groups. The rates and types of psychiatric disorders, family histories of suicidality and recent stresses are similar in countries as different as the USA (Shaffer *et al.* 1996a), Finland (Marttunen *et al.* 1991, 1993), India (Vijayakumar & Rajkumar 1999), Taiwan, in the Han Chinese and two distinct aboriginal groups (Cheng 1995).

Characteristics of suicide

Season

Contrary to popular belief, suicide is not more common during the holiday season (Lester & Beck 1975; Hillard *et al.* 1981; Bollen 1983; Phillips & Wills 1987). However, there may be a 'delayed effect', with lower suicide rates during the holiday and then higher rates immediately afterwards (Phillips & Liu 1980; Jessen & Jensen 1999). In both the northern and southern hemispheres, suicide is most common during the spring months (Lester 1979; Chew & McCleary 1995; Flisher *et al.* 1997), with a second peak in autumn (Kevan 1980; Meares *et al.* 1981; Hakko *et al.* 1998). There are similar seasonal peaks in hypomanic behaviour among individuals with bipolar illness (Eastwood & Peter 1988; Goodwin & Jamison 1990; Silverstone *et al.* 1995; Szabo & Blanche 1995). Suicide in bipolar illness is most common at the time of mood shifts, and there might be an association between the two phenomena.

Method

In the USA, the large majority of teenage boys and a smaller majority of teenage girls commit suicide with firearms, most often legally registered but inadequately secured rifles or shotguns. Only 20% of suicides committed with firearms in the USA are committed with handguns. In Great Britain, hanging is the most common method for boys, while girls are more likely to die from an overdose or fall from a height. The increase in hanging in young males in the UK and New Zealand has offset the decrease in overdose and asphyxiation deaths. Some studies have reported a relationship between diagnosis and method. Brent *et al.* (1991) found that firearms were more likely to be used by boys with substance or alcohol abuse problems, but this finding has not been consistently reported. There is some evidence that the method is largely determined by availability (Moens *et al.* 1988; Hawton *et al.* 1998a; Fisher *et al.* 2001).

Occasionally, a boy will be found having seemingly hanged himself in a state of semiundress or cross-dress, with evidence of recent orgasm and the presence at the scene of death of fetishistic objects. It is then assumed that his death was an accidental result of erotic activity (Stearns 1953; Coe 1974; Sheehan & Garfinkel 1988). Shaffer *et al.* (1996a) found that fewer than

3% of hanging deaths occurred in these circumstances. Very few published accounts of alleged auto-erotic deaths provide evidence of habitual semistrangulation, and the gender, seasonal and ethnic distribution of the victims closely resemble that of suicides. In the few psychological analyses that have been published, depression and substance abuse were common, as in suicide (Sheehan & Garfinkel 1988). Taken together, these facts suggest that, rather than many auto-erotic accidental deaths being misclassified as suicide, the reverse is equally likely.

Precipitants

Although some adolescents, predominantly girls, suffering from a major depressive disorder appear to have thought about suicide for some time and will often have made some preparation for their death, most adolescent suicides appear to be impulsive (Negron *et al.* 1997). Often they were preceded by a stress event, such as a disciplinary crisis, a ruptured relationship with a boyfriend or a girlfriend or a fight among friends (Brent *et al.* 1993b; Gould *et al.* 1996). In many instances, these stress events can be seen as a by-product of an underlying mental disorder. The events that precede a suicide often reflect the victim's underlying psychopathology. The most common precipitant is a 'disciplinary crisis', school suspension or appearance in juvenile court (Brent *et al.* 1993b; Gould *et al.* 1996). A typical situation will be that a teenager is discovered truanting or stealing and is told by the school or police that some action will be taken in the near future, e.g. parents or the court will be informed. The teenager commits suicide shortly afterward, before the anticipated response. The frequency of the situation reflects the high rate of aggressive conduct disorder in the suicidal population. By contrast, suicide victims with predominantly anxious symptomatology might commit suicide shortly before a feared event, such as an examination, starting at a new school or moving to a new neighbourhood (Shaffer 1974; Shaffer *et al.* 1996a). Suicides in the context of an acute depression might have no obvious external precipitant. A small number of suicides occur on the anniversary of a friend's death. In one study (Shaffer 1974), just over one-quarter of the children died within two weeks of their own birthdays. About half of all suicides had discussed or threatened suicide within 24 hours of their deaths.

Aetiology

Biological abnormalities

In 1976, Asberg *et al.* (1976) noted a relationship between low levels of cerebrospinal fluid 5-hydroxyindoleacetic acid (5-HIAA), the major metabolite of serotonin, and a prior suicide attempt in a group of adult patients suffering from melancholic depression. This has now become one of the most replicated findings in biological psychiatry (see Oquendo & Mann 2000 for a review). This relationship is stronger among suicides who died by firearm and hanging than in those who died from an

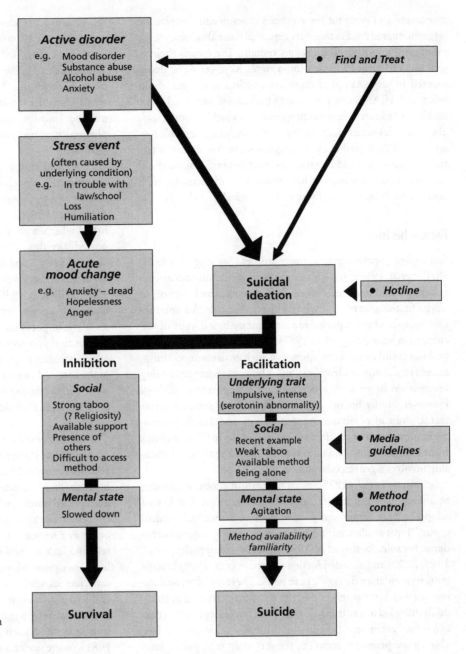

Fig. 33.3 How do suicides occur and how can they be prevented?

overdose. It is found in suicides regardless of diagnosis. However, there is as yet no information about the proportion of suicides in which serotonin abnormalities are found. Although such studies are now in progress, there are no descriptions of how suicides with evidence of serotonin dysregulation differ from those without. However, similar abnormalities have been reported in impulsive and aggressive individuals, and it is generally assumed that these behaviours distinguish the suicides with this type of biological dysregulation.

The working model (Mann 1999; Mann *et al.* 1999) is that serotinergic dysregulation is a biologically determined trait and that a mentally ill individual who possesses this trait is more likely to respond to a stressful experience in an impulsive and aggressive fashion. This response mode could lead directly to

suicide or could simply increase the stressful consequences of their behaviour, ultimately leading to their suicide (Fig. 33.3). There is some evidence that suicide attempters with low levels of cerebrospinal fluid 5-HIAA are significantly more likely to make a future attempt and/or to commit suicide (Nordstrom *et al.* 1994).

Autoradiographic studies suggest that the abnormality is presynaptic and results in compensatory upregulation of postsynaptic type-2 serotonin (5-HT2) receptors in the ventral and ventrolateral prefrontal cortex—the area of the central nervous system that is in large measure responsible for behavioural inhibition. These findings have led to an active investigation of two candidate genes: the promoter region of the serotonin transporter gene; and the gene for tryptophan hydroxylase (*TPH*), the rate-limiting enzyme for the synthesis of serotonin. Despite the large number of studies that have reported these abnormalities, a number of unanswered questions remain. The specific behavioural correlates of low serotonin states have yet to be documented in large samples; there are conflicting reports about whether 5-HIAA levels are stable or fluctuate with mental state; and it is not known in what proportion of suicide victims such abnormalities occur. If, as has been held, declining or stable low levels of 5-HIAA predict a poor prognosis, then secondary or tertiary prevention could be served by routine cerebrospinal fluid monitoring of patients who have made a suicide attempt, with special care being given to those with abnormally low levels.

Family history

Controlled psychological autopsy studies (Brent *et al.* 1996a; Shaffer *et al.* 1996a) have found that completed suicides are between two and four times more likely than matched controls to have a first-degree relative who committed suicide. A similar relationship has been reported in a community-based study of suicide attempters (Bridge *et al.* 1997a; Johnson *et al.* 1998). These findings could be the consequence of such environmental influences as imitation or identification, or be a consequence of being brought up by or with a psychiatrically ill parent or sibling. However, family history of suicidal behaviour remains a risk factor, even after accounting for parent and youth psychopathology (Brent *et al.* 1996a; Gould *et al.* 1996), and findings from both adoption and twin studies suggest that the relationship involves a genetic component.

Schulsinger *et al.* (1979), using the Danish adoption registry, found significantly higher rates of suicide in the families of adoptees who committed suicide than in a matched control group. Twin studies have found significantly greater concordance for suicide (Roy *et al.* 1991), suicide attempts (Roy *et al.* 1995, 2000) and suicide ideation (Statham *et al.* 1998) among monozygotic than dizygotic twin pairs. These findings, and the implication of dysregulation of the serotinergic system in suicidality, have led to a search for single-gene polymorphisms of two candidate genes involved in the synthesis of serotonin (see above): the promoter region of the serotonin transporter gene and the *TPH* gene—the rate-limiting enzyme for the synthesis of serotonin. Findings on these candidate genes has been inconsistent (Nielsen *et al.* 1994, 1998; Ohara *et al.* 1998; Bennet *et al.* 2000; Geijer *et al.* 2000). It is not clear whether this is because the suicide phenotype comprises many different aetiological factors, because the genetic effect is small and requires the analysis of large numbers of patients, or because the clinical importance of a single genetic variant might not be apparent unless studied with other related genes (Marshall *et al.* 1999).

Imitation and contagion

It appears that suicidal behaviour, including completed suicide, can be triggered by exposure to knowledge about other actual or fictional suicides (Velting & Gould 1997). Strong evidence for this includes case accounts of suicides that occurred shortly after a teenager saw a film or read a book or news story about a suicide (Shaffer 1974). In a quasi-experimental ABABA design, Schmidtke & Hafner (1986) showed that the showing of a fictional account of a 19-year-old male student's railway suicide was followed by a sharp but time-limited increase in similar method suicides among youth of similar age and sex. This phenomenon was repeated when the series was rebroadcast a year later.

Ecological studies have also shown a time relationship between media reports of a suicide and a subsequent increase in suicide and suicide attempt rates (Holding 1974, 1975; Gould & Shaffer 1986; Gould *et al.* 1988). None of these studies established whether an individual suicide was exposed to the purported stimulus. The excess of suicides in such circumstances lasts between 7 and 14 days, is proportional to the number of times that the news story is repeated (Phillips 1974, 1979, 1980, 1984; Bollen & Phillips 1981, 1982; Wasserman 1984) and mainly affects young people (Phillips & Carstensen 1986). Studies of the impact of a single stimulus, such as a TV programme, are not always consistent (Berman 1988; Gould *et al.* 1988). The inconsistencies might be a result of variations in the age and size of the exposed viewership and the context in which the material is seen (e.g. whether or not the programmes were accompanied by material that could direct a disturbed viewer to obtain help, etc.).

Evidence for contagion also comes from the well-documented occurrence of cluster or epidemic suicides that are estimated to account for up to 4% of all adolescent suicides in the USA and to be increasing in incidence (Gould 1990). In a suicide cluster, an unexpected number of deaths occur in a short period of time in a circumscribed community. There is no evidence that clusters occur as a response to significant changes in the community itself, and little is known about the characteristics of the suicides. In a description of one cluster (Davidson *et al.* 1989), the victims, like sporadic suicides, were predominantly male and several had a history of past suicidal attempts. Suicide clusters in time can also be triggered by publicity accorded to an unusual suicide method such as self-immolation (Ashton & Donnan 1981), or the use of a specific location such as the Golden Gate Bridge in San Francisco (Kirch & Lester 1986). The Centers for Disease Control in the USA have prepared guidelines for minimizing the problem accorded to an individual suicide, but there is as yet no evidence that applying the guidelines will reduce imitative suicides.

Associated psychiatric disorder

Almost all children and teenagers who commit suicide were suffering from a psychiatric disorder at the time of death (Marttunen *et al.* 1991, 1995; Shaffer *et al.* 1996a; Brent *et al.* 1999). In this respect, as in many others, suicide in adolescents resembles suicide in adults (Robins *et al.* 1959; Barraclough *et al.* 1974; Rich *et al.* 1988). At the time of the suicide, psychiatric disorder is usually well established and, in approximately half (Shaffer *et al.* 1996a), it has been present for 2 years or more. The most common forms in completed suicides are the following.

1 *Some form of mood disorder* in about two-thirds of all suicides. In girls this usually takes the form of an uncomplicated major depression, while in boys it is often comorbid with conduct disorder and/or substance abuse. Many of these boys are markedly irritable, impulsive and volatile, and are prone to outbursts of aggression.

2 *Substance and/or alcohol abuse*, which is present in up to two-thirds of older boys (Shaffer *et al.* 1996a; Brent *et al.* 1999) and is usually complicated by comorbid mood and or conduct problems.

3 About one-quarter to one-third have an *anxiety disorder* (Shaffer *et al.* 1996a; Brent *et al.* 1999). Performance and anticipatory anxiety are particularly prominent and might be viewed by parents as a sign of 'perfectionism'. This group of suicides will usually have gone undiagnosed and been considered to be excellent students and well liked by their peers.

4 *Conduct or oppositional* disorder is present in between one-third and one-half of suicides (Shaffer *et al.* 1996a; Brent *et al.* 1999). It is more common in males and in older suicides and is often comorbid with one of the other disorders listed above. The mechanism underlying the relationship is not known. It could reflect a common biological predisposition mediated by dysregulation of the serotinergic system; it could reflect the depression that often develops in teenagers who are in 'trouble', failing at school, unwelcome at home, and who may be distanced by their peers.

Although the rate of suicide is greatly increased in schizophrenia, because of the rarity of the condition it accounts for very few suicides in the child and adolescent age group. However, mental health professionals who care for individuals with schizophrenia should be aware of their greater risk for suicide.

About 40% of suicides have made a previous known suicide attempt (Shaffer *et al.* 1996a; Brent *et al.* 1999). Previous attempts are more common in girls and among suicides suffering from a mood disorder at the time of their death. In the New York study (Shaffer *et al.* 1996a), approximately half of all suicides had had previous contact with a mental health professional. The very few suicides who were found to be free of significant psychiatric symptomatology included a disproportionate number of prepubescent suicides.

Psychiatric disorder as risk factor

Suicides share many characteristics with other children and teenagers who have psychiatric problems and who do not commit suicide. Determining unique risk factors for suicide requires controlled comparisons, and the sizes of both the index and the control samples are small in nearly all cases. Nevertheless, certain robust findings stand out. Similar risk factors operate for both boys and girls (Shaffer *et al.* 1996a; Brent *et al.* 1999), but they differ markedly in their relative importance (Shaffer *et al.* 1996a). The most significant risk factor for girls is the presence

of major depression, which in some studies increases the risk of suicide 20-fold (Shaffer *et al.* 1996a). The most significant risk factor for boys is a previous suicide attempt, which increases risk more than 30-fold (Shaffer *et al.* 1996a; Brent *et al.* 1999). Although alcohol abuse and disruptive behaviour disorders are the most prevalent diagnoses, their base rate in the general population is high, and value for prediction is therefore low.

Family circumstances

Both large controlled psychological autopsy studies found that adolescents who committed suicide were less likely than controls to live with both of their biological parents. Whereas Brent *et al.* (1994) (*n* = 67) found that suicide victims were more likely to have been exposed to parent–child discord and residential instability, Gould *et al.* (1996) (*n* = 120) found that parent–child discord, discord between parents and divorce had only small or marginal effects. Poor parent–child communication was significantly more apparent in adolescents who committed suicide than in their matched controls, even after taking into account parent and teenage psychopathology. Socioeconomic status did not differentiate white or Hispanic adolescent suicides and controls, but African-American adolescent suicide victims had a significantly higher socioeconomic status than their matched controls (Gould *et al.* 1996).

Perinatal morbidity

Salk *et al.* (1985) examined the birth records of a large proportion of consecutive teenage suicides in Rhode Island and found significantly higher perinatal risk scores in the suicides compared with surviving controls. Jacobson *et al.* (1987) reported broadly similar findings in a Swedish birth cohort: 10% of suicides compared with 2.3% of controls experienced asphyxia at birth. The mothers of the suicides also received less antenatal care and were more likely to smoke and drink alcohol during pregnancy. These relationships could be a direct consequence of some induced neuropathy; they could reflect a 'common course', with some disturbed mothers predisposing their children to both perinatal morbidity and to later psychiatric illness; or they could be linked to one another, with the consequences of neurological damage impacting on parental competence and enhancing the likelihood of psychiatric illness.

Attempted suicide

Definition and subtypes

A suicide attempt is one of the more common psychiatric symptoms of youth. Children and teenagers who are psychotic, depressed, anxious, impulsive or, rarely, some who have no psychiatric or personality disorders at all, may think about or attempt suicide. The prognostic significance of a suicide attempt ranges from benign, with few if any negative sequelae, to malignant with later suicide. Given this heterogeneity, it is not surprising that a number of efforts have been made to define subgroups among suicide attempts.

The World Health Organization adopted the following definition of attempted suicide for its large multinational study. Attempted suicide is, 'An act with non-fatal outcome, in which an individual deliberately initiates a non-habitual behaviour that, without intervention from others, will cause self-harm, or deliberately ingests a substance in excess of the prescribed or generally recognized therapeutic dosage, and which is aimed at realizing changes which the subject desired via the actual or expected physical consequences' (Platt *et al.* 1992). What is remarkable about this lengthy definition is the careful omission of any mention of a wish to *die* and the use of the broader concept of 'self-harm'. Clinicians and parents alike are often reluctant to accept that all attempts and like behaviours are accompanied by lethal intent. This reluctance led Kreitman (1969) to coin the term *parasuicide,* which is now used loosely (Linehan *et al.* 1991) to describe overdoses or self-cutting behaviour of low medical lethality. Although parasuicidal behaviours may be repeated, they are considered to carry a low absolute risk of ultimate suicide. Another common term used by both lay individuals and professionals is a *suicide gesture.* This term assumes that the behaviour was undertaken without lethal intent and that it was intended as a 'communication'. Depending on the benevolence of the user, it can be seen as a 'cry for help', or as an act designed 'to attract attention'. Less inferential terms such as *deliberate self-poisoning* or *deliberate self-injury* (Hawton 1986) are preferable, but the avoidance of the word suicide skirts the problem of how these behaviours relate to suicide.

Because of the frequency of ideation and attempts, and the rarity of completed suicide, it is statistically reasonable to regard all attempts as benign, but the clinician needs to move beyond this actuarial position in order to assess the degree of individual risk. This is not easy. A teenager's 'intent' is very difficult to gauge after the event. Teenagers are, within certain bounds, quite naïve about the actual dangers of their behaviour. Between 30 and 50% of teenagers seen in an emergency room after an 'attempt' say that they wanted to die, but few took active precautions against being discovered (Piacentini *et al.* 1991), and their view is often at variance with that of the clinician. Hawton *et al.* (1982a) reported that examining psychiatrists confirmed lethal intent in only one-third of adolescents who said they wanted to die. How is this to be judged? Low intent cannot be inferred from the size of an overdose, because adolescents are frequently misinformed about the potential lethality of ingestions, in some instances overestimating (Piacentini *et al.* 1991) and in others underestimating (Myers 1992; Harris & Myers 1997) lethality. Piacentini *et al.* (1991) compared attempter and paediatrician estimates of the lethalness of overdoses and found that, whereas 26% of attempts were rated as having a potential to cause death by the adolescents, only 2% were considered potentially lethal by the physicians. Prior planning is a time-honoured but probably poor index of serious intent, as both suicide attempts and suicides commonly occur very shortly after a stressful event, giving little opportunity for careful planning (Shaffer *et al.* 1996a). Furthermore, the biennial Youth Risk Behaviour Survey (YRBS; Centers for Disease Control 2000), with ideation rates of between 15 and 20%, shows that 75% of teenagers who have thought about suicide have made a plan about how to commit suicide, although most will *not* go on to attempt or commit suicide.

For public health purposes, suicide attempts may be subclassified by whether or not the subject received medical treatment (Centers for Disease Control 2000). Although this is a reliable operationalized approach, it may not denote severity of intent. Medical treatment may be a function of availability and could be sought more often after an ingestion (in which the lingering presence of the ingestant requires treatment) than, say, after a failed hanging, which may indicate severe intent but leave no residual physical injury beyond a bruise. These imprecisions might not matter if the terms did not carry important implications. Parasuicide is broadly assumed to be benign, even though just under a half of completed suicides have been preceded by non-lethal ingestion or other attempts (Brent *et al.* 1993a; Shaffer *et al.* 1996a). Some patients who have made a non-lethal ingestion make a more substantial or lethal ingestion hours or days later. The unfortunate term suicide 'gesture' lends support to a causal dynamic (attention-seeking) that may not be accurate and strengthens the stigmatizing view held by many professionals and parents. Behaviour intended to obtain attention may be seen as a waste of professionals' and parents' valuable time. It may also reduce the likelihood of a subsequent referral for a psychiatric opinion.

Continuum of self-injurious behaviour

A completely different approach to the classification of suicidal behaviour is to treat it as a subcategory of a variety of behaviours that cause harm to the patient as a part of a spectrum of 'self-destructive behaviour' (Menninger 1938), such as interpersonal aggression, substance and alcohol use, compulsive gambling, unprotected sex, etc. The co-occurrence of these different behaviours is not in question (Flisher *et al.* 2000). It is possible, but by no means demonstrated, that they have in common some underlying trait such as impulsiveness (Mann *et al.* 1999), or some common prior experience such as early deprivation or abuse. It is also likely that co-occurrence reflects some sequential mechanisms, such as a suicidal response to the stresses experienced by youth with conduct disorder or secondary mood changes induced by intermittent substance and alcohol abuse (Schuckit 1995).

In summary, there is clearly a need to differentiate among the large heterogeneous group of patients who attempt suicide. The assumption that attempts are benign, although true in most instances, is dangerous because a prior suicide attempt is the single most important predictor of completed suicide (Brent *et al.* 1993a; Shaffer *et al.* 1996a). It is probably most reasonable to view a suicide attempt as a symptom or behaviour with varying aetiologies. Motivation and severity are difficult to assess, and in most instances the patient's mental state will be a better predictor of later outcome than the features and circumstances of the method (Beck 1972).

Epidemiology

Incidence

Since 1990, the USA's Centers for Disease Control has conducted biannual self-report surveys (the Youth Risk Behaviour Survey) to assess the 12-month prevalence of suicide ideation and behaviour in high-school students (Centers for Disease Control 2000). The surveys are large (sample sizes ranging between 12 000 and 16 000), and are representative of 14–17-year-old school attendees. The technique is appropriate because endorsement of questions on adolescent suicide attempts in the community is consistently higher in surveys that use a self-report method than in those given by interview (Safer 1997b). The biennial replication give these data added weight. The surveys consistently show an overall suicide attempt rate of between 8 and 9% with a rate of between 2 and 3% for attempts requiring medical attention.

Age

The YRBS shows a much higher incidence in 15–16-year-olds than in older teenagers, the age effect being strongest in girls. However, school-based studies can be misleading because a disproportionate number of suicide-prone students drop out of the last 2 years of high school.

Gender

In the YRBS, the suicide attempt rate is nearly twice as high in females (approximately 11%) as in males (approximately 6%). In many clinical populations, such as adolescents attending an emergency room, the proportion of females is significantly greater, with ratios ranging from 3 : 1 to 7 : 1 (Chung *et al.* 1987; Sellar *et al.* 1990; Piacentini *et al.* 1991). The reason for these differences could be that females use more serious methods; are more disturbed and thus more likely to seek medical treatment; that the methods used by females, e.g. a higher proportion of overdoses, are more likely to require medical attention; or assignment bias, e.g. a greater willingness among girls to seek help. Clinical experience suggests that the last two are the most likely explanations. Medical intervention is indicated for even small ingestions, the method favoured by females, whereas failure to die after one of the methods favoured by males (e.g. hanging) may not require medical intervention.

Ethnicity

In the YRBS, attempt and ideation rates are generally higher among Hispanic (approximately 13%) than among white (7%) students, with African-Americans' rates occupying an intermediate position. Reasons for the higher rate of suicidal ideation and attempt behaviour in Hispanic youth are not known. However, the risk factors for attempted suicides in African-Americans and white youths seem similar (Juon & Ensminger 1997).

Secular change

Secular changes in the suicide attempt rate in the general population have been assessed in the YRBS, which has shown a steady decline in the 1990s. These data may give a better idea of true changes than studies of clinical samples, e.g. the WHO multinational study of clinical referrals that showed an increase in Europe (Schmidtke *et al.* 1996; Hawton *et al.* 2000a). This may have resulted from changes in referral and payment procedures and may not reflect any real community change. Recent trends have not changed the fact that suicide attempters are the most common cause of hospital admission for young women (Hawton & Fagg 1992) and, as such, place a significant burden on clinical resources (Lukianowitz 1968; Leese 1969; Mattson *et al.* 1969; Pfeffer *et al.* 1980, 1984; Hawton *et al.* 1997).

Methods

In non-clinical samples of teenagers who self-report having made a suicide attempt, there are marked differences in the methods used by boys and girls. In girls, the most common attempt method is ingestion (55%), followed by cutting (31%). Among American males, the most common methods are cutting (25%), closely followed by ingestion (20%), firearms (15%) and hanging (11%) (Lewinsohn *et al.* 1996). In clinical samples, the majority of adolescents will have taken an overdose, most commonly (in North America and in Western Europe) of a non-narcotic analgesic or a psychotropic drug (Velez & Cohen 1988; Spirito *et al.* 1989; Michel *et al.* 2000).

Suicidal ideation

Suicidal ideation is very common among high-school students. In the YRBS surveys, approximately one in four females (25%) and one in six males (14%) endorse the question 'Have you seriously considered suicide in the last 12 months?' (Centers for Disease Control 2000). As with suicide attempts, ideation is more common in girls and in Hispanics.

Clinical aspects

Precipitants

Suicide attempts in young people nearly always follow some stressful event, most often a problem in a relationship, which are generally common in adolescence. Stress events that seem to have a more specific relationship to suicidal behaviour are disciplinary crises, such as a recent or anticipated arrest or court appearance, or academic failure and punishment (Lewinsohn *et al.* 1996; Beautrais *et al.* 1997). Clinical experience suggests that many of the stressors arise from the teenager's underlying psychiatric disorder or personality problem. Suicide attempters are not simply passive or chance recipients of adverse experiences. As many as one-third of adolescent attempters are unable to identify a clear precipitant (Hawton *et al.* 1982b; Kienhorst *et al.* 1995) and this should be evaluated carefully for evidence of an underlying depression.

Psychiatric disorder

Almost all adolescents who attempt suicide have a current or recent history of psychiatric illness (Andrews & Lewinsohn 1992; Beautrais *et al.* 1998; Gould *et al.* 1998b). About three-quarters will have a mood disorder, and this will often coexist with a conduct, anxiety or substance abuse disorder or, much less commonly, an eating disorder. A number of suicide attempters have what can best be described as an adjustment disorder (see Hill, Chapter 31): although they might have subthreshold symptoms, their mental state will have deteriorated abruptly in response to a stress and will recover to its former mildly abnormal level shortly after the attempt. This is in keeping with the findings from numerous studies of unreferred groups that show that suicide attempts are nearly always associated with other psychopathology (Velez & Cohen 1988; Garrison *et al.* 1991; Fergusson & Lynskey 1995; Lewinsohn *et al.* 1996; Gould *et al.* 1998b).

Personality disorders

A proneness to outbursts of aggression, anger and impulsivity is an important risk characteristic. Aggression and anger increase the likelihood of a medically severe method and later repetition (Gispert *et al.* 1985, 1987; Stein *et al.* 1998; Hawton *et al.* 1999), and high levels of impulsivity were found both in first-time attempters and repeat attempters (Stein *et al.* 1998; Kingsbury *et al.* 1999).

Cognition

Most suicide attempts in teenagers are impulsive. In one series of consecutive emergency room admissions, only 10–15% reported thinking about their attempt for more than a day (Rotheram-Borus *et al.* 1990; Piacentini *et al.* 1991; Negron *et al.* 1997). Those who made suicide attempts, compared with those who had suicidal ideation only, reported more hopelessness before the attempt and continued to have suicidal ideation after the attempt (Negron *et al.* 1997). Feelings of hopelessness are commonly reported by suicide attempters, and there is some evidence that when they occur with depression they might worsen the prognosis (Kienhorst *et al.* 1992; Morano *et al.* 1993; Steer *et al.* 1993).

Other cognitive factors that might promote suicidal behaviour include being 'problem-focused': dwelling on problems and employing wishful thinking when dealing with fantasies about interpersonal problems (Levenson 1974; Asarnow *et al.* 1987; Orbach *et al.* 1987; Rotheram-Borus *et al.* 1990). There is little evidence that a pessimistic attributional style, the most common cognitive distortion found in depression, is characteristic of suicide attempters (Asarnow *et al.* 1987; Rotheram-Borus *et al.* 1990). In one study, teenage attempters were more likely to make positive attributions than psychiatric controls (Spirito *et al.* 1991).

Family factors

Suicide attempters are more likely than controls to live in single-parent families (Groholt *et al.* 2000; Wichstrom 2000), and their parents have high rates of psychiatric illness and high levels of marital conflict and conflict with children (Taylor & Stansfield 1984; Trautman & Shaffer 1984; Asarnow 1992). Hostile, punitive, indifferent and insensitive parenting is common (Jacobs 1971; Yusin *et al.* 1972; McIntire & Angle 1973). The teenagers frequently view the relationship with their parents as more dysfunctional than the parents acknowledge (McIntire & Angle 1973; McKenry *et al.* 1982). In many instances, conflicts arise from unresolved differences about what is or is not age-appropriate behaviour for a teenager. Adolescent suicide attempters are more likely than normal, but not depressed, controls to have been sexually and/or physically abused at some time in their lives (Brand *et al.* 1996; Swanston *et al.* 1999).

Sexual orientation

Several large community studies have shown that gay, lesbian and bisexual youth are between two and seven times more likely to think about and attempt suicide than heterosexual adolescents (Faulkner & Cranston 1998; Garofalo *et al.* 1998; Remafedi *et al.* 1998; Fergusson *et al.* 1999; Lock & Steiner 1999). In these studies, gay, lesbian and bisexual youth also had higher rates of drug and alcohol use and higher rates of other psychiatric symptoms, such as major depression, generalized anxiety disorder and conduct disorder (Fergusson *et al.* 1999), and they were also more likely to have been victimized at school. Any of these features could contribute to their suicidal behaviour. However, in a study of completed suicides (Shaffer *et al.* 1996a) that included a small number of gay suicides, the precipitating events were similar to the precipitants in heterosexual suicides (interpersonal and disciplinary crises) and were not specific to the victims' homosexuality.

Death

Depending on the length of follow-up, between 0.1 and 11% of adolescent suicide attempters will eventually commit suicide (Otto 1972; Motto 1984; Goldacre & Hawton 1985; Shaffer *et al.* 1988; Spirito *et al.* 1989). Later suicide is more likely in male attempters, attempters who had been hospitalized, and teenagers who were older at the time of their initial attempt.

Otto (1972) reported that 70% of attempters who ultimately completed suicide died by methods similar to their initial attempt, the remainder using a more lethal method. Suicide attempters who would later commit suicide were much more likely than controls to be unmarried or divorced and to be listed in national registries as having criminal behaviour, alcohol problems or disability pensions.

Repeat attempts

Approximately 12–30% of adolescent suicide attempters report having made a previous attempt (White 1974; Rohn et al. 1977; Hawton et al. 1982b), and approximately 10% will go on to make another attempt within 2 years. Repeat attempts are most likely to take place during the first 3 months following the initial attempt and are more common in males; in teenagers who have a history of a prior attempt, substance abuse, previous psychotic inpatient hospitalization; those found to be less 'physically attractive' by raters (Lewinsohn et al. 1994); and in those with depressive symptomatology in which 'hopelessness' is a feature (Stanley & Barter 1970; McIntire et al. 1977; Goldacre & Hawton 1985; Gispert et al. 1987; Choquet & Menke 1989; Sellar et al. 1990; Pfeffer et al. 1991; Hawton et al. 1993, 1999; Nordstrom et al. 1995).

Evaluation and treatment

Setting

Because of the possibility of future suicidal crises, treatment should, if possible, be in a system that provides inpatient, outpatient and emergency care (Rotheram-Borus et al. 1996). Many attempters are first seen in a casualty/emergency room, where staff are not always well disposed to suicide attempters. Frequently held views are that the family is to blame for the teenager's behaviour or that the teenager is simply looking for attention. These attitudes militate against keeping later appointments (Rotheram-Borus et al. 1996, 1999) and could be modified by staff training.

Initial evaluation

After medical stabilization, the task of the psychiatrist is to decide whether the patient needs hospital admission. This will require information obtained from a parent, guardian or best friend. No adolescent who has attempted suicide should be discharged before a third party has been interviewed.

There are very few studies on the effects of hospitalization (Waterhouse & Platt 1990; King et al. 1995). Nevertheless, common sense and comparison with suicide completers (Marttunen et al. 1991; Shaffer et al. 1996a; Brent et al. 1999) suggest that admission should be considered for attempters who:

1 are male;
2 used a method other than ingestion or superficial cutting;

3 have persistent ideation or significant depressive or psychotic symptoms;
4 are reported to have had complications from alcohol or substance abuse;
5 have a history of recurrent attempts; and
6 have no adult guardian or companion to ensure the safety of the environment (remove all medications, guns, knives, etc.).
Because children under 12 years so rarely commit suicide, either suicidal ideation or suicidal behaviour should not, in itself, indicate hospitalization in that age group.

It is important not to miss the opportunity to obtain a detailed account of the events and feelings that preceded the attempt and its consequences at the first visit. This information can be invaluable for planning more definitive treatment and is best obtained while memory of the event is fresh. It will also be helpful to the clinician who will care for the youngster to have some understanding of the amount of support that will be available for the child or adolescent when they are discharged home. Treatment recommendations are more likely to be followed if they match family expectations, are affordable, and if the parent is well and available enough to support attendance.

Initial management

The parent, guardian or companion who accompanies the patient to the emergency room should be told to lock away potentially poisonous medications or firearms. When these instructions are given clearly, compliance is good (Kruesi et al. 1999; Brent et al. 2000) but, despite their obvious merits, the procedure is often overlooked (McManus et al. 1997). The accompanying parent should also be told to limit the adolescent's access to alcohol or other potentially disinhibiting substances. In the USA, it is common to require an attempter to make a *contract* with the clinician to the effect that he or she will not make a further attempt before the next clinic visit or, if they have a strong urge to do so, will first contact the clinician. There is no evidence about the impact of contracting (Reid 1998) and it should never substitute for other types of intervention, especially if the patient has a disturbed mental state. The clinician must understand that risk can persist, even if the patient agrees to a contract (Egan et al. 1997). Another common procedure is to facilitate arrangements for the teenager to contact the clinic or a clinician if he or she feels distressed or suicidal. This does not seem to affect re-attempt rates (Cotgrove et al. 1995) but it can impart a sense of support to the family.

Fewer than half of suicide attempters who present in crisis will develop a therapeutic relationship after their initial evaluation and treatment in the emergency room (Litt et al. 1983; Taylor & Stansfield 1984; Kienhorst et al. 1987; Trautman & Rotheram-Borus 1988; Spirito et al. 1989; Swedo 1989; Piacentini et al. 1991). Trautman & Shaffer (1989) and Piacentini et al. (1991) found that non-attendance was more common in attempters who were persistently suicidal and in those who had a large number of psychiatric symptoms. By contrast, maternal substance abuse, depression and poor physical health were associated with *inconsistent* compliance results. Maternal psychopathology was associated with less treatment attendance in some studies (King *et al.* 1997; Rotheram-Borus *et al.* 1999) and with greater attendance in others (Trautman & Shaffer 1989; Piacentini *et al.* 1991).

There is evidence that compliance can be improved if the clinic or clinician:

1 educates the family on the condition and psychological treatment of the patient and engages their co-operation (Rotheram-Borus *et al.* 1996);

2 addresses factors other than the patient's suicide attempt, e.g. parental conflict and other stressors;

3 develops procedures to allow emergency rooms to offer appointments directly to a family before discharge, ideally to see a specific clinician at a specific time and location; and

4 develops procedures to follow up on missed appointments.

Specific treatments

There have been few studies into the optimal treatment of suicidal behaviour in adolescents, and those tend to be small, with inadequate statistical power. For the following reasons, this is a difficult area to research.

1 *Diagnostic heterogeneity.* It seems likely that treatment findings may differ between attempters with different diagnoses or levels of severity (Verkes *et al.* 1998). Small unplanned subgroup analyses can be difficult to interpret.

2 *Outcome measures.* There is uncertainty about outcome measures. Most studies have used the rate of attempt repetition (Hawton *et al.* 2000b); however, only a small proportion of suicide attempters (between 8 and 20%) make repeat attempts (Hawton *et al.* 1982a; Spirito *et al.* 1994), and those who do differ from those who do not with respect to gender, diagnosis and cognitive status. Attempt repetition is also a poor index of seriousness. Approximately one-third of suicides are known to have made a previous attempt (Shaffer *et al.* 1996a; Brent *et al.* 1999), and of those only a minority have made repeat attempts. Finally, repeat attempts are relatively uncommon, so that a large sample is needed to show a statistically significant effect. Alternative outcome measures, such as reduced ideation, reduced impairment, fewer associated psychiatric symptoms and reduced levels of subjective distress, are all relevant but are rarely used.

3 *Exclusion from research.* It is possible that useful inferences about treatment efficacy could be drawn from treatment studies of conditions in which suicide attempts are common, such as depression or substance abuse. However, it is common that treatment studies among children and adolescents specifically exclude patients with a past history of a suicide attempt in order to minimize risk and/or liability.

4 *Unstandardized psychotherapy.* Manualized psychotherapies are only now becoming available, and, until they are, analyses of multiple studies will be difficult.

5 *Control conditions.* Many studies do not clearly delineate exactly what constitutes 'standard care' or 'treatment as usual' in their control groups.

A comprehensive meta-analysis of randomized control trials of suicide attempters of all ages (Hawton *et al.* 1998b, 2000b) examined the efficacy of several treatments on attempt repetition. These included problem-solving therapy, intensive intervention plus outreach, family interventions and antidepressants. Only two treatments showed a statistically significant reduction in attempt repetition: *dialectical-behaviour therapy* (DBT; Linehan *et al.* 1991, 1994) (see below), and the long-acting neuroleptic flupentixol (Montgomery & Montgomery 1982). Each of these has been tested in a single randomized trial of modest size. A trial of selective serotonin reuptake inhibitor (SSRI) antidepressants (Verkes *et al.* 1998) on multiple suicide attempters showed no overall effect, although suicidal ideation was reduced in a subgroup of attempters who had made fewer than five previous attempts.

In studies comparing problem-solving therapies with standard care (Gibbons *et al.* 1978; Hawton *et al.* 1987; Salkovskis *et al.* 1990; McLeavey *et al.* 1994; Evans *et al.* 1999), there were only non-significant trends toward reduction of repeat suicide attempts. Facilitating contact with a clinical service (allowing 24-hour on-demand phone contact with a therapist or admission to a hospital at the patient's request) in addition to standard care, vs. standard care alone (Hawton *et al.* 2000b), did not reduce repetition rates significantly but did increase treatment attendance (Hawton *et al.* 1981; Kerfoot & McHugh 1992; Van Heeringen *et al.* 1995; Rotheram-Borus *et al.* 1996; van der Sande *et al.* 1997; Spooren *et al.* 1998). Only a minority of first-time adolescent suicide attempters repeat their attempt in the 1- or 2-year follow-up period, and only a minority of these repeaters make multiple attempts.

A final methodological/analytical problem is the vast variety of types and delivery of treatment. There was no beneficial effect, as measured by reduced attempt repetition, in intensive intervention (often with a home-based component) vs. standard aftercare; in some therapies, between different therapists; in general admission vs. discharge; in long-term vs. short-term therapy; or in antidepressant (traditional) vs. placebo.

Harrington *et al.* (1998a) found no advantage overall between tested home-based family therapy and treatment as usual in a sample of suicidal ideators, but noted significant improvement in non-depressed attempters, and only a non-significant trend towards fewer symptoms was found in a study of the value of an 'emergency card' that expedited access to hospitalization vs. treatment as usual (Cotgrove *et al.* 1995). The absence of evidence for a 'best' therapy leaves several treatment goals that have to be addressed as well as possible by the clinician. These include:

1 treatment of any associated psychiatric disorder;

2 teaching the patient and the family to recognize and avoid or diffuse situations or events that lead to conflict, upset and suicidal behaviour (Rotheram-Borus *et al.* 1994); and

3 reducing the sense of guilt and improving the morale and sense of agency that are commonly damaged in the families of teenagers who have attempted suicide (Stuart 1980; Trautman & Shaffer 1984; Miller *et al.* 1992a).

Dialectical-behaviour therapy

Dialectical-behaviour therapy is a manualized treatment developed specifically for suicide attempters by Linehan *et al.* (1991, 1993). It assumes that the core problem in suicide attempters is an abnormality of emotional regulation such that, in a stressful environment, the patient will attempt suicide as a response to negative feelings. The suicidal behaviour is reinforced by the help it *elicits* from others and it may make the patient feel better independently of outside reinforcement (Negron *et al.* 1997).

As tested and described, DBT is a lengthy treatment (approximately 1 year) given in individual and group contexts. It employs a range of techniques to:
1 improve self-acceptance;
2 increase assertiveness in order to reduce opportunities for interpersonal conflicts;
3 train the patient to avoid situations that trigger negative moods; and
4 increase tolerance of psychological distress.

In adults, the treatment has been found to improve mental state, reduce the need for rehospitalization, and reduce the incidence of repeated attempts. It demands a significant commitment of time from the patient, numerous skills from the therapist and a generous insurance or benefits system. DBT-A is an adaptation developed for adolescents (Miller *et al.* 1997) that involves parents and is less lengthy (24 weeks). It has not yet been tested in a controlled study.

Cognitive-behaviour therapy

Cognitive-behavioural therapy, the treatment most often used for depressed adolescents (see Harrington *et al.* 1998b for a review), has generally been found to be more effective than family or supportive therapy in depressed non-suicidal adolescents over the short-term (Brent *et al.* 1997). The benefits do not seem lasting (Birmaher *et al.* 2000), and its value in the suicidal teenager has not been established.

Psychopharmacological treatment after the crisis

SSRI antidepressants

SSRI antidepressants reduce suicidal ideation in both depressed (Letizia *et al.* 1996) and non-depressed adults with cluster-B personality disorders (Verkes *et al.* 1998). SSRIs are, in general, safe and effective for adolescent depression (Emslie *et al.* 1997; Ryan & Varma 1998) and are much less dangerous in overdose than tricyclic antidepressants (Ryan & Varma 1998). Pending evidence to the contrary, it is reasonable to regard SSRIs as a first-choice medication for suicidal children and adolescents.

Lithium

Lithium treatment significantly reduces the recurrence of suicide attempts in adults with bipolar or other major affective disorders (Tondo *et al.* 1997), and when lithium is discontinued the rate of suicide attempts and the risk of suicide increase considerably. The antisuicidal effects of lithium have not been assessed in children or adolescents. Using lithium with adolescents requires careful supervision because overdoses can be fatal, and common side-effects, such as acne and cognitive dulling, are particularly troubling for teenagers.

Neuroleptics

In a controlled trial of depot flupentixol, Montgomery & Montgomery (1982) noted a significant reduction in suicide attempt behaviour in adults who had made numerous previous attempts. This study has not been replicated, and similar studies have not been carried out with adolescents.

Drug-induced suicidality

In the past decade, there has been controversy over whether SSRI antidepressants may induce suicidal ideation and/or behaviour in both adults (Teicher *et al.* 1990) and children (King *et al.* 1991). This was suggested by one meta-analysis (Mann & Kapur 1991), and a small number of adult cases have been reported in which suicidal thoughts started after treatment was begun with an SSRI, stopped after its withdrawal, but reappeared once the drug was recommenced (Rothschild & Locke 1991). Many of the case studies report that the ideation was associated with akasthisia and that it had an obsessive or ruminative quality (Hamilton & Opler 1992). These suicidogenic effects of the SSRIs are probably uncommon, and meta-analyses and re-analyses of large sets of SSRI treatment trial data of depressed, bulimic or anxious patients (Beasley *et al.* 1991; Montgomery *et al.* 1995; Letizia *et al.* 1996) suggest that the overall effect is for the medication to reduce rates of suicidal behaviour. Nevertheless, clinicians should be particularly observant during the early stages of SSRI treatment, should systematically inquire about suicidal ideation before and after treatment is started, and should, if SSRI treatment induces akasthisia, be especially alert to the possibility of suicidality.

Clinicians should be cautious about prescribing medications that can reduce self-control, such as the benzodiazapines, and phenobarbital in patients who have made a suicide attempt. Phenobarbital also has a high lethal potential if taken in overdose (Carlsten *et al.* 1996). Montgomery (1997) noted that benzodiazapines might disinhibit some individuals, who then exhibit aggression and make suicide attempts. There are indications of similar effects from the antidepressants maprotiline and amitriptyline, the amfetamines, and phenobarbital (Carlsten *et al.* 1996).

Suicide prevention

A model for prevention

For many years, the desire to commit suicide was seen by many as a logical one, arrived at after a period of consideration and, above all, open to everyone: everyone was at risk, and its prevention was comparable to finding a needle in a haystack. However, as research into the individual characteristics of suicide completers has progressed, it has become apparent that a small number of risk factors that are potentially amenable to treatment and change are present in most suicide victims. If suicide only occurs in a definable and limited population, suicide prevention should be an attainable goal.

The risk factors include specific psychiatric disorders, such as depression, alcohol abuse and a proneness to impulsive behaviour, which may in turn be caused by distinctive biological differences; adversities that are common to many types of psychopathology; and some external factors, such as exposure to media that feature suicidal behaviour. There is, in other words, a complicated chain of influences that lead to the moment when a teenager decides to commit suicide. It is likely that a small number of *necessary* and almost certainly no *sufficient* factors contribute to this fortunately unusual, but always tragic, event.

This information can be incorporated into an explanatory model (Fig. 33.3) that can be used to plan strategic prevention strategies. A factor that operates close to the execution of suicide should be a final common pathway and might be the most appropriate intervention. In practice, however, the only interventions that are appropriate for prevention are those that are modifiable. The factor that is clearly the most modifiable by clinicians is the identification and treatment of the mental disorders that are present in almost all suicide victims.

Furthermore, an active *mental disorder* is present in about 90% of adolescent suicides at the time of death and, together with *suicidal ideation* (see below), can conveniently be regarded as the closest thing we have to a *necessary* risk condition. Even though relatively few psychiatrically disturbed youths will commit suicide, aggressive case-finding and the development and provision of effective treatment for affected youth could be expected to reduce the suicide rate.

Adverse *stress events*, most often a disciplinary crisis, interpersonal loss or a perceived humiliation, often occur in close proximity to a suicide. However, such events are common during adolescence, can rarely be anticipated, and are usually beyond the influence of the clinician. They are therefore likely to be poor targets for prevention but, in many instances, these events might be a consequence of an adolescent's underlying mental disorder which, in a vicious cycle, might also deprive the teenager of parent, peer or teacher support and in other ways impede the young person's ability to cope with or seek a solution to the stress. Case-finding and treatment of psychiatric disorder would provide an effective preventive activity at this level.

These stresses are often responded to in a harmful way by the potential suicide. They may induce feelings of hopelessness or anger and a wish for revenge or intolerable affects that stimulate a need to escape or be 'better off dead'. Suicide hot lines were originally designed to operate at this point in the process (Shneidman & Farberow 1957; Litman *et al.* 1965), but their low rate of use by acutely suicidal individuals limits their value. DLT and other forms of cognitive therapy that encourage stress avoidance and that alert the adolescent to dangerous internal mental states and provide skills for dealing with them could operate at this point.

Although an underlying disorder, recent stress and inadequate support, coupled with hopelessness or preoccupation with suicide, can set the stage for suicide, we must assume that many young people experience this confluence of risk factors but only a few commit suicide. It is probably at this point that specific enhancers and inhibitors operate.

Enhancement might be mediated by a biological trait such as impulsivity or emotional volatility, drug- or alcohol-induced intoxication, or other altered mental states; by high social value being placed on suicide (as by the victim's familiarity with peers or public figures whose suicide, related by the media, carries a sense of importance or romance); by the availability of a lethal method; or by the absence of any *inhibiting* factors, such as societal or religious taboos, the presence of social support, and difficulty in accessing a method. Preventive interventions operating at this final stage would therefore include media guidelines to promote responsible reporting of suicide and to minimize contagion, promotion of a strong taboo against suicide in society, and the removal of lethal medications and weapons from the homes of suicidal youth. However, nearly all of these involve non-medical, societal or political interventions that may be beyond the scope of the clinician.

In summary, the best routine suicide prevention would seem to be the effective identification (case-finding, see below) and treatment of associated psychiatric disorders. Untreated, these operate to promote suicide in many ways, and our ability to intervene effectively with them is probably greater than our ability to bring about the societal or political changes that are needed to alter the final chance precipitants of an individual's suicide.

Case-finding

Finding teenagers who are at high risk for suicide, either because they are currently suicidal or because they have an undiagnosed depression or other predisposing condition, and who are not currently being managed by a clinician, is an important aspect of prevention. Case-finding can be undertaken by *direct* evaluation of individual, or *indirectly* by educating third parties, such as parents, teachers, and guidance personnel, to watch for and refer individuals with suggestive behaviour patterns or 'warning signs'.

Indirect case-finding

The indirect, educational approach is inexpensive and may appear cost effective. It is widely applied in suicide-awareness programmes. However, this approach is beset with problems: many suicidal adolescents show no visible symptoms or behaviours that denote risk; some of the warning signs (such as social withdrawal, irritability, and declining academic performance) are common in non-suicidal teenagers and are not strongly predictive of suicidality; and more-specific warning signs, such as giving away possessions, leaving suicidal notes for others to read, or discussing specific plans with a friend, are relatively uncommon among suicide completers (Shaffer *et al.* 1996a). Indirect case-finding is not without risk, especially if it is directed to other students who are being asked to look for signs in their peer group. It is difficult for many young people to either persuade their friends to obtain help or, if that fails, break a confidence and disclose their observations to a responsible adult. This may be why teenagers who have received systematic training in case-finding are no more likely to recommend treatment to their distressed friends than those who do not (Vieland *et al.* 1991). Finally, suicide awareness programmes directed to peers inevitably involve presenting material about suicide to youngsters who, unknown to the educator, could include past attempters or currently suicidal teens, and there is evidence that they might think more about suicide or be emotionally upset as a result of exposure to such programmes (Shaffer *et al.* 1991).

Direct case-finding

Direct case-finding determines risk from the teenagers themselves. Teenagers are clearly capable of identifying their own feelings and behaviour, and there are many self-report measures that are based on this ability (Achenbach & Edelbrock 1987; Centers for Disease Control 2000). Teenagers' self-evaluations are highly correlated with those of clinicians (Renouf & Kovacs 1994) and appear to identify a different group of troubled teenagers than those identified by teachers or parents (Kovacs 1985; Achenbach & Edelbrock 1987; Bird *et al.* 1990).

Direct screening can be carried out in primary clinicians' offices or in high schools. A typical screening programme will use some type of screening instrument to identify students with important risk factors for suicide, such as current suicidal ideation, depressed mood or a history of suicide attempts (Smith & Crawford 1986; Harkavy Friedman *et al.* 1987; Shaffer *et al.* 1996b; Goldston 2000). Some focus narrowly on suicidality and do not include many other important risk factors, such as depression or substance abuse, but others cast the net more broadly. Depending on the sensitivity and specificity of the screening instrument, students who screen positive will then be given a second-stage evaluation and, depending on the outcome of that, will be referred to a clinician (Reynolds 1991; Shaffer *et al.* 1996b). An effective screening programme will include a mechanism for facilitating referral for appropriate treatment.

A sensitive screen will identify almost all teenagers at risk for suicide (Shaffer & Craft 1999), but in the process will also identify many 'false-positives': students who are not at risk (see Fombonne, Chapter 4; Verhulst & Van der Ende, Chapter 5). In a screening of over 2000 New York teenagers (Shaffer & Craft 1999), the initial screen generated only three false-negatives (88% sensitivity), but 257 false-positives (76% specificity). If resources are abundant, the high false-positive rate might not be a problem because many of the screen-positive teenagers at low risk for suicide will be suffering from some psychiatric disorder that might be helped. However, in most instances, low specificity imposes a prohibitive financial and manpower burden and may threaten the whole programme. This problem can be addressed by giving a more specific second-stage screen to those who are positive on the initial screen. Like almost any procedure that enhances specificity, this might lower sensitivity and might miss some suicidal students but, in the final analysis, a less sensitive, two- or three-stage procedure is preferable. We routinely use a second-stage procedure that involves giving screen-positive students a more detailed assessment on a self-administered computerized diagnostic interview, such as the Voice Diagnostic Interview Schedule for Children (DISC; Shaffer *et al.* 2000), which minimizes the cost of the procedure.

A clinician, assisted by the results of a two-stage screen, can usually make a triage decision about whether the student needs to be referred for treatment or further evaluation in a relatively short time at a third and final stage of the screening process. Ideally, the clinician is assisted by a case manager who will contact the student's parents and establishes links with a clinic to facilitate treatment compliance.

Screening can be carried out in any setting attended regularly by large groups of older adolescents. An advantage of screening in a primary clinician's office is that there will be a mechanism for referring the case to a specialist when this is indicated. Because paediatricians and other primary care physicians rarely ask about suicidal ideation or behaviour (Frankenfield *et al.* 2000; Halpern-Felsher *et al.* 2000), screening for depression and suicidality is unlikely to be redundant with the practitioner's usual procedure.

School-based screening programmes can reach adolescents whose symptoms might not—for any number of reasons—be recognized by others as being clinically significant. They can reach the large number of teenagers who do not routinely attend a clinician's office or who, if they do, are not screened. Regardless of the method used, the value of case-finding may be restricted by the high base rate of some high-risk indicators, such as current suicidal ideation, a past suicide attempt, alcohol abuse and anxiety states; sparse treatment resources; and the prevailing limitations of knowledge on optimal treatment.

Crisis services

The original argument for crisis intervention (Shneidman & Farberow 1957; Litman *et al.* 1965) was that suicide intent is often associated with a critical stress event that is usually contemplated with psychological ambivalence and that arises in the context of mental disturbance. If the model of suicide presented in Fig. 33.3 is accurate, then crisis services are potentially efficient because they operate at the final common pathway to death.

Crisis services are usually provided by so-called telephone hot lines. Some are manned by teenagers (Boehm *et al.* 1991), but most by specially trained adult listeners who give information about how to access appropriate services. Some, especially those that are part of a multiservice agency, carry out more active case management, making appointments with the appropriate clinical service and following up if the appointment is not kept (Sudak *et al.* 1977). Relatively few offer direct therapy on the telephone, and most will break confidentiality if they judge that it will avert a suicide, calling parental or police help. An exception is the Samaritan organization, whose *befriending* process emphasizes acceptance, warmth and *confidentiality* (Hirsch 1981).

The efficacy of crisis intervention has usually been tested by determining whether the establishment of a service results in lower suicide morbidity in a given area. The research is inevitably ecological: there is no information on whether suicides that occurred had contacted the crisis service to no avail, or the reverse, whether highly suicidal individuals were redirected from their intended plan by the crisis service. Regardless, the balance of evidence is that crisis services have no or, at best, very limited effects on the suicide rate (Barraclough & Jennings 1977; Bridge *et al.* 1977; Jennings *et al.* 1978; Miller *et al.* 1984). Possible explanations for this (see Shaffer *et al.* 1990a for a review) are the predominance of female callers (King 1977; Boehm & Campbell 1995), who are at relatively low risk for suicide; the indifferent quality of much of the advice given (Bleach & Claiborn 1974; Apsler & Hodas 1975; Slaiku *et al.* 1975; Knowles 1979; Hirsch 1981); and the fact that a significant proportion of suicides occur when the victim is preoccupied or disorganized, under the influence of alcohol, or in an otherwise agitated state where they might not be able to summon the resources to make or benefit from an appropriate call. Only a small proportion of teenagers know how to access a hot line (Litman *et al.* 1965; Greer & Anderson 1979).

It is probably a mistake to dismiss hot lines as well-intentioned but ineffective. Hot lines are widely available in the USA (Seeley 1996; American Association of Suicidology 1999) and provide help for a needy and otherwise underserved population. King (1977) showed that only 8% of callers were currently receiving other mental health services. In a survey of high-school students who had attended a suicide education programme (Shaffer *et al.* 1988), one of the few significant effects was an increase in a declared willingness to use a hot line when experiencing emotional difficulties, there being *no increase* in willingness to use any other type of service. There is a need to develop a standardized but clinically informed screening procedure, coupled with active case-management procedures, and broaden interest in hot lines, particularly among troubled boys, with appropriately directed advertising.

Educational programmes

Educational programmes generally aim at one or more of the following goals (Shaffer *et al.* 1988; Garland *et al.* 1989).

1 *To heighten awareness of the problem* by showing taped vignettes of teenagers who have attempted suicide or by quoting disturbing statistics, e.g. that suicide is the second leading cause of death in teenagers.

2 *To promote indirect case-finding* (see above).

3 *To promote disclosure of suicidal intentions or ruminations.* This is done by presenting a model of suicide that is intended to be non-stigmatizing. Thus, the programme might state that suicide is *not* a feature of mental illness but is a response to common adolescent stress, such as pressure to succeed, family upsets, residential mobility, changing value systems, use of drugs and alcohol, etc. This might be reinforced by showing taped vignettes of attractive youngsters who have made a previous attempt for these reasons.

4 *To provide staff and students with information about mental health resources*, specifically how they operate and how they can be accessed.

Didactic school-based suicide prevention programmes can be criticized for following a low-risk strategy. The overwhelming number of adolescents who are exposed to the programmes carry no risk for suicide. Further, there is no evidence that such programmes modify attitudes about suicide or help-seeking in either normal or high-risk students (Spirito *et al.* 1988; Shaffer *et al.* 1990b, 1991; Vieland *et al.* 1991). The failure of a purely didactic approach is broadly in line with educational strategies to prevent alcohol and drug abuse (Strasburger1989) and early sexual activity (Kirby 1985). There is some suggestion that such programmes do shift students to a model of suicide that is held to be non-stigmatizing by the designers: one that renders suicide 'understandable' in the context of stress, rather than a psychopathological model (Shaffer *et al.* 1991). These programmes have not solved the dilemma of how to make suicide less shameful without, at the same time, reducing the prohibitions that might contribute to making suicide a mercifully rare event.

Educating/training primary care physicians and paediatricians

As noted above, only 20–40% of US primary care physicians and paediatricians report regularly asking about suicidal behaviours and suicide risk factors (Frankenfield *et al.* 2000; Halpern-Felsher *et al.* 2000). Those who did report screening regularly were those more likely to feel they had enough training and knowledge about suicidal risk factors, sufficient time, and the belief that they could be effective in reducing adolescent suicide (Frankenfield *et al.* 2000).

In Gotland, Sweden, a two-day course training primary care physicians to assess mood disorders and suicidality was associated with a subsequent lowering of the female suicide rate

(Rihmer *et al.* 1995; Rutz *et al.* 1995). Female suicide attempts decreased, and antidepressant prescriptions and hospitalizations for mood disorder increased. While this as yet unreplicated study of adult suicide is preliminary, and while the optimal treatment of adolescent depression is not as well understood as that of adult depression, educating all clinicians who encounter adolescents, not just mental health clinicians, in how to recognize and, if necessary, refer the suicidal child or adolescent is a worthwhile end in itself, regardless of its impact on suicide. In medical settings where, unfortunately, physicians are not given the time to take an extensive history or perform an evaluation, the case-finding screening instruments mentioned above could be administered.

Media guidelines

There is ecological evidence that media reports of suicide might induce contagion (Gould & Shaffer 1986; Velting & Gould 1997; Fekete & Macsai 1990; Ishii 1991), and so guidelines for journalists and liaison public health officials have been drafted, suggesting that reporting of suicide not be predominant and excessive, not romanticize the suicide, idealize the suicide victim, minimize the victim's multitudinous difficulties and mental illness, or provide extensive details of the method that could allow modelling (Gould *et al.* 1999; American Foundation for Suicide Prevention 2001). However, as yet, only the most preliminary ecological studies have tried to assess whether these guidelines reduce or contain the adolescent suicide rate (Etzersdorfer *et al.* 1992; Sonneck *et al.* 1994; Jobes *et al.* 1996) or which of these strategies are most helpful.

Limiting access to methods

Because youth suicide is often an impulsive act, it is reasonable to expect that limiting access to commonly used methods could prevent its occurrence in some instances. The so-called 'British experience' is a frequently cited example of how this can happen. The British suicide rate declined *pari passu* with the replacement of poisonous domestic coal gas with carbon monoxide-free natural gas (Hassall & Trethowan 1972; Kreitman 1976). Over the period of transition, British suicide rates fell by 26%, with most of the decline being attributed to a decrease in deaths from domestic-gas asphyxiation, with no compensatory increase in suicidal deaths by other methods. British rates, in contrast to those in most other countries, remained at the new lower level (Farberow 1985) for many years. Most suicides in the USA are committed with legally owned and registered firearms. It would be reasonable to expect that the early British experience could be replicated by effective firearm control in that country, but, by extension, one would only expect a similar transient effect. Whereas the recent reduction in UK suicides has been attributed to the requirement of safer catalytic converters in automobiles, analyses show that one must look to other causal factors to account for most of the decrease (McClure 2000).

'Post-vention'

Post-vention refers to a public health intervention implemented after a suicide with survivors in the victim's school or community. Post-vention can, in principle, be useful in several ways. It can provide a basis for understanding the death, and thus lighten some of the guilt and isolation frequently experienced by family survivors (Calhoun *et al.* 1982; Rogers *et al.* 1982; Henley 1984) and minimize the scapegoating that may be directed at parents, teachers, the school or particular peers. However, post-vention programmes are often implemented to reduce the probability of imitation by other teenagers, addressing abnormal symptoms of grief and depression or post-traumatic stress disorder. Emotional sequelae are common in friends of adolescents who have committed suicide, especially among those who witnessed the suicide or were told of the suicidal intent and failed to avert it (Brent *et al.* 1996b).

Because the factors that facilitate imitation are only now starting to be understood, there is no clear rationale for the most appropriate type of post-vention for this purpose. Gould (2001) has proposed that imitative suicide is most likely in those at high risk: those who are suicidal at the time of the example. If this is the case, an appropriate intervention would be to identify those teenagers by launching a screening programme in the affected high school and institute appropriate treatment.

There has only been one completed controlled study on post-vention (Hazell & Lewin 1993) that found no significant improvement in symptoms of students attending post-vention group sessions compared to controls. Those chosen for the post-vention were close friends of the teenager who committed suicide, so perhaps the controls were not matched sufficiently. Reports of reduction in guilt and sadness in a two-month volunteer-led survivors support group (Rogers *et al.* 1982) could have occurred spontaneously.

Conclusions

It is possible to view suicide, attempted suicide and suicidal ideation as part of a broad spectrum of suicidal behaviour whose prevalence is influenced by developmental factors. Suicidal ideation occurs throughout childhood, adolescence and early adulthood—and is very common in 15–17-year-olds. Suicide attempts are made relatively infrequently by prepubertal children and they increase in prevalence through adolescence, reaching a peak at around 16 years, after which they almost certainly decline (Kessler *et al.* 1999). Suicide, like suicide attempts, is rare before puberty and becomes increasingly common through late adolescence. However, unlike suicide attempts, which decline thereafter, the incidence of suicide increases until it reaches a level in early adulthood that is maintained until the end of the fifth decade.

The reason for these varying incidence patterns is not known. However, they are compatible with developmental differences in how suicidal ideation is translated into behaviour. If attempts really are attempts—if they are always associated, at some level and for some duration, no matter how brief, with a wish to die—then they could be seen as failed suicides. Failure rates are high in the young for any number of developmentally related reasons: brevity of the thought; lack of competence; lack of a sense of agency; diminished opportunity; and/or the absence of truly powerful stimuli, such as are provided by the effects of drugs and alcohol, the impact of clinical depression, and possibly some as yet unknown biological promoter that only becomes active at that age. As the youth becomes older and more competent and starts to experience these more potent stimuli to suicide, attempts are less likely to fail. However, it is possible that older teenagers also become more aware of the noxious consequences of suicide for themselves and for others they love, and develop a greater awareness, and comfort with, alternative coping strategies for common stresses. If this is the case, development could be expected to have an inhibiting effect that reduces the total amount of suicidal behaviour, redistributing it from attempts to completions and from the moderately impulsive to the seriously disturbed.

Such a model is compatible with the observation that ideation is a necessary but far from sufficient precondition of attempted and completed suicide, that the great majority of attempters will never commit suicide, and that more than half of teenage suicides have never made a known previous attempt. This model is inferred from morbidity and from retrospective data and would need to be confirmed by appropriate research. Hopefully, this would have practical benefits, perhaps in the area of suicide nosology, just as the development of heuristic models of the chain of events that lead to suicide (see Fig. 33.3) has provided a rational basis for suicide prevention.

This is not our only area of ignorance. We know little about how environmental factors operate to cause the great variability in incidence that is seen between communities and countries across time. Could these differences all be a function of imitation? Between 1960 and the late 1980s, there was a threefold increase in male adolescent suicides in the USA and similar phenomena in many developed countries (Shaffer & Hicks 1993). However, during the 1990s, there was a slow but consistent decline. Existing studies cannot confirm the suspicion that the initial increase was caused by the greater exposure of young people to drugs and alcohol, and that the recent decline was a result of the ever greater rate of prescribing the newer antidepressants to adolescents.

Given the burden of suicidality, there is an urgent need for more information on optimal treatment. The quality of psychopharmacological research on suicidality is generally poor, most studies being small and unreplicated. This is especially unfortunate because of the efficacy of psychotropic medication in other conditions, its low cost and its transportability. Well-designed studies on candidate medications need to be conducted as a matter of urgency. Psychotherapy is more demanding and costlier, but it deserves study. A form of behavioural therapy (dialectical-behaviour therapy) has been shown to be effective in adult attempters; this needs to be studied in young people, together with ways to reduce its cost and complexity.

As suicide is nearly always associated with a pre-existing psychiatric disorder, it makes the most sense to orientate prevention to identifying and effectively treating teenagers with disorders that place them at risk for suicide. The benefits of the more popular approach to prevention, through education, lacks empirical support. Furthermore, the phenomenon of suicide 'contagion' has implications about how safe it is to discuss suicide with teenagers in a group situation. No doubt, research will continue to complete this and other gaps in our knowledge in this important area of psychopathology.

Acknowledgements

This work was made possible by NIMH Research Training Grant MH 38198–11A2 and Research Training Grant MH 16434, NIMH Center Grant MH 43878 AI, the Centers for Disease Control Grant R49 CCR202598, NIMH Project Grants ROI MH 38198, ROI MH416898 and R18MH48059–02 and grants from the American Mental Health Foundation and the Leon Lowenstein Foundation.

References

Achenbach, T.M. & Edelbrock, C. (1987) *Manual for the Youth Self-Report and Profile*. Department of Psychiatry, University of Vermont, Burlington, VT.

American Association of Suicidology (1999) *Suicide Prevention and Crisis Intervention Centers*. American Association of Suicidology, Washington D.C.

American Foundation for Suicide Prevention (2001) Reporting on suicide: recommendations for the media. American Foundation for Suicide Prevention, New York City, www.afsp.org/index-1.htm.

Andrews, J.A. & Lewinsohn, P.M. (1992) Suicidal attempts among older adolescents: prevalence and co-occurrence with psychiatric disorders. *Journal of the American Academy of Child and Adolescent Psychiatry*, **31**, 655–662.

Apsler, R. & Hodas, M. (1975) Evaluating hotlines with simulated calls. *Crisis Intervention*, **6**, 14–21.

Asarnow, J.R. (1992) Suicidal ideation and attempts during middle childhood: associations with perceived family stress and depression among child psychiatric inpatients. *Journal of Clinical Child Psychology*, **21**, 35–40.

Asarnow, J.R., Carlson, G.A. & Guthrie, D. (1987) Coping strategies, self-perceptions, hopelessness, and perceived family environments in depressed and suicidal children. *Journal of Consulting and Clinical Psychology*, **55**, 361–366.

Asberg, M., Thoren, P., Traskman, L., Bertilsson, L. & Ringberger, V. (1976) Serotonin depression': a biochemical subgroup within the affective disorders? *Science*, **191**, 478–480.

Ashton, J.R. & Donnan, S. (1981) Suicide by burning as an epidemic phenomenon: an analysis of eighty-two deaths and inquests in England and Wales in 1978–9. *Psychological Medicine*, **11**, 735–739.

Barraclough, B.M. & Jennings, C. (1977) Suicide prevention by the Samaritans: a controlled study of effectiveness. *Lancet*, **2**, 237–239.

Barraclough, B., Bunch, J., Nelson, B. & Sainsbury, P. (1974) A hundred cases of suicide: clinical aspects. *British Journal of Psychiatry*, **125**, 355–373.

Beasley, C.M. Jr, Dornseif, B.E., Bosomworth, J.C. *et al*. (1991) Fluoxetine and suicide: a meta-analysis of controlled trials of treatment for depression. *British Medical Journal*, **303**, 685–692.

Beautrais, A.L., Joyce, P.R. & Mulder, R.T. (1997) Precipitating factors and life events in serious suicide attempts among youths aged thirteen through twenty-four years. *Journal of the American Academy of Child and Adolescent Psychiatry*, **36**, 1543–1551.

Beautrais, A.L., Joyce, P.R. & Mulder, R.T. (1998) Psychiatric illness in a New Zealand sample of young people making serious suicide attempts. *New Zealand Medical Journal*, **111**, 44–48.

Beck, A.T. (1972) *Depression: Clinical, Experimental, and Theoretical Aspects*, 2nd edn. University of Pennsylvania Press, Philadelphia.

Bennett, P.J., McMahon, W.M., Watabe, J. *et al*. (2000) Tryptophan hydroxylase polymorphisms in suicide victims. *Psychiatric Genetics*, **10**, 13–17.

Berman, A.L. (1988) Fictional depiction of suicide in television films and imitation effects. *American Journal of Psychiatry* **145**, 982–986.

Bird, H.R., Yager, T.J., Staghezza, B., Gould, M.S., Canino, G. & Rubio-Stipec, M. (1990) Impairment in the epidemiological measurement of childhood psychopathology in the community. *Journal of the American Academy of Child and Adolescent Psychiatry*, **29**, 796–803.

Birmaher, B., Brent, D.A., Kolko, D. *et al*. (2000) Clinical outcome after short-term psychotherapy for adolescents with major depressive disorder I. *Archives of General Psychiatry*, **57**, 29–36.

Bleach, G. & Claiborn, W.L. (1974) Initial evaluation of hot-line telephone crisis centers. *Community Mental Health Journal*, **10**, 387–394.

Boehm, K.E. & Campbell, N.B. (1995) Suicide: a review of calls to an adolescent peer listening phone service. *Child Psychiatry and Human Development*, **26**, 61–66.

Boehm, K.E., Chessare, J.B., Valko, T.R. & Sager, M.S. (1991) Teen Line: a descriptive analysis of a peer telephone listening service. *Adolescence*, **26**, 643–648.

Bollen, K.A. (1983) Temporal variations in mortality: a comparison of US suicides and motor vehicle fatalities, 1972–76. *Demography*, **20**, 45–59.

Bollen, K.A. & Phillips, D.P. (1981) Suicidal motor vehicle fatalities in Detroit: a replication. *American Journal of Sociology*, **87**, 404–412.

Bollen, K.A. & Philips, D.P. (1982) Imitative suicides: a national study of the effects of television news stories. *American Sociological Review*, **47**, 802–809.

Brand, E.F., King, C.A., Olson, E., Ghaziuddin, N. & Naylor, M. (1996) Depressed adolescents with a history of sexual abuse: diagnostic comorbidity and suicidality. *Journal of the American Academy of Child and Adolescent Psychiatry*, **35**, 34–41.

Brent, D.A., Kerr, M.M., Goldstein, C., Bozigar, J., Wartella, M. & Allan, M.J. (1989) An outbreak of suicide and suicidal behavior in a high school. *Journal of the American Academy of Child and Adolescent Psychiatry*, **28**, 918–924.

Brent, D.A., Perper, J.A., Allman, C.J., Moritz, G.M., Wartella, M.E. & Zelenak, J.P. (1991) The presence and accessibility of firearms in the homes of adolescent suicides: a case–control study. *Journal of the American Medical Association*, **266**, 2989–2995.

Brent, D.A., Perper, J.A., Moritz, G. *et al*. (1993a) Psychiatric risk factors for adolescent suicide: a case–control study. *Journal of the American Academy of Child and Adolescent Psychiatry*, **32**, 521–529.

Brent, D.A., Perper, J.A., Moritz, G. *et al*. (1993b) Stressful life events, psychopathology, and adolescent suicide: a case–control study. *Suicide and Life-Threatening Behavior*, **23**, 179–187.

Brent, D.A., Perper, J.A., Moritz, G. *et al*. (1994) Familial risk factors for

adolescent suicide: a case–control study. *Acta Psychiatrica Scandinavica*, **89**, 52–58.

Brent, D.A., Bridge, J., Johnson, B.A. & Connolly, J. (1996a) Suicidal behavior runs in families: a controlled family study of adolescent suicide victims. *Archives of General Psychiatry*, **53**, 1145–1152.

Brent, D.A., Moritz, G., Bridge, J., Perper, J. & Canobbio, R. (1996b) Long-term impact of exposure to suicide: a three-year controlled follow-up. *Journal of the American Academy of Child and Adolescent Psychiatry*, **35**, 646–653.

Brent, D.A., Holder, D., Kolko, D. *et al*. (1997) A clinical psychotherapy trial for adolescent depression comparing cognitive, family, and supportive therapy. *Archives of General Psychiatry*, **54**, 877–885.

Brent, D.A., Baugher, M., Bridge, J., Chen, T. & Chiappetta, L. (1999) Age- and sex-related risk factors for adolescent suicide. *Journal of the American Academy of Child and Adolescent Psychiatry*, **38**, 1497–1505.

Brent, D.A., Baugher, M., Birmaher, B., Kolko, D. & Bridge, J. (2000) Compliance with recommendations to remove firearms in families participating in a clinical trial for adolescent depression. *Journal of the American Academy of Child and Adolescent Psychiatry*, **39**, 1220–1226.

Bridge, T.P., Potkin, S.G., Zung, W.W. & Soldo, B.J. (1977) Suicide prevention centers: ecological study of effectiveness. *Journal of Nervous and Mental Disease*, **164**, 18–24.

Bridge, J.A., Brent, D., Johnson, B.A. & Connolly, J. (1997) Familial aggregation of psychiatric disorders in a community sample of adolescents. *Journal of the American Academy of Child and Adolescent Psychiatry*, **36**, 628–636.

Bush, J.A. (1976) Suicide and blacks: a conceptual framework. *Suicide and Life-Threatening Behavior*, **6** (4), 216–222.

Calhoun, L.G., Selby, J.W. & Selby, L.E. (1982) The psychological aftermath of suicide: an analysis of current evidence. *Clinical Psychological Review*, **2**, 409–420.

Carlsten, A., Allebeck, P. & Brandt, L. (1996) Are suicide rates in Sweden associated with changes in the prescribing of medicines? *Acta Psychiatrica Scandinavica*, **94**, 94–100.

Centers for Disease Control (2000) Youth risk behavior surveillance: United States, 1999. *Morbidity and Mortality Weekly Report*, **49**, 1–96.

Cheng, A.T. (1995) Mental illness and suicide: a case–control study in east Taiwan. *Archives of General Psychiatry*, **52**, 594–603.

Chew, K.S. & McCleary, R. (1995) The spring peak in suicides: a cross-national analysis. *Social Science and Medicine*, **40**, 223–230.

Choquet, M. & Menke, H. (1989) Suicidal thoughts during early adolescence: prevalence, associated troubles, and help-seeking behavior. *Acta Psychiatrica Scandinavica*, **81**, 170–177.

Chung, S.Y., Luk, S.L. & Mak, F.L. (1987) Attempted suicide in children and adolescents in Hong Kong. *Social Psychiatry*, **22**, 102–106.

Coe, J.I. (1974) Sexual asphyxias. *Suicide and Life-Threatening Behavior*, **4**, 171–175.

Cotgrove, A., Zirinsky, L., Black, D. & Weston, D. (1995) Secondary prevention of attempted suicide in adolescence. *Journal of Adolescence*, **18**, 569–577.

Davidson, L.E., Rosenberg, M.L., Mercy, J.A., Franklin, J. & Simmons, J.T. (1989) An epidemiologic study of risk factors in two teenage suicide clusters. *Journal of the American Medical Association*, **262**, 2687–2692.

Eastwood, M.R. & Peter, A.M. (1988) Epidemiology and seasonal affective disorder. *Psychological Medicine*, **18**, 799–806.

Eddleston, M., Sheriff, M.H. & Hawton, K. (1998) Deliberate self harm in Sri Lanka: an overlooked tragedy in the developing world. *British Medical Journal*, **317** (7151), 133–135.

Egan, M.P., Rivera, S.G., Robillard, R.R. & Hanson, A. (1997) The 'no suicide contract': helpful or harmful? *Journal of Psychosocial Nursing and Mental Health Services*, 35, 31–33.

Emslie, G.J., Rush, A.J., Weinberg, W.A. *et al.* (1997) A double-blind, randomized, placebo-controlled trial of fluoxetine in children and adolescents with depression. *Archives of General Psychiatry*, 54, 1031–1037.

Etzersdorfer, E., Sonneck, G. & Nagel-Kuess, S. (1992) Newspaper reports and suicide. *New England Journal of Medicine*, 327, 502–503.

Evans, K., Tyrer, P., Catalan, J. *et al.* (1999) Manual-assisted cognitive-behaviour therapy (MACT): a randomized controlled trial of a brief intervention with bibliotherapy in the treatment of recurrent deliberate self-harm. *Psychological Medicine*, 29, 19–25.

Farberow, N.L. (1985) Youth suicide: an international problem. In: *National Report of the Conference on Youth Suicide*, pp. 9–34. Youth Suicide National Center, Washington D.C.

Faulkner, A.H. & Cranston, K. (1998) Correlates of same-sex sexual behavior in a random sample of Massachusetts high school students. *American Journal of Public Health*, 88, 262–266.

Fekete, S. & Macsai, E. (1990) Hungarian suicidal models: past and present. In: *Suicidal Behavior and Risk Factors* (eds G. Ferrari, M. Bellini & P. Crepet), pp. 149–156. Moduzzi Editore, Bologna, Italy.

Fergusson, D.M. & Lynskey, M.T. (1995) Suicide attempts and suicidal ideation in a birth cohort of sixteen-year-old New Zealanders. *Journal of the American Academy of Child and Adolescent Psychiatry*, 34, 1308–1317.

Fergusson, D.M., Horwood. L.J. & Beautrais, A.L. (1999) Is sexual orientation related to mental health problems and suicidality in young people? *Archives of General Psychiatry*, 56, 876–880.

Fisher, P., Shaffer, D., Gould, M., Trautman, P. & Flory, M. (2001) An epidemiological study of child and adolescent suicide. *The Act of Suicide*, in preparation.

Flisher, A.J., Parry, C.D., Bradshaw, D. & Juritz, J.M. (1997) Seasonal variation of suicide in South Africa. *Psychiatry Research*, 66, 13–22.

Flisher, A.J., Kramer, R.A., Hoven, C.W. *et al.* (2000) Risk behavior in a community sample of children and adolescents. *Journal of the American Academy of Child and Adolescent Psychiatry*, 39, 881–887.

Frankenfield, D.L., Keyl, P.M., Gielen, A., Wissow, L.S., Werthamer, L. & Baker, S.P. (2000) Adolescent patients: healthy or hurting? Missed opportunities to screen for suicide risk in the primary care setting. *Archives of Pediatric and Adolescent Medicine*, 154, 162–168.

Garland, A., Shaffer, D. & Whittle, B. (1989) A national survey of school-based, adolescent suicide prevention programs. *Journal of the American Academy of Child and Adolescent Psychiatry*, 28, 931–934.

Garofalo, R., Wolf, R.C., Kessel, S., Palfrey, S.J. & DuRant, R.H. (1998) The association between health risk behaviors and sexual orientation among a school-based sample of adolescents. *Pediatrics*, 101, 895–902.

Garrison, C.Z., Jackson, K.L., Addy, C.L., McKeown, R.E. & Waller, J.L. (1991) Suicidal behaviors in young adolescents. *American Journal of Epidemiology*, 133, 1005–1014.

Geijer, T., Frisch, A., Persson, M.L. *et al.* (2000) Search for association between suicide attempt and serotonergic polymorphisms. *Psychiatric Genetics*, 10, 19–26.

Gibbons, J.S., Butler, J., Urwin, P. & Gibbons, J.L. (1978) Evaluation of a social work service for self-poisoning patients. *British Journal of Psychiatry*, 133, 111–118.

Gibbs, J. & Martin, W. (1964) *Status Integration and Suicide*. University of Oregon Press, Eugene.

Gispert, M., Wheeler, K., Marsh, L. & Davis, M.S. (1985) Suicidal adolescents: factors in evaluation. *Adolescence*, 20, 753–762.

Gispert, M., Davis, M.S., Marsh, L. & Wheeler, K. (1987) Predictive factors in repeated suicide attempts by adolescents. *Hospital and Community Psychiatry*, 38, 390–393.

Goldacre, M. & Hawton, K. (1985) Repetition of self-poisoning and subsequent death in adolescents who take overdoses. *British Journal of Psychiatry*, 146, 395–398.

Goldston, D.B. (2000) *Assessment of suicidal behaviors and risk among children and adolescents*. Technical report submitted to NIMH under Contract 263-MD-909995. (www.nimh.nih.gov/research/measures.pdf)

Goodwin, F.K. & Jamison, K.R. (1990) *Manic-Depressive Illness*. Oxford University Press, New York.

Gould, M.S. (1990) Suicide clusters and media exposure. In: *Suicide Over the Life Cycle: Risk Factors, Assessment, and Treatment of Suicidal Patients* (eds S.J. Blumenthal & D.J. Kupfer), pp. 517–532. American Psychiatric Press, Washington D.C.

Gould, M.S. (2001) Suicide and the media. In: *The clinical science of suicide prevention* (eds H. Hendin & J.J. Mann), pp. 200–224. Annals of the New York Academy of Sciences, New York.

Gould, M.S. & Shaffer, D. (1986) The impact of suicide in television movies: evidence of imitation. *New England Journal of Medicine*, 315, 690–694.

Gould, M.S., Shaffer, D. & Kleinman, M. (1988) The impact of suicide in television movies: replication and commentary. *Suicide and Life-Threatening Behavior*, 18, 90–99.

Gould, M.S., Shaffer, D. & Davies, M. (1990) Truncated pathways from childhood: attrition in follow-up studies due to death. In: *Straight and Devious Pathways from Childhood to Adulthood* (eds L. Robins & M. Rutter), pp. 3–10. Cambridge University Press, Cambridge.

Gould, M.S., Fisher, P., Parides, M., Flory, M. & Shaffer, D. (1996) Psychosocial risk factors of child and adolescent completed suicide. *Archives of General Psychiatry*, 53, 1155–1162.

Gould, M.S., Shaffer, D., Fisher, P. & Garfinkel, R. (1998a) Separation/divorce and child and adolescent completed suicide. *Journal of the American Academy of Child and Adolescent Psychiatry*, 37, 155–162.

Gould, M.S., King, R., Greenwald, S. *et al.* (1998b) Psychopathology associated with suicidal ideation and attempts among children and adolescents. *Journal of the American Academy of Child and Adolescent Psychiatry*, 37, 915–923.

Gould, M.S., Kramer, R. & Shaffer, D. (1999) *Reporting a suicide: a guide for journalists*. Pamphlet developed for the American Foundation for Suicide Prevention. The American Foundation for Suicide Prevention, New York.

Greer, S. & Anderson, M. (1979) Samaritan contact among 325 parasuicide patients. *British Journal of Psychiatry*, 135, 263–268.

Groholt, B., Ekeberg, O., Wichstrom, L. & Haldorsen, T. (2000) Young suicide attempters: a comparison between a clinical and an epidemiological sample. *Journal of the American Academy of Child and Adolescent Psychiatry*, 39, 868–875.

Hakko, H., Rasanen, P. & Tiihonen, J. (1998) Secular trends in the rates and seasonality of violent and nonviolent suicide occurrences in Finland during 1980–95. *Journal of Affective Disorders*, 50, 49–54.

Halpern-Felsher, B.L., Ozer, E.M., Millstein, S.G. *et al.* (2000) Preventive services in a health maintenance organization: how well do pediatricians screen and educate adolescent patients? *Archives of Pediatric and Adolescent Medicine*, 154, 173–179.

Hamilton, M.S. & Opler, L.A. (1992) Akathisia, suicidality, and fluoxetine. *Journal of Clinical Psychiatry*, 53, 401–406.

Harkavy Friedman, J.M., Asnis, G.M., Boeck, M. & DiFiore, J. (1987)

Prevalence of specific suicidal behaviors in a high-school sample. *American Journal of Psychiatry*, 144, 1203–1206.

Harrington, R., Kerfoot, M., Dyer, E. *et al.* (1998a) Randomized trial of a home-based family intervention for children who have deliberately poisoned themselves. *Journal of the American Academy of Child and Adolescent Psychiatry*, 37, 512–518.

Harrington, R., Whittaker, J., Shoebridge, P. & Campbell, F. (1998b) Systematic review of efficacy of cognitive behaviour therapies in childhood and adolescent depressive disorder. *British Medical Journal*, 316, 1559–1563.

Harris, H.E. & Myers, W.C. (1997) Adolescents' misperceptions of the dangerousness of acetaminophen in overdose. *Suicide and Life-Threatening Behavior*, 27, 274–277.

Hassall, C. & Trethowan, W.H. (1972) Suicide in Birmingham. *British Medical Journal*, 1, 717–718.

Hawton, K. (1986) *Suicide and Attempted Suicide Among Children and Adolescents*. Sage Publications, London

Hawton, K. & Fagg, J. (1992) Trends in deliberate self poisoning and self injury in Oxford, 1976–90. *British Medical Journal*, 304, 1409–1411.

Hawton, K., Bancroft, J., Catalan, J., Kingston, B., Stedeford, A. & Welch, N. (1981) Domiciliary and out-patient treatment of self-poisoning patients by medical and non-medical staff. *Psychological Medicine*, 11, 169–177.

Hawton, K., Cole, D., O'Grady, J. & Osborn, M. (1982a) Motivational aspects of deliberate self-poisoning in adolescents. *British Journal of Psychiatry*, 141, 286–291.

Hawton, K., O'Grady, J., Osborn, M. & Cole, D. (1982b) Adolescents who take overdoses: their characteristics, problems and contacts with helping agencies. *British Journal of Psychiatry*, 140, 118–123.

Hawton, K., McKeown, S., Day, A., Martin, P., O'Connor, M. & Yule, J. (1987) Evaluation of out-patient counseling compared with general practitioner care following overdoses. *Psychological Medicine*, 17, 751–761.

Hawton, K., Fagg, J., Platt, S. & Hawkins, M. (1993) Factors associated with suicide after parasuicide in young people. *British Medical Journal*, 306, 1641–1644.

Hawton, K., Fagg, J., Simkin, S., Bale, E. & Bond, A. (1997) Trends in deliberate self-harm in Oxford, 1985–95: implications for clinical services and the prevention of suicide. *British Journal of Psychiatry*, 171, 556–560.

Hawton, K., Fagg, J., Simkin, S., Harriss, L. & Malmberg, A. (1998a) Methods used for suicide by farmers in England and Wales: the contribution of availability and its relevance to prevention. *British Journal of Psychiatry*, 173, 320–324.

Hawton, K., Arensman, E., Townsend, E. *et al.* (1998b) Deliberate self harm: systematic review of efficacy of psychosocial and pharmacological treatments in preventing repetition. *British Medical Journal*, 317, 441–447.

Hawton, K., Kingsbury, S., Steinhardt, K., James, A. & Fagg, J. (1999) Repetition of deliberate self-harm by adolescents: the role of psychological factors. *Journal of Adolescence*, 22, 369–378.

Hawton, K., Fagg, J., Simkin, S., Bale, E. & Bond, A. (2000a) Deliberate self-harm in adolescents in Oxford, 1985–95. *Journal of Adolescence*, 23, 47–55.

Hawton, K., Townsend, E., Arensman, E. *et al.* (2000b) Psychosocial and pharmacological treatments for deliberate self harm (Cochrane Review). In: *The Cochrane Library*, 4, 2000. Update Software, Oxford.

Haynes, R.H. (1987) Suicide and social response in Fiji: a historical survey. *British Journal of Psychiatry*, 151, 21–26.

Hazell, P. & Lewin, T. (1993) Friends of adolescent suicide attempters and completers. *Journal of the American Academy of Child and Adolescent Psychiatry*, 32, 76–81.

Henley, S.H.A. (1984) Bereavement following suicide: a review of the literature. *Current Psychological Research and Reviews*, 3, 53–61.

Hillard, J.R., Holland, J.M. & Ramm, D. (1981) Christmas and psychopathology: data from a psychiatric emergency room population. *Archives of General Psychiatry*, 38, 1377–1381.

Hirsch, S. (1981) A critique of volunteer-staffed suicide prevention centres. *Canadian Journal of Psychiatry*, 26, 406–410.

Holding, T.A. (1974) The BBC 'befrienders' series and its effects. *British Journal of Psychiatry*, 124, 470–472.

Holding, T.A. (1975) Suicide and 'The Befrienders, *British Medical Journal*, 3, 751–752.

Indian Health Service (1996) *Trends in Indian health*. US Department of Health and Human Services, Rockville, MD.

Isacsson, G., Holmgren, P., Druid, H. & Bergman, U. (1997) The utilization of antidepressants: a key issue in the prevention of suicide: an analysis of 5281 suicides in Sweden during the period 1992–94. *Acta Psychiatrica Scandinavica*, 96, 94–100.

Ishii, K. (1991) Measuring mutual causation: effect of suicide news on suicides in Japan. *Social Science Research*, 20, 188–195.

Jacobs, J. (1971) *Adolescent Suicide*. Wiley Interscience, New York.

Jacobson, B., Eklund, G., Hamberger, L., Linnarsson, D., Sedvall, G. & Valverius, M. (1987) Perinatal origin of adult self-destructive behavior. *Acta Psychiatrica Scandinavica*, 76, 364–371.

Jennings, C., Barraclough, B.M. & Moss, J.R. (1978) Have the Samaritans lowered the suicide rate: a controlled study. *Psychological Medicine*, 8, 413–422.

Jessen, G. & Jensen, B.F. (1999) Postponed suicide death: suicides around birthdays and major public holidays. *Suicide and Life-Threatening Behavior*, 29, 272–283.

Jeyaratnam, J. (1990) Acute pesticide poisoning: a major global health problem. *World Health Statistics Quarterly*, 43, 139–144.

Jobes, D.A., Berman, A.L., O'Carroll, P.W., Eastgard, S. & Knickmeyer, S. (1996) The Kurt Cobain suicide crisis: perspectives from research, public health, and the news media. *Suicide and Life-Threatening Behavior*, 26, 260–269.

Johnson, B.A., Brent, D.A., Bridge, J. & Connolly, J. (1998) The familial aggregation of adolescent suicide attempts. *Acta Psychiatrica Scandinavica*, 97, 18–24.

Juon, H.S. & Ensminger, M.E. (1997) Childhood, adolescent, and young adult predictors of suicidal behaviors: a prospective study of African Americans. *Journal of Child Psychology and Psychiatry*, 38, 553–563.

Kashani, J. & Simonds, J.F. (1979) The incidence of depression in children. *American Journal of Psychiatry*, 136, 1203–1205.

Kerfoot, M. & McHugh, B. (1992) The outcome of childhood suicidal behaviour. *Acta Paedopsychiatrica*, 55, 141–145.

Kessler, R.C., Borges, G. & Walters, E.E. (1999) Prevalence of and risk factors for lifetime suicide attempts in the National Comorbidity Survey. *Archives of General Psychiatry*, 56, 617–626.

Kevan, S.M. (1980) Perspectives on season of suicide: a review. *Social Science and Medicine*, 14, 369–378.

Kienhorst, C.W., de Wilde, E.J., Diekstra, R.F. & Wolters, W.H. (1992) Differences between adolescent suicide attempters and depressed adolescents. *Acta Psychiatrica Scandinavica*, 85, 222–228.

Kienhorst, I.C., de Wilde, E.J., Diekstra, R.F. & Wolters, W.H. (1995) Adolescents' image of their suicide attempt. *Journal of the American Academy of Child and Adolescent Psychiatry*, 34, 623–628.

Kienhorst, C.W., Wolters, W.H., Diekstra, R.F. & Otte, E. (1987) A study of the frequency of suicidal behaviour in children aged five to fourteen. *Journal of Child Psychology and Psychiatry*, 28, 153–165.

King, G.D. (1977) An evaluation of the effectiveness of a telephone counseling center. *American Journal of Community Psychology*, 5, 75–83.

King, R.A., Riddle, M.A., Chappell, P.B. *et al.* (1991) Emergence of self-destructive phenomena in children and adolescents during fluoxetine treatment. *Journal of the American Academy of Child and Adolescent Psychiatry*, 30, 179–186.

King, C.A., Franzese, R., Gargan, S., McGovern, L., Ghaziuddin, N. & Naylor, M.W. (1995) Suicide contagion among adolescents during acute psychiatric hospitalization. *Psychiatric Services*, 46, 915–918.

King, C.A., Hovey, J.D., Brand, E., Wilson, R. & Ghaziuddin, N. (1997) Suicidal adolescents after hospitalization: parent and family impacts on treatment follow-through. *Journal of the American Academy of Child and Adolescent Psychiatry*, 36, 85–93.

Kingsbury, S., Hawton, K., Steinhardt, K. & James, A. (1999) Do adolescents who take overdoses have specific psychological characteristics: a comparative study with psychiatric and community controls. *Journal of the American Academy of Child and Adolescent Psychiatry*, 38, 1125–1131.

Kirby, D. (1985) Sexuality education: a more realistic view of its effects. *Journal of School Health*, 55, 421–424.

Kirch, M.R. & Lester, D. (1986) Suicide from the Golden Gate Bridge: do they cluster over time? *Psychological Reports*, 59 (3), 1314.

Knowles, D. (1979) On the tendency of volunteer helpers to give advice. *Journal of Counseling Psychology*, 26, 352–354.

Kovacs, M. (1985) The Children's Depression Inventory (CDI). *Psychopharmacology Bulletin*, 21 (4), 995–998.

Kreitman, N. (1969) Parasuicide. *British Journal of Psychiatry*, 115, 746–747.

Kreitman, N. (1976) Age and parasuicide ('attempted suicide'). *Psychological Medicine*, 6, 113–121.

Kruesi, M.J., Grossman, J., Pennington, J.M., Woodward, P.J., Duda, D. & Hirsch, J.G. (1999) Suicide and violence prevention: parent education in the emergency department. *Journal of the American Academy of Child and Adolescent Psychiatry*, 38, 250–255.

Leese, S.M. (1969) Suicide behavior in twenty adolescents. *British Journal of Psychiatry*, 115, 479–480.

Lester, D. (1979) Temporal variation in suicide and homicide. *American Journal of Epidemiology*, 109, 517–520.

Lester, D. & Beck, A.T. (1975) Suicide and national holidays. *Psychological Reports*, 36, 52.

Letizia, C., Kapik, B. & Flanders, W.D. (1996) Suicidal risk during controlled clinical investigations of fluvoxamine. *Journal of Clinical Psychiatry*, 57, 415–421.

Levenson, M. (1974) Cognitive correlates of suicidal risk. In: *Psychological Assessment of Suicidal Risk* (ed. C. Neuringer), pp. 150–163. Charles C. Thomas, Springfield, IL.

Lewinsohn, P.M., Rohde, P. & Seeley, J.R. (1994) Psychosocial risk factors for future adolescent suicide attempts. *Journal of Consulting and Clinical Psychology*, 62, 297–305.

Lewinsohn, P.M., Rohde, P. & Seeley, J.R. (1996) Adolescent suicidal ideation and attempts: prevalence, risk factors, and clinical implications. *Clinical Psychology: Science and Practice*, 3, 25–46.

Linehan, M.M., Armstrong, H.E., Suarez, A., Allmon, D. & Heard, H.L. (1991) Cognitive-behavioral treatment of chronically parasuicidal borderline patients. *Archives of General Psychiatry*, 48, 1060–1064.

Linehan, M.M., Heard, H.L. & Armstrong, H.E. (1993) Naturalistic follow-up of a behavioral treatment for chronically parasuicidal borderline patients. *Archives of General Psychiatry*, 50, 971–974.

Linehan, M.M., Tutek, D.A., Heard, H.L. & Armstrong, H.E. (1994) Interpersonal outcome of cognitive behavioral treatment for chroni-cally suicidal borderline patients. *American Journal of Psychiatry*, 151, 1771–1776.

Litman, R., Farberow, N., Shneidman, E., Heilig, S. & Kramer, J. (1965) Suicide prevention telephone service. *Journal of the American Medical Association*, 192, 107–111.

Litt, I.F., Cuskey, W.R. & Rudd, S. (1983) Emergency room evaluation of the adolescent who attempts suicide: compliance with follow-up. *Journal of Adolescent Health Care*, 4, 106–108.

Lock, J. & Steiner, H. (1999) Gay, lesbian, and bisexual youth risks for emotional, physical, and social problems: results from a community-based survey. *Journal of the American Academy of Child and Adolescent Psychiatry*, 38, 297–304.

Lukianowitz, N. (1968) Attempted suicide in children. *Acta Psychiatrica Scandinavica*, 44, 415–435.

Lynskey, M., Degenhardt, L. & Hall, W. (2000) Cohort trends in youth suicide in Australia 1964–97. *Australian and New Zealand Journal of Psychiatry*, 34, 408–412.

Mann, J.J. (1999) Role of the serotonergic system in the pathogenesis of major depression and suicidal behavior. *Neuropsychopharmacology*, 21, 99S–105S.

Mann, J.J. & Kapur, S. (1991) The emergence of suicidal ideation and behavior during antidepressant pharmacotherapy. *Archives of General Psychiatry*, 48, 1027–1033.

Mann, J.J., Waternaux, C., Haas, G.L. & Malone, K.M. (1999) Toward a clinical model of suicidal behavior in psychiatric patients. *American Journal of Psychiatry*, 156, 181–189.

Marshall, S.E., Bird, T.G., Hart, K. & Welsh, K.I. (1999) Unified approach to the analysis of genetic variation in serotonergic pathways. *American Journal of Medical Genetics*, 88, 621–627.

Marttunen, M.J., Aro, H.M., Henriksson, M.M. & Lonnqvist, J.K. (1991) Mental disorders in adolescent suicide: DSM-III-R axes I and II diagnoses in suicides among thirteen- to nineteen-year-olds in Finland. *Archives of General Psychiatry*, 48, 834–839.

Marttunen, M.J., Aro, H.M. & Lonnqvist, J.K. (1993) Precipitant stressors in adolescent suicide. *Journal of the American Academy of Child and Adolescent Psychiatry*, 32, 1178–1183.

Marttunen, M.J., Henriksson, M.M., Aro, H.M., Heikkinen, M.E., Isometsa, E.T. & Lonnqvist, J.K. (1995) Suicide among female adolescents: characteristics and comparison with males in the age group thirteen to twenty-two years. *Journal of the American Academy of Child and Adolescent Psychiatry*, 34, 1297–1307.

Mattson, A., Seese, L.R. & Hawkins, J.W. (1969) Suicidal behavior as a child psychiatric emergency. *Archives of General Psychiatry*, 20, 100–109.

May, P.A. (1987) Suicide and self-destruction among American Indian youths. *American Indian and Alaska Native Mental Health Research*, 1, 52–69.

McClure, G.M. (2000) Changes in suicide in England and Wales. 1960–97. *British Journal of Psychiatry*, 176, 64–67.

McIntire, M.S. & Angle, C.R. (1973) Psychological 'biopsy' in self-poisoning of children and adolescents. *American Journal of Disturbed Children*, 126, 42–46.

McIntire, M.S., Angle, C.R., Wikoff, R.L. & Schlicht, M.L. (1977) Recurrent adolescent suicidal behavior. *Pediatrics*, 60, 605–608.

McKenry, P.C., Tishler, C.L. & Kelley, C. (1982) Adolescent suicide: a comparison of attempters and nonattempters in an emergency room population. *Clinical Pediatrics*, 21, 266–270.

McLeavey, B.C., Daly, R.J., Ludgate, J.W. & Murray, C.M. (1994) Interpersonal problem-solving skills training in the treatment of self-poisoning patients. *Suicide and Life-Threatening Behavior*, 24, 382–394.

McManus, B.L., Kruesi, M.J., Dontes, A.E., Defazio, C.R., Piotrowski,

J.T. & Woodward, P.J. (1997) Child and adolescent suicide attempts: an opportunity for emergency departments to provide injury prevention education. *American Journal of Emergency Medicine*, **15**, 357–360.

Meares, R., Mendelsohn, F.A. & Milgrom-Friedman, J. (1981) A sex difference in the seasonal variation of suicide rate: a single cycle for men, two cycles for women. *British Journal of Psychiatry*, **138**, 321–325.

Menninger, K. (1938) *Man Against Himself*. Harcourt Brace, New York.

Michel, K., Ballinari, P., Bille-Brahe, U. *et al.* (2000) Methods used for parasuicide: results of the WHO/EURO Multicentre Study on Parasuicide. *Social Psychiatry and Psychiatric Epidemiology*, **35**, 156–163.

Miller, H.L., Coombs, D.W., Leeper, J.D. & Barton, S.N. (1984) An analysis of the effects of suicide prevention facilities on suicide rates in the United States. *American Journal of Public Health*, **74**, 340–343.

Miller, K.E., King, C.A., Shain, B.N. & Naylor, M.W. (1992a) Suicidal adolescents' perceptions of their family environment. *Suicide and Life-Threatening Behavior*, **22**, 226–239.

Miller, A.L., Rathus, J.H., Linehan, M.M., Wetzler, S. & Leigh, E. (1997) Dialectical behavior therapy adapted for suicidal adolescents. *Journal of Practical Psychology and Behavioral Health*, **3**, 78–86.

Moens, G.F., Loysch, M.J. & van de Voorde, H. (1988) The geographical pattern of methods of suicide in Belgium: implications for prevention. *Acta Psychiatrica Scandinavica*, **77**, 320–327.

Monk, M. & Warshauer, M.E. (1978) A methodologic problem in mortality studies of migrant populations. *Journal of Chronic Diseases*, **31**, 347–352.

Montgomery, S.A. (1997) Suicide and antidepressants. *Annals of the New York Academy of Sciences*, **836**, 329–338.

Montgomery, S.A. & Montgomery, D. (1982) Pharmacological prevention of suicidal behaviour. *Journal of Affective Disorders*, **4**, 291–298.

Montgomery, S.A., Dunner, D.L. & Dunbar, G.C. (1995) Reduction of suicidal thoughts with paroxetine in comparison with reference antidepressants and placebo. *European Neuropsychopharmacology*, **5**, 5–13.

Morano, C.D., Cisler, R.A. & Lemerond, J. (1993) Risk factors for adolescent suicidal behavior: loss, insufficient familial support, and hopelessness. *Adolescence*, **28**, 851–865.

Motto, J.A. (1984) Suicide in male adolescents. In: *Suicide in the Young* (eds H.S. Segdak, A.B. Ford & N.B. Rushforth), pp. 227–244. John Wright PSG, Boston.

Murphy, G.E. & Robins, E.R. (1967) Social factors in suicide. *Journal of the American Medical Association*, **199**, 303–308.

Murphy, G.E. & Wetzel, R.D. (1990) The lifetime risk of suicide in alcoholism. *Archives of General Psychiatry*, **47**, 383–392.

Myers, W.C. (1992) What treatments do we have for children and adolescents who have killed? *Bulletin of the American Academy of Psychiatry and the Law*, **20**, 47–58.

National Center for Health Statistics, Centers for Disease Control and Prevention (2000) Death rates for seventy-two selected causes, by five-year age groups, race, and sex: United States, 1979–98. Worktable GMWK 291. www.cdc.gov/nchs/datawh/statab/unpubd/mortabs.htm.

Neeleman, J. & Wessely, S. (1999) Ethnic minority suicide: a small area geographical study in south London. *Psychological Medicine*, **29**, 429–436.

Neeleman, J., Wessely, S. & Lewis, G. (1998) Suicide acceptability in African- and white Americans: the role of religion. *Journal of Nervous and Mental Disease*, **186**, 12–16.

Negron, R., Piacentini, J., Graae, F., Davies, M. & Shaffer, D. (1997) Microanalysis of adolescent suicide attempters and ideators during the acute suicidal episode. *Journal of the American Academy of Child and Adolescent Psychiatry*, **36**, 1512–1519.

Nielsen, D.A., Goldman, D., Virkkunen, M., Tokola, R., Rawlings, R. & Linnoila, M. (1994) Suicidality and 5-hydroxyindoleacetic acid concentration associated with a tryptophan hydroxylase polymorphism. *Archives of General Psychiatry*, **51**, 34–38.

Nielsen, D.A., Virkkunen, M., Lappalainen, J. *et al.* (1998) A tryptophan hydroxylase gene marker for suicidality and alcoholism. *Archives of General Psychiatry*, **55**, 593–602.

Nordstrom, P., Samuelsson, M., Asberg, M. *et al.* (1994) CSF 5-HIAA predicts suicide risk after attempted suicide. *Suicide and Life-Threatening Behavior*, **24**, 1–9.

Nordstrom, P., Samuelsson, M. & Asberg, M. (1995) Survival analysis of suicide risk after attempted suicide. *Acta Psychiatrica Scandinavica*, **91**, 336–340.

Ohara, K., Nagai, M., Tani, K., Nakamura, Y., Ino, A. & Ohara, K. (1998) Functional polymorphism of -141C Ins/Del in the dopamine D2 receptor gene promoter and schizophrenia. *Psychiatry Research*, **81**, 117–123.

Ohberg, A., Vuori, E., Klaukka, T. & Lonnqvist, J. (1998) Antidepressants and suicide mortality. *Journal of Affective Disorders*, **50**, 225–233.

Olfson, M., Marcus, S.C., Pincus, H.A., Zito, J.M., Thompson, J.W. & Zarin, D.A. (1998) Antidepressant prescribing practices of outpatient psychiatrists. *Archives of General Psychiatry*, **55**, 310–316.

Oquendo, M.A. & Mann, J.J. (2000) The biology of impulsivity and suicidality. *Psychiatric Clinics of North America*, **23**, 11–25.

Orbach, I., Rosenheim, E. & Hary, E. (1987) Some aspects of cognitive functioning in suicidal children. *Journal of the American Academy of Child and Adolescent Psychiatry*, **26**, 181–185.

Otto, U. (1972) Suicidal acts by children and adolescents: a follow-up study. *Acta Pscyhiatrica Scandinavica*, **233**, 5–123.

Pfeffer, C.R., Conte, H.R., Plutchik, R. & Jerrett, I. (1980) Suicidal behavior in latency-age children: an outpatient population. *Journal of the American Academy of Child and Adolescent Psychiatry*, **19**, 703–710.

Pfeffer, C.R., Zuckerman, S., Plutchik, R. & Mizruchi, M.S. (1984) Suicidal behavior in normal school children: a comparison with child psychiatric inpatients. *Journal of the American Academy of Child and Adolescent Psychiatry*, **23**, 416–423.

Pfeffer, C.R., Klerman, G.L., Hurt, S.W., Lesser, M., Peskin, J.R. & Siefker, C.A. (1991) Suicidal children grow up: demographic and clinical risk factors for adolescent suicide attempts. *Journal of the American Academy of Child and Adolescent Psychiatry*, **30**, 609–616.

Phillips, D.P. (1974) The influence of suggestion on suicide: substantive and theroretical implications of the Werther effect. *American Sociological Review*, **39**, 340–354.

Phillips, D.P. (1979) Suicide, motor vehicle fatalities, and the mass media; evidence toward a theory of suggestion. *American Journal of Sociology*, **84**, 1150–1174.

Phillips, D.P. (1980) Airplane accidents, murder and the mass media; towards a theory of imitation and suggestion. *Social Forces*, **58**, 1001–1004.

Phillips, D.P. (1984) Teenage and adult temporal fluctuations in suicide and auto fatalities. In: *Suicide in the Young* (eds H.S. Sudak, A.B. Ford & N.B. Rushforth), pp. 69–80. John Wright-PSG, Littleton, MA.

Phillips, D.P. & Carstensen, L.L. (1986) Clustering of teenage suicides after television news stories about suicide. *New England Journal of Medicine*, **315**, 685–689.

Phillips, D.P. & Liu, J. (1980) The frequency of suicides around major public holidays: some surprising findings. *Suicide and Life-Threatening Behavior*, 10, 41–50.

Phillips, D.P. & Wills, J.S. (1987) A drop in suicides around major national holidays. *Suicide and Life-Threatening Behavior*, 17, 1–12.

Piacentini, J., Rotheram-Borus, M.J., Trautman, P. & Graae, F. (1991) *Psychosocial correlates of treatment compliance in adolescent suicide attempters*. Presented at the Association for Advancement of Behavior Therapy Meeting, New York.

Platt, S., Bille-Brahe, U., Kerkhof, A. *et al.* (1992) Parasuicide in Europe: the WHO/EURO multicentre study on parasuicide. I. Introduction and preliminary analysis for 1989. *Acta Psychiatrica Scandinavica*, 85, 97–104.

Reid, W.H. (1998) Promises, promises: don't rely on patients' no-suicide/no-violence 'contracts'. *Journal of Practical Psychiatry and Behavioral Health*, 4, 316–318.

Remafedi, G., French, S., Story, M., Resnick, M.D. & Blum, R. (1998) The relationship between suicide risk and sexual orientation: results of a population-based study. *American Journal of Public Health*, 88, 57–60.

Renaud, J., Brent, D.A., Birmaher, B., Chiappetta, L. & Bridge, J. (1999) Suicide in adolescents with disruptive disorders. *Journal of the American Academy of Child and Adolescent Psychiatry*, 38, 846–851.

Renouf, A.G. & Kovacs, M. (1994) Concordance between mothers' reports and children's self-reports of depressive symptoms: a longitudinal study. *Journal of the American Academy of Child and Adolescent Psychiatry*, 33, 208–216.

Reynolds, W.M. (1991) A school-based procedure for the identification of adolescents at risk for suicidal behaviors. *Family Community Health*, 14, 64–75.

Rich, C.L., Fowler, R.C., Fogarty, L.A. & Young, D. (1988) San Diego Suicide Study. III. Relationships between diagnoses and stressors. *Archives of General Psychiatry*, 45, 589–592.

Rihmer, Z., Rutz, W. & Pihlgren, H. (1995) Depression and suicide on Gotland: an intensive study of all suicides before and after a depression-training programme for general practitioners. *Journal of Affective Disorders*, 35, 147–152.

Robins, E.R., Murphy, G.E., Wilkinson, R.H., Gassner, S. & Kayes, J. (1959) Some clinical considerations in the prevention of suicide based on a study of 134 successful suicides. *American Journal of Public Health*, 49, 888–899.

Rogers, J., Sheldon, A., Barwick, C., Letofsky, K. & Lancee, W. (1982) Help for families of suicide: survivors support program. *Canadian Journal of Psychiatry*, 27, 444–449.

Rohn, R.D., Sarles, R.M., Kenny, T.J., Reynolds, B.J. & Heald, F.P. (1977) Adolescents who attempt suicide. *Journal of Pediatrics*, 90, 636–638.

Rotheram-Borus, M.J., Trautman, P.D., Dopkins, S.C. & Shrout, P.E. (1990) Cognitive style and pleasant activities among female adolescent suicide attempters. *Journal of Consulting and Clinical Psychology*, 58, 554–561.

Rotheram-Borus, M., Piacentini, J., Miller, S., Graae, F. & Castro-Blanco, D. (1994) A brief cognitive-behavioral teatment for adolescent suicide attempters and their families. *Journal of the American Academy of Child and Adolescent Psychiatry*, 33, 508–517.

Rotheram-Borus, M.J., Piacentini, J., Van Rossem, R. *et al.* (1996) Enhancing treatment adherence with a specialized emergency room program for adolescent suicide attempters. *Journal of the American Academy of Child and Adolescent Psychiatry*, 35, 654–663.

Rotheram-Borus, M.J., Piacentini, J., Van Rossem, R. *et al.* (1999) Treatment adherence among Latina female adolescent suicide attempters. *Suicide and Life-Threatening Behavior*, 29, 319–331.

Rothschild, A.J. & Locke, C.A. (1991) Re-exposure to fluoxetine after serious suicide attempts by three patients: the role of akathisia. *Journal of Clinical Psychiatry*, 52, 491–493.

Roy, A., Segal, N.L., Centerwall, B.S. & Robinette, C.D. (1991) Suicide in twins. *Archives of General Psychiatry*, 48, 29–32.

Roy, A., Segal, N.L. & Sarchiapone, M. (1995) Attempted suicide among living co-twins of twin suicide victims. *American Journal of Psychiatry*, 152, 1075–1076.

Roy, A., Nielsen, D.A., Rylander, G. & Sarchiapone, M. (2000) The genetics of suicidal behavior. In: *The International Handbook of Suicide and Attempted Suicide* (eds K. Hawton & K. van Heeringen), pp. 209–221. John Wiley & Sons, Chichester.

Rutz, W., von Knorring, L., Pihlgren, H., Rihmer, Z. & Walinder, J. (1995) An educational project on depression and its consequences: is the frequency of major depression among Swedish men underrated, resulting in high suicidality? *Primary Care Psychiatry*, 1, 59–63.

Ryan, N.D. & Varma, D. (1998) Child and adolescent mood disorders: experience with serotonin-based therapies. *Biological Psychiatry*, 44, 336–340.

Safer, D.J. (1997a) Changing patterns of psychotropic medications prescribed by child psychiatrists in the 1990s. *Journal of Child and Adolescent Psychopharmacology*, 7, 267–274.

Safer, D.J. (1997b) Self-reported suicide attempts by adolescents. *Annals of Clinical Psychiatry*, 9, 263–269.

Salk, L., Lipsitt, L.P., Sturner, W.Q., Reilly, B.M. & Levat, R.H. (1985) Relationship of maternal and perinatal conditions to eventual adolescent suicide. *Lancet*, 1, 624–627.

Salkovskis, P.M., Atha, C. & Storer, D. (1990) Cognitive-behavioural problem solving in the treatment of patients who repeatedly attempt suicide. A controlled trial. *British Journal of Psychiatry*, 157, 871–876.

van der Sande, R., Buskens, E., Allart, E., van der Graaf, Y. & van Engeland, H. (1997) Psychosocial intervention following suicide attempt: a systematic review of treatment interventions. *Acta Psychiatrica Scandinavica*, 96, 43–50.

Schmidtke, A. & Hafner, H. (1986) Facilitation of suicide motivation and suicidal behavior by fictional models: sequelae of the television series 'Death of a Student'. *Nervenarzt*, 57, 502–510.

Schmidtke, A., Bille-Brahe, U., DeLeo, D. *et al.* (1996) Attempted suicide in Europe: rates, trends and sociodemographic characteristics of suicide attempters during the period 1989–92. Results of the WHO/EURO Multicentre Study on Parasuicide. *Acta Psychiatrica Scandinavica*, 93, 327–338.

Schuckit, M.A. (1995) *Drug and Alcohol Abuse: a Clinical Guide to Diagnosis and Treatment*. Plenum Medical, New York.

Schulsinger, R., Kety, S., Rosenthal, D. & Wender, P. (1979) A family study of suicide. In: *Origins, Prevention, and Treatment of Affective Disorders* (eds M. Schou & E. Stromgren), pp. 277–287. Academic Press, New York.

Seeley, M.F. (1996) Hotlines as discrete services in mental health and human service organizations. *Crisis*, 17, 100–101; 104.

Sellar, C., Hawton, K. & Goldacre, M.J. (1990) Self-poisoning in adolescents: hospital admissions and deaths in the Oxford region, 1980–85. *British Journal of Psychiatry*, 156, 866–870.

Shaffer, D. (1974) Suicide in childhood and early adolescence. *Journal of Child Psychology and Psychiatry*, 15, 275–291.

Shaffer, D. & Craft, L. (1999) Methods of adolescent suicide prevention. *Journal of Clinical Psychiatry*, 60, 70–74.

Shaffer, D. & Hicks, R. (1993) The epidemiology of child and adolescent suicide. In: *The Epidemiology of Childhood Disorders* (ed. B. Pless), pp. 339–368. Oxford University Press, New York.

Shaffer, D., Garland, A., Gould, M., Fisher, P. & Trautman, P. (1988)

Preventing teenage suicide: a critical review. *Journal of the American Academy of Child and Adolescent Psychiatry*, **27**, 675–687.

Shaffer, D., Garland, A., Fisher, P., Bacon, K. & Vieland, V. (1990a) Suicide crisis centers: a critical reappraisal with special reference to the prevention of youth suicide. In: *Preventing Mental Health Disturbances in Childhood* (ed. F.E. Goldston, C.M. Heinecke, R.S. Pynoos & J. Yager), pp. 135–166. American Psychiatric Press, Washington D.C.

Shaffer, D., Vieland, V., Garland, A., Rojas, M., Underwood, M. & Busner, C. (1990b) Adolescent suicide attempters: response to suicide-prevention programs. *Journal of the American Medical Association*, **264**, 3151–3155.

Shaffer, D., Garland, A., Vieland, V., Underwood, M. & Busner, C. (1991) The impact of curriculum-based suicide prevention programs for teenagers. *Journal of the American Academy of Child and Adolescent Psychiatry*, **30**, 588–596.

Shaffer, D., Gould, M.S., Fisher, P. *et al.* (1996a) Psychiatric diagnosis in child and adolescent suicide. *Archives of General Psychiatry*, **53**, 339–348.

Shaffer, D., Wilcox, H., Lucas, C., Hicks, R., Busner, C. & Parides, M. (1996b) The development of a screening instrument for teens at risk for suicide. *Lifesavers: The Quarterly Newsletter of the American Foundation for Suicide Prevention*, **8**, 4–7.

Shaffer, D., Fisher, P., Lucas, C.P., Dulcan, M.K. & Schwab-Stone, M.E. (2000) NIMH Diagnostic Interview Schedule for Children, Version IV (NIMH DISC-IV): description, differences from previous versions, and reliability of some common diagnoses. *Journal of the American Academy of Child and Adolescent Psychiatry*, **39**, 28–38.

Sheehan, W. & Garfinkel, B.D. (1988) Adolescent autoerotic deaths. *Journal of the American Academy of Child and Adolescent Psychiatry*, **27**, 367–370.

Shneidman, E. & Farberow, N. (1957) *Clues to Suicide*. McGraw-Hill, New York.

Silverstone, T., Romans, S., Hunt, N. & McPherson, H. (1995) Is there a seasonal pattern of relapse in bipolar affective disorders: a dual northern and southern hemisphere cohort study. *British Journal of Psychiatry*, **167**, 58–60.

Slaiku, K.A., Tulkin, S.R. & Speer, D.C. (1975) Process and outcome in the evaluation of telephone counselling referrals. *Journal of Consulting and Clinical Psychology*, **43**, 700–707.

Smith, K. & Crawford, S. (1986) Suicidal behavior among 'normal' high school students. *Suicide and Life-Threatening Behavior*, **16**, 313–325.

Sonneck, G., Etzersdorfer, E. & Nagel-Kuess, S. (1994) Imitative suicide on the Viennese subway. *Social Science and Medicine*, **38**, 453–457.

Spirito, A., Overholser, J., Ashworth, S., Morgan, J. & Benedict-Drew, C. (1988) Evaluation of a suicide awareness curriculum for high school students. *Journal of the American Academy of Child and Adolescent Psychiatry*, **27**, 705–711.

Spirito, A., Brown, L., Overholser, J. & Fritz, G. (1989) Attempted suicide in adolescence: a review and critique of the literature. *Clinical Psychology Review*, **9**, 335–363.

Spirito, A., Overholser, J. & Hart, K. (1991) Cognitive characteristics of adolescent suicide attempters. *Journal of the American Academy of Child and Adolescent Psychiatry*, **30**, 604–608.

Spirito, A., Lewander, W.J., Levy, S., Kurkjian, J. & Fritz, G. (1994) Emergency department assessment of adolescent suicide attempters: factors related to short-term follow-up outcome. *Pediatric Emergency Care*, **10**, 6–12.

Spooren, D., Van Heeringen, C. & Jannes, C. (1998) Strategies to increase compliance with out-patient aftercare among patients referred to a psychiatric emergency department: a multi-centre controlled intervention study. *Psychological Medicine*, **28**, 949–956.

Stanley, E.J. & Barter, J.T. (1970) Adolescent suicidal behavior. *American Journal of Orthopsychiatry*, **40**, 87–93.

Statham, D.J., Heath, A.C., Madden, P.A. *et al.* (1998) Suicidal behaviour: an epidemiological and genetic study. *Psychological Medicine*, **28**, 839–855.

Stearns, A.W. (1953) Cases of probable suicide in young persons without obvious motivation. *Journal of the Maine Medical Association*, **44**, 16–23.

Steer, R.A., Kumar, G. & Beck, A.T. (1993) Self-reported suicidal ideation in adolescent psychiatric inpatients. *Journal of Consulting and Clinical Psychology*, **61**, 1096–1099.

Stein, D., Apter, A., Ratzoni, G., Har-Even, D. & Avidan, G. (1998) Association between multiple suicide attempts and negative affects in adolescents. *Journal of the American Academy of Child and Adolescent Psychiatry*, **37**, 488–494.

Strasburger, V.C. (1989) Prevention of adolescent drug abuse: why 'Just Say No' just won't work. *Journal of Pediatrics*, **114**, 676–681.

Stuart, R. (1980) *Helping Couples Change: a Social Learning Approach to Marital Therapy*. Guilford Press, New York.

Sudak, H.S., Sawyer, J.B., Spring, G.K. & Coakwell, C.M. (1977) High referral success rates in a crisis center. *Hospital and Community Psychiatry*, **28**, 530–532.

Swanston, H.Y., Nunn, K.P., Oates, R.K., Tebbutt, J.S. & O'Toole, B.I. (1999) Hoping and coping in young people who have been sexually abused. *European Child and Adolescent Psychiatry*, **8**, 134–142.

Swedo, S.E. (1989) Post-discharge therapy of hospitalized adolescent suicide attempters. *Journal of Adolescent Health Care*, **10**, 541–544.

Szabo, C.P. & Blanche, M.J. (1995) Seasonal variation in mood disorder presentation: further evidence of this phenomenon in a South African sample. *Journal of Affective Disorders*, **33**, 209–214.

Taylor, E.A. & Stansfeld, S.A. (1984) Children who poison themselves. I. A clinical comparison with psychiatric controls. *British Journal of Psychiatry*, **145**, 127–132.

Teicher, M.H., Glod, C. & Cole, J.O. (1990) Emergence of intense suicidal preoccupation during fluoxetine treatment. *American Journal of Psychiatry*, **147**, 207–210.

Tondo, L., Jamison, K.R. & Baldessarini, R.J. (1997) Effect of lithium maintenance on suicidal behavior in major mood disorders. *Annals of the New York Academy of Sciences*, **836**, 339–351.

Trautman, P. & Rotheram-Borus, M.J. (1988) Cognitive therapy with children and adolescents. In: *Review of Psychiatry VII* (eds A. Frances & R. Hales), pp. 584–607. American Psychiatric Press, Washington D.C.

Trautman, P.D. & Shaffer, D. (1984) Treatment of child and adolescent suicide attempters. In: *Suicide in the Young* (eds H.S. Sudak, A.B. Ford & N.B. Rushforth). John Wright-PSG, Boston.

Trautman, P.D. & Shaffer, D. (1989) Pediatric management of suicidal behavior. *Pediatric Annals*, **18**, 134; 136; 138.

UK Office for National Statistics (2000) Health Statistics Quarterly 6. *Health Statistics Quarterly 6*.

UNICEF (1996) *The Progress of Nations*. UNICEF, New York.

Van Heeringen, C., Jannes, S., Buylaert, W., Henderick, H., De Bacquer, D. & Van Remoortel, J. (1995) The management of non-compliance with referral to out-patient after-care among attempted suicide patients: a controlled intervention study. *Psychological Medicine*, **25**, 963–970.

Velez, C.N. & Cohen, P. (1988) Suicidal behavior and ideation in a community sample of children: maternal and youth reports. *Journal of the American Academy of Child and Adolescent Psychiatry*, **27**, 349–356.

Velting, D.M. & Gould, M.S. (1997) Suicide Contagion. In: *Annual Review of Suicidology* (eds R. Maris, S. Canetto & M.M. Silverman), pp. 96–136. Guilford, New York.

Verkes, R.J., Van der Mast, R.C., Hengeveld, M.W., Tuyl, J.P., Zwinderman, A.H. & Van Kempen, G.M. (1998) Reduction by paroxetine of suicidal behavior in patients with repeated suicide attempts but not major depression. *American Journal of Psychiatry*, 155, 543–547.

Vieland, V., Whittle, B., Garland, A., Hicks, R. & Shaffer, D. (1991) The impact of curriculum-based suicide prevention programs for teenagers: an 18-month follow-up. *Journal of the American Academy of Child and Adolescent Psychiatry*, 30, 811–815.

Vijayakumar, L. & Rajkumar, S. (1999) Are risk factors for suicide universal: a case-control study in India. *Acta Psychiatrica Scandinavica*, 99, 407–411.

Wasserman, I.M. (1984) Imitation and suicide: a re-examination of the Werther effect. *American Sociological Review*, 49, 427–436.

Waterhouse, J. & Platt, S. (1990) General hospital admission in the management of parasuicide. A randomised controlled trial. *British Journal of Psychiatry*, 156, 236–242.

White, H.C. (1974) Self-poisoning in adolescents. *British Journal of Psychiatry*, 124, 24–35.

Wichstrom, L. (2000) Predictors of adolescent suicide attempts: a nationally representative longitudinal study of Norwegian adolescents. *Journal of the American Academy of Child and Adolescent Psychiatry*, 39, 603–610.

World Health Organization (1997–99) *World Health Statistic Annual*. World Health Organization, Geneva. www.who.int/whosis

Yip, P.S., Callanan, C. & Yuen, H.P. (2000) Urban/rural and gender differentials in suicide rates: east and west. *Journal of Affective Disorders*, 57, 99–106.

Yusin, A., Sinay, R. & Nihira, K. (1972) Adolescents in crisis: evaluation of a questionnaire. *American Journal of Psychiatry*, 129, 574–577.

34 Anorexia and Bulimia Nervosa

Hans-Christoph Steinhausen

Introduction

In contrast to early forms of eating disorder originating in childhood, such as rumination, failure to thrive, pica, faddiness and obesity (see Stein & Barnes, Chapter 45), the age period for the onset of anorexia nervosa and bulimia nervosa is most typically adolescence. Prepubertal onset is rare for anorexia nervosa and the first onset peak is around 15 and 19 years. The onset for bulimia nervosa is, in most cases, at the end of adolescence, peaking initially at around 19 years. Thus, anorexia nervosa is typically connected with the transition from childhood to adolescence and, in most cases, bulimia nervosa reflects the transition from adolescence to young adulthood. However, the literature for both disorders is dominated by research on adult patients with only a few reviews entirely devoted to children and adolescents with eating disorders (Lask & Bryant-Waugh 1993; Steinhausen 1995; Steiner & Lock 1998). Because of the predominance of anorexia over bulimia nervosa in children and adolescents, the two disorders will be described in unequal proportions in this chapter.

Anorexia nervosa

Clinical features

Anorexia nervosa is characterized by highly specific behavioural and psychopathological symptoms and significant somatic signs. The majority of cases are female, and the onset of the disorder is usually during adolescence, but there are also cases in which males are afflicted and cases of premenarcheal onset.

Behaviour and psychopathology

The core psychopathological feature of anorexia nervosa is the dread of fatness. There are many synonyms for this symptom, e.g. weight phobia, fear of becoming fat or drive for thinness. In the behavioural sense, it implies that the patient is deeply convinced that his or her body is too large. This pursuit of thinness may, in the classical case, persist even at times when the patient is extremely emaciated. Typically, the following pattern emerges. In the beginning, the patient starts to diet and may appear like any teenager concerned about being overweight. Sometimes, the patient is indeed slightly overweight and has been taunted by family members, schoolmates and peers. The feeling of being overweight may be related to the whole body or to particular parts, such as the thighs or buttocks.

The typical diet starts with a reduction of sweets and high-caloric, carbohydrate-rich foods, and the patient soon becomes an expert with regard to the caloric content of all sorts of food and beverages. Weeks or even months may pass before this behaviour is noticed by others. By this time, the patient may have lost control over dieting and the resulting weight loss. Usually, at this stage, the adolescent anorexic has not yet recognized the abnormal nature of her or his behaviour and denies the illness. Indeed, she or he feels better being thin and does not seek any help, despite the perceived concern of family members who feel helpless in the face of the patient's powerful behaviour.

In many of the patients, this distorted drive for thinness is associated with a disturbance in body image. Despite being emaciated, the patient does not consider herself thin or even ugly. There may also be an inability accurately to identify internal sensations, such as hunger, satiety or affective states. In addition, patients are rather vague or defensive about their feelings and are susceptible to undue influence by significant others. This in turn reinforces the bodily mistrust and the fear of loss of control. Dieting continues and may be accompanied by further efforts to reduce weight and to control bodily functions. Such efforts can include rigorous exercise, abuse of laxatives or diuretics, and vomiting, which are not only intended to promote weight loss but also serve to rigidly regulate bodily functions. From the purging and vomiting behaviour there is only a small step to binge-eating, in which the patient consumes enormous amounts of food within a very short period of time. This bulimic component is followed by either a restrictive period of fasting for several days or else vomiting to prevent weight gain. Bulimic features within the spectrum of anorexia nervosa are, however, rather infrequent during adolescence.

Aside from these very specific behavioural features of anorexia nervosa, there are further psychopathological symptoms that are shared with other psychiatric disorders. These include poor self-esteem, rigid dichotomous 'either/or' thinking, a highly restricted realm of interests and cognition that excludes almost everything but the topics of food and weight, the loss of social contacts, irritability, mood swings and insomnia. Anorexic patients rarely engage in sexual activity and, when they do, they usually experience it as being unpleasant and joyless. Many patients show signs of a depressive syndrome, including major affective disorder. (Strober 1991; Herzog *et al.* 1992). All these non-specific symptoms can be, at least partially, the result of the effects of starvation.

Many patients manifest obsessional behaviour, including compulsive behaviour and obsessional thinking about foods. This pertains not only to the peculiar eating habits, for example, eating rituals—but also to other areas, such as exercising and food and non-food-related hoarding. Comorbid obsessive-compulsive disorders are quite frequent (Råstam 1992; Thiel et al. 1995). Premorbid personality traits can be identified in the history.

Physical characteristics

Anorexic patients are apparently emaciated and show effects of downregulation of the autonomic nervous system, indicated by bradycardia, hypotension and hypothermia. In addition, complications arise as a consequence of the effects of the eating disorder on virtually every organ system and deserve careful consideration (Beumont et al. 1993, 1995; Carney & Andersen 1996).

The medical illnesses needing to be considered for differential diagnosis include: tuberculosis, acquired immune deficiency disease, primary endocrine disturbances such as anterior pituitary insufficiency, Addison's disease, hyperthyroidism, diabetes milletus, inflammatory bowel disease, hypothalamic tumours and a variety of malignancies. All of these are conditions that manifest significant and prominent weight loss but lack the psychological characteristics of anorexia nervosa (the deliberate attempt to reduce weight by exercise, purging, vomiting or dieting). There are also a variety of drugs that may produce weight loss. Binge-eating also occurs in a number of rare medical illnesses and certain chronic illnesses, such as premorbid obesity and diabetes, which in turn can act as risk factors for the development of eating disorders. Finally, there are also instances in which symptoms in patients with an eating disorder are misdiagnosed as being a medical illness.

Specific features of premenarcheal cases and of anorexia nervosa in males

The manifestation of anorexia nervosa before the age of 14 or before the menarche is rare. However, the clinical features of the prepubertal cases are essentially similar (Gowers et al. 1991; Lask & Bryant-Waugh 1993; Robin et al. 1998). Other types of closely related food refusal, selective eating and appetite loss have to be distinguished from anorexia nervosa (Lask & Bryant-Waugh 1993). Weight loss in these very young patients arrests the process of puberty and interferes with growth in stature and breast development (Russell 1992). Early diagnosis and competent treatment are therefore important for the child's development.

Anorexia nervosa in males is rare but may also be underdiagnosed. The clinical pattern is strikingly similar in the two sexes. Various studies report conflicting findings with respect to whether males show an earlier onset of the disease, atypical gender role behaviour, more grave symptomatology and poorer prognosis (Andersen 1995; Carlat et al. 1997).

Clinical assessment

A thorough examination of patients with an eating disorder requires the assessment of the history, development of the symptoms, psychopathology, family functioning and physical status (Beumont et al. 1995; Steinhausen 1997a). More specifically, the behavioural assessment of the anorexic and bulimic spectrum of symptoms should be focused upon. In addition, structural interviews and rating scales, as well as self-report questionnaires, can augment the assessment process.

The behavioural assessment should start with issues concerning food intake and eating behaviours, including thoughts and attitudes towards eating and weight. This should be followed by a systematic analysis of further significant clinical symptoms and an analysis of events and emotional states preceding food refusal or binge/purge episodes. Furthermore, the patient should be asked to report any attempts to alter eating behaviour. The assessment can be enhanced through the inclusion of one of the structured interviews designed for this purpose. These include the Eating Disorder Examination (Fairburn & Cooper 1993) and its adaptation to children (Bryant-Waugh et al. 1996), the Clinical Eating Disorder Rating Instrument (Palmer et al. 1987) and the Structured Interview for Anorexic and Bulimic Disorders (Fichter et al. 1998).

Self-report questionnaires are sometimes used for epidemiological and screening purposes, such as the Eating Attitude Test (Garner & Garfinkel 1979; Garner et al. 1982), and the Eating Disorders Inventory (Garner et al. 1983) which is an instrument that covers clinically relevant dimensions of the eating disorders. Their validity for case identification has been called into question (Steinhausen 1984; Neumärker et al. 1992; Steinhausen et al. 1992).

The assessment of body image disturbance should concentrate on the measurement of attitudinal body dissatisfaction by either questionnaire or self-ideal discrepancy measures rather than the measurement of perceptual size estimation inaccuracy. The latter is not only more expensive in terms of the employed techniques (e.g. video distortion) but was also shown to produce much less substantial effect sizes than attitudinal measures in a meta-analysis of 66 studies of body image among patients with eating disorders relative to control groups (Cash & Deagle 1997).

Finally, the variety of potential medical complications requires a careful physical assessment, including body weight and height in order to calculate the body mass index (BMI). Percentile charts appropriate for age and sex should be used because the diagnostic criteria of BMI< 17.5, as set up by the ICD-10, is inappropriate for prepubertal and most of the adolescent patients. In these age groups, large parts of the normal population fall under this criterion so that the BMI cut-offs need to be adjusted for growth. National reference data in combination with either the third or fifth percentile should be used in order to define clearly an abnormal BMI. If these data are not available, paediatric tables may be used, setting a weight commensurate to the same percentile as the patient's height as a standard of normality (Beumont *et al.* 1995).

Routine laboratory investigations should include serum electrolytes, liver enzymes, complete blood count (CBC), blood urea nitrogen (BUN), glucose, full protein and albumin, renal function, pelvic ultrasound and an electrocardiogram. Further investigations are seldom necessary. Significant abuse of laxatives might require endoscopic or roentgenographic examination to assess the extent of bowel damage. Other investigations for some selected patients may include further haematological studies, bone densitometry for chronic cases, oesophageal sphincter pressure studies for reflux, urine and blood osmolality, lactose deficiency tests for dairy intolerance, and total body nitrogen.

Classification

DSM-IV and ICD-10 share some similarities with regard to defining criteria of anorexia nervosa. These pertain to the criteria of weight loss, body image distortion, amenorrhoea, and the so-called weight phobia. However, the two systems differ to some extent with regard to the definition of these criteria. Whereas the ICD-10 makes use of Quetelets's Body Mass Index for the definition of weight and therefore considers height as well, DSM-IV uses an absolute weight threshold of 85% of expected weight loss. Both classification systems consider the special situation of prepubertal patients who fail to make the expected growth.

There are some advantages of the ICD-10 scheme as compared with those of the DSM-IV. It not only covers the criterion 'self-induced loss of weight' but also provides a clinically useful operational definition of this criterion and links the body image distortion to the main theme of psychopathology, namely, fear of becoming fat, whereas these two aspects are listed separately among the DSM-IV criteria.

Furthermore, the widespread endocrine disorder in anorexia nervosa is clearly indicated in the ICD-10 set of criteria, whereas the DSM-IV refers only to amenorrhoea. The latter criterion is more difficult to assess in young patients because of the absence of menstruation in early puberty and the sometimes irregular course soon after menarche. Finally, both ICD-10 and DSM-IV consider two different types: a restrictive type, which refers to patients who exclusively starve; and a binge-eating/purging type, which refers to patients who binge-eat and practise self-induced vomiting or misuse laxatives, diuretics or enemas.

Beyond the different eating behaviour, there are several arguments in favour of this typology: bulimic anorexic patients more frequently display premorbid overweight medical complications, various sorts of impulsive behaviours and borderline, narcissistic and antisocial personality disorders (Garfinkel *et al.* 1995). Furthermore, various outcome studies indicate a less favourable prognosis for this subtype (Steinhausen 1999). Little is currently known about whether these subtypes reflect different entities or only different indices of severity that may alternate over time in individual patients. Because of the spectrum character of the eating disorders, there are atypical cases of anorexia nervosa that do not fulfil the entire sets of criteria listed in the two major systems of classification. Atypical cases, such as where there is an absence of amenorrhoea or significant weight loss or where the key symptoms are present only to a mild degree, are explicitly considered both in the ICD-10 and the DSM-IV.

Epidemiology

Most of our current knowledge about the frequencies of eating disorders stems from incidence and prevalence studies that are based on either psychiatric case registers or medical records of hospitals in circumscribed areas. Obviously, such studies lead to an underestimation of the true incidence and prevalence because not all community cases are referred to doctors or hospitals.

An analysis of 16 incidence studies published between 1970 and 1992 shows a peak for age at onset between 15 and 19 years, a decrease in frequency at 20–24 years, and no bimodal distribution (Fombonne 1995). In five of these studies there was an increase in incidence over time, but these studies were ill-controlled for reliability and validity of diagnoses, changes in health services, demographic changes and tests of statistical significance. Also, the more recently published incidence studies provide conflicting results concerning increases in incidence rates. Some are negative (Hoek *et al.* 1995; Turnbull *et al.* 1996); others are positive (Eagles *et al.* 1995), even after correction for several register biases (Munk-Jorgensen *et al.* 1995). Another recent integrative review of 12 cumulative incidence studies covering 40 years found no increased risk over time of anorexia nervosa among teenagers, whereas a near threefold increase was observed among women in their 20s and 30s (Pawluck & Gorey 1998).

Community surveys that yield prevalence rates may circumvent some of the methodological problems of incidence studies. The 29 prevalence studies published between 1976 and 1993 provide median prevalence rates for females aged 15–2, of 1.3 in 1000 (range 0.35–2.39 in 1000) for the entire period, 1.3 in 1000 in studies published before 1985 and 1.8 in 1000 in studies published since 1985. Thus, there is no indication that prevalence rates increased over time (Fombonne 1995). A more recent study in Switzerland obtained a prevalence rate of 0.7% for the 14–17 years age range (Steinhausen *et al.* 1997).

All epidemiological data support the clinical experience that anorexia nervosa is 8–40 times more common in females than in males (Fombonne 1995; Turnbull *et al.* 1996; Pawluck & Gorey 1998). In contrast to clinical series, little evidence of anorexia nervosa being associated with higher social class has emerged from epidemiological studies. Cultural factors are clearly operative. Whereas anorexia nervosa is rarely observed among blacks in the USA, Great Britain and Africa (Andersen & Hay 1985; Pumariega *et al.* 1984; Thomas & Szmukler 1985; Silber 1986; Dolan 1991) and is almost absent in the Chinese population—with only a few cases being reported from Hong Kong (Lee &

Chiu 1989)—it is quite common in Japan (Suematsu *et al.* 1985). There is some evidence that outside Western culture, the disease may be restricted to prosperous backgrounds and the upper social strata. Reports of increasing rates of eating disorders that have been found in some cross-cultural studies may be caused by either the adoption of Western cultural values (Nasser 1988) or to conceptual errors and problems of translation of diagnostic instruments (Patton & King 1991).

Aetiology

Considering the diversity and complexity of both anorexia and bulimia nervosa, a single-factor aetiology is unlikely. Current theories emphasize multiple determinants and risk factors interacting within a developmental framework. This model is based on the following predispositions and determinants: individual, familial, sociocultural, biological factors and precipitating events (see Steiger & Stotland 1995; Steiner *et al.* 1995; for reviews of the supporting empirical evidence).

Individual factors

From a developmental point of view, anorexia emerges at a time when body fat increases and the changes in physical appearance, bodily feelings and reproductive status require reorganization and transformation of the body image (Attie *et al.* 1990).

Huon & Strong (1998) have proposed that different factors influence the initiation and the maintenance of dieting in adolescents. The initiation of dieting is most strongly affected by perceived social encouragement to diet from family members, peers and the media; with individual differences in autonomous functioning and social skill-related competencies equipping adolescent girls differently with the ability to resist those social influences. The maintenance of adolescent dieting includes a central role of motivation: dieting persists when the goals are specific and difficult; when there is a high level of commitment toward these goals; and when the reasons for dieting indicate that the adolescent is controlled. According to the theory, efficacy and personality features (such as the tendency to be autonomous) are operating only indirectly and are mediated by the proposed motivational processes.

An epidemiological study on abnormal eating attitudes in London schoolgirls (Patton *et al.* 1990) showed that dieting in the great majority of girls was a benign practice, without progression to clinical status. A previous psychiatric history and some association between general psychiatric morbidity and eating disorders in this sample gave rise to the suggestion that there is an extra set of factors that strengthens excessive dieting. Similarity, a more recent Australian epidemiological study (Patton *et al.* 1997) found psychiatric morbidity to be associated with extreme dieting only. The causal link may be bidirectional with psychopathology leading to dieting but dieting also affecting neurotransmitter systems that are involved in the regulation of mood.

Uncertainties remain about the degree to which overt anorexia nervosa (which is uncommon—see above) is on the same continuum as the much milder eating disturbances that are so frequent in adolescent girls. There is bound to be a measure of continuity because some of the same cognitive concerns (over body image and the like) are associated with both, and because some cases of anorexia nervosa must (at least for a while) exist at a subclinical level of severity. On the other hand, some discontinuity is suggested by the evidence that even severe dieting in ballet dancers and athletes is rarely accompanied by self-induced vomiting, and by the infrequency with which such dieting leads to overt anorexia nervosa (Patton *et al.* 1990). Twin studies could be informative in determining whether anorexia nervosa in one twin is associated with milder eating disturbances in the cotwin, but the sample sizes studied (see below) have been far too small for such an analysis. Follow-up studies of milder eating difficulties, similarly, could throw light on the issue but few of the investigations have presented their findings in ways that could address the question. Dieting is an early manifestation of anorexia nervosa but probably it leads to the overt disorder only in particularly susceptible individuals, perhaps in conjunction with a broader psychological disturbance.

Other possible risk factors include disturbances of self-perception of body size and of internal affective and visceral states—poor body-image (Shisslak *et al.* 1998) and poor interoceptive awareness (Leon *et al.* 1995). Furthermore, it has been speculated that the earlier heightened nutritional state in weight pathologies may lead to an earlier prepubertal maturity. This and the accompanying sexual development would require an earlier confrontation with the developmental demands of adolescence, for which the individual may be unprepared. In fact, there is some evidence that early maturity is associated with eating disorder symptoms (Atkins & Silber 1993). In addition, premorbid obesity may expose adolescents to humiliation and force them to use dieting and other weight-reducing measures. However, findings from one epidemiological study have called the aetiological relevance of premorbid obesity into question because it appeared to be more closely identified with dieting than with eating disorders (Patton *et al.* 1990).

Careful clinical history-taking often reveals a premorbid personality pattern of compliance, perfectionism and dependence. These children present few if any educational problems prior to the onset of the eating disorder. Early eating and digestive problems in childhood may also be present (Manchi & Cohen 1990). There is little evidence that psychosexual factors are involved in the causation of eating disorders. Whereas a high proportion of adverse sexual experiences in childhood has been reported in various series of anorexic women, the pathogenic relevance of these experiences to the subsequent illness is uncertain (Palmer 1995; Vanderlinden & Vandereycken 1995).

Familial factors

Empirical tests of family system models reflected in anorexic patients and their families have not supported the theoretical notion of a typical anorexia nervosa family (Kog &

Vandereycken 1988; Råstam & Gillberg 1991). There is some empirically based evidence for a significant amount of dysfunction in families of patients, not acting specifically in the development of eating disorders but rather as an indirect vulnerability to developing an eating disorder (Steiger & Stotland 1995).

Beyond the importance of communication and interaction patterns there are further family risk factors that may play a part in the multifactorial determination of eating disorders: higher incidence of weight problems and eating disorders in the family; and high incidence of physical illness, affective disorders, obsessive-compulsive disorders and alcoholism in relatives (Kog & Vandereycken 1988; Lilenfeld et al. 1998; Stein et al. 1999).

Sociocultural factors

It is possible that the pressure in Western societies to achieve, the importance of physical attractiveness and the emphasis on slimness and dieting in women may all contribute to increased risk for the development of eating disorders. The tendency in Western societies to judge self-worth in terms of shape and weight is superimposed on the need for self-control as the central feature of the disorder (Fairburn et al. 1999b). For adolescent girls, the importance of TV and magazine models and peer pressures pertaining to weight concerns have been documented (Barr Taylor et al. 1998; Shisslak et al. 1998).

Ballet dancers, some kinds of athletes and modelling students form particular risk groups for eating problems (Smolak et al. 2000) but it is less clear whether there are increased rates of anorexia nervosa. It is also an open question whether participation in these activities or sports causes eating problems or whether certain individuals with such problems are drawn to these activities. However, besides specific physical demands in terms of body shape and size and specific diets, additional risk factors result from performance pressure, including anxiety and demanding competition; from authoritarian relationships to coaches and trainers; from passive obedience to these authorities; and from visibility and public control of bodily activities. In some individuals, personality characteristics such as perfectionism may contribute both to physical performance and eating disorders.

Biological factors

There is sufficient evidence that once malnutrition and starvation have started, significant alterations occur in a broad spectrum of neurobiological parameters (Pirke & Platte 1995). These include every endocrine system, the cholinergic, norepinephric and serotonergic systems, the regulation of immune functions, and endogenous opioid activity. Once weight loss and starvation occur, the usual mechanisms for the release and inhibition of various regulators of eating behaviour change, and a new set of regulating mechanisms is established. Whereas the increased body of knowledge on these pathophysiological mechanisms has not necessarily contributed to a better understanding of the origins of anorexia nervosa, it is clear that many of the pathophysiological alterations serve to sustain the disorder.

Twin and family studies both suggest that genetic factors have a role in the liability for anorexia nervosa. Holland et al. (1988) found that 56% of monozygotic twin pairs were concordant for anorexia nervosa as compared with 5% concordance among dizygotic twins. Heritability was found to be high, especially in 'restricting' anorexia nervosa with adolescent onset, whereas it was almost non-existent among patients with bulimia nervosa (Treasure & Holland 1990). However, as Strober (1991) pointed out, direct recruitment and voluntary referral in this study may have led to potentially biased conditions of ascertainment. In any case, genetic influences may be on dispositional traits rather than the eating disorder itself.

Conflicting findings include those of the large-scale study based on the Virginia twin registry (Walters & Kendler 1995). Although cotwins of twins with anorexia nervosa were at significantly higher risk for lifetime anorexia nervosa (and bulimia nervosa, major depression and low BMI), the dizygotic proband-wise concordance rates were larger than the monozygotic rates. This pattern is contradictory to that expected for a genetic influence. Although the data suggest the presence of a familial component, it was not possible in this sample confidently to partition this component into genetic and common environmental factors and to estimate accurately a measure of heritability for anorexia nervosa. Given the very small number of concordant twins (six pairs, even with the broadest diagnostic criteria) and the possibility that the fundamental assumption of equal environments for the twins was violated, no conclusions are possible.

Precipitating events

Dieting is an antecedent of new eating disorders, and psychiatric morbidity predicts the onset of eating disorders independent of dieting status, as shown in a recent adolescent cohort study (Patton et al. 1999). As in many other psychiatric disorders, further significant events in the individual's life have been reported to have preceded the manifestation of anorexia nervosa. External precipitants have been identified in 50–100% in various studies, but the type of precipitant appears non-specific. Common initiating factors include separation and loss, disruptions of family homeostasis, new environmental demands, direct threat of loss of self-esteem and, in a small number of patients, physical illness (Atkins & Silber 1993; Robin et al. 1998). As a consequence of these threats to the patient's sense of worth and control over the world, preoccupation with the body is increased and weight-reducing measures are initiated.

Development and maintenance of the disorders

As with other psychiatric disorders it is the balance between the individual vulnerability to particular risk factors and the operation of protective factors that determines the development and maintenance of an eating disorder. Research so far has suffered from a lack of appropriate clinical control groups, and has not convincingly shown whether or not the various risk factors are specific to eating disorders. Most of the evidence stems from clinical samples instead of population studies so that a selective bias may have influenced the findings. Dieting is the first aspect to be noted in anorexia and bulimia nervosa but it is not yet the disorder. Longitudinal studies still have to show which factors have to be present in order to explain the transition from dieting to frank disorder. Both the isolation of disorder-specific risk factors in association with dieting and their timing are important research issues. The maintenance of anorexia nervosa is, at least in part, better understood. Whereas the disorder is sometimes transient, anorexia nervosa often becomes chronic. Several factors are known to sustain it. Starvation intensifies the patient's preoccupation with food and negatively affects self-concepts and mental state. It also produces a reduction of interests and social isolation. In addition, vomiting is another powerful sustaining factor. Delayed gastric emptying and chronic constipation lend the sensation of fullness after meals and serves to prolong dieting. Furthermore, distorted body perceptions may be linked with a feeling of being out of control after small increases in weight.

Certain cognitive factors continue the chain of detrimental factors, such as positive self-reinforcement resulting from weight loss or phobic avoidance of weight gain, and/or personality features such as obsessiveness, the generally restricted ability to cope with stress, and the level of impulse control. Unresolved predisposing factors from the patient's family or her own biography may also add to chronicity, unless they are addressed in psychotherapy. Secondary gain in terms of receiving considerable attention from the environment is another powerful perpetuating factor, as is the prevailing cultural emphasis on slimness.

Finally, there are also iatrogenic factors that are responsible for the perpetuation of the illness. These include rapid weight gain programmes that neglect both provisions for instituting external controls for the patient and attention to other psychosocial issues, and failure to recognize the necessity of weight gain to counteract the effects of starvation.

Treatment

Patients who suffer from anorexia nervosa require intensive professional and interdisciplinary intervention because of inherent complications and the danger of chronicity (Touyz et al. 1995; Garner & Garfinkel 1997; Steinhausen 1997a; Robin et al. 1998). Although there is a variety of treatment approaches, comparative studies evaluating the effects of treatment are scarce (Steinhausen 1999). Currently, the main psychotherapeutic approaches used with adolescent anorexic patients are individual psychotherapy, behaviour therapy and family therapy. In addition to the various psychotherapies, nutritional counselling and supervised exercise (Beumont et al. 1997) and psychoeducational measures both for the patient and the family (Garner 1997) are important components of treatment.

General principles

The treatment of anorexic patients must be based on a comprehensive and detailed assessment of both the mental and the physical status. The treating physician must then decide whether an inpatient or outpatient setting is more appropriate. This decision rests partly on rather non-specific factors, such as the availability of treatment modalities or the 'treatment philosophy' of a given centre or therapist. At many treatment centres in recent years, management has shifted increasingly from inpatient to outpatient treatment with emphasis placed on family therapy and on empowering parents as controllers of the patient's food intake. This shift may be caused by greater awareness of eating disorders both among physicians and the public, resulting in many patients presenting before they have become severely emaciated.

Unfortunately, beyond the evidence that early intervention may be a positive prognostic factor, there is a lack of solid empirical data to form a rationale for the selection of the type and setting of treatment intervention. Certain clinical criteria, e.g. severe emaciation (less than 70% of the average weight), medical complications, suicidal ideation and comorbid psychiatric conditions, are undoubtedly indices for hospital treatment. Familial factors too might tip the scales in favour of inpatient treatment; for example, in cases where conflict within a family or demoralization of the family precludes or hinders outpatient treatment. Inpatient treatment does have certain specific advantages that should be acknowledged. These include a higher degree of control and consistency, a removal of eating-related conflicts from the family, the fostering of what might otherwise be a fragile treatment alliance, greater awareness on the part of the physician of complications and/or responses to intervention, and the possibility of using—for both the patient and the family—a psychoeducational approach in which the patient's eating behaviour is modified to foster healthy nutritional attitudes and habits and to assure the maintenance of an acceptable weight.

Whereas medical and nutritional stabilization are clearly the major goals of inpatient treatment, a fuller psychiatric recovery may require subsequent outpatient psychotherapy. So far, partial hospitalization in day-treatment programmes has received little attention for young patients with eating disorders. From the beginning, outpatient treatment might be considered in cases in which purging and vomiting are not part of the clinical picture, the family is very supportive and the patient is highly motivated and co-operative. However, because anorexic patients characteristically deny that they are ill, high motivation for treatment is unusual among these patients.

The recent increase in clinical cases has affected admission rates not only in psychiatric institutions but also in paediatric and medical wards. Whereas it is evident that severely emaciated patients need intensive medical treatment, the psychological needs of the majority of these patients are better met in psychiatric wards, where it is easier to create a psychotherapeutic milieu and initiate a treatment alliance. Again, the emergence of special units and centres in many countries in the recent past is mainly because of the increase in admissions. These units are attractive in terms of accumulated clinical experience; however, there is no definite evidence that they should form the basis for service. Patients with eating disorders can also be adequately treated on adolescent psychiatric wards that treat a variety of different problems and patients.

Independent of treatment selection, weight restoration and return to physical health is the first major goal of treatment. The minimum target weight should be specified at the beginning of the treatment rather than later during the course of therapy. Although there is a lack of conformity in the literature on the degree of final weight restoration, many clinicians would agree that the goal should be set to within 10% of the recommended weight appropriate for age and height. Considering the patient's fear of losing control, a *gradual* but steady gain, averaging about 0.2 kg/day, is aimed for rather than a rapid weight gain. The patient therefore eats smaller portions but more frequent meals per day.

The regular intake of an adequate number of calories per day should start at 1500 and gradually increase to between 2000 and 3000 calories derived from four to six meals per day. With the help of a dietitian, the definite number of calories should be determined according to individual needs and whether the programme is for weight gain or for weight maintenance. Other schemes for calculating adequate calorie intake emphasize the weight at admission plus a 50% increase for activity and 50% increase every fifth day. Besides weight restoration, close monitoring of fluid and electrolyte balance, including the correction of imbalances, is an important part of the ongoing medical management. The provision of information feedback on weight gain and dietary re-education are further essential components. There are conflicting views concerning the inclusion of tube feeding, intravenous feeding or parenteral hyperalimentation for weight gain. Whereas these measures are often recommended in medical settings, many psychotherapists are concerned about the psychological side-effects: the disturbance of the fragile staff co-operation and the psychotherapeutic alliance with the patient. However, it is clear that these interventions can be life-saving in the extremely ill patient and that the various medical complications of the disorder require close collaboration with other medical disciplines.

Many clinicians consider a supportive and secure relationship with the treatment team to be the cornerstone of successful inpatient treatment. This especially applies to the nurse who is present during mealtimes and can encourage the patient to eat and to ventilate feelings related to eating. Regular weight monitoring with feedback to the patient is another essential treatment component. There is sufficient clinical evidence that improvement of the patient's weight also contributes to an improvement in his or her morbid mental state. Therefore, weight-reducing behaviours, such as hyperactivity, purging and vomiting, need to be controlled and the patient should be confronted with them in psychotherapy.

The therapeutic milieu of the ward contributes significantly to treatment, by reducing the patient's morbid fear of fatness,

establishing a sense of self-esteem and confidence, and treating concomitant psychiatric disorders such as depression. Supportive and encouraging relationships with the staff can reduce the necessity of using coercive measures, such as tube feeding or parenteral nutrition, in a small number of life-endangering situations.

The patient's individual emotional problems form another major goal of treatment and need to be met through psychotherapeutic methods, regardless of the treatment setting. Both individual and family psychotherapy may be indicated. Despite the variety of theoretical foundations that underlie the different psychotherapeutic approaches, there is a growing trend to combine therapeutic methods in the sense of multimodal approaches.

Because of the crucial role that parents play in the development and treatment of prepubertal and adolescent eating disorders, parent counselling is an intrinsic component of any intervention. In the early stages of treatment, the parents need to be relieved of self-blame and guilt feelings, and it is necessary to provide precise information on the various aspects of the eating disorder. In the middle stages of treatment, the procedure may vary according to the specific treatment modality, and in later stages the personal and partner problems of the parents should be addressed. Parent counselling is an important aspect of intervention but has not been thoroughly researched.

Clinicians differ in their views on the respective advantages and disadvantages of inpatient and outpatient approaches to treatment. The seriousness of the medical or psychological state may require hospital admission to deal with the risks involved, and sometimes this may necessitate some form of compulsion. Not surprisingly, the long-term outcome for those compulsorily admitted is worse than for those who enter hospital voluntarily (Ramsay *et al.* 1999), but this may reflect nothing more than the seriousness of their disorder. Follow-up studies have shown that there is a clear association between initial clinical severity and later outcome. Nevertheless, Gowers *et al.* (2000) found that, even after this was taken into account statistically, those admitted to hospital did worse than those treated in the community. There are inevitable doubts over whether or not their analyses took into account an adequate range of relevant variables. As Gowers *et al.* comment, there is a need for a randomized controlled trial comparing inpatient and outpatient interventions in the group for whom either could be justified (with a clinical severity sufficiently great to raise the question of admission but not so great as to require admission because of the immediate danger to life or health).

Individual psychotherapy

As with other psychiatric disorders, certain prerequisites must be fulfilled to institute individual psychotherapy with the anorexic patient, including sufficient motivation and cognitive ability. These prerequisites may be absent in cases when the patient is emaciated and manifests impaired psychological functioning; when severe depression is present; when the course of the anorexia nervosa is chronic; when severe intellectual limitations are present; when the family sabotages therapeutic efforts; or when the patient is a very young pre-adolescent.

If psychotherapy is tailored to the individual level of cognitive development and the emotional needs of the young patient, and if the adolescent can utilize empathetic support, education, problem-solving, cognitive restructuring and insight, then clinical experience suggests they may profit from this measure. Furthermore, the continuation of psychotherapy after discharge from hospital treatment may contribute to the prevention of relapses.

Behaviour therapy, including cognitive methods

The main behavioural approaches for the treatment of eating disorders are operant conditioning procedures and cognitive methods. In some instances, social skill training programmes may also be used. Whereas operant conditioning procedures may be introduced regardless of age, cognitive methods may be more suitable for the older adolescent and the adult.

Operant conditioning measures in general are more frequently employed in the hospital setting where the control of target behaviours, for example, eating behaviour and/or weight gain, is more easily accomplished. The advantages of choosing one of these target behaviours over the other have been critically reviewed by Bemis (1987). Both negative and positive reinforcement contingencies are operative. The hospital itself can be an implicit negative reinforcer in terms of being experienced as an aversive environment that can be left only through sufficient weight gain. Other negative reinforcers may include bed rest, seclusion and tube feeding. However, many of these rather coercive measures are no longer components of a standard inpatient programme. Rather, most operant programmes claim to be based mainly on positive reinforcers such as access to recreational activities, visiting privileges or freedom of movement within or outside the hospital. Critics have objected that these privileges are also negative reinforcers because they imply relief from the prior situation of being deprived from these opportunities. In addition, it has been argued that isolation and deprivation of reinforcers are not required for effective treatment.

A cognitive-behavioural approach was originally developed for adult bulimic patients but has also been advocated for the treatment of anorexic patients (Garner et al. 1997). However, the efficacy of similar strategies in anorexia nervosa and, more specifically, in adolescent patients has still to be established. Methods emphasize teaching patients to examine the validity of their beliefs on a here-and-now basis. According to Garner et al. (1997), the treatment is divided into three major phases and includes a comprehensive list of content areas.

1 Phase I mainly deals with building trust and setting treatment parameters.

2 In Phase II, the beliefs related to food and weight are changed using specific cognitive methods supplemented by an interpersonal focus in therapy and the involvement of the family. Cognitive methods include the identification of dysfunctional thoughts, schemes, and thinking patterns, the development of cognitive restructuring skills, and the modification of the self-concept.

3 Phase III aims to prevent relapse and prepare for termination of treatment.

Family therapy

Family therapy was advocated as the treatment of choice in anorexic patients for a number of years until more critical comments arose. Accordingly, some authors caution against the exclusive use of family therapy in a condition that is clearly multidetermined and object that the family therapy movement is based on personal beliefs rather than on solid research (Vandereycken et al. 1989; Vandereycken 1995). Objections pertain, for instance, to the possibility of finding no family dysfunction at all, the assumption that a family crisis is necessarily a sign of family pathology, and the uncritical use of family therapy without consideration for indications and contraindications.

Currently, there is some converging clinical agreement about the usefulness of family-orientated treatment approaches in fairly young children and adolescents who still live in intact families. However, in terms of relative contraindications for conjoint family therapy, the inexperienced family therapist should be warned with regard to chronic patients, those with delayed psychosocial development, single-parent families, broken homes, families in which one or both parents display severe psychopathology or in which a parent has physically or sexually abused the partner or a child, families with highly negative or destructive interactions, and families in which previous family therapeutic attempts failed (Vandereycken 1995).

Other limitations stem from a small number of empirical studies. Hall (1987) noted selection factors for family therapy in the treatment of anorexia nervosa. Most of her patients who underwent family therapy were younger, had a recent onset of illness and lived in an intact nuclear family with co-operative parents. In one of the few thoroughly controlled trials, family therapy was found to be superior to individual therapy in patients whose illness was not chronic and had begun before the age of 19 years, whereas individual supportive therapy tended to be more effective in older patients (Russell et al. 1987). Subsequent studies by the same group of researchers (Le Grange et al. 1992; Eisler et al. 2000) found family counselling (in which the parents and the adolescent were seen separately) to be effective as conjoined family therapy. Seeing and intervening with the entire family together was not necessary for good treatment outcomes. At a 5-year follow-up, long-term benefits of the intervention were still detectable, although the authors attributed much of the improvement to the natural outcome of the disorder (Eisler et al. 1997).

Another group of researchers compared Behavioural Family Systems Therapy (BFST) to Ego Oriented Individual Therapy (EOIT), which is a psychodynamic individual treatment with collateral sessions for the parents (Robin et al. 1999). BFST produced greater weight gain than EOIT and a higher rate of resumption of menstruation. The effects on eating attitudes, depressed affect and interoceptive awareness were equal for the two therapies. All improvements had been maintained at 1-year follow-up, with the weight gain differences disappearing between the two treatments. Furthermore, both treatments resulted in improved family relations (Robin *et al.* 1995).

A third controlled study with adolescents and young adults combined outpatient individual therapy and family therapy and compared this to inpatient treatment, outpatient group therapy, or no-treatment control (Crisp *et al.* 1991; Gowers *et al.* 1994). At the 1-year follow-up, both outpatient treatments were as effective as inpatient treatment in restoring weight, and both were superior to the control condition. The treatment effects were maintained at the 2-year follow-up. However, the design of the study did not permit the effects of individual therapy components with cognitive, behavioural and dynamic approaches to be separated from the family therapy component.

As with other child and adolescent disorders, clinical practice—especially in a residential treatment programme—should profit most from a multifaceted approach that combines diet, behavioural contracts, individual and group psychotherapy, and occupational and art therapy with family-orientated philosophy. This family-orientated approach implies that various interventions from educational guidance to counselling are used and that family therapy should be introduced when there is a clear indication to do so. In this view, the family is used as a resource that has to be mobilized to help the child or adolescent with an eating disorder. Further research is clearly needed to substantiate this pragmatic view.

Psychopharmacological treatment

Several medications have been used in the treatment of anorexia nervosa both clinically and in controlled studies. These include neuroleptics, appetite stimulants and antidepressants. Phenothiazines are still used by some clinicians, though perhaps more in the treatment of adults than adolescents. Research evidence of their usefulness, weighed against the hazards of neuroleptics and appetite stimulants, indicates that neuroleptics are generally of no clinical value in the treatment of anorexia nervosa (Heebink & Halmi 1995).

Antidepressants would seem to be indicated in anorexic patients with accompanying depression. Although controlled trials clearly show that some of the antidepressants studied (amitriptyline, clomipramine, monoamine oxidase inhibitors, lithium and fluoxetine) may have some effect on weight gain or improve dysphoria and depression, the clinical value of these findings is rather limited, especially in adolescent anorexic patients (Heebink & Halmi 1995). In contrast, the effectiveness of the more recently developed selective serotonin reuptake inhibitors (SSRIs) has been proven for adult bulimic women (see below).

Outcome and prognosis

For more than four and a half decades, a considerable body of knowledge on the outcome and prognosis of anorexia nervosa has accumulated. The following conclusions can be drawn from a total of 108 follow-up studies published in the English- and German-speaking literature from 1953 to 1996 (Steinhausen 1999) and a subset of 31 follow-up studies dealing only with adolescent and prepubertal patients (Steinhausen 1997b).

In approximately 60% of patients, weight is restored, normalization of menstruation occurs in about the same proportion, and eating behaviour returns to normal in just less than half of the patients. In the 31 studies of younger patients, the outcome was slightly better: normalization of weight occurred in 68%, in 65% for menstruation, and in 52% for eating behaviour. However, there was a wide fluctuation across studies.

Expressed in traditional terms, about half the patients with anorexia nervosa recover, nearly one-third improve but one-fifth become chronic. Mortality rates amount to 5.5% (range 0–21) for the entire series and to 2.2% (range 0–11) for the younger series of patients. After starvation, suicide is the second most common cause of death, accounting for 20% in a recent large population study of eating disorders in Denmark (Emborg 1999).

Affective disorders are noted in one-fifth of anorexic patients, anxiety disorders in one-quarter, obsessive-compulsive disorders in 1 in 8, personality disorders in 1 in 7, substance use disorders in about 1 in 7, and schizophrenia in 1 in 20. Psychosocial adaptation in terms of employment, interpersonal relationships, marriage and sexuality is the most diverse and elusive outcome parameter to study. Although close to two-thirds or even more of former patients accomplish employment and normal educational careers, only a minority enter marriage or a stable partnership.

In addition to these central trends, there is conflicting evidence on prognostic factors. According to a number of studies (frequencies in parentheses), favourable prognostic factors include: early age at onset (13), hysterical personality (8), conflict-free parent–child relationship (8), a short interval between onset of symptoms and treatment intervention (12), a short duration of inpatient treatment with no re-admissions (7), and high social status and level of education (6). However, it must be noted that the findings of a smaller number of other studies call into question the predictive value of these factors. Hyperactivity and dieting as weight-reduction strategies are prime examples of factors that many studies have found to be of no consequence with regard to outcome. The picture is even clearer for the factors that are prognostically unfavourable: vomiting (9), bulimia (10), chronicity or compulsiveness (8), and premorbid developmental or clinical abnormalities (4) have all been almost unequivocally related to poor outcome. Only very few studies have systematically tested a comprehensive list of prognostic factors in larger samples with at least an intermediate follow-up period of 5 years or more. The two studies by Strober *et al.* (1997) and by Steinhausen *et al.* (2000) found surprisingly few predictors that are associated with different facets of illness course and outcome.

There is no consistent long-term course of anorexia nervosa

(Pike 1998). In a small number of studies, there is some indication that anorexia nervosa develops into bulimia nervosa (Steinhausen 1999). In addition, recent research has shown that the offspring of mothers with eating disorders are at risk both with regard to growth and development (see Stein & Barnes, Chapter 45).

Bulimia nervosa

Clinical features

Russell (1979) introduced the term 'bulimia nervosa' to describe an ominous variant of anorexia nervosa. Within a relatively short period of time this new nosological entity received enormous attention among clinicians, researchers and the lay public.

Behaviour and psychopathology

The typical eating pattern of the bulimic patient is characterized by the rapid consumption of a large amount of food. Estimates of the caloric intake of these eating binges range from three to twenty thousand calories. These binges are often experienced as an altered state of consciousness in which the patient feels out of control. The frequency of binging varies considerably—from several times a day to less than once a week or fortnight. Binges can last from minutes to several hours and can be precipitated by feelings of anxiety, tension, boredom and loneliness. At least in the beginning, the binge itself brings temporary relief from negative mood states. However, the longer the binges continue, the more the patient experiences feelings of guilt, shame and anger.

Among the accompanying or counteracting behaviours, self-induced vomiting is not a necessary symptom for diagnosis. Whereas not all bulimics are vomiters, most vomiters are probably bulimics. Binge-eating usually precedes the vomiting. With increasing duration and severity of the disorder, patients do not require any mechanical device to induce vomiting but, rather, learn to vomit by reflex by contracting their abdominal and thoracic muscles. Purgative abuse of laxatives or other drugs are less often used than vomiting. However, most purgers also display vomiting.

Bulimic patients are not only preoccupied with constant thoughts about weight, body size and food but also the most frequently associated mental state is depression. Other personality characteristics include anxiety, emotional lability, strong needs for approval and external control, impulsiveness and compulsiveness. There is a high rate of comorbidity with other psychiatric disorders, including affective disorders, anxiety disorders, substance use disorders, and personality disorders (Mitchell *et al.* 1991; Holderness *et al.* 1994; Brewerton *et al.* 1995).

Physical characteristics

Most bulimic patients are of normal weight for their height.

Menstrual irregularities occur frequently, although amenorrhoea is not as common among bulimics as it is among anorexics. The list of medical complications associated with bulimia is a long one (Carney & Andersen 1996). Many of these complications are serious and are often overlooked; however, they may lead to the diagnosis in those patients who do not come into consultation because of bulimia. Thus, a careful physical examination of each patient suffering from bulimia nervosa is mandatory.

Specific features in males

Bulimia is rarely observed in males. Symptomatology and demographic characteristics are similar in both sexes. However, disturbances of psychosexual development, gender identity and homosexuality have been observed more frequently than in healthy males. In addition, sexual activity is more frequently inhibited in heterosexually orientated bulimic men than in those without bulimia (Fichter & Hoffmann 1990; Andersen 1995).

Clinical assessment

Because the weight of most bulimic patients is within the normal range, there is—in contrast to anorexia nervosa—no direct clinical sign of the disease. Some patients are detected by chance through careful routine physical assessment or during consultations that were made for other purposes. Thus, a high percentage of cases remain undetected unless the patients themselves report their symptoms. Diagnostic interviews and questionnaires can then be used to assist diagnosis and assessment. Examples of these measures are given in the respective section on anorexia nervosa. Further questionnaires that are designed more specifically for bulimic patients were reviewed by Fairburn *et al.* (1990).

Classification

The ICD-10 defines four major criteria.

1 A persistent preoccupation with eating, irresistible craving for food and episodes of overeating in which large amounts of food are consumed in short periods of time.

2 Attempts to counteract the fattening efforts of food with one or more of the following:

    a self-induced vomiting,

    b purgative abuse,

    c alternating periods of starvation, and

    d the use of drugs such as appetite suppressants, thyroid preparations or diuretics.

When bulimia occurs in diabetic patients, they may choose to neglect their insulin treatment.

3 A morbid dread of fatness so that the patient sets her- or himself a sharply defined weight threshold that is well below her or his premorbid weight and far below what would be clinically designated as optimal or healthy.

4 Often there is a history of an earlier episode of anorexia nervosa, the interval ranging from a few months to several years.

This episode may have been fully expressed, or may have assumed a minor cryptic form with a moderate loss of weight and/or a transient phase of amenorrhoea.

DSM-IV criteria are largely comparable with regard to the first two criteria. These criteria specify a minimum average of binge-eating and compensatory behaviours occuring twice a week for 3 months. In addition, DSM-IV states that self-evaluation is unduly influenced by body shape and weight and that these disturbances do not exclusively occur in the presence of anorexia nervosa. DSM-IV also introduces a purging type, designating patients who regularly engage in self-induced vomiting or the misuse of laxatives, diuretics or enemas, and a non-purging type. As stated above for anorexia nervosa, this distinction has some clinical relevance, whereas the validity of these two subtypes still awaits systematic studies.

Finally, both ICD-10 and DSM-IV introduce the category of atypical bulimia nervosa. It is reserved for cases in which one or more of the key features are absent. Most commonly, this applies to patients with normal or even excessive weight. Among these typical cases the DSM-IV also considers the category of binge-eating disorder with recurrent episodes of binge-eating in the absence of inappropriate compensatory behaviour characteristic of bulimia nervosa. Despite a number of questionnaire studies on the frequency of binge-eating, predominantly in adults, the nosological validity of the disorder and its potential relations to the other eating disorders in terms of continuities is yet unknown.

Epidemiology

In a review of the first studies published in the 1980s, Fairburn & Beglin (1990) concluded that consensus has increased regarding the prevalence rate among adolescents and young adult women, which is about 1%. Three recent large-scale epidemiological studies using either DSM-III-R or DSM-IV criteria support this conservative estimate. Lifetime prevalence rates were 1.1% for female subjects and 0.1% for male subjects in Ontario, Canada (Garfinkel et al. 1995), and 0.5% for females in the Virginia Twin Registry (Sullivan et al. 1998a). The 12-month prevalence rate was 0.5% in female adolescents in a Swiss canton (Steinhausen et al. 1997).

The incidence rates for case detection by GPs in the UK was 12.2 per 100 000. It was almost three times higher than that of anorexia nervosa, and the recording of bulimia nervosa increased threefold from 1988 to 1993 (Turnbull et al. 1996). Similarly, a sharp rise in incidence was observed in the Rochester Epidemiology Project in the USA from 1980 to 1983, with relatively constant rates thereafter (Soundy et al. 1995). However, the critical remarks of Fombonne (1996) have to be considered. Epidemiological studies conducted between 1980 and 1995 were partly unreliable and did not control for confounding comorbid disorders. Changes in diagnostic and referral practices were likely to account for the increase in patients seen in specialized treatment centres. Thus, there is no clear empirical evidence for secular changes in the incidence of bulimia nervosa.

Based on the findings of epidemiological studies, the following conclusions are justified. Independent of age, bulimia nervosa is more common than anorexia nervosa in non-clinical populations so that one would expect to find both more adult and more adolescent patients with bulimia nervosa than with anorexia nervosa. The majority of bulimic patients are adults with a peak onset of the disorder around the age of 19 years. Analogous to anorexia nervosa, females by far outnumber males. In contrast to epidemiological data, bulimic patients are underrepresented in clinical samples of adolescent patients with eating disorders.

Aetiology

The aetiology of bulimia nervosa shares many aspects of the model of anorexia nervosa outlined above. For the most part, the same determinants and risk factors are operative in both disorders: individual, familial, sociocultural, biological factors and precipitating events. Because these factors were extensively described above, with the exception of a few recent findings, they will not be discussed again.

A recent study found that early onset cases (at the age of 15 or below), in contrast to typical onset cases, showed premorbid overweight and parental lack of care twice as often. Deliberate self-harm was also more common in the younger patients (Schmidt et al. 1995). A large community-based case–control study on risk factors found that perfectionism and negative self-evaluation, as well as certain parental problems including alcohol use disorder, were even more common among patients with bulimia nervosa than among control subjects with other psychiatric disorders. Factors increasing likelihood of dieting were risks for bulimia, but not for anorexia. It was concluded that bulimia nervosa is the result of exposure to general risk factors for psychiatric disorders and specific factors for dieting (Fairburn et al. 1997). The same project also revealed that certain life events involving disruption of family or social relationships or a threat to physical safety may play a part in precipitating the onset of the disorder and that childhood sexual and physical abuse are also risk factors, but for psychiatric disorders in general and not bulimia specifically (Welch & Fairburn 1996; Welch et al. 1997).

Some support for the assumption that biological factors of vulnerability are important in the aetiology of bulimia nervosa comes from twin studies. Higher concordance rates for bulimia nervosa were found in monozygotic twins as compared with dizygotic twins (Fichter & Nögel 1990; Hsu et al. 1990). Statistic modelling indicated that additive genes accounted for a large proportion of the variance of a lifetime diagnosis of bulimia nervosa (Kendler et al. 1991), and the symptoms of binge-eating and vomiting (Sullivan et al. 1998b). However, the genetic influences are combined with strong individual-specific environmental factors (Bulik et al. 2000). One of the recent genetic studies found that environmental factors contribute more to the development of dietary restraint, eating concern and weight concern than genetic factors do (Wade et al. 1998). Additive genes also play an important part in the co-occurrence of bulimia nervosa and major depression, but each disorder has its own set of unique environmental risk factors (Walters *et al.* 1992).

The interpretations of the genetic findings vary among experts. Critical reviews point to the inconsistencies of findings, with estimates of the heritability of liability to bulimia nervosa ranging from 0 to 83%, and emphasize that a broad view on the aetiology of eating disorders should be maintained (Fairburn *et al.* 1999a).

Treatment

A variety of treatment strategies are available to bulimic patients. These include psychological methods (individual and group psychotherapy, cognitive and behavioural treatment) and biological approaches, such as medication and nutritional management. Self-help and support groups have also received considerable attention. Recently, the efficacy of using a self-care manual for guided self-change has also been documented (Schmidt & Treasure 1993; Treasure *et al.* 1996; Thiels *et al.* 1998).

In the past, hospitalization had been recommended by a number of experienced clinicians and experts in the field (Garfinkel & Garner 1982; Russell 1979) as a method for breaking through the vicious cycle of starvation, binge-eating and vomiting. More recently, however, others have emphasized that the vast majority of patients with bulimia nervosa can be treated on an outpatient basis (Freeman 1991; Fairburn 1995) or in a day clinic and that initially, inpatient treatment in bulimia nervosa is rarely required. The latter should be reserved for cases in which there are serious medical problems, serious concurrent psychiatric disturbances that would warrant hospitalization in their own right, and unremitting severe symptoms that have not responded to adequate trials of outpatient treatment. Individual or group approaches with bulimic patients in both inpatient and outpatient settings depend on the willingness of the patient to co-operate and on the disorder being uncomplicated (free of laxative abuse, alcohol or drugs, psychosis, suicidal or antisocial behaviour).

Practical treatment advice includes diary-keeping and self-monitoring of eating behaviour and meals, self-induced vomiting, and any abuse. In addition, dietary and eating advice must be given and educational material for implementing weight control is helpful (Freeman 1991; Garner 1997). Among the various treatment approaches, two stand out and deserve additional comments: cognitive-behavioural treatment, and psychopharmacological treatment. As in the whole field of bulimia nervosa, most experience comes from the treatment of adult patients, and there is little empirical information on controlled studies of any therapeutic intervention with adolescent patients.

Cognitive-behavioural treatment

This treatment approach and its proven efficacy and effectiveness has received the widest attention, at least among all controlled trials of psychotherapy for bulimia nervosa (Fairburn

1995; Lewandowski *et al.* 1997; Wilson *et al.* 1997; Steinhausen 1999). With the intent to disrupt the habitual binge-eating, vomiting and laxative abuse, programmes centre on the monitoring of eating, weight stimulus control, the provision of information, and education and advice regarding the normalization of eating behaviour in early stages of the treatment. Later, during the course of the therapeutic process, dysfunctional thoughts, beliefs and values that perpetuate the eating problem are identified and modified and, finally, a maintenance programme is instituted. Further characteristics of this approach are described above in the section on the treatment of anorexic patients.

Psychopharmacological treatment

A large number of psychopharmacological agents has been tested in bulimia nervosa, including anticonvulsants, antidepressants, lithium and fenfluramine. The antidepressants are the most promising agents because of their short-term effect in terms of reduced frequency of binge-eating. Nevertheless, the mechanisms underlying the effectiveness of these agents are not understood. Long-term efficacy is jeopardized by high relapse rates upon withdrawal of medication and the frequent changes of drugs required over time.

Among the various effective antidepressants, no single drug is particularly effective (Mitchell *et al.* 1993; Heebink & Halmi 1995; Walsh 1995). Fluoxetine has two advantages: its established efficacy and a relatively low rate of side-effects (Goldstein *et al.* 1995). The combination of antidepressant medication and cognitive-behavioural therapy is not superior to the latter alone. The clinical decision for the application is restricted for the following reasons.

1 The effects of treatment are still insufficient because the majority of treated patients remain symptomatic at the end of treatment.

2 Very little is known about matching patients to treatments.

3 The specific efficacy of many antidepressants in adolescents is not known.

A final caveat comes from the knowledge that, at least in affective disorders, the efficacy of antidepressants is generally lower in adolescent than in adult patients (see Harrington, Chapter 29).

Outcome and prognosis

Outcome analysis studies indicate that half fully recover from the disorder whereas one-quarter improve and another quarter run a chronic course (Steinhausen 1999). Other psychiatric disorders at outcome include affective disorders in 25%, anxiety disorders in 13%, substance use disorders in 15%, and personality disorders in almost 5%. Crude mortality rates amount to only 0.7% (range 0–6%), which is considerably lower than in anorexia nervosa, but may also partly reflect the fact that follow-up periods in bulimic patients have been shorter. In comparison with anorexia nervosa, less is known about prognostic factors. Findings are contradictory on whether either early age of onset or duration of illness are favourable or unfavourable prognostic factors. Severity has no clear prognostic value. Neither comorbidity with anorexia nervosa or substance use disorders, nor obesity as premorbid conditions influence prognosis. So far, no firm conclusions can be drawn as to the prognostic relevance of family variables and socioeconomic status. Concomitant personality disorders, suicide attempts, alcohol abuse, and low self-esteem were found to be negative predictors of outcome, whereas the role of comorbid depression was less clear.

Conclusions

The increased frequencies of eating disorders and people's awareness of these problems have greatly stimulated research. We have learned much about clinical phenomenology, epidemiology, treatment and outcome. Unfortunately, most of this knowledge stems from studies of adult patients. This is surprising because anorexia nervosa typically begins during adolescence, and more studies of this age group are needed.

As in other fields of psychiatry, rather loosely tailored aetiological models are trying to integrate a large body of diverse factors and assumptions. With the advancement of molecular genetics (see McGuffin & Rutter, Chapter 12), the identification of those individuals who are particularly vulnerable to eating disorders should be possible. This may also contribute to a revised system of classification in terms of valid subtypes. Furthermore, a longitudinal study set up in the framework of developmental psychopathology should shed more light on disorder-specific risk factors, potential protective factors within the individual and the social environment, their interaction and their timing. This approach might not only address the emergence but also the maintenance of the eating disorders and should include psychological, psychosocial and biological parameter and constructs.

There is an urgent need to tailor therapeutic interventions to the needs of young patients and to evaluate the various approaches. Given the high costs of medical treatment, regardless of setting and approach, and given the high relapse and chronicity rates, both the patients and society must have an interest in the question of which patients are most apt to profit best from certain well-evaluated treatment approaches. Studies of this kind should be connected with outcome studies that must concentrate on longer follow-up periods.

Clinical treatment rests on both inpatient and outpatient programmes with special indications and combinations of various interventions. Family involvement is essential for any intervention with children and adolescents, and psychological interventions are a part of a broader team effort that should be adjusted to the developmental level of the child or the adolescent.

Finally, greater efforts should be directed towards the prevention of eating disorders. However, given the limited knowledge on the precise aetiology and the large number of non-specific risk factors, expectations should be tempered. So far, empirical tests of several prevention studies revealed only minimal or even counterproductive results (Franko & Oroson-Weine 1998). Further research into creative and carefully designed programmes is clearly warranted.

References

Andersen, A.E. (1995) Eating disorders in males. In: *Eating Disorders and Obesity: a Comprehensive Handbook* (eds K.D. Brownell & C.G. Fairburn), pp. 177–182. Guilford Press, New York.

Andersen, E.E. & Hay, A. (1985) Racial and socioeconomic influences in anorexia nervosa and bulimia. *International Journal of Eating Disorders*, **4**, 479–488.

Atkins, D.M. & Silber, T.J. (1993) Clinical spectrum of anorexia nervosa in children. *Journal of Developmental and Behavioral Pediatrics*, **14**, 211–216.

Attie, I., Brooks-Gunn, J. & Petersen, A.C. (1990) A developmental perspective on eating disorders and eating problems. In: *Handbook of Developmental Psychopathology* (eds M. Lewis & S.M. Miller), pp. 409–420. Plenum Press, New York.

Barr Taylor, C., Sharpe, T., Shisslak, C. et al. (1998) Factors associated with weight concerns in adolescent girls. *International Journal of Eating Disorders*, **24**, 31–42.

Bemis, K.M. (1987) The present status of operant conditioning for the treatment of anorexia nervosa. *Behavior Modification*, **11**, 432–463.

Beumont, P.J., Russell, J.D. & Touyz, S.W. (1993) Treatment of anorexia nervosa. *Lancet*, **341**, 1635–1640.

Beumont, P.J.V., Lowinger, K. & Russell, J. (1995) Medical assessment and the initial interview in the management of young patients with anorexia nervosa. In: *Eating Disorders in Adolescence* (ed. H.-C. Steinhausen), pp. 221–246. Walter de Gruyter, Berlin/New York.

Beumont, P.J.V., Beumont, C.C., Touyz, S.W. & Williams, H. (1997) Nutritional counseling and supervised exercise. In: *Handbook of Treatment for Eating Disorders* (eds. D.M. Garner & P.E. Garfinkel), 2nd edn, pp. 178–187. Guilford Press, New York.

Brewerton, T.D., Lydiard, R.B., Herzog, D.B., Brotman, A.W., O'Neil, P.M. & Ballenger, J.C. (1995) Comorbidity of axis I psychiatric disorders in bulimia nervosa. *Journal of Clinical Psychiatry*, **56**, 77–80.

Bryant-Waugh, R.J., Cooper, P.J., Taylor, C.L. & Lask, B.D. (1996) The use of the eating disorder examination with children: a pilot study. *International Journal of Eating Disorders*, **19**, 391–397.

Bulik, C., Sullivan, P.F., Wade, T.D. & Kendler, K.S. (2000) Twin studies of eating disorders: a review. *International Journal of Eating Disorders*, **27**, 1–20.

Carlat, D.J., Camargo, C.A. Jr & Herzog, D.B. (1997) Eating disorders in males: a report on 135 patients. *American Journal of Psychiatry*, **154**, 1127–1132.

Carney, C.P. & Andersen, A.E. (1996) Eating disorders. guide to medical evaluation and complications. *Psychiatric Clinics of North America*, **19**, 657–679.

Cash, T.F. & Deagle, E.A. III (1997) The nature and extent of body-image disturbances in anorexia nervosa and bulimia nervosa: a meta-analysis. *Journal of Eating Disorders*, **22**, 107–125.

Crisp, A.H., Norton, K., Gowers, S. et al. (1991) A controlled study of the effect of therapies aimed at adolescent and family psychopathology in anorexia nervosa. *British Journal of Psychiatry*, **159**, 325–333.

Dolan, B. (1991) Cross-cultural aspects of anorexia nervosa and bulimia: a review. *International Journal of Eating Disorders*, **10**, 67–80.

Eagles, J.M., Johnston, M.I., Hunter, D., Lobban, M. & Millar, H.R. (1995) Increasing incidence of anorexia nervosa in the female population of northeast Scotland. *American Journal of Psychiatry*, **152**, 1266–1271.

Eisler, I., Dare, C., Russell, G.F., Szmukler, G., le Grange, D. & Dodge, E. (1997) Family and individual therapy in anorexia nervosa: a 5-year follow-up. *Archives of General Psychiatry*, **54**, 1025–1030.

Eisler, I., Dare, C., Hodes, M., Russell, G., Dodge, E. & Le Grange, D. (2000) Family therapy for adolescent anorexia nervosa: the results of a controlled comparison of two family interventions. *Journal of Child Psychology and Psychiatry*, **41**, 727–736.

Emborg, C. (1999) Mortality and causes of death in eating disorders in Denmark, 1970–93: a case register study. *International Journal of Eating Disorders*, **25**, 243–251.

Fairburn, C.G. (1995) Short-term psychological treatments for bulimia nervosa. In: *Eating Disorders and Obesity: a Comprehensive Handbook* (eds K.D. Brownell & C.G Fairburn), pp. 344–348. Guilford Press, New York.

Fairburn, C.G. & Beglin, S.J. (1990) Studies of the epidemiology of bulimia nervosa. *American Journal of Psychiatry*, **147**, 401–408.

Fairburn, C.G. & Cooper, Z. (1993) The eating disorder examination. In: *Binge Eating: Nature, Assessment, and Treatment* (eds C.G. Fairburn & G.T. Wilson), 12th edn, pp. 317–360. Guilford Press, New York.

Fairburn, C.G., Steere, F. & Cooper, P.F. (1990) Assessment of the specific psychopathology of bulimia nervosa. In: *Bulimia Nervosa: Basic Research, Diagnosis, and Therapy* (ed. M.M. Fichter), pp. 37–56. John Wiley & Sons, Chichester.

Fairburn, C.G., Welch, S.L., Doll, H.A., Davies, B.A. & O'Connor, M.E. (1997) Risk factors for bulimia nervosa: a community-based case–control study. *Archives of General Psychiatry*, **54**, 509–517.

Fairburn, C.G., Cowen, P.J. & Harison, P.J. (1999a) Twin studies and the etiology of eating disorders. *International Journal of Eating Disorders*, **26**, 349–358.

Fairburn, C.G., Shafran, R. & Cooper, Z. (1999b) A cognitive behavioural theory of anorexia nervosa. *Behaviour Research and Therapy*, **37**, 1–13.

Fichter, M.M. & Hoffmann, R. (1990) Bulimia nervosa in the male. In: *Bulimia Nervosa: Basic Research, Diagnosis, and Therapy* (ed. M.M. Fichter), pp. 99–111. John Wiley & Sons, Chichester.

Fichter, M.M. & Nögel, R. (1990) Concordance for bulimia nervosa in twins. *International Journal of Eating Disorders*, **9**, 255–264.

Fichter, M.M., Herpertz, S., Quadflieg, N. & Herpertz-Dahlmann, B. (1998) Structured interview for anorexic and bulimic disorders for DSM-IV and ICD-10: updated (third) revision. *International Journal of Eating Disorders*, **24**, 227–249.

Fombonne, E. (1995) Anorexia nervosa: no evidence of an increase. *British Journal of Psychiatry*, **166**, 462–471.

Fombonne, E. (1996) Is bulimia nervosa increasing in frequency? *International Journal of Eating Disorders*, **19**, 287–296.

Franko, D.L. & Oroson-Weine, P. (1998) The prevention of eating disorders: empirical, methodological, and conceptual considerations. *Clinical Psychology: Science and Practice*, **5**, 459–477.

Freeman, C.P. (1991) A practical guide to the treatment of bulimia nervosa. *Journal of Psychosomatic Research*, **35** (Suppl. 1), 40–49.

Garfinkel, P. & Garner, D. (1982) *Anorexia Nervosa: a Multidimensional Perspective*. Brunner/Mazel, New York.

Garfinkel, P.E., Lin, E., Goering, P. *et al.* (1995) Bulimia nervosa in a Canadian community sample: prevalence and comparison of subgroups. *American Journal of Psychiatry*, **152**, 1052–1058.

Garner, D.M. (1997) Psychoeducational principles in treatment. In: *Handbook of Treatment for Eating Disorders* (eds. D.M. Garner & P.E. Garfinkel), 2nd edn, pp. 145–177. Guilford Press, New York.

Garner, D.M. & Garfinkel, P.E. (1979) The eating attitude test: an index

of the symptoms of anorexia nervosa. *Psychological Medicine*, **9**, 273–279.

Garner, D.M. & Garfinkel, P.E. (1997) *Handbook of Treatment for Eating Disorders*, 2nd edn, pp. xv; 528. Guilford Press. New York.

Garner, D.M., Olmstead, M.P., Bohr, Y. & Garfinkel, P.E. (1982) The eating attitudes test: psychometric features and clinical correlates. *Psychological Medicine*, **12**, 871–878.

Garner, D.M., Olmsted, M.P. & Polivy, J. (1983) Development and validation of a multidimensional eating disorder inventory for anorexia nervosa and bulimia. *International Journal of Eating Disorders*, **2**, 15–34.

Garner, D.M., Vitousek, K.M. & Pike, K.M. (1997) Cognitive-behavioral therapy for anorexia nervosa. In: *Handbook of Treatment for Eating Disorders* (eds D.M. Garner & P.E. Garfinkel), 2nd edn, pp. 94–143. Guilford Press, New York.

Goldstein, D.J., Wilson, M.G., Thompson, V.L., Potvin, J.H. & Rampey, A.H. Jr (1995) Long-term fluoxetine treatment of bulimia nervosa, Fluoxetine Bulimia Nervosa Research Group. *British Journal of Psychiatry*, **166**, 660–666.

Gowers, S.G., Crisp, A.H., Joughin, N. & Bhat, A. (1991) Premenarcheal anorexia nervosa. *Journal of Child Psychology and Psychiatry and Allied Disciplines*, **32**, 515–524.

Gowers, S., Norton, K., Halek, C. & Crisp, A.H. (1994) Outcome of outpatient psychotherapy in a random allocation treatment study of anorexia nervosa. *International Journal of Eating Disorders*, **15**, 165–177.

Gowers, S.G., Weetman, J., Shore, A., Hossain, F. & Elvins, R. (2000) Impact of hospitalization on the outcome of adolescent anorexia nervosa. *British Journal of Psychiatry*, **176**, 138–141.

Hall, A. (1987) The place of family therapy in the treatment of anorexia nervosa. *Australian and New Zealand Journal of Psychiatry*, **21**, 568–574.

Heebink, D.M. & Halmi, K.A. (1995) Psychopharmacology in adolescents with eating disorders. In: *Eating Disorders in Adolescence* (ed. H.-C. Steinhausen), pp. 271–286. Walter de Gruyter, Berlin/New York.

Herzog, D.B., Keller, M.B., Sacks, N.R., Yeh, C.J. & Lavori, P.W. (1992) Psychiatric comorbidity in treatment-seeking anorexics and bulimics. *Journal of the American Academy of Child and Adolescent Psychiatry*, **31**, 810–818.

Hoek, H.W., Bartelds, A.I., Bosveld, J.J. *et al.* (1995) Impact of urbanization on detection rates of eating disorders. *American Journal of Psychiatry*, **152**, 1272–1278.

Holderness, C.C., Brooks-Gunn, J. & Warren, M.P. (1994) Co-morbidity of eating disorders and substance abuse review of the literature. *International Journal of Eating Disorders*, **16**, 1–34.

Holland, A.J., Sicotte, N. & Treasure, J. (1988) Anorexia nervosa: evidence for a genetic basis. *Journal of Psychosomatic Research*, **32**, 561–572.

Hsu, L.K.G., Chesler, B.E. & Santhouse, R. (1990) Bulimia nervosa in eleven sets of twins: a clinical report. *International Journal of Eating Disorders*, **9**, 275–282.

Huon, G.F. & Strong, K.G. (1998) The invitation and maintenance of dieting: structural models for large-scale longitudinal investigations. *International Journal of Eating Disorders*, **23**, 361–369.

Kendler, K.S., MacLean, C., Neale, M., Kessler, R., Heath, A. & Eaves, L. (1991) The genetic epidemiology of bulimia nervosa. *American Journal of Psychiatry*, **148**, 1627–1637.

Kog, E. & Vandereycken, W. (1988) The facts: a review of research data on eating disorder families. In: *The family approach to eating disorders: assessment and treatment of anorexia nervosa and bulimia* (eds. W. Vandereycken, E. Kog & J. Vanderlinden), pp. 25–67. PMA Publications, New York.

Lask, B. & Bryant-Waugh, R. (1993) *Childhood Onset Anorexia and Related Eating Disorders*. Lawrence Erlbaum, Hillsdale, NJ.

Le Grange, D., Eisler, I., Dare, C. & Russell, G.F.M. (1992) Evaluation of family treatments in adolescent anorexia nervosa: a pilot study. *International Journal of Eating Disorders*, **12**, 347–357.

Lee, S. & Chiu, H.F.K. (1989) Anorexia nervosa in Hong Kong: why not more in Chinese? *British Journal of Psychiatry*, **154**, 683–688.

Leon, G.R., Fulkerson, J.A., Perry, C.L. & Early-Zald, M.B. (1995) Prospective analysis of personality and behavioral vulnerabilities and gender influences in the later development of disordered eating. *Journal of Abnormal Psychology*, **104**, 140–149.

Lewandowski, L.M., Gebing, T.A., Anthony, J.L. & O'Brien, W.H. (1997) Meta-analysis of cognitive-behavioral treatment studies for bulimia. *Clinical Psychology Review*, **17**, 703–718.

Lilenfeld, L.R., Kaye, W.H., Greeno, C.G. et al. (1998) A controlled family study of anorexia nervosa and bulimia nervosa: psychiatric disorders in first-degree relatives and effects of proband comorbidity. *Archives of General Psychiatry*, **55**, 603–610.

Manchi, M. & Cohen, P. (1990) Early childhood eating behavior and adolescent eating disorders. *Journal of the American Academy of Child and Adolescent Psychiatry*, **29**, 112–117.

Mitchell, J.E., Specker, S.M. & de Zwaan, M. (1991) Comorbidity and medical complications of bulimia nervosa. *Journal of Clinical Psychiatry*, **52** (Suppl. 13), 20.

Mitchell, J.E., Raymond, N. & Specker, S. (1993) A review of the controlled trials of pharmacotherapy and psychotherapy in the treatment of bulimia nervosa. *International Journal of Eating Disorders*, **14**, 229–247.

Munk-Jorgensen, P., Moller-Madsen, S., Nielsen, S. & Nystrup, J. (1995) Incidence of eating disorders in psychiatric hospitals and wards in Denmark, 1970–93. *Acta Psychiatrica Scandinavica*, **92**, 91–96.

Nasser, M. (1988) Culture and weight consciousness. *Journal of Psychosomatic Research*, **32**, 573–578.

Neumärker, U., Dudeck, U., Vollrath, M., Neumärker, K.J. & Steinhausen, H.-C. (1992) Eating attitudes among adolescent patients and normal school girls in East Berlin and West Berlin: a transcultural comparison. *International Journal of Eating Disorders*, **12**, 281–289.

Palmer, R.I. (1995) Sexual abuse and eating disorders. In: *Eating Disorders and Obesity: a Comprehensive Handbook* (eds K.D. Brownell & C.G. Fairburn), pp. 230–233. Guilford Press, New York.

Palmer, R., Christie, M., Cordle, C., Davies, D. & Kenrick, J. (1987) The clinical eating disorder rating instrument (CEDRI): a preliminary description. *International Journal of Eating Disorders*, **6**, 9–16.

Patton, G.C. & King, M.B. (1991) Epidemiological study of eating disorders: time for a change of emphasis [Editorial]. *Psychological Medicine*, **21**, 287–291.

Patton, G.C., Johnson-Sabine, E., Wood, K., Mann, A.H. & Wakeling, A. (1990) Abnormal eating attitudes in London schoolgirls: a prospective epidemiological study—outcome at twelve-month follow-up. *Psychological Medicine*, **20**, 383–394.

Patton, G.C., Carlin, J.B., Shao, Q. et al. (1997) Adolescent dieting: healthy weight control or borderline eating disorders? *Journal of Child Psychology and Psychiatry*, **38**, 299–306.

Patton, G.C., Selzer, R., Coffey, C., Carlin, J.B. & Wolfe, R. (1999) Onset of adolescent eating disorders: population based cohort study over 3 years. *British Medical Journal*, **318**, 765–768.

Pawluck, D.E. & Gorey, K.M. (1998) Secular trends in the incidence of anorexia nervosa: integrative review of population-based studies. *International Journal of Eating Disorders*, **23**, 347–352.

Pike, K.M. (1998) Long-term course of anorexia nervosa: response, relapse, remission, and recovery. *Clinical Psychology Review*, **18**, 447–475.

Pirke, K.M. & Platte, P. (1995) Neurobiology of eating disorders in adolescence. In: *Eating Disorders in Adolescence* (ed. H.-C. Steinhausen), pp. 171–190. Walter de Gruyter, Berlin/New York.

Pumariega, A.J., Edwards, P. & Mitchell, C.B. (1984) Anorexia nervosa in Black adolescents. *Journal of the American Academy of Child and Adolescent Psychiatry*, **23**, 111–114.

Ramsay, R., Ward, A., Treasure, J. & Russell, G.F.M. (1999) Compulsory treatment in anorexia nervosa: short-term benefits and long-term mortality. *British Journal of Psychiatry*, **175**, 147–153.

Råstam, M. (1992) Anorexia nervosa in 51 Swedish adolescents: premorbid problems and comorbidity. *Journal of the American Academy of Child and Adolescent Psychiatry*, **31**, 819–829.

Råstam, M. & Gillberg, C. (1991) The family background in anorexia nervosa: a population based study. *Journal of the American Academy of Child and Adolescent Psychiatry*, **30**, 283–289.

Robin, A.L., Siegel, P.T. & Moye, A. (1995) Family versus individual therapy for anorexia: impact on family conflict. *International Journal of Eating Disorders*, **17**, 313–322.

Robin, A.L., Gilroy, M. & Dennis, A.B. (1998) Treatment of eating disorders in children and adolescents. *Clinical Psychology Review*, **18**, 421–446.

Robin, A.L., Sielgel, P.T., Moye, A.W., Gilroy, M., Dennis, A.B. & Sikand, A. (1999) A controlled comparison of family versus individual therapy for adolescents with anorexia nervosa. *Journal of the American Academy of Child and Adolescent Psychiatry*, **38**, 1482–1489.

Russell, G.F.M. (1979) Bulimia nervosa: an ominous variant of anorexia nervosa. *Psychological Medicine*, **9**, 429–448.

Russell, G.F.M. (1992) Anorexia nervosa of early onset and its impact on puberty. In: *Feeding Problems and Eating Disorders in Children and Adolescents* (eds P.J. Cooper & A. Stein), pp. 85–112. Harwood Academic Publishers, Chur [Switzerland]; Philadelphia.

Russell, G.F.M., Szmukler, G.I., Dare, C. & Eisler, I. (1987) An evaluation of family therapy in anorexia nervosa and bulimia nervosa. *Archives of General Psychiatry*, **44**, 1047–1056.

Schmidt, U.H. & Treasure, J.L. (1993) *Getting Better Bit(e) by Bit(e)*. Lawrence Erlbaum, London.

Schmidt, U., Tiller, J., Hoades, M. & Treasure, J. (1995) Risk factors for the development of early onset bulimia nervosa. In: *Eating Disorders in Adolescence* (ed. H.-C. Steinhausen), pp. 83–94. Walter de Gruyter, Berlin/New York.

Shisslak, C.M., Crago, M., McKnight, K.M., Estes, L.S., Gray, N. & Parnaby, O.G. (1998) Potential risk factors associated with weight control behaviors in elementary and middle school girls. *Journal of Psychosomatic Research*, **44**, 301–313.

Silber, T.J. (1986) Anorexia nervosa in Blacks and Hispanics. *International Journal of Eating Disorders*, **5**, 121–128.

Smolak, L., Murnen, S.K. & Ruble, A.E. (2000) Female athletes and eating problems: a meta-analysis. *International Eating Disorders*, **27**, 371–380.

Soundy, T.J., Lucas, A.R., Suman, V.J. & Melton, L.J. III (1995) Bulimia nervosa in Rochester, Minnesota from 1980 to 1990. *Psychological Medicine*, **25**, 1065–1071.

Steiger, H. & Stotland, S. (1995) Individual and family factors in adolescents with eating symptoms and syndromes. In: *Eating Disorders in Adolescence* (ed. H.-C. Steinhausen), pp. 49–68. Walter de Gruyter, Berlin/New York.

Stein, D., Lilenfeld, L.R., Plotnicov, K. et al. (1999) Familial aggregation of eating disorders: results form a controlled family study of bulimia nervosa. *International Eating Disorders*, **26**, 211–215.

Steiner, H. & Lock, J. (1998) Anorexia nervosa and bulimia nervosa in children and adolescents: a review of the past 10 years. *Journal of the American Academy of Child and Adolescent Psychiatry*, **37**, 352–359.

Steiner, H., Sanders, M. & Ryst, E. (1995) Precursors and risk factors of juvenile eating disorders. In: *Eating Disorders in Adolescence* (ed. H.-C. Steinhausen), pp. 95–126. Walter de Gruyter, Berlin/New York.

Steinhausen, H.-C. (1984) Transcultural comparison of eating attitudes in young females and anorectic patients. *European Archives of Psychiatry and Neurological Sciences*, **234**, 198–201.

Steinhausen, H.-C. (1995) *Eating Disorders in Adolescence*. Walter de Gruyter, Berlin/New York.

Steinhausen, H.-C. (1997a) Annotation: outcome of anorexia nervosa in the younger patient. *Journal of Child Psychology and Psychiatry*, **38**, 271–276.

Steinhausen, H.-C. (1997b) Clinical guidelines for anorexia nervosa and bulimia nervosa. *European Child and Adolescent Psychiatry*, **6**, 121–128.

Steinhausen, H.-C. (1999) Eating disorders. In: *Risks and Outcomes in Developmental Psychopathology* (eds H.-C. Steinhausen & F. Verhulst), pp. 210–230. Oxford University Press, Oxford.

Steinhausen, H.-C., Neumärker, K.J., Vollrath, M., Dudeck, U. & Neumärker, U. (1992) A transcultural comparison of the eating disorder inventory in former East and West Berlin. *International Journal of Eating Disorders*, **12**, 407–416.

Steinhausen, H.-C., Winkler, C. & Meier, M. (1997) Eating disorders in adolescence in a Swiss epidemiological study. *International Journal of Eating Disorders*, **22**, 147–151.

Steinhausen, H.-C., Boyadjieva, S., Grigoroiu-Serbanescu, M., Seidel, R. & Winkler Metzke, C. (2000) A transcultural outcome study of adolescent eating disorders. *Acta Psychiatrica Scandinavica*, **101**, 60–66.

Strober, M. (1991) Family–genetic studies of eating disorders. *Journal of Clinical Psychiatry*, **52** (Suppl.), 9–12.

Strober, M., Freeman, R. & Morrell, W. (1997) The long-term course of severe anorexia nervosa in adolescents: survival analysis of recovery, relapse, and outcome predictors over 10–15 years in a prospective study. *International Journal of Eating Disorders*, **22**, 339–360.

Suematsu, H., Kuboki, T. & Itoh, T. (1985) Statistical studies on the prognosis of anorexia nervosa. *Psychosomatics*, **43**, 104–112.

Sullivan, P.F., Bulik, C.M. & Kendler, K.S. (1998a) The epidemiology and classification of bulimia nervosa. *Psychological Medicine*, **28**, 599–610.

Sullivan, P.F., Bulik, C.M. & Kendler, K.S. (1998b) Genetic epidemiology of binging and vomiting. *British Journal of Psychiatry*, **173**, 75–79.

Thiel, A., Broocks, A., Ohlmeier, M., Jacoby, G.E. & Schussler, G. (1995) Obsessive-compulsive disorder among patients with anorexia nervosa and bulimia nervosa. *American Journal of Psychiatry*, **152**, 72–75.

Thiels, C., Schmidt, U., Treasure, J., Garthe, R. & Troop, N. (1998) Guided self-change for bulimia nervosa incorporating use of a self-care manual. *American Journal of Psychiatry*, **155**, 947–953.

Thomas, J.P. & Szmukler, G.I. (1985) Anorexia nervosa in patients of Afro-Caribbean extraction. *British Journal of Psychiatry*, **146**, 653–656.

Touyz, S.W., Garner, D.M. & Beumont, P.J.V. (1995) The inpatient management of adolescent patients with anorexia nervosa. In: *Eating Disorders in Adolescence* (ed. H.-C. Steinhausen), pp. 247–270. Walter de Gruyter, Berlin/New York.

Treasure, J. & Holland, A. (1990) Genetic vulnerability to eating disorders: evidence from twin and family studies. In: *Anorexia Nervosa* (eds H. Remschmidt & M.H. Schmidt), pp. 59–68. Hogrefe & Huber, Toronto.

Treasure, J.L., Schmidt, U.H., Troop, N., Tiller, J., Todd, G. & Turnbull, S. (1996) A randomised controlled trial of sequential treatment for bulimia nervosa incorporating a self-care manual. *British Journal of Psychiatry*, **168**, 94–98.

Turnbull, S., Ward, A., Treasure, J., Jick, H. & Derby, L. (1996) The demand for eating disorder care: an epidemiological study using the general practice research database. *British Journal of Psychiatry*, **169**, 705–712.

Vandereycken, W. (1995) The place of family therapy in the treatment of eating disorders. In: *Eating Disorders in Adolescence* (ed. H.-C. Steinhausen), pp. 287–297. Walter de Gruyter, Berlin/New York.

Vandereycken, W., Kog, E. & Vanderlinden, J. (1989) *The family approach to eating disorders: assessment and treatment of anorexia nervosa and bulimia*. PMA Publications, New York.

Vanderlinden, J. & Vandereycken, W. (1995) Sexual abuse and psychological dysfunctioning in eating disorders. In: *Eating Disorders in Adolescence* (ed. H.-C. Steinhausen), pp. 161–170. Walter de Gruyter, Berlin/New York.

Wade, T., Martin, N.G. & Tiggemann, M. (1998) Genetic and environmental risk factors for the weight and shape concerns characteristic of bulimia nervosa. *Psychological Medicine*, **28**, 761–771.

Walsh, B.T. (1995) Pharmacotherapy of eating disorders. In: *Eating Disorders and Obesity: a Comprehensive Handbook* (eds K.D. Brownell & C.G. Fairburn), pp. 313–317. Guilford Press, New York.

Walters, E.E. & Kendler, K.S. (1995) Anorexia nervosa and anorexic-like syndromes in a population-based female twin sample. *American Journal of Psychiatry*, **152**, 64–71.

Walters, E.E., Neale, M.C., Eaves, L.J., Heath, A.C., Kessler, R.C. & Kendler, K.S. (1992) Bulimia nervosa and major depression: a study of common genetic and environmental factors. *Psychological Medicine*, **22**, 617–622.

Welch, S.L. & Fairburn, C.G. (1996) Childhood sexual and physical abuse as risk factors for the development of bulimia nervosa: a community-based case–control study. *Child Abuse and Neglect*, **20**, 633–642.

Welch, S.L., Doll, H.A. & Fairburn, C.G. (1997) Life events and the onset of bulimia nervosa: a controlled study. *Psychological Medicine*, **27**, 515–522.

Wilson, G.T., Fairburn, C.G. & Agras, W.S. (1997) Cognitive-behavioral therapy for bulimia nervosa. In: *Handbook of Treatment for Eating Disorders* (eds D.M. Garner & P.E. Garfinkel), 2nd edn, pp. 67–93. Guilford Press, New York.

Obsessive-Compulsive Disorder

Judith L. Rapoport and Susan Swedo

Definition: the concept and current issues

Obsessive-compulsive disorder was once considered rare in childhood, but recent advances in diagnosis and treatment have led to recognition that the disorder is a common cause of distress for children and adolescents. Obsessive-compulsive disorder (OCD) is characterized by the presence of obsessions (unwanted repetitive or intrusive thoughts), and compulsions (unnecessary repetitive behaviours or mental activities). Because the obsessive thoughts and compulsive rituals are recognized by the child as nonsensical, they are often kept hidden for as long as possible — from both parents and practitioners. This secrecy may have contributed to the fact that until recently, OCD was unfamiliar to most child psychiatrists, even though classic descriptions of the disorder featured cases with childhood presentation (Janet 1903). The recognition that OCD was more common in adults than previously believed, and retrospective reports that one-half to one-third of adult subjects had their onset in childhood or adolescence, focused the attention of the child psychiatric community on this chronic and often disabling disorder (Karno *et al.* 1988).

Until the mid-nineteenth century, obsessive-compulsive phenomena were considered to be a variant of insanity. However, as the disorder was better defined, it came into focus as one of the neuroses. The descriptions of repetitive unwanted thoughts or rituals often characterized by magical thinking, and usually kept private by the sufferer, were relatively constant observations in those early reports. Debate about core deficits and the relative importance of volitional, intellectual and emotional impairments (all of which are in some way abnormal in OCD) have flourished for over 100 years (Berrios 1989).

Freud (1909, 1913) provided some of the most interesting and creative speculations on the similarity between obsessive-compulsive phenomena, children's games and religious rites. Although psychoanalytic theory has not added usefully to the treatment or understanding of the aetiology of severe OCD, the broad questions raised by Freud about continuity and discontinuity within individual development and OCD, as well as with secular and religious rituals, remain fascinating issues. In addition, the observations of association between certain neurological disorders and OCD have led to the most intriguing aspects of current neurobiological research: the possible localization of brain circuits mediating obsessive-compulsive behaviours, as well as mechanisms for behavioural encoding. Over the past decade, interest in these social and developmental questions,

together with increased recognition of paediatric OCD, has generated an astonishing amount of clinical observation, and basic science and clinical research (Rapoport 1989a,b; King & Scahill 1999).

Epidemiology

The Epidemiological Catchment Area (ECA) study of over 18 500 adult individuals in five different sites in the USA included OCD as a separate category and provided the first large-scale information on the prevalence of this disorder (Robins *et al.* 1981). Using the Diagnostic Interview Schedule (DIS), a structured interview designed for lay interviewers, lifetime prevalence rates ranged from 1.9 to 3.3% across the sites. Even when other disorders were excluded, the rates were 1.2–2.4%. These rates were 25–60 times greater than had been estimated on the basis of clinical populations (Karno *et al.* 1988). The mean age of onset across the sites ranged from 20 to 25 years, with 50% developing symptoms in childhood or adolescence (Karno & Golding 1990), providing further support for retrospective accounts of the frequent paediatric onset of this disorder (Black 1974).

The ECA findings have been criticized on the grounds that interviewers were not trained clinicians and the validity of the DIS is uncertain (see discussion in Karno *et al.* 1988). To address these criticisms, and assess the rates of OCD in a younger population, Flament *et al.* (1988) used trained mental health professionals and previously validated instruments to assess obsessive-compulsive symptomatology in an adolescent population. As part of a two-stage study of 5596 adolescents (Whitaker *et al.* 1990), the Leyton Obsessional Inventory was administered (together with other questionnaires on general mental health, anxiety and eating disorders) to the entire high school population of a county 80 miles from New York City (Flament *et al.* 1988). Adolescents scoring above the clinical cut-off were interviewed by child psychiatrists with extensive clinical experience with OCD. Clinical vignettes were compiled on the basis of these semistructured interviews and a high agreement for OCD, compulsive personality and subclinical OCD was obtained (overall kappa of 0.85). A total of 20 subjects received a lifetime diagnosis of OCD (18 current and two with past illness). The weighted prevalence figure (without exclusion) for OCD was 1.9%, a figure that is in close agreement with the ECA estimates for adults. Two-year follow-up demonstrated that the obsessive-compulsive symptoms were clinically significant, as the majority of subjects remained symptomatic (Berg *et al.* 1989).

In recent years, several additional epidemiological studies have been conducted (see Zohar 1999 for review), with prevalence rates ranging from 0.5 to 4% (Anderson *et al.* 1987; Lewinsohn *et al.* 1993; Reinherz *et al.* 1993; Wittchen *et al.* 1998; Rapoport *et al.*, 2000). In virtually all of these reports, the rates ascertained from direct child reports were higher than those derived from parent reports, supporting clinical data that children with OCD often hide their illness. The secrecy, and difficulties of utilizing lay interviewers, may have contributed to the low (0.5%) prevalence of OCD found by Wittchen *et al.* (1998) in a sample of 3021 adolescent subjects in Munich, Germany. Other investigators, such as Valleni-Basile *et al.* (1996) in south-eastern USA, Douglass *et al.* (1995) in New Zealand and Zohar *et al.* (1992) in Israel, used mental health interviewers and semistructured clinical interviews, and found more comparable rates of 2.9, 4.0 and 2.3%, respectively. Of note in the Israeli investigation, an additional 4% of the adolescents had subclinical obsessive-compulsive symptomatology, defined by the presence of obsessions and compulsions which were not of sufficient severity to meet DSM-III-R criteria. This group, as well as those meeting diagnostic criteria for OCD, remained symptomatic at 2-year follow-up evaluation (Zohar *et al.* 1992).

The frequency, chronicity and secrecy of paediatric OCD suggest that mental health professionals should make special efforts to question paediatric patients about symptoms of OCD.

Phenomenology and classification

OCD is defined in both ICD-10 and DSM-IV as repetitive intrusive thoughts and/or rituals that are unwanted and which interfere significantly with function or cause marked distress. The severity criteria avoid confusion with the many childhood habits which are a part of normal development, and the content and relative insight into the unreasonableness of the behaviours differentiate OCD from other disorders. The ICD and DSM-IV criteria differ in their inclusion or exclusion of comorbid psychotic disorders, such as schizophrenia. A change was made in DSM-III-R (American Psychiatric Association 1987) and continued in DSM-IV (American Psychiatric Association 1994) which allowed patients to receive a diagnosis of OCD, even in the presence of schizophrenia. This change was made because of the broad comorbidity of OCD (Karno *et al.* 1988) and convincing evidence of coexistence with schizophrenia (Lewis *et al.* 1991). DSM-IV urges the use of multiple diagnoses as appropriate, and both Karno *et al.* (1988) and our own experience (Swedo *et al.* 1989b), suggest that over 50% of OCD subjects will also merit another Axis I diagnosis, often an anxiety or affective disorder.

Current debates about diagnostic criteria — including whether obsessions are inevitably present, and what degree of insight is required concerning the irrationality of symptoms — are of particular importance for childhood OCD. Both DSM-IV and ICD-10 state that compulsions are designed to neutralize or prevent some dreaded event. This may be an error. While some children may not be willing or able to verbalize their obsessive thoughts, long-term contact has demonstrated that about 40% of children do not have obsessive thoughts — they steadfastly report the presence of only compulsive rituals accompanied by a vague sense of discomfort if the rituals are not carried out (Swedo *et al.* 1989b). In fact, over one-third of adults also deny that their compulsions are driven by an obsessive thought (Karno *et al.* 1988), suggesting that neutralization is not an essential feature of OCD at any age.

The degree of insight needed for the diagnosis is also in dispute as some patients, at least some of the time, 'believe' their obsessions. Again, children generally do not differ from adults in this respect. While in theory it might seem that young children would be particularly prone to 'believe' their obsessional thoughts, experience to date suggests that the DSM-IV adult criteria are appropriate for the diagnosis in childhood (Rapoport 1989a; Swedo *et al.* 1989b; King & Scahill 1999). It seems that for both adults and children, diagnostic criteria must acknowledge that compulsions can and do occur in the absence of obsessions, and that partial 'belief' in the necessity for these thoughts/behaviours is seen, particularly in severe cases.

Recent research has suggested that subtyping of OCD may be useful. Leckman *et al.* (1997) suggest that symptom clusters divide OCD into four phenomenological subtypes, including those with 'just right' phenomena, as well as those with primarily cognitive symptoms. The presence or absence of a comorbid tic disorder also appears to define phenomenology and symptom course; in addition, children with comorbid tics often benefit from low-dose neuroleptic augmentation of serotonin uptake inhibitors. Aetiological investigations suggest that there are at least three subtypes of OCD: familial (possibly genetic), nonfamilial and environmentally triggered (e.g. post-infectious). One example of the latter subgroup has been identified by research at the National Institute for Mental Health (NIMH) which revealed a subgroup of paediatric patients in whom symptom exacerbations are triggered by streptococcal infections; the subgroup is identified by the acronym PANDAS (paediatric autoimmune neuropsychiatric disorders associated with streptococcal infections; Swedo *et al.* 1998). The postulated aetiopathophysiology of symptoms in the PANDAS subgroup is similar to that of Sydenham chorea (the neurological manifestation of rheumatic fever), in which streptococcal infections trigger the production of antibodies which cross-react with neuronal tissue to produce an 'autoimmune' reaction situated mainly within the basal ganglia (Swedo 1994). The resulting inflammation results in a variety of neuropsychiatric symptoms, including obsessions, compulsions and tics, among others. Several clinical characteristics define the PANDAS subgroup, including prepubertal onset (mean age of 7.4 ± 2.7 year), episodic ('sawtoothed') course, presence of neurological abnormalities, such as choreiform movements or motoric hyperactivity, and a

Table 35.1 Presenting symptoms in 70 consecutive children and adolescents with primary obsessive-compulsive disorder. (Categories adapted from Goodman *et al.* 1989.)

Reported symptoms at initial interview	*n*	Percentage
Obsessions		
Concerns with dirt, germs or environmental toxins	28	40
Something terrible happening (e.g. fire, death or illness of self or loved one)	17	24
Symmetry, order or exactness	12	17
Scrupulosity (religious obsessions)	9	13
Concern or disgust with bodily wastes or secretions (urine, stool, saliva)	6	8
Lucky or unlucky numbers	6	8
Forbidden, aggressive or perverse sexual thoughts, images or impulses	3	4
Fear might harm others or self	3	4
Concern with household items	2	3
Intrusive nonsense sounds, words or music	1	1
Compulsions		
Excessive or ritualized hand-washing, showering, bathing, toothbrushing or grooming	60	85
Repeating rituals (e.g. going in or out the door, up or down)	36	51
Checking (e.g. doors, locks, stoves, appliances, emergency brake on car, paper route, homework, etc.)	32	46
Miscellaneous rituals (e.g. writing, moving, speaking)	18	26
Rituals to remove contact with contaminants	16	23
Touching	14	20
Measures to prevent harm to self or others	11	16
Ordering or arranging	12	17
Counting	13	18
Hoarding/collecting rituals	8	11
Rituals of cleaning household or inanimate objects	4	6

Multiple obsessions and compulsions are possible, thus the total exceeds 70.

temporal association between symptom exacerbations and streptococcal infections (Perlmutter *et al.* 1998; Swedo *et al.* 1998). When a young child presents with the acute onset of OCD and/or tics, consideration of a relationship between streptococcal infections and symptom onset may provide unique opportunities for intervention (see section on Investigative Treatments).

Clinical presentation

Childhood onset OCD has been documented as early as age 2, but more typically begins later in childhood or early adolescence (Despert 1955; Adams 1973; Rapoport 1989c). Children with an early age at onset (below age 6) usually begin their rituals or obsessions in easily recognizable fashion, such as excessive hand-washing or ritualized checking and repeating (Swedo 1989). However, in some cases the clinical presentation is altered by the child's developmental immaturity. For example, one 6-year-old boy, who was compelled to draw zeros repetitively, had started at age 3 to circle manhole covers on city streets. His tantrums when the circling was interrupted, his subjective distress during the behaviour and his lack of other psychosocial abnormalities (such as autism or pervasive developmental disorder) led to the diagnosis of OCD. Another child presented at age

7 with clinically significant checking compulsions, but had been evaluated previously at 3 years of age when he developed a 'compulsion' to walk only on the edges of floor tiles. Cleaning rituals in children too young to reach the water faucet might present as excessive hand-wiping or licking.

In general, the symptoms of OCD in children mirror those in adult patients, and include a wide variety of obsessive thoughts and compulsive rituals (Despert 1955; Adams 1973; Goodman *et al.* 1989; Swedo 1989; Thomsen & Mikkelsen 1991; Toro *et al.* 1992; Maina *et al.* 1999). Obsessive thoughts centre on contamination concerns, danger to self or others, symmetry or moral issues. Common compulsions include washing, checking and repeating—particularly until the child experiences a feeling of 'getting it just right'. Most children have a combination of rituals and obsessions, and 'pure' obsessives are rare compared with the more frequent 'pure' ritualizers.

The presenting symptoms of 70 children and adolescents consecutively evaluated at the NIMH are summarized in Table 35.1 (Swedo 1989). As with other OCD patients, rituals were more frequently the presenting complaint than were obsessions. Washing compulsions were by far the most common symptom in the NIMH sample, occurring at some time during the course of the illness in 85% of patients. Hand-washing was slightly more frequent than was showering, and the two activities accounted for virtually all of the washing rituals (no subject took prolonged baths), although a few children cleaned their hands with chemicals, such as alcohol or detergents, provoking eczematoid dermatitis.

Secrecy appears to be a hallmark of childhood onset OCD. The children recognize that their symptoms are nonsensical and are embarrassed by them, so they go to great lengths to hide them. Hand-washing might be disguised as more frequent voiding, and rituals are carried out in private, so that children are often symptomatic for months before their parents are aware of a problem. Teachers and peers become aware only with much greater severity. As with Tourette disorder, children may expend great effort 'controlling' their behaviours in public and 'let go' when at home. This partial voluntary control of symptoms often baffles and angers parents (see section on Family Education below).

Approximately one-third of paediatric patients report that certain stimuli trigger their rituals, and that avoidance of the trigger 'protects' them from the obsessive-compulsive symptoms (Swedo 1989). For example, a 16-year-old girl with elaborate front door touching and stepping rituals could 'sneak' into her house by a side door, avoiding the sight of the front door, and successfully avert the compulsions. Several hoarders would close their eyes to avoid seeing scraps of paper on the street that would set off the collecting urge. From an ethological perspective, the compulsions might be conceptualized as 'fixed action patterns' released by key environmental stimuli (Modell et al. 1989; Swedo 1989; Winslow 1989), perhaps mediated through the striatum (Rapoport & Wise 1988; Wise & Rapoport 1989). An ethological bias on OCD still leaves entirely open the question of what sort of innate programmes could serve to focus the developing child's attention on particular aspects of environmental stimulation that forms blocks of behavioural organization, later 'released' as OCD. Adaptive significance of such innate specification is assumed, but runs the danger of teleological argument. While evidence of selective response to certain stimuli has been demonstrated in normal infants (e.g. response to mother's voice), no studies have yet been carried out on trigger stimuli in childhood OCD. Such studies, particularly with high-risk groups, would be of great interest.

Course and natural history

There are no prospective data available to determine mean age at onset of OCD. In epidemiological studies, over 50% of adults with OCD report that their symptoms started during childhood or adolescence, with males generally having earlier onset than females (Rasmussen & Tsuang 1984). The demographics of the NIMH paediatric clinic support these retrospective data, as the mean age of onset was 10.1 (± 3.5) years in the OCD cohort, with eight of the 70 patients having symptom onset prior to age 7. Among those who had symptom onset prior to puberty, males outnumbered females by nearly 3 : 1. Of interest to our efforts to interpret retrospective data, parents of nearly half of the NIMH sample revealed that their children had displayed 'micro

episodes of OCD' several years before developing full-blown symptoms. During the episodes, excessive rigidity and repetitive rituals (e.g. wearing the same clothes for a month, refusal to take a different path through the house) were a source of concern, albeit briefly (Swedo et al. 1989b).

The clinical course of the disorder indicates some developmental influence on symptoms over time. The primary obsessions and compulsions changed over time in 90% of the NIMH paediatric patients (Rettew et al. 1992). Most children began with a single obsession or compulsion, continued with this for several months to years, and then gradually acquired different thoughts or rituals. Although the primary symptom would change (e.g. from counting to washing and then checking), the earlier symptoms often remained problematic, although at a lesser degree. The nature of the compulsive rituals also changed over time. A study of adolescents demonstrated that counting and symmetry were most prominent during grade-school years, but were replaced by washing rituals during early and mid-adolescence (Maina et al. 1999). As adolescence progressed, sexual thoughts or rituals became common; these dissipated by 18 years of age and were supplanted by more general ruminations and doubts. For a significant number of children, however, the presenting symptom continued unchanging throughout the course of the illness, such as the adolescents who report having an intrusive 'song stuck in my head' (Swedo 1989; Flament et al. 1990; Zungu-Dirwayi et al. 1999).

The clinical course of childhood onset OCD is usually described as chronic and unremitting, although epidemiological studies of adults suggest that spontaneous remissions occur in as many as one-third of patients (Karno & Golding 1990). Among children with comorbid tic disorders, symptom severity may fluctuate over time, similar to the waxing and waning course described for Tourette disorder (Leonard et al. 1992). An episodic course has also been described for the PANDAS subgroup of patients, but it is characterized as relapsing/remitting, rather than fluctuating in severity (Perlmutter et al. 1998). These variations in clinical course are intriguing, but it is not yet clear whether they reflect differences in underlying pathophysiology, or are merely the result of individual differences in clinical presentation.

The long-term prognosis of childhood onset OCD is unknown, as prospective follow-up studies are rare. Epidemiological studies suggest that symptoms remain problematic for the majority of childhood onset cases (Karno & Golding 1990). These findings are consistent with those from adult patients with childhood onset OCD, who report that their symptoms have remained problematic throughout adolescence and adulthood (Berman 1942; Warren 1965; Hollingsworth et al. 1980; Zeitlin 1986; Honjo et al. 1989; Hanna 1995). The availability of improved psychological and pharmacological therapies appears to have done little to improve the long-term outcome of childhood onset OCD. Leonard et al. (1993) carried out a 2–7 years prospective follow-up of 54 children participating in a clomipramine treatment trial. They found that 20 (37%) still met criteria for OCD and only 18 (33%) were symptom-free, despite ongoing drug treatment (Leonard *et al.* 1993). Thomsen & Mikkelsen (1991) conducted a similar longitudinal evaluation in 23 Danish children and adolescents, and demonstrated that over 50% still met severity criteria for an OCD diagnosis at 1.5–5 years follow-up.

Associated disorders

In adults, OCD has a broad range of comorbidity similar to that seen for other major Axis I disorders (Karno *et al.* 1988). The patterns of comorbidity among childhood onset cases are generally comparable to those for adult samples, with tic disorders and specific developmental disorders appearing more frequently in the paediatric populations. In the NIMH sample, only 26% of the paediatric subjects had OCD as a single diagnosis (Swedo *et al.* 1989b). Tic disorders (30%), major depression (26%) and specific developmental disabilities (24%) were most common. Rates were also increased for simple phobias (17%), overanxious disorder (16%), adjustment disorder with depressed mood (13%), oppositional disorder (11%), attention deficit disorder (10%), conduct disorder (7%), separation anxiety disorder (7%) and enuresis/encopresis (4%). Riddle *et al.* (1992) reported similar findings, with the majority of children and adolescents in their sample having comorbid diagnoses, including anxiety disorders (38%), mood disorder (29%) or tic disorder (24%).

Epidemiological studies have also found similar comorbidity patterns. Zohar *et al.* (1992) found increased rates of phobias (33%), overanxious disorder (2%) and tic disorders (8%) among adolescents with OCD identified from a population of 861 Israeli adolescents. Other community-based studies have not evaluated the rate of comorbid tic disorders, but have found increased rates of affective and anxiety disorders. In a study in the south-eastern USA, Valleni-Basile *et al.* (1996) found that the majority of adolescents with OCD had a comorbid disorder, including depression (45%), separation anxiety disorder (34%) and/or phobia (29%). Lewinsohn *et al.* (1993) noted increased rates of panic disorder (33%), overanxious disorder (33%) and social phobia (33%) in their Oregon sample, and reported that over two-thirds of the adolescents with OCD had a second anxiety disorder. Eating disorders are also increased in frequency among children and adolescents with OCD, as demonstrated in the epidemiological study by Whitaker *et al.* (1990).

Increased incidence of neurological 'soft' signs in childhood anxiety disorder has been reported by Shaffer *et al.* (1985). Early studies at the NIMH reported a lack of normal cerebral laterality and a high rate of age-inappropriate synkinesias and left hemibody signs (Rapoport et al. 1981; Behar *et al.* 1984). Subsequent studies, utilizing structured neurological examinations, revealed that over 80% of the subjects had minor neurological abnormalities, including left hemisyndrome, neurodevelopmental 'immaturity' and choreiform movements (Denckla 1989). Neuropsychological abnormalities included poor visuospatial skills and abnormal speech prosody (Cox *et al.* 1989). In a group of adult patients with OCD examined by

Hollander *et al.* (1990), increased neuropsychological abnormalities were found to correlate significantly with poor treatment response.

Choreiform movements were also found in one-third of the NIMH paediatric sample (Denckla 1989). The absence of these movements on follow-up examination 2–5 years later has been interpreted to mean that they are a marker of a pathological process aetiological to OCD (Leonard *et al.* 1993). Further support for this postulate comes from recent studies in children with infection-triggered OCD, in which over 90% demonstrated choreiform movements during periods of symptom exacerbation (Swedo *et al.* 1998).

Compulsive personality disorder appears to be less frequent (11%) among paediatric patients (Swedo 1989) than among adult patients (Rasmussen & Tsuang 1984; Black *et al.* 1988), although more systematic studies of personality disorder indicated that the prevalence of compulsive personality disorder in adult OCD patients may be less than previously believed (Joffe *et al.* 1988). Limitations of standardized instruments for assessing personality disorders and the lack of paediatric indication for this diagnosis have obscured this issue. Further, it is possible that compulsive personality disorder may develop as a secondary or adaptive response to very early onset OCD. Evidence supporting this postulate comes from follow-up to the NIMH epidemiological study, which found a number of adolescents no longer met criteria for OCD but did have features of the personality disorder—rigidity, excessive attention to details and social isolation, among others (Berg *et al.* 1989). The boundary is further obscured by a Harvard study of adult patients with OCD which demonstrated that features of the personality disorder remitted with successful treatment of the primary disorder (Ricciardi *et al.* 1992).

Case illustrations

Case 1

A 14-year-old boy, whose symptoms had begun gradually, recalls at a very early age having to wash his hands repetitively. He was unable to associate an obsessive thought with this ritual, but he felt compelled to perform it. By age 6 years he had developed an obsessive fear of tornadoes. He would repeatedly check the sky for clouds, listen to all weather reports and query his mother about approaching storms.

The tornado obsession faded over time and was replaced by a generalized fear of harm coming to himself or his family. He responded with extensive protective ritualization to keep his family safe and to protect himself. Particularly at times of separating, such as bedtime or leaving for school, the patient would be compelled to repeat actions perfectly or to check repetitively. When asked how many times he would have to repeat an action, he replied, 'It depends. The number isn't always the same, I just have to do it *right*.' When asked how he knew when it was right, he said, 'I don't know, it just *feels* right.'

As the patient entered puberty, he became obsessed with

acquired immunodeficiency syndrome (AIDS) and was convinced he would acquire it through his mouth. He began spitting in an effort to cleanse his mouth, and would spit every 15–20 s. In addition, he began extensive washing rituals. Despite these cleansing and washing compulsions, his personal appearance was slovenly and dirty. He never tied his shoelaces because they had touched the ground and were 'contaminated'; if he tied them, his hands would be 'dirty' and he would have to wash until they were 'clean' again. Remarkably, although his family was aware that 'something has been wrong for a long time', most of the content of his obsessions was kept secret. This case illustrates the contamination concerns common to adolescents, and the variety and evolution of obsessive-compulsive symptoms during development.

Case 2

A 16-year-old girl had symptoms that began abruptly, shortly after the onset of menses. She called herself 'a prisoner of my own mind'. Her obsessions centred around fear of harm to her parents. She was plagued by recurrent thoughts of her mother dying in a car accident, her father being killed by an intruder, or both her parents dying of burns received in a house fire. Always a light sleeper, she began to get up during the night to check. She spent hours checking that the doors were locked, that the coffee pot was unplugged, and that the family dog was safely ensconced in the garage. Despite her obsessions about fire, however, she did not check the smoke detector, an excellent example of the irrationality of this superficially rational disorder.

She involved her family in her rituals. Her mother made a checklist that the daughter carried to school, and both parents had to check the 24 items on the list, signing that they had done so. At night she would wake her father to help her check. The family involvement was so profound that behavioural treatment could only take place after a period of family counselling in which the parents were helped to separate from their daughter's illness.

Differential diagnosis

The broad comorbidity of OCD and array of associated features make the diagnosis in theory seem difficult; in practice, however, it is usually quite straightforward.

The diagnosis of OCD must be made only if the 'obsessive worries' are true obsessions, rather than symptoms of another disorder such as depressive ruminations or phobic avoidance. For example, when OCD is comorbid with bulimia or anorexia, the content of the obsessions or compulsions must be typical, e.g. washing, arranging, counting, and not fixed overfocused ideas about food, diet, etc. Depressive ruminations and psychotic preoccupations are also distinguished by content and associated symptomatology. Phobic disorders are not only distinguished by the content of the preoccupation (more often heights, spiders, the dark, etc.), but also by the absence of discomfort when the patient is not confronted with their phobic object. It may be more difficult to separate the obsessional concerns of OCD from the fears and worries of generalized anxiety disorder, particularly in a child with comorbid disorders (Brown *et al.* 1993). Comorbidity of OCD and other anxiety disorders is common, so assigning specific symptoms to a specific disorder may be less important than identifying the presence of OCD in a child presenting with generalized anxiety or separation anxiety disorder.

Asperger disorder can be differentiated from OCD by its lack of ego dystonicity, and in addition, by the content of the preoccupations. For example, in Asperger disorder, concerns about danger or contamination occur only rarely, while these are common among children with OCD. Autistic patients also may exhibit obsessive-compulsive symptoms, but these occur within the context of cognitive and psychosocial abnormalities, and should not be confused with symptoms of OCD.

The differential diagnosis from Tourette is the most problematic, and the relationship between the two disorders remains obscure. Distinguishing between a compulsion or a tic may be difficult, as patients with Tourette syndrome often have a complex behavioural overlay on their tics. Some 20–80% patients with clear Tourette have been reported to have obsessive-compulsive symptoms or OCD (Frankel *et al.* 1986; Pauls *et al.* 1986; Grad *et al.* 1987); while 24–67% of children with primary OCD have been observed to have comorbid tics (Leonard *et al.* 1992; Riddle 1990; Zohar *et al.* 1992). Tics are seen more often in younger patients, those with acute illness and in males (Leonard *et al.* 1992). It is unknown just how the pattern and severity of obsessive-compulsive symptoms differ between patients with Tourette syndrome and those with primary OCD, but preliminary impressions are that compulsions associated with Tourette syndrome may be more likely to involve symmetry, rubbing, staring and blinking rituals, or touching than washing and cleaning (Baer 1994; Holzer *et al.* 1994; Leckman *et al.* 1995) and may be less severe than in non-tic OCD.

The overlapping clinical profiles makes it tempting to speculate that some cases of OCD may represent an alternative form of Tourette disorder and family studies provide partial support for such a construct. In Tourette, there is an increased familial rate of OCD, independent of the presence of obsessive-compulsive symptoms in the proband (Pauls *et al.* 1995). Increased familial rates of Tourette and tics also are seen with OCD probands, particularly for their male relatives (Leonard *et al.* 1992). Any Tourette/OCD formulation, however, is likely to be oversimplified, as both tic disorders and OCD may be manifestations of basal ganglia dysfunction secondary to a number of causes, including genetic, toxic, traumatic and infectious agents.

Theories of aetiology and current research

Psychological factors

Over the past two decades, it has become clear that OCD is not caused solely by psychological factors, as had been posited by Kanner (1962) when he cited 'an "overdose" of parental perfectionism' as the source of obsessional neuroses. Instead, accumulated evidence suggests that OCD is caused by a combination of biological and psychological factors, with both nature and nurture playing a part (Esman 1989). Although no predisposing psychological factors have been identified in OCD (Anna Freud 1965), a role for psychological dysfunction is suggested by the overwhelming anxiety experienced by the patients, and the variable nature of their symptoms. For example, one 10-year-old boy developed an obsessive fear of 'doing something wrong and going to Hell' after hearing a minister preach that 'the wages of sin are eternal damnation'. Another 10-year-old attributed his obsessive fear of vomiting in public to having witnessed a classmate's humiliation. Both boys were able to pinpoint a specific event as the precipitant for their symptom onset, despite acknowledging that 'I know it won't really happen, but I can't stop worrying about it.' A particularly compelling example of post-traumatic OCD was recently reported by Boudreaux et al. (1998) who noted the onset of compulsive hand-washing and genital scrubbing in several patients following instances of rape or incest.

The effectiveness of cognitive-behaviour therapy (CBT) for OCD provides additional evidence of psychological dysfunction in the disorder. CBT is based on a conceptualization of the obsessions as intrusive and unwanted thoughts that trigger a significant and rapid increase in anxiety or distress, and compulsions as ritualized behaviours or cognitions (mental rituals) that serve to reduce the negative feelings (Piacentini 1999). In essence, the anxiety is a 'learned response' to the obsession, and the CBT is a means of teaching a new pattern of response (and 'unlearning' the old one).

Analogies have often been drawn between the obsessions and compulsions of OCD, and normal developmental rituals or superstitions, and several authors have suggested that OCD is merely 'part of typical experience' (Pollock & Carter 1999). The magical thinking and ritualistic behaviours of common superstitions, although brief, ego-syntonic and non-interfering, hold obvious features in common with OCD. Superstitious rituals before sports events are particularly similar to obsessive-compulsive rituals. However, it is not clear what such analogy really implies for OCD. Leonard et al. (1990), for example, found that superstitious beliefs or behaviours of children with OCD were no more severe or numerous than those of normal peers. Moreover, when 'micro episodes' of OCD were removed from consideration, normal childhood developmental rituals also were not exaggerated. A recent report by Evans et al. (1999) confirmed this separation between obsessive fears and 'contextual' fears of normal childhood. Obsessive-compulsive symptoms also appear to be discontinuous from normative cultural rituals and beliefs, with individuals in rural Ghana exhibiting 'typical' OCD cleaning compulsions, despite unique cultural attitudes towards hygiene (Field 1960). Thus, it would appear that OCD is not on a continuum with normal behaviours and beliefs.

Biological factors in OCD

Basal ganglia dysfunction

Understanding the aetiological role of the frontal lobe–basal ganglia circuitry in OCD is one of the most exciting challenges of psychiatry. Clues provided by historical reports of association with basal ganglia disease, brain-imaging techniques such as computed tomography (CT) and positron emission tomography (PET) and results of neurotransmitter and hormonal manipulations must be integrated into a neuropathological framework determined by basic scientific research. For reviews, see Wise & Rapoport (1989), Rapoport (1991) and Fitzgerald et al. (1999).

Association with basal ganglia disorders

The best description of neurologically based OCD comes from Constantin von Economo's treatise (1931) on post-encephalitic Parkinson disease, which followed an outbreak of encephalitis lethargica in 1916–17. Von Economo noted the 'compulsory nature' of the motor tics and ritual-like behaviours that his patients exhibited. Von Economo's patients, like OCD patients, described 'having to' act, while not 'wanting to': they experienced a neurologically based loss of volitional control. The neuropathological examinations revealed primarily basal ganglia destruction.

Basal ganglia dysfunction is also associated with OCD, as evidenced by the increased incidence of motor tics and choreiform movements in children with OCD (Denckla 1989) and the association of obsessive-compulsive symptoms with known basal ganglia disorders, such as Tourette disorder (discussed earlier) and Sydenham chorea (Swedo 1989, 1994). Sydenham chorea (SC), the neurological manifestation of rheumatic fever, is a post-streptococcal 'autoimmune' disorder which affects primarily the basal ganglia. Although the precise pathophysiology of SC is unknown, it is thought that the streptococcal bacteria induce the production of 'cross-reactive' antibodies recognizing the basal ganglia. Husby et al. (1976) demonstrated antibodies in the serum of patients with SC that not only recognized components of the streptococcus cell wall, but also reacted with the cytoplasm of the subthalamic and caudate nuclei. Kiessling et al. (1994) replicated these findings in children with OCD and tic disorders, as well as those with SC.

Osler (1894) was the first to note 'perseverativeness of behaviour' in children with SC. Over 50 years later, Chapman et al. (1958) observed obsessive-compulsive symptoms in 4 of 8 children acutely ill with SC. Grimshaw (1964) and Freeman et al. (1965) extended these findings by demonstrating an increased rate of childhood SC in patients with obsessional neuroses, as compared with other psychiatric disorders. In the late 1980s, the first systematic study of obsessive-compulsive symptoms in SC revealed significantly increased OCD and obsessive-compulsive symptoms in the 23 children with SC, as compared to a group of 14 children with rheumatic carditis (RF) (Swedo et al. 1989a). It is particularly noteworthy that the increase in

Table 35.2 Regional effects of basal ganglia disease and association with obsessive-compulsive disorder (OCD).

Disease	Cause	Basal ganglia area most affected	Most prominent signs	Association with OCD
Sydenham chorea	Autoimmune cross-reaction in streptococcus A/B	Caudate and putamen	Chorea	+++
Huntington chorea	Genetic	Caudate and putamen	Chorea	+
Wilson disease	Genetic	Putamen and caudate	Tremor and rigidity	?
Vascular disease	Vascular	Putamen	Dystonia	+
Parkinson disease				
Idiopathic	Unknown	SNC	Akinetic rigidity	−
Post-encephalitic	Infection	SNC	Akinetic rigidity	++
Seqawa dystonia	Genetic	Unknown	Dystonia	++
Tourette disorder	Genetic	Unknown	Motor/vocal tics	+++

compulsive behaviours and obsessive thoughts occurred selectively in the SC patients, as SC differs from RF only in the presence of basal ganglia dysfunction in SC and its absence in RF. Prospective studies have confirmed these findings, demonstrating obsessive-compulsive symptoms occur in two-thirds (Asbahr et al. 1999) to three-quarters of SC patients (Swedo 1994). Interestingly, the obsessive-compulsive symptoms appear to begin 2–4 weeks before the chorea appears, and wax and wane in severity in association with the choreatic movements, suggesting that the basal ganglia inflammation producing the SC also might be responsible for the OCD.

As seen in Table 35.2, a number of basal ganglia disorders are associated with OCD. Specific basal ganglia lesions in individuals also have resulted in obsessive-compulsive behaviours (Laplane et al. 1984; Rapoport 1991). Indirect evidence for basal ganglia involvement in OCD is provided by the efficacy of psychosurgical lesions which serve to disconnect the basal ganglia from the frontal cortex (Chiocca & Martuzza 1990; Mindus 1991; Jenike 1998). Currently, the preferred psychosurgeries for OCD are capsulotomy and cingulectomy. In capsulotomy, bilateral basal lesions are made in the anterior limb of the internal capsule in order to interrupt frontocingulate projections; however, the surgical target lies within the striatum, near the caudate nuclei. In order to perform a cingulectomy, the surgeon lesions the anterior portion of the cingulate gyrus, interrupting tracks between the cingulate gyrus and the frontal lobes and destroying all of the efferent projections of the anterior cingulate cortex. Both procedures result in significant reduction of obsessions and compulsions. The success of psychosurgery is not conclusive evidence of a basal ganglia defect in OCD, as the lesions could be anywhere 'upstream' from the site of treatment, but it does contribute to a biological model and focuses interest on frontostriatal tracts.

Perhaps the best evidence for basal ganglia–frontal lobe dysfunction in OCD comes from neuroimaging studies (for reviews see Rauch & Baxter 1998 or Fitzgerald et al. 1999). Structural brain imaging studies have revealed volumetric abnormalities in frontostriatal circuitry, particularly in the caudate (Luxenberg et al. 1988), putamen (Rosenberg et al. 1997) and globus pallidus (Giedd et al. 2000). Of note, Giedd et al. (2000) studied children in the PANDAS subgroup during acute symptom exacerbations and found increased volumes of the basal ganglia structures, while Luxenberg et al.'s (1988) study demonstrated decreased caudate size in a group of 10 young adult males with early childhood onset of symptoms. One possible explanation for these findings is that the early basal ganglia enlargements reflect inflammatory oedema, while the later studies are reflecting the resultant 'atrophy'. Although some evidence supporting this hypothesis is provided by a single case study which demonstrated normalization of basal ganglia volumes following immunomodulatory treatment (Giedd et al. 1996), further supportive data are needed.

Functional neuroimaging studies utilizing 18-flurodeoxyglucose positron emission tomography ([18]FDG PET) have found regional glucose metabolism in OCD to be elevated in the orbital frontal cortex, cingulate gyri and/or caudate nuclei of the OCD patient groups (see Rauch et al. 1997 for review). These metabolic abnormalities 'normalize' with successful drug or behaviour therapy (Baxter et al. 1992; Swedo et al. 1992b) and are exacerbated by tasks stimulating obsessive-compulsive symptomatology (Rauch et al. 1994, 1997). These findings are consistent with the hypothesized basal ganglia–frontal lobe dysfunction of OCD (Wise & Rapoport 1989; Insel 1992). Moreover, the findings are both replicable and the particular pattern appears specific to OCD (Baxter et al. 1987).

Although the evidence for basal ganglia–frontal lobe dysfunction in OCD is compelling, it fails to account for the behavioural specificity of the disorder—why washers wash and checkers check. It also fails to explain the varied patterns of comorbidity, ranging from generalized anxiety and depression to attention deficits and Tourette disorder. Despite these limitations, the notion of obsessive and compulsive behaviour as an expression of basal ganglia dysfunction has been most useful, accounting for a wide variety of observations and predicting others.

Genetic vulnerabilities

Despite the relatively high prevalence of OCD, and the fact

that the role of heredity in OCD has long been suspected by clinicians (Lewis 1936), genetic studies of this disorder have lagged behind those of other major neuropsychiatric disorders. The results of published twin studies are consistent in reporting substantive concordance differences between monozygotic and dizygotic twins, although the total number of twins studied is small, and there are no adoption and separation studies. There are more family studies of OCD (Lenane et al. 1990), and the two largest and most methodologically rigorous found that the risk of OCD was substantially greater in the parents of OCD probands compared to the parents of controls (16 vs. 3%) (Black et al. 1992), and that the risk of OCD was overall greater in the first-degree relatives of OCD patients compared to the relatives of psychiatrically assessed controls (10 vs. 1.9%) (Pauls et al. 1995).

There are two published segregation analyses of OCD. Nicolini et al. (1991) studied 24 families of probands with OCD and Cavalini et al. (1995, 1999) performed segregation analysis on families of 92 OCD probands. Nicolini et al. (1991) concluded that their family data are most consistent with a highly penetrant dominant major gene, although the affected phenotype under analysis included disorders other than OCD (hypothesized, but not tested, as aetiologically related to OCD). The segregation models were consistent with a gene or genes of major effect, although the mode of inheritance was not established. The findings of Cavalini et al. (1999), using a much larger sample and an analysis focused solely on OCD, were consistent with a complex genetic model which included a significant single major locus intermediate in nature (neither dominant nor recessive).

Most studies report a lack of association of candidate genetic variants with OCD (note that most of these used the relatively weak population-based design susceptible to population stratification artefacts), including one that examined the coding region of the tryptophan hydroxylase gene in OCD patients (Han et al. 1999). Another study, examining a functional variant of the catechol-O-methyltransferase (*COMT*) gene, found an association that was stronger in male than female OCD patients (Karayiorgou et al. 1997).

It is likely that the genetics of childhood onset OCD will be found to be closely related to the genetics of Tourette disorder. A number of studies have demonstrated increased rates of both OCD and tic disorders in first-degree relatives of probands with OCD (reviewed in Pauls & Alsobrook 1999), and also for relatives of probands with Tourette disorder (Pauls et al. 1991). Given this overlap, and the frequent comorbidity of tics and obsessive-compulsive symptoms, it is likely that what is 'transmitted' between generations is the OCD/Tourette disorder pattern, rather than a particular OCD subtype. In fact, Pauls et al. (1986, 1991) have hypothesized that the two disorders may not be separate, but rather are alternate expressions of the same genetic defect(s). However, a number of well-designed studies have failed to identify the gene(s) responsible. This may be caused, at least in part, by our lack of meaningful phenotypic separations. For example, the children in the PANDAS subgroup were found to have increased rates of familial OCD and tic disorders similar

to those reported for other paediatric samples (Lougee et al., 2000), despite their presumed post-infectious aetiology. The families were also notable for increased rates of immunological disorders and rheumatic fever (unpublished data), suggesting that we can expect genetic heterogeneity within the early onset cases.

Serotonin and other neurotransmitters

The serotonergic hypothesis of OCD comes from the selective efficacy of drugs that have specific serotonergic activity (Insel et al. 1985), and challenge tests with metacholorophenyl-piperazine (mCPP), a serotonergic agonist (Murphy et al. 1989; Pigott et al. 1991). Challenges with mCPP (Zohar et al. 1987, 1988; Pigott et al. 1991) show that OCD symptoms may be exacerbated by this serotonin agonist; metergoline, a serotonin antagonist, may protect against mCPP's behavioural effects (Pigott et al. 1991).

Medications that block serotonin reuptake, such as the selective serotonin reuptake inhibitors (SSRIs) fluoxetine, fluvoxamine, sertraline, paroxetine and citalopram, have been shown to be the most effective pharmacological treatments for OCD (see section on Drug Treatment). Clomipramine is a tricyclic antidepressant which is a *relatively* selective and potent inhibitor of active serotonin uptake in the brain (it also blocks histamine H_2-receptors, cholinergic and β-receptors, and has antidopaminergic properties). Its metabolite, desmethyl-clomipramine, also effectively blocks serotonin reuptake. The response of childhood OCD to clomipramine and not to the equally effective antidepressant desipramine (Leonard et al. 1989) indicates a remarkable specificity of effect for the serotonin uptake inhibitors for this condition. No unselected group of depressed patients, for example, would show such a differential response. Thus, the profile of drug response in OCD differs from that seen in depression or anxiety disorders which respond to a broad array of antidepressants and antianxiety agents and which highlight a unique role for serotonin blockers in this disorder.

Additional evidence for the serotonergic hypothesis is provided by several studies in children and adolescents with OCD. The first, conducted by Flament et al. (1985, 1987), demonstrated that response to clomipramine correlated with pretreatment platelet serotonin concentration. A high pretreatment level of serotonin was a strong predictor of clinical response and, within this sample, platelet serotonin concentrations were lower in the more severely ill patients. However, there were no differences in serotonin concentration from age- and sex-matched controls. A study of cerebrospinal fluid monoamines in 43 children and adolescents with OCD revealed that 5-hydroxyindole acetic acid, the major matabolite of serotonin, correlated most strongly with response to clomipramine therapy: the most successful responders had the highest levels of 5-hydroxyindole acetic acid in the cerebrospinal fluid (Swedo et al. 1992a). A more recent study, employing PET and serotonergic ligands, found evidence for decreased serotonin synthesis in

Table 35.3 Selected studies of cognitive-behaviour therapy for obsessive-compulsive disorder (OCD) in children and adolescents.

Study	*n*	Age range	Methods	Comments

Piacentini *et al.* (1994)	3	9–13	Psychoeducation for child and family
			Concurrent family sessions
			  to disengage family from the OCD
			10 2-h sessions weekly
				All improved
				Gains maintained at
				  1 year follow-up

March *et al.* (1994)	15	8–18	Initial education re OCD
			  as an illness
			Anxiety management
			  training + ERP
			Parent training diaries
				14 also on drug
				10/15 had ≥ 50% improvement
				3 non-responders

Scahill *et al.* (1996)	7	10–15	Visits 1–4
			Self monitoring,
			  triggering stimuli ranked,
			  hierarchy established
			Visits 5–13
			ERP (child selects provoking stimuli)
			Child and parent education weekly
			Families as cotherapists and informants
				5/7 on drug
				All improved
				  (30–90%)
				14 sessions, mostly weekly
				Booster sessions within
				  6 months post-Rx

Wever & Rey (1997)	82	7–19	Training therapists
			Family/child workbook
			Family as cotherapist
			Modified to fit patient's cognitive/
			  developmental level
			Taped exposure to obsessions
			10 sessions across 2 weeks,
			  then monthly reviews across 6 months,
			  then 6-monthly follow-ups
				57 had combined treatment of
				  which 22 (39%) weaned off
				  drugs

Franklin *et al.* (1998)	14	10–17	Non-random assignment 7: weekly Rx over 4 months 7: 18 sessions over 1 month Parental involvement or individualized	8 on concurrent drugs 12/14 had 50% reduction in Y-BOC score Both weekly and daily sessions effective Maintained at 9 months follow-up

ERP, exposure with response prevention; Y-BOC, Yale–Brown Obsessive Compulsive Scale.

the ventral prefrontal cortex and caudate nucleus in treatment naïve OCD patients aged 8–13 years (Rosenberg *et al.* 1998). The latter study provides support for both the serotonergic hypothesis of OCD, and also for dysfunction within the basal ganglia–frontal cortex circuitry.

The serotonergic hypothesis is undoubtedly too simplistic to account for the complexity of OCD. If the defect were limited to serotonergic dysfunction, clomipramine and the SSRIs should be effective in eliminating symptoms in all patients; unfortunately, this is not the case. The medications are quite effective for many patients with OCD, but usually cause only partial symptom remission. Different patients also have different patterns of response, suggesting that the non-serotonergic properties of the medications may also have key roles, and that the antiobsessional effect may actually result from an alteration in the balance of serotonin and other monoamines, and/or changes in receptor functions (Murphy *et al.* 1989).

Other neurotransmitters

Dopaminergic dysfunction in OCD is suggested not only by the obsessive-compulsive symptoms in patients with basal ganglia disorders (Table 35.3), but also by the increase in obsessive-compulsive symptoms following high-dose stimulant administration (Frye & Arnold 1981), and occasional amelioration of symptoms following dopamine-blocking agents (Goodman *et al.* 1990; McDougle 1997). High-dose stimulant administration has been thought to result in simple stereotypies, rather than in more complex compulsive or obsessive behaviour; however, 'compulsive' symptoms following high-dose amfetamines have been observed in children with attention deficit disorder and hyperactivity (ADHD; Borcherding *et al.* 1990), particularly compulsive ritualization with high-dose *d*-amfetamine (1 mg/kg) and methylphenidate (2 mg/kg) administration. For example, a 7-year-old boy spent several hours each evening vacuuming the carpet in his home, and another played with Lego blocks for 2 days, stopping only to eat and sleep. As in OCD, these children may become overly concerned with details and erase holes in their papers trying to get a single letter perfectly shaped. However, the obsessive-compulsive behaviours are not ego-dystonic in these stimulant-induced cases, leading to speculation that repetitive thoughts and behaviours (obsessions and compulsions) may result from dopaminergic overactivity and that serotonin dysregulation is required for ego dystonicity.

Tourette disorder and OCD may be at opposite ends of a spectrum of dopamine–serotonin disequilibrium. In Tourette disorder, dopaminergic overactivity overcomes serotonergic inhibition and results primarily in motor and vocal tics. By contrast, OCD is primarily a serotonergic defect. Here, a primary lack of serotonin results in an inability to inhibit normal dopaminergic activity and fixed action patterns (obsessions and compulsions) are inappropriately released. Ego dystonicity could then be related to the primary serotonin defect, or secondary to the loss of volitional control (Swedo & Rapoport 1990).

Neuroendocrine dysfunction

Although most OCD investigations concentrate on hormonal aberrations as secondary rather than primary to the disorder, case reports and anecdotal experience suggest that hormonal dysfunction and OCD may be aetiologically related (Swedo 1989). OCD symptoms often begin during early puberty, and some female patients experience an increase in obsessive thoughts and rituals immediately before their menses. Other hints at an influence of gonadal steroid on obsessive-compulsive symptomatology include the increased frequency of OCD during the post-partum period (Rasmussen & Eisen 1992), and reports of successful antiandrogen therapy for obsessive-compulsive symptoms (Casas et al. 1986). In the latter study, 5 out of 5 patients with OCD experienced a remission in their symptoms following treatment with cyproterone acetate, a potent antiandrogen. At the NIMH, two boys (ages 8 and 15) and a 14-year-old girl were treated with spironolactone, a peripheral antiandrogen particularly antitesterone agent, and testolactone, a peripheral antioestrogen medication. All experienced a temporary reduction of obsessions and compulsions, but relapsed within 3–4 months (Salzberg & Swedo 1992).

Leckman et al. (1994) have suggested that oxytocin abnormalities may be involved in OCD, citing oxytocin-mediated mating behaviours in animals as a possible model (Leckman & Mayes 1999), and finding abnormal concentrations of oxytocin in cerebrospinal fluid oxytocin from a small group of children with OCD and tic disorders. In a larger group of 43 children and adolescents studied at the NIMH (Swedo et al. 1992a), cerebrospinal fluid oxytocin levels were not significantly correlated with OCD severity, but were correlated with depressive symptoms. Interestingly, arginine vasopressin concentrations were inversely related to OCD severity, and decreased following treatment with clomipramine (Altemus et al. 1994).

At present, there is not sufficient evidence to implicate hormonal dysfunction as a direct cause of OCD. However, some intriguing data build a circumstantial case for an association between OCD and growth hormone abnormalities, perhaps through the serotonergic system. In the epidemiological study of OCD in high school students cited earlier (Flament et al. 1988), males with OCD were noted to be smaller and lighter than the community normal controls and males with other psychiatric illnesses (Hamburger et al. 1989). There were no differences in the size of females with and without OCD. The small size of the OCD males could result from an effective lack of growth hormone, or from a delay in the pubertal growth spurt, although no causality is demonstrated by the relationship. To address the issue of causality, future studies might employ direct assays, hormonal challenges or therapeutic interventions.

Treatment approaches

Family education

Treatment begins with family education about the disorder. Parents need guidance about how to handle their child's behaviours, which may be severely disruptive to family life, and how to avoid punitive responses or the alternative 'enabling' that happens when families become enmeshed in rituals. Suggested readings for families include *OCD in Children and Adolescents: a Cognitive-Behavioural Treatment Manual* (March & Mulle 1998), which is commonly used by practitioners in the USA and other countries. (The original version of this manual was entitled *How I Ran OCD Off My Land*.)

In Europe, as well as in the USA, various OCD patient groups provide information, advocacy for services, and support for both patients and parents. The groups also provide children with an opportunity to meet others with OCD, which is important in dispelling the sense that the child is the 'only one' affected by the disorder. Over the past decade, support groups have added considerably to the care of OCD and should be considered for all cases. For a model support group, see Black & Blum (1992). In the USA, the Obsessive-Compulsive Foundation (North Branford, CT) provides such information and support. On the Internet, www.ocdresource.com is a useful source of information about the disorder, including community resources and lists of relevant publications.

School

Certain perfectionistic and repeating rituals may impair school performance. For example, the need to form letters or numbers 'perfectly' or a compulsion to reread sentences or entire paragraphs may stop the child from completing assignments. In some cases, special arrangements with the school need to be made, such as allowing the child untimed tests or doing alternate projects (Shafron 1998). Occasionally, teachers may be helpful in the child's behavioural programme.

Choosing a therapy

In adults, behavioural and drug treatments have been shown to be effective for OCD, both singly and in combination. Several excellent reviews have been published recently for both behavioural treatment (Marks 1997) and drug therapy (Pato *et al.* 1998; Pigott & Seay 1999). Behavioural treatment is now being used successfully in children (March 1995; Shafron 1998), although drug treatment remains more commonly used (DeVane & Sallee 1996; Emslie *et al.* 1999).

The choice of first-line treatment will depend on the symptom pattern and severity, as well as the patient and family's preference. Whatever is tried, it is important to urge flexibility, as a combination of drug and behavioural treatment may be needed (Greist 1996; Park *et al.* 1997; Wever & Rey 1997; O'Connor *et al.* 1999; see Rapoport & Inoff-Germain 2000 for review).

Cognitive-behavioural therapy

Since an earlier review (Wolff & Rapoport 1988), there have been extensive reports on how to adapt these techniques to paediatric OCD populations. These are summarized in Table 35.3, and are discussed in relevant sections of the text.

CBT for OCD encompasses three treatment types:

1 exposure and response prevention (ERP);
2 cognitive therapy, and
3 relaxation training.

Of the three, ERP is in the forefront for effectiveness in symptom reduction (Baer & Greist 1997; Shafron 1998). Cognitive therapy (e.g. changing false beliefs regarding risk and responsibility, challenging the reality of obsessions and the necessity for compulsions; Emmelkamp & Beens 1991) is generally viewed as ineffective as a *sole* treatment for OCD, although it may be helpful in individual cases and if it encourages exposure in a broader CBT programme (Shafran & Somers 1998). Relaxation therapy is used mainly to manage affect during exposure (March 1995) but it has no direct benefits for the obsessive-compulsive symptoms.

ERP for OCD was developed in adults, and the methodology is still undergoing regular refinement (March 1995; Greist 1996). It involves:

1 daily exposure to cues avoided because of their inducing discomfort and rituals; and
2 maintaining exposure and not ritualizing for at least an hour or until the discomfort slowly subsides.

A minimal trial consists of 10–20 h of treatment with ERP (Baer & Greist 1997), with *in vivo* (as opposed to fantasy) exposure being optimal (Foa *et al.* 1985). Although gains from ERP persist beyond its discontinuation, booster treatment may help for long-term progress, and additional treatment may be needed for migration of symptoms and for lapses brought on by stress (Greist 1996).

Because most clinicians are not trained in behavioural treatment and because of its expense, interactive computer-administered self-assessment and self-help programmes for behaviour therapy (e.g. BT-STEPS; Baer & Greist 1997) may be useful (see also Clark *et al.* 1998 for a pilot study of computer-assisted ERP in adults) as it can be used by anyone having a touch telephone. No report of computer-assisted ERP with adolescents has yet appeared but, for some, this could be a particularly promising approach.

ERP has been adapted for use with children, and appears to confer similar benefits in the paediatric population as in adults (March 1995; Greist 1996; Marks 1997; King *et al.* 1998; March & Mulle 1998; Shafran 1998). The child's ability to understand the treatment and tolerate the intensity of affect are important considerations (Shafran 1998). Programmes that help the child to externalize the OCD help to empower the child and decrease his or her anxiety, as does allowing the child control over the gradient for exposure to anxiety-provoking stimuli (see March & Mulle 1998 for more details).

CBT must be tailored to specific symptoms; for example, ERP is not generally appropriate for scrupulosity and moral guilt or pathological doubt, where cognitive therapy may be helpful. Contamination fears, symmetry rituals, counting/repeating, hoarding, and aggressive urges are more amenable to ERP. Obsessional slowness appears not to respond well to either behavioural or pharmacotherapy (Wolff & Rapoport 1988). Pure obsessions are also difficult to treat with CBT, although cognitive therapy strategies that help the adolescent patient obtain benign interpretations of intrusive thoughts may be useful (Shafron & Somers 1998).

Although none of the behavioural studies described above is truly systematic and controlled, they provided sufficient evidence (March *et al.* 1994) to justify a comprehensive study of the effectiveness of CBT in paediatric OCD populations. An ongoing random-assignment collaborative treatment trial being carried out by Drs Edna B. Foa (University of Pennsylvania, PA, USA) and John March (Duke University, NC, USA) comparing CBT, drug therapy, their combination, and placebo, is now in its third year. Importantly, there will be a sizeable group without concurrent drug treatment, and outcome ratings are 'blind' to treatment condition. These data will be essential for guiding future treatment in children with OCD.

Drug treatment

The recent attention of psychiatry to drug treatment of OCD is unique in that much of the early work was carried out with children (Rapoport 1998). Subsequent adult studies demonstrated the utility of a variety of serotonergic agents for OCD. Although the paediatric trials of SSRIs have lagged behind those in adults, there is now extensive substantiation of the utility of pharmacotherapy in paediatric patients (see also Heyman & Santosh, Chapter 59).

An initial trial of a serotonin reuptake inhibitor (SRI), most often an SSRI, is the treatment of choice. If there is no or only partial response to an SSRI at 10–12 weeks, another SSRI may be tried. In adults, augmentation with other agents is effective in

Table 35.4 Pharmacological treatment for obsessive-compulsive disorder.

Drug	Adult dosage	Child/adolescent dosage from controlled study (or best available information)	Duration (weeks)
First-line agents			
Clomipramine	Up to 250 mg/day	Up to 150–200 mg/day* (3 mg/kg upper limit)	>10
Fluoxetine	Up to 100 mg/day	20 mg/day†	>10
Fluvoxamine	Up to 300 mg/day	Up to 200 mg/day‡	>10
Sertraline	Up to 200 mg/day	Up to 200 mg/day§	>10
Paroxetine	Up to 60 mg/day	Not known¶	>10
Augmenting agents			
Clonazepam	Up to 5 mg/day	Not known	>4
Haloperidol	Up to 3 mg/day	(Up to 2 mg/day)**	>3
Risperidone	(0.5–2.0 mg/day)	(1.5–2.5 mg/day)††	?

* DeVeaugh-Geiss *et al.* (1992).
† Riddle *et al.* (1992).
‡ Riddle *et al.* (1996).
§ March *et al.* (1998).
¶ Study in progress.
** J.L. Rapoport, personal communication, 1999.
†† Lombroso *et al.* (1995).

partial responders, and some reports suggest augmentors are also useful for children.

Serotonin reuptake inhibitors

Clomipramine was the first SRI antidepressant shown to be effective for OCD, with subsequent controlled trials documenting antiobsessional effects of the SSRIs—(in order of increasing selectivity), fluoxetine, fluvoxamine, sertraline and paroxetine. All have been studied in multicentre double-blind trials in adults (Pigott & Seay 1999). Citalopram has been found to be effective for OCD in adults (Montgomery *et al.* 2001), but this is not yet a labelled indication. Controlled trials with children have been carried out for clomipramine, fluoxetine, fluvoxamine and sertraline (Table 35.4). Although the comparable study of paroxetine in children is still in progress, uncontrolled reports are also positive (Emslie *et al.* 1999).

Table 35.4 gives the dosage range of SRIs for adults, the most systematically obtained dosage data for children, and the recommended duration for a treatment trial. Low initial doses, with slow upward titration, are the rule. Patients should be told that trials of more than one agent may be needed, and the possibility of augmenting agents also should be suggested early. Not only may it be necessary to switch from one serotonin inhibitor to another, but combinations of SRIs seem to help counterbalance differing adverse effects, although no systematic studies are available to document this widely held clinical belief (see below).

Augmenting strategies for partial responders

Up to 50% of child (and adult) cases show no or only partial response to initial SRI treatment, even if two different SRIs are used (Geller *et al.* 1998). Because of this, a variety of treatment modifications and augmentation strategies have evolved (see Rasmussen & Eisen 1997 for a review).

Augmentation of SRIs with other agents

There have been no randomized allocation trials of the utility of augmentation strategies for paediatric OCD. However, based on positive results in adult patients, augmentation of an SRI might be considered for paediatric patients with a partial response or intolerance to higher doses. In adults, two agents, clonazepam (Pigott *et al.* 1992) and haloperidol (McDougle *et al.* 1994) have been shown effective in controlled augmentation trials (see McDougle 1997 for a review).

Clonazepam is a benzodiazepine with anxiolytic properties and serotonergic effects (Pigott *et al.* 1992; Park *et al.* 1997; March & Leonard 1998). Clonazepam augmentation in childhood onset OCD has been described for a patient with onset of OCD symptoms at age 7 years but who, other than psychotherapy, had no treatment for OCD until age 14 (Leonard *et al.* 1994). A variety of drug treatments, including buspirone augmentation, had been tried. At age 20, clonazepam (at dosage gradually increasing to 6 mg/day) was instituted as an augmentor to fluoxetine (60 mg/day). Dramatic reduction in symptom severity was reported within 1 month and was maintained by 4 mg/day, as evaluated 1 year later.

Neuroleptic augmentation has been shown to be particularly useful in cases with comorbid tic disorders. *Haloperidol* has been reported to have significant benefits as an augmentor for adult patients with tics or a family history of tics (McDougle *et al.* 1994). Paediatric experience with haloperidol has been limited in OCD, although it is used frequently in children and adolescents with tic disorders. Because of the long-term risks of neuroleptics administration, these should only be considered if atypical antipsychotics, such as risperidone, are ineffective.

Two controlled trials have documented the utility of *risperidone augmentation* of SSRIs among adult refractory OCD patients (McDougle *et al.* 1995; Ravizza *et al.* 1996). Risperidone augmentation in paediatric OCD requires further study (Mandoki 1995). However, risperidone was used in an 11-week open trial (Lombroso *et al.* 1995) for treatment of Tourette Disorder (TD) tics in seven children and adolescents, three of whom also had OCD. One of these three had a 100% decrease in her OCD symptom severity—as measured by her endpoint Children's Yale–Brown Obsessive Compulsive Scale (CY-BOCS) score, compared to baseline—the other two had slight but not significant improvements. These three (ages: 12, 13 and 16) were given a SRI and risperidone (1.5–2.5 mg/day). The risperidone was added to their concurrent SRI at 0.5 mg orally at bedtime, with scheduled increases of 0.5 mg every 5 days as tolerated, up to a maximum of 2.5 mg/day in divided doses. The maintenance dose was generally achieved by 3 weeks and given on a twice-daily schedule. Weight gain ranging from 3.5 to 6.5 kg occurred in all patients.

Addition of a second concurrent SRI has been used as an augmenting strategy in adults (Ravizza *et al.* 1998) and, to a limited extent, in children. In an open treatment trial of six adolescents (Simeon *et al.* 1990), combined fluoxetine and clomipramine allowed lower dosage of both medicines and produced fewer side-effects. Figueroa *et al.* (1998) described an open series of seven patients, aged 9–23, given clomipramine and either fluoxetine, sertraline, fluvoxamine or paroxetine and followed through 5–22 months. Combination therapy appeared more effective than monotherapy for all cases, but double-blind controlled studies are needed.

Maintenance treatment

OCD is often chronic and long-term maintenance is to be anticipated. For example, in a 9–14 year follow-up study of 15 cases initially treated for OCD in adolescence (primarily with behaviour and family therapy), 43% still met diagnostic criteria for OCD (Bolton *et al.* 1995). In adults, long-term improvement is maintained on drugs and lower doses may suffice (Ravizza *et al.* 1998). For such patients, drug discontinuation leads to relapse in 80% of cases at 2-year follow-up (Dolberg *et al.* 1996). However, concomitant CBT may lead to medication discontinuation for some patients (Stanley & Turner 1995; Wever & Rey 1997).

In children, the need for long-term maintenance was documented by an 8-month study of 26 children and adolescents with severe OCD who had received clomipramine for a mean of 17.1 months (Leonard *et al.* 1991); a 2-month double-blind desipramine substitution resulted in 89% of the substituted (vs. 18% of the non-substituted) subjects relapsing during the substitution phase.

When discontinuation is attempted, tapering should be gradual, usually over several weeks. Long-term (indefinite) drug maintenance is suggested after 2–4 relapses.

Adverse effects of drug treatment

The SSRIs are recommended over clomipramine because of the anticholinergic, cardiovascular, sexual and sedative effects of the tricyclic. Clomipramine may be helpful when a tricyclic antidepressant may benefit other psychiatric comorbidities, and it is also less likely than SSRIs to cause insomnia, akathisia, nausea or diarrhoea (March & Leonard 1998; Riddle 1998; Thomsen 1998). Because clomipramine has the potential for tricyclic antidepressant (TCA)-related cardiotoxic effects, monitoring is recommended (Geller *et al.* 1999).

The side-effects of SSRIs are generally well-tolerated, and include drowsiness or insomnia, nausea, weight gain, agitation and a host of less common events that should be reviewed with the patient and family. While most adverse events occur within the first months of treatment, they can occur at any time. It is important for the family to be aware of this so that they remain vigilant to potentially adverse effects of the medications.

For excellent reviews on the safety of SRIs see:
Clomipramine (DeVeaugh-Geiss *et al.* 1992; Geller *et al.* 1999)
Fluoxetine (Riddle *et al.* 1992; Geller *et al.* 1995)
Fluvoxamine (Riddle *et al.* 1996; Goodman *et al.* 1997)
Sertraline (March *et al.* 1998; Alderman *et al.* 1996, 1998)
Paroxetine (Gunasekara *et al.* 1998).

Augmenting agents

There is concern over dependency on clonazepam, although at the low dosage used (see Table 35.2), this is rare. While haloperidol raises the concern of risk for tardive dyskinesia, the very low dosage (often as low as 0.5 mg/day) and yearly 6-week drug holidays reduce this risk. Atypical agents, such as risperidone, may not be quite as effective augmenting agents for OCD and have their own risks of drowsiness and weight gain (Lombroso *et al.* 1995). In paediatric cases, risperidone may be more likely to cause dystonic reactions (Lombroso *et al.* 1995).

Drug treatment and comorbidities

Mania

SSRIs can appear to trigger manic symptoms in adults (Berk *et al.* 1996) and children (Go *et al.* 1998; Diller & Avci 1999) treated for OCD. Alternately, a subgroup of OCD cases may be 'prebipolar', independent of drug treatment. Additional investigation is needed to understand when such cases reflect drug effects or the unmasking of underlying bipolar mood disorder (Berk *et al.* 1996).

Attention deficit hyperactivity disorder

The high rate of comorbid ADHD means that stimulant drug treatment may be ongoing during OCD treatment. There is some evidence that stimulants may have an adverse effect on OCD (Joffe *et al.* 1991), even triggering some compulsive or ritualistic behaviours (Borcherding *et al.* 1990). Thus, stimulants should be used with caution, and only in cases where other treatments for the ADHD symptoms are not indicated.

Psychosis

Patients with schizophrenia being treated with clozapine (Baker *et al.* 1992) or risperidone (see Saxena *et al.* 1996 and SRI augmentation section above) may have exacerbation of OCD; addition of typical neuroleptics may alleviate this complication (Baker *et al.* 1992; Patel & Tandon 1993).

Tic disorders

Tic disorders will often necessitate trials of dopamine-blocking agents. However, these may worsen anxiety symptoms (Blin 1999) and will have to be discontinued. The data on clonidine, which would be a logical alternative, are mixed (Hollander *et al.* 1991; Hewlett *et al.* 1992).

Substance abuse

OCD may be either worsened or alleviated by drugs of abuse and alcohol (Delgado & Moreno 1998; Crum & Anthony 1993; Burke *et al.* 1994; Fals-Stewart & Angarano 1994; Bolla *et al.* 1998). Where suspected or when the patient is non-responsive, substance abuse should be considered and may need to be the prime target of treatment.

Investigative treatments

Tramadol: an opioid agonist

Recent research suggests that OCD may be, in part, mediated by the opioid system (Insel & Pickar 1983; Shapira *et al.* 1997). Because the opioid antagonist naloxone exacerbates OCD in some patients, an open trial of the opioid agonist tramadol was carried out for seven treatment-refractory adult OCD patients (with a variety of comorbidities including tics or TD) (Shapira *et al.* 1997). Six of the seven cases completed at least 2 weeks of treatment, with mean dosage of 25 mg/day tramadol (in 3–4 divided doses), and all six reported a diminution in obsessive thoughts and in the urge to perform their compulsions. One, who had a history of panic attacks, discontinued medication during week 6 after experiencing a panic attack. The dose-limiting side-effect was sedation, but the drug was generally

well tolerated in this small group of adult patients. There are no paediatric data available. It is interesting that although the primary action of tramadol is as an opioid agonist, it also inhibits the reuptake of norepinephrine and serotonin, which may contribute to its effectiveness in OCD. If the results of the Shapira *et al.*'s (1997) trial are replicated, and the mechanism of action is shown to be distinct from the SRIs, tramadol may prove valuable for use in OCD.

Intravenous clomipramine

Recent research in adults (Sallee *et al.* 1997, 1998) including one placebo controlled study (Fallon *et al.* 1998) indicates that intravenous administration both speeds initial response and converts non-responders. Oral maintenance is still required. The hypothesized mechanism involves the greater bioavailability of the more serotonergic parent compound clomipramine vs. the more noradrenergic metabolite desmethylclomipramine, as a result of bypassing first-pass hepatoenteric metabolism.

In children, there have been a few small open trials of intravenous clomipramine use in adolescents with depression, or depression and OCD. In the first study, three of the five cases (age range 16–19 years) studied had OCD as well as major depressive disorder, and parenteral clomipramine infusions of up to 200 mg/dose (1 mg/min) were administered without major adverse incident (Sallee *et al.* 1989). One patient terminated the infusion as a result of nausea and vomiting. Two others had nausea after an initial 75 mg test dose during the first 15–20 min of infusion, but not during the second infusion (on night 2) of 200 mg. Drowsiness and sedation up to 18 h later were also reported. In addition to amelioration of depression, the three with concurrent OCD had an immediate decrease in obsessive-compulsive symptoms. Follow-up at 6 months (on 350 mg/day clomipramine) showed continued amelioration of OCD symptoms and no signs of depression.

In a later controlled trial, two of 16 adolescents had OCD among their comorbidities; one of these was in the single-dose 200 mg intravenous clomipramine treatment group. This case showed a decrease in depression and a 50% decrease in Y-BOCS score by the sixth day (Sallee *et al.* 1997). These reports justify systematic paediatric studies of intravenous clomipramine; however, at present, the treatment remains experimental.

Immunomodulatory therapies

For the PANDAS subgroup, the aetiology of the OCD symptoms is presumed to be related to inflammation in the basal ganglia. This postulate led to a trial of two immunomodulatory agents: intravenous immunoglobulin (IVIG) and plasma exchange (PEX) for severe acutely ill children with streptococcal-triggered OCD and tic disorders (Perlmutter *et al.* 1999). A total of 29 children (age 5–14) received IVIG ($n=9$), PEX ($n=10$), or placebo IVIG ($n=10$). At both 1 and 12 months after therapy, the results indicated striking and sustained improvement on active treatment, with virtually no placebo effect. In some cases, these improvements were paralleled by reduction in basal ganglia volume (Giedd *et al.* 2000). While these results are exciting, they await replication before being recommended as standard therapy for severely ill children in the PANDAS subgroup. Further, it should be noted that PEX produced no improvements in a group of five children and adolescents with chronic treatment-refractory OCD with *no* evidence of post-streptococcal exacerbation (Nicholson *et al.* 2000). Clearly, the immunomodulatory therapies will not be useful in all cases of childhood onset OCD, and it is unclear how many children belong in the PANDAS subgroup.

At present, the PANDAS subgroup is defined by clinical criteria—no biological markers have been identified that can reliably distinguish children with post-streptococcal OCD or tic disorders. The children in the PANDAS subgroup have an abrupt prepubertal onset of symptoms; the acuity of onset and symptom exacerbations is in striking contrast to the typical OCD patient's gradual onset and waxing and waning symptom course. Because medical records often fail to document a relationship between the neuropsychiatric symptom exacerbations and streptococcal infections, it is often necessary to follow a child for several months to determine whether or not he or she is a member of the PANDAS subgroup. The observation period should reveal that symptom relapses follow bouts of streptococcal pharyngitis or scarlet fever (or are associated with rising antistreptococcal titres) and that symptom remissions occur during intervals of streptococcal negativity. Thus, in theory, prevention of these infections should result in a decrease in antineuronal antibody titres, and a gradual improvement in neuropsychiatric symptom severity. This hypothesis led to a trial of penicillin prophylaxis, similar to that used for prevention of rheumatic fever recrudescences (Garvey *et al.* 1999). The pilot study with oral penicillin V-K (250 mg orally twice daily) failed to achieve an adequate level of streptococcal prophylaxis and was therefore inconclusive. However, for individual subjects who were adequately protected against streptococcal infections, some benefits of penicillin therapy were observed. These findings warrant further investigation but, at the present time, there is no justification for the use of penicillin prophylaxis. In fact, because a number of asymptomatic infections were documented during the pilot study, it is possible that prophylaxis might worsen neuropsychiatric symptoms by masking symptoms of pharyngitis and preventing appropriate diagnosis and treatment of the streptococcal infection.

Transcranial magnetic stimulation

Transcranial magnetic stimulation (TMS), involving non-invasive and focal stimulation of the brain, uses powerful magnetic fields to alter brain activity. It is a promising research tool and therapeutic agent for a variety of disorders involving mood and anxiety (George *et al.* 1999). In adult OCD patients (Greenberg *et al.* 1997; Cora-Locatelli *et al.* 1998), a single session of right prefrontal repetitive TMS (rTMS) decreased compulsive urges for 8 h (Greenberg & Rauch, in press). Long-term use has not yet been investigated. TMS has also not been applied to treatment refractory cases, and there are no data for children, but the preliminary data are of sufficient interest to warrant further studies.

Conclusions

In recent years, great progress has been made in the recognition and treatment of childhood onset OCD. Structured instruments, such as the CY-BOCS, allow for the accurate diagnosis of this once hidden disorder. SSRI and behaviour therapy techniques (particularly ERP), provide relief from both compulsive rituals and obsessional anxiety. Advances in neuroimaging and neurophysiological technologies have opened new vistas for understanding the biological basis of OCD, while increased knowledge of the genetics of the disorder and novel pathophysiological models hold promise for the development of better strategies for treatment and prevention of OCD. Until that time, it is important to maximize the recognition and treatment of this troublesome disorder by educating parents and primary care physicians about the symptoms of OCD, and mental health professionals about the wide range of effective therapies.

References

Adams, P.I. (1973) *Obsessive Children*. Penguin Books, New York.

Alderman, J., Wolkow, R., Chung, M. & Johnston, H.F. (1996) Sertraline treatment of children and adolescents: tolerability, efficacy, and pharmacokinetics [Abstract]. *European Neuropsychopharmacology*, 6, 11.

Alderman, J., Wolkow, R., Chung, M. & Johnston, H.F. (1998) Sertraline treatment of children and adolescents with obsessive-compulsive disorder or depression: pharmacokinetics, tolerability, and efficacy. *Journal of the American Academy of Child and Adolescent Psychiatry*, 37, 386–394.

Altemus, M., Swedo, S., Leonard, H. *et al.* (1994) Changes in cerebrospinal fluid neurochemistry during treatment of obsessive compulsive disorder. *Archives of General Psychiatry*, 51, 794–803.

American Psychiatric Association (1987) *Diagnostic and Statistical Manual of Mental Disorders*, 3rd edn, revised. American Psychiatric Association, Washington D.C.

American Psychiatric Association (1994) *Diagnostic and Statistical Manual of Mental Disorders,* 4th edn. American Psychiatric Association, Washington D.C.

Anderson, J.C., Williams, S., McGee, R. & Silva, P.A. (1987) DSM-III disorders in preadolescent children: prevalence in a large sample from the general population. *Archives of General Psychiatry*, 44, 9–76.

Asbahr, F.R., Ramos, R.T., Negrao, A.B. & Gentil, V. (1999) Case series: increased vulnerability to obsessive-compulsive symptoms with repeated episodes of Sydenham's chorea. *Journal of the American Academy of Child and Adolescent Psychiatry*, 38, 1522–1525.

Baer, L. (1994) Factor analysis of symptom subtypes of obsessive-compulsive disorder and their relationship to personality and tic disorders. *Journal of Clinical Psychiatry*, 55, 18–23.

Baer, L. & Greist, J.H. (1997) An interactive computer-administered self-assessment and self-help program for behavior therapy. *Journal of Clinical Psychiatry*, 58, 23–28.

Baker, R.W., Chengappa, K.N., Baird, J.W., Steingard, S., Christ, M.A. & Schooler, N.R. (1992) Emergence of obsessive compulsive symptoms during treatment with clozapine. *Journal of Clinical Psychiatry*, 53, 439–442.

Baxter, L.R., Phelps, M.E., Mazziotta, J.E., Guze, B.H., Schwartz, M.J. & Selin, C.E. (1987) Local cerebral glucose metabolic rates in obsessive-compulsive disorder: a comparison with rates in unipolar depression and in normal controls. *Archives of General Psychiatry*, 44, 211–218.

Baxter, L.R., Schwartz, J.M., Bergman, K.S. et al. (1992) Caudate glucose metabolic rate changes with both drug and behavior therapy for obsessive-compulsive disorder. *Archives of General Psychiatry*, 49, 681–689.

Behar, D., Rapoport, J.L. & Berg, C.J. (1984) Computerized tomography and neuropsychological test measures in adolescents with bsessive–compulsive disorder. *American Journal of Psychiatry*, 141, 363–369.

Berg, C.Z., Rapoport, J.L., Whitaker, A. et al. (1989) Childhood obsessive-compulsive disorder: a two-year prospective follow-up of a community sample. *Journal of the American Academy of Child and Adolescent Psychiatry*, 28, 528–533.

Berk, M., Koopowitz, L.F. & Szabo, C.P. (1996) Antidepressant induced mania in obsessive-compulsive disorder. *European Neuropsychopharmacology*, 6, 9–11.

Berman, L. (1942) Obsessive-compulsive neurosis in children. *Journal of Nervous and Mental Disease*, 95, 26–39.

Berrios, G.E. (1989) Obsessive-compulsive disorder: its conceptual history in France during the 19th century. *Comprehensive Psychiatry*, 30, 283–295.

Black, A. (1974) The natural history of obsessional neurosis. In: *Obsessional States* (ed. H. Beech), pp. 19–54. Methuen, London.

Black, D.W. & Blum, N.S. (1992) Obsessive-compulsive disorder support groups: the Iowa model. *Comprehensive Psychiatry*, 33, 65–71.

Black, D., Yates, W., Noyes, R., Pfohl, B., Goldstein, R. & Blum, N. (1988) Personality disorder and OCD. Presented at 137th Meeting of the American Psychiatric Association, Montreal, 12 May 1988, p. 164. American Psychiatric Press Int. Washington, D.C.

Black, D.W., Noyes, R. Jr, Godlstein, R.B. et al. (1992) A family study of obsessive-compulsive disorder. *Archives of General Psychiatry*, 49, 362–368.

Blin, O. (1999) A comparative review of new antipsychotics. *Canadian Journal of Psychiatry*, 44, 235–244.

Bolla, K.I., Cadet, J.L. & London, E.D. (1998) The neuropsychiatry of chronic cocaine abuse. *Journal of Neuropsychiatry and Clinical Neurosciences*, 10, 280–289.

Bolton, D., Luckie, M. & Steinberg, D. (1995) Long-term course of obsessive-compulsive disorder treated in adolescence. *Journal of the American Academy of Child and Adolescent Psychiatry*, 34, 1441–1450.

Borcherding, B., Keysor, C., Rapoport, J.L., Elia, J. & Amass, J. (1990) Motor vocal tics and compulsive behaviors on stimulant drugs: is there a common vulnerability? *Psychiatry Research*, 33, 83–94.

Boudreaux, E., Kilpatrick, D.G., Resnick, H.S., Best, C.L. & Saunders, B.E. (1998) Criminal victimization, post-traumatic stress disorder, and comorbid psychopathology among a community sample of women. *Journal of Trauma Stress*, 11, 665–678.

Brown, T.A., Moras, K., Zinbarg, R.E. & Barlow, D.H. (1993) Diagnostic and symptom distinguishability of generalized anxiety disorder and obsessive-compulsive disorder. *Behavior Therapy*, 24, 227–240.

Burke, J.D. Jr, Burke, K.C. & Rae, D.S. (1994) Increased rates of drug abuse and dependence after onset of mood or anxiety disorders in adolescence. *Hospital and Community Psychiatry*, 45, 451–455.

Casas, M.E., Alvarez, P., Duro, C. et al. (1986) Antiandrogenic treatment of obsessive-compulsive disorder neurosis. *Acta Psychiatrica Scandinavica*, 73, 221–222.

Cavalini, M.C., Macciardi, F., Pasquale, L., Bellodi, L. & Smeraldi, E. (1995) Complex segregation analysis of obsessive-compulsive and spectrum disorders. *Psychiatric Genetics*, 5, S31.

Cavalini, M.C., Pasquale, L., Bellodi, L. & Smeraldi, E. (1999) Complex segregation analyses for obsessive-compulsive disorder and related disorders. *American Journal of Medical Genetics (Neuropsychiatric Genetics)*, 88, 38–43.

Chapman, A.H., Pilkey, L. & Gibbons, M.J. (1958) A psychosomatic study of eight children with Sydenham's chorea. *Pediatrics*, 21, 582–595.

Chiocca, E.A. & Martuzza, R. (1990) Neurosurgical therapy of obsessive compulsive disorder. In: *Obsessive Compulsive Disorders: Theory and Management* (eds M. Jenike, L. Baer & W. Minichiello), pp. 285–294. Year Book, Littleton, MA.

Clark, A., Kirby, K.C., Daniels, B.A. & Marks, I.M. (1998) A pilot study of computer-aided vicarious exposure for obsessive-compulsive disorder. *Australian and New Zealand Journal of Psychiatry*, 32, 268–275.

Cora-Locatelli, G., Greenberg, B.D., Harmon, A. et al. (1998) Cortical excitability and augmentation strategies in OCD [Abstract]. *Biological Psychiatry*, 43, 77.

Cox, C.S., Fedio, P. & Rapoport, J.L. (1989) Neuropsychological testing of obsessive-compulsive adolescents. In: *Obsessive-Compulsive Disorder in Children and Adolescents* (ed. J.L. Rapoport), pp. 73–86. American Psychiatric Press, Washington D.C.

Crum, R.M. & Anthony, J.C. (1993) Cocaine use and other suspected risk factors for obsessive-compulsive disorder: a prospective study with data from the Epidemiologic Catchment Area surveys. *Drug and Alcohol Dependence*, 31, 281–295.

Delgado, P.L. & Moreno, F.A. (1998) Different roles for serotonin in anti-obsessional drug action and the pathophysiology of obsessive-compulsive disorder (Suppl.). *British Journal of Psychiatry*, 35, 21–25.

Denckla, M.B. (1989) The neurological examination. In: *Obsessive Compulsive Disorder in Children and Adolescents* (ed. J.L. Rapoport), pp. 107–118. American Psychiatric Press, Washington D.C.

Despert, L. (1955) Differential diagnosis between obsessive-compulsive neurosis and schizophrenia in children. In: *Psychopathology of Childhood* (eds P.H. Hoch & J. Zubin), pp. 240–253. Grune & Stratton, New York.

DeVane, C.L. & Sallee, F.R. (1996) Serotonin selective reuptake inhibitors in child and adolescent psychopathology: a review of published experience. *Journal of Clinical Psychiatry*, 57, 55–66.

DeVeaugh-Geiss, J., Moroz, G., Biederman, J. et al. (1992) Clomipramine hydrochloride in childhood and adolescent obsessive-compulsive disorder: a multicenter trial. *Journal of the American Academy of Child and Adolescent Psychiatry*, 31, 45–49.

Diller, R.S. & Avci, A. (1999) SSRI-induced mania in obsessive-compulsive disorder [Letter]. *Journal of the American Academy of Child and Adolescent Psychiatry*, 38, 6–7.

Dolberg, O.T., Iancu, I. & Zohar, J. (1996) Treatment duration of obsessive compulsive disorder. *European Psychiatry*, 11, 403–406.

Douglass, H.M., Moffitt, T.E., Dar, R. et al. (1995) Obsessive-compulsive disorder in a birth cohort of 18 year olds: prevalence and predictors. *Journal of the American Academy of Child and Adolescent Psychiatry*, 34, 1424–1431.

Emmelkamp, P.M. & Beens, H. (1991) Cognitive therapy with obsessive-compulsive disorder: a comparative evaluation. *Behavior Research and Therapy*, 29, 293–300.

Emslie, G.J., Walkup, J.T., Piszka, S.R. & Ernst, M. (1999) Nontricyclic antidepressants: current trends in children and adolescents. *Journal of the American Academy of Child and Adolescent Psychiatry*, **38**, 517–528.

Esman, A. (1989) Psychoanalysis and general psychiatry: obsessive-compulsive disorder as paradigm. *Journal of the American Psychoanalytic Association*, **37**, 319–336.

Evans, D.W., Gray, F.L. & Leckman, J.F. (1999) The rituals, fears and phobias of young children: insights from development, psychopathology, and neurobiology. *Child Psychiatry and Human Development*, **29**, 261–276.

Fallon, B.A., Liebowitz, M.R., Campeas, R. *et al.* (1998) Intravenous clomipramine for obsessive-compulsive disorder refractory to oral clomipramine: a placebo controlled study. *Archives of General Psychiatry*, **55**, 918–924.

Fals-Stewart, W. & Angarano, K. (1994) Obsessive-compulsive disorder among patients entering substance abuse treatment: prevalence and accuracy of diagnosis. *Journal of Nervous and Mental Disease*, **182**, 715–719.

Field, M. (1960) *An Ethno-Psychiatric Study of Rural Ghana*. Northwestern University Press, Evanston IL.

Figueroa, Y., Rosenberg, D.R., Birmaher, B. & Keshavan, M.S. (1998) Combination treatment with clomipramine and selective serotonin reuptake inhibitors for obsessive-compulsive disorder in children and adolescents. *Journal of Child and Adolescent Psychopharmacology*, **8**, 61–67.

Fitzgerald, K.D., MacMaster, F.P., Paulson, L.D. & Rosenberg, D.R. (1999) Neurobiology of childhood obsessive-compulsive disorder. *Child and Adolescent Psychiatric Clinics of North America*, **8**, 533–575.

Flament, M.F., Rapoport, J.L., Berg, C.J. *et al.* (1985) Clomipramine treatment of childhood compulsive disorder: a double-blind controlled study. *Archives of General Psychiatry*, **42**, 977–983.

Flament, M.F., Rapoport, J.L., Murphy, D.L., Berg, C.J. & Lake, R. (1987) Biochemical changes during clomipramine treatment of childhood obsessive compulsive disorder. *Archives of General Psychiatry*, **44**, 219–225.

Flament, M.F., Whitaker, A., Rapoport, J. *et al.* (1988) Obsessive-compulsive disorder in adolescence: an epidemiological study. *Journal of the American Academy of Child and Adolescent Psychiatry*, **27**, 764–771.

Flament, M.F., Koby, E., Rapoport, J.L. *et al.* (1990) Childhood obsessive-compulsive disorder: a prospective follow-up study. *Journal of Child Psychology and Psychiatry*, **31**, 363–380.

Foa, E.B., Steketee, G.S. & Grayson, J.B. (1985) Imaginal and *in vivo* exposure: a comparison with obsessive-compulsive checkers. *Behavior Therapy*, **16**, 292–303.

Frankel, M., Cummings, J.L., Robertson, M.M., Trimble, M.R., Hill, M.A. & Benson, D.F. (1986) Obsessions and compulsions in Gilles de la Tourette's syndrome. *Neurology*, **36**, 378–382.

Franklin, M., Kozak, M., Cashman, L.A. *et al.* (1998) Cognitive-behavioral treatment of pediatric obsessive–compulsive disorder: an open clinical trial. *Journal of the American Academy of Child and Adolescent Psychiatry*, **37**, 412–419.

Freeman, J., Aron, A.M., Collard, J. & MacKay, M.C. (1965) The emotional correlates of Sydenham's chorea. *Pediatrics*, **35**, 42–49.

Freud, S. (1909) Notes on a case of obsessional neurosis. In: *The Standard Edition of the Complete Psychological Works of Sigmund Freud*, Vol. 10 (1957) (ed. J. Strachey), pp. 153–318. Hogarth Press, London.

Freud, S. (1913) The predisposition of obsessional neurosis. In: *The Standard Edition of the Complete Psychological Works of Sigmund Freud*, Vol. 12 (1957) (ed. J. Strachey), pp. 311–326. Hogarth Press, London.

Freud, A. (1965) *Normality and Pathology in Childhood*. International University Press, New York.

Frye, P. & Arnold, L. (1981) Persistent amphetamine-induced compulsive rituals: response to pyridoxine (B_6). *Biological Psychiatry*, **16**, 583–587.

Garvey, M.A., Perlmutter, S.J., Allen, A.J. *et al.* (1999) A pilot study of penicillin prophylaxis for neuropsychiatric exacerbations by streptococcal infections. *Biological Psychiatry*, **45**, 1564–1571.

Geller, D.A., Biederman, J., Reed, E.D., Spencer, T. & Wilens, T.E. (1995) Similarities in response to fluoxetine in the treatment of children and adolescents with obsessive-compulsive disorder. *Journal of the American Academy of Child and Adolescent Psychiatry*, **34**, 36–44.

Geller, D.A., Biederman, J., Jones, J., Shapiro, S., Schwartz, S. & Park, K.S. (1998) Obsessive-compulsive disorder in children and adolescents: a review. *Harvard Review of Psychiatry*, **5**, 260–273.

Geller, B., Reising, D., Leonard, H.L., Riddle, M.A. & Walsh, B.T. (1999) Critical review of tricyclic antidepressant use in children and adolescents. *Journal of the American Academy of Child and Adolescent Psychiatry*, **38**, 513–516.

George, M.S., Lisanby, S.H. & Sackeim, H.A. (1999) Transcranial magnetic stimulation: applications in neuropsychiatry. *Archives of General Psychiatry*, **56**, 300–311.

Giedd, J.N., Rapoport, J.L., Leonard, H.L., Richter, D. & Swedo, S.E. (1996) Case study: acute basal ganglia enlargement and obsessive-compulsive symptoms in an adolescent boy. *Journal of the American Academy of Child and Adolescent Psychiatry*, **35**, 913–915.

Giedd, J.N., Rapoport, J.L., Garvey, M.A., Perlmutter, S. & Swedo, S.E. (2000) MRI Assessment of children with obsessive-compulsive disorder or tics associated with streptococcal infection. *American Journal of Psychiatry*, **157**, 281–283.

Go, F.S., Malley, E.E., Birmaher, B. & Rosenberg, D. (1998) Manic behaviors associated with fluoxetine in three 12–18-year-olds with obsessive-compulsive disorder. *Journal of Child and Adolescent Psychopharmacology*, **8**, 73–80.

Goodman, W.K., Price, L.H., Rasmussen, S.A. *et al.* (1989) The Yale-Brown Obsessive Compulsive Scale. I. Development, use and reliability. *Archives of General Psychiatry*, **46**, 1006–1011.

Goodman, W.K., McDougle, C.J., Price, L.H., Riddle, M.A., Pauls, D.L. & Leckman, J.F. (1990) Beyond the serotonin hypothesis: a role for dopamine in some forms of obsessive-compulsive disorder? *Journal of Clinical Psychiatry*, **51**, 36–43.

Goodman, W.K., Ward, H., Kablinger, A. & Murphy, T. (1997) Fluvoxamine in the treatment of obsessive-compulsive disorder and related conditions. *Journal of Clinical Psychiatry*, **58**, 32–49.

Grad, L.R., Pelcovitz, D., Olson, M., Mathews, M. & Grad, G.J. (1987) Obsessive-compulsive symptomatology in children with Tourette's syndrome. *Journal of the American Academy of Child Psychiatry*, **26**, 69–73.

Greenberg, B.D. & Rauch, S.L. (in press) Transcranial magnetic stimulation in anxiety disorders. In: *Transcranial Magnetic Stimulation in Neuropsychiatry* (eds M.S. George & R.H. Belmaker), pp. 000–000. American Psychiatric Press, Washington D.C.

Greenberg, B.D., George, M.S., Dearing, J. *et al.* (1997) Effect of prefrontal repetitive transcranial magnetic stimulation (rTMS) in obsessive-compulsive disorder: a preliminary study. *American Journal of Psychiatry*, **154**, 867–869.

Greist, J.H. (1996) New developments in behaviour therapy for obsessive-compulsive disorder. *International Clinical Psychopharmacology*, **11**, 63–73.

Grimshaw, L. (1964) Obsessional disorder and neurological illness.

Journal of Neurology, Neurosurgery and Psychiatry, **27**, 229–231.

Gunasekara, N.S., Noble, S. & Benfield, P. (1998) Paroxetine: an update of its pharmacology and therapeutic use in depression and a review of its use in other disorders. *CNS Drugs*, **55**, 85–120.

Hamburger, S.D., Swedo, S., Whitaker, A., Davies, M. & Rapoport, J.L. (1989) Growth rate in adolescents with obsessive-compulsive disorder. *American Journal of Psychiatry*, **146**, 652–655.

Han, L., Nielsen, D.A., Rosenthal, N.E. *et al.* (1999) No coding variant of the tryptophan hydroxylase gene detected in seasonal affective disorder, obsessive-compulsive disorder, anorexia nervosa, and alcoholism. *Biological Psychiatry*, **45**, 615–619.

Hanna, G.L. (1995) Demographic and clinical features of obsessive-compulsive disorder in children and adolescents. *Journal of the American Academy of Child and Adolescent Psychiatry*, **34**, 19–27.

Hewlett, W.A., Vinogradov, S. & Agras, W.S. (1992) Clomipramine, clonazepam, and clonidine treatment of obsessive-compulsive disorder. *Journal of Clinical Psychopharmacology*, **12**, 420–430.

Hollander, E., Schiffman, E., Cohen, B. *et al.* (1990) Signs of nervous system dysfunction in obsessive-compulsive disorder. *Archives of General Psychiatry*, **47**, 27–32.

Hollander, E., DeCaria, C., Nitescu, A. *et al.* (1991) Noradrenergic function in obsessive-compulsive disorder: behavioral and neuroendocrine responses to clonidine and comparison to healthy controls. *Psychiatry Research*, **37**, 161–177.

Hollingsworth, C.E., Tanguay, P.E., Grossman, L. & Pabst, P. (1980) Long-term outcome of obsessive-compulsive disorder in childhood. *Journal of the American Academy of Child and Adolescent Psychiatry*, **19**, 134–144.

Holzer, J.C., Goodman, W.K., McDougle, C.J. *et al.* (1994) Obsessive-compulsive disorder with and without a chronic tic disorder: a comparison of symptoms in 70 patients. *British Journal of Psychiatry*, **164**, 469–473.

Honjo, S., Hirano, C., Murase, S. *et al.* (1989) Obsessive–compulsive symptoms in childhood and adolescence. *Acta Psychiatrica Scandinavica*, **80**, 83–91.

Husby, G., Van de Rijn, I., Zabriskie, J.B., Abdin, Z.H. & Williams, R.C. (1976) Antibodies reacting with cytoplasm of subthalamic and caudate nuclei neurons in chorea and acute rheumatic fever. *Journal of Experimental Medicine*, **144**, 1094–1110.

Insel, T.R. (1992) Toward a neuroanatomy of obsessive-compulsive disorder. *Archives of General Psychiatry*, **49**, 739–744.

Insel, T.R. & Pickar, D. (1983) Naloxone administration in obsessive-compulsive disorder: report of two cases. *American Journal of Psychiatry*, **140**, 1219–1220.

Insel, T.R., Mueller, E.A., Alterman, I., Linnoila, M.M. & Murphy, D.L. (1985) Obsessive-compulsive disorder and serotonin: is there a connection? *Biological Psychiatry*, **20**, 1174–1188.

Janet, P. (1903) *Les Obsessions et la Psychiatrie*, 1. Felix Alan, Paris.

Jenike, M.A. (1998) Neurosurgical treatment of obsessive-compulsive disorder. *British Journal of Psychiatry*, **35**, 79–90.

Joffe, R., Swinson, R. & Regan, J. (1988) Personality features of obsessive-compulsive disorder. *American Journal of Psychiatry*, **45**, 1127–1129.

Joffe, R., Swinson, R. & Levitt, A. (1991) Acute psychostimulant challenge in primary obsessive-compulsive disorder. *Journal of Clinical Psychopharmacology*, **11**, 237–241.

Kanner, L. (1962) *Child Psychiatry*, 3rd edn. Charles C. Thomas, Springfield, IL.

Karayiorgou, M., Altemus, M., Galke, B.L. *et al.* (1997) Genotype determining low catechol-O-methyltransferase activity as a risk factor for obsessive-compulsive disorder. *Proceedings of the National Academy of Sciences of the United States of America*, **94**, 4572–4575.

Karno, M. & Golding, J. (1990) Obsessive compulsive disorder. In: *Psychiatric Disorders in America: the Epidemiological Catchment Area Study* (eds L. Robins & D.A. Regier), pp. 207–219. Free Press, New York.

Karno, M., Golding, J., Sorenson, S. & Burnam, A. (1988) The epidemiology of obsessive-compulsive disorder in five US communities. *Archives of General Psychiatry*, **45**, 1094–1099.

Kiessling, L.S., Marcotte, A.C. & Culpepper, L. (1994) Antineuronal antibodies: tics and obsessive-compulsive symptoms. *Journal of Developmental and Behavioral Pediatrics*, **15**, 421–425.

King, R.A. & Scahill, L. (1999) The assessment and coordination of treatment of children and adolescents with OCD. *Child and Adolescent Psychiatric Clinics of North America*, **8**, 577–598.

King, R.A., Leonard, H. & March, J. (1998) Practice parameters for the assessment and treatment of children and adolescents with obsessive-compulsive disorder. *Journal of the American Academy of Child and Adolescent Psychiatry*, **37**, 27S–45S.

Laplane, D., Baulac, M., Widlocher, D. & Dubois, B. (1984) Pure psychic akinesia with bilateral lesions of basal ganglia. *Journal of Neurology, Neurosurgery and Psychiatry*, **47**, 377–385.

Leckman, J.F. & Mayes, L.C. (1999) Preoccupations and behaviors associated with romantic and parental love: perspectives on the origin of obsessive-compulsive disorder. *Child and Adolescent Psychiatric Clinics of North America*, **8**, 635–665.

Leckman, J.F., Goodman, W.K., North, W.G. *et al.* (1994) The role of central oxytocin in obsessive compulsive disorder and related normal behavior. *Psychoneuroendocrinology*, **19**, 723–749.

Leckman, J.F., Grice, D.E., Barr, L.C. *et al.* (1995) Tic-related vs non-tic related obsessive-compulsive disorder. *Anxiety*, **1**, 208.

Leckman, J.F., Grice, D.E., Boardman, J. *et al.* (1997) Symptoms of obsessive-compulsive disorder. *American Journal of Psychiatry*, **154**, 911–917.

Lenane, M.C., Swedo, S.E., Leonard, H.L., Pauls, D.L., Sceery, W. & Rapoport, J.L. (1990) Psychiatric disorders in first-degree relatives of children and adolescents with obsessive-compulsive disorder. *Journal of the American Academy of Child and Adolescent Psychiatry*, **29**, 497–412.

Leonard, H.L., Swedo, S., Rapoport, J. *et al.* (1989) Treatment of childhood obsessive-compulsive disorder with clomipramine and desmethylimipramine: a double-blind crossover comparison. *Archives of General Psychiatry*, **46**, 1088–1092.

Leonard, H.L., Goldberger, E.L., Rapoport, J.L., Cheslow, D.L. & Swedo, S.E. (1990) Childhood rituals: normal development or obsessive-compulsive symptoms? *Journal of the American Academy of Child and Adolescent Psychiatry*, **29**, 17–23.

Leonard, H.L., Swedo, S., Lenane, M. *et al.* (1991) A double-blind desipramine substitution during long-term clomipramine treatment in children and adolescents with obsessive-compulsive disorder. *Archives of General Psychiatry*, **48**, 922–926.

Leonard, H.L., Lenane, M., Swedo, S., Rettew, D., Gershon, E. & Rapoport, J.L. (1992) Tics and Tourette's syndrome: a 2–7 year follow-up of 54 obsessive-compulsive children. *American Journal of Psychiatry*, **149**, 1244–1251.

Leonard, H.L., Swedo, S., Lenane, M. *et al.* (1993) A two to seven year follow-up study of 54 obsessive-compulsive children and adolescents. *Archives of General Psychiatry*, **50**, 429–438.

Leonard, H.L., Topol, D., Bukstein, O., Hindmarsh, D., Allen, A.J. & Swedo, S.E. (1994) Clonazepam as an augmenting agent in the treatment of childhood-onset obsessive-compulsive disorder. *Journal of the American Academy of Child and Adolescent Psychiatry*, **33**, 792–794.

Lewinsohn, P.M., Hops, H., Roberts, R.E., Seeley, J.R. & Andrews, J.A. (1993) Adolescent psychopathology. I. Prevalence and incidence of depression and other DSM-III-R disorders in high school students. *Journal of Abnormal Psychology*, **102**, 133–144.

Lewis, A. (1936) Problems of obsessional illness. *Proceedings of the Royal Society of Medicine*, **29**, 325–336.

Lewis, S., Chitkara, B. & Reverly, A.M. (1991) Obsessive-compulsive disorder and schizophrenia in the three identical twin pairs. *Psychological Medicine*, **21**, 135–141.

Lombroso, P.J., Scahill, L., King, R.A. *et al.* (1995) Risperidone treatment of children and adolescents with chronic tic disorders: a preliminary report. *Journal of the American Academy of Child and Adolescent Psychiatry*, **34**, 1147–1152.

Lougee, L., Garvey, M.A., Perlmutter, S., Nicholson, R. & Swedo, S.E. (2000) Rates of psychiatric disorders in first-degree relatives of children and adolescents with PANDAS. *Journal of the American Academy of Child and Adolescent Psychiatry*, **39**, 1120–1126.

Luxenberg, J.S., Swedo, S.E., Flament, M.F., Friedland, R.P., Rapoport, J.L. & Rapoport, S.I. (1988) Neuroanatomic abnormalities in obsessive-compulsive disorder detected with quantitative X-ray computed tomography. *American Journal of Psychiatry*, **145**, 1089–1093.

Maina, G., Albert, U., Bogetto, F. & Ravizza, L. (1999) Obsessive-compulsive syndromes in older adolescents. *Acta Psychiatrica Scandinavica*, **100**, 447–450.

Mandoki, M.W. (1995) Risperidone treatment of children and adolescents: increased risk of extrapyramidal side effects. *Journal of Child and Adolescent Psychopharmacology*, **5**, 49–67.

March, J.S. (1995) Cognitive-behavioral psychotherapy for children and adolescents with OCD: a review and recommendations for treatment. *Journal of the American Academy of Child and Adolescent Psychiatry*, **34**, 7–18.

March, J.S. & Leonard, H.L. (1998) Obsessive-compulsive disorder in children and adolescents. In: *Obsessive-Compulsive Disorder: Theory, Research, and Treatment* (eds R.P. Swinson, M.M. Anton, S. Rachman & M.A. Richter), pp. 367–394. Guilford Press, New York.

March, J.S. & Mulle, K. (1998) *OCD in Children and Adolescents: a Cognitive-Behavioral Treatment Manual*. Guilford Press, New York.

March, J.S., Mulle, K. & Herbel, B. (1994) Behavioral psychotherapy for children and adolescents with obsessive-compulsive disorder: an open trial of a new protocol-driven treatment package. *Journal of the American Academy of Child and Adolescent Psychiatry*, **33**, 333–341.

March, J.S., Biederman, J., Wolkow, R. *et al.* (1998) Sertraline in children and adolescents with obsessive-compulsive disorder: a multicenter randomized controlled trial. *Journal of the American Medical Association*, **280**, 1752–1756.

Marks, I. (1997) Behavior therapy for obsessive-compulsive disorder: a decade of progress. *Canadian Journal of Psychiatry*, **42**, 1021–1026.

McDougle, C.J. (1997) Update on pharmacologic management of OCD: agents and augmentation. *Journal of Clinical Psychiatry*, **58**, 11–17.

McDougle, C.J., Goodman, W.K., Leckman, J.F., Lee, N.C., Heninger, G.R. & Price, L.H. (1994) Haloperidol addition in fluvoxamine-refractory obsessive-compulsive disorder: a double-blind, placebo-controlled study in patients with and without tics. *Archives of General Psychiatry*, **51**, 302–308.

McDougle, C.J., Fleischmann, R.L., Epperson, C.N., Wasylink, S., Leckman, J.F. & Price, L.H. (1995) Risperidone addition in fluvoxamine-refractory obsessive compulsive disorder: three cases. *Journal of Clinical Psychiatry*, **56**, 526–528.

Mindus, P. (1991) *Capsulotomy in Anxiety Disorders: a Multidisciplinary Study*. Karolinska Institute Press, Stockholm.

Mindus, P., Edman, G. & Andreewitch, S. (1999) A prospective, long-term study of personality traits in patients with intractable obses-sional illness treated by capsulotomy. *Acta Psychiatrica Scandinavica*, **99**, 40–50.

Modell, J.G., Mountz, J.M., Curtis, G.C. & Greden, J. (1989) Neurophysiologic dysfunction in basal ganglia/limbic striatal and thalamocortical circuits as a pathogenetic mechanism of obsessive-compulsive disorder. *Journal of Neuropsychiatry*, **1**, 27–36.

Montgomery, S., Kasper, S., Stein, D. *et al.* (2001) Citalapram 20 mg, 40 mg and 60 mg are all effective and well tolerated compared with placebo in obsessive–compulsive disorder. *International Clinical Psychopharmacology*, **16**, 75–86.

Murphy, D., Zohar, J., Pato, M., Pigott, T. & Insel, T. (1989) Obsessive-compulsive disorder as a 5-HT subsystem behavioral disorder. *British Journal of Psychiatry*, **155**, 15–24.

Nicolini, H., Hanna, G., Baxter, L. Jr, Schwartz, J., Weissbacker, K. & Spence, M.A. (1991) Segregation analysis of obsessive-compulsive and associated disorders: preliminary results. *Ursus Medicus*, **1**, 25–28.

Nicolson, R., Swedo, S.E., Lenane, M. *et al.* (2000) An open trial of plasma exchange in childhood-onset obsessive-compulsive disorder without poststreptococcal exacerbations. *Journal of the American Academy of Child and Adolescent Psychiatry*, **39**, 1313–1315.

O'Connor, K., Todorov, C., Robillard, S., Borgeat, F. & Brault, M. (1999) Cognitive-behavior therapy and medication in the treatment of obsessive-compulsive disorder: a controlled study. *Canadian Journal of Psychiatry*, **44**, 64–71.

Osler, W. (1894) *On Chorea and Choreiform Affections*. H.K. Lewis, Philadelphia.

Park, L.T., Jefferson, J.W. & Greist, J.H. (1997) Obsessive-compulsive disorder: treatment options. *CNS Drugs*, **7**, 187–202.

Patel, B. & Tandon, R. (1993) Development of obsessive-compulsive symptoms during clozapine treatment [Letter]. *American Journal of Psychiatry*, **150**, 836.

Pato, M.T., Pato, C.N. & Gunn, S.A. (1998) Biological treatments for obsessive-compulsive disorder: clinical applications. In: *Obsessive-Compulsive Disorder. Theory, Research, and Treatment* (eds R.P. Swinson, M.A. Anthony, S. Rachman & M.A. Richter), pp. 327–348. Guilford Press, New York.

Pauls, D.L. & Alsobrook, J.P. (1999) The inheritance of obsessive-compulsive disorder. *Child Adolescent Psychiatric Clinics of North America*, **8**, 481–496.

Pauls, D.L., Raymond, C., Stevenson, J. *et al.* (1991) A family study of Gilles de la Tourette syndrome. *Human Genetics*, **48**, 154–163.

Pauls, D.L., Towbin, K.K., Leckman, J.F., Zahner, G.E.P. & Cohen, D. (1986) Gilles de la Tourette's syndrome and obsessive-compulsive disorder: evidence supporting a genetic relationship. *Archives of General Psychiatry*, **43**, 1180–1182.

Pauls, D.L., Alsobrook, J.P., Goodman, W., Rasmussen, S. & Leckman, J.F. (1995) A family study of obsessive-compulsive disorder. *American Journal of Psychiatry*, **152**, 76–84.

Perlmutter, S.J., Garvey, M.A., Castellanos, X.C. *et al.* (1998) A case of pediatric autoimmune neuropsychiatric disorders associated with streptococcal infections. *American Journal of Psychiatry*, **155**, 1592–1598.

Perlmutter, S.J., Leitman, S.F., Garvey, M.A. *et al.* (1999) Therapeutic plasma exchange and intravenous immunoglobulin for obsessive compulsive disorder and tic disorders in childhood. *Lancet*, **354**, 1153–1158.

Piacentini, J. (1999) Cognitive behavioral therapy of childhood OCD. *Child and Adolescent Psychiatric Clinics of North America*, **8**, 599–616.

Piacentini, J., Gitow, A., Jeffer, M. *et al.* (1994) Outpatient behavioral treatment of child and adolescent obsessive–compulsive disorder. *Journal of Anxiety Disorders*, **8**, 277–289.

Pigott, T.A. & Seay, S.M. (1999) A review of the efficacy of selective serotonin reuptake inhibitors in obsessive-compulsive disorder. *Journal of Clinical Psychiatry*, **60**, 101–106.

Pigott, T.A., Zohar, J., Hill, J.L. *et al.* (1991) Metergoline blocks the behavioral and neuroendocrine effects of orally administered m-chlorophenyl piperezine in patients with obsessive–compulsive disorder. *Biological Psychiatry*, **29**, 418–426.

Pigott, T.A., L'Heureux, F., Rubenstein, C.S., Hill, J.L. & Murphy, D.L. (1992) A controlled trial of clonazepam augmentation in OCD patients tested with clomipramine or fluoxetine [Abstract no. 144]. In: *New Research Program and Abstracts of the 145th Annual Meeting of the American Psychiatric Association*, p. 82. American Psychiatric Press, Washington D.C.

Pollock, R.A. & Carter, A.S. (1999) The familial and developmental context of obsessive-compulsive disorder. *Child and Adolescent Psychiatric Clinics of North America*, **8**, 461–480.

Rapoport, J.L. (1989a) *Obsessive Compulsive Disorder in Children and Adolescents*. American Psychiatric Press, New York.

Rapoport, J.L. (1989b) The neurobiology of obsessive compulsive disorder. *Journal of the American Medical Association*, **260**, 2888–2890.

Rapoport, J.L. (1989c) *The Boy Who Couldn't Stop Washing*. E.P. Dutton, New York.

Rapoport, J.L. (1991) Recent advances in obsessive-compulsive disorder. *Neuropsychopharmacology*, **5**, 1–9.

Rapoport, J.L. (1998) Child psychopharmacology comes of age. *Journal of the American Medical Association*, **280**, 1785.

Rapoport, J.L. & Wise, S.P. (1988) Obsessive–compulsive disorder: is it a basal ganglia dysfunction? *Psychopharacology Bulletin*, **1**, 27–36.

Rapoport, J. & Inoff-Germain, G. (2000) Practitioner review: treatment of obsessive–compulsive disorder in children and adolescents. *Journal of Child Psychology and Psychiatry*, **41**, 419–431.

Rapoport, J.L., Elkins, R., Langer, D. *et al.* (1981) Childhood obsessive–compulsive disorder. *American Journal of Psychiatry*, **138**, 1545–1554.

Rapoport, J.L., Inoff-Germain, G., Weissman, M.M. *et al.* (2000) Childhood obsessive-compulsive disorder in the NIMH MECA study: parent versus child identification of cases. *Journal of Anxiety Disorders*, **4**, 535–548.

Rasmussen, S.A. & Eisen, J.L. (1992) The epidemiology and differential diagnosis of obsessive-compulsive disorder. *Journal of Clinical Psychiatry*, **53**, 4–10.

Rasmussen, S.A. & Eisen, J.L. (1997) Treatment strategies for chronic and refractory obsessive-compulsive disorder. *Journal of Clinical Psychiatry*, **58**, 9–13.

Rasmussen, S.A. & Tsuang, M.T. (1984) The epidemiology of obsessive-compulsive disorder. *Journal of Clinical Psychiatry*, **45**, 450–457.

Rauch, S.L. & Baxter, L.R. (1998) Neuroimaging of OCD and related disorders. In: *Obsessive-Compulsive Disorders: Practical Management* (eds M.A. Jenike, L. Baer & W.E. Minichiello), pp. 222–253. Mosby, Boston, MA.

Rauch, S.L., Jenike, M.A., Alpert, N.M. *et al.* (1994) Regional cerebral blood flow measured during symptom provocation in obsessive-compulsive disorder using oxygen 15-labeled carbon dioxide and positron emission tomography. *Archives of General Psychiatry*, **51**, 62–70.

Rauch, S., Savage, C.R. & Alpert, N.M. (1997) The functional new anatomy of anxiety: a study of three disorders using positron emission tomography and symptom provocation. *Biological Psychiatry*, **42**, 446–452.

Ravizza, L., Barzega, G., Bellino, S., Bogetto, F. & Maina, G. (1996) Therapeutic effect and safety of adjunctive risperidone in refractory obsessive-compulsive disorder (OCD). *Psychopharmacology Bulletin*, **32**, 677–682.

Ravizza, L., Maina, G., Bogetto, F., Albert, U., Barzega, G. & Bellino, S. (1998) Long term treatment of obsessive-compulsive disorder. *CNS Drugs*, **10**, 247–255.

Reinherz, H.Z., Giaconia, R.M., Lefkowitz, E.S., Pakiz, B. & Frost, A.K. (1993) Prevalence of psychiatric disorders in a community population of older adolescents. *Journal of the American Academy of Child and Adolescent Psychiatry*, **32**, 369–377.

Rettew, D.C., Swedo, S.E., Leonard, H.L. *et al.* (1992) Obsessions and compulsions across time in 79 children and adolescents with obsessive-compulsive disorder. *Journal of the American Academy of Child and Adolescent Psychiatry*, **31**, 1050–1056.

Ricciardi, J.N., Baer, L., Jenike, M.A. *et al.* (1992) Changes in DSM-III-R axis II diagnoses following treatment of obsessive-compulsive disorder. *American Journal of Psychiatry*, **149**, 829–831.

Riddle, M. (1998) Obsessive–compulsive disorder in children and adolescents. *British Journal of Psychiatry*, **35** (Suppl), 91–96.

Riddle, M.A., Scahill, L., King, R.A. *et al.* (1992) Double-blind crossover trial of fluoxetine and placebo in children and adolescents with obsessive-compulsive disorder. *Journal of the American Academy of Child and Adolescent Psychiatry*, **31**, 1062–1069.

Riddle, M.A., Claghorn, J., Gaffney, G. *et al.* (1996) A controlled trial of fluvoxamine for OCD in children and adolescents. *Biological Psychiatry*, **39**, 568.

Riddle, M.A., Scahill, L. & King, R. (1990) Obsessive–compulsive disorder in children and adolescents: phenomenology and family history. *Journal of the American Academy of Child and Adolescent Psychiatry*, **29**, 766–772.

Robins, L., Helzer, J., Crougham, J. & Ratcliffe, K. (1981) The NIMH epidemiological catchment area study. *Archives of General Psychiatry*, **38**, 381–389.

Rosenberg, D.R., Keshavan, M.S., O'Hearn, K.M. *et al.* (1997) Fronto-striatal morphology of treatment-naive pediatric obsessive compulsive disorder. *Archives of General Psychiatry*, **54**, 831–838.

Rosenberg, D.R., Chugani, D.C., Muzik, O. *et al.* (1998) Altered serotonin synthesis in fronto-striatal circuitry in pediatric obsessive-compulsive disorder. *Biological Psychiatry*, **43**, 24.

Sallee, F.R., Pollock, B.G., Perel, J.M., Ryan, N.D. & Stiller, R.L. (1989) Intravenous pulse loading of clomipramine in adolescents with depression. *Psychopharmacology Bulletin*, **25**, 114.

Sallee, F.R., Vrindavanam, N.S., Deas-Nesmith, D., Carson, S.W. & Sethuraman, G. (1997) Pulse intravenous clomipramine for depressed adolescents: double-blind, controlled trial. *American Journal of Psychiatry*, **154**, 668–673.

Sallee, F.R., Koran, L.M., Pallanti, S., Carson, S.W. & Sethuraman, G. (1998) Intravenous clomipramine challenge in obsessive-compulsive disorder: predicting response to oral therapy at eight weeks. *Biological Psychiatry*, **44**, 220–227.

Salzberg, A. & Swedo, S.E. (1992) Oxytocin and vasopressin in obsessive-compulsive disorder [Letter]. *American Journal of Psychiatry*, **149**, 713–714.

Saxena, S., Wang, D., Bystritsky, A. & Baxter, L.R. Jr (1996) Risperidone augmentation of SRI treatment for refractory obsessive-compulsive disorder. *Journal of Clinical Psychiatry*, **57**, 303–306.

Scahill, L., Vitulano, L., Brenner, E. *et al.* (1996) Behavioral therapy in children and adolescents: a pilot study. *Journal of the American Academy of Child and Adolescent Psychopharmacology*, **6**, 191–202.

Shaffer, D., Schonfeld, I., O'Connor, P.A. *et al.* (1985) Neurological soft signs: their relationship to psychiatric disorders and intelligence in childhood and adolescence. *Archives of General Psychiatry*, **44**, 342–351.

Shafran, R. (1998) Childhood obsessive-compulsive disorder. In:

Cognitive Behavior Therapy for Children and Families (ed. P. Graham), pp. 45–73. University Press, Cambridge.

Shafran, N.A. & Somers, J. (1998) Treating adolescent obsessive-compulsive disorder: applications of the cognitive theory. *Behavior Research and Therapy*, **36**, 93–97.

Shapira, N., Keck, P.E., Goldsmith, T.D., McConville, B.J., Eis, M. & McElroy, S.L. (1997) Open-label pilot study of tramadol hydrochloride in treatment-refractory obsessive-compulsive disorder. *Depression and Anxiety*, **6**, 170–173.

Simeon, J.G., Thatte, S. & Wiggins, D. (1990) Treatment of adolescent obsessive-compulsive disorder with clomipramine-fluoxetine combination. *Psychopharmacology Bulletin*, **26**, 285–290.

Stanley, M.A. & Turner, S.M. (1995) Current status of pharmacological and behavioral treatment of obsessive-compulsive disorder. *Behavior Therapy*, **26**, 163–186.

Swedo, S.E. (1989) Rituals and releasers: an ethological model of OCD. In: *Obsessive Compulsive Disorder in Children and Adolescents* (ed. J.L. Rapoport), pp. 269–288. American Psychiatric Press, Washington D.C.

Swedo, S.E. (1994) Sydenham's chorea: a model for childhood autoimmune neuropsychiatric disorders. *Journal of the American Medical Association*, **272**, 1788–1791.

Swedo, S. & Rapoport, J.L. (1990) Neurochemical and neuroendocrine consideration of obsessive-compulsive disorders in childhood. In: *Application of Basic Neurosciences to Child Psychiatry* (eds S.I. Deutsch, A. Weizman & R. Weizman), pp. 275–284. Plenum Medical Books, New York.

Swedo, S., Rapoport, J.L. & Cheslow, D. (1989a) High prevalence of obsessive-compulsive symptoms in patients with Sydenham's chorea. *American Journal of Psychiatry*, **146**, 246–249.

Swedo, S., Rapoport, J.L., Leonard, H.L., Lenane, M. & Cheslow, D. (1989b) Obsessive-compulsive disorder in children and adolescents: clinical phenomenology of 70 consecutive cases. *Archives of General Psychiatry*, **46**, 335–341.

Swedo, S., Leonard, H.L., Kruesi, M.J.P. *et al.* (1992a) Cerebrospinal fluid neurochemistry of children and adolescents with obsessive compulsive disorder. *Archives of General Psychiatry*, **49**, 29–36.

Swedo, S., Pietrini, P., Leonard, H.L. *et al.* (1992b) Cerebral glucose metabolism in childhood-onset obsessive-compulsive disorder: revisualization during pharmacotherapy. *Archives of General Psychiatry*, **49**, 690–694.

Swedo, S., Leonard, H.L., Schapiro, M.B. *et al.* (1993) Sydenham's chorea: physical and psychological symptoms of St Vitus' Dance. *Pediatrics*, **91**, 706–713.

Swedo, S.E., Leonard, H.L., Garvey, M. *et al.* (1998) Pediatric autoimmune neuropsychiatric disorders associated with streptococcal infections (PANDAS): clinical description of the first 50 cases. *American Journal of Psychiatry*, **155**, 264–271.

Thomsen, P.H. (1998) Obsessive-compulsive disorder in children and adolescents: clinical guidelines. *European Child and Adolescent Psychiatry*, **7**, 1–11.

Thomsen, P.H. & Mikkelsen, H.U. (1991) Children and adolescents with obsessive-compulsive disorder: the demographic and diagnostic characteristics of 61 Danish patients. *Acta Psychiatrica Scandinavia*, **83**, 262–266.

Toro, J., Cervera, M., Osejo, E. & Salamero, M. (1992) Obsessive-compulsive disorder in childhood and adolescence: a clinical study. *Journal of Child Psychology and Psychiatry*, **33**, 1025–1037.

Valleni-Basile, L.A., Garrison, C.Z., Waller, J.L. *et al.* (1996) Incidence of obsessive-compulsive disorder in a community sample of young adolescents. *Journal of the American Academy of Child and Adolescent Psychiatry*, **35**, 898–906.

Von Economo, C. (1931) *Encephalitis Lethargica: its Sequelae and Treatment*. Oxford University Press, London.

Warren, W. (1965) A study of adolescent psychiatric inpatients and the outcome six or more years later. *Journal of Child Psychology and Psychiatry*, **6**, 141–160.

Wever, C. & Rey, J.M. (1997) Juvenile obsessive-compulsive disorder. *Australian and New Zealand Journal of Psychiatry*, **31**, 105–113.

Whitaker, A., Johnson, J., Schaffer, D. *et al.* (1990) Uncommon troubles in young people: prevalence estimates of selected psychiatric disorders in a non-referred adolescent population. *Archives of General Psychiatry*, **47**, 487–496.

Winslow, J. (1989) Neuroethology of obsessive-compulsive behavior. In: *Psychobiology of Obsessive Compulsive Disorder* (eds J. Zohar, S. Rasmussen & T. Insel), pp. 208–226. Springer Verlag, New York.

Wise, S. & Rapoport, J.L. (1989) Obsessive-compulsive disorder: is it basal ganglia dysfunction? In: *Obsessive-Compulsive Disorder in Children and Adolescents* (ed. J.L. Rapoport), pp. 327–347. American Psychiatric Press, Washington D.C.

Wittchen, H.U., Nelson, C.B. & Lachner, G. (1998) Prevalence of mental disorders and psychosocial impairments in adolescents and young adults. *Psychological Medicine*, **28**, 109–126.

Wolff, R. & Rapoport, J.L. (1988) Behavioral treatment of childhood obsessive compulsive disorder. *Behavioral Modification*, **12**, 252–256.

Zeitlin, H. (1986) *The Natural History of Psychiatric Disorder in Children*. Oxford University Press, New York.

Zohar, A.H. (1999) The epidemiology of obsessive-compulsive disorder in children and adolescents. *Child and Adolescent Psychiatric Clinics of North America*, **8**, 445–460.

Zohar, J., Mueller, E.A., Insel, T.R., Zohar-Kadouch, R. & Murphy, D. (1987) Serotonergic responsivity in obsessive-compulsive disorder: comparison with patients and healthy controls. *Archives of General Psychiatry*, **44**, 946–951.

Zohar, J., Insel, T. & Zohar-Kadouch, R. (1988) Serotonergic responsivity in obsessive-compulsive effects of chronic clomipramine treatment. *Archives of General Psychiatry*, **45**, 167–172.

Zohar, A.H., Ratzoni, G., Pauls, D.L. *et al.* (1992) An epidemiological study of obsessive-compulsive disorder and related disorders in Israeli adolescents. *Journal of the American Academy of Child and Adolescent Psychiatry*, **31**, 1057–1061.

Zungu-Dirwayi, N., Hugo, F., vanHeerden, B.B. & Stein, D.J. (1999) Are musical obsessions a temporal lobe phenomenon? *Journal of Neuropsychiatry and Clinical Neuroscience*, **s11**, 398–400.

36 Tic Disorders

James F. Leckman and Donald J. Cohen

Introduction

Tic disorders are transient or chronic conditions associated with difficulties in self-esteem, family life, social acceptance or school or job performance that are directly related to the presence of motor and/or phonic tics. Although tic symptoms have been reported since antiquity, systematic study of individuals with tic disorders dates only from the nineteenth century with the reports of Itard (1825) and Gilles de la Tourette (1885). Gilles de la Tourette, in his classic study, described nine cases characterized by motor 'incoordinations' or tics, 'inarticulate shouts accompanied by articulated words with echolalia and coprolalia' (Gilles de la Tourette 1885). In addition to identifying the cardinal features of severe tic disorders, his report noted an association between tic disorders and obsessive-compulsive symptoms as well as the hereditary nature of the syndrome in some families. Recently, Kushner (1999) has published a compelling account of the many 'histories' of tic disorders.

In addition to tics, individuals with tic disorders may present with a broad array of behavioural difficulties including disinhibited speech or conduct, impulsivity, distractibility, motoric hyperactivity and obsessive-compulsive symptoms (Leckman & Cohen 1998). Alternatively, a sizeable portion of children and adolescents with tics will be free of coexisting developmental or emotional difficulties. Scientific opinion has been divided on how broadly to conceive the spectrum of maladaptive behaviours associated with Tourette syndrome (Comings 1988; Shapiro *et al.* 1988). This controversy is fuelled in part by the genuine frustration that parents and educators encounter when they attempt to divide an individual child's repertoire of problem behaviours into those that are 'Tourette-related' and those that are not. Population-based epidemiological studies and family genetic studies have begun to clarify these issues, but much work remains to be done.

In this chapter, a presentation of the phenomenology and classification of tic disorders precedes a review of the aetiology, neurobiological substrates, assessment and management of these conditions. The general perspective that will be presented is that Tourette syndrome and related disorders are model neurobiological disorders in which to study multiple interactive genetic and environmental (epigenetic) mechanisms that interact over the course of development to produce a distinctive range of complex syndromes of varying severity.

Definitions and classifications

Phenomenology of tics

A tic is a sudden repetitive movement, gesture or utterance that typically mimics some aspect or fragment of normal behaviour. Usually of brief duration, individual tics rarely last more than a second. Many tics tend to occur in bouts with brief inter-tic intervals (Peterson & Leckman 1998). Individual tics can occur singly or together in an orchestrated pattern. They vary in their intensity or forcefulness. Motor tics vary from simple abrupt movements, such as eye blinking, head jerks or shoulder shrugs, to more complex purposive-appearing behaviours, such as facial expressions or gestures of the arms or head. In extreme cases, these movements can be obscene (copropraxia) or self-injurious, e.g. hitting or biting. Phonic or vocal tics can range from simple throat-clearing sounds to more complex vocalizations and speech. In severe cases, coprolalia (obscene or socially unacceptable speech) is present.

By the age of 10 years, most individuals with tics are aware of premonitory urges that may be experienced either as a focal perception in a particular body region where the tic is about to occur (like an itch or a tickling sensation) or as a generalized awareness felt throughout the body (Lange 1991; Leckman *et al.* 1993). Most patients also report a fleeting sense of relief after a bout of tics has occurred. These premonitory and consummatory phenomena contribute to an individual's sense that tics are a habitual, yet partially intentional, response to unpleasant sensory stimuli. Indeed, most adolescent and adult subjects describe their tics either as 'voluntary' or as having both voluntary and involuntary aspects. In contrast, many young children are oblivious to their tics and experience them as wholly involuntary movements or sounds. Most tics can also be suppressed for brief periods of time. The warning given by premonitory urges may contribute to this phenomenon.

Clinicians characterize tics by their anatomical location, number, frequency and duration. The intensity or 'forcefulness' of the tic can also be an important characteristic as some tics call attention to themselves simply by virtue of the exaggerated fashion in which they are performed or uttered. Finally, tics vary in terms of their 'complexity.' Complexity usually refers to how simple or involved a movement or sound is, ranging from brief meaningless abrupt fragments (simple tics) to ones that are longer more involved and seemingly more goal-directed in character (complex tics). Each of these elements has been incorporated into clinician rating scales that have proven to be useful in monitoring tic severity (Leckman *et al.* 1989).

Diagnostic categories

Diagnostic categories can be useful to families, educators and other professionals. They provide a common basis for discussion and are an essential tool in epidemiological and clinical research. Several widely used diagnostic classifications currently include sections on tic disorders. These include both the DSM-IV classification system published by the American Psychiatric Association (1994) and the ICD-10 criteria by the World Health Organization (1996). A third classification system, the Classification of Tic Disorders (CTD), has been offered by the Tourette Syndrome Classification Study Group (1993). Although clear differences exist when comparing these classification schemes, they are broadly congruent with each containing three major well-specified categories:

1 Tourette syndrome or its equivalent;
2 chronic motor or vocal tic disorder or its equivalent; and
3 transient tic disorder or its equivalent.

Current classification of tic disorders in ICD-10 includes transient tic disorder (F95.0), chronic motor or vocal tic disorder (F95.1), combined vocal and multiple tic disorder (Tourette syndrome) (F95.2) and residual categories (F95.8 and F95.9). The ICD-10 diagnostic descriptions are largely based on the diagnostic criteria contained in DSM-IV. The ICD-10 descriptions focus on the phenomenology and natural history of the disorder and are readily applied in clinical settings. Objections can be raised to the statement contained in the description of Tourette syndrome that 'tics disappear during sleep'. Based on several empirical studies, it appears that although tics are diminished during the sleep of children and adolescents with Tourette syndrome, they do not disappear (Glaze *et al.* 1983; Jankovic & Rohaidy 1987). The statement that 'symptoms [tics] frequently worsen during adolescence', is not well supported by empirical data (Leckman *et al.* 1998a). The ICD-10 description of Tourette syndrome also overlooks the frequent presence of premonitory urges, the bout-like occurrence of tics, the waxing and waning character of the disorder (with variations in the repertoire of tics occurring over weeks to months), and the usual amelioration of the condition that occurs during mid- to late adolescence and early adulthood.

With the publication of DSM-IV in 1994, a notable difference between the CTD and DSM classification schemes emerged: the DSM-IV requirement that the tic symptoms need to 'cause marked distress or significant impairment in social, occupational or other important areas of functioning'. This criterion is based on a conceptualization of mental disorder articulated by the framers of the DSM-IV and was intended to distinguish between normality and pathology. Unfortunately, in the case of tic disorders, this criterion is vague and open to varying interpretation. The DSM-IV text is currently under revision and the impairment criterion has been dropped. With this change,

less controversy will exist about who has Tourette syndrome, and individuals who have adjusted well to the presence of tics can still be considered to have the diagnosis even if their symptoms are not a major source of distress.

At present, the CTD is a rarely used system that emphasizes whether or not the tic symptoms in question have been 'witnessed by a reliable observer directly…or recorded by videotape or cinematography'. Other differences include the retention of an age of onset of 21 years or less. However, until more objective diagnostic tests are developed, differences among clinical experts are likely to persist.

To minimize error in case ascertainment and produce an instrument measuring lifetime likelihood of having had Tourette syndrome, clinical members of the American Tourette Syndrome Association International Genetic Collaboration have developed the Diagnostic Confidence Index (DCI) (Robertson *et al.* 1999). The DCI produces a score from 0 to 100 that is a measure of the likelihood of having or ever having had Tourette syndrome. However, the DCI, together with the ICD-10, DSM-IV and CTD diagnostic groupings, suffer from uncertainties on how best to categorize conditions that potentially encompass a broad range of symptoms that wax and wane in severity. As the current nosological boundaries are set by convention and clinical practice, they may not reflect true aetiological differences.

Prevalence

Transient tic behaviours are commonplace among children. Community surveys indicate that 1–13% of boys and 1–11% of girls manifest 'frequent 'tics, twitches, mannerisms or habit spasms'' (see Zohar *et al.* 1998 for a review). The instability of these estimates are in part because of the wording of items on symptom inventories, the identity of the informant and the demographic characteristics of the sample studied. Children between the ages of 7 and 11 years appear to have the highest estimated prevalence rates that are in the range of 5%. Indeed, children are 5–12 times more likely to be identified as having a tic disorder than adults (Burd *et al.* 1986a,b). Although boys are more commonly affected with tic behaviours than girls, the male : female ratio in most community surveys is less than 2 : 1. For example, in the Isle of Wight study of 10–11 year olds, approximately 6% of boys and 3% of girls were reported by their parents to have 'twitches, mannerisms, tics of face or body' (Rutter *et al.* 1970). Similar estimates have been reported from Quebec and from North Carolina (Costello *et al.* 1996; Breton *et al.* 1999). Urban living may be associated with elevated rates (Rutter *et al.* 1974). Although most reports on tics have come from European, American and Asian sources, race and socioeconomic status have not been shown to influence the point prevalence of tics.

Less is known concerning the prevalence of Tourette syndrome. Once thought to be rare, current estimates vary 100-

fold, from 2.9 in 10 000 (Caine *et al.* 1988) to 299 in 10 000 (Mason *et al.* 1998). In the largest study to date, Apter *et al.* (1993) have reported a prevalence rate of 4.5 in 10 000 for full-blown Tourette syndrome among 16–17 year olds in Israel. Using a similar design, Costello *et al.* (1996) examined 4500 children aged 9, 11 and 13 years in rural North Carolina. The children were directly examined, as was one parent and both were asked about the last 3 months. Altogether, 10 in 10 000 children met criteria for Tourette syndrome: 13 in 10 000 for boys, and 7 in 10 000 for girls.

More recently, Mason *et al.* (1998) completed a study of all pupils aged 13–14 years in a mainstream secondary school in the UK. Students were investigated using a two-stage procedure employing standardized questionnaires completed by parents, teachers and pupils. Trained personnel to identify tics carried out classroom observations. Those pupils identified as having tics underwent a semistructured interview to determine whether they had Tourette syndrome. Five subjects were identified as having Tourette syndrome, yielding a prevalence estimate of 299 in 10 000 pupils in this age group. The results of this study suggest that Tourette syndrome in the community as a whole is more common and milder than earlier population-based studies would suggest.

Clinical descriptions and natural history

With the exception of Tourette syndrome (Shapiro *et al.* 1988; Goetz *et al.* 1992; Leckman *et al.* 1998a) relatively few cross-sectional or longitudinal studies of tic disorders have been performed so that most of the information provided below is based on clinical experience and anecdotal reports.

Transient tic disorder

Almost invariably a disorder of childhood, transient tic disorder is usually characterized by one or more simple motor tics that wax and wane in severity over weeks to months. The anatomical distribution of these tics is usually confined to the eyes, face, neck or upper extremities. Transient phonic tics, in the absence of motor tics, can also occur, although more rarely. The age of onset is typically 3–10 years and boys are at greater risk. The initial presentation may be unnoticed. If medical consultation is sought, GPs, paediatricians, allergists and ophthalmologists are typically the first to see the child. Missed diagnoses are common, particularly as the symptoms may have completely disappeared by the time of the consultation. As prescribed by the prevailing diagnostic criteria, the subsequent natural history of this condition is limited to fewer than 12 consecutive months of active symptomatology. As such, this is often a retrospective diagnosis as the clinician is unable to know with certainty which children will show progression of their symptoms and which children will display a self-limiting course.

Chronic motor or vocal tic disorder

This chronic condition can be observed among children and adults. As with other tic disorders, it is characterized by a waxing and waning course and a broad range of severity. Chronic simple and complex motor tics are the most common manifestations. Most tics involve the eyes, face, head, neck and upper extremities. Although some children may display other developmental difficulties, such as attention deficit hyperactivity disorder (ADHD), the disorder is not incompatible with an otherwise normal course of childhood. This condition can also appear as a residual state, particularly in adulthood. In such instances, a predictable repertoire of tic symptoms may only be seen during periods of heightened stress or fatigue.

Chronic vocal tic disorder, by all accounts, is a rare condition. Some authors exclude 'chronic cough of adolescence' from this category (Shapiro *et al.* 1988).

Tourette syndrome

The most severe tic disorder is best known by the eponym, Gilles de la Tourette syndrome. Typically, the disorder begins in early childhood with transient bouts of simple motor tics, such as eye blinking or head jerks. These tics may initially come and go, but eventually they become persistent and begin to have adverse effects on the child and his or her family. The repertoire of motor tics can be vast, incorporating virtually any voluntary movement by any portion of the body. Although some patients have a 'rostral–caudal' progression of motor tics (head, neck, shoulders, arms, torso), this course is not predictable. As the syndrome develops, complex motor tics may appear which typically accompany simple motor tics. Often they have a 'camouflaged' or purposive appearance, e.g. brushing hair away from the face with an arm, and can only be distinguished as tics by their repetitive character. They can involve dystonic movements. In a small fraction of cases (<5%), complex motor tics have the potential to be self-injurious and to further complicate management. These self-injurious symptoms may be relatively mild, e.g. slapping or tapping, or quite dangerous, e.g. punching one side of the face, biting a wrist or gouging eyes to the point of blindness.

On average, phonic tics begin 1–2 years after the onset of motor symptoms and are usually simple in character, e.g. throat-clearing, grunting and squeaks. More complex vocal symptoms such as echolalia (repeating another's speech), palilalia (repeating one's own speech) and coprolalia occur in a minority of cases. Other complex phonic symptoms include dramatic and abrupt changes in rhythm, rate and volume of speech.

Motor and phonic tics tend to occur in bouts. Their frequency ranges from non-stop bursts that are virtually uncountable (>100 tics/min) to rare events that occur only a few times a week. Single tics may occur in isolation or there may be orchestrated combinations of motor and phonic tics that involve multiple muscle groups. The forcefulness of motor tics and the volume of phonic tics can also vary tremendously from behaviours that are not noticeable (a slight shrug or a hushed guttural noise) to strenuous displays (arm thrusts or loud barking) that are frightening and exhausting. During periods of waxing tic symptoms, clinicians may find themselves under extreme pressure to intervene medically. Although such interventions may be warranted, it is often the case that the tic symptoms will wane substantially within a few weeks.

By the age of 10, most children and adolescents have some awareness of the premonitory urges that frequently precede both motor and vocal tics (see above). These urges add to the subjective discomfort associated with having a tic disorder. They may also contribute to an individual's ability to suppress their tics for longer periods of time.

The factors that determine the degree of disability and handicap vs. resiliency are largely unknown (see below). They are likely to include the presence of additional developmental, mental and behavioural disorders; the level of support and understanding from parents, peers and educators; and the presence of special abilities (as in sports) or personal attributes (intelligence, social abilities and personality traits). The behavioural and emotional problems that frequently complicate Tourette syndrome range from impulsive, 'disinhibited' and immature behaviour to compulsive touching or sniffing. At present there are no clear dividing lines between these disruptive behaviours and complex tics on the one hand, and comorbid conditions of ADHD and obsessive-compulsive disorder (OCD) on the other. As described below, some of these conditions may be alternate expressions of the same underlying vulnerability (e.g. OCD), others may be intimately related by virtue of shared pathophysiological mechanisms (e.g. ADHD) and still others may be the consequence of having a chronic disorder that is socially disfiguring (e.g. affective and anxiety syndromes). Defining the limits of tic disorders vis-à-vis other forms of psychopathology remains one of the most controversial and difficult areas for families, clinicians and researchers. Some investigators believe that the 'spectrum' of Tourette syndrome includes attentional deficits, impulsivity, hyperactivity, disruptive behaviour, learning disabilities, pervasive developmental disorders, affective and anxiety disorders, as well as tics and OCD (Comings 1988).

Although most children with Tourette syndrome are loving and affectionate, maintaining age-appropriate social skills appears to be a particularly difficult area for many patients (Dykens et al. 1990; Stokes et al. 1991; Bawden et al. 1998). Whether this is because of the stigmatizing effects of the tics, the patient's own uneasiness, or some more fundamental difficulty linked to the neurobiology of this disorder is unknown.

Consistent with available epidemiological data, tic disorders tend to improve in late adolescence and early adulthood. In many instances, the phonic symptoms become increasingly rare or may disappear altogether, and the motor tics may be reduced in number and frequency. Complete remission of both motor and phonic symptoms has also been reported (Shapiro et

al. 1988; Goetz et al. 1992; Leckman et al. 1998a). In contrast, adulthood is also the period when the most severe and debilitating forms of tic disorder can be seen. The factors that influence the continuity of tic disorders from childhood to adolescence to adulthood are not well understood but probably involve the interaction of normal maturational processes occurring in the central nervous system with the neurobiological mechanisms responsible for Tourette syndrome, the exposure to cocaine, other central nervous system stimulants, androgenic steroids and the amount of intramorbid emotional trauma and distress experienced by affected individuals during childhood and adolescence. In addition, it should be emphasized that tic disorders may be aetiologically separable so that some of these factors, such as activation of the immune system or exposure to heat stress, may influence the pathogenesis and intramorbid course for some tic disorders but not others. Other factors, such as psychological stress, may have a more uniform adverse impact.

Coexisting conditions

The past decade has seen a renewed emphasis on the range of neurological and psychiatric symptoms seen in Tourette syndrome patients (Leckman & Cohen 1998). Symptoms associated with OCD and ADHD have received the most attention.

Obsessive-compulsive symptoms

Clinical and epidemiological studies indicate that more than 40% of individuals with Tourette syndrome experience recurrent obsessive-compulsive symptoms (Leckman et al. 1994, 1997a; Swerdlow et al. 1999). Genetic, neurobiological and treatment response studies suggest that there may be qualitative differences between tic-related forms of OCD and cases of OCD in which there is no personal or family history of tics. Specifically, compared with non-tic-related OCD, tic-related OCD has a male preponderance, an earlier age of onset, a poorer level of response to standard antiobsessional medications, and a greater likelihood of first-degree family members with a tic disorder (Miguel et al. 2001).

Symptomatically, the most common obsessive-compulsive symptoms encountered in Tourette syndrome patients are:
1 obsessions about aggression, sex, religion and the body, as well as related checking compulsions; and
2 obsessions concerning a need for symmetry or exactness, repeating rituals, counting compulsions, and ordering/arranging compulsions (Leckman et al. 1997a).

Attention deficit hyperactivity disorder

Clinical and epidemiological studies sharply differ on rates of ADHD seen among individuals with Tourette syndrome (Walkup et al. 1998). Clinical studies vary according to setting and established referral patterns, but it is not uncommon to see reports of 50% or more of referred children with Tourette syndrome diagnosed with comorbid ADHD. In contrast, epidemiological studies typically indicate a much lower rate of comorbidity (Apter *et al.* 1993). Although the aetiological relationship between Tourette syndrome and ADHD is in dispute, it is clear that those individuals with both Tourette syndrome and ADHD are at a much greater risk for a variety of untoward outcomes (Carter *et al.* 2000). Uninformed peers frequently tease individuals with Tourette syndrome. They are often regarded as less likeable, more aggressive and more withdrawn than their classmates (Stokes *et al.* 1991). These social difficulties are amplified in a child with Tourette syndrome who also has ADHD (Bawden *et al.* 1998). In such cases, their level of social skill is often several years behind their peers (Dykens *et al.* 1990).

Negative appraisal by peers in childhood is a strong predictor of global indices of psychopathology (Hinshaw 1994). This appears to be particularly true for children with Tourette syndrome and ADHD. Longitudinal studies confirm that these individuals are at high risk for anxiety and mood disorders, oppositional defiant disorder and conduct disorder (Carter *et al.* 1994, 2000). Much of this negative impact appears to be a result of the ADHD, as children who only have Tourette syndrome tend to fare far better (Spencer *et al.* 1998; Carter *et al.* 2000). Surprisingly, levels of tic severity are less predictive of peer acceptance than is the presence of ADHD (Bawden *et al.* 1998). Furthermore, the rates of subsequent psychiatric morbidity seen in Tourette syndrome plus ADHD subjects are nearly identical to those seen in prior cross-sectional and longitudinal studies of ADHD subjects who do not have tics (Greene *et al.* 1997; Mannuzza *et al.* 1998).

Other developmental disorders

Children with a range of developmental disorders appear to be at increased risk for tic disorders. Kurlan *et al.* (1994) reported a fourfold increase in the prevalence of tic disorders among children in special educational settings in a single school district in upstate New York. These children were not mentally retarded but did have significant learning disabilities or other speech or physical impairments.

Children with autism and other pervasive developmental disorders are also at higher risk for developing Tourette syndrome. In a recent survey of 447 pupils from nine schools for children and adolescents with autism, 19 children were found to have definite Tourette syndrome, yielding a prevalence rate of 4.3% (Baron-Cohen *et al.* 1999). Although this figure exceeds available population-based estimates, it should be viewed with caution. Complex motor tics can be difficult to distinguish from motor stereotypies. Differentiation among these behaviours may be especially problematic among retarded individuals with limited verbal skills. Further study is required to elucidate the relationship between Tourette syndrome and other disorders of central nervous system development.

Neuropsychological findings

Although motor and phonic tics constitute the core elements of the diagnostic criteria for Tourette syndrome, perceptual and cognitive difficulties are also common. These neuropsychological symptoms are potentially informative about the pathobiology of the disorder. Moreover, these associated difficulties can be more problematic for school and social adjustment than the primary motor symptoms (Dykens *et al.* 1998; Walkup *et al.* 1998).

Neuropsychological studies of Tourette syndrome have focused on a broad array of functions. Review of the literature suggests that the most consistently observed deficits occur on tasks requiring the accurate copy of geometric designs ('visuomotor integration') or 'visuographic' ability (see Schultz *et al.* 1998 for a review). There was no evidence to suggest that comorbid ADHD or depressive symptomatology could account for the observed group differences. Even after controlling statistically for visuoperceptual skill, intelligence and fine motor control, children with Tourette syndrome continued to perform worse than controls on the visuomotor tasks, suggesting that the integration of visual inputs and organized motor output is a specific area of weakness in individuals with Tourette syndrome.

Aetiology and pathogenesis

During the course of the past decade, Tourette syndrome and related conditions have emerged as model disorders for researchers interested in the interaction of genetic, neurobiological and environmental (epigenetic) factors which shape clinical outcomes from health to chronic disability over the life span.

Genetic factors

Twin and family studies provide evidence that genetic factors are involved in the vertical transmission within families of a vulnerability to Tourette syndrome and related disorders (Pauls & Leckman 1986). The concordance rate for Tourette syndrome among monozygotic twin pairs is greater than 50%, while the concordance of dizygotic twin pairs is about 10% (Price *et al.* 1985; Hyde *et al.* 1992). If cotwins with chronic motor tic disorder are included, these concordance figures increase to 77% for monozygotic and 30% for dizygotic twin pairs. Differences in the concordance of monozygotic and dizygotic twin pairs indicate that genetic factors have an important role in the aetiology of Tourette syndrome and related conditions. These figures also suggest that non-genetic factors are critical in determining the nature and severity of the clinical syndrome.

Other studies indicate that first-degree family members of Tourette syndrome probands are at substantially higher risk for developing Tourette syndrome, chronic motor tic disorder and OCD than unrelated individuals (Hebebrand *et al.* 1997; Pauls *et al.* 1991; Walkup *et al.* 1996). Overall, the risk to male first-degree family members approximates 50% (18% Tourette syndrome, 31% chronic motor tics and 7% OCD) while the overall risk to females is less (5% Tourette syndrome, 9% chronic motor tics and 17% OCD). These rates are substantially higher than might be expected by chance in the general population, and greatly exceed the rates for these disorders among the relatives of individuals with other psychiatric disorders except OCD.

The pattern of vertical transmission among family members has led several groups of investigators to test whether or not mathematical models of specific genetic hypotheses could be rejected. While not definitive, most segregation analyses could not rule out models of autosomal transmission (Pauls & Leckman 1986; Walkup *et al.* 1996). These studies prompted the identification of large multigenerational families for genetic linkage studies. However, subsequent efforts to identify susceptibility genes within these high-density families using traditional linkage strategies have met with little success (Barr & Sandor 1998).

More recently, non-parametric approaches using families in which two or more siblings are affected with Tourette syndrome have been undertaken (Tourette Syndrome International Consortium for Genetics 1999). This sib-pair approach is suited for diseases with an unclear mode of inheritance and has been used successfully in studies of other complex disorders, such as diabetes mellitus and essential hypertension. In this study, two areas are suggestive of linkage to Tourette syndrome: one on chromosome 4q and another on chromosome 8p. Currently, this international consortium of researchers is actively completing high-density maps of several genomic regions in an effort to refine and extend their preliminary results. In addition, several studies have implicated a region on 11q23 (Merrette *et al.* 2000; Simonic *et al.* 2001).

It is also noteworthy that none of the chromosomal regions (e.g. 3 [3p21.3], 8 [8q21.4], 9 [9pter] and 18 [18q22.3]) in which cytogenetic abnormalities have been found to cosegregate with Tourette syndrome showed any convincing evidence for linkage in the sib-pair study. It is still possible that rare susceptibility genes may be found in one or more of these regions using molecular cytogenetic techniques. Furthermore, none of the regions associated with candidate genes, such as *DRD2* [11q22] and *DRD4* [11p15], were supported by the results of the sib-pair study. Future progress is anticipated and clarity about the nature and normal expression of even a few of the Tourette syndrome susceptibility genes is likely to provide a major step forward in understanding the pathogenesis of this condition.

Neural circuits

The basal ganglia are key structures in the assembly and activation of cognitive, emotive and motor routines (habits) that are expressed in response to specific environmental cues (Graybiel 1998). The basal ganglia are subcortical nuclei that process information from the cortex before passing it along to thalamic nuclei that in turn project information back to more restricted cortical regions (Parent & Hazrati 1995). These corticostriatothalamocortical (CSTC) neural loops have long been a focus of Tourette syndrome and OCD research (see Leckman & Riddle 2000 for a review). Specifically, it has been hypothesized that Tourette syndrome and aetiologically related forms of OCD are associated with a failure to regulate sensorimotor and orbitofrontal subsets of the CSTC minicircuits, respectively (Leckman *et al.* 1991a, 1997b). Preliminary evidence in support of this hypothesis includes the ameliorative effects on tic and obsessive-compulsive behaviours following neurosurgical ablation or high-frequency electrical stimulation of thalamic nuclei and following procedures that isolate regions of the prefrontal cortex (Rauch *et al.* 1995; Lippitz *et al.* 1999; Vandewalle *et al.* 1999). In Tourette syndrome, volumetric magnetic resonance imaging (MRI) studies have also provided preliminary evidence of volume differences within the basal ganglia and cortical regions (Peterson *et al.* 1993; Peterson *et al.* 2001; Singer *et al.* 1993). Recent functional MRI studies present a more complex picture in which altered patterns of activation and/or deactivation of prefrontal cortex likely influence voluntary tic suppression or active ticking (Peterson *et al.* 1998a). If confirmed, these findings are consistent with the view that prefrontal cortex–basal ganglia circuits participate in the shaping of the inhibitory output of the basal ganglia. A similar picture has emerged in the study of individuals with OCD using functional neuroimaging techniques (Baxter *et al.* 1992).

Other aspects of the circuitry of the basal ganglia may provide important clues concerning the anatomical distribution of motor tics and the 'choice' of obsessive themes frequently encountered in forms of OCD related to Tourette syndrome. Specifically, the unidirectional input from the amygdala and the bed nucleus of the stria terminalis to widespread areas of the nucleus accumbens and ventral portions of the caudate and putamen appears to overlap those areas most affected in Tourette syndrome and related forms of OCD (Nauta 1982; Russchen *et al.* 1985). Studies in primates and humans have also shown that stimulation of the amygdala produces motor and vocal activity reminiscent of the symptoms of Tourette syndrome (McLean & Delgado 1953; Baldwin *et al.* 1954).

Reciprocal connections between midbrain sites (periaqueductal grey, substantia nigra and the ventral tegmental area), portions of the hypothalamus and structures in the basal ganglia and amygdala are likely to have a critical role in the genesis and maintenance of the symptoms of Tourette syndrome. These connections may also contribute to the stress sensitivity, including sensitivity to thermal stress observed in a limited number of subjects, and to the more frequent expression of Tourette syndrome in males than females, as many of these structures contain receptors for gonadal steroids and are responsive to alterations in their hormonal environment (see below).

Recent studies using transcranial magnetic stimulation have reported altered patterns of cortical inhibition/excitation. Specifically, following focal transcranial magnetic stimulation to the motor cortex, Ziemann *et al.* (1997) have documented that the cortical silent period was shortened and the intracortical inhibition reduced in Tourette syndrome patients. This suggests either disinhibited thalamic input or impaired intracortical inhibition directly at the level of the motor cortex.

Neurochemical and neuropharmacological data

Extensive immunohistochemical studies of the basal ganglia have demonstrated the presence of a wide spectrum of classic neurotransmitters, neuromodulators and neuropeptides (Parent 1986; Graybiel 1990). The functional status of a number of these systems has been evaluated in Tourette syndrome (see Anderson *et al.* 1998 for a review). In the following section, the current status of a select group of these compounds is reviewed with special attention to those that are related to medications currently used to treat tics and related conditions.

Dopaminergic systems

Inputs from ascending dopamine pathways originating in the substantia nigra pars compacta play a crucial role in co-ordinating the output from the striatum (Aosaki *et al.* 1994). Explicit 'dopamine' hypotheses for Tourette syndrome posit either an excess of dopamine or an increased sensitivity of D_2 dopamine receptors. These hypotheses are consistent with multiple lines of empirical evidence as well as emerging data from animal models of habit formation. Data implicating central dopaminergic mechanisms include the results of double-blind clinical trials in which haloperidol, pimozide, tiapride and other neuroleptics that preferentially block dopaminergic D_2 receptors have been found to be effective in the temporary suppression of tics for most patients (see Chappell *et al.* 1997 for a review). Tic suppression has also been reported following administration of agents such as tetrabenazine that reduce dopamine synthesis (Shapiro & Shapiro 1988 for a review). Increased tics have been reported following withdrawal of neuroleptics or following exposure to agents that increase central dopaminergic activity, such as L-dopa and central nervous system stimulants, including cocaine (see Anderson *et al.* 1998 for a review). Preliminary positron emission tomography (PET) studies of brain dopamine D_2 receptors provide some evidence that the density and/or binding of D_2 receptors in the striatum are associated with current levels of tic severity (Wolf *et al.* 1996; Wong *et al.* 1997). Post-mortem brain and ligand-based neuroimaging studies have reported alterations in the number or affinity of presynaptic dopamine carrier sites in the striatum (Singer *et al.* 1991; Malison *et al.* 1995) or the presynaptic processing of dopamine (Ernst *et al.* 1999). However, a recent assessment of the number of striatal vesicular monoamine transporter type 2 sites found no differences between Tourette syndrome patients and controls (Meyer *et al.* 1999).

In summary, while the evidence that dopaminergic pathways are intimately involved in the pathobiology of Tourette syndrome is compelling, the exact nature of the abnormality remains to be elucidated.

Excitatory amino acid systems

The excitatory neurotransmitter, glutamate, is released upon depolarization by the corticostriatal, corticosubthalamic, subthalamic and thalamocortical projection neurones. As such, these excitatory neurones are key players in the functional anatomy of the basal ganglia and the CSTC loops. While the activity of these neurones are likely to be important in Tourette syndrome, only limited data are available to evaluate their role in this disease. For example, Anderson *et al.* (1992) have hypothesized that the disinhibition of thalamocortical projection neurones may be partly caused by a failure of the subthalamic nucleus to activate the inhibitory output neurones of the basal ganglia. However, this speculation is based on the results of an examination of just four post-mortem brain specimens.

Inhibitory amino acid systems

Neurones containing inhibitory amino acid neurotransmitters, particularly gamma-aminobutyric acid (GABA), also form major portions of CSTC loops. These include GABAergic medium spiny neurones of the striatum that project to the internal segment of the globus pallidus and the pars reticulata of the substantia nigra within the 'direct pathway'. GABAergic neurones are also present in the 'indirect pathway' that relays information from the striatum to the external segment of the globus pallidus and from there to the internal segment of the globus pallidus. An imbalance between the direct and indirect pathways has been hypothesized in Tourette syndrome (Leckman *et al.* 1991a). However, there is very little direct evidence available to support this hypothesis. Clinical studies have shown that benzodiazepines, which enhance the inhibitory effects of GABA, have some value in the treatment of tics (Gonce & Barbeau 1977). But thus far, post-mortem and other studies have failed to detect any significant abnormalities in these cells compared to controls (see Anderson *et al.* 1998 for a review).

Cholinergic systems

The large aspiny interneurones found throughout the striatum are likely to be critically involved in the co-ordination of striatal response through interactions with central dopaminergic and GABAergic neurones (Aosaki *et al.* 1994). Cholinergic projections from the basal forebrain are found throughout the cortex and within key structures of the basal ganglia and mesencephalon, including the internal segment of the globus pallidus, the pars reticulata of the substantia nigra and the locus caeruleus. Evidence of cholinergic involvement in the pathobiology of Tourette syndrome concerns the reported potentiation of D_2 dopamine receptor blocking agents through the use of transdermal nicotine or nicotine gum (Sanberg *et al.* 1997) and more recent reports of the usefulness of a non-competitive cholinergic agonist, mecamylamine (Silver *et al.*, 2000). Unfortunately, the efficacy of these agents has yet to be evaluated in a double-blind trial. Further, none of the post-mortem or cerebrospinal fluid studies has detected differences between patients and controls (see Anderson *et al.* 1998 for a review).

Endogenous opioid peptides

Endogenous opioid peptides (EOPs) are localized in structures of the extrapyramidal system, are known to interact with central dopaminergic and GABAergic neurones, and are likely to be importantly involved in the gating of motor functions. Two of the three families of EOPs, dynorphin and metenkephalin, are highly concentrated and similarly distributed in the basal ganglia and substantia nigra. In addition, significant levels of opiate receptor binding have been detected in both primate and human neostriatum and substantia nigra.

EOPs have been directly implicated in the pathophysiology of Tourette syndrome. Haber *et al.* (1986) reported decreased levels of dynorphin A(1–17) immunoreactivity in striatal fibres projecting to the globus pallidus in post-mortem material from a small number of Tourette patients. This observation, coupled with the neuroanatomical distribution of dynorphin, its broad range of motor and behavioural effects, and its modulatory interactions with striatal dopaminergic systems, suggested that dynorphin might have a key role in the pathobiology of Tourette syndrome. However, subsequent studies have failed to confirm these initial observations (van Wattum *et al.* 1999; also see Anderson *et al.* 1998 for a review).

Noradrenergic systems

Noradrenergic projections from the locus caeruleus project widely to the prefrontal and other cortical regions. Noradrenergic pathways are also likely to indirectly influence central dopaminergic pathways via projections to areas near the ventral tegmental area (Grenhoff & Svensson 1989). Speculation that noradrenergic mechanisms might be relevant to the pathobiology of Tourette syndrome was based initially on the beneficial effects of α_2-adrenergic agonists including clonidine (Cohen *et al.* 1979). Although clonidine is one of the most widely prescribed agents for the treatment of tics, its effectiveness remains controversial (Goetz *et al.* 1987; Leckman *et al.* 1991b). In open trials another related α_2-adrenergic agonist, guanfacine, has also been reported to reduce tics and improve ADHD symptoms (Chappell *et al.* 1995). At the level of receptor function, clonidine has been traditionally viewed as a selective α_2-adrenoceptor agonist active at presynaptic sites, and its primary mode of action may be its ability to reduce the firing rate and the release of noradrenaline from central noradrenergic neurones. However, evidence of heterogeneity among the α_2 class of adrenoceptors and their distinctive distribution within relevant brain regions adds further complexity. Specifically, differential effects in cortical regions mediated by specific receptor subtypes may account for the differential responsiveness of particular behavioural features of this syndrome to treatment with clonidine vs. guanfacine (Arnsten 2000).

The involvement of the noradrenergic pathways may be one of the mechanisms by which stressors may influence tic severity. For example, a series of adult Tourette syndrome patients were found to have elevated levels of cerebrospinal fluid noradenaline (Leckman *et al.* 1995) and to have excreted high levels of urinary noradenaline in response to the stress of the lumbar puncture (Chappell *et al.* 1994a). These elevated levels of cerebrospinal fluid noradenaline may also contribute to the elevation in cerebrospinal fluid corticotropin releasing factor levels seen in some Tourette syndrome patients (Chappell *et al.* 1996).

Serotonergic systems

Ascending serotonergic projections from the dorsal raphe have been repeatedly invoked as playing a part in the pathophysiology of both Tourette syndrome and OCD. The most compelling evidence relates to OCD and is based largely on the well-established efficacy of potent serotonin reuptake inhibitors (SRIs) such as clomipramine and fluvoxamine in the treatment of OCD (Greist & Jefferson 1998). However, some investigators have reported that the SRIs are less effective in treating tic-related OCD compared with other forms of OCD (McDougle *et al.* 1993). It is also doubtful that treatment with SRIs diminishes tic symptoms (Scahill *et al.* 1997). Additional evidence has come from pharmacological challenge studies in which serotonergic agonists such as metachlorophenyl-piperazine (mCPP) were found to exacerbate obsessive-compulsive symptoms in some patients (Zohar *et al.* 1987). However, not all OCD patients show this response (Goodman *et al.* 1995) and this agent does not appear to exacerbate tics in Tourette syndrome patients (Cath *et al.* 1999). Finally, preliminary post-mortem brain studies in Tourette syndrome have suggested that serotonin and the related compounds tryptophan (TRP) and 5-hydroxyindoleacetic acid (5-HIAA) may be globally decreased in the basal ganglia and other areas receiving projections from the dorsal raphe (Anderson *et al.* 1992).

Gender-specific endocrine factors

Males are more frequently affected than females with Tourette syndrome (Shapiro *et al.* 1988). While this could be caused by genetic mechanisms, frequent male-to-male transmission within families appears to rule out the presence of an X-linked vulnerability gene. This observation has led us to hypothesize that androgenic steroids act at key developmental periods to influence the natural history of Tourette syndrome and related disorders (Peterson *et al.* 1992). These developmental periods include the prenatal period when the brain is being formed, adrenarche when adrenal androgens first appear at age 5–7 years, and puberty. Androgenic steroids may be responsible for these effects or they may act indirectly through oestrogens formed in key brain regions by the aromatization of testosterone.

The importance of gender differences in expression of associated phenotypes is also clear given the observation that women are more likely than men to develop obsessive-compulsive symptoms without concomitant tics (Pauls *et al.* 1991) and that boys are much more likely than girls to display disruptive behaviours (Comings & Comings 1987).

Surges in testosterone and other androgenic steroids during critical periods in fetal development are known to be involved in the production of long-term functional augmentation of subsequent hormonal challenges (as in adrenarche and during puberty) and in the formation of structural central nervous system dimorphisms (Sikich & Todd 1988). In recent years several sexually dimorphic brain regions have been described, including portions of the amygdala (and related limbic areas) and the hypothalamus (including the medial preoptic area that mediates the body's response to thermal stress) (Boulant 1998). These regions contain high levels of androgen and oestrogen receptors and are known to influence activity in the basal ganglia both directly and indirectly (Fehrbach *et al.* 1985). Indeed a proportion of Tourette syndrome patients appear to be uniquely sensitive to thermal stress such that when their core body temperature increases and they begin to sweat their tics increase (Lombroso *et al.* 1992). It is also of note that some of the neurochemical and neuropeptidergic systems implicated in Tourette syndrome and related disorders, such as dopamine, serotonin and the opioids, are involved with these regions and appear to be regulated by sex-specific factors.

Further support for a role for androgens comes from anecdotal reports of tic exacerbation following androgen use (Leckman & Scahill 1990) and from trials of antiandrogens in patients with severe Tourette syndrome and/or OCD (Casas *et al.* 1986; Peterson *et al.* 1998b; Altemus *et al.* 1999). In the most rigorous study to date, Peterson *et al.* (1998b) found that the therapeutic effects of the antiandrogen, flutamide, were modest in magnitude and these effects were short-lived, possibly because of physiological compensation for androgen receptor blockade.

Perinatal risk factors

The search for non-genetic factors which mediate the expression of a genetic vulnerability to Tourette syndrome and related disorders has also focused on the role of adverse perinatal events. This interest dates from the report of Pasamanick & Kawi (1956) who found that mothers of children with tics were 1.5 times more likely to have experienced a complication during pregnancy than the mothers of children without tics. Other investigations have reported that among monozygotic twins discordant for Tourette syndrome, the index twins with Tourette syndrome had lower birth weights than their unaffected cotwins (Leckman *et al.* 1987; Hyde *et al.* 1992). Severity of maternal life stress during pregnancy, severe nausea and/or vomiting during the first trimester have also emerged as potential risk factors in the development of tic disorders (Leckman *et al.* 1990). Whitaker *et al.* (1997) reported that premature and low birth weight children are at increased risk of developing tic disorders and ADHD. This appears to be especially true of children who had ischaemic parenchymal brain lesions. More recently, Burd *et al.* (1999) presented the results of a case–control study in which low Apgar scores at 5 min and *more* prenatal visits were associated with a higher risk of Tourette syndrome. Finally, there is limited evidence that smoking and alcohol use, as well as forceps delivery, can predispose individuals with a vulnerability to Tourette syndrome to develop comorbid OCD (Santangelo *et al.* 1994).

Post-infectious autoimmune mechanisms

It is well established that group A β-haemolytic streptococci (GABHS) can trigger immune-mediated disease in genetically predisposed individuals (Bisno 1991). Speculation concerning a post-infectious (or at least a post-rheumatic fever) aetiology for tic disorder symptoms dates from the late 1800s (Kushner 1999). Acute rheumatic fever is a delayed sequela of GABHS, occurring approximately 3 weeks following an inadequately treated upper respiratory tract infection. Rheumatical fever is characterized by inflammatory lesions involving the heart (rheumatic carditis), joints (polymigratory arthritis), and/or central nervous system (Sydenham chorea; SC). SC and Tourette syndrome, OCD and ADHD share common anatomical targets—the basal ganglia of the brain and the related cortical and thalamic sites (Husby *et al.* 1976). Furthermore, SC patients frequently display motor and vocal tics, obsessive-compulsive and ADHD symptoms suggesting the possibility that, at least in some instances, these disorders share a common aetiology (Swedo *et al.* 1989; Mercadante *et al.* 1997).

It has been proposed that paediatric autoimmune neuropsychiatric disorder associated with streptococcal infection (PANDAS) represents a distinct clinical entity, and includes SC and some cases of Tourette syndrome and OCD (Swedo *et al.* 1998). The most compelling evidence that acute exacerbations of Tourette syndrome and OCD can be triggered by GABHS comes from two independent reports demonstrating that the vast majority of patients with childhood onset Tourette syndrome or OCD have elevated expression of a stable B-cell marker (Murphy *et al.* 1997; Swedo *et al.* 1997). The D8/17 marker identifies close to 100% of rheumatic fever patients (with or without SC) but is present at low levels of expression in healthy control populations. The identity of the D8/17 epitope is not yet known, but it can be expressed by several non-B-cell types (Kemeny *et al.* 1994). Further suggestive evidence comes from Swedo *et al.* (1998) who reported that in children who met PANDAS criteria, GABHS infection was likely to have preceded neuropsychiatric symptom onset for 44% of the children, whereas pharyngitis (no culture obtained) preceded onset for another 28% of the children. There were 144 episodes of symptom exacerbation among these 50 children. In addition to tic and obsessive-compulsive symptoms, cognitive deficits, oppositional behaviours and motor hyperactivity were reported to be 'particularly common' during periods of exacerbation. Thirty-one per cent of these exacerbations were associated with documented GABHS infection, and 42% with symptoms of pharyngitis or upper respiratory infection (no throat culture obtained). While these results are intriguing, they are preliminary.

As individuals were selected for having a recent or recurrent history of GABHS infections, the magnitude of some of the reported associations may have been biased upwards.

In summary, a substantial body of circumstantial evidence exists that links post-infectious autoimmune phenomena with Tourette syndrome, OCD and ADHD. However, these data are not compelling with regard to specific immunological mechanisms (Singer *et al.* 1998), nor do they establish where in the sequence of causal events these immune changes occur. These potentially important findings require replication in independent samples and warrant more intensive investigation.

Psychological factors

Tic disorders have long been identified as 'stress-sensitive' conditions (Jagger *et al.* 1982; Shapiro *et al.* 1988; Silva *et al.* 1995; Witzum *et al.* 1996). Typically, symptom exacerbations follow in the wake of stressful life events. As noted by Shapiro *et al.* (1988), these events need not be adverse in character. Clinical experience suggests that in some unfortunate instances a vicious cycle can be initiated in which tic symptoms are misunderstood by the family and teachers, leading to active attempts to suppress the symptoms by punishment and humiliation. These efforts can lead to a further exacerbation of symptoms and further increase in stress in the child's interpersonal environment. Unchecked, this vicious cycle can lead to the most severe manifestations of Tourette syndrome and dysthymia as well as maladaptive characterological traits. Although psychological factors are insufficient to cause Tourette syndrome, the intimate association of the content and timing of tic behaviours and dynamically important events in the lives of children make it difficult to overlook their contribution to the intramorbid course of these disorders (Carter *et al.* 1994, 2000).

In addition to the intramorbid effects of stress and anxiety that have been well characterized, premorbid stress may also play an important part as a sensitizing agent in the pathogenesis of Tourette syndrome among vulnerable individuals (Leckman *et al.* 1984).

It is likely that the immediate family environment (e.g. parental discord) and the coping abilities of family members have some role (Leckman *et al.* 1990), and this may lead to a sensitization of stress-responsive biological systems such as the hypothalamic–pituitary–adrenal axis (see above, Chappell *et al.* 1994a, 1996; Leckman *et al.* 1995).

Differential diagnosis

The differential diagnosis of simple motor tics includes a variety of hyperkinetic movements: myoclonus, tremors, chorea, athetosis, dystonias, akathisic movements, paroxysmal dyskinesias, ballistic movements and hyperekplexia (see Towbin *et al.* 1998 for a review). These movements may be associated with:
• genetic conditions, such as Huntington chorea or Wilson disease;

• structural lesions, as in hemiballismus (associated with lesions to the contralateral subthalamic nucleus);
• infectious processes, as in SC;
• idiopathic functional instability of neuronal circuits, as in myoclonic epilepsy; and
• pharmacological treatments, such as acute akathisia and dystonias associated with the use of neuroleptic agents.

Differentiation between these conditions and tic disorders is usually accomplished on clinical grounds and is based on the presentation of the disorder and its natural history. For example, although aspects of tics—such as their abruptness, their paroxysmal timing or their suppressible nature—may be similar to symptoms seen in other conditions, it is rare for all of these features to be combined in the absence of a bona fide tic disorder. Occasionally diagnostic tests are needed to exclude alternative diagnoses.

Complex motor tics can be confused with other complex repetitive behaviours, such as stereotypies or compulsive rituals. Differentiation among these behaviours may be difficult, particularly among retarded individuals with limited verbal skills. In other settings where these symptoms are closely intertwined, as in individuals with both Tourette syndrome and OCD, efforts to distinguish between complex motor tics and compulsive behaviours may be futile. In cases of a tic disorder, it is unusual to see complex motor tics in the absence of simple tics. Involuntary vocal utterances are uncommon neurological signs in the absence of a tic disorder. Examples include sniffing and brief sounds in Huntington disease and involuntary moaning in Parkinson disease particularly as a result of L-dopa toxicity. Complex phonic tics characterized by articulate speech typically can be distinguished from other conditions including voluntary coprolalia. Because of their rarity in other syndromes, phonic tics can have an important role in differential diagnosis.

Anamnesis, family history, observation and neurological examination are usually sufficient to establish the diagnosis of a tic disorder. There are no confirmatory diagnostic tests. Neuroimaging studies, electroencephalography-based studies and laboratory tests are usually non-contributory, except in atypical cases.

Assessment

Once the diagnosis has been established, care should be taken to focus on the overall course of an individual's development, not simply on his or her tic symptoms. This may be a particular problem in the case of Tourette syndrome where the symptoms can be dramatic and there is the temptation to organize all of an individual's behavioural and emotional difficulties under a single all-encompassing rubric.

The principal goal of an initial assessment is to determine the individual's overall level of adaptive functioning and to identify areas of impairment and distress (Leckman *et al.* 1998b). Close attention to the strengths and weaknesses of the individual and his or her family is crucial. Relevant dimensions include the presence of comorbid mental, behavioural, developmental or physical disorders; family history of psychiatric and/or neurological disease; relationships with family and peers; school and/or occupational performance; and the history of important life events. Medication history is important, particularly if the disorder is long-standing or if medications have been prescribed for physical disorders. It may be necessary to evaluate the adequacy of the prior trials with pharmacological agents used to treat tic disorders. Inventories such as the Yale Child Study Center: Tourette Syndrome Obsessive-Compulsive Disorder Symptom Questionnaire (Leckman & Cohen 1998, Appendix 1) completed by the family prior to their initial consultation can be valuable ancillary tools to gain a long-term perspective of the child's developmental course and the natural history of the tic disorder. In addition, several valid and reliable clinical rating instruments have been developed to inventory and quantify recent tic symptoms including the Yale Global Tic Severity Scale (YGTSS; Leckman et al. 1989), the Tourette Syndrome Severity Scale (TSSS; Shapiro et al. 1988), the Hopkins Motor and Vocal Tic Scale (HMVTS), and some clinicians make regular use of standardized videotape protocols to assess current tic severity (Tanner et al. 1982; Shapiro et al. 1988; Walkup et al. 1992; Chappell et al. 1994b).

The YGTSS is a clinician-rated semistructured scale that begins with a systematic inventory of tic symptoms that the clinician rates as present or absent over the past week. Current motor and phonic tics are then rated separately according to number, frequency, intensity, complexity and interference on a 6-point ordinal scale (0, absent; 1–5 for severity) yielding three scores: Total Motor, Total Phonic and Total Tic Score. The scale concludes with an overall impairment rating. The YGTSS has shown excellent interrater agreement as well has other desirable psychometric properties (Leckman et al. 1989).

Because the YGTSS permits the clinician to incorporate direct observation with historical information, it requires both training with the instrument and clinical experience with tic disorders. At present most investigators consider the YGTSS to be state-of-the-art with regard to clinician ratings of tic severity.

Other clinician-rated scales include the TSSS (Shapiro et al. 1988); Tourette Syndrome Global Scale (TSGS; Harcherik et al. 1984); and the HMVTS (Walkup et al. 1992). Although both the TSSS and TSGS have been used in many published reports, both scales have unconventional scoring procedures and unstable psychometric properties. The HMVTS is a more recently developed instrument that combines self-report data with clinician assessment, resulting in a composite rating. This scale consists of a series of analogue scales that are tallied to yield a 1–5 score for motor, phonic and total score. This scale has shown promise as a global measure of tic severity in a preliminary study of 20 children, but has not entered into common use. When compared to other measures of tic severity, the HMVTS showed the strongest correlation with the YGTSS. In addition to clinician ratings, there are two other methods of estimating tic severity: self-reports (parent reports in the case of children) and direct observational methods, such as videotaped counts of tics for variable

periods of time. Each of these methods has advantages and disadvantages (Scahill et al. 1998). The validity of self-reports may be limited by inaccurate information about the nature of tics on the part of the child or parent leading to over- or underendorsement of symptoms. On the other hand, self-reports are efficient and potentially cost effective. At present, the most widely used self-report measure is the Tic Symptom Self-Report. It consists of a checklist of simple and complex motor and phonic tics over the prior week (Cohen et al. 1984).

Direct observational methods include videotape tic counting procedures (Chappell et al. 1994b; Goetz et al. 1999) or in vivo evaluation of tic symptoms (Nolan et al. 1994). These direct observational methods would appear to be the most objective measure of tic severity; however, the frequency of tics varies according to setting and activity. In addition, many individuals with Tourette syndrome can suppress their symptoms for brief periods of time. In practice, videotaped tic counting appears to be most useful for acute research procedures that take place over several hours. Clinically, videotaping can be quite valuable when the diagnosis is in doubt or when tics are not observed in the consultation room.

Treatment

Tic disorders are frequently chronic, if not lifelong, conditions. Continuity of care is desirable and should be considered before embarking on a course of treatment. Usual clinical practice focuses initially on the educational and supportive interventions with pharmacological treatments typically held in reserve. Given the waxing and waning course of the disorders, it is likely that whatever is done (or not done) will lead in the short term to some improvement in tic severity. The decision to employ psychoactive medications is usually made after the educational and supportive interventions have been in place for a period of months and it is clear that the tic symptoms are persistently severe and are themselves a source of impairment in terms of self-esteem, relationships with the family or peers, or the child's ability to perform at school.

Educational and supportive interventions

Educational activities are among the most important interventions available to the clinician. They should be undertaken first, not only with patients with Tourette syndrome but also with patients with milder presentations. Although the efficacy of these educational and supportive interventions has not been rigorously assessed, they appear to have positive effects by reshaping familial expectations and relationships (Cohen et al. 1988). This is particularly true when the family and colleagues have misconstrued the tic symptoms as being intentionally provocative. Families also find descriptions of the natural history comforting in that the disorders tend not to be relentlessly progressive and usually improve during adulthood. This information often contradicts the impressions gained from the available lay literature on Tourette syndrome that typically focuses on the most extreme cases. Armed with this knowledge, patients and family members and colleagues can begin to understand why waiting before beginning medical treatment makes good sense. If a patient is in the midst of a bad period of tics, it is likely that whether or not a new medication is prescribed, the tics will probably get significantly better in the near future. This insight will also help patients and their families realize why at times in the past their medications have suddenly stopped working. These dialogues can be relieving and can interrupt a vicious cycle of recrimination that leads to further tic exacerbation, and it can help aggravated parents shift the focus from blame to problem-solving.

For children, contact with their teachers can be enormously valuable. By educating the educators, clinicians can make significant progress towards securing for the child a positive and supportive environment in the classroom. If possible, teachers need to respond to outbursts of tics with grace and understanding. Repeatedly scolding a child for his or her tics can be counterproductive. The child may develop a negative attitude to authority figures and may be reluctant to attend school, and classmates may feel freer to tease the child. If tics interfere with a student's ability to receive information in the classroom, it is imperative to find alternative ways to present the material. By helping the student find a way to function even during periods of severe tics, teachers model problem-solving skills that will foster future self-esteem. It is also important for teachers to know that unstructured settings, such as the cafeteria, gym, playground and school bus, tend to be very difficult. In these situations, peers who tease or taunt tend to take advantage of the lack of adult supervision. The assignment of a paraprofessional aide to accompany the student can be remarkably beneficial—particularly in situations where there is a history of teasing. Other useful strategies that teachers may consider include: providing short breaks out of the classroom to let the tics out in private; allowing students with severe tics to take tests in private so that a child does not have the pressure to suppress tics during the test period; and being flexible with regard to the scheduling of oral presentations so that the child is not expected to make an oral presentation at a point when his or her tics are severe (Bronheim 1991). A useful compendium of educational accommodations is available on the Internet at http://www.tourettesyndrome.net.

Educated peers are equally important. Many clinicians actively encourage patients, families and teachers to help educate peers and classmates about Tourette syndrome. It is remarkable what can be tolerated in the classroom and playground when teachers and peers simply know what the problem is and learn to disregard it.

Finally, it is important for clinicians to determine the family's awareness and potential interest in advocacy organizations such as the Tourette Syndrome Association, Obsessive-Compulsive Foundation, and the Children and Adults with Attention Deficit Disorder. In the USA, these organizations have made a positive contribution to the lives of many patients and their families by providing support and information. They can also be a valuable outlet for families—to advance research and raise the general level of awareness among health care professionals, educators and the public at large. Readers are referred to their respective web sites for additional information: Tourette Syndrome Association (http://www.tsa-usa.org/); Obsessive-Compulsive Foundation (http://www.ocfoundation.org/) and Child and Adults with Attention Deficit (http://www.chadd.org/). It is likely with the expansion of the Internet that these organizations will have an increasingly important voice around the world.

Behavioural, cognitive and other psychotherapeutic treatments

The characteristic suppressibility of tic symptoms may have broad implications for treatment. Prior to seeking professional consultation, many families will have experimented with a variety of ad hoc behavioural approaches on their own. It is useful to elicit information concerning these efforts and their sequelae.

A variety of cognitive and behavioural approaches have been used with Tourette syndrome subjects (King *et al.* 1998). A battery of 'habit reversal training' techniques encompassing 'awareness' training, self-monitoring, relaxation training, competing response training (where a movement is performed that is opposite to a particular tic) and contingency management have been reported to reduce markedly tic symptoms at home and in a clinic setting (Azrin & Peterson 1990; Peterson & Azrin 1992). Additional studies are needed to confirm the effectiveness of these techniques.

The most frequently used component of this battery is some version of relaxation training which may employ tensing followed by relaxation, imagery or deep breathing. Some of these methods can be temporarily helpful; however, most families report that these techniques lose their effectiveness. Other techniques, such as massed negative practice (where the patient deliberately performs the tic movement as quickly and as forcefully as possible), have been studied with mixed results (Azrin & Peterson 1988).

Although not indicated for the treatment of tics, individual and family counselling may alleviate secondary symptoms such as low self-esteem, defiant and disruptive behaviour as well as family conflict. These interventions may also serve to reduce a significant source of psychological stress. Specifically, tic symptoms can have a powerful impact on the inner life of individuals with Tourette syndrome. They can emerge as important determinants of self-esteem and self-definition. Traditional psychotherapeutic approaches can be useful in helping patients and their families to understand and cope with their illness and to address intrapsychic conflicts that affect or result from tic symptoms.

Pharmacological treatments

The decision to begin medication is based on the level of symptoms and the clinical presentation of the individual case. Many cases of Tourette syndrome can be successfully managed without medication. When patients present with coexisting ADHD,

OCD, depression or bipolar illness it is often better to treat these 'comorbid' conditions first, as successful treatment of these disorders will often diminish tic severity.

Pharmacotherapy of tics

A variety of therapeutic agents are now available to treat tics (Chappell *et al.* 1997; Kurlan 1997; Leckman *et al.*, 2001). Each medication should be selected on the basis of expected efficacy and potential side-effects. Dopamine D_2 receptor antagonists remain the most predictably effective tic-suppressing agents in the short term. Documentation of the effectiveness of haloperidol in the early 1960s was a landmark in the history of Tourette syndrome as it called into question the prevailing view that tics were psychogenic in nature (Kushner 1998). The most widely used D_2 receptor antagonists are haloperidol, pimozide, fluphenazine and tiapride (not presently available in the USA or UK). Favourable data from double-blind clinical trials are available for haloperidol, pimozide and tiapride (Eggers *et al.* 1988; Shapiro *et al.* 1989; Sallee *et al.* 1997; Tourette Syndrome Study Group 1999). The US Food and Drug Administration has approved Tourette syndrome as an indication for haloperidol and pimozide use. Long-term experience has been less favourable, and the 'reflexive' use of these agents should be avoided (Silva *et al.* 1996; Kurlan 1997).

Typically, treatment is initiated with a low dose (0.25 mg haloperidol or 1 mg pimozide) given before sleep. Further increments (0.5 mg haloperidol or 1 mg pimozide) may be added at 7–14-day intervals if the tic behaviours remain severe. In most instances, 0.5–6.0 mg/day haloperidol or 1.0–10.0 mg/day pimozide administered over a period of 4–8 weeks are sufficient to achieve adequate control of tic symptoms. Common potential side-effects include tardive dyskinesia, acute dystonic reactions, sedation, depression, school and social phobias and/or weight gain. In many instances, by starting at low doses and adjusting the dosage upwards slowly, clinicians can avoid these side-effects. The goal should be to use as little of these medications as possible to render the tics 'tolerable'. Efforts to stop the tics completely often risk overmedication.

More recently, 'atypical' neuroleptics, including risperidone, ziprasidone and olanzapine, have been used to treat tic symptoms. These agents have potent 5-HT_2 blocking effects as well as more modest blocking effects on dopamine D_2. Initial favourable double-blind clinical trials have now been reported for both risperidone and ziprasidone, although ziprasidone is not currently available in the UK (Bruggeman *et al.* 2001; Sallee *et al.* 2000). Risperidone use often causes weight gain and complaints of sedation. Ziprasidone appears to have a more favourable side-effect profile, but more data are needed before a judgement can be made regarding its efficacy.

Clonidine is a potent α_2-receptor agonist that is thought to reduce central noradrenergic activity. Although initial open studies were favourable, subsequent double-blind clinical trials have had mixed results (Goetz *et al.* 1987; Leckman *et al.* 1991b). Clinical trials indicate that subjects can expect on average a 25–35% reduction in their symptoms over an 8–12-week period. Motor tics may show greater improvement than phonic symptoms. The usual starting dose is 0.05 mg on rising. Further 0.05 mg increments at 3–4-h intervals are added weekly until a dosage of 5 µg/kg is reached or the total daily dosage exceeds 0.25 mg. Although clonidine is clearly less effective than haloperidol and pimozide for immediate tic suppression, it is considerably safer. The principal side-effect associated with its use is sedation which occurs in 10–20% of subjects and which usually abates with continued use. Other side-effects include dry mouth, transient hypotension and rare episodes of worsening behaviour. Clonidine should be tapered and not withdrawn abruptly, to reduce the likelihood of symptom or blood pressure rebound. Initial results from a double-blind clinical trial with the closely related compound guanfacine are also promising (Scahill *et al.* 2001).

While many other medications have been used in the treatment of tics, with the exception of flutamide, an androgen receptor antagonist, none have been evaluated in double-blind randomized clinical trials (Peterson *et al.* 1998b). Promising agents include dopamine agonists that act presynaptically (pergolide) and agents that deplete presynaptic dopamine concentrations (tetrabenazine) (Gilbert *et al.* 2000; see also Carpenter *et al.* 1999 for a review). Cholinergic agents, including nicotine formulated as a patch and used in combination with a neuroleptic, have also been recommended (Sanberg *et al.* 1997). Building on its success in treating dystonia, reports concerning the benefits of botulinum toxin injections to temporarily weaken muscles associated with severe motor or vocal tics have also appeared (Jankovic 1994). Finally, GABAergic agents, particularly clonazepam, have also been widely used.

Pharmacotherapy of coexisting ADHD

The stimulants methylphenidate and dexamphetamine, are first-line agents for the medical management of ADHD (Dulcan 1997). However, the use of stimulants in ADHD associated with a tic disorder is controversial (Castellanos 1999). While many patients with both ADHD and a pre-existing tic disorder will do well on stimulants, data from clinical case reports and controlled studies indicate that some children with ADHD will exhibit tics *de novo* when exposed to a stimulant. In other cases, tics may increase to a level that warrants discontinuation of the stimulant. Commonly used non-stimulants for ADHD include:
- the tricyclic antidepressants, desipramine and nortriptyline;
- atypical antidepressants, such as bupropion;
- α_2-agonists, clonidine and guanfacine (Dulcan 1997).

Compared to clonidine, guanfacine is less sedating and has a longer duration of action as well as being more specific for α_2-receptors in the prefrontal cortex (Arnsten *et al.* 1998). Initial results from a double-blind clinical trial with guanfacine in subjects with both ADHD and coexisting tics are promising (Scahill *et al.* 2001).

Pharmacotherapy of coexisting OCD

Cognitive behavioural therapies, particularly exposure and response prevention alone or in combination with SRIs are the standard interventions for OCD (American Academy of Child and Adolescent Psychiatry 1998). Unfortunately, many patients with OCD and a coexisting tic disorder respond less well to these interventions. Investigators in controlled clinical trials have found that addition of small doses of the neuroleptic haloperidol, or the atypical neuroleptic risperidone increases the response to SRIs (McDougle et al. 1994, 2000).

Special populations: PANDAS

Post-infectious autoimmune mechanisms are likely to contribute to the pathogenesis of 10–20% of Tourette syndrome cases (Swedo et al. 1998). Preliminary evidence suggests that individuals with abrupt onset and coexisting ADHD and/or OCD may be at greater risk (Peterson et al., 2000). As in SC, the precise mechanisms are in doubt. Clarification of these mechanisms is likely to lead to improved treatment and possibly preventive interventions. Although initial results from immunomodulatory treatments, including plasma exchange, are promising, caution is warranted (Perlmutter et al. 1999). It is also premature to recommend prophylactic antibiotic treatment (Garvey et al. 1999; Shulman 1999).

Future directions

Along with a deepening appreciation of the clinical phenomenology of Tourette syndrome and related disorders, recent progress in neuroanatomy, systems neuroscience and functional in vivo neuroimaging has set the stage for a major advance in our understanding of these disorders. Success in this area will lead to the targeting of specific brain circuits for more intensive study. Diagnostic and prognostic advances can also be anticipated. Which circuits are involved and to what degree? How does that degree of involvement affect the patient's symptomatic course and outcome?

Given this potential, Tourette syndrome can be considered a model disorder to study the dynamic interplay of neurobiological systems during development. It is likely that the research paradigms utilized in these studies may lead to the development of animal models that can be exploited to develop novel interventions. Findings from these and other empirical studies will likely be relevant to other disorders of childhood onset and will enhance our understanding of normal development.

Acknowledgements

We are indebted to members of the Yale Tourette Syndrome and Obsessive-Compulsive Disorder Research Group for their support and comments on an earlier version of this review. Members of this research group include: David L. Pauls PhD, Bradley S. Peterson MD, Lawrence Scahill MSN PhD, Heping Zhang PhD, Alice S. Carter PhD, Paul J. Lombroso MD, Robert T. Schultz PhD, George M. Anderson PhD, John P. Alsobrook II PhD, Flora M. Vaccarino MD, Diane B. Findley PhD, Debra E. Bessen PhD, Syed A. Morshed MD PhD, Salina Parveen MD PhD, Robert W. Makuch PhD and Kenneth K. Kidd PhD. We are also grateful to the comments and suggestions of Yukiko Kano MD PhD, Marcos Mecadante MD PhD and Maria C. do Rosario Campos MD MS, who are currently on leave at the Child Study Center.

Portions of the research described in this review were supported by grants from the National Institutes of Health: MH18268, MH49351, MH30929, HD03008, NS16648 and RR00125, as well as by the Tourette Syndrome Association.

References

Altemus, M., Greenberg, B.D., Keuler, D., Jacobson, K.R. & Murphy, D.L. (1999) Open trial of flutamide for treatment of obsessive-compulsive disorder. Journal of Clinical Psychiatry, 60, 442–445.

American Academy of Child and Adolescent Psychiatry (1998) Practice parameters for the assessment and treatment of children and adolescents with obsessive-compulsive disorder. Journal of the American Academy of Child and Adolescent Psychiatry, 37, 27S–45S.

American Psychiatric Association (1994) Diagnostic and Statistical Manual of Mental Disorders, 4th edn. American Psychiatric Association Press, Washington D.C.

Anderson, G.M., Polack, E.S., Chatterjee, D., Leckman, J.F., Riddle, M.A. & Cohen, D.J. (1992) Postmortem analysis of subcortical monoamines and amonoacids in Tourette syndrome. In: Tourette Syndrome: Genetics, Neurobiology, and Treatment (eds T.N. Chase, A.J. Friedhoff & D.J. Cohen), pp. 253–262. Raven Press, New York.

Anderson, G.M., Leckman, J.F. & Cohen, D.J. (1998) Neurochemical and neuropeptide systems. In: Tourette Syndrome Tics, Obsessions, Compulsions: Developmental Psychopathology and Clinical Care (eds J.F. Leckman & D.J. Cohen), pp. 261–281. John Wiley and Sons, New York.

Aosaki, T., Graybiel, A.M. & Kimura, M. (1994) Effect of the nigrostriatal dopamine system on acquired neural responses in the striatum of behaving monkeys. Science, 265, 412–415.

Apter, A., Pauls, D., Bleich, A. et al. (1993) An epidemiological study of Gilles de la Tourette syndrome in Israel. Archives of General Psychiatry, 50, 734–738.

Arnsten, A.F. (2000) Through the looking glass: differential noradenergic modulation of prefrontal cortical function. Neural Plasticity, 7, 33–46.

Arnsten, A.F.T., Steere, J.C., Jentsch, D.J. & Li, B.M. (1998) Noradrenergic influences on prefrontal cortical cognitive function: opposing actions at postjunctional α_1- versus α_2-adrenergic receptors. Advances in Pharmacology, 42, 764–767.

Azrin, N.H. & Peterson, A.L. (1988) Habit reversal for the treatment of Tourette syndrome. Behaviour Research and Therapy, 11, 347–351.

Azrin, N.H. & Peterson, A.L. (1990) Treatment of Tourette syndrome by habit reversal: a waiting-list control group comparison. Behaviour Research and Therapy, 21, 305–318.

Baldwin, M., Frost, L.L. & Wodd, C.D. (1954) Investigation of primate amygdala. Neurology, 4, 586–598.

Baron-Cohen, S., Scahill, V.L., Izaguirre, J., Hornsey, H. & Robertson,

M.M. (1999) The prevalence of Gilles de la Tourette syndrome in children and adolescents with autism: a large scale study. *Psychoogical Medicine*, 29 (5), 1151–1159.

Barr, C.L. & Sandor, P. (1998) Current status of genetic studies of Gilles de la Tourette syndrome. *Canadian Journal of Psychiatry*, 43 (4), 351–357.

Bawden, H.N., Stokes, A., Camfield, C.S., Camfield, P.R. & Salisbury, S. (1998) Peer relationship problems in children with Tourette disorder or diabetes mellitus. *Journal of Child Psychology and Psychiatry*, 39, 663–668.

Baxter, L.R. Jr, Schwartz, M., Bergman, K.S. *et al.* (1992) Caudate glucose metabolic rate changes with both drug and behavior therapy for obsessive-compulsive disorder. *Archives of General Psychiatry*, 49, 681–689.

Bisno, A.L. (1991) Group A streptococcal infections and rheumatic fever. *New England Journal of Medicine*, 325, 783–793.

Boulant, J.A. (1998) Hypothalamic neurons. Mechanisms of sensitivity to temperature. *Annals of the New York Academy of Sciences*, 856, 108–115.

Breton, J.J., Bergeron, L., Valla, J.P. *et al.* (1999) Quebee child mental health survey: prevalence of DSM-IIIR mental disorders. *Journal of Child Psychology and Psychiatry*, 40, 375–384.

Bronheim, S. (1991) An educator's guide to Tourette syndrome. *Journal of Learning Disabilities*, 24, 17–22.

Bruggeman, R., van der Linden, C., Buitelaar, J.K., Gericke, G.S., Hawridge, S.M. & Temlett, J.A. (2001) Risperidone versus pimozide in Tourette syndrome: a comparative double-blind parallel group study. *Journal of Clinical Psychiatry*, 62, 50–56.

Burd, L., Kerbeshian, L., Wikenheiser, M. & Fisher, W. (1986a) Prevalence of Gilles de la Tourette syndrome in North Dakota adults. *American Journal of Psychiatry*, 143, 787–788.

Burd, L., Kerbeshian, L., Wikenheiser, M. & Fisher, W. (1986b) A prevalence study of Gilles de la Tourette syndrome in North Dakota school-age children. *Journal of the American Academy of Child Psychiatry*, 25, 552–553.

Burd, L., Severud, R., Klug, M.G. & Kerbeshian, J. (1999) Prenatal and perinatal risk factors for Tourette disorder. *Journal of Perinatal Medicine*, 27, 295–302.

Caine, E.D., McBride, M.C., Chiverton, P., Bamford, K.A., Rediess, S. & Shiao, S. (1988) Tourette syndrome in Monroe County school children. *Neurology*, 38, 472–475.

Carpenter, L.L., Leckman, J.F., Scahill, L. & McDougle, C.J. (1999) Pharmacological and other somatic approaches to treatment. In: *Tourette Syndrome Tics, Obsessions, Compulsions: Developmental Psychopathology and Clinical Care* (eds J.F. Leckman & D.J. Cohen), pp. 370–398. John Wiley and Sons, New York.

Carter, A.S., Pauls, D.L., Leckman, J.F. & Cohen, D.J. (1994) A prospective longitudinal study of Gilles de la Tourette syndrome. *Journal of the American Academy of Child and Adolescent Psychiatry*, 33, 377–385.

Carter, A.S., O'Donnell, D.A., Schultz, R.T., Scahill, L., Leckman, J.F. & Pauls, D.L. (2000) Social and emotional adjustment in children affected with Gilles de la Tourette syndrome: associations with ADHD and family functioning. *Journal of Child Psychology and Psychiatry*, 41, 215–223.

Casas, M., Alvarez, E., Duro, P. *et al.* (1986) Antiandrogenic treatment of obsessive-compulsive neurosis. *Acta Psychiatrica Scandinavica*, 73, 221–222.

Castellanos, F.X. (1999) Stimulants and tic disorders: from dogma to data. *Archives of General Psychiatry*, 56, 337–338.

Cath, D.C., Gijsman, H.J., Schoemaker, R.C. *et al.* (1999) The effect of m-CPP on tics and obsessive-compulsive phenomena in Gilles de la Tourette syndrome. *Psychopharmacology (Berlin)*, 144, 137–143.

Chappell, P.B., Riddle, M., Anderson, G. *et al.* (1994a) Enhanced stress responsivity of Tourette syndrome patients undergoing lumbar puncture. *Biological Psychiatry*, 36, 35–43.

Chappell, P.B., McSwiggan-Hardin, M.T., Scahill, L.D. *et al.* (1994b) Videotape tic counts in the assessment of Tourette syndrome: stability, reliability, and validity. *Journal of the American Academy of Child and Adolescent Psychiatry*, 33, 386–393.

Chappell, P.B., Riddle, M.A., Scahill, L. *et al.* (1995) Guanfacine treatment of comorbid attention-deficit hyperactivity disorder and Tourette syndrome: preliminary clinical experience. *Journal of the American Academy of Child and Adolescent Psychiatry*, 34, 1140–1146.

Chappell, P., Leckman, J., Goodman, W. *et al.* (1996) Elevated cerebrospinal fluid corticotropin-releasing factor in Tourette syndrome: comparison to obsessive-compulsive disorder and normal controls. *Biological Psychiatry*, 39, 776–783.

Chappell, P.B., Scahill, L.D. & Leckman, J.F. (1997) Future therapies of Tourette syndrome. *Neurologic Clinics*, 15, 429–450.

Cohen, D.J., Young, J.G., Nathanson, J.A. & Shaywitz, B.A. (1979) Clonidine in Tourette syndrome. *Lancet*, ii, 551–553.

Cohen, D.J., Leckman, J.F. & Shaywitz, B.A. (1984) Tourette syndrome and other tics. In: *Diagnosis and Treatment in Pediatric Psychiatry* (eds D. Shaffer, A.A. Ehrhardt & L. Greenhill), pp. 3–28. MacMillan Free Press, New York.

Cohen, D.J., Ort, S.I., Leckman, J.F., Riddle, M.A. & Hardin, M.T. (1988) Family functioning and Tourette syndrome. In: *Tourette Syndrome and Tic Disorders* (eds D.J. Cohen, R.D. Bruun & J.F. Leckman), p. 179. John Wiley & Sons, New York.

Comings, D.E. (1988) *Tourette Syndrome and Human Behavior*. Hope Press, Daurte, CA.

Comings, D.E. & Comings, B.G. (1987) A controlled study of Tourette syndrome. *American Journal of Human Genetics*, 41, 701–760.

Costello, E.J., Angold, A., Burns, B.J. *et al.* (1996) The Great Smoky Mountains Study of Youth: goals, design, methods, and the prevalence of DSM-III-R disorders. *Archives of General Psychiatry*, 53, 1129–1136.

Dulcan, M. (1997) Practice parameters for the assessment and treatment of children, adolescents, and adults with attention-deficit/hyperactivity disorder. *Journal of the American Academy of Child and Adolescent Psychiatry*, 36, 85S–121S.

Dykens, E., Leckman, J.F., Riddle, M.A., Hardin, M. & Schwartz, S. (1990) Intellectual, academic, and adaptive functioning Tourette syndrome with and without attention deficit disorder. *Journal of Abnormal Child Psychology*, 18, 607–615.

Dykens, E., Sparrow, S.S., Cohen, D.J., Scahill, L. & Leckman, J.F. (1998) Peer acceptance and adaptive functioning. In: *Tourette Syndrome Tics, Obsessions, Compulsions: Developmental Psychopathology and Clinical Care* (eds J.F. Leckman & D.J. Cohen), pp. 104–117. John Wiley and Sons, New York.

Eggers, C.H., Rotherberger, A. & Berghaus, U. (1988) Clinical and neurobiological findings in children suffering from tic disease following treatment with tiapride. *European Archives of Psychiatry and Neurological Sciences*, 237, 223–229.

Ernst, M., Zametkin, A.J., Jons, P.H., Matochik, J.A., Pascualvaca, D. & Cohen, R.M. (1999) High presynaptic dopaminergic activity in children with Tourette disorder. *Journal of the American Academy of Child and Adolescent Psychiatry*, 38, 86–94.

Fehrbach, S.E., Morell, J.I. & Pfaff, D.W. (1985) Identification of medial preoptic neurons that concentrate estradiol and project to the midbrain in the rat. *Journal of Comparative Neurology*, 247, 364–382.

Garvey, M.A., Perlmutter, S.J., Allen, A.J. *et al.* (1999) A pilot study of penicillin prophylaxis for neuropsychiatric exacerbations triggered by streptococcal infections. *Biological Psychiatry*, 45, 1564–1571.

Gilbert, D.L., Sethuraman, G., Sine, L., Peters, S. & Sallee, F.R. (2000) Tourette syndrome improvement with pergolide in a randomized, double-blind, crossover trial. *Neurology*, 28, 1310–1315.

Gilles de la Tourette, G. (1885) Étude sur une affection nerveuse caractérisée par de l'incoordination motrice accompagnée d'echolalie et de copralalie. *Archives de Neurologie*, 9 (19–42), 158–200.

Glaze, D.G., Frost, J.D. & Jankovic, J. (1983) Sleep in Gilles de la Tourette syndrome: disorder of arousal. *Neurology*, 33, 586–592.

Goetz, C.G., Tanner, C.M., Wilson, R.S., Carroll, V.S., Como, P.G. & Shannon, K.M. (1987) Clonidine and Gilles de la Tourette syndrome: double-blind study using objective rating method. *Annals of Neurology*, 31, 307–310.

Goetz, C.G., Tanner, C.M., Stebbins, G.T., Leipzig, G. & Carr, W.C. (1992) Adult tics in Gilles de la Tourette syndrome: description and risk factors. *Neurology*, 42, 784–788.

Goetz, C.G., Pappert, E.J., Louis, E.D., Raman, R. & Leurgans, S. (1999) Advantages of a modified scoring method for the Rush Video-Based Tic Rating Scale. *Movement Disorders*, 14, 502–506.

Gonce, M. & Barbeau, A. (1977) Seven cases of Gilles de la Tourette syndrome: partial relief with clonazepam—a pilot study. *Canadian Journal of Neurological Sciences*, 4, 279–283.

Goodman, W.K., McDougle, C.J., Price, L.H. *et al.* (1995) m-Chlorophenylpiperazine in patients with obsessive-compulsive disorder: absence of symptom exacerbation. *Biological Psychiatry*, 38, 138–149.

Graybiel, A.M. (1990) Neurotransmitters and neuromodulators in the basal ganglia. *Trends in Neuroscience*, 13, 244–254.

Graybiel, A.M. (1998) The basal ganglia and chunking of action repertoires. *Neurobiology, Learning and Memory*, 70, 119–136.

Greene, R.W., Biederman, J., Faraone, S.V., Sienna, M. & Garcia-Jetton, J. (1997) Adolescent outcome of boys with attention-deficit/hyperactivity disorder and social disability: results from a 4-year longitudinal follow-up study. *Journal of Consulting and Clinical Psychology*, 65, 758–767.

Greist, J.H. & Jefferson, J.W. (1998) Pharmacotherapy for obsessive-compulsive disorder. *British Journal of Psychiatry Supplement*, 35, 64–70.

Grenhoff, J. & Svensson, T.H. (1989) Clonidine modulates dopamine cell firing in rat ventral tegmental area. *European Journal of Pharmacology*, 165, 11–18.

Haber, S.N., Kowall, N.W., Vonsattel, J.P., Bird, E.D. & Richardson, E.P. (1986) Gilles de la Tourette syndrome: a postmortem neuropathological and immunohistochemical study. *Journal of Neurological Science*, 75, 225–241.

Harcherik, D.F., Leckman, J.F., Detlor, J. & Cohen, D.J. (1984) A new instrument for clinical studies of Tourette syndrome: a preliminary report. *Journal of the American Academy of Child Psychiatry*, 23, 153–160.

Hebebrand, J., Klug, B., Fimmers, R. *et al.* (1997) Rates for tic disorders and obsessive-compulsive symptomatology in families of children and adolescents with Gilles de la Tourette syndrome. *Journal of Psychiatric Research*, 31, 519–530.

Hinshaw, S.P. (1994) Attention Deficits and Hyperactivity in Children. Sage, London.

Husby, G., van de Rijn, I., Zabriskie, J., Abdin, Z. & Williams, R. (1976) Antibodies reacting with cytoplasm of subthalamic and caudate nuclei neurons in chorea and acute rheumatic fever. *Journal of Experimental Medicine*, 144, 1094–1110.

Hyde, T.M., Aaronson, B.A., Randolph, C., Rickler, K.C. & Weinberger, D.R. (1992) Relationship of birth weight to the phenotypic expression of Gilles de la Tourette syndrome in monozygotic twins. *Neurology*, 42, 652–658.

Itard, J.M.G. (1825) Memoire sur quelques fonctions involuntaires des appareils de la locomotion de la prehension et de la voix. *Archives Générales de Médecine*, 8, 385–407.

Jagger, J., Prusoff, B.A., Cohen, D.J., Kidd, K.K., Carbonari, C.M. & John, K. (1982) The epidemiology of Tourette syndrome: a pilot study. *Schizophrenia Bulletin*, 8, 267–277.

Jankovic, J. (1994) Botulinum toxin in the treatment of dystonic tics. *Movement Disorders*, 9, 347–349.

Jankovic, J. & Rohaidy, H. (1987) Motor, behavioral and pharmacologic findings in Tourette syndrome. *Canadian Journal of Neurological Sciences*, 14, 541–546.

Kemeny, E., Husby, G., Williams, R.C. & Zabriskie, J.B. (1994) Tissue distribution of antigen(s) defined by monoclonal antibody D8/17 reacting with B lymphocytes of patients with rheumatic heart disease. *Clinical Immunology and Immunopathology*, 72, 35–43.

King, R.A., Scahill, L., Findley, D. & Cohen, D.J. (1998) Psychosocial and behavioral treatments. In: *Tourette Syndrome Tics, Obsessions, Compulsions: Developmental Psychopathology and Clinical Care* (eds J.F. Leckman & D.J. Cohen), pp. 338–359. John Wiley and Sons, New York.

Kurlan, R. (1997) Treatment of tics. *Neurologic Clinics*, 15, 403–409.

Kurlan, R., Whitmore, D., Irvine, C., McDermott, M.P. & Como, P.G. (1994) Tourette syndrome in a special education population: a pilot study involving a single school district. *Neurology*, 44 (4), 699–702.

Kushner, H.I. (1999) *A Cursing Brain? The Histories of Tourette Syndrome*. Harvard University Press, Cambridge, MA.

Lang, A. (1991) Patient perception of tics and other movement disorders. *Neurology*, 41, 223–228.

Leckman, J.F. & Cohen, D.J., eds (1998) *Tourette Syndrome Tics, Obsessions, Compulsions: Developmental Psychopathology and Clinical Care*. John Wiley and Sons. New York.

Leckman, J.F. & Riddle, M.A. (2000) Tourette's syndrome: when habit forming units form habits of their own? *Neuron*, 28, 349–354.

Leckman, J.F. & Scahill, L. (1990) Possible exacerbation of tics by androgenic steroids. *New England Journal of Medicine*, 322, 1674.

Leckman, J.F., Cohen, D.J., Price, R.A., Minderaa, R.B., Anderson, G.M. & Pauls, D.L. (1984) The pathogenesis of Gilles de la Tourette syndrome: a review of data and hypothesis. In: *Movement Disorders* (eds A.B. Shah, N.S. Shah & A.G. Donald), pp. 257–272. Plenum, New York.

Leckman, J.F., Price, R.A., Walkup, J.T., Ort, S.I., Pauls, D.L. & Cohen, D.J. (1987) Nongenetic factors in Gilles de la Tourette syndrome. *Archives of General Psychiatry*, 44, 100.

Leckman, J.F., Riddle, M.A., Hardin, M.T. *et al.* (1989) The Yale Global Tic Severity Scale: initial testing of a clinician-rated scale of tic severity. *Journal of the American Academy of Child and Adolescent Psychiatry*, 28, 566–573.

Leckman, J.F., Dolnansky, E.S., Hardin, M.T. *et al.* (1990) Perinatal factors in the expression of Tourette syndrome: an exploratory study. *Journal of the American Academy of Child and Adolescent Psychiatry*, 29, 220–226.

Leckman, J.F., Knorr, A.M., Rasmusson, A.M. & Cohen, D.J. (1991a) Basal ganglia research and Tourette syndrome. *Trends in Neuroscience*, 14, 94.

Leckman, J.F., Hardin, M.T., Riddle, M.A., Stevenson, J., Ort, S.I. & Cohen, D.J. (1991b) Clonidine treatment of Gilles de la Tourette syndrome. *Archives of General Psychiatry*, 48, 324–328.

Leckman, J.F., Walker, D.E. & Cohen, D.J. (1993) Premonitory urges in Tourette syndrome. *American Journal of Psychiatry*, 150, 98–102.

Leckman, J.F., Walker, D.E., Goodman, W.K., Pauls, D.L. & Cohen, D.J. (1994) 'Just right' perceptions associated with compulsive behaviors in Tourette syndrome. *American Journal of Psychiatry*, **151**, 675–680.

Leckman, J.F., Goodman, W.K., Anderson, G.M. *et al.* (1995) CSF biogenic amines in obsessive-compulsive disorder and Tourette syndrome. *Neuropsychopharmacology*, **12**, 73–86.

Leckman, J.F., Grice, D.E., Boardman, J. *et al.* (1997a) Symptoms of obsessive-compulsive disorder. *American Journal of Psychiatry*, **154**, 911–917.

Leckman, J.F., Peterson, B.S., Anderson, G.M., Arnsten, A.F.T., Pauls, D.L. & Cohen, D.J. (1997b) Pathogenesis of Tourette syndrome. *Journal of Child Psychology and Psychiatry*, **38**, 119–142.

Leckman, J.F., Zhang, H., Vitale, A. *et al.* (1998a) Course of tic severity in Tourette syndrome: the first two decades. *Pediatrics*, **102**, 14–19.

Leckman, J.F., King, R.A., Scahill, L., Findley, D., Ort, S.I. & Cohen, D.J. (1998b) Yale approach to assessment and treatment. In: *Tourette Syndrome Tics, Obsessions, Compulsions: Developmental Psychopathology and Clinical Care* (eds J.F. Leckman & D.J. Cohen), pp. 285–309. John Wiley and Sons, New York.

Leckman, J.F., Cohen, D.J., Goetz, C.G. & Jankovic, J. (2001) Tourette syndrome: pieces of the puzzle. In: *Tourette Syndrome and Associated Disorders* (eds D.J. Cohen, C. Goetz & J. Jankovic), pp. 369–390. Lippincott, Williams & Wilkins, New York.

Lippitz, B.E., Mindus, P., Meyerson, B.A., Kihlstrom, L. & Lindquist, C. (1999) Lesion topography and outcome after thermocapsulotomy or gamma knife capsulotomy for obsessive-compulsive disorder: relevance of the right hemisphere. *Neurosurgery*, **44**, 452–458.

Lombroso, P.J., Mack, G., Scahill, L., King, R.A. & Leckman, J.F. (1992) Exacerbation of Tourette syndrome associated with thermal stress: a family study. *Neurology*, **41**, 1984–1987.

Malison, R.T., McDougle, C.J., van Dyck, C.H. *et al.* (1995) β-CIT SPECT imaging demonstrates increased striatal dopamine transporter binding in Tourette syndrome. *American Journal of Psychiatry*, **152**, 1359–1361.

Mannuzza, S., Klein, R.G., Bessler, A., Malloy, P. & LaPadula, M. (1998) Adult psychiatric status of hyperactive boys grown up. *American Journal of Psychiatry*, **155**, 493–498.

Mason, A., Banerjee, S., Eapen, V., Zeitlin, H. & Robertson, M.M. (1998) The prevalence of Tourette syndrome in a mainstream school population. *Developmental Medicine and Child Neurology*, **40**, 92–296.

McDougle, C.J., Goodman, W.K., Leckman, J.F., Barr, L.C., Heninger, G.R. & Price, L.H. (1993) The efficacy of fluvoxamine in obsessive-compulsive disorder: effects of comorbid chronic tic disorder. *Journal of Clinical Psychopharmacology*, **13**, 354–358.

McDougle, C.J., Goodman, W.K., Leckman, J.F., Lee, N.C., Heninger, G.R. & Price, L.H. (1994) Haloperidol addition in fluvoxamine-refractory obsessive-compulsive disorder: a double blind, placebo controlled study in patients with and without tics. *Archives of General Psychiatry*, **51**, 302–308.

McDougle, C.J., Epperson, C.N., Pelton, G.H., Wasylink, S. & Price, L.H. (2000) A double blind, placebo controlled study of risperidone addition in serotonin reuptake inhibitor-refractory obsessive-compulsive disorder. *Archives of General Psychiatry*, **57**, 794–801.

McLean, P. & Delgado, J. (1953) Electrical and chemical stimulation of frontotemporal portion of limbic system in the waking animal. *EEG and Clinical Neurophysiology*, **5**, 91–100.

Mercadante, M.T., Campos, M.C.R., Marques-Diasm, M.J., Miguel, E.C. & Leckman, J.F. (1997) Vocal tics in Sydenham' chorea. *Journal of the American Academy of Child and Adolescent Psychiatry*, **36**, 305.

Merette, C., Brassard, A. Potvin, A. *et al.* (2000) Significant linkage for

Tourette syndrome in a large French Canadian Family. *American Journal of Human Genetics*, **67**, 1008–1013.

Meyer, P., Bohnen, N.I., Minoshima, S. *et al.* (1999) Striatal presynaptic monoaminergic vesicles are not increased in Tourette syndrome. *Neurology*, **53**, 371–374.

Miguel, E.C., Rosário-Campos, M.C., Shavitt, R.G., Hounie, A.G. & Mercadente, M.T. (2001) The tic-related obsessive-compulsive disorder phenotype. In: *Tourette Syndrome* (eds D.J. Cohen, C.J. Goetz & J. Jankovic), pp. 45–55. Lippincott, Williams & Wilkins, New York.

Murphy, T.K., Goodman, W.K., Fudge, M.W. *et al.* (1997) B lymphocyte antigen D8/17: a peripheral marker for childhood-onset obsessive-compulsive disorder and Tourette syndrome? *American Journal of Psychiatry*, **154**, 402–407.

Nauta, W.J.H. (1982) Limbic innervation of the striatum. In: *Advances in Neurology, Gilles de la Tourette Syndrome* (eds A.J. Friedhoff & T.N. Chase), pp. 41–47. Raven, New York.

Nolan, E.E., Gadow, K.D. & Sverd, J. (1994) Observations and ratings of tics in school settings. *Journal of Abnormal Child Psychology*, **22** (5), 579–593.

Parent, A. (1986) *Comparative Neurobiology of the Basal Ganglia.* John Wiley and Sons, New York.

Parent, A. & Hazrati, L.N. (1995) Functional anatomy of the basal ganglia. I. The cortico-basal ganglia-thalamo-cortical loop. *Brain Research and Brain Research Reviews*, **20**, 91–127.

Pasamanick, B. & Kawi, A. (1956) A study of the association of prenatal and paranatal factors in the development of tics in children. *Journal of Pediatrics*, **48**, 596–602.

Pauls, D.L. & Leckman, J.F. (1986) The inheritance of Gilles de la Tourette syndrome and associated behaviors: evidence for autosomal dominant transmission. *New England Journal of Medicine*, **315**, 993–997.

Pauls, D.L., Raymond, C.L., Stevenson, J.F. & Leckman, J.F. (1991) A family study of Gilles de la Tourette. *American Journal of Human Genetics*, **48**, 154–163.

Perlmutter, S.J., Leitman, S.F., Garvey, M.A. *et al.* (1999) Therapeutic plasma exchange and intravenous immunoglobulin for obsessive-compulsive disorder and tic disorders in childhood. *Lancet*, **354**, 1153–1158.

Peterson, A.L. & Azrin, N.H. (1992) An evaluation of behavioral treatments for Tourette syndrome. *Behaviour Research and Therapy*, **30**, 167–174.

Peterson, B.S. & Leckman, J.F. (1998) Temporal characterization of tics in Gilles de la Tourette syndrome. *Biological Psychiatry*, **44**, 1337–1348.

Peterson, B.S., Leckman, J.F., Scahill, L. *et al.* (1992) Hypothesis: steroid hormones and sexual dimorphisms modulate symptom expression in Tourette syndrome. *Psychoneuroendocrinology*, **17**, 553–563.

Peterson, B.S., Riddle, M.A., Cohen, D.J. *et al.* (1993) Reduced basal ganglia volumes in Tourette syndrome using 3-dimensional reconstruction techniques from magnetic resonance images. *Neurology*, **43**, 941–949.

Peterson, B.S., Skudlarski, P., Anderson, A.W. *et al.* (1998a) A functional magnetic resonance imaging study of tic suppression in Tourette syndrome. *Archives of General Psychiatry*, **55**, 326–333.

Peterson, B.S., Zhang, H., Bondi, C., Anderson, G.M. & Leckman, J.F. (1998b) A double-blind, placebo-controlled, crossover trial of an antiandrogen in the treatment of Tourette syndrome. *Journal of Clinical Psychopharmacology*, **18**, 324–331.

Peterson, B.S., Leckman, J.F., Tucker, D. *et al.* (2000) Antistreptococcal antibody titers and basal ganglia volumes in chronic tic, obsessive-compulsive, and attention deficit-hyperactivity disorders. *Archives of General Psychiatry*, **57**, 364–372.

Price, A.R., Kidd, K.K., Cohen, D.J., Pauls, D.L. & Leckman, J.F. (1985) A twin study of Tourette syndrome. *Archives of General Psychiatry*, **42**, 815–820.

Rauch, S.L., Baer, L., Cosgrove, G.R. & Jenike, M.A. (1995) Neurosurgical treatment of Tourette syndrome: a critical review. *Comprehensive Psychiatry*, **36**, 141–156.

Robertson, M.M., Banerjee, S., Kurlan, R. et al. (1999) The Tourette syndrome diagnostic confidence index: development and clinical associations. *Neurology*, **53**, 2108–2112.

Russchen, F.T., Bakst, I., Amaral, D.G. & Price, J.L. (1985) The amygdalostriatal projections in the monkey: an anterograde tracing study. *Brain Research*, **329**, 241–257.

Rutter, M., Tizard, J. & Whitmore, K., eds (1970) *Education, Health, and Behaviour*. Longman, London.

Rutter, M., Yule, W., Berger, M., Yule, B., Morton, J. & Bagley, C. (1974) Children of West Indian immigrants. I. Rates of behavioural deviance and psychiatric disorder. *Journal of Child Psychology and Psychiatry*, **15**, 241–262.

Sallee, F.R., Nesbitt, L., Jackson, C., Sine, L. & Sethuraman, G. (1997) Relative efficacy of haloperidol and pimozide in children and adolescents with Tourette disorder. *American Journal of Psychiatry*, **154**, 1057–1062.

Sallee, F.R., Kurlan, R., Goetz, C.G. et al. (2000) Ziprasidone treatment of children and adolescents with Tourette syndrome: a pilot study. *Journal of the American Academy of Child and Adolescent Psychiatry*, **39**, 292–299.

Sanberg, P.R., Silver, A.A., Shytle, R.D. et al. (1997) Nicotine for the treatment of Tourette syndrome. *Pharmacological Therapeutics*, **74**, 21–25.

Santangelo, S.L., Pauls, D.L., Goldstein, J.M., Faraone, S.V., Tsuang, M.T. & Leckman, J.F. (1994) Tourette syndrome: what are the influences of gender and comorbid obsessive-compulsive disorder? *Journal of the American Academy of Child and Adolescent Psychiatry*, **33**, 795–804.

Scahill, L., Riddle, M.A., King, R.A. et al. (1997) Fluoxetine has no marked effect on tic symptoms in patients with Tourette syndrome: a double-blind placebo-controlled study. *Journal of Child and Adolescent Psychopharmacology*, **7**, 75–85.

Scahill, L., King, R.A., Schultz, R.T. & Leckman, J.F. (1998) Selection and use of diagnostic and clinical rating instruments. In: *Tourette Syndrome Tics, Obsessions, Compulsions: Developmental Psychopathology and Clinical Care* (eds J.F. Leckman & J.D. Cohen), pp. 310–324. John Wiley and Sons, New York.

Scahill, L., Chappell, P.B., Kim, Y.-S. et al. (2001) Guanfacine in the treatment of children with tic disorders and ADHD: a placebo-controlled study. *American Journal of Psychiatry*, **158**, 1067–1074.

Schultz, R.T., Carter, A.S., Gladstone, M. et al. (1998) Visual-motor integration, visuoperceptual and fine motor functioning in children with Tourette syndrome. *Neuropsychology*, **12**, 134–145.

Shapiro, A.K. & Shapiro, E.S. (1988) Treatment of tic disorders with haloperidol. In: *Tourette Syndrome and Tic Disorders* (eds D.J. Cohen, R.D. Bruun & J.F. Leckman). John Wiley & Sons, New York.

Shapiro, A.K., Shapiro, E.S., Young, J.G. & Feinberg, T.E., eds (1988) *Gilles de la Tourette Syndrome*, 2nd edn. Raven, New York.

Shapiro, E.S., Shapiro, A.K., Fulop, G. et al. (1989) Controlled study of haloperidol, pimozide, and placebo for the treatment of Gilles de la Tourette syndrome. *Archives of General Psychiatry*, **46**, 722–730.

Shulman, S.T. (1999) Pediatric autoimmune neuropsychiatric disorders associated with streptococci (PANDAS). *Pediatric Infectious Disease Journal*, **18**, 281–282.

Sikich, L. & Todd, R.D. (1988) Are neurodevelopmental effects of gonadal hormones related to sex differences in psychiatric illness? *Psychiatric Developments*, **6**, 277–310.

Silva, R.R., Munoz, D.M., Barickman, J. & Friedhoff, A.J. (1995) Environmental factors and related fluctuation of symptoms in children and adolescents with Tourette disorder. *Journal of Child Psychology and Psychiatry*, **36**, 305–312.

Silva, R.R., Munoz, D.M., Daniel, W., Barickman, J. & Friedhoff, A.J. (1996) Causes of haloperidol discontinuation in patients with Tourette disorder: management and alternatives. *Journal of Clinical Psychiatry*, **57**, 129–135.

Silver, A.A., Shyytle, R.D. & Sanberg, P.R. (2000) Mecamylamine in Tourette syndrome: a two-year retrospective study. *Journal of Child and Adolescent Psychopharmacology*, **10**, 59–68.

Simonic, I., Nyholt, D.R., Gericke, G.S. et al. (2001) Further evidence of linkage of Gilles de la Tourette syndrome susceptibility loci on chromosomes 2p11, 8q22 and 11q23–24 in South African Afrikaners. *American Journal of Medical Genetics*, **105**, 163–167.

Singer, H.S., Hahn, I.-H. & Moran, T.H. (1991) Abnormal dopamine uptake sites in postmortem striatum from patients with Tourette syndrome. *Annals of Neurology*, **30**, 558–562.

Singer, H.S., Reiss, A.L., Brown, J.E. et al. (1993) Volumetric MRI changes in basal ganglia of children with Tourette syndrome. *Neurology*, **43**, 950–956.

Singer, H.S., Giuliano, J.D., Hansen, B.H. et al. (1998) Antibodies against human putamen in children with Tourette syndrome. *Neurology*, **50**, 1618–1624.

Spencer, T., Biederman, J., Harding, M. et al. (1998) Disentangling the overlap between Tourette disorder and ADHD. *Journal of Child Psychology and Psychiatry*, **39**, 1037–1044.

Stokes, A., Bawden, H.N., Camfield, P.R., Backman, J.E. & Dooley, J.M. (1991) Peer problems in Tourette disorder. *Pediatrics*, **87**, 936–942.

Swedo, S., Rapoport, J., Cheslow, D. et al. (1989) High prevalence of obsessive-compulsive symptoms in patients with Sydenham's chorea. *American Journal of Psychiatry*, **146**, 246–249.

Swedo, S.E., Leonard, H.L., Mittleman, B.B. et al. (1997) Identification of children with pediatric autoimmune neuropsychiatric disorders associated with streptococcal infections by a marker associated with rheumatic fever. *American Journal of Psychiatry*, **154**, 110–112.

Swedo, S.E., Leonard, H.L., Garvey, M. et al. (1998) Pediatric autoimmune neuropsychiatric disorders associated with streptococcal infections: clinical description of the first 50 cases. *American Journal of Psychiatry*, **155**, 264–271.

Swerdlow, N.R., Zinner, S., Farber, R.H., Seacrist, C. & Hartston, H. (1999) Symptoms of obsessive-compulsive disorder and Tourette syndrome: a spectrum? *CNS Spectrums*, **4**, 21–33.

Tanner, C.M., Goetz, C.G. & Klawans, H.L. (1982) Cholinergic mechanisms in Tourette syndrome. *Neurology*, **32**, 1315–1317.

Tourette Syndrome Classification Study Group (1993) Definitions and classification of tic disorders. *Archives of Neurology*, **50**, 1013–1016.

Tourette Syndrome International Consortium for Genetics (1999) A complete genome screen in sib-pairs affected with Gilles de la Tourette syndrome. *American Journal of Human Genetics*, **65**, 1428–1436.

Tourette Syndrome Study Group (1999) Short-term versus longer-term pimozide therapy in Tourette syndrome: a preliminary study. *Neurology*, **52**, 874–877.

Towbin, K.E., Peterson, B.S., Cohen, D.J. & Leckman, J.F. (1998) Differential diagnosis. In: *Tourette Syndrome Tics, Obsessions, Compulsions: Developmental Psychopathology and Clinical Care* (eds J.F. Leckman & D.J. Cohen), pp. 118–139. John Wiley and Sons, New York.

Vandewalle, V., van der Linden, C., Groenewegen, H.J. & Caemaert, J.

(1999) Stereotactic treatment of Gilles de la Tourette syndrome by high frequency stimulation of thalamus. *Lancet*, **353**, 724.

Walkup, J.T., Rosenberg, L.A., Brown, J. & Singer, H.S. (1992) The validity of instruments measuring tic severity in Tourette syndrome. *Journal of the American Academy of Child and Adolescent Psychiatry*, **31** (3), 472–477.

Walkup, J.T., LaBuda, M.C., Singer, H.S., Brown, J., Riddle, M.A. & Hurko, O. (1996) Family study and segregation analysis of Tourette syndrome: evidence for a mixed model of inheritance. *American Journal of Human Genetics*, **59**, 684–693.

Walkup, J.T., Khan, S., Schuerholz, L., Paik, Y.-S., Leckman, J.F. & Schultz, R.T. (1998) Phenomenology and natural history of tic-related ADHD and learning disabilities. In: *Tourette Syndrome Tics, Obsessions, Compulsions: Developmental Psychopathology and Clinical Care* (eds J.F. Leckman & J.D. Cohen), pp. 63–79. John Wiley and Sons, New York.

van Wattum, P.J., Anderson, G.M., Chappell, P.B., Goodman, W.K., Riddle, M.A. & Leckman, J.F. (1999) Cerebrospinal fluid dynorphin A[1–8] and beta-endorphin levels in Tourette syndrome are unaltered. *Biological Psychiatry*, **45**, 1527–1528.

Whitaker, A.H., Van Rossem, R., Feldman, J.F. *et al.* (1997) Psychiatric outcomes in low-birth-weight children at age 6 years: relation to neonatal cranial ultrasound abnormalities. *Archives of General Psychiatry*, **54**, 847–856.

Witzum, E., Bar-On, R., Dolberg, O.T. & Kotler, M. (1996) Traumatic war experiences affect outcome in a case of Tourette syndrome. *Psychotherapy and Psychosomatics*, **65**, 106–108.

Wolf, S.S., Jones, D.W., Knable, M.B. *et al.* (1996) Tourette syndrome: prediction of phenotypic variation in monozygotic twins by caudate nucleus D_2 receptor binding. *Science*, **273**, 1225–1227.

Wong, D.F., Singer, H.S., Brandt, J. *et al.* (1997) D_2-like dopamine receptor density in Tourette syndrome measured by PET. *Journal of Nuclear Medicine*, **38**, 1243–1247.

World Health Organization (1996) *Multiaxial Classification of Child and Adolescent Disorders: the ICD-10 Classification of Mental and Behavioural Disorders in Children and Adolescents*, pp. 43–45. Cambridge University Press, Cambridge.

Ziemann, U., Paulus, W. & Rothenberger, A. (1997) Decreased motor inhibition in Tourette disorder: evidence from transcranial magnetic stimulation. *American Journal of Psychiatry*, **154**, 1277–1284.

Zohar, A.H., Apter, A., King, R.A., Pauls, D.L., Leckman, J.F. & Cohen, D.J. (1998) Epidemiological studies. In: *Tourette Syndrome Tics, Obsessions, Compulsions: Developmental Psychopathology and Clinical Care* (eds J.F. Leckman & J.D. Cohen), pp. 177–193. John Wiley and Sons, New York.

Zohar, J., Mueller, E.A., Insel, T.R., Zohar-Kadouch, R.C. & Murphy, D.L. (1987) Serotonergic responsivity in obsessive-compulsive disorder: comparison of patients and healthy controls. *Archives of General Psychiatry*, **44**, 946–951.

37 Schizophrenia and Allied Disorders
Chris Hollis

Introduction

Schizophrenia is one of the most devastating psychiatric disorders to affect children and adolescents. Although extremely rare before the age of 10, the incidence of schizophrenia rises steadily through adolescence to reach its peak in early adult life. An accumulating body of evidence now supports the view that schizophrenia presenting in childhood and adolescence shows continuity with the adult form of the disorder at the levels of symptoms, clinical course and underlying neurobiology. Like other disorders of presumed multifactorial origin (e.g. juvenile rheumatoid arthritis and diabetes), the early onset form of schizophrenia lies at the extreme end of a continuum of disease severity and genetic liability.

The clinical severity and poor prognosis of child and adolescent onset schizophrenia reinforces the need for early diagnosis and treatment and ultimately prevention before the onset of psychosis. The introduction of newer atypical antipsychotics has been an important recent advance with their greater efficacy against negative symptoms and a lower risk of producing extrapyramidal side-effects. The goal of early diagnosis and prevention depends on identifying clinical and biological markers that have good reliability and predictive validity. Longitudinal studies are essential here, in particular those that track the transition from high-risk status to active psychosis.

While knowledge of the fundamental causes and pathogenic mechanisms in schizophrenia remains elusive, over the last decade there have been important developments in the way the disorder is conceptualized. There is now broad support for the view that schizophrenia is a disorder of brain development. Although there has been a long-standing interest in the role of perinatal risk factors in schizophrenia, recent attention has shifted to adolescent brain development more proximal to the onset of psychosis. It is proposed that excessive synaptic elimination during adolescence may lead to abnormal neural connectivity and psychotic symptoms. There is growing evidence that symptoms of psychosis (hallucinations, delusions, disorganization of thought or behaviour) may be a final end-state for a variety of disorders including schizophrenia and represent non-specific indicators of severe mental illness. Meanwhile, the genetic and developmental vulnerability to schizophrenia may be manifest in a broader non-psychotic schizophrenic spectrum characterized by a range of subtle social and cognitive impairments. Hence, the search for the causes of schizophrenia may be better directed not at the end-state psychotic symptoms, but at the more proximal developmental and cognitive processes that predispose to psychosis. The implication is that genetic and phenotypic vulnerability to schizophrenia is distributed on a continuum in the population with only a small proportion of the highest risk individuals crossing the threshold for the expression of psychotic symptoms. The concept of schizophrenia as a discrete disease category defined essentially by the presence or absence of psychotic symptoms may actually limit our ability to detect the genetic, developmental and pathophysiological origins of the disorder.

Concepts of schizophrenia

In the late nineteenth century, Kraepelin (1919) invoked the term 'dementia praecox' to distinguish patients with a psychosis that typically began in early adult life and ran a progressive and deteriorating course from the more benign and episodic course of manic depressive illness. Bleuler (1911) reformulated dementia praecox as schizophrenia, and described four fundamental symptoms: ambivalence, disturbance of association, disturbance of affect and preference of fantasy over reality. Bleuler viewed the fundamental deficit in schizophrenia as a 'splitting' or disconnection of normally integrated cognitive functions. Interestingly, the symptoms of hallucinations and delusions which are emphasized in modern diagnostic systems (DSM-IV and ICD-10) were not seen as fundamental in Bleuler's scheme, but rather as secondary consequences of the core schizophrenic deficits.

Bleuler's development of a theory of underlying deficits in schizophrenia contrasts with Kraepelin's atheoretical empirical observations. Bleulerian definitions of schizophrenia were largely abandoned by modern diagnostic systems (DSM and ICD) because they were seen as vague and had poor reliability. Instead, modern diagnostic constructs draw largely on the Kraepelian and Schneiderian tradition that views psychotic symptoms as fundamental to schizophrenia, with Schneider's first-rank symptoms given the greatest prominence. However, there is now good evidence that first-rank symptoms are neither specific nor valid indicators of schizophrenia (Peralta & Cuesta 1999). So has diagnostic reliability been achieved at the expense of validity? One approach to improving the validity of definitions of schizophrenia has been to link groups of symptoms (symptom dimensions) to underlying neurobiological processes.

Dimensions of psychopathology in schizophrenia

Although the concept of positive and negative symptoms was first expounded by the nineteenth century neurologist, Hughlings Jackson, it was not until the 1970s that these were applied to the symptoms of schizophrenia (Strauss *et al.* 1974). Factor analytical and correlational studies have now confirmed that schizophrenic symptoms consist of at least three dimensions (Liddle 1987a; Andreasen *et al.* 1995; Johnstone & Frith 1996; Lenzenweger & Dworkin 1996).

The 'positive' symptom dimension includes hallucinations and delusions and has been linked with temporal lobe function (Liddle *et al.* 1992). The 'negative' symptom dimension includes affective blunting, avolition and alogia and has been most clearly associated with poor performance on 'frontal lobe' tasks (Liddle 1987b; Liddle & Morris 1991) and hypofunction of the dorsolateral prefrontal cortex (Weinberger *et al.* 1986). The 'disorganization' dimension includes formal thought disorder and bizarre behaviour and has been linked to functional abnormalities of the ventral prefrontal cortex (predominantly on the right) and anterior cingulate (Liddle *et al.* 1992).

Recent work suggests that these dimensions are not unique to schizophrenic patients and can be identified (with added depressive and manic dimensions) in a broad spectrum of adult psychotic patients early in the course of their illness (van Os *et al.* 1996). This finding weakens the idea of clear categorical boundaries between psychotic diagnoses both at the symptomatic and neurobiological level.

Symptom dimensions in child and adolescent onset schizophrenia

Very few studies have examined symptom dimensions in child and adolescent schizophrenia and related psychoses. The evidence so far points to a broadly similar pattern of symptom dimensions in child and adolescent onset psychotic patients (Maziade *et al.* 1996; Hollis 1999). The main difference from studies in adult patients is the higher proportion of overall symptom variance explained by the negative symptom dimension in child and adolescent onset patients (Hollis 1999). Symptom dimensions in these younger patients show some expected associations with diagnostic categories: negative symptoms are specifically associated with schizophrenia and dimensions of mania and depression with affective psychoses. In contrast, the dimensions of disorganization and positive psychotic symptoms show less clear-cut associations with any specific diagnostic category. This lack of diagnostic specificity confirms that positive symptoms cannot be regarded as pathognomonic of schizophrenia. In terms of prognosis, the dimensions of disorganization and negative symptoms predict a poor adult outcome whereas affective symptoms predict a more benign course and outcome; positive symptoms (hallucinations–delusions and passivity–thought interference) have no prognostic value.

Two other findings from the Maudsley study (Hollis 1999) are of particular interest. First, the negative symptom dimension is associated with premorbid developmental impairments, which suggests possible developmental and neurobiological continuity between these domains. Second, negative symptoms are associated with an increased familial risk of schizophrenia. Taken together, these findings suggest that negative symptoms may be the most direct expression of a genetic and developmental risk for schizophrenia. These findings also support the Bleulerian view that the fundamental features of schizophrenia are negative symptoms and cognitive deficits.

The schizophrenia spectrum: schizotypy and 'schizotaxia'

A dimensional view of a schizophrenia spectrum is consistent with multigene models in schizophrenia, yet runs counter to the categorical approach found in current diagnostic systems. Multigene models assume that multiple genes combine with one another and with environmental factors to produce schizophrenia, with the genetic liability for schizophrenia distributed on a continuum in the population. According to this model, individuals with a very high loading of risk factors may manifest schizophrenia, whereas those with a lesser loading may show signs of schizotypal personality disorder, negative symptoms or cognitive impairments. A further implication of multigene models is that those individuals with the greatest liability will develop the disorder earlier in life and will have an increased risk of schizophrenia spectrum disorders among biological relatives.

Schizotypal personality disorder is characterized by disturbances of perception and thinking that appear to represent a milder variant of schizophrenia. The biological relationship between schizotypal personality disorder and schizophrenia is supported by family and genetic studies (Kendler *et al.* 1993), similarities on measures of neuropsychological test performance (Kremen *et al.* 1994) and similar structural brain abnormalities (Cannon *et al.* 1993).

The term 'schizotaxia' was first introduced in the early 1960s (Meehl 1962) to describe the unexpressed genetic liability to schizophrenia. More recently, the concept has been reinvoked to refer to the subtle psychiatric and neurobiological features found in non-psychotic and non-schizotypal relatives of schizophrenic patients (Tsuang *et al.* 2000). These features include negative symptoms, executive cognitive impairments, deviant eye tracking and structural brain abnormalities (Faraone *et al.* 2001). Thus, schizotaxia lies on a continuum of genetic liability and neurobiological dysfunction that includes schizotypy with schizophrenia as its most extreme manifestation. It is estimated that features of schizotaxia occur in about 20–50% of first-degree relatives of patients with schizophrenia (Faraone *et al.* 1995). However, only about 10% of relatives will become psychotic and less than 10% will have schizotypal personality disorder (Battaglia & Torgersen 1996). Hence, most affected individuals with schizotaxia do not develop psychosis.

These findings are all consistent with the view that the biological risk for schizophrenia is expressed in non-schizophrenic individuals as part of a broader non-psychotic phenotype and may also be apparent before the onset of psychosis in the form of pre-morbid social and cognitive impairments. In the following sections we will consider whether a premorbid phenotype of schizophrenia can be reliably identified, if progression to psychosis can be predicted and if intervention could prevent progression to full-blown psychosis.

Clinical phases of schizophrenia

Premorbid social and developmental impairments

Child and adolescent onset schizophrenia is associated with poor premorbid functioning and early developmental delays (Alaghband-Rad et al. 1995; Hollis 1995). Similar developmental and social impairments in childhood have been reported in adult onset schizophrenia using population-based cohorts free from referral biases (Done et al. 1994; Jones et al. 1994; Jones & Done 1997; Malmberg et al. 1998). Although age of onset comparisons are plagued by methodological difficulties, premorbid developmental impairments appear to be more common and severe in the child and adolescent onset forms of the disorder. In the Maudsley study (Hollis 1999) significant early delays were particularly common in the areas of language (20%), reading (30%) and bladder control (36%). Just over 20% of cases of adolescent schizophrenia had significant early delays in either language or motor development. A history of premorbid impairments may be even more common in the very earliest onset cases. Nicholson et al. (2000) reported significant premorbid speech/language, motor and social impairments in 50% of childhood onset patients with onset of psychosis before the age of 12 years. In contrast, a similar pattern of language and motor developmental delays has been reported in only about 10% of individuals destined to develop schizophrenia in adult life (Jones et al. 1994). A consistent characteristic in the premorbid phenotype is impaired sociability. In the Maudsley study of child and adolescent onset psychoses (Hollis 1999), about one-third of cases with schizophrenia had significant difficulties in social development affecting the ability to make and keep friends. Similar, but less frequent difficulties with premorbid sociability have been noted in representative population samples of adult schizophrenia (Malmberg et al. 1998).

Premorbid IQ also appears to be lower in child and adolescent onset schizophrenia than in the adult form of the disorder. The mean premorbid IQ lies in the mid to low 80s, 10–15 IQ points lower than in most adult studies (Asarnow et al. 1994a; Spencer & Campbell 1994; Alaghband-Rad et al. 1995; Hollis 2000). In the Maudsley study (Hollis 2000), one-third of child and adolescent onset cases had an IQ below 70 (mild learning disability range).

One interpretation of these findings is that a subgroup of adolescent schizophrenic cases has abnormal premorbid development with the rest developing normally. In fact, careful analysis shows that there is no abnormal developmental subgroup—this

is simply an artefact of using rather crude categorical measures of premorbid development. Continuous IQ measures show that the whole distribution of IQ is shifted down compared to both adolescent affective psychoses and adult schizophrenia.

These findings are consistent with the view that premorbid impairments are manifestations of a genetic/developmental liability to schizophrenia. It seems clear that the premorbid phenotype does not just represent non-specific psychiatric disturbance. Subtle problems of language, attention and social relationships are typical whereas, in contrast, conduct problems are rare. However, premorbid social and behavioural difficulties are not specific to schizophrenia. Premorbid deficits also occur in adolescent affective psychoses, at a lower rate than in schizophrenia, but higher than in non-psychotic psychiatric controls (van Os et al. 1997; Sigurdsson et al. 1999).

Are premorbid impairments a risk or precursor of psychosis?

Premorbid impairments could lie on a causal pathway for psychosis or, alternatively, they could be markers of an underlying neuropathological process, such as aberrant neural connectivity which may be the cause of both premorbid social impairment and psychosis. Causality is clearly implicit in ideas of primary prevention and the risk estimates provided by population-based epidemiological studies of prepsychotic impairments (Done et al. 1994; Jones et al. 1994; Malmberg et al. 1998). Frith (1994) has speculated on the possible cognitive mechanisms that might link deficits in social cognition or 'theory of mind' in a causal pathway to both positive and negative psychotic symptoms. If these characteristics are causally related then modifying the 'primary' cognitive or social deficits may reduce the risk of psychosis. Alternatively, cognitive and social deficits, although often present, may not be necessary in the pathogenesis. The fact that individuals may develop schizophrenia without obvious premorbid impairments supports this view. In these circumstances, an intervention aimed at the neurobiological level (e.g. antipsychotic medication) may be necessary. Only a high-risk longitudinal intervention study can adequately address the issue of causality, and this would require an intervention that had benefits for the majority of individuals with the premorbid phenotype who would not develop psychosis.

Prodromal symptoms and onset of psychosis

Although some individuals show relatively stable patterns of subtle social and neurocognitive impairments, those that develop schizophrenia typically enter a prodromal phase characterized by a gradual but marked decline in social and academic functioning that precedes the onset of active psychotic symptoms. An insidious deterioration prior to onset of psychosis is typical of the presentation of schizophrenia in children and adolescents (Werry et al. 1994). In the Maudsley study of adolescent psychoses (Hollis 1999), a pattern of insidious onset was found more often in cases of schizophrenia than in affective psychoses.

Non-specific behavioural changes including social withdrawal, declining school performance, uncharacteristic and odd behaviour began, on average, over a year before the onset of positive psychotic symptoms. In retrospect, it was often apparent that non-specific behavioural changes were early negative symptoms, which in turn had their onset well before positive symptoms such as hallucinations and delusions.

Hence, early recognition of disorder can be very difficult, as premorbid cognitive and social impairments gradually shade into prodromal symptoms before the onset of active psychotic symptoms (Hafner & Nowotny 1995). Prodromal symptoms can include odd ideas, eccentric interests, changes in affect, unusual experiences and bizarre perceptual experiences. Although these are also characteristic features of schizotypal personality disorder, in a schizophrenic prodrome there is usually progression to more severe dysfunction.

Diagnosis of schizophrenia in childhood and adolescence

Historical perspective

Both Kraepelin and Bleuler believed that schizophrenia presented in a similar form, albeit more rarely, during childhood and adolescence. Kraepelin (1919) found that 3.5% of cases of dementia praecox began before the age of 10 with a further 2.7% arising between the ages of 10 and 15. Bleuler (1911) suggested that about 5% of cases of schizophrenia had their onset prior to age 15.

However, from the 1930s until the early 1970s, the concept of 'childhood schizophrenia' as a distinct category was invoked. The definition of childhood schizophrenia was broadened to encompass autism and other developmental disorders that were seen as childhood manifestations of adult schizophrenia. This lumping together of different disorders under the diagnosis of childhood schizophrenia makes most research carried out during this period very difficult to interpret.

During the 1970s the pendulum swung back to reflect Kraepelin's and Bleuler's original views. Schizophrenia in childhood and adolescence was again seen as continuous with the adult form of the disorder and presented with essentially the same clinical picture (Kolvin 1971; Rutter 1972). From ICD-9 (World Health Organization 1978) and DSM-III (American Psychiatric Association 1980) onwards, the same diagnostic criteria have been used for schizophrenia regardless of the age of onset. The current international diagnostic systems (ICD-10 and DSM-IV) have continued this tradition, with no diagnostic distinction made for schizophrenia presenting in childhood and adolescence.

Developmental issues

Although the use of the same diagnostic criteria for schizophrenia aids comparability across the age range, it does not exclude the possibility of some degree of symptom variation in childhood and adolescence. The main argument against the idea of developmental variants of schizophrenia is the finding that schizophrenia can be reliably identified in children as young as 7 years using unmodified adult diagnostic criteria (McKenna et al. 1994). However, if schizophrenia does show significant symptom variation in children and adolescents then applying unmodified adult criteria may result in a proportion of 'true' cases being missed (false-negative diagnoses). Conversely, some presentations of schizophrenia in early life could be phenocopies of adult schizophrenia (false-positive diagnoses) with a distinct aetiology and clinical course. Hence, there are two main issues to be addressed.

1 What is the validity of adult diagnostic criteria for schizophrenia when applied in childhood and adolescence?
2 Are there partial syndromes or variants of schizophrenia in childhood and adolescence that should be considered as part of a broader schizophrenic spectrum?

Diagnostic validity and stability

Good evidence for the validity of the diagnosis of schizophrenia in childhood and adolescence comes from the recent Maudsley Child and Adolescent Psychosis Follow-up Study (Hollis 2000). A DSM-IIIR diagnosis of schizophrenia in childhood and adolescence predicted a significantly worse adult outcome compared with other non-schizophrenic psychoses (American Psychiatric Association 1987). The diagnosis of schizophrenia showed a high level of stability, with 80% having the same diagnosis recorded at adult follow-up. These findings challenge the belief that adolescent schizophrenic and affective psychoses are poorly differentiated and show a high degree of diagnostic instability from adolescence into adult life (Zeitlin 1986; Werry et al. 1991).

However, there remains the problem of resolving the status of 'partial syndromes' that share some diagnostic features, or prodromal symptoms, of schizophrenia but do not meet full DSM-IV (American Psychiatric Association 1994) or ICD-10 (World Health Organization 1992) diagnostic criteria. For example, in the USA the term 'multidimensionally impaired' (MDI) (Jacobsen & Rapoport 1998; Kumra et al. 1998a) has been coined to describe children that have multiple early impairments in cognitive and social functioning and then develop transient psychotic symptoms in late childhood and early adolescence. A higher than expected rate of schizophrenia among first-degree relatives suggests that MDI children may lie on the schizophrenia spectrum, but longer follow-up studies are needed to tell if these cases progress to more typical schizophrenic presentations (Kumra et al. 1998a). At present, cases with partial or contiguous syndromes, such as MDI or schizotypal personality disorder, require careful clinical follow-up to determine if they will develop schizophrenia. The question of how best to treat these presentations (e.g. should they be given low-dose antipsychotics) remains an important but unresolved question.

Diagnostic criteria for schizophrenia

The two dominant diagnostic systems (DSM and ICD) both require the clear evidence of psychosis (in the absence of predominant affective symptoms) with minimum duration criteria. A comparison of the current DSM-IV and ICD-10 criteria for schizophrenia is presented in Table 37.1.

It may appear confusing to have different, albeit quite similar definitions for a single disorder. However, although different definitions of schizophrenia continue to exist, it is helpful that they are explicit and clearly operationalized. The existence of alternative definitions also emphasizes that these definitions are arbitrary and provisional.

ICD-10 criteria are closer to the Schneiderian concept of schizophrenia and place more reliance than DSM-IV on the presence of first-rank symptoms. In contrast, the DSM-IV definition reflects Kraepelin's concept of a psychotic disorder with a chronic and deteriorating course (Maj 1998). An example of the different approaches of the two systems can be seen in how they categorize a hypothetical patient presenting with schizophrenic symptoms but only 2 months' duration of disturbance. This patient would be given a diagnosis of schizophrenia using ICD-10 but would not fulfil the DSM-IV criteria. DSM-IV stipulates a 6-month duration of disturbance, which makes it more restrictive than the 1-month duration criteria of ICD-10. The DSM-IV category of schizophreniform disorder is used for cases with the same symptoms but an overall duration of disturbance of less than 6 months. As a result, the DSM-IIIR/DSM-IV definition of schizophrenia has greater specificity but lower sensitivity than ICD-10 in first-episode psychoses (Mason *et al.* 1997). Not surprisingly, cases of schizophrenia defined using DSM-IV have a worse prognosis than those defined using ICD-10.

DSM-IV describes various subtypes of schizophrenia defined by the most prominent symptomatology:

1 paranoid type, characterized by delusions and hallucinations;
2 disorganized type, characterized by disorganization of speech, behaviour and negative symptoms (i.e. flat or inappropriate affect);
3 catatonic type, characterized by motor abnormalities; and
4 residual type.

Clinical characteristics of schizophrenia in childhood and adolescence

Even if strict adult definitions of schizophrenia (DSM-IIIR/DSM-IV or ICD-10) are applied, there appears to be evidence of some age-dependent variations in phenomenology. Child and adolescent onset cases are characterized by a more insidious onset, negative symptoms, disorganized behaviour, hallucinations in different modalities and fewer systematized or persecutory delusions (Garralda 1984; Asarnow & Ben-Meir 1988; Green *et al.* 1992; Werry *et al.* 1994). Using the DSM-IIIR/DSM-IV scheme of subtyping schizophrenia, the disorganized subtype (hebephrenia in ICD-10) has a peak incidence

during adolescence, whereas the paranoid subtype more often presents first in adult life (Beratis *et al.* 1994).

In summary, early onset schizophrenia is characterized by greater disorganization (incoherence of thought and disordered sense of self) and more negative symptoms, whereas in later onset cases there is a higher frequency of systematized and paranoid delusions (Hafner & Nowotny 1995).

Course and outcome

Short-term course

Adolescent schizophrenia characteristically runs a chronic course with only a small minority of cases making a full symptomatic recovery from the first psychotic episode. In the Maudsley study of child and adolescent onset psychoses (Hollis 1999), only 12% of schizophrenic cases were in full remission at discharge compared with 50% of cases with affective psychoses. The short-term outcome for schizophrenia presenting in early life appears to be worse than that of first-episode adult patients (Robinson *et al.* 1999). If full recovery does occur then it is most likely within the first 3 months of onset of psychosis. In the Maudsley study, those adolescent onset patients who were still psychotic after 6 months had only a 15% chance of achieving full remission, whereas over half of all cases that made a full recovery had active psychotic symptoms for less than 3 months (Hollis 1999). The clinical implication is that the early course over the first 6 months is the best predictor of remission and that longer observation over 6 months adds relatively little new information.

Long-term outcome

A number of long-term follow-up studies of child and adolescent onset schizophrenia describe a typically chronic, unremitting, long-term course with severely impaired functioning in adult life (Eggers 1978; Werry *et al.* 1991; Schmidt *et al.* 1995; Eggers & Bunk 1997; Hollis 2000). Several common themes emerge from these studies.

1 The generally poor outcome of early onset schizophrenia conceals considerable heterogeneity. About one-fifth of patients in most studies have a good outcome with only mild impairment whereas, at the other extreme, about one-third of patients are severely impaired requiring intensive social and psychiatric support. Hence, for an individual patient, diagnosis alone is a relatively crude prognostic indicator.
2 After the first few years of illness there is little evidence of further progressive decline. This suggests that during the first 10–15 years of illness, at least, the course is relatively stable, although further progression may occur later in life.
3 Child and adolescent onset schizophrenia has a worse outcome than either adolescent onset affective psychoses or adult onset schizophrenia. This suggests that outcome and clinical severity are related to both diagnosis and the age at onset.

Table 37.1 Diagnostic criteria for schizophrenia in DSM-IV and ICD-10.

DSM-IV	ICD-10
DSM-IV requires that six separate criteria (A–F) are met for a diagnosis of schizophrenia.	A Either *at least one* of the groups of symptoms (a–d) listed under (1) *or at least two* of the groups of symptoms (a–d) listed under (2) should be present for most of the time during a psychotic episode lasting for at least *1 month*.
A Five types of 'characteristic' symptoms are listed of which at least two types must be present for at least 1 month:	1. At least *one* of the following (a–d) must be present:
(i) *Delusions* of any kind	(a) thought echo/insertion/withdrawal/broadcasting
(ii) *Hallucinations* of any kind in clear consciousness (excluding hallucinations secondary to substance misuse or an organic brain disorder)	(b) delusions of control, influence or passivity, delusional perception
(iii) *Disorganized speech/formal thought disorder*	(c) auditory hallucinations giving a running commentary on the patient's behaviour, or discussing the patient among themselves, or other types of hallucinatory voice coming from some part of the body
(e.g. frequent derailments, loosening of association or incoherence)	(d) persistent delusions of other kinds that are culturally inappropriate or completely impossible (bizarre delusions)
(iv) *Grossly disorganized or catatonic behaviour*	2. *Or* at least two of the following (a–d):
(v) *Negative symptoms*, i.e. affective flattening, alogia or avolition.	(a) Persistent hallucinations in any modality, occurring every day for at least a month, accompanied by delusions without clear affective content, or accompanied by persistent overvalued ideas
NB: A single symptom of *bizarre delusions*, or specific types of auditory hallucination (voices commenting or conversing with each other) are sufficient on their own to fulfil criterion A.	(b) Neologisms, breaks in the train of thought, resulting in incoherence or irrelevant speech
	(c) Catatonic behaviour such as excitement, posturing or waxy flexibility, negativism, mutism or stupor
B Evidence of deterioration in social or occupational functioning. In childhood and adolescence this can mean failure to reach an expected level of social, academic or occupational achievement.	(d) 'Negative' symptoms, such as marked apathy, paucity of speech, and blunting or incongruity of emotional responses (it must be clear that these are not caused by depression or neuroleptic medication)
C At least 6 *months* duration of disturbance. This period must include at least 1 month of 'active symptoms' (criterion A) and may include periods of prodromal or residual symptoms.	B Exclusion criteria:
D The exclusion of schizoaffective and other psychotic mood disorders. If affective symptoms occur, they must be relatively brief in relation to other active symptoms listed in criterion A.	(a) If the patient meets criteria for a manic or depressive episode, the criteria listed above, (1) and (2) must be present *before* the disturbance in mood developed
E Symptoms are not attributable to the effects of substance misuse, other medication or medical conditions.	(b) The disorder is not attributable to organic brain disease, or to alcohol- or drug-related intoxication, dependence or withdrawal.
F In cases with a history of pervasive developmental disorder (autism), the diagnosis of schizophrenia can only be made with at least 1 month duration of hallucinations or delusions.	

4 Social functioning, in particular the ability to form friendships and love relationships, appears to be very impaired in early onset schizophrenia.

Taken together, these findings confirm that schizophrenia presenting in childhood and adolescence lies at the extreme end of a continuum of phenotypic severity.

Prognostic factors

The predictors of poor outcome in child and adolescent onset psychoses include premorbid social and cognitive impairments (Werry & McClellan 1992; Hollis 1999), a prolonged first psychotic episode (Schmidt et al. 1995), extended duration of untreated psychosis (Hollis 1999) and the presence of negative symptoms (Hollis 1999). Premorbid functioning and negative symptoms at onset provide better prediction of long-term outcome than categorical diagnosis (Hollis 1999). This finding suggests that premorbid social and cognitive impairments and negative symptoms lie at the core of a valid clinical concept of schizophrenia.

Mortality

The risk of premature death is increased in child and adolescent onset psychoses. In the Maudsley study (Hollis 1999), there were nine deaths out of the 106 cases followed-up (8.5%). The standardized mortality ratio (SMR) was 1250 (95% CI, 170–5500), which represents a 12-fold increase in the risk of death compared to an age- and sex-matched general UK population over the same period. Of the nine deaths in the cohort, seven were male and seven had a diagnosis of schizophrenia. Three subjects suffered violent deaths, two died from self-poisoning, and three had unexpected deaths caused by previously undetected physical causes (cardiomyopathy and status epilepticus) and were possibly associated with high-dose antipsychotic medication.

The death rate in child and adolescent onset schizophrenia and other psychoses appears to be significantly higher than in the adult form of the disorder. In adults the 'all cause' SMR for schizophrenia has been reported as 157 (95% CI, 153–160) (Harris & Barraclough 1997). In a Norwegian study of adolescent psychiatric inpatients, Kjelsberg (2000) reported an SMR for psychosis of 390 in male and 1130 in female patients.

Epidemiology

Incidence and prevalence

Good population-based incidence figures for child and adolescent onset schizophrenia are notably lacking because studies have used broad categories of psychosis, without standardized assessments. Gillberg et al. (1986) calculated age-specific prevalence for all psychoses (including schizophrenia, schizophreni-

form affective psychosis, atypical psychosis and drug psychoses) in the age range 13–18 years using case-register data from Goteborg, Sweden. Of the cases, 41% had a diagnosis of schizophrenia. At age 13 years, the prevalence for all psychoses was 0.9 in 10 000, showing a steady increase during adolescence, reaching a prevalence of 17.6 in 10 000 at age 18 years.

Sex ratio

Males are overrepresented in many clinical studies of childhood onset schizophrenia (Russell et al. 1989; Green et al. 1992; Russell 1994; Spencer & Campbell 1994). However, other studies of predominantly adolescent onset schizophrenia have described an equal sex ratio (Gordon et al. 1994; Werry et al. 1994; Hollis 2000). The interpretation of these studies is complicated by the possibility of referral biases to clinical centres. In an epidemiological study of first admissions for schizophrenia and paranoia in children and adolescents there was an equal sex ratio for patients under the age of 15 (Galdos et al. 1993; Lewine 1994). The finding of an equal sex distribution with adolescent onset is intriguing as it differs from the consistent male predominance (ratio 2 : 1) reported in incident samples of early adult onset schizophrenia (Castle & Murray 1991). Clearly, future studies require population-based incident samples free from potential referral biases.

Aetiology and risk factors

Pregnancy and birth complications

Pregnancy and birth complications (PBC) have been implicated as a risk factor in schizophrenia. In a meta-analysis of 20 case–control studies, subjects that developed schizophrenia were over twice as likely to have been exposed to PBCs as controls (Geddes & Lawrie 1995). However, the findings from two other large case–control studies suggest that the link between schizophrenia and PBCs may be much weaker than previously assumed (Kendall et al. 2000). In one case–control study of childhood onset schizophrenia, Matsumoto et al. (1999) reported an odds ratio of 3.5 for PBC, suggesting a greater risk in very early onset cases. However, in the National Institute for Mental Health (NIMH) study of childhood onset schizophrenia, PBCs were no more common in cases than in sibling controls (Nicholson et al. 1999). Even if there is a significant association, it remains unclear whether there is any causal connection between PBCs and schizophrenia. There is a strong argument that PBCs are *consequences* rather than *causes* of abnormal neurodevelopment (Goodman 1988). This view is supported by the finding that schizophrenic patients have smaller head size at birth than controls (McGrath & Murray 1995), which is likely to be a consequence of either defects in genetic control of neurodevelopment or earlier environmental factors such as viral exposure.

Puberty

The close temporal association between the onset of puberty and a marked increase in the incidence of schizophrenia suggests that biological (or social) events around puberty may be related to the expression of psychotic symptoms. Galdos *et al.* (1993) reported an association between the timing of menarche and onset of psychosis in girls. However, this finding has not been supported by subsequent studies. Frazier *et al.* (1997) found no relationship between the onset of psychosis and indices of puberty in cases recruited to the NIMH study of childhood onset schizophrenia. For both boys and girls the timing of pubertal events were the same for cases and controls.

Psychosocial risks

One possible explanation for an atypically early onset of schizophrenia could be differential exposure to psychosocial adversity, such as higher levels of parental hostility and criticism ('high EE'). High levels of expressed emotion (EE) among relatives of schizophrenic adults has been shown to be a predictor of psychotic relapse and poor outcome (Leff & Vaughn 1985). Although the role of high EE in precipitating the onset of schizophrenia has not been established, it is theoretically plausible that high EE might act to 'bring forward' the onset of the disorder in a vulnerable individual. Goldstein (1987) reported that parental EE measures of criticism and overinvolvement taken during adolescence were associated with an increased risk of schizophrenia spectrum disorders in young adulthood. However, a causal link was not proven, and the association may reflect either an expression of some common underlying trait or a parental response to premorbid disturbance in the preschizophrenic adolescent. More direct comparisons between the parents of adult and childhood onset schizophrenic patients fail to support the hypothesis of higher parental EE in childhood onset cases. Asarnow *et al.* (1994b) used the Five Minute Speech Sample to measure parental EE and found that those with childhood onset schizophrenia were no more likely to have 'high EE' parents than normal controls. Overall, there seems little evidence to suggest that the onset of schizophrenia in childhood can be explained by exposure to higher levels of parental criticism and hostility than that experienced by adult onset patients. Indeed, it appears that, on average, the parents of those with childhood onset schizophrenia generally express *lower* levels of criticism and hostility than parents of adult onset patients, caused by a greater tendency to attribute their childrens' behaviour to an illness which is beyond their control (Hooley 1987).

Neurobiology of schizophrenia

Neurodevelopmental models of schizophrenia

Over the last decade the concept of schizophrenia as a neurode-

velopmental disorder has taken a strong hold, although 'neurodevelopmental' is often used with a wide range of meanings. It is possible to distinguish 'early' and 'late' neurodevelopmental models, with a third 'risk' model incorporating ideas from developmental psychopathology (Hollis & Taylor 1997).

The 'early' neurodevelopmental model emerged from the ideas of Fish (1957) who proposed that the neuropathology in schizophrenia was of perinatal origin. The 'early' neurodevelopmental model views the primary cause of schizophrenia as a static 'lesion' occurring during fetal brain development (Murray & Lewis 1987; Weinberger 1987). The putative 'lesion' could be of either neurogenetic or environmental origin (e.g. virus infection or fetal hypoxia). Two main lines of evidence support the 'early' neurodevelopmental model. First, post-mortem studies of brain morphology (Jacob & Beckman 1986) report an absence of gliosis and possible abnormalities in neuronal migration that suggest that brain abnormalities are caused by aberrant neurodevelopment rather than neurodegeneration. Second, a more indirect line of evidence includes the association of schizophrenia with premorbid social and cognitive impairments (Foerster *et al.* 1991; Done *et al.* 1994; Jones *et al.* 1994), PBCs (Lewis & Murray 1987; McNeil 1995) and minor physical anomalies (Gualtieri *et al.* 1982; Guy *et al.* 1983). According to this 'early' model, during childhood this lesion is relatively silent giving rise only to subtle behavioural symptoms (premorbid social and cognitive impairments). However, in adolescence or early adult life, the lesion interacts with the process of *normal* brain maturation (e.g. myelination of corticolimbic circuits, and/or synaptic pruning and remodelling) to manifest itself in the form of psychotic symptoms.

There are several problems with the 'early' neurodevelopmental model. First, it fails to provide a satisfactory account of the long latency between the perinatal damage/lesion and the typical onset of symptoms in late adolescence/early adult life. Second, an early neurodevelopmental insult on its own cannot account for the finding of increased extracerebral (sulcal) cerebrospinal fluid space in schizophrenia. Diffuse loss of brain tissue limited to the prenatal or perinatal periods would result in enlargement of the lateral ventricles but not increased extracerebral cerebrospinal fluid space (Woods 1998).

The 'late' neurodevelopmental model, first proposed by Feinberg (1983, 1997), argues that the key neuropathological events in schizophrenia occur as a result of *abnormal* brain development during adolescence. The current formulation of the 'late' neurodevelopmental model proposes that *excessive* synaptic and/or dentritic elimination occurs during adolescence, producing aberrant neural connectivity and psychotic symptoms (Woods 1998; McGlashen & Hoffman 2000). This 'late' model characterizes schizophrenia as a *progressive* late onset neurodevelopmental disorder in contrast to the 'early' model that proposes a *static* lesion during the perinatal period. The 'late' model predicts that progressive structural brain changes and cognitive decline will be seen in adolescence around the onset of psychosis. The excessive synaptic pruning during adolescence proposed in the 'late' model is simply an amplification of the normal process of neuronal remodelling with progressive pruning and elimination of synapses that begins in early childhood and extends through late adolescence (Huttenlocher 1979; Purves & Lichtmen 1980). These major regressive changes in adolescence with remodelling of neural connections are likely to be under genetic control, with synaptic elimination in schizophrenia representing an extreme of normal variation (Feinberg 1983). In the 'late' model, premorbid abnormalities in early childhood are viewed as non-specific risk factors rather than early manifestations of an underlying schizophrenic neuropathology.

Both the 'early' and 'late' models suppose that there is a direct and specific expression of the eventual brain pathology as schizophrenic disorder. A third viewpoint, the 'risk' model, proposes that early and/or late brain pathology acts as a risk factor rather than a sufficient cause so that its effects can only be understood in the light of an individual's exposure to other risk and protective factors (Hollis & Taylor 1997). This latter formulation provides a probabilistic model of the onset of schizophrenia in which aberrant brain development is expressed as neurocognitive impairments that interact with the environment to produce psychotic symptoms. The following sections will examine how well current neurobiological research evidence supports these competing neurodevelopmental models of schizophrenia.

Neuropathology

In the post-mortem brains of schizophrenic patients there is an absence of gliosis which is the necessary hallmark of neurodegeneration (Roberts *et al.* 1986). The prominent neuropathology in schizophrenia is not the classic form involving neuronal cell death, but instead a loss or reduction in dendritic spines and synapses which are the elements of neural connectivity (Glantz & Lewis 2000). As a result the brain in schizophrenia is characterized by increased neuronal density, decreased intraneuronal space and reduced overall brain volume. Furthermore, the decrease in dentritic spine density appears to be both region- and disease-specific, being found in the dorsolateral prefrontal cortex (layer 3 pyramidal cells), but not in the visual cortex of schizophrenic patients (Glantz & Lewis 2000). These findings are compatible with the hypothesis of reduced cortical and/or thalamic excitatory inputs to the dorsolateral prefrontal cortex in schizophrenia.

Structural brain abnormalities

Neuroimaging and post-mortem studies have shown that the brain as a whole, and the frontal and temporal cortices in particular, are smaller than in normal subjects (Andreasen *et al.* 1990; Nopoulos *et al.* 1995). Brain volume reductions in schizophrenia are specific to grey matter (Gur *et al.* 2000a), which supports neuropathological findings of increased neuronal density and reduced intraneuronal neurophil rather than neuronal loss (Selemon *et al.* 1995).

Across a range of neuroimaging studies, the volume of the hippocampus and amygdala is reduced bilaterally by 4.5–10% (Nelson *et al.* 1998; Gur *et al.* 2000a). Prefrontal grey matter volume is reduced by about 10% (Gur *et al.* 2000b). Enlargement of the third and lateral ventricles is a consistent finding, with ventricular volume increased by about 40% bilaterally (Lawrie & Abukmeil 1998). Ventricular enlargement is associated with neuropsychological impairment and negative symptoms (Vita *et al.* 1991). Studies of the basal ganglia have produced more inconsistent results, possibly as a function of the increase in basal ganglia volume associated with the use of traditional antipsychotics. Interestingly, when patients are switched to the atypical antipsychotic clozapine there is a reduction in basal ganglia volume (Chakos *et al.* 1995).

The brain changes reported in childhood onset schizophrenia appear to be very similar to those described in adult schizophrenia, supporting the idea of an underlying neurobiological continuity. In the NIMH study of childhood onset schizophrenia (onset less than 12 years of age), subjects had smaller brains than controls, with larger lateral ventricles and reduced prefrontal lobe volume (Jacobsen & Rapoport 1998). Similar to findings from adult studies, reduced total cerebral volume is associated with negative symptoms (Alaghband-Rad *et al.* 1997). The midsagittal thalamic area is decreased while the midsagittal area of the corpus callosum is increased (Giedd *et al.* 1996), suggesting that the reduction in total cerebral volume in childhood onset schizophrenia is caused by relative reduction in grey matter with sparing of white matter. Childhood onset patients have a higher rate of developmental brain abnormalities than controls, including an increased frequency of an enlarged cavum septum pellucidum (Nopoulos *et al.* 1998). Abnormalities of the cerebellum have also been found, including reduced volume of the vermis, midsagittal area and inferior posterior lobe (Jacobsen *et al.* 1997a).

Progressive brain changes

Two different types of progressive brain change have been described in schizophrenia. First, treatment with traditional antipsychotics appears to cause progressive enlargement of the basal ganglia, with these structures returning to their original size when patients are transferred to the atypical antipsychotic clozapine (Frazier *et al.* 1996). Second, there is evidence of progressive volume reductions in the temporal and frontal lobes during the first 2–3 years after the onset of schizophrenia (Gur *et al.* 1998). In the NIMH study of childhood onset schizophrenia, longitudinal repeated magnetic resonance imaging (MRI) scans through adolescence have revealed a progressive increase in ventricular volume and progressive decrease in cortical volume, with frontal (11% decrease) and temporal lobes (7% decrease) disproportionately affected (Rapoport *et al.* 1997, 1999). Both patients and controls showed progressive reductions in frontal and parietal lobe volumes, with schizophrenic subjects showing a relatively greater loss of temporal lobe volume than controls (Jacobsen *et al.* 1998). The reduction seen in temporal lobe structures may occur rather later in the illness course than the reduction in frontal lobe and midsagittal thalamic structures. Progressive changes appear to be time-limited to adolescence, with the rate of volume reduction in frontal and temporal structures declining as subjects reach adult life.

Because progressive brain changes have been described *after* the onset of psychosis, it is possible that they are a consequence of neurotoxic effects of psychosis. Evidence that progressive brain changes precede the onset of psychosis is very limited. Pantelis *et al.* (2000) have provided a preliminary report of brain MRI findings in high-risk subjects scanned before and after the transition into psychosis. For those subjects that developed psychosis there were longitudinal volume reductions in the medial temporal region (hippocampus, entorhinal cortex, inferior frontal and fusiform gyrus). There were no significant longitudinal changes in cases that remained non-psychotic. These are exciting findings and, if replicated, provide strong support for the idea that excessive developmental reductions in temporal lobe volume have a key role in the onset of psychosis.

Functional brain imaging

The emergence of functional brain imaging technology has provided a unique opportunity to link symptoms and cognitive deficits in schizophrenia to underlying brain activity. Liddle *et al.* (1992) studied the relationship between symptom dimensions (negative, positive and disorganization) in adult schizophrenic subjects and regional cerebral blood flow (rCBF) using positron emission tomography (PET). Negative symptoms (e.g. affective blunting, avolition and alogia) were associated with reduced rCBF in the dorsolateral prefrontal cortex (DLPFC). Disorganization (e.g. formal thought disorder and bizarre behaviour) was associated with reduced rCBF in the right ventrolateral prefrontal cortex and increased rCBF in the anterior cingulate. Positive symptoms (e.g. hallucinations and delusions) were associated with increased rCBF in the left medial temporal lobe, and reduced rCBF in the posterior cingulate and left lateral temporal lobe. The most consistent association in the literature, across a variety of imaging methods, has been between negative symptoms and reduced frontal activity.

In a PET study in childhood onset schizophrenia using the Continuous Performance Test (CPT), Jacobsen *et al.* (1997b) reported reduced activation compared with healthy controls in the mid and superior frontal gyrus, and increased activation in the inferior frontal, supramarginal gyrus and insula. Clearly, a simple description of 'hypofrontality' does not capture the complex pattern of changes involving interconnected frontal areas. Likewise older localizationist models, based on focal cerebral dysfunction in schizophrenia, have tended to give way to more dynamic models of cerebral 'disconnectivity' based on dysfunctional neural networks or systems. Models of cerebral connectivity view normal higher brain function as depending on the integrated activity of widely distributed neurocognitive networks, rather than the activity of discrete brain areas in isolation (Bullmore *et al.* 1997). In normal individuals, the functional anatomy of a verbal fluency task (generation of words beginning with a given letter) can be examined using PET and has consistently shown activation of the left DLPFC and reciprocal deactivation of the superior temporal gyrus (STG). A number of investigators have reported a failure of STG deactivation (disconnectivity) in schizophrenic patients during a verbal fluency task (Friston *et al.* 1995; Donlan *et al.* 1996). This left DLPFC–STG disconnectivity appears to be state-related, being only found in symptomatic patients, possibly associated with active auditory hallucinations (Spence *et al.* 2000). In contrast, schizophrenic patients in remission show reduced connectivity between the left DLPFC and anterior cingulate cortex relative to normal controls (Spence *et al.* 2000).

In summary, models of cerebral disconnectivity fit well with both neuropathological and functional neuroimaging findings. This may be one reason for inconsistent neuroanatomical findings in schizophrenia as 'lesions' in different areas of a widely distributed neural system could produce similar functional disturbance.

Magnetic resonance spectroscopy: abnormal neuronal metabolism

Magnetic resonance spectroscopy (MRS) is an imaging technique that can be used to extract *in vivo* information on dynamic biochemical processes at a neuronal level. Proton (^{1}H) MRS focuses on changes in the neuronal marker N-acetyl aspartate (NAA). Studies in adult schizophrenic patients have shown reductions in NAA in the hippocampal area and DLPFC. Similar reductions in NAA ratios specific to the hippocampus and DLPFC (Bertolino *et al.* 1998) and frontal grey matter (Thomas *et al.* 1998) have been reported in childhood onset schizophrenia, suggesting neuronal damage or malfunction in these regions.

Pettegrew *et al.* (1991) used ^{31}P MRS in first episode non-medicated schizophrenic patients and found reduced phosphomonoester (PME) resonance and increased phosphodiester (PDE) resonance in the prefrontal cortex. This result is compatible with reduced synthesis and increased breakdown of connective processes in the prefrontal cortex. A similar finding of reduced PME and increased PDE resonance has been reported in autistic adults, although they showed increased prefrontal metabolic activity which was not seen in schizophrenic subjects (Pettegrew *et al.* 1991). It is possible that excessive synaptic elimination is not specific to schizophrenia, but its timing, location and extent may have crucial implications for the development of executive functions in late childhood and adolescence.

Implications for neurodevelopmental models of schizophrenia

Taken together, the neuropathological and brain imaging findings provide considerable support for the idea of progressive neurodevelopmental changes in schizophrenia including excessive synaptic elimination resulting in aberrant neural connectivity. The progressive nature of brain volume reductions in adolescence, and the fact that reduced brain volume is not accompanied by reduced intracranial volume, suggests that a static prenatal or perinatal brain insult is insufficient to account for this process. Although early random events in fetal neuro-development (e.g. hypoxia, viruses, etc.) may affect baseline synaptic density, genetically determined excessive synaptic elimination as proposed by the 'late' neurodevelopmental model may be the neurobiological process underlying disorders in the schizophrenia spectrum (McGlashen & Hoffman 2000). What is unclear is whether excessive synaptic elimination in the prefrontal cortex (and possibly other brain regions) is a sufficient cause for psychosis to occur, or whether it provides a vulnerable neurocognitive substrate that must interact with environmental stressors (e.g. cognitive or social demands) to produce psychotic symptoms.

Genetics of schizophrenia

Multigene models of risk

Twin studies have suggested the heritability of schizophrenia to be as high as 83% (Cannon *et al.* 1998). However, one of the most significant implications of twin, adoption and family studies in schizophrenia has been the challenge the results pose to traditional qualitatively distinct categories of disorder (Rutter & Plomin 1997). Quantitative genetic studies have shown that the genetic liability to schizophrenia extends to schizotypal personality disorders and other conditions viewed as lying on the broader schizophrenia spectrum (Kendler *et al.* 1993, 1995; Erlenmeyer-Kimling *et al.* 1995). These results suggest that what is inherited in schizophrenia is unlikely to be a discrete disorder but normal dimensions of personality that determine liability to disorder. Non-psychotic relatives of schizophrenic patients show eye-tracking deficits that correlate with subtle frontal lobe dysfunction (O'Driscoll *et al.* 1999). Hence, reduced prefrontal activation may be one expression of a genetic susceptibility to schizophrenia.

While the mode of inheritance in schizophrenia remains unknown, the most widely accepted models are polygenic. These models propose that schizophrenia results from the combined action of multiple genes of small effect which confer susceptibility to the schizophrenic phenotype. Susceptibility to the disorder is expressed as a dimension in the population: the risk of schizophrenia in the population is distributed normally not binomially (a continuously distributed risk vs. a risk of 0 or 1). Because there are likely to be multiple genes involved, each conferring only a small part to the susceptibility to schizophrenia, there is little prospect of identifying 'the gene for' schizophrenia. Hence, the genetics of schizophrenia is moving away from the rather simplistic (albeit attractive) notion of finding a gene for the disorder, towards a search for genes that confer susceptibility traits (described earlier as 'schizotaxia'). Susceptibility alleles may be quite common in the population and hence the predictive value of any individual allele will be low.

Because genes affect brain development and resultant cogni-

tive function, susceptibility to schizophrenia is most likely to lie at the levels of aberrant brain development and neurocognitive deficits. According to the neurodevelopmental 'risk' model, it is the interaction of neurodevelopmental and cognitive deficits with environmental factors that will result in the expression of the schizophrenic phenotype (Hollis & Taylor 1997). It is commonly assumed that genes affecting brain development in schizophrenia are only expressed during fetal neurodevelopment. However, genes can affect 'late' as well as 'early' brain development. Hence, it is quite possible that while some susceptibility genes for schizophrenia may affect fetal brain development, other genes do not exert their effect until adolescence, possibly causing excessive or aberrant synaptic pruning with reduction in temporal and frontal lobe volume (Feinberg 1997).

Molecular genetic strategies are attempting to identify susceptibility genes for schizophrenia and current interest is focusing on chromosomes 15, 10 and 5. However, despite many claims of linkage, there has been little replication across studies (DeLisi & Crow 1999). The association between schizophrenia and chromosomal deletions offers another possible clue to the location of candidate genes. The velocardiofacial syndrome (VCFS) microdeletion on chromosome 22q11 is associated with learning difficulties, short stature, palate abnormalities, cardiac anomalies and parkinsonism (see Skuse & Kuntsi, Chapter 13). VCFS has also been associated with schizophrenia, occurring at a rate of 2% compared to 0.02% in the normal population (Karayiorgou *et al.* 1995). VCFS appears to be associated with an earlier age of onset of schizophrenia in adults (Cohen *et al.* 1999). In the NIMH study of childhood onset schizophrenia, five cases out of 47 (10.6%) had previously undetected cytogenetic abnormalities (Nicholson *et al.* 1999). These included 3 of 47 (6.3%) with VCFS, one with Turner syndrome (deletion of a long arm of one X chromosome), and one with a balanced translocation of chromosomes 1 and 7. One study has reported an association, found only in males, between childhood onset schizophrenia and an excess of CAG/CTG trinucleotide expansions (Burgess *et al.* 1998). These findings point to genetic heterogeneity in early onset forms of schizophrenia.

Genetic risk and early onset schizophrenia

If there is a continuum of transmitted liability for schizophrenia then, as with other disorders of presumed multifactorial origin, early onset cases of schizophrenia should be associated with a greater genetic loading (Childs & Scriver 1986). Pulver *et al.* (1990) found an increased morbidity risk of schizophrenia in relatives of male probands under the age of 17. Meanwhile, Sham *et al.* (1994) found an increased morbidity risk in females under age 21 compared with males or later onset females. Although both these studies suggest an inverse relationship between age at onset and transmitted liability, albeit with different gender specific effects and age cut-offs, it would be dangerous to simply extrapolate these age trends to a younger childhood onset population. Unfortunately, there is a dearth of genetic studies of childhood onset schizophrenia which have used adequate methodology. In the only major twin study of childhood onset schizophrenia, Kallman & Roth (1956) reported an uncorrected monozygotic concordance rate of 88.2% and a dizygotic concordance rate of 22.9%. Adult onset schizophrenia clustered in the families of childhood onset probands, providing support for a similar genetic aetiology. Data from family studies suggest that childhood and adolescent onset schizophrenia carries a greater familial risk of psychosis than adult onset schizophrenia. In the Maudsley study, Hollis (1999) found 20% of child and adolescent onset schizophrenia cases had at least one first-degree relative with schizophrenia, and 50% had a first-degree relative with psychosis. These rates are somewhat higher than those reported by Sham et al. (1994) for adult schizophrenia probands (13% of adult probands had a first-degree relative with schizophrenia and 23% had a first-degree relative with any psychosis). Data from the Maudsley study (Hollis 1999) also showed that the presence of negative symptoms in the proband predicted a family history of schizophrenia. This provides further support for the idea that negative symptoms may represent the genetically transmitted phenotype in schizophrenia (Tsuang 1993).

Neuropsychology of schizophrenia

Pattern of cognitive deficits

There is growing awareness that cognitive deficits in schizophrenia are a core feature of the disorder and cannot simply be dismissed as secondary consequences of psychotic symptoms (Breier 1999). The degree of cognitive impairment is greater in child and adolescent onset than in adult onset patients. A consistent finding is a mean IQ of between 80 and 85 (1 SD below the population mean), with about one-third of cases having an IQ below 70 (Jacobsen & Rapoport 1998; Hollis 1999). This represents a mean IQ score about 10 points lower than the mean IQ in adult schizophrenia. These findings raise several important questions.

1 Are the cognitive deficits specific or generalized; are some aspects of cognitive functioning affected more than others?
2 Which deficits precede the onset of psychosis and could be causal, and which are consequences of psychosis?
3 Is the pattern of deficits specific to schizophrenia or shared with other developmental and psychotic disorders?
4 Are cognitive impairments progressive or static after the onset of psychosis?

Recent research (Asarnow et al. 1994a, 1995) suggests that children with schizophrenia have specific difficulties with cognitive tasks that make demands on short-term working memory and selective and sustained attention and speed of processing. These deficits are similar to the deficits reported in adult schizophrenia (Nuechterlein & Dawson 1984; Saykin et al. 1994). Deficits of attention and of short-term and recent long-term memory have also been reported in adolescents with schizophrenia (Friedman et al. 1996). In contrast, well-established 'overlearned' rote language and simple perceptual skills are unimpaired in child and adolescent onset schizophrenia. Asarnow et al. (1991, 1995) have shown that children with schizophrenia have impairments on the span of apprehension task (a target stimulus has to be identified from an array of other figures when displayed for 50 ms). Performance on the task deteriorates markedly when increasing demands are made on information processing capacity (e.g. increasing the number of letters in the display from 3 to 10). Furthermore, evoked-potential studies using the span of apprehension task in both children and adults with schizophrenia, when compared with age-matched controls, show less negative endogenous activity measured between 100 and 300 ms after the stimulus. Similar findings of reduced event-related potentials have been found during the CPT in both childhood and adult onset schizophrenia (Strandburg et al. 1999). These findings indicate a deficit in the allocation of attentional resources to a stimulus (Strandburg et al. 1994; Asarnow et al. 1995). As with adults, children and adolescents with schizophrenia show high basal autonomic activity and less autonomic responsivity than controls (Gordon et al. 1994), with attenuated increases in skin conductance following the presentation of neutral sounds (Zahn et al. 1997). Childhood onset patients, like adults, show increased reaction times with a loss of ipsimodal advantage compared with healthy controls (Zahn et al. 1998). Abnormalities in smooth pursuit eye movements (SPEM) have also been found in adolescents with schizophrenia (mean age 14.5), which suggests continuity with the finding of abnormal SPEM in adults with schizophrenia (Iacono & Koenig 1983). Children with schizophrenia also show similar impairments to adult patients on tests of frontal lobe executive function such as the Wisconsin Card Sorting Test (WCST; Asarnow et al. 1994a).

In summary, whereas basic sensorimotor skills, associative memory and simple language abilities tend to be preserved in children with schizophrenia, deficits are most marked on tasks that require focused and sustained attention, flexible switching of cognitive set, high information processing speed and suppression of prepotent responses (Asarnow et al. 1995). Similar deficits have also been found in children genetically at 'high-risk' for schizophrenia (Erlenmeyer-Kimling & Cornblatt 1992) and non-psychotic relatives of schizophrenic probands (Park et al. 1995). This strengthens the argument that cognitive deficits cannot be simply dismissed as non-specific consequences of schizophrenic symptoms, but rather are likely to be indicators of underlying genetic and neurobiological risk.

These diverse cognitive processes have been integrated under the cognitive domain of 'executive functions', which are presumed to be mediated by the prefrontal cortical system. Executive function skills are necessary to generate and execute goal-directed behaviour, especially in novel situations. Goal-orientated actions require that information in the form of plans and expectations are held 'on-line' in working memory, and flexibly changed in response to feedback. Much of social behaviour and social development would appear to depend on these capacities as they involve integration of multiple sources of information, appreciation of others' mental states, inhibition of inappropriate prepotent responses and rapid shifting of attention.

Executive functions and onset of schizophrenia

Any cognitive theory of schizophrenia will need to explain the timing of onset during adolescence or early adulthood. Deficits in executive function and social cognition could be the developmental abnormality that predisposes to schizophrenia, as executive function deficits impinge on social skills that usually emerge in early adolescence. This period is associated with a rapid growth in abstract analytical skills, together with the development of the sophisticated social and communication abilities that underlie successful social relationships. It is during this period of development (approximately age 8–15 years) that preschizophrenic social impairments become most apparent (Done et al. 1994) and there is also relative decline in cognitive abilities in preschizophrenic subjects (Jones et al. 1994).

According to this 'risk' model of executive function deficit, the onset of psychosis would depend on the interaction between social and cognitive capacities and the demands of the environment. During adolescence, increasing academic and social demands may act as stressors on a 'high-risk' subject, pushing them over the threshold for psychosis. The greater the premorbid impairment, the earlier the age that a critical liability threshold will be passed and symptoms emerge. This model would predict that similar executive function deficits are found in non-psychotic genetically 'high-risk' relatives. However, executive functions deficits are probably not a primary cause of schizophrenia given that they also occur in other neurodevelopmental disorders including autism (Ozonoff et al. 1991; Hughes & Russell 1993) and attention deficit hyperactivity disorder (ADHD; Welsh et al. 1991; Pennington et al. 1993; Karatekin & Asarnow 1998).

Course of cognitive deficits

Kraepelin's term 'dementia praecox' implied a progressive cognitive decline as part of the disease process. Jones et al. (1994) described how academic performance becomes progressively more deviant during adolescence in those individuals destined to developed schizophrenia in adult life. There is also some tentative evidence for a possible slight decline in IQ following the onset of psychosis in childhood onset schizophrenia. In the NIMH study (Alaghband-Rad et al. 1995), the mean post-psychotic IQ was 83.7 (SD 17.3) compared with a mean prepsychotic IQ of 87.7 (SD 25.4). Although a decline in IQ during the early phase of psychosis has been reported in adults with schizophrenia (Bilder et al. 1992), in the NIMH study the decline was in both raw and scaled IQ scores and continued for up to 24–48 months after onset (Jacobsen & Rapoport 1998). There was no evidence for a decline in post-psychotic IQ raw scores repeated after 2 years, although scaled (age-adjusted) IQ scores did still decline (Bedwell et al. 1999). Russell et al. (1997) found a small non-significant IQ decline of only 2–3 points in a 20-year longi-

tudinal follow-up study of IQ in schizophrenia (about one-third of these cases had first onset of psychosis in adolescence).

In summary, when raw scores, rather than scaled scores, are analysed, there is little evidence for an absolute loss in cognitive ability in the early post-psychotic phase of schizophrenia. If a true decline does occur it is during, or before, the transition to psychosis. The small drop in IQ after the onset of psychosis could possibly be caused by the effect of psychotic symptoms on performance. Overall, the evidence points more to a premature arrest, or slowing, of normal cognitive development in child and adolescent onset schizophrenia rather than to a dementia.

Assessment

The assessment of a child or adolescent with possible schizophrenia should include a detailed history, mental state and physical examination. In addition, a baseline psychometric assessment is desirable. A detailed understanding of specific cognitive deficits in individual cases of adolescent schizophrenia can be particularly helpful in guiding education and rehabilitation. In the physical examination, particular attention should be given to detecting dysmorphic features that may betray an underlying genetic syndrome. The neurological examination should focus on abnormal involuntary movements and other signs of extrapyramidal dysfunction. Spontaneous abnormal involuntary movements have been detected in a proportion of drug-naive first-episode schizophrenic or schizophreniform patients as well as in those receiving typical antipsychotics (Gervin et al. 1998).

Developmental issues

The cognitive level of the child will influence his or her ability to understand and express complex psychotic symptoms, such as passivity phenomena, thought alienation and hallucinations. In younger children careful distinctions have to be made between developmental immaturity and psychopathology; e.g. distinguishing true hallucinations from other subjective phenomena, such as dreams, may be difficult for young children. Developmental maturation can also affect the localization of hallucinations in space. Internal localization of hallucinations is more common in younger children and makes these experiences more difficult to differentiate subjectively from inner speech or thoughts (Garralda 1984). Formal thought disorder may also appear very similar to the pattern of illogical thinking and loose associations seen in children with immature language development. Negative symptoms can appear very similar to non-psychotic language and social impairments and can also be easily confused with anhedonia and depression.

Differential diagnosis

Psychotic symptoms in children and adolescence are diagnostically non-specific, occurring in a wide range of functional psy-

Table 37.2 Differential diagnosis of schizophrenia in childhood and adolescence.

Psychoses	Affective psychoses (bipolar/major depressive disorder)
	Schizoaffective disorder
	Atypical psychosis
Developmental disorders	Autism spectrum disorders (Asperger syndrome)
	Developmental language disorder
	Schizotypal personality disorder
	'Multidimensionally impaired' disorder
Organic conditions	Drug-related psychosis (amfetamines, 'ecstasy', LSD, PCP)
	Complex partial seizures (temporal lobe epilepsy)
	Wilson disease
	Metachromatic leukodystrophy

LSD, lysergic acid diethylamide; PCP, phencyclidine.

chiatric and organic brain disorders. The differential diagnosis of schizophrenia in childhood and adolescence is summarized in Table 37.2. A summary of physical investigations in children and adolescents with suspected schizophrenia is listed in Table 37.3.

Affective, schizoaffective and 'atypical' psychoses

The high rate of positive psychotic symptoms found in adolescent onset major depression and mania can lead to diagnostic confusion (Joyce 1984). Affective psychoses are most likely to be misdiagnosed as schizophrenia if a Schneiderian concept of schizophrenia is applied with its emphasis on first-rank symptoms. Because significant affective symptoms also occur in about one-third of first-episode patients with schizophrenia, it may be impossible to make a definitive diagnosis on the basis of a single cross-sectional assessment. In DSM-IV the distinction between schizophrenia, schizoaffective disorder and affective psychoses is determined by the relative predominance and temporal overlap of psychotic symptoms (hallucinations and delusions) and affective symptoms (elevated or depressed mood). Given the difficulty in applying these rules with any precision, there is a need to identify other features to distinguish between schizophrenia and affective psychoses. Irrespective of the presence of affective symptoms, the most discriminating symptoms of schizophrenia are an insidious onset and the presence of negative symptoms (Hollis 1999). Similarly, complete remission from a first psychotic episode within 6 months of onset is the best predictor of a diagnosis of affective psychosis (Hollis 1999). Schizoaffective and atypical psychoses are unsatisfactory diagnostic categories with low predictive validity and little longitudinal stability (Hollis 2000).

Autistic spectrum and developmental language disorders

Some children on the autistic spectrum or with Asperger syn-

drome have social and cognitive impairments that overlap closely with the premorbid phenotype described in schizophrenia. Furthermore, children on the autistic spectrum can also develop psychotic symptoms in adolescence (Volkmar & Cohen 1991). Towbin et al. (1993) have labelled another group of children who seem to belong within the autistic spectrum as 'multiplex developmental disorder'. An increased risk for psychosis has also been noted in developmental language disorders (Rutter & Mawhood 1991). While some children on the autistic spectrum can show a clear progression into classic schizophrenia, others show a more episodic pattern of psychotic symptoms without the progressive decline in social functioning and negative symptoms characteristic of child and adolescent onset schizophrenia.

Often, it is only possible to distinguish between schizophrenia and disorders on the autistic spectrum by taking a careful developmental history that details the age of onset and pattern of autistic impairments in communication, social reciprocity and interests/behaviours. According to DSM-IV, schizophrenia cannot be diagnosed in a child with autism/pervasive developmental disorder (PDD) unless hallucinations/delusions are present for at least 1 month. DSM-IV does not rank the active phase symptoms of thought disorder, disorganization or negative symptoms as sufficient to make a diagnosis of schizophrenia in the presence of autism. In contrast, ICD-10 does not include autism/PDD as exclusion criteria for diagnosing schizophrenia.

Multidimensionally impaired syndrome and schizotypal personality disorder

Multidimensionally impaired (MDI) syndrome is a label applied to children who have brief transient psychotic symptoms, emotional lability, poor social skills and multiple deficits in information processing (Gordon et al. 1994). The diagnostic status of this group remains to be resolved. Short-term follow-up suggests that they do not develop full-blown schizophrenic psychosis; however, they have an increased risk of schizophrenia-spectrum disorders among first-degree relatives and the neurobiological findings (e.g. brain morphology) are similar to those in childhood onset schizophrenia (Kumra et al. 1998a). This group may possibly represent a genetically high-risk phenotype for schizophrenia rather than a prodromal state.

Children with schizotypal personality disorder (SPD) lie on a phenotypic continuum with schizophrenia and have similar cognitive and social impairments and are prone to magical thinking, mood disturbances and non-psychotic perceptual disturbances. Distinction from the prodromal phase of schizophrenia is particularly difficult when there is a history of social and academic decline without clear-cut or persisting psychotic symptoms. It has been reported that negative symptoms and attention in SPD improve with a low dose of risperidone (0.25–2.0 mg) (Rossi et al. 1997).

Table 37.3 Physical investigations in child and adolescent onset psychoses.

Investigation	Target disorder
Urine drug screen	Drug-related psychosis (amphetamines, 'ecstasy', cocaine, LSD and other psychoactive compounds)
EEG	Complex partial seizures/TLE
MRI brain scan	Ventricular enlargement, structural brain anomalies (e.g. cavum septum pellucidum)
	Enlarged caudate (typical antipsychotics)
	Demyelination (metachromatic leukodystrophy)
	Hypodense basal ganglia (Wilson disease)
Serum copper and caeruloplasmin	Wilson disease
Urinary copper	
Arylsulphatase A (white blood cell)	Metachromatic leukodystrophy
Karyotype/cytogenetics (FISH)	Sex chromosome aneuploidies, velocardiofacial syndrome (22q11 microdeletion)

EEG, electroencephalogram; FISH, fluorescent *in situ* hybridization; LSD, lysergic acid diethylamide; MRI, magnetic resonance imaging; TLE, temporal lobe epilepsy.

Epilepsy

Psychotic symptoms can occur in temporal and frontal lobe partial seizures. A careful history is usually sufficient to reveal an aura followed by clouding of consciousness and the sudden onset of brief ictal psychotic phenomena accompanied often by anxiety, fear, derealization or depersonalization. However, longer lasting psychoses associated with epilepsy can occur in clear consciousness during post-ictal or interictal periods (Sachdev 1998). In epileptic psychoses, hallucinations, disorganized behaviour and persecutory delusions predominate, while negative symptoms are rare. Children with complex partial seizures also have increased illogical thinking and use fewer linguistic-cohesive devices which can resemble formal thought disorder (Caplan *et al.* 1992). A PET study showed hypoperfusion in the frontal, temporal and basal ganglia in psychotic patients with epilepsy compared with non-psychotic epileptic patients (Gallhofer *et al.* 1985).

Epilepsy and schizophrenia may co-occur in the same individual, so that the diagnoses are not mutually exclusive. The onset of epilepsy almost always precedes psychosis unless seizures are secondary to antipsychotic medication. In a long-term follow-up of 100 children with temporal lobe epilepsy, 10% developed schizophrenia in adult life (Lindsay *et al.* 1979).

An electroencephalogram (EEG) should be performed if a seizure disorder is considered in the differential diagnosis or arises as a side-effect of antipsychotic treatment. Ambulatory EEG monitoring and telemetry with event recording may be required if the diagnosis remains in doubt.

Neurodegenerative disorders

Rare neurodegenerative disorders with onset in late childhood and adolescence can mimic schizophrenia. The most important examples are Wilson disease (hepatolenticular degeneration) and metachromatic leukodystrophy. These disorders usually involve significant extrapyramidal symptoms (e.g. tremor, dystonia, bradykinesia) or other motor abnormalities (e.g. unsteady gait) and a progressive loss of skills (dementia) that can aid the distinction from schizophrenia. Suspicion of a neurodegenerative disorder is one of the clearest indications for brain MRI in adolescent psychoses. Adolescents with schizophrenia show relative grey matter reduction with white matter sparing. In contrast, metachromatic leukodystrophy is characterized by frontal and occipital white matter destruction and demyelination. In Wilson disease hypodense areas are seen in the basal ganglia, together with cortical atrophy and ventricular dilatation. The pathognomonic Kayser–Fleischer ring in Wilson disease begins as a greenish-brown crescent-shaped deposit in the cornea above the pupil; this is most easily seen during slit lamp examination. In Wilson disease there is increased urinary copper excretion, and reduced serum copper and serum caeruloplasmin levels. The biochemical marker for metachromatic leukodystrophy is reduced arylsulphatase-A (ASA) activity in white blood cells. This enzyme deficiency results in a deposition of excess sulphatides in many tissues including the central nervous system.

Drug psychoses

Drug use is common among young people, so the co-occurrence of drug use and psychosis is to be expected, but what is less certain is the nature of any causal connection. Psychotic symptoms can occur as a direct pharmacological effect of intoxication with stimulants (amphetamines, ecstasy, cocaine), hallucinogens (lysergic acid diethylamide 'LSD', psilocybin 'magic mushrooms', mescaline) and cannabis (Poole & Brabbins 1996). The psychotic symptoms associated with drug intoxication are usually short-lived and resolve within a few days of abstinence from the drug. These drugs can have surprisingly long half-lives, with cannabinoids still measurable up to 6 weeks after a single dose. Psychotic symptoms in the form of 'flashbacks' can also occur after cessation from chronic cannabis and LSD abuse. These phenomena are similar to alcoholic hallucinosis and typically involve transient vivid auditory hallucinations occurring in clear consciousness.

It is often assumed that there is a simple causal relationship between drug use and psychosis, with any evidence of drug use excluding the diagnosis of a functional psychosis. However, drug use can also be a consequence of psychosis, with patients using drugs to 'treat' their symptoms in the early stages of a psychotic relapse. Overall, there is very little evidence to invoke a separate entity of 'drug-induced' psychosis in cases where psychotic symptoms arise during intoxication but then persist after the drug is withdrawn (Poole & Brabbins 1996). Patients whose so-called 'drug-induced' psychoses last for more than 6 months appear to have more clear-cut schizophrenic symptoms, a greater familial risk for psychosis and greater premorbid dysfunction (Tsuang et al. 1982). DSM-IV takes the sensible position that a functional psychosis should not be excluded unless there is compelling evidence that symptoms are entirely caused by drug use.

Other investigations

Whether any physical investigations should be viewed as 'routine' is debatable. However, it is usual to obtain a full blood count and biochemistry including liver and thyroid function and a drug screen (urine or hair analysis). The high yield of cytogenetic abnormalities reported in childhood onset schizophrenia (Kumra et al. 1998b; Nicholson et al. 1999) suggest the value of cytogenetic testing, including karyotyping for sex chromosome aneuploidies and fluorescent in situ hybridization (FISH) for chromosome 22q11 deletions (VCFS). The evidence of progressive structural brain changes (Rapoport et al. 1999) indicate the value of obtaining a baseline and annual follow-up MRI brain scans, although this is not a diagnostic test.

Assessment interviews and rating scales

Structured diagnostic investigator-based interviews that cover child and adolescent psychotic disorders include the Schedule for Affective Disorders and Schizophrenia for School-Age Children (Kiddie-SADS; Ambrosini 2000), the Child and Adolescent Psychiatric Assessment (CAPA; Angold & Costello 2000) and the Diagnostic Interview for Children and Adolescents (DICA; Reich 2000). The DSM and ICD definitions of schizophrenia do not provide symptom definitions so the detailed glossaries that accompany these interviews are particularly useful.

Rating scales give quantitative measures of psychopathology and functional impairment. Scales to assess positive and negative psychotic symptoms include the Scale for Assessment of Positive Symptoms (SAPS; Andreasen 1984), the Scale for As-

sessment of Negative Symptoms (SANS; Andreasen 1983) and the Positive and Negative Syndrome Scale (PANSS; Kay et al. 1987). The 30-item Kiddie Positive and Negative Syndrome Scale (K-PANSS) has been developed for use in children and adolescents, and contains three subscales: positive syndrome, negative syndrome and general psychopathology (Fields et al. 1994). The Children's Global Assessment Scale (C-GAS) provides a rating of functional impairment on a 0–100 scale (Shaffer et al. 1983; Bird et al. 1987). These scales can be used to record the longitudinal course of illness and treatment response. The Kiddie Formal Thought Disorder Story Game and Kiddie Formal Thought Disorder Scale (Caplan et al. 1989) are research instruments produced for the assessment of thought disorder in children. Assessments of extrapyramidal symptoms and involuntary movements can be made using the Abnormal Involuntary Movements Scale (AIMS; Rapoport et al. 1985) and the Simpson–Angus Neurological Rating Scale (Simpson & Angus 1970).

Treatment approaches

General principles

Although antipsychotic drugs remain the cornerstone of treatment in child and adolescent schizophrenia, all young patients with schizophrenia require a multimodal treatment package that includes pharmacotherapy, family and individual counselling, education about the illness and provision to meet social and educational needs (Clark & Lewis 1998).

Primary prevention and early detection

In theory at least, the onset of schizophrenia could be prevented if an intervention reduced the premorbid 'risk' status. However, the difficulty with the premorbid phenotype as currently conceived (subtle social and developmental impairments) is its extremely low specificity and positive predictive value for schizophrenia in the general population, assuming that these premorbid features are a causal risk factor. Future refinement of the premorbid phenotype is likely to include genetic and neurocognitive markers in order to achieve acceptable sensitivity and specificity. At present, primary prevention remains on the distant horizon.

In contrast to primary prevention, the aims of early detection are to identify the onset of deterioration in vulnerable individuals with a high predictive validity. Predictive power increases markedly in adolescence around the onset of the prodrome (Davidson et al. 1999). Recent work has attempted to identify 'high-risk' or early prodromal states with the idea of intervening to prevent the active phase of schizophrenia (McGrorry & Sing 1995; Yung et al. 1996). However, only about one-fifth of these 'high-risk' cases go on to develop frank psychosis and it has proved impossible to distinguish these 'high-risk' cases from others that remain non-psychotic. Clearly, interventions directed at 'high-risk' or prodromal states need to benefit the whole population at risk, the majority of whom will not develop schizophrenia. A pragmatic stance would be to monitor children and adolescents with a strong family history and/or suggestive prodromal symptoms to ensure prompt treatment of psychosis.

Strong claims have been made that early recognition and treatment of psychotic symptoms in schizophrenia improves outcome. The association between a long duration of untreated psychosis (DUP) and poor long-term outcome in schizophrenia (Loebel et al. 1992; Wyatt 1995; Birchwood et al. 1997) supports this view. A similar association has been found in child and adolescent onset psychoses (Hollis 1999). Whereas the association between DUP and poor outcome seems secure, the causal connection is far less certain. DUP is also associated with insidious onset and negative symptoms which could confound links with poor outcome. Although there are good a priori clinical reasons for the early treatment of symptoms to relieve distress and prevent secondary impairments, as yet it remains unproven whether early intervention actually alters the long-term course of schizophrenia.

Pharmacological treatments

Because of the very small number of trials of antipsychotics conducted with child and adolescent patients, it is necessary to extrapolate most evidence on drug efficacy from studies in adults. This seems a reasonable approach given that schizophrenia is essentially the same disorder whether it has onset in childhood or adult life. However, age-specific factors, such as the greater risk of extrapyramidal side-effects (EPS) and treatment resistance to traditional antipsychotics in younger patients (Kumra et al. 1998c), should also influence drug choice.

Antipsychotics can be broadly divided into the traditional 'typical' and newer 'atypical' drugs. The typical drugs include haloperidol, chlorpromazine and trifluoperazine which block D_2 receptors, produce catalepsy in rats, raise plasma prolactin and induce EPS. The newer atypical drugs are so-called because, while they are effective antipsychotics, they are 'atypical' in the sense that they do not produce catalepsy, do not raise prolactin levels and produce significantly fewer EPS. The atypicals have been introduced during the 1990s (clozapine was introduced in 1970 but then withdrawn following fatal blood dyscrasias) and currently include clozapine, risperidone, olanzapine, quetiapine, zotepine, amisulpiride and ziprazidone. The pharmacological profile of the atypicals is diverse, involving various combinations of 5-HT and dopamine receptor blockade. Interestingly, the therapeutic effects of clozapine (potent affinity for D_4 and $5\text{-}HT_{1,2,3}$ receptors) are independent of D_2 receptor occupancy, previously thought to be essential for antipsychotic action.

The typical antipsychotic haloperidol has been shown to be superior to placebo in two double-blind controlled trials of children and adolescents with schizophrenia (Pool et al. 1976; Spencer & Campbell 1994). It is estimated that about 70% of patients show good or partial response to antipsychotic treatment although this may take 6–8 weeks to be apparent (Clark & Lewis 1998). The main drawbacks concerning the use of high-potency typicals such as haloperidol in children and adolescents are the high risk of EPS (produced by D_2 blockade of the nigrostriatal pathway), tardive dyskinesia and the lack of effect against negative symptoms and cognitive impairment. Treatment with typical antipsychotics is also associated with enlargement of the caudate nucleus, which can be reversed with clozapine (Frazier et al. 1996). Clozapine (the prototypic atypical) has been shown to be superior to haloperidol in a double-blind trial of 21 cases of childhood onset schizophrenia (Kumra et al. 1996). Larger open clinical trials of clozapine confirm its effectiveness in child and adolescent onset schizophrenia (Siefen & Remschmidt 1986; Remschmidt et al. 1994). Similar, although less marked, benefits of olanzapine over typical antipsychotics in childhood onset schizophrenia have been reported (Kumra et al. 1998d).

Drawing together this evidence, a strong case can be made for the first-line use of atypicals in child and adolescent schizophrenia (clozapine is only licensed in the UK for treatment-resistant schizophrenia). Treatment resistance in child and adolescent patients should be defined as follows:

1 non-response with at least two conventional antipsychotics (from different chemical classes) each used for at least 4–6 weeks; and/or
2 significant adverse effects with conventional antipsychotics.

Whereas atypicals reduce the risk of EPS, they can produce other troublesome side-effects (usually dose-related) including weight gain (olanzapine), sedation, hypersalivation and seizures (clozapine). The risk of blood dyscrasias on clozapine is effectively managed by mandatory routine blood monitoring. However, knowledge of potential adverse reactions with the newest atypicals is very limited in child and adolescent patients. A further consideration is the cost of newer atypicals compared with traditional antipsychotics. In the UK, a 1-month supply of haloperidol costs less than £2, compared with £100–120 for the newer atypicals, and £200 for clozapine. Although economic studies of cost-effectiveness have suggested that the costs of the atypicals are recouped in reduced inpatient stays and indirect social costs (Aitchison & Kerwin 1997), the availability of these drugs, particularly in developing countries, may well be limited because of their high cost. In the late 1990s, the use of atypical antipsychotics by child psychiatrists in the UK was still low. Over a 2-year period, only 10% of child and adolescent psychiatrists who prescribed antipsychotics in the Trent Health Region had used an atypical drug (Slaveska et al. 1998).

Currently, there is no clear consensus about the choice of antipsychotics in children and adolescents with schizophrenia. Some authorities suggest starting with a trial of a traditional antipsychotic (e.g. haloperidol) with substitution of an atypical if the traditional antipsychotic is either not tolerated or ineffective after 6–8 weeks (Clark & Lewis 1998). However, clinical trial evidence suggests that clozapine is the most effective antipsychotic in child and adolescent onset schizophrenia, although its use is restricted to treatment-resistant cases.

A very powerful case can be made for using atypicals such as olanzapine or risperidone as a first-line treatment given that child and adolescent onset schizophrenia is characterized by negative symptoms, cognitive impairments, sensitivity to EPS and relative resistance to traditional antipsychotics.

Psychosocial and family interventions

The rationale for psychosocial family interventions follows from the association between high EE and the risk of relapse in schizophrenia (Leff & Vaughn 1985; Dixon & Lehman 1995). The overall aim is to prevent relapse (secondary prevention) and improve the patient's level of functioning by modifying the family atmosphere. Psychosocial family interventions have a number of principles in common (Lam 1991). First, it is assumed that it is useful to regard schizophrenia as an illness, so patients are less likely to be seen as responsible for their symptoms and behaviour. Secondly, the family is not implicated in the aetiology of the illness. Instead, the burden borne by the family in caring for a disturbed or severely impaired young person is acknowledged. Thirdly, the intervention is offered as part of a broader multi-modal package including drug treatment and outpatient clinical management.

Lam (1991) conducted a systematic review of published trials of psychoeducation and more intensive family interventions in schizophrenia and drew the following conclusions.
1 Education packages on their own increase knowledge about the illness but do not reduce the risk of relapse.
2 More intensive family intervention studies with high EE relatives have shown a reduction in relapse rates linked to a lowering of EE.
3 Family interventions tend to be costly and time-consuming, with most clinical trials employing highly skilled research teams. Whether these interventions can be transferred into routine clinical practice is uncertain.
4 Interventions have focused on the reduction of EE in 'high-risk' families. Whether low EE families would also benefit from these interventions is less clear. This is particularly relevant to the families of children and adolescents with schizophrenia as, on average, these parents express *lower* levels of criticism and hostility than parents of adult onset patients (Asarnow *et al.* 1994b). Hence, routine family interventions aiming to reduce high EE may be well intentioned but misguided in their focus.

Cognitive-behavioural therapy

In adult patients cognitive therapy has been used to reduce the impact of treatment-resistant positive symptoms (Tarrier *et al.* 1993). Cognitive-behaviour therapy (CBT) has been shown to improve the short-term (6-month) outcome of adult schizophrenic patients with neuroleptic-resistant positive symptoms (Turkington & Kingdon 2000). Whether CBT is equally effective with younger patients, or those with predominant negative symptoms, remains to be established.

Cognitive remediation

Cognitive remediation is a relatively new psychological treatment that aims to arrest or reverse the cognitive impairments in attention, concentration and working memory seen in schizophrenia (Hays & McGrath 2000; Wykes *et al.* 2000). The results of an early controlled trial in adults are promising, with gains found in the areas of memory and social functioning (Wykes *et al.* 2000). The relatively greater severity of cognitive impairments in child and adolescent patients suggests that early remediation strategies may be particularly important in these younger patients. Helpful advice can also be offered to parents, teachers and professionals, such as breaking down information and tasks into small manageable parts to reduce demands on working memory and speed of processing.

Organization of treatment services

It is a paradox that patients with very early onset schizophrenia have the most severe form of the disorder yet they often receive inadequate and poorly co-ordinated services. Possibly this is because the responsibility for schizophrenia is seen to lie with adult psychiatric services. In the UK, community-based child and adolescent mental health services (CAMHS) provide the first-line assessment and care for children and young adolescents with psychoses, with only about half of these cases referred to inpatient units (Slaveska *et al.* 1998). Although inpatient admission is often inappropriate, generic CAMHS services are often not well placed to provide a comprehensive assessment and treatment service for very early onset psychoses. First, the very low population prevalence of psychosis reduces the predictive value diagnosis outside specialist centres. Second, community-based services often lack familiarity with newer therapies for psychoses including atypical antipsychotics.

One possible model for the UK would be to establish specialist regional very early onset psychosis teams serving a population of about 5 million, akin to specialist cancer centres. These expert teams would be primarily outpatient-based but with access to inpatient facilities if required. Hence, the focus would be quite different from the more traditional general purpose adolescent inpatient unit. The teams could offer early diagnostic assessments for children and younger adolescents with suspected psychotic disorders and set up treatment plans in collaboration with more local child and adult psychiatric services. Ideally, these teams would be linked to a university academic centre with an interest in psychosis research and treatment evaluation.

Conclusions

The last decade has seen a dramatic growth in our understanding of the clinical course and neurobiological correlates of schizophrenia presenting in childhood and adolescence. It is now clear that adult-based diagnostic criteria have validity in this age group and the disorder has clinical and neurobiological continuity with schizophrenia in adults. Childhood onset schizophrenia is a severe variant of the adult disorder, associated with greater premorbid impairment, a higher familial risk, more severe clinical course and poorer outcome. The poor outcome of children and adolescents with schizophrenia has highlighted the need to target early and effective treatments and develop specialist services for this high-risk group. The last decade has witnessed the introduction of new atypical antipsychotics with improved side-effect profiles and efficacy, and these drugs are likely to replace the traditional antipsychotics as first-line drug therapy for schizophrenia.

However, a fundamental understanding of the underlying genetic and neurobiological bases of schizophrenia has still to be achieved. The finding of a progressive reduction in brain volume in very early onset patients and reduced synaptic density in the prefrontal cortex suggest the possibility that excessive synaptic elimination during adolescence may underlie the aetiology of schizophrenia. Although significant advances in the next decade are likely to flow from technical developments in molecular genetics and neuroimaging, advance is also limited by the defining diagnostic paradigm of schizophrenia. It is widely recognized that the clinical syndrome of schizophrenia contains considerable aetiological and clinical heterogeneity. Therefore the challenge will be to identify the genetic, neurobiological and cognitive bases of this heterogeneity. Real advance in the field will depend on a more sophisticated understanding of the interplay between genetics, neurodevelopment and environment. This will involve identifying the molecular genetic basis of neurocognitive susceptibility traits for schizophrenia. The developmental mechanisms that translate neurocognitive risks into disorder will need to be understood. Unravelling neurocognitive and clinical heterogeneity should lead to improvements in our ability to deliver individually targeted treatments, as well the ability to identify those 'at risk' in order to prevent the onset of psychosis.

References

Aitchison, K.J. & Kerwin, R.W. (1997) The cost effectiveness of clozapine. *British Journal of Psychiatry*, **171**, 125–130.

Alaghband-Rad, J., McKenna, K., Gordon, C.T. et al. (1995) Childhood-onset schizophrenia: the severity of premorbid course. *Journal of the American Academy of Child and Adolescent Psychiatry*, **34**, 1273–1283.

Alaghband-Rad, J., Hamburger, S.D., Giedd, J., Frazier, J.A. & Rapoport, J.L. (1997) Childhood-onset schizophrenia: biological markers in relation to clinical characteristics. *American Journal of Psychiatry*, **154**, 64–68.

Ambrosini, P.J. (2000) Historical development and present status of the Schedule for Affective Disorders and Schizophrenia for School-Age Children (K-SADS). *Journal of the American Academy of Child and Adolescent Psychiatry*, **39**, 49–58.

American Psychiatric Association (1980) *Diagnostic and Statistical Manual of Mental Disorders*, 3rd edn. American Psychiatric Association, Washington D.C.

American Psychiatric Association (1987) *Diagnostic and Statistical Manual of Mental Disorders*, 3rd edn revised. American Psychiatric Association, Washington D.C.

American Psychiatric Association (1994) *Diagnostic and Statistical Manual of Mental Disorders*, 4th edn. American Psychiatric Association, Washington D.C.

Andreasen, N.C. (1983) *Scale for the Assessment of Negative Symptoms* (SANS). University of Iowa, IA.

Andreasen, N.C. (1984) *Scale for the Assessment of Positive Symptoms* (SAPS). University of Iowa, IA.

Andreasen, N., Ehrhardt, J.C., Swazye, V.W. et al. (1990) Magnetic resonance imaging of the brain in schizophrenia. *Archives of General Psychiatry*, **47**, 35–44.

Andreasen, N.C., Arndt, S., Alliger, R., Miller, D. & Flaum, M. (1995) Symptoms of schizophrenia: methods, meanings and mechanisms. *Archives of General Psychiatry*, **52**, 341–351.

Angold, A. & Costello, J.E. (2000) The Child and Adolescent Psychiatric Assessment (CAPA). *Journal of the American Academy of Child and Adolescent Psychiatry*, **39**, 39–48.

Asarnow, J.R. & Ben-Meir, S. (1988) Children with schizophrenia spectrum and depressive disorders: a comparative study of premorbid adjustment, onset pattern and severity of impairment. *Journal of Child Psychology and Psychiatry*, **29**, 477–488.

Asarnow, R., Granholm, E. & Sherman, T. (1991) Span of apprehension in schizophrenia. In: *Handbook of Schizophrenia*, Vol. 5. *Neuropsychology, Psychophysiology and Information Processing* (eds S.R. Steinhauer, J.H. Gruzelier & J. Zubin), pp. 335–370. Elsevier, Amsterdam.

Asarnow, R., Asamen, J., Granholm, E., Sherman, T., Watkins, J.M. & William, M.E. (1994a) Cognitive/neuropsychological studies of children with schizophrenic disorder. *Schizophrenia Bulletin*, **20**, 647–669.

Asarnow, J.R., Thompson, M.C., Hamilton, E.B., Goldstein, M.J. & Guthrie, D. (1994b) Family expressed emotion, childhood onset depression, and childhood onset schizophrenic spectrum disorders: is expressed emotion a non-specific correlate of psychopathology or a specific risk factor for depression? *Journal of Abnormal Psychology*, **22**, 129–146.

Asarnow, R., Brown, W. & Stranberg, R. (1995) Children with schizophrenic disorder: neurobehavioural studies. *European Archives of Psychiatry and Clinical Neuroscience*, **245**, 70–79.

Battaglia, M. & Torgersen, S. (1996) Schizotypal disorder: at the crossroads of genetics and nosology. *Acta Psychiatrica Scandanavica*, **94**, 303–310.

Bedwell, J.S., Keller, B., Smith, A.K., Hamburger, S., Kumra, S. & Rapoport, J.L. (1999) Why does postpsychotic IQ decline in childhood-onset schizophrenia? *American Journal of Psychiatry*, **156**, 1996–1997.

Beratis, S., Gabriel, J. & Hoidas, S. (1994) Age at onset in subtypes of schizophrenic disorders. *Schizophrenia Bulletin*, **20**, 287–296.

Bertolino, A., Kumra, S., Callicott, J.H. et al. (1998) Common pattern of cortical pathology in childhood-onset and adult-onset schizophrenia as identified by proton magnetic resonance spectroscopic imaging. *American Journal of Psychiatry*, **155**, 1376–1383.

Bilder, R.M., Lipschutz-Broch, L., Reiter, G., Geisler, S.H., Mayerhoff, D.I. & Lieberman, J.A. (1992) Intellectual deficits in first-episode schizophrenia: evidence for progressive deterioration. *Schizophrenia Bulletin*, **18**, 437–448.

Birchwood, M., McGorry, P. & Jackson, H. (1997) Early intervention in schizophrenia. *British Journal of Psychiatry*, **170**, 2–5.

Bird, H.R., Canino, G., Rubio-Stipec, M. & Ribera, J.C. (1987) Further measures of the psychometric properties of the children's global assessment scale. *Archives of General Psychiatry*, **44**, 821–824.

Bleuler, E. (1911) *Dementia Praecox: The Group of Schizophrenias* [translated by J. Zinkin, 1950]. International Universities Press, New York.

Breier, A. (1999) Cognitive deficit in schizophrenia and its neurochemical basis. *British Journal of Psychiatry*, **174** (Suppl. 37), 16–18.

Bullmore, E.T., O'Connell, P., Frangou, S. & Murray, R.M. (1997) Schizophrenia as a developmental disorder or neural network integrity: the dysplastic net hypothesis. In: *Neuorodevelopment and Adult Psychopathology* (eds M.S. Keshervan & R.M. Murray), pp. 253–266. Cambridge University Press, Cambridge.

Burgess, C.E., Lindblad, K., Sidransky, E. *et al.* (1998) Large CAG/CTG repeats are associated with childhood-onset schizophrenia. *Molecular Psychiatry*, **3**, 321–327.

Cannon, T.D., Mednick, S.A., Parnas, J., Schulsinger, F., Praestholm, J. & Vestergaard, A. (1993) Developmental brain abnormalities in the offspring of schizophrenic mothers. II. Structural brain characteristics of schizophrenia and schizotypal personality disorder. *Archives of General Psychiatry*, **51**, 955–962.

Cannon, T.D., Kaprio, J., Lonnqvist, J. *et al.* (1998) The genetic epidemiology of schizophrenia in a Finnish twin cohort: a population-based modelling study. *Archives of General Psychiatry*, **55**, 67–74.

Caplan, R., Guthrie, D., Tanguay, P.E., Fish, B. & David-Lando, G. (1989) The Kiddie Formal Thought Disorder Scale (K-FTDS): clinical assessment reliability and validity. *Journal of the American Academy of Child and Adolescent Psychiatry*, **28**, 408–416.

Caplan, R., Guthrie, D., Shields, W.D. & Mori, L. (1992) Formal thought disorder in paediatric complex partial seizure disorder. *Journal of Child Psychology and Psychiatry*, **33**, 1399–1412.

Castle, D. & Murray, R. (1991) The neurodevelopmental basis of sex differences in schizophrenia. *Psychological Medicine*, **21**, 565–575.

Chakos, M.H., Lieberman, J.A., Alvir, J. *et al.* (1995) Caudate nuclei volumes in schizophrenic patients treated with typical antipsychotics or clozapine. *Lancet*, **345**, 456–457.

Childs, B. & Scriver, C.R. (1986) Age at onset and causes of disease. *Perspectives in Biology and Medicine*, **29**, 437–460.

Clark, A. & Lewis, S. (1998) Treatment of schizophrenia in childhood and adolescence. *Journal of Child Psychology and Psychiatry*, **39**, 1071–1081.

Cohen, E., Chow, E.W., Weksberg, R. & Bassett, A.S. (1999) Phenotype of adults with 22q11 deletion syndrome. *American Journal of Medical Genetics*, **86**, 359–365.

Davidson, M., Reichenberg, M.A., Rabinowitz, J., Weiser, M., Kaplan, Z. & Mark, M. (1999) Behavioral and intellectual markers for schizophrenia in apparently healthy male adolescents. *American Journal of Psychiatry*, **156**, 1328–1335.

DeLisi, L. & Crow, T. (1999) Chromosome workshops 1998: current state of psychiatric linkage. *American Journal of Medical Genetics*, **88**, 215–219.

Dixon, L.B. & Lehman, A.F. (1995) Family interventions for schizophrenia. *Schizophrenia Bulletin*, **21**, 631–643.

Done, J.D., Crow, T.J., Johnstone, E. & Sacker, A. (1994) Childhood antecedents of schizophrenia and affective illness: social adjustment at ages 7 and 11. *British Medical Journal*, **309**, 699–703.

Donlan, R.J., Fletcher, P., Frith, C.D. *et al.* (1996) Dopaminergic modulation of impaired cognitive activation in the anterior cingulate cortex in schizophrenia. *Nature*, **378**, 180–182.

Eggers, C. (1978) Course and prognosis in childhood schizophrenia. *Journal of Autism and Childhood Schizophrenia*, **8**, 21–36.

Eggers, C. & Bunk, D. (1997) The long-term course of childhood-onset schizophrenia: a 42-year follow-up. *Schizophrenia Bulletin*, **23**, 105–117.

Erlenmeyer-Kimling, L. & Cornblatt, B. (1992) A summary of attentional findings in the New York High-Risk Project. *Journal of Psychiatric Research*, **26**, 405–426.

Erlenmeyer-Kimling, L., Squires-Wheeler, E., Adamo, U.H. *et al.* (1995) The New York High Risk Project: psychoses and Cluster A personality disorders in offspring of schizophrenic parents at 23 years of follow-up. *Archives of General Psychiatry*, **52**, 857–865.

Faraone, S.V., Kremen, W.S., Pepple, J.R., Seidman, L.J. & Tsuang, M.T. (1995) Diagnostic accuracy and linkage analysis: how useful are schizophrenia spectrum phenotypes? *American Journal of Psychiatry*, **152**, 1286–1290.

Faraone, S.V., Green, A.I., Seidman, L.J. & Tsuang, M.T. (2001) 'Schizotaxia': Clinical Implications and New Directions for Research. *Schizophrenia Bulletin*, **27**, 1–18.

Feinberg, I. (1983) Schizophrenia: caused by a fault in programmed synaptic elimination during adolescence. *Journal of Psychiatric Research*, **17**, 319–344.

Feinberg, I. (1997) Schizophrenia as an emergent disorder of late brain maturation. In: *Neuorodevelopment and Adult Psychopathology* (eds M.S. Keshervan & R.M. Murray), pp. 237–252. Cambridge University Press, Cambridge.

Fields, J.H., Grochowski, S., Lindenmayer, J.P. *et al.* (1994) Assessing positive and negative symptoms in children and adolescents. *American Journal of Psychiatry*, **151**, 249–253.

Fish, B. (1957) The detection of schizophrenia in infancy. *Journal of Nervous and Mental Diseases*, **125**, 1–24.

Foerster, A., Lewis, S., Owen, M. & Murray, R.M. (1991) Pre-morbid adjustment and personality in psychosis. *British Journal of Psychiatry*, **158**, 171–176.

Frazier, J.A., Giedd, J.N., Kaysen, D. *et al.* (1996) Childhood-onset schizophrenia: brain magnetic resonance imaging rescan after two years of clozapine maintenance. *American Journal of Psychiatry*, **153**, 564–566.

Frazier, J.A., Alaghband-Rad, J., Jacobsen, L. *et al.* (1997) Pubertal development and the onset of psychosis in childhood-onset schizophrenia. *Psychiatry Research*, **70**, 1–7.

Friedman, L., Finding, R.L., Buch, J. *et al.* (1996) Structural MRI and neuropsychological assessments in adolescent patients with either schizophrenia or affective disorders. *Schizophrenia Research*, **18**, 189–190.

Friston, K.J., Herold, S., Fletcher, P. *et al.* (1995) Abnormal frontotemporal interactions in schizophrenia. In: *Biology of Schizophrenia and Affective Diseases* (ed. S.J. Watson), pp. 449–481. Raven, New York.

Frith, C.D. (1994) Theory of mind in schizophrenia. In: *The Neuropsychology of Schizophrenia* (eds A. David & J.S. Cutting), pp. 147–161. Lawrence Erlbaum, Hove.

Galdos, P.M., van Os, J. & Murray, R. (1993) Puberty and the onset of psychosis. *Schizophrenia Research*, **10**, 7–14.

Gallhofer, B., Trimble, M.R., Frackowiak, R., Gibbs, J. & Jones, T. (1985) A study of cerebral blood flow and metabolism in epileptic psychosis using positron emission tomography and oxygen. *Journal of Neurology, Neurosurgery and Psychiatry*, **48**, 201–206.

Garralda, M.E. (1984) Hallucinations in children with conduct and emotional disorders. I. The clinical phenomena. *Psychological Medicine*, **14**, 589–596.

Geddes, J.R. & Lawrie, S.M. (1995) Obstetric complications and schizophrenia: a meta-analysis. *British Journal of Psychiatry*, **167**, 786–793.

Gervin, M., Browne, S., Lane, A. *et al.* (1998) Spontaneous abnormal involuntary movements in first-episode schizophrenia and schizophreniform disorder: baseline rate in a group of patients from an Irish catchment area. *American Journal of Psychiatry*, **155**, 1202–1206.

Giedd, J.N., Castellanos, F.X., Rajapaske, J.C. *et al.* (1996) Quantitative analysis of grey matter volumes in childhood-onset schizophrenia and attention deficit/ hyperactivity disorder. *Society for Neuroscience Abstracts*, **22**, 1166.

Gillberg, C., Wahlstrom, J., Forsman, A., Hellgren, L. & Gillberg, J.C. (1986) Teenage psychoses: epidemiology, classification and reduced optimality in the pre-, peri- and neonatal periods. *Journal of Child Psychology and Psychiatry*, 27, 87–98.

Glantz, L.A. & Lewis, D.A. (2000) Decreased dendritic spine density on prefrontal cortical pyramidal neurones in schizophrenia. *Archives of General Psychiatry*, 57, 65–73.

Goldstein, M.J. (1987) The UCLA High Risk Project. *Schizophrenia Bulletin*, 13, 505–514.

Goodman, R. (1988) Are complications of pregnancy and birth causes of schizophrenia? *Developmental Medicine and Child Neurology*, 30, 391–406.

Gordon, C.T., Frazier, J.A., McKenna, K. *et al.* (1994) Childhood-onset schizophrenia: a NIMH study in progress. *Schizophrenia Bulletin*, 20, 697–712.

Green, W., Padron-Gayol, M., Hardesty, A. & Bassiri, M. (1992) Schizophrenia with childhood onset: a phenomenological study of 38 cases. *Journal of the American Academy of Child and Adolescent Psychiatry*, 31, 968–976.

Gualtieri, C.T., Adams, A. & Chen, C.D. (1982) Minor physical abnormalities in alcoholic and schizophrenic adults and hyperactive and autistic children. *American Journal of Psychiatry*, 139, 640–643.

Gur, R.E., Cowell, P., Turetsky, B.I. *et al.* (1998) A follow-up magnetic resonance imaging study of schizophrenia: relationship of neuroanatomical changes to clinical and neurobehavioural measures. *Archives of General Psychiatry*, 55, 145–152.

Gur, R.E., Turetsky, B.I., Cowell, P. *et al.* (2000a) Temporolimbic volume reductions in schizophrenia. *Archives of General Psychiatry*, 57, 769–775.

Gur, R.E., Cowell, P., Latshaw, A. *et al.* (2000b) Reduced dorsal and orbital prefrontal gray matter volumes in schizophrenia. *Archives of General Psychiatry*, 57, 761–768.

Guy, J.D., Majorski, L.V., Wallace, C.J. & Guy, M.P. (1983) The incidence of minor physical anomalies in adult schizophrenics. *Schizophrenia Bulletin*, 9, 571–582.

Hafner, H. & Nowotny, B. (1995) Epidemiology of early-onset schizophrenia. *European Archives of Psychiatry and Clinical Neuroscience*, 245, 80–92.

Harris, E.C. & Barraclough, B. (1997) Excess mortality of mental disorder. *British Journal of Psychiatry*, 173, 11–53.

Hays, R.L. & McGrath, J.J. (2000) Cognitive rehabilitation for people with schizophrenia and related conditions: a systemic review and meta-analysis [Abstract]. *Schizophrenia Research*, 41, 221–222.

Hollis, C. (1995) Child and adolescent (juvenile onset) schizophrenia: a case–control study of premorbid developmental impairments. *British Journal of Psychiatry*, 166, 489–495.

Hollis, C. (1999) *A study of the course and adult outcomes of child and adolescent onset psychoses*. PhD thesis, University of London.

Hollis, C. (2000) The adult outcomes of child and adolescent-onset schizophrenia: diagnostic stability and predictive validity. *American Journal of Psychiatry*, 157, 1652–1659.

Hollis, C. & Taylor, E. (1997) Schizophrenia: a critique from the developmental psychopathology perspective. In: *Neuorodevelopment and Adult Psychopathology* (eds M.S. Keshervan & R.M. Murray), pp. 213–233. Cambridge University Press, Cambridge.

Hooley, J.M. (1987) The nature and origins of expressed emotion. In: *Understanding Major Mental Disorder: the Contribution of Family Interaction Research* (eds K. Hahlweg & M.J. Goldstein), pp. 176–194. Family Process, New York.

Hughes, C. & Russell, J. (1993) Autistic children's difficulty with mental disengagement with an object: its implications for theories of autism. *Developmental Psychology*, 29, 498–510.

Huttenlocher, P.R. (1979) Synaptic density in human prefrontal cortex: developmental changes and effects of aging. *Brain Research*, 163, 195–205.

Iacono, W.G. & Koenig, W.G.R. (1983) Features that distinguish smooth pursuit eye tracking performance in schizophrenic, affective disordered and normal individuals. *Journal of Abnormal Psychology*, 92, 29–41.

Jacob, H. & Beckman, H. (1986) Prenatal developmental disturbances in the limbic allocortex in schizophrenics. *Journal of Neural Transmission*, 65, 303–326.

Jacobsen, L. & Rapoport, J. (1998) Research update: childhood-onset schizophrenia—implications for clinical and neurobiological research. *Journal of Child Psychology and Psychiatry*, 39, 101–113.

Jacobsen, L., Giedd, J.N., Berquin, P.C. *et al.* (1997a) Quantitative morphology of the cerebellum and fourth ventricle in childhood-onset schizophrenia. *American Journal of Psychiatry*, 154, 1663–1669.

Jacobsen, L., Hamburger, S.D., Van Horn, J.D. *et al.* (1997b) Cerebral glucose metabolism in childhood-onset schizophrenia. *Psychiatry Research*, 75, 131–144.

Jacobsen, L., Giedd, J.N., Castellanos, F.X. *et al.* (1998) Progressive reductions in temporal lobe structures in childhood-onset schizophrenia. *American Journal of Psychiatry*, 155, 678–685.

Johnstone, E. & Frith, C. (1996) Validation of three dimensions of schizophrenic symptoms in a large unselected sample of patients. *Psychological Medicine*, 26, 667–679.

Jones, P. & Done, J. (1997) From birth to onset: a developmental perspective of schizophrenia in two national birth cohorts. In: *Neurodevelopment and Adult Psychopathology* (eds M.S. Keshervan & R.M. Murray), pp. 119–136. Cambridge University Press, Cambridge.

Jones, P., Rogers, B., Murray, R. & Marmot, M. (1994) Child development risk factors for adult schizophrenia in the British 1946 birth cohort. *Lancet*, 344, 1398–1402.

Joyce, P.R. (1984) Age of onset in bipolar affective disorder and misdiagnosis of schizophrenia. *Psychological Medicine*, 14, 145–149.

Kallman, F.J. & Roth, B. (1956) Genetic aspects of preadolescent schizophrenia. *American Journal of Psychiatry*, 112, 599–606.

Karatekin, C. & Asarnow, R.F. (1998) Working memory in childhood-onset schizophrenia and attention deficit/hyperactivity disorder. *Psychiatry Research*, 80, 165–176.

Karayiorgou, M., Morris, M.A., Morrow, B. *et al.* (1995) Schizophrenia susceptibility associated with interstitial deletions of chromosome 22q11. *Proceedings of the National Academy of Sciences of the USA*, 92, 7612–7616.

Kay, S.R., Opler, L.A. & Lindenmayer, J.P. (1987) The Positive and Negative Syndrome Scale (PANSS) for schizophrenia. *Schizophrenia Bulletin*, 13, 261–276.

Kendall, R.E., McInneny, K., Juszczak, E. & Bain, M. (2000) Obstetric complications and schizophrenia: two case–control studies based on structured obstetric records. *British Journal of Psychiatry*, 176, 516–522.

Kendler, K.C., McGuire, M., Gruenberg, A. *et al.* (1993) The Roscommon Family Study. III. Schizophrenia related personality disorders in relatives. *Archives of General Psychiatry*, 50, 781–788.

Kendler, K.C., Neale, M.C. & Walsh, D. (1995) Evaluating the spectrum concept of schizophrenia in the Roscommon Family Study. *American Journal of Psychiatry*, 152, 749–754.

Kjelsberg, E. (2000) Adolescent psychiatric in-patients: a high risk group for premature death. *British Journal of Psychiatry*, 176, 121–125.

Kolvin, I. (1971) Studies in the childhood psychoses. I. Diagnostic criteria and classification. *British Journal of Psychiatry*, 118, 381–384.

Kraepelin, E. (1919) *Dementia Praecox* [translated by R. Barclay]. Livingstone, Edinburgh.

Kremen, W.S., Seidman, L.J., Pepple, J.R., Lyons, M.J., Tsuang, M.T. & Farone, S.V. (1994) Contributions of neuropsychology toward identifying risk indicators for schizophrenia. *Schizophrenia Bulletin*, **20**, 103–119.

Kumra, S., Frazier, J.A., Jacobsen, L.K. *et al.* (1996) Childhood-onset schizophrenia: a double blind clozapine–haloperidol comparison. *Archives of General Psychiatry*, **53**, 1090–1097.

Kumra, S., Jacobsen, L.K., Lenane, M. *et al.* (1998a) 'Multidimensionally impaired disorder': is it a variant of very early-onset schizophrenia? *Journal of the American Academy of Child and Adolescent Psychiatry*, **37**, 91–99.

Kumra, S., Wiggs, E., Krasnewich, D. *et al.* (1998b) Brief report: association of sex chromosome anomalies with childhood-onset psychotic disorders. *Journal of the American Academy of Child and Adolescent Psychiatry*, **37**, 292–296.

Kumra, S., Jacobsen, L.K., Lenane, M. *et al.* (1998c) Case series: spectrum of neuroleptic-induced movement disorders and extrapyramidal side-effects in childhood-onset schizophrenia. *Journal of the American Academy of Child and Adolescent Psychiatry*, **37**, 221–227.

Kumra, S., Jacobsen, L.K., Lenane, M. *et al.* (1998d) Childhood-onset schizophrenia: an open-label study of olanzapine in adolescents. *Journal of the American Academy of Child and Adolescent Psychiatry*, **37**, 360–363.

Lam, D.H. (1991) Psychosocial family intervention in schizophrenia: a review of empirical studies. *Psychological Medicine*, **21**, 423–441.

Lawrie, S.M. & Abukmeil, S.S. (1998) Brain abnormalities in schizophrenia: a systematic and quantitative review of volumetric magnetic resonance imaging studies. *British Journal of Psychiatry*, **172**, 110–120.

Leff, J. & Vaughn, C. (1985) *Expressed Emotion in Families: its Significance for Mental Illness*. Guilford Press, London.

Lenzenweger, M.F. & Dworkin, R.H. (1996) The dimensions of schizophrenia phenomenology: not one or two, at least three, perhaps four. *British Journal of Psychiatry*, **168**, 432–440.

Lewine, R.R.J. (1994) Comments on 'Puberty and the onset of psychosis' by P.M. Galdos *et al*. *Schizophrenia Research*, **13**, 81–83.

Lewis, S.W. & Murray, R.M. (1987) Obstetric complications, neurodevelopmental deviance and risk of schizophrenia. *Journal of Psychiatric Research*, **21**, 414–421.

Liddle, P. (1987a) The symptoms of chronic schizophrenia: a re-examination of the positive–negative dichotomy. *British Journal of Psychiatry*, **151**, 145–151.

Liddle, P. (1987b) Schizophrenic syndromes, cognitive performance and neurological dysfunction. *Psychological Medicine*, **7**, 49–57.

Liddle, P.F. & Morris, D. (1991) Schizophrenic syndromes and frontal lobe performance. *British Journal of Psychiatry*, **158**, 340–345.

Liddle, P., Friston, K.J., Frith, C.D., Hirsch, S.R., Jones, T. & Frackowiak, R.S.J. (1992) Patterns of cerebral blood flow in schizophrenia. *British Journal of Psychiatry*, **160**, 179–186.

Lindsay, J., Ounsted, C. & Richards, P. (1979) Long-term outcome of children with temporal lobe seizures. II. Marriage, parenthood and sexual indifference. *Developmental Medicine and Child Neurology*, **21**, 433–440.

Loebel, A.D., Lieberman, J.A., Alvir, J.M.N. *et al.* (1992) Duration of psychosis and outcome in first episode schizophrenia. *American Journal of Psychiatry*, **149**, 1183–1188.

Maj, M. (1998) Critique of the DSM-IV operational diagnostic criteria for schizophrenia. *British Journal of Psychiatry*, **172**, 458–460.

Malmberg, A., Lewis, G., David, A. & Allebeck, P. (1998) Premorbid adjustment and personality in people with schizophrenia. *British Journal of Psychiatry*, **172**, 308–313.

Mason, P., Harrison, G., Croudace, T., Glazebrook, C. & Medley, I. (1997) The predictive validity of a diagnosis of schizophrenia. *British Journal of Psychiatry*, **170**, 321–327.

Matsumoto, H., Takei, N., Saito, H., Kachi, K. & Mori, N. (1999) Childhood-onset schizophrenia and obstetric complications: a case–control study. *Schizophrenia Research*, **38**, 93–99.

Maziade, M., Bouchard, S., Gingras, N. *et al.* (1996) Long term stability of diagnosis and symptom dimensions in a systematic sample of patients with onset of schizophrenia in childhood and early adolescence. II. Positive/negative distinction and childhood predictors of adult outcome. *British Journal of Psychiatry*, **169**, 371–378.

McGlashen, T.H. & Hoffman, R.E. (2000) Schizophrenia as a disorder of developmentally reduced synaptic connectivity. *Archives of General Psychiatry*, **57**, 637–648.

McGrath, J. & Murray, R. (1995) Risk factors for schizophrenia: from conception to birth. In: *Schizophrenia* (eds S.R. Hirsch & D.R. Weinberger), pp. 187–205. Blackwell Science, Oxford.

McGrorry, P. & Sing, B. (1995) Schizophrenia: risk and possibility. In: *Handbook of Studies on Preventative Psychiatry* (eds B. Raphael & G. Burrows), pp. 491–514. Elsvier Science, Amsterdam.

McKenna, K., Gordon, C., Lenane, M., Kaysen, D., Fahey, K. & Rapoport, J. (1994) Looking for childhood onset schizophrenia: the first 71 cases screened. *Journal of the American Academy of Child and Adolescent Psychiatry*, **33**, 616–635.

McNeil, T.F. (1995) Perinatal risk factors and schizophrenia: selective review and methodological concerns. *Epidemiology Review*, **17**, 107–112.

Meehl, P.E. (1962) Schizotaxia, schizotypy, schizophrenia. *American Psychologist*, **17**, 827–838.

Murray, R.M. & Lewis, S.W. (1987) Is schizophrenia a neurodevelopmental disorder? *British Medical Journal*, **295**, 681–682.

Nelson, M.D., Saykin, A.J., Flashman, L.A. & Riodan, H.J. (1998) Hippocampal volume reduction in schizophrenia assessed by magnetic resonance imaging: a metaanalytic study. *Archives of General Psychiatry*, **55**, 433–440.

Nicholson, R.M., Giedd, J.N., Lenane, M. *et al.* (1999) Clinical and neurobiological correlates of cytogenetic abnormalities in childhood-onset schizophrenia. *American Journal of Psychiatry*, **156**, 1575–1579.

Nicholson, R.M., Lenane, M., Singaracharlu, S. *et al.* (2000) Premorbid speech and language impairments in childhood-onset schizophrenia: association with risk factors. *Schizophrenia Research*, **41**, 55.

Nopoulos, P., Torres, I., Flaum, M., Andreasen, N.C., Ehrhaerdt, J.C. & Yuh, W.T.C. (1995) Brain morphology in first-episode schizophrenia. *American Journal of Psychiatry*, **152**, 1721–1723.

Nopoulos, P.C., Giedd, J.N., Andreasen, N.C. & Rapoport, J.L. (1998) Frequency and severity of enlarged septi pellucidi in childhood-onset schizophrenia. *American Journal of Psychiatry*, **155**, 1074–1079.

Nuechterlain, K.H. & Dawson, M.E. (1984) Information processing and attentional functioning in the developmental course of schizophrenic disorders. *Schizophrenia Bulletin*, **10**, 160–203.

O'Driscoll, G.A., Benkelfat, C., Florencio, P.S. *et al.* (1999) Neural correlates of eye tracking deficits in first-degree relatives of schizophrenic patients: a positron emission tomography study. *Archives of General Psychiatry*, **56**, 1127–1134.

van Os, J., Fahy, T., Jones, P. *et al.* (1996) Psychopathological syndromes in the functional psychoses: associations with course and outcome. *Psychological Medicine*, **26**, 161–176.

van Os, J., Jones, P., Lewis, G. et al. (1997) Developmental precursors of affective illness in a general population birth cohort. *Archives of General Psychiatry*, **54**, 625–631.

Ozonoff, S., Pennington, B.F. & Rogers, S.J. (1991) Executive function deficits in high-functioning autistic individuals: relationship to theory of mind. *Journal of Child Psychology and Psychiatry*, **32**, 1081–1105.

Pantelis, C., Velakoulis, D., Suchling, P. et al. (2000) Left medial temporal volume reduction occurs during transition from high-risk to first-episode psychosis. *Schizophrenia Research*, **41**, 35.

Park, S., Holzman, P.S. & Goldman-Rakic, P.S. (1995) Spatial working memory deficits in the relatives of schizophrenic patients. *Archives of General Psychiatry*, **52**, 821–828.

Pennington, B.F., Groisser, D. & Welsh, M.C. (1993) Contrasting deficits in attention deficit hyperactivity disorder versus reading disability. *Developmental Psychology*, **29**, 511–523.

Peralta, V. & Cuesta, M.J. (1999) Diagnostic significance of Schneider's first-rank symptoms in schizophrenia: comparative study between schizophrenic and non-schizophrenic psychotic disorders. *British Journal of Psychiatry*, **174**, 243–248.

Pettegrew, J.W., Keshavan, M.S., Panchalingam, K. et al. (1991) Alterations in brain high energy phosphate and membrane phospholipid metabolism in first episode, drug naive schizophrenics: a pilot study of the dorsal prefrontal cortex by *in vivo* phosphorus 31 nuclear magnetic resonance spectroscopy. *Archives of General Psychiatry*, **48**, 563–568.

Pool, D., Bloom, W., Miekle, D.H., Roniger, J.J. & Gallant, D.M. (1976) A controlled trial of loxapine in 75 adolescent schizophrenic patients. *Current Therapeutic Research*, **19**, 99–104.

Poole, R. & Brabbins, C. (1996) Drug induced psychosis. *British Journal of Psychiatry*, **168**, 135–138.

Pulver, A., Brown, C.H., Wolyniec, P. et al. (1990) Schizophrenia: age at onset, gender and familial risk. *Acta Psychiatrica Scandinavica*, **82**, 344–351.

Purves, D.L. & Lichtmen, J.W. (1980) Elimination of synapses in the developing nervous system. *Science*, **210**, 153–157.

Rapoport, J.L., Conners, C. & Reatig, N. (1985) Rating scales and assessment instruments for use in pediatric psychopharmacology research. *Psychopharmacology Bulletin*, **21**, 713–1111.

Rapoport, J.L., Giedd, J., Kumra, S. et al. (1997) Childhood-onset schizophrenia: progressive ventricular change during adolescence. *Archives of General Psychiatry*, **54**, 897–903.

Rapoport, J.L., Giedd, J., Blumenthal, J. et al. (1999) Progressive cortical change during adolescence in childhood-onset schizophrenia: a longitudinal magnetic resonance imaging study. *Archives of General Psychiatry*, **56**, 649–654.

Reich, W. (2000) Diagnostic Interview for Children and Adolescents (DICA). *Journal of the American Academy of Child and Adolescent Psychiatry*, **39**, 59–66.

Remschmidt, H., Schultz, E. & Martin, M. (1994) An open trial of clozapine with thirty-six adolescents with schizophrenia. *Journal of Child and Adolescent Psychopharmacology*, **4**, 31–41.

Roberts, G.W., Colter, N., Lofthouse, R., Bogerts, B., Zech, M. & Crow, T.J. (1986) Gliosis in schizophrenia: a survey. *Biological Psychiatry*, **21**, 1043–1050.

Robinson, D., Woerner, M.G., Alvir, J.M. et al. (1999) Predictors of relapse following a first episode of schizophrenia or schizoaffective disorder. *Archives of General Psychiatry*, **56**, 241–247.

Rossi, A., Mancini, F., Stratta, P. et al. (1997) Risperidone, negative symptoms and cognitive deficit in schizophrenia: an open study. *Acta Psychiatrica Scandinavica*, **95**, 40–43.

Russell, A.T. (1994) The clinical presentation of childhood-onset schizophrenia. *Schizophrenia Bulletin*, **20**, 631–646.

Russell, A.T., Bott, L. & Sammons, C. (1989) The phenomena of schizophrenia occurring in childhood. *Journal of the American Academy of Child and Adolescent Psychiatry*, **28**, 399–407.

Russell, A.T., Monro, J.C., Jones, P.B., Hemsley, D.R. & Murray, R.M. (1997) Schizophrenia and the myth of intellectual decline. *American Journal of Psychiatry*, **154**, 635–639.

Rutter, M. (1972) Childhood schizophrenia reconsidered. *Journal of Autism and Childhood Schizophrenia*, **2**, 315–407.

Rutter, M. & Mawhood, L. (1991) The long-term psychosocial sequelae of specific developmental disorders of speech and language. In: *Biological Risk Factors for Psychosocial Disorders* (eds M. Rutter & P. Casaer), pp. 233–259. Cambridge University Press, Cambridge.

Rutter, M. & Plomin, R. (1997) Opportunities for psychiatry from genetic findings. *British Journal of Psychiatry*, **171**, 209–219.

Sachdev, P. (1998) Schizophrenia-like psychosis and epilepsy: the status of the association. *American Journal of Psychiatry*, **155**, 325–336.

Saykin, A.J., Shtasel, D.L., Gur, R.E. et al. (1994) Neuropsychological deficits in neuroleptic-naive patients with first episode schizophrenia. *Archives of General Psychiatry*, **512**, 124–131.

Schmidt, M., Blanz, B., Dippe, A., Koppe, T. & Lay, B. (1995) Course of patients diagnosed as having schizophrenia during first episode occurring under age 18 years. *European Archives of Psychiatry and Clinical Neuroscience*, **245**, 93–100.

Selemon, L.D., Rajkowska, G. & Goldman-Rakic, P.S. (1995) Abnormally high neuronal density in the schizophrenic cortex: a morphometric analysis of prefrontal area 9 and occipital area 17. *Archives of General Psychiatry*, **52**, 805–818.

Shaffer, D., Gould, M.S., Brasic, J. et al. (1983) The children's global assessment scale (CGAS). *Archives of General Psychiatry*, **40**, 1228–1231.

Sham, P.C., Jones, P.B., Russell, A. et al. (1994) Age at onset, sex, and familial psychiatric morbidity in schizophrenia. Report from the Camberwell Collaborative Psychosis Study. *British Journal of Psychiatry*, **165**, 466–473.

Siefen, G. & Remschmidt, H. (1986) Behandlungsergebnisse mit Clozapin bei schizophrenen Jungendlichen. *Zeitschift fur Kinder- und Jungendpsychiatrie und Psychotherapie*, **14**, 245–257.

Sigurdsson, E., Fombonne, E., Sayal, K. & Checkley, S. (1999) Neurodevelopmental antecedents of early-onset bipolar affective disorder. *British Journal of Psychiatry*, **174**, 121–127.

Simpson, G. & Angus, J.S.W. (1970) A rating scale for extrapyramidal side effects. *Acta Psychiatrica Scandinavica*, **212** (Suppl.), 9–11.

Slaveska, K., Hollis. C.P. & Bramble, D. (1998) The use of antipsychotics by the child and adolescent psychiatrists of Trent region. *Psychiatric Bulletin*, **22**, 685–687.

Spence, S.A., Liddle, P.F., Stefan, M.D. et al. (2000) Functional anatomy of verbal fluency in people with schizophrenia and those at genetic risk: focal dysfunction and distributed disconnectivity reappraised. *British Journal of Psychiatry*, **176**, 52–60.

Spencer, E.K. & Campbell, M. (1994) Children with schizophrenia: diagnosis, phenomenology and pharmacotherapy. *Schizophrenia Bulletin*, **20**, 713–725.

Strandburg, R.J., Marsh, J.T., Brown, W.S., Asarnow, R.F. & Guthrie, D. (1994) Information processing deficits across childhood and adult onset schizophrenia. *Schizophrenia Bulletin*, **20**, 685–696.

Strandburg, R.J., Marsh, J.T., Brown. W.S. et al. (1999) Continuous-processing ERPS in adult schizophrenia: continuity with childhood-onset schizophrenia. *Biological Psychiatry*, **45**, 1356–1369.

Strauss, J.S., Carpenter, W.T. & Bartko, J.J. (1974) The diagnosis and understanding of schizophrenia. III. Speculations on the processes that underlie schizophrenia symptoms and signs. *Schizophrenia Bulletin*, **1**, 61–69.

Tarrier, N., Beckett, R., Harwood, S., Baker, A., Yusupoff, L. & Ugartebura, I. (1993) A trial of two cognitive behavioural methods of treating drug resistant residual symptoms in schizophrenic patients. I. Outcome. *British Journal of Psychiatry*, **162**, 524–532.

Thomas, M.A., Ke, Y., Levitt, J. *et al.* (1998) Preliminary study of frontal lobe ^{1}H MR spectroscopy in childhood-onset schizophrenia. *Journal of Magnetic Resonance Imaging*, **8**, 841–846.

Towbin, K.R., Dykens, E.M., Pearson, G.S. & Cohen, D.J. (1993) Conceptualising 'borderline syndrome of childhood' and 'childhood schizophrenia' as a developmental disorder. *Journal of the American Academy of Child and Adolescent Psychiatry*, **32**, 775–782.

Tsuang, M.T. (1993) Genotypes, phenotypes and the brain: a search for connections in schizophrenia. *British Journal of Psychiatry*, **163**, 299–307.

Tsuang, M.T., Simpson, J.C. & Kronfold, Z. (1982) Subtypes of drug abuse with psychosis. *Archives of General Psychiatry*, **39**, 141–147.

Tsuang, M.T., Stone, W.S. & Faraone, S.V. (2000) Toward reformulating the diagnosis of schizophrenia. *American Journal of Psychiatry*, **157**, 1041–1050.

Turkington, D. & Kingdon, D. (2000) Cognitive-behavioural techniques for general psychiatrists in the management of patients with psychoses. *British Journal of Psychiatry*, **177**, 101–106.

Vita, A., Dieci, M., Giobbio, G.M. *et al.* (1991) CT scan abnormalities and outcome of chronic schizophrenia. *American Journal of Psychiatry*, **148**, 1577–1579.

Volkmar, F.R. & Cohen, D.J. (1991) Comorbid association of autism and schizophrenia. *American Journal of Psychiatry*, **148**, 1705–1707.

Weinberger, D.R. (1987) Implications of normal brain development for the pathogenesis of schizophrenia. *Archives of General Psychiatry*, **44**, 660–669.

Weinberger, D.R., Berman, K.F. & Zec, R.F. (1986) Physiologic dysfunction of dorsolateral prefrontal cortex in schizophrenia. *Archives of General Psychiatry*, **43**, 114–124.

Welsh, M.C., Pennington, B.F. & Groisser, D.B. (1991) A normative-developmental study of executive function: a window on pre-frontal function in children? *Developmental Neuropsychology*, **7**, 131–139.

Werry, J.S. & McClellan, J.M. (1992) Predicting outcome in child and adolescent (early onset) schizophrenia and bipolar disorder. *Journal of the American Academy of Child and Adolescent Psychiatry*, **31**, 147–150.

Werry, J.S., McClellan, J.M. & Chard, L. (1991) Childhood and adolescent schizophrenia, bipolar and schizoaffective disorders: a clinical and outcome study. *Journal of the American Academy of Child and Adolescent Psychiatry*, **30**, 457–465.

Werry, J.S., McClellan, J.M., Andrews, L. & Ham, M. (1994) Clinical features and outcome of child and adolescent schizophrenia. *Schizophrenia Bulletin*, **20**, 619–630.

Woods, B.T. (1998) Is schizophrenia a progressive neurodevelopmental disorder? Toward a unitary pathogenic mechanism. *American Journal of Psychiatry*, **155**, 1661–1670.

World Health Organization (1978) *International Classification of Diseases (ICD-9)*, 9th edn. World Health Organization, Geneva.

World Health Organization (1992) *International Classification of Diseases (ICD-10)*, 10th edn. World Health Organization, Geneva.

Wyatt, R.J. (1995) Early intervention in schizophrenia: can the course be altered? *Biological Psychiatry*, **38**, 1–3.

Wykes, T., Reeder, C., Williams, C., Corner, J., Rice, C. & Everitt, B. (2000) Cognitive remediation: predictors of success and durability of improvements [Abstract]. *Schizophrenia Research*, **41**, 221.

Yung, A.R., McGorry, P.D., McFarlane, C.A., Jackson, H.J., Patton, G.C. & Rakkar, A. (1996) Monitoring and care of young people at incipient risk of psychosis. *Schizophrenia Bulletin*, **22**, 283–303.

Zahn, T.P., Jacobson, L.K., Gordon, C.T., McKenna, K., Frazier, K. & Rapoport, J.L. (1997) Autonomic nervous system markers of pathophysiology in childhood-onset schizophrenia. *Archives of General Psychiatry*, **54**, 904–912.

Zahn, T.P., Jacobson, L.K., Gordon, C.T., McKenna, K., Frazier, K. & Rapoport, J.L. (1998) Attention deficits in childhood-onset schizophrenia: reaction time studies. *Journal of Abnormal Psychology*, **107**, 97–108.

Zeitlin, H. (1986) *The Natural History of Psychiatric Disorder in Children*. Institute of Psychiatry Maudsley Monograph, 29. Oxford University Press, Oxford.

Autism Spectrum Disorders

Catherine Lord and Anthony Bailey

Introduction

Autistic spectrum disorders are defined by the early onset of a constellation of difficulties in reciprocal social interaction and communication and restricted, repetitive behaviours or interests. They are particularly striking because of the contrast between extraordinary consistency across individuals in some behaviours, and marked differences in others. A child with autism in rural Guatemala peers out of the corner of his eye at flags made of leaves and wooden sticks in the same way that a child in suburban Chicago squints at flags made from McDonald's swizzle sticks and sweetener packets. Yet identical twins with autistic spectrum disorder may vary in IQ scores by as much as 50 points and lead very different lives, with one twin driving his own car to work and the other requiring assistance with basic hygiene.

Over the last 20 years, clinical and research emphasis has shifted from a focus on a relatively narrowly defined group of severely impaired children, to attention to a broader range of autistic disorders that share the core deficits associated with the narrower concept but in which the degree of handicap may be much less. In this chapter, we use *autism* and *autistic disorder* to refer to the narrower traditional diagnostic concept. However, when findings or implications apply more broadly, the term *autistic spectrum disorder* is used. This strategy necessarily makes for some inconsistency because, although research was often carried out only with children with autism, the implications seem likely to apply more broadly.

Clinical and epidemiological studies of autism

Early nineteenth century accounts of children described behaviours that now sound hauntingly familiar (Vaillant 1962), but it was not until nearly 150 years later that Kanner (1943) described 11 children with autism who struck him as sharing 'fascinating peculiarities'. A year later, Asperger independently described a group of children similar in many ways to Kanner's first patients (Frith 1991; Ozonoff *et al.* 1991a). At about the same time, other children who had some characteristics of the autism spectrum were described as having schizophrenia or infantile psychosis (Bender 1942; Mahler 1952). In part, confusion may have been perpetuated by the term *autism*, because of its connotations of an active withdrawal into a rich fantasy life (Bosch 1970). This is misleading, because concreteness and restricted imagination constitute one of the cardinal symptoms of the autism spectrum.

In the 1960s and early 1970s, studies confirmed that children with behaviours similar to those described by Kanner could be discriminated reliably from children with mental handicaps or with other psychiatric disorders (Rutter *et al.* 1967; DeMyer *et al.* 1972). Autism differs from schizophrenia in its much earlier onset, a greater frequency of overt neurological impairment, the relatively frequent onset of seizures in late adolescence, stronger association with mental retardation and a different pattern of cognitive deficits (Rutter 1972a; Volkmar & Nelson 1990).

The first twin study of autism led Folstein & Rutter (1977) to conclude that not only was there a high concordance rate for autism in identical twins, but that identical twins discordant for classically defined autism were usually concordant for milder but related deficits. At about the same time, Wing & Gould (1979) identified a 'triad of deficits' in reciprocal social behaviour, communication and play similar to autism that occurred in a substantial number of—mostly mentally retarded—individuals. The term 'pervasive developmental disorders' (PDD) came to be adopted in both ICD-10 (World Health Organization 1992) and DSM-IV (American Psychological Association 2000) as the umbrella term used to cover a broader range of autistic-like disorders. Recently, there has been a movement from parents and professionals to replace the term PDD with the term *autistic spectrum disorders*.

Epidemiology

The epidemiology of autistic spectrum disorders has recently become quite controversial because of disputed claims that a rise in incidence was caused by use of the mumps–measles–rubella triple vaccine (for negative findings and critique of the claim see Taylor *et al.* 1999; Dales *et al.* 2001; Kay *et al.* 2001). Large systematic epidemiological studies have shown increases in prevalence from the estimated rate of autism of 2–5 in 10 000 in the 1970s, to 6–9 in 10 000 (best estimate 7.5 in 10 000) in studies conducted since 1987 (Fombonne 1999). The same studies reported an additional 12.25 in 10 000 individuals with atypical autism/PDD, producing an overall rate of about 20 cases in 10 000 individuals. Rates for Asperger disorder, when individuals who also met criteria for autism were not included, were low, at 1–2 in 10 000. Because these studies did not focus on individuals with milder variants of the autism spectrum, it is possible that the figures for atypical autism/PDD and Asperger disorder are underestimates. A more recent study found even higher prevalence estimates of 16.8 per 10 000 for autism and 45.8 per 10 000 for other pervasive developmental disorders in a geographically defined population of preschool children (Chakrabarti & Fombonne, 2001). Several other recent studies also found higher rates (Arvidsson *et al*. 1997; Baird *et al*. 2000). At least part of the explanation for the apparent increase in incidence lies in more complete ascertainment and a broader definition of autistic spectrum disorders but the matter requires further study.

Diagnostic frameworks

The two most commonly used diagnostic frameworks, ICD-10 and DSM-IV, were intended to be identical in their representation of autism, although there are slight differences in wording and inclusiveness of disorders in the autism spectrum. Both conceptualize autistic spectrum disorders as comprising three areas of deficit—social reciprocity, communication, and restricted repetitive behaviours and interests—and also require recognition of some type of abnormality before 36 months of age. These features are described in more detail below (Le Couteur *et al*. 1989; Wing 1997a).

Clinical characteristics

Social deficits

The most characteristic aspects of the autism spectrum concern difficulties in reciprocal interaction and the ability to form relationships (Tanguay *et al*. 1998). Recent studies have stressed children's lack of automatic social responses, such as orienting to their names or to a parent's voice from across a room (Osterling & Dawson 1994; Lord 1995a). In the preschool years, children with autism can be differentiated from children who have mental retardation or language delay by their lack of interest in other children, a limited range of socially directed facial expressions, and unusual eye contact. Children with autism are less likely to comfort others (such as bringing a baby sister her blanket) and may not seek to share enjoyment in an event, such as the sight of a favourite animal. Some children with autism remain relatively uninterested in other children for many years, whereas others begin to want friends but have difficulty forming reciprocal relationships. Most children with autistic spectrum disorders do not show deficits in all these areas, and many gain some social behaviours as they grow older. Because it is within friendships that more complex social skills are often modelled and practised, children with autistic spectrum disorders are handicapped both by their disorder and their lack of opportunities to learn that result from their basic deficits.

Communication

The overlap between social skills and communication is great. Non-verbal communicative behaviours (e.g. facial expressions, gestures, eye contact) are considered to be social behaviours, but conversation and social chat, which provide the context for many non-verbal behaviours, are dealt with under communication, in ICD-10 and DSM-IV. For individuals with language, the most distinctive feature is its lack of, or unusual, social quality (Tager-Flusberg & Anderson 1991; Jarrold *et al*. 1997). Children with autism have difficulty carrying on conversations, although they may ask questions about preoccupations or forthcoming events. Some children with autistic spectrum disorders are talkative, often with repetitive speech that is more of a monologue than socially directed communication. Other children speak only rarely, primarily to ask for things (Stone & Caro-Martinez 1990).

Other characteristics of the language of children with autism include reversing pronouns (e.g. referring to themselves as 'you' or 'he'), delayed echolalia or stereotypic speech borrowed from other people or videos, sometimes with meaning, and making up words (neologisms). Abnormalities of pitch, stress, rhythm and intonation have been more difficult to quantify in research, but occur more frequently in autistic spectrum disorders than in general mental retardation (Lord *et al*. 2000). Immediate echolalia, or repeating all or part of what someone has just said, often with identical intonation, is common, especially in younger children, but is also found in other populations with limited language comprehension.

Autistic spectrum disorders are associated not only with difficulties in language but also with deficits in non-verbal communication, including use of gestures, such as pointing, nodding and showing. Thus, a child with autism who wants a drink, but cannot speak, may not use eye contact, gesture or a speech-like vocalization to communicate his or her request, but may cry or attempt physical means such as putting an adult's hand on the glass to pour it. Deficits also occur in imitation, social play (such as taking both roles in peek-a-boo or hide and seek), spontaneous imaginative role play or play with dolls or action figures (Harris 1993; Lewis & Boucher 1995).

Many children with autistic spectrum disorders have severe language delays. Unlike children with other causes of language delay, children with autism have few compensatory communication skills. Earlier estimates proposed that about 50% of children with autism did not use language as their primary method of communication and so were considered non-verbal. Recent treatment studies have suggested that, at least for children in early intensive treatment, this number may be decreasing (Rogers 1998). Autism is most often associated with lower verbal than non-verbal IQ scores (Rumsey 1992). However, in those with an IQ in the normal range, many show equal or even higher levels of verbal than non-verbal skills (Venter *et al*. 1992; Green *et al*. 2000). These are the individuals for whom the category of Asperger disorder is often used (see below; also Klin & Volkmar 1997). In addition, a significant minority of children with autism, perhaps 25%, have continuing severe language impairment. In these children, receptive and expressive language are both affected; some also have general verbal apraxia that affects their articulation, sharing features with children who have specific language impairments (Kjelgaard & Tager-Flusberg 2001).

Restricted, repetitive interests and behaviours

Stereotyped behaviours and interests include unusual preoccupations and circumscribed interests, compulsions and rituals, unusual hand and finger or whole body movements, repetitive use of objects and unusual sensory reactions or interests. Typical preoccupations include street signs, vacuum cleaners and birth dates. Circumscribed interests are age-appropriate interests carried out with unusual intensity and without a social quality, such as interests in trains or books, or fascinations with letters.

Rituals and compulsive behaviours in the autism spectrum differ from those in obsessive-compulsive disorder (OCD) (Leckman et al. 1997). Many individuals with autistic spectrum disorders are not particularly upset by their compulsive behaviours and seemingly make no effort to prevent or stop them. The most common compulsive behaviours in OCD, such as washing, checking or counting, are not typical of autism. Often the rituals in autistic disorders are arbitrary and are not linked to the prevention of an untoward event (e.g. tapping a puzzle piece before placing it). For individuals with autistic spectrum disorders who go on to develop OCD later, however, the clinical picture may be typical.

Stereotyped movements of the hands and fingers, frequently, although not always, within peripheral vision, as well as hand-flapping, often accompanied by jumping, bouncing or rocking foot to foot, are also common. Some children with autism have strong reactions, positive or negative, to sensations such as smell, touch, sight or sound. They may smell objects that do not have any obvious odour or taste objects that most people would not put in their mouths. Peering at linear patterns or objects are also common behaviours. However, as with symptoms in other areas, no child with autism shows all of these behaviours, and many show only one or two.

Although there have been arguments for the primacy of social communicative deficits in autistic spectrum disorders (Tanguay et al. 1998), the addition of a criterion concerning repetition adds significantly to the specificity of the disorder (Buitelaar et al. 1999). Earlier hypotheses that repetitive behaviours occurred primarily as a reaction to absence of social stimulation have not been supported (Romanczyk 1986). On the other hand, children and adolescents with autism are more likely to wander or do nothing at all in unstructured situations (Lord & Magill-Evans 1995; Koegel et al. 1999). Because of the lack of spontaneous creative social play, repetitive behaviours may be more noticeable and take up a larger proportion of time in autistic spectrum disorders than for other children.

One of the original descriptive criteria for autism was need for sameness. Some children with autism want to sustain their own routines and are upset by changes in subtle details of the environment that have no immediate effect on them (e.g. placement of a vase on a table). These specific difficulties are more often associated with autism than other disorders, although strong reactions to changes are relatively common in children with mental retardation as well, and many children with autistic spectrum disorders do not show these behaviours at all (Volkmar et al. 1994). Some children with autistic spectrum disorders, particu-larly those with mental retardation, hit themselves on the head or bite their wrists or arms. The factors eliciting these behaviours vary tremendously (Romanczyk 1986), from wanting attention to a response to overstimulation or an attempt to communicate. These behaviours are not diagnostic of autism but are of concern because of their possible consequences and social disruptiveness.

There is an important relationship between the autism spectrum and mental handicap, which is not yet well understood. Most earlier epidemiological studies estimated that about 75% of individuals with autism were mentally retarded, meaning that the children's strongest skills, usually in non-verbal problem-solving and daily living skills, were more than 2 SD below average (below 70 on a typical standardized test in which 100 is average). Yet not all individuals with autism have mental retardation. Newer epidemiological studies (Baird et al. 2000; Chakrabati & Fombonne 2001), and those with less narrow definitions of the autism spectrum, suggest that the proportion of non-retarded children with autistic spectrum disorders may be much higher than indicated in epidemiological studies in which subjects were recruited primarily from educational and medical services for children with severe developmental disorders.

Course of autism

Age of onset and early regression

Most children with autism are identified by their parents as showing abnormalities or delays in the second year of life, and many parents suspect problems long before this. Dates for 'onset' for children with other autistic spectrum disorders may be slightly later. Often the problems noticed are not specific autistic features, but rather concerns that the child is less 'talkative' (even before a child might normally be expected to speak) or has difficulties in settling, eating, sleeping or tantrums (Dahlgren & Gillberg 1989). Parents who have already had a child tend to recognize social deficits earlier than parents of first-borns, and social deficits are often less recognizable in very young children than when they are older (De Giacomo & Fombonne 1998). Many children under the age of 3 years who will eventually meet formal criteria for autistic spectrum disorders do not yet show clear examples of restricted or repetitive behaviours (Cox et al. 1999; Stone et al. 1999). In some cases, these behaviours may be present early on but may be difficult to differentiate from the play of normally developing toddlers.

Historically, differences in age of onset were proposed to discriminate between autism and schizophrenia at a time when both disorders were thought to represent childhood psychoses. Children with autism had developmental abnormalities in the first 3 years, whereas children with schizophrenia rarely showed abnormalities prior to later school years. Although this differentiation has been very important, in general, distinctions based on onset often confound the age of recognition with the actual onset of the disorder, a phenomenon difficult to define precisely from retrospective accounts (Volkmar et al. 1985). Recently, video studies of children at 9–12 months who were later diagnosed with autistic disorder indicated that children's responses to their names, or the number of times their parents called their names, differentiated children with autism from children with other disorders (Baranek 1999; Werner *et al.* 2000). Children with autism were also more likely to have at least one non-specific unusual sensory response, although there was considerable variability and overlap in the behaviours of children with autism and children with mental retardation without autism.

About one-quarter to one-third of parents of children with autistic spectrum disorder report a loss of speech in the first years of life (Rogers & DiLalla 1990), often, although not always, accompanied by or preceded by other changes in the child's social communication. A parent may notice that a child gradually stopped saying 'baba' for blanket, and increasingly seemed to be watching the credits on television alone in a room, even when the rest of the family had moved into another area of the house. The pattern of having a few words in the first half of the second year and then not speaking at all probably occurs more often in children with autistic spectrum disorders than in children with other developmental disorders or language impairment. Although these words may have been meaningful to the child in some cases, they were usually not part of a normal developmental trajectory of vocabulary development, but 'plateaued' very early on. The relationship between regression and prognosis in the autism spectrum is not yet clear.

Predicting adult outcome from childhood characteristics

As children with autistic spectrum disorders enter school, many are described as more flexible and socially directed. In adolescence, a small minority of youngsters with autism show marked regressions in behaviour and occasionally in cognitive skills (Gillberg & Steffenburg 1987). Although individuals with Asperger syndrome or autism, particularly those with severe mental retardation, may show violent or aggressive behaviour, this is atypical (Ghaziuddin *et al.* 1991; Howlin & Goode 1998).

Predictors of outcome from early preschool to later childhood have included joint attention (Sigman *et al.* 1999), verbal imitation (Smith & Bryson 1994) and social communicative aspects of adaptive skills (Lord & Schopler 1989a). However, non-verbal IQ and language are the two most powerful predictors. A non-verbal IQ below 50 in the preschool years (or later), provided it is based on a thorough assessment (see Rutter & Yule, Chapter 7), is associated with a reduced likelihood that the child will acquire a useful level of spoken language (Lord *et al.* 1989) and a very low probability of good social functioning in adolescence/adulthood (Lockyer & Rutter 1969). Variations in non-verbal IQ between 50 and 70 have a somewhat similar effect but those within the normal range do not. In children who are not severely retarded, language skills (and verbal IQ) are the strongest predictors of social outcome. A child who does not have fluent speech by age 5 years may still make significant gains, but the later these gains come, the less likely the child's language will be flexible and complex, and the more likely language delays of some sort may re-

duce his or her level of independence (Szatmari *et al.* 2000). Non-verbal skills are important in considering methods of teaching and preparation for employment (Venter *et al.* 1992). However, even a child with very strong visuospatial skills who has significant language delays lasting into the school years is likely to have difficulty with the social and communication demands of ordinary society (Venter *et al.* 1992; Sigman *et al.* 1999). The cut-offs of IQ 50 and no language by 5 years are arbitrary (there is no specific threshold) but they provide a general guide.

Autism in adulthood

Some adults with autistic spectrum disorders experience real behavioural and social improvements in their late 20s and early 30s (Mesibov 1984). On the other hand, autism is a lifelong disorder, and the likelihood of complete independence is limited. Individuals with both autism and severe mental retardation require supervised living and working situations throughout their lives. Opportunities for such situations within communities, rather than in institutions, have increased within the last two decades. Apart from a few notable exceptions (Grandin & Scariano 1986), most adults with autistic spectrum disorders, even those with average or greater intelligence, require some help in finding and keeping jobs and coping with responsibilities and social demands (Rutter *et al.* 1992). As discussed under Medical examination and investigations, p. 643, adolescence is a time when epileptic seizures are particularly likely to develop. Comparisons of outcome studies over the last 30 years (Howlin & Goode 1998) suggest that both educational achievement and frequency of employment, with support, have increased for individuals with average, or near average, intelligence. The independence of adults with no, or mild, cognitive delays often depends on community resources and the effort of agencies and family members in seeking vocational and residential arrangements, as much as on individuals' characteristics (Venter *et al.* 1992).

Diagnosis in adult life can be difficult and depends heavily on a developmental history. Contexts for social interaction are less uniform. Adults without mental retardation and with good verbal skills may participate in superficial social interaction relatively well, but have significant difficulties in forming relationships and coping with the demands of work. However, these difficulties are not specific to autism. Comorbid disorders, particularly depression and anxiety, are common in adults with autistic spectrum disorders (Ghaziuddin & Greden 1998). Recognition of an autistic spectrum disorder is helpful in understanding the nature of social difficulties, but it is equally important to focus on social needs and to articulate useful strategies (e.g. structured goals and motivation systems).

Differential diagnoses

Receptive-expressive language disorders

Although language delay is the most common reason for initial referral of children with autistic disorder (Siegel *et al.* 1988), autistic spectrum disorders differ from the more common varieties of developmental language disorder in the severity of receptive language impairment (Fischel *et al.* 1989; Kjelgaard & Tager-Flusberg 2001). There are non-autistic children of normal non-verbal intelligence who have a severe receptive-expressive language impairment but this is a decidedly uncommon disorder. A significant minority have undiagnosed hearing problems, so that it is important that hearing be checked routinely and expertly (Mawhood *et al.* 2000). Many have some symptoms that overlap with autistic spectrum disorders and some may fit descriptions of 'semantic-pragmatic disorder' (Bishop 1989; Boucher 1998), meaning problems with the social communicative aspects of conversational interchange. Children with semantic-pragmatic disorder or severe receptive-expressive language delay may have immediate echolalia, substantial social impairment and limited imaginative play, but unusual preoccupations and rituals are much less common than in autism.

Severe psychosocial deprivation

If a child's development has been unusual from early on, effects of severe early deprivation need to be considered. There is no evidence that 'lack of experience', such as not attending a preschool or having a rather unstimulating babysitter, causes autistic spectrum disorders. Nevertheless, children who have experienced very severe institutional deprivation can show language delay, abnormal social behaviour and marked circumscribed interests and preoccupations (Rutter *et al.* 1999; see also O'Connor, Chapter 46). In early childhood, the clinical picture is rather like autism, although there is usually more social reciprocity than typical with autism, and the course is different, so that by middle childhood it is social disinhibition and circumscribed interests that tend to predominate.

Selective mutism

Selectively mute children may be socially withdrawn and unresponsive. It has been argued that selective mutism should be considered a symptom of social anxiety or avoidance rather than a separate disorder (Dummit *et al.* 1997; Kristensen 2000). It tends to be more common in girls than boys, with an onset before age 4 years. Specific language abnormalities associated with autism (e.g. pronoun reversal, stereotyped speech, odd intonation) are uncommon. However, selective mutism is more common in children with language impairment (Kopp & Gillberg 1997). The children often have strong attachments with parents, show reciprocal social interactions and engage in spontaneous creative play, although their behaviour may be very restricted at school (Black & Uhde 1995; see also Bishop, Chapter 39).

Schizophrenia developing in childhood

Childhood schizophrenia is very rare and should be diagnosed only after other disorders have been carefully excluded (Rutter 1972b). Distinguishing schizophrenia from autism is not difficult, except in rare cases of older, high functioning children and adults with autism whose thought processes may sometimes appear paranoid or delusional (Klein & Slomkowski 1993; Nicolson & Rapoport 1999; Kumra *et al.* 2000). Often, a better understanding of the situation and the context to which the child or adolescent is referring may identify what initially sounded like a hallucination as repetitious behaviour coupled with social *naïveté* about how this behaviour may appear to others. There may be a relationship between significant receptive and expressive language problems and later development of schizophrenia (Howlin *et al.* 2000). However, most individuals with schizophrenia do not have the severe language delays or abnormalities (e.g. delayed echolalia, pronoun reversals) or the early history of deficits in social reciprocity that are typical in autistic spectrum disorders.

Differential diagnosis within the autism spectrum disorders

There is continuing uncertainty regarding the validity of differences among subtypes of autism spectrum disorder, apart from Rett syndrome (Wing 1997b). Once factors such as language and non-verbal cognition are controlled, there is more overlap than difference among subcategories (Green *et al.* 2000; Szatmari *et al.* 2000). DSM-IV and ICD-10 include priority rules that state that if an individual ever met diagnostic criteria for autism, the autism diagnosis takes precedence over any other diagnoses, except Rett syndrome and childhood disintegrative disorder. When this rule is followed, few individuals meet criteria for Asperger syndrome (Ozonoff *et al.* 1991b; Szatmari *et al.* 2000), although the numbers of children left in the non-specific general category of atypical autism remain quite high (Fombonne 1999).

Rett syndrome

Rett syndrome (Hagberg 1985; Naidu 1997) is an X-linked dominant progressive neurodevelopmental disorder that affects girls almost exclusively, with a population prevalence of about 1 in 10 000 to 15 000 females. Typically there is normal development until 6–18 months of age, then a developmental plateau followed by gradual loss of speech and of purposeful hand use, and the development of mid-line hand stereotypies often associated with social withdrawal. This presentation may be confused with autism. Subsequently, mobility becomes limited, and seizures and irregular respiration may develop. However, the range of clinical presentations is wider than at first appreciated, with both milder atypical varieties and profound mental retardation, as well as occasional cases in males (Shahbazian & Zoghbi 2001). An important clinical sign differentiating Rett syndrome from idiopathic autism is the deceleration in head growth leading to acquired microcephaly. Mutations in the *MECP2* gene (Amir *et al.* 1999), of which some 78 types have been described, have been found in 75–90% of sporadic cases and 50% of familial cases (Shahbazian & Zoghbi 2001). An animal model has now been developed (Guy *et al.* 2001) and this should facilitate elucidation of the mechanisms by which the mutations lead to the clinical syndrome.

Childhood disintegrative disorder

Childhood disintegrative disorder (CDD) refers to a syndrome in which apparently normal development over the first 2 years is followed by marked behavioural change and developmental regression. Receptive and expressive language are lost, often with loss of co-ordination and bowel or bladder function (Volkmar & Rutter 1995). Other behavioural changes include social withdrawal and the development of simple rituals, unusual sensory behaviours and hand and finger stereotypies, much like those of autism. The regression in CDD differs from that in autism in extending well beyond language; the loss of skills is usually more severe, and normal development of language and pretend play was usually clear before the regression began. Most commonly, the regression in CDD extends over several months and then plateaus, resulting in a developmental and behavioural pattern that is not distinguishable from autism with profound mental retardation (Hill & Rosenbloom 1986; Mouridsen *et al.* 1999). In some cases, deterioration continues, with increased motor dysfunction, development of seizures and localized neurological signs (Corbett *et al.* 1977). Cases have been caused by cerebral lipidoses or leukodystrophy but, in most instances, no clear cause is ever identified. Because, initial medical tests may be negative, even when neurological disorder is eventually identified, medical investigations should be repeated if there is progressive deterioration.

Landau–Kleffner syndrome

Landau–Kleffner syndrome or acquired aphasia with epilepsy (Miller *et al.* 1984; Mouridsen 1995; Deonna 2000) may also occasionally mimic autism, although the differentiation is usually straightforward. Children with this disorder have normal development and then lose receptive and then expressive language, typically in conjunction with the development of seizures or transient electroencephalogram (EEG) abnormalities (see Bishop, Chapter 39). The regression may be associated with some social withdrawal and behavioural change but family relationships are usually maintained. Non-verbal cognitive and motor functioning and adaptive skills not related to language remain intact. The outlook is better than for CDD, and sometimes language is regained.

Asperger syndrome

In the last 10 years, the concept of Asperger syndrome, as used by researchers (Gillberg 1989; Frith 1991; Klin *et al.* 2000) and clinicians (Wing 1981; Attwood 1997), has served to highlight the occurrence of autistic spectrum disorders in individuals who

are intellectually able and verbally fluent (Grandin & Scariano 1986). It has become clear that these disorders can and do occur in people who did not experience the language delay that is typical of autism. However, it has not proved easy to produce satisfactory diagnostic criteria, and differences in both definition and sampling have led to conflicting findings (Green *et al.* 2000; Klin *et al.* 2000; Szatmari *et al.* 2000). In keeping with the lack of language delay, Asperger syndrome tends to be associated with a higher verbal than non-verbal IQ (Klin *et al.* 1995). This aside, it remains uncertain whether Asperger syndrome and autism differ in pattern of neuropsychological deficit (Ozonoff *et al.* 1991b). Whether diagnosed as having Asperger syndrome or autism, individuals who are verbally fluent tend to be less impaired. However, the question arises as to whether having a history of delay in early language acquisition has a specific effect, independent of current verbal fluency (Green *et al.* 2000). Szatmari *et al.* (2000) found that, after equating for non-verbal IQ, children with autistic spectrum disorder who did not have early language delay had milder social deficits than those with language delay who had equal non-verbal intelligence. Other studies have not found an effect of language delay when current language level is controlled (Eisenmajer *et al.* 1996).

Atypical autism/PDDNOS

The terms 'atypical autism' and 'pervasive developmental disorder not otherwise specified' (PDDNOS) refer to non-specific patterns that seem to involve the same deficits as those associated with autism, although they do not fulfil all the accepted diagnostic criteria (Towbin 1997; Buitelaar *et al.* 1999). The atypicality may lie in the symptom pattern, its severity, or age of first manifestation. Epidemiological analyses (Wing & Gould 1979), clinical investigations (Fein *et al.* 1999) and family studies (Bolton *et al.* 1994) all indicate the frequency of these atypical patterns but they have been subject to little systematic research. It is likely that they reflect variations in the ways in which autistic spectrum disorders may present, rather than a separate category (Rapin 1997; Wing 1997a). The service needs are similar to those for autism, and it remains unknown whether the apparent atypicality has any implications for aetiology.

Another frequently used term in research is the broader 'autism phenotype' (see section on genetics). It refers to mild autistic-like features that are evident in some relatives but it does not necessarily imply a need for services, as discussed below.

Assessment and intervention

Screening for possible autism spectrum disorder

Screening is best considered in terms of two different questions (Filipek *et al.* 2000). The first is whether autistic spectrum disorders can be reliably identified in very young children who have not been referred for assessment and whose parents have not raised concerns about their development. One theoretically based instrument, the Checklist for Autism in Toddlers (CHAT) showed initial promise (Baron-Cohen *et al.* 1992) but its poor sensitivity at 18 months (indicating that it misses many cases) means that it cannot be relied on for screening at that age (Baird *et al.* 2000). Whether other questionnaires would do any better in children who are at a point in development when key skills are often only just emerging remains uncertain and screening at 2 years might be more practicable.

A second question concerns a different kind of 'screening' to decide which children referred to primary care clinicians, who are not experts, should be expertly evaluated for a possible autistic spectrum disorder. Several promising instruments intended for this purpose are under development (Siegel *et al.* 1996; Stone *et al.* 2000). Assessment may be indicated for children whose parents spontaneously say they seem to be 'in a world of their own' or lack social responsiveness, or have stopped speaking for more than a few weeks after having developed some language. A history of not orienting to parents' voices or not consistently understanding any words out of context by age 2 years (when motor development was unremarkable) also identified children with autistic spectrum disorders at age 2 years in one study (Lord 1995b).

Assessment and diagnostic methods

Diagnosis is based on the identification of a particular pattern of deficits, together with consideration of whether this might be fully attributable to cognitive impairment or deafness or severe neglect. Multiaxial frameworks, such as ICD-10 and DSM-IV, are well-suited to the purpose of step-by-step diagnoses, with their explicit recognition of the need to consider intellectual level, specific developmental delays, other psychiatric disorders and psychosocial factors in each decision (see Taylor & Rutter, Chapter 1).

A comprehensive psychological assessment is an important component of this diagnostic process. Several tests are available but they differ in their suitability for very young or non-verbal children, as well as in their standardization and the range of abilities they tap (Klin *et al.* 1997). The selection of appropriate tests depends on the goals of the assessment, the individual child's specific strengths and difficulties, and the psychometric properties of the test. Generally, a single test will not be sufficient. The psychologist must be knowledgeable about test selection and about ways to make the testing process more comprehensible to the child (Koegel *et al.* 1997; see also Rutter & Yule, Chapter 7). Although the use of mental ages is problematic psychometrically, the concept of approximate developmental level can be very helpful for parents and professionals, if put in perspective.

As part of an initial diagnosis, children with autistic spectrum disorders should always have a detailed skilled communication and language assessment. Articulation, language comprehension—both of single words and more complex language—and expressive language, including vocabulary, sentence structure and pragmatics, should be assessed. Aspects of non-verbal communication, including both conventional (e.g. signs) and less

formal systems (e.g. use of gaze, non-standard gestures), should also be evaluated (Wetherby & Prizant 1999). For older, higher functioning children and adolescents, individualized achievement testing that differentiates decoding (which is often an area of strength) from reading comprehension, and practical problems in arithmetic from computations, may also be important in educational and vocational planning.

Diagnostic instruments

Interview of parents or caregivers

Standardized diagnostic instruments have become a routine part of practice in the assessment of autistic spectrum disorders. The Autism Diagnostic Interview–Revised (Le Couteur *et al.* 1989, in press; Lord *et al.* 1994) is a standardized 90-min interview that provides a diagnostic algorithm for ICD-10 and DSM-IV diagnoses of autism, although not yet for other disorders within the spectrum. Separate scores are generated for socialization, communication (non-verbal and verbal) and restricted repetitive behaviours, focusing particularly on the period between 4 and 5 years of age, and on the current pattern. The Diagnostic Interview for Social and Communicative Disorders (DISCO) Handicaps Behaviour Schedule by Lorna Wing (1999) is also available. The DISCO provides a broad base of information concerning developmental and behavioural functioning. Even when standardized instruments are not used, clinicians should have a framework to gather information from the interview to ensure comprehensive coverage of important aspects of development.

The Vineland Adaptive Behaviour Scales (Sparrow *et al.* 1984) can also be helpful, not just in structuring information about everyday skills such as dressing and independent travel, but also in producing data that compare to established norms in these areas (Carter *et al.* 1998). Autism tends to be associated with very low scores on socialization, together with low scores on receptive and expressive language in the early years, and relatively higher scores in daily living skills and motor skills.

Observation/interview of the child

The goal of a clinical observation is for the clinician to be able to witness behaviours in the domains described in the interview. There are several protocols for semistructured observations of children and adults with autistic spectrum disorders including the Psychoeducational Profile (PEP-R; Schopler *et al.* 1990), for children with developmental levels between about 2 and 5 years, and the Adult–Adolescent Psychoeducational Profile (AAPEP; Mesibov *et al.* 1989). Checklists are also available that provide a framework for characterizing behaviours associated with autistic spectrum disorders. These include the Childhood Autism Rating Scale (CARS; Schopler *et al.* 1986), probably the best known and well-validated scale; the Gilliam Autism Rating Scale (GARS; Gilliam 1995); the Aberrant Behaviour Checklist (ABC; Aman & Singh 1986); and the Autism Behaviour

Checklist (ABC; Krug *et al.* 1980). These scales may be used for screening in clinical trials to evaluate behaviour but are less appropriate for diagnoses.

The Autism Diagnostic Observation Schedule (ADOS, formerly called the ADOS-G; Lord *et al.* 2000) both structures the clinician's behaviour, by providing a range of communicative demands and social 'presses' during which to observe children, adolescents and adults, and structures the observations by specifying features to rate within the context of a 30-min observation/interview. The current version of the ADOS includes four modules, each intended for children or adults with different levels of expressive language. Most children with autistic spectrum disorders appear most normal in conditions of high structure. It is not possible to evaluate a child's spontaneous social behaviour if the clinician structures the situation so well that all the child has to do is respond. Equally, in an unstructured environment (such as wandering around an office while their parents are interviewed), children with autistic spectrum disorders may show little social behaviour at all (Bartak & Rutter 1973). With younger children, an experienced clinician may observe characteristically autistic behaviours before parents recognize them as such, but with older children and adults it may be difficult to elicit these behaviours during a brief observation in an unfamiliar setting. Thus, a comprehensive diagnostic evaluation should include information from both parent interview and direct observation.

Medical examination and investigations

A comprehensive physical examination should always be undertaken to detect recognizable syndromes, particularly tuberous sclerosis, and any localizing neurological impairments (see Bailey, Chapter 10). Visual and hearing acuity should also be assessed. Even in the absence of a history or signs of identifiable syndromes, high-resolution karyotyping and molecular genetic testing for fragile X should be routine. Further investigation may be warranted when there are symptoms or signs suggestive of metabolic abnormalities. Although autism is associated with macrocephaly in a minority of cases, this sign by itself is not an indication for neuroimaging studies (Filipek *et al.* 2000). Seizures occur in perhaps one-quarter to one-third of individuals with autism, but often do not develop until adolescence (Rutter 1970; Volkmar & Nelson 1990), and clinicians need to be alert to the possibility of absence or complex partial seizures when there are sudden unexplained changes in behaviour that are not typically autistic in character. EEG abnormalities in autism are very common and are not an indication for anticonvulsant medication in the absence of symptomatology.

Aetiology

Since Kanner's original description, there have been several significant shifts in thinking about the aetiology of autistic spectrum disorders that affect our understanding of the boundaries of the disorder and the features that require explanation. Kanner (1943) initially described autism as an inborn disorder but then reconceptualized the disorder as a reaction to abnormal child-rearing (Eisenberg & Kanner 1956). In the late 1960s, the biological basis of autistic disorder became generally accepted, and autism was assumed to be a consequence of brain damage, caused by either recognized medical disorders or obstetric hazards. However, over the last 20 years or so, there has been an increasing recognition of the role of specific genetic factors in the aetiology of most cases of autistic spectrum disorders, with an appreciation of the complexity of the underlying biological and psychological processes.

Approximately 10–15% of cases of autism are associated with identifiable medical disorders (Rutter *et al.* 1994; Barton & Volkmar 1998). Although cerebral palsy and trisomy 21 are both occasionally associated with autistic spectrum disorders, these common causes of mental handicap are infrequent causes of autism. Similarly, although a wide range of chromosomal abnormalities are associated with autistic spectrum disorder (Gillberg 1998), these are only found in approximately 5% of individual, a rate substantially lower than that found in unselected mental handicap populations (Curry *et al.* 1997). The rate of fragile X anomaly is probably no higher than 4% (Dykens & Volkmar 1997), whereas the rate of tuberous sclerosis (see below) in individuals with autism is approximately 100 times higher than expected (Fombonne 1999).

A number of studies in the 1970s and 1980s reported a relationship between mild prenatal, perinatal and neonatal factors and autism (Piven *et al.* 1993). However, no association has been found between autism and the severe obstetric complications that are typically associated with a significant risk of brain damage. Twin (Bailey *et al.* 1995) and family (Bolton *et al.* 1997) genetic studies suggested that the mild obstetric difficulties sometimes associated with autistic disorders are usually a consequence of either abnormal fetal development or the genetic risk for autism rather than a cause.

Genetic influences

Interest in the genetics of the autism spectrum has recently intensified. Asperger (1944) first hypothesized that autistic psychopathy had a genetic basis which was passed from father to son. Twin studies were necessary, however, to determine whether the elevated familial recurrence risk for autism had an environmental or genetic basis. Across several twin studies, concordance rates in monozygotic (MZ) pairs have been much higher (36–91%) than in dizygotic (DZ) pairs (≈5%) (Steffenburg *et al.* 1989; Bailey *et al.* 1995). In none of these studies was concordance for autism attributable to severe obstetric hazards. The substantial difference in concordance rates between MZ and DZ twins is incompatible with a Mendelian mode of inheritance. Thus, these findings point to the likely involvement of multiple interacting genes (Bailey *et al.* 1995), with a heritability of liability to autism of >90%. The first UK twin study and several other family genetic studies of autism (reviewed by Bailey *et al.* 1998; Szatmari *et al.* 1998) have found an elevated risk for autism and other autistic spectrum disorders amongst siblings, ranging between 2 and 6%. Overall, the relative risk (the risk to relatives compared with the general population risk) is higher for autistic spectrum disorders than for just about any other genetically influenced multifactorial disorder. In practical terms, the current literature suggests a recurrence risk for a pervasive developmental disorder of about 5%, but it is not yet possible to give more precise estimates if more than one person in the family is affected.

Milder phenotypes

Folstein & Rutter's (1977) twin study was remarkable for indicating that the phenotype associated with a genetic predisposition to autistic disorder included cognitive and social difficulties extending beyond autism as traditionally diagnosed. In a follow-up into adulthood of this original sample, the majority of non-autistic MZ cotwins showed substantial social difficulties that were autistic-like but of less severity (Le Couteur *et al.* 1996). Most of the non-autistic MZ cotwins, even individuals of normal intelligence, showed social and/or cognitive abnormalities, with the most severely affected individuals having more well-defined autistic spectrum disorders (Bailey *et al.* 1995). A parallel family history study found that similar social and/or cognitive abnormalities also occurred at an increased rate amongst the relatives of probands with autism compared with the relatives of probands with trisomy 21 (Bolton *et al.* 1994). In fact, individuals with autism represented only a small proportion of all the individuals showing some phenotypic expression.

Most investigators have assumed that mild autism-related behavioural phenotypes are likely to manifest themselves as social, communicative and repetitive impairments, either alone or in combination. Some relatives of individuals with autism show a lack of interest in others or, less frequently, a lack of socioemotional responsiveness, whereas others may show socially odd behaviour (Piven *et al.* 1997a; Starr *et al.* 2001). This broad range of difficulties map onto three of the four domains of social impairment in autism in ICD-10 and DSM-IV. Amongst adult relatives, related personality traits, particularly aloofness and shyness, are also more common than in controls (Piven *et al.* 1997b). There is little evidence from these and other studies (reviewed by Bailey *et al.* 1998; Szatmari *et al.* 1998) of a sharply defined social deficit that is identical in all affected individuals. Rather, the findings point to a range of related social difficulties and personality traits that co-occur.

Most studies have found a history of language delay in a small proportion of relatives (Bailey *et al.* 1998). These individuals have lower verbal IQs than unaffected relatives (Fombonne *et al.* 1997; Folstein *et al.* 1999), indicating that language delay reflects a cognitive impairment rather than a transitory developmental lag. Some relatives show difficulties in communication planning, pragmatic and conversational ability, speech abnormalities and reading and spelling difficulties, although these have a tendency to co-occur with other language difficulties

and so their significance in isolation is at present uncertain (Fombonne *et al.* 1997; Piven *et al.* 1997b; Folstein *et al.* 1999).

Repetitive behaviours have received much less attention than social and communication impairments and are more difficult to define and measure. Bolton *et al.* (1994) identified increased rates of circumscribed interests, rigidity, obsession/compulsions and repetitive behaviours in relatives compared to controls, and Piven *et al.* (1997b) have argued that a lack of interest in seeking change may also be more common amongst relatives of individuals with autism. Abnormalities in the repetitive domain seem to be more specific to autism than social or communication impairments (Pickles *et al.* 2000). Clear-cut generational and sex differences have been found in some but not all studies (Folstein *et al.* 1999; Pickles *et al.* 2000). In contrast to the relationship between autism and milder variants of the behavioural deficits that define it, recent studies have found neither an increased rate of mental handicap amongst relatives nor a consistent pattern of cognitive discrepancies (see Fombonne *et al.* 1997 and Folstein *et al.* 1999 for contrasting findings).

Whether genetic susceptibility to autistic spectrum disorders also predisposes to the development of other psychiatric disorders is presently unclear. DeLong & Nohria (1994) suggested that autistic spectrum disorders represent the early onset of a severe, particularly bipolar, affective disease, but studies using standardized diagnostic instruments have not found an increased rate of bipolar disorder amongst relatives. Nevertheless, relatives do seem to be at increased risk for affective disease, particularly major and recurrent depressive illness, with the first depressive episode tending to occur before the birth of the child with autism (Smalley *et al.* 1995; Piven & Palmer 1999). These depressive disorders do not seem to overlap with autism-related social or language deficits, either at the individual (Piven & Palmer 1999) or familial level (Bolton *et al.* 1998), suggesting that if they are consequences of the genetic liability to the autism spectrum, some different intervening mechanisms are involved. Two studies have reported elevated rates of anxiety-related personality traits amongst adult relatives (Murphy *et al.* 2000) but there is currently no consensus about whether relatives are also at increased risk for generalized anxiety disorders or social phobia (Smalley *et al.* 1995; Bolton *et al.* 1998).

Although it is possible that Mendelian inheritance is implicated in a minority of cases of autism, the evidence suggests that most idiopathic cases arise on the basis of multiple susceptibility genes. Each susceptibility gene probably has only a weak or moderate effect and may not be sufficient to cause the full clinical phenotype. Several susceptibility genes acting together, however, confer a marked risk. Genetic heterogeneity may be assumed. Applying Risch's (1990) approach to family and twin data for autism and related phenotypes, Pickles *et al.* (1995) calculated that between two and 10 loci may be implicated in autism; models with three or four interacting loci provided the best fit.

A further question concerns the relationship between individual genetic loci and specific components of the behavioural phenotype. On the one hand, Folstein *et al.* (1999) suggested that susceptibility loci must be contributed by both parents, and that individual components of the phenotype are inherited separately and manifested independently in non-autistic family members. In contrast, Pickles *et al.* (1995) found that their data on autism and milder phenotypes was best fitted by a model in which interactions between loci contributed to a single latent trait or measure of autism, rather than individual loci predisposing to one component of the phenotype. Even when further families were added to this data set (Pickles *et al.* 2000), there was little evidence of phenotypic expression on both sides of a family, or of bilineal inheritance patterns (e.g. one parent showing social difficulties, the other language problems). Volkmar *et al.* (1998) found that relatives of individuals with Asperger syndrome showed an increased rate of autism as well as Asperger syndrome and milder phenotypes, supporting the transmission of susceptibility for a range of autistic spectrum disorders, rather than of specific disorders.

As yet, there are no clear indications that familial transmission is different for social deficits, language abnormalities or repetitive behaviours. Le Couteur *et al.* (1996) found that there was almost as much variation in IQ and in autistic symptoms within MZ twin pairs concordant for autism as there was between pairs. Starr *et al.* (2001) also found that the rates of milder phenotypes amongst relatives of probands with severe/profound mental retardation were broadly similar to those reported by Bolton *et al.* (1994) in relatives of more able probands. On the other hand, Bolton *et al.* (1994) found there was a relationship between familial loading, for milder phenotypes, and the severity of disorder in the proband, only in the families of probands with useful speech. The preponderance of males with autism (and probably also milder phenotypes) has led to the suggestion that at least some autism susceptibility loci are X-linked. However, in the UK family studies (Pickles *et al.* 2000) there was no evidence for X-linkage, sex-specific patterns of expression, imprinting effects (Skuse 2000) or higher familial loading amongst the relatives of female probands—as predicted under a multifactorial threshold model—suggesting that the sex differences are most probably a consequence of biological sex rather than X-linked genes (Pickles *et al.* 2000).

Identifying susceptibility genes

The identification of susceptibility genes should provide clues to the pathophysiology underlying autism (through identification of the functions of the encoded proteins), and should enable genetic counselling to be based on knowledge of the individual's genotype, rather than group-based risk. Several approaches are currently being used to identify susceptibility loci for autism; these include association studies of 'functional' and 'positional' candidate genes and, most promisingly, linkage studies across the whole genome (Maestrini *et al.* 2000).

Association strategies are based on identifying alleles (versions) of a gene or marker (naturally occurring variations in DNA sequence) that occur at significantly different frequencies in samples of affected and control individuals. Family-based association designs, such as the transmission disequilibrium test, use the frequencies of parental alleles that are not transmitted to affected offspring as internal controls. An association strategy can be used to examine variations in 'functional' candidate genes, genes hypothesized to be implicated in the aetiology of a disease on the basis of what is known about the underlying pathophysiology. Because of limited knowledge about the neurobiological mechanisms and the lack of specific drug effects, there are very few true functional candidate genes for autism. Most attention has focused on the serotonergic system, both because of reports of elevated platelet serotonin levels in patients and their relatives compared with controls (see below), and because of the efficacy of selective serotonin reuptake inhibitors (SSRIs) in reducing repetitive behaviour (McDougle *et al.* 1997). Several groups have examined allelic variation in the promoter of the serotonin (5-HT) transporter gene but the data are contradictory (Cook *et al.* 1997a; IMGSAC 1998), and studies of various serotonin receptor genes and other potential candidates are also equivocal (reviewed by Lamb *et al.* 2000).

Another strategy is to examine 'positional' candidate genes, brain-expressed genes that are potentially implicated because of their proximity to chromosomal abnormalities associated with autistic spectrum disorders (Maestrini *et al.* 2000). These have been reported for nearly all chromosomes (reviewed by Gillberg 1998), but most interest has focused on the reports of a rare association between an autistic-like phenotype and cytogenetic abnormalities of an unstable region of chromosome 15 (reviewed by Lamb *et al.* 2000). This region contains several imprinted genes and includes the Prader–Willi/Angelman critical region.

The most commonly observed abnormalities are interstitial duplications or a supernumerary pseudodicentric chromosome 15 (inv-dup[15]) in patients with autism spectrum disorders—often associated with severe mental retardation and seizures. When parental origin has been investigated, all of the 15q duplications associated with autism have been derived from the mother (Cook *et al.* 1997b), raising the possibility of imprinting effects. The GABA$_A$ receptor gene cluster—containing several genes of interest—lies in this region and was the initial focus of interest, although so far the evidence for association is contradictory (Cook *et al.* 1998; IMGSAC 1998). It remains to be seen whether specific genes in this region are implicated in idiopathic autism, or whether it is the increased dosage of mutant genes associated with chromosomal abnormalities that occasionally gives rise to an autistic-like picture.

Although many research groups are engaged in functional and positional candidate gene analysis, most effort is currently being expended on linkage approaches that make no prior assumptions about gene position or function. Linkage analysis is based on identifying markers that cosegregate with disease within families (Maestrini *et al.* 2000). Because the mode of inheritance of autism is not known and extended pedigrees of affected individuals are not available, most research groups use linkage methods that rely on allele sharing between two or more affected individuals within multiple nuclear families, otherwise known as multiplex families. The goal is to identify markers for which affected pairs share alleles more often than expected by chance, indicating that they may be linked to a susceptibility gene. At the time of writing, four whole genome scans have been reported in full and one in abstract form (reviewed by Lamb *et al.* 2000), with sample sizes ranging between 51 and 139 multiplex families containing two or more individuals within the autism spectrum.

So far, several chromosomal regions appear particularly promising. The strongest initial evidence for linkage was to a region on chromosome 7q (IMGSAC 1998). Subsequently, five weaker, but still positive, linkages spanning a 50-cM region including the original region of interest have been reported in other samples (reviewed by Lamb *et al.* 2000). Because none of the six groups has reported findings that meet the accepted threshold for proven linkage (Turner *et al.* 2000), it remains possible that the results simply represent the chance co-occurrence of a number of false-positives. Nevertheless, if idiopathic autism is aetiologically heterogeneous—as seems likely to be the case—and susceptibility loci are of modest effect, then overlaps in the location of linkages across multiple studies are likely to index a susceptibility locus, even if random variations in gene sharing between samples lead to modest statistical significance. In fact, the linkage in the IMGSAC sample has held up with the addition of further families (IMGSAC 2001), and a combined analysis of three other independent samples provides confirmatory evidence for linkage of autism to 7q (Santangelo *et al.* 2000), with the peak of linkage falling close to that in the IMGSAC sample.

A second region of interest lies on chromosome 2q, initially identified independently by IMGSAC (1998) and Philippe *et al.* (1999). The preliminary results were modest, but appear stronger with the addition of further families and replication by Buxbaum's group (see Lamb *et al.* 2000). Other regions currently identified by two independent groups (reviewed by Lamb *et al.* 2000) lie on 13q, 16p and 19p. Given the generally poor replicability of linkage findings in psychiatric genetics, the findings from these preliminary studies are encouraging, presumably reflecting both the strength of the genetic liability and the acceptance across research groups of well-validated diagnostic instruments (Rutter 2000). The next task is to move beyond preliminary linkage findings to cloning (identification) of genes (see McGuffin & Rutter, Chapter 12). Once a putative susceptibility gene has been identified, the next task is to establish its biochemical function, if that is not already known. Animal models may be helpful in understanding gene function; the goal is not to reproduce complex behaviours, which may occur, but to study the physiological and neuropathological consequences of particular genetic constitutions. Once a susceptibility locus is cloned, the relationship between phenotype and genotype can be re-examined, but now in the reverse direction (Turner *et al.* 2000).

Psychological studies

Although the neurobiological basis of autism is undisputed, understanding the cognitive or emotional processes that mediate abnormal behaviours is relevant for several reasons. First, these psychological mechanisms are important for clarifying the underlying brain abnormalities and their role in mental functioning. Secondly, direct psychological testing may be necessary for recognizing milder phenotypes, for elucidating the differences between behavioural traits and overt disorder, and for understanding why susceptibility alleles have persisted in the population. Thirdly, understanding the psychological mechanisms underpinning developmental psychopathology may improve early diagnosis and lead to new intervention strategies.

Over the last 15 years or so, there have been significant advances in identifying some of the cognitive abnormalities associated with autism (Happé & Frith 1996). However, there has been less progress in achieving an overall conceptualization of the relationships among different deficits, either within or across behavioural domains. Deciding which features of autism spectrum disorders require explanation is a prerequisite for judging the adequacy of theoretical accounts. For example, the co-occurrence of autism with mental retardation was frequently assumed to be caused by brain damage that impaired both specific and general cognitive processes. However, the strong genetic basis to autistic spectrum disorders suggests that any associated mental retardation is a manifestation of the underlying disease process. On a more concrete level, for older preschool and school-age children, IQ scores are as consistent across time and measures within autism as they are for language disorders or for other developmental delays (Lord & Schopler 1989b), with correlations generally above 0.65 for periods in childhood of 5–8 years. Yet this does not mean that IQ scores do not change. Several follow-up and treatment studies have shown substantial increases in IQ scores (some 15–25 points) occurring in a significant proportion of children with autism for preschool to school years and decreases in IQ scores particularly in older children who do not acquire language (Lord & Schopler 1989a; Sigman *et al.* 1999). IQ scores for children with autistic spectrum disorders should be interpreted within broad ranges and should never be used as the sole basis for placement. Whether any cognitive deficit is truly primary, with other abnormalities simply representing developmental sequelae, has been a contentious issue since psychological studies began. Wing & Wing (1971) proposed that autism might arise on the basis of more than one cognitive deficit, and Goodman (1989) has highlighted that autism and Asperger syndrome are characterized by similar social impairments but differ in the extent to which language is affected. The implication is that neither social nor language abnormalities can be construed as secondary phenomena. Although some theorists still adhere to the notion of a single primary deficit, most researchers now accept that autism arises on the basis of multiple primary cognitive deficits.

Autism has been reported in several, although not all, studies

(Starr *et al.* 2001) to be more often associated with mental retardation in females than in males (Lord *et al.* 1982), with the greatest male preponderance reported for individuals of average or greater intelligence (Volkmar *et al.* 1993). Autistic symptoms increase with more severe mental retardation for both sexes. In an epidemiological study, Wing & Gould (1979) found that about 2% of individuals with IQs of 50–69 had a triad of impairments similar to those seen in autism, in contrast to 82% of individuals with IQ scores below 20.

Effects of cognitive level on diagnosis

Diagnosis of autistic spectrum disorders can be particularly problematic at either end of the intellectual spectrum: profound mental retardation, or average and greater intelligence. The need to consider absent or limited social communicative behaviours, such as initiating joint attention, means that most standardized diagnostic instruments for autism yield high scores for many mentally retarded individuals with mental ages of less than about 12–18 months (DiLavore *et al.* 1995; Berument *et al.* 1999), despite the fact that profoundly retarded individuals with and without autism show different patterns of behaviour (De Giacomo & Fombonne 1998). Conversely, children with autistic spectrum disorders with strong intellectual and verbal skills can develop ways of engaging in social interaction that may work around some of their deficits. Two studies following children from preschool to school age found that the higher the IQ score, the greater the proportion of children who were reclassified as having PDDNOS or Asperger syndrome several years later (Eisenmajer *et al.* 1996).

Any explanatory model must account for psychological deficits at all levels of functioning. A corollary is that autism is not reducible to only those deficits found in the most able individuals, who are sometimes considered to have 'pure' autism (Minshew *et al.* 1997). Indeed, fundamental cognitive deficits may be masked in very able individuals by the availability of alternative cognitive strategies. It seems likely that what is specific about the psychological processes underlying autistic spectrum disorders is not the presence of one critical deficit, but rather the particular *combination* of abnormalities.

Several different mechanisms may be relevant for the co-occurrence of cognitive and emotional abnormalities. Abnormal development of one psychological function can affect other developmental processes. Thus, in the modular system of development of 'theory of mind' proposed by Baron-Cohen (1995), dysfunction of the shared attention mechanism is hypothesized to impair input to the theory of mind mechanism. Adequate language skills are also necessary to understand the beliefs of others. A second possibility is that deficits co-occur because they arise from abnormal functioning of a particular brain region; models of autism as a frontal lobe disorder typify this type of explanation (Pennington & Ozonoff 1996). A third possibility is that impaired cognitive and emotional processes arise on the basis of a shared, but not anatomically localized, neurobiological abnormality. Finally, behaviours that result in the selection

and restriction of individuals' environments and activities may lead to correlated psychological abnormalities and their persistence over time.

Theories emphasizing social cognitive deficits

Early psychological studies of autism focused on attention, memory and meta-cognitive processes. Studies of 'theory of mind', beginning in the mid-1980s, concern children's ability to understand that others have beliefs and desires, and to use this knowledge to predict the behaviour of others (Flavell 1999). Observations of these deficits in understanding the mental states of others in children with autism (Baron-Cohen *et al.* 1985) initially led to the conclusion that autism was a specific cognitive disorder of 'mind-blindness' (Baron-Cohen 1990). 'Theory of mind' (ToM), or mentalizing ability, was examined using tests of false belief: the ability to recognize that an individual or agent will act on the basis of his or her beliefs, not on the basis of how things really are.

Deficits in mentalizing ability have been found in individuals with autism using many experimental protocols. In a meta-analysis, Happé (1994) found that some 50% of tested individuals with autism failed a first-order ToM test. Although it is not a universal or specific deficit, ToM has been accepted as important to the understanding of autism. The social difficulties associated with ToM that characterize autism (e.g. not understanding what another person is thinking) have been attributed to impairments in general cognitive processes (e.g. attention, memory, executive functioning). Attempts to disprove the ToM hypothesis have illustrated how ToM skills are influenced by other psychological processes. Thus, Tager-Flusberg & Sullivan (1994) showed that when second-order false belief tasks are presented to individuals with autism in a way that minimizes working memory requirements, individuals who passed simpler ToM tasks could pass the more difficult tasks as well and justify their answers appropriately. Russell *et al.* (1999) demonstrated how executive factors can contribute to failure on false belief tasks. Language abilities also seem to play a critical part in ToM skills in autism. In her meta-analysis, Happé (1994) found that, for children with autism and children with mental retardation, ToM skills were related to language level but the language level necessary for success was significantly higher in the individuals with autism than those with mental retardation. Similarly, Kazak *et al.* (1997) found that ToM performance was correlated with language skills in children with autism, but not in normally developing children. One implication of these findings is that individuals with autism who pass ToM tasks may be using language-based strategies. Indeed, overall language competence is a critical factor in early social development. Thus, Lord & Pickles (1996) found that many, although not all, social and non-verbal communication impairments reported in young children with autism were also evident in individuals without autism but with severe language impairment.

Because the appearance of social abnormalities in autism typically occurs before ToM skills would even be expected to occur, and because impairments do not account for many social abnormalities in autism, such as impaired expressions of emotion (Rutter & Bailey 1993), attention has shifted to possible precursors of ToM and other social behaviours in infancy (Dawson *et al*. 1998). Modularists, such as Baron-Cohen (1995), postulate early developing modules specialized to deal with social stimuli, such as an 'eye direction detector' (EDD). Deficits in shared attentional behaviours, e.g. following another's gaze, pointing and showing, have been even more consistently documented than ToM deficits (Leekam *et al*. 1998; Sigman 1998).

Other theorists have focused on the infant's interest in facial expressions. Hobson (1993) proposed that mentalizing skills derive from children's inborn ability to perceive the affective states or attitudes of others. For Meltzoff & Gopnik (1993), the apprehension that others are like the self arises from a cross-modal mapping between the observed facial expressions and actions of others and the infant's own body movements. Although impairments have been reported in the recognition and naming of emotional expressions (Hobson *et al*. 1988), identity (Klin *et al*. 1999), holistic processing (Langdell 1978) and determination of eye gaze direction (Howard *et al*. 2000) by individuals with autism, the extent and specificity of face processing impairments and the primacy of particular cognitive processes is currently unclear and the subject of considerable scrutiny. Although facial expressions of emotion are often impaired in individuals with autistic spectrum disorders (Sigman *et al*. 1995), the relative contribution of neurological and cognitive/affective processing is not known.

Aspects of other accounts of the development of ToM may also be relevant to autistic difficulties. Russell *et al*. (1996) argued that the infant's experience of willed action is necessary for understanding the mind. Impairments in self-monitoring, as seen in impaired executive functions, were seen as critical. Moore (1996) emphasized the importance of situations in which the infant and adults were in matched psychological activity. Such opportunities may arise less frequently in autism because of other cognitive impairments. Others (Bartsch & Wellman 1995) have emphasized the role of subsequent social experience in the ongoing development of the child's ToM: opportunities that may be diminished in the lives of autistic children, who show an impaired capacity to generate social scripts (Trillingsgaard 1999).

On the other hand, able individuals with autism may eventually simulate the mental states of others based on introspection (Harris 1992). Theorizing about the acquisition of normal social behaviour has placed considerable emphasis on the role of visual input in early infant development. Nevertheless, individuals with autism are also impaired in familiar voice recognition (Boucher *et al*. 1998). Although some useful comparisons have been made with blind or deaf children (Peterson & Siegal 1997; Hobson *et al*. 1999), there is further scope for investigating the alternative cognitive strategies used to achieve social competence in the presence of sensory impairment, and examining why these are not effective in autistic individuals.

Accounting for communication deficits

One consequence of the recent focus on abnormal social development in autistic spectrum disorders has been a relative lack of interest in the mechanisms underlying abnormal language comprehension and production. Attention has mainly focused on the need to control for language level when investigating other aspects of autism (Lord & Paul 1997). This focus represents a significant shift from the earlier conceptualization of language difficulties as a core deficit (Rutter 1968). The field's focus on behaviours and cognitive processes that show diagnostic specificity may have been the major factor leading to the relative neglect of language abnormalities (and mental handicap), with the possibility raised that communication impairments were secondary consequences of impaired mentalizing abilities (Tager-Flusberg & Sullivan 1994). Nevertheless, pragmatic and conversational impairments are characteristic features of the language of individuals with both mild and severe autistic spectrum disorders.

A principal theoretical focus has been on the role of joint attentional impairments and the possibility that children who cannot achieve shared reference and understanding with others may not be motivated to learn to communicate (Mundy & Sigman 1989). Joint attention and representational play skills are strongly correlated with language skills in autistic children (Sigman 1998) but do not completely account for these language impairments. In Asperger syndrome, many aspects of language acquisition are not significantly delayed but affected individuals show some impaired joint attentional skills, albeit less than in high-functioning autism (Gilchrist *et al*. 2001). Conversely, language delay and related difficulties are found in relatives with milder phenotypes (reviewed by Bailey *et al*. 1998), although there is no suggestion that these individuals show joint attentional impairments. Even in individuals with language, although words appear to be stored with reference to their semantic properties (Tager-Flusberg 1985), retrieval in context is impaired (Happé 1997), suggesting that there are persisting abnormalities in the overall organization of the language system.

Accounting for repetitive and stereotyped behaviours

Although autistic spectrum disorders are characterized by limited imaginative play and creative activities and a tendency to stereotyped and repetitive behaviours, the relationship between limits in creativity, imagination and social communication skills and repetitive behaviours is unlikely to be simple. The intensity of interests and routines in some individuals tends to suggest that they represent a primary abnormality rather than an attempt to fill a 'creative vacuum'. An alternative explanation may be that both deficits and abnormalities are linked to a broader abnormality, such as executive functioning. Executive function refers to a set of higher cognitive abilities involved in maintaining an appropriate problem-solving network (Pennington & Ozonoff 1996). A suggestion that deficits in this area were the most likely explanation for repetitive and stereotyped behaviours first arose on the basis of comparisons with patients with acquired frontal lobe damage (Damasio & Maurer 1978). Impairments have been found in executive processes that can potentially contribute to rigid and repetitive behaviours: switching set and preservation, planning and organization, working memory, and generativity (Ozonoff 1995). Nevertheless, not all executive impairments are evident early in development (Griffith et al. 1999), suggesting that other cognitive or neurological processes are likely to be implicated.

Occasionally, intense interests and activities are associated with savant skills (Hermelin 2001). How these skills relate to other aspects of repetitive behaviours is unclear. Young & Nettlebeck (1994) found that calendrical calculators showed extreme concentration and motivation, had particularly reliable delayed recall of information, and practised regularly but applied strategies in a rigid form. Other researchers have also noted unusual perceptual processing (Plaisted et al. 1998) and increased discrimination of false memories (Beversdorf et al. 2000) in individuals with autism. One attempt to explain the coexistence of superior skills and deficits has been the suggestion that individuals with autistic spectrum disorders show weak central coherence: they have a tendency to process incoming information in context with an emphasis on detail rather than high-level meaning (Frith 1989). With the exception of studies of verbal-semantic coherence (Frith & Snowling 1983; Happé 1997), most attention has focused on studying the balance of global/local processing in visuospatial-constructional tasks, such as block design or the identification of embedded figures— an area in which individuals with autism usually show preserved abilities (reviewed by Happé 1999). Whether the same cognitive processes are relevant in language and complex social situations is not clear.

Attentional abnormalities

Information processing researchers have also investigated the role of other fundamental psychological mechanisms in autistic spectrum disorders. In the past, these were pitted against impairments in specific socioemotional processes, but lately there has been an increasing acceptance of the potential coexistence of specific and non-specific abnormalities. Attentional impairments have been the subject of theoretical accounts of autism since the late 1960s (Rimland 1964). These were motivated by the apparent highly focused attention of children with autistic disorders on minor environmental stimuli. Difficulties in visual orienting and attentional shifting have been a source of interest (Wainwright-Sharp & Bryson 1993; Townsend et al. 1999), and have been linked with putative cerebellar abnormalities (Harris et al. 1999) but not consistently (Pascualvaca et al. 1998). Sustained attention appears intact except, possibly, for individuals with autism and severe mental retardation (Burack et al. 1997). In a comprehensive study of information processing abilities in able individuals, Minshew et al. (1997) found normal or superior performance on simple attentional tasks but impair-

ments in skilled motor, complex memory, complex language and reasoning tasks. A recent study of infants with autistic spectrum disorders (Swettenham et al. 1998) found decreased looking at people compared with objects and reduced attentional shifting between objects and people, suggesting complex influences on the allocation of attentional resources.

Neurobiology

The findings from a large number of neurobiological studies have been summarized in two comprehensive books (Bauman & Kemper 1994; Gillberg & Coleman 2000). Many of the data are contradictory (Bailey et al. 1996). This area of study is problematic, partly because we know relatively little about the functioning of the normal brain and even less about the acquisition of skills during normal development. In addition, many of the features of autistic spectrum disorders that require a biological explanation, including early onset, sex ratio, association with mental handicap, and the onset of seizures in late adolescence and early adult life, have not been addressed. Also, there has been little or no study of the milder and partial phenotypes seen in some relatives.

Neuropathology

Kemper & Bauman (1998) undertook the first major neuropathological study, reporting abnormally small, densely packed neurones in the hippocampus, subiculum, mammillary body, septal nuclei and some amygdala subnuclei of nine brains. No abnormalities were noted in the cerebral cortex. In the same brains, there was evidence of decreased Purkinje cell density in the cerebellum. Findings from other comprehensive published post-mortem studies are somewhat different. Bailey et al. (1998) reported that four of seven brains were megalencephalic. Limited sampling revealed other cortical dysgenetic lesions in most of the cases. There were also obvious developmental abnormalities of the brainstem, particularly of the inferior olive. There was no apparent increase in neuronal density in the hippocampus, although decreased Purkinje cell density was identified, sometimes accompanied by gliosis. Significantly increased brain weight was also noted in the majority of individuals in the series of Kemper & Bauman (1998).

These findings have been open to various interpretations. Thus, Kemper and Bauman suggested that forebrain abnormalities underlie autistic symptomatology, whereas the decreased number of Purkinje cells together with the reported hypoplasia of cerebellar vermal lobules VI–VII (Courchesne et al. 1988) led to the suggestion of a cerebellar pathogenesis (Courchesne et al. 1994). Bailey et al. (1998) noted that autism was associated with widespread neurodevelopmental abnormalities and speculated that areas of focal cortical dysgenesis indexed a more pervasive abnormality in cortical organization. The true significance of the various post-mortem findings will have to be judged in relation to convergent evidence concerning structural and functional abnormalities.

Structural imaging studies

The many neuroimaging studies of autism have been recently reviewed (Filipek 1999; Chugani 2000; Santosh 2000). In terms of replication of post-mortem findings, increased brain volume has been reported in four studies (Howard *et al.* 2000), with some suggestion that frontal lobe volumes are not increased. Whether the underlying cause is an increase in cell number (Bailey *et al.* 1998) has yet to be confirmed. The evidence of increased head circumference (Woodhouse *et al.* 1996; Lainhart *et al.* 1997) is in keeping with the post-mortem and magnetic resonance imaging (MRI) findings, with some indications that increased head size may be a familial trait (Stevenson *et al.* 1997). With regard to the hippocampus and amygdala, these structures have been reported in different studies as unchanged, decreased and increased in size (Piven *et al.* 1998; Howard *et al.* 2000). Autism is not associated with hippocampal sclerosis.

There has been disagreement about the claims of specific hypoplasia of cerebellar vermal lobules VI and VII (Courchesne *et al.* 1988). Interpretation of the medial temporal lobe findings is problematic, both because of the relatively small size of the amygdala and hippocampus and because of the need to control for cerebral volume. Bolton & Griffiths (1997) noted an association with tubers located in the temporal lobes in individuals with tuberous sclerosis and autism, although whether these tubers primarily disrupted function of medial temporal structures or the neocortex is unclear. In terms of other structural imaging findings, there are occasional reports of localized cortical developmental abnormalities but no consistency in their site. Several studies have reported a disproportionately small corpus callosum (Piven *et al.* 1997c), raising the possibility of disturbed axonal path formation.

Studies of brain function

Along with epilepsy (Rutter 1970), one of the first indications of abnormal brain function in autism came from EEG studies. With repeated and/or extensive testing, EEG abnormalities are found in about 50% of individuals with autism (Minshew 1991). There is no evidence of regional localization of abnormalities, although regional differences in EEG power have been reported (Dawson *et al.* 1995). It has recently been suggested that autistic regression is a consequence of epileptiform activity (Lewine *et al.* 1999) but this has not been found consistently (Tuchman & Rapin 1997). Resting single photon emission computed tomography (SPECT) and positron emission tomography (PET) studies have not found consistent evidence of globally decreased or increased blood flow. There is one report (Zilbovicius *et al.* 1995) of reduced frontal perfusion in young autistic children, but it was unremarkable 3 years later, and Horwitz *et al.* (1988) reported decreased interregional correlations in metabolic rates, raising the possibility of impaired functional connectivity.

For many years, event-related potentials (ERPs) were the only means available to investigate brain function during specific cognitive tasks (Burack *et al.* 1997). The data from many of these studies are particularly contradictory, probably in part because of the low spatial resolution of EEG. The utility of studies of brain function in autistic spectrum disorders will be significantly increased with the development of functional MRI (fMRI) and magneto-encephalographic techniques. Several studies illustrate the potential of these fMRI approaches. Baron-Cohen *et al.* (1999) found that able individuals with autism or Asperger syndrome failed to activate the amygdala in an fMRI study of judging thinking or feeling from photographs of eyes. Schultz *et al.* (2000), using similar methodology, found that adults with autism or Asperger syndrome showed less activation of the right fusiform gyrus in a face recognition task. Magneto-encephalographic studies have found lack of face specificity in right fusiform gyrus (Swithenby *et al.* 2000) and impaired contextual effects in reading, possibly related to differences in the time course of representations (Bailey *et al.* in press). Other approaches to identifying neurological abnormalities are also available; Minshew *et al.* (1999) demonstrated normal cerebellar control of eye movements but impairments in cortically controlled saccades.

Neurochemical studies

Over the years, all the major neurotransmitter systems have been implicated in autistic spectrum disorders at some time but, despite the research effort in this field, many findings have not replicated (see reviews by Cook 1990; Anderson & Hoshino 1997). The most consistent findings relate to the serotonergic system. Elevated levels of whole blood serotonin have been observed in 25–33% of autistic subjects (Anderson *et al.* 1987), although more recent studies suggest that the elevation may be more prevalent in prepubertal individuals (McBride *et al.* 1998). Breakdown products are not elevated in cerebrospinal fluid, and elevated peripheral serotonin levels are also found in severe mental retardation. Hyperserotonaemia may arise on the basis of multiple mechanisms, as non-retarded relatives of hyperserotonaemic probands are also reported to show increased levels of whole blood serotonin (Cook 1996).

SSRIs have beneficial effects in the treatment of some individuals with autism, particularly reducing anxiety and obsessive-compulsive behaviours. In contrast, tryptophan depletion techniques were reported to result in a significant increase in autistic behaviours (McDougle *et al.* 1996). One PET scan study revealed decreased 5-HT synthesis in frontal cortex and thalamus, but elevated 5-HT synthesis in the contralateral dentate nucleus (Chugani *et al.* 1997). A preliminary study also found that the normal developmental process, whereby humans undergo a period of high brain 5-HT synthesis capacity until the age of 5 years, appears disrupted in children with autism (Chugani *et al.* 1999). The extent to which the observed abnormalities are primary causes of autism or simply one of the many consequences of abnormal brain development that also contribute to symptomatology is presently unclear.

The post-mortem and neuroimaging data together raise the possibility that autistic spectrum disorders affect the develop-

Table 38.1 Overall treatment programme.

Feedback to family
Diagnosis, prognosis and treatment
Genetic counselling

Medical care
Correction of hearing/vision defects
Dental care
Treatment of medical conditions (when present)

Special educational provision
Suitable class or unit or adequately supported inclusion
Extra services required
Transition planning
Vocational support and training

Treatment of child's deficits/problems
Behavioural treatments
Speech/language therapy
Social groups
Medication (when appropriate)
Other psychological therapies

Help for family
Use of behavioural/developmental methods
Counselling
Practical help
Respite
Support and advocacy groups
Books and media access

ment and function of both the cerebral cortex and subcortical structures with considerable interindividual variation. The outstanding question is whether any one of these abnormalities is truly primary, or whether the fundamental problem lies in connectivity within and between different structures.

Treatment and intervention

The specifics of treatment will necessarily vary across children and families but it is helpful to have an overall plan of areas that will always need coverage (see Table 38.1; Rutter 1985). Necessarily, this begins with feedback to the family and ensuring that medical care needs are met. An individualized plan is necessary with specific, immediate and long-term objectives appropriate to the chronological age and developmental level of the child. This should incorporate special educational provision, treatment of the child's deficits and problems, and help for the family. Working with a family is an important part of any evaluation. Clinicians must familiarize themselves with sources of information about services in their communities and work with professionals from many other disciplines in order to be effective in the treatment of autistic spectrum disorders.

Education

Education has been the most powerful source of improvement for children and adolescents with autistic spectrum disorders in the last 50 years (National Research Council 2001). With access to appropriate educational services, far fewer children are placed in long-stay institutions (Schopler & Olley 1982; Howlin & Goode 1998), rates of functional language may be higher, and there are more direct relationships between ability levels and eventual academic functioning of individuals with autistic spectrum disorders (Venter *et al.* 1992).

There is good evidence that specific behaviours and skills can be directly taught to children and adults with autism, although there are limitations to the generalization and spontaneous usage of skills learned (Lord 2000). Children with autism can be taught ToM skills, but the social benefits have been minimal (Ozonoff & Miller 1995; Hadwin *et al.* 1996). Although most studies of the effects of different methods of instruction were carried out on small samples, many have been replicated. Increasingly, the emphasis has been on teaching children proactive behaviours (e.g. learning to communicate using objects and pictures, being able to respond to a teacher's direction within a group), rather than on eliminating negative behaviours, with the assumption that many problem behaviours decrease with the child's understanding and acquisition of skills (Carr *et al.* 1999).

There have been few direct comparisons of different teaching strategies. This lack is partly caused by the heterogeneity of needs of individuals with autistic spectrum disorders, so that a programme appropriate for one child may not be relevant for another, and in part because carrying out well-controlled randomized comparisons with independent evaluations is extremely difficult in educational settings.

Gains in education have come from diverse areas (see Howlin, Chapter 68), but it is the role of early intervention that has caused the most controversy. Applied behaviour analysis (ABA) is a technique that involves one-on-one repeated presentations by an adult of materials and behaviours intended to elicit specific responses. The adult says, for example, 'Get ready. Look at me!' and the child is expected to put his or her feet on the floor, hands in his or her lap and look at the adult. Behavioural approaches include reinforcement schedules and hierarchies, methods of 'shaping' behaviours and techniques in teaching associations (Leaf & McEachin 1999). Lovaas (1987) carried out a group design study of ABA with very young preschool-age children with autism. The study included quasi-random assignment to treatment conditions and produced extraordinary results, both in the breadth of improvement of some children who were described as 'indistinguishable from normal' by school age, and in the proportion of children with autism who showed such great improvements (nearly half). In the 1990s, numerous studies, using the original ABA techniques and modified versions, replicated findings of significant but smaller improvements in intellectual skills (gains of about 20 points; Smith *et al.* 2000) but did not find the restoration of 'normal' functioning that was first reported (Leaf & McEachin 1999; Smith 1999). Overall, these findings resulted in a general increase in intensity and organization of services for preschool-age children.

There are many different 'packages' of model programmes, mostly for preschool and early school-age children with autism (Handleman & Harris 2000). Although these programmes have different emphases, they share many common features. Most of these features apply to programmes for school-age children as well (Rutter 1985). These features include entry into programmes at an early age (usually at 2 or 3 years); full-day programming (at least 25 h a week); repeated planned activities organized in small units of time (e.g. 15–20 min) with a low student : teacher ratio; inclusion of family goals and parent training; and mechanisms for ongoing assessment and changes in strategy if measurable progress does not occur within several months (Dawson & Osterling 1997; Howlin 1998; Rogers 1998; Hurth *et al.* 1999). Other features include the idea of *structure* (clearly discernible expectations and physical representations of planned activities, e.g. visual schedules; Marcus *et al.* 2000), *developmental appropriateness* (building new behaviours on behaviours the child already has), and *using strengths to support gains in weaker areas.*

More variability across programmes exists as to whether even more intensive programming (up to 40–50 h a week) should occur; where it should occur (home vs. school); the proportion of time in incidental teaching vs. highly structured, teacher-directed programming; when and how interactions with peers should be addressed; and whether a purely speech-based approach, with no use of alternative language systems, is ever appropriate. Because there are such great differences in families of children within the autism spectrum and in the resources available across school systems, decisions must be based on what is best for an individual child and family (Howlin & Rutter 1987). How best to integrate the 'active ingredients' from ABA and other well-known programmes, such as Treatment and Education of Children, Adolescents and Adults with Autism (TEACCH; Mesibov 1997; Marcus *et al.* 2000) which involves a multilevel family and community-orientated approach; more peer-orientated programmes, such as Walden School (McGee *et al.* 2000) or LEAP (Strain & Hoyson 2000); and more 'natural teaching' approaches (Greenspan & Wieder 1997; Wetherby & Prizant 1999) merits further study. In general, good evidence that specific strategies are effective (such as using schedules and visual systems and home-based parent training) is available (Howlin & Rutter 1987; Ozonoff & Cathcart 1998), but research comparing various treatments or programmes is not (Rogers 1998). Information about many different programmes is currently available on the Internet, often with extraordinary claims for outcome. This can be quite confusing for parents.

Research has suggested that when children with autism have opportunities to play with typically developing children in situations where there is skilled adult guidance, they have fewer behaviour problems and more social interaction than with peers with autism (McGee *et al.* 2000). On the other hand, in less well-supervised settings with typical children, children with autistic

spectrum disorders may have minimal interactions, little directed behaviour and significant behavioural difficulties (Guralnick 1976). The principle of seeking the least restrictive environment that is appropriate for each child offers opportunities to children who might have been excluded out of hand, but the level of structure, support and knowledge of the teaching staff is crucial. Often, plans where children with autism spend some time in highly structured individualized or small group teaching and other time where there are opportunities for positive interactions with other children are most effective. However, individualization is most important.

Help for family

Families have multiple roles in their children's lives, particularly when their child has an autistic spectrum disorder (Harris 1994). They provide emotional support and act as teachers, models of behaviour and social interaction and advocates for services. Concerns vary even within a family across time, as do the roles that parents need and want to serve for their children. The degree to which spouses are able to support each other (Bristol *et al.* 1988) and have time to spend with other children in the family are critical factors (Celiberti & Harris 1993).

Parents experience a range of emotions in response to having a child with autism, and for some families this results in considerable stress. Helping parents to accept the disappointment and fear that they feel, know that ambivalent feelings are acceptable, and that they are not alone in these feelings is part of treatment. Practical help, such as in finding respite care or dealing with social services or educational systems, may be as important as emotional support and teaching management techniques.

Parents not only need information about what they should do but how they might do this (Runco & Schreibman 1987). It is much more useful to work with parents to devise ways in which they will respond to their child's tantrums or get him or her to bed than simply to direct them to solve the problem. There is a substantial literature on working with parents in the home and in clinics (Howlin & Rutter 1987; Schopler *et al.* 1990). In order to make useful suggestions, familiarity with the child, the family and community resources is essential. Support for families is available from a wide range of agencies concerned with both autism and learning disorders. In addition, many parents take on an advocacy role for their children, which may require other new skills. Parent-based groups have made significant differences in the dissemination of knowledge, development of specific programmes (such as summer camps, social groups and residential services) and the stimulation of research funding in the UK and USA.

Specific therapies

Many different therapies are available: speech and language therapy, occupational therapy, physical therapy, cognitive-behaviour or individual psychotherapy for older high-functioning adolescents and adults, and social groups (Cohen &

Volkmar 1997), but there is little evidence on their relative efficacy (National Research Council 2001). It seems likely that it is not the profession of the therapists but what they teach, and their knowledge and abilities to teach this skill well, that make a difference. Different treatment paradigms such as auditory training (Bettison 1996), facilitated communication (Mirenda *et al.* 1983) and holding therapy (Richer & Zappella 1989) have tended to come and go over the years. However, working with an expert experienced with children with autism spectrum disorders to develop strategies for an individual child and family can be helpful. This is particularly true for communication and language, which are not only pivotal features of social and cognitive learning, but also are often extraordinarily limited in autism. The more the actual treatment can take place in the contexts in which the behaviours occur in real life, the more likely changes are to generalize and to be maintained over time. Thus, family involvement and active school or work consultation are critical to effective treatment.

Brief psychotherapy or cognitive-behaviour treatment may be helpful with adolescents and adults with sufficient verbal skills to be able to discuss their social difficulties and/or who may have cooccurring anxiety or depression. These techniques may be particularly effective when combined with social groups or consultation with a school or a job coach so that new skills can be practised in a supportive environment (Mesibov 1984; Lord 1996).

Positive behaviour support (PBS) systems address what used to be called behaviour management, by developing a comprehensive set of procedures that include changing the environment to make the problem behaviours less relevant, teaching appropriate behaviours that are more efficient than the problem behaviours in attaining the child's goals, and manipulating the consequences so that appropriate behaviours are more consistently and powerfully rewarded than are problem behaviours (for a review see Carr *et al.* 1999). Most severe behaviour problems do not go away on their own and so it is important to begin treatment early and carefully. A functional analysis that identifies the contingencies in the environment that sustain a child's problem behaviours is a crucial part of this approach (Table 38.2). The emphasis is on avoiding the use of 'aversives' or punishments and focusing on positive aspects of both the child's behaviour and the environment. *Structure* (making the environment more predictable and meaningful) often reduces the need for intense behaviour management programmes. If a non-verbal child can see from a picture schedule what his or her day's activities are, and have some choice in how he or she spends his or her free time, then he or she will be less likely to throw a tantrum when asked to do another activity.

Vocational training and support

Most individuals with autistic spectrum disorders have abilities that can be used in some type of employment although, as with other aspects of autism, there is tremendous variability across individuals. Most need help finding a place of work and support to be able to deal with social and other expectations of a job. Sys-

Table 38.2 Behavioural treatment goals.

Promotion of cognitive development and learning
    including academic and work skills
Promotion of language/communication development
    including social use of communication
Promotion of social development
    including self-help, social problem-solving and social relationships
Reduction of maladaptive behaviour
    including use of diversion, avoidance of precipitants and provision
    of coping skills

tems for providing training and ongoing support have become increasingly sophisticated (Van Bourgondien & Schopler 1990; Mawhood & Howlin 1999) but long-term support varies greatly in availability. School programmes that emphasize both general work behaviours (e.g. dealing with delays) and practice in job environments have improved the outlook for individuals with autism (Mesibov 1984; Howlin & Goode 1998).

Even for intellectually able individuals, learning appropriate work behaviours, such as respect for privacy, can be very difficult. However, great strides have been made in specific programmes to provide job coaches, 'enclaves' (where there is a core of support within a large business, such as a hotel chain, and individuals with autism work with varying degrees of support in a range of jobs) and job placement programmes (Smith *et al.* 1994). The key element for success appears to be flexibility, such as modified working hours and job requirements for individuals with autism and for their employers. With gradual training, continued support and long-term planning, it should be possible for almost every person with autism to have work in some setting. This generally requires more than simply help finding a job, but continued support on various levels from ongoing consultation to full-time staff and specialized job settings.

Many individuals with autism cannot live independently as adults. Systematic training for staff in residential programmes, from supervised apartments to group living arrangements, are available (Van Bourgondien & Schopler 1990). Many of the same features that occur in successful education characterize residential living programmes. Residential opportunities have also become much more individualized, with services ranging from supervised individual apartments to clusters of apartments and farm communities, to small-group homes. In addition, the development of leisure skills may be a long, but worthwhile, process. In many regions, there is a tremendous need for support and respite for adults with autistic spectrum disorders who are still living at home and for their families. Ongoing social groups can provide support, contact with peers with and without autism, and specific skill training beyond traditional psychiatric follow-up (Mesibov 1984; Williams 1989).

Psychopharmacology

Currently, there is no drug that has a specific ameliorative effect on autism but there is an occasional important contributory role for pharmacotherapy as an adjunct to psychological and educational interventions. Experience suggests that there are substantial variations among countries in the rate of medication use and that, outside of specialist centres, medication may quite often be the main intervention used (Aman *et al.* 1995). Injudicious medication may simply sedate a child, which, although reducing intrusive behaviours, may also diminish social interaction and the opportunity to learn. On the other hand, medication combined with behavioural analysis and appropriate psychoeducational interventions may enable a child to modify his or her behaviour in a way that would not have been possible in a drug-free state. There are several recent helpful reviews (McDougle 1997; Tsai 1999; Volkmar *et al.* 1999; see also Heyman & Santosh, Chapter 59).

Although there has been much research into the neurochemical basis of autism, pharmacotherapy is still largely based upon clinical trials rather than extrapolated from basic neurochemical findings. The majority of studies are open trials and most have been conducted in adult populations. However, clinicians may consider that a trial of medication is warranted in an individual child, even though there is no licence for use in children, and long-term safety is not yet established. In these circumstances, clinicians are advised to use medication with caution, to discuss individual cases with colleagues and to aim for as short a period of medication as is practical.

Over the years, there have been numerous claims for unusually dramatic responses to various drugs but these claims have not generally been replicated by other investigators. Probably the best-documented response has been to haloperidol (Campbell *et al.* 1990), particularly with respect to reduction in stereotypies and behavioural improvement. However, haloperidol has been associated with a high incidence of extrapyramidal side-effects, particularly when the drug is withdrawn (Campbell *et al.* 1990). Consequently, there has been much recent interest in the efficacy of the newer neuroleptics, such as risperidone and olanzapine. A double-blind placebo-controlled study of risperidone in adults with autism and other pervasive developmental disorders (McDougle *et al.* 1998) reported significant reductions in repetitive behaviour, aggression, anxiety or nervousness, and depression, although measurable changes in social behaviour and language did not occur. Open trial studies of risperidone in children have produced encouraging results (Nicolson *et al.* 1998) leading to ongoing multisite controlled studies (McDougle *et al.* 2000). Similar improvements have been reported in open trial studies of olanzapine (Potenza *et al.* 1999); nevertheless, weight gain remains a significant problem with these new drugs.

The other significant advance in the pharmacotherapy of autism and related disorders is the extent to which disabling anxiety, obsessional and repetitive behaviour and self-injury can sometimes be ameliorated by SSRIs (McDougle *et al.* 1996; Fatemi *et al.* 1998). These drugs are also an effective treatment for depression, which may be a particular problem for able individuals in adolescence. It is possible that these drugs are most effective in individuals with a family history of anxiety/depressive disorders.

Control of overactivity can often be problematic and may necessitate a trial of several different types of medication (Nicolson & Castellanos 2000). A major difficulty can be the worsening of stereotypies with stimulant use. Aman *et al.* (1995) concluded that there was little role for these medications, although others have reported beneficial effects (Quintana *et al.* 1995).

There has been some interest in the use of opiate antagonists, particularly to promote social engagement and decrease self-injurious behaviour (for a review see Tsai 1999). Naltrexone may be effective in reducing overactivity (Campbell *et al.* 1993; Willemsen-Swinkels *et al.* 1995), but other researchers have concluded that there are no positive effects (Gillberg 1995). With respect to other agents, at present there is a paucity of properly controlled clinical trials reporting consistent beneficial effects. Claims have been made for the benefits of secretin but the findings have been negative (Dunn-Geier *et al.* 2000). Similarly, although vitamin B_6 and magnesium may sometimes provide modest benefits, the results of studies do not support its regular use (Pfeiffer *et al.* 1995). Epilepsy should be managed by clinicians experienced in the use of anticonvulsant medication; the newer drugs offer significant advantages in terms of decreased cognitive impairment and long-term side-effects.

Looking to the future

Advances in understanding autistic spectrum disorders seem likely to provide important scientific and practical insights in the next few years. Standardized diagnostic measures and more appropriate measures of language and non-verbal intelligence should make replication of research across sites more straightforward and allow more systematic assessment of developmental factors. Greater collaborative efforts will allow larger samples and clearer stratification of subsets of individuals within the spectrum.

The considerable resources being expended on molecular genetic studies of autism seem likely to ensure that susceptibility loci start to be cloned in the next few years. Our understanding should accelerate rapidly once the first loci are identified, because they will point to complex pathways whose constituents will become candidates for subsequent genetic analysis. There will be much interest in whether genetic susceptibility is conferred by variation in protein-coding regions or in promoter regions or in the mechanisms that control alternative splicing of proteins. Of equal interest will be the degree of genetic heterogeneity. Identifying and understanding the mechanisms underlying genetic heterogeneity will be crucial for using genotype findings to provide improved genetic counselling.

Identification of susceptibility genes will lead directly to studies of protein function in single cell systems, if these are not already known. It might also be possible to develop an animal model of gene function. They may provide an opportunity to study the neuropathological and neurophysiological consequences of gene activity in the developing organism and to develop novel psychopharmacological strategies. There is likely to be an impact on post-mortem studies, both in terms of orientating researchers to potentially relevant pathology as well as enabling identification of more homogeneous groups of cases.

Functional imaging approaches provide a means to move beyond localization of abnormal brain activity to an understanding of the underlying mechanisms. Equally importantly, neuroimaging approaches offer one of the few opportunities to identify when normal task performance (in both affected individuals and their relatives) is mediated by abnormal mechanisms. At present, the potential of PET radioligand approaches, especially in the study of psychopharmacological mechanisms, is unclear.

There have been significant advances in our understanding of some central aspects of developmental psychopathology in autistic spectrum disorders. Nevertheless, there is still a need to identify more accurately those abnormalities that are potentially specific as well as understanding the possible interactions among different processes early in development. That task represents a considerable intellectual and practical challenge that will require a combining of many different types of approaches. The ability to identify more homogeneous groups of individuals will be advantageous, particularly in terms of understanding the mechanisms underlying effective early intervention. Increasingly, attention may shift to milder manifestations of autism spectrum disorders. Variability in phenotypic expression offers an opportunity to examine the role of specific cognitive deficits and their relationship to behavioural traits as well as establishing the extent to which these are consequences of single or multiple genes, as well as determining whether such genes are responsible for variations in similar behavioural traits in nonautistic groups.

There is a clear need for more efficient and broader mechanisms to evaluate interventions. The merging of various techniques in intervention, such as those described in ABA, developmental and TEACCH models, provides more comprehensive strategies but also makes the evaluation of critical components more difficult (National Research Council 2001). Attempts to integrate knowledge from outcomes of intervention, neurobiological research and descriptive studies are much needed. The development of statistical methods that allow quantification of individual differences within models of change or continuity may be particularly helpful.

In clinical work, difficulties in dissemination and availability of services are often even more limiting than the absence of knowledge. The strong upsurge in interest from parents' organizations in neurobiological research has had remarkable effects but should not take away from continued parent and professional advocacy for clinical and educational services. Service models should be modified to address the needs of individuals, from younger children to older adults and their families. The importance of multiple faceted individual treatment plans, specific to a particular child and family and supported by knowledgeable clinicians and educators, must continue to be recognized, as models for evidence-based and manualized interventions are disseminated. How to extend the responsibility from family and clinician to community bases is also a major challenge. Overall, there is much hope for improved understanding and the identification of neurobiological factors in the next decade. However, as these investigations proceed, the roles of clinicians and educators continue to be most likely to affect the lives of families and children with autistic spectrum disorders.

References

Aman, M.G. & Singh, M.G. (1986) *Manual for the Aberrant Behavior Checklist*. Slosson Educational Publications, East Aurora.

Aman, M.G., Van Bourgondien, M.E., Wolford, P.L. & Sarphare, G. (1995) Psychotropic and anticonvulsant drugs in subjects with autism: prevalence and patterns of use. *Journal of the American Academy of Child and Adolescent Psychiatry*, **34**, 1672–1681.

American Psychological Association (2000) *Diagnostic and Statistical Manual of Mental Disorders Revision (DSM-IV-TR)*, 4th edn. American Psychiatric Association, Washington D.C.

Amir, R.E., Van den Veyver, I.B., Wan, M., Tran, C.Q., Francke, U. & Zoghbi, H.Y. (1999) Rett syndrome is caused by mutations in X-linked MECP2, encoding methyl-CpG-binding protein 2. *Nature Genetics*, **23**, 185–188.

Anderson, G.M. & Hoshino, Y. (1997) Neurochemical studies of autism. In: *Handbook of Autism and Pervasive Developmental Disorder* (eds D.J. Cohen & F.R. Volkmar), 2nd edn, pp. 325–343. John Wiley & Sons, New York.

Anderson, G.M., Freedman, C.X., Cohen, D.J. *et al.* (1987) Whole blood serotonin in autistic and normal subjects. *Journal of Child Psychology and Psychiatry*, **28**, 885–900.

Arvidsson, T., Danielsson, B., Forsberg, P., Gillberg, C., Johansson, M. & Kjellgren, G. (1997) Autism in 3–6-year-old children in a suburb of Goeteborg, Sweden. *Autism*, **1**, 163–173.

Asperger, H. (1944) Die 'Autistischen Psychopathen' im Kindesalter. *Archiv für Psychiatrie und Nervenkrankheiten*, **117**, 76–136 (see Frith 1991 for English translation).

Attwood, T. (1997) *Asperger's Syndrome: a Guide for Parents and Professionals*. Jessica Kingsley, London.

Bailey, A., Le Couteur, A., Gottesman, I. *et al.* (1995) Autism as a strongly genetic disorder: evidence from a British twin study. *Psychological Medicine*, **25**, 63–77.

Bailey, A., Philips, W. & Rutter, M. (1996) Autism: towards an integration of clinical, genetic, neuropsychological, and neurobiological perspectives. *Journal of Child Psychology and Psychiatry*, **37**, 89–126

Bailey, A., Palferman, S., Heavey, L. & Le Couteur, A. (1998) Autism: the phenotype in relatives. *Journal of Autism and Developmental Disorders*, **28** (5), 369–392.

Bailey, A., Braeutigam, S. & Swithenby, S. (in press) Context and reading: a magnetoencephalographic study of autistic adults. *Proceedings of Biomagnetism*,

Baird, G., Charman, T., Baron-Cohen, S. *et al.* (2000) A screening instrument for autism at 18 months of age: a 6-year follow-up study. *Journal of the American Academy of Child and Adolescent Psychiatry*, **39**, 694–702.

Baranek, G.T. (1999) Autism during infancy: a retrospective video-analysis of sensorimotor and social behaviors at 9–12 months of age. *Journal of Autism and Developmental Disorders*, 29, 213–224.

Baron-Cohen, S. (1990) Autism: a specific cognitive disorder of 'mind-blindness'. *International Review of Psychiatry*, 2, 79–88.

Baron-Cohen, S. (1995) *Mindblindness: an Essay on Autism and Theory of Mind.* MIT Press, Cambridge, MA.

Baron-Cohen, S., Leslie, A.M. & Frith, U. (1985) Does the autistic child have a 'theory of mind?' *Cognition*, 21, 37–46.

Baron-Cohen, S., Allen, J. & Gillberg, C. (1992) Can autism be detected at 18 months? The needle, the haystack, and the CHAT. *British Journal of Psychiatry*, 161, 839–843.

Baron-Cohen, S., Ring, H.A., Wheelwright, S. *et al.* (1999) Social intelligence in the normal and autistic brain: an fMRI study. *European Journal of Neuroscience*, 11, 1891–1898.

Bartak, L. & Rutter, M. (1973) Special educational treatment of autistic children: a comparative study. I. Design of study and characteristics of units. *Journal of Child Psychology and Psychiatry and Allied Disciplines*, 14, 161–179.

Barton, M. & Volkmar, F. (1998) How commonly are known medical conditions associated with autism? *Journal of Autism and Developmental Disorders*, 28, 273–278.

Bartsch, K. & Wellman, H.M. (1995) *Children Talk About the Mind.* Oxford University Press, New York.

Bauman, M.L. & Kemper, T.L. (1994) *Neurobiology of Autism.* Johns Hopkins University Press, Baltimore.

Bender, L. (1942) Childhood schizophrenia. *Nervous Child*, 1, 138–140.

Berument, S.K., Rutter, M., Lord, C., Pickles, A. & Bailey, A. (1999) Autism Screening Questionnaire: diagnostic validity. *British Journal of Psychiatry*, 175, 444–451.

Bettison, S. (1996) The long-term effects of auditory training on children with autism. *Journal of Autism and Developmental Disorders*, 26, 361–374.

Beversdorf, D.Q., Smith, B.W., Crucia, G.P. *et al.* (2000) Increased discrimination of 'false memories' in autism spectrum disorder. *Proceedings of the National Academy of Sciences USA*, 97, 8734–8737.

Bishop, D.V. (1989) Autism, Asperger's syndrome and semantic-pragmatic disorder: where are the boundaries? *British Journal of Disorders of Communication*, 24, 107–121.

Black, B. & Uhde, T.W. (1995) Psychiatric characteristics of children with selective mutism: a pilot study. *Journal of the American Academy of Child and Adolescent Psychiatry*, 34, 847–856.

Bolton, P.F. & Griffiths, P.D. (1997) Association of tuberous sclerosis of temporal lobes with autism and atypical autism. *Lancet*, 349, 392–395.

Bolton, P., Macdonald, H., Pickles, A. *et al.* (1994) A case–control family history study of autism. *Journal of Child Psychology and Psychiatry*, 35, 877–900.

Bolton, P.F., Murphy, M., Macdonald, H., Whitlock, B., Pickles, A. & Rutter, M. (1997) Obstetric complications in autism: consequences or causes of the condition? *Journal of American Academy of Child and Adolescent Psychiatry*, 36, 272–281.

Bolton, P.F., Pickles, A., Murphy, M. & Rutter, M. (1998) Autism, affective and other psychiatric disorders: patterns of familial aggregation. *Psychological Medicine*, 28, 385–395.

Bosch, G. (1970) *Infantile Autism* [translated by D.J. Jordan & I. Jordan]. Springer-Verlag, New York.

Boucher, J. (1998) SPD as a distinct diagnostic entity: logical considerations and directions for future research. *International Journal of Language and Communication Disorders*, 33, 71–108.

Boucher, J., Lewis, V. & Collis, G. (1998) Familiar face and voice matching and recognition in children with autism. *Journal of Child Psychology and Psychiatry*, 39, 171–181.

Bristol, M.M., Gallagher, J.J. & Schopler, E. (1988) Mothers and fathers of young developmentally disabled and non-disabled boys: adaptation and spousal support. *Developmental Psychology*, 24, 441–451.

Buitelaar, J.K., Van der Gaag, R., Klin, A. & Volkmar, F. (1999) Exploring the boundaries of Pervasive Developmental Disorder Not Otherwise Specified: analyses of data from the DSM-IV autistic disorder field trial. *Journal of Autism and Developmental Disorders*, 29, 33–43.

Burack, J.A., Enns, J.T., Stauder, J.E., Mottron, L. & Randolph, B. (1997) Attention and autism: behavioral and electrophysiological evidence. In: *Handbook of Autism and Pervasive Developmental Disorder* (eds D.J. Cohen & F.R. Volkmar), 2nd edn, pp. 226–242. John Wiley & Sons, New York.

Campbell, M., Locascio, J.J., Choroco, M.C. *et al.* (1990) Stereotypies and tardive dyskinesia: abnormal movements in autistic children. *Psychopharmacology Bulletin*, 26, 260–266.

Campbell, M., Anderson, L.T., Small, A.M., Adams, P., Gonzalez, N.M. & Ernst, M. (1993) Naltrexone in autistic children: behavioral symptoms and attentional learning. *Journal of the American Academy of Child and Adolescent Psychiatry*, 32, 1283–1291.

Carr, E.G., Horner, R.H., Turnball, A.P. *et al.*, eds (1999) *Positive Behavior Support for People with Developmental Disabilities.* American Association on Mental Retardation Monograph Series, Washington D.C.

Carter, A.S., Volkmar, F.R., Sparrow, S.S. *et al.* (1998) The Vineland Adaptive Behavior Scales: supplementary norms for individuals with autism. *Journal of Autism and Developmental Disorders*, 28, 287–302.

Celiberti, D.A. & Harris, S.L. (1993) Behavioral intervention for siblings of children with autism: a focus on skills to enhance play. *Behavior Therapy*, 24, 573–599.

Chakrabarti, S. & Fombonne, E. (2001) Pervasive developmental disorders in preschool children. *Journal of the American Medical Association*, 285, 3093–3099.

Chugani, D.C. (2000) Autism. In: *Functional Neuroimaging in Child Psychiatry* (eds M. Ernst & J.M. Rumsey), pp. 171–188. Cambridge University Press, Cambridge.

Chugani, D.C., Muzik, O., Rothermel, R. *et al.* (1997) Altered serotonin synthesis in the dentatothalamocortical pathway in autistic boys. *Annals of Neurology*, 42, 666–669.

Chugani, D.C., Muzik, O., Behen, M. *et al.* (1999) Developmental changes in brain serotonin synthesis capacity in autistic and nonautistic children. *Annals of Neurology*, 45, 287–295.

Cohen, D.J. & Volkmar, F.R., eds (1997) *Handbook of Autism and Pervasive Developmental Disorders*, 2nd edn. John Wiley & Sons, New York.

Cook, E.H. (1990) Autism: review of neurochemical investigation. *Synapse*, 6, 292–308.

Cook, E.H. (1996) Pathophysiology of autism: neurochemistry [Brief report]. *Journal of Autism and Developmental Disorders*, 26, 221–225.

Cook, E.H., Courchesne, R., Lord, C. *et al.* (1997a) Evidence of linkage between the serotonin transporter and autistic disorder. *Molecular Psychiatry*, 2, 247–250.

Cook, E.H., Lindgren, V., Leventhal, B.L. *et al.* (1997b) Autism or atypical autism in maternally but not paternally derived proximal 15q duplication. *American Journal of Human Genetics*, 60, 928–934.

Cook, E.H., Courchesne, R.Y., Cox, N.J. *et al.* (1998) Linkage-disequilibrium mapping of autistic disorder, with 15q11–13 markers. *American Journal of Human Genetics*, 62, 1077–1083.

Corbett, J., Harris, R., Taylor, E. & Trimble, M. (1977) Progressive disintegrative psychosis of childhood. *Journal of Child Psychology and Psychiatry*, **18**, 211–219.

Courchesne, E., Yeung-Courchesne, R., Press, G.A., Hesselink, J.R. & Jernigan, T.L. (1988) Hypoplasia of cerebellar vermal lobules VI and VII in autism. *New England Journal of Medicine*, **318**, 1349–1354.

Courchesne, C., Townsend, J. & Saitoh, O. (1994) The brain in infantile autism: posterior fossa structures are abnormal. *Neurology*, **44**, 214–223.

Cox, A., Klein, K., Charman, T. *et al.* (1999) Autism spectrum disorders at 20 and 42 months of age: stability of clinical and ADI-R diagnosis. *Journal of Child Psychology and Psychiatry*, **40**, 719–732.

Curry, C.J., Stevenson, R.E., Aughton, D. *et al.* (1997) Evaluation of mental retardation: recommendations of a consensus conference: American College of Medical Genetics. *American Journal of Medical Genetics*, **72**, 468–477.

Dahlgren, S.O. & Gillberg, C. (1989) Symptoms in the first two years of life: a preliminary population study of infantile autism. *European Archives of Psychiatry and Neurological Science*, **238**, 169–174.

Dales, L., Hammer, S.J. & Smith, N.J. (2001) Time trends in autism and in MMR immunization coverage in California. *Journal of the American Medical Association*, **285**, 1183–1185.

Damasio, A.R. & Maurer, R.G. (1978) A neurological model for childhood autism. *Archives of Neurology*, **35**, 777–786.

Dawson, G. & Osterling, J. (1997) Early intervention in autism: effectiveness and common elements of current approaches. In: *The Effectiveness of Early Intervention: Second Generation Research* (ed. M. Guralnick), pp. 307–326. Brookes, Baltimore.

Dawson, G., Klinger, L.G., Panagiotides, H., Lewy, A. & Castelloe, P. (1995) Subgroups of autistic children based on social behavior display distinct patterns of brain activity. *Journal of Abnormal Child Psychology*, **23**, 569–583.

Dawson, G., Meltzoff, A.N., Osterling, J. & Rinaldi, J. (1998) Neuropsychological correlates of early symptoms of autism. *Child Development*, **69**, 1276–1285.

De Giacomo, A. & Fombonne, E. (1998) Parental recognition of developmental abnormalities in autism. *European Child and Adolescent Psychiatry*, **7**, 131–136.

DeLong, R. & Nohria, C. (1994) Psychiatric family history and neurological disease in autistic spectrum disorders. *Developmental Medicine and Child Neurology*, **36**, 441–448.

DeMyer, M.K., Barton, S. & Norton, J.A. (1972) A comparison of adaptive, verbal, and motor profiles of psychotic and nonpsychotic subnormal children. *Journal of Autism and Childhood Schizophrenia*, **2**, 359–377.

Deonna, T. (2000) Acquired epileptic aphasia (AEA) or Landau–Kleffner syndrome: from childhood to adulthood. In: *Speech and Language Impairments in Children: Causes, Characteristics, Intervention and Outcome* (eds D.V.M. Bishop & L.B. Leonard), pp. 261–272. Psychology Press/Taylor & Francis, Philadelphia.

DiLavore, P.C., Lord, C. & Rutter, M. (1995) The Pre-Linguistic Autism Diagnostic Observation Schedule. *Journal of Autism and Developmental Disorders*, **25**, 355–379.

Dummit, E.S. III, Klein, R.G., Tancer, N.K., Asche, B., Martin, J. & Fairbanks, J.A. (1997) Systematic assessment of 50 children with selective mutism. *Journal of the American Academy of Child and Adolescent Psychiatry*, **36**, 653–660.

Dunn-Geier, J., Ho, H.H., Auersperg, E. *et al.* (2000) Effects of secretin on children with autism: a randomized controlled trial. *Developmental Medicine and Child Neurology*, **42**, 796–802.

Dykens, E.M. & Volkmar, F.R. (1997) Medical conditions associated with autism. In: *Handbook of Autism and Pervasive Developmental Disorders* (eds D.J. Cohen & F.R. Volkmar), pp. 388–410. John Wiley & Sons, New York.

Eisenberg, L. & Kanner, L. (1956) Early infantile autism, 1943–55. *American Journal of Orthopsychiatry*, **26**, 556–566.

Eisenmajer, R., Prior, M., Leekam, S. *et al.* (1996) Comparison of clinical symptoms in autism and Asperger's disorder. *Journal of the American Academy of Child and Adolescent Psychiatry*, **35**, 1523–1531.

Fatemi, S.H., Realmuto, G.M., Khan, L. & Thuras, P. (1998) Fluoxetine in treatment of adolescent patients with autism: a longitudinal open trial. *Journal of Autism and Developmental Disorders*, **28**, 303–307.

Fein, D., Stevens, M., Dunn, M. *et al.* (1999) Subtypes of pervasive developmental disorder: clinical characteristics. *Child Neuropsychology*, **5**, 1–23.

Filipek, P.A. (1999) Neuroimaging in the developmental disorders: the state of the science. *Journal of Child Psychology and Psychiatry*, **40**, 113–128.

Filipek, P.A., Accardo, P.J., Ashwal, S. *et al.* (2000) Practice parameter: screening and diagnosis of autism. Report of the Quality Standards Subcommittee of the American Academy of Neurology and the Child Neurology Society. *Neurology*, **55**, 468–479.

Fischel, J.E., Whitehurst, G.J., Caulfield, M.B. & DeBaryshe, B. (1989) Language growth in children with expressive language delay. *Pediatrics*, **83**, 218–227.

Flavell, J.H. (1999) Cognitive development: children's knowledge about the mind. *Annual Review of Psychology*, **50**, 21–45.

Folstein, S. & Rutter, M. (1977) Infantile autism: a genetic study of 21 twin pairs. *Journal of Child Psychology and Psychiatry*, **18**, 297–321.

Folstein, S.E., Santangelo, S.L., Gilman, S.E. *et al.* (1999) Predictors of cognitive test patterns in autism families. *Journal of Child Psychology and Psychiatry*, **40**, 1117–1128.

Fombonne, E. (1999) The epidemiology of autism: a review. *Psychological Medicine*, **29**, 769–786.

Fombonne, E., Bolton, P., Prior, J., Jordan, H. & Rutter, M. (1997) A family study of autism: cognitive patterns and levels in parents and siblings. *Journal of Child Psychology and Psychiatry*, **38**, 667–683.

Frith, U. (1989) *Autism: Explaining the Enigma*. Blackwell Scientific, Oxford.

Frith, U. (1991) *Autism and Asperger Syndrome*. Cambridge University Press, Cambridge, MA.

Frith, U. & Snowling, M. (1983) Reading for meaning and reading for sound in autistic and dyslexic children. *British Journal of Developmental Psychology*, **1**, 329–342.

Ghaziuddin, M. & Greden, J. (1998) Depression in children with autism/pervasive developmental disorders: a case–control family history study. *Journal of Autism and Developmental Disorders*, **28**, 111–115.

Ghaziuddin, M., Tsai, L. & Ghaziuddin, N. (1991) Brief report: violence in Asperger's syndrome, a critique. *Journal of Autism and Developmental Disorders*, **21**, 349–354.

Gilchrist, A., Green, J., Cox, A., Burton, D., Rutter, M. & LeCouteur, A. (2001) Development and current functioning in adolescents with Asperger syndrome: a comparative study. *Journal of Child Psychology and Psychiatry*, **42**, 227–240.

Gillberg, C. (1989) Asperger syndrome in 23 Swedish children. *Developmental Medicine and Child Neurology*, **31**, 520–531.

Gillberg, C. (1995) Endogenous opioids and opiate antagonists in autism: brief review of empirical findings and implications for clinicians. *Developmental Medicine and Child Neurology*, **37**, 239–245.

Gillberg, C. (1998) Chromosomal disorders and autism. *Journal of Autism and Developmental Disorders*, **28**, 415–425.

Gillberg, C. & Coleman, M. (2000) *The Biology of the Autistic Syndromes*, 3rd edn. MacKeith Press, London.

Gillberg, C. & Steffenburg, S. (1987) Outcome and prognostic factors in infantile autism and similar conditions: a population-based study of

46 cases followed through puberty. *Journal of Autism and Developmental Disorders*, **17**, 273–287.

Gilliam, J.E. (1995) *Gilliam Autism Rating Scale*. Pro-Ed, Austin, TX.

Goodman, R. (1989) Infantile autism: a syndrome of multiple primary deficits? *Journal of Autism and Developmental Disorders*, **19**, 409–424.

Grandin, T. & Scariano, M. (1986) *Emergence: Labeled Autistic*. Warner Books, New York.

Green, J., Gilchrist, A., Burton, D. & Cox, A. (2000) Social and psychiatric functioning in adolescents with Asperger syndrome compared with conduct disorder. *Journal of Autism and Developmental Disorders*, **30**, 279–293.

Greenspan, S.I. & Wieder, S. (1997) Developmental patterns and outcomes in infants and children with disorders in relating and communicating: a chart review of 200 cases of children with autism spectrum diagnoses. *Journal of Developmental and Learning Disorders*, **1**, 87–141.

Griffith, E.M., Pennington, B.F., Wehner, E.A. & Rogers, S.J. (1999) Executive functions in young children with autism. *Child Development*, **70**, 817–832.

Guralnick, M.J. (1976) The value of integrating handicapped and non-handicapped preschool children. *American Journal of Orthopsychiatry*, **45**, 236–245.

Guy, J., Hendrich, B., Holmes, M., Martin, J.E. & Bird, A. (2001) A mouse Mecp2-null mutation causes neurological symptoms that mimic Rett syndrome. *Nature Genetics*, **27**, 322–326.

Hadwin, J., Baron-Cohen, S., Howlin, P. & Hill, K. (1996) Can we teach children with autism to understand emotions, belief or pretence? *Development and Psychopathology*, **8**, 345–365.

Hagberg, B. (1985) Rett's syndrome: prevalence and impact on progressive severe mental retardation in girls. *Acta Paediatrica Scandinavica*, **74**, 405–408.

Handleman, J.S. & Harris, S. (2000) *Preschool Education Programs for Children with Autism*. Pro-Ed, Austin, TX.

Happé, F.G. (1994) Current psychological theories of autism: the 'Theory of Mind' account and rival theories [Annotation]. *Journal of Child Psychology and Psychiatry and Allied Disciplines*, **35**, 215–229.

Happé, F. (1997) Central coherence and theory of mind in autism: reading homographs in context. *British Journal of Developmental Psychology*, **15**, 1–12.

Happé, F. (1999) Autism: cognitive deficit or cognitive style? *Trends in Cognitive Sciences*, **3**, 216–222.

Happé, F. & Frith, U. (1996) The neuropsychology of autism. *Brain*, **119**, 1377–1400.

Harris, N.S., Courchesne, E., Townsend, J., Caper, R.A. & Lord, C. (1999) Neuroanatomic contributions to slowed orienting of attention in children with autism. *Cognitive Brain Research*, **8**, 61–71.

Harris, P.L. (1992) From simulation to folk psychology: the case for development. *Mind and Language*, **7**, 120–144.

Harris, P.L. (1993) Pretending and planning. In: *Understanding Other Minds: Perspectives from Autism* (eds S. Baron-Cohen & H. Tager-Flusberg), pp. 228–246. Oxford University Press, Oxford.

Harris, S.L. (1994) Treatment of family problems in autism. In: *Behavioral Issues in Autism* (eds E. Schopler & G.B. Mesibov), pp. 161–175. Plenum, New York.

Hermelin, B. (2001) *Bright Splinters of the Mind*. Jessica Kingsley, London.

Hill, A.E. & Rosenbloom, L. (1986) Disintegrative psychosis of childhood: teenage follow-up. *Developmental Medicine and Child Neurology*, **28**, 34–40.

Hobson, R.P. (1993) *Autism and the Development of Mind*. Lawrence Erlbaum, Hillsdale, NJ.

Hobson, R.P., Ouston, J. & Lee, A. (1988) Naming emotion in faces and voices: abilities and disabilities in autism and mental retardation. *British Journal of Developmental Psychology*, **7**, 237–250.

Hobson, R.P., Lee, A. & Brown, R. (1999) Autism and congenital blindness. *Journal of Autism and Developmental Disorders*, **29**, 45–56.

Horwitz, B., Rumsey, J.M., Grady, C.L. & Rapoport, S.I. (1988) The cerebral metabolic landscape in autism: intercorrelations of regional glucose utilization. *Archives of Neurology*, **45**, 749–755.

Howard, M.A., Cowell, P.E., Boucher, J. *et al.* (2000) Convergent neuroanatomical and behavioural evidence of an amygdala hypothesis of autism. *Neuroreport: An International Journal for the Rapid Communication of Research in Neuroscience*, **11**, 2931–2935.

Howlin, P. (1998) Practitioner review: psychological and educational treatments for autism. *Journal of Child Psychology and Psychiatry*, **39**, 307–322.

Howlin, P. & Goode, S. (1998) Outcome in adult life for people with autism and Asperger's syndrome. In: *Autism and Pervasive Developmental Disorders* (ed. F.R. Volkmar), pp. 209–241. Cambridge University Press, Cambridge.

Howlin, P. & Rutter, M. (1987) *Treatment of Autistic Children*. John Wiley & Sons, Chichester.

Howlin, P., Mawhood, L. & Rutter, M. (2000) Autism and developmental receptive language disorder: a follow-up comparison in early adult life. II. Social, behavioural, and psychiatric outcomes. *Journal of Child Psychology and Psychiatry*, **41**, 561–578.

Hurth, J., Shaw, E., Izeman, S., Whaley, K. & Rogers, S. (1999) Areas of agreement about effective practices among programs serving young children with autism spectrum disorders. *Infants and Young Children*, **12**, 17–26.

International Molecular Genetic Study of Autism Consortium (IMGSAC) (1998) A full genome screen for autism with evidence for linkage to a region on chromosome 7q. *Human Molecular Genetics*, **7**, 571–578.

International Molecular Genetics Study of Autism Consortium (IMGSAC) (2001) Further characterisation of the autism susceptibility locus AUTS1 on chromosome 7q. *Human Molecular Genetics*, **10**, 973–982.

Jarrold, C., Boucher, J. & Russell, J. (1997) Language profiles in children with autism. *Autism*, **1**, 57–76.

Kanner, L. (1943) Autistic disturbances of affective contact. *Nervous Child*, **2**, 217–250.

Kaye, J.A., Melero-Montes, M. & Jick, H. (2001) Mumps, measles and rubella vaccine and the incidence of autism recorded by general practitioners: a time trend analysis. *British Medical Journal*, **322**, 460–463.

Kazak, S., Collis, G.M. & Lewis, V. (1997) Can young people with autism refer to knowledge states? Evidence from their understanding of 'know' and 'guess'. *Journal of Child Psychology and Psychiatry*, **38**, 1001–1009.

Kemper, T.L. & Bauman, M. (1998) Neuropathology of infantile autism. *Journal of Neuropathology and Experimental Neurology*, **57**, 645–652.

Kjelgaard, M.M. & Tager-Flusberg, H. (2001) An investigation of language impairment in autism: implications for genetic subgroups. *Language and Cognitive Processes in Developmental Disorders*, **16**, 287–308.

Klein, R.G. & Slomkowski, C. (1993) Treatment of psychiatric disorders in children and adolescents. *Psychopharmacology Bulletin*, **29**, 525–535.

Klin, A. & Volkmar, F.R. (1997) Asperger syndrome. In: *Handbook of Autism and Pervasive Developmental Disorders* (eds D. Cohen & F.R. Volkmar), pp. 94–122. John Wiley & Sons, New York.

Klin, A., Volkmar, F.R., Sparrow, S.S., Cicchetti, D.V. & Rourke, B.P.

(1995) Validity and neuropsychological characterization of Asperger syndrome: convergence with nonverbal learning disabilities syndrome. *Journal of Child Psychology and Psychiatry*, **36**, 1127–1140.

Klin, A., Carter, A.S. & Sparrow, S.S. (1997) Psychological assessment of children with autism. In: *Handbook of Autism and Pervasive Developmental Disorders* (eds D. Cohen & F.R. Volkmar), 2nd edn, pp. 418–427. John Wiley & Sons, New York.

Klin, A., Sparrow, S.S., de Bildt, A., Cicchetti, D.V., Cohen, D.J. & Volkmar, F.R. (1999) A normed study of face recognition in autism and related disorders. *Journal of Autism and Developmental Disorders*, **29**, 499–508.

Klin, A., Volkmar, F.R. & Sparrow, S.S., eds (2000) *Asperger Syndrome.* Guilford Press, New York.

Koegel, L.K., Koegel, R.L. & Smith, A. (1997) Variables related to differences in standardized test outcomes for children with autism. *Journal of Autism and Developmental Disorders*, **27**, 233–243.

Koegel, L.K., Koegel, R.L., Shoshan, Y. & McNerney, E. (1999) Pivotal response intervention. II. Preliminary long-term outcome data. *Journal of the Association for Persons with Severe Handicaps*, **24**, 186–198.

Kopp, S. & Gillberg, C. (1997) Selective mutism: a population-based study: a research note. *Journal of Child Psychology and Psychiatry*, **38**, 257–262.

Kristensen, H. (2000) Selective mutism and comorbidity with developmental disorder/delay, anxiety disorder, and elimination disorder. *Journal of the American Academy of Child and Adolescent Psychiatry*, **39**, 249–256.

Krug, D.A., Arick, J. & Almond, P. (1980) Behavior checklist for identifying severely handicapped individuals with high levels of autistic behavior. *Journal of Child Psychology and Psychiatry*, **21**, 221–229.

Kumra, S., Wiggs, E., Bedwell, J. *et al.* (2000) Neuropsychological deficits in pediatric patients with childhood-onset schizophrenia and psychotic disorder not otherwise specified. *Schizophrenia Research*, **42**, 135–144.

Lainhart, J.E., Piven, J., Wzorek, M. *et al.* (1997) Macrocephaly in children and adults with autism. *Journal of the American Academy of Child and Adolescent Psychiatry*, **36**, 282–290.

Lamb, J.A., Moore, J., Bailey, A. & Monaco, A.P. (2000) Autism: recent molecular genetic advances. *Human Molecular Genetics*, **9**, 861–868.

Langdell, T. (1978) Recognition of faces: an approach to the study of autism. *Journal of Child Psychology and Psychiatry*, **19**, 255–268.

Le Couteur, A., Bailey, A., Goode, S. *et al.* (1996) A broader phenotype of autism: the clinical spectrum in twins. *Journal of Child Psychology and Psychiatry*, **37**, 785–801.

Le Couteur, A., Rutter, M., Lord, C. *et al.* (1989) Autism Diagnostic Interview: a standardized investigator-based instrument. *Journal of Autism and Developmental Disorders*, **19**, 363–387.

Le Couteur, A., Lord, C. & Rutter, M. (in press) *The Autism Diagnostic Interview–Revised (ADI-R).* Western Psychological Services, Los Angeles, CA.

Leaf, R. & McEachin, J. (1999) *A Work in Progress: Behavioral Management Strategies and a Curriculum for Intensive Bahavioral Treatment of Autism.* Different Roads to Learning, New York.

Leckman, J.F., Grice, D.E., Boardman, J. & Zhang, H. (1997) Symptoms of obsessive-compulsive disorder. *American Journal of Psychiatry*, **154**, 911–917.

Leekam, S.R., Hunnisett, E. & Moore, C. (1998) Targets and cues: gaze-following in children with autism. *Journal of Child Psychology and Psychiatry*, **39**, 951–962.

Lewine, J.D., Andrews, R., Chez, M. *et al.* (1999) Magnetoencephalographic patterns of epileptiform activity in children with regressive autism spectrum disorders. *Pediatrics*, **104** (3, Part 1), 405–418.

Lewis, V. & Boucher, J. (1995) Generativity in the play of young people with autism. *Journal of Autism and Developmental Disorders*, **25**, 105–121.

Lockyer, L. & Rutter, M. (1969) A five- to fifteen-year follow-up study of infantile psychosis. III. Psychological aspects. *British Journal of Psychiatry*, **115**, 865–882.

Lord, C. (1995a) Facilitating social inclusion: examples from peer intervention programs. In: *Learning and Cognition in Autism* (eds E. Schopler & G. Mesibov), pp. 221–240. Plenum Publishers, New York.

Lord, C. (1995b) Follow-up of two year-olds referred for possible autism. *Journal of Child Psychology and Psychiatry*, **36**, 1365–1382.

Lord, C. (1996) Treatment of a high functioning adolescent with autism. In: *Cognitive Therapy with Children and Adolescents* (eds M.A. Reinecke, F.M. Dattilio & A. Freeman), pp. 394–404. Guilford Press, London.

Lord, C. (2000) Achievements and future directions for intervention research in communication and autism spectrum disorders [Commentary]. *Journal of Autism and Developmental Disorders*, **30**, 391–396.

Lord, C. & Magill-Evans, J. (1995) Peer interactions of autistic children and adolescents. *Development and Psychopathology*, **7**, 611–626.

Lord, C. & Paul, R. (1997) Language and communication in autism. In: *Handbook of Autism and Pervasive Developmental Disorders* (eds D. Cohen & F.R. Volkmar), 2nd edn, pp. 195–225. John Wiley & Sons, New York.

Lord, C. & Pickles, A. (1996) Language level and nonverbal social-communicative behaviors in autistic and language delayed children. *Journal of the American Academy of Child and Adolescent Psychiatry*, **35**, 1542–1550.

Lord, C. & Schopler, E. (1989a) The role of age at assessment, developmental level, and test in the stability of intelligence scores in young autistic children. *Journal of Autism and Developmental Disorders*, **19**, 483–499.

Lord, C. & Schopler, E. (1989b) Stability of assessment results of autistic and non-autistic language-impaired children from preschool years to early school age. *Journal of Child Psychology and Psychiatry*, **30**, 575–590.

Lord, C., Schopler, E. & Revicki, D. (1982) Sex differences in autism. *Journal of Autism and Developmental Disorders*, **12**, 317–330.

Lord, C., Rutter, M.L., Goode, S. *et al.* (1989) Autism Diagnostic Observation Schedule: a standardized observation of communicative and social behavior. *Journal of Autism and Developmental Disorders*, **19**, 185–212.

Lord, C., Rutter, M.L. & LeCouteur, A. (1994) Autism Diagnostic Interview–Revised: a revised version of a diagnostic interview for caregivers of individuals with possible pervasive developmental disorders. *Journal of Autism and Developmental Disorders*, **24**, 659–685.

Lord, C., Risi, S., Lambrecht, L. *et al.* (2000) The Autism Diagnostic Observation Schedule–Generic: a standard measure of social and communication deficits associated with the spectrum of autism. *Journal of Autism and Developmental Disorders*, **30**, 205–223.

Lovaas, O.I. (1987) Behavioral treatment and normal educational and intellectual functioning in young autistic children. *Journal of Consulting and Clinical Psychology*, **55**, 3–9.

Maestrini, E., Paul, A., Monaco, A.P. & Bailey, A. (2000) Identifying autism susceptibility genes. *Neuron*, **28**, 19–24.

Mahler, M.S. (1952) On childhood psychosis and schizophrenia: autistic and symbiotic psychoses. *Psychoanalytic Study of the Child*, **7**, 286–305.

Marcus, L., Schopler, E. & Lord, C. (2000) TEACCH services for preschool children. In: *Preschool Education Programs for Children with Autism* (eds J. Handleman & S.L. Harris), pp.215–232. Pro-Ed, Austin, TX.

Mawhood, L. & Howlin, P. (1999) The outcome of a supported employment scheme for high-functioning adults with autism or Asperger syndrome. *Autism*, **3**, 229–254.

Mawhood, L., Howlin, P. & Rutter, M. (2000) Autism and developmental receptive language disorder: a comparative follow-up in early adult life. I. Cognitive and language outcomes. *Journal of Child Psychology and Psychiatry*, **41**, 547–559.

McBride, P.A., Anderson, G.M., Hertzig, M.E. *et al.* (1998) Effects of diagnosis, race, and puberty on platelet serotonin levels in autism and mental retardation. *Journal of the American Academy of Child and Adolescent Psychiatry*, **37**, 767–776.

McDougle, C.J. (1997) Psychopharmacology. In: *Handbook of Autism and Pervasive Developmental Disorder* (eds D.J. Cohen & F.R. Volkmar), 2nd edn, pp. 707–729. John Wiley & Sons, New York.

McDougle, C.J., Naylor, S.T., Cohen, D.J., Volkmar, F.R., Heninger, G.R. & Price, L.H. (1996) A double-blind placebo-controlled study of fluvoxamine in adults with autistic disorder. *Archives of General Psychiatry*, **53**, 1001–1008.

McDougle, C.J., Holmes, J.P., Bronson, M.R. *et al.* (1997) Risperidone treatment of children and adolescents with pervasive developmental disorders: a prospective open-label study. *Journal of the American Academy of Child and Adolescent Psychiatry*, **36**, 685–693.

McDougle, C.J., Holmes, J.P., Carlson, D.C., Pelton, G.H., Cohen, D.J. & Price, L.H. (1998) A double-blind, placebo-controlled study of risperidone in adults with autistic disorder and other pervasive developmental disorders. *Archives of General Psychiatry*, **55** (7), 633–641.

McDougle, C.J., Scahill, L., McCracken, J.T. *et al.* (2000) Background and rationale for an initial controlled study of risperidone. *Child and Adolescent Psychiatric Clinics of North America*, **9**, 201–224.

McGee, G.G., Morrier, M.J. & Daly, T. (2000) The Walden Early Childhood Programs. In: *Preschool Education Programs for Children with Autism* (eds J. Handleman & S.L. Harris), pp. 157–190. Pro-Ed, Austin, TX.

Meltzoff, A.N. & Gopnik, A. (1993) The role of imitation in understanding persons and developing a theory of mind. In: *Understanding Other Minds: Perspectives from Autism* (eds S. Baron-Cohen, H. Tager-Flusberg & D.J. Cohen), pp. 335–366. Oxford University Press, New York.

Mesibov, G.B. (1984) Social skills training with verbal autistic adolescents and adults: a program model. *Journal of Autism and Developmental Disorders*, **14**, 395–404.

Mesibov, G. (1997) Formal and informal measures of the effectiveness of the TEACCH programme. *Autism*, **1**, 25–35.

Mesibov, G., Schopler, E. & Caison, W. (1989) The Adolescent and Adult Psychoeducational Profile: assessment of adolescents and adults with severe developmental handicaps. *Journal of Autism and Developmental Disorders*, **19**, 33–40.

Miller, J.F., Campbell, T.F., Chapman, R.S. & Weismer, S.E. (1984) Language behaviour in acquired childhood aphasia. In: *Language Disorders in Children* (ed. A. Holland), pp. 57–99. College-Hill, Cambridge.

Minshew, N. (1991) Indices of neural function in autism: clinical and biological implications. *Pediatrics*, **87** (Suppl. 5), 774–780.

Minshew, N.J., Goldstein, G. & Siegel, D.J. (1997) Neuropsychologic functioning in autism: profile of a complex information processing disorder. *Journal of the International Neuropsychological Society*, **3**, 303–316.

Minshew, N.J., Luna, B. & Sweeney, J.A. (1999) Oculomotor evidence for neocortical systems but not cerebellar dysfunction in autism. *Neurology*, **52**, 917–922.

Mirenda, P.L., Donnellan, A.M. & Yoder, D.E. (1983) Gaze behavior: a new look at an old problem. *Journal of Autism and Developmental Disorders*, **13**, 397–409.

Moore, C. (1996) Theories of mind in infancy. *British Journal of Developmental Psychology*, **14**, 19–40.

Mouridsen, S.E. (1995) The Landau–Kleffner syndrome: a review. *European Child and Adolescent Psychiatry*, **4**, 223–228.

Mouridsen, S.E., Rich, B. & Isager, T. (1999) Psychiatric morbidity in disintegrative psychosis and infantile autism: a long-term follow-up study. *Psychopathology*, **32**, 177–183.

Mundy, P. & Sigman, M. (1989) The theoretical implications of joint-attention deficits in autism. *Development and Psychopathology*, **1**, 173–183.

Murphy, M., Bolton, P.F., Pickles, A., Fombonne, E., Piven, J. & Rutter, M. (2000) Personality traits of the relatives of autistic probands. *Psychological Medicine*, **30**, 1411–1424.

Naidu, S. (1997) Rett syndrome: a disorder affecting early brain growth. *Annals of Neurology*, **42**, 3–10.

National Research Council (2001) *Educating Children with Autism*. Committee on Educational Interventions for Children with Autism. Division of Behavioral and Social Sciences Education. National Academy Press, Washington D.C.

Nicolson, R. & Castellanos, F.X. (2000) Considerations on the pharmacotherapy of attention deficits and hyperactivity in children with autism and other pervasive developmental disorders [Commentary]. *Journal of Autism and Developmental Disorders*, **30**, 461–462.

Nicolson, R. & Rapoport, J.L. (1999) Childhood-onset schizophrenia: rare but worth studying. *Biological Psychiatry*, **46**, 1418–1428.

Nicolson, R., Awad, G. & Sloman, L. (1998) An open trial of risperidone in young autistic children. *Journal of the American Academy of Child and Adolescent Psychiatry*, **37**, 372–376.

Osterling, J. & Dawson, G. (1994) Early recognition of children with autism: a study of first birthday home videotapes. *Journal of Autism and Developmental Disorders*, **24**, 247–257.

Ozonoff, S. (1995) Executive functions in autism. In: *Learning and Cognition in Autism* (eds E. Schopler & G.B. Mesibov), pp. 199–215. Plenum Publishers, New York.

Ozonoff, S. & Cathcart, K. (1998) Effectiveness of a home program intervention for young children with autism. *Journal of Autism and Developmental Disorders*, **28**, 25–32.

Ozonoff, S. & Miller, J. (1995) Teaching theory of mind: a new approach to social skills training for individuals with autism. *Journal of Autism and Developmental Disorders*, **25**, 415–434.

Ozonoff, S., Pennington, B.F. & Rogers, S.J. (1991a) Executive function deficits in high-functioning autistic children: relationship to theory of mind. *Journal of Child Psychology and Psychiatry*, **32**, 1081–1105.

Ozonoff, S., Rogers, S.J. & Pennington, B. (1991b) Asperger's syndrome: evidence of an empirical distinction from high-functioning autism. *Journal of Child Psychology and Psychiatry*, **32**, 1107–1122.

Pascualvaca, D.M., Fantie, B.D., Papageorgiou, M. & Mirsky, A.F. (1998) Attentional capacitates in children with autism: is there a general deficit in shifting focus? *Journal of Autism and Developmental Disorders*, **28**, 467–478.

Pennington, B.F. & Ozonoff, S. (1996) Executive functions and developmental psychopathology. *Journal of Child Psychology and Psychiatry*, **37**, 51–87.

Peterson, C.C. & Siegal, M. (1997) Psychological, physical, and biological thinking in normal, autistic and deaf children. In: *New Directions for Child Development*, No. 75. *The Emergence of Core Domains of Thought: Children's Reasoning About Physical and Biological Phenomena* (eds H.M. Wellman & K. Inagaki), pp. 55–70. Jossey-Bass, San Francisco, CA.

Pfeiffer, S.I., Norton, J., Nelson, L. & Shott, S. (1995) Efficacy of vitamin B6 and magnesium in the treatment of autism: a methodology review and summary of outcomes. *Journal of Autism and Developmental Disorders*, 25, 481–492.

Philippe, A., Martinez, M., Bataille-Guillot, M. *et al.* (1999) Genome-wide scan for autism susceptibility genes. Paris Autism Research International Sibpair Study. *Human Molecular Genetics*, 8, 805–812.

Pickles, A., Bolton, P., Macdonald, H. *et al.* (1995) Latent-class analysis of recurrence risks for complex phenotypes with selection and measurement error: a twin and family history study of autism. *American Journal of Human Genetics*, 57, 717–726.

Pickles, A., Starr, E., Kazak, S. *et al.* (2000) Variable expression of the autism broader phenotype: findings from extended pedigrees. *Journal of Child Psychology and Psychiatry*, 41, 491–502.

Piven, J. & Palmer, P. (1999) Psychiatric disorder and the broad autism phenotype: evidence from a family study of multiple-incidence autism families. *American Journal of Psychiatry*, 156, 557–563.

Piven, J., Simon, J., Chase, G.A. *et al.* (1993) The etiology of autism: pre-, peri- and neonatal factors. *Journal of the American Academy of Child and Adolescent Psychiatry*, 32, 1256–1263.

Piven, J., Palmer, P., Jacobi, D., Childress, D. & Arndt, S. (1997a) Broader autism phenotype: evidence from a family history study of multiple-incidence autism families. *American Journal of Psychiatry*, 154, 185–190.

Piven, J., Palmer, P., Landa, R., Santangelo, S., Jacobi, D. & Childress, D. (1997b) Personality and language characteristics in parents from multiple-incidence autism families. *American Journal of Medical Genetics*, 74, 398–411.

Piven, J., Bailey, J., Ranson, B.J. & Arndt, S. (1997c) An MRI study of the corpus callosum in autism. *American Journal of Psychiatry*, 154, 1051–1056.

Piven, J., Bailey, J., Ranson, B.J. & Arndt, S. (1998) No difference in hippocampus volume detected on magnetic resonance imaging in autistic individuals. *Journal of Autism and Developmental Disorders*, 28, 105–110.

Plaisted, K., O'Riordan, M. & Baron-Cohen, S. (1998) Enhanced discrimination of novel, highly similar stimuli by adults with autism during a perceptual learning task. *Journal of Child Psychology and Psychiatry*, 39, 765–775.

Potenza, M.N., Holmes, J.P., Kanes, S.J. & McDougle, C.J. (1999) Olanzapine treatment of children, adolescents, and adults with pervasive developmental disorders: an open-label pilot study. *Journal of Clinical Psychopharmacology*, 19, 37–44.

Quintana, H., Birmaher, B., Stedge, D. *et al.* (1995) Use of methylphenidate in the treatment of children with autistic disorder. *Journal of Autism and Developmental Disorder*, 25, 283–294.

Rapin, I. (1997) Autism. *New England Journal of Medicine*, 337, 97–104.

Richer, J. & Zappella, M. (1989) Changing social behaviour: the plus of holding. *Communication*, 23, 35–39.

Rimland, B. (1964) *Infantile Autism: The Syndrome and its Implications for a Neural Theory of Behavior*. Appleton Century Crofts, New York.

Risch, N. (1990) Linkage strategies for genetically complex traits. *American Journal of Human Genetics*, 46, 222–253.

Rogers, S.J. (1998) Empirically supported comprehensive treatments for young children with autism. *Journal of Clinical Child Psychology*, 27, 168–179.

Rogers, S. & DiLalla, D. (1990) Age of symptom onset in young children with pervasive developmental disorders. *Journal of the American Academy of Child and Adolescent Psychiatry*, 29, 863–872.

Romanczyk, R.G. (1986) Self-injurious behavior: conceptualization, assessment, and treatment. *Advances in Learning and Behavioral Disabilities*, 5, 29–56.

Rumsey, J.M. (1992) Neuropsychological studies of high-level autism.

In: *High-functioning Individuals with Autism* (eds E. Schopler & G.B. Mesibov), pp. 41–64. Plenum Press, New York.

Runco, M.A. & Schreibman, L. (1987) Socially validating behavioral objectives in the treatment of autistic children. *Journal of Autism and Developmental Disorders*, 17, 141–147.

Russell, J., Jarrold, C. & Henry, L. (1996) Working memory in children with autism and with moderate learning difficulties. *Journal of Child Psychology and Psychiatry*, 37, 673–686.

Russell, J., Saltmarsh, R. & Hill, E. (1999) What do executive factors contribute to the failure on false belief tasks by children with autism? *Journal of Child Psychology and Psychiatry*, 40, 859–868.

Rutter, M. (1968) Concepts of autism: a review of research. *Journal of Child Psychology and Psychiatry*, 9, 1–25.

Rutter, M. (1970) Autistic children: infancy to adulthood. *Seminars in Psychiatry*, 2, 643–650.

Rutter, M. (1972a) Psychiatric causes of language retardation. In: *The Child with Delayed Speech* (eds M. Rutter & J.A.M. Martin), pp. 147–160. SIMP/William Heinemann, London.

Rutter, M. (1972b) Childhood schizophrenia reconsidered. *Journal of Autism and Childhood Schizophrenia*, 2, 315–337.

Rutter, M. (1985) The treatment of autistic children. *Journal of Child Psychology and Psychiatry*, 26, 193–214.

Rutter, M. (2000) Genetic studies of autism: from the 1970s into the millennium. *Journal of Abnormal Child Psychology*, 28, 3–14.

Rutter, M. & Bailey, A. (1993) Thinking and relationships: mind and brain. In: *Understanding Other Minds: Perspectives from Autism* (eds S. Baron-Cohen, H. Tager-Flusberg & D. Cohen), pp. 481–504. Oxford University Press, Oxford.

Rutter, M., Greenfield, D. & Lockyer, L. (1967) A five to fifteen year follow-up study of infantile psychosis. II. Social and behavioural outcome. *British Journal of Psychiatry*, 113, 1183–1199.

Rutter, M., Mawhood, L. & Howlin, P. (1992) Language delay and social development. In: *Specific Speech and Language Disorders in Children: Correlates, Characteristics, and Outcomes* (eds P. Fletcher & D. Hall), pp. 63–78. Whurr, London.

Rutter, M., Bailey, A., Bolton, P. & Le Couteur, A. (1994) Autism and known medical conditions: myth and substance. *Journal of Child Psychology and Psychiatry*, 35, 311–322.

Rutter, M., Andersen-Wood, L., Beckett, C. *et al.* (1999) Quasi-autistic patterns following severe early global privation. *Journal of Child Psychology and Psychiatry*, 40, 537–549.

Santangelo, S.L., Buxbaum, J., Silverman, J., Pericak-Vance, M. & Ashley-Koch, A. (2000) *Confirmatory evidence of linkage for autism to 7q based on combined analysis of three independent data sets.* American Society of Human Genetics Meeting.

Santosh, P.J. (2000) Neuroimaging in child and adolescent psychiatric disorders. *Archives of Disease in Childhood*, 82, 412–419.

Schopler, E. & Olley, J. (1982) Comprehensive educational services for autistic children: the TEACCH model. In: *The Handbook of School Psychology* (eds C.R. Reynolds & T.B. Gutkin), pp. 629–643. John Wiley & Sons, New York.

Schopler, E., Reichler, R.J. & Renner, B.R. (1986) *The Childhood Autism Rating Scale (CARS) for Diagnostic Screening and Classification of Autism.* Irvington, New York.

Schopler, E., Reichler, R., Lansing, M. & Marcus, L. (1990) Individualized assessment and treatment for autistic and developmentally disabled children. *Psychoeducational Profile Revised (PEP-R)*, Vol. 1. Pro-Ed, Austin, TX.

Schultz, R.T., Gauthier, I., Klin, A. *et al.* (2000) Abnormal ventral temporal cortical activity during face discrimination among individual with autism and Asperger syndrome. *Archives of General Psychiatry*, 57, 331–340.

Shahbazian, M.D. & Zoghbi, H.Y. (2001) Molecular genetics of Rett syndrome and clinical spectrum of MECP2 mutations. *Current Opinion in Neurology*, **14**, 171–176.

Siegel, B., Pliner, C., Eschler, J. & Elliot, G. (1988) How children with autism are diagnosed: difficulties in identification of children with multiple developmental delays. *Developmental and Behavioral Pediatrics*, **9**, 199–204.

Siegel, D.J., Minshew, N.J. & Goldstein, G. (1996) Wechsler IQ profiles in diagnosis of high-functioning autism. *Journal of Autism and Developmental Disorders*, **26**, 389–406.

Sigman, M. (1998) The Emanuel Miller Memorial Lecture 1997. Change and continuity in the development of children with autism. *Journal of Child Psychology and Psychiatry*, **39**, 879–891.

Sigman, M., Arbelle, S. & Dissanayake, C. (1995) Current research findings on childhood autism. *Canadian Journal of Psychiatry [Revue Canadienne de Psychiatrie]*, **40**, 289–294.

Sigman, M., Ruskin, E., Arbeile, S. *et al.* (1999) Continuity and change in the social competence of children with autism, Down syndrome, and developmental delays. *Monographs of the Society for Research in Child Development*, **64**, 1–114.

Skuse, D. (2000) Imprinting, the X chromosome and the male brain: explaining sex differences in the liability to autism. *Pediatric Research*, **47**, 9–16.

Smalley, S.L., McCracken, K. & Tanguay, P. (1995) Autism, affective disorders, and social phobia. *American Journal of Medical Genetics*, **60**, 19–26.

Smith, B., Chung, M.C. & Vostanis, P. (1994) The path to care in autism: is it better now? *Journal of Autism and Developmental Disorders*, **24**, 551–564.

Smith, I.M. & Bryson, S.E. (1994) Imitation and action in autism: a critical review. *Psychological Bulletin*, **116**, 259–273.

Smith, T. (1999) Outcome of early intervention for children with autism. *Clinical Psychology: Science and Practice*, **6**, 33–49.

Smith, T., Groen, A.D. & Wynn, J.W. (2000) Randomized trial of intensive early intervention for children with pervasive developmental disorder. *American Journal of Mental Retardation*, **105**, 269–285.

Sparrow, S., Balla, D. & Cicchetti, D. (1984) *Vineland Adaptive Behavior Scales*. American Guidance Service, Circle Pines, MN.

Starr, E., Kazak, S., Pickles, A. *et al.* (2001) A family genetic study of autism associated with profound mental retardation. *Journal of Autism and Development Disorders*, **31**, 89–96.

Steffenburg, S., Gillberg, C., Helgren, L. *et al.* (1989) A twin study of autism in Denmark, Finland, Iceland, Norway, and Sweden. *Journal of Child Psychology and Psychiatry and Allied Disciplines*, **30**, 405–416.

Stevenson, R., Schroer, R., Skinner, C., Fender, D. & Simenson, R. (1997) Autism and macrocephaly. *Lancet*, **349**, 1744–1745.

Stone, W.L. & Caro-Martinez, L.M. (1990) Naturalistic observations of spontaneous communication in autistic children. *Journal of Autism and Developmental Disorders*, **20**, 437–454.

Stone, W.L., Lee, E.B., Ashford, L. *et al.* (1999) Can autism be diagnosed accurately in children under 3 years? *Journal of Child Psychology and Psychiatry*, **40**, 219–226.

Stone, W.L., Coonrod, E.E. & Ousley, O.Y. (2000) Brief report: Screening Tool for Autism in Two-year-olds (STAT): development and preliminary data. *Journal of Autism and Developmental Disorders*, **30**, 607–612.

Strain, P.S. & Hoyson, M. (2000) The need for longitudinal, intensive social skill intervention: LEAP follow-up outcomes for children with autism. *Topics in Early Childhood Special Education*, **20**, 116–122.

Swettenham, J., Baron-Cohen, S., Charman, T. *et al.* (1998) The frequency and distribution of spontaneous attention shifts between so-cial and non-social stimuli in autistic, typically developing, and non-autistic developmentally delayed infants. *Journal of Child Psychology and Psychiatry and Allied Disciplines*, **39**, 747–753.

Swithenby, S.J., Bräutigam, S.E., Bailey, A.J., Jousmäki, V. & Tesche, C.D. (2000) Comparison between the processing of static images of human faces in high functioning autistic subjects and normal controls. In: *Biomag96, Proceedings of the Tenth International Conference on Biomagnetism (Santa Fe 1996)* (eds C.J. Aine, Y. Okada, G. Stroink, S.J. Swithenby & C.C. Wood), pp. 1075–1078. Springer-Verlag, New York.

Szatmari, P., Jones, M.B., Zwaigenbaum, L. & MacLean, J.E. (1998) Genetics of autism: overview and new directions. *Journal of Autism and Developmental Disorders*, **28**, 351–368.

Szatmari, P., Bryson, S.E., Streiner, D.L., Wilson, F., Archer, L. & Ryerse, C. (2000) Two-year outcome of preschool children with autism or Asperger's syndrome. *American Journal of Psychiatry*, **157**, 1980–1987.

Tager-Flusberg, H. (1985) The conceptual basis for referential word meaning in children with autism. *Child Development*, **56**, 1167–1178.

Tager-Flusberg, H. & Anderson, M. (1991) The development of contingent discourse ability in autistic children. *Journal of Child Psychology and Psychiatry*, **32**, 1123–1134.

Tager-Flusberg, H. & Sullivan, K. (1994) A second look at second-order belief attribution in autism. *Journal of Autism and Development Disorders*, **24**, 577–586.

Tanguay, P.E., Robertson, J. & Derrick, A. (1998) A dimensional classification of autism spectrum disorder by social communication domains. *Journal of the American Academy of Child and Adolescent Psychiatry*, **37**, 271–277.

Taylor, B., Miller, E., Farrington, C.P. *et al.* (1999) Autism and measles, mumps, and rubella vaccine: no epidemiological evidence for a causal association. *Lancet*, **353**, 2026–2029.

Towbin, K.E. (1997) Pervasive developmental disorder not otherwise specified. In: *The Handbook of Autism and Other Pervasive Developmental Disorders* (eds D.J. Cohen & F.R. Volkmar), 2nd edn, pp. 123–147. John Wiley & Sons, New York.

Townsend, J., Courchesne, E., Covington, J. *et al.* (1999) Spatial attention deficits in patients with acquired or developmental cerebellar abnormality. *Journal of Neuroscience*, **19**, 5632–5643.

Trillingsgaard, A. (1999) The script model in relation to autism. *European Child and Adolescent Psychiatry*, **8**, 45–49.

Tsai, L.Y. (1999) Psychopharmacology in autism. *Psychosomatic Medicine*, **61**, 651–665.

Tuchman, R.F. & Rapin, I. (1997) Regression in pervasive developmental disorders: seizures and epileptiform electroencephalogram correlates. *Pediatrics*, **99**, 560–566.

Turner, M., Barnby, G. & Bailey, A. (2000) Genetic clues to the biological basis of autism. *Molecular Medicine Today*, **6**, 238–244.

Vaillant, G. (1962) John Haslam on early infantile autism. *American Journal of Psychiatry*, **119**, 376–376.

Van Bourgondien, M.E. & Schopler, E. (1990) Critical issues in the residential care of people with autism. *Journal of Autism and Developmental Disorders*, **20**, 391–399.

Venter, A., Lord, C. & Schopler, E. (1992) A follow-up study of high-functioning autistic children. *Journal of Child Psychology and Psychiatry*, **33**, 489–507.

Volkmar, F. & Nelson, S. (1990) Seizure disorders in autism. *Journal of the American Academy of Child and Adolescent Psychiatry*, **29**, 127–129.

Volkmar, F.R. & Rutter, M. (1995) Childhood disintegrative disorder: results of the DSM-IV autism field trial. *Journal of the American Academy of Child and Adolescent Psychiatry*, **34**, 1092–1095.

Volkmar, F.R., Stier, D.M. & Cohen, D.J. (1985) Age of recognition of pervasive developmental disorder. *American Journal of Psychiatry*, **142**, 1450–1452.

Volkmar, F.R., Szatmari, P. & Sparrow, S.S. (1993) Sex differences in pervasive developmental disorders. *Journal of Autism and Developmental Disorders*, **23**, 579–591.

Volkmar, F.R., Klin, A., Siegel, B. *et al.* (1994) Field trial for autistic disorder in DSM-IV. *American Journal of Psychiatry*, **151**, 1361–1367.

Volkmar, F.R., Klin, A. & Pauls, D. (1998) Nosological and genetic aspects of Asperger syndrome. *Journal of Autism and Developmental Disorders*, **28**, 457–463.

Volkmar, F., Cook, E.H. Jr, Pomeroy, J., Realmuto, G. & Tanguay, P. (1999) Practice parameters for the assessment and treatment of children, adolescents, and adults with autism and other pervasive developmental disorders. *Journal of the American Academy of Child and Adolescent Psychiatry*, **38** (Suppl. 12), 32–54.

Wainwright-Sharp, J.A. & Bryson, S.E. (1993) Visual orienting deficits in high functioning people with autism. *Journal of Autism and Developmental Disorders*, **23**, 1–13.

Werner, E., Dawson, G., Osterling, J. & Dinno, N. (2000) Brief report: recognition of autism spectrum disorder before one year of age—a retrospective study based on home videotapes. *Journal of Autism and Developmental Disorders*, **30**, 157–162.

Wetherby, A.M. & Prizant, B.M. (1999) Enhancing language and communication development in autism: assessment and intervention guidelines. In: *Autism: Identification, Education, and Treatment* (ed. D.B. Zager), 2nd edn, pp. 141–174. Lawrence Erlbaum, Mahwah, NJ.

Willemsen-Swinkels, S.H., Buitelaar, J.K., Weijnen, F.G. & van Engeland, H. (1995) Placebo-controlled acute dosage naltrexone

Late entry

Bailey, A., Luthert, P., Harding, B. *et al.* (1998) A clinicopathological study of autism. *Brain*, **121**, 889–905.

study in young autistic children. *Psychiatry Research*, **58**, 203–215.

Williams, T.I. (1989) A social skills group for autistic children. *Journal of Autism and Developmental Disorders*, **19**, 143–155.

Wing, L. (1981) Asperger's syndrome: a clinical account. *Psychological Medicine*, **11**, 115–129.

Wing, L. (1997a) The autistic spectrum. *Lancet*, **350**, 1761–1766.

Wing, L. (1997b) Syndromes of autism and atypical development. In: *Handbook of Autism and Pervasive Developmental Disorders* (eds D. Cohen & F. Volkmar), 2nd edn, pp. 148–170. John Wiley & Sons, New York.

Wing, L. (1999) *Diagnostic Interview for Social and Communication Disorders (DISCO)*, 10th edn. Autistic Society, London.

Wing, L. & Gould, J. (1979) Severe impairments of social interaction and associated abnormalities in children: epidemiology and classification. *Journal of Autism and Developmental Disorders*, **9**, 11–29.

Wing, L. & Wing, J.K. (1971) Multiple impairments in early childhood autism. *Journal of Autism and Childhood Schizophrenia*, **1**, 256–266.

Woodhouse, W., Bailey, A., Rutter, M., Bolton, P., Baird, G. & Le Couteur, A. (1996) Head circumference and other pervasive developmental disorders. *Journal of Child Psychology and Psychiatry*, **37**, 665–671.

World Health Organization (1992) *The ICD-10 Classification of Mental and Behavioral Disorders: Clinical Descriptions and Diagnostic Guidelines*. World Health Organization, Geneva, Switzerland.

Young, R.L. & Nettlebeck, T. (1994) The 'intelligence' of calendrical calculators. *American Journal on Mental Retardation*, **99**, 186–200.

Zilbovicius, M., Garreau, B., Samson, Y. *et al.* (1995) Delayed maturation of the frontal cortex in childhood autism. *American Journal of Psychiatry*, **152**, 248–252.

Speech and Language Difficulties

Dorothy V.M. Bishop

Introduction

The ability to communicate through language distinguishes humans from all other animals. Spoken language allows us to convey information, express our feelings and demonstrate social affiliations. It also provides a vehicle for organizing our thoughts and memories, enabling us to construct complex lines of reasoning, and to contemplate past, future and hypothetical events, rather than remaining grounded in present reality. The development of written language provides even more dramatic release from the here-and-now, making it possible to transcend space and time.

All known human cultures have language, but there is huge diversity in how languages are structured, both in terms of the sounds used to express meaning (phonemes) and the ways in which linguistic elements are combined (syntax). For instance, French has two different vowels that sound like 'oo' to a speaker of English, but which are phonemically distinct; they signal contrasts in meaning, so that 'rue' and 'roux' mean different things. In English, on the other hand, we make a phonemic contrast between the sounds 'th' and 'z' (e.g. 'bathe' vs. 'baize'), which are not distinguished in French. In tone languages, such as Chinese Mandarin, the pitch at which a word is spoken signals meaning, so that 'ba' has four completely different meanings depending on whether the pitch is rising ('to uproot'), falling ('a harrow'), changing from fall to rise ('to hold') or at a level high pitch ('eight').

Moving to grammar; in English, relationships between entities are indicated by a mixture of word order and grammatical morphemes (e.g. inflectional endings such as '-ing' or '-ed', and small function words such as 'by'). Thus it is the boy who is doing the kissing in 'the boy kisses the girl', but is the recipient of the kiss in 'the girl kisses the boy' or 'the boy is kissed by the girl'. In some languages, such as Turkish, word order generally obeys the sequence subject–object–verb, and inflectional suffixes do all the work of expressing relationships. Other languages, such as Chinese Mandarin, have virtually no inflections. Word order, particles and prepositions are used to indicate how the elements of a sentence interrelate.

Clearly, language acquisition involves far more than learning labels for things. The child must work out which speech sound contrasts are meaningful in the ambient language, and how to combine words and grammatical morphemes to express relationships between things and events. Most children master this complex skill with no explicit instruction and with relative ease,

so that the bulk of phonology and syntax is acquired by around 4 years of age. There are, however, frequent exceptions, and these are the topic of this chapter.

Delay in learning to talk is a common reason for a parent to seek advice from a family doctor or paediatrician. Because human communication is complex, assessment and diagnosis of speech and language difficulties in children is a particularly challenging problem that requires expertise in several different areas, including linguistics, audiology, child development, neuropsychology, paediatric neurology and psychiatry. This chapter will use the diagnostic flow chart shown in Fig. 39.1 to introduce a range of different conditions that can lead to speech and language difficulties in children. This depicts the sequence of decisions the clinician needs to make when first assessing a child who presents with poor communication. However, recent research suggests that this diagnostic process should not be confined to those cases where communicative impairment is the presenting complaint, but should be extended much more broadly to all children referred to psychiatric services. The reason is simple: surveys of children attending psychiatric clinics reveal that a high proportion of them have some kind of communicative impairment, and in many cases this goes unrecognized unless a formal assessment is made. Cohen (1996) summarized findings from a Canadian study in which 399 consecutive psychiatric referrals of children aged from 4 to 12 years were given a detailed language assessment. Children with autistic disorder, general developmental delay, neurological damage, hearing impairment or a non-English-speaking home background had been excluded from this sample. Around one-quarter of the children had previously identified language impairments. Of the remainder, none of whom was thought to be language-impaired, 34% met criteria for language impairment. There appeared to be two reasons why communicative difficulties had been overlooked in these children. First, they did not have such overt expressive language difficulties as children with previously identified problems, although their receptive language skills were as poor as that group. Secondly, they were more likely to have externalizing psychiatric disorders, which may have diverted attention from communication. Cohen *et al.* (1998) suggested that language function should be incorporated routinely into the assessment and treatment process for children with psychiatric impairments. Some suggestions for how to implement this recommendation are given below in the section on Assessment.

In the next section, different diagnostic entities will be reviewed, with a main focus on specific developmental language

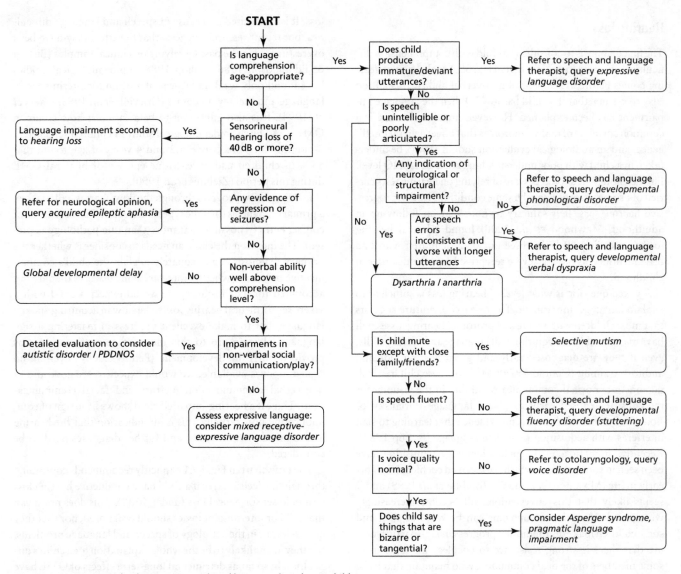

Fig. 39.1 Decision tree for diagnosing speech and language disorders in children.

disorder. Assessment procedures will briefly be reviewed in a later section.

A decision tree for diagnosis

In Fig. 39.1, the question of whether comprehension is age-appropriate is placed at the top of the decision tree. There are good reasons for this. First, whereas problems with expressive speech and language are usually fairly easy to detect on the basis of informal observation, comprehension is much harder to estimate this way. Secondly, different diagnoses need to be considered for the child with comprehension problems than for one whose problems are confined to speech output or sentence formulation.

Methods for testing comprehension are discussed at the end

of this chapter, but it is worth noting here that assessment can be difficult in children with major behavioural difficulties. It is tempting to assume that the child can understand but is unco-operative, but it is at least as likely that the behavioural difficulties stem from fear and frustration in a child who comprehends very little. If the child does not co-operate with formal comprehension testing, proceed down the decision tree on the left-hand side of the diagram.

As shown in Fig. 39.1, results from a comprehension assessment are not sufficient for a diagnosis, but they determine which diagnoses should be considered, and also help the clinician to adjust his or her language level to the child's level of understanding, for instance when conducting a psychiatric interview. Where comprehension is unimpaired, we can exclude autistic disorder and mental handicap. It is also unlikely that hearing loss or acquired epileptic aphasia is implicated.

Hearing loss

The first diagnosis to consider in a child with comprehension difficulties is hearing loss. Note that in Fig. 39.1 evaluation of hearing comes before assessment of non-verbal ability. It is all too easy to assume that if a child has low IQ then the language impairment has been explained. However, impaired hearing is a common correlate of many syndromes that affect general intelligence, and an audiological evaluation should always be undertaken in a child with poor understanding, regardless of IQ level. Furthermore, one should beware of relying on hearing tests carried out some years previously: some conditions lead to progressive hearing loss. It is salutary to note that on follow-up in adulthood, Mawhood et al. (2000) found bilateral hearing losses exceeding 40 dB in three out of 23 children who had been identified as having severe receptive language disorder in childhood.

A vexed question is what level of hearing loss is sufficient to explain language impairment. The research literature suggests that most children with severe and profound hearing losses will have major problems acquiring oral language and literacy skills, even if they are diagnosed early and given hearing aids and auditory training (Conrad 1979). Most of these children will demonstrate normal communicative ability in the visuomotor modality if exposed early to a sign language (Orlansky & Bonvillian 1985), and there is no evidence that learning to sign interferes with acquisition of spoken language (Bishop 1983). Recently, dramatic gains in spoken language acquisition have been seen in some children who have received cochlear implants early in life (Miyamoto et al. 1997; Tomblin et al. 1999) and it seems likely that this intervention will become increasingly widespread. Nevertheless, outcome can be very variable, and some children make disappointing progress. It is also worth noting that there is strong resistance to cochlear implants from some members of the deaf community, who maintain that if the child learns sign language, deafness need not be a handicap (Lane 1990).

Much less is known about the impact of mild and moderate sensorineural hearing loss on language development. The handful of studies that include children with mild or moderate hearing impairment typically find language levels intermediate between those of normally hearing and more severely hearing-impaired children (Brannon & Murry 1966). However, the average results may mask substantial variation. A recent small study of children with sensorineural hearing losses in the range of 20–70 dB HL, showed age-appropriate levels of language comprehension and expression in 78% of children (Norbury et al., 2001). All of these were attending regular classrooms, most had mild losses (20–40 dB), and most wore hearing aids. None used sign language. This suggests that mild hearing loss can act as a risk factor for language impairment, but that, given appropriate intervention, many children compensate well for their hearing difficulties.

Otitis media with effusion (OME) is a common childhood complaint that is often associated with mild conductive hearing loss. It is often cited as a cause of speech and language difficulties, but recent research suggests that the effect may have been overestimated in the past by relying on clinical samples (Bishop & Edmundson 1986; Bishop 1988). Epidemiological studies have found only weak influences, if any, on long-term speech, language and literacy outcomes (Grievink et al. 1993; Peters et al. 1994). It is also important to be aware just how common OME is. A Dutch epidemiological study of children screened at 3-monthly intervals between 2 and 4 years of age found that 55% of children had at least one episode of bilateral OME during this period (Zielhuis et al. 1990).

For simplicity, progress through the flow chart is halted when a primary diagnosis (in italic type) is arrived at. However, it is, of course, entirely possible that more than one pathology is present. The question the clinician needs to consider is whether the primary diagnosis can adequately explain the child's communicative profile, or whether there are some features that are not accounted for. For instance, we would expect a child with a severe sensorineural hearing loss to be slow in acquiring spoken language, but to make excellent progress in mastering a sign language, if exposure to this mode of communication was provided early in development (Petitto 2000). Even if no signed input is available, we would expect to see good use of non-verbal communication (gesture and facial communication). Thus, if a hearing-impaired child shows little sign of communicating non-verbally, this is an indication that the hearing loss is not the whole story, and further diagnoses need to be considered.

The flow chart in Fig. 39.1 explicitly recommends continuing through the decision tree if a child has a conductive hearing loss or a mild sensorineural loss (under 40 dB). This does not mean that mild or intermittent losses should be ignored, nor that they are irrelevant in the aetiology of speech and language problems, but they are unlikely to be the whole explanation for a child's difficulties. In so far as detrimental long-term effects of OME have been reported, they tend to occur in samples with other risk factors present, e.g. low birth weight and/or socioeconomic disadvantage (Gravel et al. 1996).

Acquired epileptic aphasia (Landau–Kleffner syndrome)

Acquired epileptic aphasia (AEA) should be suspected when language regresses after a period of normal development. Typically, the child becomes increasingly unresponsive to spoken language, sometimes over a period of months but sometimes within a matter of days. Deterioration in expressive language typically follows. Deafness may be suspected, but normal hearing thresholds are obtained. In classic Landau–Kleffner syndrome, the clinical picture is one of severe and selective receptive aphasia, with the child retaining good non-verbal intelligence (Landau & Kleffner 1957). This has also been described as an auditory agnosia, which may extend to affect perception of non-verbal as well as verbal sounds.

The epileptic basis of the disorder may be overlooked because over 50% of these children do not present with frank seizures. However, abnormal electrical activity, usually involving the temporal lobes, is evident on sleep electroencephalography (EEG), although this abnormality typically dies down by adolescence, making retrospective diagnosis difficult.

The developmental course of AEA is highly variable. In some children, the disease follows a fluctuating course, with periods of improvements followed by regression. On average, the younger the child at onset, the worse the outcome for language, but this generalization hides a great deal of variability (Bishop 1985). Many children with onset before 5 years of age have serious and lifelong difficulties in understanding spoken language. Nevertheless, a long-term case study suggests that gradual improvement of language skill can continue over many years (Van Dongen et al. 1989). Regarding seizures, the outcome is much more favourable, with these usually disappearing by adolescence.

It is particularly important that child psychiatrists are aware of this rare disorder, because the appearance of communicative difficulties in a previously normal child often prompts a psychiatric referral, especially if there are associated behavioural disturbances, as is not uncommonly the case (Appleton 1995). Differential diagnosis from deafness should be unproblematic if proper audiological assessment is carried out. AEA differs from selective mutism in that language comprehension is usually intact in the latter condition, and the child can be observed to talk normally under certain restricted conditions. Neither is true for AEA. As noted by Genton & Guerrini (1993), it is essential to conduct an EEG recording for one full sleep cycle in any child who develops an unexplained language disorder, as this will clearly demonstrate the underlying functional abnormality in the brain of the child with AEA.

As with so many of the conditions reviewed in this chapter, the boundaries of AEA are not clear-cut, and diagnosis of atypical cases poses particular problems. Cases have been described in which only expressive language is disturbed. In other children, the regression affects social interaction and adaptive behaviour as well as language, making it difficult to draw a sharp line between AEA and autistic regression (Deonna 2000).

The prevalence of AEA is hard to determine as it is a rare disorder, which is often misdiagnosed as either deafness or selective mutism (see below). Appleton (1995) noted that over 200 cases have been reported since the condition was first described in 1957, and this number is increasing as the availability of new methods of brain imaging makes it possible to discover more about the underlying abnormality (Morrell & Lewine 1994; Guerreiro et al. 1996). Most clinicians, however, can expect to see only one or two cases during a lifetime.

The aetiology of AEA remains a mystery. No structural brain lesion has been demonstrated, and magnetic resonance imaging (MRI) and computed tomography (CT) scan are usually normal, but metabolic abnormalities, predominantly in the temporal lobes, are apparent on functional imaging (Guerreiro et al. 1996; Da Silva et al. 1997). A variety of diseases, ranging from cerebral arteritis to subacute encephalitis, have been mooted but no consistent cause has been demonstrated. A pair of discordant monozygotic twins has been reported, ruling out a purely genetic aetiology (Feekery et al. 1993).

Medical interventions typically involve use of anticonvulsants to control the epileptic activity, but although this is often effective in controlling seizures, it does not necessarily normalize the underlying EEG abnormality and does not always lead to improvement in language. Some authorities have recommended aggressive treatment with corticosteroids (Lerman et al. 1991), or neurosurgical intervention in cases where it is possible to isolate the epileptic focus (Morrell et al. 1995). For both treatments, some cases of dramatic improvement have been reported, but such success is not invariable, making it difficult to weigh the risks of adverse effects against the possibility of recovery, especially in a disorder that may, in any case, follow a fluctuating course. It is generally agreed that an educational approach that relies on developing visual forms of language (written or signed) is more effective than attempting to overcome the child's auditory impairment.

There has been some debate in the literature as to whether, even after excluding those with Landau–Kleffner syndrome, there is an unusually high rate of EEG abnormality in children with language impairments (Echenne et al. 1992; Parry-Fielder et al. 1997), and whether a similar pathophysiological process might be present in children with more typical forms of developmental language disorder. For the present, this remains a speculation without firm evidence (Deonna 2000). Where a child presents with language disorders and seizures but does not have the clinical picture of AEA, it is recommended that the diagnostic process continues through the decision tree.

Global developmental delay

It is customary to make a diagnostic distinction between cases where non-verbal ability and verbal ability are equally impaired, and those where poor verbal skills are discrepant with normal non-verbal ability. Terminology in this area is something of a minefield. Clinically, the term 'global developmental delay' is used frequently, although rather imprecisely, to refer to children who function well below age level in a range of domains, including verbal and non-verbal ability, adaptive skills and motor development. Terms such as 'mental handicap' and 'intellectual retardation' are still used in some quarters to refer to children with an overall IQ below 70 (2 SD below the mean), but these labels have fallen out of favour because of negative social connotations. In the UK, the preferred term in many clinical and educational contexts is 'learning difficulty' or 'learning disability', but this has enormous potential for confusion, because outside the UK people tend to restrict the use of these terms to children with normal intelligence and a *specific* learning disability in one domain, such as specific reading disability. The term 'global developmental delay' is used here, while recognizing it is far from ideal (especially as 'delay' implies, unrealistically, that there may be subsequent catch-up).

Sadly, a diagnosis of global developmental delay is often the prelude to relative neglect of the child's language difficulties. There is a tendency to assume that the level of non-verbal ability sets some kind of limit on the level of language that can be achieved. There is evidence against this viewpoint from two sources. First, some syndromes are associated with a phenotype in which intelligence is impaired but language is an area of relative strength. The most well-known case is that of Williams syndrome. This is sometimes misleadingly described as though language is normal and other skills impaired. The reality for most children is that both verbal and non-verbal abilities are well below average but, nevertheless, skills such as verbal memory, vocabulary and syntax are far better than those seen in other children with different aetiologies who have similar levels of IQ (Morris & Mervis 1999). Furthermore, there may be relative sparing of aspects of syntax and morphology that give especial difficulty to children with developmental language disorders (Clahsen & Almazan 1998). The second point is that intervention studies suggest that in many cases children of low IQ can benefit from language intervention just as much as those of average IQ (Fey *et al.* 1994).

Although the flow chart shows global developmental delay and autistic disorder as separate entities, these disorders commonly co-occur, and so it is important to evaluate social communication, play and repetitive behaviour in children with a global developmental delay.

Autistic disorder and related conditions

Delayed language development and poor comprehension are hallmarks of autistic disorder, and the issue of differential diagnosis between autistic disorder and specific developmental language disorder frequently crops up in clinical settings. A diagnosis of autistic disorder should be suspected if the child's comprehension difficulties are accompanied by more pervasive difficulties affecting social interaction, non-verbal communication and play, or if the child shows unusual repetitive or ritualistic behaviours, or restricted interests. The clinician needs to consider whether language development is merely delayed, or whether there are deviant features that would not be regarded as normal at any age, such as repetitive use of stereotyped catch-phrases, unusual and exaggerated intonation, pronoun reversal, and a frequent failure to respond when the parent attempts to attract the child's attention. An intriguing observation in some children with autism is that scores on tests of expressive language (such as picture naming) may be higher than those on receptive tests (such as selecting a named picture). Whereas most children with communicative problems will use non-verbal means of expression, children with autism often have difficulty in both interpreting and producing appropriate non-verbal communication. Imaginative play does not develop normally in children with autism; instead there may be repetitive routines, such as forming long lines of toy cars, or the child may be preoccupied with everyday artefacts such as lights or switches, and disregards toys that most children would find attractive.

A core characteristic of autism is lack of social sensitivity. It is sometimes thought that all autistic children live in a world of their own, ignoring all other people. This is far too extreme a picture: many children with autism will enjoy cuddles and rough-and-tumble play, but they may neither seek nor offer comfort or affection. In older, verbal, high-functioning children, one may find a strong desire to interact with other people, but a severe lack of understanding of how to do this. The concept of friendship as a reciprocal emotionally supportive relationship is hard for a child with autism to grasp.

Diagnosis depends on historical information about early development as well as observation and assessment of the child's current behaviour and abilities. Specific instruments developed for the diagnosis of autistic disorder include the Autism Diagnostic Interview–Revised (ADI-R), which is a parental interview, and the Autism Diagnostic Observation Schedule (ADOS-G), which has four modules, to cover the age range from infancy to adulthood, each involving direct observation of the child or young person in situations designed to elicit autistic behaviours (Lord *et al.* 1994, 2000). Autistic disorder is covered thoroughly by Lord & Bailey (Chapter 38), so in this section I shall focus just on areas of diagnostic difficulty.

Textbook cases of autistic disorder or developmental language disorder are easy enough to recognize, but many children present with a pattern of symptoms that does not fit unambiguously in either category, while showing some features of both. Thus their difficulties extend beyond the highly selective impairment of language structure seen in developmental language disorder, but they do not have the full triad of autistic impairments in severe enough form to merit a diagnosis of autistic disorder. O'Hare *et al.* (1998) carried out an audit of 103 children referred to a speech clinic at Edinburgh Children's Hospital, and found that eight of them met diagnostic criteria for autism, but a further 14 had autistic symptomatology that fell short of meeting diagnostic criteria, in most cases because only two elements of the triad of autistic impairments were present. All but one of these children was rated as having abnormal receptive language on a speech therapy assessment. Although the diagnosis of Asperger syndrome is sometimes used in such cases, this is not appropriate if the child's language milestones are delayed.

In the UK, the term 'autistic spectrum disorder' is used quite widely, although often without clear diagnostic criteria. In the USA, and increasingly elsewhere, the DSM-IV (American Psychiatric Association 1994) term 'pervasive developmental disorder not otherwise specified' (PDDNOS) is frequently applied. However, this is not very satisfactory, as this was clearly intended as a default category to be used in rare cases when a child showed autistic symptomatology but diagnostic criteria for autistic disorder were not met. Furthermore, it provides little information about symptomatology and does not help decisions about educational placement. Bishop (2000) suggested that these difficulties probably reflect the fact that diagnostic labels impose a categorical structure on what is in reality a multidimensional space, with children varying in terms of the severity of impairments in language, social interaction and range of interests. The solution is not to force every child into the Procrustean bed of either autistic disorder or specific developmental language disorder, but rather to give the diagnosis that has the best chance of giving the child access to appropriate educational and remedial provision, while noting that the overall symptom profile may be atypical. Bishop (2000) suggested that the term 'pragmatic language impairment' might be useful for describing children who do not show repetitive behaviours and restricted interests, but whose language difficulties affect social communication and use of language in context. This label does not mean that we are dealing with a new syndrome; rather it may be helpful in characterizing that subset of children who have a symptom profile intermediate between autistic disorder and developmental language disorder, with pragmatic difficulties the most noticeable feature.

Specific developmental language disorder

In DSM-IV, an explicit contrast was drawn between specific developmental disorders and pervasive developmental disorders. Two features were important in making the distinction. The first is the specificity of the impairment: a single domain in specific developmental disorders, and multiple areas of functioning in pervasive developmental disorders. The second is the nature of the impairment: specific developmental disorder is seen as characterized by development that is delayed but not otherwise abnormal, whereas in a pervasive developmental disorder one sees behavioural deviations that are not normal for any stage of development.

In line with this dichotomy, a diagnosis of specific developmental language disorder (DLD) is appropriate when the child's language lags well behind age level, but development is proceeding normally in other respects, and when there is no obvious explanatory factor for language delay (such as grossly abnormal home environment, global developmental delay, hearing loss or acquired neurological lesion). It is important to be aware that a range of different terms has been used for this condition. Here, I follow DSM usage, but the term 'specific language impairment' is the more usual one in the research literature, whereas 'developmental dysphasia' or 'development aphasia' are now largely obsolete, although sometimes encountered in medical contexts.

Differential diagnosis

The diagnostic criteria of DSM-IV and ICD-10 (World Health Organization 1993) are similar. Both capture the notion that a developmental language disorder has three essential features.

1 Language skills are out of keeping with other aspects of intellectual development. In practice, this is often interpreted as meaning that there must be a discrepancy of at least 1 SD between a standard score on a language test and a non-verbal IQ test.

2 There should be evidence of disability associated with the language impairment: it has an adverse impact on the child's social or academic functioning.

3 The child does not meet criteria for pervasive developmental disorder.

Previous diagnostic formulations have also excluded a range of other conditions, such as intellectual retardation or sensory impairment, but these exclusions were relaxed in DSM-IV, which specifies that if they are present, the problems with language are worse than would normally be expected with such conditions.

DSM-IV draws a distinction between expressive DLD and mixed receptive–expressive DLD and this distinction is followed in the flow chart in Fig. 39.1. These are defined to be mutually exclusive, so that a diagnosis of expressive DLD is made only if criteria are not met for mixed receptive–expressive DLD. In reviewing characteristics of DLD I shall depart from the sequence of Fig. 39.1 here and treat both together, because most research studies do not distinguish between these subtypes. Furthermore, although there have been suggestions that the two subtypes are qualitatively distinct (Lahey & Edwards 1995), much of the evidence justifies treating them as points on a continuum of severity (Bishop 1979). Thus, although the distinction between receptive–expressive and pure expressive DLD may be useful clinically for educational placement and prognosis, it has yet to be shown to distinguish meaningfully between clinical entities. This is not to imply that there is a single homogeneous type of DLD: this is quite unlikely given the wide range of clinical manifestations one can observe. However, the dimensions on which children appear to differ have more to do with which components of language (e.g. morphosyntax, vocabulary, pragmatics) are affected, rather than with the expressive–receptive distinction (Bishop & Rosenbloom 1987; Rapin 1996).

The diagnostic criteria of DSM-IV and ICD-10 have come under attack in recent years. Much of the debate has centred on the question of whether it is appropriate to require a large mismatch between non-verbal ability and language level to meet diagnostic criteria for DLD. Aram *et al.* (1992) found that adoption of this discrepancy criterion overidentified normally developing children, and underidentified children who had been diagnosed as language impaired on clinical grounds. Cole *et al.* (1995) showed that the discrepancy between language and non-verbal ability was unstable, so that children tested on two occasions frequently changed category, even if the same measures were used. Bishop (1994a) found that identical twins were usually concordant for the presence of clinically significant language problems, but were often discordant in terms of meeting stringent discrepancy criteria based on DSM. Aram *et al.* (1993) compared various diagnostic criteria with the aim of improving agreement between clinical judgement and decisions based on psychometric data, and reported that the most sensitive index was one that diagnosed a DLD if the child had either a 15-point (1 SD) discrepancy between non-verbal IQ and a composite language test score, or had a mean length of utterance (MLU) more than 1 SD below age level. This definition captured 80% of clinically identified cases. Another source of criticism of the official diagnostic systems is their reliance on psychometric tests.

Research has shown that measures obtained from spontaneous speech samples are useful in identifying children who are deemed language impaired but who do not meet conventional psychometric criteria (Dunn *et al*. 1996). Unfortunately, such measures are time-consuming and not always practicable in clinical settings. Furthermore, adequate normative data are often lacking.

In the final analysis, the specific criteria adopted for identifying language impairment will depend partly on one's goals when making the diagnosis. Stringent criteria developed in research contexts are not always appropriate in clinical settings, where the goal is to provide a diagnosis that ensures the child has access to appropriate services. Here, one wants to use measures that have ecological validity—that have relevance for functioning in everyday communicative and social settings—and to identify those children who will benefit from intervention. If one requires a large discrepancy between verbal and non-verbal ability before children can be considered for special educational services, then many children with poor verbal skills are denied access, even though their linguistic problems may be identical to those of other children who do meet diagnostic criteria.

Developmental course and prognosis

A number of longitudinal studies have thrown light on the developmental course of DLD. There is general agreement that the child with significantly impaired receptive language skills has a poor prognosis, even if this diagnosis is made at a very early age. Comprehension problems do not usually appear to resolve spontaneously. On the contrary, the range of impairments seen in a child with receptive language difficulties often increases with age, extending to encompass social and psychiatric disorder (Rutter & Mawhood 1991), and impairment on non-verbal as well as verbal measures (Stothard *et al*. 1998; Johnson *et al*. 1999). There is much more debate about prognosis for preschool expressive language disorders, with some proposing that outcome is generally good and intervention is seldom warranted (Paul 2000), while others maintain that these children are at high risk for persisting difficulties that may only become apparent on detailed testing (Scarborough & Dobrich 1990; Rescorla *et al*. 1997). At least some of this controversy arises because different studies have used different follow-up periods to assess prognosis. In the longitudinal study conducted by Paul *et al*. (1996), the initial impression given by the first waves of follow-up was that 2 year olds with expressive language delays were at high risk of persisting communicative problems. However, the longer the follow-up, the smaller the proportion of children who had marked language impairment. It appears that the numbers of children with clinically significant language difficulties do shrink dramatically as children mature. It seems reasonable to conclude that a good long-term prognosis is usually seen in children identified as 'late talkers' before the age of 3 years, provided the problem is restricted to expressive language and the delay is not too severe (Whitehurst & Fischel 1994). Bishop

(1994b) offered guidelines that still seem relevant in the light of current research: children whose expressive vocabularies consist of less than 50 words at the age of 24 months should be carefully monitored, but long-term problems are unlikely in those with vocabularies of more than eight words who have good comprehension.

There are a number of longitudinal studies showing that the child whose language is significantly impaired at 4–5 years of age is at high risk of developing literacy problems (Bishop & Adams 1990; Tallal *et al*. 1997; Stothard *et al*. 1998; Johnson *et al*. 1999). Although it is commonly believed that oral language problems disappear with age to be replaced by literacy problems, this is seldom seen. Rather, the oral language problems become less obvious in casual interactions, but can be readily demonstrated on formal testing. It would be wrong to give the impression that all language-impaired 4 year olds are destined for academic failure: some children do show marked improvement. However, these tend to be children with predominantly expressive difficulties that have resolved by the age of $5\frac{1}{2}$ years (Bishop & Edmundson 1987; Bishop & Adams 1990).

DLD is associated with increased risk for psychiatric as well as language and literacy problems. The underlying nature of this association has been the cause of much speculation (Rutter & Lord 1987). Comorbidity could reflect the influence of common aetiological risk factors, or the causal effect of one condition on the other (Beitchman *et al*. 1996). For instance, for some children affective disorders and low self-esteem may be a consequence of growing awareness of communicative inadequacy.

Prevalence

Two recent epidemiological surveys, in the USA and Canada, estimated the prevalence of specific language impairment (SLI) in 5 year olds at around 7% (Tomblin *et al*. 1997; Johnson *et al*. 1999). However, it should be noted that neither study adopted the stringent 'discrepancy' criteria of DSM-IV and ICD-10, but rather diagnosed SLI if the child scored below cut-off on standardized language tests, but had a non-verbal IQ of 80 or above and no other exclusionary criteria. Furthermore, in the study by Tomblin *et al*., only 29% of those diagnosed as cases of SLI were already known by parents to have any speech or language difficulties. This estimate is likely therefore to be higher than would be the case if it were based on a definition such as DSM-IV or ICD-10, which requires both that there be a substantial discrepancy between verbal and non-verbal ability, and that the language impairment interferes with everyday or academic functioning.

Risk factors and aetiology

The principal risk factors for DLD are:
• male gender—in clinical samples, sex ratio of affected males : females is around 3 or 4 : 1 (Robinson 1991);

• family history of DLD—around 30% of affected children have an affected first-degree relative, compared with 3% of the general population (Stromswold 1998); and

• being a later-born child in a large family (Bishop 1997a).

Although much has been written about language outcomes of medical risk factors, such as otitis media and low birth weight, there is no strong evidence that these act as major risk factors for specific DLD, although they may act synergistically to cause impairment in a child who is already at risk from other causes (Bishop 1987). Although there is an association between low socioeconomic status and DLD (Fundudis *et al.* 1979), this is not strong, and there is little support for the commonly held view that parents can cause their child to become language impaired by inadequate verbal stimulation, except in the most extreme cases of abuse and neglect.

Over the past decade, there has been an explosion of research concerned with the genetic basis of DLD (see Bishop, 2001 for a review). Three twin studies have obtained closely similar findings of high heritability for this disorder (Lewis & Thompson 1992; Bishop *et al.* 1995; Tomblin & Buckwalter 1998). A molecular study of a three-generational family showing an autosomal dominant pattern of inheritance for severe speech and language disorder found clear evidence of linkage to a site on chromosome 7 (Fisher *et al.* 1998), although it is unclear how far these results will generalize to other cases of heritable language disorder.

Currently, there is considerable interest in two aspects of language functioning that have been postulated as behavioural markers of heritable SLI. The first is phonological short-term memory, typically assessed by asking the child to repeat nonsense words of increasing length, such as 'hampent' or 'blonterstaping' (Gathercole *et al.* 1994). Poor performance on this task characterizes many children with SLI, even those who had early difficulties that appear to have resolved. Furthermore, deficient performance on non-word repetition showed very high heritability in a twin study (Bishop *et al.* 1996). The second area in which many children with DLD have disproportionate difficulties concerns certain aspects of grammar. Children with DLD can have major problems in adding appropriate verb endings, such as past tense '-ed', when given an eliciting sentence frame (e.g. Q: 'Here the boy is raking the leaves. What has he just done?' A: 'Raked the leaves') (Rice 2000). Rice & Wexler (1996) have postulated an underlying impairment of an innate system that has evolved to handle specific types of grammatical rule. With the exception of non-word repetition, the measures used to assess such hypotheses are not available as standardized tests, making them unsuitable for clinical use at present. Nevertheless, the work is promising in suggesting that we may be able to develop more selective language measures that will identify homogeneous groups of children with a common aetiology. That would be a considerable improvement on the current position, where the same child may or may not receive a diagnosis of DLD depending on which tests are used to assess verbal ability.

The fact that there is strong genetic influence on DLD should not lead us to conclude that environmental factors are unimportant, or that nothing can be done to alleviate language difficulties. Provisional evidence suggests genes may act as risk factors that increase the probability that a child will have a language disorder, but the severity and persistence of language disorder can be highly variable, even within a pair of genetically identical monozygotic twins. A study by Bishop *et al.* (1999) suggested that environmental factors could impair the child's ability to process non-verbal auditory stimuli, with a subsequent small knock-on effect on language development. In children who were not at genetic risk, this negative effect was not of clinical significance, but in those who were at genetic risk, for whom language learning was a more difficult task, the combination of environmental and genetic risk factors was sufficient to lead to clinically important problems in language learning.

Intervention

Intervention is usually carried out by speech and language therapists, who use a wide range of techniques to stimulate language learning. In the past, there was a vogue for drilling children in grammatical exercises, using imitation and elicitation methods, in an attempt to have the child extract the salient grammatical regularities. Such methods fell into disuse when it became apparent that there was little generalization to everyday situations. Contemporary approaches to enhancing development of language structure are more likely to adopt 'milieu' methods, in which the intervention is interwoven into natural episodes of communication, and the therapist builds on the child's utterances, rather than dictating what will be talked about. In addition, there has been a move away from a focus solely on grammar and phonology toward interventions that develop children's social use of language, often working in small groups that may include normally developing as well as language-impaired peers (Gallagher 1996; Hayden & Pukonen 1996).

Another way in which modern approaches to remediation differ from the past is that parents are more likely to be directly involved, particularly with preschool-aged children (Girolametto *et al.* 1996). Methods such as the Hanen approach* involve videoing interactions between parent and child and then using these when working with groups of parents in a constructive way to help them facilitate communication.

A radically different approach has been developed by Tallal *et al.* (1996), who have devised a computer-based intervention, FastForword, that involves prolonged and intensive training on specific components of language and auditory processing. The theory underlying this approach maintains that language difficulties are caused by a failure to make fine-grained auditory discriminations in the temporal dimension, and the training materials are designed to sharpen perceptual acuity, in much the

---

*See website at http://hanen.velocet.ca/programs_parent.shtml

same way as has been demonstrated in animal experiments. By embedding training in attractive computerized games, children can be persuaded to participate in thousands of training trials, in a way that would simply not be possible with a standard therapist-based interaction.

For all these types of intervention, there are few adequately controlled trials that allow one to assess clinical efficacy. In general, one does not see miracle cures, but this is not to say that gains are negligible (Bryne-Saricks 1987; Law et al. 1998). A clinical trial assessing the FastForword approach showed significant gains relative to a control group (Merzenich et al. 1996), but questions remain about the persistence and generalizability of these effects. Since the initial controlled trial, the authors have gathered a large amount of data on pre- and post-intervention language test scores of children enrolled in FastForword, but this is difficult to evaluate without controls for practice and placebo effects (Tallal 2000). Furthermore, it is not possible to know which specific components of this complex intervention are most effective, or whether the whole gamut of different exercises is essential to achieve therapeutic benefits.

Developmental phonological disorder

It is customary to draw a distinction between speech, the physical act of articulating speech sounds, and language, the whole complex system of combining elements of sound at different levels of complexity to express meaning. It is possible to have a language impairment with normal speech (e.g. in cases of DLD where the child speaks clearly but does not comprehend or produce complex syntactic constructions). The converse situation is also seen, when the child has some difficulty in producing clear speech but the underlying language skills are intact, e.g. in cases of dysarthria (see below). The child who persists in using immature or deviant sound patterns but who has no physical basis for this disorder does not fit so neatly into this dichotomous view. Speech is undoubtedly the presenting problem, but the underlying impairment appears to be linguistic rather than one of motor control: a failure to learn which speech sounds are distinctive in the ambient language. Often the speech errors involve a persistence of immature patterns. For instance, sounds produced in the back of the mouth, such as 'k' and 'g' are not distinguished in the child's output from those produced in the front of the mouth, such as 't' and 'd', so that 'cat' may be pronounced as 'tat' and dog as 'dod'. The terms 'phonological disorder' (DSM-IV) and 'phonological impairment' have superseded such labels as 'functional articulation disorder' to refer to such problems. The term 'phonological' implies that the child's difficulties are linguistic rather than motoric, perhaps akin to those of an adult mastering a foreign language. Most of us have difficulty in learning to use a new set of speech sounds, not because our articulators are in any way defective, but because we have not internalized the sound distinctions that are critical in the language.

Evidence that a phonological disorder is not just a problem in articulating sounds accurately can be obtained using specialized phonological tests that require no speech from the child. Some children with phonological problems have difficulties in discriminating between similar speech sounds, such as 'pat' vs. 'cat', when asked, for instance, to select a picture to match what they have heard. However, the most common difficulty is not so much in telling sounds apart, as in recognizing that different exemplars of the same sound are indeed the same sound. So if asked to say whether 'bag' or 'boat' rhymes with 'rag', or to judge whether 'soup' or 'coat' begins with the same sound as 'Sam', the child with phonological problems may perform at chance levels (Bird et al. 1995). Such observations suggest that the difficulty is one of categorization of speech, rather than poor acuity for differences between speech sounds.

The prognosis of pure phonological disorder is much better than that of language disorder (Bishop & Adams 1990; Johnson et al. 1999), especially if the phonological difficulties resolve by the time the child starts school (Bird et al. 1995). It is difficult to estimate the prevalence of phonological problems, because studies typically do not discriminate between different types of speech problem; lisping and other deviations, specific phonological impairments, and speech problems accompanying language impairment all tend to be included together. Furthermore, prevalence appears strongly age-dependent, with speech problems declining sharply between 3 and 6 years of age (Morley 1972). After excluding children with additional handicaps, Johnson et al. (1999) obtained a prevalence estimate of 6.1% for specific speech-only impairments at 5 years of age. This figure excludes the children from this sample who had comorbid speech and language impairment. Shriberg et al. (1999) reported a prevalence of speech delay in US 6-year-olds of 3.8%, with comorbid language impairment in around 12% of these cases. Little is known about risk factors and aetiology of phonological disorders, although, as with other communication disorders, boys are at greater risk than girls (Shriberg et al. 1999). Intervention is carried out by speech-language therapists, and typically involves games and exercises to develop the child's awareness of phonemic contrasts (Dean et al. 1995).

Developmental verbal dyspraxia

Developmental verbal dyspraxia is a controversial diagnostic category that is defined differently by different experts, and not used at all by some authorities (for a review see Crary 1993). The central characteristic in most definitions is that there are difficulties in speech production that suggest an impairment of motor programming, because it is the length and complexity of what is uttered, rather than the specific speech sounds used, that is the main factor determining accuracy. In children with this diagnosis, one is likely to see speech errors that are inconsistent from one occasion to the next, that are particularly evident in polysyllabic words, and that involve transpositions of speech sounds rather than simple substitution of one sound for another. For instance, Bradford & Dodd (1996) reported a dyspraxic child whose renderings of 'elephant' on three separate occasions were 'ewint', 'wuwit' and 'uwit'.

Debate continues over the question of whether problems in sequencing non-verbal movements should be part of the diagnostic criteria: some authorities maintain that to be regarded as dyspraxic, the child should be impaired in imitating sequences of non-speech movements of the tongue and mouth. Not all children who make inconsistent phonological errors have extensive difficulties producing non-speech movements, raising the question of where they should be classified (Bradford & Dodd 1996). In addition, there is the question of whether dyspraxia should be diagnosed in a child who has broader difficulties with expressive language, or only in those with a relatively pure problem in speech output. In practice, many children who receive this diagnosis do have associated problems affecting language, literacy and phonological awareness (Stackhouse 1992).

The lack of agreed diagnostic criteria make it impossible to make generalizations about risk factors, prevalence or prognosis. The cause of developmental verbal dyspraxia remains an enigma, but it appears to be strongly familial (Morley 1972). It is also worth noting that although their grammatical difficulties have been emphasized in published accounts, the phenotype in the three-generational family mentioned in the section on DLD also involved severely dyspraxic speech (Hurst *et al.* 1990). Crary (1993) provides an overview of approaches to intervention for developmental verbal dyspraxia.

Anarthria and dysarthria

Anarthria or dysarthria is diagnosed when speech problems arise because of structural or neurological abnormalities of articulatory control. Anarthria is the term used when there is no ability to produce speech, whereas dysarthria refers to disordered articulation caused by weakness, incoordination or structural abnormalities of the articulators. It is important to distinguish these articulation problems, where speech is impaired because of problems producing articulatory movements, from developmental phonological disorders, where the child is neurologically normal and capable of producing articulatory movements (see above). Neurological conditions that can cause anarthria or dysarthria include cerebral palsy and Möbius syndrome, in which there is agenesis of cranial nerve nuclei and associated facial immobility. Structural abnormalities of articulators that can lead to dysarthric speech include cleft palate and Treacher Collins syndrome. There are a number of other genetic syndromes that are associated with unusual proportions of the articulators and/or hypotonicity which affects tongue control, e.g. Down syndrome.

Where no specific syndrome is detected, one should be alert to the possibility of dysarthria when there is poor co-ordination or weakness of facial muscles, as evidenced by drooling, feeding problems, or difficulties imitating simple oral movements such as moving the tongue from side to side or pursing the lips. Worster-Drought (1974) stressed that anarthria can occur in children in the absence of any other neurological impairment, and he gave detailed descriptions of this condition, which is known as both congenital suprabulbar paresis and Worster-Drought syndrome. However, Clark *et al.* (2000), in a recent review of 47 cases, noted that most children with this condition have additional complex impairments, including mild pyramidal tetraplegia, learning difficulties, behaviour problems and epilepsy. Crary (1993) noted that remarkably little clinical or research attention has been paid to developmental dysarthria, although it was well described by Morley *et al.* (1954) more than 40 years ago. It appears to be a strongly familial condition.

Dysarthria and anarthria involve difficulties affecting speech rather than language, and so one would expect to find normal language comprehension and normal literacy skills in pure cases. However, quite often the aetiological factors that cause articulation difficulties also lead to problems in other areas, including hearing and language.

Selective mutism

Selective mutism is diagnosed when a child is able to speak but fails to do so except in very restricted situations, such as with close family. This disorder was previously known as 'elective mutism', but the terminology was modified in DSM-IV to avoid the connotation of volitional behaviour. The diagnosis is strongly suggested when one finds mutism in a child who has no neurological or structural abnormalities of the articulators, and who has normal language comprehension, as well as a normal early history of using language. However, the crucial point that needs to be established is that the child does speak in some situations.

As Dummit *et al.* (1997) noted, this condition is more properly regarded as a form of anxiety disorder rather than a speech and language disorder. Rates of comorbid anxiety and phobic disorders are high, both in affected children and in their first-degree relatives. However, differential diagnosis can be complicated by the fact that some children with selective mutism do have developmental language disorders (Kristensen 2000), suggesting that self-consciousness about inadequate communication skills may play a part in maintaining mutism.

Persistent selective mutism affects less than 1 in 1000 children, although the frequency of transient mutism in children starting school is much higher. Girls are two to three times more likely to be affected than boys. The causes of selective mutism remain unknown. Although conventional wisdom maintains that physical or sexual abuse or other kinds of trauma may precipitate selective mutism, there is little evidence of this (Black & Uhde 1995), and the strong familial component to the disorder suggests that Dummit *et al.* (1997) may be correct in regarding this disorder as the extreme end of a biologically based continuum of temperament and social behaviour.

Behaviour modification methods have been shown to be effective in re-establishing speech (Sluckin *et al.* 1991), but the long-term prognosis of selective mutism is nevertheless poor. There is a high rate of personality disorder and psychiatric problems associated with a history of selective mutism (Kolvin & Fundudis 1981). Dummit *et al.* (1997) argued that therapeutic interventions should focus on alleviating anxiety, but there has been no systematic research on the efficacy of this approach.

Disorders of fluency

Stuttering is the popular term for dysfluent speech that is characterized by repetitions by sounds or syllables, rather than whole words. Onset is usually between 3 and 6 years of age. Campbell *et al.* (1996) noted that the high rate of spontaneous recovery in children (estimated as between 50 and 80%) makes it difficult to know when referral is appropriate, and they proposed a list of 'referral indicators' to aid clinical decision-making. Factors that should prompt clinical referral include observable tension or struggling during speech, abnormal pitch associated with dysfluency, prolongations or blocks lasting more than 1 s, and presence of distorting facial or bodily movement accompanying the stuttering.

As in most of the speech and language disorders reviewed in this chapter, the aetiology of stuttering is unknown, but it appears to be strongly familial, and boys are at considerably higher risk than girls (ratio of 3:1 according to Campbell *et al.* 1996).

Voice disorders

A voice disorder should be suspected when a child speaks with abnormal vocal quality. This includes hoarseness, deviations of pitch and abnormally loud or soft voice. These features can have profound effects on how a child is perceived by others: a grating, squeaky or whispery voice may have consequences for the child's socialization. Campbell *et al.* (1996) estimated that between 1 and 3% of school-aged children have clinically significant voice problems requiring intervention. They described unpublished data from their own survey of 203 consecutive referrals to a specialist clinic for investigation of abnormal vocal quality. Only 6% had normal laryngeal structure. The most common pathology was vocal nodules, i.e. mechanical trauma of the vocal folds usually caused by one vocal fold making extensive contact with the other. Surgical intervention is not usually used in such cases; behavioural treatment is the most effective approach, and involves training the child to use the voice more appropriately.

The child who presents with normal speech and language structure

To round off this section, it is necessary to say something about the child who has normal speech and language abilities on formal assessment. Obviously, one would expect to find large numbers of such children in the course of any routine screening programme, for instance when assessing all children attending a child psychiatry facility. However, a normal speech and language profile is occasionally seen in children who have been referred by a parent or professional because of specific concerns about communication. A striking illustration comes from a survey of 7-year-old children attending special classes for language-impaired children in the UK (Conti-Ramsden *et al.* 1997). On cluster analysis of language test scores, some 10% of children

fell in a subgroup that had little evidence of language deficit, with all language scores above the 13th centile, and word-reading and articulation above the 60th centile. One might imagine that these would be children for whom intervention had been effective who were ready to return to regular schooling but, when teacher impressions were added to the psychometric test data, a very different conclusion was reached. Quite often these were the children about whom teachers had the greatest concerns. They described them as having particular problems in the domains of semantics and pragmatics. Where a parent or teacher complains that a child gives odd, unexpected, inconsistent or over-literal interpretations to utterances, or makes tangential responses in conversation, one needs to be alert to the possibility that there may be pragmatic comprehension difficulties that will not necessarily be apparent on formal testing. In some cases, the child may speak with stereotyped intonation, as if acting a part on the stage. Where there are abnormalities in the social use of language, but early language milestones were normal, a diagnosis of Asperger syndrome should be considered (see Lord & Bailey, Chapter 38). Where there is a history of early language delay, but the child currently presents with normal test scores on measures of language structure but with odd communication, then more detailed evaluation may suggest a diagnosis of pragmatic language impairment (see section on Autistic disorder and related conditions). The next section will consider aspects of assessment, including suggestions for evaluating pragmatic competence.

Assessment

Interview with the caregiver

General guidelines for interviewing parents are given by Angold (Chapter 3), and this section will focus just on those issues that arise specifically in the context of children with speech and language difficulties.

Usually, one will place more reliance on results of standardized tests than on the caregiver's descriptions for evaluating the presence or severity of a speech or language problem. However, for very young children who may not co-operate with formal assessment, an adult who knows the child well may provide invaluable information about early language milestones, vocabulary size and typical utterance length. However, care must be taken to elicit accurate information. General questions such as 'how many words does he or she know' are unlikely to be helpful. For children around 2 years of age, the MacArthur Communicative Development Inventory (Fenson *et al.* 1994) has proved useful in identifying children with language delays. The caregiver is presented with a list of words that young children say, and simply checks off those that are produced by the child in question. Norms for passing language milestones are shown in Table 39.1. Ideally one should identify 'anchor points' in the past, such as a birthday or other special event, and ask the caregiver to provide specific examples of the kinds of things that the child said at

Table 39.1 Age (in months) at passing language milestones. (After Neligan & Prudham 1969.)

Percentile	Single words*		Sentences†	
	Boys	Girls	Boys	Girls
3rd	8.7	8.6	17.5	16.2
10th	10.0	9.8	19.1	18.4
25th	11.6	11.5	21.4	20.4
50th	12.4	12.3	23.8	22.9
75th	15.0	14.6	26.8	25.0
90th	18.0	17.3	32.5	30.8
97th	21.9	20.1	36.0+	36.0

*Three or four different words for people or objects, correctly used.
†Three or more words, strung together to make some sort of sense.

that time. It is important to establish whether the child's language development ever regressed, as this is a rare phenomenon that suggests an underlying epileptic aetiology.

The perinatal, medical and family history may provide some clues as to the aetiology, but in most cases of developmental speech and language disorder, it is difficult to identify a specific cause.

Physical examination

General aspects of examining children are covered by Bailey (Chapter 10). Where the child has abnormal speech production, it is important to assess the integrity of the articulatory apparatus. A history of difficulties with chewing, drinking from a straw, licking an ice-cream or blowing the nose should alert the clinician to the possibility of physical abnormalities, such as submucous cleft palate, and neurological impairment. Brown (1985) gives guidelines for neurological examination of speech mechanisms. Involuntary grimacing, drooling, abnormal gag reflex, and difficulties with sucking and swallowing are important upper motor neurone signs.

Motor clumsiness is a common correlate of speech and language disorder (Robinson 1991; Owen & McKinlay 1997), but one seldom finds any evidence of hard neurological signs. However, although such cases are rare, it is important to bear in mind that language delay can be the first presenting symptom of progressive diseases such as Duchenne muscular dystrophy, so it is never safe to assume that clumsiness is simply an indicator of neurodevelopmental immaturity (Kaplan & Elias 1986).

Audiological assessment

In co-operative children, behavioural audiometry provides crucial information about hearing sensitivity at different frequencies, but for some children such procedures are not feasible. A clinical audiological assessment will usually include an assess-

ment of the function of the middle ear and cochlea, with evoked response audiometry being employed if there is any doubt about the integrity of auditory pathways up to and including the brainstem. However, it is less common to have any assessment of the neural pathways from brainstem to auditory cortex. At these higher levels, auditory responsiveness is more variable and subject to attentional influences. Furthermore, the critical stimuli that elicit responses become increasingly complex. Experimental animals with bilateral ablations of auditory cortex can still detect auditory stimuli, and can learn discriminations based on changes in intensity or frequency. However, they show difficulties in discriminating between tone sequences or tone duration (Neff 1967). This raises the question of whether some children may have auditory perceptual impairments that reflect poor functioning of central auditory pathways. The concept of central auditory processing disorder (CAPD) gained momentum in the 1980s (Keith 1977), and batteries of auditory tests have been developed for diagnosing such problems as difficulty in perceiving speech in noise, or integrating inputs from two ears (Willeford 1977). Unfortunately, we still know very little about how such deficits affect language acquisition, despite several decades of research on the auditory basis of language impairments, and these methods are not in widespread clinical use.

Assessment of non-verbal ability

Where a child has impaired language, it is important to assess intelligence using methods that minimize the role of verbal expression or comprehension. It is not possible here to give a detailed review of tests, but some recommendations are offered of instruments that appear valid with language-impaired children and have adequate psychometric properties.

Probably the most widely used intelligence tests are those forming the Wechsler scales, which include a group of subtests that form a performance scale, with different versions suitable for children in the age range 3–7 years (WPPSI; Wechsler 1989) and 6–16 years (WISC-III; Wechsler 1992). The Leiter International Performance Scale–Revised (Roid & Miller 1997) has the advantage of being specifically designed for assessing intelligence without requiring any language. The examiner demonstrates what is required, rather than using verbal instruction, and the test is untimed. The revised test is considerably improved over the original version, with new norms, data on reliability and validity, and new subtests to assess attention and memory. Norms for the McCarthy Scales of Children's Abilities (McCarthy 1972) are dated, but the battery contains attractive subtests for assessing non-verbal abilities that readily engage the interest of preschool-aged children. The test is appropriate for the age range 2–8 years. The Kaufman Assessment Battery for Children (K-ABC; Kaufman & Kaufman 1983) is a well-standardized battery that includes a non-verbal scale that requires no language from tester or testee, and is suitable for ages 4–12 years. The British Ability Scales II (Elliott et al. 1996) and its US counterpart the Differential Ability Scales (Elliott 1990) consist of a battery of cognitive tests for children aged from 2 to

17 years, including some exclusively non-verbal subtests that can be combined to form a Special Non-verbal Scale.

There are a number of brief tests of non-verbal ability that are not suitable for clinical assessment, because they assess only a limited range of cognitive operations, but which are useful in research or screening settings. Raven's Matrices (Raven *et al.* 1986), which includes an easy version, Coloured Matrices, is suitable for children aged 5 years and above. This test correlates well with 'g', the principal factor that is extracted from other IQ tests. The Test of Non-verbal Intelligence, third edition (TONI-3; Brown *et al.* 1997) is a language-free measure of cognitive ability suitable for ages 5 years and above. Raven's Matrices and TONI-3 are both untimed and take around 15 min to administer. The Wechsler Abbreviated Scale of Intelligence (WASI; Wechsler 1999) includes two subtests to estimate Performance IQ and has norms from 6 years to adulthood.

Given the central importance of assessment of non-verbal ability in the DSM-IV and ICD-10 diagnoses of developmental speech and language disorders, it is perhaps surprising that there are few recommendations about which tests are most appropriate with this population. Tests can vary markedly in the cognitive functions that they assess, and in the extent to which performance may be affected by the use of verbal coding, even if no language is used explicitly. Tests involving perceptual matching or manipulation (e.g. shape matching or copying, block design, object assembly, mental rotation) seem least likely to be affected by language level. Those involving higher level conceptual matching (e.g. on the basis of number or superordinate semantic category) could conceivably be influenced by the child's ability to count, or knowledge of the verbal labels for categories. More difficult matrices tasks, which involve identifying salient information from two or more dimensions and combining this to form a solution, might well be facilitated by verbal encoding of the problem. In addition, tests vary in whether or not they stress speed as well as accuracy of performance. In the WISC-III, separate scores can be computed for Perceptual Organization and Processing Speed. Little work has been carried out to assess how these factors may influence performance of language-impaired children. In the absence of such information, one can only recommend that, in clinical contexts, a range of non-verbal tests should be administered, rather than relying solely on one or two subtests.

Speech

Speech difficulties are relatively easy to detect, but require specialized expertise to assess. Coplan & Gleason (1988) provide guidelines to help clinicians decide when to refer a child for speech assessment, on the basis of a parent's response to the question, 'How much of your child's speech can a stranger understand?':

1 less than half;
2 about half;
3 three-quarters;
4 all or almost all.

At 2 years, referral is suggested if the child is less than 50% intelligible, at 3 years if less than 75% intelligible, and at 4 years if less than 100% intelligible. Referral will usually be to a speech and language therapist, who will analyse the pattern of speech errors, and also assess how far the child has an isolated speech problem or more pervasive language difficulties. Where there is facial dysmorphology, or evidence of neurological dysfunction, referral to specialist medical services (paediatric neurology, otolaryngology, and/or clinical genetics) is warranted.

Language

Screening for language impairment

Before discussing detailed language assessment, we need to consider the question of how and when to embark on such an assessment for the child presenting with a psychiatric disorder, where a language disorder has not been suspected. We know from the work of Cohen (1996; Cohen *et al.* 1998) that a high proportion of such children do have measurable language deficits. However, in many clinical contexts, there are insufficient resources to enable every psychiatric referral to have a full language assessment. Information from parental interview and informal clinical observation can help guide the decision as to whether to refer the child for more detailed evaluation. Rutter (1987) and Cantwell & Baker (1987) provide useful clinical guidelines for evaluating the child's communicative history and current status. Where there is evidence of delayed language development, inconsistent or inadequate responses to the speech of others and, in a child above the age of 5 years, difficulty in giving simple information about a salient past event (such as a birthday party or holiday) or problems in following simple commands (e.g. 'Pick up the big ball and the spoon' from an array of objects), then this should alert the clinician to the possibility of a language problem.

The fact remains that reliance solely on clinical judgement is seldom adequate for detecting more subtle communicative difficulties. One solution is for the clinician to gain expertise in administration of simple language screening tests. Renfrew (1988) Language Scales have the advantage that they can be administered by those without specialist training, and provide an indication of level of grammatical competence, narrative skills and word-finding ability in children from 3 to 8 years of age. For older children, Cohen *et al.* (1998) found that a 30-min battery that included subtests from the Clinical Evaluation of Language Fundamentals–3 (CELF-3: Semel *et al.* 1995) provided good discrimination between children with and without language impairments. However, administration of this battery requires expertise in language assessment.

Measuring severity and nature of language impairment

More detailed investigation of speech and language problems will usually be undertaken by a speech and language therapist or specialist psychologist. In English, there are now several language test batteries to choose from, but the situation is far less satisfactory in many other languages, and it is not safe to assume that difficulty of test items will remain constant if a test is translated. The instruments that are used depend on the age of the child.

This brief review will focus predominantly on language batteries that use a range of subtests to estimate receptive and expressive language abilities. For very young children, the most suitable test is the Preschool Language Scale (PLS-3; Zimmerman *et al.* 1992), which provides norms from the ages of 2 weeks to 6 years. It has separate subscales for Auditory Comprehension and Expressive Communication. The Test of Language Development (TOLD-P3; Newcomer & Hammill 1997) has norms from over 1000 children from 4 to 8 years. It has five core subtests that are combined to give an overall Language Quotient. Tomblin *et al.* (1996) have developed an algorithm for diagnosing language impairment based on TOLD scores. The Clinical Evaluation of Language Fundamentals (CELF; Semel *et al.* 1995) is widely used by speech and language therapists in both the UK and USA to diagnose specific language impairment. Scales can be combined to yield receptive and expressive scales, and a reduced subset of tests may be used for screening. There are different versions for preschool-aged children (3–6 years) and older clients (6–21 years). The Test of Adolescent and Adult Language (TOAL-3; Hammill *et al.* 1994) provides an in-depth assessment of receptive and expressive language, including some subtests involving written language.

Pinpointing the nature of a language impairment

More specialized diagnostic tests can be used to pinpoint the nature of language difficulties more precisely. For instance, one can consider whether a child with comprehension problems has difficulty in discriminating speech sounds, in recognizing words, or in decoding complex sentences (for a review see Bishop 1997b). The Goldman–Fristoe–Woodcock Test of Auditory Discrimination (Goldman *et al.* 1970) assesses ability to discriminate speech sounds in noisy and quiet conditions in children aged 3 years and above. The British Picture Vocabulary Scale (BPVS; Dunn *et al.* 1997) or its US equivalent the Peabody Picture Vocabulary Test (PPVT-R; Dunn & Dunn 1997) assess receptive vocabulary, and the Test for Reception of Grammar (TROG; Bishop 1989) assesses understanding of grammatical contrasts. The Token Test for Children (Disimoni 1978) stresses auditory verbal memory, requiring the child to respond to commands such as, 'Pick up the big green square and the small blue circle'.

Comprehension assessment poses a particular challenge for children whose motor impairments prevent them from being able to manipulate toys or point to pictures, but it is usually possible to arrange multiple choice test materials in such a way that the child can use a communication aid, or a reliable response such as eye-pointing, to select from the alternatives.

Two points should be stressed. First, no test is a 'pure' measure of language functioning. Factors such as level of co-operation, attention, memory and executive functions may play a part in how children perform. A highly distractible child may impulsively point to a picture in an array because it is appealing or salient, without listening to instructions. Secondly, different tests that purport to measure the same functions may assess quite different underlying skills. For instance, the Wechsler scales include a subtest termed Comprehension that requires the child to respond to questions such as 'What should you do if you see thick smoke coming from the window of a neighbour's house?' Correct performance on this test requires very different skills (including reasoning ability and response formulation) from those tapped by an auditory discrimination or receptive vocabulary test. Thus, whether a child's language scores in the impaired range can depend as much on the specific tests used as on the characteristics of the child. There is evidence that 'knowledge-dependent' measures, such as vocabulary tests, exaggerate cultural and socioeconomic differences between children, whereas 'processing' measures that vary difficulty by manipulating the amount of material that has to be processed (e.g. Token Test, or non-word repetition) depend less on prior experience, and so give a culturally unbiased estimate of language ability (Campbell *et al.* 1997). Interestingly, the same processing measures also seem especially sensitive to residual language difficulties in older children and adults (Tomblin *et al.* 1992; Bishop *et al.* 1996).

Most standardized assessments focus on assessing accuracy and complexity of elicited language, or literal understanding of individual words and sentences, e.g. the child may be asked to select a picture where 'the fish is on the table'. The ability to select and interpret messages appropriately in relation to the context (pragmatics) is not adequately tapped by such tasks. The Children's Communication Checklist developed by Bishop (1998) may be helpful in obtaining information about the child's everyday use of language when pragmatic difficulties are suspected but not detected on formal assessment. In addition, it can be useful to move away from formal assessment and consider how the child behaves in a more naturalistic situation, such as toy play or, for children of 6 years and over, adult–child conversation about the child's past activities and planned future events. It is difficult and time-consuming to obtain objective indices of conversational competence from such data (Bishop *et al.* 2000) but it is possible to consider such general questions as: is the child's conversation coherent, or is it difficult to keep track of what is being talked about? Does the child go off at tangents, or keep returning to favoured topics? Does the child keep asking questions, with apparent disregard for the answers? Does speech sound stilted, over-adult, pedantic, stereotyped or robotic? Is there a tendency to give over-literal answers, such as drawing a picture when asked to 'draw the curtains'? If the answer to such questions is 'yes', this suggests one should consider a diagnosis on the autistic spectrum, and that broader evaluation of social interaction and repetitive behaviours and interests needs to be undertaken.

Conclusions

This chapter has been structured around the decision tree shown in Fig. 39.1, which was designed to facilitate clinical decision-making in this complex and difficult area. However, it is important to appreciate that this is something of an idealization, showing the steps one would follow to arrive at a primary diagnosis. In practice, few of these different disorders are mutually exclusive, and the clinician will not necessarily find all the evidence consistent with a single final diagnosis. For instance, global developmental delay often coexists with autistic disorder; selective mutism may co-occur with DLD. Speech and language difficulties often go hand in hand. Many children with dysarthria or anarthria also have some degree of hearing impairment or language impairment. Perhaps the most important message for the clinician is to remember that cases of 'pure' textbook conditions are the exception rather than the rule.

References

American Psychiatric Association (1994) *Diagnostic and Statistical Manual of Mental Disorders,* 4th edn, American Psychiatric Association, Washington D.C.

Appleton, R.E. (1995) The Landau–Kleffner syndrome. *Archives of Disease in Childhood,* **72**, 386–387.

Aram, D.M., Morris, R. & Hall, N.E. (1992) The validity of discrepancy criteria for identifying children with developmental language disorders. *Journal of Learning Disabilities,* **25**, 549–554.

Aram, D.M., Morris, R. & Hall, N.E. (1993) Clinical and research congruence in identifying children with language impairment. *Journal of Speech and Hearing Research,* **36**, 580–591.

Beitchman, J.H., Brownlie, E.B. & Wilson, B. (1996) Linguistic impairment and psychiatric disorder: pathways to outcome. In: *Language, Learning and Behavior Disorders: Developmental, Biological and Clinical Perspectives* (eds J. Beitchman, N.J. Cohen, M.M. Konstantareas & R. Tannock), pp. 493–514. Cambridge University Press, New York.

Bird, J., Bishop, D.V.M. & Freeman, N. (1995) Phonological awareness and literacy development in children with expressive phonological impairments. *Journal of Speech and Hearing Research,* **38**, 446–462.

Bishop, D.V.M. (1979) Comprehension in developmental language disorders. *Developmental Medicine and Child Neurology,* **21**, 225–238.

Bishop, D.V.M. (1983) Comprehension of English syntax by profoundly deaf children. *Journal of Child Psychology and Psychiatry,* **24**, 415–434.

Bishop, D.V.M. (1985) Age of onset and outcome in 'acquired aphasia with convulsive disorder' (Landau–Kleffner syndrome). *Developmental Medicine and Child Neurology,* **27**, 705–712.

Bishop, D.V.M. (1987) The causes of specific developmental language disorder ('developmental dysphasia'). *Journal of Child Psychology and Psychiatry,* **28**, 1–8.

Bishop, D.V.M. (1988) Technical note: otitis media and developmental language disorder. *Journal of Child Psychology and Psychiatry,* **29**, 365–368.

Bishop, D.V.M. (1989) *Test for Reception of Grammar,* 2nd edn. D.V.M. Bishop, Age and Cognitive Performance Research Centre, University of Manchester, M13 9PL.

Bishop, D.V.M. (1994a) Is specific language impairment a valid diagnostic category? Genetic and psycholinguistic evidence. *Philosophical Transactions of the Royal Society, Series B,* **346**, 105–111.

Bishop, D.V.M. (1994b) Developmental disorders of speech and language. In: *Child and Adolescent Psychiatry* (eds M. Rutter, L. Hersov & E. Taylor), pp. 546–568. Blackwell Scientific, Oxford.

Bishop, D.V.M. (1997a) Pre- and perinatal hazards and family background in children with specific language impairments: a study of twins. *Brain and Language,* **56**, 1–26.

Bishop, D.V.M. (1997b) *Uncommon Understanding: Development and Disorders of Language Comprehension in Children.* Psychology Press, Hove.

Bishop, D.V.M. (1998) Development of the children's communication checklist (CCC): a method for assessing qualitative aspects of communicative impairment in children. *Journal of Child Psychology and Psychiatry,* **39**, 879–891.

Bishop, D.V.M. (2000) Pragmatic language impairment: a correlate of SLI, a distinct subgroup, or part of the autistic continuum? In: *Speech and Language Impairments in Children: Causes, Characteristics, Intervention and Outcome* (eds D.V.M. Bishop & L.B. Leonard), pp. 99–113. Psychology Press, Hove.

Bishop, D.V.M. (2001) Genetic and environmental risks for specific language impairment in children. *Philosophical Transactions of the Royal Society, Series B,* **356**, 369–380.

Bishop, D.V.M. & Adams, C. (1990) A prospective study of the relationship between specific language impairment, phonological disorders and reading retardation. *Journal of Child Psychology and Psychiatry,* **31**, 1027–1050.

Bishop, D.V.M. & Edmundson, A. (1986) Is otitis media a major cause of specific developmental language disorders? *British Journal of Disorders of Communication,* **21**, 321–338.

Bishop, D.V.M. & Edmundson, A. (1987) Language-impaired four-year-olds: distinguishing transient from persistent impairment. *Journal of Speech and Hearing Disorders,* **52**, 156–173.

Bishop, D.V.M. & Rosenbloom, L. (1987) Classification of childhood language disorders. In: *Language Development and Disorders* (eds W. Yule & M. Rutter), pp. 16–41. Blackwell Scientific, Oxford.

Bishop, D.V.M., North, T. & Donlan, C. (1995) Genetic basis of specific language impairment: evidence from a twin study. *Developmental Medicine and Child Neurology,* **37**, 56–71.

Bishop, D.V.M., North, T. & Donlan, C. (1996) Nonword repetition as a behavioural marker for inherited language impairment: evidence from a twin study. *Journal of Child Psychology and Psychiatry,* **37**, 391–403.

Bishop, D.V.M., Bishop, S.J., Bright, P., James, C., Delaney, T. & Tallal, P. (1999) Different origin of auditory and phonological processing problems in children with language impairment: evidence from a twin study. *Journal of Speech, Language and Hearing Research,* **42**, 155–168.

Bishop, D.V.M., Chan, J., Adams, C., Hartley, J. & Weir, F. (2000) Evidence of disproportionate pragmatic difficulties in a subset of children with specific language impairment. *Development and Psychopathology,* **12**, 177–199.

Black, B. & Uhde, T.W. (1995) Psychiatric characteristics of children with selective mutism. *Journal of the American Academy of Child and Adolescent Psychiatry,* **34**, 847–856.

Bradford, A. & Dodd, B. (1996) Do all speech-disordered children have motor deficits? *Clinical Linguistics and Phonetics,* **10**, 77–101.

Brannon, J.B. & Murry, T. (1966) The spoken syntax of normal, hard-of-hearing and deaf children. *Journal of Speech and Hearing Research,* **9**, 604–610.

Brown, J.K. (1985) Dysarthria in children: neurologic perspective. In: *Speech and Language Evaluation in Neurology: Childhood Disorders* (ed. J.K. Darby), pp. 132–184. Grune & Stratton, Orlando, FL.

Brown, L., Sherbenou, R. & Johnsen, S. (1997) *Test of Nonverbal Intelligence*, 3rd edn *(TONI-3)*. Pro-Ed, Austin, TX.

Bryne-Saricks, M.C. (1987) Treatment of language disorders in children: a review of experimental studies. In: *Human Communication and its Disorders* (ed. H. Winitz), pp. 167–201. Ablex Publishing, Norwood, NJ.

Campbell, T.F., Dollaghan, C. & Felsenfeld, S. (1996) Disorders of language, phonology, fluency, and voice: indicators for referral. In: *Pediatric Otolaryngology*, Vol. 2 (eds C.D. Bluestone, S.E. Stool & M.A. Kenna), pp. 1595–1606. W.B. Saunders, Philadelphia.

Campbell, T., Dollaghan, C., Needleman, H. & Janosky, J. (1997) Reducing bias in language assessment: processing-dependent measures. *Journal of Speech, Language and Hearing Research*, **40**, 519–525.

Cantwell, D. & Baker, L. (1987) *Developmental Speech and Language Disorders*. Guilford Press, New York.

Clahsen, H. & Almazan, M. (1998) Syntax and morphology in Williams syndrome. *Cognition*, **68**, 167–198.

Clark, M., Carr, L., Reilly, S. & Neville, B.G.R. (2000) Worster-Drought syndrome, a mild tetraplegic perisylvian cerebral palsy: review of 47 cases. *Brain*, **123**, 2160–2170.

Cohen, N.J. (1996) Unsuspected language impairments in psychiatrically disturbed children: developmental issues and associated conditions. In: *Language, Learning, and Behavior Disorders* (eds J.H. Beitchman, N.J. Cohen, M.M. Konstantareas & R. Tannock), pp. 105–127. Cambridge University Press, Cambridge.

Cohen, N.J., Barwick, M.A., Horodezky, N.B., Vallance, D.D. & Im, N. (1998) Language, achievement, and cognitive processing in psychiatrically disturbed children with previously identified and unsuspected language impairments. *Journal of Child Psychology and Psychiatry*, **39**, 865–877.

Cole, K.N., Schwartz, I.S., Notari, A.R., Dale, P.S. & Mills, P.E. (1995) Examination of the stability of two methods of defining specific language impairment. *Applied Psycholinguistics*, **16**, 103–123.

Conrad, R. (1979) *The Deaf School Child*. Harper & Row, New York.

Conti-Ramsden, G., Crutchley, A. & Botting, N. (1997) The extent to which psychometric tests differentiate subgroups of children with SLI. *Journal of Speech, Language and Hearing Research*, **40**, 765–777.

Coplan, J. & Gleason, J.R. (1988) Unclear speech: recognition and significance of unintelligible speech in preschool children. *Pediatrics*, **82**, 447–452.

Crary, M.A. (1993) *Developmental Motor Speech Disorders*. Singular Publishing, San Diego.

Da Silva, E.A., Chugani, D.C., Muzik, O. & Chugani, H.T. (1997) Landau–Kleffner syndrome: metabolic abnormalities in temporal lobe are a common feature. *Journal of Child Neurology*, **12**, 489–495.

Dean, E.C., Howell, J., Water, D. & Reid, J. (1995) Metaphon: a metalinguistic approach to the treatment of phonological disorder in children. *Clinical Linguistics and Phonetics*, **9**, 1–58.

Deonna, T. (2000) Acquired epileptic aphasia (AEA) or Landau–Kleffner syndrome: from childhood to adulthood. In: *Speech and Language Impairments in Children: Causes, Characteristics, Intervention and Outcome* (eds D.V.M. Bishop & L.B. Leonard), pp. 261–272. Psychology Press, Hove.

Disimoni, F. (1978) *The Token Test for Children*. Riverside Publishing, Chicago.

Dummit, E.S., Klein, R.G., Tancer, N.K., Asche, B., Martin, J. & Fairbanks, J.A. (1997) Systematic assessment of 50 children with selective mutism. *Journal of the American Academy of Child and Adolescent Psychiatry*, **36**, 653–660.

Dunn, L.M. & Dunn, L.M. (1997) *PPVT-III: Peabody Picture Vocabulary, Test*, 3rd edn. American Guidance Service, Circle Pines, MN.

Dunn, L.M., Whetton, C. & Pintilie, D. (1997) *British Picture Vocabulary Scale*, 2nd edn. NFER-Nelson Publishing, Windsor.

Dunn, M., Flax, J., Sliwinski, M. & Aram, D. (1996) The use of spontaneous language measures as criteria for identifying children with specific language impairment: an attempt to reconcile clinical and research findings. *Journal of Speech and Hearing Research*, **39**, 643–654.

Echenne, B., Cheminal, R., Rivier, F., Negre, C., Touchon, J. & Billiard, M. (1992) Epileptic electroencephalographic abnormalities and developmental dysphasias: a study of 32 patients. *Brain and Development*, **14**, 216–225.

Elliott, C. (1990) *Differential Ability Scales*. Psychological Corporation, San Antonio, TX.

Elliott, C.D., Smith, P. & McUlloch, K. (1996) *British Ability Scales*, 2nd edn. NFER-Nelson, Windsor.

Feekery, C.J., Parry-Fielder, B. & Hopkins, I.J. (1993) Landau–Kleffner syndrome: 6 patients including discordant monozygotic twins. *Pediatric Neurology*, **9**, 49–53.

Fenson, L., Dale, P.S., Reznick, J.S., Bates, E., Thal, D.J. & Pethick, S.J. (1994) Variability in early communicative development. *Monographs of the Society for Research in Child Development*, **59**.

Fey, M.E., Long, S.E. & Cleave, P.L. (1994) Reconsideration of IQ criteria in the definition of specific language impairment. In: *Specific Language Impairments in Children* (eds R. Watkins & M. Rice), pp. 161–178. Paul H. Brookes, Baltimore.

Fisher, S.E., Vargha Khadem, F., Watkins, K.E., Monaco, A.P. & Pembrey, M.E. (1998) Localisation of a gene implicated in a severe speech and language disorder. *Nature Genetics*, **18**, 168–170.

Fundudis, T., Kolvin, I. & Garside, R. (1979) *Speech Retarded and Deaf Children: Their Psychological Development*. Academic Press, London.

Gallagher, T. (1996) Social-interactional approaches to child language intervention. In: *Language, Learning and Behavior Disorders: Developmental, Biological and Clinical Perspectives* (eds J. Beitchman, N.J. Cohen, M.M. Konstantareas & R. Tannock), pp. 493–514. Cambridge University Press, New York.

Gathercole, S.E., Willis, C., Baddeley, A.D. & Emslie, H. (1994) The children's test of nonword repetition: a test of phonological working memory. *Memory*, **2**, 103–127.

Genton, P. & Guerrini, R. (1993) What differentiates Landau–Kleffner syndrome from the syndrome of continuous spikes and waves during slow sleep? [Letter] *Archives of Neurology*, **50**, 1008–1009.

Girolametto, L., Pearce, P.S. & Weitzman, E. (1996) Interactive focused stimulation for toddlers with expressive vocabulary delays. *Journal of Speech and Hearing Research*, **39**, 1274–1283.

Goldman, R., Fristoe, M. & Woodcock, R.W. (1970) *Goldman–Fristoe–Woodcock Test of Auditory Discrimination*. American Guidance Service, Circle Pines, MN.

Gravel, J., Wallace, I. & Ruben, R. (1996) Auditory consequences of early mild hearing-loss associated with otitis-media. *Acta Oto-Laryngologica*, **116**, 219–221.

Grievink, E., Peters, S.A.F., Van Bon, W.H.J. & Schilder, A.G.M. (1993) The effects of early bilateral otitis media with effusion on language ability: a prospective cohort study. *Journal of Speech and Hearing Research*, **36**, 1004–1012.

Guerreiro, M.M., Camargo, E.E., Kato, M. *et al.* (1996) Brain single photon emission computed tomography imaging in Landau–Kleffner syndrome. *Epilepsia*, **37**, 60–67.

Hammill, D., Brown, V., Larsen, S. & Wiederholt, J.L. (1994) *Test of Adolescent and Adult Language (TOAL-3)*. Pro-Ed, Circle Pines, MN.

Hayden, D.A. & Pukonen, M. (1996) Language intervention programming for preschool children with social and pragmatic disorders. In: *Language, Learning and Behavior Disorders: Developmental, Biological and Clinical Perspectives* (eds J. Beitchman, N.J. Cohen, M.M. Konstantareas & R. Tannock), pp. 436–466. Cambridge University Press, New York.

Hurst, J.A., Baraitser, M., Auger, E., Graham, F. & Norell, S. (1990) An extended family with a dominantly inherited speech disorder. *Developmental Medicine and Child Neurology*, 32, 352–355.

Johnson, C.J., Beitchman, J.H., Young, A. *et al.* (1999) Fourteen year follow-up of children with and without speech/language impairment. *Journal of Speech, Language and Hearing Research*, 42, 744–760.

Kaplan, L.C. & Elias, E.R. (1986) Diagnosis of muscular dystrophy in patients referred for evaluation of language delay. *Developmental Medicine and Child Neurology*, 28, 110.

Kaufman, A.S. & Kaufman, N.L. (1983) *Kaufman Assessment Battery for Children*. American Guidance Service, Circle Pines, MN.

Keith, R.W., ed. (1977) *Central Auditory Dysfunction*. Grune and Stratton, New York.

Kolvin, I. & Fundudis, T. (1981) Elective mute children: psychological development and background factors. *Journal of Child Psychology and Psychiatry*, 22, 219–232.

Kristensen, H. (2000) Selective mutism and comorbidity with developmental disorder/delay, anxiety disorder, and elimination disorder. *Journal of the American Academy of Child and Adolescent Psychiatry*, 39, 249–256.

Lahey, M. & Edwards, M. (1995) Specific language impairment: preliminary investigation of factors associated with family history and with patterns of language performance. *Journal of Speech and Hearing Research*, 38, 643–657.

Landau, W.M. & Kleffner, F.R. (1957) Syndrome of acquired aphasia with convulsive disorder in children. *Neurology*, 7, 523–530.

Lane, H. (1990) Cultural and infirmity models of deaf Americans. *Journal of the Academy of Rehabilitative Audiology*, 23, 11–26.

Law, J., Boyle, J., Harris, F., Harkness, A. & Nye, C. (1998) Screening for speech and language delay: a systematic review of the literature. *Health Technology Assessment*, 2.

Lerman, P., Lermansagie, T. & Kivity, S. (1991) Effect of early corticosteroid-therapy for Landau–Kleffner syndrome. *Developmental Medicine and Child Neurology*, 33, 257–260.

Lewis, B.A. & Thompson, L.A. (1992) A study of developmental speech and language disorders in twins. *Journal of Speech and Hearing Research*, 35, 1086–1094.

Lord, C., Rutter, M. & LeCouteur, A. (1994) Autism Diagnostic Interview–Revised: a revised version of a diagnostic interview for caregivers of individuals with possible pervasive developmental disorders. *Journal of Autism and Developmental Disorders*, 24, 659–685.

Lord, C., Risi, S., Lambrecht, L. *et al.* (2000) The Autism Diagnostic Observation Schedule–Generic: a standard measure of social and communication deficits associated with the spectrum of autism. *Journal of Autism and Developmental Disorders*, 30, 205–223.

Mawhood, L., Howlin, P. & Rutter, M. (2000) Autism and developmental receptive language disorder: a comparative follow-up in early adult life. I. Cognitive and language outcomes. *Journal of Child Psychology and Psychiatry*, 41, 547–560.

McCarthy, D. (1972) *McCarthy Scales of Children's Abilities*. Psychological Corporation, New York.

Merzenich, M.M., Jenkins, W.M., Johnston, P., Schreiner, C., Miller, S.L. & Tallal, P. (1996) Temporal processing deficits of language-learning impaired children ameliorated by training. *Science*, 271, 77–81.

Miyamoto, R.T., Svirsky, M.A. & Robbins, A.M. (1997) Enhancement of expressive language in prelingually deaf children with cochlear implants. *Acta Oto-Laryngologica*, 117, 154–157.

Morley, M.E. (1972) *The Development and Disorders of Speech in Childhood*. Churchill Livingstone, Edinburgh.

Morley, M., Court, D. & Miller, H. (1954) Developmental dysarthria. *British Medical Journal*, 1, 8–10.

Morrell, F. & Lewine, J. (1994) Magnetic source imaging of spike dipole distribution in Landau–Kleffner syndrome. *Neurology*, 44, A 386.

Morrell, F., Whisler, W.W., Smith, M.C. *et al.* (1995) Landau–Kleffner syndrome: treatment with subpial intracortical transection. *Brain*, 118, 1529–1546.

Morris, C.A. & Mervis, C.B. (1999) Williams syndrome. In: *Handbook of Neurodevelopmental and Genetic Disorders in Children* (eds S. Goldstein & C.R. Reynolds), pp. 555–590. Guilford, New York.

Neff, W.D. (1967) Auditory discriminations affected by cortical ablations. In: *Sensorineural Hearing Processes and Disorders* (ed. A.B. Graham), pp. 201–206. University of Illinois Press, Urbana.

Neligan, G.A. & Prudham, D. (1969) Norms for four standard developmental milestones by sex, social class and place in family. *Developmental Medicine and Child Neurology*, 11, 413–422.

Newcomer, P. & Hammill, D.D. (1997) *Test of Language Development: Primary*, 3rd edn., Pro-Ed, Austin, TX.

Norbury, C.F., Bishop, D.V.M. & Briscoe, J. (2001) Production of verb morphology: a comparison of SLI and moderate hearing impairment. *Journal of Speech, Language and Hearing Research*, 44, 165–178.

O'Hare, A.E., Quew, R. & Aitken, K. (1998) The identification of autism in children referred to a tertiary speech and language clinic and the implications for service delivery. *Autism*, 2, 171–180.

Orlansky, M.D. & Bonvillian, J.D. (1985) Sign language acquisition: language development in children of deaf parents and implications for other populations. *Merrill-Palmer Quarterly*, 31, 127–143.

Owen, S.E. & McKinlay, I.A. (1997) Motor difficulties in children with developmental disorders of speech and language. *Child: Care, Health and Development*, 23, 315–325.

Parry-Fielder, B., Nolan, T.M., Collins, K.J. & Stojcevski, Z. (1997) Developmental language disorders and epilepsy. *Journal of Paediatrics and Child Health*, 33, 277–280.

Paul, R. (2000) Predicting outcomes of early expressive language delay: ethical implications. In: *Speech and Language Impairments in Children: Causes, Characteristics, Intervention and Outcome* (eds D.V.M. Bishop & L.B. Leonard), pp. 195–209. Psychology Press, Hove.

Paul, R., Hernandez, R., Taylor, L. & Johnson, K. (1996) Narrative development in late talkers: early school age. *Journal of Speech and Hearing Research*, 39, 1295–1303.

Peters, S.A.F., Grievink, E.H., van Bon, W.H.J. & Schilder, A.G.M. (1994) The effects of early bilateral otitis media with effusion on educational attainment: a prospective cohort study. *Journal of Learning Disabilities*, 27, 111–121.

Petitto, L.A. (2000) On the biological foundations of human language. In: *The Signs of Language Revisited: an Anthology to Honor Ursula Bellugi and Edward Klima* (ed. K. Emmorey), pp. 449–473. Lawrence Erlbaum, Mahwah, NJ.

Rapin, I. (1996) Developmental language disorders: a clinical update. *Journal of Child Psychology and Psychiatry*, 37, 643–655.

Raven, J.C., Court, J.H. & Raven, J. (1986) *Raven's Progressive Matrices and Raven's Coloured Matrices*. H.K. Lewis, London.

Renfrew, C.E. (1988) *Renfrew Language Scales*. Winslow Press, Bicester.

Rescorla, L., Roberts, J. & Dahlsgaard, K. (1997) Late talkers at 2: outcome at age 3. *Journal of Speech, Language and Hearing Research*, 40, 556–566.

Rice, M.L. (2000) Grammatical symptoms of specific language impairment. In: *Speech and Language Impairments in Children: Causes, Characteristics, Intervention and Outcome* (eds D.V.M. Bishop & L.B. Leonard), pp. 17–34. Psychology Press, Hove.

Rice, M.L. & Wexler, K. (1996) Toward tense as a clinical marker of specific language impairment in English-speaking children. *Journal of Speech and Hearing Research*, 39, 1239–1257.

Robinson, R.J. (1991) Causes and associations of severe and persistent specific speech and language disorders in children. *Developmental Medicine and Child Neurology*, 33, 943–962.

Roid, G.H. & Miller, L.J. (1997) *Leiter International Performance Scale–Revised*. Stoetling, Wood Dale, IL.

Rutter, M. (1987) Assessment: objectives and principles. In: *Language Development and Disorders* (eds W. Yule & M. Rutter), pp. 295–311. Blackwell Scientific, Oxford.

Rutter, M. & Lord, C. (1987) Language disorders associated with psychiatric disturbance. In: *Language Development and Disorders* (eds W. Yule & M. Rutter), pp. 206–223. Blackwell Scientific, Oxford.

Rutter, M. & Mawhood, L. (1991) The long-term psychosocial sequelae of specific developmental disorders of speech and language. In: *Biological Risk Factors for Psychosocial Disorders* (eds M. Rutter & P. Casaer), pp. 233–259. Cambridge University Press, Cambridge.

Scarborough, H.S. & Dobrich, W. (1990) Development of children with early language delay. *Journal of Speech and Hearing Research*, 33, 70–83.

Semel, E., Wiig, E.H. & Secord, W.H. (1995) *Clinical Evaluation of Language Fundamentals (CELF®-3)*, 3rd edn. Psychological Corporation, San Antonio, TX.

Shriberg, L.D., Tomblin, J.B. & McSweeny, J.L. (1999) Prevalence of speech delay in 6-year-old children and comorbidity with language impairment. *Journal of Speech, Language and Hearing Research*, 42, 1461–1481.

Sluckin, A., Foreman, N. & Herbert, M. (1991) Behavioural treatment programs and selectivity of speaking at follow-up in a sample of 25 selective mutes. *Australian Psychologist*, 26, 132–137.

Stackhouse, J. (1992) Developmental verbal dyspraxia. I. A review and critique. *European Journal of Disorders of Communication*, 27, 19–34.

Stothard, S.E., Snowling, M.J., Bishop, D.V.M., Chipchase, B.B. & Kaplan, C.A. (1998) Language impaired preschoolers: a follow-up into adolescence. *Journal of Speech, Language and Hearing Research*, 41, 407–418.

Stromswold, K. (1998) Genetics of spoken language disorders. *Human Biology*, 70, 293–320.

Tallal, P. (2000) Experimental studies of language learning impairments: from research to remediation. In: *Speech and Language Impairments in Children: Causes, Characteristics, Intervention and Outcome* (eds D.V.M. Bishop & L.B. Leonard), pp. 131–155. Psychology Press, Hove.

Tallal, P., Miller, S.L., Bedi, G. *et al.* (1996) Language comprehension in language-learning impaired children improved with acoustically modified speech. *Science*, 271, 81–84.

Tallal, P., Allard, L., Miller, S. & Curtiss, S. (1997) Academic outcomes of language impaired children. In: *Dyslexia: Biology, Cognition and Intervention* (eds C. Hulme & M. Snowling), pp. 167–181. Whurr, London.

Tomblin, J.B. & Buckwalter, P.R. (1998) Heritability of poor language achievement among twins. *Journal of Speech, Language and Hearing Research*, 41, 188–199.

Tomblin, J.B., Freese, P.R. & Records, N.L. (1992) Diagnosing specific language impairment in adults for the purpose of pedigree analysis. *Journal of Speech and Hearing Research*, 35, 832–843.

Tomblin, J.B., Records, N. & Zhang, X. (1996) A system for the diagnosis of specific language impairment in kindergarten children. *Journal of Speech and Hearing Research*, 39, 1284–1294.

Tomblin, J.B., Records, N.-L., Buckwalter, P., Zhang, X., Smith, E. & O'Brien, M. (1997) Prevalence of specific language impairment in kindergarten children. *Journal of Speech and Hearing Research*, 40, 1245–1260.

Tomblin, J.B., Spencer, L., Flock, S., Tyler, R. & Gantz, B. (1999) A comparison of language achievement in children with cochlear implants and children using hearing aids. *Journal of Speech, Language, and Hearing Research*, 42, 497–509.

Van Dongen, H., Meulstee, J., Blauw-van Mourik, M. & Van Harskamp, F. (1989) Landau–Kleffner syndrome: a case study with a fourteen-year follow-up. *European Neurology*, 29, 109–114.

Wechsler, D. (1989) *Wechsler Preschool and Primary Scale of Intelligence–Revised Edition*. Psychological Corporation, New York.

Wechsler, D. (1992) *Wechsler Intelligence Scale for Children*, 3rd UK edn. Psychological Corporation, London.

Wechsler, D. (1999) *Wechsler Abbreviated Scale of Intelligence*. Psychological Corporation, New York.

Whitehurst, G.J. & Fischel, J.E. (1994) Early developmental language delay: what, if anything, should the clinician do about it? *Journal of Child Psychology and Psychiatry*, 35, 613–648.

Willeford, J.A. (1977) Assessing central auditory behavior in children: a test battery approach. In: *Central Auditory Dysfunction* (ed. R.W. Keith), pp. 43–72. Grune and Stratton, New York.

World Health Organization (1993) *The ICD-10 Classification for Mental and Behavioural Disorders: Diagnostic Criteria for Research*. World Health Organization, Geneva.

Worster-Drought, C. (1974) Suprabulbar paresis: congenital suprabulbar paresis and its differential diagnosis with special reference to acquired suprabulbar paresis. *Developmental Medicine and Child Neurology*, 16 (Suppl. 30), 1–33.

Zielhuis, G.A., Rach, G.H. & Van den Broek, P. (1990) The occurrence of otitis media with effusion in Dutch pre-school children. *Clinical Otolaryngology*, 15, 147–153.

Zimmerman, I.L., Steiner, V. & Pond, R. (1992) *Preschool Language Scale–3*. Psychological Corporation, San Antonio, TX.

40 Reading and Other Learning Difficulties

Margaret J. Snowling

Introduction

The term 'learning difficulties' is widely applied to problems that pose obstacles to educational achievement. Learning difficulties can occur in the context of global delays in development or, more specifically, where there are circumscribed deficits in cognitive processes. It is conventional in clinical and educational practice to differentiate these two forms of learning disability. This chapter primarily considers specific learning difficulties, in contrast to general learning difficulties that cut across different domains, as a way of highlighting how relatively specific cognitive deficits impact upon learning processes. Moreover, the focus of the chapter is on reading difficulties. Reading difficulties (dyslexia) have attracted much more research interest than other types of learning problem and have been described at the biological, cognitive and behavioural levels. In addition, interventions to ameliorate reading problems have been evaluated. Much less is known about specific difficulties in arithmetic (dyscalculia) and about non-verbal learning disabilities, possibly because these problems can be hidden more easily in a literate society.

Specific learning difficulties

Problems of literacy

Specific reading difficulties

Following the landmark Isle of Wight studies, it became widely accepted that children who have specific reading difficulties (specific reading retardation) should be distinguished from children who have reading difficulties in the context of more general learning problems (reading backwardness) (Rutter & Yule 1975). The definition of specific reading difficulties depends upon the use of a regression approach. Thus, on the basis of the correlation between reading and IQ in children of the same age, a child is deemed to have a specific problem with reading if reading attainment is significantly below that predicted from general cognitive ability.

However, the regression approach is a statistical approach and as such it has its limitations. A key question is whether children with a disorder defined in this way are distinct from children who have the same learning difficulty in the context of low IQ (Rispens 1998). Current opinion is somewhat divided on this

issue. While there is a growing body of opinion that the causes of poor reading are similar in the two groups of children, evidence suggests that children with 'discrepancy-defined reading disorders' (specific reading retardation) differ from generally backward readers in the compensatory strategies they can use (Nation & Snowling 1998). In turn, this may influence their reading development.

The prevalence of specific reading difficulties depends upon the cut-off point taken to indicate a reading disability. Using a cut-off of 2 standard errors of measurement (SE) below their expected attainment score, Yule *et al.* (1974), reported a prevalence of specific reading retardation ranging from 3.1% among 10 year olds in the Isle of Wight to 6.3% in London, based on the discrepancy between IQ and reading accuracy. The comparable figures for specific difficulties in reading comprehension were 3.6 and 9.3%, respectively. Thus, prevalence depends both upon geographical distribution (figures were higher in an inner-city population) and also on the tests used (Rodgers 1983; Silva *et al.* 1985).

Epidemiological data also suggest that this classification of children's reading problems is not a stable entity. Shaywitz *et al.* (1992) followed the development of 414 Connecticut children and, using a cut-off of 1.5 SE below expectation as indicative of specific reading difficulties, reported prevalence rates of 5.6% in 6 year olds, 7% in 8 year olds and 5.4% in 10 year olds. Fluctuations in the numbers of children fulfilling the criteria for specific reading retardation in the different grades may partly be explained by variations in the rate of early literacy acquisition. Later on in development, the changing demands of reading can also be expected to produce variations in prevalence rate (Snowling 2000).

Epidemiological studies have typically reported an excess of males with specific reading difficulties, three to four males to every female affected, consistent with the findings from referred samples. Shaywitz *et al.* (1990) found a more even distribution of between 1:3 and 1:5 boys to every girl affected. To some extent, differences might be explained by differences in the age of the populations sampled or by differences in the cut-offs used to define specific reading problems. None the less, a bias towards boys in those children who had been referred by their schools was noted, and there was a tendency for girls to have more severe reading problems before they were referred.

A further variable that can be expected to influence prevalence rates of specific reading difficulties is the amount of time different children spend reading. A national survey conducted by McKenna *et al.* (1995) in the USA reported that attitudes to reading decline through the elementary school years, particularly for boys and for poorer readers. A disinclination to read may itself influence reading attainment and inflate the incidence of specific reading difficulties. Moreover, home factors account for large amounts of variance in the reading outcomes of children (Lundberg 1999). For this reason, it could be argued that a child should only be considered to have a specific reading deficit if they have had adequate opportunity to learn, although it is hard to put this exclusionary rule into practice.

It seems reasonable to infer that between 4 and 7% of children will have a specific reading difficulty at any one time, usually equivalent in practical terms to a retardation of some 18–24 months in reading relative to expectation based on age. However, it is noteworthy that the discrepancy definition of reading disorder typically conflates decoding problems and difficulties of reading comprehension (DSM-IV; American Psychiatric Association 1994). While it is the case that problems of decoding create a bottleneck to meaning and therefore compromise reading comprehension (Perfetti & Hogaboam 1975), it is not always the case that problems of reading comprehension are accompanied by word-level decoding difficulties. Furthermore, discrepancy definitions of reading difficulties are silent as to the signs that place a child at risk of reading failure, or that differentiate an adult with persisting difficulties in the domain of literacy who has compensated for a basic reading problem. For this reason, it is important to consider not only a child's current attainment when diagnosing a learning difficulty, but also their cognitive profile.

Normal literacy development: a framework

Before turning to a cognitive analysis of the causes of reading difficulties, it is important to make reference to normal theories of literacy development. In essence, to become literate, a child needs to integrate a system for processing written language with one that already exists for processing spoken language. In an alphabetic language such as English, the foundation of literacy is a system of mappings between orthography (the letters of printed words) and phonology (the speech sounds that make up the pronunciation of spoken words). The basic processes involved in establishing a system for word recognition are well captured by connectionist models of learning to read (Seidenberg & McClelland 1989). According to such models, reading involves the transfer of patterns of activation from orthographic input units to phonological output units for reading, and in the opposite direction for spelling. Furthermore, the transfer of activations between letter strings and pronunciations is conducted in the context of meaning (semantics). Activations from the meanings of words facilitate the decoding process by providing a top-down 'boost'. This facilitation is important for reading words that can only be partially deciphered by letter-sound translation and is particularly important for reading English that contains many exceptions to the 'rules' (Plaut *et al.* 1996). An important facet of connectionist models of reading is that, as knowledge accrues within the network of mappings, it generalizes to allow novel words to be read (e.g. non-words like 'tekwip'). The models therefore provide a parsimonious account of learning to read because a system for 'self-instruction' is part of the functional architecture.

There is now unequivocal evidence that learning to read depends upon phonological skills (Goswami & Bryant 1990). Children who can reflect on the sound structure of spoken words are well prepared to establish mappings between spoken and written words. Thus, reading and spelling achievement is strongly predicted in the school years by preschool measures of phonological awareness, even when the substantial effects of IQ are controlled (Bradley & Bryant 1983; Muter *et al.* 1997). However, a virtually exclusive focus of research on the acquisition of phonological awareness and reading skills has detracted from the important role of other language processes, such as semantic and syntactic skills, to the development of literacy. In the simple model of reading, Gough & Tunmer (1986) proposed that reading was the product of decoding and language comprehension. Children not only use knowledge of print–sound correspondences to decipher print, they also use sentence context to support this process (Share 1995). Furthermore, they must integrate the meanings of words within sentences and be able to use higher level skills, such as inference-making, to ensure text cohesion (Yuill & Oakhill 1991).

The task demands of reading are such that reading difficulties can occur for many different reasons. Broadly, reading disorders fall into two types: disorders of decoding and word identification at the word level (dyslexia); and disorders of reading comprehension that affect both single word and text comprehension. There have been a number of different typologies of reading difficulties within this framework. However, all of these leave substantial numbers of children unclassified. The main terms in current use to describe 'subtypes' of reading disorder are *phonological dyslexia* (a specific difficulty with decoding), *surface dyslexia* (a specific difficulty with the development of word recognition) and *hyperlexia* (a specific difficulty in printed word comprehension in the presence of a precocious ability to decode). However, as will become clear, these labels are used primarily to describe the surface manifestations of reading problems and do not necessarily carry implications either about aetiology or for intervention.

Word recognition and decoding deficits: the concept of dyslexia

Although in a minority of cases, problems of word identification (surface dyslexia; Coltheart *et al.* 1983) can be dissociated from problems of phonological decoding (phonological dyslexia; Seymour 1986; Castles & Coltheart 1993), the majority of children with specific reading difficulties have phonological difficulties (Manis *et al.* 1996). Within the connectionist framework outlined above, dyslexic children come to the task of learning to read with poorly specified phonological representations and deficits in both decoding (Rack *et al.* 1992) and word recognition ensue (Harm & Seidenberg 1999). In contrast, reading comprehension can be relatively good (Frith & Snowling 1983).

While the role of visual problems in dyslexia is a topic of continuing debate (Willows *et al.* 1993; Talcott & Stein 1999), most studies point to phonological deficits in dyslexic children (Brady 1997). In addition to problems with phonological awareness and limitations of verbal short-term memory, dyslexic children also have difficulties with verbal learning. These are the basis of many of their reported classroom learning problems, such as difficulty learning rote sequences like the months of the year, in mastering multiplication tables and in learning foreign languages.

The strength of the evidence pointing to the phonological deficits associated with dyslexia led to the proposal that dyslexia should be defined as a 'core' phonological deficit. Importantly, within the *phonological core–variable difference* model of dyslexia (Stanovich & Siegel 1994), poor phonology is related to poor reading performance, irrespective of IQ. Skills close to the 'core' of dyslexia include non-word reading and aspects of phonological awareness; all poor readers will tend to differ from normal readers in these skills. Children with specific reading difficulties differ from generally poor readers in skills farther from the core, including measures of working memory and listening comprehension.

An important advantage of the phonological deficit definition of dyslexia is that it makes sense in terms of what is known about the normal acquisition of reading. It also accounts well for the pattern of difficulties dyslexic people show across the life span when, although reading problems may be compensated, non-word reading and spelling impairments persist (Pennington *et al.* 1990; Bruck 1992; Snowling *et al.* 1997). These residual difficulties are often accompanied by problems of written expression.

Reading comprehension impairments

In contrast to dyslexic children who have deficits at the word level, children with specific difficulties in reading comprehension have good phonology and decode well but have problems understanding what they read. Nation & Snowling (1997) reported that 10% of a school sample of children had specific difficulties with reading comprehension. These difficulties often go unnoticed in the classroom because these children can read aloud competently. However, such children have poor vocabulary knowledge, poor syntactic skills (Stothard & Hulme 1995; Nation & Snowling 2000b) and poor working memory resources (Nation *et al.* 1999; Cain *et al.* 2000b). In the longer term, poor comprehenders have particular difficulty reading exception words that require semantic processing (e.g. 'chrome', 'aunt'). They also have difficulty using context to support their reading (Nation & Snowling 1998) and find it difficult to monitor and repair their reading errors. Although they spell well, their written composition uses a paucity of sentence structures and lacks cohesion. More generally, the problems they have making infer-

ences (Cain *et al.* 2000a) do not bode well for academic attainment across the curriculum.

Data on the longer-term outcome of poor comprehenders are lacking. A small-scale follow-up of 14 poor comprehenders studied by Stothard & Hulme (1995) suggested that, at the age of 13, some 5 years after the initial study, these children had poor reading accuracy as well as poor reading comprehension (Snowling *et al.* 1999). Similarly, Snowling *et al.* (2000) reported that children with specific language impairment who showed specific difficulties with reading comprehension at the age of 8 had general reading problems encompassing word recognition, decoding and reading comprehension skills at school leaving age. These strands of evidence suggest that there is a reciprocal interaction of component reading skills during development, such that decoding and comprehension skills, which are initially independent, support each other in the development of adult literacy.

Spelling difficulties

The spelling skills of dyslexic children are almost always impaired because they have difficulty reflecting on the sound structure of words. Although the attempts of dyslexic children to spell are phonologically motivated (Treiman 1997), a raised incidence of phonetically unacceptable errors has often been reported. A second source of spelling difficulty is poor knowledge of orthographic conventions. As English is an opaque orthography in which spelling–sound correspondences are not consistent, phonetic spelling errors are frequently seen (e.g. biscuit → biskit; chaos → kaos).

The term 'dyslexia' has sometimes been applied to individuals who have spelling difficulties in the absence of reading problems. Clinically, these children tend to have higher verbal than performance IQ and they make phonetically accurate spelling errors (Nelson & Warrington 1974). As becomes clear later, some of these children may be better characterized as having non-verbal learning disabilities rather than dyslexia.

Within a normal population, children who read well but have specific spelling problems were investigated by Frith (1980). Good readers who were poor spellers spelled phonetically; they had particular difficulty knowing when it was appropriate to double consonants (e.g. the 'n' in 'beginning') and how to represent unstressed vowels in syllables, for example the [er] sound in 'catapult'. They also found it difficult to select the correct spelling from two plausible alternatives, e.g. successful/succesful; necessary/necessery and they did less well than good spellers in proofreading and in non-word reading. It is possible therefore that a subtle reading problem can cause spelling difficulties; indeed people with poor spelling do not read in a detailed way. While a strategy of using context and partial graphic cues suffices for reading, Frith (1980) argued that it is insufficient to ensure satisfactory spelling performance. Subsequent evidence from single-case studies has confirmed a subtle difficulty with visual processing in individuals who can read but not spell well (Goulandris & Snowling 1991; Romani *et al.* 1999).

Cross-linguistic manifestations of reading disability

Languages differ in the difficulty they pose to young readers, differences that are related to the regularity or 'transparency' of their writing systems. German and Italian represent the more transparent of the European orthographies and, in these languages, letters and groups of letters (graphemes) correspond to single speech sounds (phonemes). The English writing system is, by contrast, opaque and, very frequently, a grapheme may correspond to more than one phoneme (e.g. the grapheme *e* may correspond to 'e' as in 'bed', to 'i' as in 'eve' and to 'i' as in 'believe').

A growing body of evidence indicates that children learn to read and spell more quickly in transparent languages than in opaque systems such as English (Harris & Hatano 1999). The reading and spelling symptoms of dyslexia are also different in regular orthographies. Unlike the case for English, German-speaking dyslexic children can read long unfamiliar words and also non-words as accurately as their peers, but their rate of reading is slow (Frith *et al.* 1998). Phonological awareness also develops more quickly in readers of transparent orthographies (Cossu 1999). As a consequence, the core phonological deficit of dyslexia is harder to detect in children who have learned to read in a regular orthography. In these languages, difficulties can be identified most clearly on tasks that require implicit phonological processing, such as verbal short-term memory, rapid naming and visual–verbal paired associate learning tasks (Wimmer *et al.* 1998).

Role of environmental input

Although cognitive explanations of reading disorders are compelling, it is important not to overlook the critical role of the environment in shaping a child's reading development. Indeed, social class differences in the development of reading skills are not entirely attributable to differences in reading-related phonological skills or general intelligence (Hecht *et al.* 2000). One variable that can have a significant impact on the behavioural manifestation of a reading disorder is reading practice. In the research literature, 'print exposure' is considered important for ensuring progress in an opaque reading system such as English, where there are many words that cannot be decoded using spelling–sound rules. Print exposure, measured by questionnaires that require participants to differentiate real book titles or real author's names from distracter items, and which document reading habits, accounts for variance in reading skills when other critical variables, such as IQ and phonological awareness, have been controlled (Stanovich & West 1989). It follows that clinicians need to be aware that an important source of individual differences among children with reading problems is the time they devote to reading.

Problems of numeracy

The incidence of underachievement for arithmetic (sometimes called dyscalculia) is less well documented than for reading. In the USA, the figure reported is around 6% (Baker & Cantwell 1985); in the UK, Lewis *et al.* (1994) recorded specific arithmetic difficulties of 1.3% in their epidemiological sample of 9–10 year olds; and in Israel, Gross Tsur *et al.* (1996) reported a prevalence of 6.5%, with equal numbers of boys and girls affected. It is common for arithmetic problems to co-occur with specific reading difficulties. Lewis *et al.* (1994) reported a prevalence of 2.3% for comorbid specific reading and arithmetic difficulties and Gross Tsur *et al.* (1996) reported that 17% of their sample with dyscalculia were also dyslexic.

Theoretical framework of normal development of number skills

From shortly after birth, infants can detect changes in the number of objects in visual displays of objects (Wynn 1995). This innate sense of numerosity is considered to be the foundation of later number concepts that develop rapidly during the preschool years. Gelman & Gallistel (1978) studied the development of counting from the age of around 2 years. In addition to learning the numbers and their order, children have to understand that each item in a set is labelled once and only once in the count sequence (the concept of one-to-one correspondence). The next step is to master cardinality, the knowledge that the final word in the count sequence tags its quantity. Later, children learn the principles of abstraction (that anything can be gathered together and counted) and of order irrelevance (the order in which you count things does not matter). Thus, by the time children go to school they have a foundation for the development of arithmetic skills. To become numerate demands more; children need to learn conventional systems and to use their mathematical thinking meaningfully and in logical situations (Nunes & Bryant 1996).

The earliest arithmetic skill to be taught in school is addition, a natural extension of counting skill. At first, children use a simple 'count all' strategy to solve addition problems (for a review see Geary 1993). By the age of 6, most are using a 'counting on' strategy in which they start with the smaller number and count on from this, often using fingers (MIN strategy). Later, as they learn the number bonds, they can begin to retrieve these automatically. Development involves change in the mix of strategies that are used. Importantly, the development in long-term memory of an association between the problem integers (e.g. 3+4) and the answer that is generated (7) requires practice in the execution of basic computations. With each execution, the probability of direct retrieval of that number fact or bond increases. It follows that children who have difficulty with this basic strategy will take a long time to acquire a database of number knowledge, and they may therefore fail to achieve automaticity in arithmetic skills.

While most research has been carried out on addition, analogous strategy development can be seen in subtraction, multiplication (initially approached as a set of additions) and division. Moreover, because the development of number skills is cumulative, it is easy for a child to slip behind by being unable to recover from a difficulty with a single operation that is not fully resolved before one that builds on it is introduced. Difficulty with arithmetic also causes anxiety that may compound the learning problem itself.

Classification of arithmetic difficulties

Research on number skills has distinguished between a preverbal number system (possibly in the right hemisphere) and a verbal number system acquired later (Dehaene 1992). In line with this view, children with language impairments have been reported as normal in their processing of non-verbal aspects of number, such as estimating the relative size of two blocks, but impaired on parallel verbal tasks, such as estimating the relative magnitude of two numbers (Donlan 1998). By analogy, it is likely that the arithmetic deficits of children with specific reading difficulty arise because of their verbal learning deficits (Geary et al. 1999).

Individual differences in the manifestation of number problems have been reported in the cognitive neuropsychological literature using a framework developed by McCloskey et al. (1985). Within this framework, the calculation system can be dissociated from the number processing system (Gross Tsur et al. 1996). Temple (1994) has reported single-case evidence for the existence in childhood of 'digit dyslexia', in which there is a specific difficulty in the acquisition of lexical processes within the number processing system (problems in encoding the meaning of numerals such as 348483), 'procedural dyscalculia' in which there is difficulty in learning procedures and algorithms, and 'number fact dyscalculia' in which there is specific difficulty in acquiring numerical facts. This approach is primarily descriptive and suggests neither what causes these different forms of arithmetic difficulty nor what ties them to impairments in underlying cognitive processes.

Cognitive deficits as an explanation of arithmetic problems

According to Geary (1990), children with mathematical difficulties use the same strategies as age-matched controls, but differ in the speed and skill of strategy execution. Typically, they make less use of the MIN strategy, they can retrieve fewer number facts, they are poor at monitoring their counting and they are poor at detecting computational errors (Geary et al. 1992). A slow rate of counting may contribute to their problems as may working memory deficits (Adams & Hitch 1997) or slow speed of processing (Bull & Johnston 1997).

One of the main cognitive approaches to arithmetic difficulties in children has been couched within the working memory framework of Baddeley & Hitch (1974). The working memory system has three components:

1 the central executive;
2 an attention system that controls and initiates mental operations; and
3 two slave systems
   • the phonological loop for the short-term maintenance and rehearsal of speech-based information; and
   • the visuospatial sketch pad for the storage of visual and spatial information (see Hulme & Roodenrys 1995 for a review of its application to children's learning difficulties).

It is clear that arithmetic draws on working memory resources; numbers have to be held in short-term memory during the process of mental calculation and a spatial representation of the problem to be solved can be helpful in some forms of problem-solving. Importantly, the central executive will be involved in a range of control processes, not yet well understood, but which include the selection of appropriate algorithms and the monitoring of performance (for example, checking that the solution to a problem is within the estimated range). Hitch et al., working with children who had specific arithmetic difficulties, delineated deficits in simple working memory tasks (e.g. span tasks that tap the phonological loop), on complex working memory tasks that tap the central executive (Hitch & McAuley 1991), in spatial working memory and some executive tasks (McLean & Hitch 1999). The involvement of executive processes in number work means that children with attentional difficulties are likely to be particularly at risk of failure in mathematics. A challenge for the future is to map the different forms of working memory deficit to the neuropsychological deficits observed and ultimately to the level of brain processes.

Non-verbal learning disabilities

Johnson & Myklebust (1967) were the first investigators to describe a group of children who had excellent auditory skills and spoke early in development but displayed deficiencies in visuospatial organization and non-verbal integration. These children showed normal word reading skills but reading comprehension was deficient where it involved inferential thinking, as was performance in arithmetic.

Semrud-Clikeman & Hynd (1990) noted considerable agreement among different classification schemes for non-verbal learning difficulties. Interestingly, arithmetic disabilities occurred in most reports, as did delayed reading, although decoding skills were relatively good compared to arithmetic abilities. Development of motor and visuospatial skills was reported as delayed; directional confusion was often noted as were deficits in social skills. Although described as a non-verbal syndrome, many children had associated speech–language difficulties including pragmatic deficits.

Non-verbal learning disabilities syndrome

The strongest proponent of the view that there is a syndrome of non-verbal learning disabilities (NLDS) is Rourke (1989, 1995), who described its principal clinical features in terms of neuropsychological assets and deficits. Academically, the typical strengths of a child with NLDS are in single-word reading and spelling, with deficits in handwriting (especially its acquisition), reading comprehension, mathematics and arithmetic. The principal neuropsychological asset in NLDS is the capacity to deal with information derived through the auditory modality, whereas the primary deficits are in visuoperceptual organizational abilities, complex psychomotor skills, tactile perception, and non-verbal problem-solving. From clinical experience, Rourke (1989) considered that socioemotional and adaptive deficits characterize the syndrome and can encompass extreme difficulties in adapting to novel situations and significant deficits in social competence and social interaction.

The concept of a syndrome of non-verbal learning disabilities cuts across taxonomies, such as those discussed above, that classify children according to patterns of impairment in the academic arena. An issue of considerable importance is the relationship between NLDS and disabilities on the autism spectrum. Klin et al. (1995) compared 21 subjects with Asperger syndrome and 19 with high-functioning autism in terms of the criteria for NLDS. This study used a conservative algorithm for the NLDS classification requiring concordance of 10/15 deficits and 5/7 assets from those proposed by Rourke (1989). There was a strikingly high degree of concordance between Asperger syndrome and NLDS but not between NLDS and high-functioning autism. Thus, non-verbal learning difficulties are a neuropsychological marker of Asperger syndrome.

DAMP syndrome

The term 'DAMP' is used in Nordic countries to describe children with disorders of attention and motor perception. According to Gillberg (1999), DAMP has the following clinical characteristics:

- problems of attention;
- poor gross and fine-motor skills;
- perceptual deficits; and
- speech–language impairments.

In mild forms, some of the characteristics are not present and it encompasses children with pure developmental co-ordination disorder and pervasive attention deficit. There are synergies between the syndrome of DAMP and of NLDS, although severe dyslexia is considered a symptom of DAMP but not of NLDS. The difference may reflect the manifestations of a reading impairment in the Scandinavian languages where the concept of DAMP has been used more widely than in English-speaking countries.

Although there is no doubt that children who exhibit DAMP syndrome exist, the issue whether they constitute a coherent grouping is open to debate and whether the milder and more severe variants share common core features is not clear. In the preschool years, DAMP children are usually considered hyperactive, and show motor co-ordination problems and speech–language delays although typically not sufficiently serious to warrant clinical referral. In the early school years, these children

have difficulties in concentrating and have problems learning to read and write. They are also unable to interact with their peers in an age-appropriate fashion. By the age of 10, the clinical picture can be quite different with an increase in behavioural problems and dyslexia, problems that persist into adolescence. In adulthood, criminal behaviour is not uncommon and there can be major psychiatric problems.

Cognitive deficits in non-verbal learning disabilities

The underlying causes of non-verbal learning difficulties have been under-researched. It is possible that deficits in spatial cognition, associated with poor motor skills, are at the core of the problems and account in particular for the mathematical difficulties and writing problems encountered by this group of children. Spatial deficits also lead to a range of problems in 'extracurricular' activities, such as in athletics, team games and sight-reading of music, but these difficulties are mostly of little consequence in the academic arena (Denckla 1991). However, it is clear that many children described as having non-verbal learning disabilities also show aspects of autism continuum disorder, and the role that deficits in social cognition may have requires further investigation.

Comorbid problems of attention control

The term 'comorbidity' describes the tendency for two different conditions to occur together in the same individual (Angold et al. 1999). The issue of comorbidity needs to be raised here because learning difficulties may be the result of a combination of cognitive difficulties. In particular, children with dyslexia are often reported to lack concentration and teachers complain of their poor organizational abilities. In a recent survey of a large UK primary school, Adams et al. (1999) found that 12.5% of poor readers were rated by their teachers as having a significant problem with attention. The rate was 15.6% among children with specific reading difficulties from the same school.

Pennington et al. (1993) addressed the issue of whether problems of attention are direct consequences of dyslexia or whether they reflect comorbid ADHD in a study involving three groups of children:

1 a group of dyslexic readers who did not have attentional problems (RD);
2 a group of children diagnosed with ADHD; and
3 a comorbid group who had dyslexia and ADHD (RD+ADHD).

The children completed phonological tasks chosen to tap the core deficit in dyslexia, and executive function tasks that require sustained attention, organization and planning to investigate the putative cognitive deficit in ADHD (Pennington & Ozonoff 1996). In line with expectation, the RD group performed poorly on tests of phonological processing but had no difficulty with the executive function tasks, whereas the ADHD group showed executive deficits but normal phonological processing. Importantly, the comorbid (RD+ADHD) group performed like the dyslexic group, showing phonological but not executive deficits. The resemblance of the comorbid group to the dyslexic group suggested that they had developed attention problems as a secondary consequence of their learning difficulties. This study highlights the value of cognitive tests to the diagnosis of learning difficulties; it was the lack of any deficit in executive function that set these poor readers apart from children with ADHD.

Biological bases of learning disabilities

Reading difficulties

Genetic factors

It has been known for many years that reading difficulties run in families and current estimates indicate that the risk to a son of being dyslexic if he has a dyslexic parent is 35–40%. For a daughter the risk is somewhat less, about 20%, regardless of which parent is affected (Gilger *et al.* 1991). Gene markers for dyslexia have been found on the long arm of chromosome 15 (Smith *et al.* 1983) and on the short arm of chromosome 6 in other families (Cardon *et al.* 1994). Interestingly, the markers on chromosome 6 are in the same region as the genes implicated in autoimmune diseases that have been reported to show a high degree of association with dyslexia (Geschwind & Behan 1984; Pennington *et al.* 1987).

An important contribution to understanding the causes of reading disability has come from the behaviour–genetic investigations of component reading subskills. Such analyses suggest that there is significant heritability for reading recognition and spelling deficits. In line with work by Stevenson *et al.* (1987) with a UK sample of twins, DeFries *et al.* (1997) found that heritability estimates decreased as a function of age for word recognition (0.64 vs. 0.47) but increased for spelling (0.52 vs. 0.68). There is a larger environmental contribution to reading comprehension than to word recognition, possibly because this depends on vocabulary knowledge derived through the educational and home environment (Olson *et al.* 1994). By systematically examining individual differences in reading strategy, Olson *et al.* inferred that phonological processing ability is genetically determined, and this underlies the development of both phonological decoding and orthographic reading skills (Castles *et al.* 1999), but the latter are more susceptible to environmental influence.

Children at risk of reading difficulties

With genetic studies as a backdrop, a number of studies have investigated the early precursors of dyslexia in children from high-risk families (Scarborough 1990; Lefly & Pennington 1996; Byrne *et al.* 1997; Elbro *et al.* 1998). The emerging consensus of these studies is that, in the preschool period, at-risk children who go on to become dyslexic show delayed speech and language development (Gallagher *et al.* 2000). By 4–5 years they show a characteristic pattern of poor phonological awareness and

limited letter knowledge that presages reading difficulties (Scarborough 1990). This evidence bolsters the view that children at risk of dyslexia come to the task of learning to read with poorly developed phonological skills and makes a clear argument for early intervention programmes that target the development of phonological awareness.

Dyslexia and the brain

Galaburda (Galaburda & Kemper 1978; Galaburda 1994) reported unusual symmetry of the planum temporale in the brains of dyslexic readers, and structural abnormalities (ectopias and dysplasias) throughout the perisylvian region of the left hemisphere. Findings of symmetrical plana in dyslexia have now been replicated in a number of studies using brain imaging techniques (Hynd & Hiemenz 1997). Moreover, an important study by Larsen *et al.* (1990) made a direct link between planum symmetry and phonological deficiency. More recently, functional brain imaging has confirmed differences in the pattern of brain activation between dyslexic and normal readers during phonological processing (for a review see Filipek 1999). Taken together, this evidence suggests that the behavioural findings of phonological processing deficits in dyslexia may be traced to differences in left hemisphere brain function.

An alternative hypothesis, proposed by Lovegrove *et al.* (1986), is that dyslexic readers have low-level visual impairments affecting the transient visual system (sometimes referred to as the magnocellular system). According to Lovegrove (1991) transient system deficits may affect the extraction of information to the right of fixation and naturally therefore impair reading. Moreover, the failure of transient responses to inhibit responses of the sustained visual system could obscure or mask information from later fixations (Hulme 1988). However, because visual problems co-occur with phonological processing impairments (Eden *et al.* 1996), it may be better to consider them to be a biological marker for dyslexia rather than of significance in explaining the genesis of the reading problem.

The right hemisphere hypothesis of non-verbal learning disabilities

Evidence for the biological bases of non-verbal disabilities is lacking but the most widely cited hypothesis is that these difficulties stem from disorders of the right hemisphere (Semrud-Clikeman & Hynd 1990). While the left hemisphere has specific modality areas, the right hemisphere has more association areas and specializes in intermodal integration. Thus, it is claimed that the right hemisphere is better at processing novel material and constructing schema that can then be transferred to the left hemisphere. While Rourke (1989) made use of this model to account for the syndrome of non-verbal learning disabilities, a clearer understanding of the core characteristics of NLDS and of the heterogeneity among affected cases is needed before further progress can be made towards understanding its biological substrate.

Relationship between reading and language difficulties

Studies of children with speech–language impairments frequently report a high incidence of reading difficulties and children who have problems in both oral language and phonological processing are at the greatest risk of failure (Catts *et al.* 1999). However, there is a high degree of variability in literacy outcome among children from clinical samples (Magnusson & Naucler 1990). Given the role of different language skills in the development of reading, as discussed above, this is perhaps unsurprising.

Specific language impairments

One of the most important predictors of literacy development among children with preschool specific language impairments is the status of their oral language skills at the time when they start to read (Bird *et al.* 1995). Bishop & Adams (1990) found that children whose spoken language difficulties had resolved by the age of 5.5 years had a good outcome for reading in its early stages. In contrast, children who continued to show specific language impairments at 5.5 years had widespread reading and spelling difficulties at 8.5 years.

At school leaving age, the children whose specific language impairments had resolved by 5.5 years continued to be indistinguishable from normal controls in spoken language skills. However, in spite of the good outcome for oral language, they had poorer literacy skills than controls (Stothard *et al.* 1998). Indeed, their difficulties with reading, spelling and reading comprehension were accompanied by non-word reading and spelling problems and were associated with deficits in phonological processing, resembling those seen in dyslexia. It must be stressed, however, that these children had followed a different developmental course to classically dyslexic children; they had experienced a good start with reading and their 8-year-old literacy skills had been within the normal range. A salutary finding was that, although as adolescents with resolved specific language impairments they were entered for the same number of school leaving examinations as controls (GCSEs in the UK), they obtained poorer grades in the core subjects of English language, mathematics and a foreign language (Snowling *et al.* 2001).

The literacy outcome and also the academic attainment of those with persistent specific language impairments were less good than those of the resolved group. At 15 years they performed almost as poorly as children who had been classified as generally delayed in development (with performance IQs below 70). Literacy outcomes were particularly poor for those with a performance IQ less than 100 and there had been a substantial drop in reading accuracy, relative to age, between the ages of 8.5 and 15 years (Snowling *et al.* 2000).

Reading in children with speech disorders

Although learning to read is heavily dependent upon speech processing, the relationship between speech production (expressive phonology) and phonological awareness is less than straightforward (Stackhouse 2000). Catts (1993) followed the progress of children with speech–language impairments from kindergarten through the first two years of school. As would be predicted by theories of reading acquisition, measures of kindergarten phonological awareness and rapid naming skill predicted word recognition and decoding skills at the end of first and second grade. Importantly, children with speech–articulation difficulties in kindergarten did not develop reading difficulties in first grade, while those with more widespread language impairments did. In similar vein, children with speech impairments associated with structural abnormalities, such as cleft palate, appear to have normal reading skills (Stackhouse 1982) as do those with motor speech disorders, such as dysarthria (Bishop 1985).

Taken together, these findings suggest that it is necessary to distinguish poor phonological production skills and phonological awareness as predictors of literacy outcome. Children with isolated impairments of expressive phonology do not appear to be at heightened risk of reading problems, but children who have deficits in phonological awareness are unlikely to read well.

Hyperlexia

An extreme form of poor reading comprehension is seen in the case of hyperlexic children. These children often learn to read before they receive any formal instruction, and at a rate much in excess of that to be predicted from their IQ. Hyperlexia often occurs in combination with other developmental disorders, such as autism, and is characterized by a preoccupation with reading to the exclusion of meaning (Healy 1982).

Most research on hyperlexia has been at the level of case studies which have not focused in any detail on the reading mechanisms that are involved (Nation 1999). Exceptions were two studies by Frith & Snowling (1983) and Snowling & Frith (1986) who reported that autistic children, classified as 'hyperlexic', could read words and non-words as well as reading age-matched controls and that they were sensitive to grammatical distinctions in text. However, they had more difficulty in pronouncing ambiguous words in context, such as 'bow' and 'lead', and their comprehension of the details of what they read was poorer than that of younger reading-age-matched controls. In addition to their difficulties on formal reading comprehension tests, the hyperlexic children had difficulty monitoring errors in what they read; compared with younger children of similar mental age, they had more difficulty in detecting the text anomalies, and they tended to accept implausible words as correct.

Emotional and behavioural sequelae of learning difficulties

Although it is generally believed that a significant degree of psychosocial adversity can follow from childhood learning difficulties, the evidence that substantiates this view is sparse. Moreover, the relationship between children's learning difficulties and their adult outcome will differ according to the type of learning disability they experience. The most common types of social difficulty attributed to reading difficulties (dyslexia) are behaviour problems that include offending (Jensen et al., 1999). However, the majority of poor readers do not experience mental health problems and appear to be less susceptible to psychiatric disorder than children with a history of non-verbal learning disabilities.

Psychosocial outcomes for children with reading difficulties

A considerable body of research points to an association between learning difficulties and behavioural problems (Hinshaw 1992). However, it is not clear that the relationship is a direct one (Maughan 1994). An influential hypothesis has been that behaviour problems associated with reading difficulties may be mediated by progressive school failure and lowered self-esteem (Chapman & Tunmer 1997). An alternative model of the relationship is that disruptive behaviour at school, coupled with inattentiveness, interferes with the acquisition of reading skills. However, it might be argued that both models are oversimplistic; the relationship between reading and behaviour differs according to gender and turns on the stage of development that is considered.

Williams & McGee (1994) followed a cohort of 950 children from birth to adulthood. Assessments conducted at the ages of 7, 9 and 15 years found that both reading difficulties and antisocial behaviour showed continuities over time. However, while the dimensional approach revealed no significant association between early reading and later delinquency, a categorical approach that focused on the outcomes of children 'diagnosed' as having reading difficulties (dyslexia) suggested that, at least for boys, early reading disability predicted future conduct disorder at 15 years. For girls, the association was between reading problems and anxiety, rather than conduct problems, suggesting a different outcome for reading problems between the sexes. The Dunedin study also examined the relationship between reading problems and psychosocial adjustment in young adulthood at age 18, as measured by a mental health interview. For males but not females, an index of personal disadvantage at 18 was predicted by both literacy and externalizing (behaviour) disorder at 15, as well as family disadvantage at 7 years.

Maughan et al. (1996) came to broadly similar conclusions following a study of 127 poor readers in London from the age of 10 years into early adulthood. They found there was a tendency for reading difficulties to be associated with poor attention and overactivity, which in turn placed poor readers at risk of behaviour problems (see also Fergusson & Lynsky 1997). Overall, high behaviour problem ratings at age 14 reflected earlier behaviour problems rather than reading difficulties. Social adversity was found to increase the risk of antisocial behaviour among girls but not among boys. Among boys with specific reading difficulties, increased rates of offending were associated with poor school attendance.

As young adults, aged 27–28, about 25% of this sample remained severely impaired in reading (Maughan & Hagell 1996). None the less, relatively positive self-reports suggested that many had gained employment in which there were restricted literacy demands and their reading problems were no longer of functional significance. In most areas, those with a history of specific reading difficulties were functioning comparably to peers. However, young women with a history of specific reading retardation were at increased risk of psychiatric disorder, possibly related to a high rate of relationship breakdowns. These appear to have been the consequence of leaving school without qualifications and entering early marriage or cohabitations. Male poor readers, in contrast, had more difficulty in gaining independence. However, these difficulties were the consequence of comorbid difficulties with peer relationships rather than reading problems. In the same way, alcohol problems were linked with behaviour rather than reading problems.

Socioemotional sequelae of non-verbal learning disabilities

Rourke & Fuerst (1995) used multivariate statistical methods to analyse the performance of learning disabled children on the Personality Inventory for Children. Although there was variation between studies, seven distinct subtypes emerged. Two of these subtypes showed relatively normal adjustment, three showed modest psychosocial dysfunction (mild hyperactive, mild anxiety and conduct disorder), one was associated with internalized psychopathology (depression, withdrawal anxiety and psychosis) and one with externalized psychopathology (delinquency, hyperactivity, poor social skills and emotionally unstable behaviour). However, these studies suffer from the lack of representative samples and appropriate control groups (Little 1993).

Gillberg et al. examined the psychosocial adjustment of children with DAMP syndrome by comparison to a control group selected at random for the same population (Hellgren et al. 1994). Problems of depression and feelings of low self-esteem were common during the early school years and peaked around 10 years when they coincided with conduct problems. In adolescence, the DAMP group showed three main types of psychiatric problem: depression, conduct disorder and autistic traits which were present in 50% of severe cases of DAMP. Gillberg (1999) suggested that, in the teenage years, anger and resentment may precipitate a conduct disorder that can include stealing, firesetting, lying, bullying, running away from home or drug abuse. However, it is difficult to be sure that these socioemotional difficulties were the consequences of the DAMP syndrome *per se*, because the inclusion of social and behavioural problems among the initial diagnostic criteria brings with it a degree of circularity.

Clinical implications

Early identification of reading difficulties

The convergence of evidence from studies of the normal development of reading, and from dyslexia, places practitioners in an excellent position both to identify children at risk of reading difficulties and to provide early intervention. Children who have a family history of dyslexia or a history of speech–language difficulties are at high risk, especially if the phonological system is affected and there are speech production deficits. A cautionary note is that children with preschool speech and language impairments may make a good start in learning to read but fail later as its demands increase. Careful monitoring of high-risk children is therefore advisable throughout the primary school years.

Just before school entry it is possible to detect, with reasonable accuracy, the children who will proceed to have reading difficulties by assessing performance on tests of phonological awareness and letter knowledge (Muter *et al.* 1997). Where the child cannot yet reflect upon the sound structure of spoken words, either to make judgements about rhyming pairs, or to detect their beginning sound, a programme of phonological awareness training should be implemented without delay, if possible harnessing the support of parents.

Interventions that foster the development of phonological awareness and letter knowledge have been found to have a positive effect on the subsequent reading achievement of unselected samples of children in their preschool years (Lundberg *et al.* 1988; Byrne & Fielding-Barnsley 1991, 1995). Interventions of this type also have a positive effect on children at high risk of dyslexia (Borstrom & Elbro 1997) although there is growing opinion that such children respond less well than normally developing children (Torgesen *et al.* 1994; Byrne *et al.* 1997). In order to have a substantial impact on the phonological awareness of children at risk for serious learning difficulties, it is usually recommended that training procedures go beyond those typically applied, both in terms of explicitness of phonological training and also in terms of intensity. Such interventions need to be delivered on a one-to-one basis by highly trained and supervised teachers (Torgesen *et al.*, 1999).

Assessment of reading difficulties

The most common referrals to clinicians are of children who have already failed to learn to read. Once a child has failed to learn to read, the starting point for the assessment of their difficulties should normally be an assessment of general cognitive ability, not least to identify the child's strengths and weaknesses, the specificity of the reading problem and to pinpoint any co-

morbid non-verbal learning difficulties. The assessment will have more value if it proceeds to assess the phonological skills that underlie reading development, and the reading strategies the child is currently using with a view to prescribing appropriate intervention. The assessment of reading must encompass assessment of word-level recognition and decoding skills, as well as of reading comprehension. It is also important to include a test of spelling and an assessment of expressive writing skills (Snowling & Stackhouse 1996). Attendant problems, such as with attention or fine motor control, require separate investigation and intervention.

The main priority for children who are failing is reading intervention. Contrary to the accepted clinical view that accurate assessment must be used to prescribe treatment, there is indeed some evidence that if tutoring is introduced early, it can be effective regardless of diagnosis. Vellutino *et al.* (1996) asked the teachers of 1407 children from 17 schools in the Albany area of New York state simply to rate their reading skills in the middle of first grade. The poor readers were then assigned at random into tutored or non-tutored groups. The tutored children received 30 min of individualized help daily, according to their needs, while the untutored children served as controls. Sixty-seven per cent of the tutored children gained reading scores within the normal range after only one semester. Moreover, tutored children maintained their status over time.

Although cognitive assessments from kindergarten were available for these children, they did not figure in the decision to remediate. Like other poor readers, the children who failed to progress well in the intervention were those who performed worse on tasks that tapped phonological skills including poor verbal short-term memory, poor phonological awareness and rapid naming deficits. The intransigence of the reading impairment in such 'hard-to-remediate' children is a priority for future research (Torgesen, 2000).

Interventions for poor readers

An influential approach to helping poor readers is 'reading recovery', a programme pioneered by Clay (1985) in New Zealand. The poorest readers in each school enter such programmes following screening at the age of 6 years, and leave around 20 weeks later when their reading attainment matches that of their peer group in the same schools. While the programme is generally regarded to be successful, there have been few systematic comparisons with other methods (Snowling 1996). Those that have done this have found that it is better to supplement such an approach with training in phonological awareness, involving exercises to link reading with phonology (Hatcher *et al.* 1994). In a review of such studies, Troia (1999) evaluated 39 interventions that conformed to rigorous methodological criteria. These studies showed that phonological training improves both phonological awareness and literacy skills in a relatively short time.

Evidence from the Colorado remediation project (Olson & Wise 1992) speaks to the efficacy of remedial approaches with dyslexic children. The teaching technique used in these studies involves children reading from books that are computer-presented, at the appropriate level of difficulty. Whenever the child encounters an unfamiliar word they highlight it and the computer provides feedback using synthesized speech. The outstanding issue is how best to effect successful generalization when teaching children with severe reading difficulties.

In contrast to what is known about how to teach word-level reading skills, far less is known about how to promote reading comprehension. This challenge may be tantamount to building vocabulary and other IQ-related cognitive processes (Stothard 1994). In line with this view, several recent studies have shown that IQ is a strong predictor of gains in the reading comprehension of poor readers in intervention programmes (Hatcher & Hulme 1999).

Clinical management of children with non-verbal learning disabilities

It is sensible to suppose that the management of children with non-verbal learning disabilities depends upon their careful assessment, but there are no data that speak directly to this issue. As NLDS is a multifaceted disorder, assessment of academic achievement needs to be conducted in the context of a thorough evaluation of the child's perceptual, motor and attentional skills. Like any assessment of a child who is failing, this should involve the child's caregivers and teachers in evaluating the socioemotional impact of the disorder (Gillberg 1999). Once assessment is complete, a treatment programme needs to be organized to take account of the presenting problems at the stage of development the child has reached.

Many children with NLDS require special needs support. In the primary school years, help with the acquisition of reading, writing and arithmetic skills is usually needed. Later the focus may change to assistance with self-organization and study skills. In the early years, some children with NLDS require physiotherapy but, unless motor deficits are serious, this form of intervention may not be effective in the long term because such difficulties tend to diminish with age. In short, it is important to recognize the cognitive problems of children with NLDS early in development and to provide intervention that reduces the frequency of maladaptive transactions with the environment (Fletcher 1989).

Conclusions

The field of children's learning difficulties is evolving rapidly. Understanding of the causes and characteristics of children's reading difficulties is well advanced, as is knowledge about appropriate interventions. It is striking that in this domain, cognitive models of reading acquisition have had a very positive effect on progress. Far less is known about children's arithmetic difficulties although here too the influence of cognitive models is beginning to bear fruit. An advantage of the cognitive approach to

learning difficulties is that it makes contact with what is known about normal development and an understanding of the cognitive underpinnings of disorders forges a link between brain and behaviour (Morton & Frith 1995).

In contrast, research on non-verbal learning difficulties remains syndrome-based. These children have deficits of spatial cognition that may account for their arithmetic problems, but direct relationships have not been demonstrated. It is unclear how far spatial problems can explain their difficulties in the development of motor skills, and to what extent the commonly observed psychosocial problems are a reflection of comorbid disorders of the autism spectrum rather than a consequence of the learning difficulties. Future research is needed to fractionate the so-called 'right hemisphere learning difficulties' if advances in clinical and educational management are to follow.

Acknowledgements

The author acknowledges the support of a grant from the Wellcome Trust during the preparation of this chapter and thanks Sara Bailey for help with references.

References

Adams, J.W. & Hitch, G.J. (1997) Working memory and children's mental addition. *Journal of Experimental Child Psychology*, **67**, 21–38.

Adams, J.W., Snowling, M.J., Hennessey, S.M. & Kind, P. (1999) Problems of behaviour, reading and arithmetic: assessments of comorbidity using the Strengths and Difficulties Questionnaire. *British Journal of Educational Psychology*, **69**, 571–585.

American Psychiatric Association (1994) *Diagnostic and Statistical Manual (DSM IV)*. American Psychiatric Association, Washington D.C.

Angold, A., Costello, E.J. & Erkanli, A. (1999) Comorbidity. *Journal of Child Psychology and Psychiatry*, **40**, 57–87.

Baddeley, A.D. & Hitch, G.J. (1974) Working memory. In: *The Psychology of Learning and Motivation: Advances in Research and Theory* (ed. G. Bower), pp. 47–90. Academic Press, New York.

Baker, L. & Cantwell, D.P. (1985) Developmental arithmetic disorder. In: *Comprehensive Textbook of Psychiatry* (eds H.I. Kaplan & B.J. Sadock), pp. 1697–1700. Williams & Wilkins, Baltimore.

Bird, J. & Bishop, D.V.M. & Freeman, N.H. (1995) Phonological awareness and literacy development in children with expressive phonological impairments. *Journal of Speech and Hearing Research*, **38**, 446–462.

Bishop, D.V.M. (1985) Spelling ability in congenital dysarthria: evidence against articulatory coding in translating between phonemes and graphemes. *Cognitive Neuropsychology*, **2**, 229–251.

Bishop, D.V.M. & Adams, C. (1990) A prospective study of the relationship between specific language impairment, phonological disorders and reading retardation. *Journal of Child Psychology and Psychiatry*, **31**, 1027–1050.

Borstrom, I. & Elbro, C. (1997) Prevention of dyslexia in kindergarten: effects of phoneme awareness training with children of dyslexic parents. In: *Dyslexia: Biology, Cognition and Intervention* (eds C. Hulme & M.J. Snowling), pp. 235–253. Whurr, London.

Bradley, L. & Bryant, P.E. (1983) Categorising sounds and learning to read: a causal connection. *Nature*, **301**, 419–421.

Brady, S.A. (1997) Ability to encode phonological representations: an underlying difficulty for poor readers. In: *Foundations of Reading Acquisition and Dyslexia: Implications for Early Intervention* (ed. B. Blachman), pp. 21–48. Lawrence Erlbaum, Mahwah, NJ.

Bruck, M. (1992) Persistence of dyslexics' phonological awareness deficits. *Development Psychology*, **28**, 874–886.

Bull, R. & Johnston, R.S. (1997) Children's arithmetical difficulties: contributions from processing speed, item identification and short-term memory. *Journal of Experimental Child Psychology*, **65**, 1–24.

Byrne, B. & Fielding-Barnsley, R. (1991) Evaluation of a program to teach phonemic awareness to young children. *Journal of Educational Psychology*, **83**, 451–455.

Byrne, B. & Fielding-Barnsley, R. (1995) Evaluation of a program to teach phonemic awareness to young children: a 2- and 3-year follow-up and a new preschool trial. *Journal of Educational Psychology*, **87**, 488–503.

Byrne, B., Fielding-Barnsley, R., Ashley, L. & Larsen, K. (1997) Assessing the child's and the environment's contribution to reading acquisition: what we know and what we don't know. In: *Reading Acquisition and Dyslexia: Implications for Early Intervention* (ed. B. Blachman), pp. 265–286. Lawrence Erlbaum, Hillsdale, NJ.

Cain, K., Oakhill, J.V. & Bryant, P.E. (2000a) Investigating the causes of reading comprehension failure: the comprehension matched design. *Reading and Writing*, **12**, 31–40.

Cain, K., Oakhill, J.V. & Bryant, P.E. (2000b) Phonological skills and comprehension failure: a test of the phonological processing deficit hypothesis. *Reading and Writing*, **13**, 31–56.

Cardon, L.R., Smith, S.D., Fulker, D.W., Kimberling, W.J., Pennington, B.F. & DeFries, J.C. (1994) Quantitative trait locus for reading disability on chromosome 6. *Science*, **266**, 276–279.

Castles, A. & Coltheart, M. (1993) Varieties of developmental dyslexia. *Cognition*, **47**, 149–180.

Castles, A., Datta, H., Gayan, J. & Olson, R.K. (1999) Varieties of developmental reading disorder: genetic and environmental influences. *Journal of Experimental Child Psychology*, **72**, 73–94.

Catts, H.W. (1993) The relationship between speech–language and reading disabilities. *Journal of Speech and Hearing Research*, **36**, 948–958.

Catts, H.W., Fey, M.E., Zhang, X. & Tomblin, J.B. (1999) Language basis of reading and reading disabilities: evidence from a longitudinal investigation. *Scientific Studies of Reading*, **3**, 331–361.

Chapman, J.W. & Tunmer, W.E. (1997) A longitudinal study of beginning reading achievement and reading self-concept. *British Journal of Educational Psychology*, **67**, 279–291.

Clay, M. (1985) *The Early Detection of Reading Difficulties*. Heinemann, Tadworth, Surrey.

Coltheart, M., Masterson, J., Byng, S., Prior, M. & Riccoch, J. (1983) Surface dyslexia. *Quarterly Journal of Experimental Psychology*, **35**, 469–495.

Cossu, G. (1999) Biological constraints on literacy acquisition. *Reading and Writing*, **11**, 213–237.

DeFries, J.D., Alarcon, M. & Olson, R.K. (1997) Genetic etiologies of reading and spelling deficits: developmental differences. In: *Dyslexia: Biology, Cognition and Intervention* (eds C. Hulme & M.J. Snowling), pp. 20–37. Whurr, London.

Dehaene, S. (1992) Varieties of numerical abilities. *Cognition I*, **44**, 1–42.

Denckla, M.B. (1991) Academic and extracurricular aspects of nonverbal learning disabilities. *Psychiatric Annals*, **21**, 717–724.

Donlan, C., ed. (1998) *The Development of Mathematical Skills*. Psychology Press, Hove.

Eden, G.F., VanMeter, J.W., Rumsey, J.M., Maisog, J.M., Wods, R.P. & Zeffiro, T.A. (1996) Abnormal processing of visual motion in dyslexia revealed by functional brain imaging. *Nature*, **382**, 66–69.

Elbro, C., Borstrom, I. & Petersen, D.K. (1998) Predicting dyslexia from kindergarten: the importance of distinctness of phonological representations of lexical items. *Reading Research Quarterly*, **33**, 36–60.

Fergusson, D.M. & Lynsky, M.T. (1997) Early reading difficulties and later conduct problems. *Journal of Child Psychology and Psychiatry*, **38**, 899–907.

Filipek, P.A. (1999) Neuroimaging in the developmental disorders: the state of the science. *Journal of Child Psychology and Psychiatry*, **40**, 113–128.

Fletcher, J.M. (1989) Nonverbal learning disabilities and suicide: classification leads to prevention. *Journal of Learning Disabilities*, **22**, 76–79.

Frith, U. (1980) *Cognitive Processes in Spelling*. Academic Press, London.

Frith, U. & Snowling, M.J. (1983) Reading for meaning and reading for sound in autistic and dyslexic children. *British Journal of Developmental Psychology*, **1**, 329–342.

Frith, U., Wimmer, H. & Landerl, K. (1998) Differences in phonological recoding in German and English speaking children. *Scientific Studies of Reading*, **2**, 31–54.

Galaburda, A. (1994) Developmental dyslexia and animal studies: at the interface between cognition and neurology. *Cognition*, **50**, 133–149.

Galaburda, A.M. & Kemper, T.L. (1978) Cytoarchitectonic abnormalities in developmental dyslexia: a case study. *Annals of Neurology*, **6**, 94–100.

Gallagher, A., Frith, U. & Snowling, M.J. (2000) Precursors of literacy-delay among children at genetic risk of dyslexia. *Journal of Child Psychology and Psychiatry*, **41**, 203–213.

Geary, D.C. (1990) A componential analysis of an early learning deficit in mathematics. *Journal of Experimental Child Psychology*, **40**, 363–383.

Geary, D.C. (1993) Mathematical disabilities: cognitive, neuropsychological and genetic components. *Psychological Bulletin*, **114**, 345–362.

Geary, D.C., Bow-Thomas, C.C. & Yao, Y. (1992) Counting knowledge and skill in cognitive addition: a comparison of normal and mathematically disabled children. *Journal of Experimental Child Psychology*, **54**, 372–391.

Geary, D.C., Hoard, M.K. & Hamson, C.O. (1999) Numerical and arithmetical cognition: patterns of functions and deficits in children at risk for a mathematical disability. *Journal of Experimental Child Psychology*, **74**, 213–239.

Gelman, R. & Gallistel, C.R. (1978) *The Child's Understanding of Number*. Harvard University Press, Cambridge, MA.

Geschwind, N. & Behan, P. (1984) Laterality, hormones and immunity. In: *Cerebral Dominance: the Biological Foundations* (eds N. Geschwind & A. Galaburda), pp. 211–234. Harvard University Press, Cambridge, MA.

Gilger, J.W., Pennington, B.F. & DeFries, J.C. (1991) Risk for reading disability as a function of parental history in three family studies. *Reading and Writing*, **3**, 205–218.

Gillberg, C. (1999) *Clinical Child Neuropsychiatry*. Cambridge University Press, Cambridge.

Goswami, U. & Bryant, P.E. (1990) *Phonological Skills and Learning to Read*. Erlbaum, London.

Gough, P.B. & Tunmer, W.E. (1986) Decoding, reading and reading disability. *Remedial and Special Education*, **7**, 6–10.

Goulandris, N. & Snowling, M.J. (1991) Visual memory deficits: a plausible cause of developmental dyslexia? Evidence from a single case study. *Cognitive Neuropsychology*, **8**, 127–154.

Gross Tsur, V., Manor, O. & Shalev, R.S. (1996) Developmental dyscalculia: prevalence and demographic features. *Developmental Medicine and Child Neurology*, 38, 25–33.

Harm, M.W. & Seidenberg, M.S. (1999) Phonology, reading acquisition and dyslexia: insights from connectionist models. *Psychological Review*, 106, 491–528.

Harris, M. & Hatano, G. (1999) *Learning to Read and Write: a Cross-linguistic Perspective*. Cambridge University Press, Cambridge.

Hatcher, P.J. & Hulme, C. (1999) Phonemes, rhymes and intelligence as predictors of children's responsiveness to remedial reading instruction: evidence from a longitudinal intervention study. *Journal of Experimental Child Psychology*, 72, 130–153.

Hatcher, P., Hulme, C. & Ellis, A.W. (1994) Ameliorating early reading failure by integrating the teaching of reading and phonological skills: the phonological linkage hypothesis. *Child Development*, 65, 41–57.

Healy, J.M. (1982) The enigma of hyperlexia. *Reading Research Quarterly*, 7, 319–338.

Hecht, S.A., Burgess, S.R., Torgesen, J.K., Wagner, R.K. & Rashotte, C.A. (2000) Explaining social class differences in growth of reading skills from beginning kindergarten through fourth grade: the role of phonological awareness, rate of access, and print knowledge. *Reading and Writing*, 12, 99–127.

Hellgren, L., Gillberg, I.C., Bagenholm, A. & Gillberg, C. (1994) Children with deficits in attention, motor control and perception (DAMP) almost grown up: psychiatric and personality disorders at age 16 years. *Journal of Child Psychology and Psychiatry*, 35, 1255–1271.

Hinshaw, S.P. (1992) Externalizing behaviour problems and academic underachievement in childhood and adolescence: causal relationships and underlying mechanisms. *Psychological Bulletin*, 111, 127–155.

Hitch, G.J. & McAuley, E. (1991) Working memory in children with specific arithmetical learning difficulties. *British Journal of Psychology*, 82, 375–386.

Hulme, C. (1988) The implausibility of low-level visual deficits as a cause of children's reading difficulties. *Cognitive Neuropsychology*, 5, 369–374.

Hulme, C. & Roodenrys, S. (1995) Practitioner review: verbal working memory development and its disorders. *Journal of Child Psychology and Psychiatry*, 36, 373–398.

Hynd, G.W. & Hiemenz, J.R. (1997) Dyslexia and gyral morphology variation. In: *Dyslexia: Biology, Cognition and Intervention* (eds C. Hulme & M. Snowling), pp. 38–58. Whurr, London.

Jensen, J., Lindgren, M., Meurling, A.W., Ingvar, D.H. & Levander, S. (1999) Dyslexia among Swedish prison inmates in relation to neuropsychology and personality. *Journal of International Neuropsychological Society*, 5, 452–461.

Johnson, D.J. & Mykelbust, H.R. (1967) *Learning Disabilities: Educational Principles and Practice*. Grune and Stratton, New York.

Klin, A., Volkmar, F.R., Sparrow, S.S., Cicchetti, D.V. & Rourke, B.P. (1995) Validity and neuropsychological characterization of Asperger syndrome: convergence with nonverbal learning disabilities syndrome. *Journal of Child Psychology and Psychiatry*, 36 (7), 1127–1140.

Larsen, J.P., Hoien, T., Lundberg, I. & Odegaard, H. (1990) MRI evaluation of the size and symmetry of the planum temporale in adolescents with developmental dyslexia. *Brain and Language*, 39, 289–301.

Lefly, D.L. & Pennington, B.F. (1996) Longitudinal study of children at high family risk for dyslexia: the first two years. In: *Toward a Genetics of Language* (ed. M.L. Rice), pp. 49–76. Lawrence Erlbaum, Hillsdale, NJ.

Lewis, C., Hitch, G.J. & Walker, P. (1994) The prevalence of specific arithmetic difficulties and specific reading difficulties in 9- to 10-year old boys and girls. *Journal of Child Psychology and Psychiatry*, 35, 283–292.

Little, S.S. (1993) Nonverbal learning disabilities and socioemotional functioning: a review of recent literature. *Journal of Learning Disabilities*, 26, 653–665.

Lovegrove, W. (1991) Is the question of the role of visual deficits as a cause of reading disabilities a closed one? *Cognitive Neuropsychology*, 8, 435–441.

Lovegrove, W., Martin, F. & Slaghuis, W. (1986) The theoretical and experimental case for a visual deficit in specific reading disability. *Cognitive Neuropsychology*, 3, 225–267.

Lundberg, I. (1999) Learning to read in Scandinavia. In: *Learning to Read and Write: a Cross-linguistic Perspective* (eds M. Harris & G. Hatano), pp. 157–172. Cambridge University Press, Cambridge.

Lundberg, I., Frost, J. & Petersen, O. (1988) Effects of an extensive program for stimulating phonological awareness in preschool children. *Reading Research Quarterly*, 23, 263–384.

Magnusson, E. & Naucler, K. (1990) Reading and spelling in language disordered children: linguistic and metalinguistic pre-requisites—a report on a longitudinal study. *Clinical Linguistics and Phonetics*, 4, 49–61.

Manis, F.R., Seidenberg, M.S., Doi, L.M., McBride-Chang, C. & Petersen, A. (1996) On the bases of two subtypes of developmental dyslexia. *Cognition*, 58, 157–195.

Maughan, B. (1994) Behavioural development and reading disabilities. In: *Reading Development and Disorders* (eds C. Hulme & M.J. Snowling), pp. 128–144. Whurr, London.

Maughan, B. & Hagell, A. (1996) Poor readers in adulthood: psychosocial functioning. *Development and Psychopathology*, 8, 457–476.

Maughan, B., Pickles, A., Hagell, A., Rutter, M. & Yule, W. (1996) Reading problems and antisocial behaviour: developmental trends in comorbidity. *Journal of Child Psychology and Psychiatry*, 37, 405–418.

McCloskey, M., Caramazza, A. & Basili, A. (1985) Cognitive mechanisms in number processing and calculation: evidence from dyscalculia. *Brain and Cognition*, 4, 171–196.

McKenna, M.C., Kear, D.J. & Ellsworth, R.A. (1995) Children's attitudes towards reading: a national survey. *Reading Research Quarterly*, 30, 934–956.

McLean, J.F. & Hitch, G.J. (1999) Working memory impairments in children with specific arithmetic learning difficulties. *Journal of Experimental Child Psychology*, 74, 240–260.

Morton, J. & Frith, U. (1995) Causal modelling: a structural approach to developmental psychopathology. In: *Manual of Developmental Psychopathology* (eds D. Cicchetti & D.J. Cohen), pp. 357–390. Wiley, New York.

Muter, V., Hulme, C. & Snowling, M. (1997) *Phonological Abilities Test*. Psychological Corporation, London.

Nation, K. (1999) Reading skills in hyperlexia: a developmental perspective. *Psychological Bulletin*, 125, 338–355.

Nation, K. & Snowling, M. (1997) Assessing reading difficulties: the validity and utility of current measures of reading skill. *British Journal of Educational Psychology*, 67, 359–370.

Nation, K. & Snowling, M.J. (1998) Individual differences in contextual facilitation: evidence from dyslexia and poor reading comprehension. *Child Development*, 69, 996–1011.

Nation, K. & Snowling, M.J. (2000) Factors influencing syntactic awareness in normal readers and poor comprehenders. *Applied Psycholinguistics*, 21, 229–241.

Nation, K., Adams, J.W., Bowyer-Crane, C.A. & Snowling, M.J. (1999) Working memory deficits in poor comprehenders reflect underlying language impairments. *Journal of Experimental Child Psychology*, 73, 139–158.

Nelson, H. & Warrington, E.K. (1974) Developmental spelling retardation and its relation to other cognitive abilities. *British Journal of Psychology*, 65, 265–274.

Nunes, T. & Bryant, P. (1996) *Children Doing Mathematics*. Blackwell Publishers, Oxford.

Olson, R.K., Forsberg, H. & Wise, B. (1994) Genes, environment, and the development of orthographic skills. In: *The Varieties of Orthographic Knowledge* Vol. 1, *Theoretical and Development Issues* (ed. V.W. Berninger), pp. 27–71. Kluwer Academic, Dordrecht.

Olson, R.K. & Wise, B.W. (1992) Reading on the computer with orthographic and speech feedback. *Reading and Writing*, 4, 107–144.

Pennington, B.F. & Ozonoff, S. (1996) Executive functions and developmental psychopathology. *Journal of Child Psychology and Psychiatry*, 37, 51–89.

Pennington, B.F., Smith, S.D., Kimberling, W.J., Green, P.A. & Haith, M.M. (1987) Left-handedness and immune disorders in familial dyslexics. *Archives of Neurology*, 44, 634–639.

Pennington, B.F., Orden, G.C.V., Smith, S.D., Green, P.A. & Haith, M.M. (1990) Phonological processing skills and deficits in adult dyslexics. *Child Development*, 61, 1753–1778.

Pennington, B.F., Grossier, D. & Welsh, M.C. (1993) Contrasting cognitive defects in attention deficit hyperactivity disorder vs. reading disability. *Developmental Psychology*, 29, 511–523.

Perfetti, C.A. & Hogaboam, T. (1975) Relationship between single word decoding and reading comprehension skill. *Journal of Educational Psychology*, 67, 461–469.

Plaut, D.C., McClelland, J.L., Seidenberg, M.S. & Patterson, K. (1996) Understanding normal and impaired word reading: computational principles in quasi-regular domains. *Psychological Review*, 103, 56–115.

Rack, J.P., Snowling, M.J. & Olson, R.K. (1992) The nonword reading deficit in developmental dyslexia: a review. *Reading Research Quarterly*, 27, 29–53.

Rispens, J. (1998) The validity of the category of specific developmental reading disorders. In: *Perspectives on the Classification of Specific Developmental Disorders* (eds J. Rispens, T.A. van Yperen & W. Yule), pp. 61–82. Kluwer, Dordrecht.

Rodgers, B. (1983) The identification and prevalence of specific reading retardation. *British Journal of Educational Psychology*, 53, 369–373.

Romani, C., Ward, J. & Olson, A. (1999) Developmental surface dysgraphia: what is the underlying cognitive impairment? *Quarterly Journal of Experimental Psychology*, 52, 97–128.

Rourke, B.P. (1989) *Nonverbal Learning Disabilities: The Syndrome and the Model*. Guilford Publications, New York.

Rourke, B.P., ed. (1995) *Syndrome of Nonverbal Learning Disabilities: Neuro-developmental Manifestations*. Guilford Press, New York.

Rourke, B.P. & Fuerst, D.R. (1995) Cognitive processing, academic achievement and psychosocial functioning: a neurodevelopmental perspective. In: *Manual of Developmental Psychopathology* (eds D. Cicchetti & D.J. Cohen), pp. 391–423. Wiley, New York.

Rutter, M. & Yule, W. (1975) The concept of specific reading retardation. *Journal of Child Psychology and Psychiatry*, 16, 181–197.

Scarborough, H.S. (1990) Very early language deficits in dyslexic children. *Child Development*, 61, 1728–1743.

Seidenberg, M.S. & McClelland, J. (1989) A distributed, developmental model of word recognition. *Psychological Review*, 96, 523–568.

Semrud-Clikeman, M. & Hynd, G. (1990) Right hemispheric dysfunction in nonverbal learning disabilities: social, academic and adaptive functioning in adults and children. *Psychological Bulletin*, 107, 196–209.

Seymour, P.H.K. (1986) *A Cognitive Analysis of Dyslexia*. Routledge and Kegan Paul, London.

Share, D.L. (1995) Phonological recoding and self-teaching: sine qua non of reading acquisition. *Cognition*, 55, 151–218.

Shaywitz, S.E., Shaywitz, B.A., Fletcher, J.M. & Escobar, M.D. (1990) Prevalence of reading disability in boys and girls: results of the Connecticut longitudinal study. *Journal of the American Medical Association*, 264, 998–1002.

Shaywitz, S.E., Escobar, M.D., Shaywitz, B.A., Fletcher, J.M. & Makugh, R. (1992) Evidence that dyslexia may represent the lower tail of a normal distribution of reading ability. *New England Journal of Medicine*, 326, 145–150.

Silva, P.A., McGee, R. & Williams, S. (1985) Some characteristics of 9-year-old boys with general reading backwardness or specific reading retardation. *Journal of Child Psychology and Psychiatry*, 26, 407–421.

Smith, S.D., Kimberling, W.J., Pennington, B.F. & Lubs, H.A. (1983) Specific reading disability: identification of an inherited form through linkage analysis. *Science*, 219, 1345–1347.

Snowling, M.J. (1996) Annotation: contemporary approaches to the teaching of reading. *Journal of Child Psychology and Psychiatry*, 37, 139–148.

Snowling, M.J. (2000) *Dyslexia*. Blackwell Publishers, Oxford.

Snowling, M.J. & Frith, U. (1986) Comprehension in 'hyperlexic' readers. *Journal of Experimental Child Psychology*, 42, 392–415.

Snowling, M.J. & Stackhouse, J., eds (1996) *Dyslexia, Speech and Language: a Practitioner's Handbook*. Whurr, London.

Snowling, M.J., Nation, K., Moxham, P., Gallagher, A. & Frith, U. (1997) Phonological processing deficits in dyslexic students: a preliminary account. *Journal of Research in Reading*, 20, 31–34.

Snowling, M., Nation, K. & Muter, V. (1999) The role of semantic and phonological skills in learning to read: implications for assessment and teaching. In: *Learning to Read: an Integrated View from Research and Practice* (ed. T. Nunes), pp. 195–208. Kluwer Academic, Dordrecht.

Snowling, M., Bishop, D.V.M. & Stothard, S.E. (2000) Is pre-school language impairment a risk factor for dyslexia in adolescence? *Journal of Child Psychology and Psychiatry*, 41(5), 587–600.

Snowling, M.J., Adams, J.W., Bishop, D.V.M. & Stothard, S.E. (2001) Educational attainments of school leavers with a pre-school history of speech–language impairment. *International Journal of Language and Communication Disorders*, 36, 173–183.

Stackhouse, J. (1982) An investigation of reading and spelling performance in speech disordered children. *British Journal of Disorders of Communication*, 17, 53–60.

Stackhouse, J. (2000) Barriers to literacy development in children with speech and language difficulties. In: *Speech and Language Impairments in Children: Causes, Characteristics, Intervention and Outcome* (eds D.V.M. Bishop & L. Leonard), pp. 73–97. Psychology Press, Hove.

Stanovich, K.E. & Siegel, L.S. (1994) The phenotypic performance profile of reading-disabled children: a regression-based test of the phonological-core variable-difference model. *Journal of Educational Psychology*, 86, 24–53.

Stanovich, K.E. & West, R.F. (1989) Exposure to print and orthographic processing. *Reading Research Quarterly*, 24, 402–433.

Stevenson, J., Graham, P., Fredman, G. & McLoughlin, V. (1987) A twin study of genetic influences of reading and spelling ability and disability. *Journal of Child Psychology and Psychiatry*, 28, 229–247.

Stothard, S.E. (1994) The nature and treatment of reading comprehension difficulties in children. In: *Reading Development and Dyslexia* (eds C. Hulme & M.J. Snowling), pp. 200–238. Whurr, London.

Stothard, S. & Hulme, C. (1995) A comparison of reading comprehension and decoding difficulties in children. *Journal of Child Psychology and Psychiatry*, 36, 399–408.

Stothard, S.E., Snowling, M.J., Bishop, D.V.M., Chipchase, B. & Kaplan, C. (1998) Language impaired pre-schoolers: a follow-up in adolescence. *Journal of Speech, Language and Hearing Research*, **41**, 407–418.

Talcott, J. & Stein, J. (1999) Impaired neuronal timing in developmental dyslexia: the magnocellular hypothesis. *Dyslexia*, **5**, 59–77.

Temple, C.M. (1994) The cognitive neuropsychology of the developmental dyscalculias. *Cahiers de Psychologie Cognitive*, **13**, 351–370.

Torgesen, J.K. (2000) Individual differences in response to early interventions in reading: the lingering problem of treatment resisters. *Learning Disabilities Research and Practice*, **15**, 55–64.

Torgesen, J.K., Wagner, R.K. & Rashotte, C.A. (1994) Longitudinal studies of phonological processing and reading. *Journal of Learning Disabilities*, **27**, 276–286.

Torgesen, J.K., Wagner, R.K., Rashotte, C.A. *et al.* (1999) Preventing reading failure in young children wth phonological processing disabilities: group and individual responses to instruction. *Journal of Educational Psychology*, **91**, 579–593.

Treiman, R. (1997) Spelling in normal children and dyslexics. In: *Foundations of Reading Acquisition and Dyslexia: Implications for Early Intervention* (ed. B. Blachman,), pp. 191–218. Lawrence Erlbaum, Mahwah, NJ.

Troia, G.A. (1999) Phonological awareness intervention research: a critical review of the experimental methodology. *Reading Research Quarterly*, **34**, 28–52.

Vellutino, F.R., Scanlon, D.M., Sipay, E. *et al.* (1996) Cognitive profiles of difficult-to-remediate and readily-remediated poor readers: early intervention as a vehicle for distinguishing between cognitive and experiential deficits as basic causes of specific reading disability. *Journal of Educational Psychology*, **88**, 601–638.

Williams, S. & McGee, R. (1994) Reading attainment and juvenile delinquency. *Journal of Child Psychology and Psychiatry*, **35**, 441–461.

Willows, D.M., Kruk, R.S. & Corcos, E., eds (1993) *Visual Processes in Reading and Reading Disabilities*. Lawrence Erlbaum, Hillsdale, NJ.

Wimmer, H., Mayringer, H. & Landerl, K. (1998) Poor reading: a deficit in skill-automatization or a phonological deficit? *Scientific Studies of Reading*, **2**, 321–340.

Wynn, K. (1995) Origins of numerical knowledge. *Mathematical Cognition*, **1**, 35–60.

Yuill, N. & Oakhill, J. (1991) *Children's Problems in Text Comprehension*. Cambridge University Press, Cambridge.

Yule, W., Rutter, M., Berger, M. & Thompson, J. (1974) Over and under achievement in reading: distribution in the general population. *British Journal of Educational Psychology*, **44**, 1–12.

41 Mental Retardation

Fred R. Volkmar and Elisabeth Dykens

Table 41.1 Levels of mental retardation (MR).

Introduction

Although recognized since antiquity, modern interest in mental retardation dates to the late eighteenth and early nineteenth centuries as concern for children and their development increased. Reports such as that of Itard on a supposedly feral child stimulated interest in the relative contributions of 'nature' and 'nurture' (Candland 1993). Subsequently, Seguin began to develop specific systems for intervention and training. By the latter half of the nineteenth century many training and residential facilities were developed; originally the goal was to return children to their families but gradually such institutions came to emphasize custodial care. Developments in intelligence testing and the belief, particularly in the first half of the twentieth century, in the notion of 'fixed' intelligence led to better measures of intellectual ability and, unfortunately, to a rather regressive therapeutic stance (Hunt 1961). This philosophy began to change yet again in the latter half of the twentieth century when, as a result of legislation, legal procedures and a shift in public opinion, the emphasis was on treating children in their family context and community. A second major change during this time was the remarkable progress in understanding basic aetiological factors in mental retardation (Szymanski & King 1999).

This chapter summarizes current knowledge as well as areas of research interest and, at times, of controversy. We first consider current definitions of mental retardation, then epidemiology and natural history. The aetiology of mental retardation syndromes will be discussed using specific syndromes as examples. The final sections of the chapter focus on associated behavioural and psychiatric disorders, assessment, treatment and intervention.

Definitions

ICD-10 and DSM-IV

Historically, intelligence has been defined in rather different ways, with some emphasizing more abstract cognitive abilities and others more practical 'real world' capacities for solving problems (Sternberg 2000). These two tensions are jointly embodied in the formal definition of mental retardation included in ICD-10 (World Health Organization 1993) and DSM-IV (American Psychiatric Association 1994). Both subnormal intellectual functioning and commensurate deficits in adaptive functioning (capacities for social and personal sufficiency and independence) are required. DSM-IV specifies that an appropriate standardized assessment of intelligence is generally needed, while ICD-10 does not.

The use of formal measures of intellectual functioning rests on a very substantial body of empirical work on the assessment of cognitive ability, and the reliability and stability of such measures over time (Sternberg 2000). As we discuss subsequently, the use of IQ as the *sole* criterion for mental retardation is problematic in several respects. Most importantly it includes many individuals, particularly those with IQs close to 70, who may have no actual adaptive impairment and who can cope adequately with the demands of daily life. The current approach to diagnosis is thus a compromise in which both more theoretical cognitive abilities and social adaptation must be significantly below average. Clearly, among the most severely retarded, IQ and adaptive skills are highly correlated. In contrast to more theoretical cognitive abilities, capacities for social adaptation are teachable to a greater or lesser extent, and some children with mild mental retardation lose this diagnosis in adolescence or adulthood as they become more capable of self-sufficiency (Edgerton *et al.* 1984).

American Association of Mental Retardation definition

A rather different approach to definition is embodied by the American Association of Mental Retardation (AAMR 1992) definition. In this approach, the traditional distinctions based on IQ are discarded in favour of one based on level of need for environmental support (pervasive, extensive, limited, intermittent) in each of 10 different levels of adaptive functioning. This definition allows for greater clinical judgement in that it increases the upper IQ bound to 70 or 75. What initially may appear as a small increase in IQ level actually has major implications for definition and service delivery, potentially doubling the number of cases (MacMillan *et al.* 1995). The proposed 10 areas of adaptive functioning have limited empirical support and, in practice, the AAMR definition has proven difficult to use.

Terminology

Both ICD-10 and DSM-IV continue to employ the use of various 'levels' of mental retardation grouped according to intellectual level: mild, moderate, severe and profound. DSM-IV allows

Table 41.1 Levels of mental retardation (MR)*.

Level	IQ range	Approximate mental age in adulthood (years)	Proportion of MR group (%)
Mild	50–70†	9–12	85
Moderate	35–49	6–9	10
Severe	20–34	3–6	3–4
Profound	<20	<31–2	

*Data from ICD-10 and DSM-IV.
†DSM-IV allows for some clinical judgement in the diagnosis of MR, e.g. a diagnosis could be made in an individual with IQ up to 75 who exhibits significant deficits in adaptive behaviour or a clinician could decide that an individual with IQ up to 55 might best be thought of as exhibiting moderate mental retardation.

slightly more leeway for clinical judgement. As would be expected, given the normal distribution of cognitive functioning, cases of mild mental retardation account for the majority of cases (Table 41.1). As has long been appreciated (Dingman & Tarjan 1960) there is a higher than expected proportion of severe and profound retardation, relative to the Gaussian distribution, which reflects the operation of specific biological insults.

For practical purposes the most basic distinction is probably between mild mental retardation (IQ 50–70) and more severe mental retardation (IQ < 50; this distinction was previously referred to as that between 'educable' and 'trainable'). Individuals with IQ scores in the mild range often have minimal impairments in adaptive functioning and are, on balance, more likely to come from more disadvantaged social groups (Slone *et al*. 1998). Documented medical causes for the mental retardation are less likely and family members may also exhibit lower intellectual levels. Among individuals with more severe retardation, organic factors can be documented in many cases; family members are less likely to exhibit intellectual impairment or social disadvantage; the diagnosis is made earlier; and adaptive functioning is much more impaired. As discussed below, psychiatric disorders are more common in individuals with mild mental retardation than in the general population but are fundamentally of the same type. Among those with more severe retardation, specific disorders such as autism and overactivity become more frequent and the psychiatric presentation may be more complex (Batshaw 1997; Fox & Wade 1998). In more severe retardation, cases are more likely to represent all social classes, while in mild mental retardation lower socioeconomic status is more common (McLaren & Bryson 1987; Szymanski & King 1999).

Historically, many other terms have been used, but in the UK, USA and other countries the trend recently is towards more descriptive and less pejorative terminology. Terms such as 'mental handicap' or 'mental impairment' are used. In the UK the term 'learning disability' has also been used, although this introduces potential areas of confusion with the 'specific' learning disabilities (see Snowling, Chapter 40); in this chapter we use the term 'mental retardation' to avoid this confusion. As with other conditions it is important that clinicians and researchers refer to *persons* with a disability such as mental retardation, rather than equating the individual with their disability. It must be noted that labelling may, of itself, have unfortunate negative effects (Weisz 1990) and, conversely, a failure to provide appropriate services may result from a failure to assign an appropriate label (Granat & Granat 1978).

Epidemiology

Complications for epidemiological studies of mental retardation arise from several sources. IQ does not always remain constant, and, except for the most impaired infants and young children, correlations between IQ scores obtained in infancy and later childhood are quite low; this complicates calculation of age-specific rates of mental retardation in younger individuals. As children begin formal schooling the correlations with subsequent IQ are reasonably robust, although in individual cases children may have major gains or losses in intellectual ability (Sternberg 2000). Differences in rates of intellectual development are also observed, e.g. in Down syndrome the IQ tends to decline in middle childhood (Hodapp *et al.* 1999). Identification of cases increases as children enter formal educational programmes which may themselves exhibit considerable regional or local variation (Massey & McDermott 1995). Differences in diagnostic practice or concerns regarding negative effects of labelling may complicate determination of rates based on administrative data; children with mild mental retardation might be classified as learning disabled instead. There also may be differential mortality associated with some forms of mental retardation.

The use of IQ < 70 as the sole criterion for mental retardation would result in prevalence rates of between 2 and 3%, or essentially close to what would be the expected 2.3% based on the normal curve. The use of IQ as the sole defining feature of mental retardation rests on a very solid body of work on cognitive functioning dating back to Galton (for a review see Sternberg & Salter 1982). If IQ and measures of social adaptation skills are highly correlated, the expectation would be of rates of mental retardation of about 3%. However, studies that require some degree of impairment as well as IQ < 70 report much lower rates, around 1%. This distinction has major importance for service planning, and is illustrated in the results of two studies where rates can be calculated depending either solely on IQ, or IQ and impairment (as judged by service providers). In the Isle of Wight study of 9, 10 and 11 year olds, Rutter *et al.* (1970) found that 2.5% of the children would be classified as intellectually retarded by IQ score alone but only about 1.3% were noted to have impairments sufficient to require services. Similarly, in Birch *et al.*'s (1970) study in Aberdeen, which included nearly all 8–10 year olds in both regular and special schools, the rate was 2.42% when only IQ was used but 0.92% when impairment was added.

Several factors complicate the interpretation of the differences which result when the social/adaptive impairment criterion is added. Clearly, at least some individuals with mild mental retardation may acquire better adaptive skills over time and may no longer be in need of services (McLaren & Bryson 1987; Roeleveld et al. 1997); this becomes less likely the more severe the associated intellectual impairment (Ross et al. 1985). Richardson & Koller (1992) noted a wide variation in levels of functioning and degree of impairment in adults with histories of mild mental retardation. Even when special services are not apparently required the individual may still be vulnerable and the presence of supportive family members, spouses or friends may assume particular importance (Birch et al. 1970; Granat & Granat 1978; Edgerton et al. 1984; Ross et al. 1985). In the Isle of Wight study (Rutter et al. 1970) the children in more 'mainstream' educational settings had various difficulties including lower academic skills and higher rates of neurological abnormality and psychiatric difficulty. While it is clear that the rate of mental retardation is somewhere between 1 and 3%, an exact figure cannot be determined. On the one hand it can be said that what appears to be a modest change in the threshold level for mental retardation may substantially increase prevalence; it has been proposed by some that this IQ threshold be changed to 75 which would potentially double the rate of the disorder.

As noted previously among individuals with mild mental retardation, psychosocial adversity is common. The nature of the factors leading to increased rates of mild mental retardation in children from disadvantaged, often minority, backgrounds remains the topic of much debate. Factors such as 'cultural bias' of intelligence tests (see Sergeant & Taylor, Chapter 6; Rutter & Nikapota, Chapter 16) have sometimes been invoked to account for elevated rates of mental retardation in disadvantaged groups. While such factors must be considered, it is the case that psychosocial adversity has empirically been shown to result in significantly lower IQ scores, e.g. in children adopted away to more advantaged families (Dumaret 1985). Gender differences in rates of mental retardation are observed with a male:female ratio of 1.5:1 generally reported (Richardson et al. 1986).

Course and outcome

Given the heterogeneous nature of mental retardation it is not surprising that aspects of natural history and course vary considerably depending on the severity of mental retardation and the underlying biomedical, psychological and environmental factors (Richardson & Koller 1992). Levels of communicative ability and the presence/absence of associated medical problems and psychopathology are also important determinants of adult outcome. The complex factors determining outcome can include limitations in mobility, sensory impairments and associated medical conditions such as cardiac disease or seizures. When a precise cause for the mental retardation can be established it may have important implications, e.g. individuals with Down

syndrome are at increased risk for a number of problems including cardiac difficulties and for early onset Alzheimer dementia (Aylward et al. 1997). Although traditionally the mild mental retardation group has been thought to be the one least likely to show associated organic difficulties, advances in genetics have shown that this is not always the case. For example, many females with fragile X syndrome and most individuals with Prader–Willi syndrome may function at this level. Individuals from minority groups are often over-represented in this group. One of the accomplishments of the past decade has been the substantial improvement in the quality of paediatric and general medical care and rising life expectancies of persons with mental retardation (Szymanski & King 1999).

Mild mental retardation, as expected, has the best outcome. In their systematic follow-up of cases from the Aberdeen project, Richardson & Koller (1992) noted that one-quarter of cases disappeared from services with the remainder having some degree of vulnerability, at least in certain contexts. In their analysis, IQ, evidence of brain dysfunction and family stability were found to weakly predict outcome although, of these three factors, family stability was the strongest predictor and IQ the weakest.

Individuals with moderate levels of mental retardation (IQ 40–55) have greater degrees of impairment, are more likely to be identified in the preschool years and to have some specific aetiology identified for their developmental difficulties. As might be expected, the prognosis for adult self-sufficiency and independence is more guarded for this group, although many individuals can live semi-independently and with partial support (Ross et al. 1985). For individuals with severe or profound retardation, high levels of supervision and support are generally required throughout the person's life. Goals include facilitating self-care and other skills to the extent possible; very high levels of support and supervision are typically required.

In more developed countries, various factors have acted to improve overall outcome. These factors include early diagnosis and intervention, school-based services with more emphasis on use of community-based services and resources, and adult programmes. More extensive and varied sources of support are now available to families. In both the UK and USA the recent trend, both through legislation and legal decision, has been to advocate appropriate services which are community-based with the goal of keeping individuals in, or near, their families.

Aetiological considerations

Several factors contribute to the aetiology of mental retardation: organic and sociocultural factors, and their interaction. Genetic influences can be based on specific genes that result in well-recognized syndromes, or can be more complex reflecting the operation of multiple genes or the interaction of genetic vulnerability with the environment. Studies based on twin pairs and adoption suggest that the genetic role in the transmission of intelligence is a major one, although studies that have addressed this issue in the polygenic transmission of mental retardation are uncommon (Rutter *et al.* 1996). Biological causes are most likely to be identified in the most handicapped individuals.

'Two-group' approach

Researchers have historically described two distinct groups of people with mental retardation (Zigler 1967, 1969). One group demonstrates a clear biological or 'organic' cause for their cognitive delay, and is composed of people with known prenatal, perinatal and postnatal problems. Although estimates have varied over the years, current data suggest that approximately one-half of people with mental retardation have known 'organic' aetiologies (for a review see Hodapp 1994). The second group has no clear organic cause for their mental retardation, and is postulated to account for the vast majority of persons with mild mental retardation. From its inception to the present day, this 'two-group' approach to mental retardation has dominated both theory and research.

Although a helpful classification scheme, the two-group approach has raised more questions than it has answered. Who, exactly, comprises the group of persons with non-organic aetiologies, and what is the most appropriate label for these individuals? The term 'sociocultural familial' retardation reflected a dominant view in the 1960s and 1970s that non-organic mental retardation was attributed primarily to environmental deprivation. Although impoverished chaotic environments may indeed be the culprits in a small number of individuals, this theory has generally fallen out of favour as an explanation for the entire group. Even so, a complicating factor is that disproportionately more individuals with sociocultural familial mental retardation are poor, from minority backgrounds and of low-IQ parents (for a review see Hodapp 1994).

Other views of non-organic mental retardation are reflected in additional terms used to describe this group. 'Non-specific' or 'idiopathic' mental retardation seems to best reflect the hypothesis that persons in this group have as yet unidentified biological factors associated with their delay, including undetected genetic or neurological abnormalities. With increased diagnostic precision, and with the discovery of new genetic disorders, many workers speculate that more persons with non-specific delay will receive specific genetic diagnoses in the years ahead. Progress is much slower in identifying clear neurological aetiologies in persons with unspecified mental retardation, as most neuroimaging research is conducted with persons with known genetic or other aetiologies (Robertson & Murphy 1999).

Another term for this group, 'non-organic', perhaps best represents the idea that these individuals have no organic impairment, but simply constitute the lower end of the normal Gaussian distribution of intelligence (Zigler 1967; Simonoff *et al.* 1996). Even so, multiple genetic and environmental variables are implicated in low IQ (Lee *et al.* 1993). Assuming that non-organic mental retardation is indeed the extreme end of the normal IQ distribution, then some proportion of individuals will always belong to this group, even as progress is made uncover-

Table 41.2 Selected organic causes of mental retardation.

Prenatal	Perinatal, neonatal and postnatal
Chromosome abnormalities: trisomy 21 (Down syndrome)	Fetal distress/hypoxia
Inborn errors of metabolism (phenylketonuria, Hunter syndrome)	Complications caused by prematurity
Other genetic conditions (fragile X, tuberous sclerosis)	Endocrine (hypothyroidism)
Toxins (fetal alcohol syndrome)	Trauma (central nervous system damage)
Maternal illness (pre-eclampsia, diabetes)	
Multifactorial syndromes (seizures, cerebral palsy)	Toxins (lead poisoning) Infections (meningitis)

ing genetic or neurological aetiologies for other persons at the same IQ levels.

In the organic group too, many issues remain. Early researchers lumped people together in the same group who had many different types of organic aetiologies, often comparing these heterogeneous groups to those with familial or non-specific mental retardation; it is now clear that diverse aetiologies may be involved (Table 41.2). While remarkable progress has been made in molecular genetics, researchers are now much better able to examine people with distinctive genetic aetiologies. Indeed, as many as one-third of all persons with mental retardation have already been diagnosed with a known genetic disorder (Matalainen *et al.* 1995). Further, individuals with Down syndrome, fragile X syndrome, Prader–Willi syndrome, Williams syndrome and other disorders may comprise 10–50% of individuals with mild mental retardation (Rutter *et al.* 1996).

Behavioural phenotypes: a revision of the two-group approach

In light of these advances, many workers are turning to a line of research that examines the behaviour and development of people with distinctive genetic aetiologies (Hodapp & Dykens 1994, 2001; Dykens 1995). Research on 'behavioural phenotypes' is blossoming, and these studies typically fall into one of two general categories. On the one hand, many researchers conduct between-group studies, as they are on the hunt for unique syndromic behaviours that may fast-track our understanding of gene or brain function. Promising examples of these unique behaviours include hand-wringing in Rett syndrome (Perry 1991), hyperphagia in Prader–Willi syndrome (Holm *et al.* 1993), bouts of inappropriate laughter in Angelman syndrome (Williams *et al.* 1995), the infantile cat-like cry in 5p syndrome (Gersch *et al.* 1995) and the self-hug in Smith–Magenis syndrome (Finucane *et al.* 1994). For these and other behaviours, there appears to be a strong correspondence between the behaviour and the syndrome (see Skuse & Kuntsi, Chapter 13).

Yet even these unusual behaviours are occasionally seen in people without these diagnoses. Further, the vast majority of

Table 41.3 Cognitive/linguistic profiles in selected mental retardation syndromes.

Syndrome	Genetics	Relative weaknesses	Relative strengths
Fragile X*	CGG repeat	Sequential processing Auditory–verbal short-term memory Sustaining attention, some visuospatial	Verbal long-term memory Repertoire of acquired information
Prader–Willi†	del 15q11–13 Maternal UPD	Sequential processing Auditory, visual short-term memory	Long-term memory Visual processing, jigsaw puzzles
Williams‡	del 7q11.23	Visuomotor co-ordination Spatial organization	Auditory short-term memory Semantics, syntax, facial recognition Expressive, receptive vocabulary
Down§	Trisomy 21	Auditory processing Expressive language	Visuospatial processing

For reviews see: *Dykens *et al.*, 2000; †Dykens & Cassidy (1999); ‡Mervis *et al.* (1999); and §Hodapp *et al.* (1999).

syndromic behaviour is 'partially specific', or shared across one or more conditions (Hodapp 1997). For example, sequential processing deficits characterize Prader–Willi and fragile X syndromes (Dykens *et al.* 1994; Dykens & Cassidy 1999), and inattention and hyperactivity are seen in Williams, fragile X and 5p syndromes (Baumgardner *et al.* 1995; Dykens & Clarke 1997; Einfeld *et al.* 1997). Most syndromes, then, may have distinctive but not necessarily unique behavioural features.

A second line of work stems from the view that behavioural phenotypes are not determined, but involve an increased probability or likelihood that people with a given syndrome will show certain behavioural features relative to those without the syndrome (Dykens 1995). As variability within syndromes abounds, some researchers are examining genetic, environmental, psychosocial, and subject variables that help explain individual differences in people with the same genetic disorder. Level of cognitive delay in fragile X syndrome, for example, is tied to both age and molecular genetic status (Dykens *et al.* 1994; Tassone *et al.* 1999). Similarly, in Prader–Willi syndrome, the frequency and severity of maladaptive behaviours such as skin-picking appear to vary across genetic subtypes of this disorder (Dykens *et al.* 1999).

Both between- and within-syndrome research offers many advantages over research on heterogeneous groups of persons with mental retardation (Dykens 1995; Hodapp & Dykens, 2001). In the long term, syndromic findings facilitate the search for gene–brain–behaviour relationships, as well as contribute toward a more precise science of mental retardation. In the short term, phenotypic data refine intervention and treatment (Dykens & Hodapp 1997; Dykens *et al.* 2000).

Integrating genetic disorders into the two-group approach

What, then, does this line of work on behavioural phenotypes bring to our understanding of the 'two-group' approach to mental retardation? One of the most intriguing implications of this research concerns the so-called 'similar-structure hypothesis'.

Developmentally orientated researchers hypothesize that children with familial or non-organic mental retardation show the same cognitive structures as their non-retarded counterparts (for a review see Hodapp & Zigler 1995). Other contemporary workers have expanded these basic principles to include children with genetic and other organic aetiologies (Hodapp 1998).

Historically, typically developing children and children with non-organic mental retardation were hypothesized to show even performance across various cognitive domains, reflecting Piaget's (1952) notions of 'structures d'ensemble'. In other words, children who performed at a certain level in one domain would perform at a similar level in all other cognitive domains. However, other theorists have called this all-of-a-piece view of intelligence into question, emphasizing the modularity of language (Fodor 1983), or the presence of separate multiple intelligences (Gardner 1985) among typically developing children.

Findings from people with genetic mental retardation syndromes add an additional twist to these cross-domain relations. As summarized in Table 41.3, persons with Williams, Prader–Willi, Down and other syndromes often show distinctive patterns of cognitive or linguistic strength or weakness. Many people with Williams syndrome, for example, show relative strengths in certain aspects of expressive language, even as they show pronounced deficits in visuospatial functioning. Further, despite visuospatial deficits, many have relative sparing of facial recognition. Many, although not all, persons with Prader–Willi syndrome show remarkable skills solving jigsaw puzzles, with performances that exceed those matched for chronological age (Dykens in press, a). In these various genetic aetiologies, peaks and troughs rather than all-of-a-piece functioning seem to characterize development among certain cognitive and linguistic domains.

Although such profiles can be quite pronounced, it is not yet clear to what extent specific cognitive strengths or weaknesses represent distinctive or isolated cognitive structures as opposed to uneven performance in interrelated cognitive domains. It is also not clear if profiles in these syndrome groups show areas of so-called local organization, or the idea that while some domains might be separable from others, smaller ('local') pockets of connection might nevertheless exist (Bates *et al.* 1979; Mundy *et al.* 1984). Although these issues remains unresolved, data from different syndrome groups inform our understanding of cognition in children with or without mental retardation.

Psychopathology

Prevalence

Historically, persons with mental retardation were not routinely viewed as having comorbid psychopathology or mental illness—this phenomenon has been referred to as 'diagnostic overshadowing' (Reiss *et al.* 1982). When problems were seen, clinicians typically attributed them to the intellectual deficits. Although diagnostic overshadowing is still present (White *et al.* 1995), more mental health professionals are receiving specialized training in how to assess and treat patients with mental retardation (Day 1999).

Ironically, even under the cloud of diagnostic overshadowing, one of the most robust research findings to date is that, relative to the general population, persons with mental retardation are at increased risk for psychiatric illness and severe behavioural or emotional dysfunction (Tonge 1999). Using representative samples of children with mental retardation, Rutter *et al.* (1976) found that 30% showed psychopathology, compared with just 6% of children without developmental delay. These rates are remarkably similar to Koller *et al.* (1983), who found psychopathology in 36% of children with mental retardation vs. 5% of those without developmental disabilities. Comparable figures are found among adults with and without mental retardation (Gostason 1985). Among individuals with mild mental retardation there are increased risk of various disorders including both antisocial and other disruptive behavioural disorders (Einfeld & Tonge 1996). In individuals with greater degrees of mental handicap the rates of psychiatric disorder are much higher (Corbett 1979), although in this group of individuals the application of traditional diagnostic criteria may also be more problematic and attempts have been made to clarify the nature of disorders in this group (World Health Organization 1993).

As many as 25% of persons with mental retardation may have significant psychiatric problems; these rates are much higher for behavioural difficulties (Jacobson 1999). Reported rates of psychopathology vary greatly, depending in part on the method used to ascertain subjects. For example, among 100 children with mental retardation referred to a psychiatric clinic for evaluation, as many as 87% were diagnosed with a mental disorder (Philips & Williams 1975); this is not surprising given the nature of the sample. Rates of psychopathology are lower in studies based on administrative records rather than systematic assessment, with rates as low as 10–15% reported (Jacobson 1982; Borthwick-Duffy & Eyman 1990). Rates that fall between these extremes are found in studies based on informant checklists of behaviour problems of children and adults in non-referred samples; these rates, from 30 to 40%, are probably the most accurate (Rutter *et al.* 1976; Reiss 1990; Einfeld & Tonge 1996).

Persons with mental retardation experience the same range of psychiatric problems as seen in those without developmental disabilities (King *et al.* 1994), although the distribution of disorders differs, the rates of some disorders are increased, and issues of diagnosis can be particularly complex in persons with severe mental retardation, e.g. the diagnosis of psychosis in a mute individual. Relative to the general population, people with mental retardation are more likely to show autism and related disorders, psychosis and behaviour disorders, and less likely to be diagnosed with substance abuse and affective disorders (for a review of these issues see Moss *et al.* 1997a). For example, approximately two-thirds of children with autism also exhibit mental retardation and constitute between 1 and 2% of all children with mental retardation but about 5% of a more severely retarded population; if the broader pervasive developmental disorder (PDD) category is applied, features of autism are found in perhaps 50% of cases with severe mental retardation (Wing & Gould 1979; Volkmar *et al.* 1999; see Lord & Bailey, Chapter 38).

Prevalence rates for other disorders vary widely depending, in part, on the different methods for determining 'caseness', with common approaches including record reviews, behavioural checklists and, to a lesser extent, direct interviews. Using these techniques, some researchers have examined a broad range of DSM- or ICD-based diagnoses, while others assess maladaptive features commonly seen in the general population, such as inattention or sadness. Still others focus on a more narrow range of behaviours, seen primarily in persons with mental retardation, such as stereotypies or self-injury.

Examining a few selected diagnoses, Table 41.4 illustrates this variability in prevalence rates across several studies. Rates of schizophrenia or psychosis in persons with mental retardation range from 1 to 9% among non-referred samples, and 2.8 to 24% in referred samples. Although variable, rates are clearly higher than the 0.5–1% of the general population who suffer from schizophrenia (American Psychiatric Association 1994). Similarly, rates for depression vary from 1.1 to 11% across non-referred and clinic samples of persons with mental retardation. Among children with mental retardation, rates of attention deficit disorder or attention deficit with hyperactivity disorder ranged from 7 to 15%, which contrasts with the 3–5% prevalence estimates among non-retarded children in the population at large (American Psychiatric Association 1994). While less variability is seen when comparing similar types of samples, even then the ranges are rather high (e.g. from 1 to 3–11% for depression in the clinic referred samples in Table 41.4).

Risk factors

Although refined assessment tools are needed, researchers need to address the enduring question of why persons with mental

Table 41.4 Rates (%) of three diagnoses in studies of persons with heterogeneous mental retardation. (Reprinted with permission from Dykens *et al.*, in press.)

Study	*n*	Method	Schizophrenia/psychosis	Depression	ADHD
La Malfa *et al.* (1997)*	176 adults	DSM	4.5	1.1	
Lund (1985)	302 adults	DSM	1.3/5	1.7	
Meyers (1986)*	62 adults	DSM	19/24	11.0	
Gillberg *et al.* (1986)	149 adolescents	Behaviours	1.0	10.0	11.0
Gath & Gumley (1986)	154 children–adolescents	ICD		10.0	7.0
Reid (1972)*	500 adults	ICD	3.2		
Reid (1980)*	60 children	ICD	8.3		15.0
Jacobson (1990)	42 479 children and adults	Records	6.0–7.0		
Day (1985)*	357 adults	ICD	4.2		
Grizenko *et al.* (1991)*	176 adolescents–adults	DSM	2.8/2.3	3.4	
Cooper (1997)	602 older adults	ICD	9.0	5.0–10.0	

*Clinic or hospital sample.

retardation are at increased for psychopathology. Many reasons have been discussed over the years, and most fall within the 'biopsychosocial' spectrum. Yet, in contrast to psychopathology in general, a comprehensive model is still lacking, in part because the unique qualities of those with mental retardation preclude researchers from simply applying to this population existing risk factors for psychopathology. Further, for most risk factors, the causal direction is unclear. For example, poor peer or social relations may be a precursor for psychopathology, or a consequence of disruptive behaviour. Even so, certain advances have been made, and increased risks for psychopathology have now been associated with the following.

• *Distinctive or aberrant personality styles*, including an outer-directed orientation, and being too wary or disinhibited with others, which may lead to dependency, withdrawal and impulsivity (Bybee & Zigler 1998; Dykens 1999b; Zigler & Bennett-Gates 1999).

• *Atypical motivational styles* or abnormally high or low levels of sensitivity to basic human drives, such as the need for attention or acceptance (Reiss & Havercamp 1998).

• *Increased risk of failure experiences* at school and in daily living, which may lead to learned helplessness, low expectancies for success, and depression (Weisz 1990; Zigler & Bennett-Gates 1999).

• *More global and less differentiated self concepts* that may lead to more sweeping negative evaluations of the entire self instead of not liking just one aspect of one's self (Evans 1998).

• *Reinforcement of negative behaviours*, leading to more entrenched maladaptive coping or interaction styles (Reiss & Havercamp 1997).

• *Poor communication or assertiveness skills* that may lead to increased frustration and acting out behaviour (Nezu & Nezu 1994).

• *Social strain*, or stressful social interactions, which is more strongly correlated with psychopathology than low levels of social support (Nezu *et al.* 1995; Lunsky & Havercamp 1999).

• *Social stigma*, with subsequent negative impact on daily living, vocational opportunities, adjustment and esteem (Edgerton & Gaston 1991).

• *Peer rejection and ostracism* and, among children, atypical patterns of friendship with non-retarded children marked by less shared play and laughter and more hierarchical roles (Siperstein *et al.* 1997).

• *Compromised 'social intelligence'*, or inappropriate responses to social cues, that may exacerbate stigma and isolation from others (Greenspan & Granfield 1992).

• *Heightened risks of exploitation and abuse* that may worsen behavioural or emotional problems (Ammerman *et al.* 1994).

• *Family stress, parental psychopathology* and low levels of emotional, service or financial support to families (Minnes 1998).

• *Increased rates of seizure disorders* among persons with mental retardation (Bird 1997; Caplan *et al.* 1998).

• *Abnormal neurological functioning*, which in many cases is undetected, in part because of the lack of widespread use of neuroimaging techniques among persons with idiopathic mental retardation (Peterson 1995; Robertson & Murphy 1999).

• *Biochemical or neurological anomalies* associated with unusual behaviours such as severe self-injury (King 1993).

• *Genetic aetiologies* that carry higher than usual risks for certain maladaptive or psychiatric vulnerabilities (Dykens 1999a).

Although the identification of these factors is an important first step, the field still lacks a comprehensive model that assesses the relative importance of each for the development of psychopathology. New statistical techniques, such as individual's growth modelling, as well as improved measures of pathology, hold much promise for a more specific, finely tuned 'biopsychosocial' model in the years ahead.

Genetic syndromes

Research aimed at sorting out the relative importance of these many risk factors has typically relied on heterogeneous groups of subjects with mental retardation. Yet each of the factors listed above can just as easily apply to those with or without a genetic diagnosis. Syndrome-specific work helps sort out genetic from many other biological and psychosocial risk factors. In this vein, syndromic studies allow researchers to identify the possible influence of syndromes on maladaptive behaviour or psychopathology, and may thus shed new light on genetic or other mechanisms associated with certain psychopathologies (Dykens 1995; Holland & Koot 1998).

Although a complete review of psychopathology in genetic disorders is beyond the scope of this chapter, Table 41.5 summarizes psychiatric and maladaptive features from several syndromes. In general, findings are included only if they are based on comparative studies showing increased rates of problems relative to others with mental retardation. Findings are presented for the syndromic group as a whole; individual differences in these problems abound. Indeed, identifying the genetic, developmental and psychosocial reasons for individual behavioural differences in people with the same genetic syndrome is one of the most exciting aspects of behavioural phenotype research (Dykens 1995; Dykens *et al.* 2000).

Two points are apparent from Table 41.5. First, some syndromes feature rather specific psychiatric vulnerabilities: examples include increased rates of obsessive-compulsive features in Prader–Willi syndrome (Dykens *et al.* 1996), and anxiety, fears and phobias in Williams syndrome (Dykens in press, b). Granted, people without these syndromes can be diagnosed with these conditions, but they occur with increased frequency in these syndromes. As such, studies on these syndromes hold much promise for differentiating genetic from other pathways to these psychiatric or maladaptive endpoints.

Secondly, certain problems are seen across one or more genetic syndromes, as in the inattention and hyperactivity that characterizes fragile X, 5p and Williams syndromes. Despite these common problems, important qualitative differences may exist in how these symptoms are manifest in each syndrome. Inattention in Williams syndrome, for example, may be associated with heightened anxiety and social disinhibition, while in fragile X syndrome, it may be best associated with hyperarousal and anomalies in the size of the posterior cerebellar vermis and caudate nucleus (Mostofsky *et al.* 1998).

Assessment

Cognitive assessment

Assessment of intellectual functioning is based on the administration of standardized tests of intelligence that have been shown to be reliable and valid (see Sergeant & Taylor, Chapter 6). Individuals with mental retardation may present special

Table 41.5 Psychopathology in people with selected mental retardation syndromes.

Syndrome	Salient maladaptive features
Fragile X*	Social anxiety, shyness, gaze aversion, autism/PDD, inattention, hyperactivity, depression (females)
Williams	Anxiety, fears, phobias, inattention, hyperactivity, social disinhibition, indiscriminate relating
Prader–Willi	Hyperphagia, non-food obsessions and compulsions, skin-picking, temper tantrums, lability, underactivity
5p	Infantile cat-like cry, hyperactivity, inattention, stereotypies, self-injury
Smith–Magenis	Hyperactivity, aggression, self-injury, stereotypies (often with mouth), sleep disturbance, self-hugging
Down	Non-compliance, stubbornness, inattention, overactivity, argumentative, depression and dementia among adults

*For reviews of these syndromes see Dykens *et al.*, 2000.
PDD, pervasive developmental disorder.

problems for intellectual assessment. In addition to the obvious consideration of chronological age, the individual's receptive and expressive language ability must be considered as well as any behavioural or psychiatric difficulties which may present special challenges for assessment. Other issues to be considered include the capacity of the individual to deal with challenge and frustration, particularly to timed tasks, the level of social demands placed on the individual, and any unique features present, e.g. sensory impairments. These issues are often vividly present in individuals with autism and related disorders (see Lord & Bailey, Chapter 38) many of whom also exhibit mental retardation as well as major difficulties in social interaction and communication. The examiner should be particularly sensitive to potential cultural or language issues that complicate assessment.

While some flexibility in selection and administration of standard instruments is needed, there is also the necessity to maintain standard assessments to be able to provide valid results. On the other hand, the administration of any instrument by a skilled and observant examiner will provide considerable qualitative information which may be of great relevance for developing and implementing the treatment programme. Thus, observation of the need for structure, of strategies which facilitate learning from demonstration, of coping with off-task or maladaptive behaviours, and pace of presentation are all relevant (see Sergeant & Taylor, Chapter 6).

Adaptive behaviour

Adaptive functioning refers to the capacity for personal self-sufficiency and independence in day-to-day life. Measures of adaptive ability provide the clinician with an estimate of the degree to which the individual has been able to use his or her cognitive potential in adapting to real-life settings; a large discrepancy between intellectual level and adaptive skills would suggest that the treatment should include a major focus on acquisition and generalization of adaptive skills.

Various measures of adaptive functioning have been proposed. The most widely used instrument is the Vineland Adaptive Behaviour Scales (Sparrow et al. 1984), a version of Doll's original (1935) instrument. The Vineland assesses capacities for self-sufficiency in various domains of functioning including Communication (receptive, expressive and written language), Daily Living Skills (personal, domestic and community skills), Socialization (interpersonal relationships, play and leisure time and coping skills), and Motor Skills (gross and fine). The Vineland is available in three editions: a survey form to be used primarily as a diagnostic and classification tool for normal to low functioning children or adults; an expanded form for use in the development of individual education or rehabilitative planning; and a classroom edition to be used by teachers (Sparrow et al. 1984). The survey and expanded editions utilize a semistructured interview format administered to a parent or primary caregiver. For individuals with mental retardation the expanded form is often particularly useful because it readily translates into goals for intervention planning. The other measures of adaptive functioning also typical day-to-day abilities. Other schedules (e.g. AAMR Adaptive Behaviour Scales; Lambert et al. 1993), have some different areas of emphasis, may span different age ranges and, in some cases, can be directly administered to the individual.

Assessment of psychiatric disorders

The psychiatric assessment of emotional and behavioural difficulties in the individual with mental retardation may entail some modification in usual procedures although, particularly in individuals with mild mental retardation, usual diagnostic procedures should work reasonably well. Among individuals with greater degrees of handicap, the psychiatric assessment should be comprehensive and multifocal. The presence of associated difficulties (seizures, motor impairments, sensory problems) may have important implications for assessment and treatment.

Much work has thus focused on assessing the prevalence of co-occurring mental retardation and psychiatric illness. As counting these problems depends on ways of accurately describing them, a parallel line of research has evolved on behavioural surveys and rating scales. Most of these measures are geared specifically for individuals with mental retardation, and have well-developed psychometric properties (for a review see Aman 1991). More widely used tools include the Aberrant Behaviour Checklist (Aman & Singh 1994), Reiss Screen (Reiss 1988) and Developmental Behaviour Checklist (Einfeld & Tonge 1992). While these scales are sensitive to the unique concerns of those with mental retardation, they are not necessarily compatible with DSM- or ICD-based psychiatric diagnoses. Further, each scale was designed for a slightly different purpose, and each has different sets of items and factor structures, ultimately

contributing to inconsistent findings across studies (Dykens, 2000).

In a similar vein, other researchers have raised concerns about the applicability of traditional DSM or ICD diagnoses for those with mental retardation (Sovner 1986). Many problems relate to the psychiatric interview itself, including acquiescence bias, and the more limited abilities of persons with mental retardation to express abstract thoughts and feelings, or to answer questions about the onset, duration, frequency and severity of symptoms (for a review see Moss 1999). In response to these challenges, some researchers have adapted traditional DSM or ICD criteria for those with developmental delay (King et al. 1994; Szymanski et al. 1998). Others shy away from formal diagnoses and embrace a more functional analysis of challenging behaviour (Sturmey 1999), while still others have designed interview schedules specifically for those with mental retardation, including the Psychiatric Assessment Schedule for Adults with Developmental Disability (PASS-ADD; Moss et al. 1997b). When using these options, direct interviews with both respondents and informants is best, resulting in fewer cases of missed diagnoses (Moss et al. 1996; see Angold, Chapter 3; Fombonne, Chapter 4).

Medical assessments

In individuals with mental retardation, rates of various medical conditions may be substantially increased over the general population (Ryan & Sunada 1997). Unfortunately, as with the tendency to neglect mental health needs (Einfeld & Tonge 1996), underlying medical conditions may be unappreciated. Ryan & Sunada (1997) noted that up to 75% of persons with mental retardation who had been referred for psychiatric assessment had undiagnosed or undertreated medical conditions and nearly 50% were receiving non-psychotropic medications that could have behavioural side-effects.

The medical assessment of the individual with mental retardation should include careful history (including birth, antenatal and family history). In some cases, the clinical disorder exhibits a characteristic pattern of evolution over time and the history may provide important evidence favouring a specific aetiology, e.g. Rett and Hurler syndromes (Curry et al. 1997). Physical examination should include assessment of growth and development, a search for minor physical anomalies, facial features and other neurological or psychiatric findings suggestive of a specific syndrome. Evaluation of sensory capacities may be indicated as may selected diagnostic procedures, e.g. metabolic studies, chromosome analysis (including fragile X testing), assessment of organic acids, neuroimaging and skeletal radiography (see Bailey, Chapter 10).

Treatment

Over the past decades the treatment of mental retardation has undergone a marked shift in the more developed countries (see

Bernard, Chapter 67). More individuals with mental retardation now reside with their families and in their communities. More children receive services within regular educational settings and more services are available to support them and their families. At the same time it is clear that placement in the community is not sufficient in and of itself and that the provision of adequate and appropriate support is critical.

In general, treatment planning begins with a consideration of the underlying cause, if one is known, of the intellectual disability as this, in some cases, has important implications for treatment, e.g. phenylketonuria. Many aspects of treatment planning relevant to other children also apply to children with mental retardation. All the various treatment modalities, including behaviour therapy, psychotherapy and pharmacotherapy, may be used, chosen on the basis of the specifics of the individual case. The severity of the associated mental retardation may influence the choice of treatment, e.g. for the individual with profound mental retardation who is mute, verbally based interventions are less practical although behavioural procedures and modification of the environment can be helpful (Szymanski & King 1999).

Treatment priorities should ideally be established within the context of a comprehensive view of the individual; for individuals with limited verbal skills one consideration might be the attempt to foster alternative communicative modalities. Similarly, various treatments may have synergistic effects; medications that reduce levels of self-stimulatory behaviours may make the child more amenable to educational interventions. Because various professionals and caregivers are often involved, close collaboration is essential for treatment effectiveness.

Individuals with mental retardation may present with acute psychiatric difficulties. In cases of behavioural emergency (e.g. relative to aggressive or self-injurious behaviours) the first concern should be safety of the individual and his or her caregivers. Potential medical causes for acute behavioural deterioration should always be considered and these include side-effects of medications. Environmental influences should also be considered and a treatment plan formulated.

Although data on treatment efficacy are often limited and of poor quality, there is a consensus that individuals with mental retardation can benefit from various psychosocial interventions including psychotherapy (for a review see Szymanski & King 1999). Modifications in usual procedures may include adoption of a more active therapeutic stance with careful consideration of the individual's communicative abilities. The usefulness of special education and behavioural interventions has been well established, particularly for individuals with more severe mental retardation (Reiss 1994: see Howlin, Chapter 68). Individual psychotherapy or family therapy may be useful in some cases, particularly in mild mental retardation, and cognitive-behavioural techniques can also be used, e.g. in the treatment of anxiety (Lindsay et al. 1989).

Pharmacological interventions in the management of psychiatric and behavioural problems are relatively common. In theo-ry these are not different from those in individuals without mental retardation; however, it is clear that in practice there are several important considerations. Issues of informed consent must be adequately addressed, particularly considering the potential for use of medications on a long-term basis, often by less experienced practitioners (Aman & Singh 1988; Szymanski & King 1999; see also Heyman & Santosh, Chapter 59). Medications should be one part of a broader programme of intervention and should be used only following a careful clinical assessment with due attention to sensible prescribing practices.

Neuroleptics are the most frequently prescribed medications and can be used to manage acute behavioural crises. Their potential for sedation and many recognized side-effects, such as tardive dyskinesia, are limiting factors. Lithium and other mood stabilizers have sometimes been used with success in the management of severe aggression with mixed results (Carlson et al. 1992). Stimulants can be helpful in some children with mild to moderate mental retardation who exhibit attentional problems and hyperactivity; their usefulness is more limited in individuals with severe mental retardation, and some individuals, particularly those with autism or prominent stereotyped movements, may experience an exacerbation in levels of self-stimulation (Szymanski & King 1999). There have also been some reports of behavioural disinhibition following administration of sedative hypnotics (Szymanski & King 1999). The choice of a psychopharmacological agent should encompass careful consideration of risks and benefits as part of a comprehensive treatment plan (Szymanski & King 1999). Appropriate planning, including follow-up and monitoring for side-effects, is essential. Care should be exercised in administration of multiple medications and, in general, polypharmacy should be avoided (Reiss & Aman 1998).

Prevention

Primary prevention of mental retardation is possible in some cases, e.g. with dietary treatment of phenylketonuria. For certain conditions, e.g. fragile X and Down syndromes, prenatal diagnosis is available. In other cases, mental retardation may be prevented through education of prospective parents, e.g. for the adverse effects of alcohol during pregnancy or the impact of congenital rubella (see Brent, Chapter 54; Marks et al. Chapter 51). For individuals with mild developmental delays, early intervention programmes aimed at preventing intellectual disability can be particularly helpful. The emphasis is on provision of habilitative services, family support and other services, with the goal of maximizing the individual's potential and minimizing levels of associated retardation (Rowitz 1991). Similarly, for individuals with mental retardation, attempts to diminish associated complications, through the adequate diagnosis and treatment of associated medical and mental disorders, are also helpful (Szymanski & King 1999).

Conclusions and future directions

Research on psychopathology in genetic syndromes adds to our understanding of psychopathology in people with mental retardation in general. Compared to even a decade ago, considerable progress has been made in how we assess, understand and treat psychopathology in those with mental retardation. Such insights increase dramatically as researchers apply these new understandings of assessment, treatment and risk factors to people with discrete genetic aetiologies.

Despite the progress in assessing, treating and supporting persons with mental retardation and their families, considerable work lies ahead. In the next decades, more individuals with mental retardation will live, learn and work in their local communities. Such trends highlight the need to clarify the uncertain relationship between low IQ and adaptive impairment in the definition and diagnosis of mental retardation. With advances in genetics, more persons with mental retardation will receive discrete diagnoses in the years ahead. Such diagnoses may inform treatment, yet research is needed now to identify the medical, behavioural and developmental profiles associated with these many genetic conditions. Work is also needed on the complex pathways in which experience and biological vulnerability interact in the pathogenesis of mental retardation. Finally, the field still lacks a comprehensive empirically based theory as to why people with mental retardation are at increased risk for psychopathology. Without such a model, our treatments risk being largely problem-orientated instead of preventative. Even so, researchers and clinicians have already worked together to increase substantially the quality of life for persons with mental retardation and their families.

References

Aman, M.G. (1991) *Psychopathology and Behavior Problems in Persons with Mental Retardation: a Review of Available Instruments.* US Department of Health and Human Services, Rockville, MD.

Aman, M.G. & Singh, N.N. (1988) Patterns of drug use, methodological considerations, measurement techniques, and future needs. In: *Psychopharmacology of the Developmental Disabilities* (eds M.G. Aman & N.N. Singh), pp. 1–28. Springer-Verlag, New York.

Aman, M.G. & Singh, N.N. (1994) *Aberrant Behavior Checklist: Community Supplementary Manual.* Slosson Educational Publications, East Aurora, NY.

American Association on Mental Retardation (1992) *Mental Retardation: Definition, Classification, and Systems of Support,* 9th edn. Washington D.C.

American Psychiatric Association (1994) *Diagnostic and Statistical Manual for Mental Disorders,* 4th edn. American Psychiatric Association, Washington, DC.

Ammerman, R.T., Hersen, M., Van Hasselt, V.B., Lubetsky, M.J. & Sieck, W.R. (1994) Maltreatment in psychiatrically hospitalized children and adolescents with developmental disabilities: prevalence and correlates. *Journal of the American Academy of Child and Adolescent Psychiatry,* 33, 567–576.

Aylward, E.H., Burt, D.B., Thorpe, L.U. *et al.* (1997) Diagnosis of dementia in individuals with intellectual disability. *Journal of Intellectual Disability Research,* 41, 152–164.

Bates, E., Benigni, L., Bretherton, I., Camaioni, I. & Volterra, V. (1979) *The Emergence of Symbols: Cognition and Communication in Infancy.* Academic Press, New York.

Batshaw, M., ed. (1997) *Children with Disabilities,* 4th edn. Brooks Publishing, Baltimore.

Baumgardner, T.L., Reiss, A.L., Freund, L.S. & Abrams, M.T. (1995) Specification of the neurobehavioral phenotype in males with fragile X syndrome. *Pediatrics,* 95, 744–752.

Birch, H.G., Richardson, S.A., Baird, D. *et al.* (1970) *Mental Subnormality in the Community: a Clinical and Epidemiological Study.* Williams & Wilkins, Baltimore.

Bird, J. (1997) Epilepsy and learning disabilities. In: *Seminars in the Psychiatry of Learning Disabilities* (ed. O. Russell), pp. 223–244. Gaskell, London.

Borthwick. Duffy, S.A. & Eyman, R.K. (1990) Who are the dually diagnosed? *American Journal of Mental Retardation,* 94, 586–595.

Bybee, J. & Zigler, E. (1998) Outerdirectedness in individuals with mental retardation: a review. In: *Handbook of Mental Retardation and Development* (eds J. Burack, R.M. Hodapp & E. Zigler), pp. 434–461. Cambridge University Press, New York.

Candland, D.K. (1993) *Feral Children and Clever Animals: Reflections on Human Nature.* Oxford University Press, Oxford.

Caplan, R., Arbelle, S., Magharious, W. *et al.* (1998) Psychopathology in pediatric complex partial and primary generalized epilepsy. *Developmental Medicine and Child Neurology,* 40, 805–811.

Carlson, G.A., Rapport, M.D., Pataki, C.S. *et al.* (1992) Lithium in hospitalized children at 4 and 8 weeks. *Journal of Child Psychology and Psychiatry,* 333, 411–425.

Cooper, S.A. (1997) Epidemiology of psychiatric disorders in elderly compared with younger adults with learning disabilities. *British Journal of Psychiatry,* 170, 375–380.

Corbett, J.A. (1979) Psychiatric morbidity and mental retardation. In: *Psychiatric Illness and Mental Handicap* (eds F.E. James & R.F. Smith), pp. 11–25. Gaskell, London.

Curry, C.J., Stevenson, R.E., Aughton, D. *et al.* (1997) Evaluation of mental retardation: recommendations of a Consensus Conference, American College of Medical Genetics. *American Journal of Medical Genetics,* 72, 468–477.

Day, K. (1985) Psychiatric disorder in the middle-aged and elderly mentally handicapped. *British Journal of Psychiatry,* 147, 660–667.

Day, K. (1999) Professional training in the psychiatry of mental retardation in the UK. In: *Psychiatric and Behavioural Disorders in Developmental Disabilities and Mental Retardation* (ed. N. Bouras), pp. 439–457. Cambridge University Press, Cambridge.

Dingman, H.F. & Tarjan, G. (1960) Mental retardation and the normal distribution curve. *American Journal of Mental Deficiency,* 64, 991–994.

Doll, E.A. (1935) The measurement of social competence. *American Association of Mental Deficiency,* 40, 103–123.

Dumaret, A. (1985) IQ, scholastic performance, and behaviour of sibs reared in contrasting environments. *Journal of Child Psychology and Psychiatry,* 26, 553–580.

Dykens, E.M. (1995) Measuring behavioral phenotypes: provocations from the 'new genetics'. *American Journal of Mental Retardation,* 99, 522–532.

Dykens, E.M. (1999a) Direct effects of genetic mental retardation syndromes: maladaptive behavior and psychopathology. *International Review of Research in Mental Retardation,* 22, 1–26.

Dykens, E.M. (1999b) Personality-motivation: new ties to psychopathology, etiology, and intervention. In: *Personality Development in Individuals with Mental Retardation* (eds E. Zigler & D. Bennett-Gates), pp. 249–270. Cambridge University Press, New York.

Dykens, E.M. (in press, b) *Anxiety, Fears and Phobias in Persons with Williams Syndrome. Developmental Neuropsychology.*

Dykens, E.M. (in press, a) *Are Jigsaw Puzzle Skills 'Spared' in People with Prader–Willi Syndrome? Journal of Child Psychology and Psychiatry.*

Dykens, E.M. (2000) Psychopathology in children with intellectual disabilities. *Journal of Child Psychology and Psychiatry*, 41, 407–417.

Dykens, E.M. & Cassidy, S.B. (1999) Prader–Willi syndrome. In: *Handbook of Neurodevelopmental and Genetic Disorders in Children* (eds S. Goldstein & C.R. Reynolds), pp. 525–554. Guilford Press, New York.

Dykens, E.M. & Clarke, D.J. (1997) Correlates of maladaptive behavior in individuals with 5p (cri du chat) syndrome. *Developmental Medicine and Child Neurology*, 39, 752–756.

Dykens, E.M. & Hodapp, R.M. (1997) Treatment issues in genetic mental retardation syndromes. *Professional Psychology: Research and Practice*, 28, 263–270.

Dykens, E.M., Hodapp, R.M. & Leckman, J.F. (1994) *Behavior and Development in Fragile X Syndrome.* Sage Publications, Thousand Oaks, CA.

Dykens, E.M., Leckman, J.F. & Cassidy, S.B. (1996) Obsessions and compulsions in Prader–Willi syndrome. *Journal of Child Psychology and Psychiatry*, 37, 995–1002.

Dykens, E.M., Cassidy, S.B. & King, B.H. (1999) Maladaptive behavior differences in Prader–Willi syndrome due to paternal deletion versus maternal uniparental disomy. *American Journal of Mental Retardation*, 104, 67–77.

Dykens, E.M., Hodapp, R.M. & Finucance, B.M. (2000) *Genetics and Mental Retardation Syndromes: a New Look at Behavior and Interventions.* Paul H. Brookes, Baltimore, MD.

Edgerton, R.B. & Gaston, M.A. (1991) *'I've Seen It All!': Lives of Older Persons with Mental Retardation Living in the Community.* Paul H. Brookes, Baltimore, MD.

Edgerton, R.B.M., Bollinger & Herr, B. (1984) The cloak of competence: after two decades. *American Journal of Mental Deficiency*, 88, 345–351.

Einfeld, S.L. & Tonge, B.J. (1992) *Manual for the Developmental Behavioural Checklist: Primary Carer Version.* School of Psychiatry, University of New South Wales, Australia.

Einfeld, S.L. & Tonge, B.J. (1996) Population prevalence of psychopathology in children and adolescents with intellectual disability. II. Epidemiological findings. *Journal of Intellectual Disability Research*, 40, 99–109.

Einfeld, S.L., Tonge, B.J. & Florio, T. (1997) Behavioral and emotional disturbance in individuals with Williams syndrome. *American Journal of Mental Retardation*, 102, 45–53.

Evans, D.W. (1998) Development of the self-concept in children with mental retardation: organismic and contextual factors. In: *Handbook of Mental Retardation and Development* (eds J.A. Burack, R.M. Hodapp & E. Zigler), pp. 462–480. Cambridge University Press, New York.

Finucane, B.M., Konar, D., Haas-Givler, B., Kurtz, M.D. & Scott, C.I. (1994) The spasmodic upper body squeeze: a characteristic behavior in Smith–Magenis syndrome. *Developmental Medicine and Child Neurology*, 36, 78–83.

Fodor, J. (1983) *Modularity of Mind: an Essay on Faculty Psychology.* MIT Press, Cambridge, MA.

Fox, R.A. & Wade, E.J. (1998) Attention deficit hyperactivity disorder among adults with severe and profound mental retardation. *Research in Developmental Disabilities*, 19, 275–280.

Gardner, H. (1985) The centrality of modules. *Behavioral and Brain Sciences*, 8, 12–14.

Gath, A. & Gumley, D. (1986) Behaviour problems in retarded children with special reference to Down's syndrome. *British Journal of Psychiatry*, 149, 156–161.

Gersch, M., Goodart, S.A., Pasztor, L.M. *et al.* (1995) Evidence for a distinct region causing a cat-cry in patients with 5p deletions. *American Journal of Human Genetics*, 56, 1404–1410.

Gillberg, C., Persson, E., Grufman, M. & Themmer, U. (1986) Psychiatric disorders in mildly and severely mentally retarded urban children and adolescents: epidemiological aspects. *British Journal of Psychiatry*, 149, 68–74.

Gostason, R. (1985) Psychiatric illness among the mentally retarded: a Swedish population study. *Acta Psychiatrica Scandinavica*, 71 (Suppl. 318), 1–117.

Granat, K. & Granat, S. (1978) Adjustment of intellectually below average men not identified as mentally retarded. *Scandinavian Journal of Psychology*, 19, 41–51.

Greenspan, S. & Granfield, J.M. (1992) Reconsidering the construct of mental retardation: implications of a model of social competence. *American Journal of Mental Retardation*, 96, 442–453.

Grizenko, N., Cvejic, H., Vida, S. & Sayegh, L. (1991) Behavior problems in the mentally retarded. *Canadian Journal of Psychiatry*, 36, 712–717.

Hodapp, R.M. (1994) Cultural–familial mental retardation. In: *Encyclopedia of Intelligence* (ed. R. Sternberg), pp. 711–717. Macmillan, New York.

Hodapp, R.M. (1997) Direct and indirect behavioral effects of different genetic disorders of mental retardation. *American Journal of Mental Retardation*, 102, 67–79.

Hodapp, R.M. (1998) *Development and Disabilities: Intellectual, Sensory and Motor Impairments.* Cambridge University Press, New York.

Hodapp, R.M. & Dykens, E.M. (1994) Mental retardation's two cultures of behavioral research. *American Journal of Mental Retardation*, 98, 675–687.

Hodapp, R.M. & Dykens, E.M. (2001) Strengthening behavioral research on mental retardation syndromes. *American Journal on Mental Retardation*, 106, 9–15.

Hodapp, R.M. & Zigler, E. (1995) Past, present, and future issues in the developmental approach to mental retardation and developmental disabilities. In: *Manual of Developmental Psychopathology* (eds D. Cicchetti & D.J. Cohen), pp. 299–331. John Wiley & Sons, New York.

Hodapp, R.M., Evans, D. & Gray, F.L. (1999) Intellectual development in children with Down syndrome. In: *Down's Syndrome: a Review of Current Knowledge* (eds J.A. Rondal, J. Perera & L. Nadel), pp. 124–132. Whurr, London.

Holland, A.J. & Koot, H.M. (1998) Conference report: mental health and intellectual disabilities. *Journal of Intellectual Disability Research*, 42, 505–512.

Holm, V.A., Cassidy, S.B., Butler, M.G. *et al.* (1993) Prader–Willi syndrome: consensus diagnostic criteria. *Pediatrics*, 91, 398–402.

Hunt, J.McV. (1961) *Intelligence and Experience.* Ronald, New York.

Jacobson, J.W. (1982) Problem behavior and psychiatric impairment within a developmentally delayed population. I. Behavioral frequency. *Applied Research in Mental Retardation*, 3, 121–139.

Jacobson, J.W. (1990) Do some mental disorders occur less frequently among persons with mental retardation? *American Journal of Mental Retardation*, 94, 596–602.

Jacobson, J.W. (1999) Dual diagnosis services: history, progress and perspectives. In: *Psychiatric and Behavioural Disorders in Developmental Disabilities and Mental Retardation* (ed. N. Bouras), pp. 329–358. Cambridge University Press, Cambridge.

King, B.H. (1993) Self-injury by people with mental retardation: a compulsive behavior hypothesis. *American Journal of Mental Retardation*, 98, 93–112.

King, B.H., DeAntonia, C., McCracken, J.T., Forness, S.R. & Ackerland, V. (1994) Psychiatric consultation in severe and profound mental retardation. *American Journal of Psychiatry*, 151, 1802–1808.

Koller, H., Richardson, S., Katz, M. & McClaren, J. (1983) Behavioral disturbance since childhood among a 5-year birth cohort of all mentally retarded young adults in a city. *American Journal of Mental Deficiency*, 87, 386–395.

La Malfa, G., Notarelli, A., Hardoy, M.C., Bertelli, M. & Cabras, P.L. (1997) Psychopathology and mental retardation: an Italian epidemiological study using the PIMRA. *Research in Developmental Disabilities*, 18, 179–184.

Lambert, N., Nihira, K. & Leland, H. (1993) *AAMR Adaptive Behavior Scales–School*. Pro-Ed, Austin, TX.

Lee, T., Detterman, D.K. & Plomin, R. (1993) Differences in heritability across groups differing in ability, revisited. *Behavior Genetics*, 23, 331–336.

Lindsay, W.R., Baty, F.J. & Michie, A.M. (1989) A comparison of anxiety treatments with adults who have moderate and severe mental retardation. *Research in Developmental Disabilities*, 10, 129–140.

Lund, J. (1985) The presence of psychiatric co-morbidity in mentally retarded adults. *Acta Psychiatrica Scandinavica*, 72, 563–570.

Lunsky, Y. & Havercamp, S.M. (1999) Distinguishing low level of social support and social strain: implications for dual diagnosis. *American Journal of Mental Retardation*, 104, 200–204.

MacMillan, D.L., Gresham, F.M. & Siperstein, G.N. (1995) Heightened concerns over the 1992 AAMR definition: advocacy vs. precision. *American Journal of Mental Retardation*, 100, 87–95.

Massey, P.S. & McDermott, S. (1995) State specific rates of mental retardation. *Morbidity and Mortality Weekly Report*, 45, 61–65.

Matalainen, R., Aiaksinen, E., Mononen, T., Launiala, K. & Kaariainen, R. (1995) A population-based study on the causes of severe and profound mental retardation. *Acta Pediatrica Scandinavica*, 84, 261–266.

McLaren, J. & Bryson, S.E. (1987) Review of recent epidemiological studies of mental retardation: prevalence, associated disorders, and etiology. *American Journal of Mental Retardation*, 92, 243–254.

Mervis, C.B., Morris, C.A., Bertrand, J.M. & Robinson, B.F. (1999) Williams syndrome: findings from an integrated program of research. In: *Neurodevelopmental Disorders: Contributions to a Framework from the Cognitive Sciences* (ed. H. Tager-Flusberg), pp. 65–110. MIT Press, Cambridge, MA.

Meyers, B.A. (1986) Psychopathology in hospitalized developmental disabled individuals. *Comprehensive Psychiatry*, 27, 115–126.

Minnes, P. (1998) Mental retardation: the impact on the family. In: *Handbook of Mental Retardation and Development* (eds J.A. Burack, R.M. Hodapp & E. Zigler), pp. 693–712. Cambridge University Press, New York.

Moss, S.C. (1999) Assessment: conceptual issues. In: *Psychiatric and Behavioural Disorders in Developmental Disabilities and Mental Retardation* (ed. N. Bouras), pp. 18–37. Cambridge University Press, Cambridge.

Moss, S.C., Prossner, H., Ibbotson, B. & Goldenberg, D.P. (1996) Respondent and informant accounts of psychiatric symptoms in a sample of patients with learning disability. *Journal of Intellectual Disability Research*, 40, 457–465.

Moss, S.C., Emerson, E., Buras, N. & Holland, A. (1997a) Mental disorders and problematic behaviors in people with intellectual disability: future directions for research. *Journal of Intellectual Disability Research*, 41, 440–447.

Moss, S.C., Ibbotson, B., Prosser, H., Godgerb, D.P., Patel, P. & Simpson, N. (1997b) Validity of the PAS-ADD for detecting psychiatric symptoms in adults with learning disability. *Social Psychiatry and Psychiatric Epidemiology*, 32, 344–354.

Mostofsky, S.H., Mazzocco, M.M., Aakalu, G., Warsofsky, I.S., Denckla, M.D. & Reiss, A.L. (1998) Deceased cerebellar posterior vermis size in fragile X syndrome: correlation with neurocognitive performance. *Neurology*, 50, 121–130.

Mundy, P., Seibert, J. & Hogan, A. (1984) Relationship between sensorimotor and early communication abilities in developmentally delayed children. *Merrill-Palmer Quarterly*, 30, 33–48.

Nezu, C.M. & Nezu, A.M. (1994) Outpatient psychotherapy for adults with mental retardation and concomitant psychopathology: research and clinical imperatives. *Journal of Consulting and Clinical Psychology*, 62, 34–42.

Nezu, C.M., Nezu, A.M., Rothenberg, J., DelliCarpi, L. & Groag, I. (1995) Depression in adults with mild mental retardation: are cognitive variables involved? *Cognitive Therapy and Research*, 19, 227–239.

Perry, A. (1991) Rett syndrome: a comprehensive review of the literature. *American Journal of Mental Retardation*, 96, 275–290.

Peterson, B.S. (1995) Neuroimaging in child and adolescent neuropsychiatric disorders. *Journal of the American Academy of Child and Adolescent Psychiatry*, 34, 1560–1576.

Philips, I. & Williams, N. (1975) Psychopathology and mental retardation: a study of 100 mentally retarded children. I. Psychopathology. *American Journal of Psychiatry*, 132, 1265–1271.

Piaget, J. (1952) *The Origins of Intelligence in Children*. Norton, New York.

Reid, A.H. (1972) Psychoses in adult mental defectives. I. Manic depressive psychosis. *British Journal of Psychiatry*, 120, 205–212.

Reid, A.H. (1980) Psychiatric disorders in mentally handicapped children: a clinical and follow-up study. *Journal of Mental Deficiency Research*, 24, 287–298.

Reiss, S. (1988) *The Reiss Screen for Maladaptive Behavior*. IDS Publishing, Worthington, OH.

Reiss, S. (1990) Prevalence of dual diagnosis in community-based day programs in the Chicago metropolitan area. *American Journal of Mental Retardation*, 94, 578–588.

Reiss, S. (1994) *Handbook of Challenging Behavior: Mental Health Aspects of Mental Retardation*. IDS Publishing, Worthington, OH.

Reiss, S. & Aman, M., eds (1998) *Psychotropic Medications and Developmental Disabilities: the International Consensus Handbook*. OSU Nisonger Center, Columbus, OH.

Reiss, S. & Havercamp, S.H. (1997) The sensitivity theory of motivation: why functional analysis is not enough. *American Journal of Mental Retardation*, 101, 553–566.

Reiss, S. & Havercamp, S.H. (1998) Toward a comprehensive assessment of functional motivation: factor structure of the Reiss profiles. *Psychological Assessment*, 10, 97–106.

Reiss, S., Levitan, G.W. & Szyszko, J. (1982) Emotional disturbance and mental retardation: diagnostic overshadowing. *American Journal of Mental Retardation*, 86, 567–574.

Richardson, S. & Koller, H. (1992) Vulnerabilty and resilience of adults who were classified as mildly mentally handicapped in childhood. In: *Vulnerability and Resilience in Human Development* (eds B. Tizard & V. Varma), pp. 102–119. Jessica Kingsley, London.

Richardson, S., Katz, M. & Koller, H. (1986) Sex differences in number of children administratively classified as mildly mentally retarded: an epidemiological review. *American Journal of Mental Deficiency*, **91**, 250–256.

Robertson, D. & Murphy, D. (1999) Brain imaging and behavior. In: *Psychiatric and Behavioural Disorders in Developmental Disabilities and Mental Retardation* (ed. N. Bouras), pp. 49–70. Cambridge University Press, Cambridge.

Roeleveld, N., Zielhus, G.A. & Gabreels, F. (1997) The prevalence of mental retardation: a critical review of recent literature. *Developmental Medicine and Child Neurology*, **39**, 125–132.

Ross, T.T., Begab, M.K., Dondis, E.H. *et al.* (1985) *Lives of the Mentally Retarded: a Forty-year Follow-up Study*. Stanford University Press, Stanford.

Rowitz, L. (1991) Social and environmental factors and developmental handicaps in children. In: *Handbook of Mental Retardation* (eds J. L. Matson & J. A. Mulick), 2nd edn, pp. 158–165. Pergamon Press, NY.

Rutter, M., Tizard, J. & Whitmore, K., eds (1970) *Education, Health, and Behaviour*. Longman, London.

Rutter, M., Tizard, J., Yule, W., Graham, P. & Whitmore, K. (1976) Research report: Isle of Wight studies, 1964–74. *Psychological Medicine*, **6**, 313–332.

Rutter, M., Simonoff, E. & Plomin, R. (1996) Genetic influences on mild mental retardation: concepts, findings, and research implications. *Journal of Biosocial Science*, **28**, 509–526.

Ryan, R. & Sunada, K. (1997) Medical evaluation of persons with mental retardation referred for psychiatric assessment. *General Hospital Psychiatry*, **19**, 274–280.

Simonoff, E., Bolton, P. & Rutter, M. (1996) Mental retardation: genetic findings, clinical implications, and research agenda. *Journal of Child Psychology and Psychiatry*, **37**, 259–280.

Siperstein, G.H., Leffert, J.S. & Wenz-Gross, M. (1997) The quality of friendships between children with and without learning problems. *American Journal of Mental Retardation*, **102**, 111–125.

Slone, M., Durrheim, K., Lachman, P. & Kaminer, D. (1998) Association between the diagnosis of mental retardation and socioeconomic factors. *American Journal of Mental Retardation*, **102**, 535–546.

Sovner, R. (1986) Limiting factors in the use of DSM-III with mentally ill/mentally retarded persons. *Psychopharmacology Bulletin*, **22**, 1055–1059.

Sparrow, S., Balla, D. & Cicchetti, D. (1984) *Vineland Adaptive Behavior Scales*. American Guidance Service, Circle Pines, MN.

Sternberg, R.J., ed. (2000) *Handbook of Intelligence*. Cambridge University Press, Cambridge.

Sternberg, R.J. & Salter, W. (1982) Conceptions of intelligence. In: *Handbook of Human Intelligence* (ed. R. Sternberg), pp. 3–28. Cambridge University Press, Cambridge.

Sturmey, P. (1999) Classification: concepts, progress, and future. In: *Psychiatric and Behavioural Disorders in Developmental Disabilities and Mental Retardation* (ed. N. Bouras), pp. 3–17. Cambridge University Press, Cambridge.

Szymanski, L. & King, B.H. (1999) Practice parameters for the assessment and treatment of children, adolescents, and adults with mental retardation and comorbid mental disorders. American Academy of Child and Adolescent Psychiatry Working Group on Quality Issues. *Journal of the American Academy of Child and Adolescent Psychiatry*, **38** (Suppl. 12), 5S-31S.

Szymanski, L.S., King, B.H., Goldberg, B., Reid, A.H., Tonge, B.J. & Cain, N. (1998) Diagnosis of mental disorders in people with mental retardation. In: *Psychotropic Medications and Developmental Disabilities: the International Consensus Handbook* (eds S. Reiss & M.G. Aman), pp. 3–17. Ohio State University Press, Columbus, OH.

Tassone, F.L., Hagerman, R.J., Ikle, D. *et al.* (1999) FMRP expression as a potential prognostic indicator in fragile X syndrome. *American Journal of Medical Genetics*, **84**, 250–261.

Tonge, B.J. (1999) Psychopathology of children with developmental disabilities. In: *Psychiatric and Behavioural Disorders in Developmental Disabilities and Mental Retardation* (ed. N. Bouras), pp. 157–174. Cambridge University Press, Cambridge.

Volkmar, F.R., Cook, E., Pomeroy, J. *et al.* (1999) Practice parameters for the assessment and treatment of children and adolescents with autism and pervasive developmental disorders. *Journal of the American Academy of Child and Adolescent Psychiatry*, **38**, 32S–54S.

Weisz, J.R. (1990) Cultural–familial mental retardation: a developmental perspective on cognitive performance and 'helpless' behavior. In: *Issues in the Developmental Approach to Mental Retardation* (eds R.M. Hodapp, J.A. Burack & E. Zigler), pp. 137–168. Cambridge University Press, New York.

White, M.J., Nichols, C.N., Cook, R.S., Spengler, P.M., Walker, B.S. & Look, K.K. (1995) Diagnostic overshadowing and mental retardation: a meta-analysis. *American Journal of Mental Retardation*, **100**, 293–298.

Williams, C.A., Zori, R.T., Hendrickson, J. *et al.* (1995) Angelman syndrome. *Current Problems in Pediatrics*, **25**, 216–231.

Wing, L. & Gould, J. (1979) Severe impairments of social interaction and associated abnormalities. *Journal of Autism and Developmental Disorders*, **9**, 11–29.

World Health Organization (1993) *Classification of Mental and Behavioural Disorders: Diagnostic Criteria for Research*. World Health Organization, Geneva.

Zigler, E. (1967) Familial mental retardation: a continuing dilemma. *Science*, **155**, 292–298.

Zigler, E. (1969) Developmental versus difference theories of retardation and the problem of motivation. *American Journal of Mental Deficiency*, **73**, 536–556.

Zigler, E. & Bennett-Gates, D., eds (1999) *Personality Development in Individuals with Mental Retardation*. Cambridge University Press, New York.

42 Personality and Illness

Janette Moore and Anne Farmer

Introduction

Personality refers to those personal attributes of character and temperament that make us who we are, and different from others. We use words like 'extrovert' to describe someone who is gregarious, the 'life and soul of the party', and keen to try out different hobbies or sports. We apply the term 'neurotic' to someone who is constantly fearful that things will go wrong. These human qualities or traits can be applied universally, can be detected from infancy and, until recently, were considered to be stable throughout life, irrespective of circumstance. However, as we will discuss later, recent research suggests that personality is not as immutable as previously thought. Learning, experiences and illness can all act to modify personality characteristics.

The idea that your personality can cause problems for yourself or others underpins the concept of 'personality disorder'. There are several ways in which aspects of personality can be considered pathological. For example, an extremely introverted individual may find social situations so stressful that he or she avoids them, leading to social isolation and an inability to cope with daily activities. Alternatively, certain antisocial personality characteristics can be associated with criminal behaviour or total disregard for the thoughts and feelings of others.

Disorders of personality are much discussed in psychoanalytic literature and defined operationally in the major psychiatric classifications (see J. Hill, Chapter 43). As well as being 'treated' in their own right, personality disorders are also considered to be related to some mental disorders. However, the notion that your personality can influence the type of illness, both physical and mental, from which you will suffer has its origins in antiquity.

In this chapter we review the relationship between aspects of personality (both trait and disorder), and how these relate to health and illness. In order to set the scene, we give a brief overview of the historical background and then discuss current concepts of personality, as dimensional traits. We also examine the relationship between temperament and personality and the stability and plasticity of personality over the life span. When considering the literature that examines the relationship between personality and illness, we address whether personality and the symptoms of mental disorder are part of the same spectrum, or whether certain personality attributes act as either vulnerability or protective factors for the development of mental or physical disorder. Much of the research on personality has been undertaken on adult subjects (Rutter 1987), and so where applicable we cite this literature as well as that pertaining to children and adolescents.

Brief historical background to the concept of personality

From Hippocrates in the fifth century BC until as recently as the seventeenth century (Burton 1652), it was believed that an individual's vulnerability to various physical and psychological disorders was related to the blending of four body 'humours': black and yellow bile, blood and phlegm (Maher & Maher 1994). Four characteristic personality styles were postulated, each associated with the dominance of one of the humours. Melancholic or gloomy temperament was associated with black bile, sanguine or cheerful temperament with blood, choleric or angry temperament with yellow bile, and phlegmatic or calm temperament was associated with phlegm (Porter 1997, p. 271).

By the nineteenth century, these ancient ideas had been replaced by 'phrenological theories' developed by Gall and Spurzheim (Porter 1997, p. 538). Phrenology is the study of the nature and location of bony protuberances on the head, and it was believed that these determined character and personality. Despite the somewhat implausible nature of these ideas in modern times, the phrenology movement had considerable influence and acceptance and led to improved attitudes towards, and treatment of, the mentally ill.

The modern study of personality dates from the early part of the twentieth century. Woodworth's Personal Data Sheet was possibly the first personality test (Woodworth 1919). Based on the idea of adding 'scores' on 'individual items', adopted from the IQ test model, it was used with First World War soldiers as a test to determine 'susceptibility to shock'. The test was found to differentiate between soldiers who developed 'shell shock' or 'war neurosis' (most probably labelled post-traumatic stress disorder in current terminology) and 'normal soldiers' (Winter & Barenbaum 1999).

Later in the century, several attempts were made to link personality with physical attributes. The most notable of these were the theories of Kretschmer (1936) and Sheldon *et al.* (1940, 1942), on the relationship between body build and personality. Also, Alexander (1950) and Dunbar (1943) linked personality characteristics with the development and course of disease by employing psychoanalytic concepts.

One of the most important and established associations between personality and health outcome was first reported in the

1950s. The association between 'Type A' personality and coronary artery disease (CAD) was first described by Friedman & Rosenman (1959). Type A personality was defined as a behavioural style characterized by competitiveness, hostility, impatience and achievement striving. Over subsequent decades, evidence accumulated confirming this personality type as a risk factor for CAD (Matthews 1988). Type A individuals were shown to have greater increases in heart rate, blood pressure and neuroendocrine levels of cortisol and catecholamines (Harbin 1989) in response to stress, compared with non-Type A subjects. Consequently, it was proposed that the link with CAD was the result of such heightened physiological responses to environmental demands (Friedman & Rosenman 1974). More recently, the hostility and anger-related component of Type A behaviour has been identified as being most consistently related to this outcome, in particular the behavioural expression of anger (Miller et al. 1996).

This work led to a resurgence of interest in the relationship between personality and health. An increasing number of studies explored the possibility that personality factors may increase susceptibility to or protect against the development of disease, and there have been several attempts to explain the mechanisms by which such influences may be exerted. These modern studies are reviewed later in this chapter.

Temperament and personality

There have been many debates about the definitions of temperament and personality, and the difference between the two. In the main, temperament has been conceptualized as being composed of enduring 'traits' that have a biological underpinning and that are relatively stable over time. It is also generally assumed that these 'traits' are comparatively pure in early childhood and that they become modified with increasing age by the effects of environmental, social or cultural factors. In contrast, personality is generally assumed to encompass motivational and cognitive elements as well as the dispositional aspects accounted for by temperament (Rutter 1987). Personality has been described as 'the characteristic manner in which one thinks, feels, behaves, and relates to others' (Widiger et al. 1999) or, alternatively, 'that which gives order and congruence to all the different kinds of behaviour in which an individual engages' (Hall & Lindzey 1978).

Studies of personality and temperament have often been conducted from widely varying theoretical perspectives (Bates & Wachs 1994). However, two main themes are evident: nomothetic approaches study how individuals differ from one another on a number of attributes, while the idiographic approach aims to paint a portrait of each individual as a unique and integrated whole (Deary & Power 1998). Psychoanalytic theories provide an example of the latter.

More recently, the approach has been to identify the dimensions of personal characteristics along which all individuals differ. Research has demonstrated the temporal stability, convergent validity across sources of information and predictive validity of measuring such quantitative traits (Smith & Williams 1992), although the number of dimensions proposed often vary according to different authors (Gershenfeld & Paul 1998).

Dimensions of temperament and personality in children and adults

One of the first studies to examine temperament in children was the New York Longitudinal Study (NYLS; Thomas et al. 1963). This resulted in a nine-trait classification of infant temperament. The categories proposed were activity level, regularity of biological functions, approach to or withdrawal from new stimuli, adaptability to new or altered situations, the threshold of responsiveness, the intensity of reaction, the quality of mood, distractibility and persistence/attention span. Further analyses led to the clustering of these categories into three clinically useful constellations of temperament: 'easy', 'difficult', and 'slow to warm up'. The 'easy' temperament was characterized by a combination of biological regularity, approach to new stimuli, quick adaptability and positive mood, and accounted for about 40% of the sample. In contrast the 'difficult' child displayed the reverse of these behaviours and accounted for approximately 10%. The third category, 'slow to warm up', which accounted for 15% of the study population, was characterized by withdrawal tendencies to novel stimuli, slow adaptability and frequent negative emotional outbursts of low intensity. Such children are often labelled as shy.

Two decades later, Buss & Plomin (1975) proposed four independent factors of temperament: emotionality (distress), activity (tempo and vigour), sociability and impulsivity (abbreviated as EASI). It was suggested that these factors were inherited traits that appeared early in the first year and remained stable over time, forming the foundation of later personality traits.

More recently, Kagan et al. (1988; Kagan & Snidman 1991; Kagan 1994) extensively explored the childhood trait of shyness and associated behavioural 'inhibition'. Inhibited children are typified by timidity in response to unfamiliar situations (reminiscent of the approach/withdrawal category described by Thomas and Chess), while uninhibited children are described as sociable, talkative and less fearful when confronted by the unfamiliar. 'Inhibited' children were found to have a relatively high and stable heart rate, higher salivary cortisol levels and larger eye pupils when compared with the 'uninhibited' group. Kagan speculated that this was caused by 'inhibited' children being born with a lower threshold for arousal to unexpected changes in the environment. Longitudinal studies following children from 14 months to 7 years has provided evidence for the stability of this classification over time.

As regards adult personality structure, Eysenck originally proposed that personality could be conceptualized as two uncorrelated factors: neuroticism (N) and extraversion–introversion (E) (Eysenck & Eysenck 1969). Later he also introduced a third factor, psychoticism (P) and revised his original questionnaire to provide a measure of all three (Eysenck & Eysenck 1975). These three dimensions are very broad and encompass many lower level traits. Neuroticism includes characteristics such as depression, guilt, shyness and emotionality, extraversion includes features such as sociability, liveliness, assertiveness and dominance and psychoticism includes aggressiveness, coldness, egocentricism and toughmindedness. It has been hypothesized that these personality dimensions have a biological basis. In particular, extraversion was linked to arousal and activation of the ascending reticular activating system while neuroticism was linked to the reactivity of the autonomic nervous system.

Building on this work, Cloninger (1987, 1994; Cloninger *et al.* 1993) has proposed a unified biopsychosocial theory of temperament and personality development. This model 'conceptualizes personality as a combination of heritable, neurobiologically based traits (temperament dimensions), and traits reflecting sociocultural learning (character dimensions)'. The temperament dimensions are thought to be related to activity in specific central neurotransmitter systems (Peirson *et al.* 1999) and include harm avoidance, novelty seeking, reward dependence, and persistence. Harm avoidance refers to 'a tendency to respond intensely to signals of aversive stimuli' leading to cautious, inhibited and apprehensive behaviour in high-scoring individuals. In contrast, novelty seeking is conceptualized as 'a heritable tendency toward intense exhilaration or excitement in response to novel stimuli'. The character dimensions described by Cloninger *et al.* are self-directedness, co-operativeness and self-transcendence. A self-report questionnaire (Temperament and Character Inventory) has been devised to capture these seven dimensions (Cloninger *et al.* 1993). In addition, a version for children has also been developed (Junior Temperament and Character Inventory; Luby *et al.* 1999).

Recently, another general classification of personality traits, consisting of five main dimensions, has been proposed (Costa & McCrae 1992). Termed the 'Big Five' (so named because of the breadth of features encompassed by each dimension) these dimensions were originally named to reflect the language that people use to describe personal characteristics. Consequently, they do not represent any particular theoretical perspective (John & Srivastava 1999). The five factors are usually referred to as openness, conscientiousness, extroversion, agreeableness and emotional stability (as opposed to neuroticism; acronym 'OCEAN') with each dimension encompassing a variety of more specific personality characteristics. A variety of instruments have been developed to measure the Big Five. One of the most commonly used is the NEO Personality Inventory–Revised (Costa & McCrae 1992). Originally designed to measure the three personality domains of neuroticism, extroversion and openness to experience (hence the name), it was modified to include scales for the other two dimensions of agreeableness and conscientiousness. In this scheme, extroversion measures features such as sociability, assertiveness, enthusiasm and adventurousness; agreeableness is conceptualized as encompassing forgiveness, altruistic behaviours and sympathy; conscientiousness includes orderliness, efficiency and thoroughness; emotional stability/neuroticism encompasses anxiety, anger, self-consciousness and moodiness; and openness to experience includes curiosity, imaginativeness, unconventionality and artistic traits.

Although the five-factor model (FFM) of personality appears appropriate for adult research, there is some evidence to suggest that in childhood personality structure may be somewhat more differentiated. Two independent studies have suggested that seven factors (the Big Five plus an additional two) are the most appropriate model for this age group (John *et al.* 1994; Van Lieshout & Haselager 1994). It is argued that the additional two factors of irritability and activity may become integrated into the Big Five adult personality structure over the course of adolescence (John *et al.* 1994). With the increasing consensus on the FFM of personality, there has been a resurgence of interest in the ways in which personality traits combine in individuals who share the same personality profile. Such type theories suggest that human personality variation can fit into a limited number of discrete categories. Several studies in children and adolescents have demonstrated evidence for three replicable personality types which have been generally labelled 'resilients', 'overcontrollers' and 'undercontrollers' (Van Lieshout & Haselager 1994; Caspi & Silva 1995; Robins *et al.* 1996; Hart *et al.* 1997). The resilient personality type demonstrates effective functioning on all five of the Big Five factors. Overcontrollers typically have high scores on the agreeableness and conscientiousness factors but score low on extraversion. Undercontrollers, on the other hand, have low scores on agreeableness and conscientiousness while scoring low on emotional stability. There is evidence for the validity of these personality categories in that they have been shown to be predictive of psychological adjustment, with the resilients generally demonstrating a high level of psychological adjustment.

Genetic and environmental influences on personality

Throughout the early part of the twentieth century the aetiology of both healthy and pathological psychological development was predominantly attributed to environmental forces, primarily the influence of the mother or primary caregiver. More recently, however, behavioural genetics, although confirming the importance of environmental factors, has also highlighted the importance of genetic influences. Twin studies using both self-report measures of personality (Loehlin & Nicholls 1976) and peer ratings (Riemann *et al.* 1997) have yielded consistent evidence for moderate genetic influence in most personality traits. The most extensively studied traits of extroversion and neuroticism have been investigated using a variety of behavioural genetic designs. Mathematical model fitting across studies produce heritability estimates of about 49% for extroversion and 41% for neuroticism (Loehlin 1992). In general, the net effect of genetic influences in most adult personality traits is typically in the range of 30–50%. The remainder of the variance in such studies is attributed to environmental factors, which are divided into that which is shared between family members (shared environment) and that which is uniquely experienced by individuals (non-shared environment). Research in adults has also shown that it is the non-shared environment that is the most important contribution to the variance in personality measures (Plomin & Caspi 1999). It is important to stress that this may include family experiences common to all members, such as parenting, parental separation or divorce (Hetherington & Clingempeel 1992), as these may be experienced differently by different family members.

Similarly, the relationship between personality traits and mental illness may be mediated by genetic risk factors. Kendler *et al.* (1993a) explored the relationship between neuroticism and depression using a genetic study design. The study assessed 1733 female (same sex) twins from the Virginia Twin Registry and concluded that approximately 55% of the genetic liability to major depression appeared to be shared with neuroticism, suggesting that at least part of the genetic predisposition to depression is mediated via neurotic personality traits.

Research into childhood personality and temperament, which has traditionally relied on parental ratings, often produces somewhat unusual results. Despite yielding correlations for identical twins that are typically high, fraternal twin correlations are often low or negative. These findings have been attributed to sibling competition or contrast effects (Eaves 1976; Carey 1986). Such effects may be caused by the behaviour of one twin having an inhibitory effect on the behaviour of the other (Thapar *et al.* 1995). Alternatively, parental ratings may be biased by the parent's perception that one sibling exhibits a trait to a greater degree than is the case, because he or she does so relative to his or her sibling (Neale & Stevenson 1989; Simonoff *et al.* 1998). It is also of interest that some measures of 'environment' may show genetic influence. For example, parenting style can show genetic influence as a result of the genetic characteristics of the parents, or alternatively it may reflect genetic characteristics of the children (Plomin & Caspi 1999). There is evidence from work with children and adolescents that the genetic influence on some measures of environment appears to be mediated via personality as well as other psychological factors (Pike *et al.* 1996; Saudino & Plomin 1997).

Several associations between specific genes and particular personality traits have been described. The first of these, reported by Cloninger *et al.* (1996), described an association between the D_4 dopamine receptor on chromosome 11 and novelty seeking. Alleles at this locus are associated with a varying number of trinucleotide and dinucleotide repeats. The repeat length is associated with a reduction in receptor efficiency *in vitro* as well as reduced intracellular response to dopamine (Asghari *et al.* 1994). It has been suggested that individuals with such DRD4 alleles are dopamine-deficient and seek novelty to enhance dopamine release. Despite several attempted replications of this finding (Tomitaka *et al.* 1999) the results have not been consistent (Bau *et al.* 1999).

Another allelic association has been described between neurotic traits and a functional polymorphism in the promoter region of the serotonin transporter gene on chromosome 17 (Heils *et al.* 1996; Lesch *et al.* 1996; Katsuragi *et al.* 1999).

Again, there have been inconsistent replication findings (Deary *et al.* 1999; Gustavsson *et al.* 1999; Hamer *et al.* 1999).

Change and stability of personality over the life span

In a longitudinal study of 1000 children (Caspi & Roberts 1999), first observed at the age of 3 years and followed up at the age of 18 years, moderate continuity in several temperamental styles was observed. In particular, children who exhibited restless impulsive emotional labile behaviour at 3 years tended to score highly on measures of negative emotion and low on traits reflecting constraint at 18 years. Similarly, children who were 'inhibited' at initial interview reported cautious behaviour and a preference for safe activities at follow-up; this was associated with low scores on aggression and social potency (Caspi & Silva 1995).

In contrast to this longitudinal study, the continuity between behavioural characteristics noted in infancy and those found later in the preschool years has been shown to be quite low (Caspi & Roberts 1999). To explain this apparent anomaly, the authors suggested that much of the observed variation in infant behaviour prior to the second year of life is caused by transient situational factors. However, during the second year, cognitive changes enable the child to master object permanence and begin to develop self-conscious emotions, which may be important for the development of persisting behavioural responses and the prediction of later personality differences. Although it appears that personality characteristics become increasingly stable with age (Roberts & Friend-Delvecchio 2000), there is still the possibility of change even in old age.

Although these findings suggest that there is some stability of personality across the life span, the original concept assumed that temperament was highly immutable. However, recent research evidence suggests that the stability of temperament is much more modest than originally thought and that alterations in personality can occur in response to life changes (Stewart 1996). Furthermore, it has been postulated that such changes may be influenced by genetic factors (Matheny 1984, 1989; Plomin *et al.* 1993; Cherny *et al.* 1994). For example, accentuation of already existing personality characteristics may occur during periods of social discontinuity, and personal disposition may influence behaviour most when individuals are exposed to new situations or assume new roles (Caspi 1991; Caspi & Moffitt 1991). Also, individuals select situations and companions that are compatible with their disposition, e.g. choice of spouse (Caspi & Herbener 1990). Consequently, processes of social interchange may be developed that sustain an individual's dispositional characteristics across time and circumstances. Similarly, as we will describe below, both physical and mental illnesses may also modify aspects of personality.

One explanation for the finding of only modest stability of personality characteristics over time could be measurement error. It is possible that physiological measures (e.g. pupil size, cortisol level), such as those used by Kagan *et al.* (1988; Kagan 1994; see above) to evaluate shyness in childhood, may prove to be more reliable, valid and closer to personality endophenotypes than more traditional longitudinal studies based on questionnaire measures.

Relationships between personality and illness

At the beginning of this chapter we described the links made between personality and illness, both physical and mental, throughout history. More recently, there have been many attempts to relate aspects of personality to the development of illness. Here we present the main areas of recent enquiry. First, we consider personality as a predisposing or vulnerability factor for the development of mental disorder. Secondly, we discuss personality and the symptomatology associated with mental disorders (psychopathology) as different parts of a common spectrum. Thirdly, we present recent research examining the relationships between personality and physical health and, fourthly, how aspects of personality may act as a protective factor against the development of both physical and mental illness. Fifthly, we consider evidence for a bidirectional relationship between personality and illness, and how illness may result in an alteration in personality functioning. Lastly, we speculate about future research directions.

Personality as a risk factor for psychopathology

A variety of associations between personality characteristics and psychopathology have been demonstrated, using both cross-sectional and longitudinal approaches. For example, it has been shown that high neuroticism scores are associated with a wide range of mental disorders including anxiety, major depression (Roberts & Kendler 1999; Jorm et al. 2000) and somatoform disorder (Kirmayer et al. 1994). Similarly, antisocial traits are related to the development of substance abuse (Trull & Sher 1994; Krueger et al. 1996; Gabel et al. 1999) and borderline personality traits contribute to disorders of eating, mood and impulse control (Widiger & Trull 1993). As well as neuroticism, several other personality dimensions have been consistently associated with depressive disorder. These include dependency, self-criticism, obsessionality and perfectionism (Enns & Cox 1997), traits often also seen in individuals with eating disorders. There is empirical evidence for an association between restricting anorexia and constricted, conforming and obsessional personality traits, while affective instability and impulsiveness have been described in patients with bulimia nervosa (Vitousek & Manke 1994). It has been noted that virtually all of the five main traits accounted for by the FFM are related to at least some type of mental disorder and similarly that most disorders studied are associated with at least one prominent trait of normal personality. However, as illustrated above, these relationships are generally non-specific with no one-to-one correspondence between any particular personality trait and a mental disorder. This is likely to be, at least partially, a reflection of the broad general nature of many of the traits studied, but may also be accounted for by the considerable co-occurrences among

mental disorders themselves (Watson et al. 1994). Differentiating broader personality traits according to their various facets may improve the specificity of the relationship.

Considerable attention has been focused on the relationship of neuroticism and extroversion to mental disorders, while fewer studies have explored the relationships between psychopathology and the other three factors (openness, agreeableness and conscientiousness) of the FFM (Widiger & Trull 1992). However, in one such study of adolescents, low scores on agreeableness and conscientiousness predicted juvenile delinquency; high neuroticism and low conscientiousness scores predicted internalizing disorders; while high conscientiousness and openness scores predicted school performance (John & Srivastava 1999). Children who consistently demonstrate behavioural inhibition on follow-up (stable inhibited) have been shown to suffer from significantly higher rates of anxiety disorder, while their parents have been shown to have both higher rates of childhood and continuing anxiety disorder. Further prospective studies have suggested the importance of the 'social avoidance' component of childhood behavioural inhibition in the later development of social phobia and the importance of the 'fearfulness' component for development of both social phobia and depression (Hayward et al. 1998). Evidence for the link between childhood inhibition and depressive disorder has further been provided by Caspi et al. (1996), who showed that examiner observed behavioural differences rated at 3 years were associated with adult psychiatric disorders on follow-up at 21 years. Inhibited children who were shy, fearful and easily upset were more likely to meet criteria for depression. Children rated as undercontrolled, impulsive, restless and distractible were more likely to meet criteria for antisocial personality disorder (in keeping with John & Srivastava 1999). In addition, both inhibited and undercontrolled groups had a greater risk of attempted suicide, and boys from both groups showed a greater vulnerability to alcohol-related problems (Caspi et al. 1996).

It is also possible that personality characteristics can influence the development of mental disorder indirectly. For example, certain types of severe and threatening life events are well-known risk factors for the development of major depression (Brown et al. 1973; Paykel 1978) and it has been shown that experiencing an excess of such events also runs in families (McGuffin et al. 1988; Kendler et al. 1993b). It has been postulated (McGuffin et al. 1988) that this increased familial rate of experiencing such events may be related to risk-taking, hazard-prone behaviour or threat-perceiving personality characteristics. Risk-taking is the type of behaviour associated with high scores on measures of extroversion, sensation or novelty seeking, while those who score highly on neuroticism tend to be highly threat-perceiving. Having a risk-taking personality may lead to an excess of life events that in turn could lead to the development of depression. On the other hand, it is possible that highly neurotic individuals will tend to 'make mountains out of molehills' and exaggerate the impact of life events. In a sib-pair study of life events and depression in adults, it has been shown that it is neuroticism rather than sensation-seeking behaviour that is associated with excess life events and the development of depression (Farmer *et al.* 2000, 2001).

Personality and psychopathology as parts of a common spectrum

The close relationship between psychopathology and personality traits noted above has led to speculation that personality and psychopathology are not distinct but form part of a common spectrum. Consequently, they may represent different phenotypic expressions of the same underlying aetiology. It has also been suggested that there are disease spectra that range from 'normal' personality trait, via the more extreme and 'abnormal' personality disorders, through to frank mental illness, the differences being quantitative not qualitative. Where 'personality disorder' and 'mental illness' are defined along this spectrum is somewhat arbitrary (Moore *et al.*, 2000) and this calls into question whether a categorical approach to psychiatric classification is appropriate. Some authors have suggested that categorical approaches to psychiatric classifications are merely diagnostic conventions imposed on continua of symptoms (Kendler & Gardner 1998) and that a dimensional approach would be more appropriate.

In order to demonstrate that personality traits differed only quantitatively from personality disorder, Widiger *et al.* (1994) compared ratings on the FFM (Costa & McCrae 1992) of personality traits with the definitions of personality disorders described in DSM-IV (American Psychiatric Association 2000). The results suggested that the latter can be conceptualized as maladaptive or extreme forms of normal personality traits. Similarly, the relationship between personality disorder and psychiatric illness has also been established in relation to schizophrenia. Using a twin study approach, the maximum monozygotic (MZ) to dizygotic (DZ) concordance ratio was used as a method for exploring the 'most genetic' combination of disorders within the schizophrenic spectrum (Farmer *et al.* 1984). The authors showed that by including 'affected' twins with a diagnosis of schizotypal personality disorder as well as schizophrenia improved the MZ : DZ concordance ratio, while adding in all twins with any type of Axis I mental disorder led to a reduction in the ratio. These results suggested that schizotypal personality disorder shares the same genetic diathesis as schizophrenia. Consequently, this, together with other studies, has led to schizotypal personality disorder being accepted as part of the schizophrenia spectrum (Kendler *et al.* 1995; Battaglia & Torgersen, 1996) and this personality disorder is now usually classified as a form of schizophrenia (American Psychiatric Association 1994; World Health Organization 1992).

Personality and physical illness

'Personality can be studied in relation to physical disorders, processes that culminate in physical disorders, or factors that influence health care utilization' (Contrada *et al.* 1999). In general, research has focused on two main mechanisms thought to underlie the relationship between personality and physical health: first, processes operating via direct psychophysiological pathways, and influenced by stress and, secondly, those operating at the level of specific behaviours which in turn may influence the risk of disease. It has been suggested that personality characteristics influence the frequency, intensity and duration of physiological stress responses via a variety of pathways that culminate in the development of illness (Smith & Williams 1992). It has been known for some time that psychological factors and stressful conditions can influence neuroendocrine and metabolic processes via activation of the hypothalamic–pituitary–adrenal axis (Arbuthnott 1998) and the sympathetic nervous system (Mason 1972). Both these systems direct the immune response and there is accumulating evidence that stress (Herbert & Cohen 1993), psychological states such as depression (Olff 1999), and personality factors (Borella *et al.* 1999; Miller *et al.* 1999) can influence the immune system. In particular, stress is associated with a decrease in functional immune responses, such as natural killer cell activity. It has also been noted that the immune changes are related to the duration and nature of the stressor (Herbert & Cohen 1993).

Personality can also influence health by predisposing an individual to carry out certain health-related behaviours, which may confer vulnerability to, or alternatively protection from, various disease processes. Behaviours such as smoking, a sedentary lifestyle or a poor diet have been shown to be important in the development of disorders including cancers, diabetes and CAD.

Other personality constructs suggested as having relevance for health outcomes are hardiness, dispositional optimism (both discussed in the next section), explanatory style (proposed by Peterson & Seligman 1987), emotional expressiveness (Jorgensen *et al.* 1996) and health locus of control (Wallston *et al.* 1976). Explanatory style refers to the characteristic causal attributions individuals make for life events both positive and negative. A pessimistic explanatory style is characterized by stable internal attributions for negative outcomes and external unstable attributions for positive events. It has been shown to be associated with greater reports of ill-health and visits to a doctor (Smith & Williams 1992). Personality styles that tend towards reduced emotional expressiveness, such as seen in alexithymic individuals, may also be at increased risk of physical illness. Under the health locus of control model, individuals who believe that their health is controllable are more likely to seek and comply with treatment.

As regards the FFM, there is evidence that individuals who score highly on conscientiousness lead more structured lives and that this results in better health, while individuals with low agreeableness who manifest hostility and high neuroticism appear to be at risk of poor health outcomes (John & Srivastava 1999). It is important to note, however, that although there is substantial evidence for a positive association between neuroticism and self-reports of physical illness and symptoms, there appears to be less support for a true association with actual objectively diagnosed disease. This suggests that neuroticism is associated with a reporting bias, possibly related to an increased concern about normal physical sensations (Smith & Williams

1992). Studies of adverse health behaviours, such as poor diet, smoking, drug abuse and unprotected sex in adolescents, have often highlighted the protective influence of high self-esteem and perceived self-efficacy (Breakwell & Millward 1997; Adih & Alexander 1999; Glendinning & Inglis 1999).

Caspi *et al.* (1997) explored the relationship between personality characteristics and four health-risk behaviours in young adults: alcohol dependence, violent crime, unsafe sex and dangerous driving. Adolescents who demonstrated low scores on traditionalism, harm avoidance, control and social closeness and high scores on alienation and aggression at aged 18 were significantly more likely to be involved in all four health risk behaviours at 21 years. Some personality traits were uniquely associated with specific health-risk behaviours; for example, those who scored highly on alienation were significantly more likely to be involved in violent crime and problematic alcohol use.

It is also important to note that personality and psychological factors may have an important role in the utilization of health care provision, which can affect disease course and ultimately outcome. Similarly, it has been suggested that certain personality traits may influence the diagnostic process, with physicians being more likely to label disagreeable patients as hypochondriacs (Kirmayer *et al.* 1994).

Personality as a protective factor against illness

Resilience refers to the idea that some individuals are able to withstand or rebound from adversity, and can be conceptualized as a dynamic process in which protective factors interact with risk factors to mitigate the occurrence of a negative outcome, such as becoming ill. Psychological resources deemed to have such mitigating effects can be identified in behavioural, cognitive and affective domains and include characteristics such as optimism, a sense of mastery or personal control, and certain coping styles. For example, it has been shown that belief in one's abilities and efficacy within a social or political system, in male adolescents from deprived urban areas, is associated with better self-esteem and mental health (Zimmerman *et al.* 1999). Similarly, high self-esteem in adolescents is associated with a decreased likelihood to engage in health-endangering behaviours (Gordon Rouse *et al.* 1998). However, the evidence suggests that, overall, a sense of self-efficacy, the belief that one can cope with life's challenges, may be more important than a general sense of well-being (Bandura 1995, 1997). Several studies have shown the protective effect of a positive style of planning as a reflection of a feeling of being able to control what happens to one (Quinton & Rutter 1988; Clausen 1991, 1993; Quinton *et al.* 1993; Shanahan *et al.* 1997). A style of active coping is probably important (Compas *et al.* 2001). In addition, children with chronic and disabling conditions who exhibit greater sociability and flexibility in their interactions have less emotional problems and better academic outcomes (Patterson & Blum 1996), while preschool-age children with 'easy' temperaments demonstrate fewer internalizing or externalizing behaviours when exposed to familial conflict (Tschann *et al.* 1996).

Hardiness, a personality construct first proposed by Kobasa (1979) and Kobasa *et al.* (1982), has been examined in a range of studies, including an investigation of coping in individuals with AIDS (Farber *et al.* 2000), and the factors that protect war veterans from post-traumatic stress disorder (King *et al.* 1998). In this model, hardy or stress-resistant individuals are typified by a strong sense of belief in the importance and meaningfulness of their activities and experiences (*commitment*), they believe that life events are predictable consequences of one's actions (*control*), and that change is normal and represents an opportunity (*challenge*). In general, these studies have shown that individuals with high hardiness scores tend to exhibit less psychological distress and have a better quality of life. It is likely that this influence is mediated via less threatening cognitive appraisals of the stressor and the adoption of more adaptive coping strategies. In terms of the FFM, hardy individuals score more highly on openness, conscientiousness and positive emotionality scales (Ramanaiah *et al.* 1999).

Scheier & Carver (1985) proposed that individual differences in dispositional optimism (a general and stable expectation that good things will happen) explained differences in adjustment to stressors. There is evidence that optimists, believing that positive outcomes are more likely, show more active coping strategies in the face of adversity and are less likely to respond with passive strategies, such as avoidance and denial (Scheier *et al.* 1986). Dispositional optimism also appeared to protect against a heightened physiological response to stress (Raikkonen *et al.* 1999), that may be related to better immunity (Segerstrom *et al.* 1998). It may also lead to the adoption of particular health-related behaviours such as safe sexual practices and positive behavioural changes in cardiac patients (Contrada *et al.* 1999). However, the fact that hardiness and dispositional optimism scores are both highly correlated with neuroticism has given rise to the suggestion that associations between these concepts and health outcomes might be artefactual and may in fact reflect the well-documented association between neuroticism and health discussed previously.

Whether a personality characteristic is protective or increases risk to later psychopathology may depend on the adverse situation in which the individual finds themselves, on the presence of other factors of influence and on the outcome of interest. For example, we have seen that behavioural inhibition in childhood is a risk factor for anxiety disorder; however, there is also evidence that in the children of alcoholic fathers this trait may be protective against the later development of adolescent alcohol or drug problems (Vitaro *et al.* 1999). Interestingly, it has been suggested that the well-documented relationship between socioeconomic status and health may be partially mediated by protective psychological factors, such as a sense of mastery or control. There is evidence that such factors are differentially distributed by social class, as well as being related to health outcomes. This has led to the suggestion that adverse environments which undermine personal control may have an impact on chronic arousal and thereby contribute to the development of disorders such as cardiovascular disease (Taylor & Seeman 1999). It is also of note that personality attributes that contribute to resilience are often not those that are believed to do so by the public. In a study of adolescents, it was generally held that being resilient was to be disconnected from others and isolated (Hunter & Chandler 1999).

The nature of resilience represents an important area for future research. If it becomes possible to understand what makes certain individuals resilient to the effects of adversity, it may lead to the development of strategies that promote better outcomes for the more vulnerable.

Influence of illness on personality measurement and personality on illness outcome

It is well recognized that episodes of mental disorder can distort the appearance of personality (Kerr et al. 1970), and this is particularly evident when self-report questionnaires are used to measure personality dimensions. However, the problem remains even when semistructured interviews are used as the assessment tool (Widiger et al. 1999). Difficulties in investigating the relationship between personality and physical illness can arise because of disease symptoms and treatment distorting measures of personality. Even prospective studies, which aim to assess personality before the development of disorder, may potentially be influenced by prodromal symptoms of the disease.

Conversely, there is evidence that personality can exert an influence on the presentation and course of illness. In Alzheimer disease there is evidence that premorbid personality predicts the level of personality change as rated by informants (Dawson et al. 2000) as well as other non-cognitive behavioural symptoms (Meins et al. 1998). The co-occurrence of borderline personality disorder and major depressive disorder results in a significantly higher suicide attempt rate, compared to the rates in individuals with either diagnosis alone (Lesage et al. 1994). It has also been suggested that personality dimensions can exert an influence on the outcome of schizophrenic illness through their capacity to promote adaptive mechanisms (Jorgensen & Parnas 1990). Similarly, negative affectivity (neuroticism) has been shown to be indicative of a poorer prognosis in anxiety and depressive disorders (Clark et al. 1994).

The role of personality factors in influencing response to treatment has also been explored. Cloninger et al. have suggested that depressed patients' response to antidepressant medication can be predicted from their temperament and character inventory (TCI) scores (Joyce et al. 1994; Nelson & Cloninger 1997; Tome et al. 1997). The presence of a personality disorder has been shown to detrimentally affect the outcome of cognitive-behavioural therapy in the treatment of panic disorder (Mennin & Heimberg 2000) and substance abuse (Pettinati et al. 1999). Personality change resulting from the use of medication, such as noradrenergic and serotonergic antidepressants, has also been reported (Bagby et al. 1999).

Illness resulting in a lasting alteration in personality

The 'scar hypothesis' — the possibility that episodes of mental ill-

ness result in lasting personality changes which persist beyond recovery from the disorder — has not been subjected to much study. Several investigations that have explored this possibility in relation to depressive illness have had predominantly negative (Rohde et al. 1990) or inconclusive results. Kendler et al. (1993a) found some evidence for an elevation in neuroticism scores in female twins who developed an episode of depressive illness during a 15-month follow-up period, which they suggested was related to a 'scar effect'. However, analysis of data collected as part of the National Institute of Mental Health Collaborative Program on the Psychobiology of Depression found no evidence of personality change for subjects with a prospectively observed first episode of major depression during a 6-year follow-up period (Shea et al. 1996). The results suggested a possible association between increase in emotional reliance with number of episodes, and increased introversion with length of episode. However, the findings were somewhat inconclusive, which prompted the authors to suggest the need for further research.

There is some evidence that childhood psychopathology is associated with a later diagnosis of adult personality disorder. In a follow-up of 551 youths aged 9–16 years over a 10-year period, prior disruptive disorders, anxiety disorders and major depression all significantly increased the odds of the later development of personality disorder (Kasen et al. 1999).

Both brain damage and dementia can also result in permanent changes in the manner in which individuals behave or interact with others. Typically, control of emotions, impulses, motivation and social judgement are predominantly affected (Lishman 1997).

Conclusions

It is important to appreciate that individuals can change their patterns of behaviour, thoughts and ways of interrelating as a result of intervention (Heatherton & Weinberger 1994). Consequently, although we commenced this chapter by stating that personality is largely constant throughout the life span, this is only true in a very general sense. Learning, experiences and illnesses can all modify personality characteristics. Better understanding of the nature and underlying mechanisms of personality and health relationships may well present the potential for prevention and treatment of a variety of disorders. Until relatively recently, personality and health research has been little influenced by developments in more general personality research. Many of the personality measures used have been derived with specific theoretical models in mind and, as well as issues of validity and reliability, there has been some concern about the possibility of researchers reinventing 'constructs under new labels' (Holroyd & Coyne 1987). With the general adoption of the FFM there exists an opportunity for a more integrated and ultimately applicable study of this area. Similarly, adoption of novel methods for evaluating the behavioural concomitants of personality may improve measurement and remove some of the errors associated with the questionnaire method.

Kagan's inhibition research may prove to be more productive in the future, as it avoids ratings and uses observations by trained observers in carefully described and controlled situations. This, combined with the joint study of personality concepts from different levels of personality organization, such as personal goals and cognitive processes with temperamental traits, will provide the most coherent strategy for future research.

References

Adih, W.K. & Alexander, C.S. (1999) Determinants of condom use to prevent HIV infection among youth in Ghana. *Journal of Adolescent Health*, **24**, 63–72.

Alexander, F. (1950) *Psychosomatic Medicine*. Horton, New York.

American Psychiatric Association (1994) *Diagnostic and Statistical Manual of Mental Disorders (DSM -IV)*. American Psychiatric Association, Washington D.C.

Arbuthnott, G. (1998) Neuropharmacology. In: *Companion to Psychiatric Studies* (eds E.C. Johnstone, C.P.L. Freeman & A.K. Zealley), pp. 39–80. Churchill Livingstone, Edinburgh.

Asghari, V., Schoots, O., VanKats, S. *et al.* (1994) Dopamine D4 receptor repeat: analysis of different naïve and mutant forms of the human and rat genes. *Molecular Pharmacology*, **46**, 364–373.

Bagby, R.M., Levitan, R.D., Kennedy, S.H., Levitt, A.J. & Joffe, R.T. (1999) Selective alteration of personality in response to noradrenergic and serotonergic antidepressant medication in depressed sample: evidence of non-specificity. *Psychiatry Research*, **30**, 211–216.

Bandura, A. (1995) *Self-efficacy in Changing Societies*. Cambridge University Press, Cambridge.

Bandura, A. (1997) *Self-efficacy: the Exercise of Control*. Freeman, New York.

Bates, J.E. & Wachs, T.D., eds (1994) *Temperament: Individual Differences at the Interface of Biology and Behavior*. American Psychological Association, Washington D.C.

Battaglia, M. & Torgersen, S. (1996) Schizotypal disorder: at the crossroads of genetics and nosology. *Acta Psychiatrica Scandinavica*, **94**, 303–310.

Bau, C.H., Roman, T., Almeida, S. & Hutz, M.H. (1999) Dopamine D4 receptor gene and personality dimensions in Brazilian male alcoholics. *Psychiatric Genetics*, **9**, 139–143.

Borella, P., Bargellini, A., Rovesti, S. *et al.* (1999) Emotional stability, anxiety and natural killer activity under examination stress. *Psychoneuroendocrinology*, **24**, 613–627.

Breakwell, G.M. & Millward, L.J. (1997) Sexual self-concept and sexual risk taking. *Journal of Adolescent Health*, **20**, 29–41.

Brown, G.W., Harris, T.O. & Peto, J. (1973) Life events and psychiatric disorders. II. Nature of causal link. *Psychological Medicine*, **3**, 159–176.

Burton, R. (1652) *Anatomy of Melancholy*.

Buss, A.H. & Plomin, R. (1975) *A Temperament Theory of Personality Development*. Wiley Interscience, York, NY.

Carey, G. (1986) Sibling imitation and contrast effects. *Behavior Genetics*, **16**, 319–341.

Caspi, A. (1991) Prolegomena to a model of continuity and change in behavioural development. In: *The Childhood Environment and Adult Disease. Ciba Foundation Symposium 156* (ed. D.J.P. Barker), pp. 209–219. Wiley, London.

Caspi, A. & Herbener, E.S. (1990) Continuity and change: assortative marriage and the consistency of personality in adulthood. *Journal of Personality and Social Psychology*, **58**, 250–258.

Caspi, A. & Moffitt, T.E. (1991) Individual differences are accentuated during periods of social change: the sample case of girls at puberty. *Journal of Personality and Social Psychology*, **61**, 157–168.

Caspi, A. & Roberts, B.W. (1999) Personality continuity and change across the life course. In: *Handbook of Personality: Theory and Research* (eds L.A. Pervin & O.P. John), pp. 3–27. Guilford Press, New York.

Caspi, A. & Silva, P.A. (1995) Temperamental qualities at age 3 predict personality traits in young adulthood: longitudinal evidence from a birth cohort. *Child Development*, **66**, 486–498.

Caspi, A., Moffitt, T.E., Newman, D.L. & Silva, P.A. (1996) Behavioural observations at 3 years predict adult psychiatric disorders: longitudinal evidence from a birth cohort. *Archives of General Psychiatry*, **53**, 1033–1039.

Caspi, A., Begg, D., Dickson, N. *et al.* (1997) Personality differences predict health-risk behaviours in young adulthood: evidence from a longitudinal study. *Journal of Personality and Social Psychology*, **73**, 1052–1063.

Cherny, S.S., Fulker, D.W., Corley, R.P., Plomin, R. & De Fries, J.C. (1994) Continuity and change in infant shyness from 14 to 20 months. *Behavior Genetics*, **24**, 365–379.

Clark, L.A., Watson, D. & Mineka, S. (1994) Temperament, personality, and the mood and anxiety disorders. *Journal of Abnormal Psychology*, **103**, 103–116.

Clausen, J.A. (1991) Adolescent competence and the shaping of the life course. *American Journal of Sociology*, **96**, 805–842.

Clausen, J.A. (1993) *American Lives: Looking Back at the Children of the Great Depression*. Free Press, New York.

Cloninger, C.R. (1987) A systematic method for clinical description and classification of personality variants: a proposal. *Archives of General Psychiatry*, **44**, 573–588.

Cloninger, C.R. (1994) Temperament and personality. *Current Opinions in Neurobiology*, **4**, 266–273.

Cloninger, C.R., Svrakic, D.M. & Przybeck, T.R. (1993) A psychobiological model of temperament and character. *Archives of General Psychiatry*, **50**, 975–990.

Cloninger, C.R., Adolfsson, R. & Svrakic, D.M. (1996) Mapping genes for human personality. *Nature Genetics*, **12**, 3–4.

Compas, B.E., Connor-Smith, J.K., Saltzman, H., Thomsen, A.K. & Wadsworth, M.E. (2001) Coping with stress during childhood and adolescence: problems, progress, and potential in theory and research. *Psychological Bulletin*, **127**, 87–127.

Contrada, R.J., Cather, C. & O'Leary, A. (1999) Personality and health: dispositions and processes in disease susceptibility and adaptation to illness. In: *Handbook of Personality: Theory and Research* (eds L.A. Pervin & O.P. John), pp. 576–604. Guilford Press, New York.

Costa, P.T. & McCrae, R.R. (1992) *Revised NEO Personality Inventory (NEO-PI-R) and NEO Five-factor Inventory (NEO-FFI): Professional Manual*. Psychological Assessment Resources, Odessa, FL.

Dawson, D.V., Welsh-Bohmer, K.A. & Siegler, I.C. (2000) Premorbid personality predicts level of rated personality change in patients with Alzheimer disease. *Alzheimer Disease and Associated Disorders*, **14**, 11–19.

Deary, I. & Power, M.J. (1998) Normal and abnormal personality. In: *Companion to Psychiatric Studies* (eds E.C. Johnstone, C.P.L. Freeman & A.K. Zealley), pp. 565–596. Churchill Livingstone, Edinburgh.

Deary, I.J., Battersby, S., Whiteman, M.C., Connor, J.M., Fowkes, F.G. & Harmar, A. (1999) Neuroticism and polymorphisms in the serotonin transporter gene. *Psychological Medicine*, **29**, 735–739.

Dunbar, H.F. (1943) *Psychosomatic Diagnosis*. Hoeber, New York.

Eaves, L.J. (1976) A model for sibling effects in man. *Heredity*, **36**, 205–214.

Enns, M.W. & Cox, B.J. (1997) Personality dimensions and depression: review and commentary. *Canadian Journal of Pyschiatry*, **42**, 274–284.

Eysenck, H.J. & Eysenck, S.B.G. (1969) *Personality Structure and Measurement*. Routledge & Kegan Paul, London.

Eysenck, H.J. & Eysenck, S.B.G. (1975) *Manual of the Eysenck Personality Questionnaire*. Hodder & Stoughton, London.

Farber, E.W., Schwartz, J.A., Schaper, P.E., Moonen, D.J. & McDaniel, J.S. (2000) Resilience factors associated with adaptation to HIV disease. *Psychosomatics*, **41**, 140–146.

Farmer, A.E., McGuffin, P. & Gottesman, I. (1984) Searching for the split in schizophrenia: a twin study perspective. *Psychiatry Research*, **13**, 109–118.

Farmer, A., Harris, T., Redman, K., Sadler, S., Mahnood, A. & McGuffin, P. (2000) Cardiff Depression Study: a sib-pair study of life events and familiality in major depression. *British Journal of Psychiatry*, **176**, 150–155.

Farmer, A.E., Redman, K., Harris, T., Mahmood, A., Sadler, S. & McGuffin, P. (2001) The Cardiff Depression Study: sensation seeking life events and depression. *British Journal of Psychiatry*, **178**, 549–552.

Friedman, M. & Rosenman, R.H. (1959) Association of a specific overt behavior pattern with increases in blood cholesterol, blood clotting time, incidence of arcus senilis and clinical coronary artery disease. *Journal of the American Medical Association*, **169**, 1286–1296.

Friedman, M. & Rosenman, R.H. (1974) *Type A Behavior and Your Heart*. Knopf, New York.

Gabel, S., Stallings, M.C., Schmitz, S., Young, S.E. & Fulker, D.W. (1999) Personality dimensions and substance misuse: relationships in adolescents, mother and fathers. *American Journal of Addiction*, **8**, 101–113.

Gershenfeld, H.K. & Paul, S.M. (1998) Towards a genetics of anxious temperament: from mice to men. *Acta Psychiatrica Scandinavica* (Suppl.), **393**, 56–65.

Glendinning, A. & Inglis, D. (1999) Smoking behaviour in youth: the problem of low self esteem? *Journal of Adolescent Health*, **22**, 673–682.

Gordon Rouse, K.A., Ingersoll, G.M. & Orr, D.P. (1998) Longitudinal health endangering behavior risk among resilient and nonresilient early adolescents. *Journal of Adolescent Health*, **23**, 297–302.

Gustavsson, J.P., Nothen, M.M., Jonsson, E.G. *et al.* (1999) No association between serotonin transporter gene polymorphisms and personality traits. *American Journal of Medical Genetics*, **88**, 430–436.

Hall, C.S. & Lindzey, G. (1978) *Theories of Personality*, 3rd edn. Wiley, New York.

Hamer, D.H., Greenberg, B.D., Sabol, S.Z. & Murphy, D.L. (1999) Role of the serotonin transporter gene in temperament and character. *Journal of Personality Disorder*, **13**, 312–317.

Harbin, T.J. (1989) The relationship between Type A behavior pattern and physiological responsivity: a quantitative review. *Psychophysiology*, **26**, 110–119.

Hart, D., Hoffman, V., Edelstein, W. & Keller, M. (1997) The relation of childhood personality types to adolescent behaviour and development: a longitudinal study of Icelandic children. *Developmental Psychology*, **33**, 195–205.

Hayward, C., Killen, J.D., Kraemer, H.C. & Taylor, C.B. (1998) Linking self-reported childhood behavioral inhibition to adolescent social phobia. *Journal of the American Academy of Child and Adolescent Psychiatry*, **37**, 1308–1316.

Heatherton, T.F. & Weinberger, J.L. (1994) *Can Personality Change?* American Psychological Association, Washington D.C.

Heils, A., Teufel, A., Petri, S. *et al.* (1996) Allelic variation of human serotonin transporter gene expression. *Journal of Neurochemistry*, **66**, 2621–2624.

Herbert, T.B. & Cohen, S. (1993) Stress and immunity in humans: a meta-analytic review. *Psychosomatic Medicine*, **55**, 364–379.

Hetherington, E.M. & Clingempeel, W.G. (1992) Coping with marital transitions: a family systems perspective. *Monographs of the Society for Research in Child Development*, **2** (3, Serial no. 227).

Holroyd, K.A. & Coyne, J.C. (1987) Personality and health in the 1980s: psychosomatic medicine revisited? *Journal of Personality*, **55**, 359–375.

Hunter, A.J. & Chandler, G.E. (1999) Adolescent resilience. *Image, the Journal of Nursing Scholarship*, **31**, 243–247.

John, O.P. & Srivastava, S. (1999) The Big Five Trait Taxonomy: history, measurement, and theoretical perspectives. In: *Handbook of Personality: Theory and Research* (eds L.A. Pervin & O.P. John), pp. 3–27. Guilford Press, New York.

John, O.P., Caspi, A., Robins, R.W., Moffitt, T.E. & Stouthamer-Loeber, M. (1994) The 'Little Five': exploring the nomological network of the five-factor model of personality in adolescent boys. *Child Development*, **65**, 160–178.

Jorgensen, A. & Parnas, J. (1990) The Copenhagen High-Risk Study: premorbid and clinical dimensions of maternal schizophrenia. *Journal of Nervous and Mental Disorders*, **178**, 370–376.

Jorgensen, R.S., Johnson, B.T., Kolodziej, M.E. & Schreer, G.E. (1996) Elevated blood pressure and personality: a meta-analytic review. *Psychological Bulletin*, **120**, 293–320.

Jorm, A.F., Christensen, H., Henderson, A.S., Jacomb, P.A., Korten, A.E. & Rodgers, B. (2000) Predicting anxiety and depression from personality: is there a synergistic effect of neuroticism and extraversion? *Journal of Abnormal Psychology*, **109**, 145–149.

Joyce, P.R., Mulder, R.T. & Cloninger, C.R. (1994) Temperament predicts clomipramine and desipramine response in major depression. *Journal of Affective Disorders*, **30**, 35–46.

Kagan, J. (1994) *Galen's Prophecy*. Basic Books, New York.

Kagan, J. & Snidman, N. (1991) Temperamental factors in human development. *American Psychologist*, **46**, 856–862.

Kagan, J., Reznick, J.S. & Snidman, N. (1988) Biological bases of childhood shyness. *Science*, **240**, 167–171.

Kasen, S., Cohen, P., Skodol, A.E., Johnson, J.G. & Brook, J.S. (1999) Influence of child and adolescent psychiatric disorders on young adult personality disorder. *American Journal of Psychiatry*, **156**, 1529–1535.

Katsuragi, S., Kumugi, H., Sano, A. *et al.* (1999) Association between serotonin transporter gene polymorphism and anxiety related traits. *Biological Psychiatry*, **45**, 368–370.

Kendler, K.S. & Gardner, C.O. (1998) Boundaries of major depression: an evaluation of DSM-IV criteria. *American Journal of Psychiatry*, **155**, 172–177.

Kendler, K.S., Neale, M.C., Kessler, R.C., Heath, A.C. & Eaves, L.J. (1993a) A longitudinal twin study of personality and major depression in women. *Archives of General Psychiatry*, **50**, 853–862.

Kendler, K.S., Neale, M., Kessler, R., Heath, A. & Eaves, L. (1993b) A twin study of recent life events and difficulties. *Archives of General Psychiatry*, **50**, 789–796.

Kendler, K.S., Neale, M.C. & Walsh, D. (1995) Evaluating the spectrum concept of schizophrenia in the Roscommon Family Study. *American Journal of Psychiatry*, **152**, 749–754.

Kerr, T.A., Schapira, K., Roth, M. & Garside, R.F. (1970) The relationship between the Maudsley Personality Inventory and the course of affective disorders. *British Journal of Psychiatry*, **116**, 11–19.

King, L.A., King, D.W., Fairbank, J.A., Keane, T.M. & Adams, G.A. (1998) Resilience-recovery factors in post-traumatic stress disorder among females and male Vietnam veterans: hardiness, postwar social support, and additional stressful life events. *Journal of Personality and Social Psychology*, **74**, 420–434.

Kirmayer, L.J., Robbins, J.M. & Paris, J. (1994) Somatoform disorders: personality and the social matrix of somatic distress. *Journal of Abnormal Psychology*, **103**, 125–136.

Kobasa, S.C. (1979) Stressful life events, personality, and health: an inquiry into hardiness. *Journal of Personality and Social Psychology*, **37** (1), 1–11.

Kobasa, S.C., Maddi, S.R. & Kahn, S. (1982) Hardiness and health: a prospective study. *Journal of Personality and Social Psychology*, **42** (1), 168–177.

Kretschmer, E. (1936) *Physique and Character*, 2nd edn. [Translated by W.J.H. Sprott & K. Paul Trench.] Trubner, New York.

Krueger, R.F., Caspi, A., Moffit, T.E., Silva, P.A. & McGee, R. (1996) Personality traits are preferentially linked to mental disorders: toward and framework for theory and research. In: *Personality and Depression* (eds M.H. Klein, D.J. Kupfer & M.T. Shea). Guilford Press, New York.

Lesage, A.D., Boyer, R., Grunberg, F. *et al.* (1994) Suicide and mental disorders: a case–control study of young men. *American Journal of Psychiatry*, **151**, 1063–1068.

Lesch, K.P., Bengel, D., Heils, A. *et al.* (1996) Association of anxiety-related traits with a polymorphism in the serotonin transporter gene regulatory region. *Science*, **274**, 1527–1531.

Lishman, W.A. (1997) *Organic Psychiatry*. Blackwell Science, UK.

Loehlin, J.C. (1992) *Genes and Environment in Personality Development*. Sage, Newbury Park.

Loehlin, J.C. & Nicholls, J. (1976) *Heredity, Environment and Personality*. University of Texas Press, Austin, TX.

Luby, J.L., Svrakic, D.M., McCallum, K., Przybeck, T.R. & Cloninger, C.R. (1999) The Junior Temperament and Character Inventory: preliminary validation of a child self-report measure. *Psychological Reports*, **84**, 1127–1138.

Maher, B.A. & Maher, W.B. (1994) Personality and psychopathology: a historical perspective. *Journal of Abnormal Psychology*, **103**, 72–77.

Mason, J.W. (1972) Organisation of pyschoendocrine mechanisms. In: *Handbook of Psychophysiology* (eds N.S. Greefield & R.A. Sternbach), pp. 3–121. Holt, Rinehart & Winston, New York.

Matheny, A.P. (1984) Twin similarity in the developmental transformations of infant temperament as measured in a multi-method, longitudinal study. *Acta Geneticae Medicae et Gemellologiae: Twin Research*, **33**, 181–189.

Matheny, A.P. (1989) Children's behavioral inhibition over age and across situations: genetic similarity for a trait during change. *Journal of Personality*, **57**, 215–235.

Matthews, K.A. (1988) CHD and Type A behavior: update on and alternative to the Booth Kewley and Friedman quantitative review. *Psychological Bulletin*, **104**, 373–389.

McGuffin, P., Katz, R. & Bebbington, P. (1988) The Camberwell Collaborative Depression Study. III. Depression and adversity in the relatives of depressed probands. *British Journal of Psychiatry*, **152**, 775–782.

Meins, W., Frey, A. & Theisemann, R. (1998) Premorbid personality traits in Alzheimer's disease: do they predispose to noncognitive behavioral symptoms? *International Psychogeriatrics*, **10**, 369–378.

Mennin, D.S. & Heimberg, R.G. (2000) The impact of comorbid mood and personality disorders in the cognitive-behavioral treatment of panic disorder. *Clinical Psychological Review*, **20**, 339–357.

Miller, G.E., Cohen, S., Rabin, B.S., Skoner, D.P. & Doyle, W.J. (1999) Personality and tonic cardiovascular, neuroendocrine, and immune parameters. *Brain, Behavior, and Immunity*, **13**, 109–123.

Miller, T.Q., Smith, T.W., Turner, C.W., Guijarro, M.L. & Hallet, A.J. (1996) A meta-analytic review of research on hostility and physical health. *Psychological Bulletin*, **119**, 322–348.

Moore, J., Malhi, G.S. & McGuffin, P. (2000) Depression and anxiety. In: *Analysis of Multifactorial Diseases* (eds T. Bishop & P. Sham), pp. 291–308. Bios Scientific, Oxford.

Neale, M.C. & Stevenson, J. (1989) Rater bias in the EASI temperament scales: a twin study. *Journal of Personality and Social Psychology*, **56**, 446–455.

Nelson, E. & Cloninger, C.R. (1997) Exploring the TPQ as a possible predictor of antidepressant response to nefazadone in a large multisite study. *Journal of Affective Disorders*, **44**, 197–200.

Olff, M. (1999) Stress, depression and immunity: the role of defense and coping styles. *Psychiatry Research*, **85**, 7–15.

Patterson, J. & Blum, R.W. (1996) Risk and resilience among children and youth with disabilities. *Archives of Pediatrics and Adolescent Medicine*, **150**, 692–698.

Paykel, E.S. (1978) Contribution of life events to causation of psychiatric illness. *Psychological Medicine*, **8**, 245–253.

Peirson, A.R., Heuchert, J.W., Thomalia, L., Berk, M., Plein, H. & Cloninger, C.R. (1999) Relationship between serotonin and the temperament and character inventory. *Psychiatry Research*, **13**, 29–37.

Peterson, C. & Seligman, M.E.P. (1987) Explanatory style and illness. *Journal of Personality*, **55**, 237–265.

Pettinati, H.M., Pierce, J.D., Belden, P.P. & Meyers, K. (1999) The relationship of Axis II personality disorders to other known predictors of addiction treatment outcome. *American Journal of Addiction*, **8**, 136–147.

Pike, A., McGuire, S., Hetherington, E.M., Reiss, D. & Plomin, R. (1996) Family environment and adolescent depressive symptoms and antisocial behaviour: a multivariate genetic analysis. *Developmental Psychology*, **32**, 590–603.

Plomin, R. & Caspi, A. (1999) Behavioural genetics and personality. In: *Handbook of Personality: Theory and Research* (eds L.A. Pervin & O.P. John), pp. 3–27. Guilford Press, New York.

Plomin, R., Emde, R.N., Braungart, J.M. *et al.* (1993) Genetic change and continuity from fourteen to twenty months: the MacArthur Longitudinal Twin Study. *Child Development*, **64**, 1354–1376.

Porter, R. (1997) *The Greatest Benefit to Mankind*. Harper Collins, London.

Quinton, D. & Rutter, M. (1988) *Parenting Breakdown: the Making and Breaking of Inter-Generational Links*. Avebury, Aldershot.

Quinton, D., Pickles, A., Maughan, B. & Rutter, M. (1993) Partners, peers, and pathways: assortative pairing and continuities in conduct disorder. *Development and Psychopathology*, **5**, 763–783.

Raikkonen, K., Matthews, K.A., Flory, J.D., Owens, J.F. & Gump, B. (1999) Effects of optimism, pessimism and trait anxiety on ambulatory blood pressure and mood during everyday life using experiential sampling method. *Journal of Personality and Social Psychology*, **76**, 104–113.

Ramanaiah, N.V., Sharpe, J.P. & Byravan, A. (1999) Hardiness and major personality factors. *Psychological Reports*, **84**, 497–500.

Riemann, R., Angleitner, A. & Strelau, J. (1997) Genetic and environmental influences on personality: a study of twins reared together using the self- and peer report NEO-FFI scales. *Journal of Personality*, **65**, 449–476.

Roberts, B.W., Friend-DeI. & Vecchio, W.F. (2000) The rank-order consistency of personality traits from childhood to old age: a quantitative review of longitudinal studies. *Psychological Bulletin*, **126**, 3–25.

Roberts, S.B. & Kendler, K.S. (1999) Neuroticism and self-esteem as indices of the vulnerability to major depression in women. *Psychological Medicine*, **29**, 1101–1109.

Robins, R.W., John, O.P., Caspi, A., Moffitt, T.E. & Stouthamer-Loeber,

M. (1996) Resilient, overcontrolled and undercontrolled boys: three replicable personality types? *Journal of Personality and Social Psychology*, **70**, 157–171.

Rohde, P., Lewinsohn, P.M. & Seeley, J.R. (1990) Are people changed by the experience of having an episode of major depression? A further test of the scar hypothesis. *Journal of Abnormal Psychology*, **99**, 264–271.

Rutter, M. (1987) Temperament, personality and personality disorder. *British Journal of Psychiatry*, **150**, 443–458.

Saudino, K.J. & Plomin, R. (1997) Cognitive and temperamental mediators of genetic contributions to the home environment during infancy. *Merrill-Palmer Quarterly*, **43**, 1–23.

Scheier, M.F. & Carver, C.S. (1985) Optimism, coping and health: assessment and implications of generalised outcome expectancies. *Health Psychology*, **4**, 219–247.

Scheier, M.F., Weintruab, J.K. & Carver, C.S. (1986) Coping with stress: divergent strategies of optimists and pessimists. *Journal of Personality and Social Psychology*, **51**, 1257–1264.

Segerstrom, S.C., Taylor, S.E., Kemeny, M.E. & Fahey, J.L. (1998) Optimism is associated with mood, coping and immune change in response to stress. *Journal of Personality and Social Psychology*, **74**, 1646–1655.

Shanahan, M.J., Elder, G.H. & Meich, R.A. (1997) History and agency in men's lives: pathways to achievement in cohort perspective. *Sociology of Education*, **70**, 54–67.

Shea, M.T., Leon, A.C., Mueller, T.I., Solomon, D.A., Warshaw, M.G. & Keller, M.B. (1996) Does major depression result in lasting personality change? *American Journal of Psychiatry*, **153**, 1404–1410.

Sheldon, W.H., Stevens, S.S. & Tucker, W.B. (1940) *The Varieties of Human Physique*. Harper, London.

Sheldon, W.H., Stevens, S.S. & Tucker, W.B. (1942) *The Varieties of Temperament*. Harper, London.

Simonoff, E., Pickles, A., Hervas, A., Silberg, J.L., Rutter, M. & Eaves, L. (1998) Genetic influences on childhood hyperactivity: contrast effects imply parental rating bias, not sibling interaction. *Psychological Medicine*, **28**, 825–837.

Smith, T.W. & Williams, P.G. (1992) Personality and health: advantages and limitations of the five factor model. *Journal of Personality*, **60**, 395–423.

Stewart, D.E. (1996) Women's health and psychosomatic medicine. *Journal of Psychosomatic Research*, **40**, 221–226.

Taylor, S.E. & Seeman, T.E. (1999) Psychosocial resources and the SES–health relationship. *Annals of the New York Academy of Sciences*, **896**, 210–225.

Thapar, A., Hervas, A. & McGuffin, P. (1995) Childhood hyperactivity scores are highly heritable and show sibling competition effects: twin study. *Behavior Genetics*, **25**, 537–544.

Thomas, A., Chess, S., Birch, H.G., Hertzig, M.E. & Korn, S. (1963) *Behavioral Individuality in Early Childhood*. New York University Press, New York.

Tome, M.B., Cloninger, C.R., Watson, J.P. & Isaac, M.T. (1997) Serotonergic autoreceptor blockade in the reduction of antidepressant latency: personality variables and response to paroxetine and pindolol. *Journal of Affective Disorders*, **44**, 101–109.

Tomitaka, M., Tomiatka, S., Otuka, Y. *et al.* (1999) Association between novelty seeking and dopamine receptor D4 (DRD4) exon III polymorphism in Japanese subjects. *American Journal of Medical Genetics*, **88**, 469–471.

Trull, T.J. & Sher, K.J. (1994) Relationship between the five-factor model of personaltiy and Axis I disorders in a nonclinical sample. *Journal of Abnormal Psychology*, **103**, 350–360.

Tschann, J.M., Kaiser, P., Chesney, M.A., Alkon, A. & Boyce, W.T. (1996) Resilience and vulnerability among preschool children: family functioning, temperament, and behaviour problems. *Journal of the American Academy of Child and Adolescent Psychiatry*, **35**, 184–192.

Van Lieshout, C.F.M. & Haselager, G.J.T. (1994) The Big Five personality factors in Q-sort descriptions of children and adolescents. In: *The Developing Structure of Temperament and Personality from Infancy to Adulthood* (eds C.F. Halverston, G.A. Kohnstamm & R.P. Martin), pp. 293–318. Erlbaum, Hillsdale, NJ.

Vitaro, F., Tremblay, R.E. & Zoccolillo, M. (1999) Alcoholic father, adolescent drug abuse and protective factors. *Canadian Journal of Psychiatry*, **44**, 901–908.

Vitousek, K. & Manke, F. (1994) Personality variables and disorders in anorexia nervosa and bulimia nervosa. *Journal of Abnormal Psychology*, **103**, 137–147.

Wallston, B.S., Wallston, K.A., Kaplan, G.D. & Maides, S.A. (1976) Development and validation of the Health Locus of Contol (HLC) Scale. *Journal of Consulting and Clinical Psychology*, **44**, 580–585.

Watson, D., Clark, L.A. & Harkness, A.R. (1994) Structures of personality and their relevance to psychopathology. *Journal of Abnormal Psychology*, **103**, 18–31.

Widiger, T.A. & Trull, T.J. (1992) Personality and psychopathology: an application of the five-factor model. *Journal of Personality*, **60**, 363–393.

Widiger, T.A. & Trull, T.S. (1993) Borderline and narcissistic personality disorders. In: *Comprehensive Handbook of Psychopathology* (eds P.B. Sutker & H.E. Adams), 2nd edn, pp. 371–394. Plenum Press, New York.

Widiger, T.A., Trull, T.S., Clarkin, J.F., Sanderson, C. & Costa, P.T. (1994) A description of the DSM-III-R and DSM-IV personality disorders with the five-factor model of personality. In: *Personality Disorders and the Five-factor Model of Personality* (eds P.T. Costa & T.A. Widiger), pp. 41–56. American Psychological Association, Washington D.C.

Widiger, T.A., Verheul, R. & Van Den Brink, W. (1999) Personality and psychopathology. In: *Handbook of Personality: Theory and Research* (eds L.A. Pervin & O.P. John), pp. 3–27. Guilford Press, New York.

Winter, D.G. & Barenbaum, N.B. (1999) History of modern personality theory and research. In: *Handbook of Personality: Theory and Research* (eds L.A. Pervin & O.P. John), pp. 3–27. Guilford Press, New York.

Woodworth, R.S. (1919) Examination of emotional fitness for warfare. *Psychological Bulletin*, **15**, 59–60.

World Health Organization (1992) *International Classification of Diseases*, 10th edn. World Health Organization, Geneva, Switzerland.

Zimmerman, M.A., Ramirez-Valles, J. & Maton, K.I. (1999) Resilience among urban African American male adolescents: a study of the protective effects of sociopolitical control on their mental health. *American Journal of Community Psychology*, **27**, 733–751.

43 Disorders of Personality

Jonathan Hill

Introduction

The concept of personality disorder in adult life is important and elusive. It is important because it is a major cause of burden to sufferers, to the adults and children with whom they have relationships, and to society; and because of its association with the majority of non-psychotic episodic psychiatric disorders. It is elusive because there is relatively little agreement on basic issues, such as whether there is one overarching disorder or many, and what are the core defining features of a personality disorder. Nevertheless, there is broad agreement that the concept must include stability of behaviour over substantial periods of time, and extensive or pervasive dysfunction encompassing a range of psychological, behavioural and interpersonal capacities. *Prima facie*, it seems likely that such stable and severe problems will have started before adult life, and there is evidence that in many instances analogous disorders or their antecedents do start in childhood, and that childhood experiences may affect risk for subsequent personality disorder. Accordingly, it seems crucial to consider what is known about personality disorders, with special reference to two key questions for child psychiatrists and child mental health practitioners more widely, of the extent to which there is continuity in personality disturbance between childhood and adult life, and whether it is useful to apply the diagnosis in childhood and adolescence.

Concepts of personality disorder

Attempts to classify personality types and dimensions go back to antiquity but concepts of personality disorder are of much more recent origin (Frances & Widiger 1986; Rutter 1987; Tyrer *et al.* 1991). Although there are numerous variations on the specifics, the unifying notion is the idea that there are pervasive and persistent abnormalities of overall personality functioning that cause social impairment and/or subjective distress, and that are not caused by episodic disorders of mental state. The basic assumption is that, personality disorders are different in some way from other more episodic psychiatric conditions such as schizophrenia, depression or anxiety states.

Having broadly characterized personality disorder in terms of persistent dysfunction that is not accounted for by episodic disorder, the question arises as to whether a unified concept for personality disorder (implying one set of underlying causal processes) is adequate. Several attempts to provide a unified

concept have been made, notably using the idea that personality disorder represents an extreme of normal personality. One approach, based on the proposal that there are five major domains of personality, the five-factor model (Widiger & Costa 1994), argues that 'Personality disorders are not qualitatively distinct from normal personality functioning. They are simply maladaptive, extreme variants of common personality traits.' In Cloninger's (1987) tridimensional model, personality disorder is seen to arise from a combination of extremes of temperament, each of which is thought to be influenced by different neurotransmitter systems. Some empirical support from animal and human studies for such associations have been demonstrated, and contributions of behaviour reflecting Cloninger's three dimensions of harm avoidance, novelty seeking and reward dependence have been shown to be predictive of persistence of aggression in adolescence (Kerr *et al.* 1997).

Although these frameworks are promising, it should be borne in mind that the concept of personality disorder did not originate from a model of normal personality, and indeed descriptions of different personality disorder types have come about through several contrasting routes. There are those that derive from the clinical observation that there are individuals who show enduring patterns of inflexible and seriously maladaptive behaviour that seem to fall outside the traditional criteria for mental illness or psychiatric syndrome. The need to have a term to describe these patterns of abnormal behaviour led to the concepts of psychopathy put forward by writers such as Hare (1970), Henderson (1939) and Cleckley (1941). These are the categories of personality disorder that identify individuals who are thought to be most prone to suffer from episodic mental disorders. Schneider's (1923, 1950) notion of psychopathic personality (defined quite differently from the psychopathy formulations of Hare, Henderson and Cleckley) provides the main historic notion of this approach. Many of the ICD-10 specific personality disorder categories (e.g. paranoid, anankastic and anxious) represent this tradition (World Health Organization 1992). Some categories have their origins in empirical observations of the continuities between psychopathological disorders in childhood, and pervasive social malfunction in adult lifestyle. The DSM-IV (American Psychiatric Association 1994) diagnosis of antisocial personality disorder is the obvious example of this type, with its starting point in the findings of the long-term longitudinal studies pioneered by Robins (1966, 1978) and replicated by others (see Earls & Mezzacappa, Chapter 26). Some categories stem fairly directly from theoretical, especially psychoanalytic, notions. The concept of borderline personality organization (Kernberg 1967, 1975) underlies specification of the DSM-IV diagnosis of borderline personality disorder (Gunderson *et al.* 1981). A few categories have come, at least in part, from genetic findings. Meehl (1962) coined the term 'schizotypy' to describe the postulated characteristics of schizophrenia-prone individuals. The Danish adoption study showed that the biological families of adopted schizophrenic probands included a raised rate of personality disorders that seemed to exhibit some features reminiscent of schizophrenia (Kety *et al.* 1971). Spitzer *et al.* (1979) developed more explicit criteria for this type of personality syndrome which has come to be termed 'schizotypal personality disorder'.

The differences in the origins of personality disorder have contributed to substantial heterogeneity in the balance between behaviours and psychological states that are included in the subtypes of personality disorder. DSM-IV antisocial personality disorder is based primarily on antisocial behaviours and interpersonal difficulties, and includes only one state of mind item, 'lack of remorse', which is closely tied to behaviour. By contrast, the borderline personality disorder category includes three items, 'identity disturbance', 'chronic feelings of emptiness' and 'transient paranoid ideation', referring solely to states of mind. Furthermore, within the DSM-IV framework only a subset of the total number of items is required for entry to a diagnosis, which means that criteria can be fulfilled in numerous ways.

Validation

Stability and separation from episodic disorders

It is assumed that the personality disorders should show substantial stability over time. However, there is surprisingly little evidence that this is the case. Several studies of referred adults have found low to moderate stability (Ferro *et al.* 1998). In a study of college students in the USA assessed at three time points over 4 years, Lenzenweger (1999) found moderate stability of DSM personality disorder dimensions, but the estimated prevalence of personality disorder fell from 7.6 to 2.8%.

The distinction between episodic disorders and personality disorder is enshrined in the DSM distinction between Axis I and Axis II. Axis II disorders should show persistence over a period in which there is either recovery from, or onset of, Axis I disorder. In view of this, remarkably few studies have been carried out to test the stability of personality disorder after accounting for episodic disorders. Loranger *et al.* (1991) undertook one of the few pertinent tests in their test–retest study of changes in the diagnosis of personality disorder (on a standardized interview) in a series of 84 psychiatric patients. The investigation was limited by the fact that the interval between assessments was only 1 week to 6 months, but there were major changes in mental state during this period. The key finding was that there was no effect of change in mental state on the diagnosis of personality disorder, supporting the personality disorder–episodic disorder dis-

tinction. Nevertheless, remission was associated with some fall in personality disorder symptoms and the diagnosis of personality disorder showed only moderate temporal stability (kappa = 0.55). Rutter (1977) and Rutter & Quinton (1984) tackled the issue over a longer time span by testing whether personality disorder predicted the course of handicapping symptoms in patients over a 4-year period. The results showed that personality disorder was a strong predictor of course (59% marked persistence vs. 18% in those without personality disorder), whereas duration of symptoms was unrelated to outcome in the absence of personality disorder. More recently, Quinton *et al.* (1995) examined the course of disorder in the same group of patients over a 15–20-year period. Persistent social role impairment was much more frequent in those diagnosed as showing personality disorder initially (61 vs. 17%); moreover, this difference was not accounted for by either the length or clinical severity of the initial associated episodic condition.

Although these findings support the distinction between episodic and personality disorders, the two are strongly associated. There are very high rates of personality disorder in patients with episodic disorders: nearly half in inpatient samples and 20–40% in outpatient groups (Docherty *et al.* 1986; Tyrer *et al.* 1991). These figures are much higher than the rates of 6–13% that are typical of general population samples (Casey & Tyrer 1986; Merikangas & Weissman 1986). In a study of outpatients with personality disorder referred to a private practice, the mean number of current DSM-IV Axis I disorders (mainly anxiety and depression) was 2.2, and of lifetime disorders 3.0 (Zimmerman & Mattia 1999); Zanarini *et al.* (1998a) found similarly elevated rates. The meaning of these associations is not clear. It is likely that to a certain extent they are artefacts arising from difficulties in distinguishing Axis I and Axis II items. In clinical and research practice it is often difficult to disentangle symptoms associated with episodes and those that reflect personality disorder. Furthermore, the same clinical phenomena, occurring over different time periods, can contribute either to episodic or to personality diagnoses. For instance, episodes of dysphoria lasting up to a few days contribute to the diagnosis of borderline personality disorder, while somewhat longer episodes contribute to the diagnosis of major depression.

This is unlikely to be the whole explanation. There are three mains ways in which the associations may arise. First, personality disorder may constitute a risk factor for episodic conditions. This could occur through direct mechanisms whereby a feature of the disorder, such as poor coping (Vollrath *et al.* 1994), leads to helplessness and hence depression, or through indirect mechanisms in which the personality disorder increases the likelihood of psychosocial stressors which in turn are associated with a disorder such as depression (Daley *et al.* 1998). Second, episodic conditions may create the conditions in which personality disorders develop because a chain of maladaptive behaviours and adverse environmental responses is set in motion that fosters more persistent psychopathology (Kasen *et al.* 1999). Third, both the personality disorder and the episodic disorder could reflect one underlying liability.

Most studies of comorbidity between episodic and personality disorder have been cross-sectional and therefore not well suited to distinguishing between these possibilities, and findings from prospective longitudinal studies have not provided unequivocal answers. On the one hand, there is evidence that personality disorder increases the risk of episodic disorders. In a 2-year prospective study of adolescents, personality disorder symptoms were predictive of subsequent interpersonal chronic stress which in turn increased vulnerability to depression (Daley *et al.* 1998). In a community-based longitudinal study, Johnson *et al.* (1999) found that personality disorder ascertained in adolescence predicted episodic disorders in early adult life. After controlling for episodic disorders in adolescence, the presence of personality disorder more than doubled the likelihood. By contrast, findings from the same community study indicated that the influences may run the other way. Disruptive disorders, anxiety and depression ascertained between ages 9 and 16 were all associated with personality disorder in early adult life after controlling for prior personality disorder. There could be several interpretations of these findings. In the case of disruptive disorders, they could be a function of the convention whereby antisocial behaviours in childhood are seen as indicative of an episodic disorder, but the constellation of antisocial problems seen in adult life is assessed as an antisocial personality disorder. Alternatively, different subgroups may take different routes, some starting with episodic disorders and some with personality disorder. Equally, it could be that episodic and personality disorders are so strongly associated from late childhood and early adolescence that the attempt to give causal priority to one or the other will not prove fruitful.

It might be expected that, whatever the relationship between episodic disorders and personality disorder, the combination should in some sense reflect a more severe variant, with implications for treatment outcome. However, the evidence has been mixed. Several studies have found that personality disorders are associated with a worse immediate response to treatment and a worse overall outcome for episodic mental disturbances (Docherty *et al.* 1986; Shea *et al.* 1990; Reich & Green 1991). Tyrer *et al.* (1994) found that a community-based early intervention for psychiatric emergencies had better outcomes than a hospital-based service only for patients who did not have a personality disorder. In a study of response to ECT among inpatients, personality disorder was associated with slower social recovery, but personality status was not associated with recovery from depressive symptoms (Casey *et al.* 1996). In a study of 298 psychiatric outpatients re-evaluated after 6 years, relapse of depression was predicted by the presence of borderline and dependent personality disorders (Alnaes & Torgersen 1997). However, the evidence that the presence of personality disorder predicts poorer treatment outcome has not been consistent. Studies of the effectiveness of cognitive therapy (Patience *et al.* 1995) and of fluoxetine (Nierenberg *et al.* 1999) for depression did not find associations between personality disorder and outcomes. The inconsistencies in the findings are likely to have arisen from a wide range of factors including variations in sample sizes, types of clinical problems, treatments and outcomes. Where there is an effect of personality disorder very little is known about possible mechanisms. Personality disorder may be associated with poor treatment compliance, or with greater severity of overall psychopathology, or with a greater number of psychosocial adversities and fewer interpersonal resources or with maladaptive beliefs (Kuykenetal 2001).

The conceptual distinction between personality disorders and chronic psychiatric conditions raises other difficult questions. Usually is has been assumed that the latter are more episodic in their course, do not reflect a basic characterological defect, are more amenable to change, and are ego-dystonic in the sense that they represent a difference from the person's ordinary functioning that is a source of distress to the individual and which the person wishes to change. In relation to each of these we find a blurring of the distinction. In many cases, episodic conditions such as schizophrenia and depression pursue a course in which there is relatively little evidence of discrete episodes. The idea that episodic disorders, whether chronic or acute, are not related to aspects of personality has been challenged in a number of ways. Proneness to depression is associated with the personality characteristics of neuroticism and sociotropy—a need for approval from others (Ormel & Wohlfarth 1991; Robins *et al.* 1994). The distinction does not apply with regard to genetic and biological contributions. There are substantial genetic contributions to schizophrenia, depression and personality disorder (McGuffin & Thapar 1992), and no evidence that the extent of genetic influences differs systematically between the episodic and personality disorders. Similarly, there is evidence of structural brain abnormalities in chronic episodic conditions, notably schizophrenia, and in personality disorder (Raine *et al.* 2000).

Differentiations among personality disorders

The World Health Organization (1992) classification, ICD-10, makes a basic differentiation between organic personality disorders (meaning those resulting from severe head injury, encephalitis and other forms of overt brain damage); enduring personality changes deriving from some catastrophic experience, personality abnormalities that reflect the residue of some mental illness (e.g. residual schizophrenia): and what they term personality disorders. The American Psychiatric Association (1994) scheme, DSM-IV, makes broadly comparable distinctions. This chapter is concerned with this last group of specific personality disorders because the others have only an extremely limited application in childhood and adolescence.

The ICD classification specifies nine personality disorder types, and the DSM system eleven. To a certain extent the different categories reflect the different origins referred to earlier. The DSM classification has received a lot of attention, and in spite of the operational definitions of each of the categories, the evidence for their discriminant validity is not strong. Studies have consistently shown that individuals who receive one DSM Axis II diagnosis generally receive several (Pfohl *et al.* 1986; Morey 1988; Oldham *et al.* 1992). Although there is evidence that the DSM categories cluster into three broad bands of the odd/eccentric, the dramatic/emotional/erratic and the anxious/fearful (Kass *et al.* 1985), combinations of personality disorders that cross these bands are common (Oldham *et al.* 1992).

Support for the discriminant validity of particular personality disorders would be provided if it were possible to show differential association with other psychiatric conditions, family clustering, or associations with genetic or environmental influences. Studies of the association of borderline personality disorder with other episodic and personality disorders have provided some support for its discriminant validity. Zanarini *et al.* (1998b) compared patients with borderline personality disorder and patients with other personality disorders. Those with borderline disorder had higher rates of associated paranoid, avoidant and dependent personality disorders, and higher rates of mood, anxiety and eating disorders. Zimmerman & Mattia (1999) found higher mean totals of associated episodic disorders in patients with borderline personality disorder, and increased rates of particular Axis I disorders.

The most clear-cut finding from family studies is the association between schizophrenia and a loading of schizotypal personality disorders in the biological relatives (Kendler *et al.* 1981, 1984). The evidence for a link between schizotypal personality disorder and schizophrenia is further supported by findings of similarities in magnetic resonance imaging (MRI) (Dickey *et al.* 2000) and in deficits of attention and information processing (Cadenhead *et al.* 2000). A significant but weaker association with schizophrenia has been found with paranoid personality disorders (Kendler & Gruenberg 1982; Kendler *et al.* 1985).

There are very few family and genetic data on other personality disorders (McGuffin & Thapar 1992; Maier *et al.* 1998). There is some evidence that borderline personality disorders cluster in families and also are associated with affective disorders in other family members, but it remains quite uncertain whether the family loading has a genetic basis. There is consistent evidence for genetic influences on adult antisocial behaviours (Langbehn *et al.* 1998), but not adult violence (Carey & Goldman 1997). There seems to be a genetic component to antisocial personality disorder but there is limited evidence on its strength. Most studies of the association between adverse childhood experiences and personality disorders have reported associations with a wide range of episodic and personality disorders (Johnson *et al.* 1999). There may also be more specific effects. Bezirganian *et al.* (1993) found that the combination of maternal inconsistency and high maternal overinvolvement assessed in adolescence was associated with the persistence or emergence of borderline personality disorder, and no other episodic or personality disorders. Parker *et al.* (1999) reported that dysfunctional parenting in childhood was associated with the dramatic and anxious DSM clusters, but not the odd/eccentric cluster.

In contrast to the rather sparse support for the distinctions between the majority of the different personality disorder cate-gories, recent work identifying the relevant dimensions of personality functioning has produced more consistent findings. There has been broad support for at least four factors—emotional dysregulation, dissocial behaviour, inhibitedness and compulsivity—which are identifiable in clinical as well as non-clinical samples. Distinctive genetic and environmental factors associated with these broad factors, and also with lower level more specific traits, have been identified (Livesley *et al.* 1998). This implies that there may be 'a large number of genetic building blocks each having a relatively specific effect in isolation, but also with the potential to combine to produce an almost infinite variety of configurations of personality traits and able to be expressed as "personality disorder"' (Parker & Barrett 2000).

Specific personality disorders

In view of the lack of good discriminant validity among the many specific personality disorders, only a few of the key categories that may be particularly relevant in childhood and adolescence will be discussed.

Antisocial personality disorders

Although the adjective 'antisocial' might seem to imply that the personality disorder necessarily implies criminal behaviour, it is apparent from the DSM-IV (American Psychiatric Association 1994) that this is not so. The diagnostic criteria include an inability to sustain consistent work behaviour, antisocial acts, aggression, failure to honour financial obligations, failure to plan ahead, disregard for the truth, recklessness, and a lack of remorse.

Most adults with antisocial personality disorder have shown marked conduct problems in early childhood. Conduct problems starting early in childhood carry a high risk of persistence into adolescence and adult life (Moffitt *et al.* 1996). These life-course-persistent difficulties are associated with temperamental lack of control (quick to show negative emotions when frustrated, poor impulse control), hyperactivity, lower IQ, and peer problems and adverse family backgrounds (Henry *et al.* 1996; Moffit *et al.* 1996). Although this is a high-risk group, around one-half do not go on to become antisocial adults and so identifying the predictors of persistence of conduct problems is central to understanding the causes of antisocial personality disorder. However, relatively little is known of factors and processes that predict within this vulnerable group. On the basis of retrospective reports within a large epidemiological study, Robins *et al.* (1991) found that the number of childhood antisocial problems was associated with risk of antisocial personality disorder. Studies within childhood provide some further clues regarding risk of persistence. Loeber *et al.* (1995) found that early fighting and hyperactivity predicted persistence of antisocial behaviours over a 6-year period among boys referred for conduct problems.

In a prospective study of a representative general population sample from ages 7–9 years to 14–16 years, persisters had the highest levels of family adversity, lower IQ and self-esteem; those with early conduct problems that did not persist had levels of these risk factors that were intermediate between persisters and children who lacked early behaviour problems (Fergusson *et al.* 1996). Persisters were more likely than those whose early antisocial behaviours had remitted to have a deviant peer group in adolescence. Whether this was a reflection, or a cause, of persistence is not clear; however, it is consistent with Sampson & Laub's (1993) argument that a key factor in determining persistence may be the presence or absence of social bonds and controls.

Conduct disorder in childhood leads to criminal behaviour in adult life, not so much because this is inevitable — although there are important individual influences — but rather because antisocial behaviour in childhood is likely to predispose to weak social commitments in work, friendship and marriage, and that these in turn make crime in adult life more likely. By the same token, if there are sufficiently powerful salient life events and socialization experiences of the right kind in adult life this strong indirect chain can be broken. Studies of the risk of deviant partners and the effects of quality of cohabiting relationships illustrate the point. Children who have been in care have high rates of conduct problems and have adult psychosocial difficulties typical of antisocial personality disorder. However, the risk of poor adult outcome is reduced among those who establish supportive cohabiting relationships (Rutter *et al.* 1990). Acquiring a non-deviant partner is crucial to this more benign outcome. Among individuals with conduct problems in childhood the likelihood of having a non-deviant partner was increased where they had shown evidence of planning for work before leaving school and had a non-deviant peer group in adolescence (Quinton *et al.* 1993).

Adequacy of antisocial personality disorder as a diagnosis

In common with all DSM categories, the diagnosis requires a subset of the criteria for antisocial personality disorder to be present, which means that there are numerous ways in which individuals may be identified as having the disorder. This is likely to limit precision in identifying mechanisms. Furthermore, antisocial personality disorder is no more immune from problems of multiple diagnoses than other personality disorders. A focus on particular features of the category may prove useful. Broadly speaking, it refers to antisocial behaviours, deficits in social role performance and lack of remorse. Findings from longitudinal studies in the UK have indicated that the continuity from conduct disorder in childhood to pervasive social dysfunction, affecting relationships and work, may be stronger than that of conduct disorder to antisocial behaviours (Zoccolillo *et al.* 1992), and that monozygotic twins who showed conduct disorder in childhood have greater concordance, compared with dizygotic twins, for adult social dysfunction than for anti-

social personality disorder (Simonoff 2001). It is therefore possible that difficulties in establishing and gaining from effective interpersonal, educational and work functioning not only contribute to persistence of childhood conduct problems but also constitute the core of the adult difficulties. These would, under some circumstances and in combination with additional individual vulnerabilities, be associated with antisocial behaviours, but also with a wider range of psychosocial problems.

Psychobiological mechanisms in antisocial personality disorder

It may be that conduct disorder persisters have particular biological or psychological profiles that pick them out from those who will remit. For example, a low heart rate has consistently been found to be associated with antisocial behaviours in children and adults (Farrington 1997). In a study comparing volunteer adults with antisocial personality disorder and psychiatric and normal controls, the antisocial group had lower mean prefrontal volumes and reduced autonomic activity (Raine *et al.* 2000). However, there were inconsistent associations between prefrontal volumes and autonomic measures. If these associations can be substantiated it will be important to ascertain whether remitters and persisters differ on these parameters, or whether they have the same biological vulnerabilities accompanied by other biological or social protective factors.

The role of temperament in relation to conduct disorders is reviewed by Moore & Farmer (Chapter 42) and by Earls & Mezzacappa (Chapter 26). The effects of lack of control in early childhood, as evidenced by an inability to modulate impulse expression, impersistence in problem-solving, and emotionally negative responses to stress and challenge, may be very persistent. In their prospective study of a New Zealand birth cohort, Henry *et al.* (1996) found that temperamental lack of control at ages 3 and 5 distinguished, among those who were convicted by age 18, between those with violent offences and those with non-violent offending histories.

Psychopathic disorder

Insensitivity to the feelings of others, as reflected in lack of guilt or remorse, is included as an item in DSM-IV antisocial personality disorder category. However, antisocial personality disorder and psychopathy are different concepts with different histories. Antisocial personality disorder is predominantly a behavioural description and, as many commentators have pointed out, it has substantial overlap with criminality. The concept of psychopathy, particularly as described by Cleckley (1941) and as assessed in the Psychopathy Checklist (PCL, Hare 1971), has more emphasis on inferred interpersonal and affective traits such as grandiosity, callousness, deceitfulness, shallow affect and lack of remorse. Psychopathy defines a narrower group of offenders than antisocial personality disorder. Between 50 and 80% of offenders meet DSM criteria for antisocial personality disorder, whereas the rate of psychopathy is around 15–30% (Hare *et al.* 1991; Robins *et al.* 1991). The psychopathic group is probably a subgroup of those with antisocial personality disorder. Most criminals who meet criteria for psychopathy also meet those for antisocial personality disorder, and around 30% of those with antisocial personality disorder meet criteria for psychopathy (Hart & Hare 1989). Compared with other offenders, psychopathic individuals have a lower average age of first arrest, have a higher rate of offending and are somewhat more likely to have committed violent crimes (Hare & McPherson 1984; Cooke 1995). Scores on the PCL assessment of psychopathy predict recidivism following release from prison including violent recidivism (Serin & Amos 1995).

Lack of interpersonal emotional responsiveness may be the key deficit in psychopathy. In a comparison of psychopathic and non-psychopathic prisoners, the groups did not differ in their ability to attribute correctly happiness, sadness and embarrassment to protagonists in short stories. However, in response to guilt stories, the psychopaths were more likely to attribute happiness or indifference to the protagonists (Blair *et al.* 1995). Blair *et al.* (1997) have proposed that psychopathy is associated with a failure to inhibit aggression in response to signs of distress in others, arising from a deficit in processing behavioural evidence of that distress. There is supportive evidence that, compared with other offenders, psychopathic individuals have reduced autonomic responses to distress cues (Chaplin *et al.* 1995; Blair *et al.* 1997). Several functional imaging studies have reported increased activation of the left amygdala on presentation of fearful expressions, which raises the possibility that psychopathic individuals have specific deficits in the functioning of the amygdala (Blair *et al.* 1999). It could be that psychopathy arises directly from a structural deficit, with other factors playing relatively little part. Equally, functional deficits in responsiveness to others' emotions may arise in interactions of vulnerable individuals with psychosocial adversities in childhood. In a study using a standardized investigator-based interview measure of recalled childhood experiences, psychopathic offenders reported higher rates of family adversities, such as neglect and antipathy, than non-psychopathic criminals (Marshall & Cooke 1999).

Borderline personality disorder

The overall concept of borderline personality disorder is of a pervasive pattern of instability of interpersonal relationships, self-image, affects and control over impulses. The operationalization of this concept has varied somewhat over the years, but the criteria have usually included a pattern of unstable and intense interpersonal relationships with alternating idealization and devaluation, frantic efforts to avoid real or imagined abandonment, an unstable or distorted self-image, impulsiveness, recurrent suicidal behaviour, affective instability with intense episodic dysphoria, chronic feelings of emptiness, and a lack of control over anger.

Many theories of the origins of borderline personality disorder have proposed a central role for adverse and, in particular,

traumatic experiences in childhood. If this were the case there would be a particularly important preventative role for child care and mental health professionals. Among referred individuals with borderline personality disorder, the rate of recalled sexual abuse and neglect is very high; above 90% in a study of 467 inpatients with personality disorders (Zanarini *et al.* 1997). In a comparison of borderline patients and those with other personality disorder, those in the borderline group were more likely to have been abused by a male non-caregiver, to have experienced denial of their thoughts and feelings by a male caregiver and to have experienced inconsistent treatment by a female caregiver. As we saw earlier, in a general population study of adolescents, particular patterns of mother–child interaction were associated with subsequent borderline personality disorder (Bezirganian *et al.* 1993). By contrast, in the same study, documented child sexual abuse was associated with increased symptom scores, not only for borderline functioning but also histrionic and depressive personality disorder, and neglect with a wide range of personality disorders (Johnson *et al.* 1999), suggesting a rather non-specific effect.

Although it is likely that childhood trauma and neglect have a role in the development of borderline personality disorder, very little is known regarding their importance compared with other risk factors, nor of possible causal mechanisms. In their meta-analysis covering 21 studies into possible associations between child sexual abuse and borderline personality disorder, Fossati *et al.* (1999) found there was only a moderate pooled effect size. Childhood sexual abuse and neglect are experienced by at least 20% of girls before the age of 16 (Fergusson *et al.* 2000; Hill *et al.*, 2001) and, although prevalence estimates of borderline personality disorder are lacking, it is clear that they do not come anywhere near to that level. Therefore, even if abusive or neglectful experiences were necessary for borderline personality disorder, they would not be sufficient, and it is likely that more specific aspects of childhood adversities together with other vulnerability factors need to be identified.

Identification of the role of specific aspects of childhood adversity is likely to require more precise specification of the phenomena to be explained. For example, individuals with borderline personality disorder also report more dissociative experiences (Jones *et al.* 1999). In a study of dissociative experiences among patients with borderline personality disorder, Zanarini *et al.* (2000) found that dissociative experiences were associated with particular experiences that included inconsistent behaviour by a caregiver and sexual abuse by a caregiver. There is currently no consensus on psychological mechanisms in borderline personality disorder that might provide a link with adverse experiences in childhood; however, emotional dysregulation (Linehan 1993) and failure of reflective function (Fonagy *et al.* 2000) are both promising candidates. The findings that the combination of intrusive and inconsistent mother–child interactions was associated specifically with borderline personality disorder (Bezirganian *et al.* 1993) would be consistent with a role for both of these. Intrusive parenting is likely to lead to intense affect from which the child takes evasive action to reduce affect, hence leading to the experience of extremes of emotional intensity. Inconsistent mother–child interactions are likely to inhibit the child's capacity to read the intentions or states of mind of the parent, and hence limit his or her ability to think of others' behaviours in mental state terms. If, as is often the case, the parent has also been abusive, and therefore conceiving of the parent's motives includes understanding motives for abusive behaviour, the child is likely to inhibit reflection regarding the parent, with implications for reflectiveness more generally.

Repeated self-injury, cutting, burning or hitting, is frequently observed in individuals with severe personality disorders, and is one of the diagnostic items for borderline personality disorder. It is a serious and puzzling phenomenon. There is a wide range of theories concerning the motivation for self-injury, and themes that are common to most of them are of regulation of emotions, communication and social reinforcement (Kemperman *et al.* 1997). Linehan (1993) has proposed that self-injury directly relieves painful emotions, and is reinforced by the attention and care given by others. Several studies have supported the role of self-injury in reducing painful affect. In a study of volunteers who responded to a television programme about self-harm, 66% reported that they felt better immediately after injuring themselves (Favazza & Conterio 1989). Among female offenders, those who mutilated themselves regularly were characterized by high levels of affective symptoms, and the majority reported a build-up of painful emotions prior to self-injury that were relieved by self-mutilation (Coid 1993). Kemperman *et al.* (1997) asked female inpatients with borderline personality disorder to recall changes of mood prior to, during and following self-injury, and found decreases of negative, and increases of positive, mood following self-injury. Each of these studies was limited through the use of retrospective measures with samples that in different ways were unrepresentative; however, they were consistent in finding a mood-relieving role for self-injury. However, we are left with a paradox requiring explanation, that an act that disfigures, and often is painful, improves mood. Proposals have been made that there are effects on endogenous opioids or serotonin regulation but results from a small number of investigations have been inconsistent (Kemperman *et al.* 1997).

Dissociative identity disorder

The category multiple personality disorder (MPD), renamed dissociative identity disorder (DID) in DSM-IV, has provoked considerable controversy. The diagnosis is rarely made outside of the USA and Canada (Merskey 1995), and in the USA only a minority of psychiatrists believe that DID is supported by strong evidence of scientific validity (Pope *et al.* 1999). Nevertheless, the phenomenon has been described in a range of scientific and clinical publications, and the case has been made that the symptoms can be corroborated and that in offenders there is a strong association with documented severe abuse in childhood (Lewis *et al.* 1997). It is likely that this specific manifestation of personality disorder is culturally determined and to a certain extent ia-

trogenic, but possible that disorders of similar severity and with the same risk factors are seen more widely.

Schizotypal personality disorder

The general concept of schizotypal personality disorder is that of a pervasive pattern of social and interpersonal deficits marked by acute discomfort with, and reduced capacity for, close relationships, as well as by cognitive or perceptual distortions and eccentricities of behaviour, beginning by early adulthood. It is likely that the concept of a spectrum of schizophrenic disorders, including schizotypal personality disorder, applies in the preadult years, as well as later. However, there have been only a small number of attempts to apply the criteria in childhood. One study suggested an overlap with pervasive developmental disorders, although not autism as such (Nagy & Szatmari 1986); another suggested a course similar to that of schizophrenia arising in childhood (Asarnow & Ben-Meir 1988); and a third suggested that there was a pattern of communication deficits similar to, but milder than, those found in schizophrenia (Caplin & Guthrie 1992). Olin *et al.* (1997) gathered prospective questionnaire data from teachers on 15 year olds who subsequently developed schizotypal personality disorder. Compared with a range of other groups at varying levels of risk for psychiatric disorder other than schizophrenia, the schizotypal individuals as adolescents had been more passive and unengaged and more hypersensitive to criticism.

Schizoid personality disorder

The usual concept of schizoid personality disorder is of a pervasive pattern of detachment from social relationships and a restricted range of expression of emotions in interpersonal settings (American Psychiatric Association 1994). Thus, ICD-10 criteria (World Health Organization 1992) include a lack of pleasure in activities, emotional coldness, apparent indifference to praise or criticism, a limited capacity to express either positive or negative emotions, a lack of close friends, a preference for solitary activities, a marked insensitivity to prevailing social norms and an excessive preoccupation with fantasy and introspection. The literature on the syndrome is almost confined to adults. However, since the 1970s, Wolff has pressed the case for the application of the diagnosis in childhood (Wolff & Barlow 1979). Unfortunately for comparative purposes, her criteria differ in several key respects from those generally applied with adults. She has specified increased sensitivity and paranoid ideas, whereas ICD-10 and DSM-IV indicate marked insensitivity, and she has included an unusual or odd style of communicating which would ordinarily be part of schizotypal, not schizoid, personality disorders (Wolff & Chick 1980; Wolff 1991a,b). The initial findings in childhood suggested some similarities with autism (Wolff & Barlow 1979) and the follow-up showed substantial continuity with schizotypal personality disorder in adult life (Wolff *et al.* 1991; Wolff 1995). However, a study of psychophysiological responses of adults who in childhood met Wolff's criteria for schizoid disorder failed to find abnormalities previously documented in the relatives of schizophrenic patients and adults with schizotypal personality disorder (Blackwood *et al.* 1994).

Personality disorder, development and psychopathology

It is implicit in the ideas and the findings that have been reviewed here that the set of concepts referred to broadly as personality disorder is characterized by persistent and pervasive dysfunction that is not readily accounted for by episodic disorders. Equally, the limitations of existing approaches are very evident, and the subject of substantial debate (Parker & Barrett 2000). Several issues are in particular need of investigation.

Distinction between episodic disorders and personality disorders

This distinction may, in some instances, draw the line in the wrong place. Possible reasons for the strong association between episodic (Axis I) and personality (Axis II) disorders have been reviewed above. It may be that this does not represent an association between different conditions, rather that so-called episodic disorders accompanying personality disorders are part of the same condition. Zanarini *et al.* (1998a) found that the best 'episodic' discriminator of borderline and other personality disorders was the combination of a history of disorders of mood, such as depression or anxiety, and disorders of impulse such as eating disorders. The implication could be that individuals with this combination of Axis I disorders *also* suffer from borderline personality disorder, or that this 'combination' is a reflection of underlying difficulties in affect regulation and impulsivity, both of which are probably central to borderline functioning (Linehan 1993; Links *et al.* 1999).

Concept of personality disorder

It may also be that the concept of personality disorder is not sufficiently interpersonal or developmentally sensitive. The successful development of social capabilities and attachments early in childhood are associated with a wide range of subsequent competencies, and individual competence, or lack of it, needs to be understood in relation to developmental tasks. Most current concepts and measures of personality disorder do not provide systematic approaches to interpersonal functioning or to developmental demands and this may contribute to an apparent age dependence of some personality disorders. For example, rates of offending among males decline from their 20s onwards, as do rates of antisocial personality disorder (Cloninger *et al.* 1997). However, it is possible that the interpersonal difficulties persist and that less easily detectable forms of violent behaviour, such as domestic violence, replace those seen in younger men. There may be age-related differences in the way the same underlying deficits are manifest. A focus on personality difficulties as

deficits in adult social roles may help clarify the situation. Recently, Livesley *et al.* (1998) proposed that personality disorder could be seen as a failure involving the interrelated realms of self-system, intimate relationships, and wider social and occupational interactions. This opens up the possibility that such a failure may be evident in different ways in childhood, adolescence and over adult life. This is consistent with Hill's approach to personality functioning (Hill *et al.* 1989), in which dysfunction is assessed in six domains of social role performance. Individuals with pervasive dysfunction are also likely to be judged as having personality disorder using a trait-based measure (Tyrer 1988; Hill *et al.* 2000).

Interactional features

The concepts and measures of personality disorder may not be sufficiently interactional. It is well established that children's behaviour has a powerful effect in evoking and selecting environmental experiences (see Sandberg & Rutter, Chapter 17). Although these processes have not been studied much beyond childhood, it is very likely that they apply also to adults. Some types of stressful life events have a significant heritable component because some individuals have a stable tendency to select themselves into situations that have a high probability of generating such events (Kendler *et al.* 1999). Accordingly, difficulties such as marital separation or prosecution for debts may be either (or both) stressful life events or features of personality disorder. The interplay between disordered individuals and adverse environments merits attention.

Severity of disorder

As we have seen, multiple diagnoses of personality disorder are common. Oldham *et al.* (1992) recommended that the co-occurrence of supposedly distinct personality disorders should be seen to reflect 'extensive personality disorders' implying a more severe form of disorder. The implications of severity of personality disorder have received little attention; however, a recent study of risks for alcohol dependence illustrates the issues. Bucholz *et al.* (2000) examined the extent of risk for alcohol dependence associated with severity of antisocial personality disorder symptoms contrasted with subtypes of disorder in a family genetic study of 2834 females and 3488 males. Overall, findings from both men and women did not support the existence of subtypes of antisocial personality disorder, but rather indicated a disorder distributed on a severity spectrum.

Subclinical manifestations

Patterns of persistent dysfunction falling short of the criteria for personality disorder require study. Just as variations of severity above the personality disorder threshold may be important, so may those below it. Interpersonal difficulties, which rarely amount to personality disorder, are associated with increased risk of depression (Brown *et al.* 1990; Hill *et al.* 2001). These may share childhood antecedents, and underlying biological and psychological processes, with the interpersonal difficulties seen in personality disorder.

Breadth of diagnostic category

Personality disorder may be too broad and heterogeneous a category for the investigation of some underlying causal processes. The effectiveness of the personality disorder diagnoses rests on their capacity to unify the causes, consequences or treatments of a wide range of behaviours, types of relationships and states of mind. This is clearly a possibility in some cases, but in others it may not be. For them, studies of more specific associations and processes may be needed. Examples referred to earlier include studies of the relationship between temperament and violence, neurocognitive deficits and psychopathy, and childhood experiences and dissociation.

Utility of personality disorder diagnosis in childhood and adolescence

In the light of these considerations is there an argument for applying the concept of personality disorder in adolescence or even in childhood? Given the probable heterogeneity of the personality disorders it is unlikely that there will be one answer to this question. Therefore the advantages and disadvantages will be considered in general and specific examples tested against these.

There would be a strong case if it could be shown that the category could unify diverse symptoms with a common cause, prognosis or response to treatment. It is, for example, clearly the case that the diagnosis of autism, which meets most of the requirements for personality disorder, provides an effective unifying diagnosis for diverse social and behavioural abnormalities.

Might we apply the same case in respect of conduct disorder in childhood? The case could be made that, given its strong association with poor peer relationships and educational failure, a childhood personality disorder equivalent to antisocial personality disorder in adult life should be proposed, comprising antisocial behaviours, peer problems and educational failure. There are indeed good reasons to support such a proposal. Childhood oppositional and conduct problems associated with poor peer relationships are more likely to persist (Vitaro et al. 2000), and adult antisocial outcomes are most common in children with multiple and diverse oppositional, social and educational difficulties (Stattin & Magnusson 1996).

On the other hand, the use of the personality disorder designation could introduce the limitations of the adult categories into childhood. Crucially, it would be likely to reduce our scope to investigate the links between different types of dysfunction. Vitaro et al. (2000) found that, in boys, although having a best friend who was deviant age 10 predicted delinquency at age 14, this was much less the case among those with warm relationships with their parents. Such a specific mechanism could not be investigated if poor peer relationships was an item within a childhood antisocial personality disorder. Similarly, notwithstanding the strong association of conduct disorder and attention deficit hyperactivity disorder (ADHD) and evidence that ADHD in the presence of conduct disorder increases the likelihood of persistence (Loeber et al. 1995), important genetic and neuropsychological differences would not have been identified if they had been included in a hyperactivity–conduct personality disorder.

Psychopathy in childhood

Studies paralleling those of psychopathy in adult life have identified a subgroup of antisocial children who have a high level of reported callousness and emotional indifference in their peer relationships, using a scale with similar items to those on the PCL (Frick et al. 1999). A series of studies of referred children with conduct disorder have indicated that children who are characterized as callous and unemotional differ from other children with conduct disorder in that they have lower levels of anxiety, and the extent of their antisocial problems is not associated with the quality of the parenting they receive. A recent study has reported that children who score highly on the scale of callous/unemotional characteristics have reduced psychophysiological responsiveness to distress cues (Blair 1999). At this point the identification of psychopathy in children should be regarded as promising and in need of further investigation but it is not yet clear how this group should be identified. Lynam (1998) has proposed that children comorbid for conduct problems and hyperactivity–impulsivity–attention deficits are the 'fledgling psychopaths'; however, Frick et al. argued that further identification by callous/unemotional traits is necessary (Barry et al. 2000). Compared to the volume of research on conduct disorder and ADHD, little is known about the hypothesized psychopathic group, with respect to genetic and environmental influences, or the stability of this diagnosis and its long-term outcome.

Borderline personality disorder in adolescence

Many of the studies of personality disorder in adolescence have focused on borderline personality disorder. A substantial proportion of adolescent psychiatric inpatients in the USA and the UK can be diagnosed with the disorder using adult criteria. This resembles the adult diagnosis in that there is a strong association with episodic disorders, particularly depression, and its stability is low. In adolescents, the borderline personality disorder diagnosis picks out a group who, compared with other adolescent psychiatric patients, have experienced high levels of maternal neglect and rejection, grossly inappropriate parental behaviour and a number of parental surrogates, sexual abuse (Ludolph et al. 1990) and higher levels of angry, irritable interactions in the family (James et al. 1996). Associations of inconsistent and intrusive parenting with the emergence of borderline personality disorder were found in the longitudinal study of a general population sample (Bezirganian *et al.* 1993) referred to earlier.

This study also yielded valuable findings on the relationship between episodic (Axis I) disorders and personality disorder in adolescence. Subjects with either an Axis I disorder or a personality disorder in adolescence were at increased risk for a personality disorder in adult life, but those with both were at greatly increased risk. There was evidence that the total number of episodic and personality disorders in adolescence reflected overall severity, in that the higher subjects scored on a scale of total disorders, the greater the likelihood of young adult disorder. There was some evidence that this applied particularly to the Cluster B (dramatic) disorders; however, all types were affected. These findings highlight the gains and the perils of the use of personality disorder concept in adolescence. The personality disorder assignment clearly identified dysfunction that was not reflected in the episodic disorder diagnoses. At the same time very little specificity was provided. It is possible that the episodic disorders, such as depression, contributed to social dysfunction that persisted beyond the episodes and hence increased the risk of adult personality disorder. Equally, depression may have reflected preceding family and peer difficulties, which in turn were predictive of the adult personality disorders.

Clinical implications

Clinical implications in many respects follow from these points. Children and adolescents with difficulties severe enough to merit referral frequently have multiple difficulties that go beyond the disorders currently diagnosed in childhood and early adolescence. Many of these are highly relevant to the origins, maintenance and therapeutic needs of the children's difficulties. Equally, there is a dynamic interplay between them, which blurs the edges of 'disorder'. Thus, it is important to gather information on peer and family relationships in relation to conduct problems, and yet both are likely to be consequences of the child's behaviours, and also contributors to them. In other words, the same behaviours or qualities could be seen as symptom or process, and as cause or consequence. The clinical task is to consider these various possibilities in the individual case, in order to identify areas for intervention. Similar considerations can be applied to outcome research in this area. Effectiveness must be judged not only in relation to symptomatic change, but also by whether the associated social and educational difficulties have improved.

There have not been any published studies of treatment effectiveness for personality disorders or personality dysfunction in adolescence. Studies of adult populations in relation to borderline personality disorder and chronic self-harm may provide some pointers. Perry *et al.* (1999) reviewed the results of 15 studies, and Bateman & Fonagy (2000) reviewed 25 reports of a range of psychotherapeutic approaches in adult personality disorders. Both reviews concluded that there was evidence for short- to medium-term effectiveness in a number of indices of disorder including depression and interpersonal problems, as well as personality disorder diagnosis. However, there have been very few randomized controlled studies. Linehan *et al.* (1991) carried out a randomized controlled study of outpatient dialectical behaviour therapy, a structured approach combining techniques at the level of behaviour, cognition and support. Over the year of treatment, controls were more likely to make suicide attempts and spent longer as inpatients, although these differences were not evident at 1-year follow-up (Linehan *et al.* 1993). In a recent randomized controlled trial of psychoanalytically orientated therapy, partial hospitalization for borderline personality disorder, the treated group had a lower frequency of self-harm, suicide attempts, hospital admissions, use of medication and depression, and better social adjustment over an 18-month treatment period (Bateman & Fonagy 1999). Generally, studies of effectiveness of treatment of personality disorders have used outcomes, such as service utilization or depression levels, as proxies for measures of changes in personality functioning. Tackling the difficulties associated with the current conceptualization and measurement of personality disorder should lead to improved treatment and more refined measurement of outcomes.

Bateman & Fonagy (2000) have summarized the principal features of treatments for which there is some evidence of effectiveness. The approach is active and structured with a clear focus, in the context of a strong relationship between therapist and patient over a substantial period of time. The treatment is well integrated with other services available to the patient. Effective treatments for adolescents who have extensive dysfunction, paralleling that of the adult personality disorders, may well require an approach with these features, coupled with active involvement of the family and attention to educational or vocational needs.

References

Alnaes, R. & Torgersen, S. (1997) Personality and personality disorders predict development and relapses of major depression. *Acta Psychiatrica Scandanavica*, **95**, 336–342.

American Psychiatric Association (1994) *Diagnostic and Statistical Manual of Mental Disorders DSM-IV*, 4th edn. American Psychiatric Association, Washington D.C.

Asarnow, J.R. & Ben-Meir, S. (1988) Children with schizophrenia spectrum and depressive disorders: a comparative study of pre-morbid adjustment, onset pattern and severity of impairment. *Journal of Child Psychology and Psychiatry*, **29**, 477–488.

Barry, C.T., Frick, P.J., DeShazo, T.M. *et al.* (2000) The importance of callous–unemotional traits for extending the concept of psychopathy to children. *Journal of Abnormal Psychology*, **109**, 335–340.

Bateman, A.W. & Fonagy, P. (1999) Effectiveness of partial hospitalization in the treatment of borderline personality disorder: a randomized controlled trial. *American Journal of Psychiatry*, **156**, 1563–1569.

Bateman, A.W. & Fonagy, P. (2000) Effectiveness of psychotherapeutic treatment of personality disorder. *British Journal of Psychiatry*, **177**, 138–143.

Bezirganian, S., Cohen, P. & Brook, J.S. (1993) The impact of mother–child interaction on the development of Borderline Personality Disorder. *American Journal of Psychiatry*, **150**, 1836–1842.

Blackwood, D.H., Muir, W.J., Roxborough, H.M. et al. (1994) 'Schizoid' personality in childhood: auditory P300 and eye tracking responses at follow-up in adult life. *Journal of Autism and Developmental Disorders*, **24**, 487–500.

Blair, R.J.R. (1999) Responsiveness to distress cues in the child with psychopathic tendencies. *Personality and Individual Dfferences*, **27**, 135–145.

Blair, R.J.R., Sellars, C., Strickland, I. et al. (1995) Emotion attributions in the psychopath. *Personality and Individual Differences*, **19**, 431–437.

Blair, R.J.R., Jones, L., Clark, F. & Smith, M. (1997) The psychopathic individual: a lack of responsiveness to distress cues? *Psychophysiology*, **34**, 192–198.

Blair, R.J.R., Morris, J.S., Frith, C.D., Perrett, D.I. & Dolan, R.J. (1999) Dissociable neural responses to facial expressions of sadness and anger. *Brain*, **122**, 883–893.

Brown, G.W., Bifulco, A., Veiel, H.O.S. & Andrews, B. (1990) Self-esteem and depression. *Social Psychiatry and Psychiatric Epidemiology*, **25**, 225–234.

Bucholz, K.K., Hesselbrock, V.M., Heath, A.C., Kramer, J.R. & Schuckit, M.A. (2000) A latent class analysis of antisocial personality disorder symptom data from a multi-centre family study of alcoholism. *Addiction*, **95**, 553–567.

Cadenhead, K.S., Light, G.A., Geyer, M.O. & Braff, L. (2000) Sensory gating deficits assessed by the P50 event-related potential in subjects with schizotypal personality disorder. *American Journal of Psychiatry*, **157**, 55–59.

Caplin, R. & Guthrie, D. (1992) Communication deficits in childhood schizotypal personality disorder. *Journal of the American Academy of Child and Adolescent Psychiatry*, **31**, 961–967.

Carey, G. & Goldman, D. (1997) The genetics of antisocial behaviour. In: *Handbook of Antisocial Behaviour* (eds D.M. Stoff, J. Breilling & J. Maser), pp. 243–254. Wiley, New York.

Casey, P.R. & Tyrer, P.J. (1986) Personality, functioning, and symptomatology. *Journal of Psychiatric Research*, **20**, 363–374.

Casey, P., Meagher, D. & Butler, E. (1996) Personality, functioning, and recovery from major depression. *Journal of Nervous and Mental Disease*, **184**, 240–245.

Chaplin, T.C., Rice, M.E. & Harris, G.T. (1995) Salient victim suffering and perceptual responses of child molesters. *Journal of Consulting and Clinical Psychology*, **63**, 249–255.

Cleckley, H. (1941) *The Mask of Sanity*. Henry Kimpton, London.

Cloninger, C.R. (1987) A systematic method for clinical description and classification of personality variants: a proposal. *Archives of General Psychiatry*, **44**, 573–588.

Cloninger, C.R., Bayon, C. & Przybeck, T.R. (1997) Epidemiology and Axis I comorbidity of anti-social personality. In: *Handbook of Antisocial Behaviour* (eds D.M. Stoff, J. Breiling & J.D. Maser), pp. 12–21. Wiley, New York.

Coid, J.W. (1993) An affective syndrome in psychopaths with borderline personality disorder. *British Journal of Psychiatry*, **162**, 641–650.

Cooke, D.J. (1995) Psychopathic disturbance in the Scottish prison population: cross-cultural generalisability of the Hare Psychopathy Checklist. *Psychology, Crime and Law*, **2**, 101–118.

Daley, S.E., Hammen, C., Davila, J. & Burge, D. (1998) Axis II symptomatology, depression, and life stress during the transition from adolescence to adulthood. *Journal of Consulting and Clinical Psychology*, **66**, 595–603.

Dickey, C.C., Shenton, M.E., Hirayasu, Y. et al. (2000) Large CSF volume not attributable to ventricular volume in schizotypal personality disorder. *American Journal of Psychiatry*, **157**, 48–54.

Docherty, J.P., Fister, S.J. & Shea, T. (1986) Syndrome diagnosis and personality disorder. In: *American Psychiatric Association Annual Review* (eds A.J. Frances & R.E. Hales), Vol. 5, pp. 315–355. American Psychiatric Press, Washington D.C.

Farrington, D.P. (1997) The relationship between low resting heart-rate and violence. In: *Biosocial Bases of Violence* (eds A. Raine, P.A. Brennan, D.P. Farrington & S.A. Mednick), pp. 89–105. Plenum Press, New York.

Favazza, A.R. & Conterio, K. (1989) Female habitual self-mutilators. *Acta Psychiatrica Scandinavica*, **79**, 283–289.

Fergusson, D.M. & Lynskey, M.T. & Horwood, L. (1996) Factors associated with continuity and changes in disruptive behaviour patterns between childhood and adolescence. *Journal of Abnormal Child Psychology*, **24**, 533–553.

Fergusson, D.M., Horwood, L.J. & Woodward, L.J. (2000) The stability of child abuse reports: a longitudinal study of the reporting behaviour of young adults. *Psychological Medicine*, **30**, 529–544.

Ferro, T., Klein, D.N., Schwartz, J.E., Casch, K.L. & Leader, J.D. (1998) Thirty-months' stability of personality disorder diagnoses in depressed out-patients. *American Journal of Psychiatry*, **155**, 653–659.

Fonagy, P., Target, M. & Gergely, G. (2000) Attachment and borderline personality disorder: a theory and some evidence. *Psychiatric Clinics of North America*, **23**, 103–122.

Fossati, A., Madeddu, F. & Maffei, C. (1999) Borderline personality disorder and childhood sexual abuse: a meta-analytic study. *Journal of Personality Disorders*, **13**, 268–280.

Frances, A.J. & Widiger, T. (1986) The classification of personality disorder: an overview of problems and solutions. In: *American Psychiatric Association Annual Review* (eds A.J. Frances & R.E. Hales), Vol. 5, pp. 240–258. American Psychiatric Press, Washington D.C.

Frick, P.J., Lilienfeld, S.O., Ellis, M., Loney, B. & Silverthorn, P. (1999) The association between anxiety and psychopathy dimensions in children. *Journal of Abnormal Child Psychology*, **27**, 383–392.

Gunderson, J.G., Kolb, J.E. & Austin, V. (1981) The diagnostic interview for borderline patients. *American Journal of Psychiatry*, **138**, 896–903.

Hare, R.D. (1970) *Psychopathy: Theory and Research*. John Wiley, New York.

Hare, R.D. (1971) *The Hare Psychopathy Checklist–Revised*. Multi-Health System, Toronto, Ontario.

Hare, R.D. & McPherson, L.M. (1984) Violent and aggressive behaviour by criminal psychopaths. *International Journal of Law and Psychiatry*, **7**, 35–50.

Hare, R.D., Hart, S.D. & Harpur, T.J. (1991) Psychopathy and the DSM-IV criteria for antisocial personality disorder. *Journal of Abnormal Psychology*, **100**, 391–398.

Hart, S.D. & Hare, R.D. (1989) Discriminant validity of the Psychopathy Checklist in a forensic psychiatric population. *Psychological Assessment: Journal of Consulting and Clinical Psychology*, **1**, 211–218.

Henderson, D.K. (1939) *Psychopathic States*. Norton, New York.

Henry, B., Caspi, A., Moffitt, T.E. & Silva, P.A. (1996) Temperamental and familial predictors of violent and non-violent criminal convictions: age three to eighteen. *Developmental Psychology*, **32**, 614–623.

Hill, J., Harrington, R., Fudge, H., Rutter, M. & Pickles, A. (1989) The Adult Personality Functioning Assessment: development and reliability. *British Journal of Psychiatry*, **155**, 24–35.

Hill, J., Fudge, H., Harrington, R., Pickles, A. & Rutter, M. (2000) Complementary approaches to the assessment of personality disorder: the Personality assessment Schedule and Adult Personality Functioning Assessment compared. *British Journal of Psychiatry*, **176**, 434–439.

Hill, J., Pickles, A., Burnside, E. et al. (2001) Child sexual abuse, poor parental care and adult depression: evidence for different mechanisms. *British Journal of Psychiatry*, **179**, 104–109.

James, A., Berelowitz, M. & Verker, M. (1996) Borderline personality disorder: study in adolescence. *European Child and Adolescent Psychiatry*, **5**, 11–17.

Johnson, J.G., Cohen, P., Brown, J., Smailes, E.M. & Bernstein, D.P. (1999) Childhood maltreatment increases risk for personality disorders during adulthood. *Archives of General Psychiatry*, **56**, 600–606.

Jones, B., Heard, H., Startup, M., Swales, M., Williams, J.M. & Jones, R.F. (1999) Autobiographical memory and dissociation in borderline personality disorder. *Psychological Medicine*, **29**, 1397–1404.

Kasen, S., Cohen, P., Skodol, A.E., Johnson, J.G. & Brook, J.F. (1999) Influence of child and adolescent psychiatric disorders on young adult personality disorder. *American Journal of Psychiatry*, **56**, 1529–1535.

Kass, F., Skodol, A.E., Charles, E., Spitzer, R.L. & Williams, J.B.W. (1985) Scaled ratings of DSM-III personality disorders. *American Journal of Psychiatry*, **142**, 627–630.

Kemperman, I., Russ, M.J. & Shearin, E. (1997) Self-injurious behaviour and mood regulation in borderline patients. *Journal of Personality Disorder*, **11**, 146–157.

Kendler, K.S. & Gruenberg, A.M. (1982) Genetic relationship between paranoid personality disorder and the 'schizophrenic spectrum' disorder. *American Journal of Psychiatry*, **139**, 1185–1186.

Kendler, K.S., Gruenberg, A.M. & Strauss, J.S. (1981) An independent analysis of the Copenhagen sample of the Danish Adoption Study of Schizophrenia. II. The relationship between schizotypal personality disorders and schizophrenia. *Archives of General Psychiatry*, **38**, 928–984.

Kendler, K.S., Masterson, C.C., Ungaro, O.R. & Davis, K.L. (1984) A family history study of schizophrenic related personality disorder. *American Journal of Psychiatry*, **141**, 424–427.

Kendler, K.S., Masterson, C.C. & Davis, K.L. (1985) Psychiatric illness in first-degree relatives of patients with paranoid psychosis, schizophrenia and medical illness. *British Journal of Psychiatry*, **147**, 524–532.

Kendler, K.S., Karkowski, L.M. & Prescott, C.A. (1999) The assessment of dependence in the study of stressful life events: validation using a twin-design. *Psychological Medicine*, **29**, 1455–1460.

Kernberg, O.F. (1967) Borderline personality organization. *Journal of the American Psychoanalytic Association (New York)*, **15**, 641–685.

Kernberg, O.F. (1975) *Borderline Conditions and Pathological Narcissism*. Jason Ellinson, New York.

Kerr, M., Tremblay, R.E., Pagani, L. & Vitaro, F. (1997) Boys' behavioural inhibition and the risk of later delinquency. *Archives of General Psychiatry*, **54**, 809–816.

Kety, S.S., Rosenthal, D. & Wender, P.H. (1971) Mental illness in the biological and adoptive families of adopted schizophrenics. *American Journal of Psychiatry*, **128**, 302–306.

Kuyken, W., Kuvzer, N., De Rubeis, R.J., Beck, A.T. & Brown, G.K. (2001) Response to cognitive therapy in depression: the role of maladaptive beliefs and personality disorders. *Journal of Consulting and Clinical Psychiatry*, **69**, 560–566.

Langbehn, D.R., Cadoret, R.J., Yates, W.R., Troughton, E.P. & Stewart, M.A. (1998) *Archives of General Psychiatry*, **55**, 821–829.

Lenzenweger, M.S. (1999) Stability and change in personality disorder features: the longitudinal study of personality disorders. *Archives of General Psychiatry*, **56**, 1009–1015.

Lewis, D.O., Yeager, C.A., Swica, Y., Pincus, J.H. & Lewis, M. (1997) Objective documentation of child abuse and dissociation in twelve murderers with dissociative identity disorder. *American Journal of Psychiatry*, **154**, 1703–1710.

Linehan, M.M. (1993) *Cognitive Behavioural Therapy of Borderline Personality Disorder*. Guilford Press, New York.

Linehan, M.M., Armstrong, H.E., Suarez, A. *et al.* (1991) Cognitive-behavioural treatment of chronically parasuicidal borderline patients. *Archives of General Psychiatry*, **48**, 1060–1064.

Linehan, M.M., Heard, H.L. & Armstrong, H.E. (1993) Naturalistic follow-up of a behavioural treatment for chronically parasuicidal borderline patients. *Archives of General Psychiatry*, **50**, 971–974.

Links, P.F., Heslegraver, R. & van Reekum, R. (1999) Impulsivity: poor aspect of borderline personality disorder. *Journal of Personality Disorders*, **13**, 1–9.

Livesley, W.J., Jang, K.L. & Vernon, P.A. (1998) Phenotypic and genetic structure of traits delineating personality disorder. *Archives of General Psychiatry*, **55**, 941–948.

Loeber, R., Green, S.M., Keenan, K. & Lahey, B.B. (1995) Which boys will fare worse? Early predictors of the onset of conduct disorder in a six-year longitudinal study. *Journal of the American Academy of Child and Adolescent Psychiatry*, **34**, 499–509.

Loranger, A.W., Lenzenweger, M.F., Gartner, A.F. *et al.* (1991) Trait–state artefacts and the diagnosis of personality disorders. *Archives of General Psychiatry*, **48**, 720–728.

Ludolph, P.S., Westen, D., Misle, B., Jackson, A., Wixom, M.A. & Wiss, C. (1990) The borderline diagnosis in adolescence: symptoms and developmental history. *Archives of General Psychiatry*, **147**, 470–476.

Lynam, D.R. (1998) Early identification of the fledgling psychopath: locating the psychopathic child in the current nomenclature. *Journal of Abnormal Psychology*, **107**, 566–575.

Maier, W., Franke, P. & Hawallek, B. (1998) Special feature: family-genetic research strategies for personality disorders. *Journal of Personality Disorders*, **12**, 262–276.

Marshall, L.A. & Cooke, D.J. (1999) The childhood experiences of psychopaths: a retrospective study of familial and societal factors. *Journal of Personality Disorders*, **13**, 211–225.

McGuffin, P. & Thapar, A. (1992) The genetics of personality disorders. *British Journal of Psychiatry*, **160**, 12–23.

Meehl, P.E. (1962) Schizotaxia, schizotypy, schizophrenia. *American Psychologist*, **17**, 827–838.

Merikangas, K.R. & Weissman, M.M. (1986) Epidemiology of DSM-III Axis II personality disorders. In: *American Psychiatric Association Annual Review* (eds A.J. Frances & R.E. Hales), Vol. 5, pp. 258–278. American Psychiatric Press, Washington D.C.

Merskey, H. (1995) Multiple personality disorder and false memory syndrome. *British Journal of Psychiatry*, **166**, 281–283.

Moffitt, T.E., Caspi, A., Dickson, N., Silva, P. & Stanton, W. (1996) Childhood-onset versus adolescent-onset antisocial conduct problems in males: natural history from ages three to eighteen years. *Development and Psychopathology*, **8**, 399–424.

Morey, L.C. (1988) Personality disorders in DSM-III and DSM-III-R: convergence, coverage and internal consistency. *American Journal of Psychiatry*, **145**, 573–577.

Nagy, J. & Szatmari, P. (1986) A chart review of schizotypal personality disorders in children. *Journal of Autism and Developmental Disorders*, **16**, 351–367.

Nierenberg, A.A., Keefe, B.R., Leslie, B.C. *et al.* (1999) Residual symptoms in depressed patients who respond acutely to fluoxetine. *Journal of Clinical Psychiatry*, **60**, 221–225.

Oldham, J.M., Skodol, A.E., Kellman, H.D., Hyler, S.E., Rosnick, L. & Davies, M. (1992) Diagnosis of DSM-III-R personality disorders and two structured interviews: patterns of comorbidity. *American Journal of Psychiatry*, **149**, 213–220.

Olin, S.S., Raine, A., Cannon, T.D., Parnas, J., Schulsinger, F. & Mednick, F.A. (1997) Childhood behavior predictors of schizotypal personality disorder. *Schizophrenia Bulletin*, **23**, 93–103.

Ormel, J. & Wohlfarth, T. (1991) How neuroticism, long-term difficulties and life situation change influence psychological distress: a longitudinal model. *Journal of Personality and Social Psychology*, **60**, 744–755.

Parker, G. & Barrett, E. (2000) Personality and personality disorder: current issues and directions. *Psychological Medicine*, **30**, 1–9.

Parker, G., Roy, K., Wilhelm, K., Mitchell, P., Austin, M.P. & Hadzi-Pavlovic, D. (1999) An exploration of links between early parenting experiences and personality disorder type and disordered personality functioning. *Journal of Personality Disorders*, **13**, 361–374.

Patience, D.A., McGuire, R.J., Scott, A.I. & Freeman. C.P. (1995) The Edinburgh Primary Care Depression Study: personality disorder and outcome. *British Journal of Psychiatry*, **167**, 324–330.

Perry, J.C., Bannon, E. & Ianni, F. (1999) Effectiveness of psychotherapy for personality disorders. *American Journal of Psychiatry*, **156**, 1312–1321.

Pfohl, B., Coryell, W., Zimmerman, M. & Tsangl, D.A. (1986) DSM-III personality disorders: diagnostic overlap and internal consistency of individual DSM-III criteria. *Comprehensive Psychiatry*, **27**, 21–34.

Pope, H.G., Oliva, P.F., Hudson, J.I., Bodkin, J.A. & Gruber, A.J. (1999) Attitudes toward DSM-IV dissociative disorders diagnoses among board-certified American psychiatrists. *American Journal of Psychiatry*, **156**, 321–323.

Quinton, D., Pickles, A., Maughan, B. & Rutter, M. (1993) Partners, peers, and pathways: assortative pairing and continuities in conduct disorder. *Development and Psychopathology*, **5**, 763–783.

Quinton, D., Gulliver, L. & Rutter, M. (1995) A 15–20-year follow-up of adult psychiatric patients: psychiatric disorder and social functioning. *British Journal of Psychiatry*, **167**, 315–323.

Raine, A., Lencz, T., Bihrile, S., LaCasse, L. & Colletti, P. (2000) Reduced prefrontal grey matter volume and reduced autonomic activity in antisocial personality disorder. *Archives of General Psychiatry*, **57**, 119–127.

Reich, J.A. & Green, A. (1991) Effect of personality disorders on outcome of treatments. *Journal of Nervous and Mental Disease*, **179**, 74–82.

Robins, C.J., Ladd, J., Welkowitz, J., Blaney, P.A., Diaz, R. & Kutcher, G. (1994) The personal style inventory: preliminary validation studies of new measures of sociotropy and autonomy. *Journal of Psychopathology and Behavioural Assessment*, **16**, 277–230.

Robins, L.N. (1966) *Deviant Children Grown Up*. Williams & Wilkins, Baltimore, MD.

Robins, L.N. (1978) Sturdy childhood predictors of adult antisocial behaviour: replications from longitudinal studies. *Psychological Medicine*, **8**, 611–622.

Robins, L.N., Tipp, J. & Przybeck, T. (1991) Antisocial personality. In: *Psychiatric Disorders in America: the Epidemiologic Catchment Area Study* (eds L.N. Robins & D. Regier), pp. 258–290. Free Press, New York.

Rutter, M. (1977) Prospective studies to investigate behavioural change. In: *The Origins and Course of Psychopathology* (eds J.S. Strauss, H.M. Benbabigian & N. Rolff), pp. 223–247. Plenum, New York.

Rutter, M. (1987) Temperament, personality and personality disorder. *British Journal of Psychiatry*, **150**, 433–458.

Rutter, M. & Quinton, D. (1984) Parental psychiatric disorder: effects on children. *Psychological Medicine*, **14**, 853–880.

Rutter, M., Quinton, D. & Hill, J. (1990) Adult outcome of institution-reared children: males and females compared. In: *Straight and Devious Pathways from Childhood to Adulthood* (eds L. Robins & M. Rutter), pp. 135–157. Cambridge University Press, Cambridge.

Sampson, R.J. & Laub, J.H. (1993) Crime and deviance in the life cause. *Annual Review of Sociology*, **18**, 63–84.

Schneider, K. (1923) *Diepsychopathischen Personlichkeiten*. Springer, Berlin.

Schneider, K. (1950) *Psychopathic Personalities*, 9th edn. [English Translation, 1958.] Cassell, London.

Serin, R.C. & Amos, N.L. (1995) The role of psychopathy in the assessment of dangerousness. *International Journal of Law and Psychiatry*, **18**, 231–238.

Shea, M.Y., Pilkonis, P.A., Beckham, E. *et al.* (1990) Personality disorders and treatment outcome in the NIMH treatment of depression collaborative research programme. *American Journal of Psychiatry*, **147**, 711–718.

Simonoff, E. (2001) Genetic influences on conduct disorder. In: *Conduct Disorders in Childhood and Adolescence* (eds J. Hill & B. Maughan), pp. 202–234. Cambridge University Press, Cambridge.

Spitzer, R.L., Endicott, J. & Gibbon, A.M. (1979) Crossing the border into borderline personality and borderline schizophrenia: the development of criteria. *Archives of General Psychiatry*, **36**, 17–24.

Stattin, H. & Magnusson, D. (1996) Antisocial development: a holistic approach. *Development and Psychopathology*, **8**, 617–645.

Tyrer, P., ed. (1988) *Personality Disorders: Diagnosis, Management and Course*. Right, London.

Tyrer, P., Casey, P. & Ferguson, B. (1991) Personality disorder in perspective. *British Journal of Psychiatry*, **159**, 463–472.

Tyrer, P., Merson, S., Onyett, S. & Johnson, T. (1994) The effect of personality disorder on clinical outcome, social networks and adjustment: a controlled clinical trial of psychiatric emergencies. *Psychological Medicine*, **24**, 731–740.

Vitaro, F., Brendgen, M. & Tremblay, R.E. (2000) Influence of deviant friends on delinquency: searching for moderator variables. *Journal of Abnormal Psychology*, **28**, 313–326.

Vollrath, M., Alnaes, R. & Torgersen, S. (1994) Coping and MCMI-II personality disorders. *Journal of Personality Disorders*, **8**, 53–63.

Widiger, T.A. & Costa, P.T. (1994) Personality and personality disorders. *Journal of Abnormal Psychology*, **103**, 78–91.

Wolff, S. (1991a) 'Schizoid' personality in childhood and adult life. I. The vagaries of diagnostic labelling. *British Journal of Psychiatry*, **159**, 615–619.

Wolff, S. (1991b) 'Schizoid' personality in childhood and adult life. III. The childhood picture. *British Journal of Psychiatry*, **159**, 629–635.

Wolff, S. (1995) *Loners: the Life Path of Unusual Children*. Routledge, London.

Wolff, S. & Barlow, A. (1979) Schizoid personality in childhood: a comparative study of schizoid, autistic and normal children. *Journal of Child Psychology and Psychiatry*, **20**, 29–46.

Wolff, S. & Chick, J. (1980) Schizoid personality in childhood: a controlled follow-up study. *Psychological Medicine*, **10**, 85–20.

Wolff, S., Townshend, R., McGuire, R.J. & Weeks, D.J. (1991) 'Schizoid' personality in childhood and adult life. II Adult adjustment and the continuity with schizotypal personality disorder. *British Journal of Psychiatry*, **159**, 620–628.

World Health Organization (1992). *ICD-10: the ICD-10 Classification of Mental and Behavioural Disorders. Clinical Description and Diagnostic Guidelines*. World Health Organization, Geneva.

Zanarini, M.C., Williams, A.A., Lewis, R.E. *et al.* (1997) Reported pathological childhood experiences associated with the development of borderline personality disorder. *American Journal of Psychiatry*, **154**, 1101–1106.

Zanarini, M.C., Frankenburg, F.R., Dubo, E.D. *et al.* (1998a) Axis II comorbidity of borderline personality disorder. *Comprehensive Psychiatry*, **39**, 296–302.

Zanarini, M.C., Frankenburg, F.R., Dubo, E.D. *et al.* (1998b) Axis I comorbidity of borderline personality disorder. *American Journal of Psychiatry*, **155**, 1733–1739.

Zanarini, M.C., Ruser, T.F., Frankeburg, F.R., Hennen, J. & Gunderson,

J.G. (2000) Risk factors associated with the dissociative experiences of borderline patients. *Journal of Nervous and Mental Disease*, **188**, 26–30.

Zimmerman, M. & Mattia, J.A. (1999) Axis I diagnostic comorbidity and borderline personality disorder. *Comprehensive Psychiatry*, **40**, 245–252.

Zoccolillo, M., Pickles, A., Quinton, D. & Rutter, M. (1992) The outcome of childhood conduct disorder: implications for defining adult personality disorder and conduct disorder. *Psychological Medicine*, **22**, 971–986.

44 Gender Identity Disorder
Kenneth J. Zucker

Introduction

This chapter provides an overview of seven aspects of our knowledge about gender identity disorder (GID) in children and adolescents:

1 phenomenology;
2 epidemiology;
3 diagnosis and assessment;
4 associated psychopathology;
5 aetiology;
6 long-term follow-up; and
7 treatment.

Terminology

Six terms that will be used throughout are briefly described. These are:

1 sex;
2 gender;
3 gender identity;
4 gender role (masculinity–femininity);
5 sexual orientation; and
6 sexual identity.

Sex

Sex refers to attributes that collectively, and usually harmoniously, characterize biological maleness and femaleness. In humans, the most well-known attributes that constitute biological sex include the sex-determining genes, the sex chromosomes, the H-Y antigen, the gonads, sex hormones, the internal reproductive structures, and the external genitalia (Migeon & Wisniewski 1998). Over the past couple of decades, there has also been great interest in the possibility that the human brain has certain sex-dimorphic neuroanatomical structures which, perhaps, emerge during the process of prenatal physical sex differentiation (for recent developments in understanding aspects of biological sex, see Haqq & Donahoe 1998; Vilain & McCabe 1998).

Gender

Gender is often used to refer to psychological or behavioural characteristics associated with males and females (Ruble &

Martin 1998). The use of gender as a technical term is a recent phenomenon. As late as the mid-1950s, it was not even part of the professional literature that purported to study psychological similarities and differences between males and females. In fact, the first term introduced to the literature was that of *gender role*, not gender (Money 1955).

Over the past 40 years, three major developments have occurred with regard to the usage of the terms 'sex' and 'gender'. First, there has been a tendency to conflate the use of the two terms, so that it is not always clear if one is referring to biological or psychological characteristics that distinguish males from females (Gentile 1993). Secondly, the use of the terms 'sex' and 'gender' has been related to assumptions about causality, in that the former is used to refer exclusively to biological processes and the latter is used to refer exclusively to psychological or sociological processes (for critiques of this division, see Money 1985; Maccoby 1988). As a result, some researchers who study humans employ such terms as *sex-typical*, *sex-dimorphic*, and *sex-typed* to characterize sex differences in behaviour, because terms of this kind are descriptively more neutral with regard to putative aetiology. The third development, as noted by Zucker & Bradley (1995), is that Money's original use of the term 'gender role' has been decomposed into three conceptually distinct component parts that are identified by the terms 'gender identity', 'gender role' and 'sexual orientation'.

Gender identity

Gender identity was introduced into the professional lexicon by Hooker and by Stoller in the early 1960s (Money 1985). Stoller (1964, p. 453) used the slightly different term *core gender identity* to describe a young child's developing 'fundamental sense of belonging to one sex'. This term was later adopted by cognitive-developmental psychologists, such as Kohlberg (1966), who defined gender identity as the child's ability to discriminate accurately males from females and then to identify his or her own gender status correctly—a task considered by some to be the first 'stage' in 'gender constancy' development, the end state of which is the knowledge of gender invariance (Kohlberg 1966; Eaton & Von Bargen 1981).

Gender role

Gender role has been used extensively by developmental psychologists to refer to behaviours, attitudes and personality traits that a society, in a given culture and historical period, designates as masculine or feminine, i.e. those more 'appropriate' to, or typical of, the male or female social role (Ruble & Martin 1998). It should be remembered that defining gender roles in this way assumes that they are completely arbitrary and social in origin, a view not universally shared by researchers in the field. In any case, from a descriptive point of view, the measurement of gender role behaviour in young children includes several easily observable phenomena, including affiliative preference for same-sex vs. opposite-sex peers, roles in fantasy play, toy interests, dress-up play, and interest in rough-and-tumble play. In older children, gender role has also been measured using personality attributes with stereotypic masculine or feminine connotations (Ruble & Martin 1998).

Sexual orientation

Sexual orientation is defined by a person's relative responsiveness to sexual stimuli. The most salient dimension of sexual orientation is probably the sex of the person to whom one is attracted sexually. This stimulus class is obviously how one defines a person's sexual orientation, or erotic partner preference, as heterosexual, bisexual or homosexual. In contemporary sexology, sexual orientation is often assessed by psychophysiological techniques, such as penile plethysmography or vaginal photoplethysmography (Rosen & Beck 1988), although structured interview assessments have become increasingly common, particularly when respondents do not have a compelling reason to conceal their sexual orientation.

Sexual identity

It is important to uncouple the construct of sexual orientation from the construct of *sexual identity*. A person may, for example, be predominantly aroused by homosexual stimuli, yet not regard himself or herself as 'a homosexual', for whatever reason. Sociologists, particularly those of the 'social scripting' and 'social constructionist' schools, have articulated this notion most forcefully, arguing that the incorporation of sexual orientation into one's sense of identity is a relatively recent phenomenon, culturally variable, and the result of a complex interplay of sociohistorical events (Gagnon 1990; Weeks 1991). Anthropologists, such as Herdt (1981), who have described ritualized age-structured homosexual behaviour in non-Western cultures, note that such behaviour is not at all tied to a homosexual sexual identity, but rather is a rite of passage to mature adult heterosexuality.

In contemporary Western culture, there are many individuals who are primarily or exclusively sexually responsive to same-sex persons, yet do not adopt a homosexual or 'gay' identity (Ross 1983). Moreover, there are also individuals who engage in extensive homosexual behaviour, yet who are not predominantly aroused by homosexual stimuli or do not consider themselves to 'be' homosexual, such as among male adolescents who have

sex with men for money. Thus, one must pay attention to the empirical evidence regarding disjunctions between sexual orientation and sexual identity (for a detailed analysis see Laumann *et al.* 1994).

Phenomenology

Boys and girls diagnosed with GID as described in the fourth edition of the Diagnostic and Statistical Manual (DSM-IV) (American Psychiatric Association 2000), or in ICD-10 (World Health Organization 1992), display an array of sex-typed behaviour signalling a strong psychological identification with the opposite sex. These behaviours include:

1 identity statements;
2 dress-up play;
3 toy play;
4 roles in fantasy play;
5 peer relations;
6 motoric and speech characteristics;
7 statements about sexual anatomy; and
8 involvement in rough-and-tumble play.

In general, there is a strong preference for sex-typed behaviours more characteristic of the opposite sex and a rejection or avoidance of sex-typed behaviours more characteristic of one's own sex. There are also signs of distress and discomfort about one's status as a boy or a girl, including verbal expressions of dislike or disgust about one's genital anatomy. The behaviours that characterize GID in children occur in concert, not in isolation. It is this behavioural patterning that is of clinical significance, and recognition of the patterning is extremely important in conducting a diagnostic assessment.

The onset of most of the behaviours occurs during the preschool years (2–4 years), if not earlier. Clinical referral often occurs when parents begin to feel that the pattern of behaviour is no longer a 'phase', a common initial parental appraisal, that their child will 'grow out of' (Stoller 1967; Zucker 2000a). From a developmental perspective, the onset occurs during the same period that more typical sex-dimorphic behaviours can be observed in young children (Ruble & Martin 1998). For a more detailed account of phenomenology, see Green (1974) and Zucker & Bradley (1995).

Epidemiology

Prevalence

The prevalence of GID in children has not been formally studied by epidemiological methods. Nevertheless, Meyer-Bahlburg's (1985) characterization of GID as a 'rare phenomenon' is not unreasonable. Prevalence estimates of GID in adults suggest an occurrence of 1 in 24000–37000 men and 1 in 103000–150000 women (Meyer-Bahlburg 1985). Subsequently, Bakker *et al.* (1993) inferred the prevalence of adult GID in the Netherlands from the number of persons receiving 'cross-gender' hormonal treatment at the main adult gender identity clinic in that country: 1 in 11 000 men and 1 in 30 400 women.

However, this approach suffers from at least three limitations. First, it relies on the number of persons who attend specialty clinics serving as gateways for surgical and hormonal sex reassignment, which may not see all gender-dysphoric adults. Secondly, unlike adult females with gender dysphoria, who are almost always attracted sexually to biological females, adult males with GID are about equally likely to be attracted sexually to biological males or females (Blanchard *et al.* 1987). A childhood history of GID, or its subclinical manifestation, occurs largely among gender-dysphoric adults with a homosexual sexual orientation. Estimates of the prevalence of GID in childhood inferred from the prevalence of GID in adult males should take this into account. Thirdly, the assumption that GID in children will persist into adulthood is not necessarily true (see below). It is likely therefore that the prevalence of GID is higher in children than it is in adults.

Another approach to the estimate of prevalence can borrow from normative studies of children in whom specific cross-gender behaviours were assessed (Zucker 1985, pp. 87–95). One source of information comes from the widely used Child Behavior Checklist (CBCL; Achenbach & Edelbrock 1983), a parent-report behaviour problem questionnaire with excellent psychometric properties. It includes two items (out of 118) that pertain to cross-gender identification: 'behaves like opposite sex' and 'wishes to be of opposite sex'. On the CBCL, ratings are made on a 3-point scale (0, not true; 1, somewhat or sometimes true; and 2, very true or often true). In the standardization study, endorsement of both items was more common for girls than for boys, regardless of age and clinical status (referred vs. non-referred).

As reported by Zucker *et al.* (1997a), among non-referred boys (ages 4–11 years), 3.8% received a rating of 1 and 1.0% a rating of 2 for the item 'behaves like opposite sex', but only 1.0% received a rating of 1 and 0.0% a rating of 2 for the item 'wishes to be of opposite sex.' The comparable percentages among non-referred girls was 8.3, 2.3, 2.5 and 1.0%, respectively. These findings suggest that there is a sex difference in the occurrence of mild displays of cross-gender behaviour, but not with regard to more extreme cross-gender behaviour. Similar results were obtained from the Achenbach, Connors, and Quay Behaviour Checklist (ACQ; Achenbach *et al.* 1991), which contains three items pertaining to cross-gender identification out of a total of 215 (two from the original CBCL and a third, 'Dresses like or plays at being opposite sex'; for details see Zucker *et al.* 1997a).

The main problem with such data is that they do not adequately identify patterns of cross-gender behaviour that would be of use in determining 'caseness.' Thus, such data may be best viewed as screening devices for more intensive evaluation (Pleak *et al.* 1989; Sandberg *et al.* 1993).

Incidence

Lothstein (1983) speculated, on clinical grounds, that parents who had been influenced by the cultural *Zeitgeist* to use 'non-sexist' socialization techniques may have inadvertently induced gender identity conflict in their children. However, there are no systematic data regarding changes, or the lack thereof, in the incidence of GID over the past several decades.

Sex differences in referral rates

Consistently, it has been observed that boys are referred more often than girls for concerns regarding gender identity. This has been reflected in both research and clinical reports of treatment. In our own clinic, Zucker *et al.* (1997a) reported a referral ratio of 6.6 : 1 (*n* = 275) of boys to girls.

How might this disparity be best understood? One possibility is that the sex difference in referral rates reflects a true sex difference in prevalence. Another possibility is that social factors have a role in accounting for the disparity. For example, it is well established that parents, teachers and peers are less tolerant of cross-gender behaviour in boys than in girls (Fagot 1985), which might result in a sex-differential in clinical referral (for review see Zucker & Bradley 1995). Weisz & Weiss (1991) devised a 'referability index' (RI) which reflected the frequency with which a child problem, adjusted for its prevalence in the general population, resulted in a clinic referral. All 118 items from the CBCL were analysed in a comparison of clinic-referred and non-referred children. Among parents in the USA, the 20 most referable problems (e.g. vandalism, poor schoolwork, attacks people) appeared to be relatively serious. In contrast, the 20 least referable problems (e.g. bragging, teases a lot, likes to be alone) appeared less so. Weiss (personal communication, March 4, 1992) indicated that, for boys, the CBCL item 'wishes to be of opposite sex' had an RI of 91/118 (in the upper quartile) and 'behaves like opposite sex' had an RI of 80/118. For girls, the RI was lower: 55/118 for 'wishes to be of opposite sex' and 14/118 for 'behaves like opposite sex'. Weisz & Weiss' (1991) study, together with studies from the normative literature, led us to predict that referred girls would display more extreme cross-gender behaviour than referred boys, which might account, at least in part, for the disparity by sex in referral rates. Zucker *et al.* (1997a) provided some data that supported this prediction, suggesting therefore that girls may need to display more cross-gender behaviour than boys before a referral is initiated. However, it is important to note that the sexes did not differ in the percentage who met the complete DSM criteria for GID; thus, there was no gross evidence for a sex difference in false-positive referrals.

Diagnosis and assessment

Diagnosis

DSM-IV diagnosis of gender identity disorder

In DSM-IV, there were some changes in the conceptualization of GID and in the diagnostic criteria; for example, there was a reduction of diagnostic categories from three to one between DSM-III-R (American Psychiatric Association 1987) and DSM-IV. The DSM-IV Subcommittee on Gender Identity Disorders (Bradley *et al.* 1991) took the position that the DSM-III-R diagnoses of gender identity disorder of childhood, transsexualism, and gender identity disorder of adolescence or adulthood, non-transsexual type were not qualitatively distinct disorders, but reflected differences in both developmental and severity parameters. As a result, the DSM-IV Subcommittee recommended one overarching diagnosis, gender identity disorder, that could be used, with appropriate variations in criteria, across the life cycle.

In DSM-IV, three criteria are required for the diagnosis, with one exclusion criterion. The first criterion (A) reflects the child's cross-gender identification, indexed by five behavioural characteristics, of which at least four must be present. The second criterion (B) reflects the child's rejection of his or her anatomic status and/or rejection of same-sex stereotypical activities and behaviours. The third criterion (D) specifies that the 'disturbance . . . causes clinically significant distress or impairment in social, occupational, or other important areas of functioning' (American Psychiatric Association 2000, p. 581). The exclusion criterion (C) pertains to the presence of a physical intersex condition (for discussion on this point see Meyer-Bahlburg 1994).

Reliability and validity

Can the DSM-IV diagnosis of GID be made reliably? Because the criteria have changed and because no field trials were conducted, this question cannot yet be answered; however, previous versions of the criteria have shown strong evidence for both reliability and validity (Zucker & Bradley 1995).

Distress and impairment

As noted by Zucker (1992), the DSM-III-R did not provide guidelines regarding the assessment of distress in the A criterion ('persistent and intense distress' about being a boy or a girl) or the ways in which it might be distinct from other operationalized components in the criteria (the 'desire' to be of the other sex). In the DSM-IV, this problem persists, except that it is now located in D, and there is the additional problem of defining impairment.

The inclusion of a distress/impairment criterion ('a clinical significance criterion'; American Psychiatric Association 2000, p. 8) is not unique to GID; in fact, this criterion now appears in most of the DSM-IV diagnoses. Very little empirical work preceded the introduction of the criterion (Spitzer & Wakefield 1999). Indeed, the DSM-IV states that assessment of distress and impairment 'is an inherently difficult clinical judgement' (American Psychiatric Association 2000, p. 8).

For children with GID, we need to ask two interrelated questions: are they distressed by their condition, and, if so, what is the source of the distress? Regarding these questions, there are two broad views. One view is that children with GID become distressed about their cross-gender behaviour only after it has been interfered with (Stoller 1975). Stoller argued that marked cross-gender identification (in boys) was ego-syntonic because the putative familial psychodynamics that produced it were systemically syntonic. The other view is that the distress is caused by psychopathology in the child and in the family. Coates & Person (1985) claimed that GID is a 'solution' to specific forms of psychopathology in the child, particularly separation anxiety and 'annihilation' anxiety, which were induced by familial psychopathology.

It is conceivable that both views are correct or that one or the other better fits individual cases. However, the latter view is more compatible with the notion of inherent distress, whereas the former is more compatible with the notion that social pathology creates individual pathology. Clinical experience suggests that many youngsters with GID feel a sense of discomfort regarding their status as boys or girls from a very early age, which matches nicely with the DSM notion of distress. Nevertheless, there are youngsters in whom the behavioural characteristics of GID appear to be ego-syntonic and who experience distress only when their cross-gender behaviour is interfered with. The exact manner in which we should measure the putative distress of children with GID has not been worked out (Zucker 1999a); this holds true not only for GID but also for all of the other childhood psychiatric conditions that include the distress/impairment criterion.

Regarding impairment, there are several domains that this might be manifest in children with GID. Such children seem to have more trouble than others with basic cognitive concepts concerning their gender. Zucker *et al.* (1993b) found that children with GID were more likely than controls to misclassify their own gender. Zucker *et al.* (1999b) provided additional evidence that children with GID appeared to have a 'developmental lag' in the acquisition of gender constancy. Given the ubiquity of gender as a social category, this may well lead to affective confusion in self-representation and in social interactions. There is also evidence that children with GID have poorer peer relations than controls and more general behavioural problems, possible indices of impairment (Zucker & Bradley 1995; Zucker *et al.* 1997a).

Assessment

Biomedical tests

There are no known biological markers that can identify children with GID. Gross parameters of biological sex, such as the sex chromosomes and the appearance of the external genitalia, are invariably normal. Because gender identity conflict is overrepresented among specific physical intersex conditions, particularly congenital adrenal hyperplasia (CAH) in genetic females, partial androgen-insensitivity syndrome in genetic males reared as girls, and in genetic males with cloacal exstrophy reared as girls (for review see Meyer-Bahlburg 1994; Zucker 1999b), it is important to enquire about any physical signs of these conditions; however, it is rare that these conditions have not already been diagnosed prior to a clinical assessment for GID.

Psychological tests

A number of parent-report and behavioural measures can be used to assess sex-typed behaviour in children with GID (Zucker 1992; Zucker & Bradley 1995). No one test is a replacement for a diagnosis that is established by a clinical interview that covers the behavioural signs for GID. Nevertheless, these measures have strong discriminant validity and constitute one strong line of evidence that GID is, in fact, a distinct syndrome. As reviewed elsewhere, data from psychological tests show a consistent pattern in that the percentage of false-positives appears to be lower than the percentage of false-negatives (Zucker 1992; Zucker & Bradley 1995).

One useful clinical instrument is the Gender Identity Interview for Children, shown in Table 44.1. Based on factor analysis, Zucker et al. (1993b) identified two factors: Affective Gender Confusion (questions 6–12) and Cognitive Gender Confusion (questions 1–4). Cut-off scores of either three or four deviant responses yielded high specificity rates (88.8 and 93.9%, respectively), but lower sensitivity rates (54.1 and 65.8%, respectively).

Table 44.1 Gender identity interview for children (boy version). (From Zucker *et al.* (1993b)

1 Are you a boy or a girl? BOY/GIRL
2 Are you a (opposite of first response)?
3 When you grow up, will you be a Mommy or a Daddy? MOMMY/DADDY
4 Could you ever grow up to be a (opposite of first response)? YES/NO
5 Are there any good things about being a boy? YES/NO
   If YES, say: Tell me some of the good things about being a boy (probe for a maximum of three responses)
6 Are there any things that you don't like about being a boy? YES/NO
   If YES, say: Tell me some of the things that you don't like about being a boy (probe for a maximum of three responses)
7 Do you think it is better to be a boy or a girl? YES/NO
   Why? (probe for a maximum of three responses)
8 In your mind, do you ever think that you would like to be a girl? YES/NO
   If YES, ask: Can you tell me why? (probe for a maximum of three responses)
9 In your mind, do you ever get mixed up and you're not sure if you are a boy or a girl? YES/NO
   If YES, say: Tell me more about that (probe until satisfied)
10 Do you ever feel more like a girl than like a boy? YES/NO
   If YES, say: Tell me more about that (probe until satisfied)
11 You know what dreams are, right? Well, when you dream at night, are you ever in the dream?
   If YES, ask: In your dreams, are you a boy, a girl, or sometimes a boy and sometimes a girl?
   BOY/GIRL/BOTH/NOT IN DREAMS (probe regarding content of dreams)
12 Do you ever think that you really are a girl? YES/NO
   If YES, say: Tell me more about that (probe until satisfied)

Associated psychopathology

Comorbidity (the presence of two or more psychiatric disorders) occurs frequently among children referred for psychiatric evaluation. Assuming that the putative comorbid conditions actually represent distinct disorders, it is important to know, for various reasons (e.g. prevention and treatment planning), whether one condition increases the risk for the other condition or if the conditions are caused by distinct or overlapping factors (Caron & Rutter 1991).

Among children with GID, several measurement approaches have been employed to address this matter, including standardized behaviour problem questionnaires, ratings of social behaviour in structured situations and on questionnaires, assessment of personality functioning and structure on projective tests, assessment of quality of attachment with the mother, and ascertainment of other psychiatric disorders. Most of this work has focused on boys with GID, for which a detailed summary may be found elsewhere (Zucker & Bradley 1995).

The greatest amount of information on general behaviour

problems comes from parent-report data using the CBCL and the Teacher's Report Form (Achenbach & Edelbrock 1986). On these measures, clinic-referred boys and girls with GID show significantly more general behaviour problems than their siblings and non-referred ('normal') children. Given that the siblings and non-referred children do not engage, on average, in marked cross-gender role behaviour, this might be construed as evidence for a relation between cross-gender role behaviour and general behaviour problems. The situation is clearly more complicated than this because demographically matched clinical controls (who, on average, show typical gender role behaviour) show comparable levels of behaviour problems to the children with GID (Zucker & Bradley 1995).

On the CBCL, boys with GID have a predominance of emotional difficulties, whereas girls with GID do not (Zucker & Bradley 1995). Boys with GID have also been found to show high rates of separation anxiety traits (Coates & Person 1985; Zucker et al. 1996a; Birkenfeld-Adams 1999). At present, reasons for this associated psychopathology have been best studied in boys with GID (Zucker & Bradley 1995). CBCL behaviour problems are positively associated with age, which may reflect the result of increasing social ostracism, particularly in the peer group. It is also associated with a composite index of maternal psychopathology, which may reflect generic, non-specific familial risk factors in producing behaviour problems in general. The predominance of emotional psychopathology may reflect familial risk for affective disorders and temperamental features of the boys. The extent to which aspects of the behavioural psychopathology may actually induce the emergence of the GID itself remains unresolved (see below).

Aetiological influences

Both biological and psychosocial factors have been proposed to account for the development of GID in children. In this section, I review some of the factors identified in the literature believed to be associated with an increased 'risk' for the development of GID.

Biological factors

Children with GID invariably do not show signs of a gross physical intersex condition, which would rule out a marked prenatal hormonal anomaly. Thus, the search for biological influences on the development of GID must focus on factors that are, perhaps, more subtle or at least on factors that do not affect the configuration of the external genitalia. In this regard, research strategies parallel those that have been used in the study of sexual orientation differentiation because, again, there is no evidence for the presence of gross hormonal abnormalities that would implicate the presence of a physical intersex condition (Meyer-Bahlburg 1984).

Activity level and rough-and-tumble play

Activity level (AL) is a commonly accepted dimension of temperament, with some evidence for a genetic basis (Willerman 1973; Saudino & Eaton 1991) and possibly prenatal hormonal influences (Ehrhardt & Baker 1974). Regarding children with GID, AL as a risk factor is a promising possibility, because it shows a rather strong sex difference, with boys having a higher AL than girls (Eaton & Enns 1986; Campbell & Eaton 1999). Rough-and-tumble (RT) play, another sex-dimorphic behaviour, bears some similarity to AL, in that it is often characterized by high energy expenditure; however, a distinguishing feature of RT is that it is a social interactive behaviour involving such sequences as 'play fighting' and 'chasing'. Using parent-report measures of AL, two studies found that boys with GID had a lower AL than control boys (Bates et al. 1979; Zucker & Bradley 1995). Zucker & Bradley (1995) also found that girls with GID had a higher AL than control girls; indeed, the girls with GID had a higher AL than the boys with GID, whereas for the controls the typical sex difference was observed. It is possible there-

fore that a sex-atypical AL is a risk factor that predisposes to the development of GID. For example, a low-active boy with GID may find the typical play behaviour of other boys to be incompatible with his own behavioural style (Ruble & Martin 1998), which might make it difficult for him to integrate successfully into a male peer group.

Perhaps these within-sex variations in AL are related to subtle variations in patterns of prenatal hormonal secretion and converge with recent studies in the experimental animal literature. Among female rhesus monkey offspring, it has been possible, by varying the timing of exogenous administration of hormones during the pregnancy, to alter the normal patterning of sex-dimorphic behaviour but to keep normal genital differentiation intact (Goy et al. 1988). This animal model—which shows a *dissociation* between sex-dimorphic behavioural differentiation and genital differentiation—has the most direct relevance for explaining the marked cross-gender behaviour of children with GID.

Birth weight

On average, males weigh more than females at the time of birth (Arbuckle et al. 1993). There are, of course, many factors that influence variations in birth weight. One hypothesized factor is the sex difference in prenatal exposure to androgens. In one study, girls with CAH had a higher mean birth weight than unaffected girls (Qazi & Thompson 1971). In another study, genetic males with the complete form of the androgen insensitivity syndrome were comparable in birth weight to that of genetic females (de Zegher et al. 1998).

Zucker et al. (1999a) compared the birth weights of boys with GID and clinical control boys and girls. The clinical controls showed the expected sex difference in birth weight, with an effect size of 0.29 (Cohen's d). The boys with GID had a significantly lower birth weight than the clinical control boys (d = 0.18), but did not differ significantly from the clinical control girls. Although it is not clear what factor or set of factors account for the proband-control difference in birth weight, the results are consistent with the possible role of prenatal hypoandrogenization among the GID probands.

Handedness

Slightly more males than females show a preference for using the left hand in unimanual behavioural tasks, such as writing. There is no established consensus for understanding the basis of this sex difference but genetic factors clearly have a role in determining hand preference. Another line of research implicates adverse prenatal and/or perinatal events that result in an elevation in left-handedness above the approximate gold standard of 10% in the general population.

Zucker et al. (2001) found that boys with GID (n = 205) had a significantly elevated rate of left-handedness (19.5%) when compared to three separate quasi-epidemiological samples of boys (11.8%, total n = 14 253) and with a diagnostically heterogeneous sample of clinical control boys (8.3%, $n=205$). This finding parallels studies of adult males with GID, who also appear to have an elevated rate of left-handedness (Herman-Jeglinska *et al.* 1997), as well as studies of adult men with a homosexual sexual orientation (Lalumière *et al.* 2000). At present, the explanation for the elevation remains unclear, but candidate factors have centred on some type of perturbation in prenatal development that, in some way, affects sex-dimorphic behavioural differentiation.

Sibling sex ratio and birth order

Boys with GID have an excess of brothers : sisters (sibling sex ratio) and have a later birth order (Blanchard *et al.* 1995; Zucker *et al.* 1997b). Some additional evidence shows that boys with GID are born later, primarily in relation to the number of older brothers but not sisters. In the Blanchard *et al.* study, clinical control boys showed no evidence for an altered sibling sex ratio or a late birth order. One biological explanation to account for these results pertains to maternal immune reactions during pregnancy. The male fetus is experienced by the mother as more 'foreign' (antigenic) than the female fetus. Based on studies with lower animals, it has been suggested that one consequence of this is that the mother produces antibodies that have the effect of demasculinizing or feminizing the male fetus, but no corresponding masculinizing or defeminizing of the female fetus (Blanchard & Klassen 1997). This model would predict that males born later in a sib-line might be more affected, because the mother's antigenicity increases with each successive male pregnancy, which is consistent with the empirical evidence on sibling sex ratio and birth order among GID probands. At present, however, this proposed mechanism has not been formally tested in humans.

Summary

In summary, research over the past decade has begun to identify some characteristics of children with GID, particularly in boys, that may well have a biological basis. Corresponding studies of girls have been fewer in number, largely because of problems in sample size that limit statistical power. In many respects, it has been easier to rule out candidate biological explanations, such as the influence of gross anomalies in prenatal hormonal exposure, than it has been to identify the relevant biological mechanisms that are involved in affecting sex-dimorphic behavioural differentiation but not sex-dimorphic genital differentiation. However, the identification of new potential biological markers may open up avenues for further empirical inquiry.

Psychosocial factors

Psychosocial factors, to truly merit causal status, must be shown to influence the emergence of marked cross-gender behaviour in the first few years of life. Otherwise, such factors would be better conceptualized as perpetuating rather than predisposing.

Sex assignment at birth

Because most children with GID do not have a co-occurring physical intersex condition, sex assignment at birth is invariably in accordance with the external markers of biological sex. In some physical intersex conditions, sex assignment is delayed and, on occasion, changed from the initial sex assignment. It has been argued that prolonged delay or uncertainty about the child's 'true' sex can contribute to gender identity conflict in affected individuals (Money *et al.* 1957; Meyer-Bahlburg *et al.* 1996). This does not, however, appear to be the situation for children with GID.

Parents' sexual orientation

There is little evidence to suggest that the sexual orientation of parents is related to GID in children. Studies of lesbian mothers and gay fathers have not, to date, indicated an overrepresentation of GID among their offspring. In fact, the children of gay and lesbian parents appear to have fairly typical gender identity and gender role development when compared to the children of heterosexual parents (Golombok *et al.* 1983; Green *et al.* 1986; Tasker & Golombok 1997). In our own clinic, we have not detected any convincing evidence for an elevation in the rate of a homosexual sexual orientation among the parents of both children and adolescents with GID.

Prenatal gender preference

It is common for parents to express a prenatal gender preference. Other things being equal, parents will have a child of the non-preferred sex about 50% of the time. Are parents of children with GID more likely than control parents to report having had a desire for a child of the opposite sex? The simple answer appears to be no, at least with regard to the mothers of boys with GID (Zucker *et al.* 1994). We did find, however, that the maternal wish for a girl was significantly associated with the sex composition and birth order of the sibship. Among the GID boys with only older brothers, the percentage of mothers who recalled a desire for a daughter was significantly higher than among the probands with other sibship combinations; however, the same pattern was observed in a control group (Zucker *et al.* 1994).

Social reinforcement of cross-gender behaviour

Understanding the role of parent socialization in the genesis and/or perpetuation of GID (e.g. via reinforcement principles or modelling) has been influenced by the normative developmental literature on sex-dimorphic sex-typed behaviour (Ruble & Martin 1998). It has also been influenced by the seminal observations of Money *et al.* (1957) that the rearing environment was the predominant determinant of gender identity in children with physical intersex conditions.

It should be recognized that some critics are quite sceptical of the role of parent socialization in inducing sex differences in sex-typed behaviour among ordinary children (Lytton & Romney 1991) or within-sex variations. In recent years, the importance of the rearing environment has also been questioned within the literature on physical intersex conditions (for review see Zucker 1999b). This literature has recently been discussed in relation to the long-term gender identity outcome of a normal boy whose penis was accidentally ablated during a routine circumcision at 7 months, and who was subsequently reassigned as a girl around the age of 2 years. A female gender identity was judged to have differentiated and was maintained to at least age 9 years (Money 1975). Longer term follow-up, however, revealed that the patient reverted to living as a male in early adolescence (Diamond & Sigmundson 1997), which has been interpreted by some to indicate a much stronger role for biological rather than psychosocial influences on gender identity differentiation. However, critics have pointed out that there are alternative interpretations to this case (Meyer-Bahlburg 1999a). Moreover, in another case of ablatio penis, in which a gender reassignment to female occurred at 7 months, the patient's gender identity was judged to be unequivocally female at age 26 (Bradley *et al.* 1998). It is against this backdrop of competing views on the role of socialization that the literature on GID must be appraised.

Clinicians of diverse theoretical persuasions have consistently reported that the parental response to early cross-gender behaviour in children with GID is typically neutral (tolerance) or even encouraging (for review see Zucker & Bradley 1995). Regarding boys with GID, Green (1974) assessed parental recall of such responses taken from clinical and structured interviews at the time of assessment and concluded that 'what comes closest so far to being a *necessary* variable is that, as any feminine behaviour begins to emerge, there is *no* discouragement of that behaviour by the child's principal caretaker' (p. 238, italics in original; see also Green 1987; Roberts *et al.* 1987). In our clinic, Mitchell (1991), in a structured interview study, found that mothers of GID boys were more likely to tolerate/encourage feminine behaviours and less likely to encourage masculine behaviours than were the mothers of both clinical and normal control boys. The following vignette of parents of a 4-year-old boy is illustrative.

Interviewer (I): What is the first memory that you have of Eric's interest in 'girls' things?

Mother (M): Well, when he was about 2, he started to wear my shoes. He would wear them every day.

I: What did you think about that?

M: I thought it was cute, the way he was clumping around in them.

I: What about you (to father)?

Father (F): I wasn't around much, working and all, so I didn't see much of it. She (his wife) told me about it and I said that I didn't like it, but what can you do?

I: What happened after that?

M: Well, then he got interested in my dresses (laughs) and he looked so cute, running around in the heels and my long dress. We even took pictures of him like that.

F: Yeah, right.

I: Anything else?

M: When I took him to the toddler group, he went immediately over to the girls and he got into the Barbie dolls. He seemed obsessed with their hair and we wound up buying him 3 or 4 of them. His favourite one is the Barbie with roller-blades. I asked his doctor about it when he was 3 and the doctor said that it was a phase and that he would grow out of it.

F: Yeah, and then he was pretending that he was a girl all the time and said that he would grow up and be a mommy, and then he said that he wanted to cut off his penis.

I: What happened when he said that?

M: Well, that's why we're here. I'm getting worried that he won't grow out of it…it's getting worse.

I: Before he said that he wanted to cut off his penis, how do you think you have reacted to his interest in the girls' things over the past couple of years?

M: Well, I've pretty well let him do want he wants and, anyways, the doctor told me not to worry. I thought that if he played with the Barbies, maybe he'd be a good father, but he doesn't want to be the father, he's only pretending to be me.

F: Yeah, I'm getting more worried myself, but my wife told me not to be so worried and, well, you know, she's kind of the boss when it comes to raising the kids.

Of course, the limitations of this kind of interview data need to be recognized. None the less, one aspect of these data deserves special comment. Clinicians of diverse theoretical persuasions have observed the apparent tolerance, or even encouragement, of feminine behaviour shown by parents of boys with GID. However, the fact that these parents have sought out a clinical assessment usually means that they are now concerned about their child's gender identity development (Zucker 2000a). From the standpoint of attribution theory (Weiner 1993), one might predict that parents would minimize their encouragement or tolerance of cross-gender behaviour, as it has such an obvious bearing on 'causality'. Yet a majority of the parents whom we have assessed do not recall systematic efforts to limit or redirect their child's cross-gender behaviour, particularly during the initial period of symptom onset and for various periods of time thereafter.

The reasons why parents might tolerate, if not encourage, early cross-gender behaviours appear to be quite diverse, suggesting that the antecedents to this 'end state' are multiple in origin. Some parents report being influenced by ideas regarding non-sexist child-rearing. In other parents, the antecedents seem to be rooted in pervasive conflict that revolves around gender issues. For example, a small subgroup of mothers (about 10%) of boys with GID appear to experience something akin to what we have termed *pathological gender mourning* (Zucker 1996). During the pregnancy, there is a strong desire for a girl; in all of the cases, the mother had already borne at least one other son, but no daughter — except in three instances in which the daughter was given up for adoption (one case) or had died in infancy (two cases). After the birth of the 'non-preferred' son, this wish seems to colour strongly the mother's perception and relationship with her newborn, and there are strong signs of ambivalence about his gender status. Zucker (1996) identified at least 10 possible signs of pathological gender mourning, including severe post-partum depression related to the birth of a son, recurrent nightdreams about being pregnant with a girl, delayed naming, and active cross-dressing of the boy (for further details see Zucker *et al*. 1993a; Zucker & Bradley 1995, 2000). In our clinical experience, the most common psychological trait associated with the strong wish for a daughter is the need to nurture and be nurtured by a female child, which often reflects compensatory needs originating in childhood (Gibson 1998).

Maternal emotional functioning

The role of maternal psychopathology in the genesis and perpetuation of GID has received a great deal of clinical and theoretical attention but, unfortunately, only limited empirical evaluation. At the outset, it should be noted that the available empirical studies have been delimited to the mothers of boys with GID—comparable studies are not available regarding the mothers of girls with GID (for descriptive data see Zucker & Bradley 1995, pp. 252–253).

Marantz & Coates (1991) found that the mothers of boys with GID showed more signs of psychopathology than did the mothers of demographically matched normal boys, including more pathological ratings on the Diagnostic Interview for Borderlines and more symptoms of depression on the Beck Depression Inventory.

Over the past several years, our group has collected systematic data on maternal psychopathology and marital discord, some of which was reported by Mitchell (1991) and Zucker & Bradley (1995). To date, our data show that, on average, mothers of boys with GID have levels of emotional distress and psychiatric impairment comparable to that of clinical control mothers, but higher than that of normal control mothers. We did not, however, detect between-group differences on a measure of marital discord.

On one measure—the Symptom Checklist 90–Revised—mothers of GID boys had higher scores on most of the subscales and the composites than did the mothers of the normal control boys, whereas the scores of the clinical control mothers fell in between the two other groups. The GID mothers had peak scores on the Obsessive-Compulsive, Depression, and Hostility subscales. On another measure, the Diagnostic Interview Schedule (DIS), 30% of the mothers (total $n = 140$) had two DIS diagnoses and 24% had three or more DIS diagnoses. The most common diagnoses were major depressive episode (39.6%) and recurrent major depression (32.1%). Overall, the rate of psychiatric impairment appears to be higher than our available data on mothers of both the clinical control and normal boys. Because more control group mother data are required, these results should be viewed cautiously. None the less, it is apparent by reference to epidemiological data that, on average, mothers of GID boys have a history of psychiatric disorder that is elevated.

The emerging data on emotional distress and psychiatric impairment in the mothers of boys with GID indicate that it is more common than in the mothers of normal control boys and at least comparable to the mothers of clinical control boys. Still, we are left with the problem of specificity (Garber & Hollon 1991), in that these maternal characteristics are not unique to the mothers of GID boys, but common to the mothers of clinic-referred boys in general. Accordingly, maternal emotional distress/impairment functions, at best, only as a non-specific risk factor in the development of GID. If the mother's emotional state truly is involved in the genesis of GID, then there should be evidence of psychiatric impairment prior to and during the emergence of the child's symptoms. The data are suggestive that this is the case, and that the presence of emotional difficulties in the mothers is not simply a reaction to having a child with GID (Zucker & Bradley 1995, p. 123).

Coates has argued that the presence of psychopathology renders the mothers emotionally unavailable, which results in anxiety and insecurity in the son, and that it is this state of affairs that is partly responsible for symptom onset. Indeed, Coates & Person (1985) advanced a very specific hypothesis; that the erratic and uneven emotional availability of the mothers activated separation anxiety in the boys, which, in turn, activated the symptoms of GID: 'In imitating "Mommy" [the boy] confuse[s] "being Mommy" with "having Mommy". [Cross-gender behaviour] appears to allay, in part, the anxiety generated by the loss of the mother' (p. 708). Indeed, boys with GID appear to have high rates of separation anxiety traits, as judged by maternal report on a structured interview schedule (Zucker *et al*. 1996a) and their own responses on the Separation Anxiety Test (Birkenfeld-Adams 1999).

The possible role of separation anxiety in the genesis of GID raises more general questions about the quality of the mother–son relationship. Over the past few years, our group has examined the quality of attachment to the mother among young boys and girls with GID (ages 3–6 years). Among a sample of 22 boys, Birkenfeld-Adams (1999) found that the majority (73%) were classified as insecurely attached, a rate comparable to that of an internal clinical control group and of other studies of clinical populations (Greenberg *et al*. 1991).

Because insecure attachments and separation anxiety are likely to be non-specific risk factors (many boys who have these qualities do not have GID), the crucial question that remains is why only a small minority of boys develop the 'fantasy solution' of wanting to be a girl. Various predisposing factors have been implicated, including temperamental characteristics of the child, the premorbid relationship with the mother, the position of the father in the family system, that the family psychopathology must occur during the putative sensitive period for gender identity formation (Money *et al*. 1957), and so on. However, at present the question of specificity remains unanswered in any satisfactory manner.

One possible mediating variable might be the importance of the child's gender to the mother or her attitudes towards men and masculinity in general. In this regard, pathological gender mourning, as discussed earlier, may be a potential prototype.

Pathological gender mourning appears to be part of the family history in only a small minority of cases and thus other pathways are required to account for the role of maternal impairment in the genesis of GID.

It appears therefore that there are diverse pathways that lead to how parents respond to the child's early cross-gender behaviour, either by encouraging or tolerating it. Thus, from a clinical and therapeutic point of view, it is important to identify the putative motivations with regard to the selective reinforcement of sex-typed behaviours.

Paternal emotional functioning

The role of paternal influences in the genesis and perpetuation of GID has also received a great deal of clinical and theoretical attention but, again, only limited empirical evaluation, which has been delimited to the fathers of boys with GID.

One account implicates the father's role by virtue of his absence from the family matrix. Across 10 samples of boys with GID, the rate of father absence (e.g. because of separation or divorce) was 34.5% (summarized in Zucker & Bradley 1995). It is unlikely, however, that this rate would differ significantly from the rate found in clinical populations in general, if not the general population. Green (1987) found that paternal separations occurred earlier in the families of GID boys than in normal control boys, so it is possible that timing is an additional variable to consider. Green (1987) also found that the fathers of GID boys (both father-present and father-absent) recalled spending less time with their sons than did the fathers of control boys during the second year of life, years 3–5, and at the time of assessment. The inclusion of a clinical control group would be helpful in gauging the specificity of this finding.

Unfortunately, there is little in the way of systematic research on paternal psychopathology. Wolfe (1990) conducted a small but detailed study of 12 fathers, predominantly of an upper middle-class background, of boys with GID. On the Structured Clinical Interview for DSM-III, all of the fathers received an Axis I diagnosis for either a current or past disorder (most frequently substance abuse and depression) and eight also received at least one Axis II diagnosis. Unpublished DIS data from our own clinic on 90 fathers indicate that alcohol abuse (22.2%) has been the most common diagnosis. This percentage may underestimate the prevalence of alcohol abuse in fathers of GID boys, because we were not able to interview a substantial number of fathers who were no longer part of the family matrix. On the other hand, it should be noted that about half the fathers who were interviewed did not meet criteria for any DIS diagnosis. Whatever the exact patterning of paternal emotional functioning proves to be, the same issues of interpretation discussed earlier regarding mothers apply.

Summary

In summary, data on psychosocial influences have been able to rule out some hypothesized pathways and have lent some sup-

port for others. Social reinforcement of cross-gender behaviour when it first appears in the toddler and preschool years appears to be the most common psychosocial influence on the disorder's consolidation. The role of family influences, including parental psychiatric impairment and emotional distress, appears to be an important area for further empirical inquiry.

Long-term follow-up

Green (1987) has conducted the most extensive long-term follow-up of feminine boys, the majority of whom would likely have met DSM criteria for GID. This study can be used as a benchmark for the other published follow-up reports, which have been summarized in detail elsewhere (Zucker 1985, 1990). At the moment, insufficient numbers of girls with GID have been followed prospectively to draw conclusions about long-term outcome. Green's (1987) study contained 66 feminine and 56 control boys assessed initially at a mean age of 7.1 years (range, 4–12). Forty-four feminine boys and 30 control boys were available for follow-up at a mean age of 18.9 years (range, 14–24). The majority of the boys were not in therapy between assessment and follow-up.

Sexual orientation in fantasy and behaviour was assessed by means of a semistructured clinical interview. Kinsey ratings were made on a 7-point continuum, ranging from exclusive heterosexuality to exclusive homosexuality (Kinsey et al. 1948). Depending on the measure (fantasy or behaviour), 75–80% of the previously feminine boys were either bisexual or homosexual at follow-up vs. 0–4% of the control boys. Green also reported on the gender identity status of the 44 previously feminine boys. He found that one youngster, at the age of 18 years, was gender-dysphoric to the extent of considering sex-reassignment surgery.

In a more recent study, Cohen-Kettenis (2001) reported a persistence of gender dysphoria into adolescence that appears to be considerably higher than that reported on by Green (1987). Of 129 children referred between 4–12 years, 74 had now reached adolescence. Of these, Cohen-Kettenis reported that 17 (23%) had applied for sex-reassignment. Their mean age at assessment had been at 9 years (range, 6–12), which was a couple of years older than the mean age at assessment in Green's study. About half were reported to be living full-time in the cross-gender role, six were taking puberty-blocking medication and three were taking cross-sex hormones; however, none had of yet gone through any surgical procedure. From the Cohen-Kettenis report, it is not clear if any of these youngsters had had treatment for their GID during childhood.

The prospective data are consistent with retrospective studies of adults with a homosexual sexual orientation, which have repeatedly shown that homosexual men and women recall more cross-gender behaviour in childhood than heterosexual men and women (Bailey & Zucker 1995). Thus, there is now sufficient evidence, from both retrospective and prospective studies, to conclude that childhood sex-typed behaviour is strongly associated with later sexual orientation, which represents one of the more powerful illustrations of developmental continuity to emerge from research in developmental psychiatry. Recall interviews with both adolescents and adults with GID (with a homosexual sexual orientation) almost invariably document a childhood cross-gender history. The prospective studies of children, however, show that the disorder persists into adolescence or adulthood for only a small minority. Thus, there is a marked disjunction between the prospective and retrospective studies.

How might this disjunction be explained? In some respects, the situation is comparable to that which has been found for other child psychiatric disorders. Adults with antisocial personality disorder invariably will have had a childhood history of oppositional defiant disorder and conduct disorder. Yet, the vast majority of children with oppositional defiant disorder and the majority of children with conduct disorder followed prospectively will not be diagnosed with antisocial personality disorder in adulthood (Zoccolillo *et al.* 1992; Lahey *et al.* 2000).

Regarding children with GID, then, we need to understand why, for the majority, the disorder apparently remits by adolescence, if not earlier. One possible explanation concerns referral bias. Green (1974) argued that children with GID who are referred for clinical assessment (and then therapy) may come from families in which there is more concern than is the case for adolescents and adults, the majority of whom did not receive a clinical evaluation and treatment during childhood. Thus, a clinical evaluation and subsequent therapeutic intervention during childhood may alter the natural history of GID. This is only one account of the disjunction and there may well be additional factors that might distinguish those children who are more strongly at risk for the continuation of the disorder from those who are not. Another explanation is that the diagnostic criteria for GID, at least as they are currently formulated, simply are not sharp enough to distinguish children who are more likely to show a persistence in the disorder from those who are not.

To date, very little has been done in the way of assessing the more general psychosocial and psychiatric outcomes of children with GID. This is important for at least two reasons. First, children with GID show, on average, as much general behavioural psychopathology as do demographically matched clinical controls. Whether children with GID will continue to be at risk for more general disturbances in psychiatric functioning as they mature remains an understudied area of empirical inquiry. In a recent cross-sectional study, Zucker *et al.* (2001) compared children and adolescents with GID and found that the adolescents were substantially more disturbed on the CBCL than were the children, even after co-varying for various differences in demographic characteristics. Secondly, we now know that gay and lesbian adolescents, without known GID in childhood, are at increased risk for mental health problems although the reasons for this have been largely understudied (Remafedi *et al.* 1998; Fergusson *et al.* 1999; Garofalo *et al.* 1999a,b). Presumably, some of the variance is related to the stigma of a minority sexual orientation (Meyer 1995). It could be argued, for example, that the severe social ostracism experienced by children with GID for their marked cross-gender behaviour increases the risk for general psychiatric problems (e.g. depression, suicidality), but this requires empirical verification.

Linkage between childhood sex-typed behaviour and sexual orientation

Because the linkage between GID in childhood and a later homosexual sexual orientation is so strong, understanding the connection is important, from both a theoretical and a clinical perspective. The most prominent biological explanation is that both sex-typed behaviour in childhood and sexual orientation in adolescence/adulthood are joined by some common factor or set of factors; for example, regarding genetic females with CAH, excessive prenatal exposure to androgens has been posited as the linkage factor that explains the higher rates of both behavioural masculinity during childhood (Berenbaum & Hines 1992) and bisexuality/homosexuality in adulthood (Zucker *et al.* 1996b).

Psychosocial perspectives have been varied. Green (1987) conjectured that, compared to control boys, a feminine boy's lack of close relationships with other boys and with his father might result in 'male affect starvation'. Thus, in adolescence and adulthood, homoerotic contact is used in some compensatory manner to achieve closeness with other males. This scenario is an example of accounting for a within-sex difference in a behavioural outcome (in this instance, sexual orientation); it is not clear if 'male affect starvation' during childhood would also account for a girl's later sexual attraction to males.

In Bem's (1996) developmental theory of sexual orientation, it is proposed that similar mechanisms are operative in the sexual object choice of feminine boys and feminine girls (and masculine boys and masculine girls). Bem's account is not so much a 'deficit' model, as is implied by the term 'affect starvation', but a 'difference' model. Bem proposed that variations in childhood 'temperaments' influence a child's preference for sex-typical or sex-atypical activities and peers:

> These preferences lead children to feel different from opposite-sex or same-sex peers — to perceive them as dissimilar, unfamiliar, and exotic. This, in turn, produces heightened non-specific autonomic arousal that subsequently gets eroticized to that same class of dissimilar peers (Bem 1996, p. 320).

For feminine boys and feminine girls, males are 'exotic', whereas for masculine boys and masculine girls, females are 'exotic'. Bem's (1996) theory of sexual orientation represents a prototype in trying to unite typical and atypical development. However, there are many unanswered questions and alternative interpretations raised by the theory. Bem places great emphasis on temperamental factors that affect a child's preference for sex-typical or sex-atypical activities and friendships — an emphasis that might be disputed by some developmentalists (Ruble & Martin 1998). Empirical evidence for the emergence of specific erotic feelings following 'heightened non-specific autonomic arousal' is scant, although it is quite likely that the relevant tests can be obtained through an analysis of emerging sexual interactions within the pre-adolescent peer group.

Bem's theory is intriguing in that it implies a greater potential for malleability in sexual orientation development than is apparent in some of the biological theories. If a feminine boy becomes more masculine in the course of his childhood, does this imply that the likelihood of later homoeroticism decreases? Conversely, if a feminine girl becomes more masculine in the course of her childhood, does this imply that the likelihood of later homoeroticism increases? Unfortunately, there is not much information available to answer these questions.

Green (1987) compared feminine boys who were subsequently classified as bisexual or homosexual with feminine boys who were subsequently classified as heterosexual. Although some feminine behaviours in childhood distinguished the two subgroups, a composite extent of femininity score only approached conventional levels of significance and only for the rating of sexual orientation in fantasy, not behaviour. The lack of a stronger correlation is somewhat surprising, because one might have expected an association between the degree of cross-gender identification and long-term outcome; however, Green (1987) did find that the continuation of certain feminine behaviours throughout childhood was associated with later homosexuality. Thus, it may be that the persistence of these feminine behaviours is more important than their extent during the early childhood years.

Treatment

In this section, I review some of the extant perspectives on treatment issues and what is known about the efficacy of various therapeutic interventions.

Ethical considerations

Any contemporary child clinician responsible for the therapeutic care of children and adolescents with GID will quickly be introduced to complex social and ethical issues pertaining to the politics of sex and gender in post-modern Western culture and have to think them through carefully. Is GID really a disorder or just a 'normal' variant of gendered behaviour? Is marked cross-gender behaviour inherently harmful or is it simply harmful because of social factors? If a teenager requests immediate cross-sex hormonal and surgical intervention as a therapeutic for gender dysphoria, should the clinician comply? If parents request treatment for their child with GID to divert the probability of a later homosexual sexual orientation, what is the appropriate clinical response? All of these questions force the clinician to think long and hard about theoretical and treatment issues.

Perhaps the most acute ethical issue concerns the relation between GID and a later homosexual sexual orientation. As noted earlier, follow-up studies of boys with GID, largely untreated, indicate that homosexuality is the most common long-term psychosexual outcome. Some parents of children with GID request treatment, partly with an eye towards preventing subsequent homosexuality in their child, whether this is because of personal values, concerns about stigmatization, or for other reasons.

In the 1990s, this 'rationale' for treatment was subject to intense scrutiny (Sedgwick 1991; Minter 1999). Some critics have argued that clinicians, consciously or unconsciously, accept the prevention of homosexuality as a legitimate therapeutic goal (Pleak 1999). Minter (1999) has claimed, as have others (Scholinski 1997), that some adolescents in the USA are being hospitalized against their will because of their homosexual sexual orientation but under the guise of the GID diagnosis. These allegations have not been verified in any systematic manner and I know of no such case in which this has occurred (Meyer Bahlburg 1999b). Others have asserted, albeit without direct empirical documentation, that treatment of GID results in harm to children who are 'homosexual' or 'prehomosexual' (Isay 1997). Some clinicians have raised questions about differential diagnosis, arguing that there is not always an adequate distinction between children who are 'truly' GID vs. those who are merely prehomosexual (Corbett 1996; Richardson 1996, 1999).

The various issues regarding the relation between GID and homosexuality are complex—both clinically and ethically. Three points, albeit brief, can be made. First, until it has been shown that any form of treatment for GID during childhood affects later sexual orientation, the issue is moot. From an ethical standpoint, however, the clinician has an obligation to inform parents about the state of the empirical database. Secondly, I have argued elsewhere that some critics incorrectly conflate gender identity and sexual orientation, regarding them as isomorphic phenomena (Zucker 1999c), as do some parents. Psychoeducational work with parents can review the various explanatory models regarding the statistical linkage between gender identity and sexual orientation (Bailey & Zucker 1995; Bem 1996), but also discuss their distinctness as psychological constructs. Thirdly, many contemporary clinicians emphasize that the primary goal of treatment of children with GID is to resolve the conflicts that are associated with the disorder *per se*, regardless of the child's eventual sexual orientation. Most clinicians who have worked with children and adolescents with GID believe that they experience a great deal of suffering: many such youngsters are preoccupied with gender identity issues, they experience increased social ostracism and alienation as they get older, and show evidence of other behavioural and psychiatric difficulties. Most clinicians therefore take the position that therapeutics designed to reduce the gender dysphoria, lessen the degree of social ostracism, and to reduce the degree of psychiatric comorbidity constitute legitimate goals of intervention. How, then, might one go about reaching these therapeutic goals?

Developmental considerations

One aspect of the clinical literature suggests that there are important developmental considerations to bear in mind. For example, there is some evidence to suggest that GID is less responsive to psychosocial interventions during adolescence, and certainly by young adulthood, than it is during childhood. Thus, the lessening of malleability and plasticity over time in gender identity differentiation is an important clinical consideration.

Treatment of children

For children with GID, clinical experience suggests that psychosocial treatments can be relatively effective in reducing the gender dysphoria. Therapeutic approaches have included the most commonly used interventions for children in general, including behaviour therapy, psychodynamic therapy, parent counselling, and group therapy (for detailed reviews see Zucker 1985, 1990, 2001). In considering these various therapeutic approaches, there is one important sobering fact to contemplate: apart from a series of intrasubject behaviour therapy case reports from the 1970s, one will find not a single randomized controlled treatment trial in the literature (Zucker, 2001). Thus, the treating clinician must rely largely on the 'clinical wisdom' that has accumulated in the case report literature and the conceptual underpinnings that inform the various approaches to intervention.

Treatment for children with GID often proceeds on two fronts:

1 individual therapy with the child, in which efforts are made to understand the factors that seem to fuel the fantasy of wanting to become a member of the opposite sex and then to resolve them; and

2 parent counselling, in which efforts are made to help the child, in the naturalistic environment, to feel more comfortable about being a boy or a girl.

Treatment can address several issues. For youngsters who are quite confused about their gender identity, one can focus on the mastery of basic cognitive concepts of gender, including correct identification of the self as a boy or a girl; encouragement in the development of same-sex friendships, in which areas of mutual interest can be identified; and exploration of factors within the family that might be contributing to the gender identity conflict.

With parents, treatment issues include the following:

1 limit-setting of cross-gender behaviour and encouragement of gender-neutral or sex-typical activities;

2 factors within the family matrix that may be contributing to the child's gender identity conflict; and

3 parent factors, including psychiatric impairment, that may be compromising functioning in the parental role in general.

Here, I will focus on some technical aspects of limit-setting that are often misunderstood in the clinical literature and which thus require further explication. A common error committed by some clinicians is to simply recommend to parents that they impose limits on their child's cross-gender behaviour without attention to context. This kind of authoritarian approach is likely to fail, just as it will with regard to any behaviour, as it does not take into account systemic factors, both in the parents and in the child, that fuel the 'symptom'. At the very least, a psychoeducational approach is required, but, in many cases, limit-setting needs to occur within the context of a more global treatment plan.

From a psychoeducational point of view, one rationale for limit-setting is that if parents allow their child to continue to engage in cross-gender behaviour, the GID is, in effect, being tolerated, if not reinforced. Thus, such an approach would contribute to the perpetuation of the condition. Another rationale for limit-setting is that it is, in effect, an effort to alter the GID from the 'outside in', while individual therapy for the child can explore the factors that have contributed to the GID from the 'inside out'. At the same time that one attempts to set limits, parents also need to help their child with alternative activities that might help consolidate a more comfortable same-gender identification. Encouragement of same-sex peer group relations can be an important part of such alternatives; for example, some boys with GID develop an avoidance of male playmates because they are anxious about rough-and-tumble play and fantasy aggression. Such anxiety may be fuelled by parent factors (e.g. where mothers conflate real aggression with fantasy aggression), but may also be fuelled by temperamental characteristics of the child (Zucker 2000b). Efforts on the part of parents to be more sensitive to their child's temperamental characteristics may be quite helpful in planning peer group encounters that are not experienced by the child as threatening and overwhelming. It is not unusual to encounter boys with GID who have a genuine longing to interact with other boys, but because of their shy and avoidant temperament do not know how to integrate themselves with other boys, particularly if they experience the contextual situation as threatening. Over time, with the appropriate therapeutic support, such boys are able to develop same-sex peer group relationships and begin to identify more with other boys as a result.

Another important contextual aspect of limit-setting is to explore with parents their initial encouragement or tolerance of the cross-gender behaviour. Some parents will tolerate the behaviour initially because they have been told, or believe themselves, that the behaviour is 'only a phase' that their child will grow out of. Such parents become concerned about their child once they begin to recognize that the behaviour is not merely a phase (Zucker 2000a). For other parents, the tolerance or encouragement of cross-gender behaviour can be linked to some of the systemic and dynamic factors described earlier. In these more complex clinical situations, one must attend to the underlying issues and work them through. Otherwise, it is quite likely that parents will not be comfortable in shifting their position.

Although many contemporary clinicians have stressed the important role of working with the parents of children with GID, one can ask if there is any empirical evidence that this is effective. Again, systematic information on the question is scanty. The most relevant study (Zucker et al. 1985) found some evidence that parental involvement in therapy was significantly correlated with a greater degree of behavioural change in the child at 1-year follow-up, but this study did not make random assignment to different treatment protocols, so one has to interpret the findings with caution.

Treatment of adolescents

If GID in adolescence is not responsive to psychosocial treatment, should the clinician recommend the same kinds of physical interventions that are used with adults (Harry Benjamin International Gender Dysphoria Association 1998)? Prior to such a recommendation, many clinicians usually encourage adolescents with GID to consider alternatives to this invasive and expensive treatment. One area of inquiry can therefore explore the meaning behind the adolescent's desire for sex reassignment and if there are viable alternative lifestyle adaptations. In this regard, the most common area of exploration pertains to the patient's sexual orientation. Almost all adolescents with GID recall that they always felt uncomfortable growing up as boys or as girls, but that the idea of 'sex change' did not occur until they became aware of homoerotic attractions. For some of these youngsters, the idea that they might be gay or homosexual is abhorrent. For some such adolescents, psychoeducational work can explore their attitudes and feelings about homosexuality. Group therapy, in which such youngsters have the opportunity to meet gay adolescents, can be a useful adjunct in such cases. In some cases, the gender dysphoria will resolve and a homosexual adaptation ensues (Zucker & Bradley 1995). For others, however, a homosexual adaptation is not possible and the gender dysphoria does not abate.

For adolescents in which the gender dysphoria appears chronic, the clinician can consider two main options:

1 management until the adolescent turns 18 and can be referred to an adult gender identity clinic; or

2 'early' institution of contra-sex hormonal treatment.

Regarding the latter, Gooren & Delemarre-van de Waal (1996) recommended that one option with gender-dysphoric adolescents is to prescribe puberty-blocking luteinizing hormone-releasing agonists (e.g. depot leuprolide or depot triptorelin) that facilitate more successful passing as the opposite sex. Thus, in male adolescents, such medication can suppress the development of secondary sex characteristics, such as facial hair growth and voice deepening, which makes it more difficult to pass in the female social role. Cohen-Kettenis & van Goozen (1997, 1998) reported that early cross-sex hormone treatment for adolescents under the age of 18 years, judged free of gross psychiatric comorbidity, facilitates the complex psychosexual and psychosocial transition to living as a member of the opposite sex and results in a lessening of the gender dysphoria.

Although such early hormonal treatment is controversial (Cohen-Kettenis 1994, 1995; Meyenburg 1994), it may well be the treatment of choice once the clinician is confident that other options have been exhausted. One issue that is not yet resolved concerns who are the best candidates for early hormonal treatments. Cohen-Kettenis & van Goozen (1997) have suggested that the least risky subgroup of adolescents with GID are those who show little evidence of psychiatric impairment. In my own clinic, the vast majority of adolescents with GID would not qualify on this basis (Zucker *et al.* in press). However, by adolescence, the issue is a tricky one because it is not clear to what extent the psychiatric impairment is a consequence of the chronic gender dysphoria (Newman 1970). A randomized controlled trial would be useful in resolving the matter.

Future directions

In this chapter, I have provided an overview of the literature on GID in children and adolescents. Since GID first appeared in the DSM-III in 1980, considerable advances have been made in some areas. The phenomenology of GID is now well described and extant assessment procedures are available to conduct a thorough and competent diagnostic evaluation. Like other psychiatric disorders of childhood, it is apparent that complexity, not simplicity, is the guiding rule-of-thumb in any effort to make sense of the origins of GID. It appears that both biological and psychosocial factors contribute to the disorder's genesis and we are making some progress in identifying specific markers of both processes. From an aetiological standpoint, perhaps the most vexing issue is to make progress in solving the problem of specificity. A fair bit has been learned about the 'natural history' of GID and it appears to be the case that the prospects for therapeutic intervention are more optimistic during childhood than in adolescence, perhaps not a surprising observation to developmental psychiatrists. Much remains to be learned, however, about the most efficacious forms of treatment and perhaps this will be a goal to be reached in the first decade of the new millennium.

References

Achenbach, T. & Edelbrock, C. (1983) *Manual for the Child Behavior Checklist and Revised Child Behavior Profile.* University of Vermont, Department of Psychiatry, Burlington, VT.

Achenbach, T. & Edelbrock, C. (1986) *Manual for the Teacher's Report Form and Teacher Version of the Child Behavior Profile.* University of Vermont, Department of Psychiatry, Burlington, VT.

Achenbach, T., Howell, C., Quay, H. & Conners, C. (1991) National survey of problems and competencies among four- to sixteen-year-olds. *Monographs of the Society for Research in Child Development* **56** (3, Serial no. 225).

American Psychiatric Association (1987) *Diagnostic and Statistical Manual of Mental Disorders*, 3rd edn, revised. American Psychiatric Association, Washington D.C.

American Psychiatric Association (2000) *Diagnostic and Statistical Manual of Mental Disorders*, 4th edn, text revision. American Psychiatric Association, Washington D.C.

Arbuckle, T., Wilkins, R. & Sherman, G. (1993) Birth weight percentiles by gestational age in Canada. *Obstetrics and Gynecology*, **81**, 39–48.

Bailey, J. & Zucker, K. (1995) Childhood sex-typed behavior and sexual orientation: a conceptual analysis and quantitative review. *Developmental Psychology*, **31**, 43–55.

Bakker, A., van Kesteren, P., Gooren, L. & Bezemer, P. (1993) The prevalence of transsexualism in the Netherlands. *Acta Psychiatrica Scandinavica*, **87**, 237–238.

Bates, J., Bentler, P. & Thompson, S. (1979) Gender-deviant boys compared with normal and clinical control boys. *Journal of Abnormal Child Psychology*, **7**, 243–259.

Bem, D. (1996) Exotic becomes erotic: a developmental theory of sexual orientation. *Psychological Review*, 103, 320–335.

Berenbaum, S. & Hines, M. (1992) Early androgens are related to childhood sex-typed toy preferences. *Psychological Science*, 3, 203–206.

Birkenfeld-Adams, A. (1999) *Quality of attachment in young boys with gender identity disorder: a comparison to clinic and nonreferred control boys.* PhD thesis, York University.

Blanchard, R. & Klassen, P. (1997) H-Y antigen and homosexuality in men. *Journal of Theoretical Biology*, 185, 373–378.

Blanchard, R., Clemmensen, L. & Steiner, B. (1987) Heterosexual and homosexual gender dysphoria. *Archives of Sexual Behavior*, 16, 139–152.

Blanchard, R., Zucker, K., Bradley, S. & Hume, C. (1995) Birth order and sibling sex ratio in homosexual male adolescents and probably prehomosexual feminine boys. *Developmental Psychology*, 31, 22–30.

Bradley, S., Blanchard, R., Coates, S. et al. (1991) Interim report of the DSM-IV subcommittee for gender identity disorders. *Archives of Sexual Behavior*, 20, 333–343.

Bradley, S., Oliver, G., Chernick, A. & Zucker, K. (1998) Experiment of nurture: ablatio penis at 2 months, sex reassignment at 7 months, and a psychosexual follow-up in young adulthood. *Pediatrics*, 102, E91–E95. [Available on the World Wide Web http://www.pediatrics.org/cgi/content/full/102/1/e9]

Campbell, D. & Eaton, W. (1999) Sex differences in the activity level of infants. *Infant and Child Development*, 8, 1–17.

Caron, C. & Rutter, M. (1991) Comorbidity in child psychopathology: concepts, issues and research strategies. *Journal of Child Psychology and Psychiatry*, 32, 1063–1080.

Coates, S. & Person, E. (1985) Extreme boyhood femininity: isolated behavior or pervasive disorder? *Journal of the American Academy of Child Psychiatry*, 24, 702–709.

Cohen-Kettenis, P. (1994) Die Behandlung von Kindern und Jugendlichen mit Geschlechtsidentitätsstörungen an der Universität Utrecht [Clinical management of children and adolescents with gender identity disorders at the University of Utrecht]. *Zeitschrift für Sexualforschung*, 7, 231–239.

Cohen-Kettenis, P. (1995) Replik auf Bernd Meyenburg's 'Kritik der hormonellen Behandlung Judendlicher mit Geschlechtsidentitätsstörungen' [Rejoinder to Bernd Meyenburg's 'Criticism of hormone treatment for adolescents with gender identity disorders']. *Zeitschrift für Sexualforschung*, 8, 165–167.

Cohen-Kettenis, P. (2001) Gender identity disorder in DSM? [Letter to the editor]. *Journal of the American Academy of Child and Adolescent Psychiatry*, 40, 391.

Cohen-Kettenis, P. & van Goozen, S. (1997) Sex reassignment of adolescent transsexuals: a follow-up study. *Journal of the American Academy of Child and Adolescent Psychiatry*, 36, 263–271.

Cohen-Kettenis, P. & van Goozen, S. (1998) Pubertal delay as an aid in diagnosis and treatment of a transsexual adolescent. *European Child and Adolescent Psychiatry*, 7, 246–248.

Corbett, K. (1996) Homosexual boyhood: notes on girlyboys. *Gender and Psychoanalysis*, 1, 429–461.

Diamond, M. & Sigmundson, H. (1997) Sex reassignment at birth: long-term review and clinical implications. *Archives of Pediatrics and Adolescent Medicine*, 151, 298–304.

Eaton, W. & Enns, L. (1986) Sex differences in human motor activity level. *Psychological Bulletin*, 100, 19–28.

Eaton, W. & Von Bargen, D. (1981) Asynchronous development of gender understanding in preschool children. *Child Development*, 52, 1020–1027.

Ehrhardt, A. & Baker, S. (1974) Fetal androgens, human central nervous system differentiation, and behavior sex differences. In: *Sex Differences in Behavior* (eds R.C. Friedman, R.M. Richart & R.L. Vande Wiele), pp. 33–51. Wiley, New York.

Fagot, B. (1985) Beyond the reinforcement principle: another step toward understanding sex role development. *Developmental Psychology*, 21, 1097–1104.

Fergusson, D., Horwood. L. & Beautrais, A. (1999) Is sexual orientation related to mental health problems and suicidality in young people? *Archives of General Psychiatry*, 56, 876–880.

Gagnon, J. (1990) The explicit and implicit use of the scripting perspective in sex research. *Annual Review of Sex Research*, 1, 1–43.

Garber, J. & Hollon, S. (1991) What can specificity designs say about causality in psychopathology research? *Psychological Bulletin*, 110, 129–136.

Garofalo, R., Wolf, R., Kessel, S., Palfrey, J. & DuRant, R. (1999a) The association between health risk behaviors and sexual orientation among a school-based sample of adolescents. *Pediatrics*, 101, 895–902.

Garofalo, R., Wolf, R., Wissow, L., Woods, E. & Goodman, E. (1999b) Sexual orientation and risk of suicide attempts among a representative sample of youth. *Journal of the American Medical Association*, 153, 487–493.

Gentile, D. (1993) Just what are sex and gender, anyway? A call for a new terminological standard. *Psychological Science*, 4, 120–122.

Gibson, L. (1998) *Adult attachment and maternal representations of gender during pregnancy: their impact on the child's subsequent gender-role development.* PhD thesis, City University of New York.

Golombok, S., Spencer, A. & Rutter, M. (1983) Children in lesbian and single-parent households: psychosexual and psychiatric appraisal. *Journal of Child Psychology and Psychiatry*, 24, 551–572.

Gooren, L. & Delemarre-van de Waal, H. (1996) The feasibility of endocrine interventions in juvenile transsexuals. *Journal of Psychology and Human Sexuality*, 8, 69–84.

Goy, R., Bercovitch, F. & McBrair, M. (1988) Behavioral masculinization is independent of genital masculinization in prenatally androgenized female rhesus macaques. *Hormones and Behavior*, 22, 552–571.

Green, R. (1974) *Sexual Identity Conflict in Children and Adults.* Basic Books, New York.

Green, R. (1987) *The 'Sissy Boy Syndrome' and the Development of Homosexuality.* Yale University Press, New Haven.

Green, R., Mandel, J., Hotvedt, M., Gray, J. & Smith, L. (1986) Lesbian mothers and their children: a comparison with solo parent heterosexual mothers and their children. *Archives of Sexual Behavior*, 15, 167–184.

Greenberg, M., Speltz, M., DeKlyen, M. & Endriga, M. (1991) Attachment security in preschoolers with and without externalizing behavior problems: a replication. *Development and Psychopathology*, 3, 413–430.

Haqq, C. & Donahoe, P. (1998) Regulation of sexual dimorphism in mammals. *Physiological Reviews*, 78, 1–33.

Harry Benjamin International Gender Dysphoria Association (1998) *The Standards of Care for Gender Identity Disorders*, 5th edn. Symposian Publishing, Düsseldorf.

Herdt, G. (1981) *Guardians of the Flute: Idioms of Masculinity.* McGraw-Hill, New York.

Herman-Jeglinska, A., Dulko, S. & Grabowska, A. (1997) Transsexuality and adextrality: do they share a common origin? In: *Sexual Orientation: Toward Biological Understanding* (eds L. Ellis & L. Ebertz), pp. 163–180. Praeger, Westport, CT.

Isay, R. (1997) Remove gender identity disorder in DSM. *Psychiatric News* 32, 9, 13.

Kinsey, A., Pomeroy, W. & Martin, C. (1948) *Sexual Behavior in the Human Male*. W.B. Saunders, Philadelphia.

Kohlberg, L. (1966) A cognitive-developmental analysis of children's sex-role concepts and attitudes. In: *The Development of Sex Differences* (ed. E.E. Maccoby), pp. 82–173. Stanford University Press, Stanford, CA.

Lahey, B., McBurnett, K. & Loeber, R. (2000) Are attention-deficit/hyperactivity disorder and oppositional defiant disorder developmental precursors to conduct disorder? In: *Handbook of Developmental Psychopathology* (eds A.J. Sameroff, M. Lewis & S.M. Miller), 2nd edn, pp. 431–446. Kluwer Academic/Plenum Publishers, New York.

Lalumière, M., Blanchard, R. & Zucker, K. (2000) Sexual orientation and handedness in men and women: a meta-analysis. *Psychological Bulletin*, 126, 575–592.

Laumann, E., Gagnon, J., Michael, R. & Michaels, S. (1994) *The Social Organization of Sexuality: Sexual Practices in the United States*. University of Chicago Press, Chicago.

Lothstein, L. (1983) *Female-to-male Transsexualism: Historical, Clinical, and Theoretical Issues*. Routledge & Kegan Paul, Boston.

Lytton, H. & Romney, D. (1991) Parents' differential socialization of boys and girls: a meta-analysis. *Psychological Bulletin*, 109, 267–296.

Maccoby, E. (1988) Gender as a social category. *Developmental Psychology*, 24, 755–765.

Marantz, S. & Coates, S. (1991) Mothers of boys with gender identity disorder: a comparison of matched controls. *Journal of the American Academy of Child and Adolescent Psychiatry*, 30, 310–315.

Meyenburg, B. (1994) Kritik der hormonellen Behandlung Judendlicher mit Geschlechtsidentitätsstörungen [Criticisms of hormone treatment for adolescents with gender identity disorders]. *Zeitschrift für Sexualforschung*, 7, 343–349.

Meyer, I. (1995) Minority stress and mental health in gay men. *Journal of Health and Social Behavior*, 36, 38–56.

Meyer-Bahlburg, H. (1984) Psychoendocrine research on sexual orientation: current status and future options. *Progress in Brain Research*, 61, 375–398.

Meyer-Bahlburg, H. (1985) Gender identity disorder of childhood: introduction. *Journal of the American Academy of Child Psychiatry*, 24, 681–683.

Meyer-Bahlburg, H. (1994) Intersexuality and the diagnosis of gender identity disorder. *Archives of Sexual Behavior*, 23, 21–40.

Meyer-Bahlburg, H. (1999a) Gender assignment and reassignment in 46,XY pseudohermaphroditism and related conditions. *Journal of Clinical Endocrinology and Metabolism*, 84, 3455–3458.

Meyer-Bahlburg, H. (1999b) Review of 'The last time I wore a dress: a memoir'. *Archives of Sexual Behavior*, 28, 431–434.

Meyer-Bahlburg, H., Gruen, R., New, M. *et al.* (1996) Gender change from female to male in classical congenital adrenal hyperplasia. *Hormones and Behavior*, 30, 319–332.

Migeon, C. & Wisniewski, A. (1998) Sexual differentiation: from genes to gender. *Hormone Research*, 50, 245–251.

Minter, S. (1999) Diagnosis and treatment of gender identity disorder in children. In: *Sissies and Tomboys: Gender Nonconformity and Homosexual Childhood* (ed. M. Rottnek), pp. 9–33. New York University Press, New York.

Mitchell, J. (1991) *Maternal influences on gender identity disorder in boys: searching for specificity*. PhD thesis, York University.

Money, J. (1955) Hermaphroditism, gender and precocity in hyperadrenocorticism: psychologic findings. *Bulletin of the Johns Hopkins Hospital*, 96, 253–264.

Money, J. (1975) Ablatio penis: normal male infant sex-reassigned as a girl. *Archives of Sexual Behavior*, 4, 65–71.

Money, J. (1985) The conceptual neutering of gender and the criminalization of sex. *Archives of Sexual Behavior*, 14, 279–290.

Money, J., Hampson, J. & Hampson, J. (1957) Imprinting and the establishment of gender role. *Archives of Neurology and Psychiatry*, 77, 333–336.

Newman, L. (1970) Transsexualism in adolescence: problems in evaluation and treatment. *Archives of General Psychiatry*, 23, 112–121.

Pleak, R. (1999) Ethical issues in diagnosing and treating gender-dysphoric children and adolescents. In: *Sissies and Tomboys: Gender Nonconformity and Homosexual Childhood* (ed. M. Rottnek), pp. 34–51. New York University Press, New York.

Pleak, R., Meyer-Bahlburg, H., O'Brien, J., Bowen, H. & Morganstein, A. (1989) Cross-gender behavior and psychopathology in boy psychiatric outpatients. *Journal of the American Academy of Child and Adolescent Psychiatry*, 28, 385–393.

Qazi, Q. & Thompson, M. (1971) Birthweight in congenital virilizing adrenal hyperplasia. *Archives of Disease in Childhood*, 46, 350–352.

Remafedi, G., French, S., Story, M., Resnick, M. & Blum, R. (1998) The relationship between suicide risk and sexual orientation: results of a population-based study. *American Journal of Public Health*, 88, 57–60.

Richardson, J. (1996) Setting limits on gender health. *Harvard Review of Psychiatry*, 4, 49–53.

Richardson, J. (1999) Response: finding the disorder in gender identity disorder. *Harvard Review of Psychiatry*, 7, 43–50.

Roberts, C., Green, R., Williams, K. & Goodman, M. (1987) Boyhood gender identity development: a statistical contrast of two family groups. *Developmental Psychology*, 23, 544–557.

Rosen, R. & Beck, J. (1988) *Patterns of Sexual Arousal: Psychophysiological Processes and Clinical Applications*. Guilford Press, New York.

Ross, M. (1983) *The Married Homosexual Man: A Psychological Study*. Routledge & Kegan Paul, Boston.

Ruble, D. & Martin, C. (1998) Gender development. In: *The Handbook of Child Psychology*, Vol. 3. *Social, Emotional, and Personality Development* (series ed. W. Damon; volume ed. N. Eisenberg), 5th edn, pp. 933–1016. Wiley, New York.

Sandberg, D., Meyer-Bahlburg, H., Ehrhardt, A. & Yager, T. (1993) The prevalence of gender-atypical behavior in elementary school children. *Journal of the American Academy of Child and Adolescent Psychiatry*, 32, 306–314.

Saudino, K. & Eaton, W. (1991) Infant temperament and genetics: an objective twin study of motor activity level. *Child Development*, 62, 1167–1174.

Scholinski, D. (1997) *The Last Time I Wore a Dress: A Memoir*. Riverhead Books, New York.

Sedgwick, E. (1991) How to bring your kids up gay. *Social Text*, 9, 18–27.

Spitzer, R. & Wakefield, J. (1999) DSM-IV diagnostic criterion for clinical significance: does it help solve the false positive problem? *American Journal of Psychiatry*, 156, 1856–1864.

Stoller, R. (1964) The hermaphroditic identity of hermaphrodites. *Journal of Nervous and Mental Disease*, 139, 453–457.

Stoller, R. (1967) It's only a phase': femininity in boys. *Journal of the American Medical Association*, 201, 314–315.

Stoller, R. (1975) *Sex and Gender*, Vol. 2, *The Transsexual Experiment*. Hogarth Press, London.

Tasker, F. & Golombok, S. (1997) *Growing Up in a Lesbian Family: Effects on Child Development*. Guilford Press, New York.

Vilain, E. & McCabe, E. (1998) Mammalian sex determination: from gonads to brain. *Molecular Genetics and Metabolism*, 65, 74–84.

Weeks, J. (1991) *Against Nature: Essays on History, Sexuality, and Identity*. Rivers Oram Press, London.

Weiner, B. (1993) On sin versus sickness: a theory of perceived responsibility and social motivation. *American Psychologist*, 48, 957–965.

Weisz, J. & Weiss, B. (1991) Studying the 'referability' of child clinical problems. *Journal of Consulting and Clinical Psychology*, 59, 266–273.

Willerman, L. (1973) Activity level and hyperactivity in twins. *Child Development*, 44, 288–293.

Wolfe, S. (1990) *Psychopathology and psychodynamics of parents of boys with a gender identity disorder of childhood*. PhD thesis, City University of New York.

World Health Organization (1992) *International Statistical Classification of Diseases and Related Health Problems*, 10th revision. World Health Organization, Geneva.

de Zegher, F., Francois, I., Boehmer, A. *et al.* (1998) Androgens and fetal growth. *Hormone Research*, 50, 243–244.

Zoccolillo, M., Pickles, A., Quinton, D. & Rutter, M. (1992) The outcome of childhood conduct disorder: implications for defining adult personality disorder and conduct disorder. *Psychological Medicine*, 22, 971–986.

Zucker, K. (1985) Cross-gender-identified children. In: *Gender Dysphoria: Development, Research, Management* (ed. B.W. Steiner), pp. 75–174. Plenum Press, New York.

Zucker, K. (1990) Gender identity disorders in children: clinical descriptions and natural history. In: *Clinical Management of Gender Identity Disorders in Children and Adults* (eds R. Blanchard & B.W. Steiner), pp. 1–23. American Psychiatric Press, Washington D.C.

Zucker, K. (1992) Gender identity disorder. In: *Child Psychopathology: Diagnostic Criteria and Clinical Assessment* (eds S.R. Hooper, G.W. Hynd & R.E. Mattison), pp. 305–342. Erlbaum, Hillsdale, NJ.

Zucker, K. (1996) Pathological gender mourning in mothers of boys with gender identity disorder: clinical evidence and some psychocultural hypotheses. Paper presented at the Meeting of the Society for Sex Therapy and Research, Miami Beach.

Zucker, K. (1999a) Commentary on Richardson's (1996) 'Setting Limits on Gender Health'. *Harvard Review of Psychiatry*, 7, 37–42.

Zucker, K. (1999b) Intersexuality and gender identity differentiation. *Annual Review of Sex Research*, 10, 1–69.

Zucker, K. (1999c) Gender identity disorder in the DSM-IV [Letter to the editor]. *Journal of Sex and Marital Therapy*, 25, 5–9.

Zucker, K. (2000a) Gender identity disorder. In: *Handbook of Developmental Psychopathology* (eds A.J. Sameroff, M. Lewis & S.M. Miller), 2nd edn, pp. 671–686. Kluwer Academic/Plenum, New York.

Zucker, K. (2000b) Commentary on Walters and Whitehead's (1997) 'Anorexia Nervosa in a Young Boy with Gender Identity Disorder of Childhood: A Case Report'. *Clinical Child Psychology and Psychiatry*, 5, 232–238.

Zucker, K. (2001) Gender identity disorder in children and adolescents. In: *Treatments of Psychiatric Disorders*, Vol. 2 (ed. G.O. Gabbard), 3rd edn, pp. 2069–2094. American Psychiatric Press, Washington, DC.

Zucker, K. & Bradley, S. (1995) *Gender Identity Disorder and Psychosexual Problems in Children and Adolescents*. Guilford Press, New York.

Zucker, K. & Bradley, S. (2000) Gender identity disorder. In: *Handbook of Infant Mental Health* (ed. C.H. Zeanah), 2nd edn, pp. 412–424. Guilford Press, New York.

Zucker, K., Bradley, S., Doering, R. & Lozinski, J. (1985) Sex-typed behavior in cross-gender-identified children: stability and change at a one-year follow-up. *Journal of the American Academy of Child Psychiatry*, 24, 710–719.

Zucker, K., Bradley, S. & Ipp, M. (1993a) Delayed naming of a newborn boy: relationship to the mother's wish for a girl and subsequent cross-gender identity in the child by the age of two. *Journal of Psychology and Human Sexuality*, 6, 57–68.

Zucker, K., Bradley, S., Lowry Sullivan, C., Kuksis, M., Birkenfeld-Adams, A. & Mitchell, J. (1993b) A gender identity interview for children. *Journal of Personality Assessment*, 61, 443–456.

Zucker, K., Green, R., Garofano, C. *et al.* (1994) Prenatal gender preference of mothers of feminine and masculine boys: relation to sibling sex composition and birth order. *Journal of Abnormal Child Psychology*, 22, 1–13.

Zucker, K., Bradley, S. & Lowry Sullivan, C. (1996a) Traits of separation anxiety in boys with gender identity disorder. *Journal of the American Academy of Child and Adolescent Psychiatry*, 35, 791–798.

Zucker, K., Bradley, S., Oliver, G., Blake, J., Fleming, S. & Hood, J. (1996b) Psychosexual development of women with congenital adrenal hyperplasia. *Hormones and Behavior*, 30, 300–318.

Zucker, K., Bradley, S. & Sanikhani, M. (1997a) Sex differences in referral rates of children with gender identity disorder: some hypotheses. *Journal of Abnormal Child Psychology*, 25, 217–227.

Zucker, K., Green, R., Coates, S. *et al.* (1997b) Sibling sex ratio of boys with gender identity disorder. *Journal of Child Psychology and Psychiatry*, 38, 543–551.

Zucker, K., Blanchard, R., Cavacas, A., Bradley, S., Paterson, A. & Schachter, D. (1999a) *Birthweight in children with gender identity disorder*. Poster presented at the meeting of the International Academy of Sex Research, Stony Brook, New York.

Zucker, K., Bradley, S., Kuksis, M. *et al.* (1999b) Gender constancy judgments in children with gender identity disorder: evidence for a developmental lag. *Archives of Sexual Behavior*, 28, 475–502.

Zucker, K., Beaulieu, N., Bradley, S., Grimshaw, G. & Wilcox, A. (2001) Handedness in boys with gender identity disorder. *Journal of Child Psychology and Psychiatry*, 42, 767–776.

Zucker, K., Owen, A., Bradley, S. & Ameeriar, L. (in press) Gender-dysphoric children and adolescents: a comparative analysis of demographic characteristics and behavioral problems. *Clinical Child Psychology and Psychiatry*.

Feeding and Sleep Disorders

Alan Stein and Jacqueline Barnes

Introduction

Feeding and sleeping are two areas of functioning that not only occupy a great deal of time in the young child's life but also present significant challenges to parents and children. Together, feeding and sleeping serve biological function: feeding is important in terms of basic nutrition, to survive, to thrive and to develop both physically and mentally, while sleeping serves restorative functions.

Much of early parent and infant social interaction occurs around feeding and sleeping. During mealtimes infants often learn for the first time about some of their own emerging capacities, while in sleep the infant learns about separation from carers. Through these processes the infant develops its earliest self-regulation, so critical for later development and interaction with the social world.

Although sleeping and feeding are the context for much satisfaction and pleasure for both child and caregiver, they can also be the source of much distress. Some children have physiological attributes that mitigate against the smooth developmental progression of self-regulation required for sleep, whereas others may be unable to cope with the biological processes inherent in establishing feeding. Many parents and children find that these activities then become associated with stressful, conflictual and maladaptive relationships when either parent or child does not meet with the expectations of the other. It is not surprising therefore that studies of young children's behaviour problems consistently demonstrate that disruptions in sleeping, inability to remain asleep, reluctance to feed, refusal of foods or consumption of too much food are high on the list of the most commonly reported problems.

Feeding disorders

Introduction to feeding, growth and development

Infants and young children rely on caregivers to provide their nutritional requirements. Weight gain and the proportion of energy used for growth during the first 6 months is more rapid than at any other period of development (Whitehead 1985). The social importance of feeding is also greatest in the first few months when much of a child's waking time and social contacts will be taken up with ensuring adequate intake of nutrients (Bunton *et al.* 1987). This has led to a focus on mother–infant feeding in

the psychological study of interactions (Wolke 1991). Developmental changes in feeding during the first 2 years may have a powerful influence on the development of some kinds of feeding difficulty. During that time the infant moves from a completely liquid diet, through the acceptance of smooth thickened food, then roughly chopped mixtures, to an acceptance of an approximation to adult food. Thus, classification and diagnosis of feeding and eating problems in young children and plans for their treatment need to incorporate somatic, developmental and social or behavioural factors (Budd *et al.* 1992; Chatoor 1997).

The provision of nutrition is conducted in the context of the infant's emerging social relationships, in conjunction with the development of a number of biological regulatory systems. The newborn infant has reflexes (rooting, sucking) designed to seek out and ingest food, and soon learns to signal need through crying and other forms of communication, and also learns to what extent those signals are responded to, and in what manner. This process is guided and regulated by the brain structures and physiology involved in the development of oral-motor control, taste perception, hunger, appetite, food preferences and gastric regulation (Wolke 1994).

There are three main kinds of feeding problem in infancy and childhood:

1 too little intake;

2 too much intake; and

3 highly restricted or extremely idiosyncratic diet.

Some feeding problems may be closely associated with biological rhythmicity in hunger, or biological immaturity leading to reflux. Others derive from the context of the caregiver–child relationship. Health problems can also be linked with parental feeding strategies. The early introduction of solids was found in a large Scottish sample of infants to be associated with an increased risk for respiratory illness and coughs, after adjusting for factors such as parental smoking (Forsyth *et al.* 1993).

Historical trends in infant feeding

One of the most consistent findings is the way in which patterns of feeding have changed over the twentieth century, more often reflecting the social norms of the time than any definitive knowledge about the relative impact of any type of feeding. Recently, there has been a focus on ecological intergenerational influences. Thus, among African-American adolescent mothers it is the cultural norm to introduce cereal in the bottle within the first month of life and to use other semisolid foods, contrary to most medical opinion and advice from child care books (Bentley *et al.* 1999). Grandmothers were influential in guiding feeding patterns, having extensive physical access to the infants in the context of their daughters being dependent on them for child care. The extent of a society's overall economic and social development is also relevant to the level of breastfeeding. In developing countries, mothers in rural areas are more likely to breastfeed than those in urban areas, and the more highly educated women are less likely to breastfeed, contrary to findings from many developed nations (Rogers *et al.* 1997). The wider cultural and social context is also important for understanding the development of feeding problems (Black 1999).

Epidemiology of breastfeeding

The trend in rates of breastfeeding was downwards for most of the twentieth century. In 1910, approximately 70% of mothers chose breastfeeding in the first instance (Hendershot 1984). A UK survey just after the Second World War showed that 60% of mothers breastfed when their child was 1 month of age, with the rate falling to 42% by 3 months. A study in Nottingham in the late 1950s found that the rate had dropped to 54 and 29% at 1 and 3 months, respectively. At that time the 'modern' and 'convenient' aspects of bottle-feeding were promoted at the same time that families had a higher standard of living and were thus able to afford equipment such as sterilizing units, bottles and teats (Newson & Newson 1963). Response to perceived medical wisdom is also a factor. Mothers revealed their knowledge that professionals such as health visitors preferred breastfeeding by differential responses: at 1 month 54% of mothers reported breastfeeding to their health visitor, but only 40% of the same women described breastfeeding to a university researcher (Newson & Newson 1963).

Rates of breastfeeding dropped through the 1960s to a low of 24–28% in the early 1970s, then gradually rose during the 1980s as natural childbirth became more popular. In the USA there was a similar decline from the 1950s to the 1970s, with fluctuations until the late 1990s, when the rate once again was >60% (Ryan 1997). However, by 6 months, the rate has dropped to 25%. European rates, with the exception of Ireland and Malta, are similar to or well above the UK and USA, ranging from 98% (Denmark, Sweden) to 60% (Belgium) (Meiklejohn, unpublished report, 2000). A recent community study in southwest England found that 77% of mothers intended to breastfeed at 1 month, and 58% planned to continue until at least 4 months (Barnes *et al.* 1997). National surveys have been conducted in the UK every 5 years since 1975. The two most recent surveys, completed in 1990 and 1995, found that the reported incidence of breastfeeding in the first weeks of life in England and Wales had risen slightly in those 5 years from 64 to 68% (White *et al.* 1992; Foster *et al.* 1997). There were similar rises in Scotland and Northern Ireland, but within much lower rates (Scotland 50 and 55%; Northern Ireland 36 and 45%).

Factors associated with lower rates in the UK include lower social class, living without a husband or partner, fewer years of maternal education, younger maternal age, maternal smoking, and second or later births. Among primiperous mothers aged 30 or over, 85% breastfed compared with 44% of those under 20 years; of the mothers who completed their education over the age of 18, 89% breastfed compared with 59% of those whose education was completed at 16 or younger.

Current social class differences are reversed from the pattern prior to the 1970s. Until then, breastfeeding had been more common for working class than middle class mothers, but currently it is more often the method of choice for mothers in higher social classes. A shorter duration is found in each successive social class group: in the most recent UK survey 90% of mothers in social class I breastfed at birth, compared with 57% in social class IV and 50% in social class V. By the age of 6 weeks, 73% of social class I mothers were still breastfeeding, compared with 33% in social class IV and 23% in social class V. In the USA, mothers who opt for extended nursing of their children are also likely to be from middle class backgrounds (Sugarman & Kendall-Tackett 1995).

Breastfeeding has been strongly encouraged by health professionals (Standing Committee on Nutrition of the British Paediatric Society 1994), supported by recent evidence of a variety of benefits: protection from gastrointestinal disease (Howie *et al.* 1990); less respiratory tract illness (Wright *et al.* 1989); and enhanced neurological and intellectual development throughout childhood (Lanting *et al.* 1994; Pollock 1994a; Florey *et al.* 1995; Johnson *et al.* 1996), with particular cognitive benefits for pre-term infants (Lucas *et al.* 1990, 1992, 1998). There have been suggestions that the enhanced intellectual development associated with breastfeeding is an artefact of social class (Malloy & Berendes 1998). However, a recent meta-analysis concluded that, controlling for social class and maternal education, and including both low birth weight and full-term infants, breastfeeding was associated with significantly higher scores for cognitive development than bottle-feeding (Anderson *et al.* 1999).

The reasons mothers of first babies gave in the 1995 UK survey for choosing to breastfeed reflect professional advice to a certain extent: 'best for baby' (89%); 'more convenient' (36%); 'cheaper' (23%); it helps to develop 'a closer bond between mother and baby' (21%); and for those having a second or subsequent child that it was their previous feeding method (33%). Choice of bottle-feeding was supported by reasons that include 'someone else can feed the baby' (36%), dislike of the idea of breastfeeding (27%), or embarrassment about breastfeeding (7%) (Foster *et al.* 1997).

Personal and cultural factors are also important in predicting feeding patterns, with higher rates for women who were breastfed themselves, whose friends breastfed and who did not smoke during pregnancy (Foster *et al.* 1997). Attitudes towards childrearing reflecting a child-orientated approach (e.g. always picking up a crying baby or adapting life to a baby's needs) are associated with a greater likelihood of planning to breastfeed, while socioemotional difficulties (e.g. depression or preoccupation with body weight and shape) are contraindications to breastfeeding (Barnes *et al.* 1997). Maternal depression has also been associated with early cessation of breastfeeding (Cooper *et al.* 1993). In the UK, if there was a delay of more than 12 h after the birth before mothers held their babies, they were also less likely to breastfeed (Foster *et al.* 1997). However, in some countries in Asia it is commonplace for a child not to be given the mother's colostrum, and therefore for the first feed to occur well after 24 h (Rogers *et al.* 1997). In most societies the presence of conflicting advice from health professionals and the availability of (sometimes free samples of) powdered milk decrease the likelihood that mothers will establish breastfeeding.

Sucking/suckling, weaning and introduction of solids

It is recommended that, for most infants, solids should not be introduced before the age of 4 months (DOH 1994) but the UK 1995 survey found that 7% of mothers introduced solids by 6 weeks, 13% by 8 weeks and over half (55%) by 3 months (Foster *et al.* 1997). This was strongly associated with social class and maternal smoking. By 3 months more than two-thirds (68%) of mothers in social class V had introduced solids compared with one-third (35%) of those in social class I. Weaning was also associated with feeding method in that only 1% of breastfed infants had been given solids at 6 weeks compared with 9% of bottle-fed infants. By 3 months 30% of the breastfed group had been offered solids and 63% of those given a bottle. Studies have shown that early introduction of solids is a common source of conflict between professionals and mothers (Blaxter & Paterson 1982) and the knowledge that they are acting contrary to professional advice may be a reason for not attending child health clinics (McIntosh 1986). Mothers gave reasons for introducing solids related to encouraging their baby to sleep through the night or to ease fretfulness and crying (McIntosh 1986). It has been found that boys are given solids sooner. This may be related to sociocultural factors, such as wanting them to be large and strong, or to the fact that male infants are frequently fussier and less easy to soothe (Harris 1988).

A less common concern is the late introduction of solids. Basic oral-motor patterns are dependent on maturation but a necessary prerequisite is practice in mouth opening, lip movements, chewing and swallowing. Skills related to movement of food from one side of the mouth to the other during chewing, and coping with viscous foods in addition to solids, develop gradually up to at least 8 years of age (Gisel 1988). The absence of early experiences of these actions because of late introduction of solids, highlighted by the prolonged feeding of gruel from bottles experienced by infants in Romanian orphanages, can lead to problems with feeding such as food refusal and, in extreme cases, even to failure to thrive (Skuse *et al.* 1992).

Feeding difficulties and disorders

Food refusal

Food refusal is the most common type of feeding difficulty among infants and preschool-age children. The proportion of children refusing all but a few foods is high, with as many as 30% of infants' mothers reporting feeding difficulties (Jenkins *et al.* 1980) and faddy eating (defined as refusing many foods for at least half the meals offered) reported by 12% of parents of 3 year olds (Richman *et al.* 1982). For some children the problem of food refusal can be severe, with only two or three foods eaten. This kind of behaviour may lead to children being slow to grow or to be deficient in specific nutrients, with a particular tendency to iron deficiency (Harris *et al.* 1983; Aukett *et al.* 1986). Some children will have been poor feeders from birth, others may start to limit their intake at the introduction of solids foods, and for others food refusal has its origins in illness which may or may not be related to diminished appetite or gastrointestinal disease (Harris 2000). Parents can be responsible for limiting the range of foods eaten, as a consequence of presumed food allergy (Price *et al.* 1988), cultural variations in the age of weaning or the use of many sweetened foods rather than progressing to family foods (Jones 1987). This may itself be a response to early patterns in the infant. Quite often chronic food refusers will have been poor feeders from birth, either slow to feed, with poor sucking, or frequent vomiting. Parents with such an infant may delay the onset of introducing solid foods and the later use of solids can exacerbate food refusal.

Children with food refusal frequently have acceptable behaviour outside the feeding situation but sometimes food refusal is associated with other difficulties. Chatoor *et al.* (1985) described a clinical sample in which the food refusal was seen as a component of a separation disorder; part of a broader challenge for the development of the child's autonomy in the face of parental control. This may be intensified if the parent is particularly anxious about his or her child's weight or growth, despite the fact that most food refusers do not show growth faltering. Some medical conditions, such as cerebral palsy, are associated with higher rates of food refusal. For these children oral-motor dysfunction means that they cannot manage to chew or swallow various textures which would otherwise be appropriate for their age group, leading to discomfort, gagging and ultimately to food refusal (Gisel & Patrick 1988). Children who have experienced prolonged supplementary feeding following conditions that require oesophageal surgery or those with gastrointestinal abnormalities often exhibit food refusal and gagging when textured food is offered. This may also be the case for children with conditions such as congenital heart disease and cystic fibrosis (Salzer *et al.* 1989; Thommenssen *et al.* 1992). In defining chronic food refusal, children whose behaviour can be related to a current or recent infection would be excluded.

A number of non-organic causes have also been proposed for food refusal or restriction to a narrow range of foods. Some children have small appetites, which parents may find confusing if they have had other children who were hearty eaters or if parental guidance material gives information that differs considerably from their own child's behaviour. Most children with a small appetite eat a range of foods (Harris 1997) and their management requires only growth monitoring and reassuring parents about the range on which average appetite is based. A group of, predominantly, boys who may considerably restrict the range of foods eaten has been described (Harris *et al.* 2000). They may also react if food is not the normal brand or is cooked in a different manner and react strongly to the smell and texture of foods offered. They could be exhibiting the rule-bound behaviour that is associated with a subclinical form of the autistic spectrum, and children with Asperger syndrome and autism also commonly have feeding problems as part of their wider range of symptoms (Harris *et al.* 2000). If there are no growth problems, management should focus on reducing parental anxiety and encouraging parents not to put pressure on children to accept new foods until later in childhood.

Food aversion can also be the consequence of learning. If a certain food is associated with a particularly violent episode of vomiting, which may or may not have been caused by the food in question, the single experience may be followed by absolute refusal to take the food subsequently. Dietary exposure to different tastes also has cultural variations and it has been suggested that children should be exposed to a range of salty and other savoury tastes during the preschool years, to combat their natural preference for sweet tastes (Harris *et al.* 1990). Standard behavioural management techniques, such as modelling appropriate behaviour, shaping approximations to the desired behaviour, reinforcement of appropriate eating and time out when foods are refused, can be successful (O'Brien *et al.* 1991) and parents can help to overcome children's fear of certain foods by modelling positive enjoyment and allowing use of fingers rather than insisting on utensils. However, many children are very resistant to change and coercive patterns of interaction may result (Sanders *et al.* 1993). Parents may be overanxious about their capacity to set limits and need support to help them to deal with struggles with child management and to set boundaries (Chatoor 1997).

Faddiness and selective eating

Some children persist with extreme faddiness, eating a small number of foods throughout their childhood. In particular, this may be a feature of the behavioural repertoire of autistic children (see Lord & Bailey, Chapter 38). Typically, the main foods eaten are carbohydrates, such as pasta, potatoes or bread. While they may be brought to medical attention through concern from parents, it is often the case that they are as physically healthy as their peers, with height and weight in the normal range (Bryant-Waugh & Lask 1995). Many clinicians to whom these children are referred do not usually recommend ways to increase the range of foods but instead focus on how the behaviour will influence social interactions with peers, such as attendance at parties, going on trips or staying overnight with friends. Many of these children seem to negotiate these social situations adequately, and as they move into puberty they gradually increase the range of foods eaten.

Pervasive refusal syndrome

Pervasive refusal syndrome has recently been identified as a rare condition in which refusal to eat and drink is accompanied by a more generalized refusal to walk, talk or carry out any kind of self-care activities, and is sometimes misdiagnosed as early onset anorexia nervosa. First described by Lask *et al.* (1991), it has been seen in a small number of girls, usually between the ages of 8 and 14. The marked fearful avoidance was thought to be symptomatic of post-traumatic stress disorder (PTSD), possibly following physical or sexual abuse, although there is continuing debate about both the syndrome itself and its aetiology. Two phases were conceptualized: first the trauma of abuse followed by a second phase of fear induced by intimidation about the consequences of disclosure. There has been a case report of successful treatment following the discovery of abuse, providing some support for this viewpoint (McGowan & Green 1998). Others have linked the disorder with learned helplessness (Nunn & Thompson 1996), said to be a more helpful theoretical paradigm with which to conceptualize the phenomenology, aetiology and treatment of pervasive refusal syndrome. A multidisciplinary approach has been used, taking the learned helplessness model, one particular issue of which is consent, which may very well be refused as part of the wider behavioural pattern (Nunn *et al.* 1998). However, more work needs to be conducted to allow for a fuller understanding of the condition, and its relevance to current diagnostic systems.

Non-organic failure to thrive

Failure to thrive has been given a variety of labels, including maternal deprivation syndrome, reactive attachment disorder and anorexia nervosa of infancy, and has been defined using clinical and behavioural criteria. However, there is now emerging consensus that it should be defined solely on the basis of growth (Wolke *et al.*, in press). Specifically, it has been proposed that when growth failure (defined as weight below the third percentile) in young children is identified, it will be seen as failure to thrive (FTT) and, if it cannot be attributed to organic factors or to inadequate food intake, it is referred to as non-organic failure to thrive (NOFT). Nevertheless, this definition has been criticized in that it describes a symptom rather than a disorder (Skuse 1985). A British community survey put the prevalence of FTT at 3–4% (Skuse *et al.* 1992) but problems with lack of consistency in anthropometric criteria have also been noted, such that the reported incidence may vary from 1.3 to 20.9% (Wilcox *et al.* 1989; Mayes & Volkmar 1993).

Although traditionally FTT has been thought of as caused by organic factors and NOFT by parenting that lacks nurturance, leading to poor growth despite adequate food intake, the distinction between organic and non-organic causes is not necessarily clear-cut. Oral-motor difficulties and neurological abnormalities have been found in children diagnosed as NOFT (Mathisen *et al.* 1989; Ramsey *et al.* 1993). It has been proposed more recently that, because many organic diseases including congenital heart failure and cerebral palsy lead to FTT only in interaction with poor feeding, some cases should be considered 'mixed' and the label 'non-organic' may not be appropriate (Reilly *et al.*, in press).

Although NOFT is associated with parenting problems, difficulties with the caregiver–child relationship and even child abuse, there is ongoing debate about the relevance of the role of parents (Boddy & Skuse 1994). In the past, studies have emphasized the role of the mother (Fischoff *et al.* 1971). It has been suggested that they provide insufficient nutrition either deliberately or because of financial problems, or that they are abusive, or that they are just misguided about children's nutritional requirements.

More recently, there has been a focus on the whole family and their circumstances within a multifactorial model of development in that NOFT children receive inadequate nutrition for a variety of reasons (Lieberman & Birch 1985; Drotar 1991). Family violence, environmental disorganization and social isolation have received particular attention (Bradley *et al.* 1984; Newberger *et al.* 1986; Crittenden 1987). Problems with family relationships are likely to have an adverse effect on maternal mental health and the capacity to be attentive to the infant's needs. Some clinicians have highlighted the particular impact of fathers in the development and outcome of NOFT through their participation in maladaptive patterns of parenting and/or conflicts with the child's mother (Drotar & Sturm 1987). A multidisciplinary approach to treatment is now thought to be the most beneficial, ideally including home visits, with a team of at least a child psychiatrist/paediatrician, a developmental psychologist, a speech therapist, dietician and social worker, because FTT is usually neither caused primarily by organic disease nor by the social environment (Wolke *et al.*, in press). Some infants may have insufficient diet because of disorganized meals, prolonged use of exclusive breastfeeding, errors in preparing formula, as a result of religious or cultural practices or as a consequence of distorted maternal perceptions about body weight or shape.

There is growing evidence that personal dietary choices can be relevant to children's growth if parents hold distorted beliefs about:

1 adequate nutritional requirements (Pugiliese *et al.* 1987);

2 whether infants are gaining sufficient weight (Sturm & Drotar 1991); or

3 the need to reduce fat in a child's diet (Birch 1990).

This highlights the importance of providing educational supportive intervention to families in addition to clinical treatment.

Cultural attitudes to feeding should also be taken into consideration. A UK community study conducted in a London regional health authority found that whereas 3–5% of white UK, Chinese Asian, Caribbean and mixed race infants had NOFT, the incidence was 15% for Indian Asian children and zero for African infants (Skuse *et al.* 1992). It has been suggested that the late introduction of solid foods and social isolation of the Indian Asian population may have contributed to this difference (Fenton *et al.* 1989).

The team's activities include not only an oral-motor and developmental assessment of the infant but also a history of early temperament, detailed diary of food intake, investigation of parental eating patterns, direct observation of the parent and child and a detailed caregiver interview, including a psychiatric screening. In conjunction with these investigations, information about living conditions, income, extended family support and cultural influences needs to be collected. Subsequent interventions to improve living circumstances and reduce isolation should be accompanied by therapeutic intervention directed both at maternal symptoms, such as depression, and at discordant family relationships.

Colic

Colic in infancy is characterized by paroxysmal crying and tends to follow a characteristic pattern with an onset from about 2–3 weeks of age and usually resolving by 3–4 months. There is debate about its exact definition. Clinicians have traditionally followed the 'rule of three': fussing and crying for 3 h per day on at least 3 days per week for at least 3 weeks (Wessel *et al.* 1954). More recently it has been defined for research purposes as fussing or crying of at least 2 h per day for at least 5 days out of 7, a high-pitched and pain-sounding cry and maternal report of inconsolability (Pinyerd 1992). Longitudinal investigations indicate that although disruptive and upsetting to parents in the first few months, it appears to be a transitory condition, with no discernible difference between infants with and without colic by 5 months (Stifter & Braungart 1992).

Explanations of its aetiology fall into four main types: gastrointestinal dysfunction, allergenic reactions, immaturity of the central nervous system or parental anxiety and tension (Hewson *et al.* 1987; Keefe 1988; Sampson 1989). Although colic clearly elicits much stress in parents, anxiety about separation (Humphry & Hock 1989) and strong feelings of personal inadequacy and depression (Pinyerd 1992; Stifter & Bono 1998), colic is not seen to be secondary to parental behaviour. A specific allergic reaction to the protein content of milk has been proposed (Lothe *et al.* 1982; Jakobsson & Lindberg 1983), although elimination of cows' milk from the diet of the infant—or the mother in the case of breastfed infants—has had mixed results (Wolke & Meyer 1995). Treatment strategies should take as their starting point advice on the management of crying. If that is unsuccessful then cows' milk protein intolerance may be considered, but with the proviso to parents that this does not imply lifelong allergic difficulties (Bock 1987; Wolke & Meyer 1995).

Gastro-oesophageal reflux

The involuntary return of the gastric contents into the oesophagus is particularly common in the first year of life, and takes place occasionally in many children and adults, but becomes pathological when its frequency increases. Gastro-oesophageal reflux (GOR) may also contribute to other feeding problems, such as faddiness and food refusal. The frequent reflux of the acidic gastric contents may lead to pain and skin irritation and to the infant refusing to open his or her mouth, which may persist into childhood even after the GOR has been treated.

GOR may be due to primary (anatomical or physiological) causes or to secondary causes, such as food allergy or metabolic disorders. Apart from feeding problems, many other consequences are likely: growth failure, irritability, iron-deficiency anaemia, recurrent respiratory infections, coughing and choking and, in the most severe cases, sudden infant death (Paton et al. 1988; Davies & Sandhu 1995). Infants with GOR may have laboured respiration and, in its most severe manifestation, an odd posture, holding their head on one side; the vomiting after feeds may resemble seizures with apnoea, cyanosis and stiffening (Bray et al. 1977).

Diagnosis involves 24-h pH monitoring by placing a small probe just below the oesophageal sphincter. The total number of reflux episodes can be assessed and the infant's ability to clear the reflux. Treatment includes giving thickened feeds, antacids, modifying the diet and postural adjustment, such as positioning the infant prone with their head elevated or, failing these strategies, surgical intervention (Davies & Sandhu 1995).

Rumination

Rumination is defined as the voluntary regurgitation of previously eaten food, which is then re-swallowed, persistent over at least 1 month and without any organic cause (American Psychiatric Association 1993). It appears to be pleasurable and usually self-induced through placing fingers in the mouth or contracting the tongue muscles, which distinguishes it from gastro-oesophageal reflux, which is involuntary. However, there are problems with its diagnosis in the absence of weight loss, if it is accompanied by vomiting, or in the presence of organic aetiology (Jackson & Tierney 1984). It is unrelated to acute illness or disease associated with nausea. The prevalence has been estimated at 0.7% in a sample of infants in acute paediatric hospital care and at 6–10% in children with learning disabilities, with a higher incidence in males than females (Mayes et al. 1988).

Some researchers have attributed its aetiology to family factors, specifically problems with the mother–infant relationship, such as neglect, leading the infant to develop strategies for internal gratification. For instance, a study of 20 cases aged 5–28 months suggests that psychosocial stressors, anxiety and/or depression in the primary caregiver and under- or over-stimulation were precipitating factors (Sauvage et al. 1985). Although rumination disorder, most commonly associated with developmental delay, may be long-lasting, there is evidence of 'self-limited' rumination as a reaction to situational stress during childhood (Reis 1994). Historically it was treated from a psychodynamic perspective, by extended inpatient treatment with a surrogate mother (Lavigne et al. 1981). More recently, it has been proposed that the attention received because of the behaviour serves to perpetuate it by providing positive reinforcement and behavioural strategies have been shown effective (Winton 1984). In the past, aversive punishment techniques, such as spraying lemon juice on the tongue or even electric shock, have been used to control rumination (Cunningham & Linscheid 1976) but that would not be considered ethical now, nor would parents wish to use these methods. Instead, the most common behavioural treatment strategies rely on techniques such as time out and reinforcement of retaining food (Winton & Singh 1983).

Pica

Defined by DSM-IV (American Psychiatric Association 1993) as a childhood eating disorder characterized by developmentally inappropriate and persistent eating of non-food or non-nutritive substances (e.g. dirt, starch, clay, paint, plaster) for a period of at least 1 month, pica can have serious health consequences. If the substances ingested are poisonous (e.g. contain lead or parasites) it can have serious health consequences and be life-threatening. For families living in older residences, pica has been associated with the risk of lead poisoning as many children with pica ingest flakes of paint, resulting in blood lead levels higher than even children of lead mine employees (Chiaradia et al. 1997). While this kind of indiscriminate mouthing and eating can be common in infants (eating dirt for example), its incidence declines between 1 and 4 years from 35% to ≈6% (Robischon 1971). Rates for boys and girls do not differ significantly (Marchi & Cohen 1990). There are few longitudinal studies linking early childhood eating problems with later behaviour, but a study of over 800 children in the USA found that pica before the age of 11 was a significant predictor of bulimia nervosa—but not anorexia—in the adolescent years (Marchi & Cohen 1990).

A number of causes have been suggested including nutritional deficiencies (mainly iron or zinc), infant characteristics such as developmental delay, caregiver behaviours such as deprivation or neglect, or more general deprivation of the home environment (Walker et al. 1997). Whereas there is a normative stage when mouthing of all kinds of objects is commonplace, persistence of this behaviour beyond infancy and early childhood is considered abnormal. Education of health professionals about the risks, detailed interviewing and observation of children at risk (e.g. those living in older accommodation, those with caregivers who have limited competence) and close monitoring of children can go a long way to alleviating the risks posed by pica to children's physical development (Robischon 1971). More comprehensive environmental interventions are needed to remove many of the risks and to provide support and education for parents whose children persist with the behaviour beyond infancy.

Obesity

Obesity is becoming more common in childhood (Chinn & Rona 1994; Dietz 1998; World Health Organization Consultation on Obesity 1998), in association with a rise in sedentary pursuits and greater parental protectiveness (Andersen et al. 1998). There is good evidence that childhood obesity is associated with an increased risk of adult obesity (Epstein et al. 1985; Epstein & Wing 1987). The importance of intervention is highlighted by the fact that childhood obesity, in addition to the medical risks and likelihood of persistence to adulthood (Frühbeck 2000), is likely to occur in conjunction with socioemotional difficulties such as a greater risk for bullying and other peer relationship problems, social withdrawal, and depression (Israel & Shapiro 1985; Epstein et al. 1994).

Various explanations for obesity have been put forward, including child and family factors. There is good evidence from adoption and twin studies for a genetic tendency (Sorensen et al. 1989; Cardon 1994) and the best predictor of childhood obesity is obesity in the biological parents (Meyers et al. 1990; Gallaher et al. 1991). Although no differences between children of obese and non-obese mothers can be detected by birth weight, different trajectories emerge from around 6 months onwards (Rummler & Woit 1992) at around the time that solid foods are being introduced. Children at greater risk include those with difficult temperament (Carey et al. 1988), those who are breastfed for a shorter time (Kramer et al. 1985) and those overfed during infancy (Mogan 1986). Whether obese children have a clearly defined eating disorder with features such as distorted body image, false perception of meal size or poor regulation of appetite and eating patterns is as yet unresolved (Kissileff 1989).

Behavioural treatments have proven effectiveness, and intervention effects are strengthened by parental involvement and the incorporation of exercise into the behavioural plan (Epstein & Wing 1987). There are three key settings for intervention: the family, the school and primary care (Frühbeck 2000). Work with the family has documented success, with the additional benefit of improving health and well-being of parents and other family members (Epstein et al. 1990). Nevertheless, interventions in out-of-home settings such as school may have a broader impact on children's emotional well-being, with a focus on developing self-esteem while acknowledging emotional difficulties such as depression (Little 1983).

Parental eating disorders and children's eating

Eating disorders occur commonly among women of childbearing age (Szmukler 1985; Fairburn & Beglin 1990; Hoek 1993) and the prevalence seems to be rising (Treasure et al. 1996). A concern has been that mothers' attitudes and behaviours regarding food and body shape could influence the children's feeding and eating, and ultimately their attitudes to body shape and eating. Children are particularly vulnerable during infancy, given that feeding and mealtimes take up a significant part of the day during the first months of life, and allow for close communication between parents and children. The attitudes, preoccupations and behaviours that people with eating disorders manifest may interfere with their ability to prepare meals, to sit patiently feeding their infants and, in particular, to respond appropriately to hunger and satiety cues. Their attitudes may even influence choice of infant feeding prior to the birth. A large community study found that women with the highest levels of body shape concern during pregnancy were least likely to plan breastfeeding. This relationship held even after adjustment for a wide range of factors known to influence breastfeeding preferences (Barnes et al. 1997).

Investigations of women with eating disorders who have young children have concentrated on mothers' difficulties over children's mealtimes and concerns about children's size. A Scandinavian study (Brinch et al. 1988) found that 17% of the children of women with a history of anorexia nervosa failed to thrive in the first year of life. A controlled study using direct observation of the 1-year-old children of mothers with eating disorders (Stein et al. 1994) found that, when compared with controls, the index mothers were more intrusive with their infants during both mealtimes and play, and they expressed more negative emotion (critical and derogatory remarks) during mealtimes. There was considerably more conflict between index infants and their mothers during mealtimes, and maternal responses were found to be associated with this conflict. In particular, conflict was more likely when mothers did not acknowledge their infants' signals or did not allow them to express age-appropriate needs for autonomy through self-feeding and experimentation with food (Stein et al. 1999). Furthermore, the index infants weighed less than the control infants, and infant weight was found to be independently and inversely related to the amount of conflict during mealtimes. Similar growth problems were not evident in comparison samples of mothers with postnatal depression, indicating that growth faltering was specific to the infants of mothers with eating disorders (Stein et al. 1996).

The strength and specificity of the association between maternal eating disorder psychopathology and child feeding was examined in a study using the child's feeding as the starting point. Thus, the mothers of a consecutive series of young children referred to child psychiatric clinics with feeding disorders were compared with a matched group of children with behavioural disorders and an unselected control group. Only the children with feeding disorders (defined as severe food refusal or extreme faddiness) had mothers with significantly disturbed eating habits and attitudes (Stein et al. 1995). This association has recently been confirmed in a community preschool sample (Whelan & Cooper 2000).

Although it should be emphasized that the children of parents with eating disorders are not invariably adversely affected, it is important to find out about parental characteristics, such as excessive concern about body shape and weight, as part of a thorough family assessment when a child presents with feeding problems or growth failure.

Sleep disorders

Physiological processes in sleep

Sleep is a reversible behavioural state of perceptual disengagement from, and reduced responsiveness to, the environment. This complex amalgam of physiological and behavioural processes is accompanied by characteristic electroencephalogram (EEG) changes (Carskadon & Dement 1989). A neuronal system that governs cyclic alteration between waking and sleep is situated in the core of the brain extending from the medulla through the brainstem and hypothalamus into the forebrain (Jones 1989). Within sleep, there are two different states: the non-rapid eye movement (NREM) state and the rapid eye movement (REM) state (Rechtschaffen & Kales 1968), defined on the basis of physiological parameters including EEG, muscle tone and eye movements. NREM sleep is divided into four stages: stages 1 and 2 are light sleep stages, while stages 3 and 4 represent deep sleep with a high arousal threshold. REM sleep, also called active sleep or paradoxical sleep, is characterized by EEG activation not unlike the wake state, with muscle atonia (absence of muscle tone) and intermittent bursts of rapid eye movements, from which it gets its name. Dreaming only occurs during REM sleep. The arousal threshold in REM sleep is variable. The two sleep states are interrupted throughout the night by brief arousals characterized by EEG changes towards the wake state and an increase in muscle tone with accompanying movement. Arousals vary in duration from a few seconds to several minutes. Thus, sleep is not a uniform state but is constantly changing throughout the night.

From birth onwards NREM and REM sleep alternate cyclically throughout the night. Each cycle takes about 50–60 min in the newborn and gradually increases to 90 min in older children and adults (Carskadon & Dement 1989). Sleep is entered through NREM sleep. NREM sleep stages 3 and 4 dominate the sleep cycle in the early part of the night, with only short periods of REM. As the night progresses, stages 1 and 2 of NREM sleep, as well as REM sleep, take up proportionately greater periods of each cycle, so that morning awakening occurs from REM sleep or the light stages of NREM sleep. Stages 3 and 4 sleep are maximal in young children and decrease in favour of more stage 1 and 2 sleep with age. This explains why young children can be difficult to wake from the first sleep cycle.

Despite a great deal of research, the precise function of sleep remains unresolved. The two most popular theories suggest that sleep is essential for either cerebral restitution, focusing particularly on REM sleep because of its association with dreaming (Dement & Kleitman 1957), or body replenishment because sleep with its enforced rest puts a ceiling on energy expenditure (Zepelin & Rechtschaffen 1974).

Developmental progression of sleep patterns in neonates and infants

In the first year of life, development occurs rapidly and one of the primary functions is to synchronize physiological adaptation with the primary social relationships. Sleep regulation and consolidation are amongst the most important early developmental milestones which infants need to acquire in the first year. Regulation concerns the ability of infants to make the transition smoothly from wakefulness to sleep, and consolidation concerns the infant's ability to sustain sleep in a continuous fashion for an age-appropriate period of time before fully awakening (Sadeh & Anders 1993). The internal biological 'clock' that regulates the sleep–wake cycle begins to synchronize with other internal signals, such as hunger and satiety, and with scheduled periods of social interaction, as well as with other environmental cues such as the light–dark cycle and ambient temperature.

The survival of increasingly premature babies has provided insight into some aspects of the development and maturation of the immature brain, reflected in the infants' regulation of their sleep–wake pattern. It is likely that the fetus is never truly awake but alternates between quiet sleep (QS) and active sleep (AS) which are the precursors of the NREM–REM cycle. Neonates born prior to 30 weeks' gestation spend 90% of sleep time in REM sleep (AS) compared with 50% at term. There are striking changes in the pattern of sleeping and waking in the first 16 weeks of life. Parmelee et al. (1964) found that although there was a relatively small decrease in the total hours of sleep per 24 h over the first 16 weeks from 16.3 to 14.8 h, the average daily continuous sleep period increased from 4 to 8.5 h over the 16 weeks. In conjunction with this change, the average longest daily period of wakefulness increased from 2.4 to 3.6 h. In the first week there were almost equal amounts of sleep during day and night, but by 16 weeks infants slept double the amount at night compared to the day.

There is an important relationship between two central infant activities: sleeping and feeding. Before 1 month of age the sleep–waking pattern is organized around 3–4 hourly feed times. Between 1 and 3 months of age, as the diurnal pattern begins to be established, it is also influenced by environmental and maturational factors (Kleitman & Englemann 1953). At around this time a redistribution of the sleep state takes place so that NREM sleep begins to dominate the beginning of the night and REM sleep later on (Hoppenbrouwers et al. 1982). Infants regularly experience brief periods of waking during the night but usually settle themselves back to sleep. Anders (1979) found that 2-month-old infants spent approximately 9% of the night 'sleep' awake, and this was reduced to 6% by 9 months.

Assessment of the sleep–wake cycle and sleep problems

The cornerstone of assessment is a careful history. Stores (1999a) suggested that three key screening questions should be asked about any child. Does the child experience:

1 difficulty getting to sleep or staying asleep;
2 excessive sleepiness during the day; or
3 disturbing episodes at night.

If positive answers are given for any of these, a detailed sleep history should be obtained. Careful questioning should be made of the full 24-h sleep–wake cycle (Ferber 1995; see Rutter & Yule, Chapter 7). Ferber (1995) suggested the sequence and timing of events should be obtained through each phase of the child's day in relation to sleep, beginning with the evening meal, later evening, going to bed, when asleep, waking and day time. A full history of the child's physical, emotional, health and development is also necessary. A sleep diary kept for a period of 2 weeks will provide a great deal of information which may be helpful in arriving at a clear diagnosis and in treating the problem. An assessment of the family relationships as well as the emotional state of the parents and other family members should be undertaken.

In a small number of cases physiological sleep studies, known as polysomnography, are required. These are likely to be useful in cases of excessive daytime sleepiness, complicated parasomnias and sleep apnoea (Stores 1999b). Polysomnography includes EEG, eye movement and muscle tone recordings, and from these the different sleep stages can be recognized. In children, home polysomnography is often useful rather than bringing them into a laboratory setting. An actigraph, which records body movements, is sometimes used and this can provide some basic information on sleep–wake patterns (for a review of assessment methods see Wiggs & Stores 1995).

Classification of sleep disorders in children

Sleep problems can be grouped into three main categories (Stores 1999b).
1 Sleeplessness, principally settling and night waking problems.
2 Excessive daytime sleepiness, caused by insufficient sleep, disturbed overnight sleep or increased sleep requirements.
3 Episodic disturbances of behaviour associated with sleep, known as parasomnias.

An additional section considers other conditions associated with sleep disorders. Most attention will be paid to settling and waking problems in young children, which are very common.

A comprehensive classification known as the International Classification of Sleep Disorders–Revised (American Sleep Disorders Association 1997) has been published separately from DSM and ICD and includes over 80 different conditions. It provides a number of groupings.
1 Dysomnias are primary sleep disorders which cause either difficulty getting off to sleep or remaining asleep, or excessive sleepiness during the day.
2 Parasomnias, which are subdivided according to the stage of sleep with which they are usually associated.
3 Sleep disorders associated with mental, neurological and other medical disorders.
4 Proposed sleep disorders, or conditions which require further

evaluation before being considered as sleep disorders in their own right.

Sleeplessness

Settling and night waking problems in young children

Nature and prevalence

Sleep difficulties consist of a reluctance or an inability to settle to sleep at the required time, repeated waking in the night with demands for parental attention as well as waking early in the morning. Children make very strong demands for parents to be present and become distressed if they leave (Stores 1996).

Approximately 20% of children aged 1–3 years (Richman 1981; Zuckerman *et al.* 1987) and 10% of children aged 4–5 years (Bax 1980) have significant problems in settling to sleep and waking at night. There is a significant risk that early sleeping problems will persist, with many studies finding that the best predictor of later sleeping problems is early sleeping difficulties (Richman *et al.* 1982; Jenkins *et al.* 1984; Scott & Richards 1990a; Scher 1991). Furthermore, Richman *et al.* (1982) in their large community epidemiological study found that 40% of children who had sleep problems at 8 years of age had such problems dating back to at least 3 years old. However, it should be emphasized that although there is clearly a significant risk that early sleep problems will persist, the majority do not.

Sleep problems are sometimes associated with other behavioural or emotional disturbances. Zuckerman *et al.* (1987) found that children of 3 years of age with persistent sleeping problems, compared to those with transient sleeping problems, were more likely to exhibit tantrums and behaviour management problems. Pollock (1994b), in a large epidemiological study, found that sleeping problems were associated with stomach aches, eating difficulties, headaches and temper tantrums.

Aetiological factors in settling and night waking

Many authors, such as Sadeh & Anders (1993), use a transactional model to understand children's sleep patterns, assuming that symptoms are dynamic and that there is a bidirectionality of effects. The influences on children's sleep patterns (settling and night waking in particular) can be divided into extrinsic factors (sociodemographic, cultural and parental factors) and intrinsic child factors. These factors are in turn mediated by parental caregiving interactions and the parent–child relationship.

Most reports on children's sleep patterns come from parents, whose own well-being may have been influenced by their children's difficulties. Their accounts of night waking depend on whether they have been woken themselves. Minde *et al.* (1993) compared parental diary records to videotapes of 28 children with sleep disorders and 30 controls, and found that children regarded as 'good sleepers' woke as often as 'poor sleepers', but soothed themselves back to sleep without disturbing anyone. This indicated that the critical difference between the groups was that the good sleepers had the capacity to soothe themselves back to sleep, rather than that they woke less. In addition, parents vary greatly as to whether they perceive night waking to be a problem (Scott & Richards 1990b).

Sociodemographic and cultural factors. Factors reflecting adverse living conditions, such as overcrowding and poor housing, have generally been shown to be associated with sleep problems (Chavin & Tinson 1980; Scott & Richards 1990b). However, there does not seem to be a relationship with maternal education, socioeconomic class or maternal age.

The issue of cosleeping is a rather complex one. It is not particularly sanctioned in Western countries, although it is probably relatively common, while in many communities in other countries cosleeping is probably the norm (Morelli *et al.* 1992). It appears that sleep problems are largely reported in relation to cosleeping in cultures where it is not the norm. However, as most of the data available are from developed countries it is difficult to make easy generalizable judgements. In the laboratory, cosleeping mother–infant pairs have been shown by McKenna *et al.* (1990) to have more frequent brief arousals when sleeping together than when sleeping apart. A number of studies have shown that cosleeping is associated with increased sleep problems, particularly in slightly older children (Lozoff *et al.* 1984; Schachter *et al.* 1989; Madansky & Edelbrock 1990). In a recent study comparing cosleeping patterns amongst Japanese and US families, Japanese families were more likely to cosleep (Latz *et al.* 1999). Cosleeping was strongly associated with a variety of sleep problems such as bedtime struggles and overall stressful sleep problems amongst the USA infants, but was not associated with increased sleep problems amongst Japanese infants. This study suggests that cultural factors are important in influencing whether cosleeping is related to reported sleep problems. In particular, cultural factors are likely to influence parents' expectations of infant behaviour.

There has also been considerable interest in the relationship between cosleeping and the risk of sudden infant death syndrome (see section below).

Family factors. The one family factor that has been consistently found to be important is the mother's mental state. A number of studies have reported an association between maternal mood and sleep problems (Richman 1981; Zuckerman *et al.* 1987). Zuckerman *et al.* (1987) found that maternal depression at 8 months was associated with the persistence of sleep problems from 8 months to 3 years. In a prospective study of postnatal depression, Murray (1992) found an association between maternal postnatal depression in the first few months of life and sleeping difficulties at 18 months, at which time many of the mothers were no longer depressed.

Child factors. Both Carey (1974) and Sadeh *et al.* (1992) found that infants with sleep problems had lower sensory thresholds than infants without sleep problems, and the latter study also found lower adaptability in younger children with severe night

waking problems compared to controls. Richman (1981) and Schaefer (1990) found difficult temperaments amongst children to be related to night awakenings in a community and clinical sample, respectively, and more recently Halpern *et al.* (1994) confirmed that infant sleep–wake patterns (assessed by videotape) were related to temperament. Only the study of Keener *et al.* (1988) differs in that they did not find temperamental differences between infants who cried when they woke during the night compared to those who did not. Thus, in general, infant temperament does seem to be related to sleep–wake regulation and sleep problems.

A number of other infant factors have been linked to sleep disturbance. Specific difficulties during the perinatal period as well as infant irritability in the early weeks have been found to be related to later sleep difficulties (Bernal 1973; Blurton-Jones *et al.* 1978; Richman 1981). Such difficulties include prolonged labour, poor infant state at birth (e.g. longer time to first breath and cry, poor muscle tone and reflex irritability) as well as increased frequency of crying bouts in the first 10 days. Two nonmutually exclusive mechanisms are suggested. First, infants who go on to be poorer sleepers are neurodevelopmentally more vulnerable and less adaptable and, secondly, these early perinatal difficulties may lead parents to be more attentive and responsive at night with increased handling, making the infants more susceptible to sleep difficulties (Bernal 1973).

Caregiving patterns and the parent–infant relationship. The above influences on sleep–wake patterns are mediated through the parent–infant relationship. These include interactive behaviours such as breast/bottle-feeding, parental presence at sleep time, parental cognitions and behaviours, attachment patterns and separation anxiety.

The balance of research indicates that breastfeeding has an impact on the sleep–wake cycle, with breastfed infants waking more frequently than artificially fed infants. Wright & Crow (1982), Elias *et al.* (1986) and Eaton-Evans & Dugdale (1988) all found that breastfed infants were more likely to wake at night, although some earlier studies did not find this relationship (Bernal 1973). Breastfed infants have also been found to have fewer total hours of sleep (per 24-h cycle) during the first 2 years of life (Wright *et al.* 1983; Keane *et al.* 1988). While at 2 months of age breastfed infants have large feeds early in the morning and smaller feeds at the end of the day, by 4 months this pattern changes with large meals at the end of the day (Wright & Crow 1982). This is apparently adaptive in order to allow the infant to manage the longer sleep periods without having to feed. Parents of bottle-fed infants often introduce this pattern earlier on in an attempt to reduce overnight feeds.

Both Adair *et al.* (1991) and Johnson (1991) found that parental presence when the infant goes off to sleep is associated with sleep difficulties, especially night waking. The latter study also found that active soothing at bedtime was associated with not sleeping through the night.

Parental cognitions and attitudes have also been implicated in infant sleep problems. Morrell (1999) found that certain parental cognitions were related to sleep problems, including difficulties with limit setting, resisting infant demands, as well as anger with infant demands and doubt about parenting competence. Furthermore, Scher & Blumberg (1999) found that first-born infants (although not infants born subsequently) of mothers who were rated as 'facilitators'—who feel that the baby knows best and that the environment should be adapted to the baby—had more night waking at 1 year, compared to infants of mothers who were rated as 'regulators'—who believe that the baby must adapt him or herself to the environment.

A number of authors have argued that the quality of parent–infant attachment relationships is likely to have a bearing on night settling and night waking and the development of sleep problems in young infants (Moore 1989; Anders 1994). Falling asleep alone and settling after waking during the night are said to be important aspects of early separation and individuation whereby the infant develops an autonomous self and deals with separation anxiety. A recent study by Morrell (unpublished data) examined the relationship between attachment security and persistent sleep problems by studying 100 infants, 40 with sleep problems and 60 without at 15 months and following them up 12 months later. He found that ambivalent attachment at 15 months predicted persistent sleep problems. Benoit et al. (1992) found a relationship between maternal insecure adult attachment classification and sleep disorders in young children, while Scher & Blumberg (1999) found that maternal separation anxiety from the infant was related to night waking, suggesting that the mother's own attachment status and her separation concerns have a role in infant sleep–wake regulation. Sadeh & Anders (1993), based on their clinical experience, reported that separation problems in both parent and infant are the most common relationship issues underlying persistent parent–infant difficulties in resolving sleep problems.

As mentioned above, parent–child influences are bidirectional and persistent sleep disturbance can have a considerable impact on the parents and family (Chavin & Tinson 1980), although it is often difficult to disentangle the direction of causal relationships. This complex interplay between child factors and parental factors is well illustrated in a study by Quine (1992) of mothers of children with learning difficulties who had sleep problems. These mothers were found to have particular parenting difficulties, being more irritable, using more physical punishment and being generally more negative towards their children, compared to control mothers of children with learning difficulties but without sleep problems.

Treatment

The principal aim of treatment is to help the child to fall asleep without the involvement of the parents, and, if a child wakes, to be able to soothe itself and settle back to sleep without the parents' help.

Medication. Medication is sometimes used but is not usually a first-line treatment and tends to be confined to short-term use, usually in a crisis, to allow parents and children a chance to settle before behavioural programmes are introduced. In trials evaluating the use of medication—usually antihistamine hypnotics such as trimeprazine—there were some positive effects in treating night wakings in the short term but these benefits did not seem to last once the drug was stopped (Ramchandani et al. 2000). Furthermore, there was a considerable drop-out in these drug trials.

Behavioural treatments. Generally, the procedure adopted is to encourage parents to put the child to bed awake and then left alone for progressively longer periods with repeated brief reassurances. Where night wakings occur, the same process should be followed. For further details see Douglas & Richman (1984) and France & Hudson (1993).

A number of behavioural treatments for settling problems and night waking in young children have been subjected to treatment trials (for a systematic review see Ramchandani et al. 2000).

1 Positive routines consist of a set of positive winding-down routines usually to deal with bedtime tantrums. These include enjoyable but relaxing activities for 20 minutes prior to bedtime, beginning at the time the child normally falls asleep then gradually brought forward 5–10 minutes per week, until the target bedtime is reached. After completion of the routine, any resistance from the child is dealt with by the parents saying 'It's time for sleep' and placing the child back to sleep if necessary (Adams & Rickert 1989).

2 Extinction or systematic ignoring, where parents go to the child when they hear the first cry, check that the child is not ill, change the nappy if necessary but do not pick up the child, soothe or feed in any way. Once the parent is reassured the child is not ill the parent leaves the room and does not return for the duration of the crying episode.

3 Graduated extinction (removing any reinforcing response to the child's waking behaviour) in which parents ignore bedtime tantrums for preset time intervals, the duration of which is increased each week. At the end of the interval the parents enter the room and put the child back to bed, if necessary, and tell them it is time for sleep before leaving the room again after a maximum of 15 seconds.

4 Modified extinction involves the parents ignoring the child for 20 minutes and then checking the child is not ill but not picking the child up, soothing or interacting, or feeding the child. Once reassured, the parents leave the room and only return after the child displays the settling problem, waiting for a further 20 minutes. Some parents find extinction programmes unacceptable and drop out of trials (Rickert & Johnson 1988). Support visits are often given to the parents in conjunction with modified extinction every 2 or 3 days during the first 2 or 3 weeks of treatment.

5 Scheduled wakes: following the collection of baseline data, parents are instructed to wake the child 15–60 minutes before the child usually wakes spontaneously and to resettle them in their usual manner. The number and timing of schedule wakes are then modified on a twice-weekly basis, depending on the child's sleep pattern during the previous few nights.

6 Educational booklets have also been tried (Seymour *et al.* 1989) as have sleep programmes which consist of individually tailored behavioural programmes using a variety of techniques with daily supportive telephone calls, decreasing in frequency over time, accompanied by a behavioural advice booklet.

In general, trials have shown that these specific behavioural interventions lead to improvements, with the various forms of extinction and scheduled wakenings showing reductions in night waking (Ramchandani *et al.* 2000). Adams & Rickert (1989) evaluated the effect of settling problems of two treatments: positive routines and graduated extinction. They found that both types of treatment were more effective than controls. There was some evidence that a specific educational booklet could be useful in sleeping problems (Seymour *et al.* 1989). In the trials that followed up the children (at 6 weeks or 3 months following treatment) the beneficial effects had generally been maintained.

Positive reinforcement can be used with slightly older children (3 or 4 years and above). The appropriate sleeping behaviour to be reinforced needs to be clearly defined and initially relatively easy to achieve, such as settling to bed quietly. Once achieved, the task is increased gradually until the child goes through the night without demanding parental attention. The usual reinforcers such as star charts are used. Parents are often willing to use this technique but relapses are more common.

Brief psychodynamic psychotherapy. Morrell (1999) noted that some parents dislike behavioural therapy, especially extinction techniques. This might be as a result of attachment difficulties and maternal cognitions concerning difficulty in setting limits, resisting infant demands, anger at infant demands and doubts about parenting competence. Morrell (1999) argued that this necessitates an approach that takes account of the parents' perceptions and feelings and the parent–infant relationship.

Brief psychodynamic psychotherapy for parents and their young children attempts to take account of these issues and may be more acceptable to some parents. One outcome study has shown some positive benefits for a variety of infant difficulties including sleep problems using this form of psychotherapy (Cramer 1995). Daws (1989) used a particular form of brief psychodynamic psychotherapy for parents and infants when an infant has a sleep problem and reports considerable success; however, this remains to be formally evaluated. This form of treatment deals principally with emotional and attachment issues rather than behavioural issues in trying to help parents to understand their feelings about their infant and in managing the infant's sleep. The therapist takes account of the infant's daily patterns of sleep and waking, the parents' memories of pregnancy and birth, their own past experiences and their thoughts about their relationship with the infant. In essence, the treatment links the meaning of not sleeping to deeper issues of separation and individuation between mother and infant, incorporating past and present experiences and relationships.

Sadeh & Anders (1993) used a model in which the infant is viewed as part of a system and sleep–wake is a mode of 'transaction', with attachment separation and individuation being the central issue. Their intervention also takes account of parental beliefs and expectations and enquires carefully into the way the nature of the attachment between parents and infant might relate to sleeping and waking. They provide a more focused intervention with a number of components: educational, psychodynamic (understanding the meaning of symptoms) and behavioural. However, until these forms of psychodynamic psychotherapy are subjected to formal evaluation, it is not possible to judge them in relation to other more established behavioural treatments.

Routines. One important issue, relevant to all types of intervention but particularly behavioural strategies, is that of daytime napping (Stores 1996). Two naps a day is usual at 6 months and one nap by 1 year, each nap not usually lasting more than 2–2.5 h. These naps may be taken at times of the day that complicate the sleep–wake cycle, for example, too late in the afternoon, or children may take too many naps. This may be a particular issue for children who have more than one caregiver throughout the day. The promotion of sleep 'hygiene' for children and adolescents is an important part of prevention as well as treatment. In particular, children need a sleeping environment with a comfortable familiar setting, correct temperature, a dark and quiet room, and non-stimulating, non-punitive parental behaviour. Parents should encourage bedtime or nap routines with consistent sleep and waking up times (Stores 1996). Parents often report that infants will only go off to sleep, or return to sleep, after feeding, which in turn leads to a large overnight food consumption and very wet nappies which lead to more waking. This can often be overcome by the promotion of a circadian pattern of feeding during the day and sleeping at night. This is usually most easily achieved by the reduction of night-time feeding (Stores 1996).

Impact of improving sleep patterns

There have been a number of reports indicating that where parents have been helped with the sleep problems of their young children, it can lead to improvements in maternal state, mother–child interaction and child behaviour. Wolfson *et al.* (1992), who provided parent training for infant problems, found that this led to improvements in the mother's emotional state and in her general confidence in her parenting abilities. Minde *et al.* (1994) found marked improvements following treatment, not only in sleep disturbance but in toddlers' daytime behaviour and in feeding interactions with their mothers. Thus, help for families to manage sleep disturbances can generalize to other aspects of infant behaviour and mother–infant interaction.

Sleeplessness in older preschool and school-age children

Bedtime struggles and other settling difficulties often continue in older preschool and school-aged children where children refuse or delay going to bed. The problem is often maintained by parents' continuing difficulty in establishing and consistently enforcing rules about bedtime and settling to sleep. Many of these parents find it difficult to set limits in a clear and non-punitive manner (Stores 1996).

Night-time fears are common in childhood and may be one of the causes of children's difficulty in getting off to sleep or disturbance during the night. The cause of night fears depend on children's stage of development. Children's fears include those of the dark, shadows and monsters and they require comfort and reassurance. Where severe anxiety complicates these fears, they may be associated with nightmares. If these persist a more serious cause may need to be considered, such as family disruptions and traumas, and more intensive help for the family provided.

Sometimes children are physiologically unable to go to sleep at the times the parents wish them to, as in the delayed sleep phase syndrome (DSPS). This can occur at all ages. Children and adults have a period later in the day when they are alert and tendency to sleep is at its lowest, and this is followed by a period of least alertness, ultimately leading to sleep onset. If the child's bedtime coincides with this alert period then it is likely to lead to struggles. If the child is put to bed later when obviously tired and goes off without a struggle, DSPS is the likely cause of the problem. DSPS is often associated with difficulties in waking for school or preschool because the child's sleep requirements have not been fully met. The management of this syndrome is usually to gradually advance the sleep phase by first bringing the wake time forward, then the bedtime, and this should be maintained at weekends. This is continued until the desired sleeptime is achieved (for further details see Ferber 1986).

Sleeplessness in adolescents

There are considerable changes in sleep and wakefulness and the sleep–wake cycle as adolescence is reached. The amount of slow wave sleep decreases with an apparent increase in sleep requirements and the sleep phase is delayed. These changes are a result principally of lifestyle changes, particularly going to sleep much later at night, but also because of postpubertal biological influences.

Problems of going off to sleep are very common and are often part of a DSPS, and this is associated with considerable daytime sleepiness because sleep needs have not been met. Rates of insomnia in adolescence have been described as particularly high and this may be associated with other psychological problems (Morrison et al. 1992). There are a variety of potential underlying causes of these sleep problems in adolescence and they should not simply be interpreted as normal adolescent lifestyle. These difficulties include psychological/psychiatric problems such as stress and depression, the effect of prescribed drugs, hypnotics as well as illicit drugs, some of which produce insomnia, as well as alcohol, caffeine and nicotine. In cases where adolescents have chronic sleep problems, a very careful history needs to be taken.

Excessive daytime sleepiness

Excessive daytime sleepiness is a common problem which is frequently misinterpreted as disinterest or lack of motivation on the part of the child (Stores 1999a). This sleepiness is often associated with yawning, stretching, head nodding and eye rubbing. Many children may have associated behavioural problems as well as underfunctioning educationally. In particular, in some cases, school and learning problems may be attributable to insufficient and disrupted sleep. Although children who are sleepy may have low energy levels, they are often irritable, restless and sometimes even manifest overactive behaviour (Stores 1992). Increased sleep during the day should be distinguished from fatigue or lack of energy which may be secondary to physical illnesses. There are three principal causes of such excessive daytime sleepiness.

1 Insufficient sleep, including disturbances in the sleep–wake cycle.

2 Disturbances of overnight sleep as a result of medical conditions, such as obstructive sleep apnoea or parasomnias, drugs and alcohol.

3 Increased sleep requirements including narcolepsy and the Kleine–Levin syndrome.

Insufficient sleep is the most common cause of excessive daytime sleepiness for all the reasons already described. Adolescents are particularly prone to complain of daytime sleepiness. On the one hand, there is probably a physiological postpubertal need for more sleep, yet largely for social reasons adolescents sleep less at night (Carskadon & Dement 1987; Carskadon 1990). Furthermore, DSPS may be a particular problem.

Disturbed overnight sleep occurs when both the timing and the length of sleep are sufficient but the quality of sleep is disrupted. This may be caused by a variety of medical conditions, such as obstructive sleep apnoea, nocturnal asthma and epilepsy, the parasomnias (see below) and the effects of drugs and alcohol and caffeine-containing drinks. Recent research has focused particularly on obstructive sleep apnoea (characterized by sleep-related breathing difficulties) because of the physical and psychological effects on children's functioning (Carroll & Loughlin 1995a,b). Upper airway obstruction of some degree occurs in about 1% of children (Stores 1999b). In many cases in the normal population it is secondary to enlarged tonsils and adenoids in young children, but it is also associated with a variety of conditions: Down syndrome (Silverman 1998), Prader–Willi syndrome (Clift et al. 1994), craniofacial syndromes and other conditions which affect the upper airway. Typical signs include snoring (although only 10–20% of children who snore have upper airways obstruction), other evidence of breathing difficulty during sleep, restlessness, profuse sweating and some mouth breathing. Where there is partial or complete upper airway obstruction, there is a reduction in blood oxygen levels and/or raised CO_2 levels, leading to disrupted sleep physiology and intermittent wakenings. This in turn results in daytime sleepiness and can have an impact on the child's cognitive and behavioural development and, in very severe forms, even lead to failure to thrive. In all cases careful assessment is required. Sometimes the removal of enlarged tonsils and adenoids is the key to relieving the obstruction. Where the pathophysiology is more complicated, treatment is often more difficult.

There are a number of conditions in which increased sleep requirements are part of the core pathophysiology of the condition, rather than being secondary to some other condition. The two most important conditions are narcolepsy, in which the excessive sleepiness is persistent, and the Kleine–Levin syndrome in which excessive sleepiness is intermittent.

Narcolepsy has a prevalence of about 1 in 2000 (Dement *et al.* 1973). It has a genetic predisposition, although the precise nature of the genetic susceptibility remains to be determined. The risk of a first-degree relative developing narcolepsy is 1–2% which although low is a lot higher than the general population (for a review see Mignot 1998). The condition tends to be lifelong and usually starts in adolescence. In this condition, REM sleep phenomena intrude into the awake state leading to daytime sleep attacks and hypnagogic hallucinations as a result of the dream element of REM sleep. The muscle paralysis associated with REM sleep can lead to cataplexy, when the subject suddenly loses all muscle tone and falls to the ground, as well as to sleep paralysis. The episodes of sleep last from seconds to 30 min. Overnight sleep is also disrupted by awakenings. As a result of all these disruptions children often experience serious academic problems.

Narcolepsy is often difficult to recognize in the early stages of the disorder as the characteristic sleep attacks may not be present in their full form. Support and counselling is an important part of the treatment. Medical treatment includes the use of stimulants, with modafinil usually being the treatment of choice, although methylphenidate, pemoline and sometimes tricyclic antidepressants are also used. The stimulants in particular should be used with caution. Regular sleep and good sleep routines, including planned naps during the day together with time of activities in relation to symptoms can be very helpful (Stores 1996).

Kleine–Levin syndrome is rare and typically begins following infection or some other type of stressful experience or injury in adolescent males (Stores 1996). It tends to occur in periods which last hours to weeks at intervals of weeks or months, interspersed with episodes of normality. During the episodes the subject sleeps for excessively long periods, overeats and displays hypersexual behaviour, and sometimes exhibits disturbances suggestive of a mild organic confusional state. There is a tendency towards spontaneous resolution but this may take many years. Stimulant medication may be used during episodes and positive results have been reported with lithium (Pike & Stores 1994). There are a number of conditions which are associated with excessive sleepiness, such as depression and nonconvulsive status epilepticus.

Parasomnias

The parasomnias consist of a group of disorders involving episodic disturbances of behaviour or experiences associated with sleep and are especially common in childhood. Some of the parasomnias can be very worrying to families who often believe that they indicate a serious underlying psychological problem. In childhood this is rarely the case, although there are exceptions (Stores 1999a). The parasomnias are divided into a number of types.

Partial arousal disorders

Partial arousal disorders include night terrors, sleep walking and confusional arousals. Partial arousal disorders receive their name because they occur when there is a sudden change from deep NREM sleep to a lighter stage of sleep. As the largest proportion of deep NREM occurs in the first third of the night, these disorders most commonly occur at this time. In these conditions children appear to be awake but are actually asleep.

1 During night terrors children appear particularly distressed. These tend to occur in older children and adolescents. Usually the child screams, appears terrified, sweats profusely with staring eyes. Sometimes the child jumps out of bed and rushes around. It lasts no longer than a few minutes and the episode ends abruptly with the child waking up. The child should not be woken during the episode and be guided gently back to bed when the episode is over (Stores 1996).

2 Sleep walking, another form of partial arousal disorder, is common with up to 30% of children having experienced one episode and is habitual in about 2.5% of the population (Klackenberg 1987; Handford *et al.* 1991). Sleep walking can last up to 10 min and a safe environment and protection is most important.

3 Confusional arousals usually occur in infants and toddlers and last 5–15 min. They usually begin with movements and moaning before progressing to agitation and sometimes crying. The child appears alert but does not respond to being talked to (Stores 1996). These arousals do not have a psychological significance and tend to resolve spontaneously.

The management of partial arousal disorders usually involves the need for reassurance; occasionally practical steps need to be taken to avoid any accidental injury as in sleep walking, as well as preventing overtiredness. The promotion of a relaxed attitude to bedtime and help with daytime worries can be useful. Very rarely medication is required for severe cases. Lask (1993) has described a useful intervention for night terrors: anticipatory waking 10–15 min before an episode or episodes that are consistent in their time of occurrence.

Nightmares

Nightmares are frightening dreams that arise in the course of REM sleep; they tend to occur in the later part of the night when REM is most common. In this condition children wake up and can recall the content of their frightening dream but can be comforted. The content of a nightmare may provide an indication of some underlying stress. Nightmares are common, reported as occurring in 1 in 5 children of 6–12 years in one large survey (Vela-Bueno *et al.* 1985). Treatment may be necessary if the nightmares are persistent and the child cannot be comforted. The treatment is of the underlying cause, and is especially important if the nightmares occur as part of a more serious condition, such as PTSD.

Sleep-related movements

Sleep-related head banging or other rhythmic movements are quite common, especially in children with learning difficulties, are usually benign and usually resolve spontaneously by 3–4 years of age (Stores 1999a). They are often seen as a self-comforting way of getting to sleep. Protective measures are an important part of management and occasionally behavioural treatment is required. A variety of behavioural approaches have been suggested (Balaschak & Mostofsky 1980).

There are a number of other parasomnias, including nocturnal enuresis (see P. Hill, Chapter 31) and hypnagogic and hypnopompic imagery ('hallucinations' accompanying sleep starts and sleep waking, respectively), which are common and not usually associated with any other problems.

Sleep disturbances associated with other conditions

Learning disabilities and neurodegenerative conditions

There is now considerable evidence that children with learning disabilities and neurodegenerative conditions experience high rates of disturbance which frequently go unrecognized and are often severe and persistent (Stores 1992, 1996). The origins of these difficulties tend to fall into three categories, although once the sleep disturbance has become established maintaining factors tend to be multifactorial. These causes are:
1 behavioural;
2 physical causes involving upper airway obstruction (see section on disturbed overnight sleep); and
3 central (neurological in the case of neurodegenerative conditions).

As far as behavioural causes are concerned, these often reflect parenting practices but should be seen in the context of nocturnal challenging behaviour that is often a feature of children with learning disabilities. Sleep problems are well described in a number of neurodegenerative conditions including Rett syndrome (McArthur & Budden 1998) and Angelman syndrome (Zhdanova *et al.* 1999). Nocturnal seizures may disrupt sleep but the seizures themselves should be distinguished from a primary sleep disorder (Stores 1996). It should be emphasized that, as with other sleep disorders, once the sleep disturbance is established it is likely to have an effect on daytime behaviour by exacerbating learning problems and raising the risk of daytime behavioural difficulties.

Sleep disturbance and psychiatric disorders

Disturbed sleep is a clinical feature of many psychiatric disorders and in some cases is part of the core psychopathology. Sleep disturbance in depression in children is well documented (Ryan *et al.* 1987). The difficulties include getting off to sleep, interrupted sleep and early morning waking, while a proportion of adolescents also complain of hypersomnia. One of the key features of PTSD is nightmares. These occur during REM sleep and therefore are more prominent towards the end of the night. They can be extremely persistent and disturbing.

Sleep disturbances in attention deficit hyperactivity disorder (ADHD) have been of considerable interest particularly because of the potential causal relationships involved, in that disturbed overnight sleep might lead to significant inattention during the day and even overactivity. Conversely, extreme activity and restlessness might in itself interrupt sleep. Furthermore, stimulant medication might interfere with sleep patterns. Parental reports have consistently indicated that children with ADHD have disturbed sleep, including difficulty in getting off to sleep and night waking (for a review see Corkum *et al.* 1998), with approximately 25–50% of parents of children with ADHD reporting these difficulties compared to 7% of controls. However, objective sleep studies have failed to produce consistent findings, except that children with ADHD do not differ from controls in total sleep time but do experience increased body movements during sleep. Recently, Picchietti *et al.* (1998) confirmed the increase in limb movements in sleep (with a proportion of children fulfilling criteria for period limb movement disorder) amongst children with ADHD compared to controls. Stimulant medication does affect sleep patterns by prolonging sleep latency and the length of onset to the first REM cycle but this is not thought to be at a pathological level (Corkum *et al.* 1998).

A number of studies have described both quantitative and qualitative differences in sleep patterns amongst children with autism and Asperger syndrome compared to controls (Patzhold *et al.* 1998). Children with autism are likely to experience some form of sleep difficulty at some time, such as repeated night waking, shortened night sleep and early morning waking. Richdale & Prior (1995) argue that sleep difficulties are related to the children's severe social difficulties and the consequent inability of these children to use social cues to regulate their sleep–wake cycle (Richdale & Prior 1995). There has been considerable interest in sleep difficulties in children with Tourette syndrome where both sleeplessness and parasomnias have been reported (Allen *et al.* 1992). Insufficient sleep, largely caused by extensive bedtime rituals, has been reported in association with obsessive-compulsive disorder (Rapoport *et al.* 1981).

Sudden infant death syndrome

Sudden infant death syndrome (SIDS) is the dominant cause of post-neonatal mortality in the UK and other Western countries, occurs during sleep, and accounted for 0.56 deaths in 1000 live births in 2000 in the UK (FSID 2000). The majority of deaths occur before the age of 6 months. It peaks between the ages of 2 and 4 months coinciding with a time of significant changes in sleep organization and central nervous system maturation. It is not a homogeneous condition and the diagnosis is largely by exclusion if the death cannot be explained on clinical or post-mortem grounds (CESDI 1996).

A genetic susceptibility which may interact with environmental factors is suggested by a 5.8-fold increase in recurrence of SIDS within families (Oyen *et al.* 1996). The genetic susceptibility is likely to derive from a failure to respond to cardiorespiratory challenges during sleep. Kinney *et al.* (1995) found that failure to respond to cardiorespiratory challenges during sleep may result from decreased binding muscaranic receptor in the arcuate nucleus of SIDS infants, a structure which is postulated to be involved in cardiorespiratory control. One large study of 33 000 infants found that a significant prolongation of the Q-T interval, the period of repolarization in the cardiac cycle, is strongly associated with SIDS (Schwartz *et al.* 1998). Passive smoking has also been found to be a significant modifiable risk factor in SIDS; this includes smoking during pregnancy. Interestingly, established SIDS risk factors of pre-term birth and low birth weight were found in one study to increase the risk 15-fold amongst smokers but not at all amongst non-smokers (Schellscheidt *et al.* 1997).

There is considerable evidence that SIDS is associated with some aspects of the infant's sleeping environment. In particular, it has been shown to be associated with sleeping prone, and the 'back to sleep campaign' has resulted in a significant decrease in the rate of SIDS (CESDI 1996). There has also been particular interest in the issue of cosleeping. However, because of the associated potentially confounding risk factors it has been difficult to draw firm conclusions. In a recent large population-based case–control study, using parental interview concerning sleep practices in relation to SIDS, Blair *et al.* (1999) found that infants who shared their parents' bed and were then put back in their own cot had no increased risk. There was an increased risk for infants below 14 weeks of age who shared the bed for the whole sleep or were taken to, or found in, the parental bed. The risk was particularly raised for infants who shared a sofa with a parent. Infants who slept in a separate room from their parents also had an increased risk. However, once a variety of confounding factors, including those of socioeconomic disadvantage, maternal alchohol consumption, use of duvets, parental tiredness and overcrowding, were accounted for, the risk associated with being found in the parental bed was no longer significant. This suggested that it was not bed-sharing *per se* but the circumstances in which bed-sharing occurs that carries the risk (Blair *et al.* 1999). In conclusion, whereas the aetiology of SIDS is complex and much remains to be resolved, infant sleep environment and physiology are likely to be relevant.

Conclusions

In conclusion, there are a wide range of childhood sleeping and feeding problems. At one end of the spectrum there are difficulties such as occasional night waking and refusal of some foods that could simply be construed as variations of normality, depending on the caregiver's perception. At the other end of the spectrum there are severe problems that are ultimately likely to interfere with the child's development. As many of the problems are common and treatable but are not often picked up, they represent considerable public health issues. Parents may need guidance and help in the early months of the child's life in establishing healthy patterns of feeding and sleeping, as well as with early feeding and sleeping problems. If feeding and sleeping are well managed these can be positive experiences for the child. On the other hand, if more serious problems arise specialist referral may be necessary.

References

Adair, R., Bauchner, H., Philipp, B., Levenson, S. & Zuckerman, B. (1991) Night waking during infancy: role of parental presence at bedtime. *Pediatrics*, 87, 500–504.

Adams, L.A. & Rickert, V.I. (1989) Reducing bedtime tantrums: comparison between positive routines and graduated extinction. *Pediatrics*, 84, 756–761.

Allen, R.P., Singer, H.S., Brown, J.E. & Salam, M.M. (1992) Sleep disorders in Tourette syndrome: a primary or unrelated problem? *Pediatric Neurology*, 8, 275–280.

American Psychiatric Association (1993) *Diagnostic and Statistical Manual of Mental Disorders*, 4th edn. American Psychiatric Association, Washington D.C.

American Sleep Disorders Association (1997) *International Classification of Sleep Disorders Revised: Diagnostic and Coding Manual*. American Sleep Disorders Association, Rochester, MN, USA.

Anders, T.F. (1979) Night-waking in infants during the first year of life. *Pediatrics*, 63, 860–864.

Anders, T.F. (1994) Infant sleep, night-time relationships and attachment. *Psychiatry Interpersonal and Biological Processes*, 57, 11–21.

Andersen, R.E., Crespo, C.J., Bartlett, S.J., Cheskin, L.J. & Pratt, M. (1998) Relationship of physical activity and television watching with body weight and level of fatness among children. Results from the Third National Health and Nutrition Examination Survey. *Journal of the American Medical Association*, 279, 938–942.

Anderson, J.W., Johnstone, B.M. & Remley, D.T. (1999) Breast-feeding and cognitive development: a meta-analysis. *American Journal of Clinical Nutrition*, 70, 525–535.

Aukett, M.A., Parks, Y.A., Scott, P.H. & Wharton, B.A. (1986) Treatment with iron increases weight gain and psychomotor development. *Archives of Disease in Childhood*, 61, 849–857.

Balaschak, B.A. & Mostofsky, D.I. (1980) Treatment of nocturnal head-banging by behavioural contracting. *Journal of Behaviour Therapy and Experimental Psychiatry*, 11, 117–120.

Barnes, J., Stein, A., Smith, T., Pollock, J.I. & ALSPAC Study Team (1997) Extreme attitudes to body shape, social and psychological factors and a reluctance to breast feed. *Journal of the Royal Society of Medicine*, 90, 551–559.

Bax, M. (1980) Sleep disturbance in the young child. *British Medical Journal*, 280, 1177–1179.

Benoit, D., Zeansh, C., Boucher, C. & Minde, K. (1992) Sleep disorders in early childhood: association with insecure maternal attachment. *Journal of the American Academy of Child and Adolescent Psychiatry*, 31, 86–93.

Bentley, M., Gavin, L., Black, M.M. & Teti, L. (1999) Infant feeding practices of low-income, African-American, adolescent mothers: an ecological, multigenerational perspective. *Social Science and Medicine*, 49, 1085–1100.

Bernal, J. (1973) Night waking in infants during the first fourteen months. *Developmental Medicine and Child Neurology*, 15, 760–769.

Birch, L.L. (1990) Development of food acceptance patterns. *Developmental Psychology*, 26, 515–519.

Black, M.M. (1999) Feeding problems: an ecological perspective [Commentary]. *Journal of Pediatric Psychology*, 24, 217–219.

Blair, P.S., Fleming, P.J., Smith, J.J. *et al.* & CESDI SUDI Research Group (1999) Babies sleeping with parents: case–control study of factors influencing the risk of sudden infant death syndrome. *British Medical Journal*, 319, 1457–1462.

Blaxter, M. & Paterson, E. (1982) Consulting behavior in a group of young families. *Journal of the Royal College of General Practitioners*, 32, 657–662.

Blurton-Jones, N., Rosetti Ferreira, M.C., Farquar, M. & Macdonald, B.L. (1978) The association between perinatal factors and later night waking. *Developmental Medicine and Child Neurology*, 20, 427–434.

Bock, S.A. (1987) Prospective appraisal of complaints of adverse reactions to foods in children during the first 3 years of life. *Paediatrics*, 89, 683–688.

Boddy, J.M. & Skuse, D.H. (1994) The process of parenting in failure to thrive [Annotation]. *Journal of Child Psychology and Psychiatry*, 35, 401–424.

Bradley, R.H., Casey, P.H. & Wortham, B. (1984) Home environments of low SES non-organic failure-to-thrive infants. *Merrill-Palmer Quarterly*, 30, 393–402.

Bray, P.F., Herbst, J.H., Johnson, D.G., Book, L.S., Ziter, F.A. & Condon, V.R. (1977) Childhood gastrooesophageal reflux: neurologic and psychiatric syndromes mimicked. *Journal of the American Medical Association*, 237, 1342–1345.

Brinch, M., Isager, T. & Tolstrup, K. (1988) Anorexia nervosa and motherhood: reproduction pattern and mothering behaviour of 50 women. *Acta Psychiatrica Scandinavica*, 77, 611–617.

Bryant-Waugh, R. & Lask, B. (1995) Eating disorders in children [Annotation]. *Journal of Child Psychology and Psychiatry*, 36, 191–202.

Budd, K.S., McGraw, T.E., Farbisz, R. *et al.* (1992) Psychosocial concomitants of children's feeding disorders. *Journal of Pediatric Psychology*, 17, 81–94.

Bunton, J., Bisset, E. & Harvey, D. (1987) The social experience of newborn babies in hospital. In: *Parent–Infant Relationships*, Vol. 4. *Perinatal Practice* (ed. D. Harvey), pp. 131–141. Wiley, New York.

Cardon, L.R. (1994) Height, weight, and obesity. In: *Nature and Nurture During Middle Childhood* (eds J.D. DeFries, R. Plomin & D.W. Fulker), pp. 165–172. Blackwell Science, Oxford.

Carey, W. (1974) Night waking and temperament in infancy. *Journal of Pediatrics*, 84, 756–758.

Carey, W.B., Hegvik, R.L. & McDevitt, S.C. (1988) Temperamental factors associated with rapid weight gain and obesity in middle childhood. *Developmental and Behavioural Pediatrics*, 9, 194–198.

Carroll, J.L. & Loughlin, G.M. (1995a) Obstructive sleep apnoea in infants and children: clinical factors and pathophysiology. In: *Principles and Practice of Sleep Medicine in the Child* (eds R. Ferber & M.H. Kryger), pp. 163–192. Saunders, Philadelphia, PA.

Carroll, J.L. & Loughlin, G.M. (1995b) Obstructive sleep apnoea in infants and children: diagnosis and management. In: *Principles and Practice of Sleep Medicine in the Child* (eds R. Ferber & M.H. Kryger), pp. 193–216. Saunders, Philadelphia, PA.

Carskadon, M.A. (1990) Patterns of sleep and sleepiness in adolescents. *Pediatrician*, 17, 5–12.

Carskadon, M.A. & Dement, W.C. (1987) Sleepiness in the normal adolescent. In: *Sleep and its Disorders in Children* (ed. C. Guilleminault), pp. 53–56. Raven Press, New York.

Carskadon, M.A. & Dement, W.C. (1989) Normal human sleep: an overview. In: *Principles and Practice of Sleep Medicine* (eds H. Kryger, T. Roth & W.C. Dement), pp. 3–13. W.B. Saunders, Philadelphia, PA.

CESDI (1996) *Confidential Enquiry into Stillbirth and Deaths in Infancy*. National Advisory Body of CESDI. 3rd Annual Report, 1 January–31 December 1994. Department of Health, London.

Chatoor, I. (1997) Feeding disorders of infants and toddlers. In: *Handbook of Child and Adolescent Psychiatry*, Vol. 1. *Infants and Preschoolers: Development and Syndromes* (eds S. Greespan, S. Wieder & J. Osofsky), pp. 367–386. John Wiley and Sons, New York.

Chatoor, I., Dickson, L., Schaefer, S. & Egan, J. (1985) A developmental classification of feeding disorders associated with failure to thrive: diagnosis and treatments. In: *New Directions in Failure to Thrive: Implications for Research and Practice* (ed. D. Drotar), pp. 235–258. Plenum Press, New York.

Chavin, W. & Tinson, S. (1980) The Developing Child. Children with sleep difficulties. *Health Visitor*, 53, 477–480.

Chiaradia, M., Gulson, B.L. & MacDonald, K. (1997) Contamination of houses by workers occupationally exposed in a lead–zinc–copper mine and impact of blood lead concentrations in families. *Occupational and Environmental Medicine*, 54, 117–124.

Chinn, S. & Rona, R.J. (1994) Trends in weight-for-height and triceps skinfold thickness for English and Scottish children, 1972–82 and 1982–90. *Paediatric Perinatal Epidemiology*, 8, 90–106.

Clift, A., Dahlitz, M. & Parkes, J.D. (1994) Sleep apnoea in the Prader–Willi syndrome. *Journal of Sleep Research*, 3, 121–126.

Cooper, P.J., Murray, L. & Stein, A. (1993) Psychosocial factors associated with the early termination of breast-feeding. *Journal of Psychosomatic Research*, 37, 171–176.

Corkum, P., Tannock, R. & Moldofsky, H. (1998) Sleep disturbances in children with attention-deficit/hyperactivity disorder. *Journal of the American Academy of Child and Adolescent Psychiatry*, 37, 637–646.

Cramer, B. (1995) Short-term dynamic psychotherapy for infants and their parents. *Child and Adolescent Psychiatric Clinics of North America*, 4, 649–660.

Crittenden, P.M. (1987) Non-organic failure-to-thrive: deprivation or distortion? *Infant Mental Health Journal*, 8, 51–64.

Cunningham, C.E. & Linscheid, T.R. (1976) Elimination of chronic infant rumination by electric shock. *Behavior Therapy*, 7, 231–234.

Davies, A.E.M. & Sandhu, B.K. (1995) Diagnosis and treatment of gastro-oesophageal reflux. *Archives of Disease in Childhood*, 73, 82–86.

Daws, D. (1989) *Through the Night: Helping Parents and Sleepless Infants*. Free Association Books, London.

Dement, W.C. & Kleitman, M. (1957) The relations of eye movements during sleep to dream activity: an objective method for the study of dreaming. *Journal of Experimental Psychology*, 53, 339–346.

Dement, W.C., Carskadon, M. & Ley, R. (1973) The prevalence of narcolepsy II. *Sleep Research*, 2, 147.

Department of Health (1994) *Weaning and the Waning Diet Report of the Working Group on the Weaning Diet of the Committee on Medical Aspects of Food Policy*. HMSO, London.

Dietz, W.H. (1998) Prevalence of obesity in children. In: *Handbook of Obesity* (eds G.A. Bray, C. Bouchard & W.P.T. James), pp. 93–102. Marcel Dekker, New York.

Douglas, J. & Richman, N. (1984) *My Child Won't Sleep*. Penguin, Harmondsworth.

Drotar, D. (1991) The family context of nonorganic failure to thrive. *American Journal of Orthopsychiatry*, **61**, 23–34.

Drotar, D. & Sturm, L. (1987) Paternal influences in non-organic failure to thrive: implications for psychosocial management. *Infant Mental Health Journal*, **8**, 37–50.

Eaton-Evans, J. & Dugdale, A. (1988) Sleep patterns of infants in the first year of life. *Archives of Disease in Childhood*, **63**, 647–649.

Elias, E.D., Nicolson, N.A., Bora, B.A. & Johnston, J. (1986) Sleep–wake patterns of breast-fed infants in the first two years of life. *Pediatrics*, **77**, 322–329.

Epstein, L.H. & Wing, R.R. (1987) Behavioral treatment of childhood obesity. *Psychological Bulletin*, **101**, 331–342.

Epstein, L.H., Wing, R.R. & Valoski, A. (1985) Child obesity. *Pediatric Clinics of North America*, **32**, 363–380.

Epstein, L.H., Valoski, A., Wing, R.R. & McCurley, J. (1990) Ten-year follow-up of behavioural, family-based treatment for obese children. *Journal of the American Medical Association*, **264**, 2519–2523.

Epstein, L.H., Klein, K.R. & Wisniewski, L. (1994) Child and parent factors that influence psychological problems in obese children. *International Journal of Eating Disorders*, **15**, 151–158.

Fairburn, C.G. & Beglin, S. (1990) Studies of the epidemiology of bulimia nervosa. *American Journal of Psychiatry*, **147**, 401–408.

Fenton, T.R., Bhat, R., Davies, A. & West, R. (1989) Maternal insecurity and failure to thrive in Asian children. *Archives of Disease in Childhood*, **64**, 369–372.

Ferber, R. (1986) *Solve Your Child's Sleep Problems*. Dorling Kindersley, London.

Ferber, R. (1995) Assessment of sleep disorders in the child. In: *Principles and Practice of Sleep Medicine in the Child* (eds R. Ferber & M.H. Kryger), pp. 45–53. Saunders, Philadelphia, PA.

Fischoff, J., Whitten, C. & Pettit, M. (1971) A psychiatric study of mothers of infants with growth failure secondary to maternal deprivation. *Journal of Pediatrics*, **79**, 209–215.

Florey, C.D., Leech, A.M. & Blackhall, A. (1995) Infant feeding and mental and motor development at 18 months of age in first born singletons. *International Journal of Epidemiology*, **24** (Suppl. 1), 21–26.

Forsyth, J.L., Ogston, S.A., Clark, A., Florey, C.D. & Howie, P.W. (1993) Relation between early introduction of solid food to infants and their weight and illnesses during the first 2 years of life. *British Medical Journal*, **306**, 1572–1576.

Foster, K., Lader, D. & Cheesborough, S. (1997) *Infant Feeding 1995*. HMSO, London.

FSID (2000) *Fact file 1: Cot death — facts and figures*. Foundation for the Study of Infant Deaths 2000. London.

France, K.G. & Hudson, S.M. (1993) Management of infant sleep disturbance: A review. *Clinical Psychology Review*, **19**, 635–647.

Frühbeck, G. (2000) Childhood obesity: time for action, not complacency. *British Medical Journal*, **320**, 328–329.

Gallaher, M.M., Hauck, F.R., Yang-Oshida, M. & Serdula, M.K. (1991) Obesity among Mescalero preschool children. *American Journal of Diseases of Children*, **145**, 1262–1265.

Gisel, E.G. (1988) Chewing cycles in 2- to 8-year-old normal children: a developmental profile. *American Journal of Occupational Therapy*, **42**, 40–46.

Gisel, E.G. & Patrick, J. (1988) Identification of children with cerebral palsy unable to maintain a normal nutritional state. *Lancet*, i, (8580), 283–286.

Halpern, L.F., Anders, T.F., Garcia-Coll, C. *et al.* (1994) Infant temperament: is there a relation to sleep–wake states and maternal night-time behavior? *Infant Behaviour and Development*, **17**, 255–263.

Handford, H.A., Mattison, R.E. & Kales, A. (1991) Sleep disturbances and disorders. In: *Child and Adolescent Psychiatry* (ed. M. Lewis), pp. 715–725. Williams & Wilkins, Boston.

Harris, G. (1988) Determinants of the introduction of solid food. *Journal of Reproductive and Infant Psychology*, **6**, 241–249.

Harris, G. (1997) Development of taste perception and appetite regulation. In: *Infant Development: Recent Advances* (eds G. Bremner, A. Slater & G. Butterworth), pp. 9–30. Psychology Press, Hove.

Harris, G. (2000) Developmental, regulatory and cognitive aspects of feeding disorders. In: *Feeding Problems in Children: a Guide for Health Professionals* (eds A. Southall & A. Schwartz), pp. 77–88. Radcliffe Medical Press, Abingdon.

Harris, G., Thomas, A.M. & Booth, D.A. (1990) Development of salt taste in infancy. *Developmental Psychology*, **268**, 535–538.

Harris, G., Blissett, J. & Johnson, R. (2000) Food refusal associated with illness. *Child Psychology and Psychiatry Review*, **5**, 148–156.

Harris, R.J., Armstrong, D., All, R. & Loynes, A. (1983) Nutritional survey of Bangladeshi children aged under 5 years in the London Borough of Tower Hamlets. *Archives of Disease in Childhood*, **58**, 428–432.

Hendershot, G.E. (1984) Trends in breastfeeding. *Pediatrics*, **74** (4 Pt. 2), 591–592.

Hewson, P., Oberklaid, F. & Menaham, S. (1987) Infant colic, distress and crying. *Clinical Pediatrics*, **26**, 69–76.

Hoek, H.W. (1993) Review of the epidemiological studies of eating disorders. *International Review of Psychiatry*, **15**, 346–348.

Hoppenbrouwers, T., Hodgman, J.E., Harper, R.M. & Sterman, M.B. (1982) Temporal distribution of sleep states, somatic activity and autonomic activity during the first half year of life. *Sleep*, **5**, 131–144.

Howie, P., Stewart Forsyth, J., Ogston, S.A., Clark, A. & Florey, C.duV. (1990) Protective effect of breast feeding against infection. *British Medical Journal*, **300**, 11–16.

Humphry, R.A. & Hock, E. (1989) Infants with colic: a study of maternal stress and anxiety. *Infant Mental Health Journal*, **10**, 263–272.

Israel, A.C. & Shapiro, L.S. (1985) Behavior problems of obese children enrolling in a weight reduction program. *Journal of Pediatric Psychology*, **10**, 449–460.

Jackson, H.J. & Tierney, D.W. (1984) Rumination disorder of infancy: some diagnostic issues in need of clarification. *Australia and New Zealand Journal of Developmental Disabilities*, **10**, 243–245.

Jakobsson, I. & Lindberg, T. (1983) Cow's milk proteins cause infantile colic in breastfed infants: a double-bind crossover study. *Pediatrics*, **71**, 268–271.

Jenkins, S., Bax, M. & Hart, H. (1980) Behaviour problems in pre-school children. *Journal of Child Psychology and Psychiatry*, **21**, 5–17.

Jenkins, S., Owen, C., Bax, M. & Hart, H. (1984) Continuities of common behaviour problems in pre-school children. *Journal of Child Psychology and Psychiatry*, **25**, 75–89.

Johnson, D.L., Swank, P.R., Howie, V.M., Baldwin, C.D. & Owen, M. (1996) Breast feeding and children's intelligence. *Psychological Reports*, **79** (3 Part 2), 1179–1185.

Johnson, M. (1991) Infant and toddler sleep: a telephone survey of parents in one community. *Journal of Developmental and Behavioural Pediatrics*, **12**, 108–114.

Jones, B.E. (1989) Basic mechanisms of sleep–wake states. In: *Principles and Practice of Sleep Medicine* (eds H. Kryger, T. Roth & W.C. Dement), pp. 121–138. W.B. Saunders, Philadelphia, PA.

Jones, V.M. (1987) Current infant weaning practices within the Bangladeshi community in the London Borough of Tower Hamlets. *Human Nutrition: Applied Nutrition*, 41, 349–352.

Keane, V., Charney, E., Stratus, J. & Roberts, K. (1988) Do solids help baby sleep through the night? *American Journal of Diseases of Children*, 142, 404–405.

Keefe, M.R. (1988) Irritable infant syndrome: theoretical perspectives and practice implications. *Advances in Nursing Science*, 10, 70–78.

Keener, M., Zeanah, C. & Anders, T. (1988) Infant temperament sleep organisation and nighttime parental intervention. *Pediatrics*, 81, 762–771.

Kinney, H.C., Filiano, J.J., Sleeper, L.A. *et al.* (1995) Decreased muscarinic receptor binding in the arcuate nucleus in sudden infant death syndrome. *Science*, 269, 1446–1450.

Kissileff, H.R. (1989) Is there an eating disorder in the obese? *Annals of the New York Academy of Sciences*, 575, 410–419.

Klackenberg, G. (1987) Incidence of parasomnias in children in a general population. In: *Sleep and its Disorders in Children* (ed. C. Guilleminault), pp. 99–113. Raven Press, New York.

Kleitman, N. & Englemann, T.G. (1953) Sleep characteristics in infants. *Journal of Applied Physiology*, 6, 269–282.

Kramer, M.S., Barr, R.G., Leduc, D.G., Boisjoly, C. & Pless, I.B. (1985) Infant determinants of childhood weight and adiposity. *Journal of Pediatrics*, 107, 104–107.

Lanting, C.I., Fidler, V., Huisman, M., Towen, B.C.L. & Boersma, E.R. (1994) Neurological differences between 9-year-old children fed breastmilk or formula milk as babies. *Lancet*, 344, 1319–1322.

Lask, B. (1993) 'Waking treatment' best for night terrors. *British Medical Journal*, 306, 1477.

Lask, B., Britten, C., Kroll, L., Magagna, J. & Tranter, M. (1991) Children with pervasive refusal. *Archives of Disease in Childhood*, 66, 866–869.

Latz, S., Wolf, A.W. *et al.* (1999) Cosleeping in context: sleep practices and problems in young children in Japan and the United States. *Archives of Paediatrics and Adolescent Medicine*, 153, 330–346.

Lavigne, J.V., Burns, W.J. & Cotter, P.D. (1981) Rumination in infancy: recent behavioral approaches. *International Journal of Eating Disorders*, 1, 70–82.

Lieberman, A.F. & Birch, M. (1985) The etiology of failure to thrive: an interactional developmental approach. In: *New Directions in Failure to Thrive: Implications for Research and Practice* (ed. D. Drotar), pp. 259–277. Plenum Press, New York.

Little, J. (1983) Management of the obese child in the school. *Journal of School Health*, 53, 440–441.

Lothe, L., Lindberg, T. & Jakobsson, I. (1982) Cow's milk formula as a cause of infantile colic: a double-blind study. *Pediatrics*, 70, 7–10.

Lozoff, B., Wolf, A.W. & Davis, N.S. (1984) Cosleeping in urban families with young children in the United States. *Pediatrics*, 74, 171–182.

Lucas, A., Morley, R. & Cole, T.J. (1990) Early diet in preterm babies and development status at 18 months. *Lancet*, 335, 1477–1481.

Lucas, A., Morley, R., Cole, T.J., Lister, G. & Leeson-Payne, C. (1992) Breast milk and subsequent intelligence quotient in children born preterm. *Lancet*, 339, 261–264.

Lucas, A., Morley, R. & Cole, T.J. (1998) Randomised trial of early diet in preterm babies and later intelligence quotient. *British Medical Journal*, 317, 1481–1487.

Malloy, M.H. & Berendes, H. (1998) Does breast-feeding influence intelligence quotients at 9 and 10 years of age? *Early Human Development*, 50, 209–217.

Madansky, D. & Edelbrock, C. (1990) Cosleeping in a community sample of 2- and 3-year-old children. *Pediatrics*, 86, 197–203.

Marchi, M. & Cohen, P. (1990) Early childhood eating behaviours and adolescent eating disorders. *Journal of the American Academy of Child and Adolescent Psychiatry*, 29, 112–117.

Mathisen, B., Skuse, D., Wolke, D. & Reilly, S. (1989) Oral-motor dysfunction and failure to thrive among inner city infants. *Developmental Medicine and Child Neurology*, 31, 293–302.

Mayes, L.C. & Volkmar, F.R. (1993) Nosology of eating and growth disorders in early childhood. *Child and Adolescent Psychiatry Clinics of North America*, 2, 25–35.

Mayes, S.D., Humphrey, F.J., Handford, H.A. & Mitchell, J.F. (1988) Rumination disorder: differential diagnosis. *Journal of the American Academy of Child and Adolescent Psychiatry*, 27, 300–302.

McArthur, A.J. & Budden, S.S. (1998) Sleep dysfunction in Rett syndrome: a trial of exogenous melatonin treatment. *Developmental Medicine and Child Neurology*, 40, 186–192.

McGowan, R. & Green, J. (1998) Pervasive refusal syndrome: a less severe variant with defined aetiology. *Clinical Child Psychology and Pscychiatry*, 3, 583–590.

McIntosh, J. (1986) Weaning practices in a sample of working class primiparae. *Child: Care, Health and Development*, 12, 215–226.

McKenna, J.J., Mosko, S., Dungy, C. & McAninch, J. (1990) Sleep and arousal patterns of co-sleeping human mother–infant pairs: a preliminary physiological study with implication for the study of sudden infant death syndrome (SIDS). *American Journal of Physical Anthropology*, 83, 331–347.

Meiklejohn, D. (2000) European breastfeeding rates [Unpublished report]. Baby Milk Action, Cambridge, UK.

Meyers, A.W., Klesges, R.C. & Bene, C.R. (1990) Obesity in childhood. In: *Handbook of Child and Adult Psychopathology: A Longitudinal Perspective* (eds M. Hersen & C.G. Last), 161, pp. 383–401. Pergamon Press, New York.

Mignot, E. (1998) Genetic and familial aspects of narcolepsy. *Neurology*, 5O (Suppl. 1), S16–S22.

Minde, K., Popiel, K., Leos, N., Falkner, S., Parker, K. & Handley-Derry, M. (1993) The evolution and treatment of sleep disturbances in young children. *Journal of Child Psychology and Psychiatry*, 34, 521–533.

Minde, K., Faucon, A. & Falkner, S. (1994) Sleep problems in toddlers, effects of treatment on their daytime behavior. *Journal of the American Academy of Child and Adolescent Psychiatry*, 33, 1114–1121.

Mogan, J. (1986) Parental weight and its relation to infant feeding patterns and infant obesity. *International Journal of Nursing Studies*, 23, 255–264.

Moore, M. (1989) Disturbed attachment in children: a factor in sleep disturbance, altered dream production and immune dysfunction. *Journal of Child Psychotherapy*, 15, 99–111.

Morelli, G.A., Rogoff, B. *et al.* (1992) Cultural variation in infants' sleeping arrangements: questions of independence. *Developmental Psychology*, 28, 604–613.

Morrell, J.M.B. (1999) The role of maternal cognitions in infant sleep disorder as assessed by a new instrument, the Maternal Cognitions about infant Questionnaire. *Journal of Child Psychology and Psychiatry*, 40, 247–258.

Morrell, J.M.B. (unpublished data) Attachment security and persistent infant sleeping problems: is there a link?

Morrison, D.N., McGee, R. & Stanton, W.R. (1992) Sleep problems in adolescence. *Journal of the American Academy of Child and Adolescent Psychiatry*, **31**, 94–99.

Murray, L. (1992) The impact of postnatal depression on infant development. *Journal of Child Psychology and Psychiatry*, **33**, 543–561.

Newberger, E.H., Hampton, R.L., Marx, T.J. & White, K.M. (1986) Child abuse and pediatric social illness: an epidemiological analysis and ecological reformulation. *American Journal of Orthopsychiatry*, **56**, 589–601.

Newson, J. & Newson, E. (1963) *Infant Care in an Urban Community*. Allen & Unwin, London.

Nunn, K.P. & Thompson, S.L. (1996) The pervasive refusal syndrome: learned helplessness and hopelessness. *Clinical Child Psychology and Psychiatry*, **1**, 121–132.

Nunn, K.P., Thompson, S.L., Moore, S.G., English, M., Burke, E.A. & Byrne, N. (1998) Managing pervasive refusal syndrome: strategies of hope. *Clinical Child Psychology and Psychiatry*, **3**, 229–249.

O'Brien, S., Repp, A.C., Williams, G.E. & Christopherson, E.R. (1991) Pediatric feeding disorders. *Behaviour Modification*, **15**, 394–418.

Oyen, N., Skjaerven, R. & Irgens, L.M. (1996) Population-based recurrence risk of sudden infant death syndrome compared with other infant and fetal deaths. *American Journal of Epidemiology*, **144**, 300–305.

Parmelee, A.H. Jr, Wenner, W.H. & Schulz, H.R. (1964) Infant sleep patterns: from birth to 16 weeks of age. *Journal of Pediatrics*, **65**, 576–582.

Paton, J.Y., Nanayakkhara, C.S. & Simpson, H. (1988) Vomiting and gastro-oesophageal reflux. *Archives of Disease in Childhood*, **63**, 837–856.

Patzhold, L.M., Richdale, A.L. & Tonge, B.J. (1998) An investigation into sleep characteristics of children with autism and Asperger's disorder. *Journal of Paediatrics and Child Health*, **36**, 528–533.

Picchietti, D.L., England, S.J., Walters, A.S., Willis, K. & Verrico, T. (1998) Periodic limb movement disorder and restless legs syndrome in children with attention-deficit hyperactivity disorder. *Journal of Child Neurology*, **13**, 588–594.

Pike, M. & Stores, G. (1994) Kleine–Levin syndrome: a cause of diagnostic confusion. *Archives of Disease in Childhood*, **71**, 355–357.

Pinyerd, B.J. (1992) Infant colic and maternal mental health: nursing research and practice concerns. *Issues in Comprehensive Pediatric Nursing*, **15**, 155–167.

Pollock, J.I. (1994a) Long-term associations with infant feeding in a clincally advantaged population of babies. *Developmental Medicine and Child Neurology*, **36**, 429–, 440.

Pollock, J.I. (1994b) Night waking at five years of age: predictors and prognosis. *Journal of Child Psychology and Psychiatry*, **35**, 699–708.

Price, E.E., Rona, R.J. & Chinn, S. (1988) Height of primary school children and parents' perceptions of food intolerance. *British Medical Journal*, **196**, 1696–1700.

Pugiliese, M.T., Weyman-Daum, M., Moses, N. & Lifshitz, F.M. (1987) Parental health beliefs as a cause of non-organic failure to thrive. *Pediatrics*, **80**, 175–182.

Quine, L. (1992) Severity of sleep problems in children with severe learning difficulties: description and correlates. *Journal of Community and Applied Social Psychology*, **2**, 247–268.

Ramchandani, P., Wiggs, L., Webb, V. & Stores, G. (2000) A systematic review of treatments for settling problems and night waking in young children. *British Medical Journal*, **320**, 209–213.

Ramsey, M., Gisel, E. & Boutry, M. (1993) Non-organic failure to thrive: growth failure secondary to feeding skills disorder. *Developmental Medicine and Child Neurology*, **35**, 285–297.

Rapoport, J., Elkins, R., Langer, D.H. *et al.* (1981) Childhood obsessive compulsive disorder. *American Journal of Psychiatry*, **138**, 1545–1554.

Rechtschaffen, A. & Kales, A., eds (1968) *A Manual of Standardised Terminology, Techniques and Scoring System for Sleep Stages of Human Subjects*. Brain Information Service/Brain Research Institute, UCLA, Los Angeles, CA.

Reilly, S., Skuse, D. & Wolke (in press) The nature and consequences of feeding problems in infancy. In: *Feeding Problems and Eating Disorders in Children and Adolescents* (eds P. J. Cooper & A. Stein). Harwood Press, Chur, Switzerland.

Reis, S. (1994) Rumination in two developmentally normal children: case report and review of the literature. *Journal of Family Practice*, **38**, 521–523.

Richdale, A.L. & Prior, M.R. (1995) The sleep–wake rhythm in children with autism. *European Journal of Child and Adolescent Psychiatry*, **4**, 175–186.

Richman, N. (1981) A community survey of characteristics of one- to two-year-olds with sleep disruptions. *Journal of the American Academy of Child Psychiatry*, **20**, 281–291.

Richman, N., Stevenson, J. & Graham, P. (1982) *Pre-School to School: a Behavioural Study*. Academic Press, London.

Rickert, V.I. & Johnson, C.M. (1988) Reducing nocturnal awakening and crying episodes in infants and young children: a comparison between scheduled awakenings and systematic ignoring. *Pediatrics*, **81**, 203–212.

Robischon, P. (1971) Pica practice and other hand–mouth behavior and children's developmental level. *Nursing Research*, **20**, 4–16.

Rogers, I.S., Emmett, P.M. & Golding, J. (1997) The incidence and duration of breast feeding. *Early Human Development*, **49** (Suppl.), 45–74.

Rummler, S. & Woit, I. (1992) Zur postnatalen Entwicklung von Kindern adipöser Mütter [The postnatal development of children of obese mothers]. *Deutsche Hebammen Zeitschrift*, **44**, 218–222.

Ryan, A.S. (1997) The resurgence of breastfeeding in the United States. *Pediatrics*, **99**, E12.

Ryan, D.N., Puig-Antich, J., Rabinovich, H. *et al.* (1987) The clinical picture of major depression in children and adolescents. *Archives of General Psychiatry*, **44**, 854–861.

Sadeh, A. & Anders, T.F. (1993) Infant sleep problems: origins, assessment, interventions. *Infant Mental Health Journal*, **14**, 17–34.

Sadeh, A., Lavie, P. & Scher, A. (1992) Temperament and night waking in early childhood, revisited. *Sleep Research*, **21**, 93.

Salzer, H.R., Haschke, F., Wimmer, M., Heil, M. & Schilling, R. (1989) Growth and nutritional intake of infants with congenital heart disease. *Pediatric Cardiology*, **10**, 17–23.

Sampson, H.A. (1989) Infantile colic and food allergy: fact or fiction? *Journal of Pediatrics*, **115**, 583–584.

Sanders, M.R., Patel, R.K., Grice, B.L. & Shepherd, R.W. (1993) Children with persistent feeding difficulties: an observational analysis of the feeding interactions of problem and non-problem eaters. *Health Psychology*, **12**, 64–73.

Sauvage, D., Leddet, I., Hameury, L. & Barthelemy, C. (1985) Infantile rumination: diagnosis and follow-up study of twenty cases. *Journal of the American Academy of Child Psychiatry*, **24**, 197–203.

Schachter, F.F., Fuchs, M.L., Bijur, P.E. & Stone, R.K. (1989) Cosleeping and sleep problems in Hispanic-American urban young children, *Pediatrics*, **84**, 522–530.

Schaefer, C. (1990) Night waking and temperament in early childhood. *Psychological Reports*, **67**, 192–194.

Schellscheidt, J., Oyen, N. & Jorch, G. (1997) Interactions between maternal smoking and other prenatal risk factors for sudden infant death syndrome (SIDS). *Acta Paediatrica Scandinavica*, **96**, 857–863.

Scher, A. (1991) A longitudinal study of nightwaking in the first year. *Child: Care, Health and Development*, **17**, 295–302.

Scher, A. & Blumberg, O. (1999) Night waking among 1-year olds: a study of maternal separation anxiety. *Child: Care, Health and Development*, **25**, 323–334.

Schwartz, P.J., Stramba-Badiale, M., Segantini, A. *et al.* (1998) Prolongation of the Q-T interval and the sudden death syndrome. *New England Journal of Medicine*, **338**, 1709–1714.

Scott, G. & Richards, M.P.M. (1990a) Night waking in 1-year-old children in England. *Child: Care, Health and Development*, **16**, 283–302.

Scott, G. & Richards, M.P.M. (1990b) Night waking in infants: effects of providing advice and support for parents. *Journal of Child Psychology and Psychiatry*, **31**, 551–567.

Seymour, F.W., Brock, P., During, M. & Poole, G. (1989) Reducing sleep disruptions in young chidren: evaluation of therapist-guided and written information approaches—a brief report. *Journal of Child Psychology and Psychiatry*, **30**, 913–918.

Silverman, M. (1998) Airway obstruction and sleep disruption in Down's syndrome. *British Medical Journal*, **296**, 1618–1619.

Skuse, D.H. (1985) Non-organic failure to thrive: a reappraisal. *Archives of Disease in Childhood*, **60**, 173–178.

Skuse, D., Wolke, D. & Reilly, S. (1992) Failure to thrive: clinical and developmental aspects. In: *Child and Youth Psychiatry: European Perspectives. Developmental Psychopathology* (eds H. Remschmidt & M. Schmidt) **3**, pp. 46–71. Hogrefe & Huber, Göttingen.

Sorensen, T.I.A., Price, R.A., Stankard, A.J. & Schulsinger, F. (1989) Genetics of obesity in adult adoptees and their biological siblings. *British Medical Journal*, **298**, 87–90.

Standing Committee on Nutrition of the British Paediatric Association (1994) Is breast feeding beneficial in the UK? *Archives of Disease in Childhood*, **70**, 376–380.

Stein, A., Woolley, H., Cooper, S.D. & Fairburn, C. (1994) An observational study of mothers with eating disorders and their infants. *Journal of Child Psychology and Psychiatry*, **35**, 733–748.

Stein, A., Stein, J., Walters, E.A. & Fairburn, C. (1995) Eating habits and attitudes among mothers of children with feeding disorders. *British Medical Journal*, **310**, 228.

Stein, A., Murray, L., Cooper, P. & Fairburn, C. (1996) Infant growth in the context of maternal eating disorders and maternal depression: a comparative study. *Psychological Medicine*, **26**, 569–574.

Stein, A., Woolley, H. & McPherson, K. (1999) Conflict between mothers with eating disorders and their infants during mealtimes. *British Journal of Psychiatry*, **175**, 455–461.

Stifter, C.A. & Bono, M.A. (1998) The effect of infant colic on maternal self-perceptions and mother–infant attachment. *Child: Care, Health and Development*, **24**, 339–351.

Stifter, C.A. & Braungart, J. (1992) Infant colic: a transient condition with no apparent effects. *Journal of Applied Developmental Psychology*, **13**, 447–462.

Stores, G. (1992) Annotation: sleep studies in children with a mental handicap. *Journal of Child Psychology and Psychiatry*, **33**, 1303–1317.

Stores, G. (1996) Practitioner review: assessment and treatment of sleep disorders in children and adolescents. *Journal of Child Psychology and Psychiatry*, **37**, 907–925.

Stores, G. (1999a) Sleep disorders in children and adolescents. *Advances in Psychiatric Treatment*, **5**, 19–29.

Stores, G. (1999b) Children's sleep disorders: modern approaches, developmental effects, and children at special risk. *Developmental Medicine and Child Neurology*, **41**, 568–573.

Sturm, L. & Drotar, D. (1991) Maternal attributions of etiology in nonorganic failure to thrive. *Family Systems Medicine*, **9**, 53–63.

Sugarman, M. & Kendall-Tackett, K. (1995) Weaning ages in a sample of American women who practice extended nursing. *Clinical Pediatrics*, **34**, 642–647.

Szmukler, G. (1985) The epidemiology of anorexia nervosa and bulimia nervosa. *Journal of Psychiatric Research*, **19**, 143–153.

Thommenssen, M., Heiberg, A. & Kase, B.F. (1992) Feeding problems in children with congenital heart disease: the impact on energy intake and growth outcome. *European Journal of Clinical Nutrition*, **46**, 457–464.

Treasure, J.L., Troop, N.A. & Ward, A. (1996) An approach to planning services for bulimia nervosa. *British Journal of Psychiatry*, **169**, 551–554.

Vela-Bueno, A., Bixler, E.O., Dobladez-Blanco, B., Rubo, M.E., Marrison, R.E. & Kales, A. (1985) Prevalence of night terrors and nightmares in elementary school children: a pilot study. *Research Communications in Psychology, Psychiatry and Behaviour*, **10**, 177–188.

Walker, A.R., Walker, B.F., Sookaria, F.I. & Cannan, R.J. (1997) Pica. *Journal of the Royal Society of Health*, **117**, 280–284.

Wessel, M.A., Cobb, J.C., Jackson, E.B., Harris, G.S. & Detwiler, A.C. (1954) Paroxysmal fussing in infancy, sometimes called 'colic'. *Pediatrics*, **14**, 421–434.

Whelan, E. & Cooper, P.J. (2000) The association between childhood feeding problems and maternal eating disorder: a community study. *Psychological Medicine*, **30**, 69–77.

White, A., Freeth, S. & O'Brien, M. (1992) *Infant Feeding 1990*. HMSO, London.

Whitehead, R.G. (1985) Infant physiology, nutritional requirements and lactational adequacy. *American Journal of Clinical Nutrition*, **41**, 447–458.

Wiggs, L. & Stores, G. (1995) Children's sleep: how should it be assessed? *Association of Child Psychology and Psychiatry Review and Newsletter*, **17**, 153–157.

Wilcox, W.D., Nieberg, P. & Miller, D.S. (1989) Failure to thrive: a continuing problem of definition. *Clinical Pediatrics*, **28**, 391–394.

Winton, A.S. (1984) Behavioral treatment of rumination. *Psychiatric Aspects of Mental Retardation Reviews*, **3**, 33–36.

Winton, A.S.W. & Singh, N.N. (1983) Rumination in pediatric populations: a behavioural analysis. *Journal of the American Academy of Child Psychiatry*, **22**, 269–275.

Wolfson, A., Lacks, P. & Futterman. A. (1992) Effects of parent training on infant sleeping patterns, parents' stress and perceived parental competence. *Journal of Consulting and Clinical Psychology*, **60**, 41–48.

Wolke, D. (1991) Supporting the development of low-birthweight infants [Annotation]. *Journal of Child Psychology and Psychiatry*, **32**, 723–741.

Wolke, D. (1994) Sleeping and feeding across the lifespan. In: *Development Through Life: a Handbook for Clinicians* (eds M. Rutter & D. Hay), pp. 517–557. Blackwell Scientific, Oxford.

Wolke, D. & Meyer, R. (1995) The colic debate. *Pediatrics*, **96**, 165–166.

Wolke, D., Skuse, D. & Reilly, S. (in press) The management of infant feeding problems. In: *Feeding Problems and Eating Disorders in Children and Adolescents* (eds P.J. Cooper & A. Stein). Harwood Press, Chur, Switzerland.

World Health Organization Consultation on Obesity (1998) Global prevalence and secular trends in obesity. In: *Obesity: Preventing and Managing the Global Epidemic*, pp. 17–40. World Health Organization, Geneva.

Wright, A.L., Holberg, C.J., Martinez, F.D., Morgan, W.J., Taussig,

L.M. & Group Medical Associates (1989) Breast feeding and lower respiratory tract illness in the first year. *British Medical Journal*, **299**, 946–949.

Wright, P. & Crow, R. (1982) Nutrition and feeding. In: *Psychobiology of the Human Newborn* (ed. P.M. Stratton), pp. 339–364. John Wiley & Sons, Chichester.

Wright, P., Macleod, H. & Cooper, M. (1983) Waking at night: the effect of early feeding experience. *Child: Care, Health and Development*, **9**, 309–319.

Zepelin, H. & Rechtschaffen, A. (1974) Mammalian sleep, longevity and energy metabolism. *Brain Behaviour and Evolution*, **10**, 425–470.

Zhdanova, I.V., Wurtman, R.J. & Wagstaff, J. (1999) Effects of low dose of melatonin on sleep in children with Angelman syndrome. *Journal of Pediatric Endocrinology and Metabolism*, **12**, 57–67.

Zuckerman, B., Stevenson, J. & Bailey, V. (1987) Sleep problems in early childhood: continuities, predictive factors, and behavioral correlates. *Pediatrics*, **80**, 664–671.

46 Attachment Disorders of Infancy and Childhood

Thomas G. O'Connor

Introduction

The knowledge base and currency of attachment disorders in clinical and social care settings has increased substantially in recent years. When Zeanah & Emde (1994) wrote the preceding version of this chapter in the last edition of this volume, there were very few empirical papers on attachment disorder and related behaviours and only slightly more clinical reports. Fortunately, because the concept of attachment disorder is now attracting systematic attention, we are now in a better position to evaluate its conceptual and clinical basis.

This chapter has four goals:

1 to review the history and development of the attachment disorder construct;

2 to examine the links between attachment theory and attachment disorder, and especially to identify how these ideas converge and diverge;

3 to review the evidence supporting the reliability and validity of the attachment disorders; and

4 to evaluate the limited data on intervention and clinical management.

A note on terminology is given in order to reduce the confusion concerning the concepts covered. Throughout this chapter, the term 'attachment disorder' is used to denote the diagnostic label, whereas the term 'attachment disorder behaviour' is used to denote a more general disturbance that may or may not meet diagnostic requirements. Use of the more specific terms 'disinhibited' and 'inhibited' attachment disorder (behaviour) is reserved for the particular proposed subtypes of disturbance. Finally, 'attachment theory' refers to the principles outlined by Bowlby, Ainsworth and others, whereas 'attachment behaviour' refers to the range of behaviours that form the basis of individual differences in the child–parent attachment relationship (e.g. proximity-seeking, exploration; see below); 'attachment classification' is reserved specifically for the categories of secure and insecure attachment derived from standard assessments.

---

* The terms 'disinhibited' and 'inhibited' are used throughout the chapter to refer to the two forms of attachment disorder discussed by DSM-IV and ICD-10. These terms correspond to 'reactive attachment disorder, disinhibited type' and 'reactive attachment disorder, inhibited type', respectively, in the DSM-IV and 'disinhibited attachment disorder' and 'reactive attachment disorder', respectively, in ICD-10. A diagnostic condition (disorder) is not implied unless specifically mentioned.

History and development of the attachment disorder construct

Although the first diagnostic definition of attachment disorder appeared in 1980 (DSM-III), some of the core behavioural symptoms were evident in writings on institutionalized children dating back over half a century. Indeed, one of the most remarkable features of attachment disorder behaviour is how consistent select features of the disorder have been described, despite widely varying theoretical dispositions and methodological sophistication. A second key feature underscored by a historical review is that the patterns of behaviour described did not fit existing diagnostic terms.

The consistency across reports is most evident for what DSM-IV (American Psychiatric Association 1994) and ICD-10 (World Health Organization 1992) refer to as the 'disinhibited'* form of attachment disorder (see section on detachment disorder for a more detailed discussion of symptoms and diagnostic requirements). In one of the earliest descriptions of the atypical social behaviour of (ex-)institutionalized children, Levy (1937) used the term 'superficially affectionate' to describe the behaviour of children toward others. Goldfarb (1943, 1945) also highlighted high rates of indiscriminate behaviour toward unfamiliar persons based on his observations of a sample of children in institutions in New York; he added that some institutionalized children demonstrated an 'excessive need for adult attention' that persisted long after they were placed in foster families. In their volume, *Infants without Families*, Freud & Burlingham (1946/1973) provided extensive observations of children being reared in a residential nursery without a consistent and selective attachment figure. They used the term 'indiscriminate exhibition' to convey the way in which some children eagerly approached complete strangers to show off their clothes or other belongings. The key finding was that this behaviour was found only in children 'who are emotionally starved and unattached' (Freud & Burlingham 1946/1973, p. 616). Provence & Lipton (1962) reported similar observations of 'indiscriminately friendly' behaviour toward strangers in their assessment of institutionally reared children.

Somewhat more contemporary research studies also signalled disinhibited behaviour toward strangers as a likely consequence of early institutional care, and suggested further insights into the phenomenon. In his study of 'affectionless psychopathy', Wolkind (1974) found that of the three syndromes that were linked with institutionalization, only disinhibition toward strangers was associated with *early* institutional care. A separate UK study illustrated the further point that severe and non-specific deprivation was not necessary for the development of attachment disorder behaviour. Thus, children who, apart from the lack of a consistent caregiver, received adequate care in a residential setting exhibited 'indiscriminately friendly' behaviour (Tizard & Rees 1975). This behaviour diminished by the time the children were aged 8 years, with the degree of persistence greater among children with poorer post-institutional care (Tizard & Hodges 1978).

Echoes of the above reports are evident in very recent research on children whose early experiences were characterized by severe deprivation. One of the most important sources of data on severe attachment disturbance is the investigation of children adopted into Canadian or UK families after severe and profound deprivation in institutions in Romania. Predictably, each of the three intensive studies of behavioural adjustment following adoption all reported disinhibition in a sizeable number of children (Goldberg 1997; Chisholm 1998; O'Connor *et al.* 1999). These three studies are noteworthy in several respects. First, the kinds of attachment disturbances match what was reported in prior studies. Secondly, the disturbance was apparent in observational, interview and questionnaire methods. The multimethod validation of the behavioural pattern was a new and important extension of prior studies. Thirdly, each study attempted to assess the links between attachment disorder behaviour and attachment theory. In addition, findings from these reports provide a major source of data on the reliability and validity of attachment disorder. The results of these investigations are therefore detailed in the sections on theoretical links with attachment theory and attachment disorder below.

In addition to the reports of disinhibited behaviour in Romanian adoptees, parallel reports of disinhibited behaviour or superficial friendliness toward strangers were made by investigators studying children living in comparably neglectful circumstances, such as orphans in war-torn countries such as Eritrea (Wolff & Fesseha 1999).

A second proposed form of attachment disorder according to both ICD-10 and DSM-IV, the inhibited variety, has a much less clear historical and clinical basis, and existing links are tenuous. Furthermore, no doubt because of the continuing uncertainty regarding the basic phenotype, it is not yet certain if the behaviours thought to characterize an inhibited attachment disturbance cannot be incorporated into existing diagnostic categories. A small number of children with a history of very severe maltreatment have been described as having extreme fear and even terror of strangers (Goldfarb 1943; Albus & Dozier 1999). Descriptions of children who responded with detachment, such as those reported by Bowlby *et al.* (1952) and Bowlby (1982) in their work with children separated from their parents, may also be relevant, although the source of the stress in the caregiving environment is far less severe. Also, it is likely significant that the children had already established a (presumed positive) relationship with the parent. Additionally, attempts to interpret previ-

ously reported syndromes in infancy (Spitz 1946) in attachment disorder terms has been suggested (Call 1987) although, as in the previous cases, the connection with inhibited attachment disorder is questionable.

Historically, samples of institutional children were the most common source of reports of attachment disorder behaviour. However, residential rearing of that sort is nowhere near as common as it once was. Instead, much of the current interest in the attachment disorders is based on the large and growing number of children in the adoption and foster care system. Experiences of early and severely disrupted relationships with caregivers — by which we mean the virtual absence of any consistent relationship with a caregiver rather than simply inadequate care — may put some of these children at risk for severe attachment disturbances (Howe 1995). Accordingly, it may be that the kinds of risks experienced by children in some of the more recent reports of attachment disorders differ in important respects from the earlier work in this field.

Partly because of the increased popularity and somewhat indiscriminate application of the diagnosis in diverse settings and by diverse professional and lay individuals, there is now considerable heterogeneity in the descriptions of attachment disorder behaviour — especially when considered in the context of the homogeneity of reports from several decades ago. Subsequent sections of the chapter seek to offset the increasing uncertainty about the appearance and meaning of the disturbance.

Explanations for attachment disorder behaviour

An effort to codify what was known about the effects of severely disturbed or non-existent attachment relationships, namely those behaviours described above as 'disinhibited' or 'inhibited', was made in DSM-III (American Psychiatric Association 1980). However, confusion about the manifestation of attachment disturbance(s) was apparent in the early diagnostic description. Thus, the initial definition of attachment disorder was something of a misnomer because it included symptoms separate from the child–parent attachment relationship (e.g. failure to thrive). In addition, proposed criteria were contrary to what was known about the development of child–parent relationships (e.g. the criterion that the disorder be apparent before 8 months). Further diagnostic revisions improved the face validity of the criteria (at least relative to earlier reports of institutionalized children) but, as discussed in the next section, serious problems remain in terms of the phenotypic description, general conceptualization and link with attachment theory.

Previous reports of attachment disorder behaviour have, by and large, avoided detailed discussions of the mechanisms responsible for the disturbance; neither have they proposed testable hypotheses for advancing our understanding of the meaning of attachment disorder behaviour. There is, to date, a ready acceptance that attachment theory provides an explanation (in terms of both causes and effects) for attachment disorder behaviour. It is, despite the relative lack of necessary research, the dominant and perhaps only proposed framework. An exclusive focus on attachment theory is bolstered by research on non-human primates (Kraemer 1992; Suomi 1999) and, more recently, investigations of the biological bases for relationships and their effects (Insel 1997; Carter 1998), which also draws heavily from attachment theory. These alternative lines of research reinforce the dominant position played by attachment theory and, in addition, help to anchor the behavioural disturbances within a sociobiological–ethological framework that is a hallmark of attachment theory. Given the importance of this topic, it is addressed in detail below.

Summary

A historical survey of the literature on attachment disorder behaviours reveals a remarkable degree of consistency, at least with respect to the disinhibited disturbance, but also uncertainty concerning the meaning of the behaviour and its place in psychiatric nomenclature. Several lessons are also noteworthy from prior research. Perhaps the most important of these is the need for further research on attachment disorder to focus on institutionalized populations of children or, more generally, children who lacked a selective or consistent attachment relationship from early life. Because the findings reported to date are most consistent in these populations, they provide a natural starting point and 'test case' for further conceptual and methodological study. A brief historical overview highlights parallels between the history of the concept of attachment disorder and attachment theory. Both were derived from a careful and systematic observation of children in institutional care or children whose experiences with caregivers were severely disrupted (Bowlby 1951, 1982). In addition, clinical and child care policy were the initial contexts for much of the interest in attachment theory and attachment disorders. However, while studies testing attachment theory in normal and at-risk samples proliferated in developmental and clinical psychology, attachment disorder behaviours were largely ignored. Several decades after Bowlby's initial observations, attachment theory is being reconnected to the study of development following deprivation.

Theoretical links with attachment theory

Despite the label 'attachment disorder', it is by no means a foregone conclusion that the attachment disorders represent disorders of the child–parent *attachment* relationship as defined by Bowlby and Ainsworth and elaborated in subsequent developmental research. There are several reasons for this. First, attachment disorder behaviour has not yet been adequately conceptualized in terms of attachment theory. In this regard, it is noteworthy that diagnostic formulations focus on 'social relatedness' (DSM-IV) or 'social responses' and 'selective social attachments' (ICD-10). These phrases are not easily translated into attachment theory. Assuming that a selective attachment relationship had been formed (a dubious assumption in many cases of institutionalized children), a further, more interesting

and perplexing challenge is that the prototypical 'disinhibited' or 'inhibited' behavioural patterns differ substantially from attachment theory expectations (see below). If attachment theory is to clarify the nature and meaning of attachment disorders, then it will be essential to revisit the basic principles of the theory and identify convergences and divergences between the concepts underlying attachment theory and those associated with attachment disorder.

Some rudiments of attachment theory relevant to attachment disorders

Rather than provide a detailed review of attachment theory and the research methods devised to test aspects of the theory, this chapter highlights only those features that are directly relevant to attachment disorder. Discussions of attachment theory are available from numerous sources (Marvin 1977; Sroufe & Waters 1977; Ainsworth *et al.* 1978; Bowlby 1982; Cicchetti *et al.* 1995; Rutter 1995; Thompson 1998; Cassidy & Shaver 1999).

A starting point for discussion is to note some core components of the theory and highlight what is unique about attachment relationships and attachment behaviour (Bowlby 1982; Ainsworth 1989). First, attachment is but one of several components of the child–parent relationship, and so it is important not to equate parent–child relationships with attachment relationships. The implication is that, at least in theory, there may be some positive features of the child–parent relationship in attachment disordered children (e.g. play and casual social interactions).

A second key feature is that it is essential to consider the meaning or function of the attachment behaviours according to the setting and the child's development (Bretherton & Ainsworth 1974; Bowlby 1982; Cicchetti *et al.* 1990). Thus, the meaning—in terms of attachment theory—of a child's willingness to approach a stranger will depend on such factors as the presence of the attachment figure and child's age (Rajecki *et al.* 1978). One particular application of this is that the significance of the DSM-IV symptom of indiscriminate sociability would be far greater in the absence of a current primary caregiver.

Thirdly, the development of child–parent attachment and its implications for social and personality development were constructed within what Bowlby (1982) referred to as the 'environment of evolutionary adaptedness'. Rearing environments that severely breach this condition, such as institutionalization (but perhaps not maltreatment; see Ainsworth 1978; Rajecki *et al.* 1978), may not provide the environmental input that promotes species-typical attachment. This serves to illustrate Bowlby's point that attachment evolved in a specific environmental context and, although protected from perturbations in the environment, it can nevertheless be fundamentally and critically modified. If the caregiving environment is outside the expected environment so as to severely modify or, in extreme cases, pre-empt the development of normal early selective attachment relationships, then the theory (as well as its implications for assessment and treatment) would not be expected to apply. This theme is revisited throughout the chapter.

A fourth consideration in the bridging of attachment theory with the attachment disorders concerns the ontogeny of attachment relationships. Four stages in the ontogeny of attachment were discussed by Bowlby (1982).

1 At the simplest and most immature level, the infant orientates and signals with only limited discrimination.

2 At the second stage, the infant's orientation and signals are directed towards one (or more) discriminated attachment figure(s).

3 The third stage involves the 'maintenance of proximity to a discriminated figure by means of locomotion as well as signals' (Bowlby 1982, p. 299).

4 Finally, in the preschool years, there is the formation of a 'goal-corrected partnership', which accompanies the child's emerging ability to understand, to a limited degree, the parent's feelings and motives, and is capable to attribute internal states to him or her.

This increasing differentiation and 'focusing on a figure' is what appears to be lacking in children with attachment disorder, especially in those children with the disinhibited form. In the special case of institutionally reared children this is hardly surprising because there is no one particular person towards whom the child could direct and receive interactions and attachment/ caregiving behaviours. It might therefore be tempting to view disinhibited behaviour as a 'developmental delay' in the normal ontogeny of attachment, and to assume that the formation of a new attachment relationship post infancy would proceed through the above four stages. In that instance, 'indiscriminate sociability' may be viewed as a necessary precondition for the emergence of later selective attachment relationships. Although there are no data directly relevant to this question (Provence & Lipton 1962; Shaffer 1963; Ainsworth 1967), this seems an unlikely possibility, not least because the stages of attachment are partly governed and co-ordinated by normally developing social, motor and cognitive skills (Cicchetti *et al.* 1990). Moreover, it is not yet clear how the first early signs of selective attachment behaviour would appear in preschool-aged children. Alternatively, it may be that the ontogeny of attachment behaviour in children who did not receive expectable environment/caregiving input is different from what Bowlby outlined. What is needed are systematic studies following the establishment of new attachment relationships, especially in children who experienced an absence of early care or severe maltreatment (Stovall & Dozier 2000). In addition, more detailed information on the development of attachment behaviours of infants in institutional or other forms of pathogenic care would be valuable in tracing the aberrant ontogeny of attachment relationships, although such information is naturally difficult to obtain.

A fifth consideration concerns sensitive periods in the formation of selective attachment relationships. The issue here is not whether or not early attachment relationships, once formed, have deterministic lifelong prediction—they do not (Bowlby 1988)—but instead the degree to which the *formation* of normal

selective attachment relationships requires consistent responsiveness from caregivers in infancy. A somewhat related concept is developmental programming, or the notion that experiences in early life may persistently influence how the individual responds to later experiences (Ladd *et al.* 1996). Relevant data are again limited, but extant findings indicate that 'normal' secure or insecure attachment relationships with supportive adoptive parents are less likely with prolonged periods of severe early deprivation and, more importantly, that children with such disturbances show little improvement in the short term (Chisholm 1998; O'Connor *et al.* 2000). The significance of this finding in terms of developmental theory is yet to be determined, although it is broadly in line with a sensitive period or developmental programming hypothesis. There are too few data directly relevant to sensitive periods or developmental programming for forming attachment relationships, not least because virtually all studies of attachment include children who had been reared by a biological parent since birth. Increasing applications of attachment theory to non-traditional settings will therefore provide much needed information about some of the outstanding issues for attachment theory (Rutter & O'Connor 1999).

A further issue that will need to be resolved before attachment theory and attachment disorders can be reconciled involves the assessment of whether a relationship is an *attachment* relationship. This issue is hardly relevant when children are assessed with biological parents with whom they have always lived (Ainsworth 1978), but it becomes critical in the case of children placed in the care of alternate adults beyond infancy. Interestingly, both the diagnosis (implicitly) and attachment theory (explicitly) imply that a child with attachment disorder would not have had a selective attachment relationship. A related concern is whether or not the attachment disorder is conceptualized in terms of a current relationship or instead as an effect of prior relationship experiences or, more generally, in terms of an individual or a relationship. This issue is discussed subsequently in this section. It is therefore essential to be able to define what constitutes a selective attachment relationship. Some suggestions for addressing this issue are provided in the assessment component of the section on attachment disorder.

A final issue that is relevant to creating an attachment theory-informed definition of attachment disorder is the fact that attachment theory extends beyond the particular behaviours associated with gaining proximity to, and maintaining contact with, an attachment figure. Attachment theory is also fundamentally concerned with exploration of the environment and managing and coping with fear/wariness and threat (Bowlby 1982). Indeed, the ability to describe and explain children's need for contact with caregivers as well as their tendency to leave caregivers in order to explore the environment sets attachment theory apart from rival explanations for the child–parent bond (Rajecki *et al.* 1978; Bowlby 1982).

The distinct behaviours that have received the most attention from attachment theory include attachment (gaining proximity to, and maintaining contact with, an attachment figure), fear/ wariness, sociability, and exploration (Ainsworth *et al.* 1971,

1978; Bowlby 1982; Greenberg & Marvin 1982). These behaviours are co-ordinated, such that they may inhibit or potentiate one another. Feedback mechanisms have been proposed to explain why there appears to be some degree of connection among these behaviours (Bowlby 1982). There is as yet no direct test of the feedback or 'behavioural systems' hypothesis as originally proposed, but it serves as a heuristic for defining the larger context for attachment behaviours.

The most obvious example of the links among attachment-related behaviours mentioned above is of a child who, while exploring his or her environment, perceives fear. The reaction is to curtail play and seek proximity to an attachment figure. Thus, fear inhibits exploration and leads to an increase in attachment behaviour. The experience of safety and security from the attachment figure (reduction in fear) then promotes the child's return to exploration. This behavioural pattern illustrates what is meant by the parent acting as a 'secure base' for the child's exploration, and demonstrates that an understanding of the child's attachment relationship with a caregiver requires a detailed assessment of a range of behaviours and their interrelatedness. The need to assess the interrelatedness of attachment-related behaviours may be especially important when assessing attachment disorder because it is in this area that a disturbance may be most evident.

Given that the child has (or had) formed a selective attachment relationship, then the inhibited and disinhibited patterns of behaviour present a paradox to attachment theory because they violate this basic biologically programmed patterning of behaviour. A child who wanders off with a stranger without checking back with the parent, or a child who seeks comfort from a stranger when distressed is puzzling because of the merging of apparently contradictory behaviours (e.g. fear and *lack of* attachment behaviour). In the above examples, the expected outcome is that the child would increase proximity to an attachment figure rather than to continue to wander off or seek out a stranger.

A consideration of the behaviour patterns that underlie normal attachment behaviour raises several possible explanations for attachment disorders. It may be that attachment disorder is a disorder limited to one of the attachment-related behaviours. In this regard it is noteworthy that clinical and anecdotal reports indicate that fear/wariness is often disrupted in children with attachment disturbances, such that children exhibit minimal evidence of fearfulness toward strangers, even when some degree of wariness would be developmentally appropriate. On the other hand, given that there is often a reference to problems in excessive sociability, it may be that disturbance may be confined to this behaviour. A further possibility is that there is a specific problem in attachment behaviour—seeking out of attachment figures when distressed—however, there are, at least for disinhibited children, normal instances of such behaviour (O'Connor *et al.* 2001).

It may be beneficial, both conceptually and clinically, to interpret attachment disorder behaviour according to the behaviours and behavioural patterns emphasized in attachment theory.

However, there is an obvious and important caveat to this approach; it could be a mistake to interpret behaviour in terms of a theory that may not be directly applicable. Attachment theory and its developmental and clinical implications presupposes that a child has developed an early selective attachment relationship. For those children for whom that is not the case, such as institutionalized children, there may be a danger in trying to fit attachment-related behaviour into a framework designed for children with more conventional (or species-typical) attachment histories. Accordingly, a parsimonious explanation for attachment disorder behaviour is that it is a consequence of an absence of a selective attachment relationship. Whether or not there is additive explanatory value in discussing attachment disorder behaviour in terms of the interrelatedness of behaviours remains to be seen, although there is little doubt that such a disturbance exists, as noted below.

There is substantial evidence that the patterns of behaviour found in children who did not develop an early selective attachment relationship differ radically from normal expectations. Most importantly, each of the three studies of Romanian adoptees mentioned above found that some children were classified as 'securely' attached to the main caregiver but still exhibited inappropriately friendly behaviour toward the stranger, based on either behaviour in the separation–reunion paradigm or other sources of data (Goldberg 1997; Chisholm 1998; O'Connor *et al.* 2001). In other words, several years of sensitive and responsive care from the adoptive parent may have provided the basis for the child's attachment behaviour to the adoptive parent, but the expression of apparently normal proximity-seeking and secure base behaviour may exist alongside continuing disturbance with respect to fear/wariness or sociability. On that basis, it would be a mistake, as Bowlby (1982) anticipated, to refer to these children as securely attached, not according to their behaviour toward parents *per se*, but because the organization of attachment-related behaviours is disturbed.

Although no data directly test the above explanations for attachment disorder, this approach does have some advantages over alternative proposals. It is sometimes proposed that the disinhibited behaviour of children is strategic—expressed with the intent of attracting care from potentially protective and caring adults. This explanation is possible, but has a number of drawbacks. Disinhibited behaviour is observed in very young children, including children whose cognitive capacity for such a strategic approach seems doubtful. Relatedly, many of the children with disordered behaviour exhibit marked deficits in social understanding—quite the opposite of what would be expected given the fairly sophisticated social understanding and perspective-taking that would be required to enlist strange adults to be prospective carers.

Individual or relationship disorder?

Both DSM-IV and ICD-10 require that the child's attachment disturbance be evident across social settings. Thus, the assumption made by diagnostic systems is that an attachment disorder is not a disorder confined to a particular current relationship, although it may derive from a specific pathogenic relationship in the past. This requirement is in line with general assumptions about diagnoses (e.g. that they be characteristic of the individual), but presents particular problems for integrating attachment disorders with attachment theory in young children. That is because research on child–parent attachment in young children focuses on the relationship rather than the individual as the unit of analysis. Individual children are coded as 'secure' or 'insecure' according to research methods, but it is the relationship that is so described. The relationship-specific nature of children's attachments is supported by findings indicating that a child develops different relationships with different caregivers (Anders 1989; Steele *et al*. 1996).

The relationship-specific focus of attachment theory is obviously important and has been beneficial for conceptualizing development and for designing treatments (Lieberman 1991). Both attachment-based research and clinical work with normal and at-risk populations emphasize the problems of assuming that a secure or insecure attachment can be 'localized' in the child. On the other hand, it is probably a mistake to adopt a strictly relationship-based approach to defining attachment disorder and to dismiss the diagnostic requirement that the child exhibit marked disturbances across social and relationship settings. In this context, it is important to distinguish between the qualities of the current relationship as such from the *effects* of earlier relationships on current relationships. For instance, an attachment disorder observed in a child with a foster or adoptive parent may have comparatively little to do with the current relationship and much more to do with the effects of prior experiences of deprivation or neglect. Further appreciation of the carrying forward of effects from prior relationships to current relationships must therefore figure in further diagnostic refinements. After all, one of the reasons secure or insecure attachment classifications are meaningful is that they have relevance to the child's adaptation outside the specific child–caregiver relationship context (Sroufe 1983; Cassidy *et al*. 1996).

Underlying the question of whether the attachment disturbance lies within the individual or the relationship is the further question of what explains cross-setting and cross-relationship consistency and longitudinal stability in the child's disturbed behaviour. One possibility is that the carrying forward of effects of earlier relationships (across setting or through time) is explained by an internal working model: the child's internalized cognitive schema or set of expectations for predicting others' behaviour and for making evaluations about the self and others (Bowlby 1982; Bretherton 1990). There is growing evidence for such a mechanism in normally developing and at-risk children (Bretherton & Munholland 1999). It remains for further clinical research to examine if the internal working model account provides the best explanation for cross-setting and cross-relationship disturbances found in children with attachment disorder. At present, the strongest rationale for maintaining the cross-setting/relationship criterion is that it would clearly differentiate children with potential attachment disorders from those with a more 'focused' disturbance with a particular caregiver (who may be better described in terms of a parent–child relational problem, a 'V' code in DSM-IV). What is needed is an account of this continuity that lends itself to further study.

What is the connection between attachment disorders and attachment classifications?

Initially derived from a comparatively small longitudinal study of infants in the USA (Ainsworth *et al*. 1978), the distinction between 'secure' and 'insecure-avoidant' or 'insecure-ambivalent' classifications for describing individual differences in child–parent attachment have proved to be remarkably robust (van Ijzendoorn & Sagi 1999). Nevertheless, problems with the three-way classification scheme surfaced when attachment researchers turned their attention to high-risk samples, notably maltreated children and children of parents with severe psychopathology (Radke-Yarrow *et al*. 1985; Cicchetti & Barnett 1991). A sizeable number of high-risk children did not satisfy criteria for insecure-avoidant, insecure-ambivalent or secure classification, but instead demonstrated a mixed, confused or overtly disturbed pattern (Main & Solomon 1990). The response was to define a fourth classification: 'insecure-disorganized'. A substantial literature has emerged in the past decade on this pattern in infancy and its aetiology, prevalence in high-risk samples and connection with psychopathology (Lyons-Ruth 1996; Carlson 1998; Vondra & Barnett 1999). Similarly, the preschool extension of the infant classification system (Cassidy & Marvin 1992) also makes allowances for more severe forms of insecurity, 'insecure-controlling' and 'insecure-other' classifications, in addition to 'insecure-disorganized'.

Attachment researchers resist attempts to equate an insecure attachment classification with psychopathology or disorder by emphasizing the role of attachment vis-à-vis a developmental trajectory that may be more or less likely to lead to maladaptation and psychopathology (Bowlby 1988). Nevertheless, not all authors completely reject the notion that some severe forms of attachment insecurity might be tantamount to disorder (Zeanah *et al*. 1993). The contrast between these two positions may partly stem from the substantial difficulty in assimilating attachment classifications and attachment disorder.

Importantly, most investigations indicate that the existing insecure categories adequately account for the disturbed attachment relationships found in clinical samples, even in those with well-characterized forms of developmental delay (Barnett *et al*. 1999; Waters & Valenzuela 1999). Furthermore, there is no suggestion in these lines of investigation that attachment problems can be described in terms of the atypical patterns described in children with attachment disordered behaviour. Indeed, the fact that the traditional observational assessments and coding procedures are applied, albeit with some modifications, implies that the pattern among attachment, exploration, fear/wariness and sociability behaviours is thought to be normal. Nor is there evidence yet reported that the most severe forms of insecure attachment ('disorganized' or 'controlling') are accompanied by 'indiscriminate sociability' or other hallmarks of attachment disordered children, although further research is needed to determine whether some of the atypical or 'contradictory' behaviours and sequences found in children classified as 'disorganized' are analogous to the symptoms included in DSM-IV or ICD-10. An implication of the above discussion is that insecure attachment is qualitatively different from the disturbance implied by attachment disorder. The possibility that the 'disorganized' insecure attachment might signal more severe disturbance and therefore command greater clinical and perhaps diagnostic attention is discussed in the next section.

Until recently, there were no data that directly examined the association between the standard secure and insecure classifications derived from separation–reunion procedures and attachment disorder behaviour. This gap has now been filled by findings from the three studies of Romanian adoptees referred to above. The similarities among studies, despite the different methods employed, suggest that some weight may be placed on the findings. In the current context, some of the key findings were that although some children exhibited apparently secure behaviour toward the parent, their excessively sociable and disinhibited behaviour toward the stranger undermined a secure classification; in addition, many children could not easily be classified into one of the existing categories (O'Connor et al. 2001). These findings support the previous view that there may be a qualitative difference between current attachment classifications and attachment disorder behaviour. In addition to raising obvious conceptual and clinical questions, these findings raise the equally important methodological point that very misleading conclusions might be drawn if children with attachment disorder are assessed using conventional observational assessments and coding procedures.

Summary

Considerable theoretical and empirical evidence indicates that child–parent attachment quality significantly influences the development of psychopathology (Bowlby 1977, 1988; Greenberg 1999). However, a clear distinction needs to be drawn between these research findings, derived almost entirely from children with conventional (species-typical) attachment histories, and the emerging interest in the much less well-understood concept of attachment disorder. The reason for this suggested disjunction is that the connection between attachment theory and attachment disorder is unresolved. There is the further concern that recent diagnostic formulations have explicitly attempted to resist a particular theoretical account of behaviour or a specific explanation for its origins. Trying to fit attachment disorder within the context of attachment theory—however successfully—runs counter to this approach. A key concern with the current state is that a connection between attachment theory and attachment disorder has been widely in-

ferred when, in fact, the actual fit between these concepts is weak. There is therefore a need to either reformulate attachment disorders according to attachment theory, which would require a near complete overhaul of the current diagnoses, or to make more explicit that the term 'attachment disorder' is not meant to imply any direct link with attachment theory. Given the information now available (reviewed in this and the following section), the latter approach may be preferable. Attachment theory may help elucidate the disturbed and puzzling behavioural pattern captured by attachment disorder, but for conceptual, methodological and clinical reasons it may be neither possible nor desirable to force an integration of attachment theory and the current definitions of attachment disorder. One important lesson for further research is the need for more cross-discipline research and a greater correspondence between academic attachment research and research in social work and applied settings (Rutter & O'Connor 1999).

Attachment disorder

Despite the long history of reports on disinhibited, inhibited and related disturbances and more than 20 years in the psychiatric nomenclature, we know very little about attachment disorder *per se*. Consequently, it is very difficult to review what is known about attachment disorder *qua* disorder because there are virtually no data on aetiology, comorbidity, prevalence or longitudinal course, and certainly not enough to justify a review. Accordingly, the research findings that are reviewed below are dominated by the somewhat more general disturbance of disinhibited behaviour. It remains to be established whether the findings regarding this general disturbance can be applied to the diagnosable disorder.

Phenotype and phenomenology

One notable point of agreement between DSM-IV and ICD-10 is that there are two forms of attachment disorder, although the labels used differ slightly between nosologies. As reviewed above, there is substantial support for the core behavioural element referred to as the 'disinhibited' form. In reports of institutionalized children this phenotype is most often described as 'indiscriminate friendliness', which conveys that it is not necessarily attachment behaviour that is expressed toward strangers but simply social, affectionate or excessively familiar (e.g. physical proximity-seeking) behaviour. However, the term 'indiscriminate friendliness' is misleading in other respects. The behaviour in question seems neither genuinely 'friendly' nor 'sociable', but instead superficial, impersonal, shallow and rarely reciprocal (Tizard & Rees 1975; O'Connor et al. 1999). Nor is the behaviour truly indiscriminate, although children may fail to demonstrate consistently discriminating attachment behaviour toward primary caregivers. Undoubtedly, one benefit of extending research in this area will be more precise symptom descriptions.

Diagnostic formulations of the disinhibited phenotype also require disturbed interactions with others (strangers), defined as 'indiscriminate sociability' (DSM-IV) or 'indiscriminately friendly behaviour' (ICD-10). Importantly, both DSM-IV and ICD-10 also make the additional specification that the phenotype also include disturbed *attachment behaviour* but, unfortunately, the meaning of attachment behaviour is not always clear (e.g. as noted above, behaviours as seemingly different as proximity-seeking and exploration can be viewed as attachment related). For example, in DSM-IV, evidence of 'marked inability to exhibit appropriate selective attachment' is potentially useful, but the notion of 'diffuse attachments' is not (and is an oxymoron).

The inhibited attachment disorder phenotype (or 'reactive attachment disorder' in ICD-10) is much less well developed than the disinhibited variety. Thus, the inhibited phenotype includes behaviour that ranges from 'a persistent failure to initiate or respond . . . to most social interactions' (DSM-IV) to highly ambivalent, avoidant or aggressive behaviour. The absence of relevant empirical data is hardly surprising given the diverse and contradictory ways in which this phenotype is defined. It is difficult to see how the imprecise diagnostic criteria will facilitate progress in describing and understanding the phenotype.

Both diagnostic systems are in agreement that the two attachment disorder phenotypes can be distinguished. Moreover, the almost mutually exclusive kinds of disturbance implied by the two phenotypes would suggest that there would be little overlap between the two forms. The UK study of Romanian adoptees (O'Connor *et al.* 2000) reported some of the only available data on this issue. That study supported a distinction between disinhibited and inhibited symptoms and between disinhibited and inhibited individuals, but there is a need for further research on other samples.

Several further points need to be made about the diagnostic phenotypes. First, both DSM-IV and ICD-10 specify an onset before age 5 years. Second, it must be established that the attachment disorder behaviour is not solely accounted for by developmental delay or pervasive developmental disorder. These points are generally accepted. Third, the criterion of cross-situational impairment was discussed above in the context of the debate about individual or relationship disorders. The need for modification in this instance depends on the degree of desired congruence with attachment theory. Fourth, present diagnostic proposals focus on the current behavioural abnormalities in the context of the current (presumed) attachment relationship. Symptoms not directly related to the current attachment relationship are not included. Nevertheless, consequences of early severe pathogenic care extend beyond the child's relationship with subsequent caregivers, most notably to problems in peer relationships (Rutter 1981; Hodges & Tizard 1989). It may therefore be useful to consider expanding diagnostic criteria to symptoms linked with early severe deprivation rather than strictly in terms of the current relationship. The final criterion, that there be a history of pathogenic care, is discussed below.

Alternative definitions of the phenotypes

Attachment disorders may be best viewed on a continuum of disturbance rather than as a pure categorical distinction, because evidence from studies of other forms of psychopathology supports a dimensional approach. The difficulty has been in deciding on what continuum to place attachment disorders. In particular, the section on theoretical links with attachment theory highlighted the ambiguous connection between the current definitions of attachment disorder and attachment theory, and the problems in relating the two. Lieberman & Zeanah (1995) and Boris & Zeanah (1999) sought to place attachment disorders on a continuum or spectrum with attachment classifications found in typically developing and high-risk children. This required a complete reformulation of the definition of attachment disorder. The strength of their approach is that it is anchored within attachment theory, and seeks to bridge the research on disorganized and severe forms of insecurity with attachment disorder. A key feature of their alternative definition of attachment disorder is the creation of a category of 'disorders of non-attachment' (Howe 1995). This group of children would include those who would meet the current DSM-IV and ICD-10 criteria. On the other hand, a potential liability of this approach is that it does not elucidate how, or if, the attachment theory framework described by Bowlby and others applies to children who experienced severe pathogenic care and exhibit disorders of non-attachment. It remains to be seen if this alternative definition provides conceptual, clinical or empirical advantages over the established psychiatric classifications.

A further possibility for refining current definitions of attachment disorder is to pay greater attention to the 'disorganized' insecure classification that has been subjected to rigorous study in the developmental and clinical literature. As noted above, the origins, links with psychopathology and longitudinal course of children classified as 'disorganized' in conventional assessments have been well documented (Solomon & George 1999). This is not to say that the 'disorganized' classification is tantamount to disorder or that it has any particular similarities to the existing forms of attachment disorder; neither seems to be the case. Instead, the case for focusing on 'disorganized' attachment is that it is known to be a risk for psychopathology (Greenberg 1999) and that it is often superimposed on the standard secure and other insecure categories, suggesting at least indirectly that the qualities described as disorganized may be separable from secure or insecure attachment *per se*. Furthermore, a number of authors have suggested that the links between attachment and psychopathology are greatest in the context of children classified as having a disorganized relationship (Boris & Zeanah 1999; Greenberg 1999). There are a number of limitations in attempting to extend further the connection between 'disorganized' attachment and a disorder of attachment. Not least of these is that the base rate of 'disorganized' attachment is higher than would be expected for a particular disorder of childhood and that, at least to date, a 'disorganized' classification is possible only with the use of the Strange Situation assessment

(Solomon & George 1999). Nevertheless, compared with the very limited information available on the inhibited form of attachment disorder, the clinical prospects for further research on 'disorganized' attachment are promising.

Numerous alternative approaches have been proposed to define attachment disorder, and some even include checklists and cut-off scores. Unfortunately, these other alternative definitions suffer from several severe problems, such as the absence of a clear conceptual foundation and the inclusion of separate—albeit co-occurring—symptoms, including symptoms as far afield from attachment as learning difficulties. This latter set of alternative definitions, which are much more akin to the more general and vague notion of institutional syndrome, will only lead to further confusion about the attachment disorder phenotypes.

One limitation of all proposed definitions of attachment disorder is that they focus exclusively on behaviour and on young children. Assuming that attachment disorder can persist past early childhood, what do the phenotypes look like in middle childhood or beyond? Few hints are available. In their longitudinal study, Tizard & Rees (1975) and Tizard & Hodges (1978) noted excessive talking and, from teacher reports, persistent conversation as possible markers of disturbance so there is a suggestion that there may be verbal as well as behavioural signs of disinhibition. Our own clinical observations also suggest that intrusive or personal questions and persistent questioning (without apparent genuine regard for the answer) may be important components in older children. In addition, unawareness of social boundaries and marked deficits in social understanding and interpretation of social cues may be sociocognitive features that are associated with, or part of, attachment disorders in older children. Even less is known about the more specific attachment concept of 'internal working models' of relationships in children with attachment disorder. Describing the sociocognitive underpinnings and correlates of attachment disorder is a next important stage for research, and could lead to avenues for intervention.

Finally, phenomenological accounts are all but non-existent and must await developmentally informed clinical research. Regardless of the outcome of further investigation, clinical observations attest to the significant parental concerns raised about the child's safety and about the child's difficulties in establishing relationships with others. Parents also frequently report considerable distress about the difficulty of forming a psychological connection with the child. These latter features also require research interest and clinical attention.

The remaining sections on comorbidity, prevalence, aetiology and course are concerned with the disinhibited form of attachment disorder. There is virtually no parallel or supporting evidence for inhibited attachment disorder; the implications of this for current and future diagnostic formulations are considered in the section.

Comorbidity, disorder spectrum and associated features

Attachment disorders must be distinct from other behavioural and cognitive problems if they are to be viewed as a viable clinical entity (Cantwell & Rutter 1994). The limited available evidence for disinhibited attachment disorders suggests that they are distinct from other disorders.

It is not surprising that cognitive delay figures prominently in many of the case reports of attachment disorders because the circumstances necessary for the development of attachment disorder might also lead to moderate to severe developmental delay. Fortunately, there is unambiguous evidence that disinhibited attachment behaviours are distinguishable from developmental delay. The strongest support for this position comes from the research of Tizard & Rees (1975) on ex-institutionalized children. The key feature of that research is that some children exhibited indiscriminate friendliness despite being cared for in all respects—except for the absence of a consistent caregiver—and had an IQ within the normal rage. Moreover, even in a sample of deprived children, some of whom exhibited severe cognitive delay, attachment disorder behaviour was distinguishable from cognitive delay (O'Connor et al. 2000).

There is also modest but consistent evidence that disinhibited attachment disorder behaviour overlaps with, but is not identical to, other behavioural problems in children. In the first instance, available case study material (reviewed above) indicates that although co-occurring problems are sometimes evident in children presenting with disinhibited attachment disturbances, the form of the coincident psychopathology varies. Empirical evidence is much more limited, but also indicates that the overlap between disinhibited attachment disorder behaviour and other forms of psychopathology varies from minimal to moderate. In the sample of children adopted into the UK following deprivation in Romania, a modest correlation was obtained between parent- and teacher-reported emotional and behavioural problems and disinhibited attachment disorder symptoms. An overlap with attentional/hyperactivity problems was suggested as potentially especially noteworthy (O'Connor et al. 2000). Analyses also reveal that attachment disturbances can be distinguished from co-occurring 'institutional' syndromes (Wolkind 1974; Rutter et al., 2001).

The relevance of aggressiveness as a comorbid symptom is perhaps especially controversial. In some case reports (Howe & Fearnley 1999), the authors have placed much weight on aggressiveness as a core feature of the disturbance, rather than as a co-occurring problem (see also ICD-10). Most of these reports are of children with a history of severe maltreatment. By contrast, studies of institutionalized children have not, by and large, emphasized aggressiveness as a common outcome, either on its own or in combination with attachment disorder behaviour (Tizard & Hodges 1978; O'Connor et al. 2000; Rutter et al., 2001). Indeed, passivity rather than aggressiveness has long been associated with institutional rearing (Goldfarb 1945). Consequently, at present is may be best to view aggressiveness not as part of the attachment disorder phenotype, but rather as a distinct co-occurring problem, with its roots probably in the history of severe maltreatment that preceded the disruption. Many other kinds of clinical problems are noted in reported cases, including eating problems, self-injurious behaviour and post-traumatic stress disorder, but few symptoms are consistently and systematically reported to co-occur with attachment disorder symptoms.

At present, it is best to maintain more narrowly defined definitions of attachment disorder rather than suppose that other distinct disturbances (such as conduct disorder) are part of the phenotype. However, if there is a move to extend the diagnostic boundaries of disinhibited attachment disorder, then the most likely extension would be toward including symptoms known to be associated with early severe caregiving deprivation. One commonly reported feature of children with (a history of) attachment disorder is an impairment in peer relationships (Freud & Burlingham 1973; Hodges & Tizard 1989; O'Connor et al. 1999). It is not yet clear from existing research if peer problems are an expression of a more general disturbance in social and attachment behaviour with adults, or if disturbances in peer relationships index a separate—albeit related—difficulty linked with early deprivation. Two sets of findings are noteworthy in this regard. First, there is evidence from the UK study of Romanian adoptees that problems in peer relationships could not be entirely explained by disinhibited attachment disorder behaviour (O'Connor et al. 1999). Specifically, in only a relative minority of cases did attachment disturbance extend to the peer domain. Secondly, primate research also suggests partly separate developmental lines for child–parent attachment behaviour and peer relationship behaviour (Freud & Dann 1951; Suomi 1999). Thus, although disturbance in peer relationships is a frequent characteristic of disinhibited attachment disordered children, these clinical phenomena may have somewhat different aetiologies and developmental courses. Further investigation of the sociocognitive correlates of attachment and peer problems may help to resolve this issue.

Prevalence

The rate of attachment disorder is thought to be very low, but the actual prevalence has remained a mystery since its inclusion in the psychiatric nomenclature. The diagnostic precondition that children exhibit attachment disorder in response to pathogenic care probably contributes to the uncertainty about the disorder prevalence because there is no consensus about what constitutes pathogenic care. As a result, it is not clear what population of children would need to be sampled in order to derive a prevalence estimate. If, for example, documented child maltreatment constituted 'pathogenic care', then a very sizeable number of children could be 'at risk' for the disorder. In the USA, this may involve more than 1.5 million children each year (National Research Council 1993; Sedlack & Broadhurst 1996).

Alternatively, given that most reports of disinhibited attach-

ment disorder derive from the residential, foster care and high-risk adoption settings, these may be the populations that will be informative for estimating the prevalence of attachment disorder. Even if the latter groups (or a particular subset) were thought more appropriate for a study of disinhibited attachment disorder, the scope of the problem could still be very dramatic. That is because the number of children who experienced protracted periods of foster or residential care and/or multiple care placements (usually following documented maltreatment) is large, at least in the USA and UK (Shealy 1995; Minty 1999).

The UK study of Romanian adoptees provides partial insight into the likelihood of severe disturbance following grossly pathogenic care. In a sample of 154 children (which excluded children who met criteria for pervasive developmental disorder), severe disturbance was found in 29 (19%) children at age 6 years (O'Connor et al. 2000). However, the finding that duration of exposure to deprivation was strongly associated with the rate of severe disinhibited behaviour (e.g. 7% in children adopted into the UK by age 6 months but 31% in children adopted between 24 and 42 months) further underscores the need for a clearer definition of pathogenic care. Should the definition of pathogenic care consider both severity of care and developmental timing (age)? Does severe deprivation limited to the first 2 months of life satisfy the pathogenic care criterion?

It remains for further research to reconcile the large numbers of children who may be at risk for disinhibited attachment disorder with the apparently rare occurrence. Because of the way the diagnosis is defined, research on the prevalence of this disorder cannot be separated from research on aetiology.

Aetiology

The criterion that 'pathogenic parental care' be included in the diagnosis of disinhibited attachment disorder is controversial on conceptual grounds (Zeanah 1996). One of the immediate difficulties is the failure to recognize that while poor parental care and insecure attachments are known to contribute to the development of a range of childhood disorders, from emotional problems to conduct disturbances, symptom lists for these latter disorders make no mention of parental care or causality. However, despite the problems of including pathogenic care as a symptom, few would doubt that pathogenic care has an essential aetiological role. We can draw some further aetiological conclusions from available data, although the uncertainty about what qualifies as pathogenic care pre-empts an adequate understanding of aetiology, as noted above.

First, individual differences within the normal and at-risk range of caregiving are most probably irrelevant to the origins of disinhibited attachment disorder, although perhaps not to its longitudinal course. The primary reason for suspecting that this is the case is the observation that the disinhibited attachment disorder phenotype appears qualitatively different from the attachment relationships described in normal and at-risk samples. Moreover, studies of normal and at-risk populations have not identified behaviour patterns that resemble those found in disinhibited attachment disordered children.

Second, despite the very limited evidence on the origins of inhibited attachment disturbance, some authors have suggested that the aetiologies of the disinhibited and inhibited forms of attachment disorder may be distinct. In particular, the disinhibited form of attachment disorder appears to result *only* where there has been very severely disrupted care; namely, a virtual absence of care in the early months or years of life. On the other hand, the inhibited form of the disorder may be more closely allied with severe maltreatment (e.g. 'persistent disregard' of the child's basic needs; Gaensbauer & Harmon 1982; Zeanah & Emde 1994). It seems likely that the distinction between having no caregiver and having a maltreating caregiver may be an important one in terms of the ontogeny of attachment behaviour and, in turn, the expression of attachment disordered behaviour. However, the effects of these two forms of pathogenic care may be exceptionally difficult to distinguish in clinical and social care contexts because it is increasingly common for children to experience both severe maltreatment and multiple unsuccessful placements with carers (Shealy 1995; Minty 1999).

We also need to consider whether or not maltreatment *per se* is sufficiently 'pathogenic' to meet diagnostic requirements. Careful and systematic studies of maltreated children typically do not find behavioural/emotional disturbances that resemble attachment disorder symptoms (Cicchetti *et al.* 2000). More specifically, the nature of attachment relationships of maltreated children seems adequately described by attachment theory and adequately assessed by traditional approaches (Cichhetti & Barnett 1991). These findings suggest—albeit indirectly—that most instances of maltreatment would not be expected to lead to an attachment disorder, although there is obviously a need for more direct research on this topic.

Third, the absence of a consistent caregiver appears to be sufficient for the emergence of marked disinhibition. So the tendency for clinical reports to focus on children in severe and multiple-risk settings may not be illuminating as regards aetiology. As Tizard & Rees (1975) demonstrated, attachment disorder behaviour may develop in the *absence* of economic deprivation and *despite* adequate opportunities for social interaction with adults and peers. Although necessary, pathogenic care is not sufficient to bring about severe attachment disorder behaviour. Thus, 18% of the Romanian adoptees brought into the UK after 2 years of age showed no signs of attachment disturbance when assessed at age 6 years (O'Connor *et al.* 2000).

Fourth, cognitive delay does not play a (necessary) aetiological or contributing role to the development of disinhibited attachment disorder behaviour (Tizard & Rees 1975; O'Connor *et al.* 2000). Nonetheless, very cognitively delayed children may exhibit some of the features of attachment disorder behaviour, and there may be a frequent co-occurrence of cognitive delay in children exhibiting attachment disorder behaviour (Richters & Volkmar 1994; Hinshaw-Fuselier *et al.* 1999).

Another area in need of further inquiry is whether, and to what extent, there are individual differences in children's vulnerability to developing disinhibited attachment disorder behaviours following exposure to pathogenic care. All of the studies of Romanian adoptees referred to above indicate that a sizeable minority of children do not exhibit severe disturbance despite grossly pathogenic care; the same can be said of other studies of institutionalized children. Similarly, there is, by implication, indirect evidence that many children who experienced maltreatment followed by multiple placements do not exhibit disinhibited attachment disorder.

Longitudinal course

Knowing the longitudinal course of disinhibited attachment problems would have very substantial theoretical implications (e.g. is there a sensitive period after which normal attachment patterns do not form, and will the offset of disinhibited attachment disorder behaviour coincide with the formation of a new attachment?) and clinical and practical applications (e.g. what is 'typical' progress for a child in forming attachment relationships with a foster/adoptive parents?). However, neither attachment theory nor alternative theoretical positions provide clear predictions on the longitudinal course of attachment disorder behaviour. The prevailing assumption in applied child care and clinic settings is that disinhibited attachment disorders are persistent, but this issue has not yet received systematic attention (Rushton *et al.* 1995).

Only three studies have presented systematic data on the stability or change in disinhibited attachment disorder behaviour. Two studies of children adopted from Romanian institutions (Chisholm 1998; O'Connor *et al.* 2000) found no significant change in the mean level of disinhibited behaviour over a comparatively short period, e.g. from age 4 to 6 in O'Connor *et al.* (2000). The latter study also reported stable individual differences over this time period (r = 59). The only study to report a sizeable change in the level of disturbance is by Tizard & Rees (1975) and Tizard & Hodges (1978) who assessed children at ages 4.5 and 8 years. However, although improvements were noted, in some children the level of 'overfriendly' behaviour had not returned to normal levels by age 8 years and some level of social problems persisted into adulthood (Jewitt 1998), so there were differences compared with a non-institutionalized group of children. Whether the greater reduction in problems in Tizard's study compared with the Romanian studies is explained by the longer time interval or less pervasive and severe deprivation is unknown.

One further longitudinal finding of interest is that the formation of a new attachment relationship and the expression of affectionate behaviour toward the adoptive parent are not coincident with an offset of excessively and inappropriately sociable behaviour toward strangers. As noted above, all three studies of Romanian adoptees found that some children whose behaviour toward the adoptive parent in the separation–reunion paradigm was coded as 'secure', nevertheless exhibited signs of disinhibited attachment disorder behaviour (Goldberg 1997;

Chisholm 1998; O'Connor *et al.* 2001). Tizard & Hodges' (1978) findings are also consistent with this impression. Conceptually, these findings impugn the validity of the 'secure' classification in many children, and raise doubts about the utility of conventional assessments of attachment quality. Clinically, these findings suggest that interventions need to address multiple components of the child's behaviour with others, rather than focus exclusively on the quality of the child–parent relationship.

Assessment and reliability

There is no established protocol or assessment strategy for measuring attachment disorders in a clinical or research context. This may explain why even experienced clinicians disagree when asked to apply current diagnostic guidelines to case material (Boris *et al.* 1998). Despite this parlous state of affairs, some leads for assessment can be suggested.

There are two somewhat separate issues concerning assessment: what information is essential for a diagnosis and how such information may be best obtained. As Boris *et al.*'s (1998) study showed, criteria set forth in current nosologies will not likely be sufficient for shaping clinical judgement. Thus, documenting inappropriate or 'indiscriminate sociability' toward strangers is not likely to satisfactorily distinguish children with a disinhibited attachment disorder. That is partly because accurately assessing, in this case, a disinhibited disturbance necessitates a consideration of the context of the behaviour. At present, neither diagnostic system provides leads in any direction. A further reason for expanding the assessment strategy beyond the specific symptoms is that focusing on the diagnostic criteria alone will do little to advance our understanding of the phenomena in clinical or theoretical terms.

Determining what additional clinical material should be collected may depend, in part, on the methods of collection that are available and practical. In the first instance, observations should have a central role because they have been critical in the history and development of the construct and because observations provide information that may not be readily obtained through other methods. At the very least observational assessments will be useful in identifying the core behavioural feature of disinhibited behaviour, 'excessive familiarity with relative strangers'. Structuring the observational assessment correctly may accomplish three goals.

1 Observations may be used to differentiate the level of sociable, and perhaps even comfort-seeking, behaviour directed toward a caregiver(s) compared with a stranger(s) (e.g. a clinician).

2 Detecting 'indiscriminate friendliness' toward strangers could be detected in the course of a clinical assessment; the opportunity to examine behaviour toward two separate strangers (e.g. different members of the assessment team) might well provide a reliable index of the level of disinhibition.

3 Direct interaction with the child in the course of the assessment may reveal the ways in which the child's 'indiscriminate sociability' may be manifest, e.g. physical contact-seeking, intrusive personal questions or other violation of personal boundaries in order to further define the disturbance in social behaviour and cognitions.

Thus, observational assessments can yield important confirmation of the level and severity of disinhibited behaviour.

Establishing a lack of attachment behaviour toward the caregiver is necessary to diagnose either attachment disorder. However, observing attachment behaviour or, more importantly, the lack of attachment behaviour where it would be expected, could present a substantial challenge for the clinic setting. The lesson from developmental research is that a moderately stressful situation is needed to elicit attachment behaviour from the young child (Ainsworth *et al.* 1978; Cassidy *et al.* 1992). Standard observations of child–parent interactions in the waiting room or consulting room may not therefore be very helpful for assessing attachment behaviour. The role of a parent–child separation procedure to elicit attachment behaviour may be useful but, as noted above, there may be serious limitations of using conventional assessments for deprived populations. There is the further concern that, at least with older (school-aged) children, observational assessments have not been shown to elicit attachment behaviour. It may be that observational methods may prove to be more useful for documenting disinhibition than for detecting a failure to exhibit attachment behaviour toward the caregiver, which may be more reliably obtained from the parent.

A clinical interview is a second means of collecting information on attachment disorder behaviours, and may be used with caregivers and others in a caring role (e.g. primary teachers). The interview format may be particularly useful for gathering information on the child's attachment behaviour toward the caregivers in order to determine if any of his or her relationships serves an attachment function. Particularly noteworthy would be instances in which the child sought out a caregiver when distressed or, alternatively, failed to seek out a caregiver when distressed, or was equally likely to seek comfort from a nearby stranger. Given the presence of attachment disorder behaviours, the failure of the child to seek out and derive comfort from a caregiver, in the form of physical contact or confiding, may signal a much greater disturbance and a much poorer prognosis.

The interview format may also be particularly useful for gathering information on key symptoms and further data not necessarily required for diagnosis but important nonetheless: notably the history of disturbance, the regularity of occurrence, and the circumstances in which disordered behaviours occur. In terms of history, it will be especially important to ascertain the nature of any changes in the child's responsiveness to the caregivers and in the child's disinhibited/inhibited behaviours (e.g. since placement). Furthermore, in the case of disinhibited behaviour, it will be important to document if the disturbance occurs in the absence of the caregiver or only in his or her presence. Also, if the child wanders away from caregivers without checking back, it will be important to assess the degree of dangerousness or threat to the child, if the child is equally likely to wander off in all unfamiliar settings, and what steps have been taken to modify the child's behaviour.

In the absence of an established assessment protocol, certain safeguards seem essential. The most important is the need to collect information from a variety of sources. However, having collected data from alternative sources, there is no certainty that the information collected will provide a consistent or coherent clinical picture. For example, although the case for an observational assessment seems strong, we do not know if observational assessments can reliably elicit attachment disorder-relevant behaviour. Similarly, because of the complexity of the attachment disorder phenotypes, it may be difficult to elicit reliable information in an interview format. Difficulty communicating the nature of the disturbance with parents and carers may lead to a high false-positive response. In one study, approximately 50% of adoptive parents of early placed and presumably non-deprived children reported mild symptoms of disinhibited attachment disorder behaviour (O'Connor et al. 2000). A presumed false-positive rate of 'overfriendly' behaviour (disinhibited behaviour in a non-deprived family-reared sample) was also found by Tizard & Hodges (1978), although the rate was much lower at 10%.

Summary

Two decades after entering the diagnostic lexicon, attachment disorders remain poorly understood. The few data available on the phenotype, aetiology, associated features and longitudinal course are derived from studies of a broadly and inconsistently defined disinhibited behavioural pattern using a diverse set of measurements. However, despite the methodological problems in previous studies, a reasonably compelling case can be made that disinhibited attachment disorder behaviour represents a distinct clinical phenotype. Importantly, a similar conclusion cannot be made for the inhibited form of attachment disorder, which remains difficult to define and evaluate. Although the inhibited form of attachment disorder may not withstand close scrutiny, a case may be made for greater clinical attention to the disorganized form of insecure attachment. There is certainly no suggestion that it can be used diagnostically, but it appears to be a far more promising lead for further research on attachment and psychopathology than, for instance, inhibited attachment disorder or many of the alternative definitions of disorder that have been proposed.

Intervention and clinical management

The last decade has witnessed a considerable integration of attachment theory with clinical treatment approaches, in terms of both the theoretical links and practical approaches to intervention (Lieberman 1991; van den Boom 1995; Fonagy 1999). Several groups have documented significant and clinically meaningful improvements in child behaviour and parent–child relationship quality following attachment-based interventions (van den Boom 1995; for a review see Lieberman & Zeanah

1999). Van Ijzendoorn et al.'s (1995) review of available studies provided encouraging evidence that attachment-based interventions are helpful in modifying parental sensitivity, with the effect on attachment security somewhat weaker or perhaps slower to respond to intervention.

Commonalities of established and empirically supported attachment-based interventions are discussed by Lieberman & Zeanah (1999) and van den Boom (1995). For example, there is a focus on real-life interactions between parent and child, especially concerning the parent's sensitivity; parental representations may also be assessed and integrated into the treatment. More work is needed to understand better the mechanisms underlying these interventions and whether the beneficial effects of attachment-based interventions are comparable to or greater than those found with alternative approaches. Nevertheless, there is a strong and growing empirical base supporting attachment-based interventions.

Very little is known about the form and effectiveness of interventions for children with attachment disturbances severe enough to warrant the attachment disorder label. It is natural to suppose that interventions developed for attachment disorder would build on the existing knowledge about effective attachment-based interventions, but this has not been the case. On the contrary, given the severity of disturbances found in very severely deprived children, some authors suggest, in the absence of any supporting evidence, that these children may be best served by specialist interventions that do not have much in common with the attachment-based approaches mentioned above. A consequence of this situation is a disjunction in the treatment given by clinicians in the adoption/foster care field (Levy 2000) and those in a clinical academic setting (Lieberman & Zeanah 1999). Virtually all of the attention to interventions for attachment disorder derives from the former rather than the latter.

There are some similarities among the 'alternative' approaches for treating children with attachment disorders. Although not adequately evaluated, these approaches deserve mention in this review because they are attracting increasing attention in adoption and foster care settings. Rather than attempt to review these alternative therapies, key features and limitations are provided.

Of the 'specialized' treatments for attachment disorder, so-called 'holding' therapies have attracted attention (Hughes 1999). Although described in an attachment theory context, the actual interventions prescribed bear little resemblance to attachment theory and, in many ways, the approach is antithetical to the principles underlying the formation of a secure attachment relationship. Specifically, the use of intrusive holding interventions, sometimes involving a therapist rather than a parent, contradicts the emphasis on promoting sensitive and responsive caregiving. The rationale often provided for this form of intrusive and counterintuitive treatment is that attachment disorders do not respond to traditional interventions; however, evidence for this position is lacking. It is possible that just as attachment disorder is different in kind to the types of attachment insecurity, qualitatively different treatments would be required. To date, this position has not been substantiated with systematic research. This is an important and unfortunate oversight because intensive costly inpatient treatment is not to be recommended before less intensive and less invasive approaches prove ineffective.

The very few evaluations of alternative or holding therapies (Myeroff *et al.* 1999) suffer from substantial conceptual and methodological flaws, such as small and selective samples, uncertain validity of the attachment disorder diagnosis, the absence of relevant attachment outcome data, and no comparison with other less costly and invasive treatments. There is, therefore, no evidence to support this form of intervention. Much more needs to be learned about the form and effectiveness of interventions for children with attachment disorder behaviours.

One further clinical question with notable clinical and policy implications concerns the contribution of the adoptive or foster carer to the offset of attachment disorder behaviour. In particular, are individual differences in caregiver sensitivity associated with clinical progress? Is adequate parenting 'good enough' for a clinically meaningful improvement, or is progress in attachment disordered children dependent on extraordinarily sensitive parenting? In other words, what is the caregiver's contribution to the child's progress? Available anecdotal, clinical and research reports tell us little about how the caregiver influences the child, but make clear the adverse effect of the child's attachment disturbance on the adoptive/foster caregiver. Indeed, one positive aspect of the large and growing grass roots effort to popularize attachment disorder has been to alert professionals to the particular and very distressing problems faced by a significant minority of adoptive and foster parents. What is not known is what kinds of support are helpful in reducing parents' distress. Answers to the above questions may optimize support to families and aid in determining what kinds of placements may be especially well suited to children with severe attachment disturbances.

Of course, interventions may take other forms, including therapeutic foster home and therapeutic milieu in a residential setting. It is therefore necessary that further clinical research considers a range of intervention settings (Shealy 1995) rather than assume a permanent family setting and focus exclusively on child–parent relationships.

Summary

Despite the substantial evidence supporting the use of attachment-based interventions for the treatment of even severe relationship disturbances, little is known about the effectiveness of intervention with children who exhibit attachment disorder behaviour. The lack of systematic evaluation of proposed alternative approaches, coupled with a questionable conceptual and clinical foundation of these treatments, suggest that substantial scepticism is required. One way to progress beyond the underdeveloped state of interventions for children with attachment

disorder behaviour is to foster greater co-ordination between clinicians from diverse settings, and a wider appreciation of the particular clinical issues that confront professionals working in foster care and adoption settings.

Conclusions

This chapter has sought to review the historical and theoretical basis of the attachment disorders in infancy and early childhood, and the available evidence supporting its reliability, validity and response to intervention. Based on this review, several summary statements are offered. First, the basic disturbance referred to as disinhibited attachment disturbance has a solid foundation in clinical reports dating back over half a century and an increasing number of empirical studies; the second form of attachment disorder, referred to as inhibited, lacks substantial and compelling clinical or research support. Nevertheless, there is, in general, minimal evidence of the reliability and validity of the attachment disorders as currently formulated and validating the diagnostic phenotypes will require much further research. Given the number of alternative definitions, however, there is a real danger of further diagnostic confusion and slow progress in clinical understanding and treatment. Secondly, the lack of a consistent caregiver appears to be a necessary but by no means sufficient condition for the disturbance to result. At present we know little about why some children exposed to apparently 'sufficient' pathogenic care do not develop the disorder. Thirdly, attachment theory may provide a useful framework for understanding the attachment disorder behaviour, but the concept of attachment disorder remains only loosely associated with attachment theory, and there remain some important conceptual inconsistencies. Finally, the patterns of behaviour defined as attachment disorders are relatively resistant to change, even an intervention as radical as adoption. It is not yet clear what kinds of intervention and support may promote clinical outcomes of disturbed children.

It is obvious that there are many unresolved issues surrounding the attachment disorders. Progress in resolving many of these outstanding questions will require cross-disciplinary clinical research that brings together basic scientific questions with those derived from child care policy and practice.

Acknowledgements

The author thanks Mike Rutter and Bob Marvin for their comments.

References

Ainsworth, M.D.S. (1967) *Infancy in Uganda: Infant Care and the Growth of Attachment.* Johns Hopkins University Press, Baltimore, MD.

Ainsworth, M.D.S. (1978) Comment. *Behavioural and Brain Sciences*, 3, 436–438.

Ainsworth, M.D.S. (1989) Attachments beyond infancy. *American Psychologist*, 44, 709–716.

Ainsworth, M.D.S., Bell, S.M. & Stayton, D.J. (1971) Individual differences in Strange-Situation behaviour of one-year-olds. In: *The Origins of Human Social Relations* (ed. H.R. Schaffer), pp. 17–52. Academic Press, New York.

Ainsworth, M.D.S., Blehar, M.C., Waters, E. & Wall, S. (1978) *Patterns of Attachment: A Psychological Study of the Strange Situation*. Erlbaum, Hillsdale, NJ.

Albus, K. & Dozier, M. (1999) Indiscriminate friendliness and terror of strangers in infancy: contributions from the study of infants in foster care. *Infant Mental Health Journal*, 20, 30–41.

American Psychiatric Association (1980) *Diagnostic and Statistical Manual of Mental Disorders*, 3rd edn. American Psychiatric Association, Washington D.C.

American Psychiatric Association (1994) *Diagnostic and Statistical Manual of Mental Disorders*, 4th edn. American Psychiatric Association, Washington D.C.

Anders, T.F. (1989) Clinical syndromes, relationship disturbances, and their assessment. In: *Relationship Disturbances in Early Childhood* (eds A.J. Sameroff & R.N. Emde), pp. 125–144. Basic Books, New York.

Barnett, D., Hunt, K.H., Butler, C.M., McCaskill, J.W., Kaplan-Estrin, M. & Pipp-Siegel, S. (1999) Indices of attachment disorganization among toddlers with neurological and non-neurological problems. In *Attachment Disorganization* (eds. J. Solomon & C. George), pp. 231–250. Guilford Press, New York.

Boris, N.W. & Zeanah, C.H. (1999) Disturbances and disorders of attachment in infancy: an overview. *Infant Mental Health Journal*, 20, 1–9.

Boris, N.W., Zeanah, C.H., Larrieu, J.A., Scheeringa, M.S. & Heller, S.S. (1998) Attachment disorders in infancy and early childhood: a preliminary investigation of diagnostic criteria. *American Journal of Psychiatry*, 155, 295–297.

Bowlby, J. (1951) *Maternal Care and Mental Health*. World Health Organization, Geneva, Switzerland.

Bowlby, J. (1977) The making and breaking of affectional bonds. I. Aetiology and psychopathology in light of attachment theory. *British Journal of Psychiatry*, 130, 201–210.

Bowlby, J. (1982) *Attachment and Loss: Attachment*, 2nd edn. Basic Books, New York.

Bowlby, J. (1988) Developmental psychiatry comes of age. *American Journal of Psychiatry*, 145, 1–10.

Bowlby, J., Robertson, J. & Robertson, D. (1952) A two year-old goes to hospital. *Psychoanalytic Study of the Child*, 7, 82–94.

Bretherton, I. (1990) Open communication and internal working models: their role in the development of attachment relationships. In: *Nebraska Symposium on Motivation*, Vol. 36. *Socioemotional Development* (ed. R.A. Thompson), pp. 59–113. University of Nebraska Press, Lincoln, NB.

Bretherton, I. & Ainsworth, M.D.S. (1974). Responses of one-year-olds to a stranger in a strange situation. In: *The Origins of Fear* (eds M. Lewis & L.A. Rosenblum), pp. 131–164. Wiley, New York.

Bretherton, I. & Munholland, K.A. (1999) Internal working models in attachment relationships: a construct revisited. In: *Handbook of Attachment* (eds J. Cassidy & P. Shaver), pp. 89–111. Guilford Press, New York.

Call, J.D. (1987) Psychiatric syndromes of infancy. In: *Basic Handbook of Child Psychiatry*, Vol. 5 (eds J. Call, R. Cohen, S. Harrison, I. Berlin & L. Stone), pp. 242–262. Basic Books, New York.

Cantwell, D.P. & Rutter, M. (1994) Classification: conceptual issues and substantive findings. In *Child and Adolescent Psychiatry: Modern Approaches*, 3rd edn (eds M. Rutter, E. Taylor & L. Hersov), pp. 3–21. Blackwell Science, Oxford.

Carlson, E.A. (1998) A prospective, longitudinal study of attachment disorganization/disorientation. *Child Development*, 69, 1107–1128.

Carter, C.S. (1998) Neuroendocrine perspectives on social attachment and love. *Psychoneuroendocrinology*, 23, 779–818.

Cassidy, J. & Marvin, R.S. with the MacArthur Working Group on Attachment (1992) A system for classifying individual differences in the attachment-behavior of $2\frac{1}{2}$ to $4\frac{1}{2}$ year old children. Unpublished coding manual, University of Virginia (Available as part of a training module. Outline available on request).

Cassidy, J. & Shaver, P., eds (1999) *Handbook of Attachment*. Guilford Press, New York.

Cassidy, J., Kirsch, S., Scolton, K.L. & Parke, R.D. (1996) Attachment and representations of peer relationships. *Developmental Psychology*, 32, 892–904.

Chisholm, K. (1998) A three year follow-up of attachment and indiscriminate friendliness in children adopted from Romanian orphanages. *Child Development*, 69, 1092–1106.

Cicchetti, D. & Barnett, D. (1991) Attachment organization in maltreated preschoolers. *Development and Psychopathology*, 4, 397–411.

Cicchetti, D., Cummings, E.M., Greenberg, M.T. & Marvin, R.S. (1990) An organizational perspective on attachment beyond infancy: implications for theory, measurement and research. In: *Attachment in the Preschool Years* (eds M.T. Greenberg, D. Cicchetti & E.M. Cummings), pp. 3–49. University of Chicago Press, Chicago.

Cicchetti, D., Toth, S.L. & Lynch, M. (1995) Bowlby's dream comes full circle: the application of attachment theory to risk and psychopathology. In: *Advances in Clinical Child Psychology*, Vol. 17 (eds T.H. Ollendick & R.J. Prinz), pp. 1–75. Plenum Press, New York.

Cicchetti, D., Toth, S.L. & Maughan, A. (2000) An ecological-transactional model of child maltreatment. In: *Handbook of Developmental Psychopathology*, 2nd edn (eds A.J. Sameroff, M. Lewis & S. Miller), pp. 689–722. Kluwer Academic/Plenum, New York.

Fonagy, P. (1999) Psychoanalytic theory from the viewpoint of attachment theory and research. In: *Handbook of Attachment* (eds J. Cassidy & P. Shaver), pp. 595–624. Guilford Press, New York.

Freud, A. & Burlingham, D. (1973) *The Writings of Anna Freud*, Vol. 3. *Infants Without Families*, 1939–45. International Universities Press, New York.

Freud, A. & Dann, S. (1951) An experiment in group upbringing. *The Psychoanalytic Study of the Child*, 6, 127–168.

Gaensbauer, T.J. & Harmon, R.J. (1982) Attachment in abused/neglected and premature infants. In: *The Development of Attachment and Affiliative Systems* (eds R.N. Emde & R.J. Harmon), pp. 263–280. Plenum Press, New York.

Goldberg, S. (1997) Attachment and childhood behaviour problems in normal, at-risk, and clinical samples. In: *Attachment and Psychopathology* (eds L. Atkinson & K.J. Zucker), pp. 171–195. Guilford Press, New York.

Goldfarb, W. (1943) The effects of early institutional care on adolescent personality. *Journal of Experimental Education*, 12, 106–129.

Goldfarb, W. (1945) Effects of psychological deprivation in infancy and subsequent stimulation. *American Journal of Psychiatry*, 102, 18–33.

Greenberg, M.T. (1999) Attachment and psychopathology in childhood. In: *Handbook of Attachment* (eds J. Cassidy & P. Shaver), pp. 469–496. Guilford Press, New York.

Greenberg, M.T. & Marvin, R.S. (1982) Reactions of preschool children to an adult stranger. *Child Development*, 53, 481–490.

Hinshaw-Fuselier, S., Boris, N. & Zeanah, C. (1999) Reactive attachment disorder in maltreated twins. *Infant Mental Health Journal*, 20, 42–59.

Hodges, J. & Tizard, B. (1989) Social and family relationships of ex-institutional adolescents. *Journal Child Psychology and Psychiatry*, 30, 77–97.

Howe, D. (1995) Adoption and attachment. *Adoption and Fostering*, 19, 7–15.

Howe, D. & Fearnley, S. (1999) Disorders of attachment and attachment therapy. *Adoption and Fostering*, 23, 19–30.

Hughes, D.A. (1999) Adopting children with attachment problems. *Child Welfare*, 78, 541–560.

Insel, T.R. (1997) A neurobiological basis of social attachment. *American Journal of Psychiatry*, 154, 726–735.

Jewitt, J. (1998) *The long-term outcomes of early institutional care*. Unpublished thesis, University College London.

Kraemer, G. (1992) A psychobiological theory of attachment. *Behavioural and Brain Sciences*, 15, 494–551.

Ladd, C.O., Owens, M.J. & Nemeroff, C.B. (1996). Persistent changes in corticotropin-releasing factor neuronal systems induced by maternal deprivation. *Endocrinology*, 137, 1212–1218.

Levy, D. (1937) Primary affect hunger. *American Journal of Psychiatry*, 94, 643–652.

Levy, T.M., ed. (2000) *Handbook of Attachment Interventions*. Academic Press, New York.

Lieberman, A.F. (1991) Attachment theory and infant–parent psychotherapy: some conceptual, clinical and research consideration. In: *Rochester Symposium on Developmental Psychopathology*, Vol. 3. *Models and Integrations* (eds D. Cicchetti & S. Toth), pp. 261–287. University of Rochester Press, Rochester, NY.

Lieberman, A.F. & Zeanah, C.H. (1995) Disorders of attachment. In: *Child and Adolescent Psychiatry Clinics of North America: Infant Psychiatry* (ed. K. Minde), pp. 45–76. Lippincott, Philadelphia, PA.

Lieberman, A.F. & Zeanah, C.H. (1999) Contributions of attachment theory to infant–parent psychotherapy and other interventions with infants and young children. In: *Handbook of Attachment* (eds J. Cassidy & P. Shaver), pp. 555–574. Guilford Press, New York.

Lyons-Ruth, K. (1996) Attachment relationships among children with aggressive behaviour problems: the role of disorganized early attachment patterns. *Journal of Clinical and Consulting Psychology*, 64, 64–73.

Main, M. & Solomon, J. (1990) Procedures for identifying infants as disorganized/disoriented during the strange situation. In: *Attachment in the Preschool Years: Theory, Research and Intervention* (eds M.T. Greenberg, D. Cicchetti & E.M. Cummings), pp.134–146. University of Chicago Press, Chicago.

Marvin, R.S. (1977) An ethological-cognitive model for the attenuation of mother–child attachment behaviour. In: *Advances in the Study of Communication and Affect*, Vol 3. *Attachment Behaviour* (eds T.M. Alloway, L. Krames & P. Pliner), pp. 25–60. University of Chicago Press, Chicago.

Minty, B. (1999) Outcomes in long-term foster family care [Annotation]. *Journal of Child Psychology and Psychiatry*, 40, 991–999.

Myeroff, R., Mertlich, G. & Gross, J. (1999) Comparative effectiveness of holding therapy with aggressive children. *Child Psychiatry and Human Development*, 29, 303–331.

National Research Council (1993) *Understanding Child Abuse and Neglect*. National Academy Press, Washington D.C.

O'Connor, T.G., Bredenkamp D., Rutter, M. & the English and Romanian Adoptees Study Team (1999) Attachment disturbances and disorders in children exposed to early severe deprivation. *Infant Mental Health Journal*, 20, 10–29.

O'Connor, T.G., Rutter, M. & the English and Romanian Adoptees

Study Team (2000) Attachment disorder behaviour following early severe deprivation: extension and longitudinal follow-up. *Journal of the American Academy of Child and Adolescent Psychiatry*, 39, 703–712.

O'Connor, T.G., Marvin, R.S., Rutter, M., Orlick, J.T., Britner, P.A. and the English and Romanian Adoptees Study Team (2001) Child–Parent attachment following early institutional deprivation. Manuscript submitted for publication.

Provence, S. & Lipton, R.C. (1962) *Infants Reared in Institutions*. International Universities Press, New York.

Radke-Yarrow, M., Cummings, E.M., Kuczynski, L. & Chapman, M. (1985) Patterns of attachment in two- and three-year-olds in normal families and families with parental depression. *Child Development*, 56, 884–893.

Rajecki, D.W., Lamb, M.E. & Obmascher, P. (1978) Toward a general theory of infantile attachment: comparative review aspects of the social bond. *Behavioural and Brain Sciences*, 3, 417–464.

Richters, M.M. & Volkmar, F. (1994) Reactive attachment disorder of infancy or early childhood. *Journal of the American Academy of Child and Adolescent Psychiatry*, 33, 328–332.

Rushton, A., Treseder, J. & Quinton, D. (1995) An eight-year prospective study of older boys placed in permanent substitute families: a research note. *Journal of Child Psychology and Psychiatry*, 36, 687–696.

Rutter, M. (1981) *Maternal Deprivation Reassessed*, 2nd edn. Penguin Books, Harmondsworth.

Rutter, M. (1995) Clinical implications of attachment concepts: retrospect and prospect. *Journal of Child Psychology and Psychiatry*, 36, 549–571.

Rutter, M. & O'Connor, T.G. (1999) Implications of attachment theory for child care policies. In: *Handbook of Attachment* (eds J. Cassidy & P. Shaver), pp. 823–844. Guilford Press, New York.

Rutter, M., Kreppner, J., O'Connor, T.G. on behalf of the English and Romanian Adoptees Study Team (2001). Specificity and heterogeneity in children's responses to profound institutional privation. *British Journal of Psychiatry*, 179, 97–103.

Schaffer, H.R. (1963) Some issues for research in the study of attachment behaviour. In: *Determinants of Infant Behaviour*, Vol. 2 (ed. B.M. Foss), pp. 32–75. Wiley, New York.

Sedlack, A.J. & Broadhurst, D.D. (1996) *Executive summary of the third national incidence study of child abuse and neglect*. US Department of Health and Human Services, Washington D.C.

Shealy, C.N. (1995) From boys town to Oliver Twist: separating fact from fiction in welfare reform and out-of-home placement of children and youth. *American Psychologist*, 50, 565–580.

Solomon, J. & George, C., eds (1999) *Attachment Disorganization*. Guilford Press, New York.

Spitz, R. (1946) Anaclitic depression: an inquiry into the genesis of psychiatric conditions in early childhood. *Psychoanalytic Study of the Child*, 1, 53–74.

Sroufe, L.A. (1983) Infant–caregiver attachment and patterns of adaptation in preschool: the roots of maladaptation and competence. In: *Minnesota Symposium in Child Psychology*, Vol. 19 (ed. M. Perlmutter), pp. 41–83. Erlbaum, Hillsdale, NJ.

Sroufe, L.A. & Waters, E. (1977) Attachment as an organizational construct. *Child Development*, 48, 1184–1199.

Steele, H., Steele, M. & Fonagy, P. (1996) Associations among attachment classifications of mothers, fathers and their infants. *Child Development*, 67, 541–555.

Stoval, K.C. & Dozier, M. (2000) The development of attachment in new relationships: single subject analyses for 10 foster infants. *Development and Psychopathology*, 2, 133–156.

Suomi, S. (1999) Attachment in Rhesus monkeys. In: *Handbook of*

Attachment (eds J. Casidy & P. Shaver), pp. 181–197. Guilford Press, New York.

Thompson, R. (1998) Early sociopersonality development. In: *Handbook of Child Psychology*, Vol. 3. *Social, Emotional and Personality Development*, 5th edn (series ed. W. Damon; vol. ed. N. Eisenberg), pp. 25–104. Wiley, New York.

Tizard, B. & Hodges, J. (1978) The effect of early institutional rearing on the development of eight-year-old children. *Journal of Child Psychology and Psychiatry*, **19**, 99–118.

Tizard, B. & Rees, J. (1975) The effect of early institutional rearing on the behavioural problems and affectional relationships of four-year-old children. *Journal of Child Psychology and Psychiatry*, **16**, 61–73.

van den Boon, D.C. (1995) Do first year intervention effects endure? Follow-up during toddlerhood of a sample of Dutch irritable infants. *Child Development*, **66**, 1798–1816.

van Ijzendoorn, M.H. & Sagi, A. (1999) Cross-cultural patterns of attachment: universal and contextual dimensions. In: *Handbook of Attachment* (eds J. Cassidy & P. Shaver), pp. 713–734. Guilford Press, New York.

van Ijzendoorn, M.H., Juffer, F. & Duyvesteyn, M.G. (1995) Breaking the intergenerational cycle of insecure attachment: a review of the effects of attachment-based interventions on maternal sensitivity and infant security. *Journal of Child Psychology and Psychiatry*, **36**, 225–248.

Vondra, J. & Barnett, D. (1999) Atypical attachment in infancy and early childhood among children at developmental risk. *Monographs of the Society for Research in Child Development*, **64** (3, serial no. 258).

Waters, E. & Valenzuela, M. (1999) Explaining disorganized attachment: clues from research on mild-to-moderately undernourished children in Chile. In: *Attachment Disorganization* (eds J. Solomon & C. George), pp. 265–287. Guilford Press, New York.

Wolff, P.H. & Fesseha, G. (1999) The orphans of Eritrea: a five-year follow-up study. *Journal of Child Psychology and Psychiatry*, **40**, 1231–1237.

Wolkind, S.N. (1974) The components of 'affectionless psychopathology' in institutionalized children. *Journal of Child Psychology and Psychiatry*, **15**, 215–220.

World Health Organization (1992) *The ICD-10 Classification of Mental and Behavioural Disorders: Clinical Descriptions and Diagnostic Guidelines*. World Health Organization, Geneva, Switzerland.

Zeanah, C.H. (1996) Beyond insecurity: a reconceptualization of attachment disorders of infancy. *Journal of Consulting and Clinical Psychology*, **64**, 42–52.

Zeanah, C.H. & Emde, R.N. (1994) Attachment disorders in infancy. In: *Child and Adolescent Psychiatry: Modern Approaches*, 3rd edn (eds M. Rutter, E. Taylor & L. Hersov), pp. 490–504. Blackwell Scientific, Oxford.

Zeanah, C.H., Mammen, O. & Lieberman, A. (1993) Disorders of attachment. In: *Handbook of Infant Mental Health* (ed. C.H. Zeanah), pp. 322–349. Guilford Press, New York.

47 Wetting and Soiling in Childhood

Graham Clayden, Eric Taylor, Peter Loader,
Malgorzata Borzyskowski and Melinda Edwards

Introduction

Problems of continence in childhood are common and generate a great deal of distress. Most children come, quite early in their development, to follow their caregivers' expectations for cleanness and dryness. Both maturation and learning are likely to be involved.

The course over time—with successively fewer children affected at higher ages—is suggestive of a developmental delay. Many animals control deposition of excreta so that it is done outside the places they live, so some aspects of continence can be seen as developing biological functions.

Social learning is also likely to play some part. The requirement to use lavatories is a product of civilization and organized sewage systems. Different cultures impose different expectations. For instance, the high expectations of the East African Digo produce a very different toilet training approach from the maturational readiness method that is now prevalent in the Western world (de Vries & de Vries 1977). The Digo believe that infants can learn soon after birth and begin motor and toilet training in the first weeks of life. Dryness, both by night and day, is usually accomplished by the end of the first year; it involves only walking a few steps away from living areas. In Westernized societies, by contrast, the constraints of the nappy and the lavatory make for later acquisition.

Control of excreta requires integrity of the autonomic innervation and smooth muscle of bladder and gut, together with adequate function of the spinal motor and sensory nerves. Competent defecation and micturition require more than the mechanics of control: children need to have reached the necessary cognitive level to appreciate what is required and the value of continence to their caregivers, and the motivational state to follow the expectations. In both, there is a complex interplay between these functions and the reactions of caregivers, and impairment can result from dysfunction at any of the levels. Wetting and soiling differ in detailed mechanisms and are considered separately.

Faecal incontinence

Normal development of defecation

Defecation is episodic from birth. The rectum contains faeces until there is a stimulus to release them. In infancy, the mechanism of elimination is a contraction of the rectum as a reflex response to being distended. The contracting rectum activates an inhibitory nerve impulse to relax the involuntary muscle at the anus (the internal sphincter), and the contents of the rectum are then expelled. The frequency of elimination depends on the amount of faeces, and therefore on diet and absorption. The normal range is wide—usually between three times a day and once in 3 days—and it may be as infrequent as once a week in otherwise normal people. Increasing control is acquired during development. One aspect of this control is the ability to delay defecation so that the child has time to reach the lavatory. There is a learned response to the sensation of rectal contraction and anal inhibition: to contract the voluntary part of the muscle around the anus (the external anal sphincter) and puborectalis, and thereby to defer the act of elimination. This sensation, and the relaxation of the involuntary sphincter, become more intense with increasing rectal filling. The voluntary sphincter is subject to fatigue after about 30 s in children and 60 s in adults. Other postural muscles are then used to defend faecal continence. The child needs to have developed the necessary physiological functions of the autonomic nervous system, the gut smooth muscle, and the spinal motor and sensory nerves. Children also need to have reached the necessary developmental age to appreciate what is required, and to have acquired the motivation to do so—essentially to please and be rewarded by their caregivers or avoid their displeasure, and often to take pride in achievement.

Another aspect of self-regulation is that the child learns to respond to the sensation of rectal contraction by visiting the toilet, relaxing the external sphincter and allowing the rectum to expel its contents. This is plainly complex: it must depend upon the caregiver to convey and reward the expectation. It is often accompanied by communication from the child to the parent, such as a shout, to signal their need for help. A third aspect of increasing control is learning to recognize early signals of rectal fullness and assist the process of defecation with the voluntary musculature of the abdomen, so that the toilet can be used at convenient times and before the impulse is urgent. This learning of control is also done in collaboration with parent or other caregiver—that person notices the child's physiological cues and often anticipates them; prompts and encourages the use of the pot or the lavatory; and approves of proper use and discourages elimination elsewhere. The relationship between them is the context of toilet training and is influenced by it.

Another set of challenges comes later in development, when

competence at home has to be transferred to the outside world, especially school. A new and more complex set of rules appears: longer delay between rectal fullness and elimination is usually expected, and the demand on self-control is correspondingly greater. Furthermore, the personal demands are greater: children may have to learn to assert themselves by asking to leave the classroom, and they may have to endure or outface the ridicule of other children.

What is abnormal?

Children within a culture vary considerably in the age by which continence is acquired. Large-scale studies have been conducted using parental questionnaires with a mixture of recall and current information (Bellman 1966). They indicate a steadily decreasing prevalence of incontinence with increasing age. The absence of any discontinuity is quite compatible with a sudden change in individuals; but it argues against an absolute standard of normality. Most children in Westernized societies have unreliable faecal continence in their first 2 years.

Some 10% of 3 year olds are still soiling at least once a month; by the age of 3.5–4 years the rate has dropped to less than 5%; at the age of 7 years the figure is around 1.5%. These findings, and those of other surveys such as that of preschool children in the UK by Stein & Susser (1967), led to the general adoption of a diagnostic cut-off at the fourth birthday (Quay & Werry 1972). After that time, soiling more frequently than once a month is regarded as an elimination disorder if it is not attributable to a general medical condition. In people with developmental delays, a mental age of 4 years rather than a chronological one is taken as the diagnostic threshold.

At the age of 10–12 years, soiling at a frequency of once a month or more affected 1.3% of boys and 0.3% of girls in a community survey (Rutter *et al.* 1970). Constipation and soiling problems are about the tenth most common reason for consulting a general paediatrician in the UK and contribute to 25% of the workload of a paediatric gastroenterologist. Only a small minority are referred to child mental health professionals, and these will tend to have more marked psychological problems than other children. By the age of 16, soiling is rare and no adult series have been reported. A good long-term outcome can therefore be anticipated for most.

Social expectations may be more demanding than medical ones. The 10% of 3 year olds who are soiling regularly may well find that this bars them from entrance to preschool playgroups or nurseries. A young person with intellectual impairment may well be socially handicapped by soiling. Treatment may be very useful even if a mental age of 4 has not yet been attained and a diagnosis of encopresis has therefore been withheld.

Types of faecal incontinence

Faecal incontinence is a general term embracing any sort of inappropriate deposition of faeces. There are several patterns of incontinence, and several types of possible dysfunction. The clinical pattern can give clues to the dysfunction that is involved, but does not automatically imply it.

One pattern is that of fluid faeces leaking frequently. The investigation of this pattern should be by referral to a paediatrician. When there is a medical cause of abnormal stools, then it should not be seen as an elimination disorder and it is not discussed further here. Psychological factors may sometimes be involved in the development of frequent fluid stools (Wender *et al.* 1976).

A second pattern is that of the passage of liquid or semisolid faeces into the underclothes. This is the most common pattern presented for treatment, and it points to the retentive type of dysfunction, which is considered in more detail below. The rectum is distended, and children often do not realize that soiling has taken place. The retention is a result of constipation. The term 'constipation' refers to difficulty in defecation. No precise definition is agreed and many use it to indicate an abnormal interval between episodes of defecation. A stool is often described as 'constipated' implying hardness or dryness. Most children and their families use the term if defecation is associated with pain during the passage of the stool, irrespective of the frequency.

Normally formed stools may also be passed into the underclothes in the absence of retention. This is the normal pattern of soiling in very young children, and when older children show it in the absence of retention then they may never have learned to use the toilet consistently.

Another pattern of incontinence is the deposition of normal stools in inappropriate places. Clothes are not soiled, but faeces may be found in the child's room or in other rooms; they may be obvious or concealed; they may even be wrapped and placed in the oven or the freezer. This pattern is more common in psychiatric than in paediatric practice. It is sometimes referred to as 'encopresis' but the terminology is inconsistent; in North American practice and in this chapter encopresis means faecal incontinence as defined above. The pattern of controlled but inappropriate deposition often implies that the physical functions are intact, and the reasons for the problem need to be sought in motivation and intrafamilial relationships.

It is also useful to keep in mind the distinction between primary and secondary encopresis—defined by whether or not there has ever been a period of continence. The secondary group includes that described by Anthony (1957) as 'discontinuous'—in whom good early control was followed by a pattern of inappropriate deposition, which contrasted markedly with the generally orderly, clean and obedient style that they brought to other aspects of their life.

These different patterns of incontinence have been identified by clinical descriptions (Anthony 1957; Levine 1975; Hersov 1994; Hyman & Fleisher 1994). They are not mutually exclusive, and often shade into one another. For example, a child with retention and overflow may come to deposit faeces in inappropriate places as a consequence of the shame and anger that their initial problems entailed. As another example, a child may successfully clear retained faeces, yet be left with a diminished sensitivity to rectal sensation that causes the inappropriate passage of normal stools. The same child may therefore show different patterns at different stages of development. Nevertheless, recognition of the different patterns is useful in directing the clinician's attention to the dysfunctions that are likely to be involved.

Causal pathways

Pathophysiology of retentive soiling

The majority of children referred to encopresis clinics—as many as 95%—show the pattern of functional constipation and retention with overflow (Loening-Baucke 1996). Several studies have been carried out on the alterations of function, recording changes in the pressure inside the rectum and the electrical activity of the various muscles involved (Meunier *et al.* 1979; Loening-Baucke & Cruikshank 1986; Loening-Baucke *et al.* 1987; Wald *et al.* 1986; Hatch 1988). Lack of sensitivity to rectal distension and weakness of the external anal sphincter and pelvic floor are the main findings. Some children also show an abnormal contraction of the voluntary muscles of the pelvic floor during defecation.

The reason that faecal soiling occurs when the rectum is overloaded with retained faeces is an inhibition of normal sensation. Normally, as described above, the contracting rectum both sends a sensory signal and activates an inhibitory nerve impulse to relax the internal sphincter. (This reflex is absent in Hirschsprung disease because the gut nerve network fails to reach the anus during embryonic development.) By contrast, in the child with persistent faecal loading of the rectum, the sensation of rectal filling is diminished or absent. The child is therefore not aware that the involuntary sphincter is being inhibited by the contracting rectum. Accordingly, there is no cue to contract the external sphincter and other voluntary muscles, and faecal soiling occurs. Children may fail to empty their rectums for several weeks and so soiling becomes continuous, with brief remissions occurring when the filling of the rectum is so gross that a massive stool is passed. This is often associated with pain and fear because of the size, hardness and uncontrollable nature of this massive stool. Once the retained stool is passed there may be some days of continence but the cycle of retention and then overflow soiling recurs. Children also learn that defecation is painful and so aggravate the problem by actively obstructing defecation even when they reach the point of rectal loading that produces the urge to defecate.

As the child grows older and if the problem persists, there are physical and psychological consequences. Any obstructed hollow organ of the body will tend to enlarge to accommodate the contents without risking complete obstruction to the function. (Examples can be found at all ages, from the baby of a few weeks with a hugely enlarged stomach as a result of overactivity of the stomach sphincter, to the elderly man whose bladder is chronically distended as a result of prostatic obstruction to micturition.) The rectum will likewise enlarge and the problems of faecal retention increase so that the stool may be permanently resident in the rectum with the continuous passage of looser stool around it. Even following effective clearance of the stool the sensation of the urge to defecate is often diminished for many months or even years. It is quite common for the overflow soiling to be gradually replaced by another pattern of encopresis because of this diminished sensation, especially if the child prefers to think about anything else rather than issues related to visiting the lavatory or taking medication.

The initiating causes of retention are various including painful conditions such as anal fissure, and fearful ones such as aversion to the toilet (and see below). Once retention has developed, its relief is usually a necessary condition for clinical improvement.

Genetic contributions

There are two main reasons for thinking that there may be genetic contributions to faecal soiling: it runs in families, and it is associated with other problems (such as enuresis) that are known to have genetic components in their aetiology. Bellman's (1966) data on familial incidence are notable because they are based on screening a total population of 9425 7-year-olds entering schools in Stockholm, with an excellent compliance rate (94%), and drew on detailed evaluations of the boys who soiled and comparisons with controls. Among the encopretic boys, 15% had a biological father who admitted to having soiled after the age of 7 years, and this high figure was significantly different from the zero rate in the parents of controls. There was also a 9% rate in the brothers who were old enough to show the symptom; and a zero rate in the brothers of controls. Statistically, many more of the fathers and brothers must have been prone to soiling than were prepared to admit it, so a reporting bias could have confounded the comparison, and that of other studies so far.

The transmission could be genetic or environmental. About half of the previously encopretic fathers in Bellman's series had memories of harsh punishment, and tended to pass this on to their children; half did not. The study designs that will clarify the mode of transmission—twin, adoptive and molecular genetic—are still awaited

Toilet training

There have been major changes during this century in the expectations of training. In American culture a change was captured and timed by Klatskin's (1952) survey of child care practices in New Haven around 1949, by comparison with those in Chicago around 1940 (Davis & Havighurst 1946). Sixty eight per cent of parents in the earlier study, and only 6% in the later one, had started bowel training before the age of 6 months. A directive model had been replaced by a more relaxed approach of awaiting a child's maturational readiness.

Several developmental tasks are involved in toilet training. The first is the child's learning to delay the call to stool. Like other forms of learning, this is likely to be facilitated by the setting of clear goals and the provision of consistent reinforcement.

Factors that detract from this could include a lack of parental sensitivity to the child's communication of the need (or impairment of communication in the child); disorganization within the family, witnessed by problems in acquiring other types of attainment; indulgent attitudes that do not particularly set early continence as a goal; or reluctance to foster independence in the child. Another developmental task is learning to use the toilet. This will require not only the acquisition of the skills needed, but also a willingness to employ them. If the toilet becomes aversive, then reluctance to use it may underlie both retention and the use of other places. Harsh or premature training practices might lead to the toilet becoming a place of fear and shame, and therefore being avoided.

However, empirical investigations have not yet given unequivocal support to any of these putative psychological influences. When a controlled comparison between families with and without a soiling child was carried out, there were no significant differences between the groups in the toilet practices and training provided by the parents (Borowitz et al. 1999). Bellman (1966) also found that the mothers of an epidemiologically ascertained series of encopretic boys were no more or less likely than control mothers to have started training their sons early. On the other hand, she did find that the mothers of encopretic boys expected their children to be fully trained at an earlier age than did control mothers, so there was a bigger gap between achievement and expectation—and perhaps a greater sense of failure and tension—for the encopretic. Coercive techniques and laxness of training were both more common in the parents of boys who soiled themselves. Perhaps the lack of replicated findings from group comparisons implies, not that training techniques do not influence continence, but that no *single* technique is associated with delay.

How can one summarize the confusing evidence on toilet training? Research is still needed. So far, the findings on cross-cultural variations (Oppel et al. 1968) suggest that the time of beginning training may have some influence on the average age at which continence is acquired but that the details of training do not. This is in keeping with evidence about enuresis from children reared in kibbutzim: when the caregiver started toilet training earlier, the child was dry earlier (Kaffman & Elizur 1977). The effect was not large, but the evidence is particularly useful because it separates the training function from the relationship with parents. Parental attitudes and emotions are more likely to be associated with soiling beyond the age that is normative for the culture—especially when continence has been acquired and then breaks down—but it is not yet known which is cause and which is effect.

Other psychological influences

Family factors other than the techniques of toilet training could also be involved through the developmental mechanisms previously outlined. Anthony's descriptions of discontinuous encopresis emphasized the very clean and obedient attitude of children in other parts of their life; the idea being that encopresis

might be a means of expression of resentment or rebellion when other expression is denied. Other intrafamilial factors are equally unproven, but often seem salient to clinicians. Investigators have commented on high frequencies of family disharmony and marital problems and hostile dependent relationships between child and parent (Bemporad et al. 1971). The frequency of associated problems may be high in clinical series because they have contributed to the referral rather than to the soiling. Levine's (1975) description of 102 new referrals to a paediatric clinic is worthy of note because it took some account of the issue of heterogeneity and compared 'primary encopresis' (in which incontinence had been continuous from early childhood) and 'secondary encopresis' (in which continence had been acquired and then lost). The group with secondary encopresis was more likely to come from families on welfare, and in that group the time of onset of soiling could be associated (retrospectively) with a disruptive family event—notably, the loss of a parent, a traumatic entry into school, or the birth of a sibling.

It has been hard to develop adequate control for the clinical likelihood that several different patterns may be present rather than a single cause. Clinical descriptions are a first step. Silver (1996), for example, described several family patterns based on an audit of 104 sets of clinic notes.

1 Unhappy children in families with clear difficulties (including child abuse, death of a parent, rejection, parental argument, very tense mothers), where soiling was seen as an expression of stress and unhappiness.
2 Recent family stress or traumatic events precipitating the soiling, such as the birth of a sibling, starting school or death of a grandparent.
3 Family factors that perpetuated soiling, including parents who are reluctant to control their children and who tolerate immature behaviour too well.
4 About half of the sample of families had no unusual problems and appeared warm and supportive.

As another (unvalidated) example, Anthony (1957) described prototypes of children:

1 who had never acquired continence, came from neglectful families, and who might be aggressive but seldom felt any disgust;
2 who had attained continence successfully but were overcontrolled, ashamed and compulsive, with compulsive mothers; or
3 who were 'retentive' with stubborn, battling and provocative interactions.

Chronic constipation and/or soiling may be an indicator of child sexual abuse (Oliver & Buchanan 1979). The development of encopresis may represent a defence against further anal assault, or the child may refuse to open his bowels because of an injured and painful anus (Clayden 1987).

Stressors outside the family are suggested by experience and consideration of the developmental functions involved. There may, for instance, be pressing reasons not to use the toilets at school if they become havens for bullies. Shy children, or those in repressive classroom atmospheres, may find it very difficult to convey their need to use the toilet.

Developmental delays

There are associations between encopresis and other developmental delays—enuresis (see below), sensorimotor incoordination and slow language development (Bellman 1966; Bemporad *et al.* 1971) and low IQ (Olatawura 1973). These associations are based only on parental report in referred cases, but seem consistent across studies. Several reasons are possible; the finding is compatible with the idea that some cases can be seen as showing an immaturity of development.

Associations with psychological disturbance

Most surveys of psychological problems in clinically referred children who soil are flawed by lack of representativeness in the sample, small sample sizes and lack of good control groups. The result is a contradictory set of conclusions in the literature: that behavioural problems are no more common than in a normative sample (Friman *et al.* 1988), or that emotional and behavioural problems are substantially more common (Young *et al.* 1995).

More controlled epidemiological data are needed. In the Isle of Wight surveys, it was possible to go beyond parent ratings, which are likely to include marked halo effects, and consider how far soiling reported by parents predicted psychological disorder as identified from several sources, including teacher reports (Rutter *et al.* 1970). Soiling was significantly associated with a diagnosis of psychiatric disorder, being more than three times as common in boys who soiled than in boys who did not; and more than eight times more common in girls who soiled than those who did not.

There are several good reasons why psychological disturbance might be associated with encopresis. There might be a genetic link. The family factors mentioned above might give rise both to soiling and to disturbance. We do not yet know how far it would be the case that the association between psychological disorder and encopresis would still hold for children without other types of adversity. In principle, psychological disorder might give rise to soiling. If this is the case, then it would have to apply early in development; and the many longitudinal studies of the course of children with psychiatric disorder have not identified soiling as a specific outcome in any of them. Psychological problems might also develop as a result of chronic soiling, whatever the initial cause. Faecal soiling can be very aversive to caregivers. Anthony (1957) commented that 'there is a special type of hatred reserved for the encopretic child'. The child's incontinence can be perceived—or misperceived—as intentional and rejecting; and parents may then react with anger or disgust. Physical abuse can focus around the chastisement of the supposed wickedness or dirtiness of the soiling child. Children in turn react with fear or anger; with excessive compliance or overt rebellion in other areas of life.

Other psychological consequences are also seen in clinical practice. The chronicity of the problem and its embarrassing and shaming nature lead to denial and dissociation. This intensi-

fies the problem with soiling, as children may appear to be unaware of, or uninterested in, their continence and develop an apparent indifference to personal hygiene. This denial can also lead to refusal to become involved in any routines, treatments or precautions which might reduce the social impact of the problem. As the child appears to take no interest in the soiling, it often results in parents having to become involved in coping with the incontinence. This involvement in these personal and intimate functions is very natural for parents of young children but becomes increasingly inappropriate as the child enters adolescence. This may significantly interfere with the adolescent's development of independence and ability to take on responsibilities. It puts the whole family at risk of relationships becoming frozen at too immature a level. There is even a risk that this stasis of teenage development is subtly perceived as being a benefit. There may be a gain from having a permanent 7 year old rather than confront the tensions and anxieties of being or having a teenager. Faecal incontinence provides both the reasons for children to be much more dependent on their parents and a means to continue this, especially if it leads to more time being spent at home than at school.

Management

The usual pattern of management of chronic retention and soiling is an initial paediatric assessment based on the clinical history and initial examination. In general terms, the later the child's problem presents to paediatricians, the less likely there is to be a major organic abnormality of the anatomy of the anus or rectum. Similarly, the more that soiling is described as the main problem, the less likely there is to be an obstructive anal cause, such as Hirschsprung disease. Significant faecal retention is usually detected by palpation of the child's abdomen. The anus is usually inspected to ensure its normal position and to assess whether the sphincter muscle appears to be contracting appropriately. When stools can be palpated in this way, further imaging of the gut with X-rays is unnecessary.

The first line of treatment is to evacuate residual stool if it is present. The standard method has been to use an enema, but over the last decade orally administered medications have reduced the need for this. Once the obstructing stool has been cleared maintenance laxatives need to be used for many months to prevent stools from re-accumulating. The response to medication will depend on the capacity of the rectum. In those children who can only defecate on a regular basis in response to high dosage of stimulant laxatives, such as senna, there is likely to be a degree of megarectum. In the majority of children the rectum shrinks back to its normal size slowly over time and stimulant laxatives are slowly reduced usually because their effects become unnecessarily forceful. The paediatrician judges the progress of the physical resolution by the dosage of medication needed to control the constipation.

The value of laxative medication is reasonably clear: randomized controlled trials have shown it to be preferable to no treatment (Nolan *et al.* 1991). Furthermore, the treatment is specific in that it appears not to be helpful for children who have a non-retentive pattern of soiling (van Ginkel *et al.* 2000).

Psychological treatments

Psychological aspects are always part of the management; many paediatricians have demonstrated a good understanding of psychological and family factors, and include attention to them in their approach to treatment (Garrard & Richmond 1952; Coekin & Gairdner 1960; Clayden & Agnarsson 1991). The soiling is often both the cause and the effect of a behaviour or emotional difficulty. A vicious cycle is often present, especially if parents or teachers have focused on the soiling in a negative fashion rather than having urged the child to defecate regularly to avoid accidents.

The starting point for management of the individual case should be a comprehensive assessment of the type of soiling and the mechanisms responsible for its occurrence. Different treatment approaches are required for the young child who has never been toilet trained, the child with impacted faeces and overflow soiling, the child who is frightened to defecate or to use the toilet, and the child who is intentionally defecating in inappropriate places.

Behavioural and cognitive-behavioural therapies

The most common behavioural approach is basic toilet training based on the principle of operant conditioning, with rewards for sitting on the toilet at set times and for passing stool on the toilet. Toileting after meals is good timing, because it benefits from the gastrocolic reflex. Positive reinforcement is provided by means of star charts, and appropriate rewards may be negotiated with the child and parents. This approach on its own is perhaps most suitable for children who have never established a toileting routine. Toilet training programmes are best carried out at home (Blechman 1979), but an inpatient setting can help in more complicated cases, or when the child is severely constipated and requires washout or even manual evacuation of faeces.

This simple positive reinforcement approach has mostly been evaluated in combination with medical management including laxatives. A systematic review of controlled trials by McGrath *et al.* (2000) finds it 'probably efficacious', being superior to biofeedback, to laxatives in children who are constipated, and to medical management in the non-constipated (one trial each).

More extensive behaviour therapy includes, in addition, training relaxation of the external sphincter in defecation and rewarding increases in dietary fibre intake. The McGrath *et al.* (2000) review rated this too as 'probably efficacious', but without evidence on whether it was superior to simple behavioural approaches.

Biofeedback techniques have been used to condition patients to be more sensitive to a stimulus distending the rectum and to heighten voluntary external sphincter response, with the patient watching or listening to a signal of the level of external sphincter contraction (Kamm 1998). Van der Plas *et al.* (1996) found

biofeedback to add nothing to laxative treatment in a randomized controlled trial and a long-term outcome study by Loening-Baucke (1995) came to the same conclusion.

Most therapies, whether or not this is explicitly stated, include a fundamental aspect of cognitive therapy by helping children to understand the nature of the problem and view themselves more positively. Buchanan (1992) emphasized the notion of 'demystification' of the symptoms and the importance of empowering the child with knowledge and ownership of their body. Comprehensive treatment programmes often include an educational component to help children understand the process of defecation and how they can help themselves (Levine & Bakow 1976; Clayden & Agnarsson 1991; Stark *et al.* 1997). There are very similar components in the family approach of White (1984), and art therapy may help children to express their feelings when they cannot do so verbally.

Many clinicians (Sheinbein 1975) argue that the family should always be involved in the treatment of the soiling child. In one sense, this is nearly always the case. Parents are usually involved in the development and implementation of a behavioural programme, and parallel work may be carried out with the parents (usually the mother) of a child seen in individual psychotherapy. However, the focus of therapy in these cases remains the child—whether this be with regard to the child's behaviour or his or her internal world.

Family systems therapy (see Jacobs & Pearse, Chapter 57) has a broader goal—to change patterns of family interaction that are seen as causing, or at least maintaining, the child's soiling. For example, episodes of soiling could occur when there is tension between the parents, serving to distract from marital conflict that would threaten the integrity of the family. Soiling is often treated by family therapy in the UK but accounts of this, let alone treatment trials, are poorly represented in the literature. The most influential account of family work with soiling has been provided by White (1984) who aimed to externalize the problem and join with the child in a battle against the 'sneaky poo'. Using both drama and humour, White emphasized the need to engage the child in dealing with his or her problem, with the parents having a supportive role. The work lacks outcome data but may be particularly relevant for children whose defecation is controlled but inappropriate. One retrospective audit of outcome for 108 children (aged 3–6 years) stated that White's approach gave better results than family behavioural techniques, and was rated as more helpful by parents (Silver *et al.* 1998).

Combinations of treatments

Given that childhood soiling is a multifactorial condition, involving a complex interaction at the biological, psychological, family and social levels of human functioning, it is not surprising that many workers have developed multidisciplinary and multimodal treatment programmes (Levine & Bakow 1976; Chaney 1995; Wright & Walker 1977). These include a variety of educational, psychological and medical interventions and are used in both inpatient and outpatient settings. The aims of such programmes should be to reduce the anxiety and guilt caused by the problem, restore children's self-confidence, instil hope for the future, empty the bowel of retained faeces (when relevant) and inculcate a regular toiletting regime. A combined behavioural and medical treatment programme has been shown to be superior to behaviour therapy alone, and to medical treatment with laxatives alone (Cox *et al.* 1998).

Stark *et al.* (1997) described a standard protocol for children with retentive soiling and who had failed to respond to routine medical management. Treatment consisted of separate group sessions (six in all) for children and parents, with components of the programme including psychoeducation about soiling, medical management, behavioural contracts with the child, and sticker charts/rewards for compliance. Outcome data were provided on 59 children, of whom 86% had stopped soiling by the end of treatment.

The danger of such treatment packages is that they can come to be routinely applied to all cases, and this may result in less attention being given to a comprehensive assessment. Berg & Jones (1964) pointed out that a joint approach still needs to be tailored to the individual case, with the right combination of physical and psychological interventions being employed according to need. Until the evidence is clearer, we recommend a liaison model, involving paediatricians and child mental health workers, for children who fail to respond to routine medical management (Clayden 1992).

Treatment in adolescence

Treatment in the later part of childhood and adolescence becomes more difficult because relationships within families and with friends are often profoundly affected by the bowel problem. It is unfortunately just the stage in young people's lives that they may resist engaging with agencies attempting to help them, especially if the therapist has to focus them on the areas from which they have dissociated. It is not unusual for the young people to have mixed feelings about their therapists. One of the key areas is for them to be given more and more personal responsibility for their problem. This is possible only if they are also given more autonomy in deciding which treatments to take or whether to continue therapy. It is advisable that choice and responsibility are increased, especially in teenagers, who, as a group, are very likely to opt out of their role in management if their treatment appears to be easily subsumed by another. The dilemma for those attempting to help them is that making demands on them is likely to distance them from the help which they are more likely to seek if given that autonomy and choice. It is for this reason that therapy for young people is on the basis of consensus. Some will shy away from unpleasant physical treatments, such as enemas — which they may still fear even years afterwards. Fortunately, the development over the last few years of initial treatments for constipation which are more easily tolerated should reduce the prevalence of young people who are afraid of restarting treatment.

Prognosis

Encopresis usually resolves spontaneously before adolescence (Bellman 1966), and most cases improve in the course of routine medical management. However, long-term follow-up studies are more pessimistic than the outcome results reported from major centres would suggest. They suggest that some 30–40% of cases continue to have symptoms for several years (Sutphen *et al.* 1995; Loening-Baucke 1996; Rockney *et al.* 1996), and the problem may occasionally persist into adult life (Fraser & Taylor 1986). A chronic course has serious psychosocial implications for the child and his or her family, and places a heavy burden on health care resources. Several workers have identified particular factors that suggest a poor prognosis and which point to the need for specialist treatment.

Characteristics of the child that have been found to be associated with a poor outcome include learning difficulties, hyperactivity, reading problems, particular childhood characteristics (excessive moodiness, disobedience, fearlessness), and noncompliance with treatment (Levine & Bakow 1976). The presence of behavioural problems has also been found to militate against successful treatment (Young *et al.* 1995; Stark *et al.* 1997). Rappaport *et al.* (1986) identified a high-risk group where the child demonstrated not only poor compliance but also an external locus of control. Some authors have described characteristics of the family and of parenting style that are associated with a poor outcome. These include social disadvantage (Taitz *et al.* 1986), and disorganized or chaotic families (Stark *et al.* 1990, 1997).

Urinary incontinence

Normal development of urination

Urinary continence is the function of storing urine in the bladder until it is socially appropriate to void. The volume of urine is determined by water intake, renal function and its hormonal control — which includes the secretion of vasopressin from the posterior pituitary under neural control.

The bladder performs only two functions: storage and emptying. In the normal situation the bladder fills, with very little rise in pressure, until capacity is reached. Efficient storage depends on the ability to hold a large volume of urine at low pressure. During filling the urine is held in the bladder by the bladder neck mechanism, which is composed of smooth muscle, and the distal (external) sphincter, which is composed of striated muscle and is under voluntary control. At capacity voiding is initiated. The bladder muscle (detrusor) contracts with simultaneous opening of the distal sphincter. The bladder neck is pulled open and voiding continues until the bladder is empty and the sphincters then return to their occlusive role. Children learn to use the voluntary musculature of the pelvic floor to raise the neck of the bladder and thus to defer voiding until the time and the place are appropriate; they also learn to initiate micturition voluntarily by lowering the neck of the bladder. Effective urinary storage and voiding requires intact connections between the pons, the sacral plexus via the cauda equina, the pudendal nerves (S2–4) and the hypogastric plexus (T11–L2) to innervate the bladder and sphincter. The smooth muscle of the bladder (detrusor) is innervated by parasympathetic postganglionic fibres whose ganglion cells are located in the bladder, with the preganglionic motor neurones reaching the bladder via the pudendal nerve.

Effective voiding also involves the learning and the motivation of the child. As with faecal continence, learning is involved in several stages: inhibiting micturition, making use of the consequent delay to go to the toilet, signalling to parents that they need to go there, voluntary micturition in the toilet, and visiting and using the toilet before the urge to pass urine is so strong that it can be delayed no longer.

Bladder voiding is more frequent than faecal elimination, and dryness through the night is correspondingly harder to reach than cleanness. How far nocturnal dryness is acquired by learning or by maturation has been controversial. On the one hand, some have found it hard to see how something can be learned during sleep. On the other hand, the evidence from the Israeli kibbutzim suggests that when caregivers expect dry beds earlier, the children follow suit (Kaffman & Elizur 1977).

What is abnormal?

In normal development, the age at which children acquire bladder control is variable. Most children of normal intelligence and health can successfully reach the lavatory in the daytime and use it appropriately without wetting themselves by the age of 4 years. By the fifth birthday, only about 1% of children have troublesome daytime wetting. Children generally achieve urinary control by day before night, and bedwetting is common even in later childhood. The values for the prevalence of nocturnal enuresis, in the surveys described by Butler (1998), were 15–22% for males and 7–15% for females at the age of 7 years. Even by the age of 18 years, about 1% of males (and a lower proportion of females) still have enuresis at night.

The figures from different surveys are hard to bring together because of differences in methods, populations studied and definitions of enuresis. There is no one level of frequency of wetting that is obviously abnormal, and study definitions have varied from one to 21 times a month. Further, there is no one age at which children cease to wet, but a gradual decrease in numbers with age. The diagnostic categories of nocturnal and diurnal enuresis therefore have no absolute distinction from normality, and illustrate the difficulty of imposing categories upon a dimensional distribution.

How should one decide what is abnormal? DSM-IV and ICD-10 give explicit rules. The essential feature of enuresis is the repeated voiding of urine into the bed or the clothes that is not caused by a general medical condition such as diabetes. Whether or not the voiding is involuntary is irrelevant to the diagnosis. It usually is involuntary, but it is often hard to know the exact mix of motives and awareness. The main distinctions are according to the situation in which it occurs (nocturnal only, diurnal only or both) and whether there has been continuous wetting since early childhood (primary enuresis) or wetting has reappeared after a dry period (secondary). Whether or not the diagnosis should be given depends upon severity and impact: either the enuresis should happen at least twice a week for a period of at least 3 months, or else there should be impairment as a result of the problem, such as restriction of activities, poor self-esteem or stigmatization by others.

One way of deciding on the cut-off would be by examining the frequency of bedwetting at different ages and determining whether there is a critical period during which continence is normally acquired. Verhulst et al. (1985) criticized the diagnostic definition of nocturnal enuresis with data from an epidemiological survey of 2600 Dutch children sampled from municipal registers.

The percentages of boys and girls who wet the bed at least twice a month at different ages are shown in Fig. 47.1. The suggestion is that for girls there is a rapid decline in prevalence between the fourth and sixth years and the fifth birthday is a rational cut-off, but for boys the decline in prevalence comes later, and the eighth birthday would be a better mark for them. This kind of argument from a discontinuity in development is useful; but, as discussed by Rutter & Taylor (Chapter 2), it does require rather large numbers to make the case. A difference between 6 and 2% for one gender at one age in a study of this size corresponds only to about three children and therefore may not be robust.

Another way of validating classification could be by examining the variations in course at different ages. In the second and third year of life, about 40% of children become dry in the succeeding year (Oppel et al. 1968). Thereafter, the rate of acquisition of dryness slows down. Of children who wet their beds, 15–16% experience spontaneous remission each year (Forsythe & Redmond 1974; Clark et al. 1994), and the figure is similar at all ages from 5 to 12 years. This approach has not given indication of an age beyond 4 years after which wetting is abnormal.

Another aspect of the definition of enuresis is that the child should have a developmental level corresponding to a chronological age of at least 5 years. This developmental level requirement is rather restrictive. Enuresis is more common in young people with a moderate or severe learning disability, but it is by no means universal; incontinence can make a considerable difference to the range of activities and environments that are available and to the burden on caregivers. Treatments such as the alarm can be successful in people with chronological ages higher than 5 years but mental ages well below. There is no need to wait for the arbitrary developmental milestone to be reached before offering treatment.

The implication of the uncertainties over definition is that clinicians should not base their practice slavishly upon the diagnostic manuals. The presentation of enuresis for treatment is based as much upon parental attitudes and tolerance as upon the

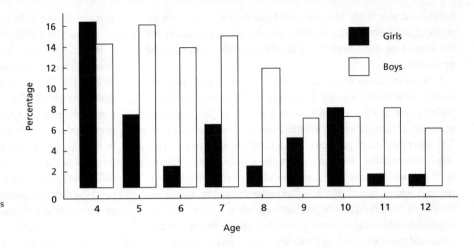

Fig. 47.1 Prevalence of bedwetting. The figure shows the percentages of boys and girls who wet the bed at least twice a month at different ages.

child's wetting; most enuretic children are never treated (see below). The decision to treat should be based on the impact of the problem rather than solely on its exact form.

Day wetting (diurnal enuresis) is far less prevalent than nocturnal enuresis and is experienced by more girls than boys (Berg 1979; Fielding & Doleys 1988). Hellstrom *et al.* (1990) reported that 3.1% of 7-year-old girls and 2.1% of boys of that age regularly wet during the day. As with nocturnal enuresis, the natural history is one of gradual resolution: each year 14% of 5–9 year olds become dry; and the corresponding rate is 10% for 10–18 year olds (Forsythe & Redmond 1974).

Types of urinary incontinence

There are several patterns of urinary incontinence which need to be established from the history (Shaffer *et al.* 1994). One—the most common—is of bedwetting (nocturnal enuresis) with no daytime problem. A second is that of diurnal enuresis, with or without bedwetting. To these three main types, other distinctions need to be added. The history may be of primary enuresis which has continued directly from the normal incontinence of early childhood. Alternatively, wetting may have started only after a period in which the child has successfully been dry (secondary enuresis).

Incontinence of urine is not usually associated with any other abnormality of micturition but, when it is, the pattern needs noting because it may well call for physical investigation of urinary function. The complaint about some children will be that they are depositing urine in inappropriate places, such as living rooms or bedrooms. As for encopresis, the pattern will direct enquiry towards motives for doing so rather than towards reasons for impairment of bladder function.

There are other sources of heterogeneity: boys compared with girls; those with psychiatric disorder compared to those without; those with developmental delays compared to those without; and those who do or do not show one of the types of pathophysiology described below. Many of the less common

types are still in need of investigation. Only one type—nocturnal enuresis without daytime wetting—has received a good deal of research.

Causal pathways

Nocturnal enuresis

The aetiology of bedwetting has attracted a good deal of research. It has been known for a long time that there is a strong tendency for it to run in families. Of children with nocturnal enuresis, 70% have a parent or sibling who was late in becoming dry (Bakwin 1971). The rate of affected parents is much higher than in a control group (Jarvelin *et al.* 1991). Bakwin (1971) found that identical twins were almost twice as likely to suffer from nocturnal enuresis as non-identical twins, suggesting strongly that there is a genetic contribution to the transmission. Molecular genetic evidence has not yet indicated a single gene. Analysis of polymorphisms of microsatellite markers has suggested possible linkage sites on chromosomes 22, 8, 12 and 13 (von Gontard *et al.* 1999a). The locus on chromosome 22, for example, was linked to enuresis in about 40% of families studied. Replication is needed before any of these loci can confidently be accepted; the most likely conclusion in present knowledge is that there is genetic heterogeneity.

Environmental factors in the aetiology have been suggested chiefly by associations found in case–control comparisons. A wide range of such associations has been found, including later initiation of toilet training, a higher rate of stressful life events (for secondary enuresis only), urinary tract infection, and constipation (reviewed by Shaffer 1994). In addition, large-scale epidemiological studies have found further associations. Children of lower socioeconomic groups and from large families living in overcrowded conditions were more at risk of enuresis (Butler 1994). Rona *et al.* (1997) described results from a national sample of nearly 15 000 children in the UK. Nocturnal enuresis was again associated with low social class (albeit in girls only), and also with African-Caribbean origin, mothers who smoked, mothers who gave birth while still teenagers, and being the second- or third-born in the family in comparison with the first-born.

In most instances the causal mechanisms that underlie these associations are not known. Fergusson *et al.* (1986) described a multivariate analysis of potential risk factors on the age of acquisition of continence in a longitudinal study of a birth cohort. The most important predictor was a family history of enuresis, and contributions also came from the child's developmental level at 1 and 3 years of age, and the child's early sleeping patterns. A wide range of psychosocial factors were measured, but they were not predictors of primary enuresis once the other influences had been taken into account. Secondary enuresis in this cohort of children was best predicted by two factors: being late to attain nocturnal bladder control, and being exposed to a high rate of adverse life events (Fergusson *et al.* 1990).

Pathophysiological mechanisms have been suggested by other associations found in case–control studies. The review by Shaffer (1994) concluded that there was evidence for lower functional bladder volume in those with enuresis, anatomical changes in the neck of the bladder, shorter stature, later puberty, worse motor co-ordination, and shorter hours of sleep as a toddler. The association with sleeping difficulties was emphasized by a questionnaire study on a national sample in Finland. Enuretic boys had more frequent nightly arousal and early morning waking than controls, while enuretic girls had more nightmares than non-enuretic girls (Moilanen *et al.* 1998). The national UK sample by Rona *et al.* (1997) also found an association between nocturnal enuresis and disturbed sleep. However, laboratory studies have found an apparent absence of association with abnormal sleep architecture (Shaffer 1994). Wetting can occur at any stage of sleep (Mikkelsen *et al.* 1980), so lack of waking to bladder cues is unlikely to be caused by altered stages of sleep, at least for most children. It may well be that people with enuresis have a normal pattern of shifting from deep to light sleep (Stage I) when the bladder gets full, but then fail to wake from light sleep (Watanabe 1995).

The neuroendocrine influences on urinary secretion have received considerable research attention. Most people show a considerable reduction of urine output at night, but some children with nocturnal enuresis produce more urine at night than controls (Norgaard 1991). Sodium excretion at night is also greater than in normal controls (Natochin & Kuznetsova 2000). This nocturia is not necessarily caused by altered secretion of the antidiuretic hormone vasopressin, for plasma levels in those with enuresis appear to be normal (Robertson *et al.* 1999); rather, there appears to be a nocturnal reduction in renal sensitivity to the antidiuretic effect of vasopressin. This research has led to the successful introduction of a synthetic analogue of vasopressin as a treatment (see below). It is not yet clear whether the response to vasopressin is predicted by vasopressin levels, but the response does seem be greater in those who do not have a reduced functional volume of the bladder (Eller *et al.* 1998; Neveus *et al.* 1999). This, if confirmed, suggests that a different mechanism

may be at work in those with diminished bladder capacity, which may be a different pathogenetic pathway.

Reviewers have often suggested that the symptom of wetting at night can be the result of several distinct disorders (Butler & Holland 2000). The evidence briefly summarized above suggests that one mechanism is either a lack of vasopressin release during sleep or a nocturnal insensitivity of renal tubules to vasopressin; that inco-ordination of voiding mechanisms, reflected in reduced functional bladder volume, is a second; and that reduced waking from light sleep in response to the sensation of a full bladder may be a third. Research is expected to clarify how far these different patterns map on to the underlying genetic and environmental influences.

Daytime wetting

Diurnal enuresis differs in several respects in its associations: the sex ratio is different; it is more likely to be associated with structural and functional disorders of the urinary tract; and less likely to predict that other family members will have shown enuresis (Hallgren 1957).

Diurnal enuresis is more likely than nocturnal enuresis to be associated with a structural abnormality. There is much less systematic research, and clinical experience guides practice. The causes include transient wetting following acute emotional stress, careless wetting as a result of poor technique and tight clothing, detrusor instability, weakness of the bladder neck, giggle incontinence, urinary tract infections, infrequent voiding, incomplete bladder emptying and anatomical abnormalities such as ectopic ureter or neuropathic bladder. The neuropathic bladder may be diagnosed late; causes include open and closed spina bifida, sacral agenesis, transverse myelitis, autonomic neuropathy, spinal cord tumour, and spinal cord trauma, as well as the more difficult to recognize occult neuropathic bladder and non-neurogenic neurogenic bladder. Sexual abuse has a recognized association with secondary wetting. Psychological factors probably play an important part in children who fail to empty their bladders effectively or frequently enough. The secondary pathophysiological changes in bladder smooth muscle and bladder function that then occur are similar to those of the megarectum that develops in children refusing to defecate. This bladder dysfunction is referred to as Hinman syndrome (Hinman & Bauman 1973) and is another good example of an incontinence problem that is best managed by a combined medical and psychological approach.

Psychological problems in children with enuresis

Psychiatric disorder is present in a significant minority of children referred because of enuresis. For instance, a recent survey of clinic attenders by von Gontard *et al.* (1999b) found that 40% of children had at least one ICD-10 diagnosis other than enuresis, with disruptive behaviour disorders outnumbering all others. Referral practices will vary from place to place but, in general, services for children with enuresis need to ensure that they have resources or collaborations to cope with comorbid problems.

The association with psychological deviance is also present when community surveys include questions about wetting and questionnaire ratings of psychological symptoms. A national health survey in the USA, involving more than 10 000 children, found a higher rate of deviance in the enuretic than the non-enuretic with an odds ratio of about 1.8 (Byrd et al. 1996). Similar degrees of association have been reported from Finland (Moilanen et al. 1998), Ireland (Devlin 1991), New Zealand (McGee et al. 1984) and the UK (Kolvin et al. 1972; Rutter et al. 1973). In the large survey by Byrd et al. (1996) the risk was similar among children with infrequent and frequent bedwetting, but greater in older than younger children, in girls than in boys, in children who wet both by day and by night, and in those with secondary enuresis by comparison with those who had never been dry. Many of these associations are replicated in other countries: enuretic girls were more disturbed than boys in Rutter et al.'s (1973) study, especially on teacher ratings; and those with secondary enuresis were more at risk than those with primary enuresis in the Kolvin et al. (1972) survey.

Of the possible reasons for the association, referral bias to clinics plainly cannot explain it all because of the robustness of the finding in unselected samples. There is a possibility of psychiatric disorder being a direct cause of enuresis; for example, by altering the motivation of affected children. Rutter et al. (1973) found that children who became secondarily enuretic were more likely to show psychological deviance before the enuresis started. This suggests that they were under more stress or that the deviance caused the enuresis. However, the latter does not seem like a complete explanation, because of the failure of treatments such as psychotherapy, anxiolytics and stimulant drugs to help enuresis.

Enuresis may sometimes cause psychiatric disorder. Feehan et al. (1990) and Fergusson & Horwood (1994) reported longitudinal studies in which there was a predictive effect of nocturnal enuresis on later adolescent disturbance; it was only a small association once potentially confounding factors had been allowed for, but it was still present. The best evidence is that specific treatments for enuresis, such as the alarm, do reduce other psychological symptoms in randomized controlled trials (Moffatt et al. 1987; Longstaffe et al. 2000); although clinically it must be said that treatment of the enuresis seldom results in a complete recovery from comorbid disorders. Clinically, too, children often present a picture in which stigmatization by others and emotional upset are direct consequences of wetting. Enuresis can be a considerable source of embarrassment often invoking ridicule or punishment. Children may suffer various adverse emotional and behavioural consequences: they may develop poor self-esteem, feeling they are dirty, lazy or smelly and isolated with their shameful secret. Restrictions to social activities, such as staying with friends/families or school trips, are not uncommon (Butler 1998) and children may be loath to develop close personal relationships for fear of being 'found out'. Ollendick et al. (1989) found that children regarded wetting in class as the third most stressful event possible (only behind 'losing a parent' or 'going blind'). Enuretic children have a lower than average sense of self-esteem (Wagner et al. 1988). An outward indifference is not uncommon (Schaefer 1979). Enuresis can also place a burden upon family relationships and resources, and is a significant financial burden (pants, washing facilities, extra sheets, etc.). It seems plausible that this kind of secondary effect could explain the disproportionate increase of risk in those where wetting would have greatest impact (teenagers rather than younger children and boys rather than girls), rather than those whose wetting is most severe.

Both enuresis and psychological disturbance may also be common consequences of a single cause, or be the consequences of causes that tend to occur together. Enuresis, as described above, is associated with other developmental delays and with social adversity and stress: it is not self-evident that these are aetiological factors, but they are known to be associated with psychiatric disorder as well. The greater risk of those with secondary enuresis is also in keeping with this view, because of the association of secondary enuresis with stressful life events that may also give rise to psychological symptoms (see Sandberg & Rutter, Chapter 17). What is not yet clear is whether the association between stress and secondary enuresis would still hold if children with overt psychological disturbance were excluded.

Clinical management of wetting

Many parents never consider that wetting is a problem and—particularly for monosymptomatic nocturnal enuresis—never seek advice. Sometimes this may reflect good coping, but sometimes the stigmatizing effects of bedwetting mean that there is avoidable impairment. One survey in France indicated that one-third of children with moderate to severe nocturnal enuresis are never presented to doctors (Lottman 1999). In the UK, only 50% of the parents consulted a doctor for enuresis in their child (Rona et al. 1997). In a survey in Ireland, enuresis was distressing for most families yet most children never saw a doctor about the problem (Devlin 1991).

Most wetting is rightly dealt with at the primary health care level, often by nurses attached to general practices or to schools. In the UK, there are a number of specialist enuresis clinics led by health visitors. Children referred to paediatricians and child mental health services have often not responded to symptomatic measures, or show signs of emotional disturbance in addition to (or as a consequence of) their wetting.

It is noteworthy that surveys of clinical practice in many countries have suggested that management commonly falls far short of that recommended by guidelines or supported by evidence. In France, 20% of doctors did not prescribe treatment, and the majority offered advice on lifestyle and diet in the first instance (Lottman 1999). When treatments were proposed, they consisted of drugs rather than the enuresis alarm. In Ireland, less than two-thirds of those assessed had a urine test and 40% of parents remained dissatisfied with the outcome of the visit to the doctor (Devlin 1991). Children were more likely to be prescribed medicine than other treatments, and the enuresis alarm was recommended for only one in 10 children. It is puzzling that medication is so often preferred to the alarm when the latter is more effective, safer and less expensive. It does not seem to be driven by parental preferences. One study from the USA reported treatment practices when families were given the option of different therapies (Schulman *et al.* 2000). Families mostly chose an alarm (31%), followed by desmopressin acetate (22%) and oxybutynin (9%). Some preferred no treatment (23%). One year after the first visit, children whose parents chose the nocturnal enuresis alarm were the most likely to be completely dry. The barrier to the use of the alarm seems likely to be in professional custom, and perhaps lack of familiarity with the technique. Whatever the reasons, the unstandard and often unsatisfactory nature of routine management suggests that specialist time may be well invested in educating and working with primary care practitioners to enhance practice.

Assessing physical factors

A careful history is the key to effective management and should include a family history of the symptoms. It is also essential to record the daytime symptoms, such as the frequency of wetting, urgency, details of bladder habits (lavatory visits) and frequency of voiding. A great deal of valuable information may be obtained from frequency-voiding and voided-volume charts. Knowledge of the bowel habits and the child's development is essential and this should include questions on gait and acquisition of walking and speech as a guide to other functions that may be affected by spinal nerve abnormalities or developmental delay.

Clinical examination should include examination of the abdomen to assess whether the bladder is palpable or percussible (which would suggest incomplete bladder emptying), the kidneys are palpable, or the child is constipated. Inspection of the spine, sacrum, perineum and legs for wasting including the reflexes for asymmetry and an absent perianal reflex and an abnormal gait may provide evidence of a neuropathic cause for the wetting. Children with spina bifida rated incontinence as one of the most distressing and challenging aspects of their condition (Lie *et al.* 1991), above problems with mobility. The perineum inspection may demonstrate an anatomical abnormality or show continuous leakage of urine. Where there is a combination of incontinence of urine and faeces it is particularly important to exclude neurological abnormality.

Urine should be sent for culture and evidence of other specific medical conditions should be sought as indicated, such as polyuria in diabetes or failure to grow at the expected velocity in chronic renal failure. Upper airways obstruction has been associated with nocturnal enuresis in children (Weider *et al.* 1991; Maizels *et al.* 1993), and nocturnal epilepsy may occasionally present with enuresis. On the whole, however, investigation is rarely indicated in children with nocturnal enuresis alone. If a child reaches 15 or 16 years and there has been little response to treatment then a videourodynamic study to assess bladder and urethral function may be indicated, even in the absence of signs or history suggestive of any other abnormality.

Children in whom abnormalities are detected in the history or examination, or who have had a urinary tract infection, should be referred to a general paediatrician who will investigate further and may decide to refer on to a specialist centre.

Assessing psychological factors

Enquiry should be made about the presence of psychiatric disorders. If they are present, the enuresis should not automatically be attributed to them. In some cases assumptions have been made about children's inability to attain continence because of their other physical problems or mental conditions (e.g. autism or learning disability) whereas with considerable perseverance and support and extended training periods continence may be achieved (Hyams 1992).

The family's social circumstances, attitudes and expectations should be asked about. Stressful events should be enquired for, such as separation from a parent, birth of a sibling, marital separation, starting school or moving house. Sexual abuse may be an underlying cause for secondary onset enuresis, but there are likely to be other indicators associated with abuse and these should be borne in mind (see Glaser, Chapter 21). The home environment (e.g. bedtime routines and access to the toilet at night) can influence nocturnal as well as daytime enuresis and should be asked about. Rigid or harsh toilet training or (conversely) complacent neglect of training may be suspected from expressed attitudes as well as from self-reports of training practices. Problems in school that might relate to stress and the effect that the wetting has on the child in the classroom are also essential information.

Treatment of urinary incontinence at night

Education and reassurance about prevalence, normal development and the low risk of a disease being the cause are essential first steps in management. Many people think that enuresis is a result of the child being lazy and this should be challenged. Reward systems and incentives are often used from an early stage of treatment. These should be based on achievable goals, records of positive gains and be valued and meaningful to the child. The child will need to see that success is possible and becoming dry has positive consequences. Possible rewards include stars, stickers and treats. It is important to motivate children by increasing their participation and responsibility for helping to minimize the consequences of wetting. This may involve devising programmes and rewards directly with them, and encouraging children to place wet items in the washing basket or change wet sheets without disturbing parents.

The treatment of nocturnal enuresis is usually successful. If common-sense methods, such as rewards for dryness or waking the child and encouraging micturition during the night, have not already been tried by parents, then they may be advised but usually there should be little delay before recommending the use of enuresis alarms. They are the most successful form of intervention. Systematic review of many random-allocation controlled trials leaves no doubt that it is a well-established therapy (Mellon & McGrath 2000). Around 60–80% of children using an alarm have achieved continence within 2–4 months of treatment (Gustafson 1993; Clark *et al.* 1994; Butler 1998). The older alarms, involving electrode sheets on the bed, have been superseded by miniaturized body alarms. A sensor is attached to underpants to detect urine as soon as it is voided; the alarm itself is attached to pyjamas, or a wristband or pocket, or can be positioned with an extension lead so as to wake the parents. The key aim is to wake the child, and he or she should then void urine appropriately.

The exact psychological mechanisms by which the alarm exerts its effects are not wholly clear, and may vary between children. A learning model is supported by the fact that the treatment is less effective if there is a delay between voiding and the alarm sounding (Collins 1973) and by the clinical observation that the course of treatment is often gradual, with the first signs of success being the shrinking of the size of the wet patch on the sheets. The original rationale was one of classical conditioning: the alarm is the unconditioned stimulus (UCS), waking and voiding appropriately is the conditioned response (CR), and the process of learning is the association of the indifferent stimuli (full bladder and the other signals for micturition) with the UCS so that they can produce the CR. However, this has not been rigorously tested. It is also possible that the alarm works through altering motivation (which is presumably responsible in those cases where the child becomes instantly dry as soon as the alarm is worn), through operant conditioning (in which the sound of the alarm is an aversive consequence), or through a beneficial focusing of parental concern.

The alarm is a safe treatment. The low risk of developing skin ulceration has been removed by the modern body alarms which work on very low voltages. There are limits to its value, some of which can be removed by good technique.

1 The treatment is troublesome: it demands time and energy from the child and caregivers, and failure of treatment is more likely in the context of a disturbed family. The alarm should always be demonstrated and explained, and doubts need to be discussed sensitively.

2 Premature termination of the therapy is quite common. It can be reduced by careful instructions about what to do and arranging follow-up; the family should be cautioned that in starting the treatment they are taking on a commitment to a 3-month course that may be only gradually successful.

3 The child may fail to wake to the alarm. This can often be answered by a louder buzzer or by arranging for the parents to wake the child.

4 There is a significant relapse rate: perhaps one-third of children who succeed initially will start to wet again. This can often be answered by a repeated course, preferably with overlearning:

after continence is acquired, the use of the alarm is continued and a fluid load is given on going to bed (Young & Morgan 1972).

Time spent in going over these details of therapy with families is rewarded by a higher success rate. Butler (1994) cautioned against the use of alarms when parents were likely to use coercive or punitive responses to them.

Other behavioural techniques have been advocated, but tend to be less effective and considerably more troublesome. Dry bed training (Azrin *et al.* 1974) involves an intensive programme of rewarding appropriate micturition at intervals through the night and practice in delaying micturition in the hope of increasing the functional capacity of the bladder ('bladder training'). Neither this nor its components have a sound evidence base.

Medication can reduce the frequency of night wetting. Desmopressin is an analogue of the naturally occurring antidiuretic hormone, with a longer duration of action and no tendency to produce vasoconstriction. It has been compared with placebo treatment in random-allocation trials, and produces significantly more dry nights (Skoog *et al.* 1997). This has been of considerable theoretical interest (see above) but its efficacy is probably not as great as the alarm, e.g. only 77 out of 399 children achieved complete dryness in an open trial by Tullus *et al.* (1999). Furthermore, relapse when desmopressin is stopped is the rule. Nevertheless, it can be a useful way of helping children who need to be dry for a short period, for instance to allow them to make a visit or a school trip, and it sometimes helps when the alarm has failed. The dose is 20–40 µg at bedtime if given as a nasal spray, 200–400 µg at bedtime if given as tablets. Its use is in general safe (provided it is not given to people with cardiac or renal disease), and a surveillance programme for more than 200 children taking it over a period of 1 year did not detect any seriously adverse effects (Tullus *et al.* 1999); in particular, hyponatraemia was not encountered. Nevertheless, there is a small risk of harm and a case of hyponatraemic convulsion has been reported after unsupervised self-administration (Apakama & Bleetman 1999), so it is important to give clear advice about avoiding overhigh doses, especially to strongly motivated young people.

Oxybutynin (dosage 2.5–5 mg three times daily with the last dose at bedtime) is an anticholinergic drug which increases bladder capacity by an action on the detrusors. Adverse effects can be troublesome, and it is not of proven value for enuresis that is nocturnal only, but some clinicians prescribe it (or other anticholinergics) for those cases in whom there is a reduced functional bladder volume secondary to detrusor instability that causes daytime wetting.

Tricyclic and tetracyclic antidepressants have a greater effect than placebo in reducing the frequency of wetting. Twenty-two trials were summarized in a systematic review (Glazener & Evans 2000). Although the quality of trials was often poor, the conclusion was clear: the drugs are more effective than placebo, comparable with desmopressin, and are associated with, on average, a reduction of wetting by about one wet night per week.

On the other hand, complete cure is not common, and even the limited gains are often lost when the treatment stops. Further, overdoses are very dangerous, although uncommon. We think these drugs should seldom be used nowadays—but they often are.

Treatment of daytime wetting

The treatment of diurnal enuresis is less well supported by an evidence base of controlled trials. Detection and treatment of associated urinary tract infection is important. The body alarm (see above) can be adapted for daytime use, but it may be equally effective to use a simple wristwatch alarm to remind the child to go to the toilet at intervals through the day (Halliday *et al.* 1987) or for a sympathetic teacher to remind and encourage the child to use the toilet at times chosen to anticipate the enuretic episodes. Management is based on clinical understanding of the reasons for the problem in the individual case. Anxiety management or problem-focused work can be used to overcome fears about using the lavatory (which include fears of the flush, the dark, general safety or dealing with aspects of privacy or bullying in using lavatories at school). Bladder training can be used when there is clinical suggestion of reduced functional volume (such as urinary frequency). It includes a regular toiletting programme, for example hourly intervals of being taken to the toilet and then increasing the time intervals between voiding when successful. Retention control, sphincter control and biofeedback techniques have been used, but sound evidence for their value is lacking (McKenna *et al.* 1999). Anticholinergic drugs, such as oxybutynin (see above), may also be useful in these circumstances. Psychotherapeutic approaches may be considered when the evidence suggests an underlying emotional conflict with enuresis as the presenting symptom or when emotional/behavioural problems coexist or are a consequence of wetting.

The isolation that many families suffer as a result of faecal or urinary incontinence can be alleviated by showing them that others are involved and interested in the conditions. Support groups are very helpful in providing information and contact points. Children and parents should be given information on the services and aids available and on support groups, such as the Enuresis Resource and Information Centre (ERIC), which has leaflets designed for children, teenagers and families, and the Continence Foundation Helpline.

Conclusions

The most common disorder of toilet function is monosymptomatic nocturnal enuresis. Considerable progress has been made in elucidating its pathophysiology. Much remains to be done, and the suggestions that different mechanisms apply to different children deserve further exploration. Nevertheless, an effective approach to therapy exists and most children can expect to be helped if it is applied. It is therefore disappointing that routine treatment in many parts of the world falls well short of best practice. The wider application of treatments known to be effective is therefore a priority for the field.

By contrast, the management of diurnal enuresis has only a slender evidence base, and the priority should be the establishment of a better understanding. The use of genetically informative designs and reliable measures of psychological and physiological change seem likely to be useful.

Most children who soil do so as part of a pattern of retention of faeces and rectal overload. The combination of paediatric management with behavioural advice is an effective model and deserves to be widely adopted. The uncommon problem of children with normal defecation who nevertheless deposit faeces in inappropriate places remains neglected by scientific investigation. There is scope and need for basic clinical research to establish a better understanding of the attitudes, motivation and abilities of affected children.

For all these disorders, it remains true that they cause a good deal of distress. The need for several perspectives makes it essential that there is good liaison between all the services available: the GP, community paediatric clinic team, the incontinence services with specialist nurses and incontinence advisors, the general paediatrician, tertiary specialist paediatric and surgical specialists, the child psychologist and the child psychiatrist. Each professional should be fully aware of the indications for further referral and joint management dependent on the severity of the symptoms and their impact upon children's lives.

References

Anthony, E.J. (1957) An experimental approach to the psychopathology of childhood encopresis. *British Journal of Medical Psychology*, **30**, 146–175.

Apakama, D.C. & Bleetman, A. (1999) Hyponatraemic convulsion secondary to desmopressin treatment for primary enuresis. *Journal of Accident and Emergency Medicine*, **16**, 229–230.

Azrin, N.H., Sneed, T.J. & Foxx, R.M. (1974) Dry-bed training: rapid elimination of childhood enuresis. *Behaviour Research and Therapy*, **12**, 147–156.

Bakwin, H. (1971) Enuresis in twins. *American Journal of Diseases of Children*, **121**, 225.

Bellman, M. (1966) Studies on encopresis. *Acta Paediatrica Scandinavica Supplement*, **170**, 1–151.

Bemporad, J.R., Pfeifer, C.M., Gibbs, L., Cortner, R.H. & Bloom, W. (1971) Characteristics of encopretic patients and their families. *Journal of the American Academy of Child Psychiatry*, **10**, 272–292.

Berg, I. (1979) Annotation: day wetting in children. *Journal of Child Psychology and Psychiatry*, **20**, 167–173.

Berg, I. & Jones, K.V. (1964) Functional faecal incontinence in children. *Archives of Disease in Childhood*, **39**, 465–472.

Blechman, E.A. (1979) Short and long term results of positive home-based treatment of childhood chronic constipation and encopresis. *Child Behaviour Therapy*, **1**, 237–247.

Borowitz, S.M., Cox, D.J. & Sutphen, J.L. (1999) Differences in toileting habits between children with chronic encopresis, asymptomatic siblings, and asymptomatic nonsiblings. *Journal of Developmental and Behavioural Pediatrics*, **20**, 145–149.

Buchanan, A. (1992) *Children Who Soil: Assessment and Treatment.* Wiley, Chichester.

Butler, R.J. (1994) *Nocturnal Enuresis: the Child's Experience*. Butterworth/Heinemann, Oxford.

Butler, R.J. (1998) Annotation: night wetting in children—psychological aspects. *Journal of Child Psychology and Psychiatry*, **39**, 453–463.

Butler, R.J. & Holland, P. (2000) The three systems: a conceptual way of understanding nocturnal enuresis. *Scandinavian Journal of Urology and Nephrology*, **34**, 270–277.

Byrd, R.S., Weitzman, M., Lanphear, N.E. & Auinger, P. (1996) Bedwetting in US children: epidemiology and related behaviour problems. *Pediatrics*, **98**, 414–419.

Chaney, C.A. (1995) A collaborative protocol for encopresis management in school-aged children. *Journal of School Health*, **65**, 360–364.

Clark, G., Fleming, C., Habel, A. *et al.* (1994) Nocturnal enuresis: a strategy for management. *Hospital Update*, (1994; no volume number) 1–11.

Clayden, G. (1987) Anal appearances and child sex abuse. *Lancet*, **8533**, 620–621.

Clayden, G.S. (1992) Management of chronic constipation. *Archives of Disease in Childhood*, **67**, 340–344.

Clayden, G.S. & Agnarsson, U. (1991) Constipation. *Current Paediatrics*, **1**, 8–12.

Coekin, M. & Gairdner, D. (1960) Faecal incontinence in children. *British Medical Journal*, **2**, 1175–1180.

Collins, R.W. (1973) Importance of the bladder-cue buzzer contingency in the conditioning treatment for enuresis. *Journal of Abnormal Psychology*, **82**, 299–308.

Cox, D.J., Sutphen, J., Borowitz, S., Kovatchev, B. & Ling, W. (1998) Contribution of behaviour therapy and biofeedback to laxative therapy in the treatment of pediatric encopresis. *Annals of Behavioural Medicine*, **29**, 70–76.

Davis, A. & Havighurst, J.R. (1946) Social class differences in child-rearing. *Annual Sociological Review*, **11**, 689–710.

Devlin, J.B. (1991) Prevalence and risk factors for childhood nocturnal enuresis. *Irish Medical Journal*, **84**, 118–120.

Eller, D.A., Austin, P.F., Tanguay, S. & Homsy, Y.L. (1998) Daytime functional bladder capacity as a predictor of response to desmopressin in monosymptomatic nocturnal enuresis. *European Urology*, **33** (Suppl. 3), 25–29.

Feehan, M., McGee, R., Stanton, W. & Silva, P.A. (1990) A 6 year follow-up of childhood enuresis: prevalence in adolescence and consequences for mental health. *Journal of Paediatrics and Child Health*, **26**, 75–79.

Fergusson, D.M. & Horwood, L.J. (1994) Nocturnal enuresis and behavioural problems in adolescence: a 15-year longitudinal study. *Pediatrics*, **94**, 662–668.

Fergusson, D.M., Horwood, L.J. & Shannon, F.T. (1986) Factors related to the age of attainment of nocturnal bladder control: an 8-year longitudinal study. *Pediatrics*, **78**, 884–890.

Fergusson, D.M., Horwood, L.J. & Shannon, F.T. (1990) Secondary enuresis in a birth cohort of New Zealand children. *Paediatric and Perinatal Epidemiology*, **4**, 53–63.

Fielding, D. & Doleys, D.M. (1988) Elimination problems: enuresis and encopresis. In: *Behavioural Assessment of Childhood Disorders* (eds E.J. Marsh & L.G. Terdak), 2nd edn, pp. 586–623. Guilford Press, London.

Forsythe, W.I. & Redmond, A. (1974) Enuresis and spontaneous cure rate: study of 1129 enuretics. *Archives of Disease in Childhood*, **49**, 259–263.

Fraser, A.M. & Taylor, D.C. (1986) Childhood encopresis extended into adult life. *British Journal of Psychiatry*, **149**, 370–371.

Friman, P.C., Mathews, J.R., Finney, J.W., Christophersen, E.R. &

Leibowitz, J.M. (1988) Do encopretic children have clinically significant behaviour problems? *Pediatrics*, **82**, 407–409.

Garrard, S.D. & Richmond, J.B. (1952) Psychogenic megacolon manifested by faecal soiling. *Pediatrics*, **10**, 474–483.

van Ginkel, R., Benninga, M.A., Blommaart, P.J. *et al.* (2000) Lack of benefit of laxatives as adjunctive therapy for functional nonretentive fecal soiling in children. *Journal of Pediatrics*, **137**, 808–813.

Glazener, C.M. & Evans, J.H. (2000) Tricyclic and related drugs for nocturnal enuresis in children (Cochrane Review). *Cochrane Database of Systematic Reviews*, **3**, CD002117.

von Gontard, A., Eiberg, H., Hollmann, E., Rittig, S. & Lehmkuhl, G. (1999a) Molecular genetics of nocturnal enuresis: linkage to a locus on chromosome 22. *Scandinavian Journal of Urology and Nephrology Supplement*, **202**, 76–80.

von Gontard, A., Mauer-Mucke, K., Pluck, J., Berner, W. & Lehmkuhl, G. (1999b) Clinical behavioural problems in day-and-night-wetting children. *Pediatric Nephrology*, **13**, 662–667.

Gustafson, R. (1993) Conditioning treatment of children's bedwetting: a follow-up and predictive study. *Psychological Reports*, **72**, 923–930.

Hallgren, B. (1957) Enuresis: a clinical and genetic study. *Acta Psychiatrica et Neurologica Scandinavica*, **32** (Suppl. 114), 1–154.

Halliday, S., Meadow, S.R. & Berg, I. (1987) Successful management of daytime enuresis using alarm procedures: a randomly controlled trial. *Archives of Disease in Childhood*, **62**, 132–137.

Hatch, T.F. (1988) Encopresis and constipation in children. *Pediatric Clinics of North America*, **35**, 257–280.

Hellstrom, A.L., Hanson, E., Hanson, S., Hjalmas, K. & Jodal, U. (1990) Micturition habits and incontinence in 7-year-old Swedish school entrants. *European Journal of Pediatrics*, **149**, 434–437.

Hersov, L. (1994) Faecal soiling. In: *Child and Adolescent Psychiatry: Modern Approaches* (eds M. Rutter, E. Taylor & L. Hersov), 3rd edn, pp. 520–528. Blackwell Science, Oxford.

Hinman, F. & Baumann, F.W. (1973) Vesicle and ureteral damage from voiding dysfunction in boys without neurologic or obstructive disease. *Journal of Urology*, **109**, 727–732.

Hyams, G. (1992) Behavioural continence training in mental handicap: a 10-year follow-up study. *Journal of Intellectual Disability Research*, **36**, 551–558.

Hyman, P.E. & Fleisher, D.R. (1994) A classification of disorders of defecation in infants and children. *Seminars in Gastrointestinal Diseases*, **5**, 20–23.

Jarvelin, M.R., Moilanen, I., Kangas, P. *et al.* (1991) Aetiological and precipitating factors for childhood enuresis. *Acta Paediatrica Scandinavica*, **80**, 361–369.

Kaffman, M. & Elizur, E. (1977) Infants who become enuretics: a longitudinal study of 161 kibbutz children. *Monographs of the Society for Research in Child Development*, **42**, 1–61.

Kamm, M.A. (1998) Faecal incontinence. *British Medical Journal*, **316**, 528–532.

Klatskin, E.H. (1952) Shifts in child care practices in three social classes under an infant care programme of flexible methodology. *American Journal of Orthopsychiatry*, **30**, 52–61.

Kolvin, I., Taunch, J., Currah, J., Garside, R.F., Nolan, J. & Shaw, W.B. (1972) Enuresis: a descriptive analysis and a controlled trial. *Developmental Medicine and Child Neurology*, **14**, 715–731.

Levine, M.D. (1975) Children with encopresis: a descriptive analysis. *Pediatrics*, **56**, 412–416.

Levine, M.D. & Bakow, H. (1976) Children with encopresis: a study of treatment outcome. *Pediatrics*, **58**, 845–852.

Lie, H.R., Lagergren, J., Rasmussen, F. *et al.* (1991) Bowel and bladder control of children with myelomeningocele: a Nordic study. *Developmental Medicine and Child Neurology*, **33**, 1053–1061.

Loening-Baucke, V. (1995) Biofeedback treatment for chronic constipation and encopresis in childhood: a long term outcome. *Pediatrics*, **96**, 105–110.

Loening-Baucke, V. (1996) Encopresis and soiling. *Pediatric Clinics of North America*, **43**, 279–298.

Loening-Baucke, V. & Cruikshank, B. (1986) Abnormal defecation dynamics in chronically constipated children with encopresis. *Journal of Pediatrics*, **108**, 562–570.

Loening-Baucke, V., Cruikshank, B. & Savage, C. (1987) Defecation dynamics and behaviour profiles in encopretic children. *Pediatrics*, **80**, 672–679.

Longstaffe, S., Moffatt, M.E. & Whalen, J.C. (2000) Behavioural and self-concept changes after six months of enuresis treatment: a randomized, controlled trial. *Pediatrics*, **105**, 935–940.

Lottmann, H. (1999) Enuresis treatment in France. *Scandinavian Journal of Urology and Nephrology Supplement*, **202**, 66–69.

Maizels, M., Gandhi, K., Keating, B. & Rosenbaum, D. (1993) Diagnosis and treatment for children who cannot control urination. *Current Problems in Pediatrics*, **23**, 402–450.

McGee, R., Makinson, T., Williams, S., Simpson, A. & Silva, R.A. (1984) A longitudinal study of enuresis from five to nine years. *Australian Pediatric Journal*, **20**, 239–242.

McGrath, M.L., Mellon, M.W. & Murphy, L. (2000) Empirically supported treatments in pediatric psychology: constipation and encopresis. *Journal of Pediatric Psychology*, **25**, 225–254.

McKenna, P.H., Herndon, C.D., Connery, S. & Ferrer, F.A. (1999) Pelvic floor muscle retraining for pediatric voiding dysfunction using interactive games. *Journal of Urology*, **162**, 1056–1062.

Mellon, M.W. & McGrath, M.L. (2000) Empirically supported treatments in pediatric psychology: nocturnal enuresis. *Journal of Pediatric Psychology*, **25**, 193–214.

Meunier, P., Marechal, J.M. & Jaubert de Beaujeu, M. (1979) Rectoanal pressures and rectal sensitivity studies in chronic childhood constipation. *Gastroenterology*, **77**, 330–340.

Mikkelsen, E.J., Rapoport, J.L., Nee, L., Gruenau, C., Mendleson, W. & Gillin, J.C. (1980) Childhood enuresis. I. Sleep patterns and psychopathology. *Archives of General Psychiatry*, **37**, 1139–1144.

Moffatt, M.E., Kato, C. & Pless, I.B. (1987) Improvements in self-concept after treatment of nocturnal enuresis: randomized controlled trial. *Journal of Pediatrics*, **110**, 647–652.

Moilanen, I., Tirkkonen, T., Jarvelin, M.R. *et al.* (1998) A follow-up of enuresis from childhood to adolescence. *British Journal of Urology*, **81** (Suppl. 3), 94–97.

Natochin, Y.V. & Kuznetsova, A.A. (2000) Nocturnal enuresis: correction of renal function by desmopressin and diclofenac. *Pediatric Nephrology*, **14**, 42–47.

Neveus, T., Lackgren, G., Tuvemo, T. & Stenberg, A. (1999) Osmoregulation and desmopressin pharmacokinetics in enuretic children. *Pediatrics*, **103**, 65–70.

Nolan, T., Debelle, G., Oberklaid, F. & Coffey, C. (1991) Randomised trial of laxatives in treatment of childhood encopresis. *Lancet*, **8766**, 523–527.

Norgaard, J.P. (1991) Pathophysiology of nocturnal enuresis. *Scandinavian Journal of Urology and Nephrology Supplement*, **140**, 1–35.

Olatawura, M.O. (1973) Encopresis: a review of thirty-two cases. *Acta Paediatrica Scandinavica*, **62**, 358–364.

Oliver, J.E. & Buchanan, A.H. (1979) Generations of maltreated children and multi-agency care in one kindred. *British Journal of Psychiatry*, **135**, 289–303.

Ollendick, T.H., King, N.J. & Frary, R.B. (1989) Fears in children and adolescents: reliability and generalizability across gender, age and nationality. *Behaviour Research and Therapy*, **27**, 19–26.

Oppel, W.C., Harper, P.A. & Rider, R.V. (1968) The age of attaining bladder control. *Pediatrics*, **42**, 614–619.

van der Plas, R.N., Benninga, M.A., Buller, H.A. *et al.* (1996) Biofeedback training in treatment of childhood constipation: a randomised controlled study. *Lancet*, **9030**, 776–780.

Quay, H.C. & Werry, J.S., eds (1972) *Psychopathological Disorders in Childhood*. Wiley, New York.

Rappaport, L., Landman, G., Fenton, T. & Levine, M.D. (1986) Locus of control as predictor of compliance and outcome in treatment of encopresis. *Journal of Pediatrics*, **109**, 1061–1064.

Robertson, G., Rittig, S., Kovacs, L., Gaskill, M.B., Zee, P. & Nanninga, J. (1999) Pathophysiology and treatment of enuresis in adults. *Scandinavian Journal of Urology and Nephrology Supplement*, **202**, 36–38.

Rockney, R.M., McQuade, W.H., Days, A.L., Linn, H.E. & Alario, A.J. (1996) Encopresis treatment outcome: long-term follow-up of 45 cases. *Journal of Developmental and Behavioural Pediatrics*, **17**, 380–385.

Rona, R.J., Li, L. & Chinn, S. (1997) Determinants of nocturnal enuresis in England and Scotland in the 90s. *Developmental Medicine and Child Neurology*, **39**, 677–681.

Rutter, M., Tizard, J. & Whitmore, K., eds (1970) *Education, Health and Behaviour*. Longman, London.

Rutter, M.L., Yule, W. & Graham, P.J. (1973) Enuresis and behavioural deviance: some epidemiological considerations. In: *Bladder Control and Enuresis, Clinics in Developmental Medicine* **48/49** (eds I. Kolvin, R.C. MacKeith & S.R. Meadow), pp. 137–147. Heinemann/Spastics International Medical Publications, London.

Schaefer, C.E. (1979) *Childhood Enuresis and Encopresis: Causes and Therapy*. Van Nostrand Reinhold, New York.

Schulman, S.L., Colish, Y., von Zuben, F.C. & Kodman-Jones, C. (2000) Effectiveness of treatments for nocturnal enuresis in a heterogeneous population. *Clinical Pediatrics*, **39**, 359–364.

Shaffer, D. (1994) Enuresis. In: *Child and Adolescent Psychiatry: Modern Approaches* (eds M. Rutter, E. Taylor & L. Hersov), 3rd edn, pp. 505–519. Blackwell Science, Oxford.

Shaffer, D.J., Gardner, A. & Hedge, B. (1994) Behaviour and bladder disturbance of enuretic children: a rational classification of a common disorder. *Developmental Medicine and Child Neurology*, **26**, 781–792.

Sheinbein, M. (1975) Treatment for the hospitalized infantile ruminator: programmed brief social behaviour reinforcers. *Clinical Pediatrics*, **14**, 719–724.

Silver, E. (1996) Family therapy and soiling. *Journal of Family Therapy*, **18**, 415–432.

Silver, E., Williams, A., Worthington, F. & Phillips, N. (1998) Family therapy and soiling: an audit of externalising and other approaches. *Journal of Family Therapy*, **20**, 413–422.

Skoog, S.J., Stokes, A. & Turner, K.L. (1997) Oral desmopressin: a randomised double-blind placebo controlled study of effectiveness in children with primary nocturnal enuresis. *Journal of Urology*, **158**, 1035–1040.

Stark, L.J., Owens-Stively, J., Spirito, A., Lewis, A. & Guevremont, D. (1990) Group behavioural treatment of retentive encopresis. *Journal of Paediatric Psychology*, **15**, 659–671.

Stark, L.J., Opipari, L.C., Donaldson, D.L., Danovsky, M.B., De Rasile, D.A.I. & Santo, A.F. (1997) Evaluation of a standard protocol for retentive encopresis: a replication. *Journal of Pediatric Psychology*, **22**, 619–633.

Stein, Z.A. & Susser, M.W. (1967) Social factors in the development of sphincter control. *Developmental Medicine and Child Neurology*, **9**, 692–706.

Sutphen, J.L., Borowitz, S.M., Hutchinson, R.L. & Cox, D.J. (1995) Long-term follow-up of medically treated childhood constipation. *Clinical Pediatrics*, **34**, 576–580.

Taitz, L.S., Wales, J.K., Urwin, O.M. & Molnar, D. (1986) Factors associated with outcome in management of defecation disorders. *Archives of Disease in Childhood*, **61**, 472–477.

Tullus, K., Bergstrom, R., Fosdal, I., Winnergard, I. & Hjalmas, K. (1999) Efficacy and safety during long-term treatment of primary monosymptomatic nocturnal enuresis with desmopressin: Swedish Enuresis Trial Group. *Acta Paediatrica Scandinavica*, **88**, 1274–1278.

Verhulst, F.C., van der Lee, J.H., Akkerhuis, G.W., Sanders-Woudstra, J.A., Timmer, F.C. & Donkhorst, I.D. (1985) The prevalence of nocturnal enuresis: do DSM III criteria need to be changed? A brief research report. *Journal of Child Psychology and Psychiatry*, **26**, 989–993.

de Vries, M.W. & de Vries, M.R. (1977) Cultural relativity of toilet training readiness: a perspective from East Africa. *Pediatrics*, **60**, 170–177.

Wagner, W.G., Smith, D. & Norris, W.R. (1988) The psychological adjustment of enuretic children: a comparison of two types. *Journal of Pediatric Psychology*, **13**, 33–38.

Wald, A., Chandra, R. & Chiponis, D. (1986) Anorectal function and continence mechanisms in childhood encopresis. *Journal of Pediatric Gastroenterology and Nutrition*, **5**, 346–356.

Watanabe, H. (1995) Sleep patterns in children with nocturnal enuresis. *Scandinavian Journal of Urology and Nephrology Supplement*, **173**, 55–56.

Weider, D.J., Sateia, M.J. & West, R.P. (1991) Nocturnal enuresis in children with upper airway obstruction. *Otolaryngology Head and Neck Surgery*, **105**, 427–432.

Wender, E.H., Palmer, F.B., Herbot, J.J. & Wender, P.H. (1976) Behavioural characteristics of children with chronic non-specific diarrhoea. *American Journal of Psychiatry*, **133**, 20–25.

White, M. (1984) Pseudo-encopresis: from avalanche to victory, from vicious to virtuous cycles. *Family Systems Medicine*, **2**, 150–160.

Wright, L. & Walker, C.E. (1977) Treatment of the child with psychogenic encopresis: an effective program of therapy. *Clinical Pediatrics*, **16**, 1042–1045.

Young, G.C. & Morgan, R.T.T. (1972) Overlearning in the conditioning treatment of enuresis. *Behaviour Research and Therapy*, **10**, 419–420.

Young, M.H., Brennen, L.C., Baker, R.D. & Baker, S.S. (1995) Functional encopresis: symptom reduction and behavioral improvement. *Journal of Developmental and Behavioral Pediatrics*, **16**, 226–232.

48 Psychiatric Aspects of Somatic Disease and Disorders

David A. Mrazek

Introduction

Severe paediatric illnesses have been shown to affect negatively the course of early emotional development in some children (Pless & Roghmann 1971; Cadman *et al.* 1987; Gortmaker *et al.* 1990; US Department of Health & Human Services 1999). The risk for diagnosable psychiatric illnesses in children with severe paediatric illnesses is approximately twice the rate of disturbance found in healthy children. Approximately 30–40% of children with severe paediatric illnesses have comorbid psychiatric illness. Clearly, the majority of children with severe medical illnesses are extremely resilient; however, in those paediatric patients with a comorbid psychiatric illness, appropriate recognition and prompt intervention are critical

The events associated with the diagnosis and treatment of a severe paediatric illness often constitute a series of negative life events. Even sensitive paediatric care involves a spectrum of illness-related challenges that are appropriately classified as a category of risk factors for early developmental psychopathology. The impact of these illness-related risk factors varies, based on a set of illness characteristics that will be discussed later in this chapter. The presence of additional biological, interpersonal or societal risk factors in physically ill children further increases the likelihood of negative psychosocial outcomes. Consequently, severely ill children should be considered a high-risk group for the development of psychopathology; they are likely to benefit from preventive interventions that can be provided in collaboration with primary care physicians.

Neurological illnesses represent a special subset of paediatric illnesses (see Goodman, Chapter 14). Epilepsy, brain tumours and other neurological disorders have an even higher degree of comorbidity with psychiatric problems when compared to paediatric illnesses that do not involve overt brain dysfunction. This is presumed to be a consequence of the direct pathophysiological effects of neurological lesions on neurotransmitter systems that ultimately result in the occurrence of both neurological signs and behavioural symptoms.

A systematic clinical approach to helping children with severe paediatric illnesses requires an understanding of the interactions among the broad set of risk factors that have been demonstrated to be associated with the onset of psychopathology. The adaptation of children to environmental stressors can be conceptualized as the product of the cumulative interactions of both risk and protective factors. The pathways involved in the expression of emotional symptomatology have not been well defined.

However, a key aspect of the mechanism almost certainly involves the expression or suppression of underlying susceptibility genes. An emotionally spontaneous child with a supportive family who has experienced a series of early successes can be expected to cope well with the early onset of a severe paediatric illness. This is not to suggest that the physical symptoms and emotional disruptions associated with the disease do not provide a challenge for both the child and the family, but rather that the child will eventually succeed in meeting these challenges. In contrast, an infant with a 'difficult' temperament is more vulnerable. Early in the life of the child who is hard to soothe, there is a high probability that parental responsivity will not be linked as strongly to an experience of comforting. Furthermore, parental positive stimulation is likely to be less frequent as well as less contingent on infant cues (Mrazek *et al.* 1985). As a consequence of these more problematic early experiences, children with difficult temperaments are more likely to develop less secure attachment relationships. For a child with few early successes and some biological limitations, the onset of a severe physical illness may prove to have serious behavioural and emotional consequences. When the onset of severe physical illness occurs simultaneously with other disruptions in the emotional homeostasis of the child, the risk for a negative outcome is further increased. The evidence that such negative reciprocal interactions are central to problems in emotional development is primarily clinical, although additive models highlighting the impact of multiple hospitalizations, particularly when associated with other risk factors, have empirical support (Quinton & Rutter 1976; Sameroff 1998).

Psychiatric considerations relevant to specific physical illnesses

It has been well recognized that similar chronic diseases have common physical limitations and emotional consequences. However, unique characteristics of a specific paediatric illness have been shown to result in variation in the relative risk for comorbid psychiatric illness. Seven severe paediatric illnesses are reviewed with the objective of highlighting aspects that result in differential risk for associated developmental psychopathology. The rationale for selection of these specific diseases is to contrast their illness-related risk factors. However, each of these paediatric illnesses represents a unique set of risk factors that help to focus the clinical approach to the patient (see also Rauch & Jellinek, Chapter 62).

Asthma

Asthma is a reversible reactive airway disease triggered by a variety of immunological, infectious, physiological and emotional triggers. There is increasing evidence that asthma is heritable, and that its expression involves multiple susceptibility genes.

Asthma is the most prevalent chronic illness of childhood. In the USA and UK, estimates of prevalence vary from approximately 3%, using questionnaires that focus on a previous diagnosis of asthma, to 12%, based on reports of episodes of wheezing in the past year. By 1994, approximately 4 million children in the USA reported having had asthma in the preceding 12 months, representing prevalence rates of 5.8% in children less than 5 years of age and 7.4% of children aged between 5 and 14 years (Mannino *et al.* 1998). The highest rates are reported in isolated populations, particularly among Pacific Islanders, where the prevalence varies between 20 and 30%. The lowest prevalence rates have been reported in Scandinavia, Switzerland, Israel and Japan, where less than 2% of children have been identified (Cookson 1987).

Three primary factors have been put forward to explain these differences. The first is that differences in genetic vulnerabilities exist in different racial and ethnic populations. This has been particularly suggested as an explanation for why small populations with a high frequency of consanguineous matings have high prevalence rates. A second factor is the variability in the methodology of ascertainment of 'caseness'. Clearly, studies that accept a history of episodic wheezing as the equivalent of the diagnosis will have elevated rates. A more recent suggestion has been that variability in the physical environment may explain increased prevalence. However, this explanation does not address the finding that some of the lowest rates were found in highly developed industrial countries with considerable air pollution.

There is strong evidence that immunoglobulin E (IgE) has a central role in the mechanism of symptom expression in allergic asthma and that the regulation of IgE antibody level is under genetic control. However, asthma, like most paediatric illnesses, is best conceptualized as a syndrome with multiple genes involved in a range of possible aetiological interactions. In this regard, it illustrates interactions that occur between physiological and psychological processes. Some children appear to have a simple form of asthma that is limited to attacks that are triggered by exposure to allergens. Conversely, some asthmatic children appear to have no allergic symptoms, but their illness is triggered by a wide variety of physical and psychological factors. The majority of children present a more complex clinical picture that involves an interaction of triggers that ultimately result in bronchial constriction. Both elevated serum IgE and early proximal emotional stressors, as measured by documented difficulties in parenting, have been shown to be predictive of the onset of asthma in children at increased genetic risk for developing the disease (Mrazek *et al.* 1999).

There is little evidence to suggest that mild asthma, defined as wheezing episodes easily controlled by inhaled bronchodilators, is associated with increased early psychopathology. However, quite severely asthmatic children, who have persistent functional disability and require multiple medications including corticosteroids to control their symptoms, have been shown to be at increased risk for emotional disturbance. Epidemiological studies have focused on the issue of severity of illness as a predictor of psychopathology (McNichol *et al.* 1973). Subsequent studies have highlighted the importance of understanding the development of emotional symptoms within the context of other risk factors for psychopathology (Steinhausen *et al.* 1983). Even preschool samples composed of very serious asthmatic children have had rates of psychopathology that have exceeded 50% (Mrazek *et al.* 1984, 1998). These high levels of disturbance can be contrasted with the relatively positive adaptation of very young asthmatic children who have less severe forms of the disease (Gauthier *et al.* 1977, 1978). In severely asthmatic older children, affective disorder is common and has serious implications for survival (Miller 1987). Both the presence of affective symptoms and disturbance in family functioning were independently associated with a higher probability of fatal episodes in very severely asthmatic children. Hypoxic seizures, a previous respiratory arrest, and rapid decrement in steroid dose were also associated with a fatal outcome (Strunk *et al.* 1985).

Families often develop idiosyncratic beliefs about the illness. Given that asthma is heritable, the diagnosis can be particularly upsetting to the parent who is asthmatic. Parents who have mild asthma virtually never consider their illness a cause for concern regarding the decision to have children. In contrast, adults with severe asthma often seriously weigh the potential risk for their offspring. The decision of a severely asthmatic woman to have a child is often complicated by her realization that her own disease may become more difficult to control while she is pregnant. Approximately one-third of asthmatic women experience some increase in their asthmatic symptoms during a pregnancy.

Given that the early physical and emotional environment of a child at genetic risk for asthma may affect the risk of illness expression, the non-affected parent is now in a position of shared responsibility regarding the child's outcome. Conversely, the successful rearing of a child at increased genetic risk for the illness is increasingly viewed as a consequence of good caregiving rather than simply 'good luck'.

The establishment of the diagnosis of asthma can be quite difficult. Controversy exists over what symptoms are sufficient to establish the diagnosis. Recurring wheezing episodes during infancy that are associated with respiratory infections resemble an asthmatic attack and have been labelled as asthma by many primary care physicians. However, the prognostic implications of infectious wheezing or wheezing bronchitis are very different from the diagnosis of asthmatic episodes in the absence of infection. The perception and response of the family will be quite different if the first wheezing attack is perceived as simply an isolated symptom associated with one of the inevitable respiratory illnesses of early childhood rather than the beginning of a chronic illness. Increasingly, there is evidence that early asthmatic attacks should be treated intensively and that such treatment will minimize the likelihood of the development of chronic asthma. A reasonable position is to consider the first attack of wheezing in a vulnerable child as possible evidence of the existence of underlying genetic vulnerability to asthma. Such a position should be accompanied by considering strategies to minimize additional symptoms through management of the child's exposure to allergens, infections and intense emotional distress.

In children with very mild asthma, there is virtually no disability. The illness can be controlled quite effectively through the use of inhaled bronchodilators. In more progressive forms of the illness chronic corticosteroids are required, and limitations on physical activity occur as a consequence of respiratory symptoms, as well as a variety of corticosteroid side-effects that can affect vision, learning and physical development. Those with mild asthma have a completely normal physical appearance. In contrast, severe debilitating disease that requires corticosteroid treatment often results in cushingoid stigmata, growth retardation and scoliosis. Children with these signs of advanced disease are at the highest risk for having problems adapting to the developmental challenges of adolescence.

Asthma tends to be an episodic illness. Consequently, most asthmatic children experience intervals without symptoms during which they can function normally. These remissions provide reasonable hope that the illness will eventually be controlled. However, for very severely asthmatic children, their prognosis is more guarded. Fatal asthmatic attacks in children have been increasing over the past two decades although there has been some suggestion that the rate has begun to stabilize (Sly & O'Donnell 1997). The risk of a fatal episode is elevated if the asthmatic child has an emotional disturbance or there is family dysfunction (Strunk et al. 1985). While these risks are most acute for severely asthmatic children who require corticosteroids to control their symptoms, rare cases of children with milder disease who have died from asthma have been reported.

In summary, asthma presents a prototype of a complex illness with multiple genetic and environmental factors interacting in a manner that ultimately results in the development of a chronic illness. Those children with severe illness are at highest risk for developing emotional and behavioural difficulties and this is particularly true if their families are having difficulties in adapting to their illness and providing appropriate support and structure.

Atopic dermatitis or eczema

Atopic dermatitis or, as it is more commonly called, eczema is an allergic skin condition that almost always begins during the first years of life. It is mediated by IgE sensitization and usually involves quite localized areas of the skin. In a minority of children with atopic dermatitis, severe lesions develop that are very distressing. The diagnosis is based on the presence of an intense pruritic rash that often begins on the face and extensor aspects of the extremities. Serum IgE levels are frequently elevated. Eczema usually resolves during childhood, but the condition can persist throughout life. Occasionally, atopic dermatitis develops in adulthood.

The incidence of atopic dermatitis in childhood is probably less than 5% (Halpern et al. 1973). Only a small number of these children suffer from the more pervasive or debilitating forms of the illness. Evidence of a genetic aetiology is supported by family studies (Ferguson et al. 1983), and the underlying heritable hypersensitive IgE response.

Studies of adults with atopic dermatitis have suggested an increased comorbidity of depression (Preston 1969). Small clinical studies have reported that exacerbations of skin lesions were associated with life stressors (Ullman et al. 1977). The paediatric clinical literature includes reports of individual children who have responded well to psychological interventions (Mirvish 1978), although systematic analyses of interventions have not been available. There is some suggestion that early avoidance of antigenic foods and prolonged breastfeeding may decrease the likelihood of the illness in at-risk samples (Matthew et al. 1977; Zeiger et al. 1989).

The care of young children with atopic dermatitis is challenging as it is necessary to support children in acute distress before they have the cognitive ability to cope with their discomfort. Parents must find a way to prevent their infants from aggravating the illness by scratching the lesions. Given that these infants are often upset and uncomfortable for prolonged periods, it is surprising that there have been no systematic studies examining the association between the early onset of severe eczema and later emotional difficulties. Furthermore, the illness often resolves in the first 2 years of life so that many children are completely amnestic for the experience. This unusual set of disease characteristics would allow an examination of the hypothesis that early disruption of the caregiving relationship, because of frustrations involved in controlling the child in order to prevent excoriation of pruritic lesions, may be associated with later interpersonal difficulties.

Atopic dermatitis is a familial illness, but one with relatively few long-term implications. Therefore, parents are generally not concerned about their children inheriting the disease. However, the primary treatment of the illness involves medicating the lesions, preventing scratching and identifying potential allergens in order to eliminate these substances from the environment of the child. Parents must therefore be alert to the behaviour of their child and be prepared to make difficult life changes. A common conflict is making the decision to give up a family pet after it is recognized that contact with the animal appears to be a primary precipitant for the skin lesions.

Differential diagnosis is not usually a problem. Seborrhoeic dermatitis may be confused with eczema, but the psychological consequences of a delay in arriving at the accurate diagnosis are minimal, as seborrhoeic dermatitis is a self-limited rash that is usually confined to the scalp and flexural areas of the extremities. One implication of making the diagnosis of atopic dermatitis is the recognition that the child is at risk for other allergic problems, such as hay fever and IgE-mediated asthma. If the child has a family history of asthmatic illness, the diagnosis of eczema can be conceptualized as an indicator of elevated risk for the later onset of allergically mediated asthma (Mrazek *et al.* 1999).

In older children with persistent and severe eczema, issues of disability and physical appearance become relevant. While it is rare that any permanent disability is created, wrapping the arm of the child to control acute episodes makes it difficult for the child to participate in sports and engage in other physical activities. When eczema spreads to the arms and face, it can be quite unattractive. The skin can become encrusted and 'weepy' if the child is allowed to scratch the skin and the excoriated lesions become secondarily infected. Supportive families are usually able to tolerate the changes in the appearance of their child with minimal difficulty. Parents who place a high value on physical appearance may experience an unattractive child as a threat to their own status and self-worth. The sudden development of overtly unattractive lesions in a previously highly valued and beautiful infant has been reported to be associated with emotional rejection of the child. Early sensitization of the parents to the negative implications of this rejection is often a sufficient intervention. Although eczema has the appearance of an infectious disease, it is not contagious. The irrational fear of contracting the disease from the child should be directly addressed while emphasizing the need to provide continued emotional support that includes physical contact.

When the lesions of the skin persist, they often have a more serious impact on the child's sense of self-esteem. In these cases, more aggressive psychiatric treatment is indicated to help the child cope with these negative self-perceptions. Throughout the process, the ultimate favourable prognosis should be stressed. This strategy is particularly effective if severe rashes have been typical for the family. Involving previously affected family members whose skin has healed is a good strategy to use with younger children who have a problem with abstract projections regarding the course of their illness into the future.

Cystic fibrosis

Cystic fibrosis is the most prevalent autosomal recessive genetic illness of childhood. In Caucasian populations, approximately 5% of adults are heterozygous for polymorphisms of the cystic fibrosis transmembrane conductance regulator gene (CFTR) (Riordan *et al.* 1989). These carriers have one normal allele that is able to code for a sufficient amount of the CFTR protein to prevent the onset of the symptoms that characterize what was once a fatal illness. Approximately 1 in 2000 children are homozygous for defective CFTR alleles and develop cystic fibrosis. Although this pattern of inheritance has been recognized for years, recent discoveries demonstrate that a wide range of defective polymorphisms result in the illness. The CFTR gene is located on the short arm of chromosome 7. The protein that is coded for by CFTR plays a part in the maintenance of the chloride permeability of chloride channels. Variations in the alleles associated with the illness are associated with variations in the production of the protein and subsequently variation in the clinical presentation of the illness. Currently, 600 polymorphisms have been reported (Davidson & Porteous 1998) which have been divided into five general classes (Zielenski & Tsui 1995). For example, one mutation may primarily affect chloride channel function in the sweat glands and pancreatic ducts while another may affect airway epithelia. Although the range of physical symptoms is broad, classic features include chronic bronchial airway obstruction that often leads to respiratory infections, and maldigestion that results from defects in the production of pancreatic enzymes. Other organs that may be affected include the liver, intestines and genitals, usually through a mechanism that involves an increase in the viscosity of secretions.

There has been a significant increase in the life span of children with cystic fibrosis. Currently, the mean age of survival has risen to approximately 40 years of age, with 90% of children with the illness reaching adulthood (Elborn *et al.* 1991). Pulmonary function assessment demonstrating a decrease in forced expiratory volume was shown to be a strong predictor of mortality in advanced patients (Kerem *et al.* 1992).

Many complications exist, including a delay in sexual development. Ninety-eight per cent of males with cystic fibrosis are sterile (Taussig *et al.* 1976). Furthermore, pregnancy in females with cystic fibrosis is a high-risk medical condition because of the likelihood of deterioration of the respiratory function later in the pregnancy. Problems in adjustment because of the limitations of the illness have been specifically reported during adolescence (Bywater 1981).

Cystic fibrosis is almost always diagnosed during infancy or in early childhood. The diagnosis should always be suspected in families in which there is a pedigree with identified affected relatives. Even in the less frequent circumstance of the marriage of two carriers with no known first- or second-degree affected relatives, a preliminary diagnosis is usually established once multiple symptoms emerge.

It is now technically possible to identify affected individuals through prenatal screening and this practice has been increasingly well accepted, with enhanced survival now being demonstrated in those children who receive intensive treatment from the first day of life (Dankert-Roelse & Meerman 1995). Traditionally, genetic counsellors have cautioned two carriers of an autosomal recessive gene about choosing to have children given that their chance of having an affected child is one in four. However, some parents are quite willing to take this level of risk. For some, the knowledge that prenatal diagnosis and the possibility that abortion are available provides them a clear strategy for eventually having unaffected children. Other families are prepared to raise a child with cystic fibrosis even when they are made aware of the very substantial emotional and fiscal burden associated with the diagnosis. However, for these decisions to be adequately informed, it is critical that potential parents receive comprehensive information regarding the pulmonary care and physical therapy that affected children require, as well as frank information regarding expected medical complications and life expectancy.

Severity of cystic fibrosis has been identified as the primary predictor of psychiatric disturbance in children with the disease (Steinhausen *et al.* 1983). Approximately one-third of the children with severe cystic fibrosis developed serious emotional disturbance and another 22% had less severe problems. However, even in children with quite advanced disease, enhanced quality of life reports were associated with positives coping strategies in both patients and their parents (Staab *et al.* 1998). Whereas a full range of psychiatric problems has been noted in children with cystic fibrosis, eating disorders have been specifically cited as developing at an increased frequency (Pumariega *et al.* 1986). The most frequent concerns in these children related to anxiety concerning the actual treatment of the disease (Steinhausen & Schindler 1981). Despite ascertaining that the probability of a shortened life span was the most difficult disease-related emotional issue for children with cystic fibrosis, these children's fears were rarely verbalized until late in the course of the illness (Petzel *et al.* 1984). This illness presents clinical problems associated with impending mortality. As the disease progresses, families and providers need support to manage their feelings of anticipated loss and the frustrations associated with the limitation of therapeutic interventions.

Previous therapeutic approaches for children with cystic fibrosis have focused on medical and emotional supportive strategies (Mrazek 1985). However, positive family and peer support appears to be an important protective factor for the emotional development of children with cystic fibrosis (Venters 1981; Graetz *et al.* 2000). Achieving medical compliance is also a key management issue (Czajkowski & Koocher 1986). Initial optimism concerning the use of gene therapy has been tempered by the relatively unsuccessful efforts to transfer intact polymorphisms able to produce normal membrane transductance in affected children (Alton & Geddes 1995; Rosenecker *et al.* 1998).

Juvenile onset insulin-dependent diabetes mellitus

Juvenile onset insulin-dependent diabetes mellitus (IDDM) is an uncommon paediatric illness in young children. It affects very few preschool-age children, and only about 1 in 500 school-age children and adolescents. IDDM is a disease of the islet cells of the pancreas, which results in a deficiency in the production of insulin. There is clear increased familial risk for the development of diabetes (Riley *et al.* 1990) and diabetic complications (Seaquist *et al.* 1989). Maternal-type diabetes, particularly in older mothers, has been demonstrated to be a risk factor for diabetes in children, together with neonatal infections, preeclampsia and caesarean section delivery (McKinney *et al.* 1999). Another recent study examining risk factors for the development of nephropathy in children with Type I diabetes found that children who had parents with Type II diabetes and nephropathy were at increased risk (Fagerudd *et al.* 1999). Al-

though the specific pattern of inheritance has not been established, progress in the identification of children at increased risk is being made through molecular genetic techniques. New evidence supporting a complex mode of inheritance has included documentation of susceptibility loci on chromosome 6 at 6p21.3 (Froguel 1997), on chromosome 11 at 11q13 and 11p15 (Hashimoto *et al.* 1994; Nakagawa *et al.* 1998; Vafiadis *et al.* 1998) and on chromosome 14 at 14q24.3 (Field *et al.* 1996).

Insulin-dependent diabetes rarely affects very early parent–child relationships because of its usual later onset. Given the probability of a normal early maternal experience, risk for relationship-related disorders should not be elevated. Given that there is minimal central nervous system involvement, neuronal dysfunction should not be considered a major risk factor for psychopathology.

Although it has been hypothesized that emotional stressors could have a role in the initial onset of the illness, Kovacs *et al.* (1985) did not find such an association in their cohort. However, a relationship between 'stressor scores' and both low serum glucose levels and triglyceride concentrations has been reported in diabetic adolescents (Chase & Jackson 1981). An association between disturbances in family interaction and overall diabetic control of adolescents as measured by elevated glycosylated haemoglobin (HbA$_1$) has also been demonstrated at the 5-year follow-up assessment after initial diagnosis (Gustafsson *et al.* 1987). Characteristics of mothers' interactions with even preschool-aged children have been shown to distinguish children who had difficulty in maintaining adequate glycaemic control from those who were easily controlled (Garrison *et al.* 1990). Diabetic patients have been reported to be at some increased risk for emotional disturbance, but modest rates have been reported (Wilkinson 1987). In Wilkinson's study of adult diabetics, 18% were diagnosed with a psychiatric disorder and these were predominantly some form of depressive or anxiety disturbances. More severe chronic diabetic samples have been shown to be at greater risk, with 51% having been identified as having a psychiatric diagnosis in a sample evaluated for pancreatic transplantation (Popkin *et al.* 1988). Much higher risk has been documented for children who have required repeat hospitalizations for ketoacidosis when compared to children with diabetes who could be controlled as outpatients. In this study, 88% of the hospitalized diabetic children met the criteria for at least one psychiatric illness as compared to 28% in the outpatient group. Additionally, the hospitalized group was reported to have lower self-esteem and social competence (Liss *et al.* 1998). A special risk in depressed diabetics is attempted suicide by the method of insulin overdose (Kaminer & Robbins 1988). Problems in adjustment to the diagnosis of diabetes in children have also been reported (Ahnsjo *et al.* 1981).

Fortunately, few physical deformities are associated with IDDM. However, Moran (1984) has reported relatively high levels of anxiety in children related to their fears of hypoglycaemic and hyperglycaemic coma as well as later vascular complications. During adolescence, it is common for teenagers to have difficulty adhering to the relatively strict dietary protocols and restrictions in their activity. The link between environmental stressors and diabetic control in children has also been studied (White *et al.* 1984). In these studies, ketoacidosis was linked to either dietary indiscretion or insulin mismanagement in only a minority of the cases (5–10%). However, in a majority of the cases family difficulties were felt to be associated with less adequate control. During adolescence, the patient must begin to assume greater responsibility for the treatment of the illness and begin to appreciate that there is a direct relationship between careful compliance and disease sequelae.

A major concern for many children with IDDM is the uncertainty that is associated with the future course of their illness. This includes both fear of severe ketoacidotic episodes and diabetic sequelae. More cognitive difficulties have been demonstrated in diabetic children with more persistent illness (Gath *et al.* 1980). Poor diabetic control was correlated with:

1 the presence of psychiatric disorder;
2 difficulties in reading; and
3 adverse psychosocial risk factors.

Cognitive difficulties in the abstract/visual reasoning subscale of the Stanford Binet Intelligence Scale have even been noted in children with relatively mild hyperglycaemia if the onset of their illness occurred before 5 years of age (Golden *et al.* 1989). Similarly, problems in cognitive processing speed, acquisition of new knowledge and conceptual reasoning ability have been documented 2 years after diagnosis. These problems may be the result of persistent hyperglycaemia (Northam *et al.* 1998).

Kovacs *et al.* (1985) described variability in the coping of diabetic children. Approximately 64% of the children in this cohort reported some social withdrawal and sadness but did not merit a diagnosis; however, 36% could be diagnosed with a psychiatric disturbance. Affective disorders were the most frequent diagnoses, but 93% of the children with these disturbances recovered over the course of the first year of their diabetic illness.

The interaction of psychiatric disturbance and the control of diabetic symptoms continues to be an area of investigation. Severe psychiatric disturbance in either the child or parent has been shown to account for approximately 44% of the variance in blood glucose level. It has also been shown to predict low glycosylated haemoglobin concentration in the children (Fonagy *et al.* 1987). In Fonagy *et al.*'s study, nearly one-third of the children had an emotional or behavioural difficulty and these children were determined to be less responsible in caring for their illness.

Juvenile rheumatoid arthritis

Juvenile rheumatoid arthritis (JRA) is characterized by chronic joint inflammation and is the most common rheumatoid disorder of children. The disease has been divided into three major categories: systemic, pauciarticular and polyarticular. While all three categories are best classified as complex diseases with an oligogenetic inheritance pattern, there is some suggestion that they each have unique genetic characteristics. Specifically, a polymorphism of the tumour necrosis factor alpha has been reported to be associated with systemic JRA but not with the other categories (Date *et al.* 1999).

The incidence of JRA has been difficult to establish definitively. Approximately 10–20 children in 100 000 have been reported in countries with reasonable ascertainment. Prevalence estimates have been as high as 400 in 100 000 in an Australian study, but are generally in the range of 100–200 in 100 000 children (Andersson 1999).

Systemic arthritis usually presents in children during the first five years of life. Immunoglobulin A (IgA) and platelet levels are usually very elevated. Liver and cardiac involvement are common. Growth retardation can be severe and complicated by the necessity of using corticosteroids (Ansell 1999). Amyloidosis is a relatively rare, but potentially fatal complication. Polyarticular disease with a positive rheumatoid factor may advance rapidly and has a relatively poor prognosis. In contrast, children with pauciarticular disease have a better outcome. Knees and ankles are more commonly involved than elbows, wrists or neck. A chronic insidious uveitis can occur with any form of the illness.

The diagnosis of JRA has proven to be challenging. Whereas fever is a non-specific feature that co-occurs with the presentation of joint pain in most patients, the pattern of the fever is variable and may occur in a prolonged spiking pattern in about 40% of children (Miller 1998). An elevated fibrin D-dimer has been reported to be present in JRA patients and associated with fever and abnormal leucocyte counts, which is predictive of the ultimate severity of the illness (Bloom *et al.* 1998). The traditional treatment of JRA continues to be pharmacological. Aspirin and corticosteroids remain the standard approach, with some children requiring gold, methotrexate or penicillamine (Ansell 1999). The importance of physical conditioning has been emphasized in children with polyarticular disease, and has been shown to decrease the severity of the joint lesions as well as enhance the functional endurance of the joints (Klepper 1991).

Not surprisingly, disease severity has been associated with the occurrence of behavioural problems as ascertained by parental questionnaire (Daltroy *et al.* 1992). A similar finding was noted in a study of young adults in which 21% of a clinical sample were assessed to be clinically depressed. The occurrence of depression was associated with the degree of disability (David *et al.* 1994). However, a recent study comparing children with JRA and chronic fatigue syndrome found that patients with chronic fatigue syndrome and their parents both reported more psychological symptoms. Of note, only two of the JRA patients had systemic disease and little detail of the severity of the illness was reported (Carter *et al.* 1999).

Children with JRA have been assessed to determine the accuracy with which they understood the nature of their illness (Berry *et al.* 1993). While the expected improvement in understanding was demonstrated with age, a surprising lack of understanding of the illness was found at all ages, suggesting a need for greater attempts to help children understand the nature of their illness.

Leukaemia

The most common paediatric malignancy is leukaemia. Nevertheless, leukaemia is a relatively rare disorder with a prevalence of less than 0.05% during childhood. The introduction of chemotherapy and irradiation therapy has continued to alter dramatically the clinical course of the illness over the past 30 years. Currently, the 10-year life expectancy of girls with acute lymphoblastic leukaemia has reached 73% and for boys it has reached 64% (Pui et al. 1999). Although these constitute a huge improvement over the recent past, many children still succumb to the disease. The term 'Damocles syndrome' has been appropriately coined to describe the chronic state of uncertainty that characterizes the lives of these children (Koocher & O'Malley 1981).

The genetic basis of leukaemia is gradually becoming more clearly defined. There are certain subtypes of the disease that appear to be familial but the majority of children with leukaemia do not have a positive pedigree for the disease. Evidence for susceptibility genes have supported the position that leukaemia has a complex genetic pattern of inheritance with gene sites on chromosome 9 at 9p21 (Faderl et al. 1999; Heerema et al. 1999), chromosome 13 at 13q14 (Coignet et al. 1999) and chromosome 17 at 17p11.2 (Stacey et al. 1999).

Leukaemia represents a disease where there is little evidence that life stressors effect the onset, although a recent report has shown that women over 35 years of age may be at increased risk of having a child with leukaemia (Hemminki et al. 1999). Furthermore, there is little to suggest that any defined parental disturbance or behaviour is associated with the onset of the disease. The emotional reactions of the family to the initial diagnosis are usually disbelief, anger and grief. A recent report has suggested that both mothers and fathers have an increase in psychiatric symptomatology immediately following diagnosis and that mothers tend to seek social support while fathers use more active coping strategies (Hoekstra-Weebers et al. 1998). For teenagers recovering from leukaemia, a somewhat paradoxical link between less family cohesion and the successful completion of treatment has been reported, which may be associated with the developmental needs of adolescents to separate successfully from their families (Rait et al. 1992).

Complications can arise in the establishment of the diagnosis of leukaemia. A primary problem is that many of the early signs of the illness, such as increased infections, lethargy and weakness, are non-specific. Once the illness is suspected, the diagnosis can be made definitively through laboratory examination. However, as it is now universally agreed that prompt and aggressive treatment is highly beneficial for the long-term survival of these patients, unnecessary delays in establishment of the diagnosis can lead to both guilt and the attribution of blame.

During the early phases of the illness, there is little physical deformity. Later, weight loss and prominent bruising can be a problem. However, the severe prognosis that is associated with the later stages of the illness usually overshadows the changes that occur in physical appearance.

There have been relatively few studies documenting elevated levels of emotional disturbance in children with leukaemia (Kupst et al. 1984; Greenberg et al. 1989). However, Sawyer et al. (1986) demonstrated elevated levels of behavioural and emotional disturbance when children with leukaemia were compared to their siblings. More leukaemia survivors were also placed in special education programmes than were their siblings, and this was particularly likely if they received cranial radiotherapy. Although these children gradually seemed to adjust to their illness over the 4-year follow-up period, they were still found to have more difficulties in school as documented by both parent and teacher reports (Sawyer et al. 1989). Longitudinal studies into early adulthood have reported no increased psychiatric morbidity in survivors of acute lymphoblastic leukaemia, but persistent problems in interpersonal relationships have been well documented (Mackie et al. 2000). Long-term survivors who had received cranial radiotherapy were less likely to enter college than their siblings (Haupt et al. 1994).

The care and treatment of leukaemia is inevitably a burden for both the child and parent. The necessity for repeated painful bone marrow biopsies as well as other invasive procedures can make these hospitalizations frightening experiences for these children (Dahlquist et al. 1995). The use of high-dose corticosteroids has been reported to be linked with decreased cognitive performance as well as lower achievement scores (Waber et al. 2000). Furthermore, the use of cranial irradiation has been shown to have a variety of negative neuropsychological sequelae, particularly if the treatment is administered before the child is 8 years of age (Moehle & Berg 1985; Anderson et al. 2000). If both cranial radiation and intrathecal methotrexate treatment are employed, a larger number of psychological sequelae are noted, as well as associated abnormal computerized tomography (CT) scans (Pavlovsky et al. 1983). Brouwers et al. (1984) also demonstrated abnormalities on CT scans as well as more frequent neuropsychological deficits and attentional disturbances in patients with documented evidence of atrophy. Eiser (1998) suggested that these attentional difficulties could play a part in decreased performance on a range of cognitive measures. Very few patients showed calcifications, but those children with calcifications demonstrated the greatest neuropsychological dysfunction. These findings are similar to results from studies that examine cognitive function in children with primary brain tumours receiving whole-brain radiotherapy (Packer et al. 1989).

Systemic lupus erythematosus

Systemic lupus erythematosus (SLE) is a chronic autoimmune disease characterized most frequently by involvement of the kidneys, skin, joints and central nervous system, but regularly affecting the heart and lungs. The key laboratory finding is an elevated serum level of immunoglobulin G (IgG) antibodies that are specifically reactive to nuclear constituents such as double-stranded DNA and chromatin (Tsao et al. 1997). The most common presentation in childhood is the occurrence of skin rash and arthritis associated with a fever, but there is considerable variability in the initial symptoms, earning the illness the colloquial name 'the great imitator'. As few as 40% of children present with the macular red facial rash that was the original basis for the name of the illness. The absence of this sign makes the disease more difficult to diagnose during childhood. The mean delay from onset of first symptoms to diagnosis is 1.2 years (Silverman 1996). Although this time can be as long as 2 years, it is reported to be much shorter in tertiary paediatric referral centres (Lacks & White 1990). In paediatric practices, the mean age of onset is approximately 12 years. The illness has been reported in infants, but rarely presents before the age of 6. Approximately 80% of paediatric patients are girls as compared to 90% of adult onset SLE. The incidence of the illness has been reported to be as high as 20 in 100 000 children, while the prevalence of this chronic illness is estimated to be 10-fold greater or 20 per 10 000. The illness occurs in all races but may be slightly more likely to occur in African-Americans and Hispanics than Caucasians.

A family history has been reported in 12.5% of children diagnosed with the illness. This pattern is typical of a complex heritable illness with an oligogenetic basis. Twin studies support this conclusion with an approximately 10-fold greater likelihood of concordance in monozygotic vs. dizygotic twins. Furthermore, the risk of a sibling developing the disease is approximately 20 times higher than the risk in the general population (Tsao & Wallace 1997). The number of candidate susceptibility genes is growing, with a prominent candidate located at 1q41–q42 (Tsao et al. 1997).

Although the prognosis of the illness has been gradually improving, relatively recent reports suggest that the 5-year survival rate is still only approximately 85% (Lacks & White 1990). Most children suffer considerable morbidity both the involvement of target organs or as the consequence of the treatment required. Arthritis occurs in almost all children with the illness. Proliferative glomerulonephritis is reported to occur in approximately 20–84% of affected children. Estimates of the comorbidity for severe neuropsychiatric complications have been reported to be between 17 and 69% and include major depression, psychosis and cognitive dysfunction (Lacks & White 1990).

The traditional treatment of the illness involves the use of salicylates or non-steroidal anti-inflammatory drugs. The focus of treatment always includes the arthritic complications and frequently includes the use of corticosteroids which have well-known neuropsychiatric sequelae. More aggressive treatment includes the use of hydroxychloroquine, methotrexate, azathioprine, cyclophosphamide and cyclosporin, which all have major side-effects (Silverman 1996).

Cognitive impairment in adult patients with non-central nervous system SLE has been reported in as many as 29% of patients, with much higher levels found in patients with documented central nervous system involvement (Kosora et al. 1996). The severity of cognitive impairment has been shown to vary over time in a manner parallel with the exacerbations and remissions of physical symptoms. This variability supports an approach of longitudinal evaluation as opposed to assessments at a single point in time (Bleiberg & Bunning 1998). A recent study of patients with SLE who had not been recognized as having psychiatric symptomatology revealed surprisingly similar rates of neuropsychological impairment, suggesting an underrecognition of psychiatric comorbidity (Sabbadini et al. 1999). The use of magnetic transfer imaging rather than the less sensitive magnetic resonance imaging identifies central nervous system involvement in patients without psychiatric symptomatology, and demonstrates that SLE patients with neuropsychiatric symptoms have more extensive brain involvement (Bosma et al. 2000). With ever-increasing capacity to demonstrate early central nervous system involvement, targeted intervention can be linked to attempts to maintain cognitive function through the initiation of earlier aggressive systemic therapeutic intervention. Whereas the occurrence of psychiatric morbidity is clearly common in young patients with SLE, there has been surprisingly little systematic assessment of emotional symptomatology in children. Adult patients without overt central nervous system involvement were reported to have elevated scores on the clinical scales of the Minnesota Multiphasic Personality Inventory (MMPI) when compared to normal controls (Kosora et al. 1996). Similarly, in an independent study, about 50% of adults with SLE were reported to meet criteria for a psychiatric disorder (Waterloo et al. 1998). Emotional distress has repeatedly been shown to be reported by patients without overt central nervous system involvement as demonstrated by traditional clinical findings (Denburg et al. 1997).

Physical symptoms without evidence of somatic aetiology

Physical symptoms commonly present in the absence of known organic disease. In the past, these problems have often been classified broadly as hysterical symptoms. More recently they have been referred to as somatization disorders, dissociation disorders or conversion disorders (Kihlstrom 1994). The diagnostic challenge related to defining this group of disorders has been the dramatic heterogeneity of symptoms. This variability has made the reliable definition of phenotypes problematic. Despite this limitation, somatization disorder has been shown to be somewhat heritable, more common in girls, and linked to alcoholism and sociopathy in male relatives (Guze 1993). Concordance of conversion symptoms in identical and fraternal twins has not been established, resulting in some uncertainty regarding the degree of heritability of this condition (Jaworowski et al. 1998).

Many of these conditions involve neurological symptoms: paralyses or incoordination (dissociative movement disorders); convulsions (pseudoseizures; see Goodman, Chapter 14); or loss of visual acuity or blindness in portions of the visual field (dissociative sensory loss). Somatoform autonomic dysfunction (characterized by diarrhoea, palpitations, hyperventilation, flushing and sweating) must be distinguished diagnostically from a wide range of medical disorders. Neurasthenia (chronic fatigue), hypochondriasis (preoccupation with the possibility of an underlying disease), and somatization disorder (multiple persistent somatic symptoms) are characterized by common symptoms that mimic the presentation of organic syndromes.

The concept of a disorder being defined chiefly by the absence of a physical explanation has always been problematic. The primary reason for this common concern is the anxiety associated with the possibility that an affected child may have an underlying physical disease that remains undiagnosed. Such concerns are justified as some children with organic brain disease have been previously diagnosed as having conversion disorders (Rivinus *et al.* 1975). Furthermore, organic symptoms regularly occur in children who also have functional symptoms. This is well illustrated by children with epilepsy who also exhibit exaggerated pseudoseizures or by the perpetuation of episodic abdominal pain that initially began as a result of a parasitic infestation. In the pursuit of possible physical causes, intensive investigations may be carried out which unfortunately carry their own iatrogenic risks.

The question facing the clinician is how aggressively to verify a negative finding when faced with an ill child and a concerned family. Sometimes the form of the symptom is in itself enough to argue strongly against a physical cause, as illustrated by diplopia appearing when one eye is covered even though in rare circumstances a dislocation of the lens can produce monocular diplopia. Similarly, if a symptom is clearly related in time to an external stressor, such as abdominal pain that is consistently linked to leaving for school, a history and examination may well be sufficient grounds on which to base a diagnosis. On the other hand, physical illness can arise even in children with psychologically determined disorders, and necessary investigations may be overlooked because of a psychiatric label. Good communication between paediatrician and psychiatrist is crucial (see Rauch & Jellinek, Chapter 62) and physical reappraisal of disorders believed to be psychogenic should be undertaken if they do not improve when a stressor believed to be responsible has been ameliorated.

Yet another issue in the interpretation of negative findings is the appreciation of the limitations of scientific knowledge and organic causes. In the past, some illnesses have been regarded as purely psychogenic that are now known to have organic contributions. Common examples are Crohn disease or narcolepsy. There is little doubt that unsuspected organic dysfunction continues to result in physical symptoms that are better described as cryptogenic than psychogenic. Such problems of definition make it difficult to obtain consistent estimates of prevalence. The most common somatic symptom attributed to psychological causes is diffuse pain that is often in the abdomen or head. Abdominal pain affected 32% of young Swedish adolescents with a frequency of at least once a month, whereas headache affected 67% of those studied (Larsson 1991). However, in this as in other surveys, there is no means of determining which cases could be confidently attributed to psychological disturbance. There is an association between somatic symptoms and

self-reports of high levels of emotional distress in psychiatrically referred children (Ryan *et al.* 1987), children with chronic illness (Wallander *et al.* 1988) and epidemiological surveys (Kashani *et al.* 1989). However, the aetiological role of specific stressors in the initiation of these symptoms has not been demonstrated.

Particular care needs to be taken in the assessment of somatic symptoms when the patient and the professional come from different cultures. Cultures vary in the types of words that are used to describe illness and in their members' readiness to seek help; e.g. Thai parents rate their children's problems as less serious and more likely to improve than do American parents (Weisz *et al.* 1991). Although a skilled translator can help to reduce linguistic barriers to understanding the nature of complaints, there may be more profound differences. Kleinman (1986) examined the Chinese concept of neurasthenia, which is defined solely in terms of somatic symptoms. He found many similarities between those affected and those Chinese who would be classified as depressed using Western criteria. The vast majority of these Chinese patients who were labelled as neurasthenic responded to antidepressant medication. The somatic terminology used by Chinese patients followed their political and social insistence that the roots of personal malaise should be sought in physical illness. This did not mean that the somatic complaints were unreal, or that the Chinese patients really had depression rather than neurasthenia. The implication is that the meaning of a somatic complaint needs to be interpreted in the light of knowledge about the culture's understanding of illness.

In the treatment of somatic symptoms, most authorities advocate an attempt to help the child and family understand why abnormal illness behaviour has developed in order to achieve a more adaptive solution to their problems (Goodyer & Taylor 1985). Suggestion and encouragement towards a gradual resumption of normal function can be useful (Dubowitz & Hersov 1976). However, systematic trials of such supportive treatment have not been conducted. While recurrent abdominal pain is regarded as having a good prognosis by many paediatricians (Graham 1986), follow-up studies of children seen for abdominal pain indicate that nearly half continue to suffer the same symptoms in adult life (Apley & Hale 1973; Christensen & Mortensen 1975). This more guarded outcome is based on studies of children who have been referred for an inpatient evaluation and is probably not generalizable to the majority of cases that are managed by primary care clinicians in outpatient settings.

Illness-related risk factors

A quantitative and analytical approach to the examination of the relationship of paediatric illness to early emotional development can be facilitated by conceptualizing the occurrence of a physical illness as a complex set of emotional stressors that have specific component characteristics. Such a frame of reference increases the precision with which variability in psychological outcomes can be examined. This strategy also provides a bridge between clinical investigators interested in studying the effects of generic chronic illness and those who have been interested in linking a specific paediatric illness with distinct behavioural outcomes. If two diseases share similar illness-related risk factors, it is logical to expect that their impact on emotional development should be similar. In contrast, if two illnesses share only a single characteristic, such as a chronic unremitting course, but have different onsets and aetiologies, it would not be reasonable to expect that such contrasting conditions would have a similar impact on the emotional adjustment of a child. The following eight illness-related risk factors represent common problems that may require clinical intervention.

Age of child at time of illness onset

To appreciate the impact of age of onset of a physical illness, it is necessary to place the onset of the illness into a developmental context (see also Rauch & Jellinek, Chapter 62). Some stressors that are particularly disruptive for toddlers will have minimal negative consequences for adolescents. Furthermore, the concept of illness for children evolves in parallel with their cognitive development (Millstein *et al.* 1981; Perrin & Gerrity 1981; Burbach & Peterson 1986).

Early studies of hospitalization suggest that separation phenomena are particularly difficult for children in their second to fourth year of life (Prugh *et al.* 1953). In examining the very early experiences of severely asthmatic children with multiple hospitalizations in the first 3 years of life, a sensitive period between 6 months and 2 years also seemed to be associated with later behavioural difficulties (Mrazek 1992). Disruptions in the formation of primary attachment relationships during the first 2 years of life have been shown to have persistent effects on later relationships. Consequently, illnesses that result in unplanned and prolonged early separations from primary attachment figures during these critical years would be predicted to have a more disruptive effect on subsequent emotional development than illnesses that have a later onset.

During the school years, illnesses that interfere with the participation of children in normal family and school events are believed to be particularly potent stressors. During this period, gender differences also begin to play a part. Boys appear to be more sensitive to illnesses that interfere with their ability to participate in athletics, while girls may be more sensitive to problems that result in their inability to take full advantage of the support provided by their school-age peer group. For example, school-age girls with chronic illnesses have been reported to have modestly higher levels of social anxiety than similarly ill school-age boys (Meijer *et al.* 2000).

In adolescence, diseases that interfere with the process of establishing greater independence are particularly problematic (Orr *et al.* 1984). Becoming a member of a peer group and developing an intimate sexual relationship become critical developmental challenges. Medical problems with sexual stigma such as venereal disease, and physical disfigurement such as facial burns, can have more dramatic emotional sequelae than more debilitating illnesses that are essentially invisible (Love *et al.* 1987).

Parental responsibility for the treatment of paediatric illness

A powerful factor related to the adaptation of a child to serious paediatric illness is the response of the family. Whereas problematic parenting should be considered a major risk factor, exceptionally sensitive and effective parenting is appropriately conceptualized as a potent protective factor. Reciprocally, the chronic illness of a child is conceptualized as a stressor that can have a negative effect on the marriage of the parents (Sabbeth & Leventhal 1984; Klinnert *et al.* 1992). Siblings of children with chronic illness have also been reported to have more behavioural problems (Tritt & Esses 1988). The link that these sibling studies suggest is that a decrease in mutual parental support can be associated with a decrease in the quality of parenting provided to both the ill and the healthy children within the family. Sibling vulnerability increases further if the care of the ill child requires a large amount of parental involvement, leaving little time for parenting a healthy brother or sister.

Given that developmental capacities shape how children perceive their illnesses, it is surprising how little empirical research has been directed towards examining the interaction of age of onset of illness and familial response on the emotional development of children with specific paediatric diagnoses. Factors that have complicated such investigations include limitations in current methods of quantitatively assessing familial protective factors. Every paediatrician knows that strong families are associated with positive clinical outcomes for their patients. A classic developmental example of family-specific variability is the range of appropriate parental support for a chronically ill teenager. These adolescents need to develop as independent individuals. A family style that supports intense commitment on the part of parents to provide physical therapy for a young child may lead to very good medical and emotional outcomes for the preschool child, but this same highly attentive and controlling behaviour may be problematic for a teenager. There must be a developmentally appropriate transition in family style to ensure that as an adolescent, the ill teenager assumes appropriate treatment responsibilities for his or her illness. More attention to the developmental implications of both the course of paediatric illness and the appropriate family responses is needed in order to clarify the significance of these developmental factors in the ultimate expression of psychological disturbance. Progress in quantification of these dimensions should lead to better studies of the specific impact of problematic parenting (Mrazek *et al.* 1995).

Unfortunately, in some circumstances, parents actually play a part in the onset of a paediatric illness through poor judgement, negligence or frank abuse. The most extreme example is Münchausen by proxy syndrome, in which a parent intentionally creates an illness in a child (see Emery & Laumann Billings,

Chapter 20). The possibility must be included in the differential diagnosis of children with a wide range of chronic paediatric conditions (Meadow 1982, 1985). The parent responsible is virtually always the mother. What is often the clue to the discovery of this form of abuse is that the mother who is inflicting the illness upon her child does not appear distressed by the persistence of the illness. From a psychological perspective, this absence of maternal concern may be more problematic for the adjustment of the child than the actual physical discomforts or disruptions associated with the medical symptoms.

Another circumstance that can influence the ability of the family to support the prescribed medical plan effectively is when a non-intentional injury occurs as a result of an action by the parent. An illustration would be the case of a father who is responsible for a vehicle collision in which he is uninjured, but his daughter sustains multiple fractures. The ability of this father to make the recovery of his daughter a primary personal goal has two positive consequences. First, the direct support of his daughter will serve as a protective factor for her emotional development. Secondly, her recovery will help him to begin to deal with his predictable feelings of guilt. Should he withdraw from participating in the provision of her care because of his sense of responsibility for her injury, this should be conceptualized as a risk factor for both father and daughter.

In other circumstances, it can be difficult to attribute responsibility. An example is a child who develops pneumonia and subsequently asthma during a period of intense family stress when his or her parents have been unavailable. In this circumstance, the parents may raise the question of whether their child being left in a large child care centre for many hours a day and exposed to many sick children could be related to the onset of the pneumonia and the subsequent onset of persistent asthma. The clinician is often tempted to provide reassurance to the parents by minimizing the links between their actions and the course of the physical illness. This clinical strategy is often supported by the belief that the parents' guilt may ultimately have a negative impact on the child and that accepting some responsibility for the occurrence of the illness is irrelevant to the subsequent management of the disease. This perspective must be counterbalanced with the knowledge that the child's risk for recurrent exposure to other illness-related risk factors may be high in this family without the benefit of an intervention designed to support appropriate parental behaviour.

Degree of heritability of the illness

A special circumstance exists related to genetic inheritance. Once parents decide to have a child, the transmission of a particular genetic trait becomes an estimated probability. Currently, parents have little control over the probability that their child will inherit a susceptibility gene for a particular illness or trait. Although this situation is likely to change (see McGuffin & Rutter, Chapter 12; Skuse & Kuntsi, Chapter 13), at present it is important that both the mother and father be made aware of any increased risk for physical illnesses that their children may have

as a consequence of their genetic make-up. When the genetic risk for an illness in their future child is remote, the decision to have a child is universally supported by family physicians and the community at large. In these cases, the occurrence of an unlikely outcome tends to have a relatively limited negative impact on the subsequent adaptation of the family. However, when the genetic risk is known to be high, as in the case of parents who previously have had a child with cystic fibrosis, there is potential for much more conflict. The decision to have another child is taken with full knowledge that there is a 25% likelihood that the next child will have the illness as well as a 50% chance that he or she will be a carrier of this well-understood autosomal recessive condition. In this case, the 'blame' is shared equally by both parents, as they are necessarily heterozygotes or carriers for cystic fibrosis.

The definition of responsible behaviour regarding the decision to have a child in light of a well-defined risk for the development of a seriously debilitating paediatric illness is beginning to change. Whereas this topic is beyond the scope of this chapter, these ethical issues are central to the care of families carrying genes associated with severe illnesses. Furthermore, when the risk for a genetic illness is well defined by the genotype of a single parent who is carrying a dominant pathological allele, the situation is further complicated by the likelihood of one parent blaming the other for passing on the gene associated with the illness of the child.

It is usually easier for families to cope with the onset of a physical illness that is perceived as the result of bad luck or the 'will of God'. In such situations, the parents are victims together with their child. However, as more is understood about environmental risk factors and genetic vulnerability, fate will become a less common aetiological explanation.

Accuracy and timeliness of the establishment of the diagnosis

The process by which the diagnosis is established can play a significant part in the ability of the child and parent to adapt to the illness. A number of factors have a role:

1 the duration of time required to come to closure on the nature of the problem;
2 the certainty with which the diagnosis can be made; and
3 the sensitivity with which the diagnosis and its implications are transmitted to the child and the family.

The diagnostic skill of the physician is important because it contributes directly to the quality of the physician–patient relationship. A strong partnership in the care of the child can ultimately affect the prognosis for the child. A rapid and accurate diagnosis can facilitate this relationship while a misdiagnosis can lead to an acutely adversarial situation.

Prompt determination of the diagnosis is the standard of care and usual parental expectation. When the determination of the diagnosis is delayed through administrative postponements in scheduling of diagnostic testing, sensitive communication with the family regarding the components of the diagnostic progress can mitigate the negative effects of a prolonged period of uncertainty.

Some illnesses are more easily recognized than others. A child who develops the classic sign of insatiable thirst coupled with an abnormal fasting serum glucose is not likely to be missed as being diabetic. In contrast, a number of illnesses can mimic asthma. These include vocal cord dysfunction, which cannot be established during the examination in the paediatrician's office as it requires direct visualization of the vocal cords that can only be observed during bronchoscopy (Christopher *et al.* 1983; Julia *et al.* 1999). Given that there is a strong association between vocal cord dysfunction and emotional disturbance, this differential diagnostic possibility should be considered carefully by a psychiatric consultant when asked to consider the role of emotional factors in children with treatment-resistant asthma.

Some illnesses, such as some of the leukaemias, can be definitively diagnosed upon inspection of the blood cells. However, prodromal symptoms can be quite vague and their significance may be minimized, delaying an appropriate work-up. Unfortunately, in cases where malignancies are discovered in relatively advanced stages, the question of why appropriate early investigations were not ordered is always difficult. Avoiding discussion of this issue may well have a negative effect on the doctor–patient relationship as well as on subsequent treatment.

A difficult responsibility is the communication to both the child and family of a confirmed grave or terminal paediatric diagnosis. Although good care involves open disclosure (British Medical Association 2001), the implications of sharing devastating information with a family in crisis is often difficult to ascertain. The entire situation can be further complicated if the physician is ambivalent about the need to share the prognosis with a relatively young child. The intensity of this conflict is illustrated by the care with which some physicians organize their practices to avoid these unhappy interactions. In these cases, a child psychiatrist can be particularly helpful by providing the paediatrician with some perspective on the emotional needs of his or her patient and the family of the child, to help ensure that they have the opportunity to explore the implications of the disease for the future of the family. Such a strategy is facilitated by the use of a multidisciplinary team approach to comprehensive care (Bingley *et al.* 1980).

One method that physicians use to cope with their paediatric patients who have terminal illnesses is to begin to focus on the treatment of the disease and avoid addressing issues related to how well the child is coping with the symptoms and prognosis. An important aspect of paediatric clinical care is to be able to help the family sustain hope for an optimal outcome while providing a realistic perspective on the medical risks that the child is facing.

Interference with function

Disability associated with chronic illness varies enormously. However, this variability in functional capacity is rarely con-

sidered as an independent variable in the analysis of risk factors associated with specific illnesses despite the clear link with long-term adaptation (Mattsson 1972; Cadman *et al.* 1987). Another factor that is rarely assessed is the substantive difference in the impact of the same disability according to the child's level of development. Although interference with intellectual processing has a negative role at all stages of development, cognitive deficits have a wider range of negative implications when the child must perform at a well-defined threshold in order to advance in school. Similarly, the inability to drive a car has no negative impact prior to the age when it is legally permitted, but can have very strong negative social connotations for older adolescents.

Disability is strongly related to the severity of the illness. An asthmatic child with easily controlled asthma may have virtually no functional disability whereas a severely asthmatic child may find it impossible to attend school consistently. Although both children may have some difficulty adapting to their illness, the probability of the occurrence of emotional difficulty is clearly higher with more severe illness (McNichol *et al.* 1973). A similar relationship between severity of renal disease and emotional adaptation has been noted (Garralda *et al.* 1988).

Impact on physical appearance

One of the most common concerns of chronically ill children is their anxiety about being physically different from their peers. This concern has often been seen to be a central aspect of a diminished sense of self-esteem (Burns & Zweig 1980). Given the importance of a positive physical appearance to the formation of a sense of self-worth, it is not surprising that disfiguring illnesses are associated with increased emotional vulnerability (Breslau & Marshall 1985).

Many illnesses result in no negative impact on physical appearance. Most asthmatic children appear to be physically normal until late in the course of their illness after long periods of respiratory compromise or as a result of physical changes secondary to treatment with chronic corticosteroids. Other illnesses, such as atopic dermatitis, can result in extensive unattractive skin lesions that are not associated with long-term physical handicap or any problems in athletic or cognitive achievement.

Again, there is a rarely appreciated association between age of illness and impact of problems in appearance. Specifically, very young children may have relatively little negative feedback regarding physical deformity from very accepting adults who care for them. However, as the peer group of a child assumes greater importance, emotional rejection based on negative response from other children can precipitate depressed mood. The classic period of peak sensitivity is adolescence, when children with severe problems of physical appearance most often show disturbances in emotional adaptation. Interestingly, little empirical evidence is available to demonstrate this frequent clinical observation.

Persistence of symptoms

Diseases vary in their pattern of symptom expression. Illnesses such as asthma and epilepsy frequently have long periods of remission in which children may have extended opportunities to interact with peers and attend school in the absence of physical reminders of their disease. Other illnesses are either unremitting or result in a gradual worsening of physical discomfort and disability.

Illnesses with more persistent or unremitting symptoms would be expected to have a more negative impact on emotional adaptation. However, there is little evidence to suggest chronicity as a primary factor. A possible alternative explanation is that some children with persistent disturbances learn to come to grips with their problems in an effective manner, while children who have intervals when they are free of symptoms continue to hope for a complete resolution of the physical difficulties. In any case, variability regarding this characteristic requires further investigation.

Hope for recovery

A brief encounter with a serious illness that results in a complete recovery is unlikely to have any negative impact on emotional development. However, children with a more uncertain prognosis have been described as having a 'Damocles syndrome' (see above). These children must come to live with considerable uncertainty about their long-term survival.

A primary concern in the treatment of children with a terminal prognosis is that they do not prematurely lose hope. Hopelessness is a cardinal symptom of clinical depression and associated with a poor prognosis. Some children are able to maintain a strong optimistic sense about their eventual recovery with little support and in the face of quite grave odds. A difficult goal that is a component of the work with children who have a terminal prognosis is to help them and their family to reach some level of acceptance of the inevitability of their impending death.

General therapeutic considerations

The role of the psychiatrist in the management of paediatric patients with serious illnesses is in transition. Traditionally, the primary therapeutic role has been to help children cope with their circumstances. Treatment has been expanded to include active interventions that involve parents and the family members as well as psychopharmacological management.

A recent development has been the increased awareness of the interactions of multiple risk factors that are frequently associated with the initial onset of many physical illnesses. Emotional stressors have been recently demonstrated to be linked to the onset of asthmatic symptoms (Mrazek *et al.* 1999), and it is hypothesized that a wide range of highly complex illnesses may involve similar mechanisms. As new knowledge about the genetic basis of specific physical illnesses is established, the challenge of developing protective early interventions will become more clinically imperative. For these interventions to be appropriately employed, new techniques involving multiple specialists will need to be developed. New intervention trials must be designed in order to test appropriate early treatments and validate their efficacy.

In the past, chronically ill children who exhibited depressive symptoms were not recognized as having a comorbid psychiatric illness (Costello *et al.* 1988). In part this was because of an expectation that children with severe physical limitations would understandably begin to show social withdrawal and signs of discouragement. It is now the standard of practice to diagnose and treat depressive illness in children with chronic paediatric disorders.

Rehabilitation efforts for chronically ill children are also now more clearly known to have multiple benefits. Although it may not be possible to completely resolve either the underlying physical illness or the psychiatric and behavioural symptoms of some patients, the objective of achieving a better overall level of emotional adaptation is a critical treatment goal. For example, the respiratory status of severely asthmatic children has been shown to improve when they participate in active exercise training (Strunk *et al.* 1989a). Furthermore, overall decrease in the medical utilization of severely asthmatic children was demonstrated after their participation in a comprehensive rehabilitation programme with active psychiatric involvement (Strunk *et al.* 1989b). Similar results may be possible for a wide range of chronic problems and should be the focus of active investigations.

Primary prevention should be a component of a comprehensive approach to the care of children at genetic risk for the development of severe paediatric illnesses. An immediate scientific objective is to begin to define the physiological and environmental factors that affect initial expression of susceptibility genes. A first step in this process is to quantify the range of potential stressors for the target disease. This is currently being achieved by carefully monitoring the initial expression and subsequent exacerbations of illnesses in vulnerable children. An alternative methodological approach is to examine carefully the recent past experience of children who have had a recent onset of a significant disease.

Using either strategy, the key research objectives must include the identification of illness-related factors. This would have the attractive feature of providing more precise insight into the mechanism of initial gene expression. Although it is possible to speculate that a particular physiological mechanism may link the symptoms of a physical illness and a set of psychiatric symptoms, there are surprisingly few models. An exception is the clinically observed association that depression is common in children with severe asthma. Three competitive neurobiological hypotheses exist. The first is that an underlying disturbance in autonomic regulation, such as a shift in the sensitivity of cholinergic receptors to parasympathetic stimulation (Cockcroft *et al.* 1977), may place a child at greater risk for environmentally triggered bronchial constriction while at the same time influencing the central nervous system in such a way as to result in increased dysphoric mood (Charney *et al.* 1981; Miller 1987; Mrazek & Klinnert 1991). A second potential mechanism could be that the contents of mast cells or basophils are released as a consequence of an immunologically mediated IgE reaction. These cells contain a wide range of substances that include both bronchial constrictors and neuropeptides (Leff 1988). Some of these neurohumoral proteins have been demonstrated to play a part in central neuroregulation of dysphoric states (Snyder 1980, 1982). A third potential mechanism could be primarily genetic, based on the possibility that a single gene is involved in the regulation of respiratory control and the regulation of central neurotransmitters. A fourth hypothesis represents a more traditional perspective that psychophysiological respiration changes are secondary to the negative subjective experiences of the asthmatic child. This explanation is based on the observation that severe episodes of respiratory insufficiency are often described as extremely frustrating and result in considerable social restrictions. The chronic experience of severe attacks subsequently becomes linked to repeated episodes of unhappiness, discouragement and depressed mood.

Only through systematic investigations will the most salient mechanism or combination of mechanisms responsible for this phenomenon become more clearly understood. Unfortunately, such investigations are difficult to conduct as a consequence of current methodological limitations. To continue the previous illustration, the study of depression in physically ill children is often confounded by the use of instruments designed to assess mood disturbance that equate physical symptoms with symptoms of affective disease (Heiligenstein & Jacobsen 1988). However, more definitive studies will become possible once reliable biological markers for affective disturbance have been clearly established.

It is ironic that partnership of paediatricians and child psychiatrists has not been more productive in designing empirically driven studies to investigate the aetiological basis of severe paediatric disease. Both specialties have a long tradition of recognizing and dealing with the emotional development of ill children. There is reason to be optimistic that renewed commitment to this shared mission will facilitate the application of new methodologies to the more comprehensive study of the complex biological processes underlying adaptation to these disorders.

References

Ahnsjo, S., Humble, K., Larsson, Y., Settergren-Carlsson, G. & Sterky, G. (1981) Personality changes and social adjustment during the first three years of diabetes in children. *Acta Paediatrica Scandinavia*, **70**, 321–327.

Alton, E.W. & Geddes, D.M. (1995) Gene therapy for cystic fibrosis: a clinical perspective. *Gene Therapy*, **2**, 88–95.

Anderson, V.A., Godber, T., Smibert, E., Weiskop, S. & Ekert, H. (2000) Cognitive and academic outcome following cranical irradiation and chemotherapy in children: a longitudinal study. *British Journal of Cancer*, **82**, 255–262.

Andersson, G.B. (1999) Juvenile arthritis: who gets it, where and when? A review of current data on incidence and prevalence. *Clinical and Experimental Rheumatology*, **17**, 367–374.

Ansell, B.M. (1999) Prognosis in juvenile arthritis. *Advances in Experimental Medicine and Biology*, **455**, 27–33.

Apley, J. & Hale, B. (1973) Children with recurrent abdominal pain: how do they grow up? *British Medical Journal*, **3**, 7–9.

Berry, S.L., Hayford, J.R., Ross, C.K., Pachman, L.M. & Lavigne, J.V. (1993) Conceptions of illness by children with juvenile rheumatoid arthritis: a cognitive developmental approach. *Journal of Pediatric Psychology*, **18**, 83–97.

Bingley, L., Leonard, J., Hensman, S., Lask, B. & Wolff, O. (1980) Comprehensive management of children on a paediatric ward: a family approach. *Archives of Diseases in Childhood*, **55**, 555–561.

Bleiberg, J. & Bunning, R. (1998) Cognitive and physical measures in rehabilitation of patients with lupus. *Current Opinion in Rheumatology*, **10**, 442–445.

Bloom, B.J., Tucker, L.B., Miller, L.C. & Schaller, J.G. (1998) Fibrin D-dimer as a marker of disease activity in systemic onset juvenile rheumatoid arthritis. *Journal of Rheumatology*, **25**, 1620–1625.

Bosma, G.P., Rood, M.J., Zwinderman, A.H., Huizinga, T.W. & van Buchem, M.A. (2000) Evidence of central nervous system damage in patients with neuropsychiatric systemic lupus erythematosus, demonstrated by magnetization transfer imaging. *Arthritis and Rheumatism*, **43**, 48–54.

Breslau, N. & Marshall, I.A. (1985) Psychological disturbance in children with physical disabilities: continuity and change in a 5-year follow-up. *Journal of Abnormal Child Psychology*, **13**, 199–216.

British Medical Association (2001) *Consent, Rights and Choices in Health Care for Children and Young People*. BMJ Books, London.

Brouwers, P., Riccardi, R., Poplack, D. & Fedio, P. (1984) Attentional deficits in longterm survivors of childhood acute lymphoblastic leukemia (ALL). *Journal of Clinical Neuropsychology*, **6**, 325–336.

Burbach, D.J. & Peterson, L. (1986) Children's concepts of physical illness: a review and critique of cognitive-developmental literature. *Health Psychology*, **5**, 307–325.

Burns, W.J. & Zweig, A.R. (1980) Self-concepts of chronically ill children. *Journal of Genetic Psychology*, **137**, 179–190.

Bywater, E.M. (1981) Adolescents with cystic fibrosis: psychosocial adjustment. *Archives of Disease in Childhood*, **56**, 538–543.

Cadman, D., Boyle, M., Szatmari, P. & Offord, D.R. (1987) Chronic illness disability, and mental and social well-being. *Pediatrics*, **79**, 805–813.

Carter, B.D., Kronenberger, W.G., Edwards, J.F., Marshall, G.S., Schikler, K.N. & Causey, D.L. (1999) Psychological symptoms in chronic fatigue and juvenile rheumatoid arthritis. *Pediatrics*, **103**, 975–979.

Charney, D., Mendes, D. & Heninger, G. (1981) Receptor sensitivity and the mechanism of action of antidepressant treatment. *Archives of General Psychiatry*, **38**, 1160–1180.

Chase, H.P. & Jackson, G.G. (1981) Stress and sugar control in children with insulin-dependent diabetes mellitus. *Journal of Pediatrics*, **98**, 1011–1013.

Christensen, M.F. & Mortensen, O. (1975) Long-term prognosis in children with recurrent abdominal pain. *Archives of Disease in Childhood*, **50**, 110–114.

Christopher, K.L., Wood, R.P., Eckert, R.C., Blager, F.B., Raney, R.A. & Souhrada, J.F. (1983) Vocal-cord dysfunction presenting as asthma. *New England Journal of Medicine*, **308**, 1566–1570.

Cockcroft, D.W., Ruffin, R.E., Dolovich, J. & Hargreave, F.E. (1977) Allergen-induced increase in non-allergic bronchial reactivity. *Clinical Allergy*, **7**, 503–513.

Coignet, L.J., Lima, C.S., Min, T. *et al.* (1999) Myeloid- and lymphoid-specific breakpoint cluster regions in chromosome band 13q14 in acute leukemia. *Genes, Chromosomes and Cancer*, 25, 222–229.

Cookson, J.B. (1987) Prevalence rates of asthma in developing countries and their comparison with those in Europe and North America. *Chest*, 91 (Suppl. 6), 97S–103S.

Costello, E.J., Edelbrock, C., Costello, A.J., Dulcan, M.K., Burns, B.J. & Brent, D. (1988) Psychopathology in pediatric primary care: the new hidden morbidity. *Pediatrics*, 82, 415–424.

Czajkowski, D.R. & Koocher, G.P. (1986) Predicting medical compliance among adolescents with cystic fibrosis. *Health Psychology*, 5, 297–305.

Dahlquist, L.M., Power, T.G. & Carlson, L. (1995) Physician and parent behavior during invasive pediatric cancer procedures: relationships to child behavioral distress. *Journal of Pediatric Psychology*, 20, 477–490.

Daltroy, L.H., Larson, M.G., Eaton, H.M. *et al.* (1992) Psychosocial adjustment in juvenile arthritis. *Journal of Pediatric Psychology*, 17, 277–289.

Dankert-Roelse, J.E. & Meerman, G.J. (1995) Long term prognosis of patients with cystic fibrosis in relation to early detection by neonatal screening and treatment in a cystic fibrosis centre. *Thorax*, 50, 712–718.

Date, Y., Seki, N., Kamizono, S. *et al.* (1999) Identification of a genetic risk factor for systemic juvenile rheumatoid arthritis in the 5′-flank region of the TNF alpha gene and HLA genes. *Arthritis and Rheumatism*, 42, 2577–2582.

David, J., Cooper, C., Hickey, L. *et al.* (1994) The functional and psychological outcomes of juvenile chronic arthritis in young adulthood. *British Journal of Rheumatology*, 33, 876–881.

Davidson, D.J. & Porteous, D.J. (1998) Genetics and pulmonary medicine. I. The genetics of cystic fibrosis lung disease. *Thorax*, 53, 389–397.

Denburg, S.D., Carbotte, R.M. & Denburg, J.A. (1997) Psychological aspects of systemic lupus erythematosus: cognitive function, mood, and self-report. *Journal of Rheumatology*, 24, 998–1003.

Dubowitz, V. & Hersov, L. (1976) Management of children with non-organic (hysterical) disorders of motor function. *Developmental Medicine and Child Neurology*, 25, 67–80.

Eiser, C. (1998) Practitioner review: long-term consequences of childhood cancer. *Journal of Child Psychology and Psychiatry*, 39, 621–633.

Elborn, J.S., Shale, D.J. & Britton, J.R. (1991) Cystic fibrosis: current survival and population estimates to the year 2000. *Thorax*, 46, 881–885.

Faderl, S., Estrov, Z., Kantarjian, H.M. *et al.* (1999) The incidence of chromosome 9p21 abnormalities and deletions of tumor suppressor genes p15 (INK4b)/p16 (INK4a)/p14 (ARF) in patients with acute lymphoblastic leukemia. *Cytokines, Cellular and Molecular Theory*, 5, 159–163.

Fagerudd, J.A., Pettersson-Fernholm, K.J., Gronhagen-Riska, C. & Groop, P.H. (1999) The impact of a family history of type II (non-insulin-dependent) diabetes mellitus on the risk of diabetic nephropathy in patients with type I (insulin-dependent) diabetes mellitus. *Diabetologia*, 42, 519–526.

Ferguson, E.M., Horwood, L.J. & Shannon, W.T. (1983) Parental asthma, parental eczema and asthma and eczema in childhood. *Journal of Chronic Disease*, 36, 517–524.

Field, L.L., Tobias, R., Thomson, G. & Plon, S. (1996) Susceptibility to insulin-dependent diabetes mellitus maps to a locus (IDDM11) on human chromosome 14q24.3–q31. *Genomics*, 33, 1–8.

Fonagy, P., Moran, G.S., Lindsay, M.K.M., Kurts, A.B. & Brown, R. (1987) Psychological adjustment and diabetic control. *Archives of Disease in Childhood*, 62, 1009–1013.

Froguel, P. (1997) Genetics of type 1 insulin-dependent diabetes mellitus. *Hormone Research*, 48 (Suppl. 4), 55–57.

Garralda, M.E., Jameson, R.A., Reynolds, J.M. & Postlethwaite, R.J. (1988) Psychiatric adjustment in children with chronic renal failure. *Journal of Child Psychology and Psychiatry*, 29, 79–90.

Garrison, W.T., Biggs, D. & Williams, K. (1990) Temperament characteristics and clinical outcomes in young children with diabetes mellitus. *Journal of Child Psychology and Psychiatry*, 31, 1079–1088.

Gath, A., Smith, M.A. & Baum, D.J. (1980) Emotional, behavioural, and educational disorders in diabetic children. *Archives of Disease in Childhood*, 55, 371–375.

Gauthier, Y., Fortin, C., Drapeau, P. *et al.* (1977) The mother–child relationship and the development of autonomy and self-assertion in young (14–30 months) asthmatic children. *Journal of the American Academy of Child Psychiatry*, 16, 109–131.

Gauthier, Y., Fortin, D., Drapeau, P. *et al.* (1978) Follow-up study of 35 asthmatic preschool children. *Journal of the American Academy of Child Psychiatry*, 17, 679–695.

Golden, M.P., Ingersoll, G.M., Brack, C.J., Russell, B.A., Wright, J.C. & Huberty, T.J. (1989) Longitudinal relationship of asymptomatic hypoglycemia to cognitive function in IDDM. *Diabetes Care*, 12, 89–93.

Goodyer, I. & Taylor, D.C. (1985) Hysteria. *Archives of Disease in Childhood*, 60, 680–681.

Gortmaker, S.L., Walker, D.K., Weitzman, M. & Sobol, A.M. (1990) Chronic conditions, socioeconomic risks, and behavioral problems in children and adolescents. *Pediatrics*, 85, 267–276.

Graetz, B.W., Shute, R.H. & Sawyer, M.G. (2000) An Australian study of adolescents with cystic fibrosis: perceived supportive and nonsupportive behaviors from families and friends and psychological adjustment. *Journal of Adolescent Health*, 26, 64–69.

Graham, P. (1986) *Child Psychiatry: a Developmental Approach*. Oxford Medical Publications, Oxford.

Greenberg, H.S., Kazak, A.E. & Meadows, A.T. (1989) Psychologic functioning in 8- to 16-year-old cancer survivors and their parents. *Journal of Pediatrics*, 114, 488–493.

Gustafsson, P.A., Cederblad, M., Ludvigsson, J. & Lundin, B. (1987) Family interaction and metabolic balance in juvenile diabetes mellitus: a prospective study. *Diabetes Research and Clinical Practice*, 4, 7–14.

Guze, S.B. (1993) Genetics of Briquet's syndrome and somatization disorder: a review of family, adoption and twin studies. *Annals of Clinical Psychiatry*, 5, 225–230.

Halpern, S.R., Sellars, W.A. & Johnson, R.B. (1973) Development of childhood allergy in infants fed breast, soy or cow's milk. *Journal of Allergy and Clinical Immunology*, 51, 139–151.

Hashimoto, L., Habita, C., Beressi, J.P. *et al.* (1994) Genetic mapping of a susceptibility locus for insulin-dependent diabetes mellitus on chromosome 11q. *Nature*, 371, 161–164.

Haupt, R., Fears, T.R., Robison, L.L. *et al.* (1994) Educational attainment in long-term survivors of childhood acute lymphoblastic leukemia. *Journal of the American Academy of Child and Adolescent Psychiatry*, 272, 1427–1432.

Heerema, N.A., Sather, H.N., Sensel, M.G. *et al.* (1999) Association of chromosome arm 9p abnormalities with adverse risk in childhood acute lymphoblastic leukemia: a report from the Children's Cancer Group. *Blood*, 94, 1537–1544.

Heiligenstein, E. & Jacobsen, P.B. (1988) Differentiating depression in medically ill children and adolescents. *Journal of the American Academy of Child and Adolescent Psychiatry*, 27, 716–719.

Hemminki, K., Kyyronen, P. & Vaittinen, P. (1999) Parental age as a risk factor of childhood leukemia and brain cancer in offspring. *Epidemiology*, 10, 271–275.

Hoekstra-Weebers, J.E., Jaspers, J.P., Kamps, W.A. & Klip, E.C. (1998) Gender differences in psychological adaptation and coping in parents of pediatric cancer patients, *Psycho-oncology*, 7, 26–36.

Jaworowski, S., Allen, R.C. & Finkelstein, E. (1998) Reflex sympathetic dystrophy in a 12-year-old twin with comorbid conversion disorder in both twins. *Journal of Paediatrics and Child Health*, 34, 581–583.

Julia, J.C., Martorell, A., Armengot, M.A. et al. (1999) Vocal cord dysfunction in a child. *Allergy*, 54, 748–751.

Kaminer, Y. & Robbins, D. (1988) Attempted suicide by insulin overdose in insulin-dependent diabetic adolescents. *Pediatrics*, 81, 526–528.

Kashani, J.H., Rosenberg, T.K. & Reide, J.C. (1989) Developmental perspective in child and adolescent depressive symptoms in a community sample. *American Journal of Psychiatry*, 146, 871–875.

Kerem, E., Reisman, J., Corey, M., Canny, G.J. & Levison, H. (1992) Prediction of mortality in patients with cystic fibrosis. *New England Journal of Medicine*, 326, 1187–1191.

Kihlstrom, J.F. (1994) One hundred years of hysteria. In: *Dissociation: Clinical and Theoretical Perspectives* (eds S.J. Lynn & J.W. Rhue), pp. 365–394. Guilford Press, New York.

Kleinman, A. (1986) *Social Origins of Distress and Disease: Depression Neurasthenia and Pain in Modern China.* Yale University Press, New Haven, CT.

Klepper, S.E. (1991) Effects of an eight-week physical conditioning program on disease signs and symptoms in children with chronic arthritis. *Arthritis Care and Research*, 12, 52–60.

Klinnert, M., Gavin, L.A., Wamboldt, F.S. & Mrazek, D.A. (1992) Marriages with children at medical risk: the transition to parenthood. *Journal of the American Academy of Child and Adolescent Psychiatry*, 31, 334–342.

Koocher, G.P. & O'Malley, J.E. (1981) *The Damocles Syndrome.* McGraw-Hill, New York.

Kosora, E., Thompson, L.L., West, S.G. & Kotzin, B.L. (1996) Analysis of cognitive and psychological deficits in systemic lupus erythematosus patients without overt central nervous system disease. *Arthritis and Rheumatism*, 39, 2035–2045.

Kovacs, M., Feinberg, T.L., Paulauskas, S., Finkelstein, R., Pollock, M. & Crouse-Novak, M. (1985) Initial coping responses and psychosocial characteristics of children with insulin dependent diabetes mellitus. *Journal of Pediatrics*, 106, 827–834.

Kupst, M.J., Schulman, J.L., Maurer, H., Honig, G., Morgan, E. & Fochtman, D. (1984) Coping with pediatric leukemia: A two-year follow-up. *Journal of Pediatric Psychology*, 9, 149–163.

Lacks, S. & White, P. (1990) Morbidity associated with childhood systemic lupus erythematosus. *Journal of Rheumatology*, 17, 941–945.

Larsson, B.S. (1991) Somatic complaints and their relationship to depressive symptoms in Swedish adolescents. *Journal of Child Psychology and Psychiatry*, 32, 821–832.

Leff, A.R. (1988) Neurohumoral regulation of airway contractile responses. *Chest*, 93, 1285–1287.

Liss, D.S., Waller, D.A., Kennard, B.D., McIntire, D., Capra, P. & Stephens, J. (1998) Psychiatric illness and family support in children and adolescents with diabetic ketoacidosis: a controlled study, *Journal of the American Academy of Child and Adolescent Psychiatry*, 37, 536–544.

Love, B., Byrne, C., Roberts, J., Browne, G. & Brown, B. (1987) Adult psychosocial adjustment following childhood injury: the effect of disfigurement. *Journal of Burn Care and Rehabilitation*, 8, 280–285.

Mackie, E., Hill, J., Kondryn, H. & McNally, R. (2000) Adult psychosocial outcomes in long-term survivors of acute lymphoblastic leukaemia and Wilms' tumour: a controlled study. *Lancet*, 355, 1310–1314.

Mannino, D.M., Homa, D.M., Pertowski, C.A. et al. (1998) Surveillance for asthma: United States, 1960–95. *Morbidity and Mortality Weekly Report, CDC Surveillance Summaries/Centers for Disease Control*, 47, 1–27.

Matthew, D.J., Taylor, B., Norman, A.P., Turner, M.W. & Soothill, J.F. (1977) Prevention of eczema. *Lancet*, i, 321–324.

Mattsson, A. (1972) Long-term physical illness in childhood: a challenge to psychosocial adaptation. *Pediatrics*, 50, 801–811.

McKinney, P.A., Parslow, R.C., Gurney, K.A., Law, G.R., Bodansky, H.J. & Williams, R. (1999) Perinatal and neonatal determinants of childhood type 1 diabetes. A case-control study in Yorkshire, UK. *Diabetes Care*, 22, 928–932.

McNichol, K.N., Williams, H.E., Allan, J. & McAndrew, I. (1973) Spectrum of asthma in children. III. Psychological and social components. *British Medical Journal*, 4, 16–20.

Meadow, R. (1982) Management of Munchausen syndrome of proxy. *Archives of Disease in Childhood*, 60, 385–393.

Meadow, R. (1985) Munchausen syndrome by proxy. *Archives of Disease in Childhood*, 57, 92–98.

Meijer, S.A., Sinnema, G., Bijstra, J.O., Mellengbergh, G.J. & Wolters, W.H. (2000) Social functioning in children with chronic illness. *Journal of Child Psychology and Psychiatry*, 41, 309–317.

Miller, B.D. (1987) Depression and asthma: a potentially lethal mixture. *Journal of Allergy and Clinical Immunology*, 80, 481–486.

Miller, J.J. (1998) Specificity of daily fever spikes for systemic arthritis in children: a test of the ILAR/WHO criteria. *Journal of Rheumatology*, 25, 1650–1651.

Millstein, S.G., Adler, N.E. & Irwin, C.E. (1981) Conceptions of illness in young adolescents. *Pediatrics*, 68, 834–839.

Mirvish, I. (1978) Hypnotherapy for the child with chronic eczema. *South African Medical Journal*, 54, 410–411.

Moehle, K.A. & Berg, R.A. (1985) Academic achievement and intelligence test performance in children with cancer at diagnosis and one year later. *Developmental and Behavioral Pediatrics*, 6, 62–64.

Moran, G.S. (1984) Psychoanalytic treatment of diabetic children. In: *The Psychoanalytic Study of the Child* (eds A.J. Solnit, R.S. Eissler & P.B. Neubauer), pp. 407–447. Yale University Press, New Haven, CT.

Mrazek, D.A. (1985) Cystic fibrosis: a systems analysis of psychiatric consequences. *Advances in Psychosomatic Medicine*, 14, 119–135.

Mrazek, D.A. (1992) Disturbed emotional development in severely asthmatic children. In: *Quality of Life in Childhood Asthma* (eds A. West & M.J. Christie), pp. 67–76. Carden, Chichester.

Mrazek, D.A. & Klinnert, M. (1991) Asthma: psychoneuroimmunological considerations. In: *Psychoneuroimmunology II* (eds R. Ader, D.L. Felten & N. Cohen), pp. 1013–1035. Academic Press, Orlando, FL.

Mrazek, D.A., Anderson, I.S. & Strunk, R.C. (1985) Disturbed emotional development of severely asthmatic preschool children. In: *Recent Research in Developmental Psychopathology* (ed. J.E. Stevenson), pp. 81–94. Pergamon Press, Oxford.

Mrazek, D.A., Mrazek, P.B. & Klinnert, M. (1995) The clinical assessment of parenting. *Journal of the American Academy of Child and Adolescent Psychiatry*, 34, 272–282.

Mrazek, D.A., Schuman, W. & Klinnert, M. (1998) Early asthma onset: risk of emotional and behavioral difficulties. *Journal of Child Psychology and Psychiatry*, 39, 247–254.

Mrazek, D.A., Klinnert, M., Mrazek, P. et al. (1999) Prediction of early onset asthma in genetically at risk children. *Journal of Pediatric Pulmonology*, **27**, 89–94.

Nakagawa, Y., Kawaguchi, Y., Twells, R.C. et al. (1998) Fine mapping of the diabetes-susceptibility locus, IDDM4, on chromosome 11q13. *American Journal of Human Genetics*, **63**, 547–556.

Northam, E.A., Anderson, P.J., Werther, G.A., Warne, G.L., Adler, R.G. & Andrewes, D. (1998) Neuropsychological complications of IDDM in children 2 years after disease onset. *Diabetes Care*, **21**, 379–384.

Orr, D.P., Weller, S.C., Satterwhite, B. & Pless, I.B. (1984) Psychosocial implications of chronic illness in adolescence. *Journal of Pediatrics*, **104**, 152–157.

Packer, R.J., Sutton, L.N., Atkins, T.E. et al. (1989) A prospective study of cognitive function in children receiving whole-brain radiotherapy and chemotherapy: 2-year results. *Journal of Neurosurgery*, **70**, 707–713.

Pavlovsky, S., Castano, J., Leiguarda, R. et al. (1983) Neuropsychological study in patients with ALL. *American Journal of Pediatric Hematology*, **5**, 79–86.

Perrin, E.C. & Gerrity, P.S. (1981) There's a demon in your belly: children's understanding of illness. *Pediatrics*, **67**, 841–849.

Petzel, S.V., Bugge, I., Warwick, W.J. & Budd, J.R. (1984) Long term adaptation of children and adolescents with cystic fibrosis: identification of common problems and risk factors. In: *Chronic Illness and Disabilities in Childhood and Adolescence* (ed. R.W. Blum), pp. 413–427. Grune & Stratton, New York.

Pless, I.B. & Roghmann, K.J. (1971) Chronic illness and its consequences: observations based on three epidomiologic surveys. *Journal of Pediatrics*, **79**, 351–359.

Popkin, M.K., Callies, A.L., Lentz, R.D., Colon, E.A. & Sutherland, D.E. (1988) Prevalence of major depression, simple phobia, and other psychiatric disorders in patients with long-standing type I diabetes mellitus. *Archives of General Psychiatry*, **45**, 64–68.

Preston, K. (1969) Depression and skin diseases. *Medical Journal of Australia*, **5**, 326–329.

Prugh, D.G., Straub, E.M., Sands, H.H., Kirschbaum, R.M. & Lenihan, E.A. (1953) A study of the emotional reactions of children and families to hospitalization and illness. *American Journal of Orthopsychiatry*, **23**, 70–106.

Pui, C.H., Boyett, J.M., Relling, M.V. et al. (1999) Sex differences in prognosis for children with acute lymphoblastic leukemia. *Journal of Clinical Oncology*, **17**, 818–824.

Pumariega, A.J., Pursell, J., Spock, A. & Jones, J.D. (1986) Eating disorders in adolescents with cystic fibrosis. *Journal of the American Academy of Child Psychiatry*, **25**, 269–275.

Quinton, D. & Rutter, M. (1976) Early hospitalization and later disturbances of behavior: an attempted replication of Douglas' findings. *Developmental Medicine and Child Neurology*, **18**, 447–459.

Rait, D.S., Ostroff, J.S., Smith, K., Cella, D.F., Tan, C. & Lesko, L.M. (1992) Lives in a balance: perceived family functioning and the psychosocial adjustment of adolescent cancer survivors. *Family Process*, **31**, 383–397.

Riley, W.J., MacLaren, N.K., Krischer, J. et al. (1990) A prospective study of the development of diabetes in relatives of patients with insulin-dependent diabetes. *New England Journal of Medicine*, **323**, 1167–1172.

Riordan, J.R., Rommens, J.M., Kerem, B. et al. (1989) Identification of the cystic fibrosis gene: Cloning and characterization of complementary DNA. *Science*, **245**, 1066–1073.

Rivinus, T.M., Jamison, D.L. & Graham, P.J. (1975) Childhood organic neurological disease presenting as psychiatric disorder. *Archives of Disease in Childhood*, **50**, 115–119.

Rosenecker, J., Schmalix, W.A., Schindelhauer, D., Plank, C. & Reinhardt, D. (1998) Towards gene therapy of cystic fibrosis. *European Journal of Medical Research*, **3**, 149–156.

Ryan, N.D., Puig-Antich, J., Ambrosini, P. et al. (1987) The clinical picture of major depression in children and adolescents. *Archives of General Psychiatry*, **44**, 854–861.

Sabbadini, M.G., Manfredi, A.A., Bozzolo, E. et al. (1999) Central nervous system involvement in systemic lupus erythematosus patients without overt neuropsychiatric manifestations. *Lupus*, **8**, 11–19.

Sabbeth, B.F. & Leventhal, J.M. (1984) Marital adjustment to chronic childhood illness: a critique of the literature. *Pediatrics*, **73**, 762–768.

Sameroff, A.J. (1998) Environmental risk factors in infancy. *Pediatrics*, **102** (5 Suppl. E), 1287–1292.

Sawyer, M., Crettenden, A. & Toogood, I. (1986) Psychological adjustment of families of children and adolescents treated for leukemia. *American Journal of Pediatric Hematology/Oncology*, **8**, 200–207.

Sawyer, M.G., Toogood, I., Rice, M., Haskell, C. & Baghurst, P. (1989) School performance and psychological adjustment of children treated for leukemia. *American Journal of Pediatric Hematology/Oncology*, **11**, 146–152.

Seaquist, E.R., Goetz, F.C., Rich, S. & Barbosa, J. (1989) Familial clustering of diabetic kidney disease. *New England Journal of Medicine*, **320**, 1161–1165.

Silverman (1996) What's new in the treatment of pediatric SLE. *Journal of Rheumatology*, **234**, 1657–1660.

Sly, R.M. & O'Donnell, R. (1997) Stabilization of asthma mortality. *Ann Allergy Asthma Immunol*, **78**, 347–354.

Snyder, S.H. (1980) Brain peptides as neurotransmitters. *Science*, **209**, 976–983.

Snyder, S.H. (1982) Neurotransmitters and CNS disease: schizophrenia. *Lancet*, **ii**, 970–974.

Staab, D., Wenninger, K., Gebert, N. et al. (1998) Quality of life in patients with cystic fibrosis and their parents: what is important besides disease severity? *Thorax*, **53**, 727–731.

Stacey, M.W., Wang, J., Byrd, R.L., Liu, J.M. & Kearns, W.G. (1999) Nuclear receptor co-repressor gene localizes to 17p11.2, a frequently deleted band in malignant disorders. *Genes, Chromosomes and Cancer*, **25**, 191–193.

Steinhausen, H. & Schindler, H. (1981) Psychosocial adaptation in children and adolescents with cystic fibrosis. *Journal of Developmental and Behavioral Pediatrics*, **2**, 74–77.

Steinhausen, H., Schindler, H. & Stephan, H. (1983) Correlates of psychopathology in sick children: an empirical model. *Journal of the American Academy of Child Psychiatry*, **22**, 559–564.

Strunk, R.C., Mrazek, D.A., Wolfson, G.S. & LaBrecque, J.F. (1985) Physiological and psychological characteristics associated with deaths from asthma in childhood: a case–controlled study. *Journal of the American Medical Association*, **254**, 1193–1198.

Strunk, R.C., Fukuhara, J.T., LaBrecque, J.F. & Mrazek, D.A. (1989b) Outcome of long term hospitalization for asthma in children. *Journal of Allergy and Clinical Immunology*, **83**, 17–25.

Strunk, R.C., Mrazek, D.A., Fukuhara, J.T., Masterson, J., Ludwick, S.K. & LaBrecque, J.F. (1989a) Cardiovascular fitness in children with asthma correlates with psychologic functioning of the child. *Pediatrics*, **84**, 460–464.

Taussig, L., Cohen, M. & Sieber, O. Jr (1976) Psychosexual and psychosocial aspects of cystic fibrosis. *Medical Aspects of Human Sexuality*, **10**, 101–102.

Tritt, S.G. & Esses, L.M. (1988) Psychosocial adaptation of siblings of children with chronic medical illnesses. *American Journal of Orthopsychiatry*, **58**, 211–220.

Tsao, B.P. & Wallace, D.J. (1997) Genetics of systemic lupus erythematosus. *Current Opinion in Rheumatology*, **9**, 377–379.

Tsao, B.P., Cantor, R.M., Kalunian, K.C. *et al.* (1997) Evidence for linkage of a candidate chromosome 1 region to human systemic lupus erythematosus. *Journal of Clinical Investigation*, **99**, 725–731.

Ullman, K.C., Moore, R.W. & Reidy, M. (1977) Atopic eczema: a clinical psychiatric study. *Journal of Asthma Research*, **14**, 91–99.

US Department of Health and Human Services (1999) *Mental Health: A Report of the Surgeon General*. US Department of Health and Human Services, Substance Abuse and Mental Health Services Administration, Center for Mental Health Services, National Institutes of Health, National Institute of Mental Health, Rockville, MD.

Vafiadis, P., Grabs, R., Goodyer, C.G., Colle, E. & Polychronakos, C. (1998) A functional analysis of the role of IGF2 in IDDM2-encoded susceptibility to type 1 diabetes. *Diabetes*, **47**, 831–836.

Venters, M. (1981) Familial coping with chronic and severe childhood illness: the case of cystic fibrosis. *Social Science Medicine* [A], **15** (3 Pt. 1), 289–297.

Waber, D.P., Carpentieri, S.C., Klar, N. *et al.* (2000) Cognitive sequelae in children treated for acute lymphoblastic leukemia with dexamethasone or prednisone. *Journal of Pediatric Hematology/Oncology*, **22**, 206–213.

Wallander, J.L., Varni, J.W., Babani, L., Banis, H.T. & Wilcox, K.T. (1988) Children with chronic physical disorders: maternal reports of their psychological adjustment. *Journal of Pediatric Psychology*, **13**, 197–212.

Waterloo, K., Omdal, R. & Mellgree, S.I. (1998) Emotional status in systemic lupus erythematosus. *Scandinavian Journal of Rheumatology*, **27**, 410–414.

Weisz, J.R., Suwanlert, S., Chaiyasit, W., Weiss, B. & Jackson, E.W. (1991) Adult attitudes toward over- and undercontrolled child problems: urban and rural parents and teachers from Thailand and the United States. *Journal of Child Psychology and Psychiatry*, **32**, 645–654.

White, K., Kolman, M.L., Wexler, P., Polin, G. & Winter, R.J. (1984) Unstable diabetes and unstable families: a psychosocial evaluation of diabetic children with recurrent ketoacidosis. *Pediatrics*, **73**, 749–755.

Wilkinson, G. (1987) The influence of psychiatric, psychological and social factors on the control of insulin-dependent diabetes mellitus. *Journal of Psychosomatic Research*, **31**, 277–286.

Zeiger, R.S., Heller, S., Mellon, M., O'Connor, R. & Hamburger, R.N. (1989) Effectiveness of dietary manipulation in the prevention of food allergy in infants. *Journal of Allergy and Clinical Immunology*, **78**, 224–238.

Zielenski, J. & Tsui, L.C. (1995) Cystic fibrosis: genotypic and phenotypic variations. *Annual Review of Genetics*, **29**, 777–807.

49 Psychiatric Aspects of HIV/AIDS in Childhood and Adolescence

Jennifer Havens, Claude Ann Mellins and Joyce S. Hunter

Epidemiological overview of the HIV epidemic as it affects children and adolescents

Because of the steadily increasing rates of HIV infection in women of child-bearing age, HIV/AIDS has become a major worldwide threat to the health and psychosocial well-being of children and adolescents. By the end of 1999, 32.4 million people were living with HIV/AIDS: 14.8 million were women and 1.2 million were children under the age of 15 years (UNAIDS 2000). Despite improved medical treatment options and ongoing prevention efforts, the death rate from AIDS continues to grow and new infections continue to emerge, particularly in women and children. In 1999, 1.1 million women and 470 000 children died from AIDS (56% of the total deaths resulting from AIDS) and 2.3 million women and 570 000 children under the age of 15 years were newly infected with HIV. Nearly half of all people who acquire HIV become infected before they are 25 and die before they are 35 from AIDS-related conditions. These numbers reflect the significant threat of AIDS for children worldwide.

In the USA, the picture is less bleak, although HIV/AIDS continues to take its toll. While the advent of new medical treatments has significantly slowed the AIDS incidence in the USA, as of June 1999, 114 612 women, 3564 youths aged 13–19 years, and 8596 children aged less than 13 years were living with AIDS (Centers for Disease Control and Prevention 1999). Furthermore, between July 1998 and June 1999, among the states with confidential HIV reporting, there were over 6300 new cases of HIV infection in adult women, 786 new cases of HIV infection in youths aged 13–24 and approximately 260 new cases of HIV in children under the age of 13 years.

Over 90% of children with HIV/AIDS worldwide acquired the virus through mother–infant (vertical) transmission from their mothers either during birth or through their mother's breast milk (Centers for Disease Control 1999; UNAIDS 2000). In a recent randomized trial in sub-Saharan Africa, the frequency of breast milk transmission of HIV was 16.2% and the use of breast milk substitutes prevented 44% of infections (Nduati *et al.* 2000). However, the infants from both groups were at similar risk for dying by the age of 2 years, reflecting the limitations of bottle-feeding in many African countries.

In the USA and other developed countries, perinatal transmission of HIV infection has been substantially reduced by the use of zidovudine (AZT) by women during pregnancy and birth. In the absence of zidovudine treatment, vertical transmission rates in the USA ranged from 15 to 30% (Centers for Disease Control 1995). Multisite studies by the Paediatric AIDS Clinical Trials Group found that rates of vertical transmission were reduced to 8% with the administration of AZT during pregnancy (Connor *et al.* 1994). In addition, several recent studies have found that elective caesarean section results in lower perinatal HIV transmission rates (Mandelbrot *et al.* 1998).

Unfortunately, standard medical treatments utilized in the developed world for the prevention of vertical transmission have not been implemented in much of the developing world, where the vast majority of new HIV infections occur. Of the 1.2 million children with HIV infection in the world, approximately 95% are in developing countries (UNAIDS 2000). In developing countries, economic conditions and health infrastructure inadequacies have limited women's access to AZT during pregnancy and thus rates of perinatal transmission continue unabated.

In addition to the direct effects of HIV infection, millions of children worldwide are affected by HIV infection and illness in their family members. By the end of 1999, 11.2 million infected and uninfected children under the age of 15 years were orphaned by their mother's death to AIDS. Many of these children also lost fathers (UNAIDS 2000). Particularly in sub-Saharan Africa, the huge numbers of children growing up without parents represents a major threat to the stability of the region.

In the USA, HIV also continues to cast a pall over a growing number of uninfected children and adolescents living with HIV infection in a parent and/or at risk of losing a parent to the disease. Recent projections are that 75 000–125 000 nationwide will have lost their mothers to AIDS by the year 2000 (Michaels & Levine 1992). While recent pharmacological advances in the treatment of HIV may reduce overall mortality, it is significant that women and ethnic minorities appear to be benefiting less from the life-prolonging impact of these new medications (Shapiro *et al.* 1999). Therefore, the children of these women are still at high risk for losing at least one parent and are clearly 'affected' by the HIV epidemic.

Also, given that at least half of HIV infections occur before the age of 25 years, adolescents remain one of the fastest growing risk groups. In the USA, among adolescent male cumulative AIDS cases, male-to-male transmission (34%) and transfusion of blood products in haemophiliac males prior to the initiation of blood screening (35%) are the most prevalent risk factors. Among adolescent female AIDS cases, heterosexual contact (52%) and intravenous drug users (IDUs; 14%) are the most prevalent risk factors (Centers for Disease Control 1999).

In the USA, children infected and affected by HIV/AIDS are disproportionately from ethnic minorities and the offspring of IDUs. Among women over the age of 13 years with AIDS, 57% are black and 20% are Latina. Intravenous drug use is the primary risk factor for HIV infection in 42% of women with AIDS in the USA; heterosexual transmission from an IDU partner is the risk factor for another 16% (Centers for Disease Control 1999).

Corresponding with the association of HIV and substance abuse in women in the USA, 53% of children under 13 years with AIDS were born to women whose risk factor for HIV infection is their own or their partner's intravenous drug use (Centers for Disease Control 1999). Also corresponding with the demographics of AIDS in women, the majority of paediatric AIDS cases are black (58%) and Latino (23%). Among adolescents ages 13–19 years, 12% of males and 33% of females have injection drug use or sex with an IDU partner as their risk factor for infection. In addition to drug use, the majority of HIV-infected women, adolescents and children live in large urban environments, such as New York City, Miami, Florida, Newark, New Jersey, and San Juan, Puerto Rico, and are typically socioeconomically disadvantaged (Boyd-Franklin et al. 1995; Centers for Disease Control 1999).

Medical treatment issues

The rate of disease progression among children with HIV varies considerably, but is typically more rapid in children than in adults, regardless of the mode of infection (Mellins et al. 1998). In the first decade of the HIV epidemic, perinatally HIV-infected children had a considerably shortened life expectancy. In 1995 in the USA, 75–90% of perinatally infected children were expected to have symptoms by 1 year of age; 25–30% would have clinical AIDS. Two relatively distinct courses were described: a rapidly progressive course occurring in 20% of children, and a more common slowly progressive course. The death rate was greatest during the first year of life (>15%), and slowed after 2 years with many children remaining stable throughout their first 10 years of life (Mellins et al. 1998).

In the USA, advances in antiretroviral therapy, such as the introduction of protease inhibitors in 1996 and the development of combination regimens with greatly superior efficacy in viral suppression, have provided substantial clinical benefits to HIV-infected children both in terms of life span and quality of life. In general, the principles of HIV treatment are the same for HIV-infected children, adolescents and adults. However, there are some unique considerations for HIV-infected infants, children and adolescents, including possible prenatal exposure to HIV and maternal antiretroviral treatment, developmental and biomedical differences in children on clinical parameters used in assessing severity of paediatric HIV disease and treat-

ment needs, and issues of adherence to treatment by children and adolescents (HIV/AIDS Treatment Information Services 2000).

The use of combination therapy, including protease inhibitors, has led to substantial improvements in neurodevelopment, growth and immunological and/or virological status. Combination therapy is now recommended for all infants, children and adolescents who are being treated with antiretroviral agents (HIV/AIDS Treatment Information Services 2000). By 1999, the median life span for perinatally HIV-infected children was 8.6–13 years; between one-third and two-thirds were expected to survive at least to 13 years of age (American Academy of Pediatrics 1999).

While treatment advances have the potential to prolong life span and reduce the incidence of vertical transmission, these advances are only available on a widespread basis to children and parents living in the developed world. On an international basis, HIV infection in children continues unabated. In the developed world, rising rates of HIV infection in women are reflected in growing numbers of children living under the shadow of parental HIV illness. This chapter provides a review of the mental health issues associated with HIV infection in children and adolescents, as well as those issues associated with living with parental HIV illness.

HIV in children and adolescents infected through vertical transmission

Neurodevelopmental sequelae of HIV infection

From the beginning of the epidemic, there have been consistent findings of significant neurological, developmental, cognitive and language deficits in HIV-infected children (Epstein et al. 1988; Brouwers et al. 1990; Mellins et al. 1994; Belman et al. 1996; Englund et al. 1996; Coplan et al. 1998; Drotar et al. 1999). In general, the severity of neurological and neuropsychological compromise increases with the severity of HIV-related illness; the children with the most significant delays have higher viral loads and the most severe non-neurological health-related symptoms (Pulsifer & Aylward 2000).

Two relatively distinct neurodevelopmental patterns have been described: progressive encephalopathy and static encephalopathy (Epstein et al. 1988; Brouwers et al. 1991). Progressive encephalopathy, corresponding with the AIDS dementia complex in adults, is characterized by the loss of developmental milestones in young children and by declining IQ scores and increasing difficulties with language, attention, concentration and memory in older children. This neurodevelopmental pattern is a direct effect of HIV on the central nervous system and is associated with a poor prognosis. Static encephalopathy, characterized by non-progressive deficits in cognitive, motor and/or language function, is not directly attributable to HIV and is most likely associated with non-HIV risk factors. For many HIV-infected children, these factors may include prenatal drug exposure, prematurity, low birth weight and heritable or environmentally mediated impairment (Epstein *et al.* 1988; Mellins *et al.* 1994).

Recent advances in antiretroviral treatment have the potential to ameliorate the development and progression of HIV-related central nervous system compromise. Zidovudine treatment alone has been shown to be associated with improvements in cognitive and neuropsychological functioning (Pizzo *et al.* 1988; Brouwers *et al.* 1990; McKinney *et al.* 1991; Brady *et al.* 1996). Current treatments, which combine several antiviral agents to achieve near total viral suppression, have the potential to reduce the prevalence and severity of central nervous system disease.

Diagnosis and treatment of AIDS encephalopathy in children

HIV-related encephalopathy is a common sequelae of HIV infection in children, reported in 21% of a cohort of 128 perinatally infected children followed in a national multisite study (Cooper *et al.* 1998). In addition to the loss of developmental milestones in young children and the declining IQ scores and increasing difficulties with language, attention, concentration and memory in older children, encephalopathic children manifest apathy, decreased social behaviour and symptoms of depression and irritability as compared to non-encephalopathic children (Moss *et al.* 1994, 1996).

Recognition of dementia-related behavioural sequelae and accurate differential diagnosis is clinically important for several reasons. First, parents and medical staff can misinterpret a child's increasing fatigue, decreased interest in and resistance to regular activities and regressive behaviour as oppositional behaviour or as depressive disorder. This can result in efforts to encourage the child to alter their behaviour when in actuality the behaviour represents sequelae of the disease process and is not within the child's control. Second, early in the presentation of AIDS dementia in children, stimulants such as methylphenidate can be very helpful to them in raising their energy level and improving their quality of life (Havens & McCaskill 1999). Third, progressive organic involvement in children is an important prognostic sign, generally accompanied by severe immunocompromise and signalling the endstage of the disease. This is an important time to shift gears in the work with children and their families to help them prepare for the final stages of the child's life.

Emotional and behavioural disorder in HIV-infected children

To date, the literature on emotional and behavioural disorders in HIV-infected children is extremely limited. In one of the few studies focusing on psychiatric disorder in HIV-infected children, Havens *et al.* (1994) found high rates of attention deficit hyperactivity disorder (ADHD): five out of 24 HIV-infected children (21%) met diagnostic criteria on a structured psychi-

atric interview. However, these rates were not different from those in a matched control group of children from similar backgrounds (children living in foster care who had been born to women who had used drugs during pregnancy).

While several other studies have also suggested a high prevalence of symptoms compatible with ADHD in HIV-infected children (Corsi *et al.* 1991; Hittleman *et al.* 1993), it is important to exclude other psychiatric disorders that may present with disruptive behaviours. Mood, anxiety and adjustment disorders in addition to bereavement reactions in children could easily mimic aspects of ADHD or may represent comorbid diagnoses. Early clinical reports suggested that HIV-infected children were at high risk for anxiety, depression, guilt and low self-esteem (Speigal & Mayers 1991; Wiener & Septimus 1991). Englund *et al.* (1996) reported that 13.3% of HIV-infected children between 3 months and 18 years of age manifested abnormalities of behaviour or affect, the most common being difficulties with social interaction. Tardieu *et al.* (1995) reported that 30% of HIV-infected children in their sample had moderate symptoms of anxiety, depression or behaviour problems. Havens *et al.* (1994) also found that HIV-infected school-aged children were found to have more symptoms of anxiety on self-report instruments than the uninfected children in their sample. Likely factors contributing to anxiety include higher levels of psychosocial stressors associated with HIV infection, such as frequent illness and hospitalization, concerns over health status, and family illnesses and instability.

It is important to note that none of the studies to date have found direct associations between HIV and emotional and behavioural problems. The complex backgrounds of HIV-infected children increase their risk for behavioural problems and also makes it difficult to establish causal relationships between HIV and behavioural outcomes, given the association of HIV with other high-risk factors (e.g. poverty, prenatal drug exposure, birth complications, family disruption). Features associated with prenatal drug exposure, such as prematurity, low birth weight and heritable parental psychopathology, may actually be more potent mediators of mental health problems in HIV-infected children than HIV itself (Havens *et al.* 1994; Mellins *et al.* 1994; Campbell 1997).

Moss *et al.* (1998) found that among a sample of 24 school-aged HIV-infected children, the majority had depression, anxiety and behavioural problem scores in the normal range. However, those who experienced more negative life events showed more psychological and behavioural problems. In the USA, the fact that the majority of HIV-infected children reside in inner-city environments suggests that they are at risk for significant life events including economic hardships, inadequate housing, inner-city violence and social discrimination (Levenson & Mellins 1992) and so related emotional and behavioural outcomes. Regardless of causality, there is clearly a constellation of factors associated with HIV infection in children that place them at risk for mental health problems and that need to be considered by mental health and education providers.

Psychotherapeutic issues in helping children cope with HIV illness

Communication about health

Children's age and/or developmental level dictate their capacity to understand the meaning of their HIV illness. Preschool-aged and young school-aged children generally cannot grasp the concept of chronic illness and understand episodes of HIV-related illness as discrete and unconnected events. Because of the stigma associated with HIV infection and young children's inability to contain information discretely, they are usually not informed by family members or health care providers about their HIV infection. As children age, communication about the nature of their health problems becomes more important, both to secure their participation in their health regimes and to facilitate the adjustment to living with HIV. Often, older school-aged children who are not directly informed of their diagnosis will deduce it from clues presenting in the medical care environment or elsewhere. A lack of open communication in these cases serves to isolate the child from adult help with issues related to HIV. These issues include coping with secrecy, stigma and potential rejection by peers, coping with chronic illness, and anxiety about the future (Boyd-Franklin et al. 1995).

Parents or other family caregivers often resist communication with the HIV-positive child about his or her health in an effort to protect the child from emotional distress (Mellins & Ehrhardt 1994). Often entangled with this motivation are one or more other factors: the adult's own fear of experiencing more intense pain about the child's diagnosis; parental fears about disclosing their own HIV infection through disclosure of the child's infection and/or parental guilt about having transmitted the virus to the child and their own HIV risk behaviours (e.g. sexual behaviour, drug use); and concerns that the child will disclose family secrets about HIV in undesirable ways.

While for adult family caregivers and health care providers the specific diagnosis of HIV is often a highly charged overwhelming element in their efforts to communicate to the child about health issues, it is in fact only a single component. The child may be more concerned about medications, medical appointments and procedures associated with a chronic health condition, or with impingement on functioning. Establishment of effective communication with the child on the broad range of health-related issues is of great importance. When the efforts of family caregivers and health professionals are not achieving this goal, a therapist may need to intervene. The starting point must be listening to the child to ascertain what the child knows and fears, and what information he or she actually wants. Often the child is seeking an admixture of medical data and affective material. One useful technique is to work with the child on making a list of questions. These questions provide a structure for adult responses, and help to assure that the child's needs frame the communication process.

Adherence to medical regimens

HIV-infected children, like those with many other chronic illnesses, may need to adhere to complicated medication regimens, attend numerous medical appointments and undergo frequent diagnostic procedures. While the use of antiretroviral therapies has resulted in improved life expectancy for HIV-infected children (Abrams & Nicholas 1998), these therapies require patients to follow arduous regimens that can interfere with everyday lifestyle (Katzenstein 1997). In a recent clinical trial of protease inhibitors, 30% of participating children discontinued the prescribed medications (Falkenberg 1999). Little is known about treatment adherence in HIV-infected children, although these results correspond with studies in other chronic diseases, including adult HIV. Typically, 40–50% of children do not use medications as prescribed (Becker et al. 1972). Even brief episodes of missed medication doses can permanently undermine HIV treatment (Macilwain 1997).

In studies of other childhood chronic diseases (e.g. asthma, cancer, diabetes) a combination of child, caregiver and provider psychosocial characteristics has been associated with adherence, including caregiver health, parenting style, child and caregiver knowledge of disease and treatment, family functioning and resources, satisfaction with medical care, provider–patient relationships, and child emotional and behavioural problems (Johnson 1980; Manne et al. 1993; Auslander et al. 1997; Bender et al. 1998).

Given the potential threats to each of these areas among HIV-infected children, they are at risk for non-adherence to treatment. Furthermore, the stigma and discrimination experienced by an HIV-infected child and their family may further complicate adherence to medications that must be taken throughout the day, often when the child is in school (Armistad et al. 1998). Many HIV-infected children are not told their diagnosis, which can further impede their co-operation with treatment. Moreover, HIV medications often have unpleasant tastes or side-effects. Engaging in a behaviour with noxious consequences for future health benefits is difficult for many adults; it is even harder for young children who are functioning at a concrete level of thinking, with limited future orientation.

Effective communication with the child about his or her health is the best foundation for securing the child's participation in these activities. Many families will need considerable support to administer the complexly scheduled medication for the child, and in managing the child's potential opposition to taking medication. Behaviour modification techniques, and especially positive reinforcement, may be very helpful to families in dealing with these issues. Offering the child as much control as possible ('Which pill do you want to take first?') may also minimize struggles over medication.

Promotion of optimal development

As is the case for adults, the mental health issues for infected children change over the course of the disease. There are an increasing number of HIV-infected children who remain relatively symptom-free for long periods of time. They may not know their diagnosis and their lives may be relatively unaffected by illness. However, they may be very stressed by the illness of a parent, by substance abuse in the family, by disrupted placements and ruptured attachments, or any of the other problems which so often plague the families at highest risk for HIV (see below). Interventions for these problems and attention to promotion of the child's optimal development may be of more relevance in his or her mental health care than a narrow focus on HIV (Rosen *et al.* 1997; Ryan *et al.* 1997).

Educational issues

Part of optimal development is capacity for adequate school functioning. All too often, the various systems that should serve the HIV-infected child—the family, child welfare agencies, foster agencies, school and health care institutions—fail to assure that the child's education needs are met. Given the prevalence of HIV-related encephalopathy, neuropsychological problems and multiple medical appointments that interfere with school attendance, HIV-infected children are at high risk for school-related problems. HIV-infected children require regular psychoeducational evaluations—to monitor possible deterioration. Teachers may not always know about a child's HIV infection, given rules of confidentiality. They may misinterpret frequent absence and potential lack of motivation as reflecting a lack of interest or commitment to school. HIV-infected children may require considerable special education resources. As their health deteriorates, home-based education may be necessary (Haike *et al.* 1991). It is important to the general well-being of these children that as normal an education experience as possible, including social experiences, be maintained.

Issues in adolescence

For HIV-infected children who live to adolescence, the normal developmental challenges of this stage, including puberty, sexuality and the desire to 'fit in' or be 'normal' are seriously complicated by HIV disease. The detrimental effects of HIV on growth and pubertal development pose significant challenges for the growing number of congenitally infected young people living into their teenage years. Nevertheless, as congenitally infected children move through adolescence and become sexually active, they require significant support in managing the complex issues of integrating healthy sexual development with their HIV infection. Open and honest communication around patterns of sexual behaviour, disclosure to sexual partners and strategies for the prevention of the spread of HIV are essential.

Therapeutic support for the child and family as death approaches

With disease progression, children must confront the physical and mental decline associated with AIDS. As they approach late stage illness, they and their families must confront the terminal nature of the disease. Often, families are overwhelmed at this stage and have difficulty communicating with the child about issues related to prognosis and death. Sensitive mental health intervention by clinicians with an ongoing relationship with the child and their family can provide a place for a child to express the inevitable anxieties and fears about separation from family members and dying, and to help the child, if old enough, to communicate their wishes about medical treatment. Special attention must be paid to issues in pain management at this stage, particularly for young children with limited ability to communicate information to health care providers effectively (Havens *et al.* 1999).

As children approach the end of life, they may experience confusion and great anxiety. Parents or other adult family caregivers, and perhaps even medical and nursing staff, frequently find communicating with the child about the approach of death so difficult and overwhelming that they avoid it. Despite this, dying children need a venue in which the impending death can be discussed. They require an opportunity to express their thoughts and fears, and to receive reassurance. For many pre-adolescent children, separation from family, and especially from a primary attachment figure, is the most worrisome aspect of death. A therapist may be able to draw on elements in the family's spiritual or religious belief system to sustain hope of continuity of attachment between the deceased and surviving family members (Ryan *et al.* 1997; Havens *et al.* 1999).

Psychopharmacological management in HIV-infected children and adolescents

Psychopharmacological management of psychiatric disorder, delirium and dementia in HIV-infected children is often a necessary component of adequate treatment. However, it is complicated by drug–drug interactions with antiretroviral medications used to treat HIV disease (an issue in all HIV-infected children undergoing such treatment) and potential central nervous system impairment secondary to HIV infection (a particular issue in those children with advanced HIV disease). Guidance with psychotropic medications in paediatric HIV tends to be analogous to geriatric psychopharmacology, where dosage should be initiated at doses lower than standard treatment and titration upward should be slow and carefully monitored.

When evaluating children with behavioural syndromes who are treated with antimicrobial, antifungal and/or antiviral agents, potential neuropsychiatric side-effects must be included in the differential diagnosis, because many drugs commonly used in the management of HIV disease have such side-effects. When planning pharmacological treatment of HIV-infected children on antiretroviral medication, potential drug interactions must be taken into consideration (Sahai 1996). Of particular importance in drug interactions is the family of cytochrome P450 isoenzymes, which are responsible for the metabolism of many psychotropic medications and antiretrovirals, especially the protease inhibitors. Other HIV-related medications, including antimicrobial and antifungal medications used in treatment and prophylaxis, also interact with cytochrome P450 isoenzymes. It is important when initiating treatment with psychoactive medications to review the metabolism of the medication(s) with the entire treatment regimen to identify interactions and contraindications. Unfortunately, the paediatric psychopharmacologist treating HIV-infected children is often in unexplored and undocumented territory, so treatment should proceed cautiously and with frequent monitoring (Heylen & Miller 1996a,b; Fauci et al. 1999; Oleske et al. 1999).

In a case series, Havens & McCaskill (1999) described the psychostimulant treatment of 12 HIV-infected children and adolescents, eight with ADHD and four with HIV-related dementia. Two-thirds of the children tolerated psychostimulants with good efficacy as measured by the Efficacy Index of the Clinical Global Impressions. The maintenance dosage of methylphenidate ranged from 0.2 to 1.2 mg/kg, and the one child on dexamphetamine required 0.6 mg/kg. Four of the 12 children treated (three out of the ADHD sample) experienced adverse side-effects precluding their continuation of the methylphenidate. While the neuropsychiatric adverse effects argue for caution in the psychostimulant treatment of this population, such treatment should not be withheld when clinically indicated. Two out of the three children who could not tolerate methylphenidate were managed with clonidine. The successful use of clonidinde in the treatment of behavioural symptoms in a preschool-aged child with HIV encephalopathy was also described in a case study (Cesena 1995).

Acquired HIV infection in adolescence

The fact that a large number of HIV-infected adults learn of their diagnosis in their 20s suggests primary HIV infection occurs during adolescence (Centers for Disease Control 1999). There are several groups of adolescents who are at particularly high risk for HIV infection. These include teenagers living in poverty in inner-city environments where substance abuse is endemic; adolescents with substance abuse problems; gay and bisexual youth; youth with psychiatric disorders; and homeless and street youth. Adolescents acquiring HIV are at risk for a range of mental health problems related to their specific risk factors for HIV infection, premorbid conditions, and ramifications of having the disease itself. Risk factors for HIV infection in adolescence are described below as well as the corresponding mental health issues.

Inner-city racial and ethnic minority teenagers

In economically depressed areas of inner cities, teenagers of colour living in poverty have been overrepresented among AIDS cases, particularly young heterosexual females (Centers for Disease Control 1999b,c; New York City Department of Health 1999). Many inner-city adolescents engage in unsafe sexual behaviour, such as inconsistent contraceptive use and concurrent substance use. Risk factors that have been associated with ado-

lescent risky sexual behaviour include poverty, stress, family disruption, exposure to substance use, and early onset of sexual activity (Hogan & Kitagawa 1983; Hofferth et al. 1987; Walter et al. 1991). Early onset of sexual intercourse among adolescents of colour is well documented. Studies of inner-city youth have estimated sexual initiation at a mean age of 12–14 years (Brooks-Gunn & Frustenberg 1989; Orr et al. 1989; Keller et al. 1991; Paikoff 1995), with more than half of high school students having engaged in sexual intercourse prior to graduation (Kann et al. 1998). Engaging in sexual activity before the age of 15 has been related to unprotected sex, multiple partners, exposure to sexually transmitted diseases (STDs) and pregnancy (Walter et al. 1991; Smith 1997). Immaturity of the reproductive organs and immune systems of adolescents increases their risk of contracting STDs including HIV (Morris et al. 1993); adolescents now account for one-third of STD cases reported nationally (Kann et al. 1998). High rates of unprotected intercourse and STDs are both linked to an increased risk of contracting HIV (Wasserheit 1992).

Substance use

Drug use also tends to begin early in ethnic minority inner-city youth, often before the age of 14; in one study, 13 and 14 year olds reported using an average of three to four different drugs (Adger 1992). As adolescents mature, the proportion who experiment with sex and drugs increases. Substance use is considered to be part of a cluster of problem behaviours that occur during adolescence (Jessor & Jessor 1977) and therefore is likely to be related to behaviours that put adolescents at risk for HIV disease. For example, substance use increases the risk of HIV both directly, in the case of injected drugs, and indirectly, through disinhibition leading to unsafe sexual behaviours. Roger et al. (1998), in the REACH study of HIV-infected adolescents, reported that 14% of females and more than 25% of males reported drinking alcohol during the past 3 months, and 7% of females and 20% of males reported using hard drugs during that same period.

Homelessness

Many HIV-infected adolescents are homeless or living on the streets (Clatts & Davis 1999). In the USA, according to the US General Accounting Office (1989), it is estimated that 1–2 million youth are living on the streets. Many of the youth spend their time in and around bus terminals and known cruising areas (both heterosexual and homosexual). On the streets, with no employable skills and with their bodies as their only commodity, many homeless girls and boys often become part of the street economy and turn to prostitution in order to survive. Many of them are gay, lesbian or bisexual. Many use drugs and alcohol to cope with working in the sex trade and manage the constant stresses of day-to-day living on the streets (Hunter & Schaecher 1992). A vicious cycle is then established as they begin to trade in risky sex for drugs (Hunter & Schaecher 1992; Hunter &

Haymes 1997), increasing their risk for poor health outcomes, such as hepatitis, tuberculosis, STDs and HIV infection.

Gay and bisexual youth

Among 13–24-year-old males, 51% of all AIDS cases in 1998 were among young men who have sex with men (Centers for Disease Control 1999); gay and bisexual youth are overrepresented in this group (Centers for Disease Control 1999). Gay and bisexual male youth are at risk for HIV infection, not only because of the high prevalence of HIV among potential sexual partners, but also because heterosexism and homophobia and, for youth of racial and ethnic minority, racism make the process of identity development for gay and bisexual youth extremely difficult. Difficulties with identity development have been associated with risk behaviour in gay and bisexual youth, and therefore with HIV infection itself (Rotheram-Borus et al. 1995; Rosario et al. 1997).

An essential part of adolescence for all youth is the development of a personal and social identity, which includes the development of sexual identity (D'Augelli 1996; Hunter 1996; Hunter & Mallon 2000). Most self-identified gay and bisexual youth come into awareness of their sexual orientation in early adolescence. For gay youth, the process of developing a sense of self, coming out, and finding a supportive group of peers is extremely difficult and, for those who become infected, is further compounded by the stigma of HIV/AIDS itself.

Recent school-based studies have found high rates of suicide among gay, lesbian and bisexual youth (Garofalo et al. 1998; Remafedi et al. 1998). Youth who choose not to hide their sexual orientation or whose sexual orientation is discovered are often faced with negative responses: verbal harassment, sexual assault and sometimes violent reactions from family, friends, peers or strangers (Hunter & Schaecher 1987; Hunter 1990). Having limited options when they need support, many of these young people turn to alcohol and drug use as a means to cope with isolation and rejection.

Youth with psychiatric disorders

A number of research studies have found that self-esteem, self-efficacy and mental health are directly related to early onset of sexual activity, unsafe sex and the inability to change behaviours in HIV prevention programmes (Hofferth et al. 1987; Rotheram-Borus et al. 1991, 1995; Walter et al. 1991). Among non-clinical samples of urban teenagers, higher rates of depression were associated with early sexual activity (Smith 1997). Adolescents with psychiatric disorders are at increased risk for HIV infection because of impaired judgement, poor problem-solving ability, impulsivity, low self-esteem, self-destructive behaviours, drug and alcohol use, increased sexual activities and poor interpersonal relationships (Brown et al. 1997). Thus, many youth engaged in risk behaviours associated with their HIV-infection because of premorbid mental health problems (Hoffman et al. 1999).

Psychosocial issues for HIV-infected adolescents

In working with all HIV-infected youth, a solid understanding of adolescent development is critical (Hoffman et al. 1999). It has been well documented that adolescent development is characterized by substantial physical growth, cognitive change and transformation, as well as social and cultural challenges. During this period, youth are adjusting to physical, emotional and sexual maturation, ranging from the onset of puberty and the emergence of secondary sexual characteristics to the achievement of full maturity. This is a period that elicits a wide range of emotions (Brooks-Gunn & Paikoff 1993), as youth must master a series of developmental tasks in order to proceed to the next stage of development. These tasks include development of self-esteem and interpersonal skills, as well as the management of social and sexual roles. Mastery of these tasks is essential for an adolescent's well-being. Furthermore, as youth move through this period towards adulthood, their basic developmental and psychosocial needs include being valued as a member of a group, receiving social support, participating in caring relationships, acquiring skills to cope adaptively with everyday life, and believing in a future with real opportunities (Hamburg 1990). For youth who enter this period under adverse circumstances with prior deprivation or for whom there is any interference with the developmental process at this stage, this period can be problematic, with negative behaviours such as school drop-out, drug abuse, early or unintended pregnancy, mental health problems and suicide (Hamburg 1990).

Many HIV-infected adolescents have already experienced significant hardships prior to their diagnosis, including poverty, violence and abandonment (Balfer et al. 1988; Falloon et al. 1989; Ryan et al. 1997). They are at high risk for mental health problems and difficulties negotiating adolescent developmental tasks. HIV infection itself can then pose another challenge to each area of adolescent development.

Development of a healthy self-identity is challenged by HIV infection for many adolescents. Clinical reports indicate that many HIV-infected adolescents see themselves as infectious people, feel contemptuous of themselves for this reason, and thus struggle with low self-esteem (Hunter & Schaecher 1992; Hunter & Haymes 1997). A normative adolescent development task is a healthy separation and individuation from parents. For HIV-infected youth, the process of developing an adult identity gets distorted and delayed. Reliance on parents or other adult family members for health care may lead to regression and difficulty seeing oneself as a young adult.

For young people, disclosing their status to others can be traumatic. They have to decide who to tell and when, if they have that choice. Many HIV-infected youth fear rejection from family, peers and friends more than they do the illness itself (Wiener et al. 1998). For gay youth, disclosing their HIV status can be threatening because it may mean coming out as gay; for others, disclosure of drug use or pregnancy may be the issue.

While HIV among young gay men of racial and ethnic minority is still increasing (Valleroy et al. 2000), the face of the

HIV/AIDS epidemic is changing, with more heterosexual young females becoming infected. Clinical data reveal that many adolescent girls with HIV infection are identified during screening for pregnancy or when they give birth (Rotheram-Borus *et al.* 1996). While the challenge for them is the same as for other youth living with HIV (e.g. coping with a potentially fatal illness and the stigma of HIV/AIDS disease) these girls must also cope with the social stigma and burden of teenage pregnancy. The role of motherhood at an early age generates stress, for which the young mother lacks coping and parenting skills in order to deal with the multitude of issues which arise and which often lead to negative consequences. Even though she may be physically mature enough to have baby at this time, social, emotional and cognitive development are still underway. Adolescent girls will need to access and negotiate a health care system, not only for themselves but, if they are pregnant or have a baby, for the child as well. Teenage HIV-infected parents must deal with issues of illness, death and child custody at a time when they are only just developing more basic coping skills.

All infected youth, whether they have physical symptoms or not, will need help in understanding the nature of the virus, their illness and the importance of adhering to medical regimens. However, many adolescents are still largely in concrete stages of cognitive development and have difficulty understanding the full implications of their infection. They may deny the presence of the disease and its symptoms (Hunter & Schaecher 1992). Furthermore, many are not ready for the responsibility of caring for their health, particularly adhering to medication regimens. For adolescents, impulsivity and the desire to fit in with peers often leads to poor adherence to medication for many chronic illnesses including asthma and diabetes. Unfortunately, the HIV medication regimens are particularly arduous. HIV-infected adolescents are at particular risk for non-adherence and poor health care (Wiener *et al.* 1998).

Psychiatric disorders

While it has been recognized that HIV-infected adolescents are at risk for experiencing many stressful events as they negotiate this period of their lives, and that many of the factors that placed them at risk for HIV infection in the first place also place them at risk for future psychiatric disorders and problems with psychosocial functioning, the literature on psychiatric aspects of HIV disease in adolescents, as in children, is extremely limited. Clinical reports suggest that HIV-infected adolescents are at high risk for mental health problems (Ryan *et al.* 1997; Wiener *et al.* 1998). Case studies of HIV-positive adolescents indicate a high prevalence of anxiety, depression and bipolar disorder (Hoffman *et al.* 1999). Studies of HIV-infected adolescents reveal rates of affective disorder ranging from 25 to 44% and histories of sexual abuse ranging from 26 to 50% (Kissinger *et al.* 1997; Pao *et al.* 2000). It is also important to note that the mental health issues described above for perinatally HIV-infected children (e.g. central nervous system and neuropsychological ef-fects of HIV disease, issues of death and dying, etc.) are also present for adolescents.

Regardless of mode of transmission, one of the major goals in working with youth who live with HIV is to encourage a better quality of life by helping them develop strategies to deal with their illness and the stressful life events that they experience and will encounter in the future, and by helping them develop a support system. Eventually, these young people may have to address specific planning around death and coping with the end-stage disease.

Secondary prevention among HIV-infected youth must also be addressed, so that these youth do not reinfect themselves or infect others. Issues for young people with HIV/AIDS, such as sexual behaviour, communication and negotiation, are very important in secondary prevention. HIV prevention education must address the underlying reasons for unsafe behaviours and focus on ways of motivating youth to engage in preventive behaviours (Hunter & Haymes 1997).

Mental health issues in children living with parental HIV illness

Mental health issues related to familial HIV illness

Children and adolescents, both infected and uninfected, are often also 'affected' by HIV disease in a family member. The uninfected children of HIV-infected parents are typically ignored by health care systems, even though they are at significant risk for their own mental health problems. The mental health issues associated with HIV illness in families evolve over the dynamic course of HIV illness, which moves through specific predictable psychosocial stages, roughly paralleling the natural history of the disease (Havens *et al.* 1996). These stages begin with diagnosis of HIV infection and continue through illness progression, late-stage illness, death and reconfiguration of the family with the children in new care arrangements.

Children may exhibit a variety of responses to parental HIV diagnosis, illness or loss at any stage in this process. These responses may be characterized as one or more of the following:

1 normative responses requiring supportive counselling and/or increased access to existing social supports;

2 responses complicated by developmental histories of poor or disrupted attachment and/or trauma (particularly common in children also affected by parental drug addiction), indicating a need for individual and/or family psychotherapy; and

3 exacerbations of pre-existing psychiatric disorder or precipitations of new onset disorder, in which syndrome-specific treatment must be among the interventions (Ryan *et al.* 1997; Havens *et al.* 1999).

Issues in differential diagnosis within the stage model of HIV illness will be reviewed below.

Mental health care of children through stages of HIV illness in the parent

Diagnosis and disclosure of HIV

When a diagnosis of HIV infection is made, it typically engenders anxiety about health and anticipatory grief for a potentially foreshortened future. When the diagnosed individual is a parent, these issues are compounded by concerns about the care of children in the future and by questions of communication with children and adolescents about HIV.

Infected parents frequently withhold information about their HIV diagnosis from their children. Most do not tell children prior to early or mid-adolescence (Mellins & Ehrhardt 1994). Even in the absence of direct communication, many children and teenagers develop their own suspicions about the parent's health problems from clues such as medications, symptoms or multiple medical appointments. Children may experience a great deal of distress, suspecting that a parent is struggling with HIV-related illness, yet because they are not 'supposed to know' they remain unable to reach out for adult support and reassurance.

Disclosure of a family member's HIV status to a child is often misunderstood as a discrete event that can be accomplished as a single communication. It is more appropriately handled as an ongoing process, with new information provided with any change in parental health status. Not only the content of the information communicated to the child but also the emotional tone with which it is conveyed will have an effect on the young person's understanding of the meaning of the information (Havens *et al.* 1996).

Moreover, the child's developmental level may limit ability to absorb complex affectively laden material. A school-aged child will normatively cope with difficult information about a parent's illness by denial, and may opt 'not to know' this threatening fact much of the time. Under stress, the school-aged child may revert to magical thinking that the virus can be wished away. Adolescents do not normatively defend themselves against knowledge of parental HIV by magical thinking or absolute denial, but may rigidly compartmentalize this information so as not to have to face it (Ryan *et al.* 1997).

Parents and other adult caregivers of the HIV-affected child should be counselled about the importance of developmentally appropriate communication about the parent's health. The child's need for the information and readiness to receive it must be accorded priority in deciding what information to communicate and when to disclose it. It is important for the adult to be honest, while respecting the child's coping mechanisms, including adaptive denial. The family's established style of communication about emotionally charged information may not be sufficiently flexible to allow for complete disclosure, but may be able to tolerate communication of part of the truth without specifying the precise diagnosis ('Mommy has an infection in her blood. She's taking medicine to keep her healthy'). Adults should be counselled to provide children with realistic reassurance about the parent's health, and about their own future care and security. HIV-negative children may worry that they themselves are infected because their parent is, and should be assured that they and their siblings are uninfected. In cases where there is uncertainty about a child's serostatus or where additional reassurance is indicated, HIV testing can be very helpful.

Other therapeutic issues that arise for children and adolescents learning about their parent's HIV diagnosis include fear for the parent's health, and anxiety about potential separation from or loss of their parent. Shame and a sense of social isolation caused by the stigmatization of HIV are also common responses. Because the child's self-esteem is often dependent on identification with the parent, the HIV diagnosis may be felt by the child as detracting from his or her own self-worth. It is important to explore carefully with children their understanding of the meaning of parental illness and to provide ongoing support to help them cope effectively with parental HIV infection (Ryan *et al.* 1997).

Progression of HIV illness

As parental HIV disease progresses, children are confronted with deterioration in the parent's ability to function and separations because of hospitalizations. At this stage, children and adolescents manifest one or more normative emotional and behavioural responses to parental illness progression. In general, the distinction of normative from problematic responses is the extent of the response and its effect on the child's functioning. For a toddler, some increase in separation protest may be normative, while a more intensified inability to separate would be problematic; some increase in tantrums is to be expected, while extremely disruptive behaviour is a warning sign. Similarly, school-aged children may experience a minimal to moderate decline in school performance, but a precipitous decline is an indicator of more significant difficulty in coping with the parent's illness.

The importance of communication with children and adolescents about parental illness and its impact on family life increases as HIV disease progresses. Normative emotional and behavioural responses can be complicated when children experience a parent's physical, cognitive or functional decline without accurate information about illness and prognosis. The normal sadness, anger and/or anxiety experienced by children living with an ill parent can be exacerbated by the need to manage these feeling without support from adults who are unable to allow open communication about their illness.

Given the high-risk backgrounds of many HIV-affected families, children's responses to the parent's illness may also be complicated by underlying psychiatric disorder, developmental difficulties in the child's attachment to parent, and/or difficulties in family environment. When working with families affected by both drug use and HIV, it is important to assess carefully children presenting with symptoms in response to parental illness; the attribution of symptomatology to HIV-related stressors alone is often clinically inappropriate (Havens *et al.* 1996).

With the pressure of increasing parental illness, the child or adolescent may experience and express intense ambivalence toward the parent, particularly if the risk factor for the parent's HIV infection is understood by the child to be a negative behaviour (for example, drug use or selection of a drug-abusing partner). In these circumstances, the child or adolescent may be both sad and anxious about the parent and angry. This is often the case when children perceive that the behaviour which impaired past parenting (e.g. drug use) is leading to further erosion in capacity as illness progresses and perhaps ultimately to abandonment of the child when the parent dies an early death. Extreme ambivalence toward the parent is perhaps the most difficult psychotherapeutic issue in working with HIV-affected children because it greatly complicates the bereavement process (Rosen et al. 1997; Ryan et al. 1997).

Permanency planning

With HIV progression in the parent, caregivers may require counselling about planning for the placement of children following parental death. Communication about HIV illness and permanency planning tend to be closely intertwined, with difficulties in one area being reflected in the other. Family-based permanency planning that actively involves the children, particularly teenagers, is more likely to have a successful outcome than that which excludes the affected young people. Effective permanency planning can be undermined by active substance abuse and untreated psychiatric disorder in family members, as well as by family dynamics related to substance abuse.

Optimally, parents with progressive HIV illness have begun the permanency planning process prior to the final stage of parental HIV illness and other adults are available to provide care and support for affected children. However, some parents, particularly those struggling unsuccessfully with mental illness and/or substance abuse, present to medical care settings in end-stage AIDS without having addressed these issues. In clinical experience, these are usually the most disorganized families with the highest burden of psychiatric and substance abuse disorder. In these families, careful attention to the mental health needs of the children and adolescents is essential. Both the lack of family preparation and factors associated with that lack of preparation flag increased risk for mental health problems in these children.

Bereavement and family reconfiguration

Death of a parent in childhood ruptures the child's parental attachment before the child has completed the developmental tasks necessary for functioning as an independent adult. A wide array of emotional and behavioural problems may be observed over time following the loss: irritable mood in younger children and sadness in older ones; behavioural difficulties ranging from increased tantrums and fighting with siblings to conduct disorders; and decreased school performance (Rutter 1966; Kranzler et al. 1990). Studies of long-term sequelae, in particular depres-

sion in adulthood, have reported mixed findings, probably because of numerous confounding variables. A positive relationship between the parents prior to the death and a strong surviving parent to keep the family intact have been identified as protective against elevated risk of mental health problems (Harris et al. 1986; Kranzler et al. 1990). Among the predictors of complicated bereavement are child emotional and behavioural factors predating the loss, including prior emotional difficulties, emotional lability and poor impulse control (Kranzler et al. 1990). Many of the factors associated with complicated bereavement in childhood are present in HIV-affected children and adolescents, including emotional difficulties and negative relationships with parents prior to loss and absence of a surviving parent to provide adequate parenting after death.

Grieving HIV-affected children and adolescents most commonly move into reconfigured families with extended family members also mourning the loss of the loved one. In countries with well-developed health services, the social and concrete service supports available to the families by virtue of the parent's AIDS diagnosis generally diminish or disappear following the parent's death. Generally, children and adolescents orphaned by AIDS are moving from one situation of poverty to another, with the responsibility for the care of these children falling on financially limited and often overwhelmed extended family members. In those cases where children and adolescents move into non-relative foster care, they must make the difficult adaptation to new family members and often very different family lifestyles.

An important issue that may occur in the assessment of a bereaved child is differentiation of illusory phenomena related to grief from hallucinations. Children and adolescents frequently experience visual or auditory perceptions of a deceased parent in the period immediately after the death, or sometimes for months or years following. It is important to differentiate illusory phenomena associated with bereavement from hallucinations associated with a psychotic or affective disorder. The more benign perceptions may involve the parent calling the child's name or appearing in a familiar location in the home or neighbourhood. Particularly when the family's religious or cultural context provides reinforcement for such experiences, these perceptions of the deceased parent may be comforting to the child. When the child lacks cultural supports for these experiences, they may cause confusion. It is often helpful to probe gently with the grieving child to determine whether they are experiencing such perceptions and, if so, to reassure the child and assist him or her to understand the experience.

Education for the grieving child and counselling for his or her adult caregivers are very useful in many families. It is helpful to distinguish the usual course of mourning by adults (a sustained period of dysphoria, followed by a gradual return to normal mood) from that more typical of children, especially pre-adolescents (immediate periods of dysphoria punctuated by apparently normal play or socializing, with periods of grieving throughout the developmental trajectory). When a child's deceased parent has been absent or otherwise deficient in their role with the child, adult caregivers may be puzzled by the child's mourning over the loss: they need an explanation that the loss of inadequate parenting may in fact complicate rather than minimize the child's grieving process.

Mental health issues related to parental substance abuse

For children with drug-abusing parents, risk factors for mental health problems cluster in two areas. The first area relates to the sequelae of parenting deficiencies associated with parental substance abuse (neglect, abuse, discontinuity of attachments and disruption of placement); the second to the biological risks associated with parental drug addiction (prenatal drug exposure, heritable parental psychiatric disorder).

Neglect, abuse and disrupted attachment associated with parental drug addiction

One of the most devastating effects of substance abuse is the erosion of parenting capacities essential to children's development and well-being. Children living with substance-abusing parents are at increased risk for neglect, abuse, exposure to domestic violence and disruption of attachments (Rodning et al. 1989; Kelley 1992; Singer et al. 1992), all of which have been shown to increase children's risk for mental health problems (Cicchetti & Carlson 1989; McLeer et al. 1994; Pelcovitz et al. 1994).

Biological risks associated with parental drug addiction

Prenatal drug exposure

Several studies have described the developmental and behavioural problems of children exposed to prenatal drug abuse (Coles et al. 1993; Griffith et al. 1994; Wilens et al. 1995). Methodological problems in much of the research on drug-exposed children limit definitive conclusions regarding the link between specific drug exposures and behavioural or cognitive outcomes (Hutchings 1993; Gonzalez & Campbell 1994). However, it is clear that maternal drug use during pregnancy with its associated problems, such as inadequate prenatal care, premature birth and low birth weight, may act to increase children's risk for developmental, cognitive and mental health problems.

Heritable psychiatric disorders

Adults with substance abuse disorders have high rates of psychiatric comorbidity, particularly affective and anxiety disorders and childhood histories of ADHD (Regier et al. 1990; Carroll & Rounsaville 1993; Haller et al. 1993). Children born to adult substance abusers are at increased risk for mental health problems because of the heritable nature of these psychiatric disor-

ders (Weissman et al. 1984; Goodman & Stevenson 1989; Biederman et al. 1990).

HIV illness commonly strikes families already struggling with substance abuse and its associated problems, including impairment of parenting capacities and psychiatric disorder. When a child's parent is substance abusing and HIV-positive, the HIV disease may play a less significant part in the child's mental health problems than do issues related to the substance abuse.

Conclusions

Almost 20 years into the HIV epidemic, HIV/AIDS continues to affect millions of children and adolescents worldwide. In the developed world, medical advances both in antiretroviral treatment and prevention of vertical transmission has decreased morbidity and mortality in infected children and in their infected family members. In the developing world, the cost of antiretroviral treatment and health infrastructure inadequacies make widespread implementation of treatment advances difficult, leaving millions of children and adolescents without parents and at risk for their own HIV infection and illness. While clinical trials are underway, there is no currently available vaccine against HIV (D'Souza et al. 2000). Continued targeted prevention efforts, more equitable distribution of health care resources and meaningful therapeutic interventions to address the mental health consequences of individual and/or familial HIV disease are essential elements in the uphill fight against HIV/AIDS.

References

Abrams, E.J. & Nicholas, S.W. (1998) Optimism at the millennium's end: the outlook for pediatric HIV infection. *Insights in HIV Disease Management*, 6, 9–88.

Adger, H. (1992) Alcohol and other drug use and abuse in adolescents. In: *Adolescents at Risk: Medical and Social Perspectives* (eds D.E. Rogers & E. Ginzberg), pp. 80–95. Westview Press, San Francisco.

American Academy of Pediatrics (1999) Disclosure of illness status to children and adolescents with HIV infection. *Pediatrics*, 103, 164–166.

Armistead, L., Forehand, R., Steele, R. & Kotchick, B. (1998) Pediatric AIDS. In: *Handbook of Child Psychopathology*, (eds T.H. Ollendick & M. Hersen), 3rd edn, pp. 463–481. Plenum Press, New York.

Auslander, W.F., Thompson, S.J., Dreitzer, D. & Santiago, J.V. (1997) Mothers' satisfaction with medical care: perceptions of racism, family stress, and medical outcomes in children with diabetes. *Health and Social Work*, 22, 190–199.

Balfer, M.L., Krener, P.K. & Black Miller, F. (1988) AIDS in children and adolescents. *Journal of the American Academy of Child and Adolescent Psychiatry*, 27, 147–151.

Becker, M.H., Drachman, R.H. & Kirscht, J.P. (1972) Predicting mothers' compliance with pediatric medical regimens. *Medical Care*, 81, 843–854.

Belman, A.L., Muenz, L.R., Marcus, J.C. *et al.* (1996) Neurologic status of human immunodeficiency virus 1-infected infants and their controls: a prospective study from birth to 2 years. *Pediatrics*, **98**, 1109–1118.

Bender, B., Milgrom, H., Rand, C. & Ackerson, L. (1998) Psychological factors associated with medication nonadherence in asthmatic children. *Journal of Asthma*, **35**, 347–353.

Biederman, J., Faraone, S.V., Keenan, K. *et al.* (1990) Family-genetic and psychosocial risk factors in DSM-III attention deficit disorder. *Journal of the American Academy of Child and Adolescent Psychiatry*, **29**, 526–533.

Boyd-Franklin, N., Steiner, G.L. & Boland, M.G., eds (1995) *Children, Families, and HIV/AIDS*. Guilford Press, New York.

Brady, M.T., McGrath, N., Brouwers, P. *et al.* (1996) Randomized study of the tolerance and efficacy of high- versus low-dose zidovudine in human immunodeficiency virus-infected children with mild to moderate symptoms (AIDS Clinical Trial Group 128). *Journal of Infectious Disease*, **173**, 1097–1106.

Brooks-Gunn, J. & Frustenberg, F.F. (1989) Adolescent sexual behavior. *American Psychologist*, **44**, 249–253.

Brooks-Gunn, J. & Paikoff, R.L. (1993) Sex is a gamble, kissing is a game: adolescent sexuality and promotion. In: *Promoting the Health of Adolescents: New Directions for the Twenty-First Century* (eds S.G. Millstein, A.C. Petersen & E.O. Nightingale), pp. 180–208. Oxford University Press, New York.

Brouwers, P., Moss, H., Wolters, P. *et al.* (1990) Effect of continuous infusion zidovuine therapy on neuropsychologic functioning in children with symptomatic human immunodeficiency virus infection. *Journal of Pediatrics*, **117**, 980–985.

Brouwers P., Belman A.L., Epstein, L.G. (1991) Central nervous system involvement: manifestations and evaluation. In: *Pediatric AIDS: the Challenge of HIV Infection in Infants, Children and Adolescents* (eds P. Pizzo & C. Wilfert), pp. 318–335. Williams & Wilkins, Baltimore, MD.

Brown, L.K., Danovsky, M.B., Lourie, K.J., DiClemente, R.J. & Ponton, L.E. (1997) Adolescents with psychiatric disorders and the risk of HIV. *Journal of the American Academy of Child and Adolescent Psychiatry*, **36**, 1609–1617.

Campbell, T. (1997) A review of the psychological effects of vertically acquired HIV infection in infants and children. *British Journal of Health and Psychology*, **2**, 1–13.

Carroll, K.M. & Rounsaville, B.J. (1993) History and significance of childhood attention deficit disorder in treatment-seeking cocaine abusers. *Comprehensive Psychiatry*, **34**, 75–82.

Centers for Disease Control (1995) US Public Health Service recommendations for human immunodeficiency virus counseling and voluntary testing for pregnant women. *Morbidity and Mortality Weekly Report*, **44** (no. RR-7).

Centers for Disease Control and Prevention (1999a) *HIV/AIDS Surveillance Report*. Midyear edition, 11.

Centers for Disease Control and Prevention (1999b) *CDC Update: National Data on HIV Prevalence Among Disadvantaged Youth in the 1990s*. Website. http://www.cdc.gov

Centers for Disease Control and Prevention (1999c) *CDC Update: HIV/AIDS among African Americans*. Website: http://www.cdc.gov

Cesena, M., Douglas, L.O., Cebollero, A.M. & Steingard, R.J. (1995) Case study: Behavioral symptoms of pediatric HIV-1 encephalopathy successfully treated with clonidine. *Journal of the American Academy of Child and Adolescent Psychiatry*, **34**, 302–306.

Cicchetti, D. & Carlson, V., eds (1989) *Child Maltreatment: Theory and Research on the Causes and Consequences of Child Abuse and Neglect*. Cambridge University Press, New York.

Clatts, M.C. & Davis, W.R. (1999) A demographic and behavioral profile of homeless youth in New York City: implications for AIDS outreach and prevention. *Medical Anthropology Quarterly*, **13**, 365–374.

Coles, C., Platzman, K., Smith, I.E., James, M.E. & Falek, A. (1993) Effects of cocaine and alcohol use in pregnancy on neonatal growth and neurobehavioral status. *Neurotoxicity and Teratology*, **15**, 289.

Connor, E.M., Spreling, R.S., Gelber, R. *et al.* (1994) Reduction of maternal–infant transmission of human immunodeficiency virus type 1 with zidovudine treatment. *New England Journal of Medicine*, **331**, 1173–1180.

Cooper, E.R., Hanson, C., Diaz, C. *et al.* (1998) Encephalopathy and progression of human immunodeficiency virus disease in a cohort of children with perinatally acquired human immunodeficiency virus infection. *Journal of Pediatrics*, **132**, 808–812.

Coplan, J., Contello, K.A., Cunningham, C.K. *et al.* (1998) Early language development in children exposed to or infected with human immunodeficiency virus. *Pediatrics*, **102**, 8.

Corsi, A., Albizzati, A., Cervini, R., Grioni, A., Musetti, L. & Saccani, M. (1991) Hyperactive disturbance in the behavior of children with congenital HIV infections. In: *Abstracts of the Seventh International AIDS Conference*. Vol. 2, W.D.4280, Florence, Italy.

D'Augelli, A.R. (1996) Lesbian, gay and bisexual development during adolescence and young adulthood. In: *Textbook of Homosexuality and Mental Health* (eds R.P. Cabay & T. Stein), pp. 267–268. American Psychiatric Press, Washington D.C.

Drotar, D., Olness, K., Wiznitzer, M. *et al.* (1999) Neurodevelopmental outcomes of Ugandan infants with HIV infection: an application of growth curve analysis. *Health Psychology*, **18**, 114–121.

D'Souza, M.P., Cairnes, J.S. & Plaeger, S.F. (2000) Current evidence and future directions for targeting HIV entry: therapeutic and prophylactic strategies. *Journal of the American Medical Association*, **284**, 215–222.

Englund, J.A., Baker, C.J., Raskino, C. *et al.* (1996) Clinical and laboratory characteristics of symptomatic, human immunodeficiency virus-infected infants and children. *Pediatric Infectious Disease Journal*, **15**, 1025–1036.

Epstein, L.G., Sharer, L.R. & Goudsmit, J. (1988) Neurological and neuropathological features of human immunodeficiency virus infection in children. *Annals of Neurology*, **23**, S19–S23.

Falkenberg, J. (1999) The longest triple-drug combination trial reported in HIV-infected children. *Women's Treatment News*, **1**, 3–4.

Falloon, J., Eddy, J., Wiener, L. & Pizzo, P.A. (1989) Human immunodeficiency virus infection in children. *Journal of Pediatrics*, **114**, 1–30.

Fauci, A.D., Bartlett, J.G., Goosby, E.P. *et al.* (5 May 1999) Guidelines for the use of antiretroviral agents in HIV-infected adults and adolescents. *Panel of Clinical Practices for Treatment of HIV infection, The Living Document*. May 5, 1999, www.hivatis.org/trtgdlns.html.

Garofalo, R., Wolf, R.C., Kessel, S., Falfrey, J. & DuRant, R.H. (1998) The association between health risk behaviors and sexual orientation among a school-based sample of adolescents. *Pediatrics*, **101**, 895–902.

Gonzalez, N.M. & Campbell, M. (1994) Cocaine babies: does prenatal drug exposure to cocaine affect development. *Journal of the American Academy of Child and Adolescent Psychiatry*, **33**, 16–19.

Goodman, R. & Stevenson, J. (1989) A twin study of hyperactivity. II. The aetiological role of genes, family relationships, and perinatal adversity. *Journal of Child Psychology and Psychiatry*, **30**, 691–709.

Griffith, D.R., Azuma, S. & Chasnoff, I. (1994) Three-year outcome of children exposed prenatally to drugs. *Journal of the American Academy of Child and Adolescent Psychiatry*, **33**, 20–27.

Haike, Hernandze, Minz & Boland (1991) School-aged HIV-infected children and access to education. *Pediatric AIDS and HIV Infection: Fetus to Adolescent*, **2**, 74–79.

Haller, D.L., Knisely, J.S., Dawson, K.S. & Schnoll, S.H. (1993) Perinatal substance abusers: psychological and social characteristics. *Journal of Nervous and Mental Disease*, **181**, 509–513.

Hamburg, B.A. (1990) *Life Skills Training: Preventive Interventions for Young Adolescents*. Carnegie Council on Adolescent Development: Working Papers, Carnegie Corporation, New York.

Harris, T., Brown, G.W. & Bifulco, A. (1986) Loss of parents in childhood and adult psychiatric disorder: the role of lack of adequate parental care. *Psychological Medicine*, **16**, 641–659.

Havens, J.F. & McCaskill, E.O. (1999) Psychostimulants in HIV-infected children and adolescents: a case series. In: *Ritalin Theory and Practice* (eds L.L. Greenhill & B.B. Osman), 2nd edn, pp. 165–173. Mary Ann Liebert, Larchmont, NY.

Havens, J., Whitaker, A., Feldman, J. & Ehrhardt, A. (1994) Psychiatric morbidity in school-age children with congenital HIV-infection: a pilot study. *Journal of Developmental and Behavioral Pediatrics*, **15**, S18–S25.

Havens, J., Mellins, C.A. & Pilowski, D. (1996) Mental health issues in HIV-affected women and children. *International Review of Psychiatry*, **8**, 217–225.

Havens, J., Ryan, S. & Mellins, C.A. (1999) Child psychiatry: areas of special interest/psychiatric sequelae of HIV and AIDS. In: *Comprehensive Textbook of Psychiatry* (eds H. Kaplan & B. Saddock), 7th edn, pp. 2897–2902. Lipincott Williams & Wilkins, Philadelphia, PA.

Heylen, R. & Miller, R. (1996a) Adverse effects and drug interactions of medications commonly used in the treatment of adult HIV positive patients. *Genitourinary Medicine*, **72**, 237–246.

Heylen, R. & Miller, R. (1996b) Adverse effects and drug interactions of medications commonly used in the treatment of adult HIV positive patients: part II. *Genitourinary Medicine*, **73**, 6–11.

Hittleman, J., Nelson, N., Shah, V., Gong, J. & Peluso, F.S. (1993) Neurodevelopmental disabilities in infants born to HIV-infected mothers. *AIDS Reader*, July/August, 126–132.

HIV/AIDS Treatment Information Services (1999) Website: http://hivatis.org.

Hofferth, S.L., Kahn, J.R. & Baldwin, W. (1987) Premarital sexual activity among US teenage women over the past three decades. *Family Planning Perspectives*, **19**, 46–53.

Hoffman, N. Futterman, D. & Myerson, A. (1999) Treatment issues for HIV positive adolescents. Massachusetts Medical Society. *AIDS Clinical Care*, **11**, 3.

Hogan, D.P. & Kitagawa, E.M. (1983) *Family factors in the fertility of black adolescents*. Paper presented at the annual meeting of the Population Association of America. Cited in National Research Council.

Hunter, J. (1990) Violence against lesbian and gay male youths. *Journal of Interpersonal Violence*, **5**, 295–300.

Hunter, J. (1996) *Emerging from the shadows: lesbian, gay, and bisexual adolescents—personal identity achievement, coming out and sexual risk behaviors*. Dissertation, City University of New York.

Hunter, J. & Haymes, R. (1997) It's beginning to rain: gay/lesbian/bisexual adolescents and AIDS. In: *Pride and Prejudice: Working with Lesbian, Gay and Bisexual Youth* (ed. M.S. Schneider) pp. 137–163. Central Toronto Youth Services, Toronto, Canada.

Hunter, J. & Mallon, G. (2000) Lesbian, gay and bisexual adolescent development: dancing with your feet tied together. In: *Education, Research, and Practice in Lesbian, Gay, Bisexual, and Transgendered Psychology: a Resource Manual*, Vol. 5 (eds B. Green & G.L. Croom), pp. 226–243. Sage Publications, Thousand Oaks, CA.

Hunter, J. & Schaecher, R. (1987) Stresses on lesbian and gay adolescents in schools. *Social Work in Education*, **9**, 180–188.

Hunter, J. & Schaecher, R. (1992) Adolescents and AIDS: coping issues.

In: *Living and Dying with AIDS* (ed. P. Ahmed), pp. 35–45. Plenum Press, New York.

Hutchings, D. (1993) The puzzle of cocaine's effects following maternal use during pregnancy: are there reconcilable differences? *Neurotoxicology and Teratology*, **15**, 281–286.

Jessor, S.L. & Jessor, R. (1977) *Problem Behavior and Psychosocial Development*. Academic Press, New York.

Johnson, S.B. (1980) Psychosocial factors in juvenile diabetes: a review. *Journal of Behavioral Medicine*, **3**, 95–116.

Kann, L., Kinchen, S.A., Williams, B.I. *et al.* (1998) Youth risk behavior surveillance: United States. *Morbidity and Mortality Weekly Report, CDC Surveillance Summaries*, **47**, 1–89.

Katzenstein, D.A. (1997) Adherence as a particular issue with protease inhibitors. *Journal of the Association of Nurses in AIDS Care*, **8** (S1), 10–17.

Keller, S.E., Bartlett, J.A., Schleifer, S.J., Johnson, R.L., Pinner, E. & Delaney, B. (1991) HIV-relevant sexual behavior among a healthy inner-city heterosexual adolescent population in an endemic area of HIV. *Journal of Adolescent Health*, **12**, 44–48.

Kelley, S. (1992) Parenting stress and child maltreatment in drug-exposed children. *Child Abuse and Neglect*, **16**, 312–328.

Kissinger, P., Fuller, C., Clark, R.A. & Abdalian, S.E. (1997) Psychosocial characteristics of HIV-infected adolescents in New Orleans. *Journal of Adolescent Health*, **20**, 258.

Kranzler, E.M., Shaffer, D., Wasserman, G. & Davies, M. (1990) Early childhood bereavement. *Journal of the American Academy of Child and Adolescent Psychiatry*, **29**, 513–520.

Levenson, R.L. Jr & Mellins, C.A. (1992) Pediatric HIV/AIDS: what psychologists need to know. *Professional Psychology: Research and Practice*, **23**, 410–415.

Macilwain, C. (1997) Better adherence vital in AIDS therapies. *Nature*, **392**, 431.

Mandelbrot, L., LeChenadec, J., Berrebi, A. *et al.* (1998) Perinatal HIV-1 transmission: interaction between zidovudine prophylaxis and mode of delivery in the French Perinatal Cohort. *Journal of the American Medical Association*, **280**, 55–60.

Manne, S.L., Jacobsen, P.B., Gorfinkle, K., Gerstein, F. & Redd, W.H. (1993) Treatment adherence difficulties among children with cancer: the role of parenting style. *Journal of Pediatric Psychology*, **18**, 47–62.

McKinney, R.E., Maha, M.A., Connor, E.M. *et al.* (1991) A multicenter trial of oral zidovuine in children with advanced human immunodeficiency disease. *New England Journal of Medicine*, **324**, 1018–1025.

McLeer, S., Callaghan, M., Delmina, H. & Wallen, J. (1994) Psychiatric disorders in sexually abused children. *Journal of the American Academy of Child and Adolescent Psychiatry*, **33**, 313–319.

Mellins, C.A. & Ehrhardt, A.A. (1994) Families affected by pediatric AIDS: sources of stress and coping. *Journal of Developmental and Behavioral Pediatrics (Supplement)*, **15**, S54–S60.

Mellins, C.A., Levenson, R.L., Zawadzki, R., Kairam, R. & Weston, M. (1994) Effects of pediatric HIV infection and prenatal drug exposure on mental and psychomotor development. *Journal of Pediatric Psychology*, **19**, 617–628.

Mellins, C.A., Havens, J. & Arpadi, S.M. (1998) Children. In: *Encyclopedia of AIDS: a Social, Political, Cultural, and Scientific Record of the Epidemic* (ed. R.A. Smith), pp. 128–132. Fitzroy-Dearborn, Chicago and London.

Michaels, D. & Levine, C. (1992) Estimates of the number of motherless youth orphaned by AIDS in the United States. *Journal of the American Medical Association*, **268**, 3456–3461.

Morris, L., Warren, C.W. & Aral, S.O. (1993) Measuring adolescent sexual behaviors and related health outcomes. *Public Health Reports*, **108**, 31–36.

Moss, H.A., Brouwers, P., Wolters, P.L., Wiener, L., Hersh, S. & Pizzo, P.A. (1994) The development of a Q-sort behavioral rating procedure for pediatric HIV patients. *Journal of Pediatric Psychology*, **19**, 27–46.

Moss, H.A., Wolters, P.L., Brouwers, P., Hendricks, M.L. & Pizzo, P.A. (1996) Impairment of expressive behavior in pediatric HIV-infected patients with evidence of CNS disease. *Journal of Pediatric Psychology*, **21**, 379–400.

Moss, H.A., Bose, S., Wolters, P. & Brouwers, P. (1998) A preliminary study of factors associated with psychological adjustment and disease course in school-age children infected with human immunodeficiency virus. *Journal of Developmental and Behavioral Pediatrics*, **19**, 18–25.

Nduati, R., John, G., Mboir-Ngacha, D. *et al.* (2000) Effect of breast-feeding and formula feeding in the transmission of HIV-1. *Journal of the American Medical Association*, **283**, 1167–1174.

New York City Department of Health, Office of AIDS Surveillance (1999) *AIDS Surveillance Update*, 4th quarter.

Oleske, J., Scott, G.B. *et al.* (15 April 1999) 1999 Guidelines for the use of antiretroviral agents in pediatric HIV infection: working group on antiretroviral therapy and medical management of HIV-infected children. *The Living Document*, www.hivatis.org/trtgdlns.html.

Orr, D.P., Wilbrandt, M.L., Brack, C.J., Rausch, S.P. & Ingersoll, G.M. (1989) Reported sexual behaviors and self-esteem among young adolescents. *American Journal of Diseases of Children*, **143**, 86–90.

Paikoff, R.L. (1995) Early heterosexual debut: situations of sexual possibility during the transition to adolescence. *American Journal of Orthopsychiatry*, **65**, 389–401.

Pao, M., Lyon, M., D'Angelo, L.J., Schuman, W.B., Tipnis, T. & Mrazek, D.A. (2000) Psychiatric diagnoses in adolescents seropositive for the human immunodeficiency virus. *Archives of Pediatric Adolescent Medicine*, **154**, 240–244.

Pelcovitz, D., Kaplan, S., Goldenberg, B., Mandel, F. & Lehane, J. (1994) Guarrera post-traumatic stress disorder in physically abused adolescents. *Journal of the American Academy of Child and Adolescent Psychiatry*, **33**, 305–312.

Pizzo, P., Eddy, J., Fallon, J. *et al.* (1988) Effect of continuous intravenous infusion of zidovudine (AZT) in children with symptomatic HIV infection. *New England Journal of Medicine*, **319**, 889–896.

Pulsifer, M.B. & Aylward, E.H. (2000) Human immunodeficiency virus. In: *Pediatric Neuropsychology: Research, Theory, and Practice* (eds K.O. Yeates, M.D. Ris & H.G. Taylor), pp. 381–402. Guilford Press, New York.

Regier, D.A., Farmer, M., Rae, D.S. *et al.* (1990) Co-morbidity of mental disorders with alcohol and other drugs of abuse. *Journal of the American Medical Association*, **264**, 2511–2518.

Remafedi, M.D., French, S., Story, M., Resnick, M.D. & Blum, R. (1998) The relationship between suicide risk and sexual orientation: results of a population-based study. *American Journal of Public Health*, **88**, 57–60.

Rodning, C., Beckwith, L. & Howard, J. (1989) Characteristics of attachment organization and play organization in prenatally drug-exposed toddlers. *Development and Psychopathology*, **1**, 277–289.

Roger, A.S. *et al.* (1998) The REACH project of the Adolescent Medicine HIV/AIDS Research Network: design, methods and selected characteristics of participants. *Journal of Adolescent Health*, **22**, 300–311.

Rosario, M., Hunter, J. & Gwadz, M. (1997) Exploration of substance use among lesbian, gay and bisexual youth: prevalence and correlates. *Journal of Adolescent Research*, **12**, 454–476.

Rotheram-Borus, M., Koopman, C., Haignere, C. & Davies, M. (1991) Reducing HIV sexual risk behavior among runaway adolescents. *Journal of the American Medical Association*, **266**, 1237–1241.

Rotheram-Borus, M.J., Hunter, J. & Rosario, M. (1995) Coming out as lesbian or gay in the era of AIDS. In: *AIDS, Identity, and Community: the HIV Epidemic and Lesbians and Gay Men* (eds G.M. Herek & B. Greene), pp. 150–168. Sage Publications, Thousand Oaks, CA.

Rotheram-Borus, M.J., Murphy, D. & Miller, S. (1996) Intervening with adolescent girls living with HIV. In: *Women and AIDS* (eds A. O'Leary & L. Sweet Jemmott), pp. 87–108. Plenum Press, New York.

Rutter, M. (1966) *Children of Sick Parents*. Oxford University Press, London.

Ryan, S., Havens, J. & Mellins, C. (1997) Psychotherapy with HIV-affected adolescents. In: *Psychotherapy and AIDS* (ed. L. Wicks), pp. 143–164. Taylor & Francis, Washington D.C.

Sahai, J. (1996) Risks and synergies from drug interactions. *AIDS*, **10**, S21–S25.

Shapiro, M.F., Morton, S.C., McCaffrey, D.F. *et al.* (1999) Variations in the care of HIV-infected adults in the United States: results from the HIV cost and services utilization study. *Journal of the American Medical Association*, **281**, 2035–2315.

Singer, L., Farkas, K. & Kliegman, R. (1992) Childhood medical and behavioral consequences of maternal cocaine use. *Journal of Pediatric Psychology*, **17**, 389–406.

Smith, C.A. (1997) Factors associated with early sexual activity among urban adolescents. *Social Work*, **42**, 334–346.

Speigal, L. & Mayers, A. (1991) Psychosocial aspects of AIDS in children and adolescents. *Pediatric Clinics of North America*, **38**, 153–167.

Tardieu, M., Mayaux, M.J., Seibel, N. *et al.* (1995) Cognitive assessment of school-aged children infected with maternally transmitted human immunodeficiency virus type 1. *Journal of Pediatrics*, **126**, 375–379.

UNAIDS (2000) *AIDS Epidemic Update, December 2000*. World Health Organization, Joint United Nations Programme on HIV/AIDS, UNAIDS.

United States General Accounting Office (1989) *Homeless and Runaway Youth Receiving Services at Federally Funded Shelters*. US General Accounting Office, Washington D.C.

Valleroy, L.A., MacKellar, D.A., Karon, J.M. *et al.* (2000) HIV prevalence and associated risks in young men who have sex with men. *Journal of the American Medical Association*, **284**, 198–204.

Walter, H.J., Vaughan, R.D. & Cohall, A.T. (1991) Psychosocial influences on acquired immunodeficiency syndrome-risk behaviors among high school students. *Pediatrics*, **88**, 846–852.

Wasserheit, J.N. (1992) Epidemiological synergy: interrelationships between human immunodeficiency virus infection and other sexually transmitted diseases [Review]. *Sexually Transmitted Diseases*, **19**, 61–77.

Weissman, M.M., Gershon, E.S., Kidd, K.K. *et al.* (1984) Psychiatric disorders in the relatives of probands with affective disorders. *Archives of General Psychiatry*, **41**, 13–21.

Wiener, L. & Septimus, A. (1991) Psychosocial consideration and support for the child and family. In: *Pediatric AIDS: the Challenge of HIV Infection in Infants, Children and Adolescents* (eds P.A. Pizoo & C.M. Wilfert), pp. 577–594. Williams & Wilkins, Baltimore, MD.

Wiener, L., Septimus, A. & Grady, C. (1998) Psychosocial support and ethical issues in pediatric AIDS. In: *Pediatric AIDS* (eds P.A. Pizzo & C. Wilfert), 3rd edn, pp. 703–727. Lippincott Williams & Wilkins, Baltimore.

Wilens, T.M., Biederman, J., Kiely, K., Bredin, E. & Spencer, T.J. (1995) Pilot study of behavioral and emotional disturbance in the high risk children of parents with opioid dependence. *Journal of the American Academy of Child and Adolescent Psychiatry*, **34**, 779–785.

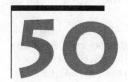

Psychiatric Aspects of Specific Sensory Impairments

Peter Hindley and Tiejo van Gent

Introduction

Sensory impairments alone do not increase children's vulnerability to mental health problems. However, the consequences of being sensorially impaired in a world orientated to the needs of hearing and sighted people do increase children's vulnerability. Understanding why and how that is the case throws light onto both normal development and psychopathology. In this chapter, we focus primarily on children with the most severe sensory impairments. In addition, we discuss the effects of otitis media with effusion (OME) and the mental health of hearing children of deaf parents. Given that 90–95% of deaf children and 99% of blind children are born into hearing and sighted families, the response of their parents is likely to be particularly important. For deaf children (meaning severe hearing impairment, HI), the major challenge is accessing meaningful communication. For many, visuospatial language will be the most effective route. For blind children (meaning severe visual impairment, VI), the challenge is how to access information relating to non-verbal communication and spatial orientation. For many children this will be accomplished by building a narrative picture of the world. Children with multisensory impairment (MSI) face challenges that are often greater than the sum of the HI and VI because sensory information needs to be integrated. Their main difficulties lie in accessing experience *per se* and that experience often has to be mediated through adults.

Hearing impairment

Epidemiology of hearing impairment

In the UK, approximately 1.2 in 1000 children have permanent bilateral HI of moderate or greater severity (Davis *et al.* 1995). In most cases, the HI is a result of genetic causes (Gorlin *et al.* 1995) or severe prematurity. Congenital rubella is a less frequent cause than it used to be; the introduction of vaccination for meningitis is likely similarly to reduce its role as a cause of deafness. Acute otitis media is probably the most common reason for consultation with GPs in the preschool years (Haggard & Hughes 1991). It is usually a time-limited condition that does not cause HI, but the complication of OME can lead to fluctuating HI. Approximately 10–30% of 2–7-year-old children will have fluctuating HI from middle ear disease (Haggard & Hughes 1991).

HI is often accompanied by other impairments, particularly in vision, motor function (resulting from brain damage) and intelligence (Freeman *et al.* 1975; Sinkkonen 1994). These additional impairments are least likely when the HI is genetically determined. An important exception is Usher syndrome, the co-occurrence of sensorineural deafness and VI caused by retinitis pigmentosa. The occurrence of additional impairments means that early screening for them is essential.

Cultural aspects

Meadow-Orlans & Erting (2000), in their comprehensive introduction to a sociocultural view of deafness, suggested that deaf culture had three characteristic elements: a primarily visual experience of the world; membership of an oppressed minority; and the use of sign language. However, the move towards more inclusive forms of education is changing the situation. Because most deaf children have hearing parents, membership of the deaf community is mainly acquired outside the family. To varying degrees, deaf people are effectively bilingual and bicultural (Padden 1996), identifying with both their sign language community and the spoken language community—in addition to subcommunities according to ethnicity or sexual orientation (Parasnis 1996).

Sign languages

Sign languages appear to develop naturally wherever groups of deaf people come together (Groce & Whiting 1988). They differ according to national groups, not necessarily relating to the dominant spoken language. British Sign Language (BSL) and American Sign Language (ASL) have little in common at a lexical level, whereas ASL and Langue des Signes Françaises (LSF) do. Nevertheless, all sign languages have in common the expression of semantic and grammatical concepts by movements of the hands, face and upper body. Most sentence structure follows a topic–comment construction, and most sign languages use a system in which verbs or subjects are represented by a limited number of hand shapes or classifiers (Sutton-Spence & Woll 1999).

The educational status of native sign languages has changed dramatically in the last 20 years with the development of bilingual/bicultural programmes in Sweden (Heiling 1995), USA (Strong 1995), UK (Young 1999) and many other countries. At the same time, the introduction of cochlear implants (see below) has led to increasing tension between the deaf community and the audiological establishment (Hindley 1997). The study of sign language provides insights into the ontology of language (Stokoe 1998) and the neuropsychological processes that underpin language function (Corina 1999). The latter are similar to those of spoken language except that the brain areas involved in proprioception are also involved (Corina 1999).

Deaf children of deaf parents

The language development of deaf children of deaf parents is comparable to that of hearing children (Caselli & Volterra 1989; Pettito & Marentette 1991). Deaf parents tend to have greater sensitivity to the early communicative efforts of their infants than do hearing parents of deaf infants (Smith-Gray & Koester 1995), and deaf infants are more likely to use bodily movements than auditory signals to attract their mothers' attention. In turn, deaf mothers are more likely to perceive these signals as attempts to communicate and so reciprocate.

Deaf mothers use a variety of methods to gain their infant's attention (Harris 2001) and to make communication salient and contingent upon the child's activity. These include signing in the child's signing space, moving objects into the child's visual field before signing and waiting to obtain the child's visual attention before signing. Deaf parents adapt their signs in ways that are reminiscent of hearing parents' spoken 'motherese' (Erting *et al.* 1989; Masataka 1992). They show greater sensitivity in regaining their child's attention (Koester *et al.* 1998) and greater capacity for repair and discourse maintenance (Prendergast & McCollum 1996). This seems to improve the children's development.

Deaf children of deaf parents appear to outperform both deaf children of hearing parents and hearing children on false-belief tasks (Courtin & Melot 1998). This may be a consequence of early exposure to visual perspective-taking (a central feature of sign language). Braden (1994), reporting a meta-analysis, noted that deaf children of deaf parents have the highest mean IQ (108) of all groups of deaf children. Their educational achievements are also superior (Meadow 1968; Balow & Brill 1972).

Hearing parents of deaf children

The vast majority of hearing parents of deaf children will not have had prior contact with deaf people and experience considerable shock on realizing that their child is deaf (Freeman *et al.* 1975; Stein & Jabaley 1981). However, when they have had prior suspicions, there may also be an initial feeling of relief when the diagnosis is confirmed (Gregory 1991). In areas where deafness is conceptualized in cultural terms, they then have to come to terms with their child as different, not disabled (Young 1999). Many parents come to embrace this positive construction of deafness but many struggle with the notion as much as with disability (Hindley 1999). The use of cochlear implants (electro-assistive devices that transmit a signal direct to the cochlea) with younger children is raising parental expectations about their children's potential to develop spoken language, and

thereby clashes with the 'culturally different' concept. The family response reflects their coping skills and their social network (Danek 1988). However, many parents come to rely increasingly on professional networks (Quittner *et al.* 1990). Neonatal screening for life-threatening conditions has raised concerns that it may increase parental anxiety, with a deleterious effect on parent–infant relationships (Martineau 1993); this does not seem to apply to neonatal screening for deafness (Watkin *et al.* 1998).

Interaction between deaf children and hearing parents

Deafness affects the interaction between parents and their children (Brinich 1981; Vaccari & Marschark 1997; Marschark 1993). Although the mechanisms involved remain unclear, two seem to be involved: the emotional impact of deafness on the parents' perception of the child (Schlesinger & Meadow 1972); and the consequences of deafness for communication between child and parents. Schlesinger & Meadow (1972) suggested that parental depression following diagnosis can lead to decreased parental interaction. Meadow-Orlans (1995) found that mothers of children with HI experienced greater emotional distress than fathers, perceiving their children as inattentive.

Hearing mothers of deaf infants are less responsive than either deaf mothers of deaf infants or hearing mothers of hearing infants (Spencer & Meadow-Orlans 1996). This diminished responsiveness seems to stem from a lesser sensitivity to the deaf infants' visual signals (Spencer *et al.* 1992; Prendergast & McCollum 1996; Harris 2000) and is likely to have implications for the children's language development.

Parents of deaf children also tend to be more directive and controlling in their interactions with their deaf children when compared with hearing:hearing dyads and with deaf:deaf dyads (Marschark 1993). This could derive from difficulties in managing divided attention (Harris 2000) but could also be a response to the children's delayed language development (see below). Interestingly, despite these interactive features, deaf children do not show an increased vulnerability to anxious attachments (Greenberg & Marvin 1979; van Ijzendoorn *et al.* 1992; Hadadian 1995).

Language development in deaf children

There are two features of the language that hearing parents use with their deaf children (Marschark 1993). First, hearing parents tend to simplify both their spoken and signed language and, in the case of sign language, drop important function signs. As a result, communication is frequently impoverished. Secondly, interactions between deaf children and hearing parents tend to be shorter, less complex and contain fewer questions and self-references.

Much the same applies to teacher–child interactions (Wood *et al.* 1986; Power *et al.* 1990). Teachers tend to be more controlling, use more conversational repair strategies and initiate fewer interactions. This controlling style was associated with fewer questions from pupils and less elaborated answers from them.

In a meta-analysis of early intervention programmes, Meadow-Orlans (1987) found that preschool-age deaf children enrolled in oral language programmes had spoken language some 2–3 years behind their hearing peers; very few had gone beyond the 10-word stage at 2.5 years. Two-thirds of the children that Gregory studied in the 1970s were using some form of sign language by the time they reached late adolescence, and one-sixth had such poor language that they could not participate in the study (Gregory et al. 1995). Deaf children using spoken language appear to have particular difficulty in understanding wh-questions, relative clauses and embedded questions (De Villiers et al. 1994). This may lead to poor understanding even when their spoken language is reasonable. Geers & Nicholas (1997) found that 'heuristic' communication functions (questions and answers rather than repetitions and imitations) at age 3 predicted better language development at 5 years in deaf children.

Two recent developments are affecting the course of deaf children's spoken language. First, early ascertainment (below 6 months) is associated with better receptive and expressive spoken language development (Yoshinaga-Itano & Apuzzo 1998). Secondly, the use of cochlear implants also leads to significant gains in language development for some children (Meyer et al. 1998).

Children exposed to gesture but not to formal sign tend to develop their own gestural systems, often called 'homesign'. These appear to convey second language learning advantage when formal sign language is encountered later in life (Morford 1998). When deaf children are presented with signed versions of spoken language, their expressive signing increasingly approximates to native sign language, particularly in the use of spatial grammatical principles (Supalla 1991). When deaf children of hearing parents receive good-quality sign input, their sign language development mirrors spoken language development in hearing children in sequence, but not always rate (Marschark 1993).

Some early intervention programmes provide mentorship from a deaf person; their support with respect to communication and to cultural awareness about deafness seems to foster the children's language development (Watkins et al. 1998; Young 1999).

Cognitive development

Historically, deafness has been seen as an opportunity to study cognitive development in the 'absence of language' but this fails to appreciate the relevance of sign language (Marschark & Everhart 1997). The possible risk factors for cognitive development in children with HI include restriction of experience (both as a result of deafness per se and because of residential schooling); the effects of signing rather than spoken language; central nervous system damage; and lack of exposure to sound (Marschark 1993). The last could have an effect because of its effect on the integration of distal and proximal events (Campbell 1998).

An increasing awareness, from the 1950s onwards, of the effects of language on cognitive assessment led to the development of specific non-verbal tests (Snijders Oomans, Leiter, Hiskey Nebraska) for children with HI, as well as the performance scales from instruments such as the Wechsler Intelligence Scale for Children (WISC). Nevertheless, even on non-verbal tests deaf children tend to show small but significant deficits when compared with same-age hearing children (Marschark 1993). Zwiebel (1987) found that genetically deaf children of hearing parents showed deficits, whereas deaf children of deaf parents had mean IQs that were significantly above hearing norms. Overall better language is associated with better cognitive performance. Subtest performance suggests that deaf children rely more than hearing children on visuoperceptual thinking and visual memory, and less on abstract thinking.

Deaf children lag behind hearing children by approximately 2–4 years in their development of conservation. Language seems to have an important function in allowing explicit and implicit acquisition of categories and concepts (Marschark 1993); bootstrapping processes in deaf children may also be impaired (Campbell 1998).

HI seems, in addition, to be associated with deficits in short- and long-term memory, perhaps because of the lesser reliance on temporal sequential strategies (Marschark 1993). Linguistic creativity seems to be impaired if assessed through inappropriate spoken language tests, but not perhaps if assessed using sign language.

Academic achievement in deaf children

Deaf children significantly underachieve, especially in reading and writing (Gregory & Powers 1998), and also in mathematical concepts (Nunes & Monero 1998). It is probably relevant that most deaf children learn to read and write in what is effectively a second language. For some deaf children there is no basic problem with phonological coding but there is restricted vocabulary knowledge and syntactical ability. Their reduced working memory capacity (Marschark 1993) and diminished experience of the interaction among the semantic, syntactic and pragmatic components of spoken language (Campbell 1998) may be influential.

Approaches to improving deaf children's reading and writing skills include accessing reading through sign language (Hoffmeister et al. 1997; Prinz & Strong 1998) and presenting spoken language by presenting phonological code in the form of hand shapes presented alongside the face (Campbell 1998). Hoffmeister et al. (1997) suggested that detailed knowledge of ASL syntax enhances children's meta-linguistic skills and so enables them to decode English. However, many children with HI need further 'bridging' skills (Prinz & Strong 1998) such as enhancing recognition of phonological code (Campbell 1998) and recognizing letter–word patterns through the use of finger spelling and sign initialization (Padden & Ramsey 1998). Marschark (1993) suggested that the best outcomes for literacy in deaf children occur when children experience both signed and spoken language in early intervention programmes.

Social and emotional development

Deaf infants appear to show the same range of emotional states as hearing infants (Snitzer Reilly *et al.* 1989) but, as they develop, they tend to have smaller emotional vocabularies and are less good in recognizing other people's emotional states (Greenberg & Kusche 1989, 1993). Lederberg & Mobley (1990) found that deaf children showed less social initiative, less compliance, creativity and enjoyment in their interactions with their mothers and more misbehaviour. Harris (1978) found that deaf children of deaf parents showed less impulsive, and more reflective, cognitive styles than deaf children of hearing parents.

Although preschool friendship patterns do not differ between deaf and hearing children (Lederberg *et al.* 1986), deaf preschool-age children are more likely to use linguistic and non-linguistic visual communication with their deaf than with their hearing peers (Lederberg *et al.* 1986). As deaf children pass though the early years of mainstream school there are few initial peer difficulties (Hindley 2000) but later on they are increasingly likely to be socially isolated. Interventions based on promoting integrated activities rather than social skills appear to have short-term positive effects on deaf–hearing peer relationships (Antia *et al.* 1993).

Gregory & Mogford (1982) found that deaf children's play was less well elaborated than that of hearing children. Spencer & Deyo (1993) found that imaginative play was closely related to language level but Spencer & Meadow-Orlans (1996) suggested that maternal sensitivity rather than children's language predicts the emergence of representational play.

It has been suggested that deaf children will have difficulty in passing false-belief tasks because of delayed language and a lack of conversations about mental states (Gale *et al.* 1996; Peterson & Siegal 1998). Because deaf children of deaf parents appear to develop theory of mind earlier (Courtin & Melot 1998), it is likely that conversational experience is the relevant risk factor. However, methodological concerns (e.g. giving false-belief tests through interpreters) mean that there is some uncertainty regarding the validity of the theory of mind findings in children with HI.

Visual impairment

Severe VI is estimated to affect 81 in 100 000 children in industrialized societies (Bryars & Archer 1977), with over one-third of these completely blind (Cullinan 1987; Baird & Moore 1993). VI is more common in developing countries (Chirambo *et al.* 1986; Bard & Moore 1993), mainly because of retinol deficiency, measles and other acquired causes.

Over the last decade there has been growing awareness of cortical blindness (Jan & Freeman 1998). Children with cortical blindness can present with puzzling pictures of apparently inconsistent or variable visual functioning; also there may be significant improvements over time in visual functioning.

Additional impairments are very common among children with VI. In a clinic-based study, one-half had intellectual impairments and two-fifths had other disabilities, such as cerebral palsy, epilepsy and HI (Hill *et al.* 1986). Additional impairments are common, even in general population samples (Jan *et al.* 1977). As with children with HI, screening for associated problems is crucial.

Cultural aspects

The notion of a sociocultural perspective on blindness is a relatively recent development. Fogel (1997) suggested that the central experience of blindness involves construction of the world as a narrative rather than a gestalt, and that this constituted essential strength of the blind person. The only published study of the interaction between a blind mother and her blind infant (Rowbury 1991) suggested that, when compared with a hearing dyad, the blind mother used more spoken language and touch to maintain contact with her baby.

Family response to visual impairment

Jan *et al.* (1977) found that one-third of parents reacted with shock and disbelief to the diagnosis of VI (usually in infancy); one-half said that they did not want to have any more children. Some parents experience considerable distress, and it has been suggested that parental depression can lead to decreased interaction between child and parent (Fraiberg 1977; Warren 1994). The process of communication between children with VI and their parents may sometimes be affected adversely but positive interaction has also been found (Als *et al.* 1980).

It appears that the presence of VI affects the quality of language used by parents. In one study (Kekelis & Andersen 1984), parents were more directive and made more imperative statements and more requests. They also made fewer elaborations and fewer statements about events and people in the here-and-now. They may also be less contingent in their interaction with their children (Webster & Roe 1998).

Groenveld (1993) warned that multiple professional involvement with families of babies with VI could adversely affect parents' intuitive parenting style. However, that need not occur (Sonksen *et al.* 1991), although it is important to make appropriate use of the families' existing social networks and their inherent coping skills (Nixon 1994).

Language development

It is noteworthy that many blind people use gestures with spoken language in the same way that hearing people do (Iverson 1998). For children with VI but without additional impairments, language probably develops at about the usual time (Landau 1997; but see Adelson 1983 and Dunlea 1989 for a contrary view). However, there is evidence that they are delayed in their use of referential language such as 'I' and 'You' (Warren 1994). It is unclear whether this is as a result of difficulties in processing visuospatial information (Mulford 1980) or a more profound difficulty in understanding interpersonal relationships because of a lack of visual interaction (Hobson *et al.* 1997). Longitudinal studies of the early development of children with VI suggest that attachment formation may be significantly affected but there is a lack of systematic research (Warren 1994). In a small-scale study, McAlpine & Moore (1995) found that children with VI were significantly delayed in their understanding of theory of mind. Failing false-belief tasks correlated with severity of VI and was not related to mental age. Given the child's dependence on gaining information through language, maintaining a stream of language appears important (Recchia 1997); it is important that this should be responsive to the child's activities and interests (Rowland 1983; Peters 1994).

Cognitive development

A commonly adopted strategy in assessing cognitive functioning in children with VI is to use just the verbal scale or to rely on adaptations of verbally loaded scales, such as the Stanford–Binet (Davis 1980). However, it is desirable to assess non-verbal skills in addition (Warren 1994), through the use of VI-appropriate performance items (Ohwaki *et al.* 1960), developing VI-appropriate aptitude tests such as the Blindness Aptitude Test (Newland 1979), or using a specific intelligence test designed for children with VI—the Intelligence Test of Visually Impaired Children (ITVIC; Dekker & Koole 1992). The ITVIC is explicitly based on Thurstone's (1938) model of intelligence and has been extensively assessed and normed. Factor analysis has revealed four main factors: orientation, reasoning, spatial ability and verbal ability. Of these, only the spatial ability factor correlates with degree of useful vision.

The degree of VI (in the absence of other disabilities) does not have a significant effect on cognitive skills apart from spatial ability. There is some suggestion that specific aetiologies may play a part with retinoblastoma being associated with both significantly raised and diminished IQ scores (Warren 1994). Retinopathy of prematurity has generally been associated with lowered IQ, this is most likely a reflection of concomitant central nervous system damage.

Warren (1994) reviewed the development of classification in children with VI. He concluded that development in both areas 'generally proceeds along a normal path'. However, he added that there is considerable within-sample variability and that IQ, visual experience and the range of the children's experience with the materials in the test will all have an effect. His comments should act as a caution to those using standardized tests with children with VI to ensure that the test materials themselves are within the children's experience. It appears that the development of abstract concepts is delayed in children with VI, but Warren pointed out that the studies do not exclude IQ and age as possible confounding factors.

As with deaf children, there has been considerable interest in the development of conservation in children with VI. They appear to develop conservation of weight and substance between 8 and 11 years and conservation of volume between 12 and 14 years (Warren 1994). Development of conservation of volume is clearly affected by degree of VI. Other important factors include IQ, institutional setting and direct experience of the materials used.

VI does not appear to have significant effect on either short-term or long-term memory. There is a debate as to whether or not visual imagery facilitates language learning with children with VI. It appears that there is considerable individual variation, visual imagery enhancing learning for some and interfering with learning for others (Warren 1994). There is a debate as to whether or not VI affects cognitive style. Some research suggests that the presence of VI leads to a more global (diffuse and unstructured) rather than articulated (structured) cognitive style (Warren 1994) but this is disputed by other research. VI does not appear to have an effect on children's creativity. Finally, research into the processing of phonological and tactile information in children with VI suggests that the two are separate but interdependent (Warren 1994). This is particularly important with respect to the reading of Braille.

Academic achievement

Research into the academic achievements of children with VI is far more limited. Warren cited one study (Coker 1979) that suggested that children with VI, in both public and special schools, match the academic achievements of their sighted peers up to 8–9 years of age. From this point onwards children in mainstream schools fell behind, whereas children in special schools maintained progress with sighted peers. In contrast to studies in sighted children which found positive correlations between internal locus of control and academic achievement, one study of children with VI has found the reverse—that external locus of control correlated with higher academic achievement (Jones & McGhee 1972). Freeman *et al.*'s (1991) long-term follow up of the grown-up children and young people in their original study found better than expected academic outcomes, with 76% having completed secondary education and 19% having attended or attending university.

Braille reading appears to develop as a result of a range of converging processes. Warren (1994) suggested that phonological decoding and tactile–spatial decoding function separately but interdependently. Millar (1997) suggested a complex process involving phonological, lexical and syntactic processes interacting with progressively organized hand movements which provide spatial referencing cues and verbal information.

Social and emotional development

Studies of the social and emotional development of children with VI have come to widely divergent conclusions about the impact of VI (Fraiberg 1977; McGurk 1983; Hobson *et al.* 1997). Mulford (1983) found that by the ages of 5–6 most blind children had established a range of verbal and non-verbal communication strategies for establishing referential communication.

Preisler (1995; 1997) noted that children related much more to adults; they extended their interaction with peers in structured play but continued to have difficulty in free play settings (Rogers & Puchalski 1984); and expressed feelings of loneliness. Freeman *et al.* (1991), in their follow-up of children with VI into adult life, found half had a romantic relationship and 20% were in partnerships, all with sighted people.

Multisensory impairment

Epidemiology

Best (1983) estimated that 1 in 100 000 children have MSI but this is likely to be an underestimate. In the past, congenital rubella has accounted for one-third to one-half of cases (Trybus 1985) but this has fallen as a result of universal rubella immunization in many countries. Genetic conditions, such as Usher syndrome, and brain abnormalities associated with very low birth weight are now likely to account for the majority. Additional impairments are very common, with intellectual impairment in one-third to one-half and brain abnormalities in one-quarter (Trybus 1985).

Cultural aspects

In areas where there is high incidence of Usher syndrome, such as in the Cajun community of Louisiana, USA, deaf-blind communities have formed. A similar community has formed in Seattle, Washington, primarily through migration. Miner (1999) provided essential guidance on therapeutic techniques when working with deaf-blind people (see also the deaf-blind website: www.deafblind.com).

Impact of multisensory impairment

MSI is one of the most devastating (Adler 1987) and least understood (McInnes & Treffry 1982) of handicapping conditions. However, its impact on children and their families is influenced by the severity of the sensory impairments and the nature and severity of associated impairments (Jenkins & Chess 1996). Responses to sensory losses may include feelings of anxiety, isolation, denial, resentment or distortion of body image. Children with MSI demand a tremendous amount of effort and adaptation of approach from their parents (Freeman 1975, 1985). In the case of Usher syndrome, many parents appear devastated and unable to imagine the future life of their child when they are informed that their already deaf child may well go progressively blind (Miner 1995). More frequently than in the examination or treatment of children with HI and VI, the clinician will encounter dependency needs. The differential diagnostic problems are the same as for children with VI and HI, but with a particular concern not to miss sensory impairments when there is a complex multicausal neuropsychiatric syndrome combined with serious communicative problems.

Psychiatric aspects of hearing impairment

Most studies have shown that the rate of psychopathology is increased in children with HI compared with the general population, although the majority do not have a mental disorder (Hindley 1997). However, comparisons across studies are difficult because only three used a clinical interview with the child (Rutter *et al.* 1970; Hindley *et al.* 1994; van Gent, in preparation); only four were based on the general population (Rutter *et al.* 1970; Freeman *et al.* 1975; Sinkkonen 1994); and only three used instruments specifically designed for deaf children (Hindley *et al.* 1994; Vostanis *et al.* 1997; van Gent, in preparation).

The range of psychiatric disorders is the same as in hearing children (Hindley *et al.* 1994) but deaf children are exposed to a range of additional risk factors including communication problems, central nervous system disorders, physical health problems and intellectual impairment (Kammever & Hütsch 1988a, 1988b; Hindley 1997). This may explain why pervasive developmental disorders are more common amongst deaf children (Table 50.1). Although there is a greater proportion of disruptive than emotional disorders amongst children referred to specialist services (van Gent & Hendricks 1994; Hindley & van Gent 2000), high rates of emotional disorders are found in a school population of deaf children in comparison to hearing children (van Eldik 1998). Findings are contradictory on whether disorder is more common amongst children with HI in mainstream or special schools. Smith & Sharp (1994) found that deaf children in mainstream schools were particularly likely to be bullied. On the other hand, deaf children in residential schools are vulnerable to abuse (Sullivan *et al.* 2000).

Psychiatric assessment

Deaf children rely on visual communication. When interviewing them, the room needs to be uncluttered and well lit but without a bright light, such as a window behind the interviewer. Lip-reading requires a clear view of the lips; bushy beards and moustaches can cause problems. No more than 25% of spoken language is seen through lip patterns alone (Conrad 1979). Deaf people have to make educated guesses when lip-reading (Beck & de Jong 1990), and a strong foreign accent can make that more difficult.

When clinicians have limited signing skills, their efforts to engage signing deaf children can blunt their capacity to detect subtle affective signals, thereby missing affective disorders (Hindley *et al.* 1993). It is better to engage a professional sign language interpreter, preferably with experience of child mental health and with an opportunity to meet the child prior to the interview and for debriefing afterwards. This is particularly important because the interpreter will have the child's eye contact and may have picked up subtle emotional cues (Turner *et al.* 2000). The coexistence of deafness and psychiatric disorder can lead clinicians to

Table 50.1 Prevalence of psychiatric disorders in children and adolescents with hearing impairment (HI) and hearing controls.

Study	Number of children with HI	Range of HI	Prevalence of disorder	
			HI group (%)	Control (%)
Rutter et al. (1970)	13	Moderate–profound	15	7
Schlesinger & Meadow (1972)	512	Severe–profound	31	10
Freeman et al. (1975)	120	Severe–profound	22	—
Fundudis et al. (1979)	54	Moderate–profound	Profound: 54*	18
			Moderate: 28†	
Aplin (1985)	61	Profound	36	—
Aplin (1987)	42	Mild–profound	17	—
Hindley et al. (1994)	81	Moderate–profound	Profound: 42	—
			Moderate: 61	
Sinkkonen (1994)	379	Funct. deaf	Profound: 19	16
			Moderate: 25	
Vostanis et al. (1997)	84	Profound	Deaf: 40	—
van Gent (in preparation)	60	Severe–profound	27	16

*Profound: severe to profound, early onset hearing impairment.

†Moderate to profound acquired hearing impairment.

an unwarranted assumption that deafness explains all—the phenomenon of 'diagnostic shadowing' (Kitson & Thacker 2000).

Psychological assessments

Caution is needed in interpreting psychological test findings in deaf children because most tests have been validated exclusively in hearing populations. A knowledge of developmental and cultural aspects of deafness is also helpful (Orr et al. 1987; Blennerhassett 2000).

Autism and related disorders

Two studies of deaf children attending audiology clinics found autism and related disorders to be more common than in hearing children. Juré et al. (1991) estimated a prevalence of 5.3% and Rosenhall et al. (1999) 3.5%. In the latter study, intellectual impairment did not account for the raised rate. One of the assumed causes of an increased prevalence of autism in deaf children is a common underlying cause arising from brain damage caused by agents such as intrauterine rubella (Chess 1977) and cytomegalovirus (Stubbs 1978; see van Gent et al. 1997).

The age of diagnosis of autism is frequently later in deaf children (Juré et al. 1991), in part reflecting 'diagnostic shadowing' (see above). This is despite the fact that the basic impairments associated with autism are qualitatively different from what is seen in other deaf children. Nevertheless, poor language skills stemming from deafness may be associated with delayed but not impaired imaginative play. Unusual communication patterns and passivity are more common in deaf children with intellectual impairment who do not have autism. Also, even clinicians with good signing skills can have difficulty in detecting language

disorder in sign. Further, some deaf children with autism show significant improvements in social functioning when educated in signing environments (Juré et al. 1991; Roberts & Hindley 1999).

Disruptive behaviour

The overrepresentation of HI children with disruptive behaviour among those referred to clinics may partially reflect referral patterns. However, there may also be associations with brain pathology that occur with some types of deafness (Kelly et al. 1993). In a longitudinal study of children affected by congenital rubella, Chess et al. (1971) and Chess & Fernandez (1980) found that early impulsiveness in those with deafness alone disappeared as the children acquired language and self-control skills. By contrast, impulsiveness persisted in deaf children with additional impairments. Oppositional behaviour can be an expression of underlying feelings of impotence, anxiety or sadness, or an expression of frustration with difficulties of communication (Kelly et al. 1993). Symptoms of distractibility and overactivity may reflect a distracting visual environment, or poor language matching in the classroom leading to boredom (Hindley & Kroll 1998), or undetected intellectual language impairments, seizure disorders or the side-effects of drugs (Kelly et al. 1993).

Emotional disorders

The underrepresentation of emotional disorders in children with HI seen in the specialist services runs counter to the epidemiological evidence. Using the Child Behaviour Checklist (CBCL; Achenbach 1991), van Eldik (1998) found significantly higher scores on the anxious/depressive scale among deaf teenagers than among hearing peers. Emotional problems may be missed because poor signing skills prevent parents and teachers recognizing the mood disturbance.

The display of emotion used to illustrate narratives in sign must not be confused with an affective disorder. The latter is pervasive and persistent, whereas the former changes rapidly and is congruent with the narrative (Roberts & Hindley 1999). Behavioural problems that have distinct beginnings and endings, with no clear response to changes in circumstance may derive from depression (Kitson & Thacker 2000).

Schizophrenia and other psychoses

Psychotic disorders are not more common in deaf young people (Kitson & Thacker 2000). Because the syntax of sign language is very different from spoken language, disorders of thinking can be misattributed (Evans & Elliott 1987; Jenkins & Chess 1996). Equally, accurate assessments of thought disorder and abnormal experiences can be difficult (Kitson & Thacker 2000). Nevertheless, phenomena such as clang associations and flight of ideas have been clearly identified in deaf adults with psychotic disorders (Fraunhofer & Kitson 1991; Kitson & Thacker 2000).

Intervention

In the early 1960s, Rainer & Altschuler (1966) described the then revolutionary service for deaf adults in New York State; and more recently Sleeboom-van Raaij (1991) offered her experience in setting up a similar unit in the Netherlands. Specialist services for children and adolescents with HI and their families are still few but are better developed in the Netherlands, Sweden and the UK than in most other countries. In the Netherlands an inpatient and outpatient service was started in 1993. In the UK, an outpatient service was started in 1991 and a national inpatient unit opened in 2001. Sweden has a national outpatient service. All these services emphasize the importance of the sociocultural model of deafness, consultation with the deaf community and parents of children with HI, and a combined team of deaf and hearing professionals. Hearing professionals are expected to achieve high levels of sign language proficiency (Hindley & van Gent 2000).

After initial assessment, the same range of outpatient treatments are provided as for hearing children and their families (Hindley 2000). Treatment often has to be organized nearer to the child's home because of the distance to the specialized service. Because of their scarcity, specialized services are often brought in as consultants to local clinics (van Gent 1999).

Elliott et al. (1987) described specific pitfalls in the psychotherapy of children with HI as well as the value of deaf therapists. Interpreters in family and group therapy may become incorporated into transference relationships (Harvey 1989; Hoyt et al. 1981). Medication may involve effects that impede communication because they influence the skills needed for signing or lip-reading (Sleeboom-van Raaij 1997). Also, children

with HI are sometimes unable to describe the effects and side-effects of the medication prescribed. The inpatient treatment of children with HI usually involves a highly structured programme tailored to the individual child within a small and well-organized community and the wider deaf community (teachers, social workers, etc.).

Specialist or generic services

Specialist services exist in only a few countries and, where present, may not be geographically accessible to all. Specialist services for deaf children do not fit neatly into tiered models of services. Unlike other specialist services, their specialism is not in a particular group of disorders, but in communication—a fundamental aspect of all service provision. Two considerations should guide referral to specialist services: the communication needs of the child and the complexity of the case. Where there are no specialist services, clinicians will need help with signing from interpreters but should also be prepared to use non-verbal means of communication.

Otitis media with effusion

Otitis media with effusion can lead to transient, but sometimes severe, conductive hearing impairment. Early reports suggested that this could result in impaired language skills and behavioural difficulties (McGee et al. 1982; Chalmers et al. 1989). However, the weight of evidence now indicates that although the recurrent hearing impairment may lead to some minor impairments in language functioning, it less often causes a serious language disorder (Haggard et al. 1990; Bennett & Haggard 1999).

Hearing children of deaf parents

Knowledge on the development of hearing children of deaf parents is relatively limited (Meadow-Orlans 1995; Singleton & Tittle 2000). The most comprehensive report is an anthropological study of 150 grown-up children of signing deaf parents (Preston 1994). Most deaf parents are competent and caring but they experience stresses as a result of being deaf in a hearing world (Singleton & Tittle 2000). Hearing children of deaf parents are at the centre of interaction between deaf and hearing cultures. Although use of sign language is a central component of being deaf and often a source of pride, some deaf people see their sign language as less valued than spoken language and may experience shame when using sign outside their deaf community. This may lead some to choose not to use sign with their hearing child and to rely on inadequate spoken language. In other circumstances hearing children are drawn into the role of communicator/interpreter for their parents. These experiences can be seen as adverse, 'parentifying' the child at an early age, but to others these experiences lead to 'greater adaptiveness, resourcefulness, curiosity and "worldliness" ' (Singleton & Tittle 2000). Deaf parents may have difficulty in accessing information about parenting, and their own childhood within a hearing family may not have provided them with good models of parenting. This may lead to their feeling unconfident or incompetent as parents (Singleton & Tittle 2000). In some respects, the experience of deaf parents of hearing children can be compared to that of parents raising children from ethnic backgrounds different from their own (Singleton & Tittle 2000). Some lessons about 'cultural brokering' may be relevant.

Most of the grown-up hearing children of deaf parents studied by Preston (1994) acknowledged some difficulties in their childhood but attributed these as much to the hearing society's response to their parents as to their parent's failings. Their roles as interpreters and advocates were linked to experiences that were both fulfilling and hurtful. In a similar vein, many described loyalties that were divided between their deaf parents and their hearing grandparents.

Little is known about the psychological well-being of hearing children of deaf parents but perhaps a characteristic pattern should not be expected. Clinical experience suggests that emotional difficulties may be more common than in children with HI but whether this applies to non-referred children is not known.

Mental health aspects of cochlear implantation

Advocates for cochlear implants in congenitally deaf children argue for 'the unique possibility of restoring some hearing to the deaf' and claim long-term postoperative gains with respect to hearing, language and scholastic achievements at school (Van den Broek et al. 1998). Critics (including most organizations for the deaf) express ethical objections on the grounds that the implants constitute a serious invasion, and denial, of the cultural identity of deaf people and they query both the consistency and validity of the supposed benefits (Hindley 2000). Adequate psychological evaluations have yet to be undertaken but they are much needed.

Adult psychotherapy

A community survey of deaf adults (Checinski 1993) has suggested that the rate of psychiatric disorder is increased, with perhaps one-third experiencing an episode of depression. In London, referral for depression and for anxiety disorder have increased recently, as a result of improvements in service provision (Kitson & Thacker 2000). In line with our clinical experience with adolescents, there has been some increase in drug use (Austen & Checinski 2000) and abuse (Vernon & Daigle-King 1999) amongst deaf adults.

Psychiatric aspects of visual impairment

Epidemiology

Jan et al. (1977) studied a heterogeneous total population of blind and partially sighted children and young people aged 0–20 years, using questionnaires and interviews and a neighbourhood control group matched for age and sex. Of 86 children with VI, 57% showed psychiatric or cognitive disorder. Mental retardation or a developmental disorder was present in one-third of the children, and the psychiatric diagnoses spanned adjustment reaction, personality disorder and behaviour disorder. More children with VI were prescribed more psychotropic medication, and more had sleep and nutritional problems.

Van Hasselt et al. (1986) found that male adolescents with VI had higher mean scores than sighted controls on the parent, teacher and self-report versions of the CBCL (Achenbach & Edelbrock 1983). Those attending a residential school had higher mean scores than those attending a mainstream day school. In a study of preschool-age children with severe VI and mental retardation, one-third of the group showed social withdrawal, lack of relationships with other children, self-injurious behaviour and/or poor compliance at bedtime (Kitzinger & Hunt 1985). Ollendick et al. (1985) noted a pattern of fears in adolescents with VI that reflected the dangers they faced in their everyday world. Huure & Aro (1998), in a study of adolescents with VI in mainstream schools, found an increased rate of loneliness and difficulties making friends, but not of depression, compared with controls. Thus, the evidence suggests that VI is accompanied by a raised rate of psychopathology that, to some extent, follows a possibly slightly different pattern from that found in sighted children (although there were marked similarities in the study by Schnittjer & Hirshoren 1981).

Yoshida et al. (1998) found an excess of emotional disorders in young adults with VI but there have been reports of increased depression and anxiety among adults who became blind at a later age (De Leo et al. 1999). Also, blind people may be at a greater risk of developing chronic post-traumatic stress disorder because of their difficulty in reconstructing a mental image of the initiating traumatic event (McFarlane 1988).

As with HI, psychiatric disorder in children with VI is more likely when there are additional impairments. Probably, congenital blindness has a more pervasive effect on psychological development but acquired VI may lead to a greater sense of loss for both parents and children (Jan et al. 1997). Early visual experience can have a positive effect on the acquisition of skills such as Braille reading (Sampaio & Philip 1995). Although VI can have a powerful impact, children vary in their response, and there is no such thing as a 'blind personality' (Vander Kolk 1987).

Psychiatric assessment

The assessment of children with VI and their families is comparable to that of children with HI, except that it does not involve the need for an interpreter. Given the impact of VI on early mother–child interaction, a careful account of this period should be obtained from parents. Early sleep difficulties (Tabandeh et al. 1998) may reflect circadian cycle disturbances stemming from lack of visual feedback (Sasaki et al. 1992) or perception of social cues relating to sleep (Sadeh et al. 1995).

Separation anxiety may be increased in young children with VI (Burlingham 1972; Fraiberg 1977), and in adolescence over-protection may make the development of personal and sexual relationships more difficult (Scholl 1974).

The psychiatric interview should take place in a room adapt-ed to the child with VI. Obstacles should be few, lighting should be good if the child has any vision, and children need to be given time to explore and adapt to the new environment (Hansen *et al.* 1982). The clinician must be prepared to have much more phys-ical contact than with sighted children, to take the time to de-scribe and respond to questions about the contents of the room and the toys, and about the purposes and procedures of the as-sessment (Jenkins & Chess 1996). Many children with VI use touch and oral manipulation to become familiar with toys and test objects. Clinicians must be aware of their own reactions to the child with VI; one study showed that there was a tendency to make a more favourable assessment of cognitive and social capacities when the blind child used gaze direction (Raver-Lampman 1990). In view of the frequency of additional impair-ments, it is essential that clinical appraisal should include an adequate physical assessment.

Psychological assessment

Blindness affects children's variety of experiences, their ability to get about, and their control of the environment (Lowenfeld 1948). These need to be considered when interpreting test find-ings (Warren 1977). A focus more on the functional skills used and on style of problem-solving may be as informative as scores on tests designed for sighted children (Hansen *et al.* 1982). Such tests can be useful, however, if used to assess patterns of per-formance (Groenveld & Jan 1992). There are some tests spe-cifically designed for use with children with VI (e.g. the Reynell–Zinkin; Reynell 1979). Others have been translated into Braille or large print, but appropriate modifications of stan-dard tests may allow them to be used (Van Hasselt & Sisson 1987), although care is needed in relation to implications re-garding comparisons with standardization data (see Sergeant & Taylor, Chapter 6). As with children with HI, the testing of chil-dren with VI tends to take somewhat longer than that of sighted children.

Autism and related disorders

Children with severe congenital VI not infrequently show autis-tic-like features (Cass 1998); one-quarter did so in the study by Brown *et al.* (1997). These features include echolalia, pronomi-nal reversal and delayed emergence of symbolic play (Fraiberg 1977), and stereotyped behaviours, or 'blindisms', such as repetitive body-rocking, hand-flapping, toe-walking, eye-pressing, rubbing or poking, eye flicking with fingers and light gazing. The latter may derive from early lack of sensory ex-periences (Jan *et al.* 1977), giving rise to compensatory self-stimulation (Warren 1984). The autistic qualities may also reflect failures in psychological perspective-taking (Hobson *et al.* 1999). Autistic patterns are much more frequent when VI is accompanied by mental retardation (Brown *et al.* 1997) and they may also stem from brain pathology associated with some forms of VI (Chase 1972).

In summary, autism in children with severe VI may reflect shared risk factors but also VI may give rise to 'blindisms' that carry a somewhat different meaning. They may be influenced by interventions and usually gradually disappear but may reappear with anxiety, lack of sufficient stimulation or in new stressful situations.

Interventions

There are far fewer specialized psychiatric inpatient and outpa-tient services for children and adolescents with VI than for those with HI. The usual range of therapeutic modalities are appli-cable but styles of therapist–child interaction may need some modification (see Frailberg 1977; Van Hasselt *et al.* 1983; Warren 1984; Erin *et al.* 1991; Sisson 1992). Therapists must appreciate that VI will impair children's ability to perceive communicative cues conveyed through posture and facial expressions and they must be willing to translate their responses into words. Also, VI may alter the child's use of directed gaze, facial expression and posture to convey feelings. The presence of a guide dog some-times complicates matters, if it becomes protective of its owner through awareness of negative emotions. In insight-directed therapy, the child may express contradictory feelings and desires regarding dependence and independence, when memories of helplessness and of the significance of the VI re-emerge (Johnson 1989). Therapists may take a more active protective attitude than they would towards sighted children. Particularly in the final phases of treatment, intense separation anxiety may recur, reflecting early fears of losses. Parenting a child with VI can be extremely stressful and approaches to reduce parental stress have been developed (Kirkham *et al.* 1986; Van Hasselt *et al.* 1987; Webb 1990). As with children with HI, careful monitor-ing of the effects and side-effects of medication is very important in relation to possible influences on sensory functioning.

Adult outcome

Freeman *et al.* (1991) followed the heterogeneous sample of children with VI previously studied by Jan *et al.* (1977) into early adult life. Mannerisms had almost disappeared (except in those with multiple handicaps), and several individuals who exhibited stereotypies when they were alone were able to control this be-haviour in public. A worse psychiatric outcome was found in those with mental retardation and in those whose vision deteri-orated. It was striking that one-third of the women and one in nine of the men reported that they had been sexually molested or abused. Also, nearly three-quarters said they had been cruelly teased at school. Misunderstandings tended to be worse for the partially sighted students, whose visual abilities were more difficult to comprehend. There was a strong tendency for the partially sighted to want to pass as normal. Employment outcomes were poor, with three out of five out of work.

Conclusions

Our knowledge of the developmental pathways of sensory impaired children, and of their differences from hearing and sighted children, continues to grow. However, on the whole, we know more about the effects of HI than of VI, and services for children with VI are less well developed than for those with HI. This is impeding both our understanding of psychopathological factors and our care of these young people. Uncertainties remain about the optimal balance between specialist and local services. Until recently, the main psychological focus has been on the effects of HI and VI on key developmental experiences and on the effects of society's response to sensory deficits. These remain important but opinions are divided on the extent to which sensory impairments should be viewed as a cultural difference rather than as a disability. The improvements that are likely in medical interventions, such as cochlear implants, will make resolution of this issue both more difficult and more important. There is also a growing awareness that some of the psychopathological problems found in children with HI or VI stem from associated neurodevelopmental impairment or cognitive deficits. An integrated approach to mental health issues will continue to be crucial.

References

Achenbach, T.M. (1991) *Integrative Guide for the 1991 CBCL/4–18, YSR and TRF Profiles*. University of Vermont Department of Psychiatry, Burlington, VT.

Achenbach, T.M. & Edelbrock, C.S. (1983) *Manual for the Child Behavior Checklist and Revised Behavior Profile*. University of Vermont Department of Psychiatry, Burlington, VT.

Adelson, E. (1983) The role of vision in early development. In: *Language Acquisition in the Blind Child: Normal and Deficient* (ed. A.E. Mills), pp. 1–12. Croom-Helm, London.

Adler, M.A. (1987) Psychosocial interventions with deaf-blind youths and adults. In: *Psychosocial Interventions with Sensorially Disabled Persons* (eds B.W. Heller, L.M. Flohr & L.S. Zegans), pp. 187–207. Grune & Stratton, London.

Als, H., Troninck, E. & Brazelton, T.B. (1980) Affective reciprocity and the development of autonomy: the study of a blind infant. *Journal of the American Academy of Child Psychiatry*, **19**, 22–40.

Antia, S.D., Kreimeyer, K.H. & Eldridge, N. (1993) Promoting social interaction between young children with hearing impairments and their peers. *Exceptional Children*, **60**, 262–275.

Aplin, D.Y. (1985) Social and emotional adjustments of hearing-impaired children in special schools. *Journal of the British Association of Teachers of the Deaf*, **9**, 84–94.

Aplin, D.Y. (1987) Social and emotional adjustments of hearing-impaired children in ordinary and special schools. *Educational Research*, **29**, 56–64.

Austen, S. & Checinski, K. (2000) Addictive behavior and deafness. In:

Mental Health and Deafness (eds P. Hindley & N. Kitson), pp. 232–252. Whurr, London.

Baird, G. & Moore, A.T. (1993) Epidemiology of childhood blindness. In: *The Management of Visual Impairments in Childhood, Clinics in Developmental Medicine No. 128* (eds A. Fielder, A. Best & M. Bax), pp. 1–8. MacKeith Press, London.

Balow, I.H. & Brill, R.G. (1972) *An evaluation study of leading academic achievement levels of sixteen graduating classes of the Californian School for the Deaf*. Mimeo Report Contract No 4566 with the State of California, Department of Education, Riverside, CA.

Beck, G. & de Jong, E. (1990) *Opgroeien in een Horende Wereld*. van Tricht, Twello, NL.

Bennett, K.E. & Haggard, M.P. (1999) Behaviour and cognitive outcomes from middle ear disease. *Archives of Disease in Childhood*, **80**, 28–35.

Best, C. (1983) The 'new' deaf-blind? Results of a national survey of deaf-blind children in ESN (S) and hospital schools. *British Journal of Visual Impairment*, **1**, 11–13.

Blennerhassett, L. (2000) Psychological assessments. In: *Mental Health and Deafness* (eds P. Hindley & N. Kitson), pp. 185–205. Whurr, London.

Braden, J.P. (1994) *Deafness, Deprivation and IQ*. Plenum Press, New York.

Brinich, P.M. (1981) Application of the metapsychological profile to the assessment of deaf children. *Psychoanalytic Study of the Child*, **36**, 3–32.

Brown, R., Hobson, R.P., Lee, A. & Stevenson, J. (1997) Are there 'autistic' features in congenitally blind children? *Journal of Child Psychology and Psychiatry*, **38**, 693–703.

Bryars, J.H. & Archer, D.B. (1977) Aetiological survey of visually handicapped children in Northern Ireland. *Transactions of the Ophthalmological Societies of the United Kingdom*, **97**, 26–29.

Burlingham, D. (1972) *Psychoanalytic Studies of the Sighted and the Blind*. International University Press, New York.

Campbell, R. (1998) Read the lips: speculation on the nature and role of lipreading in cognitive development of deaf children. In: *Relations of Language and Thought* (eds M. Marschark, P. Siple, D. Lillo-Martin, R. Campbell & V. Everhart), pp. 110–146. Oxford University Press, Oxford.

Caselli, M.C. & Volterra, V. (1989) From communication to language in hearing and deaf children. In: *From Gesture to Language in Hearing and Deaf Children* (eds V. Volterra & C.J. Erting), pp. 263–277. Springer-Verlag, Berlin.

Cass, H. (1998) Visual impairment and autism: current questions and future research. *Autism*, **2**, 117–138.

Chalmers, D., Stewart, I., Silva, P. & Mulvena, A. (1989) Otitis media with effusion in children: the Dunedin Study. *Clinics in Developmental Medicine*, **108**, MacKeith Press, London.

Chase, J.B. (1972) *Retrolental Fibroplasia and Autistic Symptomatology*. New York American Foundation for the Blind, New York.

Checinski, K. (1993) *An estimate of the point prevalence of psychiatric disorder in prelingually deaf adults living in the community*. MD thesis, Cambridge University.

Chess, S. (1977) Follow-up report on autism in congenital rubella. *Journal of Autism and Childhood Schizophrenia*, **7**, 69–81.

Chess, S. & Fernandez, P. (1980) Do deaf children have a typical personality? *Journal of the American Academy of Child Psychiatry*, **19**, 654–664.

Chess, S., Korn, S.J. & Fernandez, P.B. (1971) *Psychiatric Disorders of Children with Congenital Rubella*. Brunner & Mazel, New York.

Chirambo, M.C., Tielsch, J.M., West, K.P. Jr *et al.* (1986) Blindness and visual impairment in southern Malawi. *Bulletin of the World Health Organization*, **64**, 567–572.

Coker, C. (1979) A comparison of self-concepts and academic achievement of visually handicapped children enrolled in a regular school and in a residential school. *Education of the Visually Handicapped*, **11**, 67–74.

Conrad, R. (1979) *The Deaf Schoolchild*. Harper & Row, London.

Corina, D.P. (1999) Neural disorders of language and movement: evidence from American Sign Language. In: *Gesture Speech and Sign* (eds L. Messing & R. Campbell), pp. 27–44. Oxford University Press, Oxford.

Courtin, C. & Melot, A.M. (1998) Development of theories of mind in deaf children. In: *Psychological Perspectives of Deafness 2* (eds M. Marshark & M.D. Clarke), pp. 79–102. Lawrence Erlbaum, Mahwah, NJ.

Cullinan, T.R. (1987) [cited in Baird, G. & Moore, A.T. (1993)] Epidemiology of childhood blindness. In: *The Management of Visual Impairments in Childhood, Clinics in Developmental Medicine* (eds A. Fielder, A. Best & M. Bax), **128**, pp. 1–8. MacKeith Press, London.

Danek, M.M. (1988) Deafness and family impact. In: *Family Interventions Throughout Chronic Illness and Disability*, (eds P. Power, A. Dell Orto & M. Gibsons), pp. 120–135. Springer, New York.

Davis, A., Wood, S., Healy, R., Webb, H. & Rowe, S. (1995) Risk factors for hearing disorders: epidemiological evidence of change over time. *UK Journal of the American Academy of Audiology*, **6**, 365–370.

Davis, C.J. (1980) *Perkins–Binet Tests of Intelligence for the Blind*. Perkins School for the Blind, Watertown, MA.

Dekker, R. & Koole, F.D. (1992) Visually impaired children's visual characteristics and intelligence. *Developmental Medicine and Child Neurology*, **34**, 123–133.

De Leo, D., Hickey, P.A., Meneghel, G. & Cantor, C.H. (1999) Blindness, fear of sight loss, and suicide. *Psychosomatics*, **40**, 339–344.

De Villiers, J.E., de Villiers, P. & Hoban, E. (1994) The central problem of functional categories in the English syntax of oral deaf children. In: *Constraints on Language Acquisition: Studies of Atypical Children* (ed. H. Tager-Flusberg), pp. 9–47. Lawrence Erlbaum, Hillsdale, NJ.

Dunlea, A. (1989) *Vision and the Emergence of Meaning*. Cambridge University Press, New York.

Elliott, H., Bell, B., Langholtz, D., Ngoyen, M. & Peters, L. (1987) Assessment from the perspective of the deaf therapist. In: *Mental Health Assessment of Deaf Clients* (eds H. Elliott, L. Glass & J.W. Evans), pp. 143–152. Little, Brown, San Diego.

Erin, J.N., Dignan, K. & Brown, P.A. (1991) Are social skills teachable? A review of the literature. *Journal of Visual Impairment and Blindness*, **85**, 58–61.

Erting, C.J., Prezioso, C. & O'Grady Hynes, M. (1989) The interactional context of deaf mother–infant interactions. In: *From Gesture to Language in Hearing and Deaf Children* (eds V. Volterra & C.J. Erting), pp. 97–106. Springer Verlag, Berlin.

Evans, J.W. & Elliott, H. (1987) The mental status examination. In: *Mental Health Assessment of Deaf Clients. A Practical Manual* (eds H. Elliott, L. Glass & J.W. Evans), pp. 83–92. Little, Brown, San Diego.

Fogel, A. (1997) Seeing and being seen. In: *Blindness and Psychological Development* (eds V. Lewis & G.M. Collis), pp. 86–98. BPS Books, Leicester.

Fraiberg, S. (1977) *Insights from the Blind: Comparative Studies of Blind and Sighted Children*. Basic Books, New York.

Fraunhofer, N. & Kitson, N. (1991) A study of Evans' and Elliott's criteria in mental state assessment of schizophrenia in the prelingually profoundly deaf. In: *Proceedings of the Mental Health and Deafness Conference*, pp. 54–56. St. George's Hospital Medical School, London.

Freeman, R.D., Malkin, S.F. & Hastings, J.O. (1975) Psychological problems of deaf children and their families: a comparative study. *American Annals of the Deaf*, **120**, 275–304.

Freeman, R.D., Goetz, E., Richards, D.P. *et al.* (1991) Defiers of negative prediction: a 14-year follow-up study of legally blind children. *Journal of Visual Impairment and Blindness*, **85**, 365–370.

Fundudis, T., Kolvin, I. & Garside, R. (1979) *Speech Retarded and Deaf Children: Their Psychological Development*. Academic Press, London.

Gale, E., de Villiers, P., de Villiers, J. & Pyers, J. (1996) Language and theory of mind in oral deaf children. In: *Proceedings of the 20th Annual Boston University Conference on Language Development*, Vol. 1 (eds A. Stringfellow, D. Cahana-Amitay, E. Hughes & A. Zukowski), pp. 213–224. Cascadilla Press, Somerville, MA.

Geers, J.G. & Nicholas, A.E. (1997) Communication of oral deaf and normally hearing children at 36 months of age. *Journal of Speech, Language and Hearing Research*, **40**, 1314–1327.

Gorlin, R.J., Toriello, H.V. & Cohen, M.M., eds (1995) *Hereditary Hearing Loss and its Syndromes*. Oxford University Press, New York.

Greenberg, M.T. & Kusche, C. (1989) Cognitive, personal and social development of deaf children and adolescents. In: *The Handbook of Special Education: Research and Practice*, Vol. 1 (eds M.C. Wang & M. Reynolds), pp. 95–129. Pergamon Press, Oxford.

Greenberg, M.T. & Kusche, M.T. (1993) *Promoting Social and Emotional Development in Deaf Children: the PATHS Project*. University of Washington Press, Seattle, WA.

Greenberg, M.T. & Marvin, R.S. (1979) Patterns of attachment in profoundly deaf preschool children. *Merrill-Palmer Quarterly*, **25**, 265–279.

Gregory, S. & Mogford, K. (1982) The development of symbolic play in young deaf children. In: *The Acquisition of Symbolic Play* (eds D. Rogers & J. Sloboda), pp. 221–231. Plenum Press, New York.

Gregory, S. (1991) Challenging motherhood: mothers and their deaf children. In: *Motherhood: Meanings, Practices and Ideologies* (eds A. Phoenix, A. Woolett & E. Lloyd), pp. 123–142. Sage, London.

Gregory, S. & Powers, S. (1998) *The educational achievements of deaf children: a literature review*. DFEE Research Report No 65. University of Birmingham & E.D. Thoutenhoofd, University of Durham.

Gregory, S., Bishop, J. & Sheldon, L. (1995) *Deaf Young People and their Families: Developing Understanding*. Cambridge University Press, Cambridge.

Groce, N.E. & Whiting, M. (1988) *Everyone Here Spoke Sign Language: Hereditary Deafness on Martha's Vineyard*. Harvard University Press, Cambridge, MA.

Groenveld, M. (1993) Effects of visual disability on behaviour and the family. In: *The Management of Visual Impairments in Childhood, Clinics in Developmental Medicine No. 128* (eds A. Fielder, A. Best & M. Bax), pp. 64–77. MacKeith Press, London.

Groenveld, M. & Jan, J.E. (1992) Intelligence profiles of low vision and blind children. *Journal of Visual Impairment and Blindness*, **86**, 68–71.

Hadadian, A. (1995) Attitudes toward deafness and security of attachment relationships among young deaf children and their parents. *Early Education and Development*, **6**, 181–191.

Haggard, M. & Hughes, E. (1991) *Screening of Children's Hearing: a Review of the Literature and the Implications of OM*. HMSO, London.

Haggard, M.P., Birkin, J.A. & Pringle, D.P. (1990) Consequences of otitis media for speech and language. In: *Practical Aspects of Audiology: Pediatric Audiology 0–5 Years* (ed. B. McCormick). Whurr, London.

Hansen, R., Young, J. & Ulrey, G. (1982) Assessment considerations with the visually handicapped child. In: *Psychological Assessment of Handicapped Infants and Young Children* (eds G. Ulrey & S. Rogers), pp. 108–114. Thieme-Stratton, New York.

Harris, M. (2000) Social interaction and early language development in deaf children. *Deafness and Education International*, **2**, 1–11.

Harris, M. (2001) It's all a matter of timing: sign visibility and sign reference in deaf and hearing mothers of 18-month-old children. *Journal of Deaf Studies & Deaf Education*, **6**, 177–185.

Harris, R.I. (1978) The relationship of impulse control to parent hearing status, manual communication and academic achievement in deaf children. *American Annals of the Deaf*, **123**, 52–67.

Harvey, M.A. (1989) *Psychotherapy with Deaf and Hard of Hearing Persons: A Systemic Model.* Lawrence Erlbaum, Hillsdale, NJ.

Heiling, K. (1995) *The development of deaf children. International Studies on Sign Language and Communication of the Deaf*, Vol. 30. Signum, Hamburg.

Hill, A.E., McKendrick, P., Poole, J.J., Pugh, R.E., Rosenbloom, L. & Turnbull, R. (1986) The Liverpool Visual Assessment Team: 10 years experience. *Child: Care, Health and Development*, **12**, 37–51.

Hindley, P.A. (1997) Psychiatric aspects of hearing impairments. *Journal of Child Psychology and Psychiatry*, **38**, 101–117.

Hindley, P.A. (1999) The cultural–linguistic model of deafness: response by a psychodynamic family psychiatrist specialising in work with families which include a deaf child. *Journal of Social Work Practice*, **13**, 174–176.

Hindley, P.A. (2000) Child and adolescent psychiatry. In: *Mental Health and Deafness* (eds P. Hindley & N. Kitson), pp. 42–74. Whurr, London.

Hindley, P.A. & Kroll, L. (1998) Theoretical and epidemiological aspects of attention deficit and overactivity in deaf children. *Journal of Deaf Studies and Deaf Education*, **3**, 64–72.

Hindley, P. & van Gent, T. (2000) Mental health in deaf children and adolescents: an Anglo-Dutch collaborative study. *Poster Presentation at the Fourth European Conference of the Association for Child Psychology and Psychiatry, London*.

Hindley, P.A., Hill, P.D. & Bond, D. (1993) Interviewing deaf children, the interviewer effect: a research note. *Journal of Child Psychology and Psychiatry*, **34**, 1461–1467.

Hindley, P.A., Hill, P.D., McGuigan, S. & Kitson, N. (1994) Psychiatric disorder in deaf and hearing impaired children and young people: a prevalence study. *Journal of Child Psychology and Psychiatry*, **35**, 917–934.

Hobson, R., Brown, R., Minter, E.M. & Lee, A. (1997) Autism 'revisited': the case of congenital blindness. In: *Blindness and Psychological Development in Young Children* (eds V. Lewis & G. Collis), pp. 99–115. BPS Books, Leicester.

Hobson, R.P., Lee, A. & Brown, R. (1999) Autism and congenital blindness. *Journal of Autism and Developmental Disorders*, **29**, 45–56.

Hoffmeister, R., De Villiers, P., Engen, E. & Topol, D. (1997) English reading achievement and ASL skills in deaf students. In: *Boston University Conference on Language Development, 21 Proceedings* (eds R. Hoffmeister, P. de Villiers, E. Engen *et al.*), pp. 307–318. Cascadilla Press, Somerville, MA.

Hoyt, M.F., Siegelman, E.Y. & Schlesinger, H.S. (1981) Special issues regarding psychotherapy with the deaf. *American Journal of Psychiatry*, **138**, 807–811.

Huure, T.M. & Aro, H.M. (1998) Psychosocial development among adolescents with visual impairment. *European Child and Adolescent Psychiatry*, **7**, 73–78.

Iverson, J.M. (1998) Gesture when there is no visual model. *New Directions for Child Development*, **79**, 89–100.

Jan, J.E. & Freeman, R.D. (1998) Who is a visually impaired child? *Developmental Medicine and Child Neurology*, **40**, 65–67.

Jan, J.E., Freeman, R.D. & Scott, E.P. (1977) *Visual Impairment in Children and Adolescents*. Grune & Stratton, New York.

Jenkins, I.R. & Chess, S. (1996) Psychiatric evaluation of perceptually impaired children: hearing and visual impairments. In: *Child and Adolescent Psychiatry: a Comprehensive Textbook* (ed. M. Lewis), 2nd edn, pp. 526–534. Williams & Wilkins, Baltimore.

Johnson, C.L. (1989) Group counseling with blind people: a critical review of the literature. *Journal of Visual Impairment and Blindness*, **83**, 202–207.

Jones, R.L. & McGhee, P.W. (1972) Locus of control, reference group and achievement in blind children. *Rehabilitation Psychology*, **19**, 18–26.

Juré, R., Rapin, I. & Tuchman, R.F. (1991) Hearing impaired autistic children. *Developmental Medicine and Child Neurology*, **33**, 1062–1072.

Kammerer, E. & Hütsch, M. (1988a) Deafness from a child- and youth-psychiatric point of view. I. Medical aspects, epidemiology, and aspects of developmental psychology. *Praxis der kinderpsychologie und kinderpsychiatrie*, **37**, 167–175.

Kammerer, E. & Hütsch, M. (1988b) Deafness from a child- and youth-psychiatric point of view. II. Social and emotional development, child-psychiatric morbidity, significance of family and social environments. *Praxis der Kinderpsychologie und Kinderpsychiatrie*, **37**, 204–212.

Kekelis, L.S. & Andersen, E.S. (1984) Family communication styles and language development. *Journal of Visual Impairment and Blindness*, **78**, 54–65.

Kelly, D., Forney, J., Parker-Fischer, S. & Jones, M. (1993) The challenge of attention deficit disorder in children who are deaf or hard of hearing. *American Annals of the Deaf*, **138**, 343–348.

Kirkham, M.A., Schilling, R.R., Norelius, K. & Schinke, S.P. (1986) Developing coping styles and social support networks: an intervention outcome study with mothers of handicapped children. *Child: Care, Health and Development*, **12**, 313–323.

Kitson, N. & Thacker, A. (2000) Adult psychiatry. In: *Mental Health and Deafness* (eds P. Hindley & N. Kitson), pp. 75–98. Whurr, London.

Kitzinger, M. & Hunt, H. (1985) The effect of residential setting on sleep and behaviour patterns of young visually-handicapped children. In: *Recent Research in Developmental Psychopathology* (ed. J.E. Stevenson), pp. 73–80. Pergamon Press, Oxford.

Koester, L.S., Karkowski, A.M. & Traci, M.A. (1998) How do deaf and hearing mothers regain eye contact when their infants look away? *American Annals of the Deaf*, **143**, 5–13.

Landau, B. (1997) Language and experience in blind children: retrospective and perspective. In: *Blindness and Psychological Development* (eds V. Lewis & G.M. Collis), pp. 86–98. BPS Books, Leicester.

Lederberg, A. & Mobley, C. (1990) The effect of hearing impairment on the quality of attachment and mother toddler interaction. *Child Development*, **61**, 1596–1604.

Lederberg, A., Ryan, H.B. & Robbins, B.L. (1986) Peer interaction in young deaf children: the effect of partner hearing status and familiarity. *Developmental Psychology*, **22**, 691–700.

Lowenfeld, B. (1948) Effects of blindness on the cognitive functions of children. *Nervous Child*, **7**, 45–54.

Marschark, M. (1993) *Psychological Development of Deaf Children*. Oxford University Press, Oxford.

Marschark, M. & Everhart. V. (1997) Relations of language and cognition: what do deaf children tell us? In: *Relations of Language and Thought* (eds M. Marschark, P. Siple, D. Lillo-Martin, R. Campbell & V. Everhart), pp. 3–23. Oxford University Press, Oxford.

Martineau, T. (1993) Psychological consequences of screening for Down's Syndrome. *British Medical Journal*, **307**, 26–28.

Masataka, N. (1992) Motherese in a signed language. *Infant Behaviour and Development*, **15**, 453–460.

McAlpine, L.M. & Moore, C. (1995) The development of social understanding in children with visual impairments. *Journal of Visual Impairment and Blindness*, **89**, 349–358.

McFarlane, A.C. (1988) Posttraumatic stress disorder and blindness. *Comprehensive Psychiatry*, **29**, 558–560.

McGee, R., Silva, P.A. & Stewart, I.A. (1982) Behaviour problems and otitis media with effusion: a report from the Dunedin Multidisciplinary Child Development Study. *New Zealand Medical Journal*, **95**, 655–657.

McGurk, H. (1983) Affective motivation and development of communication competence in blind and sighted children. In: *Language Acquisition in the Blind Child: Normal and Deficient* (ed. A.E. Mills), pp. 108–113. Croom-Helm, London.

McInnes, J.M. & Treffry, J.A. (1982). *Deaf-Blind Infants and Children: a Developmental Guide*. Open University Press, Milton Keynes.

Meadow, K.P. (1968) Early manual communication in relation to the deaf child's intellectual, social and communicative functioning. *American Annals of the Deaf*, **113**, 29–41.

Meadow-Orlans, K.P. (1987) An analysis of the effectiveness of early intervention programs for hearing impaired children. In: *The Effectiveness of Early Intervention for at Risk and Handicapped Children* (eds M. Guralnick & F. Bennett), pp. 325–362. Academic Press, Orlando, FL.

Meadows-Orlans, K.P. (1995) Sources of stress for mothers and fathers of deaf and hard of hearing infants. *American Annals of the Deaf*, **140**, 352–357.

Meadow-Orlans, K. (1995) Parenting with a sensory or physical disability. In: *Handbook of Parenting*, Vol. 4. *Applied and Practical Considerations* (ed. M. Borstein), pp. 57–84. Erlbaum, Hillsdale, NJ.

Meadow-Orlans, K.P. & Erting, C. (2000) Deaf people in society. In: *Mental Health and Deafness* (eds P. Hindley & N. Kitson), pp. 3–24. Whurr, London.

Meyer, T.A., Svirsky, M.A., Kirk, K.I. & Miyamoto, R.T. (1998) Improvements in speech perception by children with profound hearing loss: effects of device, communication, mode and chronological age. *Journal of Speech, Language and Hearing Research*, **41**, 846–848.

Millar, S. (1997) Reading without vision. In: *Blindness and Psychological Development* (eds V. Lewis & G.M. Collis), pp. 86–98. BPS Books, Leicester.

Miner, I.D. (1995) Psychosocial implications of Usher syndrome, type I, throughout the life cycle. *Journal of Visual Impairment and Blindness*, **89**, 287–296.

Miner, I.D. (1999) Psychotherapy for people with Usher syndrome. In: *Psychotherapy with Deaf Clients from Diverse Client Groups* (ed. I.W. Leigh), pp. 302–327. Gallaudet University Press, Washington D.C.

Morford, J.P. (1998) Gesture when there is no speech model. *New Directions for Child Development*, **79**, 101–116.

Mulford, R. (1980) *Talking without seeing: some problems of semantic development in blind children*. Doctoral dissertation, Stanford University.

Mulford, R.C. (1983) Referential development in blind children. In: *Language Acquisition in the Blind Child: Normal and Deficient* (ed. A.E. Mills), pp. 89–107. Croom-Helm, London.

Newland, T.E. (1979) The blind aptitude test. *Journal of Visual Impairment and Blindness*, **73**, 134–139.

Nixon, H.L. (1994) Looking sociologically at family coping with visual impairment. *Journal of Visual Impairment and Blindness*, **88**, 329–337.

Nunes, T. & Monero, C. (1998) Is hearing impairment a cause of difficulties in learning mathematics. In: *The Development of Mathematical Skills* (ed. C. Donlan), pp. 227–253. Psychology Press, Hove.

Ohwaki, Y., Tanno, Y., Ohwaki, M., Hariu, T., Hayasaka, K. & Miyake, K. (1960) Construction of an intelligence test for the blind. *Tohoku Psychologia Folia*, **18**, 45–63.

Ollendick, T.H., Matson, J.L. & Helsel, W.J. (1985) Fears in visually impaired and normally-sighted youths. *Behavior Research and Therapy*, **23**, 375–378.

Orr, F.C., De Matteo, A., Heller, B., Lee, M. & Nguyen, M. (1987) Psychological assessment. In: *Mental Health Assessment of Deaf Clients: a Practical Manual* (eds H. Elliott, L. Glass & J.W. Evans), pp. 93–106. Little, Brown, Boston.

Padden, C. (1996) From the cultural to the bicultural: the modern deaf community. In: *Cultural and Language Diversity and the Deaf Experience* (ed. I. Parasnis), pp. 76–98. Cambridge University Press, Cambridge.

Padden, C. & Ramsey, C. (1998) Reading ability in signing deaf children. *Topics in Language Disorders: ASL Proficiency and English Literacy Acquisition: New Perspectives*, **18**, 30–46.

Parasnis, I. (1996) On interpreting the deaf experience within the context of cultural and language diversity. In: *Cultural and Language Diversity and the Deaf Experience* (ed. I. Parasnis), pp. 3–19. Cambridge University Press, Cambridge.

Peters, A.M. (1994) The interdependence of social, cognitive and linguistic development: evidence from a visually impaired child. In: *Constraints on Language Acquisition: Studies of Atypical Children* (ed. H. Tager-Flusberg), pp. 195–219. Lawrence Erlbaum, Hillsdale, NJ.

Peterson, C. & Siegal, M. (1998) Changing focus on the representational mind: deaf, autistic and normal children's concepts of false photos, false drawings and false beliefs. *British Journal of Developmental Psychology*, **16**, 301–320.

Pettito, L.A. & Marentette, P.F. (1991) Babbling in the manual mode: evidence for the ontogeny of language. *Science*, **251**, 1493–1496.

Power, D.J., Wood, D.J. & Wood, H.A. (1990) Conversational strategies of teachers using three methods of communication with deaf children. *American Annals of the Deaf*, **135**, 9–13.

Preisler, G.M. (1995) The development of communication in blind and in deaf infants: similarities and differences. *Child: Care, Health and Development*, **21**, 79–110.

Preisler, G. (1997) Social and emotional development of blind children: a longitudinal study. In: *Blindness and Psychological Development in Young Children* (eds V. Lewis & G. Collis), pp. 69–85. BPS Books, Leicester.

Prendergast, S.G. & McCollum, J.A. (1996) Let's talk: the effect of maternal hearing status on interactions with toddlers who are deaf. *American Annals of the Deaf*, **141**, 11–18.

Preston, P. (1994) *Mother Father Deaf*. Harvard University Press, Cambridge, MA.

Prinz, P. & Strong, M. (1998) ASL proficiency and English literacy within a bilingual deaf education model of instruction. *Topical Language Disorders*, **18**, 47–60.

Quittner, A.L., Glueckauf, R.L. & Jackson, D.N. (1990) Chronic parenting stress: moderating versus mediating effects of social support. *Journal of Personality and Social Psychology*, **59**, 1266–1278.

Rainer, J.D. & Altshuler, K.Z. (1966) *Comprehensive Mental Health Services for the Deaf*. Department of Medical Genetics, New York State Psychiatric Institute.

Raver-Lampman, S.A. (1990) Effect of gaze direction on evaluation of visually impaired children by informed respondents. *Journal of Visual Impairment and Blindness*, **84**, 67–70.

Recchia, S.L. (1997) Play and concept development in infants and young children with severe visual impairments: a constructivist's view. *Journal of Visual Impairment*, **91**, 401–406.

Reynell, J. (1979) *Manual for the Reynell–Zinkin Developmental Scales for Young Visually-Handicapped Children. Part I*. NFER, Windsor.

Roberts, C. & Hindley, P. (1999) Practitioner review: the assessment and treatment of deaf children with psychiatric disorders. *Journal of Child Psychology and Psychiatry*, 40, 151–167.

Rogers, S.J. & Puchalski, C.B. (1984) Social characteristics of visually impaired infants' play. *Topics in Early Childhood Special Education*, 3, 52–56.

Rosenhall, U., Nordin, V., Sandström, M., Ahlsen, G. & Gillberg, C. (1999) Autism and hearing loss. *Journal of Autism and Developmental Disorders*, 29, 349–357.

Rowbury, C. (1991) Referential communication between a blind mother and a blind child. *Paper Presented at the British Psychological Society Developmental Section. Annual Conference September, 1991, Cambridge*. BPS, Leicester.

Rowland, C. (1983) Patterns of interaction between three blind infants and their mothers. In: *Language Acquisition in the Blind Child* (ed. A.E. Mills), pp. 114–132. Croom-Helm, London.

Rutter, M., Graham, P. & Yule, W. (1970) A Neuropsychiatric Study in Childhood. *Clinics in Developmental Medicine Nos. 35/36*. Spastics International Medical Publications, London.

Sadeh, A., Klitzke, M., Anders, T.F. & Acebo, C. (1995) Case study: sleep and aggressive behavior in a blind, retarded adolescent—a concomitant schedule disorder? *Journal of the American Academy of Child and Adolescent Psychiatry*, 34, 820–824.

Sampaio, E. & Philip, J. (1995) Influences of age at onset of blindness on Braille reading performances with left and right hands. *Perceptual and Motor Skills*, 81, 131–141.

Sasaki, H., Nakata, H., Murakami, S., Uesugi, R., Harada, S. & Teranishi, M. (1992) Circadian sleep–wake rhythm disturbance in blind adolescence. *Japanese Journal of Psychiatry and Neurology*, 46, 209.

Schlesinger, H.S. & Meadow, K.P. (1972) *Sound and Sign: Childhood Deafness and Mental Health*. University of California Press, Berkeley.

Schnittjer, C.J. & Hirshoren, A. (1981) Factors of problem behavior in visually-impaired children. *Journal of Abnormal Child Psychology*, 9, 517–522.

Scholl, G.T. (1974) The psychosocial effects of blindness: implications for program planning in sex education. *New Outlook for the Blind*, 68, 210–215.

Singleton, J.L. & Tittle, M.D. (2000) Deaf parents and their hearing children. *Journal of Deaf Studies and Deaf Education*, 5, 221–236.

Sinkkonen, J. (1994) *Hearing impairment, communication and personality development*. PhD thesis, University of Helsinki.

Sisson, L.A. (1992) Positive behavioral support: new foci in the management of challenging behaviors. *Journal of Visual Impairment and Blindness*, 86, 364–369.

Sleeboom-van Raaij, I. (1991) Issues of importance to be considered in setting up new mental health services for the deaf. In: *Proceedings of the Second International Congress of the European Society for Mental Health and Deafness*, pp. 139–143. La Bastide, Namur.

Sleeboom-van Raaij, I. (1997) Psycho-pharmacological treatment and deafness, hazards and highlights. In: *Services for Mental Health and Deafness. European Perspectives. Overview, Reports and Occasional Papers from the MADE project* (eds N. Keane & B. Clowes), pp. 120–123. ESMHD, Ireland.

Smith, P.K. & Sharp, S. (1994) *School Bullying: Insights and Perspectives*. Routledge, London.

Smith-Gray, S. & Koester, L.S. (1995) Defining and observing social signals in deaf and hearing infants. *American Annals of the Deaf*, 140, 422–427.

Snitzer Reilly, J., McIntire, M.L. & Bellugi, U. (1989) Faces: the relationship between language and affect. In: *From Gesture to Language*

in *Hearing and Deaf Children* (eds V. Volterra & C.J. Erting), pp. 128–141. Springer-Verlag, Berlin.

Sonksen, P.M. (1983) The assessment of 'Vision for Development' in severely visually handicapped babies. *Acta Ophthalmologica Supplement*, 157, 82–91.

Sonksen, P.M., Petrie, A. & Drew, K.J. (1991) Promotion of visual development of severely visually impaired babies: evaluation of a developmentally based programme. *Developmental Medicine and Child Neurology*, 33, 320–355.

Spencer, P.A., Bodner-Johnson, B.A. & Gutfreund, M. (1992) Interacting with infants with a hearing loss: what can we learn from mothers who are deaf? *Journal of Early Intervention*, 16, 64–78.

Spencer, P.E. & Deyo, D.A. (1993) Cognitive and social aspects of deaf children's play. In: *Psychological Perspectives on Deafness* (eds M. Marschark & M.D. Clark), pp. 65–92. Lawrence Erlbaum, Hillsdale, NJ.

Spencer, P.E. & Meadow-Orlans, K.P. (1996) Play, language and maternal responsiveness: a longitudinal study of deaf and hearing infants. *Child Development*, 67, 3176–3191.

Stein, L.K. & Jabaley, T. (1981) Early identification and parent counseling. In: *Deafness and Mental Health* (eds L.K. Stein, E.D. Mindel & T. Jabaley), pp. 23–35. Grune & Stratton, New York.

Stokoe, W. (1998) A very long perspective. In: *Psychological Perspectives on Deafness 2* (eds M. Marschark & M.D. Clarke), pp. 1–18. Lawrence Erlbaum, Mahwah, NJ.

Strong, M. (1995) A review of bilingual/bicultural programs for deaf children in North America. *American Annals of the Deaf*, 140, 84–94.

Stubbs, E.G. (1978) Autistic symptoms in a child with congenital cytomegalovirus infection. *Journal of Autism and Childhood Schizophrenia*, 8, 37–43.

Sullivan, P., Brookhouser, P. & Scanlan, M. (2000) Maltreatment of deaf and hard of hearing children. In: *Mental Health and Deafness* (eds P. Hindley & N. Kitson), pp. 148–184. Whurr, London.

Supalla, S. (1991) Manually coded English: the modality question in signed language development. In: *Theoretical Issues in Sign Language Research*, Vol. 2. *Psychology* (eds P. Siple & S.D. Fischer), pp. 86–109. University of Chicago Press, Chicago, IL.

Sutton-Spence, R. & Woll, B. (1999) *The Linguistics of British Sign Language: an Introduction*. Cambridge University Press, Cambridge.

Tabandeh, H., Lockley, S.W., Buttery, R. *et al.* (1998) Disturbance of sleep in blindness. *American Journal of Ophthalmology*, 126, 707–712.

Thurstone, L.L. (1938) Primary mental abilities. *Psychometric Monographs*, 1, ix–121.

Trybus, R.J. (1985) Demographics and population character research in deaf-blindness. In: *State of the Art: Research Priorities in Deaf-Blindness* (eds J.E. Stahlecker, L.E. Glass & S. Machalow). Center on Deafness, UCSF, California.

Turner, J., Klein, H. & Kitson, N. (2000) Interpreters in mental health settings. In: *Mental Health and Deafness* (eds P. Hindley & N. Kitson), pp. 297–310. Whurr, London.

Vaccari, C. & Marschark, M. (1997) Communication between parents and deaf children: implications for social-emotional development. *Journal of Child Psychology and Psychiatry*, 38, 793–801.

Van den Broek, P., Vermeulen, A., Brokx, J. & Snik, A. (1998) Cochlear implantation in deaf children. *Nederlands Tijdschrift Voor Geneeskunde*, 142, 2581–2586.

Vander Kolk, C. (1987) Psychosocial assessment of visually impaired persons. In: *Psychosocial Interventions with Sensorially Disabled Persons* (eds B. Heller, L. Flohr & L. Zegans), pp. 33–52. Grune & Stratton, Orlando.

Van Eldik, T. (1998) *Mental health problems, family stress, family func-*

tioning and stressful life events of deaf children. PhD thesis, Erasmus Universiteit, Rotterdam.

van Gent, T. (1999) Factors complicating psychiatric assessment and treatment of deaf and severely hard of hearing children. In: *1st European Symposium on Deaf Children and Mental Health of the ESMHD Children and Families Special Interest Group.* Pathfinder National Deaf Services, Danbury.

van Gent, T. (in preparation) *Psychological well-being and psychiatric disorders in deaf children and adolescents.* PhD thesis, University of Leyden.

van Gent, T. & Hendriks, S. (1994) Psychiatric disorders in children and adolescents referred to the first psychiatric clinic for deaf and severely hard of hearing children and adolescents in the Netherlands. In: *European Society for Mental Health and Deafness Third International Congress Workshops Abstracts, Paris.* ESMHD, Paris.

van Gent, T., Heijnen, C.J. & Treffers, Ph.D.A. (1997) Autism and the immune system. *Journal of Child Psychology and Psychiatry,* **38,** 337–349.

Van Hasselt, V.B. & Sisson, L.A. (1987) Visual impairment. In: *Psychological Evaluation of the Developmentally and Physically Disabled* (eds V.B. Van Hasselt & M. Hersen). Grune & Stratton, New York.

Van Hasselt, V.B., Hersen, M., Kazdin, A.E. & Mastantuono, A.K. (1983) Training blind adolescents in social skills. *Journal of Visual Impairment and Blindness,* **7,** 203.

Van Hasselt, V.B., Kazdin, A.E. & Hersen, M. (1986) Assessment of problem behavior in visually handicapped adolescents. *Journal of Clinical Child Psychology,* **15,** 134–141.

Van Hasselt, V.B., Sisson, L.A. & Aach, S.R. (1987) Parent training to increase compliance in a young multihandicapped child. *Journal of Behavior Therapy and Experimental Psychiatry,* **18,** 275–283.

Van Ijzendoorn, M.H., Goldberg, S., Kroonenberg, P.M. & Frenkel, O.J. (1992) The relative effects of maternal and child problems on the quality of attachment: a meta-analysis of attachment in clinical samples. *Child Development,* **63,** 840–858.

Vernon, M. (1982) Multihandicapped deaf children: types and causes. In: *The Multihandicapped Hearing Impaired: Identification and Instruction* (eds D. Tweedie & E.H. Shroyer), pp. 11–28. Gallaudet College Press, Washington D.C.

Vernon, M. & Daigle-King, B. (1999) Historical overview of inpatient care of mental patients who are deaf. *American Annals of the Deaf,* **144,** 51–61.

Vostanis, P., Hayes, M., Du Feu & Warren, J. (1997) Detection of behavioural and emotional problems in deaf children and adolescents: comparison of two rating scales. *Child: Care, Health and Development,* **23,** 233–246.

Warren, D.H. (1977) *Blindness and Early Childhood Development.* American Foundation for the Blind, New York.

Warren, D.H. (1984) *Blindness and Early Childhood Development,* 2nd edn. American Foundation for the Blind, New York.

Warren, D.H. (1994) *Blindness and Children: An Individual Differences Approach.* Cambridge University Press, Cambridge.

Watkin, P.M., Baldwin, M., Dixon, R. & Beckman, A. (1998) Maternal anxiety and attitudes to universal hearing screening. *British Journal of Audiology,* **32,** 27–37.

Watkins, S., Pitman, P. & Walden, B. (1998) The deaf mentor experimental project for young children who are deaf and their families. *American Annals of the Deaf,* **143,** 29–34.

Webb, B. (1990) Mutual support for families of children with eye cancer. *Child: Care, Health and Development,* **16,** 319–329.

Webster, A. & Roe, J. (1998) *Children with Visual Impairments: Social Interaction, Language and Learning.* Routledge, London.

Wood, D., Wood, H., Griffiths, A. & Howarth, I. (1986) *Teaching and Talking with Deaf Children.* John Wiley, Chichester.

Yoshida, T., Ichikawa, T., Ishikawa, T. & Hori, M. (1998) Mental health of visually and hearing impaired students from the viewpoint of the University Personality Inventory. *Psychiatry and Clinical Neurosciences,* **52,** 413–418.

Yoshinaga-Itano, C. & Apuzzo, M.-R.L. (1998) The development of deaf and hard of hearing children identified early through the high-risk registry. *American Annals of the Deaf,* **143,** 416–424.

Young, A.M. (1999) Hearing parents adjustment to a deaf child: the impact of a cultural linguistic model of deafness. *Journal of Social Work Practice,* **13,** 157–172.

Zwiebel, A. (1987) More on the effects of early manual communication on the cognitive development of deaf children. *American Annals of the Deaf,* **134,** 16–22.

51 Implications for the Infant of Maternal Puerperal Psychiatric Disorders

Maureen N. Marks, Alison E. Hipwell and R. Channi Kumar

Introduction

Maternal psychopathology in the puerperium is associated with increased risk for subsequent impairments in cognitive, social and emotional development in offspring. There are multiple pathways to these effects: physiological, genetic and environmental. We describe associations observed between maternal psychopathology and subsequent infant outcome and concentrate attention on links between these associations and the maternal environment provided for the infant by the mentally ill mother. This environment will depend not only on the nature of her disorder but also on a variety of other environmental factors, some of which in turn may be causes or consequences of maternal psychopathology.

Maternal mental illness

The extent to which maternal psychopathology might have an impact on the child will depend not only on primary diagnosis but also on other characteristics of the illness, e.g. comorbidity, severity of illness, the course of illness during pregnancy and after the infant's birth and the timing of the infant's exposure to it (Rutter 1989).

Mother's parenting style

Associations between maternal mental illness and the mother–infant relationship and/or infant development may be the indirect consequence of disturbances in the mother's parenting style (Bornstein 1995) rather than mental illness *per se*. An important contributor to a how a mother parents her child will be the parenting she herself received as a child. Research across generations has demonstrated significant concordance between mothers' 'working models' of their own early relationships and their children's security of attachment (Fonagy *et al.* 1991; for a review of studies see Fonagy *et al.* 1994). There is also evidence for intergenerational continuities in a number of behaviours, e.g. smoking, antisocial behaviour, aggression, social withdrawal and violence by young men to their partners. Whereas intergenerational associations such as these may sometimes be related to parenting practices (Patterson & Dishion 1998), other factors could account for or mediate them, such as genetic transmission of temperamental traits, or continuities of social conditions (e.g. poverty), across generations (for a discussion of these issues see Patterson 1998; Rutter 1998).

The child's father

A husband or partner can sometimes influence the course of maternal postnatal psychiatric illness (Brown *et al.* 1990; Marks *et al.* 1992, 1996) and it is likely that he will have some effect on infant development, either directly through his relationship with the child, or indirectly via his relationship with the infant's mother (Egeland *et al.* 1988; Cabrera *et al.* 2000). Family structure, in particular the place of the infant's father in the family, is also likely to be important (Marks & Lovestone 1995; Lamb 1999).

Social adversity

The presence of social stress not only increases the likelihood of maternal mental illness, but also exacerbates negative parent–infant interactions (Hamilton *et al.* 1993) and has a direct impact on infant function (Adrian & Hammen 1993). Poverty in particular is linked with depressed mood in parents, conflict between the parents, more negative parental interactions with offspring, an increase in emotional and behavioural problems in children (Conger *et al.* 1994) and a negative impact on their academic performance (Brody *et al.* 1994).

Infant factors

The infant's outcome will depend to some extent on the infant's inherent characteristics. There are gender differences in infants' vulnerability to environmental adversity. Male infants appear to be more vulnerable to death by injury (accidental or non-accidental) and by homicide (Marks 1996); to the impact of maternal postnatal depression (Sharp *et al.* 1995); and to elicit more adverse parental responses (Murray *et al.* 1993). In an examination of findings in some studies, but not in others, that boys seem to be more adversely affected by parental divorce than girls, Zaslow (1988, 1989) has commented on some methodological problems. Outcome measures may not be sensitive to girls' possible adverse responses and the context within which outcome has been assessed may have contributed to the differences observed (e.g. in the divorce studies, when post-divorce family form is taken into account, it is remaining with a mother who does not remarry that is the most adverse outcome for boys).

The infant's temperament can also have an impact on the parent. Research has shown how infant characteristics influence

858

parental behaviours (Papousek & Papousek 1997). Infant factors may also influence the mother's mental health (Field *et al.* 1988; Whiffen & Gotlib 1989; Murray *et al.* 1996).

Genetics

Clearly, any or all of the above may be influenced directly or indirectly by genetic factors and the task of future research will be to delineate how genes and environment interact (see Rutter *et al.* 1997 for a discussion of current key findings and future research strategies). There is no doubt that psychiatric disorders in parents are associated with increased risk of psychiatric illness in their children. The evidence suggests that there is a genetic component to the development of schizophrenia and bipolar disorder but that depressive illnesses in offspring are largely determined by environmental factors. Even when there is good evidence that genes play a part, associations are weak and often diagnoses of offspring are not the same as those of the parents; the non-specificity suggests that influences other than genetic ones are likely to have contributed. More recently, it has become evident that environmental experience can sometimes alter genetic material. Caldji *et al.* (1998) found that maternal care of neonatal rat pups altered the genetic expression of behavioural responses to stress and that this alteration was then passed on to the next generation.

Pregnancy

Few systematic prospective studies have examined either the prevalence or course of substantial mental health problems during pregnancy, or the risk for relapse in women with prior psychiatric histories who discontinue medication when they become pregnant. Nevertheless, it is known that women who experience clinically significant psychiatric symptoms during pregnancy are at risk of inadequate antenatal care, poor nutrition and obstetric complications (Gotlib *et al.* 1991; Steer *et al.* 1992; Perkin *et al.* 1993; O'Hara 1995; Orr & Miller 1995). Altshuler *et al.* (1998) also suggested that the potential impact of hypothalamic–pituitary–adrenal dysregulation associated with maternal depression on fetal well-being may be of theoretical concern.

The maternal psychological state, particularly in the later stages of pregnancy (Hedegaard *et al.* 1993), may have a significant impact on the physical outcome for the newborn. Maternal anxiety, perceived stress, and life-event distress have been shown to be associated with lower infant birth weight and reduced gestational age at birth (Lobel *et al.* 1992; Wadwa *et al.* 1993; Lou *et al.* 1994). Maternal anxiety in the last trimester of pregnancy has been found to be associated with increased risk of emotional and behavioural problems in the children when they are 4 years old (O'Connor *et al.* in press). Recent evidence (Gitau *et al.* 1998; Gitau *et al.* 2001) has suggested that there may be two possible mechanisms by which these characteristics of maternal mood during pregnancy have their effect on the fetus:

1 by direct transport of cortisol across the placenta; and
2 by impaired blood flow through the uterine arteries.

One of the possible major hazards for the fetus of mothers who have histories of severe psychiatric illness or who experience an episode of illness during pregnancy is exposure to psychotropic medication. At present studies are few and limited in terms of sample size, fetal outcome measures and period of follow-up (for a review see Altshuler *et al.* 1996). For women treated with antipsychotic medication, there is some evidence of an increased risk of congenital abnormalities when phenothiazines are administered in the first trimester, but for high-potency neuroleptics, such as haloperidol, or the newer antipsychotic drugs, such as clozapine, little is known. There are case reports of mostly transient (lasting up to 10 days) perinatal syndromes in neonates of mothers who took neuroleptics in pregnancy (e.g. motor restlessness, tremor, hypertonicity, abnormal movements). There is no evidence for any association between fetal exposure to tricyclic antidepressants and congenital abnormalities, suggesting that these are relatively safe drugs for pregnant women, although neonates have shown withdrawal syndromes (jitteriness, irritability, convulsions). With regard to serotonin selective reuptake inhibitors, fluoxetine has also been found, on the basis of preliminary data, to be relatively safe. The data for sertraline, paroxetine and fluvoxamine are either insufficient or non-existent. Likewise, there is little information available about monoamine oxidase inhibitors. First trimester exposure to lithium is associated with an increased risk of cardiovascular malformations. While there have been case reports of neonatal toxicity in infants exposed to lithium, a study of bipolar women maintained on lithium during pregnancy found no evidence for this. First trimester exposure to benzodiazepines and to carbamazepine increases the risk of a congenital malformation.

The clinician has to weigh up the potential risk to the fetus from drug exposure with the risk to mother and infant of not medicating a seriously ill mother or of discontinuing medication. The relative risks of *in utero* exposure to psychotropic medication compared with the risks of untreated psychiatric disorder are still unclear and further research is urgently needed (Oates 1997; Cohen & Rosenbaum 1998).

Postnatal period

Psychiatric disorders occurring postpartum may or may not have aetiological links with childbirth and may or may not be exacerbated by childbirth. Diagnoses such as postpartum depression and postpartum psychosis are frequently referred to in clinical practice and in psychiatric research investigations, but neither DSM-IV nor ICD-10 (World Health Organization 1992) refer to them as formal diagnostic categories, although DSM-IV provides for a postpartum *onset* specifier for mood disorders and for brief psychotic disorder. Many episodes of postpartum depression begin during pregnancy or even before pregnancy (Gotlib *et al.* 1991; Marks *et al.* 2000) as do episodes of bipolar disorder (Brockington *et al.* 1990). Other disorders occurring in the puerperium, some of which may constitute a relapse of a previous disorder (e.g. anxiety disorders) or may be associated with an increase in severity of symptoms (e.g. obsessive-compulsive disorder) and some of which have long-standing and chronic courses with no increase or decrease in symptoms (e.g. schizophrenia), tend not to be given the label postpartum, but none the less are likely to have an impact on the mother's parenting of her child.

Thus, postpartum illnesses are defined by their temporal proximity to child-bearing. In general, symptomatology and clinical course are similar to illnesses occurring at other times. On this basis, Brockington (1996) dismissed the scientific value of the concept of postnatal depression but argued the case for a 'pure' postpartum psychosis as a specific disease entity when episodes of the illness occur only after childbirth and recur after subsequent pregnancies. A similar case could be made for depressions or other illnesses that occur only in the context of childbirth.

Unipolar (non-psychotic) depression

Inconsistencies in the time frame used to delineate the postpartum period—ranging from 4 weeks to 6 months after delivery—make the literature on the impact of postnatal depression on the child difficult to interpret. Studies have fairly consistently reported rates of depression of 12–16% during the 6–12 weeks after delivery (O'Hara & Swain 1996). A range of psychosocial risk factors for postpartum mood disorder have been identified, including prior postpartum depression (Wisner et al. 1993), depressive symptomatology during pregnancy and family or personal histories of major depression, as well as stressful newborn-associated events such as health problems and infant irritability (Kumar & Robson 1984; Gotlib et al. 1991; Beck 1996; Murray et al. 1996; O'Hara & Swain 1996).

In the last decade there has been considerable research into the impact of mothers' depressions on their children (for overviews of research to date see Murray & Cooper 1997; Radke-Yarrow 1998). Weinberg & Tronick (1998) summarized the extent to which the quantity, quality and timing of depressed mothers' social and affective behaviour with their infants are compromised in ways that are associated with impairments in infant functioning. In the first few months of life, infants of depressed mothers have been shown to have difficulties engaging in social and object interactions, and show less positive and more negative affect, lower activity levels, and greater physiological reactivity as evidenced by higher heart rate and cortisol levels than the infants of non-depressed control mothers (Campbell & Cohn 1991; Field 1995). They may also show compromised ability to regulate their affective and behavioural states which are present from the newborn period, often in the form of irritability and inconsolable crying (Zuckerman et al. 1990). This suggests that prenatal factors (e.g. neuroendocrine changes associated with the mothers' depression) may have had an impact on the infant's behaviour. In addition, there is growing evidence from prospective studies that the adverse effects on social, emotional and cognitive development continue well after the mother's symptoms have remitted (Stein et al. 1991; Murray 1992; Campbell et al. 1995; Sharp et al. 1995; Murray et al. 1999). Murray (1992) demonstrated that children of mothers with postnatal depression were less likely to form secure attachments to their mothers at 18 months, performed worse on object concept tasks, and showed more mild behavioural difficulties. Whereas this study reported no overall effect of depression on more general measures of cognitive development, postnatal depressive disorders seemed to have potentiated the adverse effects of low social class. Field et al. (1988) demonstrated that infants of depressed mothers generalized a withdrawn and avoidant interactional style to other adults, which clearly has implications for the child's social development.

There is fairly consistent evidence that male infants may be at greater risk from maternal depression than females. On a measure of general cognitive functioning, Sharp et al. (1995) reported that the 4-year-old boys of postnatally depressed women were performing at a mean of 1 SD lower than that of boys of well mothers but no such differences were found for the girls in that study. In a recent follow-up of the same children at the age of 11 years, the same finding was reported (Hay et al. 2001). Boys of women who have experienced an episode of postnatal depressive illness also appear to be at risk of subsequent behavioural and emotional difficulties. During the transition to school, for example, teachers have described these children as showing signs of hyperactive and distractible behaviour. In contrast, the girls whose mothers had been depressed in the postnatal period were not only perceived as extremely well behaved, but more prosocial and diligent than the control group girls (Sinclair & Murray 1998). While there is insufficient research to draw any conclusions about the mechanisms that might be involved in these observed differences within clinical samples, the fine-grained observations of early mother–infant interactions in non-clinical samples have suggested that males rely more on maternal support to regulate their affective state and take longer to repair 'interactive errors' than female infants in interaction with their mother (Weinberg & Tronick 1998). Thus, these social demands that may be characteristic of male infants in the postnatal period are likely to be especially difficult for mothers to cope with if they are also feeling depressed at this time, and may set in train a pattern of relating that is maintained over time despite remission of the mother's symptoms.

Although studies of postnatal depression have reported significant differences in mother and infant functioning on the group level, it is clear that the behaviour of depressed mothers is heterogeneous and therefore will be experienced by infants in a variety of ways. Some depressed mothers disengage and withdraw when they are with their infants, others may become intrusive and overtly hostile during interactions, whereas others are able to mobilize a normal range of behaviour and affect (Lyons-Ruth et al. 1986; Cohn & Tronick 1989). Cohn & Tronick (1989) reported that, in turn, the infants' affective states are specifically related to their mothers' style of interaction. These investigators found that the infants of withdrawn depressed mothers spend most of their time fussing and crying, whereas the infants of intrusive depressed mothers rarely cried but avoided looking at, and interacting with, the mother. The infants of depressed mothers who were able to respond within the normal range behaved similarly to control group infants. These results highlight the need to consider the mother's affective style in addition to her diagnostic status, which is likely to have specific implications for therapeutic intervention.

Weissman & Paykel (1974) and Frankel & Harmon (1996) noted the disparity between the mother's perception of her ability to parent and the quality of the mother–infant interaction. They highlighted the need to address difficulties in the mother–infant relationship in the course of therapeutic intervention rather than aim to treat the mother alone. This need is further indicated by the reciprocal nature of interactions and the infant's active role in shaping relationships (Weinberg & Tronick 1994). Furthermore, 'the infant who functions well can be used as a therapeutic ally to increase the mothers' sense of competence as a parent' (Weinberg & Tronick 1998, p. 59).

Anxiety disorders

More recently, researchers have begun to recognize the postpartum period as a time of increased vulnerability to symptoms of anxiety such as panic and obsessionality (Metz et al. 1988; Sichel et al. 1993; Cohen et al. 1994; Northcott & Stein 1994; Williams & Koran 1997). In a prospective study, Cohen et al. (1996) reported that 90% of patients with panic disorder (some of whom had experienced a reduction in symptoms during pregnancy) were actively symptomatic in the first 1–3 months postpartum. The 10% of patients remaining well were taking anxiolytic medication. Furthermore, Wisner et al. (1999) reported that women who develop postnatal depression are more likely to experience disturbing aggressive obsessional thoughts or images than women whose depression occurs outside the postpartum period. There was also a significant association between aggressive obsessions and checking compulsions that were primarily focused on the baby.

Relatively little is known about the impact of maternal anxiety in the postnatal period on infant functioning. Most studies have focused on older children, and on panic disorder to the exclusion of other anxiety disorders. However, as with depression, there may be important developmental effects on children. Mullen et al. (1993) found that 10–15% of children in their US sample were described as 'inhibited' and predisposed to be irritable as infants, and shy, fearful and introverted at older ages. Children of mothers with panic disorder also have a higher rate of insecure attachment to the mother than non-clinical samples (Manassis et al. 1994). Eighty per cent of the preschool-age children in this study were classified as insecurely attached to their mother, with 65% being judged as 'disorganized'. The mothers of securely attached children differed from mothers of insecure

preschool-age children in reporting fewer depressive symptoms, fewer stressful life events and an increased sense of parenting competence. However, this study was based on a relatively small sample in which the children ranged in age from 18 to 59 months. In addition, there were some methodological problems as a result of modest reliability coefficients for the attachment ratings and observers who were not 'blind' to maternal diagnosis. These findings must therefore be considered as preliminary and treated with caution.

More longitudinal observational studies are clearly needed to confirm some of these initial findings and to evaluate the importance of these risk factors in the development of psychopathology.

Affective psychosis

The rate of postpartum relapse in women who suffer from bipolar illness has been estimated at 33–50% (Reich & Winokur 1970; Kendell et al. 1987; Marks et al. 1992), and many of these women present with postpartum psychosis. Although postpartum psychosis can present with delirium-like symptoms and confusion that distinguish it from a typical manic episode (Brockington et al. 1981), several follow-up studies of women with postpartum psychosis noted recurrence of episodes of bipolar disorder (Benvenuti et al. 1992; Videbech & Gouliaev 1995) or schizoaffective illness (Klompenhouwer & Van Hulst 1991).

Postpartum psychosis is considered a psychiatric emergency that typically requires inpatient treatment with mood stabilizers and antipsychotic medication in order to avoid placing the mother and infant at risk of harm. Rates of infanticide associated with untreated puerperal psychosis have been estimated to be as high as 4% (Davidson & Robertson 1985).

Compared with well women, those experiencing an episode of psychosis in the postpartum period tend to demonstrate poorer quality caregiving at the time of the illness (Kumar & Hipwell 1994), although there may be substantial improvement with recovery (Thiels & Kumar 1987). Preoccupation with hallucinations and psychotic ideation, blunting of affect, increased irritability, etc., may lead the parent to be unresponsive to the child's emotional and physical needs. The form of disturbance in caregiving has been found to vary according to whether the episode is schizoaffective, manic-depressive, or a severe form of unipolar depression. Hipwell & Kumar (1996) found nurses' ratings to differ significantly according to diagnostic status, mothers with schizophrenic symptoms being rated the most impaired, followed by those with manic, bipolar and, finally, depressive symptoms.

It is somewhat counterintuitive therefore that adverse effects on the developing child have not been consistently demonstrated. McNeil et al. (1988) reported that, compared with the children of well controls and mothers with a history of psychosis but no symptoms postnatally, the children of puerperally psychotic mothers were no more impaired on measures of attachment to the mother and maternal perceptions of infant temperament at 1 year. Furthermore, at the age of 6, there were no differences on measures of cognitive development and mental disturbance. Similar negative findings had previously been reported by Grunebaum *et al.* (1975) when comparing the developmental quotients of 1 year olds admitted to hospital with their mentally ill mothers, with those infants of well mothers. There have even been reports of superior functioning in some children of psychotic mothers (Kauffman *et al.* 1979). In contrast, DeMulder & Radke-Yarrow (1991) reported that two-thirds of 24 children of mothers with bipolar illness in their study showed insecure patterns of attachment when they were aged 15–52 months of age, most of whom were classified as insecure-disorganized. This proportion was significantly more than the 42% of insecurity reported for the offspring of mothers with unipolar depression or no mental health problems. However, 13 of the fathers of these 24 children were diagnosed as having unipolar depression, and the mothers with bipolar disorder were significantly more impaired in terms of their functioning during the child's lifetime than the mothers in the other groups.

Although some reports suggest that there is little detrimental effect of puerperal affective psychosis on infant development, many of the infants in the index groups had experienced significant separations from their mother during her illness. Hipwell *et al.* (2000) suggested that the absence of adverse outcome in these children may well arise because the infant's exposure to the maternal illness was limited, rather than because there were genuinely no detrimental effects. In this study, there was no excess of insecure attachment in the 1 year olds of mothers experiencing postpartum mania, in spite of the early interactions being rated as poor. By contrast, infants of unipolar depressed mothers whose interactions were rated as much less impaired were more likely to be insecurely attached. Examination of clinical management suggested that infants of mothers with manic symptoms were more often separated from their mothers and cared for by nursing staff than were infants of women with unipolar depressive episodes who may therefore have been less protected from the adverse effects of the mother's illness. However, there was also evidence that those suffering from manic episodes made a more complete recovery than those with depression, and the different infant outcome in these two groups could reflect current maternal functioning, rather than the protective effects of separating mother and infant. Another explanation may be that infants of mothers with bipolar illness show a different developmental course from the offspring of women with unipolar disorders such that emotional and affective difficulties are not apparent until later in childhood, when the direct and indirect effects of exposure to the mother's illness have become chronic. Using an accelerated longitudinal research strategy to examine the developmental pathways of 22 children whose mothers had been diagnosed with bipolar illness, Radke-Yarrow *et al.* (1992) reported that during the preschool period (age 1.5–3.5 years) the children of mothers with bipolar disorder appeared to be competent and without problems; they were able to separate from their mother without anxiety and related easily with a

stranger. But, by middle to late childhood, children exposed to maternal bipolar illness demonstrated significant symptoms of depression and anxiety. This early 'maturity' in the preschool phase may have represented a precarious method of coping with chaotic mothering.

One of the major hazards for children of mentally ill parents is that resulting from discontinuity of care because of separate admission of the mother to hospital. Alternative care that is both stable and personalized, e.g. from the child's father or grandmother, is sometimes preferable to that provided by a highly disturbed mother. However, separation from the mother frequently involves placements with a series of unfamiliar foster parents (see Rushton & Minnis, Chapter 22) and this can have profound effects on the development of attachments and serious consequences for the children both during childhood and as adults (Bowlby 1973; Rutter & Quinton 1984; Brown 1988). The role of the other parent (Webster 1990) or extended family is therefore crucial in providing continuity of care and the necessary support to the mother so that her hospitalization can be kept short.

Schizophrenia

For women with schizophrenia, rates of relapse or symptomatology do not appear to be exacerbated by childbirth (McNeil 1986; Davies *et al.* 1995). In contrast to the acute episodes of psychotic relapse that are typical for women with a history of bipolar illness, outcome studies from mother-and-baby units that admit women with chronic schizophrenia with their infants for treatment and assessment show that the prognosis for their ability to care for their infant is poor, particularly if they are single and have no social support to assist in providing consistent care for their child (Appleby & Dickens 1993; Davies *et al.* 1995; Kumar *et al.* 1995). The best predictor of the ability to parent successfully with a diagnosis of chronic schizophrenia appears to be the best level of functioning before the child was born (Oates 1996).

Children born to schizophrenic parents are at increased risk of impaired cognitive, sensorimotor and neurological development compared with the offspring of parents with other psychiatric disorders and with those of normal controls (Ragins *et al.* 1975; Fish 1977; Weintraub 1987; Wynne *et al.* 1987; Fish *et al.* 1992; McNeil *et al.* 1993; Sameroff *et al.* 1997). These differences have been found as early as the first few days or months of life and have sometimes been linked to obstetric complications and/or low birth weight (Mednick *et al.* 1971; Marcus *et al.* 1981; Yoshida *et al.* 1999).

One of the aims of studies of the offspring of parents with schizophrenia has been to determine early indicators of the development of schizophrenia in the children. The general conclusion of such studies has been that because impairments have appeared early in the infant's life they are probably largely genetically determined. However, the impairments may also have been in part a consequence of the intrauterine environment or the quality of parental care received by the developing infant.

Sacker et al. (1995) studied obstetric complications in schizophrenic cases identified in the British Perinatal Mortality Survey birth cohort. They reported that the increased risk of obstetric complications in those with schizophrenia may result from the physique/lifestyle of their mothers. Their mothers were more likely to have smoked, to have attended fewer antenatal clinics, to have had more previous pregnancies and to have been attended by untrained people at the birth. They concluded that the increased vulnerability of infants thought to have the potential to develop schizophrenia, obstetric insult and low birth weight may be an epiphenomenon of their mothers' chaotic lifestyles rather than a genetic characteristic. Further evidence for this is provided by Goodman & Emory (1992) who compared the prenatal care received by schizophrenic, depressed and control women. Having schizophrenia increased the likelihood of both receiving inadequate prenatal care and having obstetric complications.

Inadequacies in the prenatal environment are likely to continue postpartum. In the Stony Brook high-risk project (Weintraub 1987) the lifestyles of families with a schizophrenic parent were described as characterized by increased marital discord, family conflict, financial problems, and poorer ratings of family solidarity and household facilities compared with normal control families.

Goodman (1987), who assessed the children of schizophrenic, depressed and well mothers, from birth to 5 years of age, reported that the offspring of women with schizophrenia showed more deficits on social competence and had lower IQs than the other children. These deficits were linked to the child-rearing environment provided by their mothers. Schizophrenic mothers were rated as providing the poorest overall environment (less play stimulation, fewer learning experiences, less emotional and verbal involvement) and were also rated as less affectively involved and less responsive than well mothers.

Bergman et al. (1997) examined the interaction between parental psychiatric status and child maltreatment on neuromotor functioning in the children of parents with schizophrenia, with other psychiatric diagnoses or with no psychiatric diagnoses. Children who had been maltreated performed worse than those who had not. There was no main effect of psychiatric diagnosis.

In summarizing the Israeli high-risk study, Marcus et al. (1987) provided data showing that the parenting provided by mothers with schizophrenia was an important factor in the child's psychosocial development and the subsequent development of illness in the offspring. Of the schizophrenic offspring who showed early neurobehavioural deficits in this study, 15/24 (63%) also received poor parenting compared to 4/26 (15%) of the offspring who did not show early behavioural deficits. Further, only children who had experienced poor parenting subsequently became schizophrenic.

Observational studies of the schizophrenic mother's parenting of her infant have reported that these women are more likely to be 'grossly disturbed and inadequate' (Sobel 1961; Ragins et al. 1975). Schizophrenic mothers touch and play less with their 4-month-old infants than controls (Garmezy 1974). Psychotic hospitalized mothers, particularly schizophrenics, have been described as being more likely to perceive their infants as passive creatures and to interpret their cues, such as smiles, as 'accidental grimaces' compared with mothers in a control group (Cohler et al. 1970). Separation from their infants during the acute phase of their illnesses may have contributed to these disturbed patterns of behaviour. By contrast, Schachter et al. (1977) observed schizophrenic mothers to be more responsive and affectionate, and to play more with their 14-month-old infants than did controls. However, all the participants in this latter study were informed of the study's hypothesis, which may have differentially increased anxiety and motivation among the schizophrenic mothers to perform well.

Gamer et al. (1976) investigated cognitive and emotional outcome in the infants of 15 women who had been hospitalized in the puerperium. These investigators found that infants of mothers with schizophrenia tended to perform worst on tests of object constancy at age 1 year. They were also less likely to approach their mothers and interact positively with them after a brief separation, which, it could be argued, is suggestive of insecure attachment to the mother. These infants were also more likely to have had multiple caregivers during the mother's illness.

McNeil et al. (1983) carried out a major longitudinal study of infants of mothers with histories of various kinds of psychotic illnesses. They found consistently less social contact between schizophrenic mothers and their infants in comparison with healthy mothers up to 6 months. Subsequently at 1 year, these children were more likely to show anxious attachment using a modified version of the Strange Situation Test (Ainsworth & Wittig 1969; Näslund et al. 1984), and were less likely to be afraid of strangers. At 1 year, their mothers also displayed greater tension and a higher frequency of vocal discrepancy (positive intonation combined with negative content) in a feeding and play situation. By contrast, Sameroff et al. (1982) reported no difference in attachment security between infants of mothers with schizophrenia and either those of mothers with non-psychotic depression or personality disorder or those of healthy controls.

McNeil et al. (1984) suggested that the infants of mothers with schizophrenia may contribute to non-optimal maternal behaviour as a result of being temperamentally more difficult and more reactive to stimulation. Other kinds of infant factors may also precipitate and/or maintain problematic interactional style. Gamer et al. (1976) reported that these infants were more inhibited. Similarly, Ragins et al. (1975) described infant characteristics such as less spontaneity and a lesser tendency to imitate, less responsivity to verbal stimulation and heightened distress to separation from the mother than healthy control infants. However, these studies could not disentangle the bidirectional effects of disturbed mother–infant interactions.

The Finnish Adoptive Family Study of Schizophrenia (Tiernari et al. 1994; Wahlberg et al. 1997) assessed the interaction between genetic risk and rearing-family risk. Findings suggested that the adult offspring of schizophrenics may have a genetically determined hypersensitivity to the family environment. They fared better than controls in an adequate family situation and worse than controls in a disturbed one. The findings have yet to be replicated but they suggest hypotheses for future research. For example, if a mother is suffering from schizophrenia, then it is likely that the family environment of her infant will be somewhat disturbed, either because the infant is more likely to be separated from the mother and placed in institutional care or given multiple alternative carers, or because her mothering skills are likely to be less than adequate in the first place, and it may be that this environment, as much as, or in interaction with, the infant's inheritance, is linked to impairments in subsequent development.

These studies demonstrated the need for further longitudinal observational studies of the mother–infant relationship when mothers have schizophrenia, starting during pregnancy, to disentangle the impact on the infant of the schizophrenic mother–infant relationship, and the environment she provides for her child, from those genetic factors which place the infant at risk.

Eating disorders

The literature on the impact of maternal eating disorders on the fetus and infant is sparse. Evidence is mixed whether maternal symptoms diminish during pregnancy but return to prepregnancy levels postpartum (Lacey & Smith 1987; Lemberg & Phillips 1989) or worsen during pregnancy and postpartum (Stewart et al. 1987). This may be because of differences in the course of symptoms associated with the type of eating disorder. A recent prospective study (Blais et al. 2000) found that women with bulimia showed a decrease in symptoms during the pregnancy and this decrease was sustained for the 9 months they were followed up. Women with anorexia also showed decreased symptomatology during the pregnancy but their symptoms had returned to prepregnancy levels by 6 months postpartum.

Although the evidence concerning the course of eating disorders during the perinatal period is mixed, having an eating disorder during pregnancy does appear to pose risk for the fetus. Perinatal deaths in women with eating disorders are six times the expected rate (Brinch et al. 1988), twice the rate of fetal loss in women with bulimia compared with controls (Mitchell et al. 1991) and a 10% lower birth rate in a mixed group of anorexia and bulimia (Blais et al. 2000). Newly born infants of women with eating disorders have lower birth weights and smaller lengths than control group infants (Waugh & Bulik 1999). The mothers of full-term infants who are small for gestational age are three times more likely to have eating disorders than mothers of premature infants and six times more likely than mothers of control infants (Conti et al. 1998).

It is not known whether these infants are at risk in the long term for impaired growth and its neurodevelopmental sequelae. Lacey & Smith (1987) raised concern that mothers with bulimia may try to slim their infants down during the first year of life, de-

spite their weights being in the normal range. However, this phenomenon was observed in only three of the 20 mothers in their study. Similarly, Woodside & Shekter-Wolfson (1990), in their sample of 12 mothers or fathers with anorexia or bulimia nervosa, described many examples of highly distorted parent–child relationships. Two of the parents had abandoned their children altogether as a result of their eating disorder, while in other families the children had become extremely involved in their parent's illness by cooking for them or dieting in response to parental weight loss. In some families the parent was wearing the children's clothes. Brinch et al. (1988) reported that 17% of a group of 50 mothers with a history of anorexia nervosa described their children as failing to thrive during the first year postpartum. However, the mothers were interviewed between 4 and 22 years after their children were born and these retrospective findings must be interpreted with caution. Nevertheless, other reports (van Wezel-Meijler & Wit 1989) also raised concerns about inadequate child nutrition and care within their samples of mothers with eating disorders.

In a controlled observational study of 1-year-old infants, Stein et al. (1994) found that mothers with eating disorders were more intrusive and expressed more negative emotion towards their infants during meals compared with controls. They were also more intrusive but not more negative during play. In addition, the infants of index mothers were lighter than those of controls; infant weight was related to the degree of conflict between mother and infant that was observed during mealtimes and to the extent of the mother's concern about her shape. A later study (Stein et al. 1996) also found evidence for growth faltering in the children of women with eating disorders. They compared children of women with eating disorders with those of women with postnatal depression and with those of controls. Infants of mothers with eating disorders were smaller (weight for length and weight for age) than infants in both comparison groups.

The mechanism whereby maternal eating disorder pathology affects the infant's growth is as yet unclear and there is a need for further research to elucidate the psychic or behavioural factors that are involved.

Substance abuse

A comprehensive and comparative review of adverse effects of different kinds of substance abuse is beyond the scope of this chapter. Instead, the general characteristics and effects of maternal substance abuse are illustrated by reference to selected studies of alcohol, opioid and cocaine abuse.

Maternal substance abuse is associated with increased rates of complications during pregnancy, labour and delivery and is believed to have a wide range of effects on the fetus and infant that are dependent on the dosage, timing and conditions of exposure (West 1986). Infants of substance abusers are at greater risk of sudden infant death syndrome (Kandall et al. 1993) and the children of addicted parents are at increased risk for later dysfunctional behaviours (Fergusson et al. 1998; Yates et al. 1998; Weissman et al. 1999).

A longitudinal prospective study carried out in Sweden by Aronson *et al.* (1985) shed some light on the risks involved for the fetus. The offspring of alcoholic mothers who had been reared by foster parents showed hyperactivity, inattention and poor motor skills, and were also found to have lower IQ scores than their controls despite showing no signs of fetal alcohol syndrome (Jones & Smith 1973). Streissguth *et al.* (1984) reported that the 4-year-old children born to heavy drinkers displayed attention and reaction time abnormalities compared with children born to light and infrequent drinkers. Similar findings have been reported in several studies (for an overview of research see Streissguth & Kanter 1997), although there is some discussion as to the existence of a threshold of safe exposure, or whether abnormalities of balance in particular are observed among 'social drinking' mothers (Streissguth *et al.* 1984; Barr *et al.* 1990). In O'Connor *et al.*'s (1987) study of primiparous middle-class mothers, an increase in attachment insecurity was observed among infants of moderate-to-heavy drinkers compared with the offspring of abstinent or light drinkers.

It is known that many infants who are prenatally exposed to opioids undergo some degree of withdrawal after delivery (for overviews of research findings see Mayes & Bornstein 1997; Kosofsky 1999) which may last up to 6 months and is manifested as irritability, high-pitched crying, tenseness of muscles, tremulousness, regurgitation (Kron *et al.* 1975) and also rejection of their mothers' attempts to console them (Strauss *et al.* 1975). Chasnoff & Griffith (1991) have also reported that cocaine-exposed neonates have low thresholds for overstimulation and significant difficulty with self-regulation when these thresholds are exceeded, which is likely to have far-reaching effects in a range of contexts if this difficulty continues over several years (Howard *et al.* 1989). In the early postnatal period therefore such infant behaviours are likely to be primarily associated with problems in infant–caregiver interaction patterns. However, Jeremy & Bernstine (1984) reported no differences in patterns of mother–infant interaction between the 4 month olds of mothers maintained on methadone during pregnancy compared with infants of control mothers. The mothers who abused drugs showed worse interaction and communication with their infants but this was related more to lack of current maternal resources than to drug use *per se*.

Substance-abusing mothers have also been described as being at high risk for difficulties in parenting, including child neglect and abuse (Lawson & Wilson 1979). Thus, there are separate and interactive implications for the child of maternal abuse, e.g. alcohol, during or after pregnancy because of the likely associations between alcohol consumption and maternal personality characteristics, physical and mental health, intelligence, social circumstances, multigenerational and/or multiple substance abuse, and the impact of being reared in a drug- or alcohol-seeking environment. It is clear that many kinds of psychological stressors are associated with the environments of children whose parents abuse drugs or alcohol, and it is particularly difficult to tease out the effects on the fetus from those occurring postnatally on the infant (for a discussion of these issues see

Kaltenbach 1994). A study that compared substance-abusing women in the context of high and low levels of social adversity found that women in the high adversity group had poorer scores on parenting attitude scales (Kettinger *et al.* 2000). In another study, the effect of maternal opioid use on parenting behaviour was accounted for by effects of comorbid personality disorder (Hans *et al.* 1999).

Studies of the effects of drug abuse are beset by numerous methodological difficulties, such as the confounding effects of nutritional deficits, concurrent infections, multiple drug use, differential effects of motivation and sample attrition, the chaotic lifestyle of substance-abusing mothers and other mental health problems such as clinical depression and anxiety or personality characteristics such as low tolerance to frustration and neediness for immediate gratification. It is therefore not possible to predict the developmental outcomes for these high-risk children until more is known about the additive and interactive effects of the multiple risk factors to which they are exposed.

Infanticide

The younger the infant, the more likely the risk the child will become the victim of homicide and the more likely the perpetrator will be a parent (Marks & Kumar 1993, 1996).

The characteristics and causes of the homicide of infants within 24 h of their birth (neonaticide) are very different from those of the homicide of children older than 1 day. Compared with parents who kill older infants, neonaticidal mothers are more likely to be young (under 20), single, and often still living at home with parents. The pregnancy is often the first, unintentional and concealed. The motivation to kill is usually because the child was unwanted (Resnick 1970) and the infant's death is more likely to have resulted from inaction rather than the violent action that often characterizes the killing of older infants: nearly half die from neglect (Marks & Kumar 1993). In addition, the mothers are rarely mentally ill (D'Orban 1979). Mothers who kill their neonates are treated comparatively leniently by the legal system in the UK; a major proportion are never indicted and those who are usually receive infanticide convictions (Marks & Kumar 1993).

The most frequent observation about women who commit neonaticide is that the pregnancy had been denied (Brozovsky & Falit 1971; Green & Manohar 1990). In some cases the woman may 'know' she is pregnant but to all intents and purposes behaves as if she were not. This state of affairs is usually the consequence of an unconscious belief: if you do not think about it, then the pregnancy will, magically, disappear. Sometimes the woman does not seem to acknowledge even to herself that she is pregnant. In either case the woman does not seek medical help and makes no preparation for the delivery. After the child is born and disposed, the mother returns immediately to her normal daily life.

The denial in these concealed pregnancies is sometimes so powerful that it seems also to influence the perceptions of other people as well as the pregnant woman. This may be related to the fact that the biological manifestations of pregnancy sometimes become attenuated; for example, there may be reduced change in body contour, continuation of menstrual bleeding during pregnancy and no complaints of pregnancy such as nausea or increased urinary frequency. Brozovsky & Falit (1971) report a neonaticidal mother who during the pregnancy had convinced her physician, after a positive pregnancy test and at 5 months, that she was no longer pregnant.

The labours are often rapid: the woman thinks she has colic or menstrual pain and may interpret the contractions as a need to defecate and the delivery itself as a bowel movement. The arrival of the baby is thus experienced as a traumatic shock and puts an end to the denial and the woman is then confronted with the overwhelming fear that made the denial so necessary and effective in the first place. Anxiety of such intensity sometimes leads to ego disorganization, especially when the ego is less than resilient in the first place, which is typical of these women, and in this disorganized or dissociated state the woman kills the child or leaves it to die.

The overrepresentation of naive young women in studies of neonaticide may be in part a consequence of their naivety. It is generally considered that reported rates of neonaticide underestimate true rates. This is because many neonaticides remain undiscovered. It may be that more mature worldly women are more able to conceal successfully an unwanted pregnancy and dispose of the newly delivered infant in such a way that it remains undiscovered. Funayama & Sagisaka (1988) report 12 recorded cases of mothers in Japan who had carried out multiple neonaticides (three or more in each case). Eleven of the women were married and their ages ranged from 31 to 45 years.

Sakuta & Saito (1981) distinguished between two different kinds of neonaticide, which they described as the 'mabiki' and 'anomie' types. 'Mabiki' is a Japanese term that means 'thinning out' and is also used to refer to neonaticide when it is used as a form of population control, which was once culturally acceptable in Japan. The mabiki type of neonaticidal mother is typically married, has several children and does not wish to have more. In contrast, the 'anomie' type of mother is characteristically unmarried, this is her first child and the reasons for the infanticide are 'avoiding ill-repute' or 'loss of psychological support'. It may be that a similar, if less clear-cut, distinction also applies to neonaticides that occur in Western countries today.

Paternal neonaticide is rare. Kaye et al. (1990) reviewed four cases, one of which involved an infant with severe congenital abnormalities, two men with a psychiatric disorder (schizophrenia) and one man with an intellectual impairment.

In contrast with neonaticide, infanticide is usually attributed to either mental illness or child abuse; the parent who has killed his or her child is generally considered to be either 'mad' or 'bad'. In England and Wales there is an Infanticide Act, particular legislation which applies to a woman who has killed her child under 1 year of age. Implicit in this legislation is the idea that childbirth may sometimes have a destabilizing impact on mothers' minds, that the infant homicide may have occurred under these unsta-

ble psychological conditions, and that therefore there may be a case for diminished responsibility for the crime. In contrast, in Scotland and in the USA, mothers who kill their children are charged as for any other homicide offence with the possibility that the infanticidal mother can plead diminished responsibility within the usual terms of each country's homicide legislation. Despite these differences in legislation, in most Western countries the younger the infant, the greater the likelihood that the offence will be attributed to some form of mental illness and the perpetrator convicted of a less serious offence and given a lighter sentence. This is particularly so for mothers who kill their infants. In England and Wales most mothers who kill their infants are convicted of infanticide and given probation sentences. This is in contrast to fathers who kill their infants, who are usually given prison sentences (Marks & Kumar 1993). Despite there being no infanticide act in Scotland the outcome is similar. Most mothers who kill infants receive non-custodial sentences, either probation or hospital orders, and most fathers are sent to prison (Marks et al. 1996).

Studies in the USA have not examined differential sentencing of mothers and fathers but Crittenden & Craig (1990) reported that in Florida, the younger the infant, the more likely the offence will be ascribed to parental mental illness, and the less serious the conviction and lighter the sentence.

Public records provide limited information about the details surrounding these offences and so it is difficult to know if sentencing reflects the circumstances and severity of the crime. The Scottish Office computer records include the motive for the offence. Mothers are usually recorded as having killed their infant because of their mental state, whereas the most frequent attribution given to fathers is that of rage (Marks & Kumar 1996). However, it is impossible to assess how these motivations are ascribed and whether the difference between mothers and fathers is because of the circumstances surrounding the offence or to the effects of gender on the attributions about the causes of events.

In a systematic study of maternal filicides, D'Orban (1979) studied 89 women admitted to Holloway prison during 1970–75, who had been charged with the killing or attempted murder of 109 children. This constituted almost the total sample remanded in custody during the period in London and the south-east of England, since during that time all mothers charged with the killing or attempted murder of their children were remanded to Holloway for some period before trial.

D'Orban found that the most frequent category of perpetrator was that of the 'battering mothers': the mother had lost her temper with some aspect of the child's behaviour, e.g. the child's crying, feeding or incontinence. Only 14/89 women in D'Orban's study were psychotic at the time of the offence and he concluded that puerperal psychotic illness is a relatively rare cause of maternal filicide. However, about half the offences in D'Orban's study had been against children aged 1 year or more: they had occurred sometime after the postpartum period by which time the risk of maternal mental illness has substantially declined (Kendell et al. 1987; Cox et al. 1993). In addition, a further proportion had involved neonaticide, which is unlikely to be related to either battering or mental illness.

In a later reanalysis of D'Orban's data (Marks & Kumar 1996), the relative contribution of mental illness to offences that occurred nearer the infant's delivery (when the mother was more likely to have a postnatally related psychological illness) was assessed. The effect of the time since delivery on the contribution of mental illness to the mother's impulse to kill was examined by comparing infants aged between 1 day and under 6 months old, with those aged between 6 months and under 1 year and those aged 1 year or more. Neonaticides were excluded from this analysis. The results indicated that maternal mental illness was more likely to be implicated in the killing of *older* children. Women who killed children between 1 day and under 6 months were most frequently categorized as 'battering' mothers, whereas mothers who had killed or attempted to kill older infants were most frequently categorized as mentally ill. Although maternal mental illness had contributed to some of the homicides of the younger aged infants, more often infants had been killed, or nearly killed, because the mother had suddenly lost her temper with the child.

Likewise, in Australia, Wilkey *et al.* (1982) concluded that the largest group of homicide of children were those occurring as the end result of non-accidental injury assaults. Similar results have been reported in studies in the USA. A study of all victims 12 years of age or less, during 1956–82, in Florida (Copeland 1985) found that 45% of all deaths were caused by fatal child abuse. This study notes that the younger the child the more likely the death was a consequence of child abuse; 91% of the child abuse fatalities occurred in children aged 3 or less, whereas non-child abuse cases were more evenly distributed throughout the age range. Copeland also found that male children were more likely to be child abuse fatalities.

Crittenden & Craig (1990) reported that children between 1 month and 5 years were more than twice as likely to be killed as a result of injuries inflicted by parents responding to noxious behaviour (e.g. incessant crying or disobedience) than were neonates or older children (52% compared to 17% of neonates and 21% of school-aged children). They also found that in 60% of children aged between 1 month and under 5 years there was evidence of present or past abuse or neglect, e.g. marks on the child's body, a service record of maltreatment or an eyewitness report. Only 7% of neonates and 10% of school-aged children had any evidence of abuse or neglect.

Although there are many individual case examples published, few studies have systematically examined the circumstances surrounding filicide where the parent's mental state was the main precipitating factor. McGrath (1992) studied a cohort of 115 women who were in Broadmoor Hospital, and who had killed their child, during 1956–69. For 46% of the sample the diagnosis was affective psychosis, and for 37% it was schizophrenia. Only 5% were categorized as having personality disorder. Seventy-five per cent had a history of previous psychiatric illness and 49% had attempted suicide at the time of the offence. In many cases the claimed motivation was altruistic, to relieve the child of suffering, although only one victim had severe disability. However, Broadmoor is a high-security hospital to which only the more severely ill and dangerous patients are admitted and so the psychiatric characteristics observed in this sample are likely to be typical of Broadmoor's patient population in general rather than being peculiar to women who had killed their child.

The sample studied by D'Orban (1979) was more representative. In this study, 54% of mothers who had been categorized as having killed their child as a direct consequence of mental illness had a history of previous psychiatric illness requiring inpatient or outpatient treatment and 88% suffered from psychiatric symptoms prior to the offence. Two-thirds had attempted or contemplated suicide at the time of the offence. Usually the murder and suicides were simultaneous acts. In the majority, the conscious motive was primarily self-destruction, and the killing of the child was an extension of the suicide act. Less often the killing was a result of some delusional idea.

D'Orban (1979) reported that many of the women categorized by him as 'battering' also had psychiatric diagnoses, although these diagnoses were not implicated in the offence. Forty-seven per cent had personality disorder and a further 33% were depressed at the time of the offence.

A high proportion of women who have killed a child, as a consequence of abuse, are also likely to be suffering from some kind of psychiatric disorder, either depression or personality disorder, particularly the latter. In turn, it is the case that both personality disorder and depression are more likely to be associated with either high levels of hostility or a reduction in the capacity to inhibit the expression of hostility, or both. In fact, personality disorders are defined by these features: the DSM-IV criteria for personality disorder include abnormalities in cognition (ways of perceiving and interpreting), affectivity, interpersonal functioning and impulse control (American Psychiatric Association 1994). Individuals with personality disorder by definition experience difficulties in all areas of interpersonal functioning and these will apply in their relationships with their children as much as, if not even more so given the emotional intensity of family life, in any social domain. It would appear that while such diagnoses may not usually be directly linked to infant homicide, they are likely to contribute indirectly in that they may make the task of containing aggressive feelings, which all parents sometimes feel towards their infants, difficult, if not impossible for some.

In assessing risk to future children when a mother has killed a child, there are no studies that have followed up this client group to assess outcome in subsequent pregnancies. Each case therefore has to be considered individually, and the usual methods of assessing parenting and risk for the children applied as discussed in the parenting assessment section later in this chapter. As with assessing the risk of violence in psychiatric patients generally, there are difficulties in assessing the risk of filicide in a mentally ill parent. The risk of being killed by a parent as a direct

Table 51.1 Maternal psychiatric disorders. Some questions to ask when a woman with a history of mental illness becomes pregnant and decides to keep the baby.

Pregnancy	
Antenatal clinic	Has she booked in?
	Do obstetricians and midwives know of her psychiatric history?
Family doctor, health visitor and psychiatrist	Do they know she is pregnant?
	Have they seen her recently?
Social Services	Is a planning meeting necessary to discuss possible concerns about child protection?
	Does she need counselling and practical help, e.g. about housing?
	Does she need an allocated social worker?
Medication	Has it been reviewed since her pregnancy became known?
Labour, delivery and early puerperium	
Admission	Will she see staff she has met before?
	Is there a contact number for the liaison psychiatrist?
	Have arrangements been made, if needed, to call upon a psychiatric nurse to 'special' her, after delivery?
	Do the obstetric and paediatric teams know what medication she is taking?
Postnatal management	Is the baby staying with her or in a nursery?
	How long is the planned stay on the postnatal ward and where is she going from there?
	Has an assessment by a psychiatrist been organized?
	Are Social Services convening a child protection conference, and have they got all the relevant clinical data?
Discharge separately from baby	If she is being separated from the baby, has she been prepared for this and does she know her rights?
	What part are her partner and her family playing?
	Where is she going, and do receiving staff know about her needs?
	Who will organize access to the baby?
Discharge with baby	What level of supervision, if any, is needed?
	Have Social Services assessed her need for facilities such as day nursery, home help, etc.?
	Who will organize reviews of the child's welfare and what information is required for such reviews?
	Who is responsible for the mother's clinical management?

consequence of the parent's mental illness is unrelated to the child's age. Most parents with mental illness do not harm their children. When they do, the most frequent scenario involves a parent who is suicidal and who believes the child will also be better off dead.

Jacobson & Miller (1998) presented three examples of detailed, systematic and extensive assessments of future parenting risk when a mentally ill mother had killed someone previously: a neonaticidal mother, a 'battering' mother who had killed a 1-year-old child and a mother who had killed an adult friend during a psychotic episode. As a result of the assessments, all three were deemed to be at *low* risk for future child maltreatment and violence. This article well illustrates the highly complex and multifaceted issues involved in making assessments of parents at risk of filicide.

Clinical management

A particular feature of the management of perinatal women is the protection of the infant. From a practical clinical perspective, the prevention of possible harm to the child begins in preg-

nancy and depends upon effective liaison. The checklist of questions in Table 51.1 is intended as an *aide-mémoire*—it is neither comprehensive nor are all the items relevant to every patient. It has been prepared in the hope that going through such a list and acting upon the information available or lack of it may obviate some of the crises that occur on postnatal wards or at home after discharge from the obstetric unit.

Non-psychotic disorders

Most child-bearing women with mental disorders do not come to the attention of psychiatric services. Epidemiological and case register studies (Nott 1982; Oates 1989) show contact rates between 4 and 15 per 1000 deliveries, of which about 2 per 1000 represent admission (Meltzer & Kumar 1985; Kendell *et al.* 1987). The prevalence of depression after childbirth is at least 10% and therefore about 90% of depressed mothers remain exclusively under the care of their family doctors. To this number may be added cases of other pre-existing non-psychotic disorders, such as phobias and obsessive-compulsive disorders, many of which may also not have been referred for specialist assessment and treatment. The majority of postnatal depressions are self-limiting and resolve within 6 months but, for about one-quarter of those affected, childbirth marks the beginning of chronic and persistent depression (Pitt 1968; Watson *et al.* 1984) and, for a similar proportion, the start of recurrent, remitting and relapsing depressive disorder (Kumar & Robson 1984). Studies of child-bearing women in the community have shown that about half of those meeting operational clinical criteria for caseness remain undetected by family doctors (Kumar & Robson 1984; Sharp 1992) or by health visitors (Briscoe 1986).

The first priority therefore is to improve the detection of women with non-psychotic postnatal psychiatric disturbances and a very significant step in this direction has been made by the development of screening questionnaires such as the Edinburgh Postnatal Depression Scale (Cox *et al.* 1987). Such methods allied with the introduction of systematic psychiatric liaison for obstetrics (Appleby *et al.* 1988; Cox *et al.* 1992) may greatly improve detection rates. However, an essential next step is to develop indices that will help in picking out women most in need of interventions, such as counselling (Holden *et al.* 1989), pharmacotherapy (Henderson *et al.* 1991; Appleby *et al.* 1997) or measures specifically targeted at improving the quality of interaction between mother and infant (Seeley *et al.* 1996; Cooper & Murray 1997).

The childbirth experience in the present context is best summarized as reflecting discontinuities of care. As the mother passes from family doctor to student midwife or to junior obstetricians for subsequent antenatal visits, then meets new faces in the delivery suite and subsequently in the postnatal ward where she must undergo checks from obstetricians and paediatricians before leaving hospital to go back into the care of the community midwives, health visitors and her family doctor, it is not surprising that changes in her mental state may be missed. Even when vigorous attempts are made to detect women at risk, or those already suffering with psychiatric problems in antenatal clinics and postnatal wards (Appleby *et al.* 1988), a significant proportion—nearly 30%—fail to keep clinic appointments. It is possible that many such non-attenders are also the most needy; they may be overwhelmed by the problems of coping with other small children without support from their partners or others and cannot contemplate travelling to a hospital clinic while feeling depressed and run down with an infant and toddlers in tow. There is a need for a co-ordinated policy of care based upon links between hospital and community primary health care services, Social Services and voluntary agencies. Such resources, to be effective, must also be capable of being delivered at home and the contribution of child psychiatrists to the development and shaping of these services seems indispensable.

Psychosis

Admission of a mother to a psychiatric hospital may mean separation from her infant at a time when their relationship is starting to develop. The practice of joint mother-and-infant admissions has become relatively widespread (Buist *et al.* 1990;

Margison 1990), especially in the UK, since it was first proposed by Main (1948). Joint admission was initiated as a consequence of the work of Bowlby (1977) who argued that prolonged separation of mothers and children may be detrimental to the psychological development of the child as well as to the ongoing process of attachment. However, later work (Robertson & Robertson 1971) has indicated that the quality of substitute parenting, rather than separation from the mother *per se*, may be the key factor which influences child outcome.

Studies carried out over the last 30 years have provided support for the feasibility of specialized mother-and-baby units in as much as the burden on nursing staff is manageable, there is no clearly increased risk of physical injury to the child and there appears to be no adverse effect on the mental health of the mother. Baker *et al.* (1961) reported that joint admission of mothers and babies resulted in shorter hospital stays, lower relapse rates and a greater likelihood of the mother adequately caring for her child. However, these findings have not always been supported by other studies (Glaser 1962; Bardon *et al.* 1968; Stewart 1989). Nevertheless, it is generally accepted that the mother's recovery is hastened by the practice of joint admission, as a result of either the continued contact with her infant and the associated confidence in her role as a mother or the particularly supportive and structured environment that is created by grouping women together with similar illnesses. The mother may learn by direct observation of other adult–infant interactions how to care for and play with her baby. Destructive, ambivalent and guilty feelings, obsessional thoughts and misinterpretations can be detected by staff and dealt with promptly. Joint admission may also facilitate attachment by allowing breastfeeding for infants whose mothers are taking certain psychotropic drugs. Mothers who become ill as a result of environmental difficulties but with no obvious problem in their feelings for their baby will also benefit from joint admission by the very fact that separation from the child and the ensuing effects on their relationship will only add to the crisis that brought them into hospital.

However, assessing the positive value of joint admission is complicated by variations in admission criteria between units. Systematic studies have yet to test the validity of claims about the benefits for the mother or, even more surprisingly, for the developing child. In the latter case, another methodological puzzle presents itself. In an attempt to ascertain the potential advantages and disadvantages for the infant of joint admission with a psychotic mother, how can one separate out the effects of the mother's illness from the fact that the pair have been placed in an institution with the influences of multiple caregivers or risks from other patients in addition to the child's own mother?

A feature of mother-and-baby units, like that of neonatal intensive care units, is that caregiving is carried out by a large number of different people, not all of whom are able to learn individual characteristics of a particular baby; their interventions therefore may not always be sensitive to the infant's current mood or activity and may interfere with the normal development of infant self-regulation (Minde & Benoit 1991). Grunebaum *et al.* (1975) described a study of seven infants of mentally ill mothers who were jointly admitted to hospital, seven babies of mentally ill mothers not treated in hospital and 14 babies of normal mothers. Although the social development of the children in the former two groups was judged to be impaired at 18 months compared with controls, the 'joint admission' children attained markedly higher developmental quotients than the other groups, mainly as a result of higher scores on expressive language development. It was suggested that the infant's experience of multiple caregivers and heightened and varied environmental stimulation in the hospital proved to be beneficial to cognitive development at this time.

A number of factors may further heighten the risk of maladaptation of infants whose mothers become psychotic in the puerperium. These include the mother's own difficulties in establishing patterns of mutually responsive interaction with her infant because of heavy sedation from antipsychotic drugs; discontinuation of breastfeeding; and some degree of limited access to the baby as a result of staff concerns about safety and competence of care. Another important consideration that will indirectly affect the mother and infant's long-term outcome is the impact of their joint admission on the quality of the marital or familial relationship (Harvey & McGrath 1988; Lovestone & Kumar 1993), the concerns felt by the family about the baby's safety and the difficulty that the partner/father may experience in getting to know the newborn.

Assessment of risk for the infant must be the most important consideration in the provision of joint care. In community-based samples, researchers have repeatedly tried to identify factors arising before and after childbirth that could indicate mothers who are at high risk for child abuse or neglect. In one of the few prospective studies carried out, Gray *et al.* (1979) identified such a wide range of maternal characteristics and social problems potentially associated with risk for the child that clinical decision-making was not made any easier. Systematic measures of current and future risk among inpatient populations of mentally ill mothers and their infants, however, remain to be defined. A detailed psychiatric history would go some way of raising awareness about the functioning of particular patients who have shown violent or impulsive behaviour in the past or who have experienced command hallucinations or persecutory delusions. A measure that could formally assess characteristics such as maternal motivation and competence to care safely for the infant both during psychiatric illness and after remission of symptoms in an acute episode would clearly be invaluable from a clinical point of view. The development of measures such as the Bethlem Mother–Infant Interaction Scale that was devised in the course of clinical observation on a specialized mother-and-baby unit are likely to provide a useful adjunct in predicting caregiving difficulties from observations in the early weeks of joint admission (Hipwell & Kumar 1996; Kumar & Hipwell 1996). Such measures intended to assess risk should only be one part of the decision-making process of experts and their routine use could clearly have serious consequences where false-negatives or false-positives occur.

Joint care thus poses a number of specific problems: assessment of risk, regulation of access and support in developing an appropriate mother–infant relationship. The practice of domiciliary care of carefully selected severely depressed or manic mothers has recently been shown to be a viable alternative to admission to a mother-and-baby unit (Oates 1988). In this study, the women were managed at home if they were free from active suicidal or infanticidal ideas, lived within reach of the base hospital in case of emergency, were not living alone and had the support of family and friends. The minimal disruption to the family and, the individuality of care provided by the community nurse, encouraging maternal self-confidence and autonomy in her own home, were described as particular benefits of this type of management. No major difference in the clinical recoveries of 17 patients who had been admitted previously with an episode of puerperal psychosis was reported, although these women felt their recovery had been faster when managed at home.

Assessment of parenting

Child psychiatrists may be invited to assess a mentally ill mother who is contesting actions by Social Services under child protection procedures. Most mentally ill mothers are competent parents and colleagues can manage adequately if appropriate support is provided. The difficulty lies in defining criteria and thresholds for what is deemed to be adequate in the context of maternal mental illness, not only currently, in the case of infants, but also stretching into the future as the child's needs change and develop. Conflict between the child's welfare and the mother's parental rights is explicitly recognized by the Children Act and this conflict can begin when a woman suffering from severe mental illness becomes pregnant. There are often lapses and delays in recognizing potential or actual risk to infants, and relatively little attention has been paid to detecting and evaluating threats to welfare that may apply, particularly in the case of infants.

Although there are methods and frameworks for assessing safety and adequacy of parenting and potential risk to older children (Steinhauer 1983; Adcock & White 1985; Kennedy 1991; Reder & Lucey 1995; Budd & Holdsworth 1996; Goepfert *et al.* 1996; Louis *et al.* 1997), the evaluation of risk to infants, in the presence of maternal mental illness, is less well established. There are several key areas that have to be addressed. These involve not only the mother's mental illness and its impact on her capacity to nurture her child, but also the social and physical environment within which mother and child are located (Rutter 1988). Parenting assessments need to be multidimensional and include an evaluation of the following.
- *Caregiving.* Attachment to infant, warmth, sensitivity and responsivity, knowledge and expectations about children, attitudes to being a parent, commitment, competence and consistency in routine care, planning, safety and prevention of risk.
- *Social situation.* Social support, marital relationship, other relationships, violence in relationships, social adversity.
- *History of parenting.* Immediate past with other children and the mother's own experience of being parented.

• *Infant factors*. The baby's health, temperament, difficulties with crying, feeding, etc.
• *Psychiatric issues*. Severity and chronicity of illness, presence of delusions and hallucinations and whether the infant is incorporated in maternal psychopathology, insight about the illness and its impact on the infant, acceptance of and responsiveness to interventions and treatment, including compliance with medication.

Conclusions

Over the past 20 years there has been a convergence of interest by clinicians and researchers investigating the impact of maternal psychiatric disorders on parenting ability, and those whose primary focus of investigation has been the sensitivities of infants to the emotional states of their primary caregivers. This has led to a better understanding of some of the mechanisms involved in the effects of maternal psychopathology on the developing infant and has important and hopeful implications — parenting attitudes and behaviours can sometimes be changed — but highlights the need for the development and evaluation of strategies for early intervention for families at risk.

A review of the current literature on maternal psychiatric illness and child adjustment and development is complicated by the diversity of questions asked and methods used. The merits and drawbacks of a variety of procedures to assess mother–infant interaction were discussed by Melhuish *et al.* (1988), who concluded that an integration of methods is essential for future research and clinical practice. Ideally, highly detailed observations of short duration that describe the interactive roles and behaviours of mother and infant should be combined with longer observations in naturalistic settings that provide a more typical, although global, account. Such systematic assessments in the early postpartum months may then be placed in the context of long-term longitudinal investigations of developmental outcome for the child and its network of relationships.

Another major problem with almost all studies to date concerns the confounding of diagnosis with other predisposing factors, not only genetic, but also, for example, the downward social mobility that accompanies serious psychiatric illness (Yoshida *et al.* 1999) or pre-existing dysfunctional relationship patterns which can co-occur with, but independently of, diagnosis (De Mulder *et al.* 1995) or when the infant's and mother's temperaments have a poor fit, to name but a few. Then there is the possible impact of different management strategies, e.g. was the mother admitted to hospital, with her baby or not, or was she looked after at home? Not all children are affected by their mother having a puerperal psychiatric illness. When maternal postnatal depression has been found to have an impact on the infant it may be perhaps only when other factors are also present, e.g. when the mother's attachment to her infant is compromised (Kumar 1997) or the depression occurs in the context of pre-existing disturbed patterns of family relationships or when the baby is irritable. Relatively recently developed methods for the

design and analysis of longitudinal studies (Willet *et al.* 1998) allow for more sophisticated projects which would take into account not only factors such as those discussed above but also the changes over time that occur in individual behaviour. Multicentred studies to obtain adequate sample sizes together with the use of these newer methods of design and analyses would allow us to begin to disentangle effects and their mediators.

One of the most important clinical developments in the last decade or so has been the consequence of a shift in emphasis from parental rights to the rights of the child and parental responsibility in ensuring that these are adequately met. In the UK, the passing and implementation of the Children Act (1989) has resulted in important changes in practice. The key feature of this act is that the welfare of the child is paramount. This means that where there is conflict the child's needs take precedence over those of the parent.

The work of Bowlby and subsequent attachment theory research has had two consequences. On the one hand, it has highlighted the importance of the development of secure attachments to caregivers in infants for their later psychological development. On the other hand, in emphasizing the difficulties for the infant of separations from the mother, rather than the importance of the stability and quality of care, whoever the carer may be, mother and infant may have been kept together perhaps sometimes under inappropriate circumstances when the best outcome for the infant might have been separation as early as possible with view to placement in a permanent and stable situation.

There is always sympathy and concern for a woman who has a severe psychiatric disorder. Often she herself has been the victim of grossly inadequate parenting from which society failed to protect her. Under these circumstances the woman's carers may find it difficult to keep both mother and baby's sometimes conflicting needs in mind. A frequently expressed, and understandable, view is that all mothers need to be given a chance. A society that asserts and legislates for the primacy of the child's welfare ensures that it is the baby who is given a chance. This may be through therapeutic intervention aimed at helping a mother to better protect, care for and understand her child, or where necessary through separation and safe and secure placement. The improvement in, and systematization and testing of, methodology for assessing adequacy of parenting and risk to the infant, not only in the context of severe maternal mental illness but also in the community, will be an important next step.

References

Adcock, M. & White, R., eds (1985) *Good Enough Parenting: a Framework for Assessment*. British Association for Adoption and Fostering, London.
Adrian, C. & Hammen, C. (1993) Stress exposure and stress generation in children of depressed mothers. *Journal of Consulting and Clinical Psychology*, 61, 354–359.
Ainsworth, M. & Wittig, B. (1969) Attachment and exploratory behav-

iour of one-year-olds in a strange situation. In: *Determinants of Infant Behaviour* (ed. B. Foss), pp. 113–136. Methuen, London.

Altshuler, L.L., Cohen, L., Szuba, M.P., Burt, V.K., Gitlin, M. & Mintz, J. (1996) Pharmacologic management of psychiatric illness during pregnancy: dilemmas and guidelines. *American Journal of Psychiatry*, **153**, 592–606.

Altshuler, L., Hendrick, V. & Cohen, L. (1998) Course of mood and anxiety disorders during pregnancy and the postpartum period. *Journal of Clinical Psychiatry*, **59**, 29–33.

American Psychiatric Association (1994) *Diagnostic and Statistical Manual of Mental Disorders*, 4th edn. American Psychiatric Association, Washington D.C.

Appleby, L. & Dickens, C. (1993) Mothering skills of women with mental illness. *British Medical Journal*, **306**, 348–349.

Appleby, L., Fox, H., Shaw, M. & Kumar, R. (1988) The psychiatrist in the obstetric unit: establishing a liaison service. *British Journal of Psychiatry*, **154**, 510–515.

Appleby, L., Warner, R., Whitton, A. *et al.* (1997) A controlled study of fluoxetine and cognitive-behavioural counselling in the treatment of postnatal depression. *British Medical Journal*, **314**, 932–936.

Aronson, M., Kyllerman, M., Sabel, K., Sandin, B. & Olegard, R. (1985) Children of alcoholic mothers: developmental, perceptual and behavioural characteristics as compared to matched controls. *Acta Psychiatrica Scandinavica*, **74**, 27–35.

Baker, A., Morison, M., Game, J. & Thorpe, J. (1961) Admitting schizophrenic mothers with their babies. *Lancet*, **ii**, 237–239.

Bardon, D., Glaser, Y., Protheroe, D. & Weston, D. (1968) Mother and baby unit: psychiatric survey of 115 cases. *British Medical Journal*, **2**, 755–758.

Barr, H., Streissguth, A., Darby, B. & Simpson, P. (1990) Prenatal exposure to alcohol, caffeine, tobacco, and aspirin: effects on fine and gross motor performance in 4-year-old children. *Developmental Psychology*, **26**, 339–348.

Beck, C. (1996) A meta-analysis of predictors of postpartum depression. *Nursing Research*, **45**, 297–303.

Benvenuti, P., Cabras, P., Servi, P., Rosseti, S., Marchetti, G. & Pazzagli, A. (1992) Puerperal psychosis: a clinical case study with follow-up. *Journal of Affective Disorders*, **26**, 25–30.

Bergman, A.J., Wolfson, M.A. & Walker, E.F. (1997) Neuromotor functioning and behaviour problems in children at risk for psychopathology. *Journal of Abnormal Psychology*, **25**, 229–237.

Blais, M.A., Beeker, A.E., Burwell, R.A. *et al.* (2000) Pregnancy: outcome and impact on symptomatology in a cohort of eating-disordered women. *International Journal of Eating Disorders*, **27**, 140–149.

Bornstein, M.H., ed. (1995) *Handbook of Parenting*. Lawrence Erlbaum, Mahwah, NJ.

Bowlby, J. (1973) *Attachment and Loss: Attachment*. Basic Books, New York.

Bowlby, J. (1977) The making and breaking of affectional bonds. I. Aetiology and psychopathology in the light of attachment theory. *British Journal of Psychiatry*, **130**, 201–210.

Brinch, M., Isager, T. & Tolstrup, K. (1988) Anorexia nervosa and motherhood: reproduction pattern and mothering behaviour of 50 women. *Acta Psychiatrica Scandinavica*, **77**, 611–617.

Briscoe, M. (1986) Identification of emotional problems in postpartum women by health visitors. *British Journal of Psychiatry*, **292**, 1245–1247.

Brockington, I. (1996) *Motherhood and Mental Health*. Oxford University Press, Oxford.

Brockington, I., Cernik, K., Schofield, E., Downing, A., Francis, A. & Keelan, C. (1981) Puerperal psychosis: phenomena and diagnosis. *Archives of General Psychiatry*, **38**, 829–833.

Brockington, I.F., Oates, M. & Rose, G. (1990) Prepartum psychosis. *Journal of Affective Disorders*, **19**, 31–35.

Brody, G.H., Stoneman, Z., Flor, D., McCrary, C., Hastings, L. & Conyers, O. (1994) Financial resources, parent psychological functioning, parent co-caregiving, and early adolescent competence in rural two-parent African-American families. *Child Development*, **65**, 590–605.

Brown, G.W. (1988) Causal paths, chains and strands. In: *Studies of Psychosocial Risk: the Power of Longitudinal Data* (ed. M. Rutter), pp. 285–314. Cambridge University Press, Cambridge.

Brown, G.W., Bifulco, A. & Andrews, B. (1990) Self-esteem and depression. III. Aetiological issues. *Social Psychiatry and Psychiatric Epidemiology*, **25**, 235–243.

Brozovsky, M. & Falit, H. (1971) Neonaticide: clinical and psychodynamic considerations. *Journal of the American Academy of Child Psychiatry*, **10**, 673–683.

Budd, K.S. & Holdsworth, M.J. (1996) Issues in clinical assessment of minimal parenting competence. *Journal of Clinical Child Psychology*, **25**, 2–14.

Buist, A., Norman, T. & Dennerstein, L. (1990) Breastfeeding and the use of psychotropic medication: a review. *Journal of Affective Disorders*, **19**, 197–206.

Cabrera, N., Tamis-LeMonda, C., Bradley, R., Hofferth, S. & Lamb, M.E. (2000) Fatherhood in the twenty-first century. *Child Development*, **71**, 127–136.

Caldji, C., Tannenbaum, B., Sharma, S., Francis, D., Plotsky, P.M. & Meaney, M.J. (1998) Maternal care during infancy regulates the development of neural systems mediating the expression of fearfulness in the rat. *Neurobiology*, **95**, 5335–5340.

Campbell, S. & Cohn, J. (1991) Prevalence and correlates of postpartum depression in first-time mothers. *Journal of Abnormal Psychology*, **100**, 594–599.

Campbell, S., Cohn, J. & Meyers, T. (1995) Depression in first-time mothers: mother–infant interaction and depression chronicity. *Developmental Psychology*, **31**, 349–357.

Chasnoff, I. & Griffith, D. (1991) Maternal cocaine use: neonatal outcome. In: *Theory and Research in Behavioural Paediatrics*, Vol. 5 (eds H. Fitzgerald & B. Lester), pp. 1–17. Plenum Press, New York.

Cohen, L. & Rosenbaum, J. (1998) Psychotropic drug use during pregnancy: weighing the risk. *Journal of Clinical Psychiatry*, **59** (Suppl. 2), 18–28.

Cohen, L., Sichel, D., Dimmock, J. & Rosenbaum, J.F. (1994) Postpartum course in women with pre-existing panic disorder. *Journal of Clinical Psychiatry*, **55**, 289–292.

Cohen, L., Sichel, D., Faraone, S., Robertson, L., Dimmock, J. & Rosenbaum, J. (1996) Course of panic disorder during pregnancy and the puerperium: a preliminary study. *Biological Psychiatry*, **39**, 950–954.

Cohler, B.J., Weiss, J. & Grunebaum, H. (1970) Child-care attitudes and emotional disturbances in mothers of young children. *Genetic Psychological Monographs*, **82**, 3–47.

Cohn, J. & Tronick, E. (1989) Specificity of infants' response to mothers' affective behaviour. *Journal of the American Academy of Child and Adolescent Psychiatry*, **28**, 242–248.

Conger, R.D., Ge, X., Elder, G.H. Jr, Lorenz, F.O. & Simons, R.L. (1994) Economic stress, coercive family process, and developmental problems of adolescents. *Child Development*, **65**, 541–561.

Conti, J., Abraham, S. & Taylor, A. (1998) Eating behaviour and pregnancy outcome. *Journal of Psychosomatic Research*, **44**, 465–477.

Cooper, P. & Murray, L. (1997) The impact of psychological treatments of postpartum depression on maternal mood and infant development. In: *Postpartum Depression and Child Development* (eds L. Murray & P. Cooper), pp. 201–220. Guilford Press, New York.

Copeland, A.R. (1985) Homicide in childhood: the Metro-Dade County experience from 1956 to 1982. *American Journal of Forensic Medicine and Pathology*, 6, 21–24.

Cox, J.L., Holden, J. & Sagovsky, R. (1987) Detection of postnatal depression: development of the Edinburgh Postnatal Depression Scale. *British Journal of Psychiatry*, 150, 782–786.

Cox, J.L., Kumar, R., Oates, M., Foreman, D. & Anderson, H. (1992) Report of the General Psychiatry Section working party on postnatal mental illness. *Psychiatric Bulletin*, 16, 519–522.

Cox, J.L., Murray, D. & Chapman, G. (1993) A controlled study of the onset, duration and prevalence of postnatal depression. *British Journal of Psychiatry*, 163, 27–31.

Crittenden, P. & Craig, S.E. (1990) Developmental trends in the nature of child homicide. *Journal of Interpersonal Violence*, 5, 202–216.

Davidson, J. & Robertson, E. (1985) A follow-up study of postpartum illness, 1946–78. *Acta Psychiatrica Scandinavica*, 71, 451–457.

Davies, A., McIvor, R. & Kumar, R. (1995) Impact of childbirth on a series of schizophrenic mothers: a comment on the possible influence of oestrogen on schizophrenia. *Schizophrenia Research*, 16, 25–31.

DeMulder, E. & Radke-Yarrow, M. (1991) Attachment with affectively ill and well mothers: concurrent behavioural correlates. *Development and Psychopathology*, 3, 227–242.

DeMulder, E.K., Tarulla, L.B., Klimes-Dougan, B. *et al.* (1995) Personality disorders of affectively ill mothers: links to maternal behaviour. *Journal of Personality Disorders*, 9, 199–212.

D'Orban, P. (1979) Women who kill their children. *British Journal of Psychiatry*, 134, 560–571.

Egeland, B., Jacobvitz, D. & Sroufe, L.A. (1988) Breaking the cycle of abuse. *Child Development*, 59, 1080–1088.

Fergusson, D., Woodward, L. & Horwood. L.J. (1998) Maternal smoking during pregnancy and psychiatric adjustment in late adolescence. *Archives of General Psychiatry*, 55, 721–727.

Field, T. (1995) Infants of depressed mothers. *Infant Behaviour and Development*, 18, 1–13.

Field, T., Healy, B., Goldstein, S. *et al.* (1988) Infants of depressed mothers show 'depressed' behaviour even with non-depressed adults. *Child Development*, 59, 1569–1579.

Fish, B. (1977) Neurobiologic antecedents of schizophrenia in children. *Archives of General Psychiatry*, 34, 1297–1313.

Fish, B., Marcus, J., Hans, S.L., Auerbach, J.G. & Perdue, S. (1992) Infants at risk for schizophrenia: sequelae of a genetic neurointegrative defect—a review and replication analysis of pandysmaturation in the Jerusalem Infant Development Study. *Archives of General Psychiatry*, 49, 221–235.

Fonagy, P., Steele, H. & Steele, M. (1991) Maternal representations of attachment during pregnancy predict the organization of infant–mother attachment at one year of age. *Child Development*, 62, 891–905.

Fonagy, P., Steele, M., Steele, H., Higgitt, A. & Target, M. (1994) The theory and practice of resilience. *Journal of Child Psychology and Psychiatry*, 35, 231–259.

Frankel, K. & Harmon, R. (1996) Depressed mothers: they don't always look as bad as they feel. *Journal of the American Academy of Child and Adolescent Psychiatry*, 35, 289–298.

Funayama, M. & Sagisaka, K. (1988) Consecutive infanticides in Japan. *American Journal of Forensic Medicine and Pathology*, 9, 9–11.

Gamer, E., Gallant, D. & Grunebaum, H.U. (1976) Children of psychotic mothers. *Archives of General Psychiatry*, 33, 311–317.

Garmezy, N. (1974) Children at risk: the search for the antecedents of schizophrenia. II. Ongoing research programmes and intervention. *Schizophrenia Bulletin*, 9, 55–125.

Gitau, R., Cameron, A., Fisk, N.M. & Glover, V. (1998) Fetal exposure to maternal cortisol [Letter]. *Lancet*, 352, 707–708.

Gitau, R., Fisk, N.M., Cameron, A., Teixeira, J., Glover, V. (2001) Fetal HPA stress responses to invasive procedures are independent of maternal responses. *Journal of Clinical Endocrinology and Metabolism*, 86, 104–109.

Glaser, Y.I.M. (1962) A unit for mothers and babies in a psychiatric hospital. *Journal of Child Psychology and Psychiatry*, 3, 53–60.

Goepfert, M., Webster, J. & Seeman, M.V., eds. (1996). *Parental Psychiatric Disorder: Distressed Parents and Their Children*. Cambridge University Press, Cambridge.

Goodman, S.H. (1987) Emory University project on children of disturbed parents. *Schizophrenia Bulletin*, 13, 411–423.

Goodman, S.H. & Emory, E.K. (1992) Perinatal complications in births to low socioeconomic status schizophrenic and depressed women. *Journal of Abnormal Psychology*, 101, 225–229.

Gotlib, I., Whiffen, V., Wallace, P. & Mount, J. (1991) Prospective investigation of postpartum depression: factors involved in onset and recovery. *Journal of Abnormal Psychology*, 100, 122–132.

Gray, J.D., Cutler, C., Dean, J. & Kempe, C.H. (1979) Prediction and prevention of child abuse. *Seminars in Perinatology*, 3, 85–90.

Green, C.M. & Manohar, S.V. (1990) Neonaticide and hysterical denial of pregnancy. *British Journal of Psychiatry*, 156, 121–123.

Grunebaum, H.U., Weiss, J.L., Cohler, B.J., Hartman, C.R. & Gallant, D.H. (1975) *Mentally Ill Mothers and Their Children*. University of Chicago Press, Chicago, IL.

Hamilton, E.B., Jones, M. & Hanimen, C. (1993) Maternal interaction style in affective disordered, physically ill and normal women. *Family Process*, 32, 329–340.

Hans, S.L., Berstein, V.J. & Henson, L.G. (1999) The role of psychopathology in the parenting of drug-dependent women. *Developmental Psychopathology*, 11, 957–977.

Harvey, I. & McGrath, G. (1988) Psychiatric morbidity in spouses of women admitted to a mother and baby unit. *British Journal of Psychiatry*, 152, 506–510.

Hay, D., Pawlby, S., Sharp, D., Asten, P., Mills, A. & Kumar, R. (2001) Intellectual problems shown by 11 year-old children whose mothers had postnatal depression. *Journal of Child Psychology and Psychiatry*, 42, 871–890.

Hedegaard, M., Henriksen, T.B., Sabroe, S. & Secher, N.J. (1993) Psychological distress in pregnancy and preterm delivery. *British Medical Journal*, 307, 234–239.

Henderson, A.F., Gregoire, A., Kumar, R. & Studd, J.W.W. (1991) Treatment of severe postnatal depression with oestradiol skin patches. *Lancet*, 338, 816–817.

Hipwell, A. & Kumar, R. (1996) Maternal psychopathology and prediction of outcome based on mother–infant interaction ratings (BMIS). *British Journal of Psychiatry*, 169, 655–661.

Hipwell, A., Goossens, F., Melhuish, E. & Kumar, R. (2000) Severe maternal psychopathology and infant–mother attachment. *Development and Psychopathology*, 12, 157–175.

Holden, J., Sagovsky, R. & Cox, J. (1989) Counselling in a general practice setting: controlled study of health visitors' intervention in treatment of postnatal depression. *British Medical Journal*, 298, 223–226.

Howard, J., Beckwith, L., Rodning, C. & Kropenske, V. (1989) The development of young children of substance-abusing parents: insights from 7 years of intervention and research. *Zero to Three*, 9, 8–12.

Jacobson, T. & Miller, L.J. (1998) Mentally ill mothers who have killed: three cases addressing the issue of future parenting capability. *Psychiatric Services*, 49, 650–657.

Jeremy, R.J. & Bernstine, V.J. (1984) Dyads at risk: methadone-maintained women and their 4-month-old infants. *Child Development*, 55, 1141–1154.

Jones, K.L. & Smith, D.W. (1973) Recognition of the fetal alcohol syndrome in early infancy. *Lancet*, **ii**, 999–1001.

Kaltenbach, K.A. (1994) Effects of *in utero* opiate exposure: new paradigms for old questions. *Drug and Alcohol Dependence*, **36**, 83–87.

Kandall, S.R., Gaines, J., Habel, L., Davidson, G. & Jessop, D. (1993) Relationship of maternal substance-abuse to subsequent sudden infant death syndrome in offspring. *Journal of Pediatrics*, **123**, 120–126.

Kauffman, C., Grunebaum, H., Cohler, B. & Gamer, E. (1979) Superkids: competent children of psychotic mothers. *American Journal of Psychiatry*, **136**, 1398–1402.

Kaye, N.S., Borenstein, N.M. & Donnelly, S.M. (1990) Families, murder and insanity: a psychiatric review of paternal neonaticide. *Journal of Forensic Sciences*, **35**, 133–139.

Kendell, R., Chalmers, J. & Platz, C. (1987) Epidemiology of puerperal psychosis. *British Journal of Psychiatry*, **150**, 662–673.

Kennedy, R. (1991) Parental responsibility. *Psychiatric Bulletin*, **15**, 129–132.

Kettinger, L.A., Nair, P. & Schuler, M.E. (2000) Exposure to environmental risk factors and parenting attitudes among substance abusing women. *American Journal of Drug and Alcohol Abuse*, **26**, 1–11.

Klompenhouwer, J. & Van Hulst, A. (1991) Classification of postpartum psychosis: a study of 250 mother and baby admissions in the Netherlands. *Acta Psychiatrica Scandinavica*, **84**, 255–261.

Kosofsky, B.E. (1999) Effects of alcohol and cocaine on brain development. In: *Neurobiology of Mental Illness* (eds D.S. Charney, E.J. Nestler & B.S. Bunney), pp. 601–615. Oxford University Press, New York.

Kron, R.E., Kaplan, S.L., Finnegan, L.P., Litt, M. & Phoenix, M.D. (1975) An assessment of the behavioural change in infants undergoing narcotic withdrawal: comparative data from clinical and objective methods. *Addictive Diseases*, **2**, 257–275.

Kumar, R. (1997) 'Anybody's child': severe disorders of mother-to-infant bonding. *British Journal of Psychiatry*, **171**, 175–181.

Kumar, R. & Hipwell, A. (1994) Implications for the infant of maternal puerperal psychiatric disorders. In: *Child and Adolescent Psychiatry: Modern Approaches* (eds M. Rutter, E. Taylor & L. Hersov), pp. 759–775. Blackwell Science, Oxford.

Kumar, R. & Hipwell, A. (1996) Development of a clinical rating scale to assess mother–infant interaction in a psychiatric mother and baby unit. *British Journal of Psychiatry*, **169**, 18–26.

Kumar, R. & Robson, K. (1984) A prospective study of emotional disorders in childbearing women. *British Journal of Psychiatry*, **144**, 35–47.

Kumar, R., Marks, M., Platz, C. & Yoshida, K. (1995) Clinical survey of a psychiatric mother and baby unit: characteristics of 100 consecutive admissions. *Journal of Affective Disorders*, **33**, 11–22.

Lacey, H.J. & Smith, G. (1987) Bulimia nervosa: the impact of pregnancy on mother and baby. *British Journal of Psychiatry*, **150**, 777–781.

Lamb, M.E. (1999) Noncustodial fathers and their impact on the children of divorce. In: *The Postdivorce Family: Children, Parenting and Society* (eds R. Thompson & P. Amato), pp. 105–125. Sage, Thousand Oaks, CA.

Lawson, M.S. & Wilson, G.S. (1979) Addiction and pregnancy: two lives in crisis. *Social Work in Health Care*, **4**, 445–457.

Lemberg, R. & Phillips, J. (1989) The impact of pregnancy on anorexia nervosa and bulimia nervosa. *International Journal of Eating Disorders*, **8**, 285–295.

Lobel, M., Dunkel-Schetter, C. & Scrimshaw, S. (1992) Prenatal maternal stress and prematurity: a prospective study of socioeconomically disadvantaged women. *Health Psychology*, **11**, 32–40.

Lou, H., Hansen, D., Nordenloft, M. & Pryds, O. (1994) Prenatal stressors of human life affect fetal brain development. *Developmental Medicine and Child Neurology*, **36**, 826–832.

Louis, A., Condon, J., Shute, R. & Elzinga, R. (1997) The development of the Louis MACRO (Mother and Child Risk Observation) forms: assessing parent–infant–child risk in the presence of maternal mental illness. *Child Abuse and Neglect*, **21** (7), 589–606.

Lovestone, S. & Kumar, R. (1993) Postnatal psychiatric illness: the impact on spouses. *British Journal of Psychiatry*, **163**, 210–216.

Lyons-Ruth, K., Zoll, D., Connell, D. & Grunebaum, H. (1986) The depressed mother and her one-year-old infant: environment, interaction, attachment, and infant development. In: *Maternal Depression and Infant Disturbance: New Directions for Child Development*, Vol. 34 (eds E. Tronick & T. Field), pp. 61–82. Jossey-Bass, San Francisco, CA.

Main, T.F. (1948) Mothers with children in a psychiatric hospital. *Lancet*, **ii**, 845–847.

Manassis, K., Bradley, S., Goldberg, S., Hood, J. & Price Swinson, R. (1994) Attachment in mothers with anxiety disorders and their children. *Journal of the American Academy of Child and Adolescent Psychiatry*, **33**, 1106–1113.

Marcus, J., Auerbach, J., Wilkinson, L. & Burack, C.M. (1981) Infants at risk for schizophrenia: the Jerusalem Infant Development Study. *Archives of General Psychiatry*, **38**, 703–713.

Marcus, J., Hans, S.L., Nagler, S., Auerbach, J.G., Mirsky, A.F. & Aubrey, A. (1987) Review of the NIMH Israeli Kibbutz–City Study and the Jerusalem Infant Development Study. *Schizophrenia Bulletin*, **13**, 425–438.

Margison, F. (1990) Infants of mentally ill mothers: the risk of injury and its control. *Journal of Reproductive and Infant Psychology*, **8**, 137–146.

Marks, M.N. (1996) Characteristics and causes of infanticide in Britain. *International Review of Psychiatry*, **8**, 99–106.

Marks, M.N. & Kumar, R. (1993) Infanticide in England and Wales. *Medicine, Science and the Law*, **33**, 329–339.

Marks, M.N. & Kumar, R. (1996) Infanticide in Scotland. *Medicine, Science and the Law*, **36**, 299–305.

Marks, M.N. & Lovestone, S. (1995) The role of the father in parental postnatal mental health. *British Journal of Medical Psychology*, **68**, 157–168.

Marks, M.N., Wieck, A., Checkley, S.A. & Kumar, R. (1992) Contribution of psychological and social factors to psychotic and nonpsychotic relapse after childbirth in women with previous histories of affective disorder. *Journal of Affective Disorders*, **29**, 253–264.

Marks, M.N., Wieck, A., Checkley, S.A. & Kumar, R. (1996) How does marriage protect women with histories of affective disorder against post-partum relapse? *British Journal of Medical Psychology*, **69**, 329–342.

Marks, M.N., Siddle, K. & Warwick C. (2000) A randomised controlled trial to assess the effect of specialist midwifery care on rates of postnatal depression in high risk women. *Archives of Women's Health*, **3**, 103–104.

Mayes, L. & Bornstein, M.H. (1997) The development of children exposed to cocaine. In: *Developmental Psychopathology: Perspectives on Adjustment Risk and Disorder* (eds S.S. Luthar, J.A. Burciek, D. Cicchetti & J.R. Weisz), pp. 166–168. Cambridge University Press, Cambridge.

McGrath, P.G. (1992) Maternal filicide in Broadmoor hospital, 1916–69. *Journal of Forensic Psychiatry*, **3**, 271–297.

McNeil, T.F. (1986) A prospective study of postpartum psychoses. I. Clinical characteristics of the current postpartum episodes. *Acta Psychiatrica Scandinavica*, **74**, 205–216.

McNeil, T.F., Kaij, L., Malmquist-Larsson, A. *et al.* (1984) Offspring of women with nonorganic psychoses: progress report. In: *Children at Risk for Schizophrenia: a Longitudinal Perspective* (eds N. Watt, E.J. Anthony, L. Wynne & J. Rolf), pp. 465–481. Cambridge University Press, New York.

McNeil, T.F., Kaij, L., Malmquist-Larsson, A. *et al.* (1983) Offspring of women with nonorganic psychosis: development of a longitudinal study of children at high risk. *Acta Psychiatrica Scandinavica*, **68**, 234–250.

McNeil, T., Persson-Blennow, L., Binett, B., Harty, B. & Karyd, U. (1988) A prospective study of postpartum psychoses in a high-risk group. VII. Relationship to later offspring characteristics. *Acta Psychiatrica Scandinavica*, **78**, 613–617.

McNeil, T.J., Harty, B., Blennow, G. & Cantor-Graae, E. (1993) Neuromotor deviation in offspring of psychotic mothers: a selective development deficiency in two groups of children at heightened psychiatric risk? *Journal of Psychiatric Research*, **27**, 39–54.

Mednick, S.A., Mura, M., Schulzinger, F. & Mednick, B. (1971) Perinatal conditions and infant development in children with schizophrenic parents. *Social Biology*, **18**, S103–S113.

Melhuish, E., Gambles, C. & Kumar, R. (1988) Maternal mental illness and the mother–infant relationship. In: *Motherhood and Mental Illness*, Vol. 2. *Causes and Consequences* (eds R. Kumar & I. Brockington), pp. 191–211. Wright/Butterworth, London.

Meltzer, E.S. & Kumar, R. (1985) Puerperal mental illness, clinical features and classification: a study of 142 mother-and-baby admissions. *British Journal of Psychiatry*, **147**, 647–654.

Metz, A., Sichel, D.A. & Goff, D. (1988) Postpartum panic disorder. *Journal of Clinical Psychiatry*, **49**, 278–279.

Minde, K. & Benoit, D. (1991) Infant psychiatry: its relevance for the general psychiatrist. *British Journal of Psychiatry*, **159**, 173–184.

Mitchell, J.E., Seim, H.C., Glotter, D., Soll, E.A. & Pyle, R.L. (1991) A retrospective study of pregnancy in bulimia nervosa. *International Journal of Eating Disorders*, **10**, 209–214.

Mullen, N., Snidman, N. & Kagan, J. (1993) Free play behavior in inhibited and uninhibited children. *Infant Behavior and Development*, **16**, 383–389.

Murray, L. (1992) The impact of postnatal depression on infant development. *Journal of Child Psychology and Psychiatry*, **33**, 543–561.

Murray, L. & Cooper, P.J., eds (1997) *Postpartum Depression and Child Development*. Guilford Press, New York.

Murray, L., Kempton, C., Woolgar, M. & Hooper, R. (1993) Depressed mothers' speech to their infants and its relation to infant gender and cognitive development. *Journal of Child Psychology and Psychiatry*, **34**, 1083–1101.

Murray, L., Fiori-Cowley, A., Hooper, R. & Cooper, P. (1996) The impact of postnatal depression and associated adversity on early mother–infant interactions and later infant outcome. *Child Development*, **67**, 2512–2526.

Murray, L., Sinclair, D., Cooper, P., Ducournau, P., Turner, P. & Stein, A. (1999) The socioemotional development of 5-year-old children of postnatally depressed mothers. *Journal of Child Psychology and Psychiatry*, **40**, 1259–1271.

Näslund, B., Persson-Blennow, L., McNeil, T., Kaij, L. & Malmquist-Larsson, A. (1984) Offspring of women with organic psychosis: infant attachment to the mother at one year of age. *Acta Psychiatrica Scandinavica*, **69**, 231–241.

Northcott, C. & Stein, M. (1994) Panic disorder in pregnancy. *Journal of Clinical Psychiatry*, **55**, 539–542.

Nott, P. (1982) Psychiatric illness following childbirth in Southampton: a case register study. *Psychological Medicine*, **12**, 557–561.

O'Connor, M.J., Sigman, M. & Brill, N. (1987) Disorganisation of attachment in relation to maternal alcohol consumption. *Journal of Consulting and Clinical Psychology*, **6**, 831–836.

O'Connor, T.G., Heron, J., Golding, J., Beveridge, M. & Glover, V. (in press) Maternal antenatal anxiety and children's behavioral/emotional problems at 4 years. *British Journal of Psychiatry*.

O'Hara, M. (1995) Childbearing. In: *Psychological Aspects of Women's Reproductive Health* (eds M. O'Hara, R. Reiter, S. Johnson, A. Milburn & J. Engeldinger), pp. 26–48. Springer, New York.

O'Hara, M.W. & Swain, A.M. (1996) Rates and risk of postpartum depression: a meta-analysis. *International Review of Psychiatry*, **8**, 37–54.

Oates, M. (1988) The development of an integrated community oriented service for severe postnatal mental illness. In: *Motherhood and Mental Illness*, Vol. 2 (eds R. Kumar & I. Brockington), pp. 133–158. Wright, London.

Oates, M. (1989) Management of major mental illness in pregnancy and the puerperium. *Bailliere's Clinical Obstetrics and Gynaecology*, **3**, 905–920.

Oates, M. (1996) Psychiatric services for women following childbirth. *International Review of Psychiatry*, **8**, 87–98.

Oates, M. (1997) Patients as parents: the risk to children. *British Journal of Psychiatry*, **170** (Suppl. 32), 22–27.

Orr, S. & Miller, C. (1995) Maternal depressive symptoms and the risk of poor pregnancy outcome: review of the literature and preliminary findings. *Epidemiological Review*, **17**, 165–171.

Papousek, H. & Papousek, M. (1997) Fragile aspects of early social integration. In: *Postpartum Depression and Child Development* (eds L. Murray & P. Cooper), pp. 35–53. Guilford Press, New York.

Patterson, G.R. (1998) Continuities: a search for causal mechanisms [Comment]. *Developmental Psychology*, **34**, 1263–1268.

Patterson, G.R. & Dishion, T.J. (1998) Multilevel family process models: traits, interactions, and relationships. In: *Relationships Within Families: Mutual Influences* (eds R.A. Hinde & J. Stevenson-Hinde), pp. 283–310. Clarendon Press, Oxford.

Perkin, M., Bland, J.M., Peacock, J.L. & Anderson, H.R. (1993) The effect of anxiety and depression during pregnancy on obstetric complications. *British Journal of Obstetrics and Gynaecology*, **100**, 629–634.

Pitt, B. (1968) Atypical depression following childbirth. *British Journal of Psychiatry*, **114**, 1325–1335.

Radke-Yarrow, M. (1998) *Children of Depressed Mothers*. Cambridge University Press, New York.

Radke-Yarrow, M., Nottelmann, E., Martinez, P., Fox, M. & Belmont, B. (1992) Young children of affectively ill parents: a longitudinal study of psychosocial development. *Journal of the American Academy of Child and Adolescent Psychiatry*, **31**, 68–77.

Ragins, N., Schachter, J., Elmer, E., Preisman, R., Bowes, A. & Harway, V. (1975) Infants and children at risk for schizophrenia: Environmental and developmental observations. *Journal of the American Academy of Child Psychiatry*, **14**, 150–177.

Reder, P. & Lucey, C., eds (1995) *Assessment of Parenting*: Psychiatric and Psychological Contributions. Routledge, New York.

Reich, T. & Winokur, G. (1970) Postpartum psychosis in patients with manic depressive disease. *Journal of Nervous and Mental Disease*, **151**, 60–68.

Resnick, P.J. (1970) Murder of the newborn: a psychiatric review of neonaticide. *American Journal of Psychiatry*, **126**, 1414–1420.

Robertson, J. & Robertson, J. (1971) Young children in brief separation: a fresh look. In: *The Psychoanalytic Study of the Child*, **26**, pp. 264–315. Hogarth Press, London.

Rutter, M. (1988) *Studies of Psychosocial Risk: the Power of Longitudinal Data*. Cambridge University Press, Cambridge.

Rutter, M. (1989) Psychiatric disorder in parents as a risk factor for children. In: *Prevention of Psychiatric Disorders in Child and Adolescent: the Project of the American Academy of Child and Adolescent Psychiatry. OSAP Prevention Monograph 2* (eds D. Shaffer, I. Philips, N. Enver, M. Silverman & V.Q. Anthony), pp. 157–189. Office of Substance Abuse Prevention, US Department of Health and Human Services, Rockville, MD.

Rutter, M. (1998) Some research considerations on intergenerational continuities and discontinuities [Comment]. *Developmental Psychology*, **34**, 1269–1273.

Rutter, M. & Quinton, D. (1984) Parental psychiatric disorder: effects on children. *Psychological Medicine*, **14**, 853–880.

Rutter, M., Dunn, J., Plomin, R. *et al.* (1997) Integrating nature and nurture: implications of person–environment correlations and interactions for developmental psychopathology. *Development and Psychopathology*, **9**, 335–364.

Sacker, A., Done, D.J., Crow, T.J. & Golding, J. (1995) Antecedents of schizophrenia and affective illness. *British Journal of Psychiatry*, **166**, 734–741.

Sakuta, T. & Saito, S. (1981) A socio-medical study of 71 cases of infanticide in Japan. *Keio Journal of Medicine*, **30**, 155–168.

Sameroff, A., Seifer, R. & Zax, M. (1982) Early development of children at risk for emotional disorder. *Monographs of the Society for Research in Child Development*, **47**, 1–82.

Sameroff, A., Seifer, R. & Bartko, W. (1997) Environmental perspectives on adaptation during childhood and adolescence. In: *Developmental Psychopathology: Perspectives on Adjustment, Risk and Disorder* (eds S. Luthar, J. Burack, D. Cicchetti & J. Weisz), pp. 507–526. Cambridge University Press, New York.

Schachter, J., Elmer, E., Ragins, N. & Wimberley, F. (1977) Assessment of mother–infant interaction: schizophrenic and non-schizophrenic mothers. *Merrill-Palmer Quarterly*, **23**, 193–205.

Seeley, S., Murray, L. & Cooper, P. (1996) The outcome for mothers and babies of health visitor intervention. *Health Visitor* **69**, 135–138.

Sharp, D. (1992) *Childbirth related emotional disorders: a prospective longitudinal study in primary care*. PhD thesis, University of London.

Sharp, D., Hay, D., Pawlby, S., Schmücker, G., Allen, H. & Kumar, R. (1995) The impact of postnatal depression on boys' intellectual development. *Journal of Child Psychology and Psychiatry*, **36**, 1315–1337.

Sichel, D., Cohen, L., Rosenbaum, J. & Driscoll, J. (1993) Postpartum onset of obsessive-compulsive disorder. *Psychosomatics*, **34**, 277–279.

Sinclair, D. & Murray, L. (1998) Effects of postnatal depression on children's adjustment to school: teacher's reports. *British Journal of Psychiatry*, **172**, 58–63.

Sobel, D. (1961) Children of schizophrenic patients: preliminary observations on early development. *American Journal of Psychiatry*, **118**, 512–517.

Steer, R.A., Scholl, T.O., Hediger, M.L. & Fischer, R.L. (1992) Self-reported depression and negative pregnancy outcomes. *Journal of Clinical Epidemiology*, **45**, 1093–1099.

Stein, A., Gath, D., Bucher, J., Bond, A., Day, A. & Cooper, P. (1991) The relationship between postnatal depression and mother–child interaction. *British Journal of Psychiatry*, **158**, 46–52.

Stein, A., Woolley, H., Cooper, S.D. & Fairburn, C.G. (1994) An observational study of mothers with eating disorders and their infants. *Journal of Child Psychology and Psychiatry*, **35**, 733–748.

Stein, A., Murray, L., Cooper, P. & Fairburn, C.G. (1996) Infant growth in the context of maternal eating disorders and maternal depression: a comparative study. *Psychological Medicine*, **26**, 569–574.

Steinhauer, P.D. (1983) Assessing for parenting capacity. *American Journal of Orthopsychiatry*, **53**, 468–481.

Stewart, D.E. (1989) Psychiatric admission of mentally ill mothers with their infants. *Canadian Journal of Psychiatry*, **34**, 34–37.

Stewart, D.E., Raskin, J., Garfinkel, P.E., MacDonald, O.L. & Robinson, G.E. (1987) Anorexia nervosa, bulimia, and pregnancy. *American Journal of Obstetrics and Gynecology*, **157**, 1194–1198.

Strauss, M.E., Lessen-Fireston, J.K., Starr, R.H. & Ostrea, E.M. (1975) Behavior of narcotics-addicted newborns. *Child Development*, **46**, 887–893.

Streissguth, A.P. & Kanter, J. (1997) *The Challenge of Fetal Alcohol Syndrome: Overcoming Secondary Disabilities*. University of Washington Press, Seattle.

Streissguth, A.P., Martin, D.C., Barr, H.M. & Sandman, B.M. (1984) Intrauterine alcohol and nicotine exposure: attention and reaction time in 4-year-old children. *Developmental Psychology*, **20**, 533–541.

Thiels, C. & Kumar, R. (1987) Severe puerperal mental illness and disturbances in maternal behaviour. *Journal of Psychosomatic Obstetrics and Gynaecology*, **7**, 27–38.

Tiernari, K.A., Wynne, L.C., Mosing, J. *et al.* (1994) The Finnish Adoptive Family Study of Schizophrenia: implications for family research. *British Journal of Psychiatry*, **164** (Suppl. 23), 20–26.

Videbech, P. & Gouliaev, G. (1995) First admission with postpartum psychosis: 7–24 years of follow-up. *Acta Psychiatrica Scandinavica*, **91**, 167–173.

Wadwa, P., Sandman, C. & Porto, M. (1993) The association between prenatal stress and infant birth weight and gestational age at birth: a prospective investigation. *American Journal of Obstetrics and Gynecology*, **169**, 858–865.

Wahlberg, K.-E., Wynne, L.C., Oja, H. *et al.* (1997) Gene–environment interaction in vulnerability to schizophrenia: findings from the Finnish Adoptive Family Study of Schizophrenia. *American Journal of Psychiatry*, **154**, 355–362.

Watson, J., Elliott, S., Rugg, A. & Brough, D. (1984) Psychiatric disorder in pregnancy and the first postpartum year. *British Journal of Psychiatry*, **144**, 453–462.

Waugh, E. & Bulik, C.M. (1999) Offspring of women with eating disorders. *International Journal of Eating Disorders*, **25**, 123–133.

Webster, D. (1990) Women and depression (alias co-dependency). *Family and Community Health*, **13**, 58–66.

Weinberg, K. & Tronick, E. (1994) Beyond the face: an empirical study of infant affective configurations of facial, vocal, gestural and regulatory behaviours. *Child Development*, **65**, 1503–1515.

Weinberg, M. & Tronick, E. (1998) The impact of maternal psychiatric illness on infant development. *Journal of Clinical Psychiatry*, **59**, 53–61.

Weintraub, S. (1987) Risk factors in schizophrenia: the Stony Brook high-risk project. *Schizophrenia Bulletin*, **13**, 439–449.

Weissman, M. & Paykel, E. (1974) *The Depressed Woman: a Study of Social Relationships*. University of Chicago Press, Chicago.

Weissman, M.M., Warner, U., Wickramavatne, P.J. & Kandel, D.B. (1999) Maternal smoking during pregnancy and psychopathology in offspring followed to adulthood. *Journal of the American Academy of Child and Adolescent Psychiatry*, **38**, 892–899.

West, J.R. (1986) *Alcohol and Brain Development*. Oxford University Press, London.

van Wezel-Meijler, G. & Wit, J.M. (1989) The offspring of mothers with anorexia nervosa: a high risk group for undernutrition and stunting? *European Journal of Paediatrics*, **149**, 130–135.

Whiffen, V. & Gotlib, I.H. (1989) Infants of postpartum depressed mothers: temperament and cognitive status. *Journal of Abnormal Psychology*, **98**, 274–279.

Wilkey, I., Pearn, J., Petrie, G. & Nixon, J. (1982) Neonaticide, infanticide and child homicide. *Medicine Science and the Law*, 22, 31–34.

Willett, J.B., Singer, J.D. & Martin, N.C. (1998) The design and analysis of longitudinal studies of development and psychopathology in context: statistical models and methodological recommendations. *Developmental Psychopathology*, 10, 395–426.

Williams, K.E. & Koran, L.M. (1997) Obsessive-compulsive disorder in pregnancy, the puerperium and the premenstruum. *Journal of Clinical Psychiatry*, 58, 330–334.

Wisner, K., Peindl, K. & Hanusa, B. (1993) Relationship of psychiatric illness to childbearing status: a hospital-based epidemiologic study. *Journal of Affective Disorders*, 28, 39–50.

Wisner, K., Peindl, K., Gigliotti, T. & Hanusa, B. (1999) Obsessions and compulsions in women with postpartum depression. *Journal of Clinical Psychiatry*, 56, 176–180.

Woodside, D.B. & Shekter-Wolfson, L.F. (1990) Parenting by parents with anorexia nervosa and bulima nervosa. *International Journal of Eating Disorders*, 9, 303–309.

World Health Organization (1992) *The ICD-10 Classification of Mental and Behavioural Disorders: Clinical Descriptions and Diagnostic Guidelines*. World Health Organization, Geneva.

Wynne, L.C., Cole, R.E. & Perkins, P. (1987) University of Rochester child and family study: risk research in progress. *Schizophrenia Bulletin*, 13, 463–476.

Yates, W.R., Cadaret, R.J., Troughton, E.P., Stewart, M. & Giunta, T.S. (1998) Effect of fetal alcohol exposure on adult symptoms of nicotine, alcohol, and drug dependence. *Alcoholism, Clinical and Experimental Research*, 22, 914–920.

Yoshida, K., Marks, M.N., Craggs, M., Smith, B. & Kumar, R. (1999) Sensorimotor and cognitive development of infants of mothers with schizophrenia. *British Journal of Psychiatry*, 175, 380–387.

Zaslow, M.J. (1988) Sex differences in children's response to parental divorce. I. Research methodology and postdivorce family forms. *American Journal of Orthopsychiatry*, 58, 355–378.

Zaslow, M.J. (1989) Sex differences in children's response to parental divorce. II. Samples, variables, ages, and sources. *American Journal of Orthopsychiatry*, 59, 118–141.

Zuckerman, B., Bauchner, N., Parker, S. & Cabral, H. (1990) Maternal depressive symptoms during pregnancy and newborn irritability. *Journal of Developmental and Behavioral Pediatrics*, 11, 190–194.

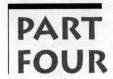

PART FOUR

Approaches to Treatment

Prevention

David R. Offord and Kathryn J. Bennett

Introduction

Identifying and treating children with psychiatric disorder on a one-to-one basis cannot be expected to produce a substantial reduction in the suffering from such disorders. There are several reasons. First, the number of children with clinically important psychiatric disorders far exceeds, sometimes by factors of 10–20, the ability of clinical services to assess and treat them (US Congress 1986; Boyle & Offord 1988). This is no doubt an overestimate because, even though community surveys indicate that the prevalence of one or more psychiatric disorders is about 20% (Costello 1989; Costello *et al.* 1996), many of these children would not necessarily require specialized mental health services. However, lowering the prevalence rate to include only those children with psychiatric disorders of sufficient severity and impairment to require clinical services (estimated at 10–12%) (Institute of Medicine 1994) would still produce numbers of children far exceeding clinical resources. Secondly, compliance is a troublesome issue. In families who begin treatment because their child has a mental disorder, 40–60% withdraw from treatment prematurely (Kazdin 1996). Further, many parents of children at high-risk for emotional or behavioural problems do not enroll in parent training programmes even when they are widely available (Cunningham *et al.* 1995, 2000; O'-Donnell *et al.* 1995). Thirdly, the time interval, between parents seeking help and actually receiving treatment, may be considerable. The child, and his or her family, can be expected to suffer during this period, and the disorder and associated impairment may worsen and become more entrenched. Fourthly, although considerable progress is being made in discovering effective treatments for child psychiatric disorders (Kazdin & Weisz 1998), for many disorders, e.g. early onset conduct disorders, little evidence of effective treatments is available (Offord & Bennett 1994; Kazdin 1997).

The marked limitations of clinical work alone in alleviating the suffering from child psychopathology has motivated researchers, policy makers and even clinicians to examine carefully the possibilities of developing and evaluating prevention efforts (Institute of Medicine 1994; Durlak & Wells 1997). The finding that, for some disorders (e.g. marked antisocial behaviour in adulthood), there are recognizable childhood antecedents before the onset of adult disorder suggest that high-risk groups can be identified for prevention, so that risk modifications can be carried out (Loeber & Farrington 1997).

Definitions

Historically, prevention initiatives were classified as *primary*, *secondary* or *tertiary* (Caplan 1964; Cowen 1983). *Primary prevention* programmes aim at reducing the incidence or number of new cases of a disorder. The goal of *secondary prevention* is to lower the prevalence of disorder by early identification and effective treatment, while *tertiary prevention* centres on rehabilitation aimed at reducing the severity of the impairment associated with an established disorder. A major problem with this classification is that the distinction between the presence or absence of disorder (and thus between primary and secondary prevention) is blurred because determining the threshold for disorder is difficult and arbitrary when the frequency and severity of symptoms occur on a continuum (Offord 1987).

More recent conceptualizations have moved away from the determination of whether the prevention is primary, secondary or tertiary towards a classification system centring on who is offered the intervention (Institute of Medicine 1994; Offord *et al.* 1998). In a *universal* programme, all residents in a geographical area as large as an entire country, or a smaller setting (e.g. community or school) are offered the intervention. The individuals do not actively seek help, and no one, within the population, is singled out for the intervention. The setting itself may be a psychopathological high-risk one but, if the intervention is not targeted at specific children and youth, then the intervention is classified as universal. In a *targeted* programme, again potential recipients do not seek help, but rather individuals within the population are singled out for the intervention. Targeted interventions can be divided into two subtypes: *selective preventive* and *indicated preventive* (Institute of Medicine 1994). In *selective preventive* interventions, the target group is individuals or a population subgroup where there is an increased risk for developing a psychiatric disorder. An example would be the offspring of parents who are on social assistance (Offord *et al.* 1987a). In *indicated preventive* interventions, the high-risk group is identified on the basis of having mild symptoms or even a biological marker of an established disorder. An example of such a high-risk group would be children who have mild antisocial symptoms and, although they do not qualify for conduct disorder, are at increased risk for it (Lipman *et al.* 1998).

The trade-offs between universal and targeted programmes have been described in detail elsewhere (Offord *et al.* 1998). The advantages of universal programmes include the absence of labelling or stigmatization, the inclusion of the middle class who demand that the programme be well run, and the sensitizing of the setting or 'tilling the soil' for targeted interventions. Some of the disadvantages of universal programmes are that they will have a small benefit to the individual, will be seen as being unnecessarily expensive, and may have their greatest effect on those at lowest risk, thus increasing inequality between the high- and low-risk subgroups within the population.

The targeted approach can address problems early on and is potentially efficient if the targeting can be done accurately. The disadvantages are several and include the possibility of labelling and stigmatization; the difficulties with ongoing screening including the cost and commitment; the challenge that the compliance with the screening manoeuvre will be least amongst those at highest risk; and the difficulty of targeting accurately. It is a formidable task to identify accurately individuals for targeted interventions (Bennett et al. 1998, 1999; Bennett 2000). Whereas clinicians are primarily interested in the positive predictive value of an early identification instrument (e.g. what proportion of children have a clinical disorder at follow-up), the policymaker is concerned not just with the positive predictive value but also with the sensitivity (e.g. what proportion of children who have the disorder at follow-up were identified by the screen earlier on) (Bennett et al. 1998; Lipman et al. 1998). There is always a trade-off between positive predictive value and sensitivity. An additional limitation of the targeted approach is that more cases of disorder will be attributable to the large number of persons at low risk, not the relatively small number at high risk. Data from the Ontario Child Health Study, a large community study of the prevalence and distribution of selected psychiatric disorders in children of 4–16 years of age (Boyle et al. 1987; Offord et al. 1987b), revealed that children living in families with an annual income under $Can10 000 were at high risk for developing psychiatric disorders, the prevalence rate being 36.3%. However, only 7.3% of children in Ontario lived in families in this income category. Thus, economically disadvantaged children account for only 14.5% of those with psychiatric disorder. By contrast, children who lived in families with a higher annual income ($Can25 000 or more) accounted for more than one-half (59%) of children with psychiatric disorder. The risk of psychiatric disorder was much lower in this relatively well-off population than in the poorest population, but the large number of children in the non-poor group means that their contribution to the population of children with disorder was far greater than that of the economically disadvantaged children. An implication of this finding is that one targeted programme, even if effective, cannot be expected to have marked beneficial effects at the population level.

Approaches

There are two quite different approaches to developing and evaluating preventive programmes. The first can be termed Preventive Science (PS) and this perspective was favoured in the In-

stitute of Medicine (IOM) report (Institute of Medicine 1994). A series of five steps were outlined in setting up a prevention programme:

1 identification of a problem or disorder;
2 the identification of risk and protective factors;
3 carrying out pilot efficacy studies;
4 launching and evaluating large-scale effectiveness trials; and
5 dissemination of the programme in a variety of community settings.

Usually, expert personnel from academic settings are in charge of such programmes, and participation by community members in planning and carrying out the studies is not emphasized.

The second contrasting model is termed the Collaborative Community Action Research (CCAR) model where community members are participants throughout the whole prevention initiative (Kelly 1988; Tolan et al. 1990). The resulting prevention programme will be community-specific, if not in terms of causes, almost certainly in terms of solutions, and the programme will not necessarily be suitable for dissemination to other communities. Because of the limitations of the design, the strength of the scientific evidence supporting the effectiveness of these programmes cannot be strong (Canadian Task Force on the Periodic Health Examination 1979). The advantages and disadvantages of these two approaches were reviewed recently (Weissberg & Greenberg 1998), with suggestions for melding the two approaches.

There are two somewhat different but overlapping groups of initiatives in the field of the prevention of child and adolescent psychiatric disorders (Institute of Medicine 1994). The first focuses on preventing specific psychiatric disorders, such as conduct disorder and depression. The second centres not so much on preventing illness but on promoting health, and enhancing competence across many domains including psychological, social, physical and spiritual.

This chapter first covers selected contributions of developmental psychopathology to prevention, and then moves on to review what is known about the prevention of three child and adolescent psychiatric disorders: conduct disorder, anxiety disorder and depressive disorder. Two risk situations (child abuse and children of divorce) are taken up next. Brief summaries are provided of prevention in low-income countries, the issue of environmental contaminants and barriers to prevention, and the chapter ends with concluding comments.

Selected contributions of developmental psychopathology to prevention

Developmental psychopathology, which emerged in the 1980s, is concerned with factors that influence the onset and course of emotional and behavioural disorders in children and adolescents (Stroufe & Rutter 1984). The hallmark of this field of inquiry is the integration of knowledge and research methodologies from several complementary disciplines, most notably developmental psychology, clinical psychology, psychiatry and epidemiology. Numerous significant contributions are now available that have important implications for prevention practice and research. In this section we summarize these contributions under four headings:

1 risk and protective factors;
2 multiplicity, specificity and timing;
3 theories of development and life-course studies; and
4 causal models.

Risk and protective factors

Developmental psychopathology has increased our understanding of the risk and protective factors associated with emotional and behavioural problems in children. A risk factor is a characteristic of the individual or his or her environment and must meet the following criteria:

1 the factor must be present prior to the onset of disorder; and
2 increase the likelihood of future disorder in individuals exposed to the factor, compared to those who are not.

A risk factor is considered causal when additional scientific criteria are satisfied. Ideally, evidence for causation is derived from experimental studies wherein exposure to the putative causal factor is determined in a bias-free manner using random assignment. However, when experimental evidence cannot be obtained for ethical reasons, or is not yet available, a 'case for causation' can be made using evidence of temporality; documentation of a risk increase when the putative causal factor is present; evidence of a dose–response relationship; specificity of cause and effect; consistency of findings between different studies conducted using different methods; and epidemiological and biological sense (Hill 1965; Kraemer *et al.* 1997).

Risk factors for psychiatric disorder can be either internal or external to the individual. A large number have been identified (Institute of Medicine 1994) and they can be grouped into five levels:

1 individual characteristics (e.g. gender, temperament);
2 parent and family factors (e.g. psychopathology, marital discord, socioeconomic status);
3 peer group characteristics (e.g. deviance);
4 school characteristics (e.g. leadership, academic); and
5 community or neighbourhood qualities (e.g. 'poor' neighbourhoods, social support).

It is essential to distinguish causal risk factors from correlates, markers and non-causal risk factors for disorder (Kraemer *et al.* 1997; Offord & Kraemer 2000). Prevention interventions that focus on causal risk factors will have a high likelihood of achieving their intended goal—a reduction in the incidence or severity of a future disorder. Interventions that focus on correlates, markers or non-causal risk factors have little or no impact on disorder. For example, correlates of disorder may be associated with disorder but may contribute little or nothing to its occurrence. In fact, the disorder may cause the correlate. Markers, which are fixed variables such as race or gender, are not modifiable and should not be the focus of intervention. Non-causal risk factors for disorder are modifiable variables that precede disor-

		Conduct disorder (CD)	
		Present	Absent
Early aggressive symptoms	Present	4 (a)	7 (b)
	Absent	6 (c)	83 (d)
		10	90	100

Odds ratio = (a)(d)/(c)(b) = (4)(83)/(6)(7) = 332/42 = 7.9
Population attributable risk

= $\dfrac{\text{Rate of CD in population} - \text{Rate of CD among those without symptoms}}{\text{Rate of CD in the population}}$

= $\dfrac{10/100 - (6/89)}{10/100}$

= $\dfrac{0.1 - 0.0674}{0.1}$

= 0.326 or 33%

Fig. 52.1 Measures of risk (data hypothetical for illustrative purposes only).

der but, if they are not causally related to disorder, changing them will have no impact on outcomes.

Protective factors precede the occurrence of disorder and can reduce its likelihood in the presence of a risk factor or situation. Again, it is important to distinguish causal from non-causal protective factors. Characteristics of the individual, the nature of their relationships with others and environmental characteristics have been proposed as possible causal protective factors (Rutter 1985; Rae-Grant *et al.* 1989; Weissberg & Greenberg 1998). However, two problems continue to plague this area: the first concerns what distinguishes a risk factor from a protective factor; the second concerns their mechanism of action or how a causal protective factor reduces or ameliorates risk. Despite this lack of clarity, substantial evidence exists that only a proportion of children exposed to conditions of adversity develop psychiatric symptoms (Werner & Smith 1982; Rutter 1985). Further work is needed to understand the processes that lead to variation in outcome in this group of children.

The strength of the relationship between a risk factor and future psychiatric disorder can be expressed using measures such as the odds ratio and population attributable risk. Simply put, the odds ratio tells us the increase in risk associated with a particular factor. It is defined formally as the likelihood of the outcome in those exposed to a risk factor compared to those not exposed (Streiner & Norman 1996). In contrast, population attributable risk helps us understand the contribution of a specific risk factor to the occurrence of a specific disorder in the population. The formal definition is the percentage of all cases of disorder in a population that are attributable to a specific risk factor (Kelsey *et al.* 1996). The higher the percentage, the more important the risk factor, if it is indeed causal.

Figure 52.1 shows some hypothetical study results relating the presence of antisocial behaviour symptoms in childhood to conduct disorder in adolescence. The odds ratio for disorder in adolescence given the presence of early antisocial symptoms is 7.9, so children with early symptoms are almost eight times

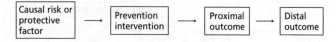

Fig. 52.2 The prevention model.

more likely than children without to develop conduct disorder in adolescence. The population attributable risk for these data is 33%. This means that if we could eliminate early aggressive behaviour symptoms in this population, the proportion of children with conduct disorder in adolescence would be reduced by approximately one-third, if indeed early aggressive behaviour symptoms are a causal risk factor for conduct disorder.

Figure 52.2 provides a simple model that links risk and protective factors to the design of programmes to prevent psychiatric disorder in children and adolescents. Four components—a causal risk or protective factor, a prevention intervention, a proximal outcome and a distal outcome—make up the model and are explained in the following. Under ideal circumstances, the prevention intervention consists of a set of actions that decrease the effects of a causal risk factor or increase the effects of a causal protective factor and, consequently, causes the proximal outcome to occur. The proximal outcome is a causal risk or protective factor that is known, or assumed, to cause the distal outcome to occur. The distal outcome might be the incidence of one or more psychiatric disorders. For example, social skills training is a competence-enhancing prevention intervention that is offered to young children to prevent conduct disorder. Figure 52.2 can be used to illustrate the theory behind this prevention strategy—how it is thought to exert its effect. The risk factor being addressed is poor social skills, the proximal outcome targeted by social skills training is an increase in prosocial skills, e.g. sharing and taking turns. The underlying logic is that by teaching children prosocial behaviours, and how to apply them in particular social situations, responses characterized by externalizing behaviour symptoms (a risk factor for conduct disorder, the distal outcome) will be minimized or eliminated.

Another example of a prevention intervention strategy is parent management training for parents with poor parenting skills (Webster-Stratton 1991). The objective is to reduce or eliminate this causal risk factor for conduct disorder in a group of parents who have it. The intervention teaches parents ways to improve how they monitor their children's behaviour and respond to aggression and non-compliance. Improved parenting skills are the proximal outcome, which in turn are thought to decrease the risk for conduct disorder.

Multiplicity, specificity and timing

Developmental psychopathology has increased our awareness of three important aetiological principles: multiplicity, specificity and timing. First, the onset of psychiatric disorder in children and adolescents is multifactorial in nature (Institute of Medicine 1994). The risk of disorder is thought to depend on the number of causal risk factors present and to accumulate over time (Yoshikawa 1994). Very little risk increase is evident when only one or two factors are operating. However, when three or more factors are present the risk of disorder is increased significantly. Secondly, there has been very little progress in demonstrating the specificity of causal risk factors—that certain risk factors are associated with one disorder and not another. In contrast, most of the evidence suggests the existence of common causal risk factors for multiple outcomes—a lack of specificity. For example, parental psychopathology has been shown to be a causal risk factor for conduct disorder, depression and anxiety disorders (Institute of Medicine 1994). Thirdly, the influence of a particular causal risk or protective factor depends upon timing or the developmental stage of the individual. For example, poor parenting is thought to exert much more of an influence in younger than in older children (Reid & Eddy 1997).

Theories of development and life-course studies

Theories of child development aim to explain how cognitive, emotional and behavioural characteristics emerge and evolve over time. Developmental psychology has focused primarily on understanding the processes of normal development, whereas clinical psychology, psychiatry and epidemiology have been concerned with the onset and clinical course of emotional and behavioural disorders. Developmental psychopathology has shown that longitudinal studies of representative populations, which identify individuals early in life and follow them up into adulthood, are needed to understand the aetiology and outcome of child and adolescent psychopathology. Several excellent reviews of the major longitudinal studies are available elsewhere (Institute of Medicine 1994; Loeber & Farrington 1997). Collectively, these studies have produced a number of findings that have had a major influence on the field.

Longitudinal studies have shown that there are both continuities and discontinuities in the onset and persistence of psychiatric symptoms and disorder (Rutter 1995). For example, for some individuals there is a high level of stability in clinically important antisocial behaviour symptoms across the life-course (Moffitt 1993; Loeber & Farrington 1997). However, it is also evident that children with high levels of symptoms early in life may not possess them in adolescence and/or adulthood (Nagin & Tremblay 1999).

Longitudinal studies have also introduced the concept of developmental trajectory and helped us to understand its relationship to possible causal risk and protective factors (Kellam & VanHorn 1997). The result has been a shift away from research models that focus on identifying increases in the rate of future discrete events to new approaches that describe and explain differences in the rate of growth of a particular emotional or behavioural trait over time. Figure 52.3 illustrates this concept using hypothetical data. The rate of decline of externalizing symptoms following entry to elementary school is compared between groups of children who have been classified according to their parents' level of parenting skills. As can be seen, the down-

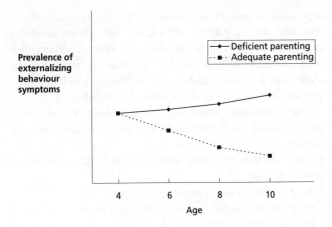

Fig. 52.3 Developmental trajectories (data hypothetical for illustrative purposes only).

ward slope is greater for children whose parents have adequate parenting skills; very little change is evident for children whose parents are deficient. This difference in the rate of change reflects the different developmental trajectories of the two groups of children.

Longitudinal studies have helped us understand that the links between an early risk factor and future psychiatric disorder may be indirect and depend upon other mediating variables. A recent study (Fergusson & Horwood 1998) showed that the link observed between early conduct disorder symptoms and two important adolescent psychosocial outcomes (educational attainment and unemployment) may be mediated by certain behaviours in adolescence (peer affiliations, substance use, truancy and problems with school authority).

Causal models

A major challenge facing child mental health researchers concerns how causal risk and protective factors work to exert their influence on child psychiatric disorders. Causal chains or pathways have been used as a simple way to explain the sequence of events associated with the onset and persistence of disorder. For example, one causal pathway into conduct disorder proposes that early learning problems lead to disruptive behaviour symptoms which result in problems in school, association with a deviant peer group, school failure and antisocial behaviour (Offord & Fleming 1996). However, several authors have called for a deeper analysis of the role that specific risk factors have in producing disorder (Baron & Kenny 1986; Baronowski et al. 1997; Holmbeck 1997). They have distinguished mediating factors from moderating factors and provided useful examples to illustrate why we need to increase the clarity and consistency with which these concepts are operationalized in the design and analysis phase of studies. A mediating factor is a variable that links an independent variable to an outcome: the independent variable causes the mediator, which then causes the outcome

(Shadish & Sweeny 1991). For example, marital conflict may exert its effect on psychiatric symptoms through an effect on the quality of parenting. Moderating factors, on the other hand, interact with or moderate the influence of an independent variable on outcome so the effect of the independent variable on the outcome depends upon the level of the moderating factor present. Family structure (e.g. intact vs. divorced) might moderate the relationship between marital conflict and psychiatric symptoms, with the relationship being present for divorced families but not for intact families.

Two final points concern the dynamic nature of variables with respect to their role as a mediator or moderator; and the limits to intervention impact that are imposed by mediating variables. The evidence suggests that a specific variable may act as a mediator in one instance and a moderator in another. For example, in one context poor parenting skills may mediate the relationship between an independent variable and the occurrence of psychiatric symptoms. However, in another context, poor parenting skills may interact with the independent variable. In this instance, the influence of the independent variable depends upon the level of parenting skills present.

The strength of the association between a mediating variable and an outcome will limit the impact of an intervention. This is because most interventions exert their influence through a mediating variable (Baronowski et al. 1997). Social skills and parent management training programmes exert their influence on conduct disorder by modifying proximal risk factors that are thought to be causal (poor social skills or poor parenting skills). However, although these risk factors are correlated with future conduct disorder, the relationship is not one-to-one. Consequently, the magnitude of the link between each one and future conduct disorder places an upper limit on the impact of intervention on conduct disorder.

Prevention of psychiatric disorders

In this section, a selective summary is presented of what is known about effective strategies to prevent conduct disorder, anxiety disorder and depressive disorder. Most of what is known concerns conduct disorder and antisocial behaviour and has been derived from studies of programmes designed to measure the competence of the child, the parent, or both. Relatively few programmes that target the prevention of specific psychiatric disorders have been tested to date. For each programme reviewed the following issues are discussed: the target population; whether the programme was universal or targeted; whether the intervention was designed to prevent a specific psychiatric disorder or to exert a more generalized competence-enhancing effect (cognitive, emotional and/or behavioural–social); the domains addressed; the findings to date, including the strength of the research design. Almost all of the prevention strategies reviewed here have been evaluated in randomized controlled trials. This design, when executed rigorously, provides the greatest number of safeguards against biased estimates of programme effectiveness (Jadad 1998). For simplicity, for conduct disorder, age is used to organize the programmes into three groups (the under 5s; ages 5–11; and older than age 11).

Conduct disorder

Programmes for children under 5

Nurse home visitation has been shown to prevent antisocial behaviour in a programme designed for poor unmarried pregnant women. Olds et al. (1998a,b) followed up children at age 15 whose mothers received home visits by a nurse (during pregnancy and up to the age of 2), as part of the Elmira randomized trial of nurse home visitation. When these adolescents were compared to children who had not received the full programme of home visitation, the authors found (based on youth self-report) lower rates of arrests (56% reduction), convictions and violations of probation (81% reduction), running away (60% reduction), lifetime sexual partners (63% reduction) and alcohol consumption (56% reduction). Parents also reported lower rates of behaviour problems associated with alcohol and other drugs (56% reduction) for these adolescents. This same preventive intervention initiative is reviewed in more detail in the section on child abuse.

Findings from the Perry Preschool Project show that compensatory preschool education exerted an effect on the incidence of antisocial behaviour (Schweinhart & Weikert 1988, 1989). The programme was designed in the 1960s for poor black 3- and 4-year-old children and aimed to improve academic and social outcomes. The intervention was 2 years in duration and included a daily preschool programme (90-min classes, 5 days per week) and a weekly home visit provided by highly trained teachers. The preschool component was designed to promote academic, social and physical development. The home visits were designed to help parents reinforce the preschool curriculum. Programme effectiveness was evaluated in a randomized controlled trial and the children were followed up into adulthood; 58 children were assigned to the experimental group and 65 to the control group. Early results showed that initial IQ gains in the experimental group were lost. However, long-term follow-up at ages 19 and 27 showed important differences on measures of antisocial behaviour including fewer lifetime arrests (31% in the experimental group vs. 51% in the control group) and a substantially reduced rate of being arrested five or more times (5% in the experimental group vs. 35% in the control group). Cost–benefit analyses have demonstrated that the benefits of the programme exceed the costs (Barnett 1998).

The Carolina Abecedarian Project also evaluated the effects of compensatory preschool education in an extremely high-risk group of children born to poor African-American mothers (Campbell & Ramey 1994). The intervention began in the first year of life and was very intensive. The birth-to-age-5 programme included a range of services offered through a daycare centre: daycare curriculum to enhance cognitive, language, perceptuomotor and social development; medical care; social

services; some home visits; parent groups and toy lending. Once the child entered primary school, the intervention consisted of a home–school resource teacher who assisted parents with supplementary individualized educational activities for the child to do at home. This was delivered through 15 home visits per year, beginning in kindergarten and ending in grade 2.

The Abecedarian approach was evaluated in a randomized trial, in which the outcomes of four groups of children were compared:
Group 1: birth to age 5 programme plus kindergarten to grade 2 programme ($n = 25$);
Group 2: birth to age 5 programme only ($n = 22$);
Group 3: kindergarten to grade 2 programme only ($n = 21$);
Group 4: no programme ($n = 22$).

The results showed that children who received the full programme did better than children in the other three groups on measures of IQ and school achievement. The results also showed that intervention before age 5 in this high-risk group was more effective than intervention in the early school years. IQ and school achievement in children who received the birth-to-age-5 programme only were superior to those of children who received the kindergarten to grade 2 programme only, when they were followed up at age 8 (conclusion of the programme) and age 12. Unfortunately, antisocial outcomes were not assessed. However, given the nature of the intervention and the positive effects found on academic outcomes, this intervention would appear to hold promise as a prevention strategy for antisocial behaviour.

In summary, there is evidence that prevention strategies offered before age 5 to extremely high-risk groups of poor predominantly black children are effective in preventing antisocial behaviour. The focus of these programmes is on risk and protective factors related to early family supports, parental caregiving skills and child cognitive outcomes. At present, the mechanisms by which these programmes exert their effects are not entirely clear and there is a need for a more coherent conceptual and theoretical basis for these types of programmes (Yoshikawa 1994; Ramey & Ramey 1998). In general, it is thought that early intervention increases school readiness through a set of developmental priming mechanisms (Ramey & Ramey 1998). The effect is to increase the ability of the child to meet academic expectations and to adapt behaviourally to the school setting. This in turn sets in motion a series of mediating mechanisms that protect against a wide range of negative health and social outcomes.

Finally, there is a need to evaluate these approaches in other populations of children. The results to date have been collected on small samples of extremely deprived African-American children, particularly in the case of compensatory education strategies. Consequently, the magnitude of benefit that can be expected in populations at less extreme levels of risk and material deprivation is not known. It seems likely that the benefit will be less than that observed to date. Further evidence of costs and effects is therefore needed to guide policy decisions about the provision of these types of programmes to other groups of children.

Programmes for children aged 5–11

Most of the programmes evaluated for children in this age group have been offered through schools to groups of children at elevated risk for conduct disorder and antisocial behaviour. Four types of strategies are reviewed in this section:

1 single-factor approaches;
2 multicomponent approaches;
3 competence-enhancement approaches; and
4 school development approaches.

Prevention strategies that focus on a single risk or protective factor in a single context have been evaluated in randomized trials and shown to have small to moderate effects on antisocial symptoms. An evaluation was carried out of a violence prevention programme for elementary school children in a randomized trial involving 7 and 8-year-old students in 12 elementary schools (Grossman *et al*. 1997). The intervention, called Second Step, consists of 30 social skills lessons that address anger management, impulse control and empathy and are provided in the classroom by the teacher. Observational measures showed a moderate reduction in aggressive behaviour and an increase in prosocial behaviour 2 weeks after the conclusion of the intervention; some effects persisted 6 months later. No effects were found on teacher and parent reports of behaviour.

The Good Behaviour Game (GBG) is another single-component strategy and consists of a classroom management strategy (Kellam *et al*. 1994) wherein the teacher divides the classroom into teams, and monitors the rate of disruptive events (physical disruption, verbal disruption, out-of-seat without permission, non-compliance). Any team whose number of disruptive events does not exceed four during the game period wins a reward. Over time, the frequency and duration of the game period is increased; at the same time, the teacher begins to initiate the game without announcements and delays the provision of rewards to winners. The GBG approach has been evaluated in a randomized trial. Schools were randomized to provide the GBG or not for 6 and 7-year-old students. Results at the end of the school year for 6 and 11-year-old students suggest that children from classrooms who received the GBG had lower levels of aggressive behaviour and that the effect is more pronounced for males with high levels of aggressive behaviour at the outset.

Peer mediation is another single-component strategy. In this approach students are trained in conflict mediation skills and then assigned to act as peer-mediators on the school playground. Their job is to identify conflict in the early stages, to intervene within 10 s and to carry out mediation according to a standard protocol. This approach has been shown to be effective in resolving playground conflicts; physically aggressive playground behaviour was reduced by 51–65% and the effects were maintained at a 1-year follow-up (Cunningham *et al*. 1998).

Multicomponent strategies that address multiple risk and protective factors operating at several levels have also been designed and evaluated to determine their impact on behavioural maladjustment and antisocial behaviour. The Montreal Longitudinal Experimental Study evaluated a targeted intervention for high-risk kindergarten males (Tremblay *et al*. 1995). The intervention was designed to address two risk factors for conduct disorder: one at the child level (social skills training) and one at the family level (parenting skills). All boys in 53 Montreal schools who scored above the 70th percentile on the Social Behaviour Questionnaire and whose parents were French-speaking and had less than 14 years of formal education were randomized to one of three treatment groups.

1 A 2-year intervention programme consisting of school-based social skills training and home-based parent training sessions. In the parent training component, parents were taught how to monitor their child's behaviour, give positive reinforcement, to discipline effectively without using harsh or punitive strategies and to manage family crises. The maximum number of sessions was 46 over the 2-year period; the mean number attended was 17.4. Social skills training was taught in a lunchtime session at the boy's school by members of the study professional team. Small groups included two study boys and six prosocial peers; 9 sessions were held in year 1 and 10 sessions in year 2.
2 An attention-control group.
3 A control group.

Overall, the intervention seems to have had little or no lasting effect beyond the elementary school period. Initial results in elementary school showed that intervention boys did better on measures of school adjustment. However, by age 15, 6 years after the conclusion of the programme, intervention group members were not different from that of the control group. Gains, measured in terms of whether the boy was in an age-appropriate regular class, disappeared after age 13. Teacher-rated disruptive behaviour did not differ between the two groups over the follow-up period to age 15. The intervention group reported statistically significantly fewer delinquent acts, but there was no difference between intervention and control boys when juvenile court records were compared over the follow-up period from age 10 to 15.

The Tri-Ministry Helping Children Adjust Project was designed as a universal programme to address three risk factors for emotional–behavioural maladjustment in childhood: poor reading skills, poor social skills and poor parenting skills (Boyle *et al*. 1999). The initial intervention plan called for a reading partners programme, a social skills programme and a parent management programme, alone or in combination, to be provided to children at entry to primary school. However, consistent with other investigators, the uptake of the parent management programme was very poor and this programme element had to be dropped after the first year of the evaluation. Consequently, three programme groups were compared in a randomized trial: reading partners alone, social skills training alone and a combination of both reading partners and social skills training. Sixty schools were selected from 11 school boards in a defined geographical area and were randomly allocated to receive one of the three programmes or the control condition. Programme duration was a minimum of two school terms. The results, after 1.5–3.5 years of follow-up, showed that the effects of the intervention were modest at best. Playground observations revealed statistically significant increases in prosocial behaviour and there was some evidence that externalizing symptoms were reduced (Hundert *et al.* 1999).

Fast Track is another multicomponent approach. It was designed specifically to address risk and protective factors for antisocial conduct problems (Conduct Problems Prevention Reseach Group 1999a,b). The intervention model focuses on multiple levels (child, family, school, peer group, community) and factors (academic skills, social skills, parenting skills, family support) and includes a universal and targeted component. The programme begins in grade 1 and is planned to continue through middle school. The universal programme is offered at the classroom level to all children in the school and consists of the Promoting Alternative Thinking Strategies (PATH) curriculum that teaches skills in self-control, emotional awareness and social problem-solving. The targeted component consists of the following.

1 A weekly 2-hour enrichment session for high-risk children (selected on the basis on high levels of externalizing behaviour symptoms) and their families. The sessions include parent groups, child social skills training and academic tutoring and are held on Saturdays or in the evening.

2 Home visits held approximately every other week in grade 1. The purpose is to provide individualized help and to support generalization of the skills learned in the enrichment session.

Fast Track is currently being evaluated in a large randomized trial involving 54 schools in four geographically distinct sites in the USA. The unit of allocation is the school. Results based on outcomes at the end of grade 1 showed the following.

1 In the high-risk sample, positive effects were found on children's social, emotional and academic skills, peer interactions, social status, conduct problems and special education use. Parents also reported positive effects on parenting outcomes (less physical discipline needed; greater parenting satisfaction; more appropriate and consistent parenting; more warmth/positive involvement and more involvement with the school).

2 In the full sample, the universal social skills programme combined with the targeted intervention for the high-risk children resulted in statistically significant effects on peer ratings of aggression, hyperactive-disruptive behaviour and observer ratings of classroom atmosphere.

It is too early to tell whether the Fast Track approach will translate into clinically and policy significant reductions in conduct problem rates as the children move into adolescence and adulthood. Moreover, the approach is extremely intensive and cost-effectiveness analyses are needed to determine whether the cost is justified in relation to the benefits achieved. Finally, it is possible that the apparent early benefits will be lost when adolescent outcomes become available, as was the case in the Montreal Longitudinal Experimental Study. As already noted above, the results of the Montreal study showed little or no lasting effect beyond the elementary school period as, at age 15, no between-group differences were found on measures of teacher-reported disruptive behaviour and court reports of delinquent behaviour.

Competence-enhancing intervention strategies have also shown effects on antisocial behaviour. The rationale is to promote social competence rather than reduce psychopathology. The Seattle Social Development Project consists of three components that aim to improve child bonding to their family and school and, consequently, social competence:

1 teacher training in classroom instruction and management;

2 child social skills development in grade 1 and drug resistance skill development in grade 6; and

3 parent training.

The programme is offered from grades 1–6. The results of a nonrandomized controlled trial showed that, at age 18, adolescents who had participated in the programme self-reported fewer delinquent acts (19% reduction), less heavy drinking (40% reduction), fewer sex partners (19% reduction) and pregnancies (35% reduction) compared to control students (Hawkins *et al.* 1999).

The Social Competence Promotion Program for Young Adolescents is another approach to competence enhancement (Weissberg & Greenberg 1998). The programme consists of 45 classroom sessions designed to promote a set of social competencies: self-control; stress-management; responsible decision-making; social problem-solving; and communication skills. Self-reported antisocial and delinquent behaviour was shown to be reduced among middle school students who received this programme for 2 years, compared to others who received no training or less than 1 year of training. Both of these strategies would benefit from further evaluation in a randomized trial design to minimize the influence of bias on estimates of effect size, in particular overestimates of intervention effectiveness (Jadad 1998).

Finally, school development strategies have been applied in elementary schools and may have a role to play in reducing the rate of antisocial behaviours. The School Development Program developed by Comer *et al.* is made up of three components.

1 A school planning and management team composed of school administrators, teachers, support staff and parents who identify school problems and develop and implement appropriate solutions.

2 A mental health team responsible for prevention initiatives and addressing the needs of individual teachers and students.

3 A parent programme that involves parents in all aspects of school life, including problem identification and the design and implementation of solutions.

This approach differs from the other methods already described in that it consists of a mechanism (or process) to support change. The specific content of the programme is not defined, but left up to the school management and mental health teams. The overall goal is to modify and enhance school policies and programmes so that school climate is improved, positive behaviours are promoted and negative health and social outcomes are prevented or minimized. The Comer approach has been evaluated in a non-randomized controlled study. Children who attended schools using the approach had superior educational outcomes to children attending non-programme schools

(Comer 1985). Again, further evaluation in a randomized design is needed.

In summary, over the past decade a number of promising conduct disorder prevention approaches have been developed and applied in the elementary school setting. Clearly, this is an important venue for prevention programmes. Schools have a central role in behavioural and social development and it is well recognized that they function *de facto* as the primary mental health care service for children and adolescents (Mortimore *et al.* 1988; Sylva 1994; Hoagwood & Erwin 1997).

The single-component approaches have the advantage of being simple and rather straightforward to implement. However, when evaluated against our understanding of the aetiology of conduct disorder this model is clearly weak and unlikely to have a major impact on the incidence and severity of disorder. Multicomponent approaches, which address multiple risk and protective factors at the level of the child, family, peer group, school and community, are consistent with current causal models. However, this programme approach is complex and expensive, and the magnitude of benefit in relation to cost is uncertain at this time (Hundert *et al.* 1999).

Competence-enhancement approaches have the advantage of targeting multiple risk and protective factors. However, the impact of this approach depends upon the strength of the link between the mediating factors targeted (social skills, self-control, coping and stress management) and the occurrence of disorder. School development approaches make theoretical sense because they address the environmental supports needed to support and sustain adaptive behaviours (Bronfenbrenner & Morris 1998). However, this is a relatively new area with respect to rigorous evaluation of promising strategies.

Programmes for children over 11

Prevention programmes in older children are less prominent for conduct disorder because the emphasis is primarily on treatment in this age group. Two programmes are summarized here, one that shows promise and one that has been shown to be ineffective.

The PATHE programme (Positive Action Through Holistic Education) is a school development model that has been applied in this age group and shown to influence antisocial outcomes. The programme consists of organizational change strategies and the provision of services to high-risk students as follows.

1 A school team responsible for reviewing and revising school policies and for supporting shared decision-making between school and community agencies and parents.

2 Development of school and classroom goals (academic and behaviour) followed by staff training in how to implement them through classroom management strategies and student participation.

3 School-wide academic innovations.

4 School-wide climate innovations.

5 Mental health and academic services for high-risk students.

This approach has been evaluated in a non-equivalent comparison group design. Student reports suggested that the programme results in fewer delinquent acts, lower rates of drug use and school suspensions (Gottfredson 1986). Further work on this promising school reform strategy is warranted.

Finally, the Cambridge Somerville Study deserves comment. In this programme, which was initiated in the 1930s, boys around the age of 11 were randomized to be assigned or not to a social worker (McCord 1992). The role of the social worker was to build a close personal relationship with the boy and to provide assistance to both the boy and his family. Follow-up in adulthood (when participants were 40–50 years of age) showed that the treatment group boys had worse outcomes (convicted of a crime; death before age 35; received a diagnosis of alcoholic, schizophrenic or manic-depressive) than the controls, and that the treatment had in fact been harmful. The reasons why the programme failed are not entirely clear.

Anxiety disorders

The literature on the prevention of anxiety disorders is sparse (Spence 1994). Although there has been a discussion of various universal interventions that could be used in the prevention of childhood fears (e.g. classroom-based intervention for prevention of fears of the dark) (Robinson *et al.* 1991), no well-controlled experiments have been conducted. There is literature on the prevention of fears in specific situations, such as attending the dentist and subsequent avoidance of dental treatment (Melamed *et al.* 1975a,b; Milgrom *et al.* 1992); preventing fear and anxiety relating to medical procedures (Jay *et al.* 1987); test anxiety (Tryon 1980; Van der Ploeg-Stapert & Van der Ploeg 1986); and facilitating the transition to a new school (Felner & Adan 1988).

A programme addressing this latter issue, entitled the School Transition Environment Project (STEP; Felner & Adan 1988), focused on children making the transition from elementary to high school, and included three components: organizing the physical plan of the school into units with homerooms, the availability of a 'homeroom' staff member who can provide counselling for academic and behavioural problems, and the provision of a co-ordinated liaison between teaching and school counselling staff. The overall aims of the programme were to increase meaningful relationships between pupils and staff, and to create smaller environments within the overall larger school environment. Evaluations of the STEP programme, using a randomized controlled design, showed that programme participants compared to control children had greater improvements in academic performance and self-esteem, better school attendance and lower drop-out rates. A particular strength of the programme is that its positive effects have been replicated in various school settings with children from different backgrounds. Although this intervention is not designed specifically to prevent fears or anxiety disorders in the students, it illustrates an approach aimed at reducing the severity of a stressor experience in order to prevent the development of emotional and be-havioural difficulties.

A randomized controlled trial aimed at preventing the onset and development of anxiety problems in children, the Queens-land Early Intervention and Prevention of Anxiety Project (Dadds & Spence 1997), screened 1786 children representing all children between 7 and 14 years of age in grades 3–7 in eight preselected primary schools in the metropolitan area of Brisbane, Australia. These children participated in a compli-cated and extensive four-stage screening procedure using both teacher nominations and children's self-report. Children who met criteria for DSM-IV anxiety disorder, but were not rated as the most severe in terms of impairment, were included in the study as were those who did not meet criteria but had fea-tures of anxiety disorder, or were particularly shy and sensitive based on parent reports. Children exhibiting primarily external-izing problems were excluded. Of the 1786 children screened, 121 (6.8%) entered the trial. Children selected were allocated to the intervention and control groups on the basis of school. Schools matched on size, sociodemographics and socioeco-nomics were randomly assigned to the intervention or control groups.

The intervention was based on *The Coping Koala: Prevention Manual* (unpublished data) and consisted of 1–2-h sessions with the children over 10 weeks with group sizes ranging from 5 to 12 children. Children were taught strategies for coping with anxiety using a congnitive-behavioural approach. In addition, parent sessions were conducted at weeks 3, 6, 7 and 9 and fo-cused on child management skills, and how to employ these skills to manage their child's anxiety. Attendance at the interven-tion sessions for the children themselves was approximately 80%, while parents attended approximately 58% of the ses-sions. By the 6-month follow-up, only five children had with-drawn from the trial: two from the intervention group and three from the control group. At that follow-up, children in the inter-vention group had lower rates of anxiety disorder than those in the initial group and, of those who had features but not full dis-order, at pretreatment (*n*=33) 56% progressed to a diagnosable disorder in the control group at the 6-month follow-up com-pared with 16% in the intervention group. The authors con-cluded that the intervention was successful both in reducing rates of disorder in children with mild to moderate anxiety dis-orders, and preventing the onset of anxiety disorders in children with early features of the disorders. A 2-year follow-up (Dadds *et al.* 1999) revealed that at 1 year the rates of anxiety disorder were similar in the intervention group (37%) and the control group (42%), but at 2 years the rates had diverged, as they did at the 2-month follow-up, with rates of anxiety disorders in the experimental and control groups of 24 and 37%, respectively. Severity of pretreatment diagnoses, female gender and parental anxiety predicted poor initial response to intervention, but pre-treatment severity was the only predictor of chronicity at 2 years. This preventive intervention is promising in that it showed that a school-based targeted intervention for children can produce sustained reductions in anxiety problems. How-ever, the labour-intensive four-stage screen is a barrier to wide adoption of the programme.

Depressive disorder

There are no examples of universal programmes that have been shown to be effective in preventing the onset of depressive symp-toms or depressive disorders (Harrington 1997). Suggestions of which risk factors could be addressed in universal programmes include the provision of good-quality parenting, prevention of bullying, and increasing social competence and positive atti-tudes. There are several targeted programmes, both of the indicated and selective types, that have focused on depressive disorder aimed at preventing future depressive symptoms.

In one indicated targeted intervention (Jaycox *et al.* 1994), school-aged children, 10–13 years of age, were identified on the basis of self-reports of both elevated levels of depressive symptomatology and parental conflict. The 143 children were assigned to one of three 12-week treatment conditions (cogni-tive treatment only, social problem-solving skills only, or both) or to one of two control groups (waiting list and no participa-tion). The cognitive component emphasized challenging nega-tive beliefs about the self, present circumstances and the future, and the social problem-solving skills component taught children goal-setting, perspective-taking, information-gathering, devel-oping action alternatives, decision-making and self-instruction. Because at post-test no important differences were observed between the three treatment conditions, they were collapsed into one group, as were the two control groups. The results re-vealed statistically and clinically important differences in the re-duction and prevention of depressive symptoms in the treatment compared to the control groups, both at the end of treatment and at the 6-month and 2-year follow-ups (Gillham *et al.* 1995). Because the differences between the treatment and control groups widened over time, it suggests that the intervention may have immunized children against future depressive episodes. Weaknesses of the study include the very poor re-sponse rate in both the intervention and control schools. Of the approximately 900 children in the initial pool in the interven-tion schools, 174 (19%) returned consent forms, and in the con-trol schools the numbers were 88 (13%) of 700. Further, there was no evaluation of the psychometric properties of the screen-ing procedure.

Three additional indicated targeted interventions were car-ried out, using randomized controlled trials, by the same group of investigators. In the first two (Gillham *et al.* 1995), educa-tional interventions ranging from three lectures on the symp-toms, causes and treatment of depression in the first study to five sessions designed to increase the daily rate of their pleasant ac-tivities in the second study did not produce positive results. In the third study (Clarke *et al.* 1995), the quality and power of the intervention were increased. Of 1652 adolescents screened in two stages, 150 were identified as experiencing depressive symp-toms but did not meet the criteria for depression, and they agreed to participate in the study. The intervention consisted of a 15-session cognitive-behavioural intervention (three sessions per week for 5 weeks) and data were collected at post-treatment and at follow-up at 6 and 12 months. The preventive intervention emphasized training adolescents in cognitive-restructuring skills to allow them to reduce mild levels of negative cognitions before they reach depressive symptoms of clinical proportions. Overall, the total incidence of either major depression or dysthymia at follow-up was 14.5% for the treated group and 25.7% for the control group—a statistically significant difference.

Beardslee et al. (1993, 1996, 1997a,b) have been involved for several years in selective type targeted prevention programmes, where children aged 8–15 are identified, on the basis of having a parent with a recent episode of affective disorder, as being at increased risk for depressive disorder themselves. Children were randomly assigned to one of two psychoeducational interventions (clinician-facilitated or lecture group discussion), both of which were designed to prevent childhood depression and other related problems through decreasing the effects of risk factors and promoting resiliency. The two interventions were similar in content but differed in intensity, with the clinician-facilitated intervention having a greater children's involvement and a greater linking of the educational material to the families' individual life experiences. The intervention had a strong cognitive orientation and a primary goal was to increase family members' understanding of the illness experience. It included individual sessions with the parents, an individual session with each child, and one or two family meetings. The lecture group discussion consisted of two 1-hour lectures, while the mean number of clinician-facilitated intervention sessions was 7.7. The most recent article (Beardslee et al. 1997a) reports on data gathered from the first 37 families who completed the initial assessment, and the immediate post-intervention assessment. Nineteen families had been randomly assigned to the clinician-facilitated intervention and 18 to the lecture intervention. Not unexpectedly, positive results were more marked in the clinician-facilitated group. They reported a significantly larger number of overall changes, with more parents and children reporting that they gained a better understanding of the parents' illness, and higher levels of change regarding communications about the illness. It should be pointed out that it will not be known for some period of time whether or not these interventions actually reduce the level of depressive disorder and other morbidities in these high-risk children.

Risk situations

There are many examples where children are at increased risk for psychiatric disorders and where attempts have been made to either reduce the risk itself or modify the effects of the risk. Some of the markers or indicators of increased risk are intrinsic variables (within the child), and others are extrinsic (outside the child) (Offord et al. 1998). Examples of the former include low birth weight, developmental delay, brain damage, epilepsy, difficult temperament, mental retardation and chronic medical illness. Examples of the latter are parents with psychiatric disorder, violent and dysfunctional families, physical and sexual abuse, divorce, marked economic disadvantage and crowded inner-city neighbourhoods. Because of space limitations, this chapter covers only three risk situations: child abuse (see Emery & Laumann Billings, Chapter 20; Glaser, Chapter 21), parental divorce (see Friedman & Chase-Lansdale, Chapter 15) and environmental contaminants.

Child abuse

The prevention of child abuse is especially appealing for two reasons. First, there is limited success in the treatment of children and their families once abuse has occurred (Cohn 1979a,b). Secondly, the prevalence of child maltreatment in the general population is surprisingly high. The Mental Health Supplement to the Ontario Health Survey was a general population survey involving a random sample of almost 10 000 residents, aged 15 years and older (MacMillan et al. 1997). Based on a self-administered questionnaire, 31.2% of males and 21.0% of females reported a history of child physical abuse, while sexual abuse in childhood was reported by 12.8% of females and 4.3% of males.

Prevention studies can be classified into two main categories: those that focus on the prevention of physical abuse and/or neglect; and those that centre on the prevention of sexual abuse and/or abduction (MacMillan et al. 1994a). In the first category, there are both universal and targeted programmes (Leventhal 1996). Universal programmes include the provision of general services, such as satisfactory housing and financial support, quality childcare, and the availability of child development and parenting resource centres for children aged 0–5 years and their families. It is known that the availability of these resources for selected groups of impoverished preschool-age children results in improved health and well-being (McCain & Mustard 1999). Although it would be expected that providing the universal programmes outlined above, especially to vulnerable populations, would decrease rates of physical abuse and neglect, there are no clinical trials that have examined the efficacy of these types of services in decreasing maltreatment (Leventhal 1996).

The targeted interventions have focused on home visiting and there is evidence that extended home visitation can prevent physical abuse and neglect among disadvantaged families (MacMillan et al. 1994b; MacMillan 2000; MacMillan & Canadian Task Force on Preventive Health Care 2000). The Prenatal and Early Childhood Nurse Home Visitation Program is a model that has been tested in two randomized controlled trials in Elmira, New York and Memphis, Tennessee (Olds et al. 1993, 1997, 1998a,b, 1999; Kitzman et al. 1997; Karoly et al. 1998). The intervention consists of nurse home visitors working intensively with families to achieve three broad goals: improvement of pregnancy outcomes, improvement of the child's health and development, and improvement of the parental life-course. Positive results have been reported in each of these areas; for example, in the intervention compared to the control groups, there were significant reductions in cigarette smoking during pregnancy among women who smoked cigarettes at registration (25% reduction); rates of child maltreatment from birth through the child's 15th year (79% reduction); and unmarried mothers' behavioural problems caused by alcohol and drug abuse over the 15 years following programme enrollment (44% reduction).

There are essential ingredients of home visiting programmes if they are to be successful (Leventhal 1996). Services should begin early, preferably during the prenatal period or right after birth, and extend through the first couple of years of a child's life. The visits must be frequent enough so that a trusting relationship is formed between the home visitor and the family. The home visitor should develop a therapeutic relationship with the parents, keep a watchful eye on the home, be able to model effective parenting, not lose sight of the child's needs, and be able to provide concrete services to the family.

Further work needs to be done to address the limitations of existing home visitation programmes (Leventhal 1996; Guterman 1997). They include developing effective strategies to deal with fathers and boyfriends as well as mothers, formulating and evaluating intervention approaches in cases involving parental substance and alcohol abuse, developing culture-specific interventions, and focusing on improving the parent's feelings of powerlessness. Two further points should be emphasized. It cannot be expected that leaner, cheaper, watered-down interventions will have the same beneficial effects as those effective interventions reported in the literature. A major challenge in the prevention of child abuse and neglect is to discover strategies to move from small demonstration studies to large-scale dissemination projects with proven effectiveness.

The literature on the prevention of child sexual abuse is not nearly as extensive as that on physical abuse and neglect. The central finding is that there is evidence that educational programmes, usually delivered in the school setting, can improve safety skills and knowledge about sexual abuse, but no study has produced results that education actually reduces the occurrence of sexual abuse (MacMillan et al. 1994a; MacMillan 2000; MacMillan & Canadian Task Force on Preventive Health Care 2000). The effect sizes attained in these programmes vary as a function of both programme and child characteristics (Rispens et al. 1997). Programmes of longer duration that focus on skill training, and permit a long enough time for children to integrate self-protection skills into their cognitive repertoire, are more likely to be effective. Younger children (less than 5.5 years) and economically disadvantaged children derive a greater benefit from these programmes, although these differential effects fade over time as do the overall programme effects. The implication here is that it makes sense to repeat the programmes at regular intervals.

Children of divorce

Divorce involves large numbers of children. The proportion of

children growing up in homes with two biological married parents has dropped from almost 90% in the 1960s to about 50% of children in the UK and 40% in the USA (Wadsworth 1986). Escalating rates of divorce, out-of-wedlock child-bearing and cohabitation are the major contributors to these changes. In the USA in 1996, divorces and annulments involved over 1 million children (National Center for Health Statistics 1997). In most instances the divorce is followed by remarriage or cohabitation, and thus many children are exposed to a sequence of change in their family members, relationships and roles (Cherlin & Furstenberg 1994; Bumpass & Raley 1995). The effects of divorce on the psychosocial adjustment of children have recently been reviewed (Hetherington & Stanley-Hagan 1999). Many children experience adjustment difficulties in the months immediately following parental divorce, especially in the externalizing behaviour domain, and to a lesser extent in the internalizing area. For many children, the problems lessen over time, but a meta-analysis of 95 studies confirmed that, on average, children of divorced parents are less well adjusted socially, emotionally and academically than children of non-divorced parents (Amato & Keith 1991). Even in those cases where children have shown no upset, or only short-term problems immediately following their parents' divorce, difficulties in adjustment can arise as a result of the divorce in adolescence and even in adult life. However, it should be emphasized that children's reactions to divorce vary widely, and the vast majority of children do not show severe and enduring behaviour problems (Hetherington et al. 1992; Hetherington 1993).

Interventions for divorced parents and their children have been reviewed (Grych & Fincham 1992; Emery et al. 1999; Hetherington & Stanley-Hagan 1999) and the interventions are of three types: child-focused, parent-focused and those centring on the legal system. Adequate research in this area is scarce. Interventions for children are usually school-based, involve groups of children of divorced parents, consist of both educational and therapeutic activities, and are of short duration.

The most extensively evaluated school-based programme is the Children of Divorce Intervention Project (Pedro-Carroll & Cowen 1985; Pedro-Carroll et al. 1986; Alpert-Gillis et al. 1989; Pedro-Carroll & Alpert-Gillis 1997). This intervention attempts to foster feelings of support, clarify divorce-related misconceptions (e.g. that the children are responsible for the divorce), and develop effective coping skills to deal with the stressors associated with divorce. In the initial evaluation (Pedro-Carroll & Cowen 1985), 75 grade 4–6 children from four suburban schools were randomly assigned to either an immediate 12-week intervention or a delayed intervention initial group. Positive findings were reported by teachers, parents, group leaders and the children themselves in anxiety behaviours and in school-related problems, but not in perceived self-competence. In subsequent studies of urban children with diverse ages, ethnicities and socioeconomic backgrounds (Pedro-Carroll & Cowen 1985; Pedro-Carroll et al. 1986) and of kindergarten and first-grade teachers (Pedro-Carroll & Alpert-Gillis 1997), gains were reported for the intervention group compared to the comparison group in the emotional–behavioural area and in school-related competencies. One child-focused intervention programme that has been widely disseminated (Kalter *et al.* 1984, 1988) showed few positive results on ratings of children's adjustment before and after participation in the group, and, in addition, there was a lack of a comparison group.

Parent-focused interventions employ group therapy to enable parents to deal more effectively with the stresses of divorce, increase their coping skills and adjustment, and only secondarily are aimed at improving parenting and family relationships (Hetherington & Stanley-Hagan 1999). Although the average effect size of parent-focused programmes on the adjustment of parents is 0.80 SD, the interventions are associated with minor or no improvement in child adjustment (Emery *et al.* 1999). One of the more promising programmes grew out of the Oregon Divorce Study (Forgatch & DeGarmo 1999). Results of this randomized controlled trial, where the intervention programme consisted of 14 parent group sessions, showed that the mothers in the intervention group reported significant improvements in maternal discipline; in addition, significant improvements in teachers' ratings of children's behaviour were reported.

The third type of intervention focuses on legal issues: mediation and coparenting (Emery *et al.* 1999). Although there may be a number of advantages of mediation for divorcing couples compared to an adversarial settlement (Kelly 1989), there is no evidence that it improves the adjustment of the children. Further, there are no consistent findings of an association between type of custody and children's adjustment (Grych & Fincham 1992).

The intervention literature on the children of divorced parents has several important flaws. There are very few well-conducted randomized controlled trials, the informants providing the outcome measures were not blind to the intervention status of the children, and the follow-up periods were brief. Further, because only a proportion of the children of divorce will exhibit adjustment problems, many of the children receiving the intervention did not need it, and it may even have been harmful because of labelling and stigmatization. In addition, for any intervention to show significant differences between the experimental and control groups, it will have to have a marked beneficial effect on the subgroup of children exhibiting adjustment problems. It should be kept in mind that the most these interventions have been shown to do in the emotional and behavioural area is to reduce symptoms slightly, and certainly not decrease emotional and behavioural disorders *per se*.

Environmental contaminants

Because there is evidence that environmental pollutants can adversely affect children's health (Environment Leaders of the Eight 1998), lessening or eliminating them is an important universal prevention initiative. Children are especially vulnerable to these environmental agents because of their early reliance on breast milk which can become contaminated (Sonawane 1995),

and because of the short stature and early crawling activities of young children who spend approximately 90% of their time indoors (Chance & Harmsen 1998). Further, because of their disadvantaged housing arrangements and neighbourhoods, children of poverty experience a disproportionate impact from environmental health threats (Mott 1995; Chaudry 1998).

There are virtually no data on the effects of long-term low-level exposure to pesticides (which are designed to be neurotoxic), despite the fact that many are persistent in the environment and are routinely detected in human tissue. However, methylmercury has resulted in episodes of frank neurotoxic poisoning in humans (Rice 1998). Further, there is epidemiological and experimental evidence that exposure to phencyclidine hydrochlorides (PCPs) in the developmental years produces impairment in cognition functioning and attention (Ware *et al.* 1986; Stern *et al.* 1994). In addition, air pollution has been associated with increased rates of low birth weight in China (Wang *et al.* 1997) and reduced lung function in many countries (Brunekreef *et al.* 1997; Raizenne *et al.* 1998).

The most studied neurotoxicant is lead. It has been clearly established that exposure of fetuses and children to amounts of lead routinely observed as a consequence of environmental contamination produces deficits in IQ (Schwartz 1994; Needleman 1998). It has been reported that a 2.6 decrease in IQ score is associated with an increase in blood level from 10 to 20 μg/dL in a meta-analysis of eight studies (Schwartz 1994). It has been noted that lead has other detrimental effects on children in addition to IQ, including attentional problems, language function and, perhaps, social adjustment (Rice 1998). It is clear that the elimination of environmental contaminants would improve the health of children. In particular, the elimination of lead poisoning would reduce cognitive and attentional deficits in children (Needleman 1998). The beneficial effects of such a manoeuvre for individual children would be small, with the greatest impact occurring among the economically and socially disadvantaged populations of children. The removal of lead from gasoline in 1990 in the USA has been heralded as one of the public health triumphs of the twentieth century. Between 1976 and 1994, the mean blood lead concentration in US children was reduced by almost 80%, in direct proportion to the amount of tetraethyl lead produced (Needleman 1998).

Low-income countries

Although there have been substantial improvements in children's survival over the past several decades and in physical health and education, children's mental health has probably worsened (Desjarlais *et al.* 1995). Millions of children grow up in unbearable circumstances as refugees, displaced persons, street children, casualties of war or victims of child labour. The prevention of mental disorders in populations of these children requires major societal changes in these countries where the well-being of children, not just their survival, becomes a high priority. It cannot be assumed that effective interventions in wealthy countries will necessarily be effective in poor ones (Dans *et al.* 1998; Rahman *et al.* 2000).

However, there are universal interventions that show promise of enriching the lives of children and decreasing mental health problems even in these severely economically disadvantaged circumstances. The first is to improve maternal education (Caldwell 1986; Hobcraft 1993). It has been reported that the status of women in most, but not all, low-income countries, as reflected by their literacy rate, is a more important predictor of the well-being of children than are economic indicators such as the gross national product (GNP; Caldwell 1986). Possible mechanisms by which more maternal education may translate into increased child well-being have been suggested (Hobcraft 1993). Women with more education marry later, have their first child later, have fewer children, are much less likely to die in childbirth, and are more responsive to modern hygienic practices.

The factors that appear to confer advantages to the offspring of better educated mothers lead to a second universal intervention: better family planning. The more numerous and closely spaced the pregnancies of a mother, the greater risks for not only maternal and infant mortality but for poor developmental and mental health outcomes (Desjarlais *et al.* 1995). A third universal intervention that is capturing the interest in the developing world is to enrich the lives of the first 5 years of children (Young 1997). The provision of adequate nutrition, and early child development and parenting programmes will have both short-term and long-term beneficial effects on the lives of these children (McCain & Mustard 1999). The last universal prevention programme to be mentioned is to increase the percentage of children enrolled in schools. In low-income countries this has increased from under 30% in 1960 to over 70% in the 1980s (Carnegie Commission 1992) but many of them drop out in the elementary school grades. Obviously, the topic of the prevention of emotional and behavioural problems in children in poor countries is an important and complex one, and only a brief summary of selected issues is presented here.

Barriers

There are obstacles to carrying out prevention studies but there are two that are particularly relevant to child psychiatrists. The first is that in many instances, particularly in North America, child psychiatrists are funded on a fee-for-service basis. Thus, there is no remuneration for activities related to planning and carrying out prevention projects that do not involve direct clinical contact. A second obstacle is that child psychiatrists are usually not trained to do prevention work (Group for the Advancement of Psychiatry 1999); their expertise lies in individual clinical work. At a minimum, one could argue that child psychiatrists should know the prevention literature thoroughly so that they can advise groups planning and launching prevention projects (Rae-Grant 1991; Harrington 1997; Group for the

Advancement of Psychiatry 1999; Offord *et al.* 1999). Further, child psychiatrists should be at home in making use of the epidemiological perspective in their clinical work, e.g. if a child psychiatrist is having to deal with a spate of similar referrals from one school, it should suggest to the child psychiatrist that intervening at the school level needs to be considered.

A second potential barrier to prevention initiatives is an uncivic community, one in which the community, or an entire country, is so disorganized that prevention initiatives would have little chance of success (Offord *et al.* 1999), e.g. launching a social skills training programme in a school has little chance of success if the school is disorganized and demoralized.

A third issue is that effective primary prevention programmes are not guaranteed widespread implementation. In the case of childhood lead poisoning, a strong national effort to eliminate the disease developed in the early 1990s in the USA (Needleman 1998). As mentioned earlier, the effort was successful in eliminating lead from gasoline, but not lead from paint. By 1998, 7 years after publication of the prevention plan, it had been abandoned because of the roles and attitudes of several powerful institutions.

Conclusions

Our knowledge about what works to prevent child psychiatric disorders has grown in important ways over the past two decades. However, a number of challenges remain to be dealt with. The first concerns efficacy vs. effectiveness (Tugwell *et al.* 1985). Most of the evaluations to date are efficacy evaluations: the programmes are designed and evaluated in the context of ideal conditions. These ideal conditions include highly skilled programme personnel, high levels of motivation on the part of the individuals and organizations involved, and high levels of resources. Whether or not the effects observed can be obtained when the same programmes are applied in a field setting, where conditions are less than ideal, is uncertain and probably unlikely in the absence of special supports. The expansion of an efficacious small demonstration to a large-scale effective programme disseminated to many settings has not been successfully accomplished.

A second issue concerns implementation and the fidelity with which an intervention is applied (Moncher & Prinz 1991). The impact of programmes to prevent emotional and behavioural disorder has been shown to be directly related to the fidelity of implementation (Botvin *et al.* 1995). Manualization of programme content and procedures, and regular inservicing of programme staff have been recommended as strategies to maximize implementation rigour and fidelity (Durlak 1995).

Thirdly, the impact of prevention programmes may be dependent on individual characteristics, such as gender, socioeconomic status, culture and/or the level of the symptomatology already present. As a result, effect sizes, which reflect the average benefit for the average person, may mask significant variation in benefit that exists between individuals. Stoolmiller *et al.* (2000) have shown that the effect of a universal conduct disorder prevention programme was dependent on the level of aggressive symptoms present at the outset—the most aggressive children benefited most from the programme.

Fourthly, there are particular problems in demonstrating the effectiveness of universal programmes and they have been discussed in detail (Hundert *et al.* 1999). One of the difficulties is that by the time there is the will to evaluate universal programmes, they are already widespread in some form or another and, in addition, participation in a study may stimulate diffusion of programmes to the comparison group. In the Tri-Ministry Study, interventions similar to the ones being implemented in the experimental schools were present in the comparison schools. Further, during the course of the study, the percentage of teachers in comparison schools stating that social skills was taught as a special subject increased from 35.7% in the year prior to the study to over 50.0% in the fourth year of implementation. The social skills programme in the experimental schools was pitted against existing social skills programmes in the comparison schools, thus setting the bar high to show effectiveness of the programme in the experimental schools.

Fifthly, effective programmes tend not to be maintained, let alone disseminated (Offord 1996). Their cost, acceptability and requirement of a charismatic leader for their success are some of the barriers preventing sustainability of efficacious and effective programmes.

Finally, there is a disturbing trend that prevention programmes without proven effectiveness end up being widely disseminated (Kalter *et al.* 1984, 1988). Certainly, as suggested previously, one of the important functions of child psychiatrists in the prevention field is to inform policymakers and colleagues about the strength of scientific evidence supporting the effectiveness and ineffectiveness of various preventive initiatives.

Activity in the preventive field has grown enormously over the past two decades. In the second edition of this textbook, published in 1985 (Rutter & Hersov 1985), there was no chapter devoted to prevention nor were the terms 'prevention' or 'primary prevention' mentioned in the index. There are some promising leads now in the prevention field, but much work remains to be done. More precise knowledge is needed from small studies about what works in which populations, under what conditions, and what the mechanisms are by which the intervention has its effects, and how large these effects are. It is important to work out that if an intervention were shown to be efficacious in a demonstration project, what are the chances of it being successfully widely disseminated.

A final point. It makes no sense for the prevention and treatment enterprises to be seen as being antagonistic, competitive and separate from each other. There is much room for collaboration between prevention and treatment personnel in initiatives, such as discovering strategies to prevent comorbidity, the so-called primary prevention of secondary disorders (Kessler & Price 1993). The burden of suffering from child and adolescent psychiatric disorders is so high that both effective treatment and prevention programmes are needed to reduce this burden substantially.

References

Alpert-Gillis, L.J., Pedro-Carroll, J.L. & Cowen, E.L. (1989) The children of divorce intervention program: development, implementation, and evaluation of a program for young urban children. *Journal of Consulting and Clinical Psychology*, 57, 583–589.

Amato, P.R. & Keith, B. (1991) Parental divorce and the well-being of children: a meta-analysis. *Psychological Bulletin*, 110, 24–46.

Barnett, W.S. (1998) Longterm cognitive and academic effects of early childhood education on childhood poverty. *Preventive Medicine*, 27, 204–207.

Baron, R.M. & Kenny, D.A. (1986) The moderator–mediator variable distinction in social psychological research: conceptual, strategic and statistical considerations. *Journal of Personality and Social Psychology*, 51, 1173–1182.

Baronowski, T., Lin, L.S., Wetter, D.W., Resnicow, K. & Hearn, M.D. (1997) Theory as mediating variables: why aren't community interventions working as desired? *Annals of Epidemiology*, S7, 89–95.

Beardslee, W.R., Salt, P., Porterfield, K. *et al.* (1993) Comparison of preventive interventions for families with parental affective disorder. *Journal of the American Academy of Child and Adolescent Psychiatry*, 32, 254–263.

Beardslee, W.R., Wright, E., Rothberg, P.C., Salt, P. & Versage, E. (1996) Response of families to two preventive intervention strategies: long-term differences in behavior and attitude change. *Journal of the American Academy of Child and Adolescent Psychiatry*, 35, 774–782.

Beardslee, W.R., Versage, E., Wright, E. *et al.* (1997a) Examination of preventive interventions for families with depression: evidence of change. *Development and Psychopathology*, 9, 109–130.

Beardslee, W.R., Wright, E., Salt, P. *et al.* (1997b) Examination of children's responses to two preventive intervention strategies over time. *Journal of the American Academy of Child and Adolescent Psychiatry*, 36, 196–204.

Bennett, K.J. (2000) Accurate screening tools for externalizing behaviour problems in normal populations. *Journal of the American Academy of Child and Adolescent Psychiatry*, 39, 1341–1343.

Bennett, K.J., Lipman, E.L., Racine, Y. & Offord, D.R. (1998) Do measures of externalising behaviour in normal populations predict later outcome: implications for targeted interventions to prevent conduct disorder [Annotation]. *Journal of Child Psychology and Psychiatry*, 39, 1059–1070.

Bennett, K.J., Lipman, E.L., Brown, S., Racine, Y., Boyle, M.H. & Offord, D.R. (1999) Predicting conduct problems: can high-risk children be identified in kindergarten and grade 1? *Journal of Consulting and Clinical Psychology*, 67, 470–780.

Botvin, G.J., Baker, E., Dusenbury, L., Botvin, E.M. & Diaz, T. (1995) Long-term follow-up results of a randomized drug abuse prevention trial in a white middle-class population. *Journal of the American Medical Association*, 272, 1106–1112.

Boyle, M. & Offord, D.R. (1988) Prevalence of childhood disorder, perceived need for help, family dysfunction and resource allocation for child welfare and children's mental health services in Ontario. *Canadian Journal of Behavioural Science*, 20, 374–388.

Boyle, M.H., Offord, D.R., Hofmann, H.G. *et al.* (1987) Ontario Child Health Study. I. Methodology. *Archives of General Psychiatry*, 44, 826–831.

Boyle, M.H., Cunningham, C.E., Heale, J. & Hundert, J. (1999) Helping children adjust: a Tri-Ministry study. I. Evaluation methodology. *Journal of Child Psychology and Psychiatry*, **40**, 1051–1060.

Bronfenbrenner, U. & Morris, P.A. (1998) The ecology of developmental processes. In: *Handbook of Child Psychology*, Vol. 1. *Theoretical Models of Human Development* (eds W. Damon, I.E. Sigel & K.A. Renninger), 5th edn, pp. 993–1028. John Wiley & Sons, New York.

Brunekreef, B., Janssen, N.A.H., de Hartog, J., Harssema, H., Knape, M. & van Vliet, P. (1997) Air pollution from truck traffic and lung function in children living near motorways. *Epidemiology*, **8**, 298–303.

Bumpass, L.L. & Raley, R.K. (1995) Redefining single-parent families: cohabitation and changing family reality. *Demography*, **32**, 97–109.

Caldwell, J.C. (1986) Routes to low mortality in poor countries. *Population and Development Review*, **12**, 171–220.

Campbell, F.A. & Ramey, C.T. (1994) Effects of early intervention on intellectual and academic achievement: a follow-up study of children from low-income families. *Child Development*, **65**, 684–698.

Canadian Task Force on the Periodic Health Examination (1979) The periodic health examination. *Canadian Medical Association Journal*, **121**, 3–45.

Caplan, G. (1964) *Principles of Preventive Psychiatry*. Basic Books, New York.

Carnegie Commission (1992) *Partnerships for Global Development: The Clearing Horizon*. Carnegie Commission on Science, Technology and Government, New York.

Chance, G. & Harmsen, E. (1998) Children are different: environmental contaminants and children's health. *Canadian Journal of Public Health*, **89**, S9–S13.

Chaudry, N. (1998) Child health, poverty and the environment: the Canadian context. *Canadian Journal of Public Health*, **89**, S26–S30.

Cherlin, A.J. & Furstenberg, F.F. (1994) Stepfamilies in the United States: a reconsideration. In: *Annual Review of Sociology* (eds J. Blake & J. Hagan), pp. 359–381. Annual Reviews, Palo Alto, CA.

Clarke, G.N., Hawkins, W., Murphy, M., Sheeber, L.B., Lewinsohn, P.M. & Leeley, J.R. (1995) School-based primary prevention of depressive symptomatology in adolescents: findings from two studies. *Journal of the American Academy of Child and Adolescent Psychiatry*, **34**, 312–321.

Cohn, A.H. (1979a) An evaluation of three demonstration child abuse and neglect treatment programs. *Journal of the American Academy of Child Psychiatry*, **18**, 283–291.

Cohn, A.H. (1979b) Essential elements of successful child abuse and neglect treatment. *Child Abuse and Neglect*, **3**, 491–496.

Comer, J.P. (1985) The Yale–New Haven primary prevention project: a follow-up study. *Journal of the American Academy of Child and Adolescent Psychiatry*, **24**, 154–160.

Conduct Problems Prevention Reseach Group (1999a) Initial impact of the Fast Track prevention trial for conduct problems. I. The high-risk sample. *Journal of Consulting and Clinical Psychology*, **67**, 631–647.

Conduct Problems Prevention Reseach Group (1999b) Initial impact of the Fast Track prevention trial for conduct problems. II. Classroom effects. *Journal of Consulting and Clinical Psychology*, **67**, 648–657.

Costello, E.J. (1989) Developments in child psychiatric epidemiology. *Journal of the American Academy of Child and Adolescent Psychiatry*, **28**, 836–841.

Costello, E.J., Angold, A., Burns, B.J. *et al.* (1996) The Great Smoky Mountain Study of Youth: goals, design, methods, and the prevalence of DSM-III-R disorders. *Archives of General Psychiatry*, **53**, 1129–1136.

Cowen, E.L. (1983) Primary prevention in mental health: past, present, and future. In: *Preventive Psychology: Theory, Research, and Practice* (eds R.D. Felner, A. Jason, J.N. Moritsugu & S.S. Farber), pp. 11–25. Pergamon Press, New York.

Cunningham, C.E., Bremner, R. & Boyle, M. (1995) Large group community-based parenting programs for families of preschoolers at risk for disruptive behaviour disorders: utilization, cost effectiveness and outcome. *Journal of Child Psychology and Psychiatry*, **36**, 1141–1159.

Cunningham, C.E., Cunningham, L.J., Martorelli, V., Tran, A., Young, J. & Zacharias, R. (1998) The effects of primary division, student-mediated conflict resolution programmes on playground aggression. *Journal of Child Psychology and Psychiatry*, **39**, 653–662.

Cunningham, C.E., Boyle, M., Offord, D.R. *et al.* (2000) Correlates of school-based parenting course utilization. *Journal of Consulting and Clinical Psychology*, **68**, 928–933.

Dadds, M.R. & Spence, S.H. (1997) Prevention and early intervention for anxiety disorders: a controlled trial. *Journal of Consulting and Clinical Psychology*, **65**, 627–635.

Dadds, M.R., Holland, D.E., Laurens, K.R., Mullins, M. & Barrett, P.M. (1999) Early intervention and prevention of anxiety disorders in children: results at 2-year follow-up. *Journal of Consulting and Clinical Psychology*, **67**, 145–150.

Dans, A.L., Dans, L.F., Guyatt, G.H. & Richardson, S. (1998) Users' guides to the medical literature. XIV. How to decide on the applicability of clinical trial results to your patient. *Journal of the American Medical Association*, **279**, 545–549.

Desjarlais, R., Eisenberg, L., Good, B. & Kleinman, A. (1995) *World Mental Health: Problems and Priorities in Low-income Countries*. Oxford University Press, New York.

Durlak, J.A. (1995) *School-based Prevention Programmes for Children and Adolescents*. Sage, London.

Durlak, J.A. & Wells, A.M. (1997) Primary prevention mental health programs for children and adolescents: a meta-analytic review. *American Journal of Community Psychology*, **25**, 115–151.

Emery, R.E., Kitzmann, K.M. & Waldron, M. (1999) Psychological interventions for separated and divorced families. In: *Coping with Divorce, Single Parenting and Remarriage: a Risk and Resiliency Perspective* (ed. E.M. Hetherington), pp. 323–344. Lawrence Erlbaum Associates, Mahwah, NJ.

Environment Leaders of the Eight (1998) 1997 Declaration of the environment leaders of the eight on children's environmental health. *Canadian Journal of Public Health*, **89** (Suppl. 1), S5–S8.

Felner, R.D. & Adan, D. (1988) The School Transition Environment Project: an ecological intervention and evaluation. In: *Fourteen Ounces of Prevention: a Case Book for Practitioners* (eds R.H. Price, E.L. Cowen, R.P. Lorion & J. Ramos-McKay), pp. 111–122. American Psychological Association, Washington D.C.

Fergusson, D.M. & Horwood. L.J. (1998) Early conduct problems and later life opportunities. *Journal of Child Psychology and Psychiatry*, **39**, 1097–1108.

Forgatch, M.S. & DeGarmo, D.S. (1999) Parenting through change: an effective prevention program for single mothers. *Journal of Consulting and Clinical Psychology*, **67**, 711–724.

Gillham, J.E., Reivich, K.J., Jaycox, L.H. & Seligman, M.E.P. (1995) Prevention of depressive symptoms in school children: a two-year follow-up. *Psychological Science*, **6**, 343–351.

Gottfredson, D. (1986) An empirical test of school-based environmental and individual interventions to reduce the risk of delinquent behaviour. *Criminology*, **24**, 705–731.

Grossman, D.C., Neckerman, H.J., Koepsell, T.D. *et al.* (1997) Effectiveness of a violence prevention curriculum among children in elementary school. *Journal of the American Medical Association*, **277**, 1605–1611.

Group for the Advancement of Psychiatry, Committee on Preventive Psychiatry (1999) Violent behavior in children and youth: preventive intervention from a psychiatric perspective. *Journal of the American Academy of Child and Adolescent Psychiatry*, 38, 235–241.

Grych, J.H. & Fincham, F.D. (1992) Interventions for children of divorce: toward greater integration of research and action. *Psychological Bulletin*, 111, 434–454.

Guterman, N.B. (1997) Early prevention of physical child abuse and neglect: existing evidence and future directions. *Child Maltreatment*, 2, 12–34.

Harrington, R. (1997) The role of the child and adolescent mental health service in preventing later depressive disorder: problems and prospects. *Child Psychology and Psychiatry Review*, 2, 46–57.

Hawkins, J.D., Catalano, R.F., Kosterman, R., Abbott, R. & Hill, K.G. (1999) Preventing adolescent health-risk behaviours by strengthening protection during childhood. *Archives of Pediatric and Adolescent Medicine*, 153, 226–234.

Hetherington, E.M. (1993) An overview of the Virginia longitudinal study of divorce and remarriage with a focus on early adolescence. *Journal of Family Psychology*, 7, 1–18.

Hetherington, E.M. & Stanley-Hagan, M. (1999) The adjustment of children with divorced parents: a risk and resiliency perspective. *Journal of Child Psychology and Psychiatry*, 40, 129–140.

Hetherington, E.M., Clingempeel, W.G., Anderson, E.R. *et al.* (1992) *Coping with marital transitions: a family systems perspective.* Serial no. 227, edn. 57, 2–3. Monographs of the Society for Research in Child Development, Chicago: University of Chicago Press.

Hill, A.B. (1965) The environment and disease: association or causation? *Proceedings of the Royal Society of Medicine*, 58, 295–300.

Hoagwood, K. & Erwin, H.D. (1997) Effectiveness of school-based mental health services for children: a 10-year research review. *Journal of Child and Family Studies*, 6, 435–451.

Hobcraft, J. (1993) Women's education, child welfare and child survival: a review of the evidence. *Health Transition Review*, 3, 159–175.

Holmbeck, G.N. (1997) Toward terminological, conceptual and statistical clarity in the study of mediators and moderators. *Journal of Consulting and Clinical Psychology*, 65, 599–610.

Hundert, J., Boyle, M.H., Cunningham, C.E. *et al.* (1999) Helping children adjust: a Tri-Ministry Study. II. Program effects. *Journal of Child Psychology and Psychiatry*, 40, 1061–1073.

Institute of Medicine (1994) *Reducing Risks for Mental Disorders: Frontiers for Preventive Intervention Research.* National Academy Press, Washington D.C.

Jadad, A. (1998) *Randomized Trials.* BMJ Books, London.

Jay, S.M., Elliot, C.H., Katz, E. & Siegel, S.E. (1987) Cognitive-behavioral and pharmacologic interventions for children's distress during painful medical procedures. *Journal of Consulting and Clinical Psychology*, 55, 860–865.

Jaycox, L.H., Reivich, K.J., Gillham, J. & Seligman, M.E.P. (1994) Prevention of depressive symptoms in school children. *Behavior Research and Therapy*, 32, 801–816.

Kalter, N., Pickar, J. & Lesowitz, M. (1984) School-based developmental facilitation groups for children of divorce: a preventive intervention. *American Journal of Orthopsychiatry*, 54, 613–623.

Kalter, N., Alpern, D., Falk, J. *et al.* (1988) *Children of divorce: facilitation of development through school-based groups.* Michigan Department of Mental Health, Lansing, MI.

Karoly, L.A., Greenwood, P.W., Everingham, S.S. *et al.* (1998) *Investing in our children: what we know and don't know about the costs and benefits of early childhood interventions.* Rand Corporation, Santa Monica, CA.

Kazdin, A.E. (1996) Dropping out of child psychotherapy: issues for research and implications for practice. *Clinical Child Psychology and Psychiatry*, 1, 133–156.

Kazdin, A.E. (1997) Practitioner review: psychosocial treatments for conduct disorder in children. *Journal of Child Psychology and Psychiatry*, 38, 161–178.

Kazdin, A.E. & Weisz, J.R. (1998) Identifying and developing empirically supported child and adolescent treatments. *Journal of Consulting and Clinical Psychology*, 66, 19–36.

Kellam, S.G. & VanHorn, Y.V. (1997) Life course development, community epidemiology and preventive trials: a scientific structure for prevention research. *American Journal of Community Psychology*, 25, 177–188.

Kellam, S.G., Rebok, G.W., Ialongo, N. & Mayer, L.S. (1994) The course and malleability of aggressive behavior from early first grade into middle school: results of a developmental epidemiologically based preventive trial. *Journal of Child Psychology and Psychiatry*, 35, 259–281.

Kelly, J.G. (1988) *A Guide to Conducting Prevention Research in the Community: First Steps.* Haworth Press, Binghamton, NY.

Kelly, J.B. (1989) Mediated and adversarial divorce: respondents' perceptions of their processes and outcomes. *Mediation Quarterly*, 24, 71–88.

Kelsey, J.L., Whittemore, A.S., Evans, A.S. & Thompson, W.D. (1996) *Methods in Observational Epidemiology.* Oxford University Press, New York.

Kessler, R.C. & Price, R.H. (1993) Primary prevention of secondary disorders: a proposal and agenda. *American Journal of Community Psychology*, 21, 607–633.

Kitzman, H., Olds, D.S., Henderson, C.R. Jr, *et al.* (1997) Effect of prenatal and infancy home visitation by nurses on pregnancy outcomes, childhood injuries, and repeated childbearing: a randomized controlled trial. *Journal of the American Medical Association*, 278, 644–652.

Kraemer, H.C., Kazdin, A.E., Offord, D.R., Kessler, R.C., Jensen, P.S. & Kupfer, D.J. (1997) Coming to terms with the terms of risk. *Archives of General Psychiatry*, 54, 337–343.

Leventhal, J.M. (1996) Twenty years later: we do know how to prevent child abuse and neglect. *Child Abuse and Neglect*, 20, 647–653.

Lipman, E.L., Bennett, K.J., Racine, Y. & Mazumdar, R. (1998) What does early antisocial behaviour predict: a follow-up of 4- and 5-year-olds from the Ontario Child Health Study. *Canadian Journal of Psychiatry*, 43, 605–613.

Loeber, R. & Farrington, D.P. (1997) Strategies and yields of longitudinal studies on antisocial behavior. In: *Handbook of Antisocial Behavior* (eds D.M. Stoff, J. Breiling & J.D. Maser), pp. 125–139. Wiley, New York.

MacMillan, H.L. (2000) Child maltreatment: what we know in the year 2000. *Canadian Journal of Psychiatry*, 45, 702–709.

MacMillan, H.L. & Canadian Task Force on Preventive Health Care (2000) Preventive health care, 2000 update: prevention of child maltreatment. *Canadian Medical Association Journal*, 163, 1451–1458.

MacMillan, H.L., MacMillan, J.H., Offord, D.R., Griffith, L. & MacMillan, A.B. (1994a) Primary prevention of child sexual abuse: a critical review. II. *Journal of Child Psychology and Psychiatry*, 35, 857–876.

MacMillan, H.L., MacMillan, J.H., Offord, D.R., Griffith, L. & MacMillan, A.B. (1994b) Primary prevention of child physical abuse and neglect: a critical review. I. *Journal of Child Psychology and Psychiatry*, 35, 836–856.

MacMillan, H.L., Fleming, J.E., Boyle, M.H. *et al.* (1997) Prevalence of child physical and sexual abuse in the community: results from the

Ontario Health. *Journal of the American Medical Association*, **278** (Suppl.), 131–135.

McCain, M.N. & Mustard, J.F. (1999) *Reversing the Real Brain Drain: Early Years Study, Final Report*. Ontario Children's Secretariat, Toronto, Ontario.

McCord, J. (1992) The Cambridge–Somerville Study: a pioneering longitudinal experimental study of delinquency prevention. In: *Preventing Antisocial Behaviour* (eds J. McCord & R.E. Tremblay), pp. 196–206. Guilford Press, New York.

Melamed, B.J., Hawes, R.R., Heiby, E. & Glick, J. (1975a) Use of filmed modeling to reduce uncooperative behavior of children during dental treatment. *Journal of Dental Research*, **54**, 791–801.

Melamed, B.J., Weinstein, D., Hawes, R.R. & Katin-Borland, M. (1975b) Reduction of fear-related dental management problems with use of film modeling. *Journal of the American Dental Association*, **90**, 822–826.

Milgrom, P., Vignehsa, H. & Weinstein, P. (1992) Adolescent dental fear and control: prevalence and theoretical implications. *Behavior Research and Therapy*, **30**, 367–375.

Moffitt, T.E. (1993) Adolescence-limited and life-course-persistent antisocial behaviour: a developmental taxonomy. *Psychological Review*, **100**, 674–601.

Moncher, F.J. & Prinz, R.J. (1991) Treatment fidelity in outcome studies. *Clinical Psychology Review*, **11**, 247–266.

Mortimore, P., Sammons, P., Stoll, L., Lewis, D. & Ecob, R. (1988) *School Matters*. University of California Press, Berkeley, CA.

Mott, L. (1995) The disproportionate impact of environmental health threats on children of color. *Environmental Health Perspectives*, **103**, 33–35.

Nagin, D. & Tremblay, R. (1999) Trajectories of boys' physical aggression, opposition, and hyperactivity on the path to physically violent and nonviolent juvenile delinquency. *Child Development*, **70**, 1181–1196.

National Center for Health Statistics (1997) *Births, marriages, and deaths for 1996*. Monthly statistics report. **45**, 12. National Center for Health Statistics, Hyattsville, MD.

Needleman, H.L. (1998) Childhood lead poisoning: the promise and abandonment of primary prevention. *American Journal of Public Health*, **88**, 1871–1877.

O'Donnell, J., Hawkins, J.D., Catalano, R.F., Abbott, R.D. & Day, L.E. (1995) Preventing school failure, drug use, and delinquency among low-income children: long-term intervention in elementary schools. *American Journal of Orthopsychiatry*, **65**, 87–100.

Offord, D.R. (1987) Prevention of behavioral and emotional disorders in children. *Journal of Child Psychology and Psychiatry*, **28**, 9–19.

Offord, D.R. (1996) The state of prevention and early intervention. In: *Preventing Childhood Disorders, Substance Abuse, and Delinquency* (eds R.D. Peters & R.J. McMahon), pp. 329–344. Sage, Thousand Oaks, CA.

Offord, D.R. & Bennett, K.J. (1994) Long-term outcome of conduct disorder and interventions and their effects. *Journal of the American Academy of Child and Adolescent Psychiatry*, **33**, 1069–1078.

Offord, D.R. & Fleming, J.E. (1996) Epidemiology. In: *Child and Adolescent Psychiatry: a Comprehensive Textbook* (ed. M. Lewis), 2nd edn, pp. 1166–1178. Williams & Wilkins, Philadelphia, PA.

Offord, D.R. & Kraemer, H.C. (2000) Risk factors and prevention. *Evidence-Based Mental Health*, **3**, 70–71.

Offord, D.R., Boyle, M.H. & Jones, B.R. (1987a) Psychiatric disorder and poor school performance among welfare children in Ontario. *Canadian Journal of Psychiatry*, **32**, 518–525.

Offord, D.R., Boyle, M.H., Szatmari, P. *et al.* (1987b) Ontario Child Health Study II: six-month prevalence of disorder and rates of service utilization. *Archives of General Psychiatry*, **44**, 832–836.

Offord, D.R., Kraemer, H.C., Kazdin, A.E., Jensen, P.S. & Harrington, R. (1998) Lowering the burden of suffering from child psychiatric disorder: trade-offs among clinical, targeted, and universal interventions. *Journal of the American Academy of Child and Adolescent Psychiatry*, **37**, 686–694.

Offord, D.R., Kraemer, H.C., Kazdin, A.E., Jensen, P.S., Harrington, R. & Gardner, J.S. (1999) Lowering the burden of suffering: monitoring the benefits of clinical, targeted, and universal approaches. In: *Developmental Health and the Wealth of Nations: Social, Biological and Educational Dynamics* (eds D.P. Keating & C. Hertzman), pp. 293–310. Guilford Press, New York.

Olds, D.L., Henderson, C., Phelps, C., Kitzman, H. & Hanks, C. (1993) Effects of prenatal and infancy nurse home visitation on government spending. *Medical Care*, **31**, 155–174.

Olds, D.L., Eckenrode, J., Henderson, C.R. Jr *et al.* (1997) Long term effects of home visitation on maternal life course and child abuse and neglect: 15-year follow-up of a randomized trial. *Journal of the American Medical Association*, **278**, 637–643.

Olds, D.L., Henderson, C.R. Jr, Cole, R. *et al.* (1998a) Long-term effects of nurse home visitation on children's criminal and antisocial behavior: 15-year follow-up of a randomized trial. *Journal of the American Medical Association*, **280**, 1238–1244.

Olds, D.L., Henderson, C.R., Kitzman, H. *et al.* (1998b) Prenatal and infancy home visitation by nurses: a program of research. In: *Advances in Infancy Research* (eds C. Rovee-Collier, P. Lipsitt & H. Hayne), pp. 79–130. Ablex, Stamford, CT.

Olds, D.L., Henderson, C.R., Kitzman, H., Eckenrode, J., Cole, R.E. & Tatelbaum, R.C. (1999) Prenatal and infancy home visitation by nurses: recent findings. *Future of Children*, **9**, 44–65.

Pedro-Carroll, J. & Alpert-Gillis, L. (1997) Preventive interventions for children of divorce: a developmental model for 5- and 6 year-old children. *Journal of Primary Prevention*, **18**, 5–23.

Pedro-Carroll, J.L. & Cowen, E.L. (1985) The children of divorce intervention program: an investigation of the efficacy of a school-based prevention program. *Journal of Consulting and Clinical Psychology*, **53**, 603–611.

Pedro-Carroll, J., Cowen, E.L., Hightower, A.D. & Guare, J.C. (1986) Prevention intervention with latency-aged children of divorce: a replication study. *American Journal of Community Psychology*, **14**, 277–289.

Rae-Grant, N.I. (1991) Primary prevention. In: *Child and Adolescent Psychiatry: a Comprehensive Textbook* (ed. M. Lewis), pp. 918–929. Williams & Wilkins, Baltimore, MD.

Rae-Grant, N., Thomas, H., Offord, D.R. & Boyle, M.H. (1989) Risk, protective factors, and the prevalence of behavioral and emotional disorders in children and adolescents. *Journal of the American Academy of Child and Adolescent Psychiatry*, **23**, 262–268.

Rahman, A., Harrington, R., Mueser, K.T. & Gaudet, N. (2000) Developing child mental health services in developing countries [Annotation]. *Journal of Child Psychology and Psychiatry*, **41**, 539–546.

Raizenne, M., Dales, R. & Burnett, R. (1998) Air pollution exposures and children's health. *Canadian Journal of Public Health*, **89**, S43–S48.

Ramey, C.T. & Ramey, S.L. (1998) Early intervention and early experience. *American Psychologist*, **53**, 109–120.

Reid, J.B. & Eddy, J.M. (1997) The prevention of antisocial behaviour: some considerations in the search for effective interventions. In: *Handbook of Antisocial Behaviour* (eds D.M. Stoff, J. Breiling & J.D. Maser), pp. 343–356. John Wiley and Sons, Toronto.

Rice, D.C. (1998) Issues in developmental neurotoxicology: interpretation and implications of the data. *Canadian Journal of Public Health*, **89**, S31–S38.

Rispens, J., Aleman, A. & Goudena, P.P. (1997) Prevention of child sexual abuse victimization: a meta-analysis of school programs. *Child Abuse and Neglect*, **21**, 975–987.

Robinson, E.H., Rotter, J.C., Fey, M.A. & Robinson, S.L. (1991) Children's fears: towards a preventative model. *School Counselor*, **38**, 187–202.

Rutter, M. (1985) Resilience in the face of adversity. *British Journal of Psychiatry*, **147**, 598–611.

Rutter, M. (1995) Relationships between mental disorders in childhood and adulthood. *Acta Psychiatrica Scandinavica*, **91**, 73–85.

Rutter, M. & Hersov, L. eds (1985) *Child and Adolescent Psychiatry: Modern Approaches*, 2nd edn. Blackwell Scientific, Oxford.

Schwartz, J. (1994) Low-level lead exposure and children's IQ: a meta-analysis and search for a threshold. *Environmental Research*, **65**, 42–55.

Schweinhart, L.J. & Weikert, D.P. (1988) The High/Scope Perry Preschool Program. In: *12 Ounces of Prevention: a Casebook for Practitioners* (eds R.H. Price, R.P. Cowen, R.P. Lorion & J. Ramos-McKay), pp. 53–65. American Psychological Association, Washington D.C.

Schweinhart, L.J. & Weikert, D.P. (1989) The High/Scope Perry Preschool Study: implications for early childhood care and education. *Prevention in Human Services*, **7**, 109–132.

Shadish, W.R. & Sweeny, R.B. (1991) Mediators and moderators in meta-analysis: there's a reason we don't let dodo birds tell us which psychotherapies should have prizes. *Journal of Consulting and Clinical Psychology*, **59**, 883–893.

Sonawane, B.R. (1995) Chemical contaminants in human milk: an overview. *Environmental Health Perspectives*, **103**, 197–205.

Spence, S.H. (1994) Preventative strategies. In: *International Handbook of Phobic and Anxiety Disorders in Children and Adolescents* (eds T.H. Ollendick, N.J. King & W. Yule), pp. 453–474. Plenum Press, New York.

Stern, B.R., Raizenne, M.E., Burnett, R.T. *et al.* (1994) Air pollution and childhood respiratory health: exposure to sulfate and ozone in 10 Canadian rural communities. *Environmental Research*, **66**, 125–142.

Stoolmiller, M., Eddy, J.M. & Reid, J.B. (2000) Detecting and describing preventive intervention effects in a universal school-based randomized trial targeting delinquent and violent behaviour. *Journal of Consulting and Clinical Psychology*, **68**, 296–306.

Streiner, D.L. & Norman, G.R. (1996) *PDQ Epidemiology*, 2nd edn. Mosby, Toronto.

Stroufe, L.A. & Rutter, M. (1984) The domain of developmental psychopathology. *Child Development*, **83**, 173–189.

Sylva, K. (1994) School influences on children's development. *Journal of Child Psychology and Psychiatry*, **35**, 135–170.

Tolan, P., Keys, C., Chertok, F. & Jason, L. (1990) *Researching Community Psychology: Issues of Theories and Methods*. American Psychological Association, Washington D.C.

Tremblay, R.E., Kurtz, L., Mûsse, L.C., Vitaro, F. & Pihl, R.O. (1995) A bimodal preventive intervention for disruptive kindergarten boys: its impact through mid-adolescence. *Journal of Consulting and Clinical Psychology*, **63**, 560–568.

Tryon, G.S. (1980) The measurement and treatment of test anxiety. *Review of Educational Research*, **50**, 343–372.

Tugwell, P., Bennett, K.J., Haynes, R.B. & Sackett, D.L. (1985) The measurement iterative loop: a framework for the critical appraisal of needs, benefits and costs of health interventions. *Journal of Chronic Disease*, **38**, 339–351.

US Congress (1986) *Children's Mental Health: Problems and Services. A Background Paper*. US Government Printing Office, Washington D.C.

Van der Ploeg-Stapert, J.D. & Van der Ploeg, H.M. (1986) Behavioral group treatment of test anxiety: an evaluation study. *Journal of Behavior Therapy and Experimental Psychiatry*, **17**, 255–259.

Wadsworth, M.E.J. (1986) Grounds for divorce in England and Wales: a social and demographic analysis. *Journal of Biosocial Science*, **18**, 127–153.

Wang, X., Ding, H., Ryan, L. & Xu, X. (1997) Association between air pollution and low birth weight: a community-based study. *Environmental Health Perspectives*, **105**, 514–520.

Ware, J.H., Ferris, B.G., Dockery, D.W. *et al.* (1986) Effects of ambient sulfur oxides and suspended particles on respiratory health of preadolescent children. *American Review of Respiratory Disease*, **133**, 834–842.

Webster-Stratton, C. (1991) Strategies for helping families with conduct disordered children [Annotation]. *Journal of Child Psychology and Psychiatry*, **32**, 1047–1062.

Weissberg, R.P. & Greenberg, M.T. (1998) School and community competence-enhancement and prevention programs. In: *Handbook of Child Psychology*, Vol. 4. *Child Psychology in Practice* (eds I.E. Sigel & K.A. Renninger), 5th edn, pp. 877–953. John Wiley & Sons, New York.

Werner, E.E. & Smith, R.S. (1982) *Vulnerable But Invincible: a Longitudinal Study of Resilient Children and Youth*. McGraw-Hill, New York.

Yoshikawa, H. (1994) Prevention as cumulative protection: effects of early family support and education on chronic delinquency and its risks. *Psychological Bulletin*, **115**, 28–54.

Young, M. (1997) *Early Child Development: Investing in Our Children's Future*. Elsevier, New York.

Behavioural Therapies

Martin Herbert

Introduction

The plural 'behavioural therapies' in the title of this chapter reflects the growing sophistication and range of applications that have come about in the half century since operant and classical conditioning principles of learning were first applied systematically to the clinical problems of children and adolescents. The names of the various therapies, which, to varying degrees, are rooted in behaviourism, represent milestones on a journey of ever-increasing conceptual elaboration and theoretical inclusiveness: applied behaviour analysis, behaviour modification, behaviour therapy, cognitive-behaviour therapy, behavioural family therapy, functional family therapy, behavioural casework and cognitive-behavioural psychotherapy.

Theoretical background

Behaviour therapy starts from a clear objective of producing planned goal-directed change. It represents a theory — indeed, a philosophy — of treatment and behaviour modification, rooted in broad empirically based theories of learned human behaviour. The central assumption of behavioural work is that much abnormal behaviour and cognition in children is on a continuum with normal (non-problematic) behaviour and thought. These phenomena do not differ, by and large, from their normal counterparts in their development, their persistence and the way in which they can be altered. The laws of learning that apply to the acquisition and changing of normal functional (e.g. socially approved) behaviour and attitudes are assumed to be relevant to the understanding of dysfunctional actions and cognitions. Unfortunately, and it is the case with all forms of learning, the very processes that help the child adapt to life can, under certain circumstances, contribute to maladaptation. An immature child who learns by imitating an adult does not necessarily comprehend when it is undesirable (deviant) behaviour or distorted thinking that is being modelled. The youngster who learns adaptively on the basis of classical and instrumental conditioning processes to avoid or escape from dangerous situations can also learn in the same way (maladaptively) to avoid school or social gatherings. A caregiver may unwittingly reinforce antisocial coercive behaviour by attending, or giving in, to it.

Of course, there is much more to both adaptive and maladaptive learning than is conveyed by these examples. There may be learned behavioural, cognitive or affective overlays to problems that have an organic basis (conditions such as epilepsy and the Lesch–Nyhan syndrome, or an adverse temperamental predisposition), which are therefore accessible to some alleviation by behavioural methods. In addition, the application of behavioural principles based on a model of normal learning may not always be clinically apposite. The process of learning for some children may be altered by anomalies of brain function, as may be the case with attention deficit hyperactivity disorder (ADHD), where it is hypothesized that the learning situation can be complicated by a rapid delay-of-reward gradient. Such an aberration might require a treatment plan that arranges for a sufficiently speedy delivery of reinforcers to produce, and maintain, change (for a discussion of these and similar issues see Taylor 1994).

Levels of intervention

Behaviour therapy based on the one-to-one (dyadic) or behavioural family therapy (systemic) model tends to take place in the clinic. Behavioural training based on the triadic or behavioural consultation model (using significant caregivers or teachers as mediators of change) often takes place in the home, or is located in a school. When it involves group work it may take place in a community centre. Although the distinction between treatment and training is at times blurred, the treatment model is most appropriate to the emotional disorders of childhood (e.g. fears and phobias), the training model to the longer term problems (e.g. antisocial behaviour and pervasive developmental disorders). At least four levels of intervention need to be implemented in concert in order to meet long-term goals (Evans 1989):

1 altering the immediate consequences of the undesirable behaviour and/or belief;

2 reducing the probability of the behaviour or belief occurring by rearranging the environment;

3 facilitating (teaching, reinforcing, shaping) the emergence of alternative skills and attitudes; and

4 designing long-term prevention through imparting new patterns of behaviour and/or attitudes.

At the simplest level (point 1, above) there are three basic learning tasks that are commonly encountered in child therapy:

1 the acquisition (learning) of a desired response in which the individual is deficient (e.g. compliance, self-esteem, self-control, bladder and bowel control, fluent speech, social or academic skills);

2 the reduction or elimination (unlearning) of an unwanted response in the child's repertoire (e.g. self-deprecatory self-talk, aggression, temper tantrums, stealing, facial tics, phobic anxiety, compulsive eating); or

3 the exchange of one response for another (e.g. social approach behaviour in place of excessively shy withdrawal).

Each of these tasks (and potential ameliorative methods) may be served by either one or a combination of the major types of learning: operant and classical conditioning, observational, and cognitive learning.

Behaviour modification

Early behavioural theorists, in reaction to the subjectivism of psychoanalysis, sought a positivist approach to the therapeutic treatment and training of severely handicapped and disturbed children. It involved the systematic application of response-contingent (operant) principles of learning to the problems of autistic and mentally handicapped patients (Ferster & De Myer 1962). They attended to the functional relationship between precisely defined and observable actions (targets for modification) and clearly specified environmental contingencies, thereby achieving an overt, if restricted, conceptual formulation of behaviour change.

Operant conditioning

In essence, operant behaviour (mainly under voluntary control) is defined by the manner it changes the environment; it is behaviour that is maintained by its consequences. Actions are increased or strengthened—and thus shaped—by having consequences that are rewarding (positive reinforcement) or that lead to the avoidance of, or escape from, punishment (negative reinforcement). They are reduced or eliminated by punitive sanctions (fines, penalties, etc.) that follow, contingently, their unwanted performance. The term 'operant' refers also to behaviours that have an identical effect on the environment. A child may find that he or she can get his or her parent to delay or forgo an unwelcome command to go to bed (a rewarding outcome) by a variety of operants: screaming, crying or pleading. The parent, by giving in, escapes the aversive behaviour (also a rewarding outcome). The repeated consequence of such submissive and coercive behaviours reinforces them, in other words increases the probability of their occurrence by parent and child in future situations of a similar kind. This illustration of positive and negative reinforcement for child and parent, respectively, is familiar to clinicians treating oppositional-defiant problems.

Functional analysis

A careful observation-based analysis of the positive and negative reinforcing stimuli that produce or maintain fearful, antiso-cial or other unwanted behaviours is referred to as a 'functional analysis'. The analysis leads to procedures that bring about the systematic manipulation of a behaviour's consequences so as to modify its subsequent performance. With their individual learning histories, their experience as they grow up, of attention, approval, disapproval or neglect, children have unique reinforcement profiles. An event that functions as a reinforcer for one child may not do so for another. Similarly, a reinforcer for an individual in one situation may not have the same effect in another (for detailed accounts of the theoretical and practical aspects of behavioural analysis see Gambrill 1977; Herbert 1987a; Sturmey 1996). The functional analysis is also referred to as an 'applied behaviour analysis'. It became the source of the formulation in the earliest single-case studies that were published in a newly founded *Journal of Applied Behavior Analysis* (Baer *et al.* 1968). The term 'behaviour modification' was applied to this form of behavioural work.

Although early practitioners reported successful interventions, their emphasis on short-term gains often neglected developmental, diagnostic and generalization issues, the need for follow-up, and the possibility of negative concurrent effects such as disruptions to family relationships.

Behaviour therapy

Classical conditioning

At about the same time as these advances in operant technology (the late 1950s and early 1960s), behavioural therapy began to come into its own in the treatment of clinical patients, notably those with anxiety disorders. The early theorists and practitioners in this development (Wolpe 1958; Eysenck 1960) were impressed by the therapeutic possibilities of stimulus-contingent reinforcement, and preferred to call their approach 'behaviour therapy' to emphasize the clinical application of this principle of learning. The essence of stimulus-contingent reinforcement, a model of learning called classical or respondent conditioning developed by Ivan Pavlov (1927), is that a stimulus (the unconditioned stimulus) is presented to the organism and reflexly elicits a response. A previously neutral stimulus repeatedly paired with the unconditioned stimulus gradually acquires its response-eliciting properties. The response of the organism is now conditioned to the second stimulus (the conditioned stimulus). Emotional reactions of phobic intensity can be evoked directly by classical conditioning, a fact demonstrated in a distasteful experiment on a young child (Little Albert) by Watson & Rayner (1920).

The most often quoted account of a prescient and more benign therapeutic use of classical conditioning, referred to as counter-conditioning, is Mary Cover Jones' successful treatment of Little Peter's fear of a rabbit (Jones 1924). She used guided re-exposure to the anxiety-eliciting rabbit in a systematic but gradual manner and in the presence of food (conceptualized as a stimulus that would produce an incompatible positive response). Mowrer & Mowrer (1938) invented the urine alarm ('bell-and-pad') for the treatment of nocturnal enuresis. A pad, when moistened with urine during the night, closed a circuit and rang a bell. It was arranged that when that happened, someone would wake the child, take him or her to the toilet, and change the bed and night clothes. This conditioning technique was and, in updated versions, continues to be very effective.

Some 20 years later, a curious gap in the development of such promising therapeutic procedures, Wolpe (1958) was to make a major contribution to the rationale for using respondent conditioning in the establishment, maintenance and 'cure' of anxiety states: the development of systematic desensitization. He relied primarily on relaxation as the competing, and therefore, inhibitory response, calling the process 'reciprocal inhibition'. Researchers have sought, by a process of experimental deconstruction, the active and necessary therapeutic ingredients of systematic desensitization. Despite disagreements (some practitioners question the need for relaxation), it remains an effective procedure for a variety of anxiety disorders of childhood and adolescence. Mowrer (1947), in a further theoretical advance, described the interaction of stimulus-contingent and response-conditioned learning in the development of phobic anxiety. He suggested that the intense fear of stimuli associated with a distressing event was established by classical conditioning, while responses that remove the individual from the fear-eliciting stimuli (escape/avoidance) are reinforced by relief, the operant process of fear (drive) reduction.

Observational learning (vicarious conditioning)

Stimulus–response theories of learning and their various clinical applications continue to be acknowledged for their undoubted usefulness. However, learning theory moved on, influenced in large part by the innovative work of Bandura (1977). His concept of vicarious conditioning, or learning by observation, is central to the child's rapid acquisition of much complex and novel behaviour, and also its modification. Watching and imitating the behaviour of exemplary models is considered by social learning theorists to be the cornerstone of learning for socialization (an issue we return to).

Emotional responses can be conditioned observationally by witnessing the affective reactions of others undergoing painful or pleasurable experiences. Fearful and avoidance behaviour can similarly be extinguished. Modelling has been used to reduce 'normal' fears, such as the dark, animals and spiders, as well as more serious symptoms of anxiety disorder. Children are encouraged to observe other children (or adults) approaching and coping with (rather than mastering) the feared object, or engaging in anxiety-reducing strategies they have been taught.

Cognitive-behavioural therapy

The critical role of cognition in childhood learning (Bruner 1975) led to a sometimes reluctant reappraisal by many behaviour therapists of the significance of 'private events', and the cog-

nitive mediation of problematic behaviour. Thus, we arrive at an acceptance in the 1980s and 1990s, in what came to be known as cognitive-behavioural therapy (CBT), of the phenomenology of problems as primary data. It is proposed that cognitions (e.g. schemata, attributions, opinions) require investigation in order to understand children's emotional and behavioural difficulties (Kendall & Gosch 1994). These might include self-statements describing fears, such as those reported by Zatz & Chassin (1983) in test-anxious children. Their cognitions not only encompass many self-denigrating statements (e.g. 'I'm doing poorly; I don't do well on tests like this; everyone usually does better than me'), they also make use of few facilitative, coping statements (e.g. 'I am bright enough to do this; I am doing the best that I can; I do well on tests like this').

Cognitive-behavioural therapy focuses on goal-setting and self-directed behaviour by the child, also targeting divergent thinking as a way of encouraging inventive solutions to personal difficulties. The techniques used have their roots in cognitive therapy (e.g. Socratic questioning, persuasion, challenging, debate, hypothesizing, cognitive-restructuring, verbal self-instruction and internal dialogue). Others are drawn from behaviour therapy (e.g. operant procedures, desensitization, exposure training, social-skills training, role-play, behaviour rehearsal, modelling, relaxation exercises, redefinition, self-monitoring). The methods share a common assumption: that children can be taught to eliminate some of their maladaptive behaviours by challenging their irrational beliefs and faulty logic, by getting them to instruct themselves in certain ways, or to associate wanted behaviour with positive self-statements and unwanted ones with negative self-statements.

A recent development which is an adaptation of cognitive therapy as it was originally applied to adults is cognitive-behavioural play therapy (CBPT): a developmentally sensitive treatment for young children that relies on flexibility, decreased expectation of verbalization by the child, and increased reliance on experiential approaches (Knell 1998, p. 28). There is a need to reach preschool-age children whose conceptual language is still too immature to benefit from traditional cognitive strategies, but whose positive response to play and play therapy is well established (Axline 1947; Webb 1991).

Applied social learning theory

Social learning theory

Cognitive-behavioural therapy, which, as we have seen, goes well beyond the earlier epistemological position of radical behaviourists, finds much of its rationale in the development of social learning theory (SLT). There is an emphasis on the crucial fact that rewards and punishments, and other events, are mediated by human agents and within attachment and social systems, and are not simply the impersonal consequences of behaviour. Children do not simply respond to stimuli; they interpret them. They relate to, interact with, and learn from people who have meaning and value for them. They feel antipathetic to some, attached by respect and/or affection to others, and thus may perceive an encouraging word from the latter as rewarding (positively reinforcing), but from the former as valueless, perhaps even aversive. Stimuli influence the likelihood of particular behaviours through their predictive function; contingent experiences create expectations rather than stimulus–response connections (Bandura 1977). The failure of children to comprehend such meanings, which is the case in semantic-pragmatic disorder or Asperger syndrome, is devastating in its effects.

Behavioural family therapy

Behavioural family therapy and parent management programmes draw on applications of social learning, cognitive, and family theory (Herbert 1998c; Patterson 1982; Herbert & Wookey 1998; Webster-Stratton 1991; Webster-Stratton & Herbert 1994; Sanders 1996). They typically address themselves to the fact that parents of children with behaviour problems tend to flounder because they issue so many commands, provide attention following deviant behaviour, and are unlikely to perceive deviant behaviour as deviant. There is a tendency to get embroiled frequently in extended coercive hostile interchanges. They give vague commands, and are generally ineffectual in bringing their children's deviant behaviour to a halt. A typical programme is described later in the chapter.

Functional family therapy

Alexander & Parsons (1982) have integrated aspects of structural and strategic family therapy with behavioural family therapy in a promising approach to delinquency and related problems. Patients are trained in communication and problem-solving skills, contingency contracting and self-regulation skills, such as relaxation.

Psychodynamic influences

The drift of behaviour therapy to a cognitive mode is paralleled by a noticeable, if modest, leaning of cognitive therapy towards psychodynamic thinking (Power 1991). The psychoanalysts' exegesis of the mysteries of intrapsychic life and their preoccupation with motivation are precisely where, in Wachtel's opinion, they have much to offer behaviour therapists as they investigate the 'what' and 'why' questions of clinical problems (Wachtel 1977, 1997). Hersen (1981), an eminent behaviour therapist, has acknowledged that his fellow professionals often rely, perhaps unwittingly, on techniques associated with traditional psychotherapy in overcoming resistance to therapy, by utilizing support, interpretation and reality confrontation.

It is generally recognized that the insights that arise from intrapsychic exploration and interpretation do not necessarily lead to changes in behaviour; behaviour change, in turn, does not necessarily lead to an insightful understanding of personal

difficulties. Nevertheless, there is a sense in which a functional analysis can achieve this. At its simplest, behaviour is a function of certain contingent stimuli, originating in the person's internal and external environment. Here, the important questions are: 'What triggers (elicits) the phobia?' or 'What is the pay-off (reinforcement) the child obtains when behaving in this antisocial way?' At a more interpretative level, the child's behaviours may have the function of solving (or attempting to solve) a developmental or life problem. They serve a purpose; they are functional (dysfunctional though they may appear to the parental or professional eye) for the individual. An example of this is the 'pay-off' of attention, guilt-reduction, nurturance, or some other reinforcement that maintains what otherwise appears to be incomprehensible self-injurious behaviour (Oliver & Head 1993).

It is suggested that psychodynamic ideas constitute a semantic theory about meanings, rather than a scientific model of practice, and as such may contribute to a broader, more integrated perspective for the psychological therapy of children. This contribution to therapy is not the scientific one of elucidating the causes of children's choices and actions, but the semantic one of making sense of them (Rycroft 1970, p. 328).

Transition and change: a developmental perspective

Learning, like growth and development in children, is essentially about change. Parents too—and indeed their family—are locked into a developmental life cycle, with its stage-related life-tasks. The nature, sources and consequences of parents' ideas about development (Goodnow & Collins 1990), and the ramifications of transition and change in family life, are important in the assessment of children's problems.

In the early stages of behaviour therapy's history there was little or no communication between clinical practitioners and developmental psychologists. There have been attempts to integrate findings between the two disciplines since the 1970s (Achenbach 1974; Herbert 1974). The evaluation of normality and abnormality within a developmental framework requires a familiarity with general principles of development (Herbert 1998a; 2001). For Cicchetti et al. (1983), to take one example, abnormal patterns of behavioural adaptation (as represented by clinical problems such as hyperactivity and failure to thrive) are most fruitfully construed and formulated in terms of a series of stage- and age-related tasks. The issue of competence is common to all of them and, as the child gets older, his or her self-esteem. If the child fails to develop skills and social competence, he or she is likely to suffer, among other problems, a sense of inadequacy. There is evidence not only of the power of parents to facilitate or hinder the child's mastery of developmental tasks, but to do this unwittingly (Cicchetti et al. 1983).

These matters become important themes in parenting skills programmes, most of which set themselves the task of increasing parents' sense of 'self-empowerment' (Herbert & Wookey

Table 53.1 Sources of increased self-empowerment.

	Content	Process
Knowledge		
Child development	Developmental norms and tasks	Discussion
Behaviour management	Behavioural (learning) principles	Books/pamphlets to read
Individual and temperamental differences	Child management (disciplinary strategies)	Modelling (videotape, live role play, role reversal, rehearsal)
	Relationships (feelings)	Metaphors/analogies
	Self-awareness (self-talk, schema, attributions)	Homework tasks
		Networking
	Interactions (awareness of contingencies, communications)	Developmental counselling
		Videotape viewing and discussion
	Resources (support, sources of assistance)	Self-observation/recording at home
	Appropriate expectations	Discussing records of parents' own data
	Parent involvement with children	Teaching, persuading
Skills		
Communication	Self-restraint/anger management	Self-reinforcement
Problem-solving (including problem analysis)	Self-talk (depressive thoughts)	Group and therapist reinforcement
	Attend–ignore	Self-observations of interactions at home
Tactical thinking (use of techniques/methods)	Play–praise–encourage	Rehearsal
	Contracts	Participant modelling
Building social relationships	Consistent consequences	Homework tasks and practice
Enhancing children's academic skills	Sanction effectively (time out, loss of privileges, natural consequences)	Video modelling and feedback
		Self-disclosure
	Monitoring	Therapist use of humour/optimism
	Social/relationship skills	Relaxation training
	Problem-solving skills	Stress management
	Fostering good learning habits	Self-instruction
	Self-assertion/confidence	Visual cues at home
	Empathy for child's perspective	
	Ways to give and get support	
Values		
Strategic thinking (working out goals, philosophy of child rearing, beliefs)	Treatment/life goals	Discussion/debate
	Objectives (targeted child behaviours)	Sharing
	Ideologies	Listening
	Rules	Respecting/accepting
	Roles	Negotiating
	Relationships	Demystifying
	Emotional barriers	Explaining/interpreting
	Attributions	Reframing
	Prejudices	Resolving conflict
	Past history	Clarifying
		Supporting
		Adapting

1998; Webster-Stratton & Herbert 1994). This rather vague concept can be operationalized in terms of knowledge, skills and values (see Table 53.1).

There are far-reaching benefits for the enhancement and timing of interventions to be had from an appreciation of the development of different pathways to adult antisocial behaviour (Frick 1998) and the relevance of attachment theory and parental responsiveness to family behaviour therapy (Rutter 1995; Wahler & Meginnis 1997). Also helpful is an understanding of the causes and consequences of any 'mismatches' in the parents' and children's ideas and expectations that arise from differences in conceptual level, and which promote conflict (Goodnow & Collins 1990).

Behavioural assessment and formulation

Rigorous assessment is the sine qua non of effective behavioural

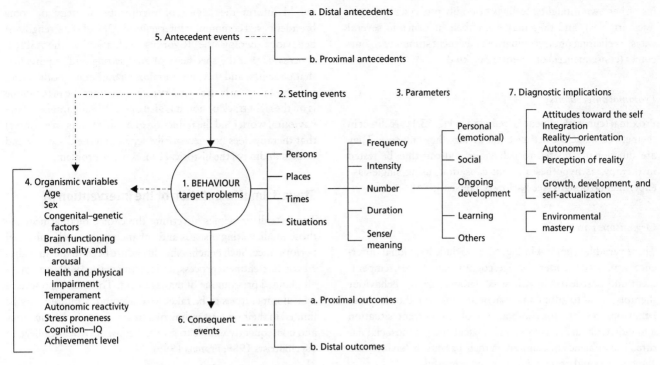

Fig. 53.1 A conceptual framework for an assessment of behaviour problems.

treatment. The strategy is to begin with a broad-based assessment of the child and his or her environment (e.g. family, school, peers) and then to obtain information regarding specific stimulus features, response modes, antecedents and consequences, severity, duration and pervasiveness of the particular problems. The assessment utilizes a multimethod problem-solving approach to obtain as complete a picture of the child and the family as is possible. When the collection of sufficient data allows, there is a behavioural formulation, a set of explanatory hypotheses describing the determinants, historical and current, of the problem. A conceptual framework for gathering data for assessment and a clinical formulation is provided in Fig. 53.1.

The formulation of the client's problem bridges the assessment, the treatment plan and implementation, and is arrived at in several stages summarized by the mnemonic ASPIRE (Sutton & Herbert 1992).

Stage 1: Assessment (AS)

The what and why questions are directed towards the precise identification of the antecedent (A), consequent (C), and symbolic conditions which control the targeted behaviours and/or beliefs (B) which are problematic. This linear analysis is elaborated into a recursive sequence such that Cs become As, which generate new Cs, and thus ramify to affect the actions of others in the vicinity of the main protagonists (say, parents and child). The main assessment tasks are twofold: to identify target problems and to identify controlling variables.

Identifying target problems

Point 1 in Fig. 53.1 underlines the importance of a developmental context for evaluating (say) a child's fearfulness or aggressiveness. The judgement arises from the essential normality of these emotions, universal responses and normal adaptations to a wide range of life events, and which are therefore functional in the sense of having survival and reward value. The parameters that separate behaviours defined as problematic from the anxieties, avoidance, aggression, indecision and obsessions shown by all children at one time or another are, *inter alia*, their rate and intensity (point 3 in Fig. 53.1). The persistence (duration) with which they are manifested, their pervasiveness, and the sheer number of problems with which they are associated are also important diagnostic criteria.

Their implications for the individual's well-being and effective functioning at home and in the wider world (e.g. school) provide further diagnostic guidelines for the therapist (point 7 in Fig. 53.1). The meaning of the problems, the sense made of them, the pay-off they provide for the child, and indeed for the family, constitute vital elements of the overall assessment.

Identifying controlling variables

Two categories are generally considered when identifying controlling variables: current environmental variables (antecedent and consequent events; points 5 and 6 in Fig. 53.1) and organismic variables (point 4 in Fig. 53.1). The contemporary causes of problem behaviour may exist in the client's environment or in his or her own thoughts, feelings or bodily processes (organismic variables), and they may exert their influence in several ways: as eliciting or discriminative antecedent stimuli or as outcomes (consequences) of a reinforcing kind.

Proximal antecedents

Proximal (current) influences (point 5b in Fig. 53.1) are direct in their effects and close in time to the actions they influence. They are functionally related to behaviour and can thus be tested in therapy, as hypotheses about causation, using single-case experimental designs (see Barlow & Hersen 1984).

Organismic variables

These variables (point 4 in Fig. 53.1) include individual differences produced by, *inter alia*, age, cognitive structures, temperament and past learning (Chess & Thomas 1995). Behaviour therapists tend to adopt a transactional position, the view that behaviour results from interaction of the current situation and individual differences of a biological and psychosocial nature. The influence of children on their parents' behaviour and choices, past and present, is active and powerful.

Brown & Harris (1989) use the term 'life structure' for the interface of the internal and external worlds of the individual and to reflect the transitions and changes in the child's family life, his or her moods, regrets and attitudes. This moves the assessment on from a consideration of current antecedent influences to an inquiry into distal (historical) antecedents (point 5a in Fig. 53.1).

The analysis of the problems may be assisted by information about the patient's past (e.g. attachments, health, reinforcement history, attitudes, life-events) (point 5 in Fig. 53.1), but the information is gathered primarily as a source of clues to contemporary conditions that influence the elicitation and maintenance of symptoms rather than as primary treatment objectives in themselves. The behaviour therapist places most emphasis on providing the patient with new learning experiences. The past may haunt the present in the sense that it may influence current attitudes. An adolescent boy may try, by means of offensive behaviour, to sabotage his mother's relationship with his stepfather, because she has 'betrayed' a deceased father and husband. Some parents harbour guilty attributions about past child care 'mistakes' that, in turn, engender overprotective actions toward their children. It may be necessary, before programmatic work can begin, to lay such 'ghosts' to rest, by discussing past events and possibly changing attitudes to them, using techniques such as cognitive restructuring ('reframing').

Stage 2: Planning (P)

The strategic treatment plan and the tactical specification of methods/techniques for bringing about change, the 'how' questions, generally flow from the assessment of the determinants or causes of the problem(s). In an ideal world this formulation would inform the choice of therapeutic strategy or some broader based community intervention. One of the strengths of behaviour therapy (the 'Rigorous Evaluation' in the ASPIRE process) is that the specificity of goal-setting and requirement that patient(s) and therapist monitor change allow both parties to judge fairly early in the intervention whether the programme is on the right track or not. It is also one of the advantages of behavioural work (and the reduction of phobic fear is an example) that therapy does not necessarily depend on the discovery and understanding of the historical causes of the problem.

Stage 3: Implementation of the intervention (I)

The overall principles governing the choice of treatment are those of alleviating distress and enhancing personal and social performance. Such benefits should endure beyond the immediacies of the treatment process, and treatment used within an overall planned programme of management. There are also several ethical imperatives to be taken into account. Children may be limited in their understanding of a treatment or its implications and consequently unable to give full consent (Royal College of Psychiatrists 1989; Francis 1999).

Non-specific conditions

Relationship and other therapeutic process variables cannot be overlooked in behaviour therapy any more than in other forms of psychotherapy. They are necessary but usually not sufficient conditions of change. Positive expectations about the outcome of treatment and attitudes towards the therapist are important elements in determining the success or failure of programmes, yet parents often complain that professionals simply do not understand, or attend to, their personal concerns. Prior to therapy, parents of conduct problem children, for example, often feel as if they are 'under siege'. The child's hyperactivity, distractibility, developmental problems and unpredictability drain the parents and lead to many ripple effects. Their relationships with other family members, friends and people in the community (notably at school) are quite likely to be adversely affected. Marital discord and depression are common (Webster-Stratton & Hammond 1999).

A collaborative approach to therapy designed to address these difficulties is described by Webster-Stratton & Herbert (1993, 1994). They suggest that the first role of the therapist in the collaborative process is to build a supportive relationship with the parents. This is often achieved through appropriate use of self-disclosure, humour and optimism, as well as actively advocating for parents (such as at the child's school). A second role is to empower parents, through reinforcing and validating parents' insights, helping them to modify powerless thoughts, promoting self-efficacy (knowledge, skills and values) and building family and group supports. A third role is to teach by persuading, explaining, suggesting, adapting, giving assignments, reviewing, summarizing, ensuring generalization, using videotape examples and role-playing. A fourth role is to interpret or 'translate' the cognitive, behavioural and developmental concepts into words that the parents can understand and apply. This includes the use of analogies and metaphors, reframing, and making connections between the parents' own childhood or other life experiences and those of the child. A fifth role is to lead and challenge, including setting limits (especially in groups), pacing the sessions, and dealing with resistance.

Bandura (1977) is of the opinion that success depends on the degree to which the interventions create or strengthen the client's expectations of personal efficacy, hence the concentration on 'doing' (e.g. behaviour rehearsal, modelling, role-play, homework tasks) in behavioural parent training.

Clinical applications

It is an indication of the versatility of modern behaviour therapy that it is possible here to mention only a small sample of psychiatric, psychiatry/health liaison, and school-based problems to which behavioural methods have been applied. Behavioural methods have been evaluated in different ways. Some have compared behavioural interventions, at termination and follow-up, with other therapeutic approaches, and with no-treatment (e.g. waiting list) patient groups, as controls (Blagg & Yule 1984). Others have tested the ability of behavioural methods to reduce deviant, neurotic and other behaviours/symptoms to within normal limits (Bernal et al. 1980). Psychometric instruments are often used to measure change in symptomatology. The contribution of a behavioural component to a multisystemic or multimodal programme may be 'teased out' (unpublished data). The deconstruction of particular methods, experimentally 'stripping' out aspects that are therapeutically inert or redundant in relation to the desired outcome of therapy (a feature of early research on systematic desensitization), is an important validation procedure. Cost-effectiveness studies comparing group vs. individual interventions are also carried out (Christenson et al. 1980; Cunningham et al. 1995).

Emotional disorders

Anxiety disorders

Cognitive-behavioural therapy

The primary goals of CBT with anxious children, in the light of what has been established theoretically, are:
1 management of the anxiety;
2 reduction of the child's distress; and
3 increasing mastery and coping skills.
Children are helped to detect early signs and triggers of anxious arousal, and then to utilize these cues as signals for initiating active cognitive and behavioural coping strategies. Treatment gains have been maintained at 3-year follow-up assessments (Kendall & Southam-Gerow 1996). Probably the most fre-

quently used cognitive approach with anxious children is verbal self-instruction training (Kanfer et al. 1975).

Ronan & Deane (1998) have described in detail their FEAR plan in which children combine these individual skills within an integrated 'coping template'—a programme that outcome studies suggest is effective (Kendall 1994). The inclusion of parents in this and other approaches is recommended, the Family Anxiety Management (FAM) programme being an example of how to enhance the individual programme for children with anxiety disorder. Barrett et al. (1991) demonstrated, in a study of 79 children aged 7–14 years, the advantage of adding to a CBT approach a family management treatment condition (dealing with parents' interactions with their children during anxiety attacks, emotional upsets and family communication plus exercises in problem-solving), as compared with CBT on its own and a waiting list control group. At the end of treatment (individual) 57% of cases were clinically improved, rising to 70% a year later. However, the combined treatment resulted in an 84% improvement at termination, rising to 96% at 1-year follow-up.

Systematic desensitization

This tends to be the preferred intervention for children exhibiting simple and social phobias (Ollendick & King 1998). The method consists of three basic steps:
1 progressive relaxation training;
2 development of a fear-provoking stimuli hierarchy; and
3 the systematic graduated pairing of situations in the hierarchy with relaxation.
A vast array of controlled and uncontrolled single-case studies and a number of group studies have evaluated systematic desensitization applied to a variety of phobias. They have established its credibility as a 'probably efficacious' method. However, it is not the method of choice for those phobias, that occur because of a lack of skills, or inadvertent rejection by significant others (King et al. 1988). Younger children appear to have difficulty in acquiring muscular relaxation and in being able to image clearly the fear-producing stimuli (Rosentiel & Scott 1977). As a result, in vivo desensitization and emotive imagery have become increasingly popular, especially in working with young children. Methods used in children manifesting night-time fears include the use of engaging stories and images of heroic characters to build up positive affect with which fear-eliciting stimuli are gradually interwoven and 'defeated'.

Eye movement desensitization and reprocessing

It has been said that eye movement desensitization and reprocessing (EMDR) has greater rapidity of treatment effects relative to other exposure methods. However, Muris et al. (1998) found that EMDR in the treatment of phobic children was less effective than traditional exposure techniques.

Operant methods

The exposure-training described earlier for anxiety reduction has also been referred to as reinforced practice, as developed by Leitenberg & Callahan (1973). It combines a number of operant components. Children's avoidance behaviours are treated by reinforcing graduated approaches to the feared stimulus. The components of reinforced practice are:

1 repeated and graduated *in vivo* practice at approaching the phobic stimuli;
2 social reinforcement for small improvements;
3 trial-by-trial feedback on performance; and
4 the therapist's communication to the child of expectations of gradual success.

Panic disorder

Panic attacks and panic disorders are common in adolescence (Ollendick 1998). Little is known, relatively speaking, about these disorders or their treatment for children and young adults. However, adolescents have been successfully treated using CBT procedures (Ollendick 1995) with gains maintained at a 6-month follow-up. Further evaluations of CBT with adolescents, and studies of its application to children, are required.

School refusal

School refusal is a heterogeneous problem, notorious for its conceptual complexities. All of the methods described above have been recruited in the daunting challenge of returning an adamant school-refuser back to the classroom. Fortunately, as attested to by an extensive clinical literature, behavioural strategies, embedded in individually tailored programmes, are highly effective in this task. A functional analysis—both contingency analysis and assessment of the broader functions of school refusal—is central to whichever methods, ranging from operant to cognitive procedures, are used (Blagg 1987; Kearney & Silverman 1990; King *et al.* 1995; Elliott 1999).

Blagg & Yule (1984) compared the effectiveness of family-based behaviour therapy (FBT), a hospital-based multimodal inpatient programme (MIT), and home tuition/psychotherapy (HT/P). FBT (taking, on average, 3 weeks and about 6 sessions) led to a far more rapid resolution of school attendance difficulties associated with school phobia and separation anxiety than the MIT and HT/P conditions (both taking, on average, 1 year). The psychotherapy programme, involving daily tuition, fortnightly individual psychotherapy and concurrent parent counselling, did least well. At 1-year follow-up 93% of the FBT children were successful in returning to school, compared with 38 and 10% for the MIT and HT/P programmes, respectively.

Post-traumatic stress disorder

Almost all treatment strategies for post-traumatic stress disorder (PTSD) focus on re-exposing the individual to traumatic cues under safe conditions, so as to encourage approach behaviour in addition to emotional processing of traumatic memories. Systematic desensitization, imaginal and *in vivo* exposure methods are vital components incorporating reparative and mastery elements. Methods for treating PTSD are described in detail by Smith *et al.* (1998) and Joseph *et al.* (1997); a CBT package incorporating prolonged therapeutic exposure, cognitive restructuring, and work with parents is, in their opinion, the treatment of choice for PTSD in childhood. King *et al.* (1999) evaluated the efficacy of child and caregiver participation in the CBT treatment of 36 sexually abused children aged 5–17 years who were suffering from PTSD. They reported significant improvements in PTSD symptoms and self-reports of fear and anxiety compared with controls. Maintenance of improvements was evident at a 12-week follow-up. In general, the involvement of parents did not enhance the efficacy of CBT. As is generally observed, there remains much research to be conducted on this disorder.

Obsessive-compulsive disorder

Studies of the results of using behaviour therapy for the once seemingly intractable symptoms of obsessive-compulsive disorder (OCD) have established its pre-eminence in work with adults (Foa & Meadows 1997). Despite less systematic evaluative research on children and (particularly) adolescents, it is probably fair to arrive at a similar, if guarded, verdict for them (Apter *et al.* 1984; Berg *et al.* 1989).

The essence of the method is that the patient voluntarily confronts the feared object or ideas, either directly or in imagination. At the same time he or she is strongly encouraged to refrain from ritualizing, with support provided by the therapist, and possibly by others (e.g. parents). A compulsive hand-washer may be encouraged to touch an object believed to be contaminated, and then urged to avoid washing for several hours until the anxiety provoked has decreased. Treatment then proceeds on a step-by-step basis, guided by the patient's ability to tolerate the anxiety and control the rituals. A more cognitively based therapeutic perspective emphasizes changing the patient's beliefs and thought patterns. The phenomenology of the disorder incorporates cognitive distortion involving risk appraisal and responsibility (Rachman 1993). It is suggested that obsessions persist as long as such misinterpretations continue. A review of the literature is available in Francis & Gragg (1996) and March & Mulle (1998).

Depression

The need for a broad-based intervention with depressive problems seems to be the conclusion of available studies (Kazdin 1990). Tricyclic medication, behaviour therapy, counselling, psychotherapy and cognitive therapy appear to be the main options, singly or in combination. Depressed patients tend to manifest a high rate of intrusive negative thoughts, including selective ruminations about past events that were unhappy, thoughts about the hopelessness of the future, and their own helplessness. It would therefore seem plausible as a therapeutic strategy to combine cognitive-behavioural methods (which enhance their self-esteem and self-empowerment) with drugs, where indicated. The evidence certainly suggests that this is indeed the case (Butler *et al.* 1980; Stark *et al.* 1987; Kazdin 1990; Moore & Carr 2000a,b). However, many of the treatment outcome studies on depressed children involve non-referred children manifesting depressive symptoms. When compared with non-treatment controls, cognitive behavioural methods are beneficial in reducing these symptoms. Cognitive restructuring, role-playing, self-control training and problem-solving tend to predominate in these studies, but what the necessary and/or sufficient 'therapeutic ingredients' are in such multiple component programmes remains uncertain (Kazdin 1990). It is also unclear how these approaches would generalize to clinical populations.

When it comes to adolescence, changing life-tasks and levels of cognitive, emotional and social maturity call for age-appropriate developmental perspectives when confronting depression (Reynolds & Coats 1986; Lewinsohn *et al.* 1990). A multimethod approach (usually involving CBT and, not infrequently, medication), both chosen on the basis of a comprehensive clinical assessment, remains currently the most successful way of dealing with adolescent depression.

Disruptive behaviour disorders

Oppositional/non-compliance problems

Problems of disobedience are commonplace in children as they grow up. However, there is a typical developmental progression in which certain children start to show extreme oppositional and argumentative behaviour early in life, and then gradually progress up a figurative pyramid of increasingly more severe patterns of aggressive, nonconformist, disruptive behaviour (Frick 1998). There are prognostic and treatment implications arising from two developmental pathways to the fully fledged condition:

1 the children mentioned above (with childhood onset conduct disorders); and
2 a substantial number of young people who begin showing antisocial behaviour as they approach adolescence, with little or no history of oppositional behaviour during childhood.
The young people who begin showing conduct problems in adolescence are less likely to persist in their antisocial behaviour in adulthood (Farrington 1995).

Positive parenting practices, notably appropriate and timely transactions between mothers and their young children, are the key to a child's willingness to comply with the demands of the socialization process (Dix 1991). Failure is costly to parents and a blight, in the long run, on the lives of seriously uncontrolled children who suffer from oppositional-defiant disorder (Loeber &

Hay 1997; Herbert 2000). Here then is a powerful incentive to intervene early with effective remedial or preventive programmes.

Oppositional-defiant disorder

Positive parenting is commonly assessed by behaviour therapists within the framework of reinforcement theory: the provision of information, attention or approval presented following the child's prosocial actions, but withheld following inappropriate actions (Herbert 1987b). Those with reasonably obedient children give more so-called alpha commands that are characterized by being specific and direct, given one at a time and followed by a wait of 5 s. Parents of children with oppositional-defiant disorder (ODD), who give more negative commands than parents of 'normal' youngsters, can be taught to use these alpha commands rather than their ineffectual beta variety which include chain commands, vague commands and question commands (Forehand & McMahon 1981).

Developmental theorists emphasize a more general influence on socialization drawn from social attachment theory, namely the concept of 'responsiveness'. Behavioural theorists have interpreted this construct within an expanded reinforcement framework (Wahler & Meginnis 1997). There is experimental evidence indicating the weakness of maternal praise as a positive reinforcer for compliance from children with conduct problems. Wahler & Megginis (1997) are of the opinion that the potential impact of maternal feedback is inherently governed by the mother's general responsiveness, and that praise and mirroring are simply components of this attribute. It is suggested that the dual operation of specific positive reinforcement (praise) and responsive feedback are required in reducing non-compliance in children, with or without more serious conduct problems. As yet no proven method for encouraging responsiveness is available. However, programmes attending to the needs of parents alongside discussion of the needs of their children show some promise (Herbert & Wookey 1998).

Mealtime and bedtime difficulties

Oppositional mealtime activities that cause concern are refusing food, fiddling with it, leaving the table, producing a tantrum, crying and complaining. The effectiveness of a range of behavioural treatment procedures has been demonstrated for reducing such disruptive activity and the duration of meals, while increasing food intake (Ireton & Guthrie 1972). Serketich & Dumas (1996) conducted a meta-analysis of over 100 studies of behavioural parent training and found it a highly effective intervention for childhood oppositional behaviour problems.

Behavioural management techniques applied to settling and waking difficulties have been found to be successful in 90% of children between 1 and 5 years old (Richman *et al.* 1985). Douglas & Richman (1984) produced a manual for bedtime problems that has been successfully used by health visitors and in community clinics. Individual or group behavioural programmes attending to both antecedents (commands) and consequences (reinforcement) in the ABC equation illustrated in Fig. 53.1, produce better generalization of effects. Attention to each side of the equation provides the parent with constructive skills (Forehand & McMahon 1981).

Guidelines for setting up behavioural programmes for the oppositional/non-compliance problems associated with mealtimes and bedtime difficulties, respectively, have been prepared for practitioners and parents by Herbert (1996a).

Conduct disorders

Children with conduct disorders, with their extremes of aggressive antisocial behaviour, are capable of wreaking havoc in their own and other people's lives, and their prevalencies are probably on the increase, creating a need for a therapeutic service that outstrips the resources available (Herbert 1995). A large percentage of the 'early starter' children with conduct problems are likely to remain circulating through the revolving door of the social services, mental health agencies and criminal justice systems (Loeber & Hay 1997). Many different types of intervention have been applied to children and adolescent youths with conduct disorders. But, as Kazdin (1998) observed, little outcome evidence exists for most of the techniques. Four treatments, in his opinion, with the most promising evidence to date are problem-solving skills training, functional family therapy, multisystemic therapy, and parent management training (also known as behavioural parent training).

Behavioural parent training

With regard to behavioural parent training (BPT), the developmental literature provides some useful guidelines to supplement behavioural theory in parent consultation work. Factors that facilitate prosocial behaviour include a rich supply of positive reinforcement for positive behaviour, 'fuelled' by a strong attachment to a caregiver with whom a child can therefore identify; firm moral demands made by parents upon their offspring; the consistent use of sanctions; techniques of punishment that are psychological rather than physical (methods which signify or threaten withdrawal of approval); and an intensive use of inductive methods, such as reasoning and explanations.

Today there is less emphasis in BPT on the contingency management of specific target behaviours, and more on broad principles of child management. Attention is also paid to enhancement work on the interpersonal interactions of members of the family, the perceived efficacy of parents and the marital relations which are often fraught. Parents, individually or in groups, are encouraged and guided to increase their positive interactions with their children through the use of play and other special/quality time activities, and by looking for the positives in their actions. They are encouraged to reinforce their children's appropriate behaviour with praise, encouragement and other rewards; also to introduce the child to behaviours that are either intrinsically reinforcing, or which make previously unattainable reinforcements available. Homework practice tasks help parents to limit unnecessary commands, to increase the clarity of their house rules and the consistency with which they follow them through. Parents are guided to implement brief mild non-aggressive sanctions, such as judicious ignoring, time-out, loss of privileges and logical consequences. They are provided with the means of understanding and analysing problematic behaviour; in addition, they role-play negotiation and problem-solving strategies in order to avoid what were previously corrosive confrontational situations. The techniques studied and rehearsed in groups include planned ignoring, time-out, alpha commands, praise, differential attention, response-cost, logical consequences, and use of tokens and recording charts. Parents are encouraged to monitor their children's activities effectively (Dishion & McMahon 1998).

Behavioural parent training programmes have been put under the microscope of many validational studies (for reviews of highly successful applications see Webster-Stratton 1991; Kazdin 1998; Brestan & Eyberg 1998). Brestan & Eyberg (1998), applying rigorous evaluative criteria, identified two particularly 'well-established' treatments: Patterson & Gullion's (1968) *Living With Children* programme, and Webster-Stratton's (1988) Group Discussion Video Modelling Programme, the latter providing videotapes with examples of multiethnic American parents with their 'problematic' children 'doing it right' and 'getting it wrong', the vignettes leading to group discussions and homework exercises.

Other behaviourally based approaches include behavioural marital therapy (Jacobson & Margolin 1979; Baucom *et al.* 1998); behavioural casework (Herbert 1993), and treatment fostercare (Chamberlain 1994). Cognitive marital therapy focuses on helping couples challenge negative beliefs and attributions in their relationships. There is evidence that low general marital satisfaction is correlated with a variety of child outcomes, in particular for conduct problems of childhood (Sanders 1996; Browne & Herbert 1997; Webster-Stratton & Hammond 1999). Dadds *et al.* (1987) demonstrated that although couples who were high or low in marital discord showed similar levels of improvements with child management training, couples high in marital discord had greater difficulty maintaining the gains made unless they received partner support training as well. This is where behavioural marital therapy or couple therapy may be useful. Meta-analyses of behavioural and cognitive marital therapy indicate that the average treated case fares better than between 79 and 83% of untreated controls (Hahlweg & Markman 1988; Dunn & Schwebel 1995).

Operant methods

Behavioural approaches using reinforcement of desired behaviour in the classroom and home have been repeatedly demonstrated to lead to beneficial changes, albeit usually short-term and situation-specific, in disruptive behaviour, aggression, poor co-operation with peers and poor school attendance (Patterson 1982). Academic performance also responds to classroom reinforcement programmes (O'Leary & O'Leary 1977; Goldstein 1995).

Direct work with adolescents

The issue of parent training gives rise to a conceptual boundary problem. At what stage in childhood-onset conduct disorders does the practitioner shift the therapy paradigm from the so-called triadic model that involves caregivers as primary mediators of change to one that more appropriately deals with an individual in his or her own right (as in dyadic or group-based cognitive behaviour therapy)? A growing number of theorists acknowledge the significance of the cognitive representation of events and experiences in the development of conduct and delinquent disorders (Hollin 1990; Kendall & Hollon 1994).

Children and adolescents with these disorders tend to have difficulty anticipating consequences of their behaviour, attribute other's behaviour in ambiguous situations to their hostile intentions and underperceive their responsibility for early stages of dyadic conflict. These distortions are addressed in individual or group work with cognitive behavioural strategies (Herbert 1998b). For example, there are anger-management programmes designed specifically for adolescents (Feindler & Ecton 1986). Most of them consist of three stages, cognitive preparation, skill acquisition and application training, the intention being to lower the likelihood of aggressive behaviour by increasing awareness of the signs of incipient hostile arousal and by encouraging self-control.

Attention deficit hyperactivity disorder

There are several commonly used approaches in dealing with ADHD, a problem often associated (comorbid) with conduct disorders in childhood:

1 creating and maintaining a well-structured ('prosthetic') environment to compensate for poor stimulus control;

2 behaviour therapy (notably operant techniques to shape up prosocial behaviour);

3 CBT to enhance poor information processing and self-control; and

4 stimulant medication, which can be combined with each of the above.

Multiple problems are the rule, and demand the sort of multimodal assessment and treatment that, in turn, requires co-operation between child psychiatry, psychology, paediatrics and education (Richters et al. 1995). The heterogeneity of ADHD makes it imperative to assess a variety of underlying causes, such as family conditions (physical, social, psychological), attachment difficulties, emotional problems, learning disabilities and physical impairments.

Behavioural parent and teacher training programmes, and structured programmes of contingency management, are the main and most successful psychosocial interventions, especially when combined with medication (methylphenidate). Nolan & Carr (2000) have reported a review of 20 multimodal programmes. A CBT component usually entails a stop–think–do training programme conducted by the therapist or parents. There have been many favourable reports promoting this method (Braswell & Bloomquist 1991; Kendall 1994; Kendall & Gosch 1994). See Barkley (1995) and Taylor (1997) for parent-friendly guides to the management of this daunting problem.

Ecological approaches

Structural causes that undermine parenting and family life, such as poor housing, inner-city deprivation and alienation, contribute to the development of conduct disorders. An example of a broadband ecological approach is the Early Alliance Programme conducted by Dumas et al. (1999). They describe an integrated set of four preventive interventions which are delivered across multiple domains of functioning and across multiple social settings, designed to promote competence and reduce risk of early-onset conduct disorder, substance abuse, and school failure (see also Borduin et al. 1995 on the multisystemic treatment of juvenile offenders).

Delinquency

Although not all young persons adjudicated as delinquent suffer from conduct disorders, nor the reverse, there is a substantial overlap and the antisocial groups treated by behavioural methods tend often to merge. Major reviews of behavioural interventions suggest that individual behaviour therapy is not a popular option for practitioners dealing with offender populations. However, there have been reports of limited successes (Herbert 1987b; Kazdin et al. 1992).

Therapists have drawn on communication skills as one of their treatment targets within multimodal interventions. The package might involve communication training, feedback, positive interruptions, problem-solving and decision-making skills, providing rationales, happy talk, positive requests, non-blaming communication, negotiation skill-training, didactic dialogue and family games. The behavioural methods are likely to include self-correction, overcorrection, positive practice, observation and recording behaviour, self-management, cognitive restructuring, positive reinforcement, differential attention, response-cost, time-out, and the use of symbolic rewards (tokens and points). Contracts are drawn up defining goals and mutual obligations (Alexander & Parsons 1982). Among the best known multimodal cognitive-behavioural programmes is Aggression Replacement Training (ART; Glick & Goldstein 1987), which includes three main approaches to changing behaviour: structured life-skills learning (social skills and social problem-solving), anger control training and moral education. Outcome studies indicate that the programmes have led to improved skills, improved self-control and more acceptable institutional behaviour. A programme based on ART by Leeman *et al.* (1993) was successful in improving conduct problems and reducing recidivism.

There are encouraging demonstrations on a variety of quantitative and qualitative outcome measures (notably behavioural indices, cognitive functioning, family relationships, and different academic and social skills) that short-term changes can be achieved by using techniques like these. However, there is less room for optimism about the longer term benefits and, in the case of delinquent youngsters, about any significant generalization from general disruptive behaviour to specifically offending activities.

Developmental problems

Enuresis

Butler (1998) comments on one of the reasons why enuresis provides such an interesting challenge: the fact that with its clearly defined dependent variable (a 'cure' rather than the usual 'improvement' criterion of success) it offers an ideal opportunity to test out particular theories and models. The evidence for the superiority of the urine alarm method (with rates of remission between 80 and 90%) over no treatment and other treatment control procedures is well documented for nocturnal enuresis (Doleys 1977, 1978). Doleys' (1977) review of data, based on over 600 subjects, revealed an average relapse rate of 40%; but nearly 60% of these returned to continence after booster sessions. Less specific psychotherapeutic interventions, such as individual or family therapy, have proved to be no more effective than no-treatment control conditions or other forms of treatment (Ondersma & Walker 1998). However, a meta-analysis by Houts *et al.* (1994), in reporting that the highest success rates for psychological programmes were those using urine alarms, found them no more effective than the medical treatments (e.g. tricyclics) at post-treatment, although they were significantly superior at follow-up.

Butler (1998) provides a helpful review of the advantages of the enuresis alarm, and some of the practical difficulties that hinder the realistic expectation of success. Many clinicians prefer to begin treatment with the use of incentive sticker charts, adding components such as the urine alarm if the child does not respond. A detailed description of behavioural and combined methods of treating nocturnal and diurnal enuresis has been prepared for practitioners and parents by Herbert (1996b).

Encopresis (soiling)

Encopresis has been treated by a variety of methods, but not with comparable success. Family therapy has not proved useful without the addition of behavioural, dietary and/or a medical intervention (Walker 1995). Individual psychotherapy has not

been demonstrated to be more effective than no therapy (Doleys 1977). Doleys (1978), in his review of treatment studies, reported that 93% of cases were successfully treated by the use of behavioural methods. Researchers have recommended the combination of behavioural techniques and laxatives in the common 'retention with overflow' cases of encopresis (Firestonean & Koplewicz 1992; Herbert 1996b). This short-term treatment protocol involves an assessment of possible fear elements (constipation may make toileting painful), an initial clean-out phase (usually with laxatives), psychoeducational input, scheduled toilet sittings, cleanliness training, mild penalties for inappropriate behaviour, and positive reinforcement of appropriate toileting behaviour (e.g. for 'effort') and for not soiling. Fibre intake and other dietary issues are aspects of treatment (for reports of successful programmes see also Stark *et al.* 1990; Nolan *et al.* 1991).

Psychophysiological disorders

Anorexia and bulimia nervosa

The operant paradigm generally applied to this potentially life-threatening disorder includes, *inter alia*, restricting the anorexic patient to his or her room and making activities and privileges contingent on weight gain. Those who advocate operant methods claim that they produce faster and larger weight gains during hospitalization than do other medically or psychiatrically orientated techniques. Some of the most painstaking outcome studies have investigated operant procedures aimed at rapid weight restoration. What emerges (see review by Harris & Phelps 1987) is that behavioural interventions focusing solely on this goal are not sufficient to accommodate the many-sided subtlety and complexity of this puzzling condition, and are not particularly effective in the longer term. Short-term gains may be made more durable by interventions that address issues such as interpersonal problem-solving and the dynamics of low self-esteem (e.g. cognitive-restructuring, conversational therapy). Systematic desensitization has been used to mitigate the anorexic individual's extreme fear of obesity (Ollendick 1979). Ollendick combines systematic desensitization with cognitive restructuring (see also Garner & Bemis 1985).

Treatment approaches to bulimia have involved group therapy (Boskind-Lodahl & White 1978), interpersonal therapy (Fairburn 1995) and behaviour therapy interventions (Fairburn 1980, 1981; Linden 1980; Mizes 1995). Results indicated that bulimic individuals exhibiting the most severe symptoms over the longest periods of time were (unsurprisingly) the least responsive to treatment. Cognitive-behavioural treatments appear to be the most effective, with little relapse after improvement (see review by Mizes 1995). In general, patients reduce their frequency of bingeing and purging by 75–80%, with 30–40% ceasing altogether to binge and purge.

Child abuse

Azar & Wolfe (1989) have described several factors that make the treatment of children with abusing families difficult. One is the tendency to focus on eliminating a circumscribed problem when, in fact, the abusive events are highly complex (Wolfe & Birt 1995; Babiker & Herbert 1998). Interventions with parents usually involve elements of self-control training (e.g. anger management), problem-solving, and the encouragement of proximity-seeking and attachment behaviour (Iwaniec *et al.* 1988). Of necessity, they usually need to tackle wider systemic (family) issues. The treatment targets might include the following.

1 *Characteristics of the parents*: alcohol abuse; deficits in bonding and child-rearing skills, faulty expectations of the child; low self-esteem; ineffective communication; poor reinforcement skills; punitive attitudes, and failure to supervise the child.

2 *Characteristics of the child*: problems involving hyperactivity, non-compliance and aggression; incontinence; inappropriately inflexible responses to different situations; disability.

3 *Unique interactions of the child and his or her parents*: coercive/aversive communications; mutual avoidance; inappropriate, inconsistent or non-contingent reinforcement/punishment.

4 *Significant others in the family*: interference, subversion of maternal authority by grandparent; sexual/physical abuse by relative/lodger, etc.

5 *Environmental factors*: poverty, overcrowding, social isolation.

Specific techniques to implement these goals are detailed in Herbert (1987a, 1993) and Deblinger & Heflin (1996). The findings from several studies of BPT in child-protection work have indicated improved child care and management, and/or a reduction in the reoccurrence of child abuse. Wolfe & Wekerle (1993) concluded on the basis of a review that cognitive-behavioural approaches enjoyed a consistent success rate at helping maltreating parents improve several of the conditions that predispose them to abusive and neglectful treatment of their children. All such programmes produced improvements in parenting skills; for example, in their ability to interact positively with their children and control behaviour without over-reliance on negative physically coercive child management techniques. Reassessment after treatment and at follow-up (generally 3 months–1 year) tended to support the maintenance and generalization of these changes. Abuse or neglect did not recur among treatment families in those studies reporting significant outcome data.

King *et al.* (1999) made the point that among the plethora of psychological symptoms that appear in the wake of child sexual abuse, several are characteristic of PTSD. Their review of the cognitive-behavioural treatment of sexually abused children, drawing on case studies, open clinical trials, multiple baseline investigations and randomized clinical trials, suggests that the efficacy findings are 'encouraging'.

The characteristics of the dysfunctional thoughts of abused children that lead to anxiety are that they repetitively construe events as harmful or dangerous, that they cannot be 'reasoned away', and that they become readily attached to a wide range of stimuli that can elicit them. Jehu (1992) has demonstrated clearly how important negative schemas are in the long-term sequelae of sexual abuse, explaining why some young females develop severe anxiety disorders that persist into adulthood, while others remain relatively unscathed. Here would seem to be the opportunity to do remedial and/or preventive cognitive-behavioural work with maltreated children and adolescents.

Stevenson's (1999) review of meta-analytic studies of controlled trials for mental health treatments in child abuse cases indicated that the mean effect sizes have a range from 0.45 for the impact of family therapy on family interaction to 0.96 for the efficacy of behavioural treatments (Stevenson 1999, p. 96). He states that '. . . the same treatments that are most efficacious (behavioural and cognitive methods) and least efficacious (non-behavioural methods) with adults (Shapiro & Shapiro 1982) are also, respectively, the most and least efficacious for children' (Stevenson 1999, p. 97).

Can we simply treat the problems of abused children as complex disorders regardless of their particular causal path? Holmes' (1995) finding that, within a group of adults being treated for anxiety and depression, the various psychological therapies being applied were very effective for patients without a history of abuse but ineffective for those with such a history makes such an assumption somewhat questionable.

Discussion

Unanswered questions

There are many content and process issues in behavioural work that require clarification by future researchers. The questions are not only concerned with the effective strategies in behavioural therapy, but also the impact of treatment style of working. Does a collaborative style of working achieve better and longer lasting results than the expert model? And, if so, under what circumstances and by utilizing what particular strategies? What are the sufficient and necessary therapeutic elements that make a particular method effective? What can be done to mitigate the learned helplessness of some patients or overcome resistance to therapy? What is required to reduce high attrition rates or modify intractable attributions that effectively exculpate parents from accepting that they have any influence on, or responsibility for, their offspring's actions? These are but a few of the issues that await answers.

Status of behavioural therapy

We have seen examples of the wide range of methods, and the diversity of child and family problems, to which contemporary behavioural therapies are applied. They incorporate, in addition to the original aetiologically simplistic conditioning theories, procedures and principles derived from more complex conceptual models, such as social and developmental psychology and cognitive science (Kazdin 1978).

Nevertheless, behavioural therapy has maintained a surprising degree of cohesiveness, perhaps because of its steadfast commitment to the importance of empirical validation. The behavioural therapies have been investigated and evaluated more intensively than any other psychological interventions, but it is a moot point as to which ones meet all the requirements set out in Paul's (1967) criteria. As he describes them: 'What treatment, by whom, is most effective for this individual with that specific problem, and under which set of circumstances' (Paul 1967, p. 111). Yet Taylor & Biglan (1998) considered that behavioural family therapy methods are, along with other behavioural interventions, highly compatible with the emerging trends towards time-limited treatments which are empirically supported and which painstakingly document programme gains (Taylor & Biglan 1998, p. 49; see also Carr 2000 and Target & Fonagy 1996). Comparisons with client-centred methods, psychodynamic therapy, systemic and structural family therapy, Adlerian methods, and Parental Effectiveness Training indicate the advantage of giving priority to behavioural parent training and behavioural family therapy (Webster-Stratton 1991; Brestan & Eyberg 1998). The consideration paid to a child's social and interpersonal context (vital features in parent management training and behavioural family therapy, when dealing with externalizing disorders) appears to be equally significant in the treatment of internalizing (e.g. anxiety) conditions. Here there is also an encouragingly high success rate (Kendall 1998; Ollendick *et al*. 1998).

Future directions

Kazdin (1997) acknowledged that among the important questions yet to be addressed (his remarks apply to the conduct disorders but they have wider clinical relevance) are the magnitude of change and durability of treatment effects. These give rise to issues about how to evaluate treatment and about the status of any particular intervention. As he put it:

> We cannot yet say that one intervention can ameliorate conduct disorder and overcome the poor long-term prognosis. On the other hand, much can be said. Much of what is practised in clinical settings is based on psychodynamically orientated treatment, general relationship counselling, family therapy and group therapy (with antisocial youths as members). These and other procedures, alone and in various combinations in which they are often used, have not been evaluated carefully in controlled trials. Of course, absence of evidence is not tantamount to ineffectiveness. At the same time, promising treatments have advanced considerably and a very special argument might be needed to administer treatments that have neither basic research on their conceptual underpinnings in relation to conduct disorder nor outcome evidence from controlled clinical trials on their behalf. (Kazdin 1997, p. 175).

One might add that there is an ethical imperative that patients should not be exposed to invalid or unvalidated therapies.

Kazdin (1988) stated that to ensure progress, those processes that are considered to be responsible for therapeutic change ought to be assessed directly and to a high level of specificity, and codified ideally in treatment manual format. Replication in research and clinical practice requires knowing precisely the details of a treatment programme. There has to be a balance of clear manual guidelines, possibilities for improvization, and space for individual therapist differences: a challenging task. Kazdin (1998) is of the opinion that difficult though it may be, it would be a mistake to think that facets of treatment and their implementation ought not (or cannot) be made explicit and codified. In today's health and other services, with their growing demand for empirically supported treatment procedures, simultaneous efforts are needed in order to educate practitioners and policymakers about what constitutes proper empirical validation (Taylor & Biglan 1998).

Most outcome research involves demonstrations of efficacy rather than demonstrations of effectiveness or clinical utility. Efficacy studies are directed at establishing whether a particular intervention works (e.g. reduces symptoms, increases adaptive functioning) and they are usually conducted under tightly controlled conditions. Effectiveness, or clinical utility studies, are directed at establishing how well a particular intervention works in the environments, and under the conditions, in which treatment is typically offered (Lonigan *et al*. 1998). Such studies, unfortunately, are in short supply.

Search for integrative concepts

The search for theoretical coherence for contemporary behaviour therapy, with its wide conceptual base, remains unresolved (Power 1991). Kendall & Lochman (1994) claimed that CBTs present a broader convergence of concepts in their rationale than is achieved in most other approaches. They state that: '. . . they integrate cognitive, behavioural, affective, social and contextual strategies for change . . . the cognitive-behavioural model includes the relationships of cognition and behaviour to the affective state of the organism and the functioning of the organism in the larger social context' (Kendall & Lockman 1994, p. 844). Where, however, do we find a theoretical framework to integrate the models drawn from various branches of experimental psychology referred to above, or to accommodate ideas from the growing alliance of family therapy, cognitive therapy, psychotherapy, and behaviour therapy? It is not enough simply to link up, without definition, the names (e.g. 'behavioural cognitive psychotherapy') of somewhat disparate approaches. There is a risk that practice degenerates into an atheoretical ragbag of ad hoc techniques.

A rationale for many practitioners, at its broadest level, derives from the fact that all therapy is about change, and change implies learning. In that sense all therapies contain an element of learning in the form of workable applications. Goldstein *et al*. (1966, p. 63) propose that, whatever else it is, psychotherapy must be considered a learning enterprise involving specific behaviours, attitudes or even, possibly, a whole new outlook on life. Such an overinclusive definition can be made to explain everything, but predict (as is the case with psychoanalytic theory) nothing. Nor, unfortunately, does it serve to bind together into a theoretically coherent system, the many elements that make up contemporary behavioural practice.

Role of psychotherapy

Because of the remit of this chapter I have not been able to do justice to any of the interventions that come under the rubric of psychotherapy. Reviews of psychotherapy suggest that many of its concepts have been validated, and that it is better than no treatment for a large number of childhood problems (Lee & Herbert 1970; Kazdin 1988; Tuma 1989; Fonagy & Moran 1990; Weisz & Weiss 1993). Traditional psychotherapy is not a natural science, whereas behavioural work differs from psychotherapeutic traditions in finding its origins in controlled laboratory experiments on learning processes (Pavlov 1927; Skinner 1953; Ferster & De Myer 1962) rather than clinical casework (Freud 1916). It is an article of faith for behaviourally orientated psychologists who call themselves 'applied scientists' that explanations dealing with complex aspects of human functioning which tend to be more intuitive, literary or semantic than 'scientific' hinder the discovery of valid treatment methods.

This argument fails to impress those who are antipathetic to behaviour therapy. A scientific approach to treatment is rejected by some critics as impersonal, political and mechanistic. The putative ethical relativism of behaviour therapists is thought to imply an undue influence on the client towards received societal values. They are also regarded as disingenuous to claim an unswerving commitment to an epistemological model confined exclusively to learning theory (Erwin 1978; Power 1991). Wilson & Evans (1983) found that 22% of a sample ($n=118$) of members of the American Association for the Advancement of Behaviour Therapy formulated three written case-descriptions introducing psychodynamic and intrapsychic terminology.

Systemic thinking

A further objection arises from an obsolete view that behaviour therapy is very much a method of treatment aimed at the individual child, and therefore out of step with current systemic thinking. In fact, the systemic philosophy of family theory has had a significant influence on the development of behavioural practice. It was important for therapists to be more aware of the dynamics of family life, their contribution to the causation of childhood psychopathology, the role of children as family scapegoats ('symptom-carriers') and, when formulating the reasons for a member's behaviour, the fact that a family is more than the sum of its parts. Where non-behavioural family therapy has had modest results in dealing with children's psychological problems, the addition of a behavioural perspective has enhanced the success rate significantly, notably in dealing with externalizing

(disruptive) disorders (Gurman *et al.* 1986; Webster-Stratton 1991; Herbert 1998c).

What does not work?

Because the frontiers of behavioural therapy are still expanding it is difficult to answer the question: 'Which problems are not amenable to a behavioural approach?' The range of problems now tackled has been, and continues to be, broadened by its enlarged theoretical base. In terms of therapeutic process the more directive and performance-orientated style of the behavioural approach may simply not provide an appropriate universe of discourse for those who wish to discuss, in depth and in conversational mode, some personal problem. Given such a case, can judgements about what constitutes a 'successful' outcome be defined by conventional clinical criteria? According to humanistic ideologies, which feature often in counselling and psychotherapeutic work, the concerns on which the counsellor and client focus are precisely those excluded from scientific method.

Despite behavioural therapists' predilection for explicit and objective methods, Sloane *et al.* (1975) found that patients rated them at least as highly on interpersonal factors, such as warmth and empathy, as non-behavioural therapists. Bandura (1969) insists that the emphasis of behavioural therapy on explicit negotiated objectives and self-direction as therapeutic goals gives patients access to self-empowering knowledge and skills, which also represent a liberating therapeutic philosophy. A collaborative therapeutic process, as described by Webster-Stratton & Herbert (1994), underpins such a viewpoint.

Conclusions

This chapter has described contemporary behavioural therapies, bringing them (with their developmental, cognitive and systemic elaborations) up to date from their early behaviourist origins. It is now possible to claim with some confidence that in relation to child and adolescent mental health problems, such as anxiety, depression, ODD, conduct disorders, ADHD, OCD, and developmental problems such as enuresis and encopresis, behavioural programmes are among the favoured interventions. For these and other conditions (notably learning disability, anorexia and autism) there are circumstances, following a comprehensive assessment, where a multimodal or multisystemic programme is likely to be enhanced by a behavioural component. There is, inevitably, a continuing need for good programme designs based, because so many clinical child disorders are heterogeneous in nature, on multimodal assessment procedures and appropriate (quantitative and qualitative) outcome measures. Other requirements are built-in strategies to facilitate temporal and other forms of generalization.

Behavioural therapy research and service delivery programmes are conducted too often by inappropriately trained or minimally experienced individuals. Such a question mark over programme and professional 'integrity' reflects the need for agreed standards of competence in behavioural work, which means, in turn, the establishment of accredited multidisciplinary training courses. Some do exist, but they are few in number and do not meet the need for nationally organized training programmes.

The nature of systemic family work involves a partnership with family members, much discussion and debate. The inner life and subjective experiences of caregivers and children (beliefs, attributions, attitudes) are acknowledged to be important in the assessment and treatment of problems. In a very real, if informal sense, parents use behavioural methods in order to teach, influence and change the children in their care. Although parents are unfamiliar with the 'small print' and terminology of learning theory, behavioural methods, when explained carefully, do tend to have face validity for them. For those who believe in the advantages of a partnership model in work with families, this demystification of the therapeutic process is welcome.

For the author, behavioural therapy is a 'craft', an amalgam of applied science and art. There is, in fact, an impressive empirical knowledge base. However, the application of science is only part of the story. Because of the exigencies of clinical work it requires the 'spirit' of scientific method, rather than the restrictive 'letter' of what might be called 'scientism'. There should be room for creativity and divergent thinking. There is the art of teaching children, the skill of devising and using imaginative materials to capture their interest, and by means of a shared therapeutic alliance, the intuition to unravel complex problems with parents and their offspring, and the empathy to boost their confidence and self-esteem.

References

Achenbach, T.M. (1974) *Developmental Psychopathology.* Ronald Press, New York.

Alexander, J. & Parsons, B. (1982) *Functional Family Therapy.* Brooks Cole, Monterey, CA.

Apter, A., Berhout, E. & Tyano, S. (1984) Severe obsessive-compulsive disorder in adolescence: a report of eight cases. *Journal of Adolescence*, 1, 349–358.

Axline, V.M. (1947) *Play Therapy: The Inner Dynamics of Childhood.* Houghton Mifflin, Boston, MA.

Azar, S.T. & Wolfe, D. (1989) Child abuse. In: *Treatment of Childhood Disorders* (eds E.J. Marsh & R.A. Barkley). Guilford Press, New York.

Babiker, G. & Herbert, M. (1998) Critical issues in the assessment of child sexual abuse. *Clinical Child and Family Psychology Review*, 1, 231–252.

Baer, D.M., Wolf, M.M. & Risly, T.R. (1968) Some current dimensions of applied behavior analysis. *Journal of Applied Behavior Analysis*, 1, 91–97.

Bandura, A. (1969) *Principles of Behavior Modification.* Holt, Rinehart & Winston, New York.

Bandura, A. (1977) Self-efficacy: toward a unifying theory of behavioural change. *Psychological Review*, 84, 191–215.

Barkley, R. (1995) *Taking Charge of ADHD: The Complete Authoritative Guide for Parents.* Guilford Press, New York.

Barlow, D.H. & Hersen, M. (1984) Single-case experimental designs.

Strategies for Studying Behavior Change, 2nd edn. Pergamon, New York.

Berg, C.Z., Rapoport, J.L. & Wolff, R.P. (1989) Behavioral treatment for obsessive-compulsive disorder in children. In: *Obsessive Compulsive Disorder in Children and Adolescents* (ed. J.L. Rapoport). American Psychiatric Association, Washington D.C.

Bernal, M. & Klinnert, M. & Schultz, L. (1980) Outcome evaluation of behavioural parent training and client-centred parent counselling for children with conduct problems. *Journal of Applied Behavior Analysis*, 3, 677–691.

Blagg, N.R. (1987) *School Phobia and its Treatment.* Croom-Helm, London.

Blagg, N.R. & Yule, W. (1984) The behavioural treatment of school phobia: a comparative study. *Behaviour Research and Therapy*, 22, 119–127.

Borduin, C., Mann, B., Cone, L. *et al.* (1995) Multisystemic treatment of serious juvenile offenders. *Journal of Consulting and Clinical Psychology*, 63, 569–578.

Boskind-Lodahl, M. & White, W.C. (1978) The definition and treatment of bulimia in college women: a pilot study. *Journal of American College Health Association*, 27, 84–97.

Braswell, L. & Bloomquist, M. (1991) *Cognitive Behavioural Therapy for ADHD Children: Child, Family and School Interventions.* Guilford Press, New York.

Brestan, E.V. & Eyberg, S.M. (1998) Effective psychosocial treatment of conduct-disordered children and adolescents: 29 years, 82 studies, 5275 children. *Journal of Clinical Child Psychology*, 27, 180–189.

Brown, G.W. & Harris, T.O. (1989) *Life Events and Illness.* Unwin Hyman, London.

Browne, K. & Herbert, M. (1997) *Preventing Family Violence.* Wiley, Chichester.

Bruner, J.S. (1975) *Beyond the Information Given.* Allen and Unwin, London.

Butler, L., Miezitis, S., Friedman, A. & Cole, E. (1980) The effect of two school-based intervention programs on depressive symptoms in pre-adolescents. *American Educational Research Journal*, 17, 111–119.

Butler, R. (1998) Night wetting in children: psychological aspects [Annotation]. *Journal of Child Psychology and Psychiatry*, 39, 453–463.

Carr, A., ed. (2000) *What Works With Children and Adolescents?: A Critical Review of Psychological Interventions with Children, Adolescents, and Their Families.* Routledge, London.

Chamberlain P. (1994) *Family Connections: A Treatment Foster Care Model For Adolescents With Delinquency.* Eugene, Castalia, OR.

Chess, S. & Thomas, A. (1995) *Temperament in Clinical Practice.* Guilford Press, New York.

Christenson, A., Johnson, S. & Glasgow, R. (1980) Cost effectiveness in behavioral family therapy. *Behavior Therapy*, 11, 208–226.

Cicchetti, D., Toth, S. & Bush, M. (1983) Developmental psychopathology and incompetence in childhood: suggestions for intervention. In: *Advances in Clinical Child Psychology* (eds B.B. Lahey & A.E. Kazdin), Vol. 11. Plenum Press, New York.

Cunningham, C., Bremmer, R. & Boyle, M. (1995) Large groups community based parenting programmes for families of preschoolers at risk of disruptive behaviour disorders. *Journal of Child Psychology and Psychiatry*, 36, 1141–1160.

Dadds, M., Schwartz, S. & Sanders, M. (1987) Marital discord and treatment outcome in behavioural treatment of child conduct disorders. *Journal of Consulting and Clinical Psychology*, 55, 396–403.

Deblinger, E. & Heflin, A. (1996) *Treating Sexually Abused Children and their Non-offending Parents: A Cognitive-behavioral Approach.* Sage, Thousand Oaks, CA.

Dishion, T.J. & McMahon, R.J. (1998) Parental monitoring and the prevention of child and adolescent problem behavior: a conceptual and empirical formulation. *Clinical Child and Family Psychology Review*, **1**, 61–75.

Dix, T. (1991) Effective organizing of parenting: adaptive and maladaptive processes. *Psychological Bulletin*, **110**, 3–25.

Doleys, D.M. (1977) Behavioral treatments for nocturnal enuresis in children: a review of the recent literature. *Psychological Bulletin*, **84**, 30–54.

Doleys, D.M. (1978) Assessment and treatment of enuresis and encopresis in children. In: *Progress in Behavior Modification* (eds M. Hersen, R.M. Eisler & P.M. Miller*)*, Vol. 6. Academic Press, New York.

Douglas, J. & Richman, N. (1984) *My Child Won't Sleep*. Penguin, Harmondsworth.

Dumas, J.E., Prinz, R.J. & Phillips Smith, E. & Laughlin, J. (1999) The Early Alliance Prevention Trial: an integrative set of interventions to promote competence and reduce risk for conduct disorder, substance abuse, and school failure. *Clinical Child and Family Psychology Review*, **2**, 37–53.

Dunn, R. & Schwebel, A. (1995) Meta-analytic review of marital therapy outcome research. *Journal of Family Psychology*, **9**, 58–68.

Elliott, J.G. (1999) School refusal: Issues of conceptualisation, assessment and treatment. *Journal of Child Psychology and Psychiatry*, **40**, 1001–1012.

Erwin, E. (1978) *Behaviour Therapy: Scientific, Philosophical and Moral Foundations*. Cambridge University Press, Cambridge.

Evans, I.M. (1989) A multi-dimensional model for conceptualizing for the design of child behavior therapy. *Behavioural Psychotherapy*, **17**, 237–251.

Eysenck, H.J. (1960) The conditioning model of neurosis. *Behavioural and Brain Science*, **2**, 155–199.

Fairburn, C.G. (1980) Self-induced vomiting. *Journal of Psychosomatic Research*, **24**, 193–197.

Fairburn, C.G. (1981) A cognitive-behavioral approach to the treatment of bulimia. *Psychological Medicine*, **11**, 707–711.

Fairburn, C.G. (1995) *Overcoming Binge Eating*. Guilford Press, New York.

Farrington, D. (1995) The Twelfth Jack Tizard Memorial Lecture. The development of offending behaviour from childhood. *Journal of Child Psychology and Psychiatry*, **36**, 929–964.

Feindler, E.L. & Ecton, R.B. (1986) *Adolescent Anger Control: Cognitive-behavioral Techniques*. Pergamon Press, Elmsford, NY.

Ferster, C.B. & De Myer, M.K. (1962) A method for the experimental analysis of the behavior of autistic children. *American Journal of Orthopsychiatry*, **32**, 89–98.

Firestonean, G. & Koplewicz, H.S. (1992) Short-term treatment of children with encopresis. *Journal of Psychotherapy Practice and Research*, **1**, 64–71.

Foa, E.B. & Meadows, E.A. (1997) Psychosocial treatments for post-traumatic stress disorder: a critical review. *Annual Review of Psychology*, **48**, 449–480.

Fonagy, P. & Moran, G.S. (1990) Studies of the efficacy of child psychoanalysis. *Journal of Consulting and Clinical Psychology*, **58**, 684–695.

Forehand, R. & McMahon, R. (1981) *Helping the Noncompliant Child: A Clinician's Guide to Parent Training*. Guilford Press, New York.

Francis, G. & Gragg, R. (1996) *Obsessive Compulsive Disorder*. Sage, Thousand Oaks, CA.

Francis, R.D. (1999*) Ethics for Psychologists: A Handbook*. British Psychological Society (BPS) Books, Leicester.

Freud, S. (1916*) Introductory Lectures on Psychoanalysis*, Vol. 16.

Standard Edition of Sigmund Freud's Works (ed. J. Strachey). Hogarth Press/Institute of Psychoanalysis, London.

Frick, P.J. (1998) Conduct disorders. In: *Handbook of Child Psychopathology* (eds T.H. Ollendick & M. Hersen), 3rd edn. Plenum Press, New York.

Gambrill, E. (1977) *Behavior Modification*. Jossey-Bass, New York.

Garner, D.M. & Bemis, K.M. (1985) Cognitive therapy for anorexia nervosa. In: *Handbook of Psychotherapy for Anorexia and Bulimia* (eds D. Garner & P.E. Garfinkel). Guilford Press, New York.

Glick, B. & Goldstein, A.P. (1987) Aggression replacement training. *Journal of Counseling and Development*, **65**, 356–367.

Goldstein, B.P., Heller, H. & Sechrest, L.B. (1966) *Psychotherapy and the Psychology of Behavior Change*. Wiley, New York.

Goldstein, S., ed. (1995) *Understanding and Managing Children's Classroom Behaviour*. Wiley, New York.

Goodnow, J.J. & Collins, A.W. (1990) *Development According to Parents: The Nature, Source and Consequences of Parents' Ideas*. Erlbaum, Hillsdale, NJ.

Gurman, A.S., Kniskern, D.P. & Pinsof, W.M. (1986) Research in the process of marital and family therapy. In: *Handbook of Psychotherapy and Behavior Change* (eds S.L. Garfield & A.E. Beergin), 3rd edn. Wiley, New York.

Hahlweg, K. & Markman, H. (1988) Effectiveness of behavioral marital therapy: empirical status of behavioral techniques for preventing and alleviating marital distress. *Journal of Consulting and Clinical Psychology*, **56**, 440–447.

Harris, F.C. & Phelps, C.F. (1987) Eating disorders. In: *Cognitive-behavioural Treatment of Anxiety Disorders* (eds L. Michelson & M. Archer). Guilford Press, New York.

Herbert, M. (1974) *Emotional Problems of Development in Children*. Academic Press, London.

Herbert, M. (1987a) *Behavioural Treatment of Children with Problems: A Practice Manual*, 2nd edn. Academic Press, London.

Herbert, M. (1987b) *Conduct Disorders of Childhood and Adolescence*, 2nd edn. Wiley, Chichester.

Herbert, M. (1993) *Working With Children and the Children Act*. British Psychological Society (BPS) Books, Leicester.

Herbert, M. (1995) A collaborative model of training for parents of children with disruptive behaviour disorders. *British Journal of Clinical Psychology*, **34**, 325–342.

Herbert, M. (1996a) *Coping with Children's Feeding Problems and Bedtime Battles*. British Psychological Society (BPS) Books, Leicester.

Herbert, M. (1996b) *Toilet Training, Bedwetting and Soiling*. British Psychological Society (BPS) Books, Leicester.

Herbert, M. (1998a) *Clinical Child Psychology: Social Learning, Development and Behaviour*, 2nd edn. Wiley, Chichester.

Herbert, M. (1998b) Cognitive behaviour therapy of adolescents with conduct disorders. In: *Cognitive Behaviour Therapy for Children and Adolescents* (ed. P. Graham*)*. Cambridge University Press, Cambridge.

Herbert, M. (1998c) Family treatment. In: *Handbook of Child Psychopathology* (eds T. Ollendick & M. Hersen*)*, 3rd edn. Plenum Press, New York.

Herbert, M. (2000) Children in control. In: *Family Support: Direction from Diversity* (eds J. Canavan, P. Dolan & J. Pinkerton). Croom-Helm, London.

Herbert, M. (2001) *Typical and Atypical Development: From Conception to Adolescence*. Blackwell Publishers, Oxford.

Herbert, M. & Wookey, J. (1998) *Childwise Parenting Skills Manual* (Revised edn.). Impact Publications, Exeter.

Hersen, M. (1981) Complex problems require complex solutions. *Behaviour Therapy*, **12**, 15–29.

Hollin, C.R. (1990) *Cognitive-behavioral Interventions with Young Offenders*. Pergamon, New York.

Holmes, T.R. (1995) History of child-abuse: a key variable in client response to short-term treatment. *Families in Society: the Journal of Contemporary Human Services*, 76, 349–359.

Houts, A.C., Berman, J.S. & Abramson, H. (1994) Effectiveness of psychological and pharmacological treatments for nocturnal enuresis. *Journal of Child Psychology and Psychiatry*, 39, 307–322.

Ireton, C.L. & Guthrie, H.A. (1972) Modification of vegetable eating behavior in pre-school children. *Journal of Nutrition Education*, 4, 100–103.

Iwaniec, D., Herbert, M. & Sluckin, A. (1988) Helping emotionally abused children who fail to thrive. In: *Early Prediction and Prevention of Child Abuse* (eds K. Brown, C. Davies & P. Stratton). Wiley, Chichester.

Jacobson, N. & Margolin, G. (1979) *Marital Therapy: Strategies Based on Social Learning and Behavioural Exchange Principles*. Brunner Mazel, New York.

Jehu, D. (1992) Adult survivors of sexual abuse. In: *Assessment of Family Violence: a Clinical and Legal Source Book* (eds R.T. Ammerman & M. Hersen). Wiley, New York.

Jones, M.C. (1924) A laboratory study of fear: the case of Peter. *Journal of Genetic Psychology*, 31, 308–315.

Joseph, S., Williams, R. & Yule, W. (1997) *Understanding Post-traumatic Stress: A Psychosocial Perspective on PTSD and Treatment*. Wiley, Chichester.

Kanfer, F.H., Karoly, P. & Newman, A. (1975) Reduction of children's fear of the dark by competence-related and situational threat-related verbal cues. *Journal of Consulting and Clinical Psychology*, 43, 251–258.

Kazdin, A.E. (1978) *History of Behavior Modification*. University Park Press, Baltimore.

Kazdin, A.E. (1988) *Child Psychotherapy: Developing and Identifying Effective Treatments*. Pergamon Press, Oxford.

Kazdin, A.E. (1990) Childhood depression. *Journal of Child Psychology and Psychiatry*, 31, 121–160.

Kazdin, A.E. (1998) Psychosocial treatments for conduct disorder in children. In: *A Guide to Treatments That Work* (eds P. Nathan & J. Gorman). Oxford University Press, New York.

Kazdin, A.E., Siegel, T.C. & Bass, D. (1992) Cognitive problem-solving, skills training and parent management training in the treatment of antisocial behavior in children. *Journal of Consulting and Clinical Psychology*, 60, 733–747.

Kearney, C. & Silverman, W. (1990) Measuring the function of school refusal behaviour: the school refusal assessment scale (SRAS). *Journal of Clinical Child Psychology*, 22, 85–96.

Kendall, P.C. (1994) Treating anxiety disorders in children: Results of a randomized clinical trial. *Journal of Consulting and Clinical Psychology*, 62, 100–110.

Kendall, P.C. (1998) Empirically supported psychological therapies. *Journal of Consulting and Clinical Psychology*, 66, 3–6.

Kendall, P.C. & Gosch, E.A. (1994) Cognitive-behavioural interventions. In: *International Handbook of Phobic and Anxiety Disorders in Children and Adolescents* (eds T.H. Ollendick, W. Yule & N.J. King). Plenum Press, New York.

Kendall, P.C. & Hollon S.D, eds (1994) *Cognitive-behavioral Interventions: Theory, Research and Procedures*. Academic Press, New York.

Kendall, P.C. & Lochman, J. (1994) Cognitive-behavioural therapies. In: *Child and Adolescent Psychiatry: Modern Approaches* (eds M. Rutter, E. Taylor & L. Hersov). Blackwell Scientific, Oxford.

Kendall, P.C. & Southam-Gerow, M. (1996) Long-term follow-up of

treatment for youths with anxiety disorders. *Journal of Consulting and Clinical Psychology*, 64, 724–730.

King, N.J., Hamilton, D.I. & Ollendick, T.H. (1988) *Children's Phobias: A Behavioural Perspective*. Chichester, Wiley.

King, N.J., Ollendick, T.H. & Tonge, B.J. (1995) *School Refusal: Assessment and Treatment*. Allyn and Bacon, London.

King, N.J., Tonge, B.J., Mullen, P., Myerson, N., Heyne, D. & Ollendick, T.H. (1999) Cognitive-behavioral treatment of sexually abused children: a review of research. *Behavioral and Cognitive Psychotherapy*, 27, 295–309.

Knell, S.M. (1998) Cognitive-behavioural play therapy. *Journal of Child Psychology and Psychiatry*, 27, 28–33.

Lee, S.G. & Herbert, M. (1970) *Freud and Psychology*. Penguin Books, Harmondsworth.

Leeman, L.W., Gibbs, J.C. & Fuller, D. (1993) Evaluation of a multi-component group treatment program for juvenile delinquents. *Aggressive Behavior*, 19, 281–292.

Leitenberg, H. & Callahan, E.J. (1973) Reinforced practice and reduction of different kinds of fears in adults and children. *Behaviour Research and Therapy*, 11, 19–30.

Lewinsohn, P., Clarke, G., Hops, H. & Andrews, J. (1990) Cognitive behavioral treatment for depressed adolescents. *Behaviour Therapy*, 21, 385–401.

Linden, W. (1980) Multi-component behavior therapy in a case of compulsive binge-eating followed by vomiting. *Journal of Behavior Therapy and Experimental Psychiatry*, 11, 297–300.

Loeber, R. & Hay, D.F. (1997) Key issues in the development of aggression and violence from childhood to early adulthood. *Annual Review of Psychology*, 48, 371–410.

Lonigan, C.J., Elbert, J.C. & Johnson, S.B. (1998) Empirically supported psychosocial interventions for children: an overview. *Journal of Clinical and Child Psychology*, 27, 138–145.

March, J.S. & Mulle, K. (1998) *OCD in Children and Adolescents: A Cognitive Behavioral Treatment Manual*. Guilford Press, New York.

Mitchell, M. & Carr, A. (2000) Anorexia and bulimia. In: *What Works with Children and Adolescents?* (ed. A. Carr). Routledge, London.

Mizes, J.S. (1995) Eating disorders. In: *Advanced Abnormal Child Psychology* (eds M. Hersen & R.T. Ammerman). Lawrence Erlbaum, Hillsdale, NJ.

Moore, M. & Carr, A. (2000a) Anxiety disorders. In: *What Works with Children and Adolescents?* (ed. A. Carr). Routledge, London.

Moore, M. & Carr, A. (2000b) Depression and grief. In: *What Works with Children and Adolescents?* (ed. A. Carr). Routledge, London.

Mowrer, O.H. (1947) On the dual nature of learning: a reinterpretation of 'conditioning and problem solving'. *Harvard Educational Review*, 17, 102–148.

Mowrer, O.H. & Mowrer, W. (1938) Enuresis: a method for its study and treatment. *American Journal of Orthopsychiatry*, 8, 436–447.

Muris, P., Merckelbach, H., Holdrinet, I. & Sijsenaar, M. (1998) Treating phobic children: effects of EMDR versus exposure. *Journal of Consulting and Clinical Psychology*, 66, 193–198.

Nolan, M. & Carr, A. (2000) Attention deficit hyperactivity disorder. In: *What Works with Children and Adolescents?* (ed. A. Carr). Routledge, London.

Nolan, T., Debelle, G. & Oberklaid, F. & Coffey, C. (1991) Randomized trial of laxatives in treatment of childhood encopresis. *Lancet*, 338, 523–527.

O'Leary, K.D. & O'Leary, S.G. (1977) *Classroom Management: The Use of Behavior Modification*, 2nd edn. Pergamon Press, Oxford.

Oliver, C. & Head, D. (1993) Self-injurious behavior: Functional analyses and interventions. In: *Challenging Behavior and Intellectual Dis-*

ability: a Psychological Perspective (eds R.S.P. Jones & C.B. Eyeres). BILD Publications, Clevedon, UK.

Ollendick, T.H. (1979) Fear reduction techniques with children. In: *Progress in Behavior Modification*, Vol. 8 (eds M. Hersen, R.M. Eisler & P.M. Miller). Academic Press, New York.

Ollendick, T.H. (1995) Cognitive-behavioral treatment of panic disorder with agoraphobia in adolescents: a multiple baseline design analysis. *Behavior Therapy*, **26**, 517–531.

Ollendick, T.H. (1998) Panic disorder in children and adolescents: new developments, new directions. *Journal of Child Psychology and Psychiatry*, **27**, 234–245.

Ollendick, T.H. & King, N.J. (1998) Empirically supported comprehensive treatments for children with phobic and anxiety disorders. *Journal of Clinical Child Psychology*, **27**, 156–167.

Ollendick, T.H., King, N. & Yule, W., eds (1998) *International Handbook of Phobic and Anxiety Disorders in Children and Adolescents*. Plenum Press, New York.

Ondersma, S.J. & Walker, C.E. (1998) Elimination disorders. In: *Handbook of Child Psychopathology* (eds T.H. Ollendick & M. Hersen), 3rd edn. Plenum Press, New York.

Patterson, G. (1982) *Coercive Family Process*. Castalia, Eugene, OR.

Patterson, G. & Gullion, E. (1968) *Living With Children: New Methods for Parents and Teachers*. Research Press, Champaign, IL.

Paul, G.L. (1967) Outcome research in psychotherapy. *Journal of Consulting Psychology*, **31**, 109–118.

Pavlov, I. (1927) *Conditioned Reflexes* [Translation by G.V. Anrep]. Clarendon Press, Oxford.

Power, M.J. (1991) Cognitive science and behavioural psychotherapy: where behaviour was there shall cognition be. *Behavioural Psychotherapy*, **19**, 20–41.

Rachman, S. (1993) Obsessions, responsibility and guilt. *Behaviour Research and Therapy*, **31**, 149–154.

Reynolds, W.M. & Coats, K.J. (1986) A comparison of cognitive-behavioral therapy and relaxation training for the treatment of depression in adolescents. *Journal of Consulting and Clinical Psychology*, **54**, 653–660.

Richman, N., Douglas, J., Hunt, H. *et al.* (1985) Behavioural methods in the treatment of sleep disorders – a pilot study. *Journal of Child Psychology and Psychiatry*, **26**, 581–590.

Richters, J.E., Arnold, L.E., Jensen, P.S. *et al.* (1995) NIMH collaborative multisite multimodal treatment study of children with ADHD: I. Background and rationale. *Journal of the American Academy of Child and Adolescent Psychiatry*, **34**, 987–1000.

Ronan, K.R. & Deane, F.P. (1998) Anxiety disorders. In: *Cognitive Behaviour Therapy for Children and Families* (ed. P. Graham). Cambridge University Press, Cambridge.

Rosentiel, S.K. & Scott, D.S. (1977) Four considerations in imagery techniques with children. *Journal of Behaviour Therapy and Experimental Psychiatry*, **8**, 287–290.

Royal College of Psychiatrists (1989) *Report of the Working Party to Produce Guidelines in the Use of Behavioural Treatments*. Approved by Council, October, London.

Rutter, M. (1995) Clinical implications of attachment concepts: retrospect and prospect. *Journal of Child Psychology and Psychiatry*, **36**, 549–571.

Rycroft, C. (1970) Causes and meaning. In: *Freud and Psychology* (eds S.G. Lee & M. Herbert). Penguin, Harmondsworth.

Sanders, M.R. (1996) New directions in behavioral family interventions with children. *Advances in Clinical Child Psychology*, **18**, 284–330.

Serketich, W. & Dumas, J. (1996) The effectiveness of behavioral parent training to modify antisocial behavior in children. *Behavior Therapy*, **27**, 171–186.

Shapiro, D.A. & Shapiro, D. (1982) Meta-analysis of comparative ther-

apy studies: a replication and refinement. *Psychological Bulletin*, **92**, 581–604.

Skinner, B.F. (1953) *Science and Human Behavior*. Free Press, New York.

Sloane, R.B., Staples, F.R., Cristol, A.H. *et al.* (1975) *Psychotherapy Versus Behavior Therapy*. Harvard University Press, Cambridge, MA.

Smith, P., Perrin, S. & Yule, W. (1998) Post-traumatic stress disorder. In: *Cognitive Behaviour Therapy for Children and Adolescents* (ed. P. Graham). Cambridge University Press, Cambridge.

Stark, K.D., Reynolds, W.R. & Kaslow, N.J. (1987) A comparison of the relative efficacy of self-control therapy and a behavioral problem-solving therapy for depression in children. *Journal of Abnormal Child Psychology*, **15**, 91–113.

Stark, L.J., Owens-Stively, J. & Lewis, A.V. & Guevremont, D. (1990) Group behavioral treatment of retentive encopresis. *Journal of Pediatric Psychology*, **15**, 659–671.

Stevenson J. (1999) The treatment of the long-term sequelae of child abuse. *Journal of Child Psychology and Psychiatry*, **40**, 89–112.

Sturmey, P. (1996) *Functional Analysis in Clinical Psychology*. Wiley, Chichester.

Sutton, C. & Herbert, M. (1992) *Mental Health: A Client Support Resource Pack*. National Foundation of Educational Research/Nelson, Windsor.

Target, M. & Fonagy, P. (1996) The psychological treatment of child and adolescent psychological disorders. In: *What Works for Whom?: a Critical Review of Psychotherapy Research* (eds A. Roth & P. Fonagy). Guilford Press, New York.

Taylor, E. (1997) *Understanding Your Hyperactive Child*. Vermilion, London.

Taylor, E. (1994) Syndromes of attention deficit and overactivity. In: *Child and Adolescent Psychiatry: Modern Approaches* (eds M. Rutter, E. Taylor & M. Hersov), 3rd edn. Blackwell Scientific, Oxford.

Taylor, T.K. & Biglan, A. (1998) Behavioral family interventions for improving child-rearing: a review of the literature for clinicians and policy makers. *Clinical Child and Family Psychology Review*, **1**, 41–60.

Tuma, J.M. (1989) Traditional therapies with children. In: *Handbook of Child Psychopathology* (eds T.H. Ollendick & M. Hersen), 2nd edn. Plenum Press, New York.

Wachtel, P.L. (1977) *Psychoanalysis and Behavior Therapy*. Basic Books, New York.

Wachtel, P.L. (1997) *Psychoanalysis, Behavior Therapy and the Relational World*. American Psychological Society, Washington D.C.

Wahler, R.G. & Meginnis, K.L. (1997) Strengthening child compliance through positive parenting practices: what works? *Journal of Clinical Child Psychology*, **26**, 433–440.

Walker, C.E. (1995) Elimination disorders: Enuresis and encopresis. In: *Handbook of Pediatric Psychology* (ed. M.C. Roberts). Guilford Press, New York.

Watson, J.B. & Rayner, R. (1920) Conditioned emotional reactions. *Journal of Experimental Psychology*, **3**, 1–14.

Webb, N.B. (1991) *Play Therapy with Children in Crisis*. Guilford Press, New York.

Webster-Stratton, C. (1988) *Parents and Children Videotape Series: Basic and Advanced Programs*, 1–7. 1411, 8th Avenue West, Seattle, WA 98119, USA.

Webster-Stratton, C. (1991) Strategies for helping families with conduct disordered children [Annotation]. *Journal of Child Psychology and Psychiatry*, **32**, 104–1062.

Webster-Stratton, C. & Hammond, M. (1999) Marital conflict management skills, parenting style and early conduct problems: processes and pathways. *Journal of Child Psychology and Psychiatry*, **40**, 917–927.

Webster-Stratton, C. & Herbert, M. (1993) What really happens in parent training? *Behavior Modification*, 17, 407–456.

Webster-Stratton, C. & Herbert, M. (1994) *Troubled Families: Problem Children. Working with Parents: A Collaborative Process.* Wiley, Chichester.

Weisz, J. & Weiss, B. (1993) *Effects of Psychotherapy With Children and Adolescents.* Sage, London.

Wilson, F.E. & Evans, I.M. (1983) The reliability of target behavior selection in behavioural assessment. *Behavioral Assessment*, 5, 15–23.

Wolfe, D.A. & Wekerle, C. (1993) Treatment strategies for child physical abuse and neglect: a critical progress report. *Clinical Psychology Review*, 13, 473–500.

Wolfe, V. & Birt, J. (1995) The psychological sequelae of child sexual abuse. In: *Advances in Clinical Child Psychology* (eds T.H. Ollendick & R. Prinz), Vol. 17, pp. 233–263. Plenum Press, New York.

Wolpe, J. (1958) *Psychotherapy by Reciprocal Inhibition.* Stanford University Press, Stanford, CA.

Zatz, S. & Chassin, L. (1983) Cognitions in test-anxious children. *Journal of Consulting and Clinical Psychology*, 51, 526–534.

54 Cognitive-behavioural Approaches to the Treatment of Depression and Anxiety

David A. Brent, Scott T. Gaynor and V. Robin Weersing

Introduction

In this chapter, we review the efficacy of cognitive-behavioural therapy (CBT) for the treatment and prevention of child and adolescent depression, anxiety, post-traumatic stress disorder (PTSD), and obsessive-compulsive disorder (OCD). In general, our review is restricted to randomized controlled trials, but when treatment development is at a relatively early stage, as is the case in the treatment of PTSD and OCD, open trials are also included. Prior to reviewing the extant literature, we provide some background on the development of CBT, the common elements to cognitive-behavioural treatments, some general principles in the administration of CBT, and developmental considerations in the use of this approach for children and adolescents.

General description

Cognitive-behavioural therapy includes a wide range of therapeutic techniques predicated upon the principle that there is a close interrelationship among thoughts, feelings and behaviour. Modification of distressing feeling states and problematic behaviours can therefore be accomplished by alteration in patterns of thinking that are associated with vulnerability to disorder. These pathogenic forms of thinking are often termed 'cognitive distortions' or 'automatic thoughts'. Most cognitive therapies identify cognitive distortions through some type of mapping procedure, by which one identifies the association of cognitions with certain affects and expectations, and then attempts to determine if those cognitions are grounded in reality or, rather, represent distortions. By understanding expectable patterns of distortions, anxious or depressed individuals can learn to anticipate typical responses to a given situation, and be prepared to counter those distortions with more rational and adaptive self-talk, coping and countervailing ideas.

Cognitive-behavioural therapy model of depression

Beck, one of the founders of cognitive therapy, proposed that depression was manifested by a negative cognitive triad: distorted thinking about oneself, about the future, and the world (Beck *et al.* 1979). Certainly, in adults, prospective studies have demonstrated the power of hopelessness about the future to predict suicide (Beck *et al.* 1985) and, in children, hopelessness predicts drop-out from therapy (Brent *et al.* 1998). Moreover, there are studies indicating that cognitive distortions, more broadly, are a risk factor for the development of depressive symptomatology in children and adolescents (Garber & Hilsman 1992; Garber *et al.* 1993; Lewinsohn *et al.* 1994). On the other hand, it has been argued that cognitive distortions, while useful to track clinically, are simply epiphenomenal to psychopathology. Murphy *et al.* (1984) compared the change in hopelessness in depressed adults treated with a tricyclic antidepressant to those treated with CBT. Pharmacotherapy was just as effective as CBT in relieving hopelessness, a cognitive 'cause' of depression. A recent study assessing the specificity of depressotypic cognitions to depression in adolescents concluded that pessimistic thinking and helpless attributional style were 'weakly' specific to depression; depressotypic cognitions were most strongly associated with the depressed group, but were also significantly associated with the non-mood disordered (clinical) control group. No significant associations were noted with the non-disorder control group (Lewinsohn *et al.* 1997).

The behavioural component of CBT has several origins. For the treatment of depression, this component is based on the recognition that a psychomotor-retarded patient lying in bed ruminating is not going to recover unless his or her level of activity is restored, the sleep cycle is normalized and the person begins to interact with his or her surroundings in an enjoyable way. In fact, increase in pleasurable activities is correlated with decrease in depression symptomatology (Lewinsohn *et al.* 1996). Subsequently, the 'behavioural' component has broadened to include a range of structured interventions that impact skills in child contracting, negotiation and problem-solving, social skills and assertiveness training, and in emotional regulation and distress tolerance.

Cognitive-behavioural therapy model of anxiety

In anxiety disorders, cognitive distortions appear to focus more on overestimation of the probability of unlikely but dangerous events, general perceptions of the world as risky and unsafe, and the inability to cope with these threats. It is hypothesized that individuals experience anxiety when certain situations trigger overly fearful thoughts, accompanied by defeatist self-statements and further automatic danger-focused cognitions. This cycle spirals pathogenically because such individuals lack skills to cope with anxious thoughts and feelings, and because significant others in the environments (e.g. parents) may actually model poor coping behaviour and encourage avoidance.

With regard to anxiety disorders, PTSD and OCD, the behavioural component is coequal to cognitive restructuring, and involves exposure to feared thoughts, situations and sensations, and prevention of avoidance or compulsive responses. In general, the initial phases of treatment for the anxiety disorders include generating a graded hierarchy of anxiety-provoking experiences and learning techniques to manage and contain anxiety. This is followed by gradual exposure to the hierarchy of increasingly anxiogenic situations while harnessing cognitive techniques for anxiety management. In addition, parents can be trained in behaviour management in order to help facilitate courageous behaviour and extinguish anxious behaviour.

Cognitive-behavioural therapy structure and therapeutic stance

What are the elements of CBT that distinguish it from other therapeutic approaches? First, the treatment is goal-orientated, focused and time-limited. One of the most critical tasks for a cognitive-behavioural therapist is to help the patient and family operationalize their goals. The therapist then works with the patient to achieve these agreed goals. The beginning of every session in CBT starts with the generation of an agenda. This agenda helps to guide the patient and therapist as to the topics and priorities for a particular treatment session.

Secondly, the therapist is active and directive. Passivity will lead to certain defeat with depressed individuals who, without prodding and structure, have difficulty setting or pursuing therapeutic goals. Similarly, directiveness is required for the child with school refusal, or the individual with social phobia who avoids every novel social situation. Given the central role of avoidance in the genesis of anxiety disorders, it is critical for the therapist to gently insist that exposure take place.

The third characteristic of CBT is that of collaborative empiricism, meaning that the therapist and patient examine issues and the evidence supporting a particular viewpoint or strategy, collaboratively. In many CBT models with children, the therapist is introduced as a 'coach'. The therapist is actively didactic and socializes the patient to the model so that the patient understands exactly what is expected to happen and the rationale for each particular intervention. Collaborative empiricism also means that concepts are operationalized in a concrete manner, by asking questions like, 'How will we know when you're better and we've reached our goal?'

Adaptation of cognitive-behavioural therapy to younger populations

There are several elements of cognitive therapy that require adaptation for its use in younger populations. Children's experiences are embedded in a family context, and they rarely seek treatment on their own (Weisz et al. 1998). Therefore, involvement of the family is critical in socialization, education and goal-

setting, all of which have the potential to reduce the drop-out rate dramatically (Brent et al. 1993). For younger children, involvement of the family members may be helpful to reinforce, or actually deliver, CBT (Barrett et al. 1996; Cohen & Mannarino 1996a). There is evidence that a family anxiety management component greatly enhances CBT outcome for younger anxious children (Barrett et al. 1996). Moreover, relief of parental distress is important, in so far as parental emotional difficulties may interfere with otherwise credible treatments and result in poor outcome (Cohen & Mannarino 1996a,b, 1998a; Brent et al. 1998; Southam-Gerow et al. 2001). In addition, related familial constructs, such as discord, lack of support and lack of cohesion, may interfere with the outcome of otherwise efficacious treatments (Cohen & Mannarino 1996b; Kolko 1996; Brent et al. 1998; Birmaher et al. 2000).

Younger populations show a wide variability of developmental maturity. This makes it incumbent upon the therapist to assess cognitive development, and to explain the principles and concepts of treatment in language that the child can grasp. Children may also lack the ability to decentre, and take the perspective of others—a key element of CBT and a challenge in adapting CBT for very young patients (Weisz & Weersing 1999). A related issue is the importance of differentiating between a cognitive distortion and a cognitive deficit. A child may complain about having difficulty in school because of depression, but alternatively, he or she may have a learning disability. Another patient may complain about lacking friends because of the cognitive distortions accompanying depression, because of actual loss of friends as a result of social withdrawal and irritability, or because of a deficit in the social skills essential to the development and maintenance of intimate friendships.

Children and adolescents often show attendant difficulties with decision-making, problem-solving, emotional regulation and impulsivity, in addition to mood and anxiety disorders. In fact, poor decision-making and problem-solving often get these patients into difficulties that lead to increased anxiety, depression and self-destructive behaviour such as self-cutting or suicide attempts. Therefore, it is important to assess and remediate these difficulties, because otherwise these patients will continue getting into interpersonal difficulties with painful and often self-destructive consequences.

It is rare for a child or adolescent to initiate a request for treatment. Instead, treatment is usually requested by the parent, the school or a referring health professional. It is vital to try to educate and socialize the young patient as to the nature of his or her illness, the nature of psychotherapy in general, and CBT specifically, and to address any concerns and distortions that might sabotage engagement in a successful working alliance. It is important to recognize the adolescent's need for autonomy, which can be reflected by telling the patient that the goal of treatment is to teach him or her how to become his/her own therapist. The collaborative empirical approach is usually quite well received by most adolescent patients, as it requires that the patient take a major role in setting the agenda and determining the goals of treatment. At the same time, parents must be involved and informed; the therapist must avoid getting trapped into promises of confidentiality that not only cannot be kept, but do not constitute good care.

Cognitive-behavioural therapy of youth depression

In this section, we review controlled clinical trials to treat child and adolescent depressive disorders. As previously discussed, the defining features of cognitive-behavioural approaches toward youth depression have focused on the identification and modification of negativistic thought patterns, and improvements in disturbed behavioural self- and social-regulation skills thought to underlie the aetiology of depression. In youth depression treatment, these foci have been addressed through the application of cognitive and behavioural techniques such as:

1 mood monitoring;
2 cognitive restructuring;
3 behavioural activation, pleasant activity scheduling, and goal-setting strategies;
4 relaxation and stress management;
5 social skills and conflict resolution training; and
6 training in general problem-solving skills (for discussion, see Kaslow & Thompson 1998; Kazdin & Weisz 1998).

Although the total number of youth depression studies is small, and different investigations have used different combinations of these CBT techniques, preliminary evidence suggests that, overall, CBT packages have beneficial effects on youth depression symptoms. In two recent meta-analyses of treatment of adolescent depression, mean effects of CBT were estimated to be quite large, 1.02 and 1.27 post-treatment, respectively (Reinecke et al. 1998; Lewinsohn & Clarke 1999).

To date, there have been 13 randomized studies of CBT with depressed youth, four with depressed children and nine with depressed adolescents. In addition to differences in developmental level, youth in these studies have differed with respect to referral source (clinical vs. school or advertisement) and presence of a diagnosable depressive disorder (vs. presence of subclinical symptoms). These two domains are, obviously, not unrelated. Most studies rely on samples of depressed youth recruited from school or community settings who have mild to moderate symptoms of depression, as assessed by dimensional screening instruments, and they are discussed only briefly herein. However, within the past 5 years, several investigative teams have published controlled trials in youth who met diagnostic criteria for depression, and often were clinically referred. We will begin our discussion with these more recent and well-developed treatment programmes, and then more briefly review historical work with subclinical samples of community youth. For all studies, basic study characteristics (sample size, measures) and clinical response are summarized in Table 54.1.

Studies on clinical samples

Wood et al. (1996) compared the impact of five to eight sessions of CBT intervention with a comparable period of relaxation training in the treatment of early to middle adolescent outpatients with depressive disorders, with 54% of the CBT group and 26% of the relaxation group remitting by the end of treatment. Similar results were obtained on self-report measures of depressive symptoms, self-esteem and general psychosocial adjustment. Upon 6-month follow-up, the groups had converged, as a result of continued improvement in the relaxation group and symptomatic relapse in the CBT group. Younger age of diagnosis and higher level of functioning at intake were associated with better outcome (Jayson et al. 1998). The addition of a median of 6-monthly booster CBT sessions after acute treatment resulted in a much lower relapse rate than acute treatment alone (20 vs. 50%; Kroll et al. 1996).

Using a similar CBT treatment package to Wood et al. (1996), Vostanis et al. (1996a,b) randomized depressed outpatients to either individual CBT or an attention-placebo condition—nonfocused intervention (NFI). CBT and NFI were equivalent with regard to the proportion not meeting depressive criteria at the end of treatment (87 vs. 75%) and at 9-month follow-up (71 vs. 75%). However, 46% of patients across conditions reported experiencing a 'depressive episode' at some point during the follow-up period (Vostanis et al. 1996b). On average, patients in both the CBT and NFI conditions attended six sessions with a therapist, but the range of sessions was from two to nine, occurring over a 1–5-month period.

Brent et al. (1997) tested CBT, derived from Beck et al. (1979), against systemic behaviour family therapy (SBFT) and a nondirective supportive therapy (NST), using a primarily clinically referred sample (two-thirds vs. one-third from newspaper advertisements) of depressed adolescents. In comparison to Wood et al. and Vostanis et al. these treatments were much longer and more regular (12–16 weekly sessions). At post-treatment assessment, significantly fewer of those subjects receiving CBT (17%) than NST (42%) continued to have diagnosable major depressive disorder (MDD). Remission, as defined by the absence of MDD and at least three consecutive Beck Depression Inventory (BDI) scores <9, was more common in the CBT cell (60%) than in either SBFT (38%) or NST (39%). Reductions in suicidality and improvements in general psychosocial adjustment were not different across groups. CBT resulted in greater change in cognitive distortions than did either SBFT or NST, although changes in depressive symptoms were not mediated by changes in cognitive style (Kolko et al. 2000). Across treatment cells, poorer response was predicted by greater cognitive distortion, more severe depression at intake, and referral via an advertisement rather than by clinical referral. The latter finding was mediated in part by lower hopelessness in those who were referred to the study via advertisement (Brent et al. 1998). Removal from the study and drop-out were predicted by double depression (depression comorbid with dysthymia) and greater hopelessness, respectively (Brent et al. 1998).

Table 54.1 Cognitive-behavioural therapy (CBT) treatment of youth depression.

Author	n	Attrition (%)	Age (years)	Interventions	Number of sessions	Clinical response	Proportion responding at post-treatment (%)	Proportion responding at first follow-up (%)	Proportion responding at second follow-up (%)	Remarks
Clinical samples										
Brent et al. (1997)	107	10	15.6	CBT package Family Supportive	12.1 10.7 11.2	No mood diagnosis and normal BDI	60 38 39	94 77 74 24 months		CBT most 'robust' to adverse predictors of outcome (comorbid anxiety, more severe depression) (Brent et al. 1998)
Vostanis et al. (1996a,b)	63/57	26	12.7	CBT package Supportive	6 6	No mood diagnosis	86 75	71 75 9 months		
Wood et al. (1996)	53/48	9	14.2	CBT package Relaxation	6.4 6.2	'Clinical remission'	54 21	45 23 3 months	56 36 6 months	CBT most effective for younger and less impaired patients (Jayson et al. 1998)
Diagnosed community samples										
Clarke et al. (1999)	123	22	16.2	CBT package CBT + parents Waiting list	16 16 + 9 –	No mood diagnosis	65 69 48			CBT booster sessions may be useful for patients not recovered at post-treatment
Lewinsohn et al. (1990)	69/59	14	16.2	CBT package CBT + parents Waiting list	14 14 + 7 –	No mood diagnosis	43 47 5			CBT most effective with younger, less depressed, less anxious more rational, more activated patients Parent involvement in CBT also positively related to outcome (Clarke et al. 1992)
Rosselló & Bernal (1999)	71	19	14.7	CBT IPT Waiting list	12 12 –	Normal CDI	59 82 –			Only investigation of CBT with minority youth

Study	n	%	Mean age	Conditions	No. of sessions	Categorical measure	% responding	% responding at follow-up	Follow-up
Symptomatic community samples									
Butler et al. (1980)	56	2	11.5	Cognitive Role-play Attention Waiting list	10 10 10 —	No categorical measure			
Clarke et al. (1995)	150	17	15.3	Cognitive Community	15 Variable	Categorical measure only available at follow-up		85 74	12 month
Kahn et al. (1990)	68	0	12.1	CBT package Relaxation Self-modeling Waiting list	12 12 12 —	Normal CDI	88 76 59 29	76 65 41	1 month
Liddle & Spence (1990)	31	0	9.2	CBT package Attention No treatment	8 8 —	No categorical measure			
Reynolds & Coats (1986)	30	20	15.7	CBT package Relaxation Waiting list	10 10 —	Normal BDI	83 75 0	100 100 44	1 month
Stark et al. (1987)	29	21	11.2	Self-control Problem-solving Waiting list	12 12 —	Normal CDI	78 60 11	88 67	2 months
Weisz et al. (1997)	48	0	9.6	CBT package No treatment	8 —	Normal CDI	50 16	62 31	9 months

Percentage responding is cumulative for entire period of follow-up

Abbreviations: BDI, Beck Depression Inventory; CDI, Children's Depression Inventory; IPT, interpersonal therapy.

925

Comorbid anxiety was associated with more robust response to CBT, and maternal depressive symptoms were associated with a poorer response to CBT. At post-treatment, CBT continued to be superior to NST and SBFT, even in the presence of multiple adverse predictors, suggesting that CBT may be the most efficacious intervention for use in real world service settings with clinically complex cases. At 2-year follow-up, differences between treatment groups on the presence of current MDD were not significant (Birmaher et al. 2000), although the descriptive data again favour CBT (6%) over SBFT (23%) and NST (26%). Recurrence of depression over the 2-year follow-up period was predicted by greater severity of depression symptoms at intake, and by higher levels of parent–child conflict (Birmaher et al. 2000).

Diagnosed community samples

The following set of studies used community samples of youth with diagnostic depression recruited either from schools or via advertisements.

Lewinsohn et al. (1990) randomized 59 participants to either, Coping with Depression–Adolescent Version (CWD-A) alone, CWD-A plus the parent group (consisting of seven weekly sessions), or a waiting list control (WLC). CWD-A consists of 14 2-h psychoeducationally orientated group sessions delivered over 7 weeks. The focus of CWD-A is on increasing social skills, pleasant events/activities, and problem-solving and conflict resolution skills, while reducing anxious and depressive cognitions. At the conclusion of treatment, 43% of the adolescent-only group and 48% of the adolescent-plus-parent group no longer met diagnostic criteria compared to only 5% of the WLC subjects. Significantly decreased scores on abbreviated self-report depression measures were also obtained for both treatment groups relative to the WLC group. In addition, treatment gains persisted at 1-, 6-, 12- and 24-month follow-up. The adolescent-plus-parent group did not result in better outcomes than the adolescent-only condition. Poor outcome was associated with greater depressive symptomatology, comorbid anxiety symptoms and greater cognitive distortions at intake (Clarke et al. 1992).

Clarke et al. (1999) replicated these results, with 65, 69 and 48% of subjects in the adolescent-only, adolescent-plus-parent and WLC conditions, respectively, no longer meeting diagnostic criteria for MDD or dysthymia post-treatment. In this trial, there was a rerandomization to a one to two session booster condition that did not reduce the rate of depression recurrence for those who had remitted by the end of treatment. However, for patients who had not yet recovered from depression at the end of the acute treatment phase, booster sessions did accelerate their rate of recovery. Across both studies assessing the effects of CWD-A with diagnosed samples, a positive treatment response was predicted by a less severe initial depression, higher initial engagement in and enjoyment of pleasant activities, and fewer irrational thoughts (Clarke et al. 1992; Lewinsohn et al. 1996).

Rosselló & Bernal (1999) compared the efficacy of a 12-week, individually administered CBT programme to a similar dose of interpersonal therapy (IPT) and WLC in adolescents with diagnosed MDD and/or dysthymia referred by school personnel. Both active interventions were adapted to be culturally appropriate for use with Puerto Rican youth (Rosselló & Bernal 1999). Attendance problems occurred in both treatments as only 68% of IPT cases and 52% of CBT cases completed over seven treatment sessions. To assess outcome, a clinical cut-off was selected on the Children's Depression Inventory (CDI) that was approximately three points lower than the mean intake CDI score for the sample. Using this criteria for clinically significant change (Jacobson & Truax 1991), 59% of adolescents in the CBT condition and 82% of IPT cases achieved clinically significant improvement in depression symptoms by post-treatment; data were not provided for the WLC condition. Using an unspecified normative cut-off point for the CDI, the authors indicated that 56% of the IPT cases, 48% of the CBT cases, and 61% of the WLC were 'severely depressed' at intake. At post-treatment, these percentages were 11, 24 and 34%, respectively, and 17 and 18% at 3-month follow-up for IPT and CBT, respectively. While this investigation has several methodological difficulties (e.g. substantial attrition and no intent-to-treat analyses conducted), these results provide some of the first information on the efficacy of CBT for depressed Latino youth and the only extant comparison of CBT and IPT in adolescent depression.

Symptomatic community samples

There are several community-based studies of symptomatic children and adolescents in which CBT is compared to other active treatments (e.g. relaxation treatment, self-control, modelling) as well as a WLC (Butler et al. 1980; Reynolds & Coats 1986; Stark et al. 1987; Kahn et al. 1990; Liddle & Spence 1990; Weisz et al. 1997). In general, all active interventions are superior to WLC and the impact is sustained on follow-up but, with few exceptions, CBT showed no differential impact compared to the other active interventions. These studies are important because they are some of the only CBT studies of depressive symptoms in children, are usually delivered in a group format, and therefore may guide future efforts to prevent early-onset depression.

Prevention

Clarke et al. (1995) tested the efficacy of an adaptation of CWD-A in preventing diagnosable depression in adolescents with sub-syndromal depressive symptoms, but without a diagnosable depressive disorder. One hundred and fifty high school students, who scored highly on the Center for Epidemiological Studies–Depression scale (CES-D) but failed to meet diagnostic criteria for a current depressive disorder, were randomly assigned to the 15-session CWD or 'usual care'. At 12 months post-intervention, fewer cases of depressive disorder (15%) had developed in the CWD group than in the control group (26%).

Summary of cognitive-behavioural therapy for youth depression

Taken together, results from these three tiers of studies suggest that CBT for youth depression appears to be more efficacious than no treatment, WLC, or attention placebo controls, and some studies, especially in clinically referred samples, indicate that CBT can produce better results than alternative active treatments (Wood *et al.* 1996; Brent *et al.* 1997). Data from Brent *et al.* (1998) suggest that CBT may also be 'robust' to many of the adverse clinical indicators in depression treatment. Efficacy also appears to be robust to format (group vs. individual), emphasis (behavioural vs. cognitive), and dose (5–16 sessions).

While these results are promising, many patients continue to have clinically significant levels of depression at post-treatment, and near majorities of patients experience at least one recurrence of depression within 2 years of treatment termination. It is perhaps not surprising that many patients (estimates range from 29 to 48%) seek additional services following acute CBT (Brent *et al.* 1999).

These studies provide some clues with regard to the improvement of depression using CBT. CBT did more poorly in the face of maternal depressive symptoms, greater severity, and double depression; family discord also retarded recovery and predicted recurrence. Therefore, additional interventions that target maternal depression and family discord may well augment outcome. Moreover, particularly refractory and chronic conditions, such as double depression, may respond better to combinations of medication and CBT than to either monotherapy alone, as is suggested by comparable data in adults with chronic depression (Keller *et al.* 2000). We currently have very little information on the treatment of serious depression in pre-adolescents, and it is unclear how CBT may need to be adapted to take into account the more concrete cognitive style and greater dependence on parents seen in most pre-adolescent as compared to adolescent, patients (Weisz & Weersing 1999).

Cognitive-behavioural therapy of anxiety disorders

In this section, we review controlled clinical trials to treat childhood anxiety disorders: separation anxiety, generalized anxiety disorder, and simple and social phobia. No studies have specifically focused on panic disorder. Studies of the treatment of PTSD and OCD are reviewed in separate sections. Table 54.2 outlines key features and outcomes of these clinical trials, which are described in further detail below.

Coping Cat studies and variants

Kendall (1994) reported the first controlled trial of a manualized CBT, the Coping Cat programme, for anxiety disorders in children. Forty-seven youths were randomized to either 16–20 sessions of individual CBT or an 8-week WLC, after which youths were offered CBT. Four essential components were included:

1 recognition of cognitive, emotional, and somatic manifestations of anxiety;

2 recognition of cognitive distortions that are anxiogenic;

3 development of a plan to cope with anxiety-provoking situations; and

4 learning how to evaluate one's performance in potentially anxiety-provoking situations, and to reward desirable performance.

Children were liberally reinforced by therapists for participating in the therapeutic activities, and especially for successful coping, with the goal to transform from a 'scaredy cat' to a 'coping cat'. A summary of a session-by-session treatment from Kendall (1994) is noted in Table 54.3.

The proportion of youths who no longer met diagnostic criteria for an anxiety disorder was much higher in CBT than WLC (64 vs. 5%). Furthermore, a significant strength of this study was the multimodal measurement of anxiety through parent and self-report, and behaviour observation, with remarkably consistent treatment-by-time interactions greatly favouring CBT. Given the high rate of comorbid depression (32%), it is salient to note that CBT, although it did not specifically target depression, resulted in a significant reduction in self-reported depression.

Follow-up at 1 and 3.4 years later showed preservation of the gains that occurred during treatment (Kendall 1994; Kendall & Southam-Gerow 1996). When, as part of the long-term follow-up, participants were asked to recall which aspects of treatment were most relevant and helpful, subjects stressed the therapeutic relationship, games and activities, and the discussion of problems. However, recall of specific skills in coping with anxiety, *in vivo* exposure, and relaxation exercises were all related to positive outcomes in anxiety, ability to cope, and reduction in anxiogenic cognitions (Kendall & Southam-Gerow 1996).

Kendall *et al.* (1997) replicated and extended these results in a larger clinical trial of Coping Cat vs. WLC for 94 youths with anxiety disorder. Again, CBT was overwhelmingly superior to WLC with regard to proportion no longer meeting criteria for anxiety disorder at post-treatment (46–53 vs. 4%). Group differences were also detected for self-reported coping statements, anxiogenic cognitions, and self-reported, parent-reported and behaviourally observed anxiety symptoms.

As in the first trial, the WLC group received CBT after 8 weeks of treatment, allowing for a comparison of the differential efficacy of 8 vs. 16 weeks of CBT. The effects of the full 16 weeks of CBT were vastly superior, suggesting that the initial skill-building component alone is not efficacious without the addition of the exposure component. Gains in the treatment programme may occur through decreases in subjects' anxious self-talk (Treadwell & Kendall 1996). In a 1-year follow-up, there was strong evidence for the maintenance of initial therapeutic effects across measures of anxiety.

Barrett *et al.* (1996) adapted and extended Kendall's treatment model (termed 'Coping Koala') and tested the additive

Table 54.2 CBT treatment of anxiety disorders.

Author	n	Age (years)	Diagnosis	Interventions	Number of sessions	Proportion without anxiety disorder at follow-up (%)	Proportion without anxiety disorder at 1 year (%)	Remarks
Kendall (1994)	47	9–13	Anxiety	CBT WLC	16–22 –	64 5	69*	
Kendall et al. (1997)	94	9–13	Anxiety	CBT WLC	16 –	46–53† 4	Gains maintained‡	
Barrett et al. (1996)	79	7–14	Anxiety	CBT+FAM CBT WLC	12 12 –	84 57 26	70 96 –	CBT+FAM was particularly effective for younger and for female children
Last et al. (1998)	56	6–17	School phobia Mixed anxiety disorders	CBT SET	12 12	65 50	– –	
Hayward et al. (2000)	35	Adolescent female (15.8 = M)	School phobia	Group CBT WLC	16 –	45 4	60 44	
Dadds et al. (1997)	128	7–14	25% at risk 75% with anxiety disorder	Group CBT+FAM WLC	10+3 –	73 59	73§ 44	
King et al. (1998)	34	5–15	School refusal anxiety (76)	CBT + parent training WLC	6+5 –	88¶ 29	82‖ –	

*75% without anxiety disorder at 3.35 year follow-up.
†From child and parent interviews, respectively.
‡Diagnosis not reported.
§6-month follow-up.
¶Percentage attending school >90% of days.
‖12-week follow-up.
Abbreviations: CBT, cognitive-behavioural therapy; FAM, family anxiety management; SET, supportive-expressive therapy; WLC, waiting list control.

Table 54.3 Outline of Kendall's Coping Cat CBT treatment by session (Kendall 1994).

Session	
1	Build rapport, gather information about anxiety-provoking situations and how child responds
2	Learn to identify two types of feelings
3	Develop a hierarchy of anxiety-provoking situations and responses
4	Relaxation training with personalized cassette
5	Recognize self-talk, reduce anxiogenic self-talk
6	Recognition and development of coping strategies (e.g. self-talk)
7	Learn how to self-evaluate and self-reward coping behaviour
8	Review of concepts and skills
9	Practice of new skills (e.g. coping self-talk, relaxing imagery) in low-anxiety situations
10–13	Exposure to imagined and real situations with increasing levels of anxiety, test recognition of anxiety, self-coping, and evaluation of performance
14–15	Practice in very stressful situations
	Development of 'infomercial' aimed at informing other children how to cope with anxiety
16	Review of therapy experience, skills, and consideration about application in future anxiogenic situations
17–20	Generalization, biweekly sessions (optional)

Table 54.4 Family anxiety management (FAM) for parents (Barrett *et al.* 1996).

Sessions	
1–4	*Contingency management*
	Rewarding coping and courageous behaviour
	Ignoring excessive anxiety and initial empathetic response
5–8	*Management of own anxiety*
	Awareness of anxiety in stressful situations
	Learn problem-solving and coping behaviour to mitigate anxiety
	Model positive coping for children
9–12	*Communication and problem-solving*
	Responding to conflict, especially around dealing with child's anxious behaviour
	Encouragement of daily discussion and improved communication between parents
	Training in problem-solving skills

efficacy of a family anxiety management (FAM) component. FAM consisted of three components:

1 education of the parents in contingency management to reinforce courageous and to ignore anxious behaviour;
2 teaching the parents to manage their own anxiety and model positive coping; and
3 training in communication and problem-solving (detailed in Table 54.4).
In this study, anxious youth were randomized to one of three cells: CBT alone, CBT+FAM, and WLC. Those selected for CBT alone received 12 60–80-min sessions, whereas those se-

lected for CBT+FAM received approximately 30 min on CBT and 40 min on FAM.

Overall, both CBT+FAM and CBT alone were markedly superior to WLC in the proportion of children without a diagnosable anxiety disorder post-treatment (89, 51 and 26%, respectively). The combination of CBT+FAM appeared to be particularly helpful for younger girls, for whom the rate of no longer having an anxiety disorder diagnosis was much lower than in those who received CBT alone (100 vs. 55%; 84 vs. 37%). In contrast, among older participants (aged 11–14), both active treatments resulted in a 60% remission rate with respect to the proportion no longer meeting diagnostic criteria for an anxiety disorder. Similarly, in males the results were closely comparable in the CBT+FAM (84%) and CBT alone (65%) groups. The authors speculated that the age effect might be a natural consequence of the greater dependence of younger children on their parents, whereas the sex difference is less easy to explain.

This same research group randomized 128 youths (three-quarters of whom had significant anxiety, the remainder at risk for the development of an anxiety disorder) to either a modified version of the Coping Koala (10-week group CBT with three FAM sessions) or WLC (Dadds *et al.* 1997). There were significant treatment effects, both at the end of treatment and 6 months later on parent and clinician rating of child adjustment, anxiety, avoidance and functioning. Diagnostically, no differences in the rates of disorder were noted at the end of treatment, but a significant difference emerged by 6 months after the intervention (see Table 54.2; 56 vs. 27% rate of anxiety in WLC vs. intervention), both in the at-risk and fully symptomatic subgroups. This might have been caused by a 'sleeper' effect or the timing of the follow-up assessment, which coincided with the beginning of next school year, when symptoms might have re-emerged. Therefore, group CBT+FAM was more efficacious than WLC for both treating anxiety disorder and decreasing the incidence of anxiety disorder in those with subclinical symptoms.

Programmes for school refusal and social anxiety in children and adolescents

Last *et al.* (1998) examined the relative efficacy of 12 weekly sessions of CBT vs. supportive-expressive therapy (SET) for children and adolescents with 'school phobia', who most commonly met diagnostic criteria for simple or social phobia (58%) or separation anxiety disorder (32%). Both treatments resulted in a significant improvement in school attendance with no major between-group differences. Specifically, the proportion of children who had reached 95% school attendance by the end of treatment was 65% in the CBT cell vs. 48% in the comparison cell, a non-significant difference. There was evidence of differential attrition, with all nine subjects who dropped out having been randomized to the CBT cell. On re-entry to school the next academic year, both groups demonstrated similar rates of having mild or no difficulty returning to school (70 vs. 71%). Level of school attendance at the end of treatment was inversely related to difficulty returning to school on follow-up. Both treatments were more efficacious for younger participants and for those who showed better school attendance at baseline.

In another study of CBT for school refusal, King *et al.* (1998) randomized school-refusing children and adolescents aged 5–15 to either six sessions of CBT plus five parent sessions in contingency-setting and child management delivered over 4 weeks, or a WLC group. Approximately two-thirds of subjects had at least one diagnosable anxiety disorder. CBT resulted in dramatically improved school attendance compared to the WLC condition (proportion attending >90% of school days, 88 vs. 29%), with this improved attendance maintained at 12-week follow-up (82%).

Bernstein *et al.* (2000) reported on the efficacy of CBT+imipramine vs. CBT+placebo for the treatment of school refusal in adolescents. Therefore, this study was designed to test the efficacy of imipramine added to CBT, but not CBT *per se*. In contrast to all of the above-noted studies, all of the subjects were adolescents and had both depression and anxiety. The CBT intervention was an adaptation of the model of treatment used by Last *et al.* (1998), with a reduced number of sessions (eight rather than 13). The imipramine+CBT was superior to the placebo+CBT with regard to school attendance (70 vs. 28% attendance), the proportion attending at least 75% of classes (54 vs. 17%) and rate of decrement in depressive symptoms. The poor outcome in the CBT+placebo cell, relative to a previous application of this CBT intervention (Last *et al.* 1998), could be brought about by the older age of the subjects, their greater clinical complexity (depression and anxiety) or lower dose of treatment received.

Hayward *et al.* (2000) reported on a clinical trial of group CBT vs. WLC condition in 35 female adolescents with social phobia. Those 12 subjects randomized to group CBT received 16 sessions, consisting of education about anxiety (sessions 1 and 2), development of coping strategies, assertiveness, and cognitive restructuring skills (sessions 3–8), and simulated and *in vivo* exposure (sessions 9–16). At the end of treatment, a lower proportion of those randomized to CBT met full diagnostic criteria for social phobia (55 vs. 96%). While these gains were sustained upon 1-year follow-up, the WLC group also improved spontaneously, so that the two groups were no longer different with respect to rates of social phobia (40 vs. 56%). There was also some limited support that the intervention might be helpful in preventing the recurrence of depression in those who had a prior depressive episode, as only 17% of the CBT-treated subjects with a previous depressive episode had another depressive episode over follow-up, whereas 64% of the previously depressed WLC group experienced a recurrent depressive episode.

Summary of anxiety disorder studies

There is strong and consistent evidence that a structured CBT intervention, either individual or group, is more helpful than WLC in reduction of anxiety symptoms and restoration of functionality, and that these improvements are sustained over follow-up. At the same time, a high proportion of those treated still reported continued anxiety symptomatology, which suggests either the need for longer or more intensive treatment, or the combination of pharmacotherapy with CBT in those with residual symptomatology. The addition of a family anxiety management component appears to boost the response rate of CBT, especially for female and for younger patients. CBT also appears to be helpful in the prevention of anxiety in those with subdiagnostic manifestations of anxiety; also, treatment of anxiety may relieve or even prevent further depression. However, almost all the above-cited studies compare CBT to WLC; in the one study that compares CBT to another credible treatment, the two treatments were equivalent. While decrements in anxious self-talk are related to improvement in CBT, it is unclear whether CBT is truly a specific treatment for anxiety disorder. Also, this series of studies did not use intent-to-treat analyses, although attrition was generally low. Finally, an additional caveat is that the majority of the subjects for these studies came via advertisements, which may attract more treatment-responsive subjects (Brent *et al.* 1998).

Cognitive-behavioural therapy of maltreatment and post-traumatic stress disorder

Sexual abuse

With regard to the treatment of sexually abused youth, Finkelhor (1990) noted four contributors to anxious symptomatology, inappropriate behaviours and impairment following sexual abuse: traumatic sexualization, stigmatization, powerlessness and betrayal. Cohen & Mannarino (1996a,b) subsequently demonstrated that these four factors are related to symptom formation, and therefore are particularly important to address in psychotherapy. Inappropriate sexual behaviour following abuse may result from modelling the behaviour of the abuser, cognitive distortions about what is appropriate sexual behaviour, and reinforcement from seductive and coercive adults. Thus, therapy would need to focus on relearning appropriate behaviour and restructuring cognitive distortions. Stigma can be examined by trying to understand the victim's cognitions about the abuse, such as thinking of oneself as 'damaged' or dirty. Powerlessness and betrayal can be addressed by helping the child to understand what are the limits to which these inferences should be generalized, and what steps to take should a similar situation arise again. The preceding description serves as a backdrop for evaluating the five randomized treatment trials for sexually abused youngsters and the one dealing with physically abused youth.

Cohen & Mannarino (1996a) randomized sexually abused preschool-age children to 12 sessions of either CBT or NST. Both treatments targeted both the parent and child. Parental issues addressed in the CBT model were ambivalence about belief in the abuse, attributions about the abuse, concerns that the child was now 'damaged', provision of appropriate support to the child, issues dealing with a personal history of abuse (if applicable), and legal issues. Topics focused on with the child included safety education and assertiveness, identification of appropriate and inappropriate touching, attributions about the abuse and the abuser, and attendant anxiety symptoms. NST provided support through active listening, clarification of affect, and affirmation, but without a focus on specific skills or problem-solving, thereby controlling for attention and treatment credibility. CBT was more efficacious than NST in reducing symptomatology from the clinical to non-clinical range for parent-reported total and for internalizing problems (56 vs. 22%, 60 vs. 11%). In addition, six of those in NST vs. none in the CBT group had to be removed from treatment because of sexually inappropriate behaviour. Parental negative reaction to disclosure and parental depression predicted behavioural and emotional difficulties of the child at the end of treatment, independent of treatment assessment (Cohen & Mannarino 1996b). The CBT group showed sustained improvement upon 1-year follow-up (Cohen & Mannarino 1998a) with continued problems with inappropriate sexual and externalizing behaviour predicted by the degree of parental support.

Cohen & Mannarino (1998b) compared 12 sessions each of CBT to NST for sexually abused children and adolescents and their parents. A much greater proportion of youth in CBT vs. NST moved from the clinical to non-clinical range for self-reported depression, inappropriate sexual behaviour, parent reported social competence, and total behaviour problems. A higher proportion of youth in NST ($n=7$, 27%) were removed for inappropriate sexual behaviour, or dropped out, relative to those assigned to CBT ($n=2$, 6%). Child cognitions about the abuse were related to post-treatment anxiety, anger, depression,

PTSD and dissociation (Cohen & Mannarino, 2000). Family support and adaptability were related to post-treatment anxiety, depression and PTSD.

Deblinger et al. (1996) randomized 100 sexually abused school-aged children to one of four conditions: community care, child CBT, a non-offending parental intervention, or child CBT + parental intervention, in a 2×2 factorial design. The child CBT intervention consisted of 12 45-min sessions delivered weekly, as did the parental intervention; the combined intervention lasted 80–90 min per week. The child intervention included gradual exposure, modelling, education, coping and body safety skills training. The gradual exposure was designed to help the child unlink associations made between the triggers for PTSD and abuse-related cognitive and external reminders. The parental intervention involved teaching the parent therapeutic ways to respond to their children's fears and avoidance through modelling, gradual exposure, coping and child management skills (e.g. contingency management, negotiation, communication and problem-solving skills). There was a treatment-by-time effect favouring the child CBT intervention for its impact on PTSD. There was also a treatment-by-time effect favouring the parental intervention for child-reported depressive symptoms, improvement in parental skills, and parent-reported externalizing symptoms. Among children whose parents reported them as above the clinical cut-off for externalizing problems, only 26% of those assigned to a parental intervention were still at or above the cut-off post-treatment, as compared to 80% of the child and community treatment groups. Although there were no parent-by-child intervention interactions detected, the complementary effects of the two treatment components suggest that the combined treatment may be the most efficacious, especially in children who present with both internalizing and externalizing difficulties.

Berliner & Saunders (1996) randomly assigned sexually abused children to one of two 10-week group treatments: 'conventional abuse treatment' vs. conventional abuse treatment + stress-inoculation training and gradual exposure. Treatment analyses were restricted to the subjects who completed treatment and a 2-year follow-up, whereas nearly twice that number were initially recruited into the study. Groups were stratified by age, and the two older age groups were homogeneous for gender. The conventional treatment was highly structured and didactic, focusing on different aspects of the abuse experience, including self-esteem, body awareness and sexuality, impact of exposure, and reaction of family and friends. The experimental intervention also taught children about identification of anxiety, relaxation and thought-stopping coping exercises, and gradual exposure (in vivo). There were significant decreases in self-reported anxiety, sexual abuse-related anxiety, depression, inappropriate sexual behaviour, and parent-related internalizing and externalizing scores across the course of both treatments but, contrary to hypotheses, there were no differences between the two treatments. At 2-year follow-up, 20–40% of the group remained improved; however, 20% had deteriorated. The lack of a differential intervention effect was attributed to the relatively low levels of PTSD and anxiety symptomatology at intake, lack of substantive difference between the two treatments, and insufficient dosage of important cognitive elements.

Celano *et al.* (1996) compared the efficacy of 8 weeks of CBT vs. treatment as usual for African-American sexually abused girls aged 8–13. Each child in the CBT intervention received two individual 30-min sessions dedicated to each of the four domains from the model of Finkelhor (designed to decrease stigmatization and blame, feelings of betrayal, traumatic sexualization, and powerlessness/anxiety); safety education was also provided. A parental component followed the same topics in parallel. The treatment as usual was less structured, but involved discussion with both parent and child about abuse-related feelings and symptomatology, self-esteem, peer and family issues, parent–child communication, feelings about the perpetrator, and reaction to disclosure.

Thirty-two subjects completed treatment; the higher drop-out rate in the experimental treatment (10 vs. 5 drop-outs from treatment as usual) makes the findings difficult to interpret. For the most part, both treatments resulted in significant decrements in symptomatology, similar to the findings of Berliner & Saunders (1996). Differential effects were found favouring the experimental intervention with regard to increasing parental support, and decreasing parent self-blame; treatment as usual had greater impact than the experimental treatment on depression.

Physical abuse

Kolko (1996) compared the treatment outcome of physically abused children randomly assigned to individual child and parent CBT, family therapy, or routine community services. Each intervention consisted of around 18 h of treatment delivered over a 16-week period. The CBT programme was delivered to parents and children by separate therapists. The parental CBT programme focused on teaching intrapersonal and interpersonal skills, including anger control and cognitive coping skills, and appropriate punishment and contingency management. CBT for children focused on their views of family stressors and violence, coping, self-control, safety skills, and social skills training (e.g. enhancing social support, assertion, negotiation). Family therapy consisted of three phases:
1 gaining an understanding of family roles and interactions and developing a no-violence contract with each family member;
2 teaching problem-solving and communication skills; and
3 establishment of problem-solving as routine family alternatives to coercion and physical violence.
The community service component was more heterogeneous, but consisted of case management, risk assessment, teaching of family skills, provision of parenting information, and referral to support groups.

Family therapy was associated with a greater reduction in child-reported parent-to-child violence, and both CBT and family interventions were associated with greater reduction in child-reported child-to-parent violence. Both interventions were also associated with greater impact on child abuse potential, individual child externalizing symptoms and parental general distress and depression, and family cohesion and conflict. The rates of reabuse were higher in community care (30%) than in CBT (10%) and family therapy (12%), although these results escaped statistical significance. This study demonstrates the relative advantage of both CBT and family therapy over routine community care for physically maltreated youth and their families, and supports the importance of including the parents, either in a structured CBT or a family therapy intervention.

In summary, studies of maltreated (mostly sexually abused) children support the efficacy of CBT interventions over non-directive supportive treatment, and over standard community treatment. Modification in abuse-related cognitions appears to be related to relief of internalizing symptomatology. Perhaps because of the difficulties inherent in working with these populations, the drop-out rate in several of these studies was substantial and, unfortunately, none of the studies appeared to have utilized an intent-to-treat data analytic approach. The importance of involving the parent in the cognitive treatment was demonstrated in several of the above-noted studies, and the role of parental distress and support in predicting child outcome is consistent with these findings.

Natural disasters

Several research groups have studied CBT approaches to the treatment of trauma caused by unpredictable catastrophic environmental events. Galante & Foa (1986), in the aftermath of a disastrous Italian earthquake, provided a seven-session group treatment programme to children in some affected villages and not others. The group treatment involved expression of fears about the earthquake, discussion of erroneous beliefs about earthquakes, focus on grief and rebuilding for the future, and role-playing about taking an active role in one's survival. A greater reduction in the proportion of children at risk on the Rutter Teacher Children's Questionnaire was found in those villages where the children received the treatment programme.

Goenjian *et al.* (1997) treated early adolescent students in two schools 18 months after a devastating earthquake in Armenia. Subjects were randomized to trauma/grief-focused psychotherapy or no treatment. The intervention consisted of four 30-min classroom-based group psychotherapy sessions, and an average of 2–4 1-h individual sessions. Five content areas were addressed:
1 cognitive distortions and avoidance related to trauma;
2 identification of traumatic reminders, and enhancing toleration for these reminders by exposure, seeking external support, and cognitive restructuring;
3 mastering interpersonal problem-solving skills to deal with losses and other adversities and promote adaptation to the post-disaster environment;
4 helping the bereaved person attain a non-traumatic representation of the deceased person (when applicable); and
5 promotion of normal development, in the light of missed

developmental opportunities because of loss, and collapse, of family and community infrastructure.

Therefore, this intervention contains a mixture of cognitive, supportive-expressive, and interpersonal dynamic elements.

Eighteen months after the conclusion of treatment, a reduction in PTSD symptomatology was noted for the active intervention, and an increase in PTSD symptomatology was observed in the non-intervention group, with parallel findings for depression. Three years after the earthquake, and 18 months after the intervention, 28% of the intervention group and 69% of the non-intervention group still exceeded the clinical cut-off for PTSD, and 46% of the intervention group and 75% of the non-intervention group were over the clinical cut-off for depression. Of particular significance in this study is the worsening of the course of the untreated group over time, both with regard to PTSD and depression. These results provide support for the utility of a brief intervention directed at those who have been exposed to natural disasters, as exposees are at high risk for PTSD and depressive disorders that become increasingly prevalent over time without intervention.

March et al. (1998a) reported on a group CBT intervention for PTSD after a single-incident stressor, termed multi-modality trauma treatment (MMTT). In MMTT, PTSD is conceptualized as an aversive emotional response to a traumatic stressor, resulting from a severe traumatizing stressor interacting with pre-existing personal vulnerability to the effects of trauma (e.g. anxiety disorder or anxious temperament). Subsequently, cues reminiscent of the traumatic event can elicit the alterations in arousal, memory and affect that comprise PTSD. Over time, it is hypothesized that persons with PTSD develop 'fear structures', which are sequences of trauma-related cues, thoughts, affects and memories. To evaluate the efficacy of MMTT, March et al. (1998a) treated 17 subjects screened for PTSD whose precipitant was a 'single incident'. Four groups received MMTT, with two of the four groups lagged 4 weeks behind the other two groups, allowing for experimental control for time effects.

Of the 17 subjects, 14 completed the treatment and three were lost to follow-up. At the end of treatment, 57% no longer met criteria for PTSD, and by 6 months after the completion of treatment, 86% no longer met criteria for PTSD. There were also significant effects with respect to self-rated anxiety, depression, trait anger, and a change from external to internal locus of control; the latter noted only at the 6-month follow-up. MMTT appears to have promise and should be evaluated in larger clinical trials that control for the attention and support of psychotherapy.

Obsessive-compulsive disorder

The initial treatment studies for paediatric OCD involved the serotonergic antidepressant clomipramine and, more recently, the selective serotonin reuptake inhibitor (SSRI) sertraline (Flament et al. 1985; DeVeaugh-Geiss et al. 1992; Riddle et al. 1992; March et al. 1998b). However, in both sets of studies,

while it was recognized that there was significant improvement relative to placebo, subjects at the end of these medication trials often remained significantly symptomatic. Therefore, psychosocial interventions, either alone or in combination with medication, hold promise for resulting in more complete restoration of functionality in this serious and potentially debilitating disease.

March et al. (1994) reported on a structured CBT protocol for the treatment of OCD. The essence of this treatment approach is the encouragement of the child to externalize the disease, OCD, into a 'nasty name' that is to be run off the child's land. In this way, the child is to become the 'boss' of OCD. The child is to make a 'map' of OCD on the basis of situational triggers and subsequent OCD symptoms (obsessions and compulsions). This map identifies triggers that the child can manage easily, those that are still under the control of the 'OCD' and those in-between. The in-between, or 'transition zone', represents the substrate for constructing a hierarchy of tasks for exposure and response prevention, with the ultimate aim to expand the amount of 'land' (self) that the child is now the 'boss' of, relative to OCD. CBT techniques for achieving this goal include management of the anxiety associated with obsessions and compulsions, and graduated exposure to more and more 'compelling' triggers which, in turn, will allow the child to gain back more 'land'. March et al. (1994) reported on the CBT treatment of 15 subjects ranging in age from 8 to 18, with all but one receiving concurrent medication. Of the 15 subjects, 10 (67%) showed >50% decline in the Yale–Brown Obsessive Compulsive Scale (Y-BOCS), and three were considered non-responders. According to the Clinical Global Improvement (CGI), 9/15 (60%) were judged to be asymptomatic at follow-up.

Franklin et al. (1998) treated 14 children and adolescents with OCD with a similar CBT protocol to that described by March et al. (1994), with the exception that the latter treatment omitted anxiety management training and focused exclusively on exposure and response prevention, with half receiving all their sessions in 1 month and half receiving them as weekly treatments. The vast majority (12/14, 86%) were at least 50% improved on the Y-BOCS, with treatment improvement sustained over the 9-month follow-up. Both fear and engagement in rituals declined significantly over time. The intensive and weekly treatment groups were compared, and the effect sizes were somewhat larger in the weekly group, although not statistically so. CBT appeared to be as effective and durable in those who were treated with concomitant medication as in those who were not.

De Haan et al. (1998) have reported on the only randomized controlled trial of 12 weekly sessions of CBT (similar to the Franklin et al. 1998 model) vs. medication (clomipramine) in paediatric OCD. The average dosage of clomipramine was 2.5 mg/kg, slightly lower than the planned target of 3 mg/kg, because of the emergence of side-effects. Behavioural treatment produced a greater decrease in OCD symptoms than did clomipramine. Non-responders who accepted a combination of medication and behaviour therapy achieved further symptomatic improvement.

These data indicate that CBT has a role in the management of paediatric OCD. The simpler exposure and response prevention may be as efficacious as the more elaborate protocol articulated by March *et al.* (1994), and has been shown in one randomized trial to be as, or even more, efficacious than medication. Further research is indicated to examine the individual and combined effects of CBT and pharmacotherapy for paediatric OCD.

Conclusions

The CBT approaches reviewed in this chapter cover a wide range of techniques, from cognitive restructuring, to social skills programmes, to exposure and response prevention. While these specific techniques may vary in their points of emphasis and placement along the cognitive-behavioural continuum, they emerge from a common tradition emphasizing the interrelatedness of thoughts, feelings and actions.

Overall, the research literature suggests that CBT for youth depression and anxiety is more efficacious than a WLC condition. For both youth depression and for treatment of sexually traumatized youth, there is a growing body of evidence suggesting that CBT may also be more efficacious than attention placebo controls or alternative active treatments. CBT may also be a robust intervention for depression even in the face of adverse clinical indicators. CBT treatment of anxiety may also ameliorate or even prevent depression.

Although these results are promising, many young patients with either depression or anxiety remain symptomatic or, worse, do not improve after an acute course of CBT. While the effects of CBT on anxiety appear enduring (Kendall 1994; Kendall & Southam-Gerow 1996), the recurrence of depression does not seem to be differentially affected by participation in CBT in the absence of additional booster sessions (Kroll *et al.* 1996; Wood *et al.* 1996; Clarke *et al.* 1999; Birmaher *et al.* 2000). A substantial portion of anxious youths also remain clinically impaired at post-treatment, and little information is available on the long-term recurrence of diagnosable levels of anxiety after acute CBT treatment (for a notable exception see Kendall 1994; Kendall & Southam-Gerow 1996).

Examining predictors of success in CBT may provide clues for how to boost response for treatment-resistant youths. In both depression and anxiety treatment, younger patients appear to respond better than older adolescents, arguing for an emphasis on early identification and CBT intervention for internalizing symptomatology among youths. It may also be useful to augment traditional child-focused CBT packages with family focused interventions in younger children, as this combination of family anxiety management with CBT has been demonstrated to be particularly efficacious in the treatment of anxiety in preadolescent children (Barrett *et al.* 1996). Maternal depression had a deleterious effect on CBT for youth depressive disorders. Therefore, identification and treatment of parental depression may boost the efficacy of CBT for the treatment of adolescent depression.

There have been a paucity of studies comparing medication treatment to CBT or evaluating the combination. SSRIs are now the second most prescribed class of psychotropic agents in youth (Weisz & Jensen, 1999), and there is growing evidence of their utility for youthful depression, anxiety and OCD (Emslie *et al.* 1997; March *et al.* 1998b). Because there appears to be significant symptomatic residual after either CBT or pharmacological interventions (Brent *et al.* 1997; Emslie *et al.* 1997; Pine 2000), combination treatment may be indicated, particularly for those with more chronic and severe conditions. Studies of chronic depression in adults confirm the clinical impression that the combination of CBT and pharmacotherapy is superior to either monotherapy (Keller *et al.* 2000). Even though the overall efficacy of the two types of interventions appears comparable, SSRIs may have the advantage of cost and time savings, whereas CBT may have an impact on functional status more broadly defined than just by symptoms (e.g. improved social skills and self-esteem).

Relatively little is known about the mechanism of action of CBT. Kolko *et al.* (2000) showed specificity of CBT vs. other psychosocial treatments with regard to change in cognitive distortions, but failed to demonstrate that changes in cognitions mediate change in depression. Southam-Gerow *et al.* (2000) showed a relationship between negative self-talk and levels of anxiety symptomatology. Cohen & Mannarino (1996b, 1998a, 2000) found a relationship between child cognitions about abuse and outcome in sexually abused youth. Therefore, the extant data, scant as they are, do support a key role for alteration of cognitions in ameliorating internalizing symptomatology. However, the assessment of cognitive distortion has usually derived from a paper-and-pencil measure that is highly correlated with depression or anxiety. Other related domains, such as measures of mood regulation (Flett *et al.* 1996; Catanzaro 1997), tendency to ruminate or distract in the face of negative emotion (Nolen-Hoeksema & Morrow 1993), ability to acknowledge negative affect (McFarland & Buehler 1997), and ability to access positive memories to regulate negative mood (Rusting & DeHart 2000). Laboratory measures of cognitive and emotional regulation may also be helpful in understanding the relationship between information processing, working memory, attention and emotional regulation (Gotlib & McCann 1984; Power *et al.* 1996). More precisely targeted studies, using laboratory-based tasks, may help to inform us of the mechanisms of action of CBT and at the same time may allow more precise treatment development and treatment prescription. It may not be far-fetched to imagine that a treatment plan will be developed that combines neuroimaging and emotional regulation paradigms to pinpoint critical issues to target in treatment.

It would also be desirable to have additional information about the effectiveness of CBT in conditions more representative of typical clinical practice (Weisz *et al.* 1998). The findings on the robustness of CBT for the treatment of depression in the face of clinically complicating conditions may bode well for the effectiveness of the techniques in practice. Efforts to transport standard CBT protocols to anxious and depressed youth in community settings are now ongoing. It is quite likely that effects of CBT will be more modest in real-world samples of youth that may be characterized by parental histories of depression and substance abuse, high life stress and current chaos, single-parent or step-parent living situations, and multiple comorbid conditions (Hammen *et al.* 1999). However, such empirical transportability studies are needed because they will help us to understand overall efficacy in community settings, identify predictors of treatment response, and help provide guidance as to what aspects of CBT will need to be adapted to maximize effectiveness in real-world settings.

A related research agenda is the role of CBT in large-scale prevention. There is evidence that CBT can prevent the onset of depression and anxiety, but such findings need to be replicated. In addition, it is critical to evaluate the cost-efficiency of such an effort.

Overall, CBT has a strong track record as an intervention for youth with depression, anxiety and exposure to trauma. Future work on its use in combination with medication in complex and refractory cases, in extending its efficacy to efforts in the prevention of anxiety and depression, and in understanding its mechanisms of action should all enhance the utility of this intervention for paediatric anxiety and depression in the future.

Acknowledgements

This work was supported by NIMH grants MH18269, MH46500 and MH55123. It should be noted that the second and third authors contributed equally to this manuscript. The assistance of Beverly Sughrue in preparation of the manuscript is appreciated.

References

Barrett, P.M., Dadds, M.R. & Rapee, R.M. (1996) Family treatment of childhood anxiety: a controlled trial. *Journal of Consulting and Clinical Psychology*, 64, 333–342.

Beck, A.T., Rush, A.J., Shaw, B.F. & Emery, G. (1979) *Cognitive Therapy of Depression*. Guilford Press, New York.

Beck, A.T., Steer, R.A., Kovacs, M. & Garrison, B. (1985) Hopelessness and eventual suicide: a 10-year prospective study of patients hospitalized with suicidal ideation. *American Journal of Psychiatry*, 142, 559–563.

Berliner, L. & Saunders, B.E. (1996) Treating fear and anxiety in sexually abused children: results of a controlled 2-year follow-up study. *Child Maltreatment*, 1, 294–309.

Bernstein, G.A., Borchardt, C.M., Perwien, A.R. *et al.* (2000) Imipramine plus cognitive-behavioral therapy in the treatment of school refusal. *Journal of the American Academy of Child and Adolescent Psychiatry*, 39, 276–283.

Birmaher, B., Brent, D.A., Kolko, D. *et al.* (2000) Clinical outcome after short-term psychotherapy for adolescents with major depressive disorder. *Archives of General Psychiatry*, 57, 29–36.

Brent, D.A., Poling, K., McKain, B. & Baugher, M. (1993) A psychoeducational program for families of affectively ill children and adoles-

cents. *Journal of the American Academy of Child and Adolescent Psychiatry*, 32, 770–774.

Brent, D.A., Holder, D., Kolko, D. *et al.* (1997) A clinical psychotherapy trial for adolescent depression comparing cognitive, family, and supportive treatments. *Archives of General Psychiatry*, 54, 877–885.

Brent, D.A., Kolko, D., Birmaher, B. *et al.* (1998) Predictors of treatment efficacy in a clinical trial of three psychosocial treatments for adolescent depression. *Journal of the American Academy of Child and Adolescent Psychiatry*, 37, 906–914.

Brent, D.A., Kolko, D., Birmaher, B., Baugher, M. & Bridge, J. (1999) A clinical trial for adolescent depression: predictors of additional treatment in the acute and follow-up phases of the trial. *Journal of the American Academy of Child and Adolescent Psychiatry*, 38, 263–270.

Butler, L.F., Meizitis, S. & Friedman, R.J. (1980) The effect of two school-based intervention programs on depressive symptoms in preadolescent children. *American Education Research Journal*, 17, 111–119.

Catanzaro, S.J. (1997) Mood regulation expectancies, affect intensity, dispositional coping, and depressive symptoms: a conceptual analysis and empirical reanalysis. *Personality and Individual Differences*, 23, 1065–1069.

Celano, M., Hazzard, A., Webb, C. & McCall, C. (1996) Treatment of traumagenic beliefs among sexually abused girls and their mothers: an evaluation study. *Journal of Abnormal Child Psychology*, 24, 1–17.

Clarke, G., Hops, H., Lewinsohn, P.M., Andrew, J. & Williams, J. (1992) Cognitive-behavioral group treatment of adolescent depression: prediction of outcome. *Behavioral Therapy*, 23, 341–354.

Clarke, G.N., Hawkins, W., Murphy, M., Sheeber, L.B., Lewinsohn, P.M. & Seeley, J.R. (1995) Targeted prevention of unipolar depressive disorder in an at-risk sample of high school adolescents: a randomized trial of a group of cognitive intervention. *Journal of the American Academy of Child and Adolescent Psychiatry*, 34, 312–321.

Clarke, G.N., Lewinsohn, P.M., Rohde, P., Hops, H. & Seeley, J.R. (1999) Cognitive-behavioral group treatment of adolescent depression: efficacy of acute group treatment and booster sessions. *Journal of the American Academy of Child and Adolescent Psychiatry*, 38, 272–279.

Cohen, J.A. & Mannarino, A.P. (1996a) A treatment outcome study for sexually abused preschool children: initial findings. *Journal of the American Academy of Child and Adolescent Psychiatry*, 35, 42–50.

Cohen, J.A. & Mannarino, A.P. (1996b) Factors that mediate treatment outcome of sexually abused preschool children. *Journal of the American Academy of Child and Adolescent Psychiatry*, 35, 1402–1410.

Cohen, J.A. & Mannarino, A.P. (1998a) Interventions for sexually abused children: initial treatment outcome findings. *Child Maltreatment*, 3, 17–26.

Cohen, J.A. & Mannarino, A.P. (1998b) Factors that mediate treatment outcome of sexually abused preschol children: six- and 12-month follow-up. *Journal of the American Academy of Child and Adolescent Psychiatry*, 37, 44–51.

Cohen, J.A. & Mannarino, A.P. (2000) Predictors of treatment outcome in sexually abused children. *Child Abuse and Neglect*, 24, 983–994.

Dadds, M.R., Spence, S.H., Holland, D.E., Barrett, P.M. & Laurens, K.R. (1997) Prevention and early intervention for anxiety disorders: a controlled trial. *Journal of Consulting and Clinical Psychology*, 65, 627–635.

Deblinger, E., Lippmann, J. & Steer, R. (1996) Sexually abused children suffering posttraumatic stress symptoms: initial treatment outcome findings. *Child Maltreatment*, 1, 310–321.

DeVeaugh-Geiss, J., Moroz, G., Biederman, J. *et al.* (1992)

Clomipramine hydrochloride in childhood and adolescent obsessive-compulsive disorder: a multicenter trial. *Journal of the American Academy of Child and Adolescent Psychiatry*, 31, 45–49.

Emslie, G., Rush, J.A., Weinberg, W.A. *et al.* (1997) A double-blind, randomized placebo-controlled trial of fluoxetine in depressed children and adolescents. *Archives of General Psychiatry*, 54, 1031–1037.

Finkelhor, D. (1990) Early and long-term effects of child sexual abuse: an update. *Professional Psychology: Research and Practice*, 21, 325–330.

Flament, M., Rapoport, J., Berg, C.J. *et al.* (1985) Clomipramine treatment of childhood obsessive-compulsive disorder: a double-blind controlled study. *Archives of General Psychiatry*, 42, 977–983.

Flett, G.L., Blankstein, K.R. & Obertynski, M. (1996) Affect intensity, coping styles, mood regulation expectancies, and depressive symptoms. *Personality and Individual Differences*, 20, 221–228.

Franklin, M.E., Kozak, M.J., Cashman, L.A., Coles, M.E., Rheingold, A.A. & Foa, E.B. (1998) Cognitive-behavioral treatment of pediatric obsessive-compulsive disorder: an open clinical trial. *Journal of the American Academy of Child and Adolescent Psychiatry*, 37, 412–419.

Galante, R. & Foa, D. (1986) An epidemiological study of psychic trauma and treatment effectiveness for children after a natural disaster. *Journal of the American Academy of Child and Adolescent Psychiatry*, 25, 357–363.

Garber, J. & Hilsman, R. (1992) Cognitions, stress, and depression in children and adolescents. *Mood Disorders*, 1, 129–167.

Garber, J., Weiss, B. & Shanley, N. (1993) Cognitions, depressive symptoms, and development in adolescents. *Journal of Abnormal Psychology*, 102, 47–57.

Goenjian, A.K., Karayan, I., Pynoos, R.S. *et al.* (1997) Outcome of psychotherapy among early adolescents after trauma. *American Journal of Psychiatry*, 154, 536–542.

Gotlib, E.H. & McCann, C.D. (1984) Construct accessibility and depression: an examination of cognitive and affective factors. *Journal of Personality and Social Psychology*, 47, 427–439.

de Haan, E., Hoogduin, K., Buitelaar, J.K. & Keijsers, G. (1998) Behavior therapy versus clomipramine for the treatment of obsessive-compulsive disorder in children and adolescents. *Journal of the American Academy of Child and Adolescent Psychiatry*, 37, 1022–1029.

Hammen, C., Rudolph, K., Weisz, J., Rao, U. & Burge, D. (1999) The context of depression in clinic-referred youth: neglected areas in treatment. *Journal of the American Academy of Child and Adolescent Psychiatry*, 38, 64–71.

Hayward, C., Varady, S., Albano, A.M., Thienemann, M.L., Henderson, L. & Schatzberg, A. (2000) Cognitive-behavioral group therapy for social phobia in female adolescents: results of a pilot study. *Journal of the American Academy of Child and Adolescent Psychiatry*, 39, 721–726.

Jacobson, N.S. & Truax, P.A. (1991) Clinical significance: a statistical approach to defining meaningful change in psychotherapy research. *Journal of Consulting and Clinical Psychology*, 59, 12–19.

Jayson, D., Wood, A., Kroll, L., Fraser, J. & Harrington, R. (1998) Which depressed patients respond to cognitive-behavioral treatment? *Journal of the American Academy of Child and Adolescent Psychiatry*, 37, 35–39.

Kahn, J.S., Kehle, T.J., Jenson, W.R. & Clark, E. (1990) Comparison of cognitive-behavioral relaxation, and self-modeling interventions for depression among middle-school students. *School Psychology Review*, 19, 196–211.

Kaslow, N. & Thompson, M. (1998) Applying the criteria for empirically supported treatments to studies of psychosocial interventions for child and adolescent depression. *Journal of Clinical Child Psychology*, 27, 146–155.

Kazdin, A.E. & Weisz, J.R. (1998) Identifying and developing empirically supported child and adolescent treatments. *Journal of Consulting and Clinical Psychology*, 66, 19–36.

Keller, M.B., McCullough, J.P., Klein, D.N. *et al.* (2000) A comparison of nefazodone, the cognitive behavioral-analysis system of psychotherapy, and their combination for the treatment of chronic depression. *New England Journal of Medicine*, 342, 1462–1470.

Kendall, P.C. (1994) Treating anxiety disorders in children: results of a randomized clinical trial. *Journal of Consulting and Clinical Psychology*, 62, 100–110.

Kendall, P.C. & Southam-Gerow, M.A. (1996) Long-term follow up of a cognitive-behavioural therapy for anxiety-disordered youth. *Journal of Consulting and Clinical Psychology*, 64, 724–730.

Kendall, P.C., Flannery-Schroeder, E., Panichelli-Mindel, S.M., Southam-Gerow, M.A., Henin, M. & Warman, M. (1997) Therapy for youths with anxiety disorders: a second randomized clinical trial. *Journal of Consulting and Clinical Psychology*, 65, 366–380.

King, N.J., Tonge, B.J., Heyne, D. *et al.* (1998) Cognitive-behavioral treatment of school-refusing children: a controlled evaluation. *Journal of the American Academy of Child and Adolescent Psychiatry*, 37, 395–403.

Kolko, D.J. (1996) Individual cognitive behavioral treatment and family therapy for physically abused children and their offending parents: a comparison of clinical outcomes. *Child Maltreatment*, 1, 322–342.

Kolko, D., Brent, D., Baugher, M., Bridge, J. & Birmaher, B. (2000) Cognitive and family therapies for adolescent depression: treatment specifity, mediation and moderation. *Journal of Consulting and Clinical Psychology*, 68, 603–614.

Kroll, L., Harrington, R., Jayson, D., Fraser, J. & Gowers, S. (1996) Pilot study of continuation cognitive-behavioral therapy for major depression in adolescent psychiatric patients. *Journal of the American Academy of Child and Adolescent Psychiatry*, 35, 1156–1161.

Last, C.G., Hansen, C.R. & Franco, N. (1998) Cognitive-behavioral treatment of school phobia. *Journal of the American Academy of Child and Adolescent Psychiatry*, 37, 404–411.

Lewinsohn, P.M. & Clarke, G.N. (1999) Psychosocial treatments for adolescent depression. *Clinical Psychology Review*, 19, 329–342.

Lewinsohn, P.M., Clarke, G.N., Hops, H. & Andrews, J. (1990) Cognitive-behavioral treatment for depressed adolescents. *Behavior Therapy*, 21, 385–401.

Lewinsohn, P.M., Roberts, R.E., Seeley, J.R., Rohde, P., Gotlib, I.H. & Hops, H. (1994) Adolescent psychopathology. II. Psychosocial risk factors for depression. *Journal of Abnormal Psychology*, 103, 302–315.

Lewinsohn, P.M., Clarke, G.N., Rohde, P., Hops, H. & Seeley, J.R. (1996) A course in coping: a cognitive-behavioral approach to the treatment of adolescent depression. In: *Psychosocial Treatments for Child and Adolescent Disorders: Empirically Based Strategies for Clinical Practice* (eds E.D. Hibbs & P.S. Jensen), pp. 109–135. American Psychiatric Association, Washington D.C.

Lewinsohn, P.M., Gotlib, I.H. & Seeley, J.R. (1997) Depression-related psychosocial variables: are they specific to depression in adolescents? *Journal of Abnormal Psychology*, 106, 365–375.

Liddle, B.J. & Spence, S.H. (1990) Cognitive-behavior therapy with depressed primary school children: a cautionary note. *Behavioural Psychotherapy*, 18, 85–102.

March, J.S., Mulle, K. & Herbel, B. (1994) Behavioral psychotherapy for children and adolescents with obsessive-compulsive disorder: an open trial of a new protocol-driven treatment package. *Journal of* the *American Academy of Child and Adolescent Psychiatry*, **33**, 333–341.

March, J.S., Amaya-Jackson, L., Murray, M.C. & Schulte, A. (1998a) Cognitive-behavioral psychotherapy for children and adolescents with posttraumatic stress disorder after a single-incident stressor. *Journal of the American Academy of Child and Adolescent Psychiatry*, **37**, 585–593.

March, J.S., Biederman, J., Wolkow, R. *et al.* (1998b) Sertraline in children and adolescents with obsessive-compulsive disorder: a multicenter randomized controlled trial. *Journal of the American Medical Association*, **280**, 1752–1756.

McFarland, C. & Buehler, R. (1997) Negative affective states and the motivated retrieval of positive life events: the role of affect acknowledgment. *Journal of Personality and Social Psychology*, **73**, 200–214.

Murphy, G.E., Simons, A.D., Wetzel, R.D. & Lustman, P.J. (1984) Cognitive therapy and pharmacotherapy: singly and together in the treatment of depression. *Archives of General Psychiatry*, **41**, 33–41.

Nolen-Hoeksema, S. & Morrow, J. (1993) Effects of rumination and distraction on naturally occurring depressed mood. *Cognition and Emotion*, **7**, 561–570.

Pine, D. (2000) *The RUPP anxiety study: design and results.* 40th Annual New Clinical Drug Evaluation Unit Program Meeting, May, 2000.

Power, M.J., Cameron, C.M. & Dalgleish, T. (1996) Emotional priming in clinically depressed subjects. *Journal of Affective Disorders*, **38**, 1–11.

Reinecke, M.A., Ryan, N.E. & DuBois, L. (1998) Cognitive-behavioral therapy of depression and depressive symptoms during adolescence: a review and meta-analysis. *Journal of the American Academy of Child and Adolescent Psychiatry*, **37**, 26–34.

Reynolds, W.M. & Coats, K.I. (1986) A comparison of cognitive-behavioral therapy and relaxation training for the treatment of depression in adolescents. *Journal of Consulting and Clinical Psychology*, **54**, 653–660.

Riddle, M.A., Scahill, L., King, R.A. *et al.* (1992) Double-blind, crossover trial of fluoxetine and placebo in children and adolescents with obsessive-compulsive disorder. *Journal of the American Academy of Child and Adolescent Psychiatry*, **31**, 1062–1069.

Rosselló, J. & Bernal, G. (1999) The efficacy of cognitive-behavioral and interpersonal treatments for depression in Puerto Rican adolescents. *Journal of Consulting and Clinical Psychology*, **67**, 734–745.

Rusting, C.L. & DeHart, T. (2000) Retrieving positive memories to regulate negative mood: consequences of mood-congruent memory. *Journal of Personality and Social Psychology*, **78**, 737–752.

Southam-Gerow, M.A., Kendall, P.C. & Weersing, V.R. (2001) Examining outcome variability: correlates of treatment response in a child and adolescent anxiety clinic. *Journal of Clinical Child Psychology*, **30**, 422–436.

Stark, K.D., Reynolds, W.M. & Kaslow, N.J. (1987) A comparison of the relative efficacy of self-control therapy and a behavioral problem-solving therapy for depression in children. *Journal of Abnormal Child Psychology*, **15**, 91–113.

Treadwell, K.R. & Kendall, P.C. (1996) Self-talk in youth with anxiety disorders: states of mind, content specificity, and treatment outcome. *Journal of Consulting and Clinical Psychology*, **64**, 941–950.

Vostanis, P., Feehan, C., Grattan, E. & Bickerton, W. (1996a) A randomised controlled out-patient trial of cognitive-behavioural treatment for children and adolescents with depression: 9-month follow-up. *Journal of Affective Disorders*, **40**, 105–116.

Vostanis, P., Feehan, C., Grattan, E. & Bickerton, W. (1996b) Treatment for children and adolescents with depression: lessons from a controlled trial. *Clincal Child Psychology and Psychiatry*, **1**, 199–212.

Weisz, J.R. & Jensen, P.S. (1999) Efficacy and effectiveness of child and adolescent psychotherapy and pharmacotherapy. *Mental Health Services Research*, **1**, 125–158.

Weisz, J.R. & Weersing, V.R. (1999) Psychotherapy with children and adolescents: efficacy, effectiveness, and developmental concerns. In: *Rochester Symposium on Developmental Psychopathology*, Vol. 9. *Developmental Approaches to Prevention and Intervention* (eds D. Cicchetti & S.L. Toth), pp. 341–386. University of Rochester Press, Rochester, NY.

Weisz, J.R., Thurber, C.A., Sweeney, L., Proffitt, V.D. & LeGagnoux, G.L. (1997) Brief treatment of mild-to-moderate child depression using primary and secondary control enhancement training. *Journal of Consulting and Clinical Psychology*, **65**, 703–707.

Weisz, J.R., Huey, S.M. & Weersing, V.R. (1998) Psychotherapy outcome research with children and adolescents: the state of the art. In: *Advances in Clinical Child Psychology* (eds T.H. Ollendick & R.J. Prinz), Vol. 20, pp. 49–92. Plenum Publishing, New York.

Wood, A., Harrington, R. & Moore, A. (1996) Controlled trial of a brief cognitive-behavioural intervention in adolescent patients with depressive disorders. *Journal of Clinical Child Psychology*, **37**, 737–746.

# 55

Problem-solving and Problem-solving Therapies

Bruce E. Compas, Molly Benson, Margaret Boyer,
Thomas V. Hicks and Brian Konik

Introduction

The capacity to solve social and interpersonal problems is an integral feature of adaptive development. Conversely, deficits in problem-solving are related to both internalizing and externalizing disorders in childhood and adolescence. Problem-solving skills and deficits are implicated in social information processing models of aggression and disruptive behaviour disorders (Crick & Dodge 1996), cognitive models of depression (Lewinsohn & Gotlib 1995), the development of social competence (Rudolph & Heller 1997), self-regulatory processes (Eisenberg *et al.* 1997) and coping with stress and adversity (Compas *et al.*, 2001). The apparent significance of problem-solving skills is further evident in its prominence in many forms of cognitive-behavioural interventions for children and adolescents, including the treatment of anxiety, depression, conduct disorder and family conflict. The centrality of problem-solving skills in psychological treatment is reflected in a subset of therapies that are explicitly labelled 'problem-solving therapy' (Dujovne *et al.* 1995; Mynors-Wallis *et al.* 1997; Nezu *et al.* 1998).

In spite of the pervasive role of problem-solving skills in child/adolescent psychopathology and treatment, much of the research on, and application of, these skills has dealt with them in isolation from other forms of self-regulation. Problem-solving skills can be best understood as a component of a larger set of adaptive self-regulatory skills that are involved in successfully managing stressful and adverse situations, circumstances and events. In this chapter we examine problem-solving skills in the context of the more general processes of self-regulation and coping, the current role of problem-solving in the treatment of child/adolescent psychopathology, and consider future directions for increasing our understanding of the importance of problem-solving in child/adolescent psychopathology.

Conceptual models of problem-solving

Definitions of problem-solving

Problem-solving is broadly defined as a cognitive and behavioural process involved in managing and mastering the challenges and difficulties encountered in everyday living (D'Zurilla & Goldfried 1971; D'Zurilla & Sheedy 1991). Problem-solving encompasses both a cognitive-motivational orientation and a set of cognitive and behavioural skills used in responding to and overcoming daily problems. The primary components of problem-solving skills as outlined by D'Zurilla & Nezu (1990) include:

1 problem definition and formulation;
2 generation of alternative solutions;
3 decision-making and selection of a solution; and
4 implementation and evaluation of a solution.

Problem definition and formulation involves obtaining relevant, factual information about the problem, clarifying the nature of the problem and delineating a set of realistic problem-solving goals. Generation of alternative solutions includes the identification, discovery or creation of as many alternative solutions as possible in order to maximize the likelihood that the best possible solution or solutions will be among them. Decision-making involves the evaluation and comparison of the different alternatives and the selection of the best overall solution for the particular problematic situation. Finally, implementation and evaluation of a solution includes self-monitoring and assessment of the outcome of the solution that has been implemented.

Shure & Spivack (1971), in their conceptualization of interpersonal cognitive problem-solving, highlighted the following three related skills.

1 *Alternative thinking*: the generation of alternative solutions to a given problem.
2 *Consequential thinking*: the ability to imagine the short- and long-range outcomes of particular solutions.
3 *Means–ends thinking*: the ability to plan a sequence of specific goal-directed actions in order to avoid obstacles and solve problems in a desirable timely manner.

Problem-solving skills are often described as synonymous with problem-focused coping strategies: strategies for coping with stress that are orientated toward managing or dealing with the problem that is the source of stress (D'Zurilla & Chang 1995). As such, problem-solving skills are orientated toward resolving a problem in the social environment or a problematic situation and are distinct from the skills that are used in managing emotional distress and arousal (typically referred to as emotion-focused coping). Problem-solving responses are instrumental and involve engagement with the problem at hand, as opposed to disengagement or avoidance of the problem.

Problem-solving skills are related to higher social competence and adaptive functioning in children and adults, and deficits in problem-solving skills have been documented in children and adolescents with disruptive behaviour disorders, anxiety disorders, depression and interpersonal conflict. Both well-adjusted and poorly adjusted children generate socially undesirable solutions to problems, such as aggressive retaliation, but only well-adjusted children also identify positive solutions and probable outcomes to various alternative solutions (Spivack *et al.* 1976). Problem-solving skills are also related to other psychological variables among children and adolescents, including family conflict and communication skills (Robin *et al.* 1990), externalizing disorders (Kazdin 1997) and internalizing disorders (Sacco & Graves 1984).

Problem-solving, self-regulation and coping

In spite of the well-established relationships between problem-solving skills and both social competence and psychopathology, it is important to place problem-solving in a broader context. Specifically, problem-solving skills are one component of broader processes of self-regulation and coping with stress. Self-regulation refers to the capacity of the individual to initiate, terminate, delay, modify the form or content, or modulate the amount or intensity of a thought, emotion, behaviour or physiological reaction; or redirect thought or behaviour toward a new target (Compas *et al.*, 2001). Coping further refers to a subset of self-regulatory processes that are volitionally and intentionally enacted specifically in response to stress (Compas *et al.* 1999). Specifically, coping involves conscious volitional efforts to regulate emotion, cognition, behaviour, physiology and the environment in response to stressful events or circumstances (Compas *et al.* 2001).

Coping processes, including problem-solving skills, are controlled and volitional in nature, as contrasted with other responses to stress that are automatic and involuntary. The basis for the distinction between controlled voluntary and automatic involuntary responses is based on extensive research from cognitive, social, developmental and clinical psychology. This includes research on associative conditioning and learning (Shiffrin 1997); research on strategic/controlled and automatic cognitive processes in emotions and emotional disorders (Mathews & MacLeod 1994; McNally 1995); research distinguishing some involuntary aspects of temperamental characteristics from intentional behaviour and cognitive processes (Rothbart 1991); and research on automaticity in social cognition (Bargh 1997; Mischel 1997). Both voluntary and involuntary stress responses can be further distinguished as engaging with a stressor or one's responses to the stressor, or disengaging from the stressor and one's responses. The origins of the engagement–disengagement dimension can be found in the concept of the fight (engagement) or flight (disengagement) response (Cannon 1933, 1934; Gray 1991), and in the contrast between approach and avoidance responses (Krohne 1996). Problem-solving skills are an important aspect of engagement orientated coping responses.

Problem-solving skills have frequently been described as an example of the broader category of problem-focused coping strategies within a framework that contrasts problem-focused with emotion-focused coping (D'Zurilla & Chang 1995). How-

ever, recent research with children and adolescents has shown that the problem- and emotion-focused model does not adequately reflect the characteristics of the ways that children and adolescents cope with stress. Specifically, using confirmatory factor analyses to contrast different conceptual models of child and adolescent coping, both Ayers *et al.* (1996) and Connor-Smith *et al.* (2000) found that a problem- and emotion-focused model of coping did not achieve an adequate fit with self-reports of coping from large samples of children and youth. In contrast, results of confirmatory factor analyses suggest that three categories of coping may warrant further analysis (Ayers *et al.* 1996; Walker *et al.* 1997; Connor-Smith *et al.* 2000). The first involves active coping efforts that are intended to achieve some degree of personal control over the stressful aspects of the environment and one's emotions. This factor has been labelled 'active coping' by Ayers *et al.* (1996) and Walker *et al.* (1997), and we have used the label of 'primary control coping' (Connor-Smith *et al.* 2000). In our recent factor analytic studies, problem-solving coping loads on the primary control factor along with coping responses representing emotion regulation and emotional expression (Connor-Smith *et al.* 2000). This provides some evidence that problem-solving skills are closely related to other important aspects of self-regulation, including the regulation of emotion and arousal. Active or primary control coping is distinguished from accommodative or secondary control coping (e.g. acceptance, distraction, cognitive restructuring), and from disengagement coping (e.g. avoidance, denial, wishful thinking), the second and third coping categories.

Because coping involves conscious volitional regulatory efforts, it is a subset of executive functions or processes governed by the frontal cortex. Executive functions include the cognitive processes for future goal-directed behaviour that involve achieving and maintaining a problem-solving set, and include processes such as planning, organizational skills, selective attention and inhibitory control (Morgan & Lilienfeld 2000). The executive functions of the frontal cortex have been hypothesized to have a central role in response control or inhibition, and other aspects of self-regulation (Dempster 1992; Fox 1994; Barkley 1998). Furthermore, coping processes, including problem-solving, are strongly influenced by linguistic function, and some of the more complex aspects of coping include cognitive processes, such as generating plans or solutions to a problem, cognitively reframing a stressful situation, distracting oneself with pleasant thoughts, and accepting circumstances as they are. Thus, problem-solving skills are likely to emerge over the course of development in early and middle childhood. Tapert *et al.* (1999) found that neurocognitive abilities (as reflected in a measure of general intelligence) interacted with coping skills in predicting relapse to alcohol and drug use. These processes can be contrasted with involuntary responses to stress that are hypothesized to be controlled by more primitive aspects of the brain and central nervous system, including the amygdala and aspects of the limbic system (Kagan *et al.* 1992). These include the sympathetic and parasympathetic arms of the autonomic nervous system that control stress reactivity and recovery (Grossman

1992; Porges *et al.* 1994; Berntson *et al.* 1997). Although autonomic nervous system processes can be brought under conscious control to some degree (e.g. through biofeedback), they are triggered by automatic or involuntary responses to threat or challenge.

Problem-solving therapy

We now turn our attention to the role of problem-solving in the treatment of child and adolescent psychopathology. Early reviews of problem-solving interventions presented support for these programmes in effecting positive behavioural changes in children (Urbain & Kendall 1980; Pellegrini & Urbain 1985). The reported effects of problem-solving interventions included decreases in aggression and impulsivity, as well as increases in prosocial behavior and cognitive abilities. These early reviews also found several shortcomings in intervention programmes, such as small effect sizes, small sample sizes and the lack of control groups (Urbain & Kendall 1980; Pellegrini & Urbain 1985). Although these prior reviews represented an important contribution to the field, they were limited in several ways. First, the initial reviews were conducted over 15 years ago, limiting the conclusions that can be drawn about the current status of problem-solving interventions. Second, previous reviews have highlighted only certain aspects of problem-solving, such as focusing primarily on interventions based on Spivack & Shure's model (Pellegrini & Urbain 1985).

The present review is designed to provide a contemporary look at the effects of child/adolescent therapies that involve problem-solving, and to consider the development of problem-solving skills as contrasted with other components of these interventions. We approach the literature by examining therapies for four different problems: anxiety disorders, depression, disruptive behaviour disorders, and parent–adolescent conflict. The present review is not intended to be comprehensive, but rather to highlight certain interventions in which the teaching of problem-solving skills plays a central part. Although there are other models for the treatment of these disorders, comparative studies of problem-solving therapies with other approaches have been rare, an issue to which we return in the final section of this chapter.

Anxiety disorders

Problem-solving in the treatment of child/adolescent anxiety is best exemplified by the work of Kendall *et al.* (1990) in the development of a cognitive-behavioural therapy. This manualized treatment, the 'Coping Cat', was identified as a 'probably efficacious' treatment by Kazdin & Weisz (1998) in their review of empirically supported child and adolescent treatments.

Primary components

The Coping Cat is a 16-session treatment that involves several behavioural methods for the treatment of anxiety including exposure exercises, relaxation training, modelling, role-plays, and positive reinforcement contingencies. These behavioural methods are combined with several cognitive techniques aimed at addressing the information-processing factors believed to underlie excessive anxious arousal. Cognitive techniques incorporated into Kendall's approach include the identification and modification of maladaptive self-talk, and the development of cognitive strategies for reducing unwanted physiological arousal. The Coping Cat treatment programme is divided into two sections. The first eight sessions are aimed at skill development and training, and the final eight sessions focus on skill implementation and practising the acquired coping strategies in anxiety-provoking situations.

Problem-solving components

Although the Coping Cat programme is not explicitly defined as a problem-solving approach to childhood anxiety, there are a number of problem-solving features incorporated into the programme. Through a series of lessons and exercises, children are taught to use a four-step plan for coping with unwanted anxiety. In order to help them remember these steps in challenging situations, children in Kendall's programme refer to this four-step plan using the acronym FEAR. The first step in the FEAR plan ('Feeling frightened?') helps children to identify the somatic signs and symptoms of their anxiety. The second step ('Expecting bad things to happen?') focuses on identifying negative cognitions that may be contributing to unwanted anxious arousal. This second step also serves to assist children in identifying an important aetiological component of their problem by examining 'anxious self-talk'. The third step in the FEAR plan ('Attitudes and actions that will help?') encourages children to generate alternative solutions to their problem and then consider which of those alternatives would be the most effective given the situation. This third step therefore involves not only the generation of possible solutions to the problem, but also a consideration of the consequences of each of the choices available. The final step of the FEAR plan ('Results and rewards?') asks children to evaluate the results of the methods they used to cope with the anxiety-provoking situation. After evaluating the results of their actions, children in the Coping Cat programme are encouraged to reward themselves for success or partial success in dealing with their anxiety.

The four-step FEAR plan central to Kendall's treatment package has a great deal in common with conceptualizations of the problem-solving process. The problem-solving strategies conveyed through the FEAR plan in Kendall's programme are consistent with the essential problem-solving skills identified by D'Zurilla & Goldfried (1971) and D'Zurilla (1988): problem definition and formulation; generation of alternative solutions; decision-making; and solution implementation and verification. Furthermore, this programme incorporates all three of the fundamental skills outlined in Spivack & Shure's (1976) model: alternative thinking; means–end thinking; and consequential thinking. Thus, the Coping Cat treatment can be viewed as an attempt to teach effective problem-solving strategies to children in order to cope with unwanted anxious arousal.

Treatment outcome research

The effectiveness of this cognitive-behavioural treatment for child anxiety has been demonstrated in a series of empirical studies. Kendall (1994) conducted a randomized clinical trial of 47 children (aged 9–13 years) with a primary anxiety disorder diagnosis to compare his cognitive-behavioural intervention to a waiting list control condition. Based on child and parent reports, as well as behavioural observations, it was found that children in the treatment condition showed significantly more improvement at post-treatment as compared to children in the waiting list condition. Furthermore, these differences represented clinically significant improvement and treatment effects were maintained at both 1- and 3-year follow-ups (Kendall & Southam-Gerow 1996). A second randomized clinical trial of 94 children with a primary diagnosis of an anxiety disorder replicated and confirmed these results (Kendall et al. 1997). This second study again showed that treatment gains were maintained at 1-year follow-up.

Additional support for Kendall's cognitive-behavioural treatment can be found in research conducted in Australia by Barrett et al. (1996). By shortening the initial skill development and training section of the programme, these investigators modified Kendall's 16-session Coping Cat treatment to create a very similar 12-session cognitive-behavioural programme (the Coping Koala). In a study of 79 children with a primary anxiety disorder diagnosis, Barrett et al. (1996) found that their modified version of Kendall's programme produced both statistically and clinically significant change relative to a waiting list control. Treatment gains were maintained at 6- and 12-month follow-ups. In addition to the support provided by this Australian adaptation of Kendall's therapy, it is worth noting that other authors have provided evidence that Kendall's approach can be modified to create an effective group cognitive-behavioural treatment for anxiety disorders in children (Barrett 1998; Silverman et al. 1999).

Given the impressive empirical data supporting Kendall's approach, the next logical question involves the identification of the essential active ingredients within the Coping Cat programme. Specifically, is the acquisition of problem-solving skills essential to the effectiveness of Kendall's method? Addressing this question requires components analysis, and unfortunately only a single preliminary examination of treatment segments has been conducted to explore active ingredients within Kendall's Coping Cat therapy (Kendall et al. 1997). Mid-treatment assessment data were obtained in the second randomized clinical trial of the treatment in order to compare the effects of the first half of the programme, which focuses on education, to the second half of the programme, which focuses on exposure and skill implementation. Kendall et al. found that changes generated by the first half of treatment were not significantly different from the waiting list control condition. In contrast, changes

that occurred during the second half of treatment were significantly different from the waiting list control.

This preliminary examination suggests that an intervention limited to education regarding the nature of anxious arousal combined with learning a systematic approach to problem-solving in anxiety-provoking situations does not produce significant behavioural change. This suggests that not only learning but also practising problem-solving skills is important for behaviour change. However, as Kendall et al. (1997) noted, because the order of the treatment segments was not counterbalanced, an analysis of the effects of the second half of treatment is actually an analysis of the effects of both treatment segments combined. In other words, the effectiveness of this second half of the treatment may not simply be brought about by effects of imaginal and in vivo exposure, but rather by exposure that occurs while the child uses the systematic FEAR problem-solving strategy acquired during the first half of the programme.

Both Kendall et al. (1997) and Kazdin & Weisz (1998) have emphasized the need to 'unpack' cognitive-behavioural treatments for child anxiety disorders in order to identify treatment components that are essential to creating lasting behavioural change. This type of components analysis will also be necessary in order to clarify the importance of acquiring effective problem-solving skills for dealing with fear and anxiety. Although Kendall et al.'s preliminary examination of treatment segments seems to imply that simply educating children in effective problem-solving is not enough to effect significant change, it is not yet clear how essential problem-solving skills are when combined with exposure. Future studies are necessary to compare the effectiveness of an intervention that is limited to imaginal and in vivo exposure with a programme combining these exposure elements with education in effective problem-solving strategies.

Depression

Cognitive-behavioural treatment programmes targeting depressed children and adolescents have extensively utilized components of problem-solving training. One treatment protocol for depressed youth, the Adolescent Coping with Depression course for adolescents (Clarke et al. 1990), includes sessions that specifically focus on problem-solving. Research on this treatment programme indicates that the intervention effectively reduces symptoms of depression in adolescents diagnosed with dysthymia or major depressive disorder (Lewinsohn et al. 1985, 1990; Clarke et al. 1999).

Primary components

The Adolescent Coping with Depression programme (Clarke et al. 1990) is a 16-session cognitive-behavioural and psychoeducational treatment designed for adolescents aged 14–18 years. Sessions focus on relaxation training, pleasant events scheduling, cognitive restructuring, and building social skills, communication skills and problem-solving skills. The treatment protocol is designed for a group format, although it can be adapted for individual treatment. Therapist-led groups include didactic presentations, group discussions, role-playing and in-group practice of specific skills. Adolescents complete weekly homework assignments focused on monitoring and practice of skills learned in group sessions. The programme includes optional parent groups that can be run simultaneously with the adolescent groups for nine sessions. Although these groups are run separately, two sessions of problem-solving included in the adolescent treatment manual are designed for joint parent–child group interactions.

Problem-solving components

The 16-session treatment includes four sessions that specifically focus on problem-solving and communication skills. Clarke *et al.* (1990) included problem-solving in the treatment protocol based on the hypothesis that the inability to resolve family conflicts may contribute to and maintain adolescent depression. Clarke *et al.* (1990) based their model of problem-solving and negotiation techniques on those developed by Gottman *et al.* (1976), Robin (1979) and Forgatch & Patterson (1989). The sessions draw on Robin's (1979) model of a four-step problem-solving process: problem definition; brainstorming alternative solutions; selection of a solution through negotiation; and specification of details for implementation of solution. Problem-solving and negotiation are the final skills taught and practised as part of the overall treatment programme.

The first session dedicated to problem-solving introduces rules for defining a problem and involves in-session practice of problem-solving and active listening through role-playing techniques. Adolescents are asked to practice these skills as homework before the next session. In the subsequent session, youths are introduced to brainstorming techniques. This includes structured guidelines for evaluating solutions and writing detailed contracts for implementation of the chosen solution. Adolescents then practice role-playing the process of problem definition, solution generation, evaluation and implementation. Participants are assigned homework involving the completion of the Issues Checklist (Robin & Weiss 1980) and practice of the skills learned in-session. The final two sessions dedicated to problem-solving address in-session interactions between youths and their parents. In the absence of parents, adolescents role-play with other group members in dyads that are closely supervised by therapists. These final two sessions address actual problems defined by the adolescents and their caregivers on the Issues Checklist. In-session, adolescents utilize the skills they have learned to practise problem-solving these issues. In addition, time is spent reviewing how to explain this process to parents and how to explore more distressing issues in the future.

Treatment outcome research

Outcome studies of the Adolescent Coping with Depression course have demonstrated statistically and clinically significant changes in symptoms of depression at post-treatment and follow-up (Lewinsohn *et al.* 1990; Clarke *et al.* 1999). Patients in Lewinsohn *et al.*'s (1990) study were assigned to an adolescent only, adolescent–parent, or waiting list control group. Compared to participants in the waiting list group, adolescents in both treatment groups reported significantly fewer symptoms of depression on the Beck Depression Inventory (BDI) and the Center for Epidemiological Studies–Depression Scale (CES-D) post-treatment. Similarly, they reported a significant decrease in the number of participants meeting diagnostic criteria for depression, as determined by the Schedule for Affective Disorders and Schizophrenia for School-Age Children (Kiddie-SADS) interview in the treatment groups following the intervention. Differences between the two treatment groups were not significant, indicating that the parent group did not have a differential effect on the youth's self-report of depressive symptoms. Scores reflecting internalizing and externalizing symptoms on the Child Behaviour Checklist (CBCL; Achenbach 1991) completed by parents, on the other hand, were significantly lower for adolescents in the adolescent–parent group as compared with the adolescent only group at post-treatment. However, behaviours reported by parents of participants in the adolescent only group continued to decrease so that CBCL scores were equivalent by 6-month follow-up. Participants in both treatment conditions maintained treatment gains over a 2-year follow-up period.

These clinically and statistically significant reductions in depressive symptoms were replicated by the Clarke *et al.* (1999) study. This second study expanded the intervention by providing booster sessions and follow-up assessments. The results indicated that booster sessions did not reduce unipolar depression recurrence rates in the follow-up period, but did accelerate recovery in adolescents who were still depressed at the end of the intervention trial (Clarke *et al.* 1999).

Components analysis

Although no studies to date have looked at a components analysis of the problem-solving element of this intervention, Lewinsohn *et al.*'s (1990) study did investigate outcomes related to specific issues addressed by the treatment components. Measures were used to assess depressive cognitions, pleasant events, social skills and conflict resolution. The Issues Checklist (Robin & Weiss 1980), which contains 44 issues that are typically problematic for adolescents and their parents, was used to assess conflict resolution. Although this is not a precise measure of problem-solving skills, the components of the intervention that addressed problem-solving and negotiation also utilized this checklist. Therefore, outcome data on this measure are likely to reflect specific skills gained during treatment. However, the results indicated no significant differences post-treatment between the treatment and waiting list conditions on scores on the Issues Checklist (Lewinsohn *et al.* 1990). Nevertheless, scores on the Issues Checklist did improve over time, resulting in a significant difference between post-treatment and 6-month follow-up scores (Lewinsohn *et al.* 1990).

Disruptive behaviour disorders

Problem-solving therapies for disruptive behaviour disorders have been developed to train children and adolescents to identify effectively potential problem situations, to create alternative solutions to the problem, to evaluate the different possible results of each alternative and choose the most effective one. Early studies showed that non-clinical samples of oppositional and defiant children could improve their abilities to create alternative solutions to problems as well as display some limited improvement in overall problem-solving abilities (Gresham 1985). Building on this early work, Kazdin et al. (1987a,b, 1989, 1992) have demonstrated that these same problem-solving strategies can result in reductions in problem behaviours with clinical samples.

Kazdin et al. have developed a specific variation of problem-solving therapy, Problem-solving Skills Training (PSST), which incorporates aspects of self-instructional procedures similar to those in early problem-solving interventions (Camp & Bash 1981). Based on the work of Luria (1961), Vygotsky (1962) and Meichenbaum & Goodman (1971), it has been hypothesized that problem-solving skills training could lead to the reduction of impulsive behaviours (Spence 1994). In PSST the primary goal is to bolster the interpersonal problem-solving skills that are considered to be deficient in children with conduct disorder.

Primary components

Kazdin (1996) describes five essential features of PSST. First, the emphasis in PSST is on the process that the child uses in choosing behaviours, rather than on the behaviours themselves. The second essential feature of PSST involves teaching the strategy of a step-by-step analysis of interpersonal situations. In this phase, self-instructional features are used to direct the child's attention to critical elements of the process that can lead to a successful and appropriate resolution of a conflict. Third, although problem-solving skills are eventually applied to real world situations, PSST begins with the application of problem-solving skills to simulated situations presented in the form of games, academic tasks and stories. When efficacy is established in these simulations, the skills are progressively applied to real-world situations. The fourth component of PSST is the active role that the therapist takes in the treatment. The therapist not only teaches the skills, but also models the use of self-instruction and provides feedback and rewards for effective use of the skills. The use of a wide array of methods to teach problem-solving skills, such as modelling, role-play and positive reinforcement, is the final distinguishing component of PSST.

Problem-solving components

PSST was designed as a manualized treatment conducted over a minimum of 16 sessions over 4–5 months. The process of problem-solving has been broken down into five different steps.

Each of the following five problem-solving steps is linked to a self-instruction statement.
1 Step 1 requires a child to identify a problem.
2 Step 2 involves the child arriving at solutions to the problem.
3 Step 3 asks the child to evaluate the generated solutions.
4 Step 4 asks the child to choose the answer thought to be the most correct.
5 Step 5 requires the child to verify whether or not the answer was correct or appropriate, and the child is asked to determine whether the choice was self-reinforcing.

A central component in problem-solving skills therapy is the use of contingencies. Social reinforcement in the form of verbal, non-verbal and affectionate attention is used to facilitate skill development. A token system is used in PSST for two purposes: first to reduce the frequency of errors in problem-solving tasks and strategies; and secondly to reduce impulsive behaviour. Following a basic response–cost model, the child is given a specific number of tokens at the beginning of each session. When the child acts impulsively by moving too quickly through a task, or makes a mistake by improperly using a problem-solving skill, the child is fined a token. The child is able to earn additional tokens by accurately self-evaluating his or her performance at the end of a session. At the end of each therapy session the child is able to use these tokens to purchase a prize from a reward menu.

Treatment outcome research

Kazdin has conducted the majority of outcome studies on the effects of PSST in children with conduct disorder. In a series of studies, PSST has been compared against a non-directive relationship therapy (RT) and a waiting list control in the treatment of children exhibiting severe antisocial childhood behaviour. Kazdin et al. (1987a) examined the effects of PSST on children in the study who met diagnostic criteria for conduct disorder (69% of the sample), and children with scores in the clinical range on the Aggression or Delinquency scales of the CBCL. PSST was shown to reduce externalizing and aggressive behaviours significantly more than RT or no intervention. There were also significant reductions, as compared to RT and controls, in overall problem behaviours at school and home for the PSST group (Kazdin et al. 1987a).

In a subsequent study in which 75% of the participants met criteria for conduct disorder, PSST alone was compared to PSST with in vivo practice (PSST-P) that extended therapy and training to situations outside of treatment (Kazdin et al. 1989). Children in the PSST-P group were given tasks that involved applying skills learned to treatment in real-life situations where their problem behaviours often occurred. PSST and PSST-P groups were compared to RT groups and controls. Children in the PSST and PSST-P groups showed significantly greater reductions in antisocial behaviour and overall behaviour problems, and an increase in prosocial behaviour as compared to the RT and control groups. All differences between PSST and PSST-P groups were absent at follow-up (Kazdin et al. 1989).

More recent outcome studies have focused on comparing the benefits of combining PSST and other cognitive therapies such as parent management training (PMT; Kazdin *et al.* 1987b, 1992). The combined effects of PSST and PMT have been shown to be more effective at reducing externalizing and aggressive behaviours then either PSST or PMT alone (Kazdin *et al.* 1987b, 1992).

Clinical significance

Even though the children in these outcome studies showed a decrease in antisocial behaviour, the PSST intervention has not yet demonstrated high levels of clinically significant change. For example, in Kazdin's study investigating the effects of PSST in conjunction with PMT for children with conduct disorder, the total behaviour score on the CBCL was 10 points lower at follow-up but still had an average T score of 68.4, a level higher than 95% of the normative sample on this measure (Kazdin *et al.* 1987a). Kazdin's study comparing PSST to RT found similar results, with 1-year follow-up scores of total behaviour problems at a mean T score of 68.5 (Kazdin *et al.* 1987b). Kazdin *et al.* (1992) found reportedly stronger effects in a 1992 study combining PSST and PMT in which the mean total behaviour problem scores for children with conduct disorder was a T score of 63.9, but this still falls at a level greater than 90% of the normative sample on the CBCL. More research is needed to parcel out how PSST affects children with conduct disorder differently from other cognitive therapies, and to determine what other steps are needed to reach the ultimate goal of these children achieving normative levels of problem behaviours.

Parent–adolescent conflict

Problem-solving training has been used in interventions with parents and adolescents experiencing high levels of conflict and relationship difficulties (Patterson & Forgatch 1987; Foster & Robin 1989). From a skills-deficit viewpoint, parent–adolescent conflict results from a family's inability to solve difficult issues productively, and that directly teaching these skills will lead to less conflict and greater accord in families (Foster & Robin 1998). The most extensive research on problem-solving with this population has been conducted by Foster & Robin (1989), who designed an intervention called Problem-solving Communication Training (PSCT) for conflicting families.

Problem-solving components

PSCT involves 8–12 sessions usually conducted with the entire family present, in which therapists teach specific problem-solving methods as well as guide families in using these skills to solve actual problems they experience. Therapists use modelling, direct instruction and feedback, role-play, taped models of other families and written outlines to convey the problem-solving information.

In general, the conceptualization of problem-solving in this intervention reflects the four- or five-step cognitive-behavioural process originally outlined by D'Zurilla & Goldfried (1971) and D'Zurilla (1988). First, parents and adolescents are taught to define problems in a concise and non-defensive manner. Secondly, they learn to generate solutions for particular problems, using specific brainstorming methods that emphasize the inclusion and non-evaluation of several possible solutions. In the next stage, solutions are evaluated for their potential effectiveness, following which a particular solution is chosen and implemented. The final step involves the evaluation of the chosen solution, and the possible choice of another solution if the original one is found to be ineffective.

In addition to teaching basic problem-solving skills, the PSCT treatment and similar interventions for parent–adolescent conflict incorporate training in communication skills, including active listening, non-verbal attention, expressing praise, and asking questions of the speaker (Patterson & Forgatch 1987; Foster & Robin 1989). The inclusion of communication skills in the intervention reflects the hypothesis that adolescents, when compared to younger children, have developed some of the higher order linguistic and interpersonal skills important for mastering these techniques.

Treatment outcome research

The effectiveness of PSCT has been examined in a series of studies. In one study, researchers trained 24 pairs of teenagers and their mothers in communication and problem-solving, using both hypothetical and real problems (Robin *et al.* 1977). Inclusion criteria included no psychiatric history, as well as a history of 'excessive disagreement'. After the five-session training, observed communication between parents and teenagers improved significantly, but reports of conflict at home remained unchanged.

In another study with a slightly different version of PSCT, 33 families experiencing disagreements were assigned to one of three groups: a waiting list control group, a best-alternative treatment group, or PSCT with a cognitive restructuring component (Robin 1981). Results indicated that both treatment groups showed decreases in anger intensity and improved relationship functioning, whereas only the PSCT group showed improvements in specific problem-solving and communication skills. A 3-month follow-up showed that both treatment groups maintained improved communication, despite increases in anger intensity.

Investigators have compared different versions of PSCT to assess which form of the intervention renders it most effective. In one study, evaluators compared traditional PSCT, PSCT with generalization training including homework, and a waiting list control group (Foster *et al.* 1983). The treatment consisted of seven sessions, and the training for the 28 participant families included both mothers and fathers. Results showed no change in observed communication in any of the groups, but the two treatment groups demonstrated improvements in questionnaire reports of familial relationship functioning, including decreases in maternal anger. In addition, the generalization group appeared to show no enhanced performance of problem-solving skills outside of the therapy office and, in fact, appeared at 2-month follow-up to show relative declines in skills compared to the non-generalization group.

Stern (1984) evaluated whether the addition of anger management techniques increased the effectiveness of PSCT, by comparing basic PSCT to PSCT with anger and stress control instruction with a group of conflicting families. Results indicated that both groups showed enhanced communication and decreased insults in mothers and teenagers, as well as less anger intensity and fewer issues of conflict rated by mothers. Only teenagers in the anger management group showed decreases in anger intensity and fewer conflict-producing issues. Both groups showed improved communication and problem-solving skills, with anger management adding slight benefits.

Nayar (1985) compared PSCT with and without cognitive restructuring to a waiting list control group, using a small group of conflicting families who were trained in groups over seven sessions. Results indicated that both groups were more effective than the control group, and that the additional cognitive restructuring yielded decreases in maternal self-blame and distortion.

Clinical significance

A preliminary study of the clinical significance of problem-solving interventions revealed that this training produces some important changes for parents and teenagers in conflict (Robin & Foster 1989). Examining changes in communication, anger and number of conflict-producing issues, the investigators compared 45 families receiving PSCT with 29 control group families. On a measure of communication, 68% of treated parents and 39% of treated teenagers showed gains after treatment, compared to 24% of teenagers and 24% of parents in the control groups. On a measure of anger intensity and conflict, 54% of treated parents and 27% of treated teenagers showed improvements, compared to 24% of parents and 31% of teenagers in the control groups.

It should be noted that most studies of PSCT have generally involved families in which overall psychological functioning is fairly high, and changes in diagnosed psychopathology because of the intervention are usually not tracked. In preliminary studies of children with specific psychological disorders, PSCT has shown mixed and even negative results. One recent study, for instance, has shown that PSCT is not effective and may even decrease functioning in families in conflict where adolescents have attention deficit hyperactivity disorder (Barkley *et al.* 1992). In order to determine the clinical significance of PSCT, additional research is needed to assess the effectiveness of PSCT in conflicting families in which adolescents manifest psychological disorders, such as conduct disorder or depression.

Drawing clear conclusions about the effectiveness of PSCT is somewhat limited by methodological and measurement inconsistencies across studies, as well as by small sample sizes. Nevertheless, in several studies PSCT has yielded significant improvements in the functioning of conflicting families. The addition of anger management training appears to increase the effectiveness of PSCT, whereas some evidence indicates that generalization of the skills through homework assignments produces no additional change. In terms of component analyses, it may be difficult to parcel out whether or not problem-solving skills are the effective component of the PSCT intervention, because these skills make up the majority of the treatment. Nevertheless, future research could measure whether the communication training adds significantly to the intervention, or if any of the specific steps of problem-solving (e.g. identifying the problem or generating solutions) are more important than others.

Summary and future directions

Deficiencies in problem-solving skills have been implicated in internalizing disorders (anxiety, depression), externalizing disorders (oppositional-defiant disorder, conduct disorder), and family conflict in childhood and adolescence. Furthermore, treatments designed to increase problem-solving skills have been shown to be associated with both statistically and clinically significant improvement in all of these problem areas.

In several instances, cognitive-behavioural treatments that teach problem-solving skills meet the stringent criteria for empirically supported treatments outlined by Chambless & Hollon (1998). The effects of the treatments have been evaluated in controlled clinical trials in comparison to either a no treatment control condition or an alternative intervention, and the effects have been replicated by independent groups of investigators (Kazdin & Weisz 1998). For example, cognitive-behavioural interventions for the treatment of childhood anxiety disorders, which include elements of problem-solving training, have been shown to be effective in controlled outcome studies by Kendall *et al.* (1997) and effects of a similar intervention have been reported by Dadds *et al.* (1999). These studies provide relatively strong evidence for the efficacy of this treatment package that is superior to no treatment and is independent of effects of a single investigator. Other interventions that include problem-solving components can be classified as probably efficacious at this time, as they have been shown to be superior to either no treatment or to an alternative treatment, but these effects have not been replicated across more than one investigative team (Lewinsohn *et al.* 1990; Kazdin 1996; Clarke *et al.* 1999).

In spite of the significant progress that has been made in the development, implementation and evaluation of therapies involving problem-solving skills, four significant problems remain. First, there is little or no evidence that the teaching of problem-solving skills *per se* is an essential and active ingredient in these therapies. We did not find any research that included components analysis of cognitive-behavioural therapy supporting the role of problem-solving skills as essential to producing behaviour change in the treatment of either internalizing or externalizing problems. In the absence of studies that break treatments into their component parts, the effects of problem-solving cannot be clearly delineated. A high priority for future research will involve the use of research designs that allow for specificity in determining the contribution of problem-solving skills as compared to other elements in comprehensive cognitive-behavioural treatments.

A second limitation of this research is the failure to consider problem-solving skills as a component of a broader range of skills of coping and self-regulation. Problem-solving skills are only one important aspect of the skills that are needed for the regulation of cognition, emotion, behaviour and physiological arousal. The usefulness of problem-solving skills may depend on the ability to first soothe and regulate emotional arousal, including the management of fear, anxiety, anger and dysphoria. Furthermore, problem-solving skills may be augmented by other regulatory skills, including those involved in adapting to problem situations (secondary control coping responses). Adaptational skills include the ability to distract or shift attention away from threatening stimuli, accept problems that may be uncontrollable, and cognitively reframe problems to view them in a more positive light.

Third, there has been little comparison or integration of problem-solving methods with other models of treatment. For example, behavioural treatments for disruptive behaviour disorders that emphasize working with parents to change parenting skills and the use of contingencies to manage children's externalizing behaviour problems have been shown to be effective (Webster-Stratton & Hammond 1997; Webster-Stratton & Hancock 1998). The integration of problem-solving therapies with these other treatment methods remains relatively unexplored.

Finally, there is little evidence of individual differences that may be associated with positive or negative response to problem-solving therapy. Child characteristics that may influence treatment response to problem-solving therapy may include general cognitive or intellectual skills, temperamental characteristics and comorbid conditions. Similarly, characteristics of children's social environments, especially the quality of parent–child relationships, may influence the efficacy of interventions that enhance children's problem-solving skills.

In spite of these limitations, significant progress has been made in the development and evaluation of problem-solving therapies for a number of disorders of childhood and adolescence. These interventions offer relatively powerful empirically based methods to professionals to use in the treatment of anxiety, depression, disruptive behaviour disorders and parent–adolescent conflict. Future research will be important in refining these interventions to enhance their efficacy and increase specificity in their application to problems of childhood and adolescence.

References

Achenback, T.M. (1991) *Manual for the Child Checklist and 1991 Profile.* University of Vermont, Department of Psychiatry, Burlington, VT.

Ayers, T.S., Sandler, I.N., West, S.G. & Roosa, M.W. (1996) A dispositional and situational assessment of children's coping: testing alternative models of coping. *Journal of Personality,* 64, 923–958.

Bargh, J.A. (1997) The automaticity of everyday life. In: *The Automaticity of Everyday Life: Advances in Social Cognition* (ed. R.S. Wyer), 10, pp. 1–61. Erlbaum, Mahwah, NJ.

Barkley, R.A. (1998) *Attention Deficit Hyperactivity Disorder.* Guilford Press, New York.

Barkley, R.A., Guevremont, D.C., Anastopoulos, A.D. & Fletcher, K.E. (1992) A comparison of three family therapy programs for treating family conflicts in adolescents with attention-deficit hyperactivity disorder. *Journal of Consulting and Clinical Psychology,* 60, 450–462.

Barrett, P.M. (1998) An evaluation of cognitive-behavioral group treatments for childhood anxiety disorders. *Journal of Clinical Child Psychology,* 64, 333–342.

Barrett, P.M., Dadds, M.R. & Rapee, R.M. (1996) Family treatment of childhood anxiety: a controlled trial. *Journal of Consulting and Clinical Psychology,* 64, 333–342.

Berntson, G.G., Bigger, T., Eckberg, D.L. *et al.* (1997) Heart rate variability: origins, methods, and interpretive caveats. *Psychophysiology,* 34, 623–648.

Camp, B. & Bash, M.A.S. (1981) *Think Aloud: Increasing Social and Cognitive Skills—A Problem-Solving Approach.* Research Press, Champaign, IL.

Cannon, W. (1933) *The Wisdom of the Body.* Norton, New York.

Cannon, W. (1934) The significance of emotional level. *Scientific Monthly,* 38, 101–110.

Chambless, D.L. & Hollon, S.D. (1998) Defining empirically supported therapies. *Journal of Consulting and Clinical Psychology,* 66, 7–18.

Clarke, G., Lewinsohn, P.M. & Hops, H. (1990) *Instructors Manual for the Adolescent Coping with Depression Course.* Castalia Press, Eugene, OR.

Clarke, G., Rohde, P., Lewinsohn, P.M., Hops, H. & Seeley, J.R. (1999) Cognitive-behavioral treatment of adolescent depression: efficacy of acute group treatment and booster sessions. *Journal of the American Academy of Child and Adolescent Psychiatry,* 38, 272–279.

Compas, B.E., Connor, J.K., Thomsen, A.H., Saltzman, H. & Wadsworth, M. (1999) Getting specific about coping: effortful and involuntary responses to stress in development. In: *Stress and Soothing* (eds M. Lewis & D. Ramsey), pp. 229–256. Cambridge University Press, New York.

Compas, B.E., Connor-Smith, J.K., Saltzman, H., Thomsen, A.H. & Wadsworth, M.E. (2001) Coping with stress during childhood and adolescence: progress, problems, and potential. *Psychological Bulletin,* 127, 87–127.

Connor-Smith, J.K., Compas, B.E., Wadsworth, M.E., Thomsen, A.H. & Salzman, H. (2000) Responses to stress in adolescence: measurement of coping and involuntary responses to stress. *Journal of Consulting and Clinical Psychology,* 68, 976–992.

Crick, N.R. & Dodge, K.A. (1996) Social information-processing mechanisms on reactive and proactive aggression. *Child Development,* 67, 993–1002.

D'Zurilla, T.J. (1988) Problem-solving therapies. In: *Handbook of Cognitive-Behavioral Therapies* (ed. K.S. Dobson), pp. 85–135. Guilford Press, New York.

D'Zurilla, T.J. & Chang, E.C. (1995) The relations between social problem-solving and coping. *Cognitive Therapy and Research,* 19, 547–562.

D'Zurilla, T.J. & Goldfried, M.R. (1971) Problem-solving and behavior modification. *Journal of Abnormal Psychology,* 78, 107–126.

D'Zurilla, T.J. & Nezu, A.M. (1990) Development and preliminary evaluation of the social problem-solving inventory. *Psychological Assessment: A Journal of Consulting and Clinical Psychology*, **2**, 156–163.

D'Zurilla, T.J. & Sheedy, C.F. (1991) Relation between social problem-solving ability and subsequent level of psychological stress in college students. *Journal of Personality and Social Psychology*, **61**, 841–846.

Dadds, M.R., Holland, D.E., Laurens, K.R., Mullins, M., Barrett, P.M. & Spence. S.H. (1999) Early intervention and prevention of anxiety disorders in children: results at 2-year follow-up. *Journal of Consulting and Clinical Psychology*, **67**, 145–150.

Dempster, F.N. (1992) The rise and fall of the inhibitory mechanism: toward a unified theory of cognitive development and aging. *Developmental Review*, **12**, 45–75.

Dujovne, V.F., Barnard, M.U. & Rapoff, M.A. (1995) Pharmacological and cognitive behavioral approaches in the treatment of childhood depression: a review and critique. *Clinical Psychology Review*, **15**, 589–611.

Eisenberg, N., Fabes, R.A. & Guthrie, I. (1997) Coping with stress: the roles of regulation and development. In: *Handbook of Children's Coping with Common Stressors: Linking Theory, Research, and Intervention* (eds J.N. Sandler & S.A. Wolchik), pp. 41–70. Plenum, New York.

Forgatch, M. & Patterson, G. (1989) *Parents and Adolescents Living Together: Family Problem Solving Therapy*, Vol. 2. Castalia Publishing, Eugene, OR.

Foster, S.L. & Robin, A.L. (1989) *Negotiating Parent and Adolescent Conflict: a Behavioral-Family Systems Approach*. Guilford Press, New York.

Foster, S.L. & Robin, A.L. (1998) Parent–adolescent conflict and relationship discord. In: *Treatment of Childhood Disorders* (eds E.J. Mash & R.A. Barkley), 2nd edn, pp. 601–646. Guilford Press, New York.

Foster, S.L., Prinz, R.J. & O'Leary, K.D. (1983) Impact of problem-solving communication training and generalization procedures on family conflict. *Child and Family Behavior Therapy*, **5**, 1–23.

Fox, N.A. (1994) Dynamic cerebral processes underlying emotion regulation. *Monographs of the Society for Research in Child Development*, **59**, 152–166; 250–283.

Gottman, J.M., Notarius, C., Gonso, J. & Markman, H. (1976) *A Couple's Guide to Communication*. Research Press, Champaign, IL.

Gray, J.A. (1991) The neuropsychology of temperament. In: *Explorations in Temperament: International Perspectives on Theory and Measurement* (eds J. Strelau & A. Angleitner), pp. 105–128. Plenum, New York.

Gresham, F.M. (1985) Utility of cognitive-behavioral procedures for social skills training with children: a critical review. *Journal of Abnormal Child Psychology*, **13**, 411–423.

Grossman, P. (1992) Respiratory and cardiac rhythms as windows to central and autonomic biobehavioral regulation: selection of window frames, keeping the panes clean and viewing the neuroal topography. *Biological Psychology*, **34**, 131–161.

Kagan, J., Snidman, N. & Arcus, D.M. (1992) Initial reactions to unfamiliarity. *Current Directions in Psychological Science*, **1**, 171–174.

Kazdin, A.E. (1996) Problem-solving and parent management in treating aggressive and antisocial behavior. In: *Psychological Treatments for Child and Adolescent Disorders: Empirically Based Strategies for Clinical Practice* (eds E.D. Hibbs & P.S. Jensen), pp. 377–407. American Psychological Association, Washington D.C.

Kazdin, A.E. (1997) Practitioner review: psychosocial treatments for conduct disorder in children. *Journal of Child Psychology and Psychiatry*, **38**, 161–178.

Kazdin, A.E. & Weisz, J.R. (1998) Identifying and developing empirically supported child and adolescent treatments. *Journal of Consulting and Clinical Psychology*, **66**, 19–36.

Kazdin, A.E., Esveldt-Dawson, K., French, N.H. & Unis, A. (1987a) Problem-solving skills training and relationship therapy in treatment of antisocial child behavior. *Journal of Consulting and Clinical Psychology*, **55**, 76–85.

Kazdin, A.E., Esveldt-Dawson, K., French, N.H. & Unis, A. (1987b) Effects of parent management training and problem-solving skills training combined in the treatment of antisocial child behavior. *Journal of the American Academy of Child and Adolescent Psychiatry*, **26**, 416–424.

Kazdin, A.E., Bass, D., Siegel, T. & Thomas, C. (1989) Cognitive-behavioral therapy and relationship therapy in the treatment of children referred for antisocial behavior. *Journal of Consulting and Clinical Psychology*, **57**, 522–535.

Kazdin, A.E., Seigel, T.C. & Bass, D. (1992) Cognitive problem-solving skills training and parent management training in the treatment of antisocial behavior in children. *Journal of Consulting and Clinical Psychology*, **60**, 733–747.

Kendall, P.C. (1994) Treating anxiety disorders in children: results of a randomized clinical trial. *Journal of Consulting and Clinical Psychology*, **62**, 100–110.

Kendall, P.C. & Southam-Gerow, M.A. (1996) Long-term follow-up of a cognitive-behavioral therapy for anxiety-disordered youth. *Journal of Consulting and Clinical Psychology*, **64**, 724–730.

Kendall, P.C., Kane, M., Howard, B. & Siqueland, L. (1990) *Cognitive-Behavioral Treatment of Anxious Children: Treatment Manual*. (Available from the authors: Department of Psychology, Temple University, Philadelphia, PA 19122.)

Kendall, P.C., Flannery-Schroeder, E., Panichelli-Mindel, S.M., Southam-Gerow, M., Henin, A. & Warman, M. (1997) Therapy for youths with anxiety disorders: a second randomized clinical trial. *Journal of Consulting and Clinical Psychology*, **65**, 366–380.

Krohne, H.W. (1996) Individual differences in coping. In: *Handbook of Coping: Theory, Research, and Application* (eds M. Zeidner & N.S. Endler), pp. 381–409. Wiley, New York.

Lewinsohn, P.M. & Gotlib, I.H. (1995) Behavioral theory and treatment of depression. In: *Handbook of Depression* (eds E.E. Beckam & W.R. Leber), pp. 352–375. Guilford Press, New York.

Lewinsohn, P.M., Hoberman, H., Teri, L. & Hautzinger, M. (1985) An integrative theory of depression. In: *Theoretical Issues in Behavior Therapy* (eds S. Reiss & R. Bootzin), pp. 331–359. Academic Press, New York.

Lewinsohn, P., Clarke, G., Hops, H. & Andrews, J. (1990) Cognitive-behavioral treatment for depressed adolescents. *Behavior Therapy*, **21**, 385–401.

Luria, A. (1961) *The Role of Speech in the Regulation of Normal and Abnormal Behaviors*. Liveright, New York.

Mathews, A. & MacLeod, C. (1994) Cognitive approaches to emotion and emotional disorders. *Annual Review of Psychology*, **45**, 25–50.

McNally, R.J. (1995) Automaticity and the anxiety disorders. *Behavior Research and Therapy*, **33**, 747–754.

Meichenbaum, D. & Goodman, J. (1971) Training impulsive children to talk to themselves: a means of developing self control. *Journal of Abnormal Psychology*, **77**, 115–126.

Mischel, W. (1997) Was the cognitive revolution just a detour on the road to behaviorism? On the need to reconcile situational control and personal control. In: *The Automaticity of Everyday Life: Advances in Social Cognition* (ed. R.J. Wyer), **10**, pp. 181–186. Erlbaum, Mahwah, NJ.

Morgan, A.B. & Lilienfeld, S.O. (2000) A meta-analytic review of the relation between antisocial behavior and neuropsychological measures of executive function. *Clinical Psychology Review*, **20**, 113–156.

Mynors-Wallis, L., Davies, I., Gray, A. *et al.* (1997) A randomised controlled trial and cost analysis of problem-solving treatment for emotional disorders given by community nurses in primary care. *British Journal of Psychiatry*, **170**, 113–119.

Nayar, M. (1985) *Cognitive factors in the treatment of parent–adolescent conflict*. Doctoral dissertation, Wayne State University.

Nezu, A.M., Nezu, C.M., Friedman, S.H., Faddis, S. & Houts, P.S. (1998) *Helping Cancer Patients Cope: A Problem-solving Approach*. American Psychological Association, Washington D.C.

Patterson, G. & Forgatch, M. (1987) *Parents and Adolescents Living Together: the Basics*, Vol. 1. Castalia Publishing, Eugene, OR.

Pellegrini, D.S. & Urbain, E.S. (1985) An evaluation of interpersonal cognitive problem-solving training with children. *Journal of Child Psychology and Psychiatry*, **26**, 17–41.

Porges, S.W., Doussard-Roosevelt, J.A. & Maiti, A.K. (1994) Vagal tone and the physiological regulation of emotion. In: *The Development of Emotion Regulation: Biological and Behavioral Considerations* (ed. N.A. Fox). Monographs of the Society for Research in Child Development, Serial no. 240, **59**, 167–186.

Robin, A.L. (1979) Problem-solving communication training: a behavioral approach to the treatment of parent-adolescent conflict. *American Journal of Family Therapy*, **7**, 69–82.

Robin, A.L. (1981) A controlled evaluation or problem-solving communication training with parent–adolescent conflict. *Behavior Therapy*, **12**, 593–609.

Robin, A.L. & Foster, S.L. (1989) *Negotiating Parent–Adolescent Conflict: a Behavioral-Family Systems Approach*. Guilford Press, New York.

Robin, A.L. & Weiss, J.G. (1980) Criterion-related validity of behavioral and self-report measures of problem-solving communication skills in distressed and nondistressed parent–adolescent dyads. *Behavioral Assessment*, **3**, 339–352.

Robin, A.L., Kent, R.N., O'Leary, K.D., Foster, S. & Prinz, R.J. (1977) An approach to teaching parents and adolescents problem-solving communication skills: a preliminary report. *Behavior Therapy*, **8**, 639–643.

Robin, A.L., Koepke, T. & Moye, A. (1990) Multidimensional assessment of parent–adolescent relations. *Psychological Assessment*, **2**, 451–459.

Rothbart, M.K. (1991) Temperament: a developmental framework. In: *Explorations in Temperament: International Perspectives on Theory and Measurement* (eds J. Strelau & A. Angleitner), pp. 61–74. Plenum Press, New York.

Rudolph, K.D. & Heller, T.L. (1997) Interpersonal problem solving, externalizing behavior, and social competence in preschoolers: a knowl-edge-performance discrepancy? *Journal of Applied Developmental Psychology*, **18**, 107–117.

Sacco, W.P. & Graves, D.J. (1984) Childhood depression, interpersonal problem-solving, and self-ratings. *Journal of Clinical Child Psychology*, **13**, 10–15.

Shiffrin, R.M. (1997) Attention, automatism, and consciousness. In: *Scientific Approaches to Consciousness* (eds J.D. Cohen & J.W. Schooler), pp. 49–64. Erlbaum, Mahwah, NJ.

Shure, M.B. & Spivack, G. (1971) *Solving interpersonal problems: a program for four-year-old nursery school children*. Training script. Hahnemann Medical College Department of Mental Health Science, Philadelphia.

Silverman, W.K., Kurtines, W.M., Ginsburg, G.S., Weems, C.F., Lumpkin, P.W. & Carmichael, D.H. (1999) Treating anxiety disorders in children with group cognitive-behavioral therapy: a randomized clinical trial. *Journal of Consulting and Clinical Psychology*, **67**, 995–1003.

Spence, S.H. (1994) Cognitive therapy with children and adolescence: from theory to practice [Practitioner review]. *Journal of Child Psychology and Psychiatry*, **35**, 1191–1228.

Spivack, G. & Shure, M.B. (1976) *Social Adjustment of Young Children*. Jossey-Bass, San Francisco.

Spivack, G., Platt, J. & Shure, M.B. (1976) *The Problem-solving Approach to Adjustment*. Jossey-Bass, San Francisco, CA.

Stern, S. (1984) *A group cognitive-behavioral approach to the management and resolution of parent–adolescent conflict*. Doctoral dissertation, University of Chicago.

Tapert, S.F., Brown, S.A., Myers, M.G. & Granholm, E. (1999) The role of neurocognitive abilities in coping with adolescent relapse to alcohol and drug use. *Journal of Studies on Alcohol*, **60**, 500–508.

Urbain, E.S. & Kendall, P.C. (1980) Review of social-cognitive problem-solving interventions with children. *Psychological Bulletin*, **88**, 109–143.

Vygotsky, L. (1962) *Thought and Language*. Wiley, New York.

Walker, L.S., Smith, C.A., Garber, J. & Van Slyke, D.A. (1997) Development and validation of the Pain Response Inventory for Children. *Psychological Assessment*, **9**, 392–405.

Webster-Stratton, C. & Hammond, M. (1997) Treating children with early-onset conduct problems: a comparison of child and parent training interventions. *Journal of Consulting and Clinical Psychology*, **65**, 93–109.

Webster-Stratton, C. & Hancock, L. (1998) Training for parents of young children with conduct problems: content, methods, and therapeutic processes. In: *Handbook of Parent Training: Parents as Cotherapists for Children's Behavior Problems* (eds J.M. Briesmeister & C.E. Schaefer), 2nd edn, pp. 98–152. John Wiley & Sons, New York.

Parent Training Programmes

Stephen Scott

Introduction

Parent training programmes teach behavioural principles of child management by following a specific curriculum over several weeks. Parent training delivered in this structured way is the most widely researched psychological intervention in child and adolescent mental health. It is the single most effective intervention for the treatment of conduct problems in children, and is solidly based on extensively researched models of parent–child interaction. From early beginnings that focused on techniques for managing child misbehaviour at home, it has spread to include the promotion of child problem-solving skills, improvement of peer relationships, and the enhancement of literacy and school relationships. The content of programmes now goes beyond behaviour to address beliefs, emotions and the wider social context, and addresses issues that can impair parents' effectiveness, such as poor self-confidence, depression, an unsupportive partner and social isolation. Yet despite being highly effective and well received by parents, parent training is not routinely available as a treatment in any country in the world. This chapter will examine developments in parent training mainly in connection with child conduct problems, for which there is most evidence.

Distinction from other approaches

Some characteristics of parent training programmes are given in Table 56.1. They differ from other psychological interventions in important ways. A *psychoeducational* approach is used by many clinicians, where parents are informed about the nature of their child's difficulties and advised on management but are not expected to practise specific skills. *Individual behavioural work* is used by many clinicians for a wide range of presenting conditions (Herbert 1987). It has the advantage of flexibility, so that content, pace and duration can be tailored to the specific needs of a family. However, it may not match the range and depth of coverage of techniques found in a systematic programme. *Counselling* of a Rogerian type (Rogers 1961) is widely used in non-medical settings, with an emphasis on non-judgemental positive regard and respect for the parent. Listening well to parents helps engagement and is popular, but unless there are other elements such as helping them to find new solutions to their difficulties, as for example in the Parent Adviser Model (Davis & Spurr 1998), the gain for child mental health may be little.

Family therapy shares with parent training an interactional view of the maintenance of child behaviour problems. Exploration of families' beliefs and interrelationships may lead them to greater understanding of their predicament. Skills are not as a rule imparted, the theoretical model is not usually made explicit to the family and has less research backing, and there are fewer evaluations (Chamberlain & Rosicky 1995). *Humanistic parenting programmes* often focus on the improvement of parent–child relationships, particularly how to talk and communicate with a child (see review by Smith 1996). A strength of these programmes is that they are often delivered by voluntary sector organizations in community settings which can make them more accessible and acceptable than clinic services (Cunningham *et al.* 1995). A disadvantage is that sometimes staff are less well trained, and the programmes have seldom been rigorously evaluated using child outcomes.

Theoretical considerations

History

Parent training originated in the USA in the 1960s and drew on two traditions. The first was behavioural learning theory. This was developed by Skinner (1953) and others in the 1950s and led to its use in much adult clinical work, including the running of whole hospitals on token economies to increase desired behaviours. In the 1960s the learning theory framework was elaborated to include social learning. A logical application was to teach parents to manage the contingencies around child social behaviour. This was developed by, amongst others, Wahler *et al.* (1965) in Tennessee, and Patterson *et al.*, who founded the Oregon Social Learning Centre (Patterson 1969). The second tradition, less often acknowledged, was play therapy. Constance Hanf in Portland, Oregon developed an unpublished parent programme based on non-directive play (Hanf 1969) that greatly influenced the parent training programmes of Forehand (Forehand & McMahon 1981), Eyberg (Eyberg 1988; Hembree-Kigin & McNeil 1995), and Webster-Stratton (1981a, 1984). Since these foundations, parent training has incorporated a range of other concepts from child development and psychological treatment research, while paying less attention to others that are also relevant, as discussed below.

Table 56.1 Characteristics of effective parent training programmes.

Content

Structured sequence of topics, introduced in set order over 8–12 weeks

Subjects include play, praise, incentives, setting limits and discipline

Emphasis on promoting sociable self-reliant child behaviour and calm parenting

Constant reference to parent's own experience and predicament

Theoretical basis informed by extensive empirical research and made explicit

Detailed manual available to enable replicability

Delivery

Collaborative approach acknowledging parents' feelings and beliefs

Difficulties normalized, humour and fun encouraged

Parents supported to practise new approaches during session and through homework

Parent and child seen together in individual family work; just parents in some group programmes

Crèche, good quality refreshments, and transport provided if necessary

Therapists supervised regularly to ensure adherence and to develop skills

Parenting styles and child behaviour

A note of caution before examining the association between child-rearing styles and child behaviour! Some pundits confidently assert the 'right' and 'wrong' ways to bring up children. However, judging by the changes in the last 100 years, what we assert today may be dramatically overturned in future. For example, in Victorian Britain it was stated that children should be 'seen and not heard' and a popular motto was 'spare the rod and spoil the child', whereas today emphasis is on listening to children, and there is pressure to make any physical punishment illegal. Parenting beliefs and practices vary over time and across cultures, and research findings need to be interpreted bearing this in mind. The work of Deater-Deckard *et al.* (1996) suggests that while for white Americans not smacking children is associated with the lowest rates of conduct problems, in African-Americans not smacking is associated with an *increase* in antisocial behaviour. None the less, a strong association has repeatedly been found between particular styles of parenting and child antisocial behaviour. Harsh, inconsistent discipline, high criticism, rejection and neglect are implicated for children at all ages, with lack of supervision becoming especially important as the young person spends more time out of the home (Patterson *et al.* 1992). Longitudinal studies indicate that these factors are predictive of later antisocial behaviour even after allowing for the initial level of aggression (Patterson *et al.* 1992), suggesting a possible causal role, although other explanations are possible. The role of positive parenting practices has more recently been shown to make an independent contribution, with warmth, involvement in children's activities, praise and encouragement being associated with lower levels of antisocial behaviour (Pettit *et al.* 1997). Once a moderate level of positive parenting prac-

tices is present, however, it appears to be the presence of negative parenting that seems most influential.

Operant learning theory

Despite the many influences on child socialization, an overarching principle in parent training has been operant conditioning. Patterson's detailed observational work (Patterson 1982) showed that in families with an antisocial child, two processes maintained aversive child behaviour. First, it was frequently reinforced by parental attention, usually negative remarks such as nagging and criticism. A pattern of negative coercive interactions between parent and child led to escalation by both sides. Secondly, having made repeated unpleasant threats, the parents often failed to carry them through and would retreat, thus reinforcing the child's escalation by stopping being unpleasant. Detailed sequential observational analyses showed that within parent–child dyads, when parents behaved coercively (as defined above) child antisocial behaviour became more frequent, whereas when parents desisted from this, difficult child behaviour diminished (Patterson 1982; Snyder & Patterson 1986). Therapeutic programmes were therefore developed to encourage parents to extinguish unwanted behaviour through selectively ignoring it, and to follow through calmly on punishments, which might include withdrawal of privileges and 'time out' from any positive reinforcement.

In tandem with the need to reduce unwanted behaviour, learning theory stressed the need to promote appropriate behaviour. Attention and rewards for desired behaviour are a major part of training programmes, encapsulated by the motto 'catch your child being good' (Becker 1971). More recent observational studies confirm that parents who reward prosocial behaviour have children with fewer behaviour problems (Gardner 1987), even when controlling for harsh parenting (Pettit *et al.* 1997).

Classical learning theory and the antecedents of child behaviour

Operant learning theory is more concerned with the *responses* to a spontaneously emitted behaviour than with the prior setting events that may *elicit* a behaviour. Classical learning theory puts more emphasis on stimuli that trigger behaviour. From this perspective, antisocial behaviour may not simply develop from being unwittingly rewarded once it has occurred, but may have been precipitated by antecedent events, regardless of consequences. This approach is reflected in behavioural manuals that refer to *stimulus control*. They encourage parents to keep a diary of their child's problem behaviour, so that with the therapist they can look for precipitants and make suitable changes (Herbert 1987). Surprisingly, many parent training programmes make little use of structuring the day and planning ahead with routines to avoid trouble. Yet most parents and clinicians would see this as an essential part of effective parenting, e.g. giving active children opportunity to run around after school, avoiding demanding tasks when children are tired or hungry, taking toys or books to occupy the child when a long wait is likely, and so on. Involving children in constructive pastimes within the home such as painting or cooking, and outside such as football or swimming, can offer the opportunity to enhance confidence and build social skills, thus reducing the likelihood of oppositional behaviour. The development of instruments to measure such activity is underway, e.g. the Parent–Child Joint Activity Scale (Chandani *et al.* 2000).

Social learning theory

Processes other than stimulus–response psychology are involved in the integration of a child into the social world, such as imitation in early childhood and identification in middle childhood (Bandura 1977). These mechanisms of social learning have seldom explicitly been drawn upon in parent training. However, some recent programmes address parents' own aggressive behaviour with each other and teach them to solve their own problems, so their children can learn from them via imitation, aided by direct modelling (Webster-Stratton 1994a).

Cognitive processes

The behaviourist approach is mainly concerned with the external events impinging on an individual, and takes less account of how they may be thinking or feeling. Indeed, a central tenet is the lack of a need for introspection or understanding of what is in the 'black box' inside an organism (Skinner 1953). This has made it especially useful for dealing with animals and babies, but ignores the fundamentally human phenomena of language and thought. In contrast, over the last 30 years particular cognitive styles have been shown to be characteristic of children and young people with disorders such as depression and conduct problems. In interpersonal encounters, the latter are more likely to perceive the intentions of others as hostile, generate fewer solutions to conflicts, and to believe an aggressive solution will be more effective (Dodge & Schwartz 1997). Individual cognitive and problem-solving programmes have been developed (Lochman & Wells 1996), and can be used with parent training programmes, as discussed below.

Less work has been carried out mapping the cognitive processes of parents with disruptive children. Unsurprisingly, parents of antisocial children have more negative beliefs about them and attribute more negative intentions to them; rates of depression amongst mothers are high (Sanders & McFarland, 2000). Some parent training programmes incorporate techniques from cognitive therapy. Parents may be encouraged to monitor their own 'self-talk' or 'inner voice' and to check on hopeless and defeatist cognitions, and be helped to find ways of replacing these with more positive statements that facilitate coping (Webster-Stratton & Hancock 1998).

However, parents of children with behaviour problems may not just think differently, they may perceive events differently too. Experiments showing videotapes found that these parents not only failed to see many episodes of positive child behaviour

but, surprisingly, also saw fewer episodes of *negative* child behaviour. This suggests that rather than just being biased to see child behaviour in a bad light, these parents are also less attuned to perceiving *any* child behaviour accurately, and hold global non-specific negative feelings towards their children (Wahler & Dumas 1989). The implication for parent training may be that parents need to be helped to perceive their children's behaviour more accurately, and become more attuned to nuances of their child's mental state, rather than just being offered management skills. Parent training programmes that use videotaped sequences of parent–child interaction incorporate this.

Peers and academic influences on child outcome

Longitudinal studies have shown that independent of the initial level of antisocial behaviour and parenting quality, deviant peer associations (Fergusson *et al.* 1999; Poulin *et al.* 1999) and lower IQ and academic underachievement further influence antisocial behaviour (Hinshaw 1992; Patterson *et al.* 1992; Fergusson & Lynskey 1997; Rutter *et al.* 1998). While some programmes aimed at antisocial outcomes have added on components to address these issues, e.g. by promotion of prosocial peer affiliation (Conduct Problems Prevention Research Group 1992; Dishion & Andrews 1995) and special tuition (Conduct Problems Prevention Research Group 1992; Barkley *et al.* 2000), parents also can have some influence on these processes, which could be incorporated into parenting programmes. This would envisage a model of parenting that goes beyond a good interactional style and prudent management within the home, to playing a part in helping the child cope with the outside world. This may include programme elements to enable the parent to negotiate with school (Webster-Stratton & Hancock 1998), to coach better peer relationships through 'play dates' (Frankel *et al.* 1997), or to raise child literacy through training parents to use specific reading techniques with their child (Scott & Sylva 1997). At a broader level, parents can help select the environment to which the child is exposed, by encouraging certain friendships to flourish and discouraging others, by choosing an appropriate school for the child's needs, and by helping learning through providing a facilitative home environment. These aspects of parenting are seldom parts of parent training programmes, although they feature in some 'self-help' books on parenting.

Natural history, genes and environment

Studies of the natural history of serious antisocial behaviour used to suggest that it peaks in late teenage or young adulthood, when most offending occurs. However, as Tremblay (2000) has pointed out, the age when physical aggression is maximal is around 22 months (and not 22 years!). From this perspective, it may be pertinent to ask not what causes antisocial behaviour to develop, but rather, why did the usual peak at around 2 years not reduce? What are the usual mechanisms that cause antisocial behaviour to diminish after this age? They may turn out to be the same mix of parent and child factors already identified, but studies are needed to see whether antisocial schoolchildren were more disruptive than others before the age of 2, or only after.

Better characterization of antisocial behaviour has revealed at least two reliable subtypes. In one, antisocial behaviour is manifest early, typically by 3 years of age, carries on throughout life ('early onset–lifetime persistent' pattern; Moffitt 1993), and is associated with hyperactivity, impulsiveness, irritability and emotional problems, and lower IQ. In the other, antisocial behaviour begins in adolescence often as part of peer group rebelliousness, and desists in adulthood ('adolescence-limited' type). The early onset pattern appears to have a substantially higher heritability than the adolescence-limited type, where environmental influences, especially shared ones, are more prominent. More complex typologies of antisocial behaviour usually include a type with multiple comorbid psychopathology and neuropsychological deficits, where the heritability can be as high as 96% (Silberg *et al.* 1996). Some might conclude that changing the parental environment will have little effect where genetic influence is high.

This is erroneous for several reasons. First, the cause of a problem and solutions to ameliorate it may operate through quite different mechanisms, e.g. phenylketonuria is a genetically caused condition but responds to environmental manipulation, namely a low-phenylalanine diet. Second, genetic studies measure the variation in environment occurring naturally in the study population, which may not be very great for most members, whereas intervention often allows the level to be experimentally changed to a greater extent. Thus, early onset type antisocial behaviour might not vary much across the range of environments found in most families, but if very different environments are applied (as obtained, say, in treatment foster-care or an inpatient unit) it may change substantially. Thirdly, there is now good evidence of an interaction between child predisposition to antisocial behaviour and rearing environment. Infants with more negative temperaments (assessed independently from their parents) are more susceptible to poor parenting as shown by the development of more externalizing problems by age 3 than would be predicted from just adding the effects of temperament and parenting (Belsky *et al.* 1998). Likewise, adoption studies suggest that children with higher genetic risk (as indexed by parental criminality, antisocial personality or substance misuse) are far more likely to develop criminal behaviour in families with difficulties (e.g. criminal, psychiatric or legal problems) than predicted by just adding the genetic and rearing risks (Cadoret *et al.* 1995; Bohman 1996). The implication for parent training is that rather than being *less* effective for children with severe types of antisocial behaviour with high genetic liability, it may be *more* effective for them.

Taylor *et al.* (1996) conducted a community study of 7-year-old children with hyperactivity who were followed up aged 17. Subsequent analyses have shown that the 7-year-old hyperactive children whose parents were highly critical had developed far higher levels of conduct problems by 17 than those whose parents were not unduly critical. This suggests that children with disruptive behaviour that has a substantial inherited component can nevertheless be parented in a way that makes a considerable difference to their psychosocial outcome.

Parental factors that influence parenting

Not all parents start with the same level of skills for parenting, and not all are able to change to the same degree. A number of risk factors are relevant, and the question arises whether outcome is better if they are addressed through adding specific components to parenting programmes.

Generalized learning disability

There is no intrinsic reason why people with IQs under 70 should parent poorly, although as IQ gets lower, especially below 60, general impairment of social functioning becomes more and more evident (Scott 1994). Empirical evidence is patchy, but children deemed by local authorities to be at risk from parental abuse or neglect are more likely to have parents of lower IQ (Dowdney & Skuse 1993). Parental IQ has not been studied as a predictor of outcome in parent training although, as with any new learning task, it is likely to have a moderating effect.

Parental mental disorder

Any mental disorder of moderate or severe degree may interfere with parenting ability. However, harm does not appear to be done through the parent having a mental disorder unless it leads to poorer care for the child (Rutter & Quinton 1994). Conversely, ameliorating the disorder will not necessarily lead to a great improvement in parenting skills, unless they were at a good enough level previously. Maternal depression leads to less sensitive responding and less cognitive stimulation for the child (Murray & Cooper 1997) but, unless severe, is not a contraindication to parent training. Indeed, some studies have shown significant improvement in depression levels compared with controls after parent training (Sanders & McFarland, 2000). One mechanism may be the increased sense of self-efficacy and reduced helplessness about child management that parents report after programmes (Sanders *et al.*, 2000a).

Interparental discord

Cross-sectional studies have found that interparental discord adds to the prediction of child antisocial behaviour, over and above parenting practices (Webster-Stratton & Hammond 1999). While genetic transmission of aggressiveness may well be a component, the child is also likely to learn antisocial habits of conflict resolution and see fewer examples of prosocial skills and negotiation. Therefore gains from a parenting programme may be limited if the child is still exposed to interparental conflict.

Some programmes have a specific component to address inter-parental relationships, as reviewed below.

Poor living conditions

In the UK there is a gradient of increasing prevalence of child disorders with lower social class as defined by occupation of chief breadwinner in the household (Meltzer *et al.* 2000). This gradient is especially marked for conduct problems. The extent to which this has a direct effect on children, or is a marker for other mechanisms, is not fully resolved. In some studies, once quality of parenting is allowed for, poor living conditions are not associated with further levels of disorder (reviewed in Rutter *et al.* 1998). However, such an analysis does not allow for the possibility that poor conditions *lead to* poorer parenting. It is not difficult to imagine that living in adverse housing conditions with few facilities and no money to buy practical support, such as child-minding, could disrupt calm and constructive parenting, especially for, say, a lone parent with a mental heath problem. Studies indicate that child psychopathology increases with psychosocial adversity (Rutter 1995), and Patterson *et al.* (1992) showed a strong association between deprivation and poor parenting. Improving living conditions is usually beyond parenting programmes, although some offer practical support to help parents engage with housing and benefits agencies.

Social isolation

Social isolation is associated with poorer parenting and with a worse response to parent training (Dumas & Wahler 1983). Amongst what Wahler termed 'insular mothers', most adult contacts were with official agencies and their own mothers who were critical and negative. On days when this occurred, the mothers' harsh and inconsistent parenting of the children rose severalfold. Moreover, while they did as well as non-insular mothers in the immediate outcome of parent training, at follow-up nearly all the gains had been lost. Attempts have been made to add social support systems to parent training programmes (Dadds & McHugh 1992), and to address their despondent cognitions and narratives about themselves (Wahler *et al.* 1993), as discussed below.

Parents who experienced poor parenting as children

Many neglectful or abusing parents experienced little good care themselves, so have little experience to draw upon with their own children. However, this does not mean that they inevitably are unable to become good enough parents. Quinton & Rutter (1988) studied girls who had been brought up in children's homes who subsequently became mothers. Their own experience of parenting had been poor in two ways: first, the reason they were in the homes was their parents' inability to care for them adequately; and, secondly, at the time children's homes were run on very institutional lines without a great deal of close personal contact between staff and children, and a high turnover of staff made the development of long-term trusting relationships with them unlikely. Despite this and probable associated genetic risk factors, half the women with this background were parenting satisfactorily as judged by interview and direct observation measures. Current attachment research, using the Adult Attachment Interview, is linking parents' own attachment status to the quality of their upbringing (Main 1996). There do not appear to be studies using parents' own upbringing (as opposed to parents' attachment status) as a predictor of intervention outcome.

Particular beliefs about one child

So far, parenting has been discussed as a general ability. However, the quality of relationship between the same parent and different children in the family varies. Adoption studies show that children who were scapegoated in comparison to their siblings in their family of origin do especially badly in terms of outcome (Rushton *et al.* 2000). While some of this may be because of inherent characteristics of the child which led them to become criticized or scapegoated, it is likely that the negative environment further added to their difficulties, particularly in light of the evidence of the interaction between child vulnerability and harsh parenting described above. In clinical practice it is not uncommon to uncover resentments around what the child represents, e.g. an antisocial boy who is seen by his mother to resemble his father whom she hates because he beat her. The implication for intervention is that, in addition to imparting skills, beliefs about the child need to be explored and attempts made to help the parent view the child more positively.

Programme delivery

Engaging families

A sympathetic and effective approach to engaging families is crucial if parenting programmes are to work. This is a major issue for providers of mental health services, because the populations that may benefit the most are often the most reluctant to attend. Several approaches have been taken to improve acceptability and accessibility of programmes. First, the general approach now preferred is to form a *collaborative* relationship characterized by working with parents to achieve their goals by recognizing and building on their existing strengths. This is in contrast to an instructional relationship whereby after an assessment where they are informed of what 'the matter' is with their child, and what is 'wrong' with their handling, parents are 'told' the 'right' way to bring up children. Features of a collaborative approach include asking about child strengths as well as difficulties, praising parents for good aspects of parenting, respecting them as the expert on the individual characteristics of their child, listening carefully to, and showing understanding of, their beliefs about their child's behaviour, working on solutions parents generate themselves, and normalizing the problem behaviour where possible (Herbert 1995).

Secondly, many practical steps can be taken, e.g. home visits to parents, holding the groups in the local community setting, providing transport, offering a crèche, holding the sessions outside working hours, rewarding parents for attendance through payment or prize draws, telephoning parents between sessions to check on progress and give encouragement, getting parents to ring each other between sessions for support, sending cards to parents who miss sessions, encouraging parents to bring their partner or a friend to sessions, etc.

Format of programmes

Individual work

Here the parent(s) and child are seen together, as in traditional psychological therapies. This has the advantage of allowing the therapist to go at the pace of the parent, observe precisely how they are relating to their child, and modify the intervention accordingly. This can be especially helpful where the child responds differently from the majority with conduct problems, e.g. if he or she is hyperactive, has a hearing or learning disability, or has autistic traits. An individualized approach enables the therapist to do some in-depth work on other issues impinging on parenting, such as interparental consistency, sibling relationships, coming to terms with abuse in the parent's own childhood, etc. In sessions at the Maudsley Hospital, we spend about half of each session addressing such personal issues, and about half working on the behavioural programme. For hard-to-engage families, the programme can be delivered in the family home.

Group work

In the last two decades there has been a strong movement towards parenting groups, and much recent research has been using this format (Barlow 1999). Usually the parents of 6–10 children are seen without their children being present. Therefore therapists have to rely on parents' descriptions of what goes on and cannot practise new approaches 'live'. However, parents can role-play any situation, and report this as being a highly effective component of change. In groups there is less opportunity to explore deeper personal issues but, against this, other parents can offer experience and solutions that are usually more credible than those from professional therapists, an there is often considerable support offered by group members to each other. More intensive programmes may include an element of coaching parents 'live' with their children in addition to parenting groups (Puckering et al. 1994; Conduct Problems Prevention Research Group 1999), or may offer a group for the children simultaneously with a group for their parents (Webster-Stratton & Hammond 1997). Contrary to the notion

that individualized treatment would be best, head-to-head comparisons suggest that they are equally effective, as described below.

Written materials, videotapes, broadcasts and self-administered programmes

Most of the well-known programmes have a written manual for therapists, and hand-outs or a book for parents (Webster-Stratton et al. 1988; Forehand & Long 1996; Barkley 1997). Some use professionally made videotaped vignettes of parents and children in life-like situations to help parents become sensitive to patterns of behaviour and to show them alternatives (Webster-Stratton 1981b; Sanders et al. 1996; Sharry & Fitzpatrick 1999).

Content of a typical programme

Most basic programmes take 8–12 sessions lasting 1.5–2 h each. For details, see manuals by Forehand & McMahon (1981), Barkley (1997), Sanders & Dadds (1993), Webster-Stratton & Herbert (1994) or Hembree-Kigin & McNeil (1995). The programme used for individual work at the Maudsley Hospital is fairly typical and runs as follows.

Part 1: Techniques for promoting a child-centred approach

First session: play

The programme starts with this fundamental aspect of improving the relationship with the child. Parents are asked to follow the child's lead rather than impose their own ideas. Instead of giving directions, teaching and asking questions during play, parents are instructed simply to describe what the child is doing, to give a running commentary on their child's actions. The target is to give at least four of these 'descriptive comments' per minute. If the parent has difficulty in getting going, the practitioner suggests precisely what they should do, e.g. by saying 'I'd like you to say to Johnny "You've put the car in the garage."' As soon as the parent complies, the practitioner gives feedback, 'that was a good descriptive comment'.

After 10–15 min, this directly supervised play ends and the parent is 'debriefed' for half an hour or more alone with the clinician. How the parent felt while doing it is explored, and reservations and difficulties that arose are addressed. The effect of their behaviour on the child during the training session is usually soon observed by the parent. Experiencing this close non-judgemental attention is surprisingly powerful for children, who at best feel they are 'the apple of their parent's eye'. For cases where virtually all communication with the child has become nagging and complaining, play is an important first step in mending the relationship. It often helps the parent to have fun with the child and begin to have some positive feelings towards him or her. Parents are asked to practise these techniques for 10 min every day.

Second session: checking progress with homework; elaboration of play skills

For the first 20 min, the previous week's 'homework' of playing at home is discussed with the parent in considerable detail. Often there are practical reasons for not doing it ('I have to look after the other children', 'I've got no help') and parents are then encouraged to solve the problem and find ways around the difficulty (solutions arrived at might include doing the play after the younger sibling has gone to bed, getting the oldest child to look after the baby while the parent plays with the toddler, etc.). For some parents there may be emotional blocks ('It feels wrong—no one ever played with me as a child') that need to be overcome before they feel able to practise the homework.

After this discussion, live practice with the child is carried out. This time the parent is encouraged to go beyond describing the child's behaviour and to make comments describing the child's likely mood state, e.g. 'You're really trying hard making that tower', or 'That puzzle is making you really fed up.' This process has benefits for both the parent and the child. The parent gets better at observing the fine details of the child's behaviour, which makes them more sensitive to the child's mood. The child gradually gets better at understanding and labelling his or her own emotional states, a crucial step in gaining self-control in frustrating situations.

Subsequent sessions

These follow the same pattern of:
1 reviewing the previous week's homework;
2 direct training of interaction with the child; and
3 discussion afterwards of how it went.
The speed at which the content is covered depends on progress. Later sessions cover the following ground.

Part 2: Increasing acceptable child behaviour

Praise and rewards

The parent is required to praise their child for lots of simple everyday behaviours, such as playing quietly on their own, eating nicely, getting dressed the first time they are asked, and so on. In this way the frequency of desired behaviour increases. However, many parents find this difficult. First, they may say, 'But he *should* be doing these things anyway, without being praised for it—there's really no need.' Second, when their child has misbehaved earlier in the day they are still cross, and this prevents them praising good behaviour when it occurs. Third, some parents find that even when they want to praise their child, the whole process feels alien to them as often they never experienced praise themselves as a child but, with directly coached practice,

it usually becomes easier. Later sessions go through the use of reward charts.

Part 3: Setting clear expectations

Commands

A hallmark of ineffective parenting is a continuing stream of ineffectual nagging demands for the child to do something. In the programme, parents are taught to reduce the number, but make them much more authoritative. This is done through altering both the manner in which they are given, and what is said. The manner should be forceful (not sitting down, timidly requesting from the other end of the room; instead, standing over the child, fixing him or her in the eye, and in a clear firm voice giving the instruction). The emotional tone should be calm, without shouting and criticism. The content should be phrased directly ('I want you to . . .') and not indirectly or as a question ('Wouldn't you like to . . .'). It should be specific, labelling the desired behaviour which the child can understand, so it is clear to the child when he or she has complied ('Keep the sand in the box') rather than vague ('Do be tidy'). It should be simple (one action at a time, not a chain of orders), and performable immediately. Commands should be phrased as what the parent *does* want the child to do, not as what he should *stop* doing ('Please speak quietly' rather than 'Stop shouting'). If a child is in the middle of an activity, rather than abruptly ordering a stop, a warning should be given ('In two minutes you'll have to go to bed'). Rather than threatening the child with vague dire consequences ('You're going to be sorry you did that'), *when–then* commands should be given ('When you've laid the table, then you can watch TV').

Part 4: Reducing unacceptable child behaviour

Consequences for disobedience

Consequences for disobedience should be applied as soon as possible. They must always be followed through—children quickly learn to calculate the probability they will be applied, and if a sanction is only given every third occasion, a child is being taught he or she can misbehave the rest of the time. Simple logical consequences should be devised and enforced for everyday situations. If water is splashed out of the bath, the bath will end; if a child refuses to eat dinner, there will be no pudding, etc. The consequences should 'fit the crime', should not be punitive, and should not be long term (no bike riding for a month), as this will lead to a sense of hopelessness in the child who may see no point in behaving well if it seems there is nothing to gain. Consistency of enforcement is central.

Ignoring

This sounds easy but is a hard skill to teach parents. Whining, arguing, swearing and tantrums are not dangerous to children and other people and can usually safely be ignored. The technique is very effective. Children soon realize they are getting no pay-off for the behaviours and soon stop and vice versa; if acting this way gets them attention and shows them they can annoy and wind-up their parents, they will continue to hone their skills in so doing. Ignoring means avoiding discussion, avoiding eye-contact and turning away, but staying in the room to monitor. As soon as the child begins to behave appropriately, it is essential to attend and give praise. This is central to shaping desirable behaviour. Many parents find this difficult as they are often still angry with the child.

Time out from positive reinforcement

The point here is to put the child in some boring place, away from a reasonably pleasant context. This will not be the case if the home is generally negative, when being sent to a room alone will be a relief and not a punishment. Equally, if the room has lots of interesting toys it will also not be a punishment. Time out should be for a previously agreed reason (hitting, breaking things, etc., not minor infringements) for a short time (say, 1 min for each year of age). However, the child must be quiet for the last minute—if the child is still screaming, he or she stays in for as long as it takes until he or she has been quiet for a minute. Parents must resist responding to taunts and cries from the child during time out, as this will reinforce the child by giving attention. Time out provides a break for the adult to calm down too.

Part 5: Strategies for avoiding trouble

These include *planning ahead* to avoid troublesome times of day and situations, *negotiating* with the child how to accommodate their wishes while fitting in with the family goals, and *developing a problem-solving approach with the child* to promote independence, along the lines of problem-solving approaches taught directly by professionals to children (Petersen & Gannoni 1992).

Effectiveness

Methodological considerations

Several general issues are relevant before discussing particular trials (Kazdin 2001). First, different measurement methods and informants will give different effect sizes (Scott, in press). As a rule, teacher-rated questionnaire ratings of child antisocial behaviour are more predictive of later antisocial behaviour than those that are parent-rated, and methods that use objective standardized criteria, such as semistructured interviews or direct observation, are more predictive than questionnaires (Bank *et al.* 1993; Patterson & Forgatch 1995).

Second, statistical significance does not equate to clinical significance. The latter can be assessed from the original dimensional measure of psychopathology statistically in terms of the *effect size* (the mean change in the treated group minus

the change in the control group, divided by the pooled pre-treatment standard deviation; according to Cohen's (1988) guidelines that are widely accepted, an effect size of 0.2 SD is small, one of 0.5 SD moderate, and one of 0.8 SD is large; or by the proportion of the groups that improve by more than 30% (Webster-Stratton 1989), or by more complex formulae that compare the change in the treated sample with general population means (Jacobson & Truax 1991). Clinically significant change can also be assessed in terms of the proportion of the sample who no longer meet criteria for a diagnosis, or by using a measure that assesses the impact of the problem on social functioning or quality of life (Gowers *et al.* 2000). Clinical significance has only relatively recently become reported in studies, but for most described below it was possible to calculate an effect size.

Third, there is usually substantial attrition in trials with families of children with conduct problems. Two reporting strategies artificially inflate effectiveness: only reporting those who attend the majority of treatment sessions, and dropping those who are lost to assessment after entering the trial. The former is becoming less common, but the latter is still widespread. It should be mandatory to at least publish both the results for all those on whom data was collected, and a second analysis including those on whom post-treatment data is missing but adjustments made, e.g. assuming no change since the last data point. Otherwise it is impossible to estimate how much change one can expect if a treatment modality is introduced to a service.

Fourth, the sample used is crucial. Volunteers who respond to advertising campaigns are more likely to be motivated, to have space to think about and implement programmes, and be better off financially. Those referred to specialist parenting clinics may also have been deemed suitable by the referrer, or be self-referred. Some university-based trials exclude children with significant comorbidity, thus dropping those who are likely to do worst. This is in contrast to those referred to generic mental health clinics, who may be more multiply disadvantaged and have more severe and comorbid symptoms (Woodward *et al.* 1997). Even these clinics may miss the most disadvantaged. This is particularly important now that services are starting to target whole populations.

Lastly, many of the cited trials have taken place in university clinics run by highly motivated originators of programmes who supervise carefully chosen therapists intensively in demonstration projects. In the meta-analysis of child psychotherapy trials by Weisz *et al.* (1995) those conducted in university clinics had a large mean effect size of 0.7 SD, whereas all the clinic-based studies reviewed since 1950 did not have any significant effects. It might be concluded that 'the good news is that child psychotherapies work, but the bad news is that they don't work in real life'. Therefore, to be considered robust, findings need to be replicated in ordinary clinical settings by therapists who are part of the routine service and independent of the originator of the programme (Weisz & Hawley, 1998), as occurred in the replication of the Webster-Stratton programme by Scott *et al.* (2001a).

Outcome studies

Individual parent training programmes

For the programmes given individually, several well-designed studies showed substantial changes in observed parent practices and in reported and observed child oppositional behaviour, in comparison to untreated controls (Patterson & Reid 1973; Wells *et al.* 1980; Eyberg & Robinson 1982; Webster-Stratton 1984; Sanders *et al.*, in press). Improvements have typically been of the order of 0.5–0.6 SD on direct observation measures, and 0.6–0.9 SD on parent-report measures. The gains have been substantially maintained at follow-up 1 year later (Patterson 1974; Kazdin *et al.* 1992; Webster-Stratton *et al.* 1989) and over the longer term; Forehand & Long (1988) reported follow-ups of 4–10 years, and Long *et al.* (1993) reported a 14-year follow-up with no relapse of antisocial behaviour.

Group parent training programmes

For group programmes, again there are several good studies. The meta-analysis by Serkitch & Dumas (1996) calculated a mean effect size of 0.86 SD for child behaviour change; that by Hoag & Burlingame (1997) 0.69 SD. The systematic review by Barlow (1999) found 255 studies of group parent training, but only 16 were of a high standard methodologically. In these, the mean effect size of child behaviour change compared to waiting list controls rated by *parents* ranged from 0.4 to 1.0 SD. *Direct observation* showed an effect size of 0.4–0.6 SD, somewhat smaller than parent-report results. Surprisingly, none of these studies used semistructured interviews or structured ones. Follow-up at 1–3 years has shown that significant gains remain, with rather little loss in most programmes. Drop-out rates were typically in the range of 10–20%, lower than the usual 30% plus or so found in usual clinical practice. Weisz *et al.* (1995) have pointed out the lack of effectiveness studies in 'real-life' clinics, but the multicentre trial by Scott *et al.* (2001a) found an effect size of 1.06 SD for clinically referred cases using regular clinic staff to administer the intervention.

Self-administered programmes

Sending parents a book and then offering regular telephone advice led to reasonable gains on parent questionnaires and direct observation in two small studies by Sutton (1992, 1995). In a larger study, Webster-Stratton (1984) invited parents to come into the clinic regularly and follow the self-administered version of her videotape series with clinicians on hand to offer help if requested. Gains of around 1 SD compared with waiting list controls were found on parent-report, which was as great a gain as in the clinician-led comparison group. However, on direct observation there was no change, whereas the clinician-led group did 0.4 SD better than controls.

Multilevel programmes

Sanders *et al.* in Brisbane, Australia (Sanders 1999) have developed a comprehensive set of ways of delivering their Positive Parenting Programme (Triple P). Level 1 comprises a universal strategy of providing an entire population with information through television advertisements and entertaining TV programmes specifically made to reinforce good parenting practice, with the opportunity to call for a tip sheet. Level 2 comprises brief (one or two 20-min consultations) with a primary health care worker who has 3 days' training, reinforced for the parent with four videotapes on parenting and tip sheets. Level 3 is similar but offers more consultations in primary care. Level 4 offers a fuller 10-week traditional parenting programme that can be delivered as self-administered, individualized at clinic, or group. The self-administered programme comprises a book of instruction and a workbook of exercises, which can be supplemented by telephone calls. Level 5 (enhanced) is a further 10-week programme added on to the individually administered clinic programme that comprises addressing in an individualized way parental factors that get in the way of effective parenting, and addresses marital communication, mood management and stress coping skills. It is given to those who have not progressed sufficiently with lower levels of intervention, and includes home visits.

Evaluation of the different ways of delivering the standard Level 4 programme has been carried out in a trial with 305 3 year olds (Sanders *et al.*, 2000a). Participants were volunteers screened to meet criteria that included having an elevated score on the Eyberg Child Behaviour Inventory and at least one index of family adversity; parents were predominantly lower class, but mostly not highly disadvantaged. They were allocated to receive the standard basic clinician-administered 10-week programme, self-administered, or an abbreviated version of the enhanced programme. The results showed that, on direct observation, only the enhanced condition reduced antisocial behaviour (ES = 0.5 SD) compared to waiting list controls. However, on the Eyberg questionnaire all treatment conditions produced an improvement, with a trend towards a larger effect in the enhanced (enhanced 1.0 SD, basic 0.7 SD, self-administered 0.5 SD). However, the self-administered programme showed improvements on only two out of five child behaviour measures. One-year follow-up showed further improvements in all three treatment groups, but there were no controls at this stage.

A possible problem when interpreting this study was the differential attrition rates in post-intervention data collection between treatment and control groups. The attrition rates were enhanced 40%, basic 29%, self-administered 31%, but controls 8%. Careful analysis was carried out that showed attrition to be more likely in children with more severe behaviour problems, and mothers who were more depressed and had worse relationships with their partners. These are some of the risk factors associated with less change. The difference in attrition rates of 32% between the reportedly most effective intervention (enhanced) and the controls could be disguising a much smaller treatment effect, if the missing 32% changed less than those followed-up.

Sanders *et al.* (2000b) evaluated an innovative 13-episode television series ('Families') that included elements of the Triple P programme interwoven into an 'infotainment'. The series had been broadcast to millions in New Zealand. In this study, however, volunteers with children aged 2–8 in Australia were allocated to watch the programmes on video at home, or were allocated to a waiting list. Parents were reasonably advantaged. Evaluation was by questionnaire only, and showed an effect size of 0.4–0.5 SD in antisocial behaviour, increased sense of parenting competence, and no loss at 6-month follow-up. Attrition was not reported.

In conclusion, there is reasonable evidence that self-administered programmes may help some families. Further research is needed to see whether more disadvantaged families benefit. This mode of delivery has the potential to be a cost-effective way of disseminating parent training widely.

Humanistic programmes

There have been a number of methodologically acceptable studies of humanistic programmes, although they have tended to use volunteer samples with better motivated parents and less severe child problems than in clinical samples. Sheeber & Johnson (1994) studied 3–5 year olds with 'difficult temperaments' and compared a parenting group based on understanding of child characteristics with waiting list controls and found no difference in Child Behaviour Checklist (CBCL) scores on externalizing behaviour, but an effect size of 0.6 SD on internalizing problems. Freeman (1975) compared an Adlerian group with a 'traditional' mothers' discussion group and a no-treatment control, and found that both treatment groups had significant reductions in total CBCL scores, but were not significantly different. These studies used volunteer samples with moderate levels of child difficulty; none used interviews or direct observation to evaluate outcome.

Direct comparison of behaviourally based with humanistic programmes

In head-to-head comparisons of humanistic vs. behavioural programmes, findings are mixed. Pinsker & Geoffrey (1981) compared a behavioural group with Parent Effectiveness Training (PET), a humanistic approach. They found that on parent-report the behavioural group showed a significant reduction in child problem behaviour, whereas PET and controls did not, but on direct observation both treatment groups did better than controls. Bernal *et al.* (1980) compared client-centred group with behavioural management and waiting list controls and found on parent-report the behavioural group did better than the other two, but on direct observation no group changed. Frasier & Matthes (1975) compared behavioural with Adlerian parenting groups and had a no-treatment

control and found on parent-report that none of the groups changed significantly. Again, all these studies used volunteer samples.

In contrast, Nicol *et al.* (1988) studied 38 families referred by local social services for active physical abuse and allocated them to individual play therapy for the child plus support from social worker for the mother (a traditional child guidance approach), or home-based work that offered elements of parent training plus parent support through 'casework'. Drop-out was high in both groups at 45%, but the intervention with parent training led to a greater reduction in parental coerciveness and aversive behaviour towards their children, measured using direct observation. Overall, the evidence for humanistic programmes is weak.

Generalization to home, siblings and school

Several studies used direct observation to show generalization of parent training from clinic to home (Peed *et al.* 1977; Forehand & McMahon 1981; Boggs *et al.* 1990) confirming parental reports of improved behaviour. Moreover, studies suggest that parents use the newly learned parenting behaviours with other children in the family, as well as the index child (Humphries *et al.* 1978; Eyberg & Robinson 1982; Eyberg *et al.* 1995).

Studies looking for transfer of improved behaviour to the school setting have been inconsistent. Cox & Matthews (1977), Horn *et al.* (1987), Webster-Stratton *et al.* (1988) and McNeil *et al.* (1991) all found reduced antisocial behaviour in the school setting following parent training, whereas Johnson *et al.* (1976), Forehand *et al.* (1979), Webster-Stratton *et al.* (1989), Kazdin *et al.* (1992), Webster-Stratton & Hammond (1997), Taylor *et al.* (1998) and Webster-Stratton (1998) found no change. This is important because, if only questionnaires are used, teacher-reports predict later antisocial behaviour better than parent ones (Bank *et al.* 1993). Therefore, in the development of programmes to prevent antisocial behaviour, school-based elements are now often included (Conduct Problems Prevention Research Group 1999).

Adding behavioural components to increase parental adherence

Studies suggest that adding explicit teaching of social learning principles to a programme (McMahon *et al.* 1981), or adding explicit monitoring of the achievement of parenting goals followed by self-reward (Wells *et al.* 1980), improves the change in parental behaviour and child compliance on direct observation.

Programmes that address factors interfering with effective parenting

General approaches

Wahler *et al.* (1993) developed an adjunctive treatment called 'synthesis training' for isolated mothers. Parents are guided to identify and label their reactions to stressful events, understand their own reactions and feelings and the way they explain events to themselves, and change the way they treat their children accordingly. Studies suggest that this is an effective treatment and prevents drop-off in gains seen in insular mothers offered standard programmes. Blechman & McEnroe (1985); Blechman (1998) included communication skills and step-wise problem-solving to help identify and resolve problems arising from broad extrafamilial factors that interfere with parenting. Pfiffner et al. (1990) found a similar intervention enhanced the maintenance of gains with moderately aggressive children.

Multisystemic therapy (MST) was developed by Henggeler et al. (1998). It is a home-based clinical intervention that is intensive (only three to four clients per therapist), relatively short (3 months) and highly supervised. Therapy is given according to the 'system' that is assessed as showing weaknesses, e.g. parent–child, marital, peer relationship or social. The precise form of intervention may vary, but the approach incorporates many elements of structural family therapy. Brunk et al. (1987) compared MST with group parent training for abusive and neglectful families. Both interventions were associated with improvements in parental psychiatric symptoms and overall stress, and identified problems. Those receiving MST showed more improvement on observed parent–child interactions, whereas those receiving parent training showed more reduction in social problems, which the authors attributed to the group format. The parent training offered was described by the authors as 'mechanistic' and had no role-play element, sticking strictly to parental management. Therefore it would seem useful to take the best elements of both approaches, and offer MST with a major parent training component.

Maternal depression

Sanders & McFarland (2000) took 47 families with a depressed mother and a child with conduct disorder. They were allocated to either 12 sessions of individual standard behavioural parent training, or the same intervention but including cognitive therapy elements for depression. Both interventions reduced maternal depression and improved child behaviour, but the effects on maternal depression were stronger for the cognitive condition, with 72% as opposed to 35% moving into the non-clinical range; there was no difference in child behaviour improvement.

Partner discord

Griest et al. (1982) randomly assigned 17 families to basic parent training or basic plus an adjunctive treatment that included work on personal and marital adjustment and extrafamilial relationships. Greater changes were seen for the adjunctive treatment in child compliance and deviant behaviour, and for several specific parental behaviours. In an elegantly designed study,

Dadds et al. (1987) compared the addition of partner communication and support to basic individual parent training in 12 maritally discordant families and 12 non-discordant families, all of whom had children with conduct problems. Each condition received the same amount of therapist contact. The adjunctive treatment led to substantially enhanced gains at 6-month follow-up in the maritally discordant families but not in the non-discordant families. This suggests that intervention should be tailored to the presenting problem, and that a 'one-size fits all' preventive approach may not be efficient.

Adult social skills

Webster-Stratton noted that parents' own difficulties in their partner relationship was one of the most potent predictors of failure to improve parenting, so devised her 'advanced' programme to address adult relationship skills (Webster-Stratton 1994). She studied the outcome of her basic 12-week programme in comparison to the basic plus the advanced 14-week programme. While observed partner communication and child-generated solutions to hypothetical social problems improved more in the advanced group, directly observed parenting behaviour and all measures of behaviour improved equally in both groups.

Puckering et al. (1994) found a group intervention that provided mother support improved self-esteem, depression and social isolation, but not parenting style (Cox et al. 1990). They therefore developed an additional parenting skills component: Mellow Parenting. It was specifically devised to help highly disadvantaged mothers. The programme runs for a whole day a week over 16 weeks, and has three components. In the morning, a psychotherapeutic group is run for the mothers on their own that addresses past and current relationships and present feelings, and encourages members to reflect on how these link to being a parent. At lunch, mothers and children eat together, then the mothers are asked to become involved with their children in an activity, such as cooking or arts and crafts, and may be helped by staff. In the afternoon, mothers review videotapes of themselves with their children in everyday situations at home and work on specific parenting skills. Outcome using direct observation and questionnaires showed large improvements in reducing negative affect, promoting child autonomy and increasing maternal sensitivity (Puckering et al. 1994). Of the families on the local Child Protection Register, 83% were subsequently deregistered because their children were no longer judged to be at risk of abuse.

Social isolation

Dadds & McHugh (1992) offered a group parent management training programme to 22 lone parents recruited as volunteers but with substantial child behaviour problems. One group received a basic 8-week programme, called Child Management Training. The other group received the same 8-week management training course, but were asked to recruit an *ally* who was present at the first meeting, whose role was to:

1 be available to offer support when needed;

2 communicate regularly with the parent and listen to them; and

3 be involved in problem-solving and solution implementation.

This arm of the trial was named Child Management Training plus Ally Support Training. The results showed that parents in the combined condition did indeed use their allies to offer support, listen to them and help in problem-solving. However, although both groups made large improvements in child behaviour, the gains of the ally support group were no greater. This may be because although the parents carried out the support procedures, measures of *perceived* support did not increase. Whichever treatment was received, those parents who perceived they received substantial support from friends showed considerably grater improvement in child outcome. This confirms the importance of support as a predictor, but suggests it is not easy to increase it substantially in brief programmes. Equally, lack of support may well also be an indicator of less ability to create and maintain good relationships of all kinds.

Predictors of drop-out and response

Predictors of drop-out

Drop-out rates are typically high in families with children who behave antisocially, e.g. 45–65% in the review by Pekarik & Stephenson (1988). Even at dedicated centres of excellence it is often high, e.g. 37% in the series of 397 children described by Kazdin & Wassell (2000). Kazdin *et al.* (1994) and Kazdin & Mazurick (1994) found that pretreatment variables predicting drop-out in the *child* were more severe antisocial symptomatology, poorer peer relations and lower IQ. In the *parent*, demographic predictors of higher drop-out rates were younger mothers, lone-parent families, those on low incomes and of low socioeconomic status, and those from ethnic minorities. Parental psychiatric predictors included more negative life events, greater perceived stress, an antisocial history in mothers and more adverse parenting of the child. Unfortunately, many of these variables are intercorrelated, and it is not clear which are most important.

Prinz & Miller (1994) addressed retention of parents in treatment experimentally by comparing standard individual parent training with enhanced parent training that addressed wider family issues and feelings. Using a strict definition of drop-out as missing any session, the standard treatment had a 47% drop-out, whereas the enhanced 29%. However, they did not report whether the enhanced condition led to any better child outcomes for those who remained in treatment, nor give figures for less strictly defined drop-out.

Predictors of response

Child factors

Adolescents are generally found to do less well in parenting programmes. Bank *et al.* (1991) from Oregon Social Learning Centre (OSLC) found a far smaller effect size when using parent training with adolescents than with younger children at the same institution; Irvine *et al.* (1999) offered a parent training programme for 12 year olds and got inconsistent changes. More generally, the meta-analysis of 443 studies of a range of interventions for juvenile delinquency by Lipsey (1995) found the effectiveness was 'perilously close to zero'. However, there is a possibility that studies on adolescents have only the most severe persistent cases. This notion is supported by the findings of Ruma *et al.* (1996) who compared response to treatment using the parent CBCL score for groups in early childhood (2–5 years), middle childhood (6–11 years) and adolescence (12–16 years). The adolescent group did slightly less well, but the difference disappeared on multiple regression analysis that showed that greater initial severity was the only significant predictor of poorer response. Within the prepubertal age group, Dishion & Patterson (1992) had expected to find parent training more effective for younger (2.5–6.5 years) than older children (6.5–12.5 years) assessed by direct observation. However, they found it was of similar effectiveness for both age groups, although drop-out was higher in the older age group. The meta-analysis by Serkitch & Dumas (1996) found that *across* 36 studies, effectiveness was greater in older children, within the range 3–10 years. These studies would appear to indicate that parent training is reasonably effective across the age range from 3 to 10 or perhaps 12, but that after this it may be less effective for severely antisocial adolescents, for whom more studies are needed.

Boys are as likely to improve as girls (Webster-Stratton 1996; Scott & Spender, submitted). More severe initial antisocial behaviour is often believed to reduce the size of change, and the study of Ruma *et al.* (1996) found this. However, Scott & Spender (submitted) found that the more severely antisocial children made similar improvements, whereas those with substantial hyperactivity did less well.

Parent factors

No effect was found for socioeconomic status in the meta-analysis by Serkitch & Dumas (1996) or in other studies (Webster-Stratton 1992; Ruma *et al.* 1996; Scott & Spender, submitted). Lone parenthood was found to be predictive by Webster-Stratton (1992) and by Ruma *et al.* (1996), but not by Scott & Spender (submitted). It is not necessarily synonymous with social isolation, which is generally predictive of worse outcomes (Dumas & Wahler 1983; Dadds & McHugh 1992). Likewise, maternal depression is associated with poorer outcomes (Webster-Stratton 1992; Sanders & McFarland, 2000), as is interparental discord (Dadds *et al.* 1992; Webster-Stratton & Hammond 1999). Parents' expectations of what will happen during treatment influences outcome (Morrissey-Kane & Prinz 1999).

Combining parent training with other interventions

Parent training and child social skills training

There are several reasons to compare child social skills training with parent training. First, because the referred patient is the child, trying to alter their behaviour directly is logical. Second, it has shown to be reliably effective in reducing antisocial behaviour in adolescents (Lochman *et al.* 1993; Lechman & Wells 1996; Lochman *et al.* 2000; Kendall 1998), although initial trials showed it to be less effective with younger children, say under 6 years (Denham & Almeida 1987; Coie & Koeppl 1990). Third, some parents are either unable to change their parenting style, or are unwilling to attend sessions, yet may be prepared to put their children forward for treatment because they believe something is 'wrong' with them. Fourth, although parent training improves children's relationships with their parents, it does not reliably improve their behaviour at school, nor with their peers.

Kazdin *et al.* (1987) compared a programme of combined individual parent management training plus individual child problem-solving skills training vs. general discussion sessions of comparable duration in a sample of 40 7–12 year olds who were psychiatric inpatients because of antisocial behaviour. Results showed good improvements in the combined treatment group over controls, not only on parent-report (ES = 1.5 SD) but also on teacher-report (ES = 1.0 SD). No direct observations were made. There was no significant loss of effectiveness at 1-year follow-up. A subsequent paper (Kazdin *et al.* 1992) teased out the effectiveness of each component by comparing parent training alone, child social skills training alone, and both combined. All groups improved substantially, with improvements seen not only by parents at home, but also by teachers at school and self-reported offending by the young people. However, the combined treatment had greater effectiveness on nearly all measures, notably 0.5–1.1 SD greater effect than parent training alone on antisocial behaviour.

Webster-Stratton & Hammond (1997) used a group format with videotapes to compare parent training only with child training only, parent training plus child training, and a waiting list control group. Ninety-seven children aged 4–8 years specifically referred to a parenting clinic were studied with a thorough set of measures including direct observation at home, and observation of interaction with a friend. The intervention was relatively long (22 weekly sessions of 2 h) and attendance was excellent, with all cases attending at least half the sessions and most attending nearly all. There were no drop-outs. There were several important findings. First, on parent questionnaire, children in all three intervention conditions did considerably better than waiting list controls who did not improve significantly. The fact that *child training alone* led to improvements in child be-

haviour is important practically because there will always be some parents who are unable or unwilling to attend for intervention. Secondly, all interventions had an effect in reducing observed directive parenting behaviour. From a theoretical standpoint, it is interesting that child training led to less coercive parenting behaviour, confirming the hypothesis that for children with clinically significant antisocial behaviour (as for non-clinical children) child as well as parent factors are involved in driving parenting style; it shows that the coercive cycle of negative parenting and child defiance can be interrupted from either end.

Thirdly, parent training led to greater changes in parent-reported child behaviour problems than child training, whereas child training led to better improvements in the ratio of positive to negative strategies used by children when interacting with a friend on direct observation, and on laboratory tests of social problem-solving. Fourthly, the combined parent plus child intervention led to similar effect sizes as one would predict from either intervention alone in the domain in which they were most effective, but did not act synergistically. Thus, parent-rated child behaviour was no more improved in the combined condition than for child training alone, and observed child–peer behaviour was no more improved in the combined condition than with parent training alone. The exception was observed antisocial behaviour in the home at 1-year follow-up, where the combined condition had a greater effect than either alone. Unfortunately, although in all intervention conditions there was a good effect compared to controls for observed reduction in child behaviour at home (ES = 0.7–0.8, total deviant behaviour reduced to half original levels whereas controls did not change), the variance was large (standard deviations greater than means in all cases) so none was significant.

Fifthly, all gains were maintained at 1-year follow-up, suggesting that the reduction in antisocial behaviour is lasting. Unfortunately, further follow-up to test longer term persistence of benefits will not be possible from this study as the control group were treated after the waiting period for ethical reasons. Finally, no intervention made any difference to teacher-rated child behaviour in either the short or longer term. This was partly because some of the children had no significant problems at school, but it nevertheless suggests that child behaviour may be fairly context-specific. This supports an interactional framework, whereby the contingencies and expectations in a situation influence child behaviour. Given that child behaviour at school is also a major predictor of later child antisocial behaviour, and that classroom disruption is a major issue for teachers because of its impact on other pupils, findings such as this have fuelled the search for interventions that include a teacher element.

Parent training and classroom intervention

Barkley *et al.* (2000) screened 3100 5-year-old children in kindergarten and selected the top 9.3% with attention deficit hyperactivity disorder (ADHD) and conduct symptoms. They were allocated to group parent training only, special treatment classroom only, combined parent training and classroom treatment, or to no-treatment control. The parent training used Barkley's protocol (Barkley 1997) and lasted 10 weeks in the autumn term, followed by monthly boosters and was held at a medical centre. The special treatment classroom children spent a year at another school in a class that consisted of about 15 other similarly selected disruptive children. Teachers were highly trained and supervised in behaviour management techniques, and also were trained to deliver an accelerated curriculum aimed to advance academic skills; close supervision was provided. Children allocated to either of the classroom intervention conditions effectively received the full planned intervention in that context, but of those allocated to a condition with parent training, take-up was low: one-third of the parents did not attend at all, and only 42% attended five sessions or more. Crucially, the results of this study that targeted a whole high-risk population were analysed on an intention-to-treat basis. The outcomes showed no difference on parent-rated measures for any condition, and no difference on observed parent–child interaction or observed child attending ability. There were improvements in the classroom conditions on some teacher-rated measures, e.g. on the Teacher Report Form (Achenbach 1991) aggression and attention subscales, but not on the delinquency subscale or any of the internalizing subscales; some other scales measuring rather similar behaviours also showed no change. Direct observation of classroom behaviour showed reasonable (0.3–0.5 SD) improvements in externalizing behaviour. The authors attribute the failure of the parenting programme to low attendance at the parenting group, but do not give a dose–response curve or analyse the results of those parents who attended, say, half or more sessions. The classroom intervention had useful effects on some but not other measures. There were no cross-context or synergistic effects.

Parent training, child social skills and classroom intervention

The FasTrack project (Conduct Problems Prevention Research Group 1999) is a 'state of the art' multimodal intervention study. Five year olds in kindergarten were screened and the top 10% with antisocial behaviour selected. A total of 891 children were allocated to a multimodal intervention or to no intervention. The intervention included the following.

1 A universal element given to all pupils in the classroom that consisted of two to three lessons per week of recognizing emotions, friendship skills, self-control skills, social problem-solving skills, plus classroom management consultation for the teachers.

2 Parent training for 2 h per week over 22 weeks for which the parents were paid $15 per session; for half an hour a reading tutor worked with the child on reading skills while parents watched.

3 Child social skills group for 1 h per week for 22 weeks.

4 Child reading skills for three 30-min sessions a week with a special tutor.

5 Home visits fortnightly, alternating with telephone calls to develop a close relationship with the parents and promote generalization of parenting skills.

6 A peer friendship promotion programme that paired the index child with another, low-risk child from the class for 30 min per week of constructive play time together.

Parental participation was relatively high: 72% received more than half of the sessions, and 81% received at least half the home visits.

Given this massive input of resources, and thorough coverage of theoretical risk factors, the outcomes were very modest. Antisocial behaviour was assessed on eight measures: on all but one, there was no significant change; the mean effect size across all was 0.11 SD. Only two of the five social behaviour measures changed significantly, with a mean effect size across all of 0.18 SD. Social cognition tests showed gains on four of five measures (mean ES = 0.28). Reading attainment scores showed no improvement, although a reading process test ('word attack') did, and grades for language arts improved (mean effect size for all three was 0.33). As for parental behaviour harsh discipline did not change on questionnaire or observation, although did on a hypothetical test of responses to vignettes; appropriate and consistent discipline did not improve according to parental report or event-recorded observation, though did on coder impression of the observation. Warmth increased on direct observation but not according to parental report. Thus, of the eight measures of parenting behaviour, three changed significantly (mean effect size for all eight was 0.17 SD). The intervention is ongoing and the hope must be that the children will show bigger changes later, although such a comprehensive, prolonged and intensive intervention is likely to be too expensive to replicate.

Conclusions

Effectiveness

Parent training has moved on a long way from its origins 40 years ago. Programmes have become more responsive to parents' own views, and can now address contextual and mental health issues that impair 'good enough' parenting. Scores of careful studies attest that programmes lead to improvements in the way parents relate to their children *and* to reduced antisocial behaviour in the children themselves, thus giving them access to more satisfying relationships and better chances for successful adjustment. Combining parent training with child social skills training appears to increase the benefits outside the home. However, problems remain in making programmes acceptable to the most needy parents, and population-based prevention programmes have so far shown only modest benefits.

Future research

While the effectiveness of parent training in referred cases is firmly established, the precise mode of action is not. From the evidence reviewed above, it seems likely that humane empathetic interpersonal skills are necessary to engage and retain parents, but good inculcation of behavioural skills is necessary to bring about changes in parenting style and child behaviour. Studies suggest that parental mood, beliefs about the child, expressed emotion towards the child, and behaviour all change. Which is the active ingredient, or are changes in all necessary? Which aspects of parenting are most crucial: sensitive responding and communication, encouragement of prosocial behaviour, setting of clear boundaries, or effective punishment for misbehaviour? Does child attachment status become more secure as parenting is improved? Is the child's capacity for empathy increased, and is the likelihood of developing antisocial personality reduced? One hopes that future studies may answer these questions.

Service delivery

Children with antisocial behaviour cost society a great deal of money. An economic analysis found that those with conduct disorder aged 10 cost 10 times as much as controls by age 27 (Scott, *et al.* 2001b). Therefore there is a strong financial incentive to invest in these children's futures, as well as a humanitarian one. In the USA and the UK there is considerable governmental interest in early prevention. However, to stand a chance of being effective, several characteristics need to be in place. In addition to choosing empirically supported interventions (which is far from always the case), staff need to be supervised to deliver them to a high standard, otherwise efficacy is lost (Henggeler *et al.* 1997). Management needs to be good, with reasonable staff morale and training. A total population has to be targeted, not just those who are motivated to turn up; an assertive outreach strategy needs to be pursued to reach the most needy families. Currently, group parent training is more cost-effective than individual work. Scott *et al.* (2001a) found that a 12-week programme cost £571 per child, no more than standard individual treatment for six sessions.

Given that, say, 5% of children have conduct disorder with impairment (Meltzer *et al.* 2000), and up to 20% have DSM-IV oppositional-defiant disorder (Kazdin 1995), parenting programmes could not possibly be delivered by mental health professionals to most of the population who would benefit. A change in the culture around parenting is necessary, plus a stepped approach to intervention. The broadcast programmes of Sanders *et al.* suggest that this might be achieved, backed up by a carefully graded range of services, starting with self-administered programmes and only working up to intensive approaches for those who do not respond. Schools will need to focus more on children's behavioural and social development and implement approaches shown to work. If this occurs and the culture changes towards more informed and effective parenting, there is a prospect of making a considerable reduction in children's misery and of helping them to achieve a balanced way of life integrated with their family, friends and school.

References

Achenbach, T.M. (1991) *Manual for the Child Behavior Checklist/4–18 and 1991 Profile*. Department of Psychiatry, University of Vermont, VT.

Bandura, A. (1977) *Social Learning Theory*. General Learning Press, New York.

Bank, L., Marlowe, J.H., Reid, J.B., Patterson, G.R. & Weinrott, M.R. (1991) Imparative evaluation of parent-training interventions for families of chronic delinquents. *Journal of Abnormal Child Psychology*, **19**, 15–33.

Bank, L., Duncan, T., Patterson, G.R. & Reid, J. (1993) Parent and teacher ratings in the assessment and prediction of antisocial and delinquent behaviours. *Journal of Personality*, **61**, 693–709.

Barkley, R. (1997) *Defiant Children: a Clinician's Manual for Assessment and Parent Training*, 2nd edn. Guilford Press, New York.

Barkley, R.A., Shelton, T.L., Crosswait, C. *et al.* (2000) Multi-method pyscho-educational intervention for preschool children with disruptive behaviour: preliminary results at post-treatment. *Journal of Child Psychology and Psychiatry*, **41**, 319–332.

Barlow, J. (1999) *Systematic Review of the Effectiveness of Parent-training Programmes in Improving Behaviour Problems in Children Aged 3–10 Years*, 2nd edn. A review of the literature on parent-training programmes and child behaviour outcome measures. Health Services Research Unit, University of Oxford.

Becker, W.C. (1971) *Parents Are Teachers: a Child Management Programme*. Research Press, Champaign, IL.

Belsky, J., Hsieh, K.-H. & Crnic, K. (1998) Mothering, fathering, and infant negativity as antecedents of boys' externalizing problems and inhibition at age 3 years: differential susceptibility to rearing experience? *Development and Psychopathology*, **10**, 301–319.

Bernal, M.E., Klinnert, M.D. & Schultz, L.A. (1980) Outcome evaluation of behavioural parent-training and client-centered parent counseling for children with conduct-problems. *Journal of Applied Behaviour Analysis*, **13**, 677–691.

Blechman, E.A. (1998) Parent training in moral context: pro-social family therapy. In. *Handbook of Parent Training: Parents as Co-therapists for Children's Behavior Problems* (ed. J.M. Breismeister), 2nd edn, pp. 508–548. John Wiley & Sons, New York.

Blechman, E. & McEnroe, M.J. (1985) Effective family problem solving. *Child Development*, **56**, 429–437.

Boggs, S.R., Eyberg, S. & Reynolds, L.A. (1990) Concurrent validity of the Eyberg Child Behavior Inventory. *Journal of Clinical Child Psychology*, **19**, 75–78.

Bohman, M. (1996) Predisposition to criminality: Swedish adoption studies in retrospect. In: *Genetics of Criminal and Antisocial Behaviour: Ciba Foundation Symposium 194* (eds G. Bock & J. Goode), pp. 99–114. John Wiley & Sons, Chichester.

Brunk, M., Henggeler, S.W. & Whelan, J.P. (1987) A comparison of multisystemic therapy and parent training in the brief treatment of child abuse and neglect. *Journal of Consulting and Clinical Psychology*, **55**, 311–318.

Cadoret, R.J., Yates, W.R., Troughton, E. & Woodworth, G. (1995) Genetic environmental interaction in the genesis of aggressivity and conduct disorders. *Archives of General Psychiatry*, **52**, 916–924.

Chamberlain, P. & Rosicky, J.G. (1995) The effectiveness of family therapy in the treatment of adolescents with conduct disorders and delinquency. *Journal of Marital and Family Therapy*, **21**, 441–459.

Chandani, K., Prince, M.J. & Scott, S. (2000) Development and initial validation of the Parent–Child Joint Activity Scale: a measure of joint engagement in activities between parent and pre-school children. *International Journal of Methods in Psychiatric Research*, **8**, 219–228.

Cohen, J. (1988) *Statistical Power Analysis for the Behavioral Sciences*. Lawrence Erlbaum Associates, Hillsdale, NJ.

Coie, J.D. & Koeppl, G.K. (1990) Adapting intervention to the problems of aggressive and disruptive rejected children. In: *Peer rejection in childhood: Cambridge Studies in Social and Emotional Development* (eds S.R. Asher & J.D. Coie), pp. 309–337. *Cambridge University Press*, New York.

Conduct Problems Prevention Research Group (1992) A developmental and clinical model for prevention of conduct disorder. *Development and Psychopathology*, **4**, 509–527.

Conduct Problems Prevention Research Group (1999) Initial impact of the fast track prevention trial for conduct problems. I. The high-risk sample. *Journal of Consulting and Clinical Psychology*, **67**, 631–647.

Cox, A.D., Puckering, C., Pound, A., Mills, M. & Owen, A.L. (1990) *The Evaluation of a Home Visiting and Befriending Scheme*. NewPin, London.

Cox, W.D. & Matthews, C.O. (1977) Parent group-education: what does it do for the children? *Journal of School Psychology*, **15**, 358–361.

Cunningham, C.E., Bremner, R. & Boyle, M. (1995) Large group community-based parenting programs for families of preschoolers at risk for disruptive behaviour disorders: utilization, cost effectiveness, and outcome. *Journal of Child Psychology and Psychiatry*, **36**, 1141–1159.

Dadds, M.R. & McHugh, T.A. (1992) Social support and treatment outcome in behavioral family therapy for child conduct problems. *Journal of Consulting and Clinical Psychology*, **60**, 252–259.

Dadds, M.R., Schwartz, S. & Sanders, M.R. (1987) Marital discord and treatment outcome in behavioral treatment of child conduct disorders. *Journal of Consulting and Clinical Psychology*, **55**, 396–403.

Davis, H. & Spurr, P. (1998) Parent counselling: an evaluation of a community child mental health service. *Journal of Child Psychology and Psychiatry*, **39**, 365–376.

Deater-Deckard, K., Dodge, K.A., Bates, J.E. & Pettit, G.S. (1996) Physical discipline among African American and European American mothers: links to children's externalizing behaviors. *Developmental Psychology*, **32**, 1065–1072.

Denham, S.A. & Almeida, M.C. (1987) Children's social problem-solving skills, behavioral adjustment, and interventions: a meta-analysis evaluating theory and practice. *Journal of Applied Developmental Psychology*, **8**, 391–409.

Dishion, T. & Andrews, D. (1995) Preventing escalation in problem behaviors with high-risk young adolescents: immediate and 1-year outcomes. *Journal of Consulting and Clinical Psychology*, **63**, 538–548.

Dishion, T.J. & Patterson, G.R. (1992) Age effects in parent training outcome. *Journal of Behavior Therapy*, **23**, 719–729.

Dodge, K. & Schwartz, D. (1997) Social information processing mechanisms in aggressive behavior. In. *Handbook of Antisocial Behavior* (eds D. Stoff, J. Breiling & J. Maser), pp. 171–180. J. Wiley & Sons, New York.

Dowdney, L. & Skuse, D. (1993) Parenting provided by adults with mental retardation. *Journal of Child Psychology and Psychiatry*, **34**, 25–47.

Dumas, J.E. & Wahler, R.G. (1983) Predictors of treatment outcome in parent training: mother insularity and socio-economic disadvantage. *Behavioural Assessment*, **5**, 301–313.

Eyberg, S.M. (1988) Parent–child interaction therapy: integration of traditional and behavioural concerns. *Child and Family Behaviour Therapy*, **10**, 33–46.

Eyberg, S.M. & Robinson, E.A. (1982) Parent–child interaction training: effects on family functioning. *Journal of Clinical Child Psychology*, **11**, 130–137.

Eyberg, S.M., Boggs, S.R. & Agina, J. (1995) New developments in psychosocial, pharmacological and combined treatments of conduct disorders in aggressive children. Parent–child interaction therapy: A psychosocial model for the treatment of young children with conduct problem behaviour and their families. *Psychopharmacology Bulletin*, **31**, 83–91.

Fergusson, D.M. & Lynskey, M.T. (1997) Early reading difficulties and later conduct problems. *Journal of Child Psychology and Psychiatry*, **38**, 899–907.

Fergusson, D.M., Woodward, L.J. & Horwood, L.J. (1999) Childhood peer relationship problems and young people's involvement with deviant peers in adolescence. *Journal of Abnormal Child Psychology*, **27**, 357–369.

Forehand, R. & Long, N. (1988) Outpatient treatment of the acting out child: procedures, long term follow-up data, and clinical problems. *Journal of Advanced Behavioural Research Therapy*, **10**, 129–177.

Forehand, R.L. & Long, N. (1996) *Parenting the strong-willed child: The clinically proven five week program for parents of two to six-year olds*. Contemporary Books, Chicago.

Forehand, R.L. & McMahon, R.J. (1981) *Helping the Noncompliant Child: a Clinician's Guide to Parent Training*. Guilford Press, London.

Forehand, R., Sturgis, E.T., McMahon, R.J. *et al.* (1979) Parent behavioral training to modify child noncompliance: treatment generalization across time and from home to school. *Journal of Behavior Modification*, **3**, 3–25.

Frankel, F., Myatt, R., Cantwell, D.P. & Feinberg, D.T. (1997) Parent-assisted transfer of children's social skills training: effects on children with and without attention-deficit hyperactivity disorder. *Journal of the American Academy of Child and Adolescent Psychiatry*, **36**, 1056–1064.

Frasier, F. & Matthes, W.A. (1975) Parent education: a comparison of Adlerian and behavioral approaches. *Elementary School Guidance and Counseling*, **10**, 31–38.

Freeman, C. (1975) Adlerian mother study groups and traditional mother discussion groups: effects on attitudes and behavior. *Journal of Individual Psychology*, **31**, 37–50.

Gardner, F.M.E. (1987) Positive interaction between mothers and conduct-problem children: is there training for harmony as well as fighting? *Journal of Abnormal Child Psychology*, **15**, 283–293.

Gowers, S., Bailey-Rogers, S.J., Shore, A. & Levine, W. (2000) The health of the nation outcome scales for child and adolescent mental health. *Child Psychology and Psychiatry Review*, **5**, 50–56.

Griest, D.L., Forehand, R., Rogers, T., Breiner, J., Furey, W. & Williams, C.A. (1982) Effects of parent-enhancement therapy on the treatment of outcome and generalization. *Behavior Research and Therapy*, **20**, 429–436.

Hanf, C. (1969) *A Two Stage Program for Modifying Maternal Controlling During Mother–Child (M–C) Interaction*. Western Psychological Association, Vancouver, British Columbia.

Hembree-Kigin, T.L. & McNeil, C.B. (1995) *Parent–Child Interaction Therapy*. Plenum Press, New York.

Henggeler, S.W., Melton, G.B., Brondino, M.J., Scherer, D.G. & Hanley, J.H. (1997) Multisystemic therapy with violent and chronic juvenile offenders and their families: The role of treatment fidelity in successful dissemination. *Journal of Consulting and Clinical Psychology*, **65**, 821–833.

Henggeler, S.W., Schoenwald, S.K., Borduin, C.M., Rowland, M.D. & Cunningham, P.B. (1998) *Multisystemic Treatment of Antisocial Behavior in Children and Adolescents*. Guildford Press, New York.

Herbert, M. (1987) *Behavioural Treatment of Children with Problems: a Practice Manual*, 2nd edn. Academic Press, London.

Herbert, M. (1995) A collaborative model of training for parents of children with disruptive behaviour disorders. *British Journal of Clinical Psychology*, **34**, 325–342.

Hinshaw, S. (1992) Externalizing behaviour problems and academic underachievement in childhood and adolescence: causal relationships and underlying mechanisms. *Psychological Bulletin*, **111**, 127–155.

Hoag, M.J. & Burlingame, G.M. (1997) Evaluating the effectiveness of child and adolescent group treatment: a meta-analytic review. *Journal of Clinical Child Psychology*, **26**, 234–246.

Horn, W.F., Ialongo, N., Popovich, S. & Peradotto, D. (1987) Behavioral parent training and cognitive-behavioral self-control therapy with ADD-H children: comparative and combined effects. *Journal of Clinical Child Psychology*, **16**, 57–68.

Humphries, L., Forehand, R., McMahon, R. & Roberts, M. (1978) Parent behavioral training to modify child noncompliance: effects on untreated siblings. *Journal of Behavior Therapy and Experimental Psychiatry*, **9**, 235–238.

Irvine, A.B., Biglan, A., Smolkowski, K., Metzler, C.W. & Ary, D.V. (1999) The effectiveness of a parenting skills program for parents of middle school students in small communities. *Journal of Consulting and Clinical Psychology*, **67**, 811–825.

Jacobson, N.S. & Truax, P. (1991) Clinical significance: a statistical approach to defining meaningful change in psychotherapy research. *Journal of Consulting and Clinical Psychology*, **59**, 12–19.

Johnson, S.M., Bolstad, O.D. & Lobitz, G.K., eds (1976) *Generalization and Contrast Phenomena in Behavior Modification with Children, Behavior Modification and Families*. Brunner Mazel, New York.

Kazdin, A.E. (1995) Conduct disorder. In: *The Epidemiology of Child and Adolescent Psychopathology* (ed. F.C.K. Verhulst), pp. 258–290. Oxford University Press, New York.

Kazdin, A.E. (2001) Treatment of conduct disorders. In: *Conduct disorders in childhood and adolescence. Cambridge Child and Adolescent Psychiatry* (eds J. Hill & B. Maughan), pp. 408–448. Cambridge University Press, New York.

Kazdin, A.E. & Mazurick, J.L. (1994) Dropping out of child psychotherapy: distinguishing early and late dropouts over the course of treatment. *Journal of Consulting and Clinical Psychology*, **62**, 1069–1074.

Kazdin, A.E. & Wassell, G. (2000) Therapeutic changes in children, parents, and families resulting from treatment of children with conduct problems. *Journal of the American Academy of Child and Adolescent Psychiatry*, **39**, 414–420.

Kazdin, A.E., Esveldt-Dawson, K., French, N.H. & Unis, A.S. (1987) Effects of parent management training and problem-solving skills training combined in the treatment of antisocial child behavior. *Journal of the American Academy of Child and Adolescent Psychiatry*, **26**, 416–424.

Kazdin, A., Siegel, T. & Bass, D. (1992) Cognitive problem-solving skills training and parent management training in the treatment of antisocial behavior in children. *Journal of Consulting and Clinical Psychology*, **60**, 733–747.

Kazdin, A.E., Mazurick, J.L. & Siegel, T.C. (1994) Treatment outcome among children with externalizing disorder who terminate prematurely versus those who complete psychotherapy. *Journal of the American Academy of Child and Adolescent Psychiatry*, **33**, 549–557.

Kendall, P.C. (1998) Empirically supported psychological therapies. *Journal of Consulting and Clinical Psychology*, **66**, 3–6.

Lipsey, M.W. (1995) What do we learn from 400 research studies on the effectiveness of treatment with juvenile delinquents? In: *What Works: Reducing Re-offending: Guidelines from Research and Practice* (ed. J. McGuire), pp. 63–78. John Wiley & Sons, Chichester.

Lochman, J. & Wells, K. (1996) A social-cognitive intervention with aggressive children: prevention effects and contextual implementation issues. In: *Preventing Childhood Disorders, Substance Abuse and Delinquency* (eds R. Peters & R. McMahon), pp. 111–143. Sage, Thousand Oaks, CA.

Lochman, J.E., Coie, J.D., Underwood, M.K. & Terry, R. (1993) Effectiveness of a social relations intervention program for aggressive and nonaggressive, rejected children. *Journal of Consulting and Clinical Psychology*, **61**, 1053–1058.

Lochman, J.E., Whidby, J.M. & FitzGerald, D.P. (2000) Cognitive-behavioral assessment and treatment with aggressive children. In: *Child and Adolescent Therapy: Cognitive-behavioral Procedures* (ed. P.C. Kendall), 2nd edn, pp. 31–87. Guilford Press, New York.

Main, M. (1996) Introduction to the special section on attachment and psychopathology: overview of the field of attachment. *Journal of Consulting and Clinical Psychology*, **64**, 237–243.

McMahon, R.J., Forehand, R. & Griest, D.L. (1981) Effects of knowledge of social learning principles on enhancing treatment outcome and generalization in a parent training program. *Journal of Consulting and Clinical Psychology*, **49**, 526–532.

McNeil, C.B., Eyberg, S., Eisenstadt, T.H., Newcomb, K. & Funderburk, B. (1991) Parent–child interaction therapy with behavior problem children: generalization of treatment effects to the school setting. *Journal of Clinical Child Psychology*, **20**, 140–151.

Meltzer, H., Gatward, R., Goodman, R. & Ford, T. (2000) *The Mental Health of Children and Adolescents in Great Britain*. Office of National Statistics, London.

Moffitt, T. (1993) Adolescence-limited and life-course persistant antisocial behaviour: a developmental taxonomy. *Psychology Review*, **100**, 674–701.

Morrissey-Kane, E. & Prinz, R.J. (1999) Engagement in child and adolescent treatment: the role of parental cognitions and attributions. *Clinical Child and Family Psychology Review*, **2**, 183–198.

Murray, L. & Cooper, P.J. (1997) *Postpartum Depression and Child Development*. Guilford Press, New York.

Nicol, A.R., Smith, J., Kay, B., Hall, D., Barlow, J. & Williams, B. (1988) A focused casework approach to the treatment of child abuse: a controlled comparison. *Journal of Child Psychology and Psychiatry*, **29**, 703–711.

Patterson, G.R. (1969) Behavioural techniques based upon social learning: an additional base for developing behaviour modification technologies. In: *Behaviour Therapy: Appraisal and Status* (ed. C. Franks). McGraw Hill, New York.

Patterson, G.R. (1974) Interventions for boys with conduct problems: multiple settings, treatments and criteria. *Journal of Consulting and Clinical Psychology*, **42**, 471–481.

Patterson, G.R. (1982) *Coercive Family Process, a Social Learning Approach*. Castalia, Eugene, OR.

Patterson, G.R. & Forgatch, M.S. (1995) Predicting future clinical adjustment from treatment outcome and process variables. *Psychological Assessment*, **7**, 275–285.

Patterson, G. & Reid, J. (1973) Intervention for families of aggressive boys: A replication study. *Behaviour Research and Therapy*, **11**, 383–394.

Patterson, G.R., Chamberlain, P. & Reid, J.B. (1982) A comparative evaluation of a parent-training program. *Behavior Therapy*, **13**, 638–650.

Patterson, G.R., Reid, J.B. & Dishion, T.J. (1992) *Antisocial Boys*. Castalia, Eugene, OR.

Peed, S., Roberts, M. & Forehand, R. (1977) Evaluation of the effectiveness of a standardized parent-training programme in altering the interaction of mothers and their noncompliant children. *Behavior Modification* **1**, 323–350.

Pekarik, G. & Stephenson, L.A. (1988) Adult and child client differences in therapy dropout research. *Journal of Clinical Child Psychology*, **17**, 316–321.

Petersen, L. & Gannoni, A.F. (1992) *Manual for Social Skills Training in Young People with Parent and Teacher Programmes: Stop, Think, Do.* Australian Council for Educational Research, Hawthorn, Victoria.

Pettit, G.S., Bates, J.E. & Dodge, K.A. (1997) Supportive parenting, ecological context, and children's adjustment: a seven-year longitudinal study. *Child Development*, **68**, 908–923.

Pfiffner, L.J., Jouriles, E.N., Brown, M.M. & Etscheidt, M.A. (1990) Effects of problem-solving therapy on outcomes of parent training for single-parent families. *Child and Family Behavior Therapy*, **12**, 1–11.

Pinsker, M. & Geoffrey, K. (1981) A comparison of parent-effectiveness training and behavior modification training. *Family Relations*, **30**, 61–68.

Poulin, F., Dishion, T.J. & Haas, E. (1999) The peer influence paradox: friendship quality and deviancy training within male adolescent friendships. *Merrill-Palmer Quarterly*, **45**, 42–61.

Prinz, R.J. & Miller, G.E. (1994) Family-based treatment for childhood antisocial behavior: experimental influences on dropout and engagement. *Journal of Consulting and Clinical Psychology*, **62**, 645–650.

Puckering, C., Rogers, J., Mills, M., Cox, A.D. & Mattsson-Graff, M. (1994) Process and evaluation of a group intervention for mothers with parenting difficulties. *Child Abuse Review*, **3**, 299–310.

Quinton, D. & Rutter, M. (1988) *Parenting Breakdown: the Making and Breaking of Inter-generational Links.* Avebury, Aldershot.

Rogers, C.R. (1961) *On Becoming a Person.* Constable, London.

Ruma, P.R., Burke, R.V. & Thompson, R.W. (1996) Group parent training: is it effective for children of all ages? *Behavior Therapy*, **27**, 159–169.

Rushton, A., Dance, C. & Quinton, D. (2000) Findings from a UK based study of late permanent placements. *Adoption Quarterly*, **3** (3), 51–72.

Rutter, M. (1995) *Challenges Psychosocial Disturbances in Young People for Prevention.* Cambridge University Press, New York.

Rutter, M. & Quinton, D. (1994) Parental psychiatric disorder: effects on children. *Psychological Medicine*, **14**, 853–880.

Rutter, M., Giller, H. & Hagell, A. (1998) *Antisocial Behavior by Young People.* Cambridge University Press, New York.

Sanders, M.R. (1999) Triple P-Positive Parenting Program: towards an empirically validated multilevel parenting and family support strategy for the prevention of behavior and emotional problems in children. *Journal of Clinical Child and Family Psychology Review*, **2**, 71–89.

Sanders, M.R. & Dadds, M.R. (1993) *Behavioral family intervention.* Allyn & Bacon, Needham Heights, MA.

Sanders, M.R. & McFarland, M.T. (2000) Treatment of depressed mothers with disruptive children: A Controlled Evaluation of Cognitive Behavioral Family Intervention, *Behavior Therapy*, **31**, 89–112.

Sanders, M.R., Markie-Dadds, C. & Turner, K.M.T. (Producers/Directors) (1996) *Every parent's survival guide* (videotape and booklet). Families International, Brisbane.

Sanders, M.R., Markie-Dadds, C., Tully, L.A. & Bor, W. (2000a) The Triple P-Positive Parenting Program: a comparison of enhanced, standard and self-directed behavioral family intervention for parents of children with early onset conduct problems, *Journal of Consulting and Clinical Psychology*, **68**, 624–640.

Sanders, M.R., Montgomery, D.T. & Brechman-Toussaint, M.L. (2000b) The mass media and the prevention of child behavior problems: the evaluation of a television series to promote better child and parenting outcomes, *Journal of Child Psychology and Psychiatry*, **41**, 939–948.

Scott, S. (1994) Mental retardation. In: *Child and Adolescent Psychiatry: Modern Approaches* (eds M. Rutter, E. Taylor & L. Hersov), 3rd edn, pp. 616–646. Blackwell Science, Oxford.

Scott, S. (1998) Aggressive behaviour in childhood. *British Medical Journal*, **316**, 202–206.

Scott, S. (in press) Deciding whether interventions for antisocial behaviour work: Principles of outcome assessment and practice in a multicentre trial. *European Child and Adolescent Psychiatry*, **10**.

Scott, S. & Spender, Q. (submitted) Which families benefit from parenting programmes? Predictors of outcome from a multicentre trial.

Scott, S. & Sylva, K. (1997) *Enabling parents: Supporting specific parenting skills with a community programme.* Department of Health, London.

Scott, S., Knapp, M., Henderson, J. & Maughan, B. (2001b) Financial cost of social exclusion: Follow-up study of antisocial children into adulthood. *British Medical Journal*, **323**, 191–194.

Scott, S., Spender, Q., Doolan, M., Jacobs, B. & Aspland, H. (2001a) Multicentre controlled trial of parenting groups for child antisocial behaviour in clinical practice. *British Medical Journal*, **323**, 194–197.

Serketich, W.J. & Dumas, J.E. (1996) The effectiveness of behavioral parent training to modify antisocial behavior in children: a meta-analysis. *Journal of Behavior Therapy*, **27**, 171–186.

Sharry, J. & Fitzpatrick, C. (1999) *Parents plus programmes: practical and positive support for parents* [Video]. Department of Child and Family Psychiatry, Mater Hospital, Dublin.

Sheeber, L.B. & Johnson, J.H. (1994) Evaluation of a temperament-focused, parent-training programme. *Journal of Clinical Child Psychology*, **23**, 249–259.

Silberg, J., Meyer, J., Pickles, A. *et al.* (1996) Heterogeneity among juvenile antisocial behaviours: Findings from the Virginia Twin Study of Adolescent Behavioral Development. In: *Genetics of criminal and antisocial behaviour. CIBA Symposium No. 194* (eds. G. Bock & J. Goode), pp. 76–86. John Wiley & Sons, Chichester & New York.

Skinner, B.F. (1953) *Science and Human Behaviour.* MacMillan, New York.

Smith, C. (1996) *Developing Parenting Programmes.* National Children's Bureau, London.

Snyder, J.J. & Patterson, G.R. (1986) The effects of consequences on patterns of social interaction: a quasi-experimental approach to reinforcement in natural interaction. *Child Development*, **57**, 1257–1268.

Sutton, C. (1992) Training parents to manage difficult children: a comparison of methods. *Journal of Behavioural Psychotherapy*, **20**, 115–139.

Sutton, C. (1995) Parent training by telephone: a partial replication! *Behavioural and Cognitive Psychotherapy*, **23**, 1–24.

Taylor, E., Chadwick, O., Heptinstall, E. & Danckaerts, M. (1996) Hyperactivity and conduct problems as risk factors for adolescent development. *Journal of the American Academy of Child and Adolescent Psychiatry*, **35**, 1213–1226.

Taylor, T.K., Schmidt, F., Pepler, D. & Hodgins, C. (1998) A comparison of eclectic treatment with Webster-Stratton's parents and children series in a children's mental health center: a randomized controlled trial. *Journal of Behavior Therapy*, **29**, 221–240.

Tremblay, R.E. (2000) The development of aggressive brain behaviour during childhood: What have we learned in the past century? *International Journal of Behavioural Development*, **24**, 129–141.

Wahler, R.G. & Dumas, J.E. (1989) Attentional problems in dysfunctional mother–child interactions: an interbehavioral model. *Psychological Bulletin*, **105**, 116–130.

Wahler, R.G., Winkel, G.H., Peterson, R.F. & Morrison, D.C. (1965) Mothers as behaviour therapists for their own children. *Behaviour Research and Therapy*, **3**, 113–124.

Wahler, R.G., Cartor, P.G., Fleischman, J. & Lambert, W. (1993) The impact of synthesis teaching and parent training with mothers of conduct-disordered children. *Journal of Abnormal Child Psychology*, **21**, 425–440.

Webster-Stratton, C. (1981a) Modification of mothers' behaviours and attitudes through videotape modelling group discussion. *Behaviour Therapy*, **12**, 634–642.

Webster-Stratton, C. (1981b) *Parents and Children Video Series.* Castalia, Eugene, OR.

Webster-Stratton, C. (1984) A randomized trial of two parenting training programmes for families with conduct disordered children. *Journal of Consulting and Clinical Psychology*, **52**, 666–678.

Webster-Stratton, C. (1989) Systematic comparison of consumer satisfaction of three cost-effective parent training programs for conduct problem children. *Behaviour Therapy*, **20**, 103–115.

Webster-Stratton, C. (1992) *The incredible years: A trouble-shooting guide for parents of children aged 3–8.* Umbrella Press, Toronto, Ontario.

Webster-Stratton, C. (1994) Advancing videotape parent training: a comparison study. *Journal of Consulting and Clinical Psychology*, **62**, 583–593.

Webster-Stratton, C. (1998) Preventing conduct problems in Head Start children: Strengthening parenting competencies. *Journal of Consulting and Clinical Psychology*, **66**, 715–730.

Webster-Stratton, C. & Hammond, M. (1997) Treating children with early-onset conduct problems: a comparison of child and parent training interventions. *Journal of Consulting and Clinical Psychology*, **65**, 93–109.

Webster-Stratton, C. & Hammond, M. (1999) Marital conflict management skills, parenting style, and early-onset conduct problems: processes and pathways. *Journal of Child Psychology and Psychiatry*, **40**, 917–927.

Webster-Stratton, C. & Hancock, L. (1998) Training for parents of young children with conduct problems: content, methods and therapeutic processes. *Handbook of Parent Training*, 98–152.

Webster-Stratton, C. & Herbert, M. (1994) Working with parents who have children with conduct disorders: a collaborative process. In: *Troubled Families, Problem Children* (ed. C. Webster-Stratton), pp. 105–167. John Wiley & Sons, Chichester.

Webster-Stratton, C., Kolpacoff, M. & Hollinsworth, T. (1988) Self-administered videotape therapy for families with conduct-problem children: comparison with two cost-effective treatments and a control group. *Journal of Consulting and Clinical Psychology*, **56**, 558–556.

Webster-Stratton, C., Hollinsworth, T. & Kolpacoff, M. (1989) The long-term effectiveness and clinical significance of three cost-effective training programs for families with conduct-problem children. *Journal of Consulting and Clinical Psychology*, **57**, 550–553.

Weisz, J.R. & Hawley, K.M. (1998) Finding, evaluating, refining and applying empirically supported treatments for children and adolescents. *Journal of Clinical Child Psychology*, **27**, 206–216.

Weisz, J.R., Donenberg, G.R. & Han, S.S. (1995) Bridging the gap between laboratory and clinic in child and adolescent psychotherapy. *Journal of Consulting and Clinical Psychology*, **63**, 688–701.

Wells, K.C., Griest, D.L. & Forehand, R. (1980) The use of a self-control package to enhance temporal generality of a parent training program. *Journal of Behavioural Research and Therapy*, **18**, 347–353.

Family Therapy

Brian W. Jacobs and Joanna Pearse

Introduction

For the non-specialist, family therapy and systems theory can be infuriating. It is steeped in theory that does not articulate well with what actually works and there has been fierce rivalry over the years both with other approaches and internally. Despite this, it has some successes in empirical research and is seen as an important approach in child mental health treatments because the child has to live in the context of their family, affects it and is affected by the behaviour and beliefs of other family members. This sets the context for treatments and for this chapter.

The purposes of this chapter are to outline the approaches taken by family therapists, to provide access for those that wish to inquire further into the literature and to provide a brief review of what seems to be effective from research carried out thus far.

Gorrell Barnes (1998) succinctly summarized the aims of family therapy. It examines *current context*, what is going on in people's lives now as well as earlier. It 'listens to the ways in which current relationships, as well as former relationships, come to form patterns and conversations in people's minds and therefore influence their daily beliefs and practices'. Notice that she immediately linked behavioural and belief systems in this framing of family therapy. She stated that 'the practice of family therapy encompasses a number of different activities in relation to these ideas of context and mind:

1 a philosophy of how to observe and frame relational events;
2 methods of description that explicitly make connections between people and their wider social context;
3 a relational approach to treating dilemmas and problems in families; and
4 a number of therapeutic methods addressing these, with particular skills devolving from each approach' (Gorrell Barnes 1998).

The development of a systemic family therapy needs to be understood historically. It originally rejected oversimplistic and reductionist accounts; but in the mean time mainstream child psychiatry has produced increasingly complex interactional models of the development of disorders.

It is worth remembering that, in common with many new fields of endeavour, the proponents of systemic family therapy had to define themselves as essentially different from what had gone before. This led to a rejection of previous thinking and a reframing of concepts, often with their own new vocabulary and tiresome jargon. It seems to take some decades for the new

thinking to allow itself to re-examine what has been rejected, to begin to integrate concepts and approaches that have previously found to be useful. This process of integration now seems to be happening to an extent in the field of systemic thinking, both internally between different schools of thinking and therapy (Sprenkle *et al.* 1999), and externally with other approaches to thinking about child mental illness and family distress. However, the process is still fluid.

Definitions

Gorrell Barnes (1998) listed characteristics of the systemic approach as follows.
• People in families are intimately connected, and focusing on these connections and the beliefs different members hold about them can be a more valid way of understanding and promoting change on problem-related behaviour than focusing on the perspective of any one individual.
• People living in close proximity over time set up patterns of interaction made up of relatively stable sequences of speech and behaviour.
• The patterns of interaction, beliefs and behaviour that therapists observe and engage with can be understood as the 'context' of the problem and be considered as both the 'cause' and 'effect', acting as feedback loops that create the 'fit' between problem and family. These are often referred to as 'circular patterns of interaction', in contrast with the cause and effect 'linear' thinking of the psychology from which early systems thinkers were trying to break free. Such patterns involve mutual influence and mutually regulated learning.
• Problems within patterns of family life are often related to dilemmas in adapting to some environmental influence or change.
• The minute details of the ways in which families describe such changes—the language within which constructions of problems, both past and anticipated, are generated—are of key importance in understanding the nuances of family thinking; the 'discourses' or discussions about family life and its problems and solutions. These take place both within individuals and between them. All the adults who form part of the family may carry different discourses in their minds which, while often unspoken in the room, nevertheless carry powerful imperatives for action or restraint in their thinking about themselves and the processes they are engaged in.

Other definitions have been offered by Gurman *et al.* (1986) and Reimers & Street (1993). The latter is particularly inclusive of all therapies aiming to bring about change in a family. This is helpful in some ways but it makes defining the boundaries of research into this domain of therapeutic endeavour difficult. Perhaps a wider overview of the field suggests that it should call itself 'systemic psychotherapy' to acknowledge that practitioners now work both with individuals and with organizations as well as working with families. In each case the interpersonal connectedness of individuals in the system is an organizing principle of the work.

Beginnings

Family therapy has evolved considerably since its inception about the middle of the twentieth century. Its beginnings were rooted in the era after the Second World War on the West coast of the USA in the Palo Alto project headed by Bateson *et al.* From a variety of disciplines, they began to observe family interactions and to analyse the patterns they saw. They noticed that these patterns could be seen as repetitive in some families. There appeared to be difficulties that they came to regard as redundant communications. Later it was realized that repeating patterns of interactions can be seen in all families and that difficulties can occur when these patterns are inflexible in the face of new information.

The concepts presented below have been important in the evolution of systems thinking and lie behind many of the intervention styles that have been conceived.

General systems theory

At its heart, systemic thinking rejects a simplistic view of causality: that one thing directly causes another to happen. Hoffman (1981) gave a typical account of the rejection of linear models, as they were seen by systemic theorists to apply to psychiatric approaches to mental illness during the middle part of the twentieth century. She wrote:

Mental illness has traditionally been thought of in linear terms, with historical, causal explanations for the distress. Efforts to explain symptomatic behaviour have usually been based on either a medical or psychodynamic model. The former compares emotional or mental distress to a biological malfunction or illness. Treatment consists of finding an "aetiology" of the so-called illness (a typically linear construct) and then instituting a treatment, such as administering drugs or devising other means of altering or blocking those bodily processes which are considered responsible for the patient's state. The people in charge of this treatment would of course be doctors, and the setting would often be hospitals.

She gave a similar account of the psychodynamic approach to mental distress and then went on to say, 'These two models typically see symptomatic distress as a malfunction arising either from biological or physiological causes, or from a repressed event in the past. In both models the individual is the locus of the malfunction and the aetiology is connected with an imperfection in his genes, biochemistry, or intrapsychic development.'

A useful account of general systems theory was given by Watzlawick *et al.* (1967). This description was written as the theoretical model was being developed for application to the domain of family interactions. The concept was proposed by von Bertalanffy (1950). It defines a system as 'a set of objects together with relationships between the objects and their attributes in which the objects are the components or parts of the system, attributes are the properties of the objects and relationships "tie the system together"'. Hall & Fagan (1956) distinguished between closed (sealed and self-contained) as against open systems, with the latter characterized by an exchange of energies and information with the environment.

In summary, Watzlawick characterized an open system as being more than the sum of its parts; that change in any part of the system at one time or over time produces change elsewhere in the system to balance it. There are feedback loops operating and the system exchanges information with the outside world. This brings us to the second group of important influences — observations on communication and the theory that evolved to explain them.

Communication theory and practice

At many places in the USA an interest by clinicians and others in studying families in their homes and then through the use of the one-way mirror in clinical settings seemed to blossom during the 1950s and 1960s (Riskin & Faunce 1972; Bateson 1979; Hoffman 1981). Work with families where there was supposedly a schizophrenic member produced the concept of the double bind (a situation where there were two different levels of communication in conflict with one another, e.g. verbal and non-verbal, in the same interaction). It led to a rapid growth of observations of communication patterns in such families (Jackson 1967a,b; Watzlawick *et al.* 1972).

There were a number of difficulties with this work, not least the later realization that the definitions of schizophrenia used at that time in the USA were unhelpful. They were abandoned for much narrower ones. The dyadic model of double bind communication was too simplistic for family communications (Weakland 1976). Bateson extended this approach to talking about inherently unstable patterns of alliances in the communication patterns in families with a schizophrenic member (Bateson 1973). One outcome from this work was that of Vaughan & Leff (1976) on expressed emotion. For our purpose, although the double bind hypothesis for the aetiology of schizophrenia was wrong (Hirsch & Leff 1975), it was influential in bringing about a paradigm shift to thinking about communication patterns within families as having an aetiological or maintaining role in mental distress.

Psychodynamic origins

A third important strand in systemic thinking came from the

psychoanalytic field. Family therapy emerged in opposition to psychoanalytic thinking, which had a particularly firm stronghold on the thinking of therapists in the USA in the 1950s. Nevertheless, many early leaders in the family therapy field came from a background of psychoanalytic training (Dreikurs 1949). They variously incorporated their previous training into their subsequent practice or ostentatiously rejected it. This use sometimes went unacknowledged. It has taken about two decades for a better assimilation of the strengths of the psychoanalytic models into systemic work. Interestingly, this has been a two-way process, at least conceptually, as psychoanalysts have promoted the interpersonal aspects of their work (Casement 1985).

Psychoanalytic theory has addressed the couple relationship and the interacting mutual projective identifications that are involved (Giovacchini 1958; Dicks 1963; Zinner & Shapiro 1976). This is relevant to family life (Bowen 1965; Boszormenyi-Nagy 1967; Framo 1970; Box et al. 1981) as the complex interaction between unconscious and conscious processes continue around family formation and development. In essence they are describing variants of projective identification (Klein 1946; Hinshelwood 1989). This can be generalized to family development. Dare (1988) suggested that psychoanalytic theories, 'all have in common a view of a person as having mental structures that transport personal history with them as important organizers of present and future personal relationships. Parents may in daydream or unconscious fantasy seek to set a child up as of equal or more importance than the co-parent in conflict with the interparental relationship.'

The notion of fixation points has also been used in psychoanalytic family therapy to describe the concept of unmet or painful relationship experiences which tend to repeat in subsequent phases of life. Family life can get stuck at transitions when these systems become activated in the minds of individual family members and are then enacted between them (Skynner 1981; Nichols & Schwartz 1991).

Kernberg (1966) described pathological processes in which splitting of the ego leads to marked compartmentalization of different ego states (or partial objects). These can be triggered by perceived threat and result in the expression of two mutually conflicting patterns of behaviour formed either side of the unresolved internal conflict. For example, a parent may unexpectedly acquiesce in the face of their child's assertive behaviour but equally may react the next time with unpredictable rage. Whatever the explanation, such patterns are quite often seen and produce an atmosphere of anxiety and uncertainty in a family.

Boszormenyi-Nagy & Ulrich (1981) wrote of the concept of ethical accountability within families—fair and responsible behaviour by parents tending to engender loyalty in the children. However, one parent can demand unfair conflicts of loyalty and invisible loyalties can be demanded or offered at the expense of the child's developing autonomy. Nichols & Schwartz (1991) suggested that the 'sick' or identified child in such families is 'chosen because of a trait that makes them a target for the parents' projected emotions. These children should not be thought of as helpless victims. In fact, they collude in the projected iden-

tification in order to cement attachments, assuage unconscious guilt or preserve the parents' shaky marriage.' Such views are not proven but they fit with the way that families describe themselves in treatment in their scripts, family stories and myths (Ferreira 1963; Byng-Hall 1995).

Family typologies

An idea that has been disproved but that led to serious research was that particular types of family difficulties would be associated with particular ways of family functioning. This idea probably arose from the study of schizophrenic families but extended rather more widely (Lewis et al. 1976). Later research suggested that there were broad aspects of family functioning that were associated with certain ways of being in families. This research approach also showed that it was very difficult to tease apart the *causal* factors from those *maintaining* the pattern. Helpfully, this research led to description of factors (Lewis et al. 1976; Skynner 1981) that seem to be indicative of family health. They include:

• a clear but flexible power structure in the family, with parents collaborative and in charge but consulting their children increasingly as they get older;
• spontaneous, open, honest and clear communication;
• relationships characterized by trust, mutual satisfaction and tolerance of ambivalence;
• self-image of family consistent with that of other's view of them;
• a positive emotional atmosphere with low levels of criticism and hostility; and
• tolerance of change over time as the life cycle progresses and a transcendent family value system.

Two questions arise from these beginnings in systemic thinking: first, how did these influences link with developing practice in family and systemic therapies; and, secondly, is there any evidence that any of this is more than theoretical hot air? The first question can be more completely answered at the moment than the second, although evidence for efficacy of family therapeutic approaches is accumulating (see below).

In essence, family therapy thinking has developed in three phases, reflecting changes in the therapist's supposed position in relation to his or her clients and, perhaps more importantly, reflecting changes in society's requirements and acceptance concerning the position of therapists, doctors and other healers. The first phase was characterized by the therapist as expert observer and manipulator to produce systemic change. The second and third phases see a gradual shift to a less hierarchical, expert position.

Influential approaches in family therapy

Within the first phase of development of family therapy the Mental Research Institute (MRI) at Palo Alto was particularly important. They developed a brief therapy based on the ideas of general systems theory but also on the ideas of Gregory Bateson. He had observed factors producing stability and sudden change in Iatmul culture in New Guinea (Bateson 1958; Hoffman 1981, pp. 38–40).

The rationale for this approach was that change in interactions between people in one part of a family would usually produce one or more compensating changes elsewhere that in effect cancelled out the effect of any innovation (Jackson 1957). At other times patterns of interactions amplified change, producing real discontinuous change in the relationship with a breaking of the overarching rule, so-called 'second order change'. More commonly, the amplification would build to a certain level and then abort. They wished to harness this tendency to lasting change. Labelling a family member as being unwell with a diagnosis counteracted potential for change in their view. It had unhelpful consequences for the development of the 'sick' individual (Hoffman 1981, p. 64). The attempted solutions of the family had become part of the problem, inadvertently helping to maintain it.

Fisch et al. set up the Brief Therapy Centre at MRI. They set themselves a limit of 10 sessions with a family, focusing on the interactions around the target behaviour and the underlying rules governing these patterns. They set tasks between sessions, often reframing the symptomatic behaviour as helpful, to try to unbalance the crucial family rules that seemed to be maintaining the symptoms. They focused on removing the symptomatic behaviours.

What would such a therapist do? He or she concentrated on the problem as presented and did not overtly aim to alter the family structure. The therapist might see only part of the family living at home at a time. He or she might set mutually conflicting tasks for different members or subgroups of the family and try to utilize the current experience of different family members to lend momentum for changed interactional patterns. The therapist would focus on the presented problem and withdrew once that changed. He or she would offer ingenious rationales for asking people to try different behaviours or to try to get them to act in opposition to his or her suggestions.

Structural family therapy

This was the next major influence in the early development of family therapy. As with other early approaches, there was no question who was in charge of the therapy—the therapist or often the supervisor behind the one-way screen.

Minuchin et al. (1967) began working in poor Puerto Rican families where there was a degree of disorganization and delinquency. They developed a way of working with these families that was in part educational, providing them with information and encouraging links between them and others in the community, and partly it was a very active series of techniques to improve the communication skills between members of the family. These techniques formed the basis of what was later called the structural approach. They were extended in work with other family problems at the Philadelphia Child Guidance Clinic resulting in three influential books (Minuchin 1974, 1978; Minuchin & Fishman 1981). A colleague (Aponte 1976), regarded these families as underorganized rather than disengaged.

The aim and rationale for this approach is based on a normative model, characterized by distinct but permeable boundaries between the parents and children with a clear hierarchy. Similarly, there will be boundaries between siblings and their parents and there will be functional effective boundaries between the family, the wider family network and the outside world. Minuchin, as others, emphasized the changing family life cycle and the changes in family structure that are necessary to accommodate the different stages within this. Minuchin viewed behavioural patterns as reflecting structure in the family. Changed behaviour would lead to structural change (persistent relationship changes).

How would such a therapist work to achieve change? In the clearest account of the techniques that they used, Minuchin & Fishman (1981) described techniques for taking small elements of interaction in the therapeutic interview and using them to achieve change by strongly encouraging family members, often parents, to make them happen differently then and there. The view was that by changing such small elements of behavioural interaction a new interactional pattern could be enabled. Minuchin used other techniques to increase the flexibility of the belief system in which the behaviours were embedded. For example, a father may come to believe that he is peripheral in the family and that that is the fate of all boys. He may apparently be uninvolved with his son but be covertly encouraging his young adolescent son to be rebellious and difficult with the child's mother. In the course of therapy a structural therapist might speak positively of the father's covert encouragement of his son's behaviour, talking of it as helping the son not to drift out of his mother's mind. The therapist might encourage the father to do more of this. He would hope that the father would react against this at some point. The therapist would choose his moment to encourage the mother to draw in the father to help her parent their son more directly. Through this the therapist hopes to help the family re-establish a healthier pattern of functioning, strengthening the parental alliance. The therapist would be trying to get the parents to change their pattern of behaviour around the son in the room by setting agreed rules and sanctions in the session. There would be homework for the family to demonstrate to themselves and the therapist their 'newly learned' skills. Minuchin would see himself as re-establishing the parental boundaries, amending the current family belief systems and opening new realities for them through expanding their interactional repertoire.

Minuchin believed that the family's constructed story of their beliefs for why certain things happen at home and in relation to the outside world should be linked using their language. This should be reformulated using their beliefs as justification for the new behaviours. Many of the ways of working with families help them find alternative belief systems. For Minuchin it is an active harnessing of beliefs to push for changes that the therapist thinks are necessary in the structures and hierarchies in the family and the associated communication patterns between family members.

The structural approach does not concentrate only on communication patterns, but rather on the permitted relationships in which these patterns come to form and in which they are embedded. Much skill and some delicacy of touch is required from the therapist to ensure that the approach is helpful and not experienced as coercive.

Variations of the structural approach were also adopted by Bowen (1965), Haley (1973, 1976) and Madanes (1981, 1984, 1990).

Psychodynamic approaches to family therapy

A parallel but rather separate stream of development in family therapy came from psychodynamically trained therapists who saw benefit in sustaining a concern with unconscious processes and the internal worlds of each family member. The rationale of such therapy was described by Nichols & Schwartz (1991) as being 'to free family members of unconscious restrictions so that they will be able to interact with one another as a whole, healthy persons on the basis of current realities rather than unconscious images of the past'. Some took the view that the therapy needs to uncover deep material, especially that which is hidden, unconscious and from the past (Framo 1970; Nichols & Schwartz 1991). Such therapists try to apply the detailed listening skills of psychoanalysts to the family therapy situation. This nondirective style may be more applicable in marital therapy with adult couples (Dicks 1963, 1967).

Others, including Dare (1988), took the view that therapy should be limited in time and scope, using much more active techniques. It can be usefully informed by psychoanalytic concepts such as those intended to guide the family formulation.
- *The structural qualities of the family*: coalitions and alliances; family hierarchy; distances of family members from each other; quantity, quality and direction of communication; boundaries within and around the family; control, organization and affective tone.
- *Some identifiable 'functions' for the symptoms*: usually the protection of aspects of the family organization from the change consequent on life cycle developmental and other crises of loss or addition.
- *Thoughts about what might be the 'risk' to the family of losing the symptoms*: fear of dissolution of the family; pain at the loss of special closeness; dread of responsibility having to be taken for past disasters.

These ideas were based on a related but distinct formulation developed by Bentovim & Kinston (1981), Bentovim & Jacobs (1988) and Bentovim (1992). Such therapists assemble observations from short detailed behavioural sequences. They build through descriptions of subsystem relations to the development of meaning systems. They will craft their interventions to attend to the holistic formulation: they will try to attend to behaviour and meaning systems as well as their view of unconscious elements that may be working to sustain the present family

dynamics. They will want to provide a forgiving rationale for the present situation while outlining alternative possibilities to the family.

Milan systemic family therapy

The so-called second wave of family therapy styles was heralded by the Milan approach. This group of therapies became more collaborative in their style with the family but still maintained the hierarchy of the therapist being the expert.

The rationale for this therapy was to address the belief systems that operate between family members, often across several generations, and that shape current interpersonal behaviour patterns (Selvini Palazzoli *et al.* 1978). Two key facets of this approach were a highly ritualized series of steps in each session and a particular style of questioning. Each session would follow the form of a pre-session discussion of the therapy team to produce a hypothesis for that session; the interview itself; and then a break. Feedback, with the purpose of construing the symptomatic behaviours in a positive light in the context of the family belief systems, was finally followed by a case discussion once the family had left. Sessions were commonly spaced at 4–6-week intervals as the therapy team had the idea that the family would often produce its own solution to the tensions between the current symptoms and the uncovered beliefs concerning their relationships with each other (Selvini Palazzoli *et al.* 1980; Boscolo *et al.* 1987; Cecchin 1987).

The team originally thought that the crucial element in their practice was the intervention message. However, they, and others (Penn 1982), came to believe that the style of questioning was a powerful intervention in its own right. This format was intended to be overtly neutral throughout the session. The style of circular questioning asks questions of one person about the relationship between two other people in the family around a particular issue, event or behaviour pattern. The answers to such questions then form the basis of subsequent questioning in the same style. Making unspoken beliefs explicit elicits further curiosity in the family about their relationships and can be a strong force for change. The method of using the interview itself as a form of intervention was further delineated by Tomm (1987a, 1987b, 1988) in a series of articles. This style has been influential in the UK (Campbell *et al.* 1983, 1991; Campbell & Draper 1985). Elsewhere it has influenced many and was part of the movement that led to what came to be called 'second order' family therapy (Hoffman 1985).

This style of work has also proved useful in considering other complex systems, such as work organizations and teams and the way in which they perform their core tasks (Campbell 1985; Coppersmith 1985; Lindsey 1985; Nitzberg *et al.* 1985). Many clinicians experience this as a much more respectful approach to families than directive problem-solving procedures. The approach emphasizes the inclusion of the therapist him or herself as an active participant during the elaboration of the therapy.

There is not a body of empirical research that directly examines the effectiveness of the Milan approach, but a style of therapy partly based on this approach has been used in some family research where there are teenage problems, such as drug abuse, and has proven effective (Quinn *et al.* 1988; Joanning *et al.* 1992).

Solution-focused therapy

In 1969 de Shazer *et al.* at the Milwaukee Brief Family Therapy Centre started developing the brief problem focused model of the MRI group and devised their own brand of brief solution-focused therapy.

De Shazer initially retained the exploration of the problem but moved on to concentrate much more stringently on the times when the problem was not occurring, believing that careful analysis of these exceptions and their behavioural sequences would highlight where the solutions lay. Identifying exceptions allowed the clients to repeat successful behaviours and take control of their problems (de Shazer 1985, 1991; de Shazer & Berg 1992).

De Shazer has, unlike others, attempted quantitative evaluation of his work (Fisher 1984; de Shazer *et al.* 1986). Using a self-report form (with the weaknesses that entails), they found that 72% of clients either met their own goals for therapy or felt significant improvements had occurred so that therapy was no longer necessary.

Constructivist and social constructionist systemic therapy

The third wave in family therapy began in the early 1980s. The changes were fuelled from a variety of sources within the social, scientific and biological realms. The objective certainty of 'reality' was challenged, and Capra (1983), a physicist, suggested that one can only approximate objectivity in measuring reality. With Maturana (1978) and Maturana & Varela (1980) this led to the idea that biology would constrain the ways in which information could be used. Some, rather optimistically, applied this to family systems.

Mendez *et al.* (1988) proposed that family systems could not be taught or directed to change. This view opposed the directive style of the time and suggested to some a very different therapeutic style, one in which change was evolved through a mutual construction between client and therapist. Social constructionism (Gergen 1982, 1985) correspondingly focused more on social interaction, e.g. 'Problems are stories people have agreed to tell themselves' (Hoffman 1990). In retrospect, these trends can be seen in a societal context in which there has been increasing distrust of experts. Perhaps they provided the 'logical' rationale for a stepping down from the teacher position, with a certain amount of shedding of assumed hierarchical power of the therapist over the client. With the acceptance of the possibility of multiple 'truths' it became much harder for professionals to hold on to the position that their views or 'truths' are superior to those of their clients. Other theorists supported

this view from various perspectives (Von Foerster 1981; Von Glaserfield 1984).

Therapists began to ask: 'How can specific techniques be employed with the hope of a specific outcome if there is no way of predicting how an individual or family unit may respond?' The task of the constructivist therapist became to perturb the system with the hope of producing but not being able to predict the direction in which that change might occur. For the social constructionist, the task became the art of the narrative therapeutic conversation (see below).

The 'observing systems' perspective brought a need for self-reflexivity and an examination by the therapist of what issues they were bringing to the therapy with what value systems? There was a return to thinking about things in ways that were not dissimilar to the ideas of identification, projection, transference and counter-transference used in psychoanalytic therapy but which systemic therapists had long ago rejected.

The writings of feminists were influential at this time, and there was an increasingly strong voice of women within the family therapy field (Goldner 1985; Boss & Weiner 1988; Perelberg & Miller 1990). In particular, issues of power and gender became a focus with a need to look at working with families and acknowledging the power differential between men and women. This provided an influential perspective on, among other issues, sexual abuse and family violence (Goldner *et al.* 1990; Gorrell Barnes & Henesy 1994).

Narrative therapy

Narrative approaches drew strongly on the work of Gregory Bateson. An important premise informing these schools is that we do things, not because we are driven, but because we see no alternatives. Information that does not fit within a particular belief system is discarded. Alternatives, which may hold the solution to problems, can often not be incorporated into the family's thinking because the difference is too great. Only as a rigid system becomes perturbed to the point of discontinuous change can it accept new information to enable it to change, so-called 'news of a difference'. The therapeutic task in this framework then becomes how to make the difference big enough to make a difference, but not so different that it is rejected.

Solution-focused therapists tackle the problem behaviourally but show that the difference can be tolerated because actually it is being done already and it is simply a case of recognizing the different successful behavioural sequences and increasing them. The Milan school attempted to make space for the difference by trying to change belief systems so that they were more in line with the difference, and the difference could then safely be incorporated.

Narrative approaches (Anderson *et al.* 1986; Andersen 1987, 1990; White & Epston 1990; Hoffman 1993; White 1995) are based on the idea that human beings make sure of their lives by telling the story of their experiences. The only way we tell our stories and the way in which stories become dominant or subjugated depends on such factors as culture, gender, family and social norms. Once these narratives have been formed it can be difficult to see alternatives. Eventually they are not only an account of our lives but they also begin to dictate what happens in our lives. This effects a constraint.

Individual stories are always heavily influenced by the more dominant societal stories: what we are told to believe by society (Foucault 1980). Those in helping professions often uphold these dominant discourses. They can inadvertently marginalize members of the community who may hold different beliefs.

The narrative theory of change suggests that people are likely to encounter difficulties and thus seek therapeutic help when the narrative they hold about themselves no longer 'fits' all or a certain aspect of their lived experience. The therapeutic aim is then to form a collaborative respectful alliance. The therapist works with the client first to deconstruct the constraining narrative and then to 're-story' or 're-author' their experiences in such a way as to highlight success already present or change the meaning of their experiences, so that these experiences have a better 'fit' within the client's larger narrative. This style of therapy is another one that works at the level of family belief systems rather than at a behavioural intervention level.

Anderson & Goolishian (1988, 1992) also put forward the 'not knowing position' in which therapists subsumed their expertise in order to allow clients to reclaim their own knowledge. In Norway, Andersen (1987) developed the idea of the 'reflecting team', a process whereby the therapy team will discuss hypothesis and their construction of what happened in the therapy session in front of the family. The purpose of this is to demystify the therapist's position by making their work transparent. It also ensures that therapists always speak in respectful empowering ways when they discuss families, instead of slipping into the all too familiar pathology-riven professional jargon that sometimes abounds. Families that have been interviewed about the therapeutic process prefer this and feel included, both in hearing the discussion and in being able to ask their own questions of the team.

Byng-Hall has had an interest in family scripts that predates the narrative movement, although much of his current work is influenced by the ideas of Michael White and others. He was initially interested in theories of attachment and worked closely with Bowlby. His ideas developed into an interest in the ways in which family patterns and behaviours were transmitted linguistically. His early work centred on ideas of myths and legends in families (Byng-Hall 1973, 1995). He also saw the relevance of Main's work on adult attachment to this style of intervention (Main *et al.* 1985).

Behavioural family therapy

Behavioural techniques have become quite widely used in family therapy. A helpful account of the applications of behavioural methods to family therapy can be found in Nichols & Schwartz (1991). Observations of the family interactions and behaviours become part of the structural family therapy approach, with the use of manoeuvres to achieve within-session changes in behav-

iour followed by tasks for the family between sessions. Similarly, strategic family therapists use a problem-solving approach, concentrating on altering the behaviours between family members. However, both schools make active use of the belief systems in the family as a lever for change and recognize them as potential blocks to change. By contrast, behavioural family therapists focus on the behaviours and are not concerned with the metaphorical meanings of these behaviours (Crowe 1982). They adopt a psychoeducational approach but try to mobilize the efforts of the family to solve the particular behavioural difficulties.

Patterson developed behavioural interventions for use in the classroom and at home which he delivered as a form of behavioural family therapy (Patterson 1971a,b). This work has evolved into various forms of parent training and working with oppositional-defiant children and children with conduct disorder (Webster-Stratton 1984; Kazdin *et al.* 1992). Contingency contracting was utilized early by Stuart (1971) in his work with delinquent adolescents and has become a feature of many subsequent programmes.

Alexander & Parsons (1982), working with delinquent adolescents, used the family systems' conceptual framework to assess the function of the target behaviours for the family as a whole, as well as for the individual family members. They used very recognizable behavioural techniques to effect change. In their functional family therapy model, they worked to alter the contingencies at home in response to wanted and unwanted behaviours from the young person, as well as working on the expectations and attributions in the family, introducing a cognitive element to the treatment. Kazdin (1997), in reviewing the literature, came to the conclusion that functional family therapy, parent management training and multisystemic therapy are among the more promising treatments for adolescent conduct disorder.

A behavioural family therapy approach was found to be an effective treatment of school refusal (Blagg & Yule 1984). Others (Barrett *et al.* 1996) used behavioural techniques, such as tokens, verbal reinforcement and planned ignoring within a family therapy context as part of their programme for the treatment of anxiety in childhood.

Special topics

Separation, divorce and step-families

The effects on family relationships of separation, divorce and the evolution of step-families are increasingly becoming a norm in modern Western society. More than a half of children whose parents separate before they are 16 years old will come to live in a step-family while they are still growing up. Cockett & Tripp (1994) found that fewer than half of children had continuing contact with their non-resident parent 2 years after a separation. Agreement and continued conversation may often be impossible between ex-partners. Simpson *et al.* (1995) found that this was the case for over one-quarter of 400 families in their Newcastle study.

Gorrell Barnes & Dowling (1997) and Gorrell Barnes *et al.* (1998) have written in some detail about the transitions that take place in family life through these processes and the repercussions down the subsequent years. As they pointed out, children are also required to keep secrets, to 'not know' and, at times, are subject to uncertainty about the end of the relationship and what arrangements there will be for parenting them for considerable lengths of time (Gorrell Barnes 1998). These can easily lead to distress and the keeping alive of quite unreal expectations. Family therapists have developed clinical approaches to helping divorcing and divorced families (Robinson 1997) but the research in this area seems to focus mainly on behavioural, parent management training and helping children with problem-solving training rather than systemic family therapy approaches (O'Halloran & Carr 2000).

Difference and the need for self-reflexivity

Britain is no longer a predominantly homogeneous society with variations mainly in socioeconomic and regional differences. There is now a huge diversity in the population, including differences in race, ethnicity, religion and also differences in family forms with large increases in lone-parent families, reconstituted families and families headed by same sex couples. Although culture is often associated with race and ethnicity, many of the above groups also have distinct culturally defined norms and expectations.

Cultural differences must therefore be taken into account when trying to understand areas as diverse as customs, food preferences, gender roles, child-rearing practices and the expression of emotion. Self-reflection becomes paramount as the therapist recognizes that they are as culturally influenced as their clients and that cultural issues affect us all and are not purely located in minority groups. Family therapists have acknowledged the need to become aware of their culturally determined biases and prejudices, to ensure that 'difference' does not become equated with 'abnormal'. There must also be a recognition of the large differences in power that various groups have and how this affects their ability to have their norms acknowledged and validated. It is very easy for a lack of understanding of different cultural norms and experiences to lead to a pathologizing of the unknown; examples include family governance, appropriate individuation or closeness in family networks and the effects of racism.

Falicov & Brudner-White (1983) have described how dominant dyads vary greatly from culture to culture. In Western culture there is a view that the parental couple should have an executive function, but in other cultures the executive position may be held by mother and son, or father and son. These cross-generational alliances could easily be seen as pathological if seen through a Westernized/Eurocentric lens.

Similarly, beliefs about appropriate levels of closeness and individuation are very culturally determined. Western views hold that the successful completion of the adolescent phase of the life cycle results in the young person individuating, and becoming independent and autonomous, whereas many cultures view success as the acceptance of continued involvement in, and responsibility for, the family. If these beliefs are not taken into account, families can often be pathologized as enmeshed, undifferentiated or overprotective.

Societal context is also relevant. Closeness and protectiveness may be very appropriate responses to living in a hostile environment.

It is important that differences are acknowledged, because attitudes seeking to 'treat everyone the same' will lead to everyone being judged by the current dominant social norms, which may not be applicable.

Cultural specificity involves identifying discrete cultural groups and then attempting to describe their norms, customs and beliefs. McGoldrick *et al.*'s (1996) study contained detailed culture-specific information about working with a large variety of different cultural groups. This approach has been useful as it has challenged the idea that there can be universal family norms. However, it also carries a risk of stereotyping and it must be remembered that there is always considerable intercultural diversity (Ho 1987).

Multiculturalism proposes that therapists adopt a culturally sensitive position with every family, even those that appear to be of similar culture to their own. The aim of this approach is to reduce the risk of making false assumptions. The family will be the best guide as to what is or is not appropriate for them. The maintenance of a respectful interested position on the part of the therapist is likely to produce the most accurate source of information. For instance, rather than trying to learn the cultural norms of black families—within which there is obviously a huge diversity—it may be more useful to have an awareness of some of the likely shared experiences that minority ethnic groups face such as language barriers, cultural shock, living with prejudice and discrimination, feelings of powerlessness sometimes resulting in hopelessness, depression, rage and suspicion.

Similarly, when working with gay and lesbian couples, a recent survey showed that the following were areas in which couples felt that therapists should be sensitive.

- The invisibility of their relationship.
- Having to deal with 'coming out' whether it be in their personal lives or working environment.
- Having to live with homophobia and the fear of verbal or physical attack purely on the basis of their sexual orientation (Long 1996).

However, in all considerations of cultural issues there can remain a tension between avoiding creation of 'pathology' and the overlooking or minimizing of problems by seeing them purely as cultural differences.

Family therapy and psychosomatic illness

Family therapy has been an approach of choice in the treatment of anorexia nervosa and bulimia nervosa for the past two decades. This has probably come about because two influential approaches within family therapy suggested specific ways to treat such cases (Minuchin 1978; Selvini Palazzoli 1978). Anorexia has been increasingly recognized and has worried professionals and families because of its life-threatening nature and because previous styles of treatment, involving rigid behavioural approaches in inpatient settings, were thought to be ineffective in the longer term, although they could achieve immediate weight gain, and such treatments became unacceptable as an intervention style. The family typology proposed by Minuchin has been refuted (Kog *et al.* 1985, 1987) but this work served as the stimulus to therapeutic advances and there has amassed a significant research evidence-base that involving the family in the treatment of child and adolescent cases of anorexia nervosa improves outcome (see below) although this is less clear in adult cases. For bulimia nervosa there are few trials of family therapy that have been included in recent meta-analyses (Hartmann *et al.* 1992; Wilson & Fairburn 1998).

Research on the family

Regrettably, the development of family therapies has occurred without much attention to empirical research findings. Nevertheless, such findings are relevant. Four main issues need to be considered. First, despite claims to the contrary, there is substantial evidence that family adversities of various kinds provide an important environmentally mediated psychopathological risk (Rutter 2000; see also Friedman & Chase-Lansdale, Chapter 15) that is best demonstrated with respect to family discord and negativity, a lack of continuity in personalized caregiving, and a deviant social ethos. Secondly, the reality of social group processes, both within the family and outside (Bronfenbrenner 1979), is well established (Rutter 1999a). That is, the functioning of families has to be considered in dynamic terms with the interaction between any two individuals having an effect on others in the group (Patterson 1982) and with each person's behaviour affected by who else is present (Clarke-Stewart 1978; Dunn & Kendrick 1982; Hinde & Stevenson-Hinde 1988). Thirdly, it is clear that risk and protective processes involve individual as well as family features; accordingly, it would seem that therapeutic interventions should be able to consider both (Rutter 1999b; see also Jacobs, Chapter 58; Brent *et al.*, Chapter 54). Fourthly, there is a paucity of evidence on whether the specifics of family therapy strategies constitute the most effective means of providing a remedy for the family risk processes. Thus, a systematic randomized controlled trial provided convincing evidence that family therapy was superior to individual psychotherapy in the treatment of anorexia nervosa in adolescents, although not in adults (Russell *et al.* 1987; Eisler *et al.* 1997). Nevertheless, a small-scale randomized control study by the same researchers seemed to show that comparable benefits were obtained by family counselling (Le Grange *et al.* 1992). The question is less whether family therapy can be effective (because there is reasonable evidence that it can; see below) but, rather, in which circumstances it is the treatment of choice and in which it is not. Even more crucially, we lack good evidence on which elements of family therapy constitute the essential agents of change.

Efficacy of family therapy

In a major meta-analysis of family and marital therapy, Shadish (1992) and Shadish *et al.* (1993) examined 163 studies, recruiting subjects until 1988 of marital ($n=62$) and family therapy ($n=101$) with random assignment of participants. They found an overall effect size of 0.47 compared with untreated controls ($n=44$ studies of family therapy). Family therapy was effective for 'general childhood conduct disorders' and for childhood aggression but it was ineffective for delinquency. They also found evidence for the effectiveness of this form of treatment for global family problems, communication/problem-solving, with some evidence for efficacy in phobias, schizophrenia and 'global psychiatric symptoms'. They did not find that different theoretical orientations with family therapy approaches made a difference to outcome.

Manualization of the treatment appeared to improve the outcome (Shadish *et al.* 1995). They found very few studies of effectiveness in a general clinical setting as opposed to the efficacy in university research settings. In the later review they also found a different result with regard to interventions for conduct disorder and school problems, with individual approaches proving more effective than a family therapy approach.

Carr (2000) recently reviewed family therapy research from an evidence-based perspective, examining several areas of child mental health practice. He pointed out that there are now a number of studies validating family therapy as an approach to treatment of child mental health problems. Most of the examples (apart from anorexia nervosa and substance abuse) involve behavioural and cognitive methods applied in a family setting. He also emphasized that a multisystemic approach is effective in many circumstances. This approach, pioneered by Henggeler & Borduin (1990), links a variety of different approaches to treatment in a tailored package over time for the particular needs of the family and child's situation. Thus, a child may need individual attention to improve coping mechanisms. His parents may need teaching cognitive behavioural skills as a couple or in the whole family setting and a programme may need to be introduced into the school setting that goes beyond the usual liaison skills practised in child mental health. Work may need to be undertaken to improve peer group skills, to enable the child to move away from a dysfunctional group of peers to a healthier set. Carr saw this attention to detail as illustrating a family and systemic perspective. The other area that he highlighted throughout this review is the attention of a family therapy perspective to communication between family members. Whether this is between parents in improving their discipline strategies or between parents and the identified child in improving negotiation of boundaries and a sense of fairness, this is probably a contribution that the family therapy perspective has contributed to treatments in child mental health.

Emotional disorders are responsive to family approaches, sometimes combined with other interventions including medication. For example, obsessional-compulsive disorder has been treated with a combination of clomipramine and a family therapy approach based on the work of White (1989). This uses his technique of 'externalization of the symptoms' in a programme called *How I ran OCD out of my land* (March & Mulle 1998). They found that they could produce a clinically significant improvement in 80% (12/15 cases showed a 30% improvement on Yale–Brown Obsessive Compulsive Scale with no relapses at an 18-month follow-up) of cases (March *et al.* 1994). The programme included coaching the children with anxiety management and relaxation training to work with their difficulties in a hierarchical approach, together with helping the parents to avoid reinforcing the rituals.

Blagg & Yule (1984) found that a behavioural hierarchical desensitization family-based programme produced a better outcome than an inpatient treatment programme (93 vs. 38% successful outcome at 1-year follow-up). The outpatient treatment programme was provided on an intensive basis with negotiation with the school to ensure a rapid return.

Other studies for specific anxieties and for generalized anxiety disorder (Graziano & Mooney 1980; Barrett *et al.* 1996) have taken a family approach. Those studies reported quantitatively have tended to use behavioural components applied in the family context.

Grief reactions following the death of a parent have been treated with home-based family therapy and showed both short-term and longer term improvements (Black 1987; Sandler *et al.* 1992).

With regard to psychosomatic problems, family-based approaches have been found to be effective in several areas. Thapar *et al.* (1992) reviewed the treatments for encopresis and found that a combination of dietary fibre increase, medication and behavioural family therapy was the most effective approach. White (1989) developed a treatment in which the soiling is characterized as another individual who is trying to subvert the child and family. The aim of therapy is to overcome and defeat this character. The programme was researched by Silver *et al.* (1998) and was found to be more effective than a purely behavioural approach.

Family therapy has been found to be useful as an adjunct to medication in the treatment of several disorders, including asthma (Lask & Matthew 1979; Gustafsson *et al.* 1986), attention deficit hyperactivity disorder (ADHD) (with other components of a multimodal treatment; Barkley 1990; Barkley *et al.* 1992; Hinshaw *et al.* 1998) and obsessive-compulsive disorder (March *et al.* 1994; March & Mulle 1998).

The effectiveness of family therapy interventions in the treatment of physical illness has been reviewed by Campbell & Patterson (1995). Methodologically poorer studies of family therapy intervention have not used control groups but have

shown changes with intervention for asthma (Liebman *et al.* 1974; Minuchin *et al.* 1975) and for conversion symptoms (Turgay 1990). Better studies included those by Lask and Gustafsson already cited. Psychoeducational approaches working with the family have been better researched and shown to be effective for compliance for diabetic control, management of asthma, recurrent abdominal pain and helping families manage chronic physical illnesses.

Psychoeducational approaches have also been found to be useful in preventing relapse in schizophrenia (Leff *et al.* 1982; Leff & Vaughan 1985; Goldstein & Miklowitz 1995). This is based on pioneering work by Vaughan and Leff's earlier studies of factors leading to relapse in schizophrenia (Vaughan & Leff 1976). This work has been applied to early onset schizophrenia in adolescence although its impact on relapse has not yet been properly researched.

In a series of trials (Russell *et al.* 1987; Le Grange *et al.* 1992; Eisler *et al.* 1997; Robin *et al.* 1999), family therapy has been found to be a treatment of choice for anorexia nervosa. Structural and Milan systemic family therapy approaches have formed the basis of family treatments provided, but they have been modified with time to take account of the acute sensitivity of such families to expressed emotion and critical comments. For some families, this has meant that a more effective approach has been to provide separated family therapy in which the parents are seen separately from the adolescent but a systemic stance is maintained with both (Eisler *et al.* 1997).

In reviews where parent management training (PMT) has been included in the broad definition of family therapy, it has repeatedly been found to be effective for oppositional-defiant disorder and childhood conduct disorder. (Estrada & Pinsof 1995; Kazdin 1998). The latter authors also concluded from their review of the literature that PMT reduces the non-compliance and aggression in children with ADHD but that it does not really improve the core symptomatology of the disorder. Satterfield *et al.*'s (1981, 1987) studies were the exception to this finding in that the addition of family therapy to a pharmacological intervention did improve the outcome in their cohort.

Chamberlain & Rosicky (1995) reviewed several recent studies' use of family therapy approaches to adolescent conduct disorder. They emphasized the importance of a manualized approach. All the recent studies seemed to involve a social behavioural learning approach (Bank *et al.* 1991), a structural family therapy approach (Szapocznik *et al.* 1989) or one that combined the social learning approach with other individual components for the young person to improve social cognitive appraisal and other peer-related processes (Chamberlain 1990; Henggeler *et al.* 1992). They referred to the latter as multi-target ecological treatment (MET). They discussed two types of study. The first involves the youngster spending time with a specially trained foster family while their own parents undertake a course of parent management training and a reintegration of the young person to the family. Very close attention is paid to managing the child's contact with school and peers during this programme. It has been successful in preventing young people being incarcerated and in reducing their subsequent antisocial behaviour (Chamberlain & Reid 1991; Chamberlain 1994).

The second approach reviewed by these authors, the family preservation services (FPS) model, has the young person remain at home with their parents but with very intensive home-based and community interventions. Taking place over 2–4 months, it requires many hours of professional time each week. It has a mixed outcome (reviewed by Rivera & Kutash 1994). The latter authors also pointed out that a significant proportion of conduct disordered families drop out of treatment. Families that drop out typically show high rates of various risk factors such as stress, maternal depression, social isolation, low socioeconomic status and were referred for treatment by an external agency.

In substance-abusing adolescents, reviews by Waldron (1996) and by Cormack & Carr (2000) indicate that family therapy approaches are more effective than individual or group approaches and at least as or more effective than parent training. The approaches used included a structural family therapy and strategic approach. Liddle & Dakof (1995) reviewed 10 studies of family-based approaches to adolescent drug abuse. All showed positive findings, both in terms of engaging families and subsequent outcome. Two studies indicated a better outcome when comparing this with a peer-based approach. Henggeler *et al.* (1991) showed a reduction in drug-related offences in a 4-year follow-up study of a multisystemic approach that included family therapy.

Hampson & Beavers (1996) asked which families respond best to which family therapy approach. In general, they found that underorganized families do better with more structured directive approaches while families that are relatively well functioning benefit from more narrative/social constructionist approaches.

Conclusions

Family therapy has come a long way since its beginnings. There is a research literature developing but it is still far too sparse for comfort. There is a dearth of process research and the outcome research is slanted towards behaviourally based interventions at present. This can lead to the 'truth' that only this type of family interventions work. It may just be that it is largely investigators with this background that have carried out the studies thus far. One of the difficulties that the field faces is the rapidity with which theoretical ideas move on, to be followed apace by clinical self-reinvention. This means that there is rarely time for the development of manualized treatment approaches, let alone randomized clinical trials before the next 'leap forward' occurs.

Despite these reservations, family therapy can take pride that many of its ideas have become incorporated into the thinking of child and adolescent mental health practice so that many other professionals take for granted a systemic approach to their work even if they are not practising family therapists.

There is a recognition among family therapists that there are

links between elements of behaviour through increasingly complex ways of assembling these to individual belief systems, family scripts and societal ones. The choice then becomes at what levels interventions can and may be made. With this synthesis it becomes much more possible to integrate thinking about families. It allows the use of elements from behavioural approaches through interpersonal narrative ones and to include psychodynamic thinking to produce a more holistic formulation. This could appear muddled but there does appear to be benefit from the family's viewpoint of the giving up of territorial wars and the harnessing of skills from many domains—psychosocial and biological—in the treatment of families.

There is a recognition among clinicians that a rather more structural behavioural-based approach is taken with the problems of families that involve younger children while a shift to more inclusion of belief systems of both adults and youngsters occurs as the child reaches adolescence. This can be seen in the greater evidence for such styles in working with those with anorexia nervosa and young people who are substance abusers.

The one thing that is striking but often forgotten is that the family and child that we treat are the same whatever spectacles we choose to view them through. We may elicit different aspects of their world but all the aspects are there to be understood.

It is sad that in a recent family therapy journal review of the research, Carr (2000) felt it necessary to insert paragraphs justifying an evidence-based approach in the context of a current preoccupation with a social constructionist view of systemic thinking. Surely an aim for the future must be to work beyond the constraints of acceptable theory at any one point in time.

References

Alexander, J.F. & Parsons, B.V. (1982) Short term behavioral interventions with delinquent families: impact on family process and recidivism *Journal of Abnormal Psychology*, 81, 219–225.

Andersen, T. (1987) The reflecting team. *Family Process*, 26, 415–428.

Andersen, T. (1990) *The Reflecting Team.* W.W.Norton, New York.

Anderson, H. & Goolishian, H.H. (1988) Human systems as linguistic systems: preliminary and involving ideas about the implications for clinical theory. *Family Process*, 27, 371–393.

Anderson, H. & Goolishian, H.H. (1992) *The Client Is the Expert: A Not Knowing Approach to Therapy as a Social Construction.* Sage, Newbury Park, CA.

Anderson, H., Goolishian, H.H. & Winderman, L. (1986) Problem-determined systems: towards transformation in family therapy. *Journal of Strategic and Systemic Therapies*, 5, 1–13.

Aponte, H. (1976) Underorganisation in the poor family. In: *Family Therapy: Theory and Practice* (ed. P. Guerin), pp. 249–283. Gardner Press, New York.

Bank, L., Marlowe, J.H., Reid, J.B., Patterson, G.R. & Weinrott, M.R. (1991) A comparative evaluation of parent training interventions for families of chronic delinquents. *Journal of Abnormal Child Psychology*, 19, 15–33.

Barkley, R. (1990) *Attention Deficit Hyperactivity Disorder: a Handbook for Diagnosis and Treatment.* Guilford Press, New York.

Barkley, R., Guevremont, D., Anastopoulos, A. & Fletcher, K. (1992) A comparison of three family therapy programs for treating family conflicts in adolescents with ADHD. *Journal of Consulting and Clinical Psychology*, 60, 450–462.

Barrett, P., Dadds, M. & Rappee, R. (1996) Family treatment of childhood anxiety: a controlled trial. *Journal of Consulting and Clinical Psychology*, 64, 333–342.

Bateson, G. (1958) *Naven*. Stanford University Press, Stanford, CA.

Bateson, G. (1973) *Steps to an Ecology of Mind*. Paladin, St Albans.

Bateson, G. (1979) *Mind and Nature*. Wildwood House, London.

Bentovim, A. (1992) *Trauma-organized Systems: Physical and Sexual Abuse*. Karnac, London.

Bentovim, A. & Jacobs, B.W. (1988) Children's needs and family therapy: the case of abuse. In: *Family Therapy in Britain* (eds E. Street & W. Dryden), pp. 217–239. Open University Press, Milton Keynes.

Bentovim, A. & Kinston, W. (1981) Brief focal family therapy when the child is the referred patient. In: *Developments in Family Therapy* (ed. S. Walrond-Skinner), pp. 202–245. Routledge & Kegan Paul, London.

von Bertalanffy, L. (1950) An outline of general system theory. *British Journal of the Philosophy of Science*, 1, 134–165.

Black and Urbanowicz (1987) Family intervention with bereaved children. *Journal of Child Psychology and Psychiatry*, 23, 467–476.

Blagg, N. & Yule, W. (1984) The behavioural treatment of school refusal: a comparative study *Behaviour Research and Therapy*, 2, 119–127.

Boscolo, L., Cecchin, G., Hoffman, L. & Penn, P. (1987) *Milan Systemic Family Therapy*. Basic Books, New York.

Boss, P. & Weiner, P. (1988) Rethinking assumptions about women's development and family therapy. In: *Family Transitions: Continuity and Change Over the Life Cycle* (ed. C.J. Falicov), pp. 235–251. Guilford Press, New York.

Boszormenyi-Nagy, I. (1967) Relational modes and meaning. In: *Family Therapy and Disturbed Families* (eds Zuk, G.H. & Boszormenyi-Nagy, I.), pp. 58–73. Science and Behavior Books, Palo Alto.

Boszormenyi-Nagy, I. & Ulrich, D.N. (1981) Contextual family therapy. In: *Handbook of Family Therapy* (eds A.S. Gurman & D.P. Kniskern), pp. 159–186. Brunner/Mazel, New York.

Bowen, M. (1965) Family psychotherapy with schizophrenia in the hospital and in private practice. In: *Intensive Family Therapy* (eds I. Boszormenyi-Nagy & J.L. Framo), pp. 213–244. Harper & Row, New York.

Box, S., Copley, B., Magagna, J. & Moustaky, E. (1981) *Psychotherapy with Families*. Routledge, Kegan & Paul, London.

Bronfenbrenner, U. (1979) *The Ecology of Human Development: Experiments by Nature and Design*. Harvard University Press, Cambridge, MA.

Byng-Hall, J. (1973) Family myths used as defence in conjoint family therapy. *British Journal of Psychology*, 46, 239–250.

Byng-Hall, J. (1995) *Rewriting Family Scripts: Improvisation and Systems Change*. Oxford University Press, Oxford.

Campbell, D. (1985) The consultation interview. In: *Applications of Systemic Family Therapy: the Milan Approach*, Vol. 3 (eds D. Campbell & R. Draper), pp. 193–202. Grune & Stratton, London.

Campbell, D. & Draper, R. (1985) *Applications of Systemic Family Therapy: the Milan Approach*, .Grune & Stratton, London.

Campbell, D., Reder, P., Draper, R. & Pollard, D. (1983) *Working with the Milan Method: Twenty Questions*. Institute of Family Therapy, London.

Campbell, D., Draper, R. & Huffington, C. (1991) *Second Thoughts on the Theory and Practice of the Milan Approach to Family Therapy*. Karnac, London.

Campbell, T.L. & Patterson, J.M. (1995) The effectiveness of family interventions in the treatment of physical illness. *Journal of Marital and Family Therapy*, 21, 545–583.

Capra, F. (1983) *The Tao of Physics*. Flamingo, Fontana, London.

Carr, A. (2000) Evidence-based practice in family therapy and systemic consultation. *Journal of Family Therapy*, 22, 29–60.

Casement, P. (1985) *On Learning from the Patient*. Tavistock, London.

Cecchin, G. (1987) Hypothesising, circularity and neutrality revisited: an invitation to curiosity *Family Process*, 26, 405–513.

Chamberlain, P. (1990) Comparative evaluation of specialized foster-care for seriously delinquent youths: a first step. *Community Alternatives: International Journal of Family Care*, 2, 21–36.

Chamberlain, P. (1994) *Family Connections*, Castalia, Eugene, OR.

Chamberlain, P. & Reid, J. (1991) Using a specialized foster-care treatment model for children and adolescents leaving the state mental hospital. *Journal of Community Psychology*, 19, 266–276.

Chamberlain, P. & Rosicky, J.G. (1995) The effectiveness of family therapy in the treatment of adolescents with conduct disorders and delinquency. *Journal of Marital and Family Therapy*, 21, 441–459.

Clarke-Stewart, K.A. (1978) And Daddy makes three: the father's impact on mother and young child. *Child Development*, 49, 466–478.

Cockett, M. & Tripp, J. (1994) *The Exeter Study*. Joseph Rowntree Foundation, London.

Coppersmith, E.I. (1985) Families and multiple helpers: a systemic perspective. In: *Applications of Systemic Family Therapy: the Milan Approach*, Vol. 3 (eds D. Campbell & R. Draper), pp. 203–212. Grune & Stratton, London.

Cormack, C. & Carr, A. (2000) Drug abuse. In: *What Works with Children and Adolescents: a Critical Review of Psychological Interventions with Children, Adolescents and Their Families* (ed. A. Carr), pp. 155–177. Routledge, London.

Crowe, M. (1982) The treatment of marital and sexual problems. In: *Family Therapy: Complementary Frameworks of Theory and Practice*, Vol. 1 (eds A. Bentovim, G. Gorell Barnes & A. Cooklin), pp. 257–284. Academic Press, London.

Dare, C. (1988) Psychoanalytic family therapy. In: *Family Therapy in Britain* (eds E. Street & W. Dryden), pp. 23–50. Open University Press, Milton Keynes.

Dicks, H.V. (1963) Object relations theory and marital studies *British Journal of Medical Psychology*, 36, 125–129.

Dicks, H.V. (1967) *Marital Tensions*. Basic Books, New York.

Dreikurs, R. (1949) Counselling for family adjustment. *Individual Psychology Bulletin*, 7, 119–137.

Dunn, J. & Kendrick, C. (1982) *Siblings: Love, Envy and Understanding*. Harvard University Press, Cambridge, MA.

Eisler, I., Dare, C., Russell, G., Szmuckler, G., Le Grange, D. & Dodge, E. (1997) Family and individual therapy in anorexia nervosa: a 5 year follow-up. *Archives of General Psychiatry*, 54, 1025–1030.

Estrada, A.U. & Pinsof, W.M. (1995) The effectiveness of family therapy for selected behavioural disorders of childhood. *Journal of Marital and Family Therapy*, 21, 403–441.

Falicov, C. & Brudner-White, L. (1983) The shifting family triangle: the issue of cultural and contextual relativity. In: *Cultural Perspectives in Family Therapy* (ed. L. Falicov), pp. 51–67. Aspen Systems, Rockville, MD.

Ferreira, A.J. (1963) Family myth and homeostasis. *Archives of General Psychiatry*, 9, 457–463.

Fisher, S.G. (1984) Time-limited brief therapy with families: a one-year follow up study. *Family Process*, 23, 101–106.

Foucault, M. (1980) *Power/Knowledge: Selected Interviews and Other Writings*. Pantheon Books, New York.

Framo, J.L. (1970) Symptoms from a family transactional viewpoint. In: *Family Therapy in Transition* (ed. N. Ackerman), pp. 125–171. Little, Brown, Boston.

Gergen, K. (1982) *Toward Transformation in Social Knowledge*. Springer-Verlag, New York.

Gergen, K.J. (1985) The social constructionist movement in modern psychology. *American Psychologist*, **40**, 266–275.

Giovacchini, P. (1958) Mutual adaptation in various object relations. *International Journal of Psycho-analysis*, **39**, 547–554.

Goldner, V. (1985) Feminism and family therapy. *Family Process*, **24**, 31–47.

Goldner, V., Penn, P., Sheinberg, M. & Walker, G. (1990) Love and violence: gender paradoxes in volatile attachments. *Family Process*, **29**, 343–364.

Goldstein, M.J. & Miklowitz, D.J. (1995) The effectiveness of psychoeducational family therapy in the treatment of schizophrenic disorders. *Journal of Marital and Family Therapy*, **21**, 361–376.

Gorrell Barnes, G. (1998) *Family Therapy in Changing Times*. Macmillan, London.

Gorrell Barnes, G. & Dowling, E. (1997) Rewriting the story: mothers, fathers and children's narratives following divorce. In: *Multiple Stories: Narratives in Systemic Family Psychotherapy* (eds R. Papadooulos & J. Byng-Hall), pp. 184–205. Duckworth, London.

Gorrell Barnes, G. & Henesy, S. (1994) Re-claiming a female mind from the experience of sexual abuse. In: *Gender, Power and Relationships* (eds C. Burck & B. Speed), pp. 69–85. Routledge, London.

Gorrell Barnes, G., Thompson, P., Daniel, G. & Burchardt, N. (1998) *Growing Up in Step-families*. Clarendon Press, Oxford.

Graziano, A.M. & Mooney, K.C. (1980) Family self-control instruction and children's night time fear reduction. *Journal of Consulting and Clinical Psychology*, **48**, 206–213.

Gurman, A.S., Kniskern, D.P. & Pinsof, W.M. (1986) Research on the process and outcome of marital and family therapy. In: *Handbook of Psychotherapy and Behaviour Change: an Empirical Analysis* (eds S.L. Garfield & A.E. Bergin), pp. 817–902. John Wiley, New York.

Gustafsson, P., Kjellman, N. & Cederbald, M. (1986) Family therapy in the treatment of severe childhood asthma. *Journal of Psychosomatic Research*, **30**, 369–374.

Haley, J. (1973) *Uncommon Therapy: the Psychiatric Techniques of Milton A. Erickson M.D.* W.W. Norton, New York.

Haley, J. (1976) *Problem Solving Therapy*. Jossey Bass, San Francisco, CA.

Hall, A.D. & Fagan, R.E. (1956) Definition of system. In: *General Systems: Yearbook of the Society for the Advancement of General Systems Theory* (eds L. von Bertalanffy & A. Rapoport), pp. 18–28. American Association for the Advancement of Science, Ann Arbor, MI.

Hampson, R.B. & Beavers, R.W. (1996) Family therapy and outcome: relationships between therapist and family styles. *Contemporary Family Therapy*, **18**, 345–370.

Hartmann, A., Herzog, T. & Drinkman, A. (1992) Psychotherapy of bulimia nervosa: what is effective? A meta-analysis. *Journal of Psychosomatic Research*, **36**, 159–167.

Henggeler, S.W. & Borduin, C.M. (1990) *Family Therapy and Beyond: a Multisystemic Approach to Treating the Behaviour Poblems of Children and Adolescents*. Brooks Cole, Pacific Grove, CA.

Henggeler, S.W., Borduin, C.M., Melton, G.B. *et al.* (1991) Effects of multisystemic therapy on drug use and abuse in serious juvenile offenders: a progress report from two outcome studies. *Family Dynamics Addiction Quarterly*, **1**, 40–51.

Henggeler, S.W., Melton, G.M. & Smith, L.A. (1992) Family preservation using multisystemic therapy: an effective alternative to incarcerating serious juvenile offenders. *Journal of Consulting and Clinical Psychology*, **60**, 953–961.

Hinde, R.A. & Stevenson-Hinde, J., eds (1988) *Relationships Within Families: Mutual Influences*. Oxford Scientific Publications. Oxford University Press, Oxford.

Hinshaw, S., Klein, R. & Abikoff, H. (1998) Childhood attention hyperactivity disorder: nonpharmacological and combination approaches. In: *A Guide to Treatments That Work* (eds P. Nathan & J. Gorman), pp. 26–41. Oxford University Press, New York.

Hinshelwood, R.D. (1989) *A Dictionary of Kleinian Thought*. Free Association Books, London.

Hirsch, S.R. & Leff, J.P. (1975) *Abnormalities in the Parents of Schizophrenics*. Oxford University Press, Oxford.

Ho, M.K. (1987) *Family Therapy with Ethnic Minorities*. Sage, Newbury Park, CA.

Hoffman, L. (1981) *Foundations of Family Therapy: a Conceptual Framework for Systems Change*. Basic Books, New York.

Hoffman, L. (1985) Beyond power and control: towards a 'second order' family systems therapy *Family Systems Medicine*, **3**, 381–396.

Hoffman, L. (1990) Constructing realities: an art of lenses. *Family Process*, **29**, 1–12.

Hoffman, L. (1993) *Exchanging Voices*. Karnac Books, London.

Jackson, D. (1957) The question of family homeostasis. *Psychiatric Quarterly* (Suppl.), **31**, 79–90.

Jackson, D.D., ed. (1967a) *Communication, Family and Marriage*. Science and Behaviour Books, Palo Alto, CA.

Jackson, D.D., ed. (1967b) *Therapy, Communication and Change*. Science and Behaviour Books, Palo Alto, CA.

Joanning, H., Quinn, W., Thomas, F. & Mullen, R. (1992) Treating adolescent drug abuse: a comparison of family systems therapy, adolescent group therapy and family drug education. *Journal of Family and Marital Therapy*, **18**, 345–356.

Kazdin, A. (1997) Psychosocial treatments for conduct disorder. *Journal of Child Psychology and Psychiatry*, **38**, 161–178.

Kazdin, A. (1998) Psychosocial treatments for conduct disorder in children. In: *A Guide to Treatments That Work* (eds P. Nathan & J. Gorman), pp. 65–89. Oxford University Press, Oxford.

Kazdin, A.E., Siegel, T.C. & Bass, D. (1992) Cognitive problem solving skills training and parent management training in the treatment of antisocial behavior in children. *Journal of Consulting and Clinical Psychology*, **60**, 733–747.

Kernberg, O.F. (1966) Structural derivatives of object relationships. *International Journal of Psycho-analysis*, **47**, 236–253.

Klein, M. (1946) Some notes on schizoid mechanisms. *International Journal of Psycho-analysis*, **27**, 99–110.

Kog, E., Vandereyecken, W. & Vertommen, H. (1985) Towards a verification of the psychosomatic family model: a pilot study of ten families with an anorexia/bulimia patient. *International Journal of Eating Disorders*, **4**, 525–538.

Kog, E., Vertommen, H. & Vandereyecken, W. (1987) Minuchin's psychosomatic family model revised: a concept validation study using a multitrait-multimethod approach. *Family Process*, **26**, 235–253.

Lask, B. & Matthew, D. (1979) Childhood asthma: a controlled trial of family psychotherapy. *Archives of Diseases in Childhood*, **55**, 116–119.

Leff, J. & Vaughan, C.E. (1985) *Expressed Emotion in Families*. Guilford Press, New York.

Leff, J., Kuipers, L., Berkowitz, R., Eberlein-Vries, R. & Sturgeon, D. (1982) A controlled trial of social intervention in the families of schizophrenic patients. *British Journal of Psychiatry*, **141**, 121–134.

Le Grange, D., Eisler, I., Dare, C. & Russell, G. (1992) Evaluation of family treatments in anorexia nervosa: a pilot study. *International Journal of Eating Disorders*, **12**, 347–357.

Lewis, J.M., Beavers, W.R., Gossett, J.T. & Phillips, V.A. (1976) *No Single Thread: Psychological Health in Family Systems*. Brunner/Mazel, New York.

Liddle, H.A. & Dakof, G.A. (1995) Efficacy of family therapy for drug abuse: promising but not definitive. *Journal of Marital and Family Therapy*, **21**, 511–543.

Liebman, R., Minuchin, S. & Baker, L. (1974) The use of structural family therapy in the treatment of intractable asthma. *American Journal of Psychiatry*, **131**, 535–540.

Lindsey, C. (1985) Consultations with professional and family systems in the context of residential and fostering services: 'in and out of care'. In: *Applications of Systemic Family Therapy: the Milan Approach*, Vol. 3 (eds D. Campbell & R. Draper), pp. 221–227. Grune & Stratton, London.

Long, J. (1996) Working with lesbians, gays and bisexuals: addressing heterosexism in supervision. *Family Process*, **35**, 377–388.

Madanes, C. (1981) *Strategic Family Therapy*. Jossey-Bass, San Francisco, CA.

Madanes, C. (1984) *Behind the One-way Mirror*. Jossey-Bass, San Francisco, CA.

Madanes, C. (1990) *Sex, Love and Violence: Strategies for Transformation*. Norton, New York.

Main, M., Kaplan, N. & Cassidy, J. (1985) Security in infancy, childhood and adulthood: a move to the level of representation. In: *Monograph of the Society for Research in Child Development*, Volume Serial No. 209, 50: Nos. 1–2 (eds I. Bretherton & E. Waters), pp. 66–104. University of Chicago Press, Chicago.

March, J. & Mulle, K. (1998) *OCD in Children and Adolescents: a Cognitive-behavioural Treatment Manual*. Guilford Press, New York.

March, J., Mulle, K. & Herbel, B. (1994) Behavioural psychotherapy for children and adolescents with OCD: an open trial of a new protocol-driven treatment package. *Journal of the American Academy of Child and Adolescent Psychiatry*, **33**, 333–341.

Maturana, H. (1978) Biology of language: the epistemology of reality. In: *Psychology and Biology of Language and Thought: essays in honor of Eric Lenneberg* (eds G.A. Miller & E. Lenneberg), pp. 27–63. Academic Press, New York.

Maturana, H. & Varela, F. (1980) *Autopoiesis and Cognition: the Realization of the Living*. Reidel, Dordrecht, Holland.

McGoldrick, M., Giordano, J. & Pearce, J.K. (1996) *Ethnicity and Family Therapy*. Guilford Press, New York.

Mendez, C.L., Coddou, F. & Maturana, H.R. (1988) The bringing forth of pathology. *Irish Journal of Psychology*, **9**, 144–172.

Minuchin, S. (1974) *Families and Family Therapy*. Harvard University Press, Cambridge, MA.

Minuchin, S. (1978) *Psychosomatic Families*. Harvard University Press, Cambridge, MA.

Minuchin, S. & Fishman, H.C. (1981) *Family Therapy Techniques*. Harvard University Press, Cambridge, MA.

Minuchin, S., Montalvo, B., Guerney, B.G.J., Rosman, B.L. & Schumer, F. (1967) *Families of the Slums*. Basic Books, New York.

Minuchin, S., Baker, L., Rosman, B.L., Liebman, R., Milman, L. & Todd, T.C. (1975) A conceptual model of psychosomatic illness in children. *Archives of General Psychiatry*, **32**, 1031–1038.

Nichols, M.P. & Schwartz, R.C. (1991) *Family Therapy: Concepts and Methods*. Allyn & Baker, Boston.

Nitzberg, L., Patten, J., Spielman, M. & Brown, R. (1985) In-patient hospital systemic consultation: providing team consultation in in-patient hospital settings where the team is part of the system. In: *Applications of Systemic Family Therapy: the Milan Approach* (eds D. Campbell & R. Draper), 3rd edn, pp. 213–220. Grune & Stratton, London.

O'Halloran, M. & Carr, A. (2000) Adjustment to parental separation and divorce. In: *What Works with Children and Adolescents? a Critical Review of Psychological Interventions with Children, Adolescents and Their Families* (ed. A. Carr), pp. 280–299. Routledge, London.

Patterson, G.R. (1971a) Behavioral intervention procedures in the classroom and in the home. In: *Handbook of Psychotherapy and Behavior Change: an Empirical Analysis* (eds A.E. Bergin & S.L. Garfield), pp. 751–775. Wiley, New York.

Patterson, G.R. (1971b) *Families: Application of Social Learning Theory to Family Life*. Research Press, Champain, IL.

Patterson, G.R. (1982) *Coercive Family Process: A Social Learning Process*. Castalia, Eugene, OR.

Penn, P. (1982) Circular questioning. *Family Process*, **21**, 267–280.

Perelberg, R.J. & Miller, A.C., eds (1990) *Gender and Power in Families*. Routledge, Tavistock, London.

Quinn, W., Kuehl, B., Thomas, F. & Joanning, H. (1988) Families of adolescent drug abusers: systemic interventions to obtain drug free behavior. *American Journal of Drug and Alcohol Abuse*, **14**, 65–87.

Reimers, S. & Street, E. (1993) Using family therapy in child and adolescent services. In: *Using Family Therapy in the 90s* (eds J. Carpenter & A. Treacher), pp. 32–56. Blackwell, Oxford.

Riskin, J. & Faunce, E. (1972) An evaluative review of family interaction and research. *Family Process*, **11**, 365–455.

Rivera, V.R. & Kutash, K. (1994) *Components of a System of Care. What Does the Research Say?* University of South Florida Mental Health Institute, Research and Training Center for Children's Mental Health, Tampa, FL.

Robin, A.L., Siegel, P.T., Moye, A.W., Gilroy, M., Dennis, A.B. & Sikand, A. (1999) A controlled comparison of family versus individual therapy for adolescents with anorexia nervosa. *Journal of the American Academy of Child and Adolescent Psychiatry*, **38**, 1482–1489.

Robinson, M. (1997) *Divorce as Family Transition*. Karnac, London.

Russell, G., Szmuckler, G., Dare, C. & Eisler, I. (1987) An evaluation of family therapy in anorexia nervosa and bulimia nervosa. *Archives of General Psychiatry*, **44**, 1047–1056.

Rutter, M. (1999a) Social context: meanings, measures and mechanisms. *European Review*, **7**, 139–149.

Rutter, M. (1999b) Resilience concepts and findings: implications for family therapy. *Journal of Family Therapy*, **21**, 119–144.

Rutter, M. (2000) Psychosocial influences: critiques, findings, and research needs. *Development and Psychopathology*, **12**, 375–405.

Sandler, I.N., West, S.G., Baca, L. *et al.* (1992) Linking empirically based theory and evaluation: the family bereavement program. *American Journal of Community Psychology*, **20**, 491–521.

Satterfield, J.H., Satterfield, B. & Cantwell, D.P. (1981) Three-year multi-modality study of 100 hyperactive boys. *Journal of Pediatrics*, **98**, 650–655.

Satterfield, J.H., Satterfield, B. & Schell, A.M. (1987) Therapeutic interventions to prevent delinquency in hyperactive boys. *Journal of the American Academy of Child and Adolescent Psychiatry*, **26**, 56–64.

Selvini Palazzoli, M. (1978) *Self-starvation: From Individual to Family Therapy in the Treatment of Anorexia Nervosa*. Jason Aronson, New York.

Selvini Palazzoli, M., Boscolo, L., Cecchin, G. & Parata, G. (1978) *Paradox and Counterparadox*. Aronson, New York.

Selvini Palazzoli, M., Boscolo, L., Cecchin, G. & Parata, G. (1980) Hypothesising–circularity–neutrality: three guidelines for the conductor of the session. *Family Process*, **19**, 3–12.

Shadish, W.R. (1992) Do family and marital psychotherapies change what people do? A meta-analysis of behavioral outcomes. In: *Meta-analysis for Explanation: a Casebook* (eds T.D. Cook, H.M. Cooper, D.S. Cordray *et al.*), pp. 129–208. Sage, New York.

Shadish, W.R., Montgomery, L.M., Wilson, M.R., Bright, I. &

Okwumabua, T. (1993) Effects of family and marital psychotherapies: a meta-analysis. *Journal of Consulting and Clinical Psychology*, **61**, 992–1002.

Shadish, W.R., Ragsdale, K., Glaser, R.R. & Montgomery, L.M. (1995) The efficacy and effectiveness of marital and family therapy: a perspective from meta-analysis *Journal of Marital and Family Therapy*, **21**, 345–360.

de Shazer, S. (1985) *Keys to Solution in Brief Therapy*. W.W. Norton, New York.

de Shazer, S. (1991) *Putting Difference to Work*. W.W. Norton, New York.

de Shazer, S. & Berg, I.K. (1992) Doing therapy: a post-structural revision. *Journal of Marital and Family Therapy*, **18**, 71–81.

de Shazer, S., Berg, I.K., Lipschik, E. *et al.* (1986) Brief therapy: focussed solution development. *Family Process*, **25**, 207–222.

Silver, E., Williams, A., Worthington, F. & Phillips, N. (1998) Family therapy and soiling: an audit of externalizing and other approaches. *Journal of Family Therapy*, **20**, 413–422.

Simpson, B., McCarthy, J. & Walker, J. (1995) *Being There: Fathers After Divorce*. Relate, University of Newcastle, Newcastle.

Skynner, A.C.R. (1981) An open-systems, group-analytic approach to family therapy. In: *The Handbook of Family Therapy*, Vol. 1 (eds A. Gurman & D. Kniskern), pp. 39–84. Brunner/Mazel, New York.

Sprenkle, D.H., Blow, A.J. & Dickey, M.H. (1999) Common factors and other nontechnique variables in marriage and family therapy. In: *The Heart and Soul of Change: What Works in Therapy* (eds M.A. Hubble, D.L. Barry & S.D. Miller), pp. 329–359. American Psychological Association, Washington D.C.

Stuart, R.B. (1971) Behavioral contracting within the families of delinquents. *Journal of Behavior Therapy and Experimental Psychiatry*, **2**, 1–11.

Szapocznik, J., Rio, A., Murray, E. *et al.* (1989) Structural family therapy versus psychodynamic therpay for problematic Hispanic boys. *Journal of Consulting and Clinical Psychology*, **57**, 571–578.

Thapar, A., Davies, G., Jones, T. & Rivett, M. (1992) Treatment of childhood encopresis: a review. *Child: Care, Health and Development*, **8**, 343–353.

Tomm, K. (1987a) Interventive interviewing: I. *Family Process*, **26**, 3–13.

Tomm, K. (1987b) Interventive interviewing. II. *Family Process*, **26**, 167–183.

Tomm, K. (1988) Interventive interviewing. III. Intending to ask lineal, circular, strategic or reflexive questions. *Family Process*, **27**, 1–15.

Turgay, A. (1990) Treatment outcome for children and adolescents with conversion disorder. *Canadian Journal of Psychiatry*, **35**, 585–588.

Vaughan, C.E. & Leff, J. (1976) The influence of family and social factors on the course of psychotic illness. *British Journal of Psychiatry*, **129**, 125–137.

Von Foerster, H. (1981) *Observing Systems*. Intersystems Publications, Seaside, CA.

Von Glaserfield, E. (1984) An introduction to radical constructivism. In: *The Invented Reality* (ed. P. Watzlawick), pp. 17–40. W.W. Norton, New York.

Waldron, H.B. (1996) Adolescent substance abuse and family therapy outcome: a review of randomized trials. *Advances in Clinical Child Psychology*, **19**, 199–234.

Watzlawick, P., Bavelas, J.B. & Jackson, D.D. (1967) *Pragmatics of Human Communication: a Study of Interactional Patterns, Pathologies and Paradoxes*. W.W. Norton, New York.

Watzlawick, P., Weakland, J. & Fisch, R. (1972) *Change*. Norton, New York.

Weakland, J. (1976) The 'double bind' hypothesis of schizophrenia and three party interaction. In: *Double Bind, the Foundation of the Communication Approach to the Family* (eds C. Slucki & D. Ransom), pp. 23–38. Grune and Stratton, New York.

Webster-Stratton, C. (1984) Randomized trial of two parent training programs for families with conduct disordered children. *Journal of Clinical and Consulting Psychology*, **52**, 666–678.

White, M. (1989) The externalising of the problem and the re-authoring of lives and relationships. In: *Selected Papers* (ed. M. White), pp. 5–28. Dulwich Centre, Adelaide, South Australia.

White, M. (1995) *Re-authoring Lives: Interviews and Essays*. Dulwich Centre, Adelaide, South Australia.

White, M. & Epston, D. (1990) *Narrative Means to Therapeutic Ends*. W.W. Norton, New York.

Wilson, T. & Fairburn, C. (1998) Treatments for eating disorders. In: *A Guide to Treatments That Work* (eds P. Nathan & J. Gorman), pp. 501–530. Oxford University Press, Oxford.

Zinner, J. & Shapiro, R. (1976) Projective identification as a mode of perception and behaviour in families of adolescents. *International Journal of Psycho-analysis*, **53**, 520–530.

58 Individual and Group Therapy

Brian W. Jacobs

Introduction

This chapter considers individual and group treatments that are used directly with children and adolescents and that are based on psychodynamic principles, relationship concepts or social skills approaches. The starting point is that, whatever the style of therapy, there are basic considerations that will influence clinical delivery. Therapists often feel pressed to break new ground and to emphasize how what they do is different from anything that has gone before. This tension over the need to differentiate among treatments that appear to have much in common has led some commentators to note the 'non-specific' effects of psychological therapies. In the adult field, some have claimed that the largest effects derive from the therapist–client relationship rather than from any specific intervention components (Lambert 1992; Hubble *et al.* 1999). Similar considerations may be applicable to treatments of children, with the additional complication that children rely on adults for both access to treatment and understanding of the treatment processes.

Although the claims regarding the predominant importance of non-specific effects seem overstated, clearly it is the case that treatment methods involving personal interaction will depend on the skills of empathy, of pacing, of responsiveness to cues and of active listening that span different approaches. To different degrees, and in varying ways, all psychotherapies bring together interpersonal microelements, behavioural patterns, conscious and unconscious applied to recurring or new situations, and belief systems about their own and others' actions. Treatments differ on the levels on which they focus and differ even more on the elements they emphasize as crucial. Psychoanalytic psychotherapy stresses the importance of unconscious thought processes and the extent to which the present is shaped by the past, but therapist–client interactions will be subject to the behavioural influences that constitute the central justification of behaviour therapies. Similarly, modern behaviour therapies recognize the role of thought processes, of thinking patterns that derive from past experiences, and they make use of qualities in the therapeutic relationship. This is most apparent with cognitive behaviour therapies (see Brent *et al.* Chapter 54) but it applies also to other behavioural methods (see Herbert, Chapter 53).

Individual psychodynamic approaches

Aims and history

Psychodynamic psychotherapy seeks to help children process the cognitive and affective components of memories that may be distortions of actual events or which are one-sided in their focus. Children are helped to obtain some sense of mastery and understanding of their lives and learn to manage themselves without having to resort to troublesome defensive (self-protective) strategies. The aim is to restore 'normal' psychological development when this has gone awry and to strengthen internal psychological resources. Psychodynamic approaches all accept the idea of unconscious parts of the mind where normal everyday logic does not apply and where quirky links are made among thoughts, feelings and memories in odd idiosyncratic ways.

Psychodynamic theory may sometimes appear rather opaque. In part this may reflect outmoded theory, but in large degree it stems from the difficulty of describing the feeling states and fluctuations in feelings attached to memories that constitute the heart of the therapeutic process. The complex patterns of communication between child and therapist are perhaps more akin to music than to language.

A particular problem for psychoanalytic theory has been that it was mostly developed in work with adult patients looking back towards childhood, providing a very different perspective from that of the child looking forwards. Classical psychoanalytic theory has undergone many changes over the years (Spillius 1988; Rayner 1990; Tyson & Tyson 1990; Sandler *et al.* 1992). Although the concept of 'drives' (a central feature of early psychoanalysis) may have some validity, its limitations are now widely accepted.

Object relations theory has been helpful in thinking about the internal world of the child and of the people — distorted through the child's own defence mechanisms — that inhabit that world. These defence mechanisms are important to the child in helping him or her to obtain mastery and some sense of control in phases of life when he or she has very limited actual control, but they can become a liability. The development of object relations theory was charted by Greenberg & Mitchell (1990), and its modifications in relation to children by Sandler *et al.* (1980) and by Spillius (1988, particularly Vol. 2, part 3).

Increasing attention has been paid to the findings that have emerged from developmental psychology. The writings of

Brazelton, Emde and Stern (Stern 1985) have been particularly influential. Very much briefer accounts of psychodynamic theory, as applied to work with children, have been provided by Lanyado & Horn (1999) and by Jacobs (1997).

In essence, psychoanalytic theory is increasingly taking into account the findings of the developmental psychology of early life. This requires a rethink of many concepts; for example, it is now evident that newborn infants are sentient beings with thought processes and learning that show rapidly increasing complexity over the early childhood years. This was not realized in earlier psychodynamic writing.

Another important element in the modernization of psychodynamic thinking as applied to children has been the development of attachment theory and its helpfulness in bringing a theoretical framework that can more easily be tested empirically (see O'Connor, Chapter 46). This latter framework has led to the development of instruments that are thought to measure activation of the attachment system, normal and abnormal, at various ages from early to middle childhood (Bretherton et al. 1990; Goldwyn et al. 2000; Green et al. 2000). Although not yet well tested, these instruments offer the potential to measure changes in attachment patterns and, in particular, the degree of attachment disorganization (Hesse & Main, in press) that takes place with various approaches to treatment of childhood disorders.

The replication in therapy of emotional scripts that are enacted outside therapy and that often seem to have a history from early in the child's development provides much of the material for the therapy. Gradually enabling a child to feel less threatened and more able to relax rigid defence patterns, to become more flexible in the way that he or she understands and approaches, and reacts to approaches from others, forms much of the work of therapy. This, together with reducing the child's need to use defences that have become developmentally outdated is one central aim of child psychotherapy.

Working with parents to enable them to support the child's therapy is seen as an essential component of the work. Sometimes this work may be more intensive in its own right; at other times group work with parents seems more appropriate. It has been found to be particularly useful when the parent is isolated in reality or through a sense of failure with their child. Meeting others in a similar predicament can be very supportive (Rustin 1999; Tsiantis 1999).

Therapeutic strategy

Parents need to understand and support the nature of the therapeutic contract for a child to be brought to therapy on a regular basis. Interruptions in therapy are very disruptive, particularly those occurring at short notice. Most child psychotherapists see children at fixed times each week for sessions lasting about 45 min. These times may be reduced for younger children. The therapist provides a range of toys to allow the child to build an imaginary world with animals (wild and domestic) and people (Hartnup 1999). Many therapists prefer not to have construc-

tional toys or board games. These can easily lead to a child 'avoiding' an engagement with their inner world that is more likely to occur through less structured activities. Other therapists, it has to be said, have found that constructional toys can be helpful to anxious children and that in due course the child comes to use them in fantasy to represent other things. Most therapists will provide each child with their own box of toys and play materials including paper, glue, plasticene, drawing materials, etc. For adolescents, a more adult setting is usually demanded (Wilson 1991) but it can be helpful to have creative materials available.

It is important that therapists negotiate their role with the child or adolescent including the knotty issue of confidentiality. Complete confidentiality cannot be offered; issues of child abuse may arise in therapy. How such matters are dealt with need careful negotiation with the child so that they can feel supported safely rather than being betrayed. Equally, adults who bring children for therapy must feel reassured about the issues of confidentiality but also understand its importance for the child and therapist in the normal working of therapy. Reviews of therapy are commonly built into the method and form part of the process of deciding how and when to end treatment.

In sessions the therapist generally takes the stance of an interested observer. Periodically, he or she will ask questions about what is happening in the child's play and will make comments about possible links to other elements in the play and, perhaps later in the therapy, to issues in the child's own life. Depending on the style of psychodynamic therapy, some therapists will make more interpretations about possible links to conflicts in the child's inner world and oppositions between wishes, desires and fears. The therapist hopes to induce a curiosity in the child about why he or she thinks, feels and behaves as he or she does and whether he or she wants to continue thus or decide to change these patterns.

Therapists will be careful to monitor their own behaviour towards the children they see and the effect that each child has upon the therapist. Combined with information arising from the child's activities and behaviour in the session, this will provide some insight into how the child sees the external world through the distorting lens of his or her own internal world. This can give a lead as to how the therapist might intervene to try to describe this process and through this to begin to 'challenge' it.

A therapist must be able to tolerate 'not knowing' the meaning of a child's play or behaviour for some time until it becomes clear. Prematurely putting the matter into words can distort the real meaning and lead to a loss of confidence by the child or the creation of false memories.

The child psychotherapist must be able to accept and tolerate intense feelings generated by the child. Tolerating these projections that often are generated non-verbally, sometimes in silence with little action, can require considerable containment and ability for self-reflection by the therapist. Not acting at such times but reflecting and gradually trying to come to understand the meaning of such 'feeling storms' can be crucial to the outcome of therapy.

Applications

Child psychotherapy in the UK has had to adapt to the NHS framework, with children being seen once or twice weekly. The indications for such work and its limitations are well described by Parsons et al. (1999). Only a small number of children are seen intensively (Green 1999). Child psychotherapists carry out significant consultation work with other professionals in social services (Hughes 1999; Hunter 1999), education and therapeutic communities (Flynn 1999; Wilson 1999). In addition, they are increasingly working directly with youngsters who are in the local authority care system. This has been a new venture for child psychotherapists as there was a time when the lack of stability of placement for such children was seen as an insuperable impediment for any work except brief consultation (Hunter 2001).

Child psychotherapists have found a place in specialist paediatric departments and provide direct assessment and on-going work with patients as well as support for the staff who are often working with children who have emotionally distressing conditions. Ramsden (1999) gave a helpful account of such work with several clinical examples. Some empirical evidence for such work is described below (Fonagy & Moran 1990; Moran et al. 1991).

Empirical review

Overall, there is evidence that psychodynamic approaches to treatment are effective, although there are disputes about the degree of effectiveness and their relative efficacy compared with other psychological treatments for children and adolescents.

An early empirical review (Levitt 1957) was not encouraging, suggesting that child psychotherapy was no more effective than the passage of time. This was challenged on the basis that the studies showing improvement without treatment were poor and the definitions of the children's symptomatology were inadequate by today's standards (Kolvin et al. 1988; Roth & Fonagy 1996, p. 279). By the early 1980s there was weak evidence in favour of child psychotherapeutic approaches (Kashudin 1974; Tramonata 1980, p. 32; Rutter 1982).

One careful meta-analytic review (Kazdin 1990) has described effect sizes of 0.88 comparing those who receive any child psychological treatment against those receiving no treatment. This reduced to an effect size (ES) of 0.77 when there was a placebo control treatment. Others (Casey & Berman 1985) have found much smaller effect sizes (0.21) for child psychotherapy compared with a client centred approach (ES = 0.49) or a behavioural approach (ES = 1.00).

However, this low effect size for child psychotherapy was based on five studies only, largely (75%) non-clinic referrals (Saxe et al. 1986). The behavioural treatments were assessed using measures that are similar to the intervention leading to the possibility of 'training' (Casey & Berman 1985). Here and elsewhere (Weisz et al. 1987), removing studies that use outcome measures that closely relate to the therapy task from the analysis shows behavioural and non-behavioural interventions to have similar effect sizes.

Shirk & Russell (1992) also demonstrated an allegiance effect and the importance of relating the treatment to actual clinical practice. They reanalysed data from Weisz et al. (1987), looking at the 24 studies with 29 treatments that involved non-behavioural methods. They showed that many studies had three or more significant methodological flaws (62%). The more rigorous studies had double the effect size (0.6 vs. 0.3) and those non-behavioural studies carried out by therapists with an allegiance to non-behavioural approaches had an effect size of 0.56 compared with 0.17 when behaviourists tried to carry out non-behavioural therapies (often as control/comparisons for their own behavioural treatments).

Furthermore, in other studies (Koocher & Pedulla 1977; Silver & Silver 1983; Snow & Paternite 1986; Kazdin et al. 1990), group treatments for non-behavioural approaches seemed to be frequently used while such approaches were rarely reported in clinical practice with children. The effect size from these group-based treatments was also much less than when the child saw a therapist individually (0.27 vs. 0.8).

The studies also failed to show evidence of efforts to maintain treatment integrity; only six of 29 samples showed such efforts. The brief non-behavioural interventions contrast with longer term individual psychotherapy that was a common approach at the time of the study. Finally, the research populations used in the 29 samples differed in their origin from most clinical samples; a disproportionate number of studies came from institutional settings rather than outpatient clinics.

When can individual psychodynamic psychotherapy with children help?

There are several studies that suggest that intensive psychodynamic psychotherapy with children can be of benefit. These have included single case methodology and small group comparisons. Lush et al. (1991) and Boston & Lush (1994) have shown that it is possible to develop a methodology to examine psychoanalytic psychotherapeutic treatment for severely deprived children in local authority care, asking whether it improved their adjustment in family placements. The result suggested, in a very preliminary way, that this might be a group of youngsters who can benefit from a psychotherapeutic approach.

Moran & Fonagy carried out several investigations of the treatment of brittle insulin-dependent diabetes mellitus with child psychoanalysis in conjunction with the physical management of the illness (Fonagy & Moran 1990; Moran et al. 1991). This small series of case studies showed that it was possible to produce operational definitions of a set of conflicts and psychological symptom categories specific to the patient. Independent ratings over a 3-year psychoanalysis offered some support to their hypothesis that brittle diabetes is related to unconscious conflicts. Improvements in diabetic control were clearly followed 1–3 weeks later by increased psychological symptomatology. Conversely, themes of conflict often foreshadowed periods of improvement in the diabetic control. In a subsequent small group comparison study using glycosylated haemoglobin (HbA$_1$) as a marker for diabetic control and a less intensive psychodynamic psychotherapeutic approach, it was found that the group offered psychoanalytically informed psychotherapy showed a significant ($P < 0.01$) reduction in HbA$_1$ that largely persisted at 1-year follow-up. While the possibility remains that it was the therapeutic attention that these children received rather than the specific therapy that was the important factor, these studies do suggest that this approach warrants further investigation for what can be an intractable and dangerous situation.

The final small but elegant study used an experimental design in three single cases of brittle diabetes with significant growth retardation. Growth was used as a biological outcome. An increase in growth velocity leading to increased predicted adult height of 5–10 cm was observed to accompany psychodynamic treatment. These findings were associated with improvements in HbA$_1$ levels. Again, although this work was on a small scale, it was rather suggestive that psychodynamic psychotherapy can have a role in the management of brittle diabetes.

Systematic examination of the case notes of the Anna Freud Clinic in London also provide some clues as to which children may benefit from intensive or less intensive psychodynamic psychotherapy. In an uncontrolled study, Fonagy & Target (1994) and Target & Fonagy (1994) found that younger children with behaviour or emotional disorders did better than older ones. Intensive treatment seemed to be important in establishing change for the younger behaviourally disturbed children. This was untrue for the emotionally disturbed youngsters. For the disruptive children the length of treatment and the presence of an emotional disorder were positively linked to improved outcome. Comorbidity of anxiety and behaviour disorder improved the outcome for these children whereas other diagnoses worsened the outcome. As anxiety has not generally been associated with a good outcome in oppositional-defiant disorder and conduct disorder, this may be a feature of the psychoanalytic intervention.

Contextual factors are important in the treatment of behavioural disorders. Those that the Anna Freud Clinic could address were parental support during therapy and admission of high-risk children to their nursery at a young age. The holding of the family in longer term treatments has also been found to be an important element in other centres, e.g. Satterfield in his work with boys with attention deficit hyperactivity disorder (ADHD) where those who were engaged in various treatments for 2 years or longer had a much improved outcome (Satterfield *et al.* 1981, 1987).

Of the emotionally disordered patients, depressed youngsters were significantly less likely to show remission, measured by a persisting dysfunctional Childrens' Global Assessment Scale (C-GAS) score. Children with anxiety disorder, depression or mixed disorders of conduct and emotion did better with the more intensive treatments. Equally, when the children were divided into severe cases and less severe cases the former group did

better in the more intensive treatment while for the latter cases this seemed less important.

Non-random assignment of cases that is likely to have occurred clinically makes this result only suggestive at this stage. For example, it is possible that those children with less stable home settings/in care but who had severe problems might be differentially placed in less intensive treatment because of the worry that the treatment might be prematurely stopped. Intensive treatment was also associated with a reduction in the proportion of cases where there was no change or deterioration over the course of treatment.

Taken together, the studies suggest (but remembering that they are uncontrolled and non-random in assignment) that psychoanalysis can be an effective intervention for some situations in childhood. Given the high cost in morbidity and financial costs to families and to society of some of the disorders, particularly in the behavioural disorders spectrum, it may be a justifiable intervention, particularly with younger children with behavioural difficulties. However, the costs of this treatment are high and there may be more effective ways of using limited financial resources. It is not yet clear whether there are particular cases of mixed disorders of conduct and emotion in younger children that may benefit from this resource that will not benefit from less costly interventions.

In the educational field, Heinicke (1969) and Heinicke & Ramsey-Klee (1986) studied children who had educational difficulties of a degree that required supplementary help; some subjects had been held back in school. They met criteria for anxiety with attention deficit and half of the children were also hyperactive. In this very small study, they showed that the group of children having once weekly individual therapy made greater gains during the study. However, boys exposed to four times weekly psychodynamic psychotherapy for 1 year as part of the 2-year treatment made the greatest gains in reading by the time of the 1-year follow-up. The authors offered tentative evidence that the boys who had four times a week therapy made greater gains in effective adaptation, self-esteem, their capacity for relationships, their ability to tolerate frustration and ability to work (weak evidence) and in flexible adaptation. The number of measures, the qualitative nature of the assessments and few subjects mean that caution must be taken in interpreting statistically significant results. None the less, the results accord with those of Fonagy & Target in suggesting the gains that may be made from intensive child psychotherapy. They also, incidentally, are an example of effects appearing during follow-up that were previously masked. This seems to be occurring more frequently in child mental health studies and challenges the scepticism that had built up in the research community regarding so-called 'sleeper effects'.

Thus, as summarized by Roth & Fonagy (1996, pp. 285–6) as the result of their meta-analytic review of the literature, the evidence shows 'consistent differences between treatments in terms of effect size. Behavioural treatments show significantly larger effect sizes than non-behavioural ones, humanistic/existential and family based treatments obtaining somewhat better effect sizes than individual psychodynamic interventions.' They also conclude that 'Between treatment differences are seriously confounded by the use of measures to assess outcome that favour behavioural treatment. There are very few studies of psychodynamic interventions in the pool available for meta-analysis, and these are unrepresentative of practice because of their brevity and the predominance of group-based treatments.' They emphasize the difficulty of investigator allegiance and that of the gap between so-called laboratory-based studies with convenience samples and clinic-based studies with more severe cases. A later meta-analytical review by Carr (2000) for a number of areas in child and adolescent psychological treatments does little to alter this situation.

Richardson (1998) discussed the hurdles of evidence-based medicine, pointing out that child psychotherapy is not alone in not yet meeting the standards of evidence demanded by the clinical effectiveness agenda. He illustrated a fallacy of this approach in which good research can fail to be included in a meta-analysis because it fails to meet one particular criterion of the reviewer's selection system, e.g. the degree to which the diagnostic group is defined. Other methodologically flawed research is included because it does meet all the selection criteria. This is a general point about the meta-analytical approach and highlights the crucial stage of setting the initial inclusion criteria.

In summary, psychodynamic treatments are beginning to show some evidence for their effectiveness, with effect sizes between 0.5 and 0.6, producing benefit relative to an untreated population in 69–73% of cases. There is still a dearth of controlled studies with random assignment. The conditions in which it is the treatment of choice have still to be delineated and a strategy that used less intensive resources *in the first instance* would currently be sensible, although there should still be room for clinical judgement. Well-conducted clinical trials to determine the specific uses of a psychodynamic approach are urgently needed. Work such as that by Moran may well be justified because of the life- and health-threatening nature of brittle diabetes and its frequent resistance to more ordinary approaches.

Place of psychodynamic psychotherapy in training

It would be far too early to consign psychodynamic approaches with children to a few specialist centres; the evidence does not support this. In the present author's view, it is important for trainees to get experience of treating children psychodynamically under supervision from fully trained child psychotherapists. This experience will help to teach the trainee the skills that are necessary to deliver this specific therapy, as well as skills that are applicable in other modes of therapy that they are more likely to use themselves during their careers. It can improve their empathic abilities and other technical skills as well as providing a unique opportunity to experience the emotional forces that a child can muster. The effects on trainees are both expected and unexpected and their capacity to think when offering supervised child psychotherapy is revealing for them. Such experience provides an insight into ways in which children's minds operate,

which can be very valuable throughout a child mental health career. Adults, including professionals, too often forget the child's perspective in producing compromises that work for adults.

A gradual realization that there are many more links between behavioural approaches to treatment and the more psychodynamic approaches is likely to produce benefit for the evolution of therapeutic styles in the next few decades.

Interpersonal therapy for adolescents

Interpersonal therapy (IPT) was developed for adult use by Klerman *et al.* (1984), and was adapted for use in adolescents (ITP-A) by Mufson *et al.* (1993, 1996). The therapy is designed as a once weekly therapy carried out individually with the adolescent over 12 weeks. The originators describe three phases of treatment. During sessions 1–4 the aim is to assess the depression, the family and social context for the adolescent and then negotiate a treatment contract. The responsible parent is used as a resource during the assessment. In the second phase, the therapist works with the patient and, where necessary, conjointly with other family members to address one or two of the problems identified earlier. These may include grief, role disputes or transitions, interpersonal deficits and the particular difficulties of living in a single-parent family.

The style of the therapy is that of a collaborative approach to problem-solving. However, there are links to a brief focused psychodynamic approach, as well as differences (Fombonne 1998; Markowitz *et al.* 1998). The patient is allowed a limited 'sick role' to reduce self-blame and criticism from other family members while at the same time encouraging the adolescent to maintain as many social roles as possible and engage in activities from their previous lifestyle. The final phase of therapy (sessions 9–12) mainly addresses relinquishing the therapist and establishing a sense of competence to deal with future problems.

The evidence for the efficacy of IPT-A is increasing. Robbins *et al.* (1989) tried using adult IPT with adolescents in an open trial for depression among adolescent inpatients and found that 47% made clinically significant improvements. Adding tricyclic antidepressants to the treatment protocol for non-responders obtained a final response rate of 92%. An open clinical trial (Mufson *et al.* 1994) showed good attendance by the adolescents, with significant decreases in depressive symptomatology. Symptoms of physical and psychological distress reduced accompanied by improvement in psychosocial functioning.

This team have now completed a randomized control trial (Mufson *et al.* 1999) in which patients were offered the active treatment or were assigned to clinical monitoring. Therapists were given a brief treatment manual instructing them to refrain from advice-giving or skills training, and to use the 30-min sessions to review depressive symptoms, school attendance, assess suicidal ideation, and just listen supportively. An intention-to-treat analysis revealed that the IPT-A group had significantly fewer symptoms on the Hamilton Scale for Depression at the end of therapy while the self-rated Beck Depression Inventory failed to reach significance at the same time point. They showed better problem-solving skills at the end of the therapy than the clinical monitoring group and they rated their social adjustment as better in relation to peers and dating; there were no self-rated differences between the groups in family relationships or their school adjustment at termination. Unfortunately, no follow-up data are reported and the data must be regarded as preliminary still because of the sample size, the attrition rate in the control group, the exclusion of most comorbid disorders except anxiety, and the population treated (mainly older adolescent female Puerto Ricans). None the less, this individual psychological treatment continues to look promising.

Group therapy

Group therapies have been surprisingly limited in their application and in the research associated with them in child and adolescent psychiatry. Surveys of clinicians in the USA have found that they do not think of group approaches as their preferred methods of treatment of children and adolescents (Koocher & Pedulla 1977; Kazdin *et al.* 1990), yet some investigators have shown that they can be effective interventions (Kolvin *et al.* 1981).

Early history

Kymissis (1997) provided an interesting history of the development of group therapy for children and adolescents from the beginnings in 1932 in Vienna (Dreikurs 1959). Slavson, in the mid-1930s, used *activity group therapy* in which he thought that the patient's 'ego could be repaired through self-directing and self-generating participation by patients in the group' (Slavson & Schiffer 1975). Aichorn (1935) treated delinquent youngsters using groups with a psychoanalytic approach, defining the therapist's role as neutral and non-punitive with unconditional acceptance of group members. This type of approach continues today (Reid 1999) although very clear limits are set around acceptable behaviour in the room.

Overarching theoretical considerations

Attempts have been made to classify the factors that may be operating in the group approach as used with adults (Corsini & Rosenberg 1955; Evans 1998). Nine groups are evident: acceptance, altruism, universalization, reality testing, ventilation, spectator therapy, transference, interaction and intellectualization. This work was taken further for adult groups by Yalom's (1985) delineation of 'curative factors'.

The lack of empirical evidence means that we have to rely more upon theoretical positions and the comments of clinicians who use a group approach about the advantages and dangers that they have found in working with groups of children and adolescents.

Reid (1999), writing about psychodynamic style groups

for children and adolescents, described helpful aspects of group therapy that may be useful for adolescents:
- acceptance by therapist and peers;
- the safety of group boundaries;
- the opportunity to make friends in a protected setting;
- observation of the strengths and weaknesses of other group members as a yardstick to assess oneself;
- enhancing of self-worth;
- observation of and feedback about the effects of one's behaviour on others;
- modelling;
- realization that one's difficulties are not unique;
- the opportunity to treat some youngsters who could not tolerate an individual treatment;
- an increase in self-responsibility through peer interactions;
- the opportunity to take treatment to the child in a variety of settings where it would otherwise be very difficult; and
- economy of treating several young people at once.

Some groups have been designed for youngsters trying to come to terms with specific issues, such as sexual abuse. Bentovim *et al.* (1988) wrote of group work that avoided replication of the secrecy of the abusive experience. The group offers specific support around the conflicts engendered by such abuse. The experience of not being alone in having been abused is thought to be important for these youngsters. A separate psychoeducational function in these groups is to help the young people distinguish between needs for affection/care and sexual feelings, and to help them learn to manage their urge towards sexual 'acting-out'. The group provides peer-based social support, an opportunity to work out what they want to achieve in their relationship with their parents and, finally, to help them to improve their self-esteem.

In all the descriptions of group psychotherapy as applied to children and adolescents, one finds adaptations of content and process to the appropriate developmental stage of the young people concerned. In this regard, groups should probably have a restricted age range because of developmental issues (Kymissis 1997). For adolescents, some suggest that groups should be composed of same sex members because the anxiety of heterosexual issues may interfere with the group climate (Kennedy 1989). This latter position would not be accepted by all.

In summary, where they have been used in psychotherapeutic work, groups use the interpersonal peer and social learning opportunities in addition to the common psychotherapeutic factors that run through most forms of psychotherapy and the specific focus engendered by a particular psychotherapeutic approach.

Psychodynamic groups and non-directive relationship-based therapies in groups

These are considered together because the theoretical frameworks within which they operate have drawn together in many ways over the years. Strict psychoanalytical interpretations are less commonly used now, although consideration by the group leader of unconscious processes within the group is common. A clearer focus on current interactions is common.

Strategies for relationship-based groups

Thinking about the needs of group members and some aspects of group processes using a psychodynamic developmental framework can be useful (Evans 1998). In his active analytic group therapy, Evans has been concerned with both the impact of stressors on the youngster and their maladaptive (defence-driven) responses.

There is a need to balance overall accessibility with the style best adapted for a particular youngster. A practical consideration is that adolescents tend to lose their impetus for change unless they get a quick response. Thus, an active analytic group therapy can offer a pragmatic and responsive style. Its aims include the following.

1 Achievement of age-appropriate tasks:
- development of a viable adult identity or sense of self;
- achievement of a level of independence of parents no more and no less than is appropriate for their age and culture;
- coming to terms with strong sexual feelings; and
- making optimal and effective use of their increasingly powerful assertive (aggressive) drives.

2 Improved object relations through acquiring the resources to abandon immature style of relating to people. This will lead to greater empathy and ability to form trusting relationships.

3 Improved coping mechanisms and defences with reduction of anxieties: learning to notice the styles that they use and to encourage the use of more mature styles of managing stress.

4 Improving their capacity to tolerate anxieties and frustrations.

5 Improved reality testing.

6 Removal of fixations: ceasing to use patterns of behaviour that have become age-inappropriate.

7 Recovery of repressed memories. In general, this is less important for adolescents but for particular youngsters it can be very helpful.

Kymissis (1997) gave guidance on selection and exclusion criteria for children and adolescents in psychodynamic groups, suggesting that 'strong indications for candidacy include children with separation anxiety, poor self-image and poor social and interpersonal skills or non-assertive and isolated youngsters'. Exclusion criteria may include:
- patients who actively insist on using chemical substances or alcohol are not ready to join the group;
- those who have active psychotic symptoms (delusions, hallucinations) may not be able to develop a cohesive bond with the group;
- patients who are actively suicidal may become a threat and present a difficult issue to deal with in the group setting; and
- violent, aggressive or impulsive patients need to be carefully evaluated for inclusion in the group, and should only be accepted on the condition that they will be able to comply with the group rules.

Young people may sometimes instigate a coherent attack on the group's function. This can prove too exciting to be resisted by the rest of the group. If one child's difficulties are too different from the group norm then the flexibility offered by an individual approach may be preferable for that child.

The techniques used in children's groups include drawing, painting puppets and group games. Adolescent groups may use fewer accessory materials. The group therapist must attend to certain group processes. Failure to do so can easily result in an ineffective group and a poor outcome. The conductor should carry out the following.

- Act to develop good group cohesion recognizing that there are two complementary but separate meaning systems at work: first, one relating to developmental strivings for the children or adolescents in everyday life and, secondly, a therapeutic group culture collaboratively created by the youngsters and the therapist. The latter often is only achieved after much resistance over many sessions.
- Establish a work group that does focus on the difficulties of its members rather than a work-avoidant group. This requires some skill and an attention to diversions, recognizing them as such.
- Be willing to set limits to acceptable behaviour. A permissive style is inappropriate when lacking clear boundaries in children's and adolescent groups.
- Provide a setting in which individual identities can develop.
- Encourage coherence and individuation in the group discussion and activities. Evans (1998) aptly likened this to the complexity of music in harmony and in contrapuntal sections.

Client reports and therapist observations suggest that interpretations of patient behaviour and transference in groups in terms of childhood experiences is less useful and much less appreciated than understandings based on current situations (Corder *et al.* 1981).

Empirical evidence

The number of studies of child and adolescent psychodynamic groups is few. Very few studies have used random assignment in well-controlled studies to compare relationship-based group treatments with 'general child and adolescent services' for referred clinical cases. Those that have (Trowell *et al.* 2000) tended to focus on particular issues, such as child sexual abuse, rather than study the heterogeneous psychodynamic groups that have been run in various clinical settings for some decades. Reviews of psychodynamic and non-directive relationship-based group therapies for children and adolescents include those by Abramowitz (1976) and Henry & Kilmann (1979). Tillitski (1990), in a meta-analysis of individual vs. group therapy, suggested that individual therapy was more effective with children whereas a group approach is more effective for adolescents. Against this should be set the findings of Mulvey *et al.* (1993), who noted in their review that group treatment for adolescents with conduct disorders and delinquency can make matters worse. They suggested that this occurs because of the opportunity for maladaptive group learning. It may be particularly relevant for institutional settings for delinquent adolescents. The finding needs to be treated seriously and is a particular reason for limiting the numbers of such children in relationship-based group therapy.

However, it can be overinterpreted to suggest that such youngsters should not be included in a heterogeneous group. As will be seen from the above account, this is possible with care over group composition and with skill in the management of the group. Further, Kazdin (1994) reviewed the issue of relationship-based groups with some alternative conclusions. He highlighted a study of group therapy with delinquent adolescent girls showing it to be more effective than normal treatment in the institution (Truax et al. 1966). Similarly, with delinquent boys, Persons & Pepinsky (1966) and Persons (1966, 1967) showed that delinquent boys randomly assigned to a treatment group involving weekly individual therapy and twice weekly group therapy (in a style that was initially non-directive and accepting but which gradually became more directive during the therapy) showed fewer parole violations over the next year than the control group that received the usual institutional management. The therapy used appeared to be something of a hybrid but also an effort was made to produce anxiety at the prospect of performing any antisocial activity.

Another inpatient group-based study, with younger children, was carried out by Kazdin et al. (1987). They were able to produce some improvements in antisocial behaviour, but not as great as those produced in cognitive-behavioural approaches. Abramowitz et al. (1974) addressed the issue of directive or non-directive group styles for internalizing and externalizing disorders.

In summary, there is only limited evidence on the effectiveness of group psychodynamic or relationship-based therapies for children and adolescents. This should lead to care and caution in setting up such groups in clinical settings. A clear theoretically informed framework for case selection and mode of running the group that involves clear boundaries and careful processing of interventions by the young people and the group therapist is necessary. A 'here and now' perspective is appropriate rather than a historical one that focuses on early childhood. It is wise, too, for anyone running child or adolescent groups to seek to appreciate the perspectives of the young people in the group.

Social skills groups (and problem-solving skills training)

History

Social skills training for children and adolescents developed during the early 1970s. Early attempts included both the teaching of micro-skills of social interaction (eye contact, smiling, body posture, etc.) (Argyle 1969; Spence & Marzillier 1979) and a focus on the macro-patterns of interactions (Spivack et al. 1976; Shure & Spivack 1978). In general, those programmes that focused on larger sequences of interaction seemed to be more accessible and more useful to children. Accordingly, elements of the micro-interactions have become subsumed into the larger sequence style of social skills programmes.

At the same time as social skills programmes were developing, another strand of work led to the various social problem-solving programmes that currently exist (see Compas et al., Chapter 55). Many programmes now use elements from both social skills training and from social problem-solving.

Rationale

Both social skills training and social problem-solving training accept that there are deficits in a child's or adolescent's ability to interact with their peers. There has been some disagreement in relation to claims that the primary deficit is in the child's abilities to analyse the nature of a social interaction and to activate successful prosocial strategies. Alternatively, it has been argued that children can understand the social situation but lack the skills to take part in a way in which they will gain the liking and respect of their peers. A third view has held that much of the difficulty experienced by children is their lack of ability to understand and process emotional cues, both internal and external.

Applications to oppositional-defiant disorder and conduct disorder

Children with behavioural difficulties seem to:
• generate fewer solutions to social problems;
• develop solutions that tend to be aggressive;
• tend to misinterpret positive and neutral cues from others as negative ones;
• attend only to immediate consequences—longer-term ones are ignored;
• are apparently relatively insensitive to interpersonal conflict; and
• fail to recognize the causes of other children's and adults' behaviour
(Spivack et al. 1976; Shure & Spivack 1978; Spivack & Shure 1982; Asarnow & Callan 1985; Dodge 1985). However, these children also have poor abilities to label emotions, they show labile and intense emotions and they come from families where there is also a diminished vocabulary concerning feelings. They have poor empathic skills (Ellis 1982).

Social skills group programmes, such as the Dinosaur School curriculum (Webster-Stratton & Hammond 1997) have been developed for the younger age group. These include elements to develop:
• relaxation techniques;
• recognition of emotions and empathy training;
• social problem-solving skills (as per problem-solving skills training, PSST);
• anger management;
• friendship skills;
• communication skills; and
• managing in the classroom setting.

For example, the friendship skills part of the Dinosaur programme (Webster-Stratton 1996) is delivered over three to four sessions of 2 h each. The first session concentrates on the concepts of helping with the aims of learning what friendship means and of understanding ways of helping others. The second session in this part of the programme concentrates upon sharing and learning the relationship between helping and sharing. The third session moves to 'teamwork at school' through learning about teamwork, learning to understand the benefits of sharing, helping and teamwork and practising friendship skills. The final element of this part of the whole programme concentrates on 'teamwork at home' extending the ideas from the three previous sessions.

In the communication skills section of the programme (two to three sessions) children:
• learn how to ask questions and tell something to a friend;
• learn how to listen carefully to what a friend is saying;
• learn why it is important to speak up about something that is bothering them;
• understand how and when to give an apology or compliment;
• learn how to enter into a group of children who are already playing;
• learn how to give suggestions rather than commands; and
• practise friendship skills.

The methods used throughout this programme use many ways to help the children overlearn the ideas. This is a particularly rich and child-attractive multimodal social skills programme. Other programmes aimed at children with behavioural difficulties use many of the elements seen here, combining them in slightly different ways.

Social skills approaches to helping children with behaviour problems in groups and individually have been reviewed recently by Taylor *et al.* (1999). They took three age ranges: young children up to age 7 years, studies covering the 6–13 years age range, and adolescents. In the youngest age group, the only randomized control study to date was carried out with the Dinosaur curriculum (Webster-Stratton & Hammond 1997). This showed a reduction in aggressive behaviour at home and an improvement in peer social skills, as reported by parents and observed in interaction tasks. These changes persisted until 1-year follow-up. Even greater changes were achieved when the programme was combined with a parenting group. The teachers in school did not report changes. This may reflect a lack of generalization, as noted in other social skills programmes. It may be overcome by a more detailed collaborative approach involving the teachers heavily from the outset. This finding has led to further developments in Webster-Stratton's intervention programmes.

There were more studies in middle childhood. Most concerned school samples rather than clinical referrals. The results of interpersonal skills training for primary school children when applied in groups have been disappointing. Kazdin *et al.* (1992) and Kazdin (1996) achieved moderate success using an individual problem-solving training approach (see Compas *et al.*, Chapter 55) in middle childhood, supplemented by parenting programmes delivered to the parents of each child rather than a group approach. This study did involve children with clinical levels of disturbed behaviour. Change was produced in the school setting as well as at home, with effects persisting 1 year later. However, many of their children still scored in the clinical range for disturbed behaviour despite significant improvements.

Lochman *et al.* (1991) developed an anger-coping programme for children in middle childhood that addressed both cognitive and affective processes to remediate skills deficits in conflict situations. The programme was highly structured and was delivered in group format. Specific goals were to 'increase children's awareness of internal cognitive, affective and physiological phenomena related to anger arousal; enhance self-reflection and self-management skills; facilitate alternative, consequential and means–end thinking in approaching social problems and increase children's behavioural repertoire when facing social conflict'. The programme was broader than a pure PSST approach and used a range of social skills methods as well as some that were specific to this programme, e.g. concentration on physiological cues. Their social skills programme has been shown to have some lasting effect in school-selected populations, both in teacher ratings and in observer ratings (Lochman *et al.* 1984, 1989, 1993).

Interpersonal skills training for adolescents has been disappointing when delivered in group format for aggressive behaviour-disordered adolescents. Feindler *et al.* (1984) found some effect for mild problems (arguing, shoving and cursing) but they have found no effects upon fighting, property damage and severe verbal abuse. Others have found similar negative results (Huey & Rank 1984; Guerra & Slaby 1990). Byrnes *et al.* (1999) were more optimistic. Their data showed a substantial reduction in criminal recidivism that correlated with the hours spent in a group or individual treatment, but not in family therapy, as part of an intensive day and residential programme. However, this was not a controlled trial but a review of the population that took part in the programme over a 4-year period. The style was eclectic, using cognitive-behavioural techniques as well as a more traditional group therapy approach. The study is therefore open to selection and other biases because not all clients entered each therapy.

Application to attention deficit hyperactivity disorder

ADHD is associated with social skills deficits (Whalen & Henker 1985). School observations suggest that children with ADHD are similar to their peers in terms of positive and neutral interactions but differ in being more bossy, intrusive and aggressive (Abikoff & Hechtman 1996). In the light of these observations, various attempts have been made to develop social skills training programmes. Meichenbaum & Goodman's (1971) original individual self-instructional programme has been expanded to include social skills elements and is used by some as a group programme. One review concluded that it worked best if the therapy focuses both on academic and social tasks and involves therapy-based contingency management (Baer & Nietzel 1991).

Abikoff & Hechtman (1996) developed group social skills programmes from two programmes developed in the 1980s: *Getting Along With Others: Teaching Social Effectiveness to Children* (Jackson *et al.* 1983) and the Walker Social Skills programme (ACCEPTS) (Walker *et al.* 1983).

Nolan & Carr (2000) concluded that self-instructional training and social skills training have positive effects on preadolescent school children with ADHD. Social skills training over 12 sessions supplemented with therapy-based contingency management and parental psychoeducation is probably effective in reducing home- and school-based behaviour problems. However, the studies reviewed did not address the long-term effects of such interventions. The recent MTA trial did not find an additional benefit to medication to be derived from the social skills programme that was a part of that trial (MTA Group 1999). This suggests that there is further work to be done to make the social skills interventions currently in use more specific and to improve their generalization.

Application to drug abuse

One trial (Liddle & Dakof 1995) suggested that multisystemic family therapy that included group and individual approaches to social skills and social problem-solving training was better than group therapy alone.

Application to sexually abused girls

McGain & McKinzey (1995) found that group therapy was better than no treatment for girls who had suffered sexual abuse. Trowell *et al.* (2000) studied the comparative effect of individual psychodynamic psychotherapy (up to 30 sessions) with a weekly psychotherapeutic/psychoeducational group of up to 18 sessions. Girls who had been subject to sexual abuse (age 6–14 years) were randomly allocated to the two treatments. Girls treated with either form of therapy improved in mental health (as rated by reduction of psychopathology and reduction of C-GAS scores). Re-experiencing of the trauma was differentially improved by the individual psychodynamic therapy.

Application to anxiety disorders

Albano & Barlow (1996) developed a cognitive-behavioural group treatment for socially phobic adolescents. This included an important social skills component, although it was not the central thrust of the programme. Social skills approaches do not seem to have been much developed for this group of disorders.

Application to depression

Social skills components are included in group cognitive-behavioural therapy programmes such as that developed by Lewinsohn *et al.*'s (1996) Coping With Depression–Adolescent (CWD-A) course. It is based on a social learning view of depression and focuses on training the youngsters in social skills

throughout the course as well as dealing with the specific cognitions of depression on the basis of work showing that depressed people have deficits in social skills. Butler *et al.* (1980), in a school-based programme lasting 10 sessions, found that a social skills approach may be more useful in that setting compared with a cognitive-behavioural approach. However, Fine *et al.* (1991) found that supportive group therapy was better than their social skills programme for clinically presenting depressed adolescents, although the differences disappeared over a 9-month follow-up, because the youngsters who had been treated with a social skills programme continued to show improvements.

Application to separation and divorce

Several studies have shown that group support for children combined with social skills and problem-solving skills training leads to better coping and better adjustment in school than found in control conditions (Roseby & Deutsch 1985; Alpert-Gillis *et al.* 1989). Some of the programmes also specifically help children with stress management (Pedro-Carroll *et al.* 1992). There is an impact on behaviour at home and in school as well as mood state. Methods include discussion, instruction, therapist and video modelling, role-play and rehearsal, together with social skill homework assignments.

As a salutary warning, another popular programme in which the children are offered support groups which has been in widespread use in the USA has been shown to be ineffective (Skitka & Frazier 1995).

Groups for parents

In many of the programmes cited in this section, parallel parent groups are conducted to help them support their children in the work. This seems to be an important issue for generalization, as does close liaison with schools if school-related behaviours are being targeted.

Groups in schools

Groups have been run in school settings, both for specific school-related problems and for more generalized difficulties. Several of the studies cited above have sampled their populations from schools. In such cases there is always the question as to whether these children and adolescents are similar to clinically referred cases or whether they differ in type or severity. One advantage in running groups in schools is that of the captive audience. It does not rely on parents bringing the children to clinics. However, there is the risk of poor generalization of effects because typically parents are not involved very much. Group interventions have been given to youngsters withdrawn from classes or as universal interventions as a prevention measure. Such interventions include bullying programmes.

More recently, teacher training programmes that aim to improve behavioural classroom management such as the Assertive

Discipline Programme (Canter & Canter 1992) and that of Webster-Stratton (see above) have been tried. The latter is intended to articulate with her parenting programme delivered as a universal intervention and later with introducing an adaptation of her Dinosaur school to whole classroom settings for infant school children (4–8 years).

Kolvin et al. (1981) reviewed psychotherapeutic school intervention programmes. Of the many studies he reviewed, he found only two with positive outcome that had adequate follow-up data (Mezzano 1968; Warner 1971). More work has been carried out subsequently but the field is still quite limited (Walker et al. 1983; Bierman 1989; Frankel et al. 1996).

Kolvin et al. developed a non-directive group therapy (four to five children, mixed sex groups) for 7 year olds based on Rogerian principles and drawing on the work of Axline (1947) and Ginott (1961). A similar client-centred Rogerian approach was used with older children (12 year olds, single sex groups) but the groups were based on discussions rather than activities. The therapists were given a moderately intensive training in the methods that they were to use in the schools over 1 year prior to the start of the trial. Nearly 600 of the 4300 children screened were selected for presence of social, psychiatric or learning difficulties in mainstream schools at age 7–8 years and at 11–12 years. The children were randomly allocated to one of the treatment approaches or to the control group.

Group therapy for the primary school children (PG) and for those of secondary school (SG) were compared with no intervention (ARC), to individual nurture work in the younger age group only, to behaviour modification (BM) in the older group, and to parent counselling/teacher consultation (JPC and SPC) in both groups. All treatments except PG and SG were delivered individually. Interestingly, an attempt was made to involve parents in the BM approach, although apparently not as a central plank from the outset. It failed through lack of interest on the part of the parents (for alternative approaches see Scott, Chapter 56).

Of the younger children with neurotic disorders, those who received nurture work or the play group treatment showed improvement at 18 months that was maintained at the 3-year follow-up. For those with antisocial disorders the effect was similar, but the benefit was not seen until the 3-year assessment. Those who had been offered teacher/parent counselling showed less improvement, as did the no-treatment controls.

For the older children with neurotic difficulties, both behaviour modification and the group therapy brought benefits by 18 months. At the 3-year assessment both showed benefits compared with parent/teacher counselling or no treatment. For those with antisocial problems, group treatment was better than both parent/teacher counselling and behaviour modification at 18 months. At 3 years, all three treatments showed more improvement than the no-treatment controls. Treatment benefits generally were greater in the older children.

More recently, Frankel et al. (1996) developed a social skills programme conducted in schools for peer-rejected children aged 7–12 years. Their treatment plan aimed to:

1 reduce the negative effect of the child's current reputation with his or her peers;
2 reduce the importance of the peer-rejecting group by helping the child to expand his or her social network;
3 instruct parents and children how to work together to make having a friend over to play work more successfully; and
4 improve the child's non-aggressive responses to teasing and conflicts with children and adults to reduce the ability of peers to provoke the child.

Children were seen in groups of six to nine pupils over 12 sessions of 1 h. Their parents were seen separately in a concurrent group. The sessions were divided into four sections with feedback of homework assignments, didactic teaching of a new skill, practice in coached play and then a new social skills homework task.

Children were taught the do's and don'ts of group entry, slipping into games and rejection, learning to praise others and negotiating changes of game, being a good host, confrontations with adults, e.g. inappropriate accusations of cheating, coping with teasing (through good humour), being a good winner and avoiding physical fights.

The programme has yielded promising results including those for children with ADHD, particularly when the parent component was enhanced with some generalization to the school setting. The published results for the children who had oppositional-defiant disorder were less encouraging.

Efficacy vs. effectiveness — a challenge

Weisz et al. (1995) have had a particular concern with the difference between studies carried out in expert academic research settings (efficacy studies), sometimes with convenience samples, and those carried out in clinical centres (effectiveness studies). Much larger effects of treatment have been found in the efficacy studies. There were far fewer clinic-based studies—they could only find six conducted since 1960 and three before then, as opposed to more than 100 efficacy studies. Cases presenting to clinics tend to be more complex and severe and the resources available to treat them may be less. The physical conditions in which the efficacy studies were carried out were better and there was more use of behavioural approaches than in the effectiveness studies. Other factors, such as specific therapist training, the possibility of greater skill among research therapists, more specificity of treated problems in the efficacy studies and the greater structure of research therapy did not seem to play a part in explaining the results. The effect of this review and other work has been to increase pressure on investigators to conduct therapeutic research in clinical settings with more typical patients.

Conclusions

Over the past decade substantial advances have been made in the delineation of the types of individual and group interventions that can work for children and adolescents. Some indications of the effectiveness and limitations of a psychodynamic approach to child and adolescent therapy have begun to be clarified. The research into psychodynamic groups remains rather more limited. There is an urgent need to define the modifications that have been made clinically to the methods of running adult psychotherapy groups and then to provide controlled trials of the method as a whole and of modifications to it.

In the domain of social skills training, the picture is at present mixed. Some programmes appear to work but when large-scale trials take place the results seem to be much more uncertain. This may form part of the widespread issue of efficacy vs. effectiveness. Further work is needed to define the specific elements of such programmes that are effective, how they can efficiently be combined and how generalization can be ensured. Kazdin's model of behaviour disorders as resembling chronic medical illnesses in their requirement of periodic intervention needs further investigation. If he is correct, what are the appropriate interventions and when will they have most effect? Tantalizing suggestions of sleeper effects in various social skills programmes continue to appear and are then treated with scepticism by others in the research community.

In the domain of social skills training, the relationship between behaviour patterns that can be learnt and the belief systems of the child, parents and teacher remains largely unexplored. This may be appropriate but it would gainsay experience from individual and family approaches where there seem to be creative links across the domains that might be usefully explored to increased effect in this area of treatment and research. Equally, the echoes of disturbed early parent–child relationships are largely ignored in the pragmatic 'here and now' approaches of the skills deficit models but they may need to be addressed at times to provide a context in which a belief in successful change can occur. Such pieces of work can be taken up in multimodal therapies but they are easily ignored in programmatic treatment trials. This is not an argument for a return to long-term individual non-directive therapy for parents or children, but rather a clinical request for short-term focused pieces of integrated work. As ever, much remains to be done.

References

Abikoff, H., B. & Hechtman, L. (1996) Multimodal therapy and stimulants in the treatment of children with attention deficit hyperactivity disorder. In: *Psychosocial Treatments for Child and Adolescent Disorders: Empirically Based Strategies for Clinical Practice* (eds E.D. Hibbs & P.S. Jensen), pp. 341–369. American Psychological Association, Washington D.C.

Abramowitz, C.V. (1976) The effectiveness of group therapy with children. *Archives of General Psychiatry*, **33**, 320–326.

Abramowitz, C.V., Abramowitz, S.I., Roback, H.B. & Jackson, C. (1974) Differential effectiveness of directive and non-directive group therapies as a function of client internal–external control. *Journal of Consulting and Clinical Psychology*, **42**, 849–853.

Aichorn, A. (1935) *Wayward Youth*. Viking, New York.

Albano, A.M. & Barlow, D. (1996) Breaking the vicious cycle: cogni-tive-behavioral group treatment for socially anxious youth. In: *Psychosocial Treatments for Child and Adolescent Disorders: Empirically Based Strategies for Clinical Practice* (eds E.D. Hibbs & P.S. Jensen), pp. 43–62. American Psychological Association, Washington D.C.

Alpert-Gillis, L., Pedro-Carroll, J. & Cowen, E. (1989) The children of divorce intervention program: development, implementation and evaluation of a program for young children. *Journal of Consulting and Clinical Psychology*, **57**, 583–589.

Argyle, M. (1969) *Social Interaction*. Methuen, London.

Asarnow, J.R. & Callan, J.W. (1985) Boys with peer adjustment problems: social cognitive processes. *Journal of Consulting and Clinical Psychology*, **53**, 113–149.

Axline, V.M. (1947) *Play Therapy*. Houghton Mifflin, Boston.

Baer, R. & Nietzel, M. (1991) Cognitive and behavioral treatments of impulsivity in children: a meta-analytic review of the outcome literature. *Journal of Clinical and Consulting Psychology*, **20**, 400–412.

Bentovim, A., Elton, A., Hildebrand, J., Tranter, M. & Vizard, E. (1988) *Child Sexual Abuse Within the Family: Assessment and Treatment*. Wright, London.

Bierman, K.L. (1989) Improving peer relationships of rejected children. In: *Advances in Clinical Child Psychology*, Vol. 12 (eds B.B. Lahey & A.E. Kazdin), pp. 53–85. Plenum Press, New York.

Boston, M. & Lush, D. (1994) Further considerations for methodology of evaluating psychoanalytic psychotherapy with children: reflections in the light of research experience. *Journal of Child Psychotherapy*, **20**, 205–229.

Bretherton, I., Ridgeway, D. & Cassidy, J. (1990) Assessing internal working models of the attachment relationship: an attachment story completion task for 3 year-olds. In: *Attachment in the Preschool Years: Theory, Research and Intervention* (eds M. Greenberg & D. Cicchetti), pp. 273–308. University of Chicago Press, Chicago, IL.

Butler, L., Miezitis, S., Friedman, R. & Cole, E. (1980) The effect of two school-based intervention programs on depressive symptoms in preadolescents. *American Educational Research Journal*, **17**, 111–119.

Byrnes, E.I., Hansen, K.G., Malloy, T.E., Carter, C. & Curry, D. (1999) Reduction in criminality subsequent to group, individual and family therapy in adolescent residential and day treatment settings. *International Journal of Group Psychotherapy*, **49**, 307–321.

Canter, L. & Canter, M. (1992) *Assertive Discipline: Positive Behaviour Management for Today's Classroom*. Canter, Santa Monica, CA.

Carr, A., ed. (2000) What works with children and adolescents? A critical review of psychological interventions with children. *Adolescents and Their Families*. Routledge, London.

Casey, R. & Berman, J. (1985) The outcome of psychotherapy in children. *Psychological Bulletin*, **98**, 388–400.

Corder, B.F., Whiteside, L. & Haizlip, T.M. (1981) A study of curative factors in group psychotherapy with adolescents. *International Journal of Group Psychotherapy*, **31**, 345–354.

Corsini, R.J. & Rosenberg, B. (1955) Mechanisms of group therapy: processes and dynamics. *Journal of Abnormal and Dynamic Psychology*, **51**, 406–411.

Dodge, K. (1985) Attributional bias in aggressive children. In: *Advances in Cognitive-behavioral Research and Therapy*, Vol. 4 (ed. P.C. Kendall), pp. 75–110. Academic Press, New York.

Dreikurs, R. (1959) Early experiments with group psychotherapy. *American Journal of Psychotherapy*, **13**, 882–891.

Ellis, P.L. (1982) Empathy: a factor in antisocial behavior *Journal of Abnormal Child Psychology*, **10**, 123–133.

Evans, J. (1998) *Active Analytic Group Therapy for Adolescents*, Jessica Kingsley, London.

Feindler, E.L., Marriott, S.A. & Iwata, M. (1984) Group anger control training for junior high school delinquents. *Cognitive Therapy and Research*, 8, 299–311.

Fine, S., Forth, A., Gilbert, M. & Haley, G. (1991) Group therapy for adolescent depressive disorder: a comparison of social skills and therapeutic support. *Journal of the American Academy of Child and Adolescent Psychiatry*, 30, 79–85.

Flynn, D. (1999) The challenges of in-patient work in a therapeutic community. In: *The Handbook of Child and Adolescent Psychotherapy: Psychoanalytic Approaches* (eds M. Lanyado & A. Horne), pp. 167–182. Routledge, London.

Fombonne, E. (1998) Interpersonal psychotherapy for adolescent depression. *Child Psychology and Psychiatry Review*, 3, 169–175.

Fonagy, P. & Moran, G. (1990) Studies on the efficacy of child psychoanalysis *Journal of Consulting and Clinical Psychology*, 58, 684–695.

Fonagy, P. & Target, M. (1994) The efficacy of psychoanalysis for children with disruptive disorders. *Journal of the American Academy of Child and Adolescent Psychiatry*, 33, 45–55.

Frankel, F., Cantwell, D. & Myatt, R. (1996) Helping ostracized children: social skills training and parent support for socially rejected children. In: *Psychosocial Treatments for Child and Adolescent Disorders: Empirically Based Strategies for Clinical Practice* (eds E.D. Hibbs & P.S. Jensen), pp. 595–617. American Psychological Association, Washington D.C.

Ginott, H. (1961) *Group Psychotherapy with Children*. McGraw-Hill, New York.

Goldwyn, R., Green, J.M., Stanley, C. & Smith, V. (2000) The Manchester child attachment story task: relationship with parental AAI, SAT and child behaviour. *Attachment and Human Development*, 2, 65–78.

Green, J.M., Stanley, C., Smith, V. & Goldwyn, R. (2000) A new method of evaluating attachment representations on young school age children: the Manchester child attachment story task. *Attachment and Human Development*, 2, 42–64.

Green, V. (1999) Intensive psychotherapy. In: *The Handbook of Child and Adolescent Psychotherapy: Psychoanalytic Approaches* (eds M. Lanyado & A. Horne), pp. 199–214. Routledge, London.

Greenberg, J.R. & Mitchell, S.A. (1990) *Object Relations in Psychoanalytic Theory*. Harvard University Press, Cambridge, MA.

Guerra, N.G. & Slaby, R.G. (1990) Cognitive mediators of aggression in adolescent offenders. II. Intervention. *Developmental Psychology*, 26, 269–277.

Hartnup, T. (1999) The therapeutic setting: the people and the place. In: *The Handbook of Child and Adolescent Psychotherapy: Psychoanalytic Approaches* (eds M. Lanyado & A. Horne), pp. 93–104. Routledge, London.

Heinicke, C.M. (1969) Frequency of psychotherapeutic session as a factor affecting outcome: analysis of clinical ratings and test results. *Journal of Abnormal Psychology*, 74, 553–560.

Heinicke, C.M. & Ramsey-Klee, D.M. (1986) Outcome of child psychotherapy as a function of frequency of sessions. *Journal of the American Academy of Child and Adolescent Psychiatry*, 4, 561–588.

Henry, S.E. & Kilmann, P.R. (1979) Student counselling groups in senior high school settings: an evaluation of outcome. *Journal of School Psychology*, 17, 27–46.

Hesse, E. & Main, M. (in press) Disorganization in infant and adult attachments: descriptions, correlates and implications for developmental psychology. *Journal of the American Psychoanalytic Association*, in press.

Hubble, M.A., Duncan, B.L. & Miller, S. (1999) *The Heart and Soul of Change: What Works in Therapy*. American Psychological Association, Washington D.C.

Huey, W.C. & Rank, R.C. (1984) Effects of counsellor and peer-led group assertiveness training on Black adolescent aggression. *Journal of Counselling Psychology*, 31, 95–98.

Hughes, C. (1999) Deprivation and children in care: the contribution of child and adolescent psychotherapy. In: *The Handbook of Child and Adolescent Psychotherapy: Psychoanalytic Approaches* (eds M. Lanyado & A. Horne), pp. 293–310. Routledge, London.

Hunter, M. (1999) The child and adolescent psychotherapist in the community. In: *The Handbook of Child and Adolescent Psychotherapy: Psychoanalytic Approaches* (eds M. Lanyado & A. Horne), pp. 127–139. Routledge, London.

Hunter, M. (2001) *Psychotherapy in Young People*. Routledge, London.

Jackson, N.F., Jackson, D.A. & Monroe, C. (1983) *Getting Along with Others: Teaching Social Effectiveness to Children*. Research Press, Champaign, IL.

Jacobs, B.W. (1997) Some aspects of theories of the mind: a psychodynamic perspective. How might they help a judge? In: *Rooted Sorrows: Psychoanalytic Perspectives on Child Protection, Assessment, Therapy and Treatment* (ed. N. Wall), pp. 9–16. Family Law, Jordan Publishing, Bristol.

Kashudin, A. (1974) *Child Welfare Services*. Macmillan, New York.

Kazdin, A. (1990) Childhood depression. *Journal of Child Psychology and Psychiatry*, 31, 121–160.

Kazdin, A. (1994) Psychotherapy for children and adolescents. In: *Handbook of Psychotherapy and Behaviour Change* (eds A. Bergin & S. L. Garfield), pp. 543–594. John Wiley & Sons, New York.

Kazdin, A.E. (1996) Problem solving and parent management in treating aggressive and antisocial behavior. In: *Psychological Treatments for Child and Adolescent Disorders: Empirically Based Strategies for Clinical Practice* (eds E.D. Hibbs & P.S. Jensen), pp. 377–407. American Psychological Association, Washington D.C.

Kazdin, A., Esveldt-Dawson, K., French, N.H. & Unis, A.S. (1987) Problem-solving skills training and relationship therapy in the treatment of antisocial child behaviour. *Journal of Clinical and Consulting Psychology*, 55, 76–85.

Kazdin, A., Siegel, T. & Bass, D. (1990) Drawing on clinical practice to inform research on child and adolescent psychotherapy: survey of practitioners. *Professional Psychology: Research and Practice*, 21, 189–198.

Kazdin, A.E., Seigel, T.C. & Bass, D. (1992) Cognitive problem solving skills training and parent management training in the treatment of antisocial behavior in children. *Journal of Consulting and Clinical Psychology*, 60, 733–747.

Kennedy, J.F. (1989) The heterogeneous group for chronically physically ill and physically healthy but emotionally disturbed children and adolescents. *International Journal of Group Psychotherapy*, 39, 105–125.

Klerman, G., Weissman, M., Rounsaville, B. & Chevron, E. (1984) *Interpersonal Therapy of Depression*. Basic Books, New York.

Kolvin, I., Garside, R.S., Nicol, A.R., MacMillan, A., Wolstenholme, F. & Leitch, I.M. (1981) *Help Starts Here: the Maladjusted Child in the Ordinary School*. Tavistock, London.

Kolvin, I., MacMillan, A. & Wrate, R. M. (1988) Psychotherapy is effective. *Journal of the Royal Society of Medicine*, 81, 261–266.

Koocher, G.P. & Pedulla, B.M. (1977) Current practices in child psychotherapy. *Professional Psychology*, 8, 275–287.

Kymissis, P. (1997) Group therapy. *Child and Adolescent Psychiatric Clinics of North America*, 6, 173–184.

Lambert, M.J. (1992) Implications of outcome research for psychotherapy integration. In: *Handbook of Psychotherapy Integration* (eds J.C. Norcross & M.R. Goldfried), pp. 92–129. Basic Books, New York.

Lanyado, M. & Horn, A., eds (1999) *Child and Adolescent Psychotherapy: Psychoanalytic Approaches*. Routledge, London.

Levitt, E.E. (1957) The results of psychotherapy with children: an evaluation. *Journal of Consulting Psychology*, **21**, 186–189.

Lewinsohn, P.M., Clarke, G.N., Rohde, P., Hops, H. & Seeley, J.R. (1996) A course in coping: a cognitive-behavioral approach to the treatment of adolescent depression. In: *Psychosocial Treatments for Child and Adolescent Disorders: Empirically Based Strategies for Clinical Practice* (eds E.D. Hibbs & P.S. Jensen), pp. 109–135. American Psychological Association, Washington D.C.

Liddle, H. & Dakof, G. (1995) Efficacy of family therapy for drug abuse: promising but not definitive. *Journal of Marital and Family Therapy*, **21**, 511–543.

Lochman, J.E., Burch, P.R., Curry, J.F. & Lampron, L.B. (1984) Treatment and generalization effects of cognitive behavioral and goal-setting interventions with aggressive boys. *Journal of Consulting and Clinical Psychology*, **52**, 915–916.

Lochman, J.E., Lampron, L.B., Gemmer, T.C. & Harris, S.R. (1989) Teacher consultation and cognitive-behavioral interventions with aggressive boys. *Psychology in the Schools*, **26**, 179–188.

Lochman, J.E., White, K.J. & Wayland, K.K. (1991) Cognitive-behavioral assessment and treatment with aggressive children. In: *Child and Adolescent Therapy: Cognitive Behavioral Procedures*, Vol. 4 (ed. P.C. Kendall), pp. 25–65. Guilford Press, New York.

Lochman, J.E., Coie, J.D., Underwood, M.K. & Terry, R. (1993) Effectiveness of a social relations intervention program for aggressive and nonaggressive, rejected children. *Journal of Consulting and Clinical Psychology*, **61**, 1053–1058.

Lush, D., Boston, M. & Grainger, E. (1991) Evaluation of psychoanalytic psychotherapy with children: therapist's assessments and predictions *Psychoanalytic Psychotherapy*, **5**, 191–234.

Markowitz, J.C., Svartberg, M. & Swartz, H.A. (1998) Is IPT time-limited psychodynamic psychotherapy? *Journal of Psychotherapy Practice and Research*, **7**, 185–195.

McGain, B. & McKinzey, R. (1995) The efficacy of group treatment in sexually abused girls. *Child Abuse and Neglect*, **19**, 1157–1169.

Meichenbaum, D. & Goodman, J. (1971) Training impulsive children to talk to themselves: a means of developing self-control. *Journal of Abnormal Psychology*, **77**, 115–126.

Mezzano, J. (1968) Group counselling with low-motivated male high school students: comparative effects of two uses of counsellor time. *Journal of Educational Research*, **61**, 222–224.

Moran, G.S., Fonagy, P., Kurtz, A., Bolton, A. & Brook, C. (1991) A controlled study of the psychoanalytic treatment of brittle diabetes. *Journal of the American Academy of Child and Adolescent Psychiatry*, **30**, 926–935.

MTA Group (1999) A 14-month randomized clinical trial of treatment strategies for attention-deficit/hyperactivity disorder. The MTA Cooperative Group. Multimodal Treatment Study of Children with ADHD. *Archives of General Psychiatry*, **56**, 1073–1086.

Mufson, L., Moreau, D. & Weissman, M. (1993) *Interpersonal Psychotherapy for Depressed Adolescents*. Guilford Press, New York.

Mufson, L., Moreau, D., Weissman, M.M., Wickramaratne, P., Martin, J. & Samoilov, A. (1994) The modification of interpersonal psychotherapy with depressed adolescents (IPT-A): Phase I and II studies. *Journal of the American Academy of Child and Adolescent Psychiatry*, **33**, 695–705.

Mufson, L., Moreau, D. & Weissman, M. (1996) Focus on relationships: interpersonal psychotherapy for adolescent depression. In: *Psychosocial Treatments for Child and Adolescent Disorders: Empirically Based Strategies for Clinical Practice* (eds E.D. Hibbs & P.S. Jensen), pp. 137–155. American Psychological Association, Washington D.C.

Mufson, L., Moreau, D., Weissman, M.M. & Garfinkel, R. (1999) Effi-

cacy of interpersonal psychotherapy for depressed adolescents. *Archives of General Psychiatry*, **56**, 573–579.

Mulvey, E., Arthur, M. & Reppucci, N. (1993) The prevention and treatment of juvenile delinquency. *Clinical Psychology Review*, **13**, 133–167.

Nolan, M. & Carr, A. (2000) Attention deficit hyperactivity disorder. In: *What Works with Children and Adolescents? A Critical Review of Psychological Interventions with Children, Adolescents and Their Families* (ed. A. Carr), pp. 65–101. Routledge, London.

Parsons, M., Radford, P. & Horne, A. (1999) Non-intensive psychotherapy and assessment. In: *The Handbook of Child and Adolescent Psychotherapy: Psychoanalytic Approaches* (eds M. Lanyado & A. Horne), pp. 215–232. Routledge, London.

Pedro-Carroll, J., Alpert-Gillis, L.J. & Cowen, E.L. (1992) An evaluation of the efficacy of a prevention intervention for 4th to 6th grade urban children of divorce. *Journal of Primary Prevention*, **13**, 115–130.

Persons, R.W. (1966) Psychological and behavioural change in delinquents following psychotherapy. *Journal of Clinical Psychology*, **22**, 337–340.

Persons, R.W. (1967) Relationship between psychotherapy with institutionalised boys and subsequent community adjustment. *Journal of Consulting Psychology*, **31**, 137–141.

Persons, R.W. & Pepinsky, H.B. (1966) Convergence in psychotherapy with delinquent boys. *Journal of Counselling Psychology*, **13**, 329–334.

Ramsden, S. (1999) The child and adolescent psychotherapist in a hospital setting. In: *The Handbook of Child and Adolescent Psychotherapy: Psychoanalytic Approaches* (eds M. Lanyado & A. Horne), pp. 141–158. Routledge, London.

Rayner, E. (1990) *The Independent Mind in British Psychoanalysis*. Free Association Books, London.

Reid, S. (1999) The group as a healing whole: group psychotherapies with children and adolescents. In: *Child and Adolescent Psychotherapy: Psychoanalytic Approaches* (eds M. Lanyado & A. Horne), pp. 247–260. Routledge, London and New York.

Richardson, P. (1998) *Factsheet on Psychotherapy Outcome Research*. Tavistock Clinic Foundation, London.

Robbins, D., Allessi, N. & Colfer, M. (1989) Treatment of adolescents with major depression: Implications of the DST and the melancholic subtype. *Journal of Affective Disorders*, **17**, 99–104.

Roseby, V. & Deutsch, R. (1985) Children of separation and divorce: effects of social role-taking group intervention on fourth and fifth graders. *Journal of Clinical Child Psychology*, **14**, 55–60.

Roth, A. & Fonagy, P. (1996) *What Works With Whom? A Critical Review of Psychotherapy Research*. Guilford Press, New York.

Rustin, M. (1999) Parental consultation and therapy. In: *Child and Adolescent Psychotherapy: Psychoanalytic Approaches* (eds M. Lanyado & A. Horne), pp. 87–92. Routledge, London.

Rutter (1982) Psychological therapies in child psychiatry: issues and prospects. *Psychological Medicine*, **12**, 723–740.

Sandler, J., Kennedy, H. & Tyson, R. (1980) *The Technique of Child Analysis: Discussions with Anna Freud*. Hogarth Press, London.

Sandler, J., Dare, C., Holder, A. & Dreher, A.U. (1992) *The Patient and the Analyst: the Basis of the Psychoanalytic Process*. International Universities Press, Madison, CT.

Satterfield, J.H., Satterfield, B.T. & Cantwell, D.P. (1981) Three-year multimodality treatment study of 100 hyperactive boys. *Journal of Pediatrics*, **98**, 650–655.

Satterfield, J.H., Satterfield, B.T. & Schell, A.M. (1987) Therapeutic interventions to prevent delinquency in hyperactive boys. *Journal of the American Academy of Child and Adolescent Psychiatry*, **26**, 56–64.

Saxe, L., Cross, T. & Silverman, N. (1986) *Children's mental health:*

problems and services. Background paper, US Government Printing Office, Washington D.C.

Shirk, S.R. & Russell, R.L. (1992) A re-evaluation of estimates of child therapy effectiveness *Journal of the American Academy of Child and Adolescent Psychiatry*, **31**, 703–709.

Shure, M.B. & Spivack, G. (1978) *Problem-solving Techniques in Child Rearing.* Jossey-Bass, San Francisco, CA.

Silver, L. & Silver, B. (1983) Clinical practice of child psychiatry: a survey. *Journal of the American Academy of Child and Adolescent Psychiatry*, **22**, 573–579.

Skitka, L. & Frazier, M. (1995) Ameliorating the effects of parental divorce: do small group interventions work? *Journal of Divorce and Remarriage*, **24**, 159–179.

Slavson, S.R. & Schiffer, M. (1975) *Group Psychotherapies for Children: a Textbook.* International Universities Press, Madison, CT.

Snow, J. & Paternite, C. (1986) Individual and family therapy in the treatment of children. *Professional Psychology: Research and Practice*, **17**, 242–250.

Spence, S. & Marzillier, J.S. (1979) Social skills training with adolescent male offenders. I. Short term effects. *Behaviour Research and Therapy*, **17**, 7–16.

Spillius, E.B., ed. (1988) *Melanie Klein Today.* Routledge, London.

Spivack, G. & Shure, M.B. (1982) The cognition of social adjustment: interpersonal cognitive problem-solving thinking. In: *Advances in Clinical Psychology*, Vol. 5 (eds B.B. Lahey & A.E. Kazdin), pp. 323–372. Plenum, New York.

Spivack, G., Platt, J.J. & Shure, M.B. (1976) *The Problem-solving Approach to Adjustment.* Jossey-Bass, San Francisco, CA.

Stern, D. (1985) *The Interpersonal World of the Infant.* Basic Books, New York.

Target, M. & Fonagy, P. (1994) Efficacy of psychoanalysis for children with emotional disorders *Journal of the American Academy of Child and Adolescent Psychiatry*, **33**, 361–371.

Taylor, T.K., Eddy, J.M. & Biglan, A. (1999) Interpersonal skills training to reduce aggressive and delinquent behavior: limited evidence and the need for an evidence-based system of care. *Clinical Child and Family Psychology Review*, **2**, 169–182.

Tillitski, C.J. (1990) A meta-analysis of estimated effect sizes for control treatment. *International Journal of Group Psychotherapy*, **40**, 215–224.

Tramonata, M. (1980) Critical review of research on psychotherapy outcome with adolescents 1967–77. *Psychological Bulletin*, **88**, 429–450.

Trowell, J., Kolvin, I., Weerhmanthri, T. *et al.* (in press) Psychotherapy for sexually abused girls: psychopathology outcome findings and patterns of change. *British Journal of Psychiatry*.

Truax, C.B., Wargo, D.G. & Silber, L.D. (1966) Effects of group psychotherapy with high accurate empathy and nonpossessive warmth upon female institutionalised delinquents. *Journal of Abnormal Psychology*, **71**, 267–274.

Tsiantis, J. (1999) *Working with Parents of Child and Adolescents Who Are in Psychoanalytic Psychotherapy.* Karnac Books, London.

Tyson, P. & Tyson, R. (1990) *Psychoanalytic Theories of Development: an Integration.* Yale University Press, New Haven.

Walker, H.M., McConnell, S., Holmes, D., Todis, B., Walker, J.L. & Golden, N. (1983) *A Curriculum for Children's Effective Peer and Teacher Skills (ACCEPTS).* Pro-Ed Publishers, Austin, TX.

Warner, R.W. (1971) Alienated students: six months after receiving behavioral group counselling. *Journal of Counselling Psychology*, **18**, 426–430.

Webster-Stratton, C. (1996) Early intervention with videotape modelling: programs for families of children with oppositional defiant disorder or conduct disorder. In: *Psychosocial Treatments for Child and Adolescent Disorders: Empirically Based Strategies for Clinical Practice* (eds E.D. Hibbs & P.S. Jensen), pp. 435–474. American Psychological Association, Washington D.C.

Webster-Stratton, C. & Hammond, M. (1997) Treating children with early onset conduct problems: a comparison of child and parent training interventions. *Journal of Consulting and Clinical Psychology*, **65**, 93–109.

Weisz, J., Weiss, B., Alicke, M. & Klotz, M. (1987) Effectiveness of psychotherapy with children and adolescents: meta-analytic findings for clinicians. *Journal of Consulting and Clinical Psychology*, **55**, 542–549.

Weisz, J.R., Donenberg, G.R., Han, S.S. & Weiss, S.S. (1995) Bridging the gap between laboratory and the clinic in child and adolescent psychotherapy. *Journal of Consulting and Clinical Psychology*, **63**, 688–701.

Whalen, C.K. & Henker, B. (1985) The social worlds of hyperactive children. *Clinical Psychology Review*, **5**, 1–32.

Wilson, P. (1991) Psychotherapy with adolescents. In: *Textbook of Psychotherapy in Psychiatric Practice* (ed. J. Holmes), pp. 443–467. Churchill-Livingstone, New York.

Wilson, P. (1999) Therapy and consultation in residential care. In: *The Handbook of Child and Adolescent Psychotherapy: Psychoanalytic Approaches* (ed. M. Lanyado & A. Horne), pp. 159–166. Routledge, London.

Yalom, I.D. (1985) *The Theory and Practice of Group Psychotherapy.* Basic Books, New York.

59 Pharmacological and other Physical Treatments

Isobel Heyman and Paramala Santosh

Role of pharmacological treatment in child psychiatry

Drug treatment represents a powerful way of altering the behaviour and mental states of children. There are large differences in prescribing practices between countries, and current usage includes drugs that may be ineffective or even hazardous. In the USA, the use of medication tends to exceed what has been validated by objective evidence for safety and efficacy (Jensen *et al.* 1999). In the UK, the reverse situation may exist: underprescribing for children whose conditions could be effectively treated with drugs. There is an understandable worry about medication in children, particularly in terms of possible long-term side-effects, yet there are few data on whether children really are more vulnerable to side-effects. Some children are denied treatment with medication, either because of ideological opposition to this form of therapy, or lack of knowledge. Medication has an important place in child psychiatric treatment, and expertise in the theoretical and practical aspects of drug use should be available in all child mental health services.

In recent years, the emphasis on evidence-based practice has led to a more rational evaluation of the use of drugs in child psychiatry. While there remain few definitive randomized controlled trials of the use of medication in child psychiatry, for some conditions, such as obsessive-compulsive disorder and hyperactivity, child psychiatry has led the way in evidence-based practice in psychiatry (Rapoport 1998). Although a controlled trial may show that a particular treatment is, on average, more effective than a control therapy for a specific indication, the decision about whether or not to prescribe for a particular child is clearly more complex. The potential prescriber should ask the following:

• Does the child have a condition known to be responsive to medication?
• How severe is this disorder, and what is the outcome target for this child?
• Which aspects of the child's condition are likely to be improved by medication and which will be unaffected?
• What is the chance of response (from trial evidence and from case judgement)?
• What is the balance of benefits and risks, both short- and long-term?
• How will response and outcome be monitored?
• Is monitoring for hazards required?

In almost every case, pharmacological treatment for children with psychiatric disorder should be just one part of a package of psychological, social and educational intervention. Even in conditions where drug treatment plays a significant part, and there are many where it does not (see Tables 59.1 and 59.2), drug treatment will nearly always only be a component of a multimodal treatment plan. For example, the tics of Tourette syndrome may be highly responsive to treatment with dopamine antagonists, and this may be an important part of the treatment, although it carries a significant risk of side-effects. However, for the majority of children, a knowledge of the natural history of Tourette syndrome and a suitable psychoeducational intervention can obviate the need for treatment of the tics with drugs (Peterson & Leckman 1998; Leckman & Cohen, Chapter 36).

In this chapter, the evidence for rational prescribing of psychopharmacological agents in young people will be reviewed, together with brief accounts of the basic pharmacology, pharmacokinetics and toxicology. Clinical guidelines for the use of drugs in the management of individual child and adolescent psychiatric disorders is given in the chapters on individual disorders, although some brief guidance is given for specific disorders. There are several good manuals available for clinical guidance on disease management, drug doses and other clinical details, in particular Werry & Aman (1999), Kutcher (1997) and Walsh (1998). Where possible, reference is made to recent review articles on individual drugs groups or management of specific disorders (March & Vitello 2001; Riddle *et al.* 2001).

General considerations in prescribing for children

Clinical observation and clinical trials

The history of psychopharmacology is characterized by chance findings, and paediatric psychopharmacology is no exception. Use of stimulants to treat hyperactivity was based on the unexpected discovery that children treated with amphetamines for post-lumbar puncture headache were less hyperactive and irritable (Bradley 1937). Clinical observation has provided many such clues for drug treatments in child psychiatry, and usually then leads to more formal scientific study. Controlled trials, the assessment of behavioural and neurochemical effects in animal models, and an experimental analysis of effects on

Table 59.1 Summary of child psychiatric disorders in which drug treatment plays a significant role.

Disorder	First-line drugs	Second-line drugs
Psychosis	Atypical antipsychotics Risperidone Olanzapine Amisulpiride	Typical antipsychotics Haloperidol Chlorpromazine Clozapine
Hyperactivity	Stimulants Methylphenidate Dexamphetamine	Imipramine Clonidine Venlafaxine
Obsessive-compulsive disorder	SSRIs Sertraline Fluoxetine Paroxetine Fluvoxamine Citalopram	Clomipramine
Tourette syndrome/tic disorders	Clonidine Risperidone Sulpiride	Pimozide Haloperidol SSRIs
Depression	SSRIs Sertraline Fluoxetine Paroxetine Citalopram Fluroxamine	Tricyclic antidepressants Imipramine Amitriptyline Clomipramine Atypical antidepressants

Table 59.2 Child and adolescent disorders which rarely require drug treatment

Mental retardation
Autism
Conduct disorders
Eating disorders
Sleep disorders
Anxiety disorders
Enuresis

psychological processes all contribute to the evaluation of drug efficacy.

Because of the inherent difficulties of experimental studies in children, much of the knowledge of drug effects has been extrapolated from adult studies. However, children differ from adults developmentally as well as pharmacologically, so caution is needed until appropriate efficacy studies are carried out in children (Tosyali & Greenhill 1998). However, the commonly held idea that drugs are more hazardous in young people is not necessarily true. For example, antipsychotic-induced akathisia seems to be less common in children and adolescents, but acute dystonias seems to be more common in adolescent males (Keepers *et al.* 1983).

Regulatory controls and procedures: medicolegal issues

Until about 30 years ago, treatments were chosen on the basis of clinical judgement rather than on objective testing. Many drugs now in use have never been subjected to controlled clinical trials, although all newly introduced drugs must be before a licence is granted. For a particular drug to be licensed for use for a specific indication and in a particular age group, regulatory authorities demand that the appropriate studies must be carried out. In the USA it has been estimated that approximately 80% of drug use in paediatrics is unlicensed or 'off-label' (Jensen *et al.* 1999). This means that it is prescribed with the clinician's judgement. In some cases there is published clinical trial evidence for efficacy, and this greatly strengthens a clinical decision to prescribe 'off-label' for a child.

A controlled clinical trial aims to compare the response of a *test group* of patients receiving a new treatment to that of a *control group* receiving an existing standard treatment. If there is no current treatment, the control group may receive no treatment or a *placebo*. To avoid bias, clinical trials should be randomized and double-blind. Jensen *et al.* (1999) classified evidence supporting the use of psychotropic medication in children into three levels. Level A denotes support by two or more randomized controlled trials, level B denotes support from at least one randomized controlled trial and level C is supported only by uncontrolled trials or clinical opinion. These ratings for eight psychotropic drug groups were then compared with the frequency with which the drugs were prescribed. With the exception of attention deficit hyperactivity disorder (ADHD) treatment with stimulant drugs, there was little association between frequency of use and clinical trial evidence of efficacy.

Patterns of drug use in different countries and settings

There are marked differences in prescribing practices in different countries, although these differences have had little objective measurement. The management of ADHD in the USA and the UK provides a striking example of cultural differences in both diagnosis and treatment.

In the USA, one child in 20 meets the DSM-IV diagnostic criteria for ADHD. The prevalence in Europe seems to be much lower, about one in 200, mainly because European psychiatrists use the narrower ICD-10 diagnosis of hyperkinetic disorder (HD). Children with similar symptoms are more often labelled as having conduct disorder in the UK, as opposed to ADHD in the USA. The result is that clinicians in the UK tend to use psychosocial treatments without medication, unlike their counterparts in the USA who use medication as the first line of treatment. In some countries in Europe, especially in the UK and France, there has been widespread public hostility to the use of psychotropic medication for this purpose. In certain countries such as India, stimulants are not available and hence second-line medications, such as tricyclic antidepressants (TCAs) and clonidine, are used as first-line drugs. It is therefore difficult to formulate uniform guidelines for the management of even very common disorders.

Other demographic variables may show associations with variation in medical treatment. A recent retrospective analysis of prescriptions for psychotropic drugs in US youths aged 5–14 years reported that African-American youths were less likely than Caucasian youths to have been prescribed psychotropic medications, especially methylphenidate (Zito *et al.* 1998). This is an important finding and needs to be investigated further to find out whether youths with similar symptoms receive different diagnosis (conduct disorder instead of ADHD) leading to different treatment.

Differences between children and adults

Pharmacokinetics

Much less is known about the pharmacokinetics of psychotropic medications in children than in adults. Generally, drug response may vary with age, weight, sex, disease-state, absorption, distribution, metabolism and excretion; thus developmental factors that influence these are important to consider. Although the extent of drug absorption for most medication is similar in children and adults, the rate of absorption may be faster in children, and peak levels are reached earlier. Absorp-

tion is also dependent on the form in which it is administered (liquid vs. tablet) and levels peak faster for liquid preparations.

Hepatic metabolism is highest during infancy and childhood (1–6 years), approximately twice the adult rate in prepuberty (6–10 years), and equivalent to adults by the age of 15 (Bourin & Couetoux du Tertre 1992). This is clinically important, as younger children may require higher milligram/kilogram dosages of hepatically metabolized medications than older children or adults (Wilens *et al.* 1992). In addition, a transient decrease in metabolism for some medications has been reported in the few months before puberty, which is believed to be caused by the competition for hepatic enzymes with sex hormones. Protein binding and volume of distribution affect the pharmacokinetics of medications. These parameters differ in children and have practical clinical implications, such as the fraction of drug that is active (unbound). Body fat increases during the first year, then gradually falls, until puberty. Substantial fat stores slow elimination of highly liposoluble drugs from the body (e.g. fluoxetine, pimozide).

Pharmacodynamics

The pharmacodynamic properties of a drug are the mechanisms and responses that are mediated by binding to one or more target molecules, which are commonly receptors, ion channels, enzymes or carrier molecules. Little is known about differences in pharmacodynamics throughout development but, as neural development is better understood, it is becoming clearer that children may have different target molecule distributions or subtypes, and indeed that brain development continues into adult life.

A clinical puzzle is that TCAs seem relatively ineffective in depressed children (Hazell *et al.* 1995). Possible explanations have included differences in pharmacokinetics and pharmacodynamics, including the hormonal milieu of the brain or incomplete maturation of neurotransmitter systems involved in the control of affect. There may be clinical selection biases, such as inclusion of adolescents who will over time turn out to have bipolar illness.

The maturation of autonomic cardiac control may have an important influence on psychotropic related cardiotoxicity in children. Vagal modulation of heart rate increases during the first decade of life, peaks sometime during the second decade, then declines gradually with age to the sixth decade of life. Sympathetic modulation follows a similar pattern, but rates of maturation of the two branches are not the same. Furthermore, there is considerable variation between individuals of similar age in autonomic maturation. The relative loss of vagal modulation associated with TCA use may be accentuated in some younger subjects because of these maturational factors (Mezzacappa *et al.* 1998), leading to cardiotoxicity.

Main classes of drugs used in child psychiatry

Stimulants

Basic pharmacology and mechanism of action

Stimulant drugs, including methylphenidate, dexamphetamine and pemoline, are widely used and effective in the treatment of ADHD. There are many published reviews of the clinical efficacy literature; for example, Greenhill *et al.* (1999) report that by 1996 there were 161 randomized controlled trials of these drugs, constituting the largest body of treatment literature on any child psychiatric disorder. Despite this extensive clinical and pharmacological knowledge, the basis for their efficacy in ADHD remains unclear. The recent review of stimulant medication by Santosh & Taylor (2000) gives a detailed account of the existing prescription practice of stimulants, neurological basis of stimulant action, evidence base for use of stimulants, prescription guidelines, their use in ADHD with comorbidity and other indications, and cost-effectiveness.

Stimulants act by releasing monoamines from nerve terminals in the brain. Noradrenaline and dopamine are the most important mediators, but serotonin release also occurs. They increase intrasynaptic concentrations of dopamine by blocking the dopamine transporter, and by displacement of monoamines from synaptic vesicles. Human functional imaging studies are beginning to allow us to measure these processes more directly (Volkow *et al.* 1998). The core behavioural response in hyperactive children seems to be an improved ability to 'inhibit', and

Table 59.3 Summary table of drugs and their indications.

Drug class (specific examples)	Main indications	Possible indications
Stimulants		
Methylphenidate	ADHD, narcolepsy	Resistant depression
Dexamphetamine		
Antipsychotic and antimanic drugs		
Chlorpromazine, thioridazine, trifluoperazine and other phenothiazines	Schizophrenia, Tourette syndrome/tic disorders	Psychotic features in affective disorders, acute aggression
Haloperidol, droperidol, pimozide, sulpiride	Schizophrenia, Tourette syndrome/tic disorders	Psychotic features in affective disorders, acute aggression, PDD
Atypical antipsychotics: clozapine, olanzapine, amisulpiride, risperidone	Schizophrenia, Tourette syndrome/tic disorders	Psychotic features in affective disorders, acute aggression, PDD
Lithium	Mania, bipolar disorder	
Carbamazepine	Mania, bipolar disorder	
Sodium valproate	Mania, bipolar disorder	
Antidepressants		
Tricyclic and related antidepressants: amitriptyline, clomipramine, imipramine, trimipramine, dothiepin	ADHD (especially those with anxiety and/or tics), OCD	Enuresis
SSRIs and related antidepressants: fluoxetine, fluvoxamine, paroxetine. sertraline, citalopram, venlafaxine	OCD, depression	Panic disorder, anorexia and bulimia, PDD
MAOIs	Resistant depression	Resistant ADHD
Anxiolytics, sedatives and miscellaneous drugs		
Benzodiazepines	Sedation	Acute aggression
Antihistamines	Sedation	Anxiety disorder
Anticonvulsants	Epilepsy	Sleep problems
Clonidine	ADHD, tics	Repetitive self-injury in PDD
Naltrexone		

Abbreviations: ADHD, attention deficit hyperactivity disorder; MAOI, monoamine oxidase inhibitor; PDD, pervasive developmental disorder; SSRI, selective serotonin reuptake inhibitor.

Table 59.4 Dosage range of psychotropic medication used in children and adolescents.

Drug	Dose range
Stimulants	
Methylphenidate	5–60 mg/day
Dexamphetamine	2.5–40 mg/day
Pemoline	37.5–112.5 mg/day
Antidepressants	
Tricyclic antidepressants	
Imipramine, desipramine	10–20 mg/day in <6 year olds
	10–75 mg/day in >6 years (prepubertal)
	50–150 mg/day postpubertal
Clomipramine	10–200 mg/day
Selective serotonin reuptake inhibitors (SSRIs)	
Fluoxetine	10–60 mg/day
Fluvoxamine	50–300 mg/day
Sertraline	25–150 mg/day
Paroxetine	10–60 mg/day
Citalopram	10–60 mg/day
Serotonin noradrenaline reuptake inhibitors (SNRIs)	
Venlafaxine	37.5–150 mg/day
Antipsychotics	
Haloperidol	0.5–8 mg/day (prepubertal)
	1–16 mg/day (postpubertal)
Sulpiride	25–500 mg/day
Clozapine	50–600 mg/day
Pimozide	1–12 mg/day
Olanzapine	2.5–20 mg/day
Risperidone	0.25–6 mg/day
Amisulpiride	25–1000 mg/day
Sertindole	2–16 mg/day
Ziprasidone	40–120 mg/day
Quetiapine	25–500 mg/day
Antiepileptic medication	
Carbamazepine	5–10 mg/L (serum level)
Sodium valproate	50–100 mg/L (serum level)
Clonazepam	0.5–4 mg/day
Others	
Lithium carbonate	0.4–1.0 mEq/L (serum level)
Clonidine	0.05–0.25 mg/day
Buspirone	10–45 mg/day
Naltrexone	12.5–50 mg/day

therefore enhance persistence in motor and cognitive functions, but the pharmacological mechanisms underlying this remain obscure (Solanto 1998). Genetic, neuroimaging and neuropsychological findings all suggest that the brain abnormalities in ADHD are neurodevelopmental in origin (Zametkin & Liotta 1998). Susceptibility to ADHD may be increased by variation in genes encoding components of the dopamine system, such as receptors and transporters (reviewed by Faraone & Biederman 1998). The catecholamine-rich frontosubcortical systems appear to be dysfunctional in some children with ADHD, perhaps suggesting a link with sites of stimulant drug action, although no consistent abnormalities in peripheral catecholamines have been found.

Pharmacokinetic issues

Stimulants are rapidly absorbed following oral administration, show low plasma protein binding and are eliminated from the body within 24 h following hepatic metabolism. One study has suggested that the behavioural response is sustained even after drug discontinuation (Gillberg *et al.* 1997) but, in general, the effects cease when the drug is stopped.

The different stimulants have slightly different half-lives, and this may be important in clinical practice (Barkley *et al.* 1999). Methylphenidate has the most rapid onset of action (1–3 h) and shortest half-life (2–3 h), so that clinical effects wear off after 4–6 h. Slow-release preparations may be useful in children who develop rebound hyperactivity, or in whom frequent dosage is impractical. There is little evidence for the development of tolerance in children taking stimulants for treatment of ADHD (Safer & Allen 1989), although clinically there are reports of decreased efficacy after prolonged administration.

Side-effects and toxicity

Although the stimulants are safe, dose-dependent side-effects may occur, and are similar for all stimulants. The most common side-effects are delay of sleep onset, reduced appetite, stomachache, headache, jitteriness and dysphoria (Barkley *et al.* 1990). They often wear off spontaneously, or may be reduced by lowering the dose. Persistent or severe side-effects may require changing drugs. Growth retardation may occur during acute treatment (Klein *et al.* 1988), but in longer follow-up, adolescents show no significant growth impairment (Vincent *et al.* 1990), although studies into adult life are needed. There is also a suggestion that children with ADHD may have slower growth rates independent of stimulant use, perhaps as a component of the neurodevelopmental disorder itself (Spencer *et al.* 1996a).

Sleeplessness can be a problem and it is clinically important to distinguish those children whose insomnia is an unwanted effect of the drug from those children whose insomnia may be caused by the recurrence (or worsening) of the behavioural difficulties as the medication effect subsides. There is little evidence that stimulants produce a decrease in the seizure threshold (Crumrine *et al.* 1987) or that addiction results from the prescription of stimulants for ADHD. Clinical experience suggests that the euphoriant response to stimulants that is evident in adult life, and which predisposes to recreational usage and dependence, is much less usual in childhood. Similarly, the effects of amphetamine in predisposing to a paranoid psychosis (Connell 1958), so prominent in the abuse of this drug in adult life, has not been a feature in childhood. Unfortunately, systematic studies of age-related differences in response seem to be lacking.

The long-term use of pemoline has been associated with abnormalities in liver function tests and, in some cases, liver failure (Berkovitch *et al.* 1995). This has led to it being withdrawn from licence in the UK (although it may be prescribed on a named-patient basis), and being used only as a second-line treatment in the USA.

Main indications including trial data or other evidence of efficacy

There is abundant evidence for the short-term beneficial effects of stimulants for the treatment of ADHD. A review of clinical trials by Greenhill *et al.* (1999) summarized the findings from 5899 patients recruited to clinical trials; 65–75% showed improvement in response to stimulants, compared with only 4–30% in response to placebo.

A recent study of methylphenidate and dexamphetamine found that 96% improved behaviourally in response to one or other drug (Elia *et al.* 1991). Contrary to common assumptions, stimulants have a wide variety of social effects in addition to improving the core symptoms of inattention, hyperactivity and impulsivity. Stimulant effects on attentional, academic, behavioural and social domains, however, are highly variable between individuals (Rapport *et al.* 1994). Greater hyperactivity, inattention and clumsiness in the absence of emotional disorder predict greater positive response to methylphenidate (Taylor *et al.* 1987). Stimulant medication remains effective over many years as indicated by short-term measures, but it remains unclear whether, in the long term, treatment of ADHD in childhood has an impact on adult functioning.

Despite this strong clinical trial evidence for efficacy, there are many clinical issues which the trial data do not answer. The threshold level of ADHD symptoms for initiation of treatment has not been defined, so the diagnosis alone serves as the main criterion for starting treatment. There is no good association between plasma levels and behavioural response, so dosage regimes continue to be clinically judged. There are few good predictors of individual variability in response. Clinical experience suggests an important role for parent training, or school-based interventions, but controlled trials have shown little additional effect of these interventions over medication alone (MTA Cooperative Group 1999). There is extensive discussion in the literature about aspects of study design that may predispose to a differentially positive outcome for drug treatment. Pelham (1999) suggests that the measurement of outcome after the ending of behavioural treatment, but while medication treatment was still continuing, may have biased the findings. Another interesting finding from the MTA study was the improved response to methylphenidate in the research protocol group compared with those in the 'standard' community treatment

group. This may be because the research group protocol involved a very detailed initial evaluation of the optimal dose of stimulant necessary for each child (involving a 4-week period of using various doses of stimulant and placebo), and subsequent close monitoring of drug dosage. In contrast, the community group received standard dose regimens, less specifically tailored to the individual child. A commentary by Taylor (1999) concluded that services for children with ADHD should always incorporate the option of treatment with medication, as behavioural treatment alone is unlikely to be effective. He also notes that while the MTA study did not show significant additional value of behavioural treatment, its beneficial effects may emerge in longer term study, or for specific subgroups of patients.

The presence of a comorbid condition may alter the response to stimulant medication. There is disagreement as to whether response to stimulants is reduced in children and adolescents with comorbid anxiety disorders. Low doses of methylphenidate have been shown to produce an elevation of heart rate in children with ADHD with comorbid anxiety (Tannock *et al.* 1995). Pliska (1989) found fewer stimulant responders amongst subjects with ADHD and comorbid anxiety and some had a placebo response as large as the stimulant response itself. Other studies find that children with comorbid anxiety respond as well as those without anxiety to stimulants (Livingston *et al.* 1992); it is currently generally accepted that stimulants are the first-line drugs in this group, although TCAs may represent a useful alternative if anxiety is exacerbated or response is poor (Spencer *et al.* 1996b).

There are concerns about stimulants precipitating or exacerbating tics, and some studies have found worsening of tics in 25–30% of patients (Spencer *et al.* 1996b). For children who have Tourette disorder or chronic tics, low to moderate doses of methylphenidate often improve attention and behaviour without significantly worsening the tics (Gadow *et al.* 1999; Law & Schachar 1999). The current consensus is that cautious treatment with stimulants may be both tolerable and useful to many children with tics and ADHD (Castellanos 1999). Pliska *et al.* (2000) have published expert opinion-based algorithms in the management of ADHD in the presence of comorbid tics, aggression and anxiety/depression.

Stimulants should be used with caution in autism with comorbid ADHD. Quintana *et al.* (1995) report good stimulant response in a double-blind placebo controlled study in this comorbid group. However, it is not unusual in clinical practice to note a worsening in repetitive behaviours.

For drugs with such well-established therapeutic efficacy, and a high safety margin, it is remarkable that such a level of controversy exists about stimulant use in children. Greenhill *et al.* (1999) point out that no evidence of long-term harm has been revealed in nearly 30 years of evaluated use. They conclude that stimulants should not be withheld from children with ADHD, or limitations placed on the chronicity of use, but rather that practice standards should be high, including careful initial diagnosis and optimum monitoring of the response to treatment.

Antipsychotic drugs

Basic pharmacology and mechanism of action

The antipsychotic drugs are all dopamine receptor antagonists, although many of them also act on other targets, such as serotonin, noradrenaline and glutamate receptors. A robust finding from adult studies of schizophrenia is the strong association between D_2 receptor binding activity, and antipsychotic potency (Seeman et al. 1976). Antipsychotics may take days or weeks to be effective, suggesting that secondary effects, such as altered numbers of D_2 receptors in limbic structures, may be more important than the direct receptor blockade. There is no reason to suppose that juvenile forms of the psychoses have specific differences in the mechanisms of response to drug treatment, although general differences related to developmental immaturity in neurotransmitter systems may apply. Dopamine antagonism is also likely to be the mechanism of action of antipsychotics in Tourette syndrome, where they are effective in diminishing tics. The antipsychotic drugs are also widely used in a range of behavioural emergencies, and in some instances in child psychiatry for less acute behavioural disturbance, particularly in the context of autism and mental retardation. There is evidence for efficacy in these conditions, although it is not known whether dopamine blockade is the key mechanism of action.

The main categories of antipsychotic drugs are the *classical* or *typical* antipsychotics, and the newer drugs that are often called *atypical*. The classical group includes chlorpromazine, haloperidol and thioridazine. Relatively new drugs in this group include pimozide and sulpiride. The 'atypical' or 'newer' antipsychotics have different pharmacological profiles (serotonin–dopamine antagonism), generally have fewer extrapyramidal side-effects, and may be effective in groups of patients resistant to treatment with the classical antipsychotics. Clozapine was the first atypical antipsychotic agent introduced and remains the only one to be therapeutically superior to other antipsychotics in efficacy (in resistant schizophrenia). The other atypical antipsychotics include risperidone, olanzapine, amisulpride, quetiapine and ziprasidone. The behavioural effects of all antipsychotics are similar, but their side-effects differ.

Pharmacokinetics

In children as in adults, there is huge individual variation in plasma drug levels, with little correlation between drug dosage and blood levels (Ernst et al. 1999). In general, children eliminate drugs more rapidly than adults, and the antipsychotics are no exception; for example, chlorpromazine has a shorter half-life in younger children (Furlanut et al. 1990).

Side-effects and toxicity

Antipsychotic drugs have the potential to produce significant side-effects (for a review see Campbell et al. 1999), in particular extrapyramidal side-effects (including acute dystonias, akathisia, parkinsonism and dyskinesias), sedation and, rarely, neuroleptic malignant syndrome (Silva et al. 1999). The dyskinesias are the most serious of these, and the prevalence in children ranges from 8 to 51% (Gualtieri et al. 1984). This includes both tardive dyskinesia and withdrawal dyskinesia. Withdrawal dyskinesia may occur with either gradual or sudden cessation of antipsychotic agents, with one-third or more of children developing these movements when the drug is abruptly withdrawn. Withdrawal dyskinesia is usually reversible, whereas tardive dyskinesia may persist even if the antipsychotic agent is discontinued. 40 of 118 (33.9%) autistic children receiving haloperidol over a 15-year period (for hyperactivity, tantrums, aggression, withdrawal, self-injurious behaviour and stereotypies) developed drug-related dyskinesias (Campbell et al. 1997). They were predominantly drug withdrawal dyskinesias and the risk was increased with duration of exposure to drug, cumulative drug dose and the female gender.

The atypical antipsychotics are less likely to cause extrapyramidal side-effects, although there are case reports of risperidone-induced dyskinesias in children (Demb & Nguyen 1999). Clozapine induces little if any dyskinesia in adults, but can cause blood dyscrasias, especially in children (reviewed by Wahlbeck et al. 1999).

Main indications of antipsychotic drugs

Psychosis

Antipsychotic medication continues to be the only specific treatment of documented efficacy for psychosis, although most of the evidence for efficacy in children is an extrapolation from the adult literature. Differences between early onset and adult schizophrenia seem at most to be only quantitative and developmental, and it is reasonable to assume that data from adult studies should form the basis for the treatment of early onset cases. The effectiveness of antipsychotic drugs in adults with schizophrenia has been shown in more than 100 double-blind randomly assigned controlled studies, but there are few studies with adolescents and children (Realmuto et al. 1984; Spencer & Campbell 1994). Clinical experience, and one systematic study (Rapoport et al. 1980a), suggests that children with schizophrenia may respond less well to antipsychotics than do adults, although one of the few controlled studies suggests that the response is similar (Spencer et al. 1992). With the exception of clozapine, there is no evidence to suggest that any one antipsychotic agent is superior in the treatment of schizophrenia. The choice of medication should be based on the agent's relative antidopaminergic potency and side-effects spectrum, and the patient's history of medication response. Currently, most clinicians would recommend the use of an atypical antipsychotic for first-line maintenance therapy in psychosis, although many use the more conventional group for acute behavioural control, often in conjunction with a benzodiazepine.

Clozapine (Frazier et al. 1994; Kumra et al. 1996) is recommended mainly in patients with early onset schizophrenia who are either non-responsive to typical antipsychotics or have developed tardive dyskinesia, although there are theoretical arguments for its first-line use in young patients. It has been found to be effective in at least 30% of adult patients with treatment-resistant schizophrenia (reviewed by Wahlbeck *et al.* 1999). It can only be prescribed in conjunction with a blood-monitoring programme, because of the risk of blood dyscrasias. Newer antipsychotics, such as risperidone or olanzapine, are being used in open clinical trials currently, with encouraging results (Kumra *et al.* 1998), although they do not share clozapine's property of having additional effects in resistant psychosis. The major advantage of the newer antipsychotics is their improved side-effect profile, and in particular the reduced risk of extrapyramidal side-effects, less sedation and resultant improved compliance.

Autism

Antipsychotic drugs are quite widely used in autistic spectrum disorder, in an attempt to reduce repetitive and aggressive behaviours. Campbell *et al.* (1999) reviewed the clinical trials of haloperidol in the treatment of these behaviours, and reported evidence of statistically significant therapeutic efficacy. Despite the improvement noted with haloperidol, about one-third of the children developed dyskinesia as a side-effect (either withdrawal or tardive dyskinesia) (Campbell *et al.* 1997), which suggests that typical antipsychotic agents should be used infrequently and with caution in autism. Open trials of the atypical antipsychotics, e.g. risperidone (McDougle *et al.* 1997) and olanzapine (Potenza *et al.* 1999), reported improvements in angry and labile affect, sleep, interfering repetitive behaviour, aggression, impulsivity and self-injury in children and adolescents with autism (for a review see Santosh & Baird 1999). Significant side-effects of both drugs include major weight gain, hypotension and sedation. A double-blind placebo controlled trial of risperidone reported similar improvements in older individuals with autism (McDougle *et al.* 1998).

Tourette syndrome

Antipsychotic drugs are the most effective treatment for motor and vocal tics, although side-effects of these drugs may limit their usefulness in long-term treatment. Haloperidol has proved effective in controlled trials (Shapiro *et al.* 1989) and a more recent study suggested that pimozide may be superior to haloperidol (Sallee *et al.* 1997). Atypical antipsychotics are being increasingly used in tic disorders, and preliminary studies with ziprasidone (Sallee *et al.* 2000), sulpiride and risperidone show promising results.

Aggression

Antipsychotic drugs have been used for the treatment of aggression in the context of conduct disorder or learning disability

(mental retardation). In neither case is there clear evidence for efficacy. In adults with mental retardation, a recent meta-analysis found no clinical trial evidence for efficacy of antipsychotics in the treatment of challenging behaviour (Brylewski & Duggan 1999). Nevertheless, in clinical practice these drugs are widely used, and behavioural improvement is reported by clinicians and families (for a review see Campbell *et al.* 1999).

Many other medications have been tried in the treatment of behavioural disorders including conduct disorder, aggression and delinquency, but the consensus is that psychopharmacological treatment alone is insufficient (Campbell 1992).

Attention deficit hyperactivity disorder

Antipsychotics, as well as many other psychotropic medications, have been tried in the treatment of ADHD; there are no systematic data supporting their use, or the use of fenfluramine, benzodiazepines or lithium in ADHD (Green 1995). Dopamine-blocking agents may seem an illogical combination with stimulants, but there is some trial evidence for an increased benefit for methylphenidate plus thioridazine over methylphenidate alone—especially in behaviour as seen at home rather than at school (Gittelman-Klein *et al.* 1976). This must be set against the known toxicity of antipsychotic drugs, and cautious practice will only use the combination in rare and extreme circumstances. In principle, the advent of atypical antipsychotics with fewer hazards may have altered the ratio of risk:benefit. Risperidone, for example, is coming into frequent use before trials have been completed, on the basis of a reputation for fewer extrapyramidal hazards. It is not free of adverse effects, sedation and weight gain being prominent, and it may antagonize some of the actions of methylphenidate (such as those mediated by D_2 receptors). In general, the combination of stimulants and antipsychotics—like most other forms of polypharmacy—should only be tried by a specialist service, and that in those exceptional cases where it is to be used, an atypical antipsychotic should be chosen.

Lithium

Basic pharmacology and mechanism of action

The psychotropic effects of lithium were discovered in 1949 by Cade, and this inorganic cation is still a mainstay in the prophylaxis of manic-depressive (bipolar) illness in adults. Its mechanism of action is uncertain, although it is known to interfere with two important second messenger systems, and thus to have widespread and complex effects on neurotransmitter function.

Pharmacokinetic issues

Lithium is given orally, usually as the carbonate salt, and its elimination is almost entirely dependent on renal excretion.

Children tend to have a higher glomerular filtration rate and a higher proportion of body water than adults, which may mean that higher doses of lithium, relative to body weight, are needed to achieve therapeutic levels, and steady state may be achieved more rapidly (Vitiello *et al.* 1988). Apart from this higher excretion rate, lithium pharmacokinetics is overall similar to that in adults.

Side-effects and toxicity

Lithium is generally well tolerated in children and adolescents, although younger children with neurological problems may be more vulnerable to side-effects (Campbell *et al.* 1991). Common side-effects in children are nausea, tremor, polyuria and enuresis. Other potential side-effects which are documented in adults include weight gain, acne, hypothyroidism and impaired renal function. In younger children (aged 4–6 years) more neurological side-effects have been reported, including tremor, drowsiness, ataxia and confusion, especially at the beginning of treatment (Hagino *et al.* 1995), suggesting that a strong clinical indication would be needed to justify lithium use in such young children. Lithium has a narrow therapeutic index and monitoring of the plasma concentration is an essential part of treatment (Tueth *et al.* 1998). Acute lithium toxicity can cause coma, convulsion and death, and may need treatment with plasmapheresis.

Main indications including trial data or other evidence of efficacy

The main indication for lithium use in young people, as in adults, is for the prophylaxis of bipolar disorder, and the treatment of acute mania. There have been very few good studies in children, and in general use of lithium in children is based on evidence from adult studies (Ryan *et al.* 1999). There is some evidence for efficacy in the treatment of aggression, and little evidence for efficacy in the treatment of ADHD and conduct disorder.

Mood stabilization

There are few randomized controlled trials of lithium in young people. One study in substance-dependent adolescents with co-morbid bipolar illness showed significant benefit of lithium treatment, in terms of global impairment and illicit drug use (Geller *et al.* 1998). Other small cross-over and open studies have given variable results. Strober *et al.* (1990) showed greater rates of relapse in adolescents with bipolar disorder who discontinued lithium treatment.

In summary, open trials of lithium in adolescents appear to give similar response rates to adults. Its usefulness in younger children seems less clear, particularly as this group seems more prone to adverse effects. A study in children less than 12 years showed little apparent benefit of lithium (Carlson *et al.* 1992).

Aggression and conduct disorder

Several open studies have shown lithium to be useful in the treatment of extreme aggressiveness, particularly in the context of mental retardation (DeLong & Aldershof 1987). There have been small studies suggesting positive effects of lithium in conduct disorder (Campbell *et al.* 1995) and others with negative results (Rifkin *et al.* 1997).

Antidepressant drugs

Basic pharmacology and mechanisms of action

Antidepressant drugs comprise a diverse group, and new agents frequently appear on the market, reflecting the recognized shortcomings of those that are currently available. The main shortcomings (see below) are limited clinical efficacy, delayed onset of action and prevalence of side-effects.

The pharmacological rationale for these drugs rests mainly on the monoamine theory of depression, which holds that depression results from a functional deficit of monoamine transmitters—particularly noradrenaline and serotonin. Current thinking about the action of antidepressant drugs, and a look ahead, are given in reviews by Frazer (1997) and Nestler (1998).

Currently, the main types of antidepressant drugs are the following.
• TCAs (e.g. imipramine, amitriptyline, clomipramine, desipramine).
• Selective serotonin reuptake inhibitors (SSRIs, e.g. fluoxetine, fluvoxamine, paroxetine, sertraline, citalopram). These widely used drugs appear to be as efficacious as TCAs (and possibly more so in children, see below) with fewer side-effects.
• Monoamine oxidase inhibitors (MAOIs, e.g. phenelzine, tranylcypromine, moclobemide).
• 'Atypical' antidepressants (e.g. maprotiline, bupropion, venlafaxine, trazodone, nefazodone, mianserin, mirtazapine). This is a heterogeneous group. Maprotiline inhibits noradrenaline uptake, and resembles the TCAs, although its chemical structure and side-effects are different. Venlafaxine inhibits both serotonin and noradrenaline reuptake, and has weaker receptor blocking actions than TCAs. The mechanism of action of bupropion is unclear. The others act mainly as antagonists of various monoamine receptors, including presynaptic adrenoceptors and serotonin receptors.

Despite their pharmacological differences, the different groups appear to be indistinguishable with respect to clinical efficacy in adults. However, they differ in their side-effects, which may be the main basis for the choice of which drug to prescribe in individual cases.

Pharmacokinetics

Detailed information about these drugs has been obtained in adults, the few studies in children being confined to TCAs. In adults, all of the drugs are well absorbed orally. Their plasma half-lives vary widely between drugs, and also between individuals. Thus, imipramine (relatively short-acting) has a half-life of 6–24 h, while fluoxetine (long-acting) has a half-life of 24–200 h. For several reasons, there is generally little correlation between plasma concentration and clinical response.

• Many antidepressants give rise to long-lived active metabolites.

• The clinical response usually takes 2–4 weeks to develop after treatment has started. The reason for this delay is not known, but it suggests that the clinical effect reflects a secondary adaptation to the primary action of the drug.

Comparison of TCA half-lives in children and adults suggests that they are generally two- to three-fold shorter in children, and equi-effective doses, on a body weight basis, are correspondingly larger in children. Despite the wide variation in half-life between different drugs and different individuals, most of these drugs are given once daily.

Side-effects and toxicity

1 TCAs and drugs classified as atypical antidepressants are active as antagonists at several different monoamine receptors, notably muscarinic cholinoceptors, histamine (H$_1$) receptors and noradrenaline (α_1) receptors, as well as various different serotonin receptors, and these actions account for many of their side-effects:

• sedation (mainly amitriptyline, trazodone, clomipramine, maprotiline, uncommon with bupropion);

• anticholinergic side-effects (dry mouth, blurred vision, constipation, urinary retention—mainly TCAs, maprotiline, rare with other atypical antidepressants);

• postural hypotension (mainly TCAs, maprotiline, trazodone), paradoxically, hypertension at rest sometimes occurs, particularly with imipramine;

• weight gain (mainly TCAs);

• seizures (especially bupropion, but also reported with TCAs);

• cardiotoxicity, evident as a slowing of conduction and tachycardia, which can progress to ventricular dysrhythmias, is the most serious adverse effect of TCAs, and sudden deaths have been reported in children (Biederman 1991). Other antidepressants are much safer in this respect.

2 SSRIs. The side-effects appear to be associated with the primary mechanism of action of these drugs, and there is little evidence that individual SSRIs differ significantly from each other; venlafaxine has a similar profile:

• agitation and insomnia;

• headache;

• nausea and vomiting, mainly at the beginning of treatment.

Sexual dysfunction, a major problem associated with SSRIs in adults, is inconsequential in young children but may be important in adolescents.

3 MAOIs. The serious side-effects of first-generation MAOIs, especially hypertensive crisis ('cheese reaction'), greatly limited their clinical utility, particularly in children. The newer MAO-A-specific and reversible compounds, such as moclobemide, overcome some of these problems, but have not yet gained wide acceptance for use in children.

Clinical uses and efficacy

Depression

A depressive disorder starting in childhood or adolescence is a serious psychiatric condition that may become a chronic illness. The prevalence of major depressive disorder and dysthymia increases dramatically in adolescents, reaching close to adult levels in late teenage years. Treatment of depression includes effective resolution of the current episode and effective prophylaxis to prevent further episodes or to reduce their morbidity if they do occur. Medication should be used in conjunction with interventions designed to improve interpersonal, social and academic functioning.

There is increasing evidence that SSRIs are effective in child and adolescent depression, and should generally be the first choice of medication (Emslie et al. 1999). Commonly used SSRIs include fluoxetine and paroxetine, with accumulating experience with sertraline and fluvoxamine. The evidence from a few controlled studies and numerous open trials show that around 60–70% of cases will show some improvement. A more recent randomized controlled trial of fluoxetine showed a 56% rating in improvement in the drug treatment group, compared with 33% in the placebo group (Emslie et al. 1997).

In contrast, TCAs are probably relatively ineffective in children. A large double-blind, placebo-controlled trial of desipramine hydrochloride showed no benefit compared to placebo, regardless of the type of outcome measure used or subtype of the major depressive disorder (Kutcher et al. 1994). A meta-analysis of the efficacy of TCAs in the treatment of childhood depression concluded that there was no evidence they were more effective than placebo (Hazell et al. 1995). The total numbers of children studied are small, and in general childhood depression has many similarities with adult depression; however, current evidence does not support the general use of TCAs in childhood depression, although they may be useful in individual cases (Geller et al. 1999).

There are preliminary findings with atypical antidepressants, but numbers remain very small. A small study of refractory childhood depression showed positive responses to nefazodone (Wilens et al. 1997) but a small controlled study of venlafaxine failed to show significant difference between drug and placebo (Mandoki et al. 1997), although clinical anecdote suggests that this may be a useful drug in the younger age group. There is little evidence that the typical MAOIs, such as tranylcypromine or phenelzine, are effective treatments for depressed children or adolescents. The dangers of traditional MAOIs are well known and the special dietary requirements that accompany their use make them difficult to use in children and problematic in adolescents. Ryan *et al.* (1988) concluded that it was risky to use MAOIs in adolescents, although this was before the introduction of reversible MAOIs, such as moclobemide, which have yet to be evaluated in children but might prove useful in resistant depression.

In childhood depression that is non-responsive to an SSRI, a trial of another SSRI is advisable. If this is ineffective, a trial of a drug with added noradrenergic impact, such as venlafaxine, may be used. If the patient continues to remain symptomatic, review diagnosis—if depression remains the diagnosis, augmentation with lithium or buspirone should be tried. Continued non-response should lead to the use of atypical antidepressants such as bupropion, nefazedone, reboxetine, or the use of a reversible MAOI drug, such as moclobamide. Non-response to this strategy should lead one to contemplate the use of electro-convulsive therapy (ECT) if impairment remains significant. Psychological intervention, such as cognitive-behavioural therapy and environmental manipulation, should be attempted together with the pharmacotherapy in all resistant cases. ECT will need to be contemplated earlier if the patient is in depressive stupor, very suicidal or severely impaired. A low dose of one of the atypical antipsychotics (such as olanzapine) should be added to the antidepressant if there are psychotic symptoms. It is advisable that resistant childhood depression be managed in a specialist centre.

Obsessive-compulsive disorder

The treatment of obsessive-compulsive disorder (OCD) with clomipramine is probably the best established use of a TCA in childhood, with the serotonin reuptake properties of clomipramine being an essential part of its efficacy. Leonard *et al.* (1991) found a very high relapse rate in children and adolescents following substitution of clomipramine with desipramine in a cross-over study. In another double-blind placebo controlled multicentre study of 60 adolescent patients with OCD, treated for 8 weeks, a mean reduction of 37% in total obsessive-compulsive score was seen in the clomipramine group compared to 8% in the placebo group (DeVeaugh-Geiss *et al.* 1992). However, the SSRIs have now largely superseded clomipramine as a first-line treatment for OCD in young people, because of their improved side-effect profiles. There is controlled clinical trial evidence of SSRI efficacy and safety for fluoxetine and fluvoxamine (reviewed by Grados *et al.* 1999) and more recently for sertraline (March *et al.* 1998). Although the effect sizes are relatively small, they are generally equivalent to clomipramine, and are consistent with findings from adult studies. Over 75% of the children and adolescents treated in an open trial of citalopram showed a moderate to marked improvement in OCD symptoms with only minor and transient adverse effects (Thomsen 1997). Medication treatment for childhood OCD may need to be long term; Leonard *et al.* (1993) reported that response to treatment with clomipramine in childhood or adolescence predicted a better outcome 2–7 years later. However, only

11% were totally asymptomatic, 43% still met diagnostic criteria for OCD and 70% were on psychoactive medication at follow-up, including the asymptomatic patients. As in adults, up to 80% of young people with OCD relapse on discontinuation of medication, but there is clinical suggestion that remissions may be prolonged if medication is combined with cognitive-behavioural therapy.

A double-blind placebo-controlled cross-over trial of fixed dose fluoxetine (20 mg/day) in Tourette syndrome showed that fluoxetine had no effect on tics but produced a modest decrease in obsessive-compulsive symptoms. The most common side-effect was transient behavioural activation which occurred in about half of the subjects and was more common in children (Riddle *et al.* 1990).

Attention deficit hyperactivity disorder

Although far less studied than stimulants, controlled trials of TCAs in both children and adolescents demonstrate efficacy in the treatment of ADHD (Popper 1998). Despite the narrow margin of safety, they may be used as second-line drugs for stimulant-resistant ADHD, and for those who develop significant depression or other side-effects on stimulants, and for patients with comorbid tics or Tourette disorder, anxiety disorder or depression. The long duration of action of TCAs averts the need for a dose at school and rebound is not a problem. Efficacy in improving cognitive symptoms does not appear as great as for stimulants.

Desipramine is effective in both children and adolescents (Biederman *et al.* 1989), but is more cardiotoxic than imipramine. Consequently, imipramine is probably the first choice amongst TCAs in the treatment of prepubertal children with ADHD. In two open trials of children and adolescents, many of whom had a poor response to stimulants, TCAs increased attention span and decreased impulsivity (Wilens *et al.* 1993).

There have been some studies of atypical antipressants in the treatment of ADHD. An open study of venlafaxine suggested efficacy (Olvera *et al.* 1996). Bupropion may decrease hyperactivity and aggression and perhaps improve cognitive performance of children with ADHD and conduct disorder (Conners *et al.* 1996) and was found to be as effective as methylphenidate in a double-blind controlled trial (Barrickman *et al.* 1995). Its most serious side-effect is a decrease in seizure threshold and it may exacerbate tics.

Although used safely in some contexts, the combination of imipramine and methylphenidate has been associated with a syndrome of confusion, affective lability, marked aggression and severe agitation (Grob & Coyle 1986). A double-blind controlled cross-over study of 16 hospitalized children with ADHD, mood disorder, or both, and with either conduct disorder or oppositional-defiant disorder, treated with a combination of desipramine and methylphenidate showed that the combination was significantly better than either drug alone although clinically the benefits were modest. In this carefully monitored setting there were no untoward side-effects (Carlson *et al*. 1995).

Anxiety disorders

Four placebo-controlled studies of TCAs for separation anxiety disorder, with and without school refusal, provide contrasting results. The inconsistencies may be explained by differences in dosages and comorbidity patterns and lack of control of concurrent therapies. In the original studies of Gittelman-Klein & Klein (1971, 1973), 35 children receiving imipramine were significantly more successful in returning to school than those on placebo (81% on imipramine and 47% on placebo). Although recent studies have failed to replicate these results (Berney *et al*. 1981; Bernstein *et al*. 1990; Klein *et al*. 1992), clinical experience suggests that some children and adolescents with anxiety-based school refusal improve on TCAs, and they may also be effective in treating panic disorder in children and adolescents (Ballenger *et al*. 1989; Black & Robbins 1990).

Literature is starting to emerge about the use of SSRIs for children with anxiety disorders. Open trials of fluoxetine have demonstrated significant effect in children and adolescents with social phobia, overanxious disorder or separation anxiety disorder (Birmaher *et al*. 1994). Similarly, case reports (Wright *et al*. 1995), an open trial (Dummit *et al*. 1996) and a controlled study (Black & Uhde 1995) indicate that fluoxetine (10–40 mg/day) may be beneficial in the treatment of elective mutism. A recent randomised controlled trial has shown efficacy of fluroxamine for a range of child anxiety disorders (The Research Unit on Pediatric Psychopharmacology Anxiety Study Group 2001).

Pervasive developmental disorders

SSRIs, such as fluoxetine (Cook *et al*. 1992) and sertraline (Steingard *et al*. 1997), have been used in autistic children with encouraging improvements in aggression, repetitive and maladaptive behaviour, social relatedness and self-injurious behaviour in the short term. Fluvoxamine in a double-blind placebo-controlled study has also produced similar improvements in adults with pervasive developmental disorders (PDD) (McDougle *et al*. 1996).

Enuresis

Imipramine is well established in the treatment of enuresis. It may act by decreasing the deepest stages of sleep to lighter sleep, by stimulating secretion of antidiuretic hormone (ADH) indirectly or by peripheral mechanisms. A study that compared imipramine, desipramine, methscopolamine and placebo showed that both TCAs were superior to placebo or methscopolamine but did not differ from each other (Rapoport *et al*. 1980b). Despite a lack of comparative clinical trials, desmopressin (a synthetic analogue of ADH) is now considered a safer,

more effective and better tolerated alternative to the use of TCAs for treating enuresis.

Anxiolytics, sedatives and miscellaneous drugs

Basic pharmacology, pharmacokinetics and side-effects

A wide variety of psychoactive drugs have been tried in many different psychiatric disorders, sometimes in combination, in adults and in children. With a few exceptions, there is little systematic evidence for efficacy and safety. The main drugs which have been usefully deployed in child and adolescent psychiatry are summarized in Table 59.5, and the subsequent section reviews the evidence for clinical usefulness. A more detailed review by Riddle *et al*. (1999) considered all of the drugs mentioned in this section, including benzodiazepines, buspirone, clonidine and naltrexone.

Clonidine

An α_2-adrenoceptor agonist has been shown in placebo controlled trials to attenuate significantly hyperactivity and disruptive behaviours in children with ADHD. A recent meta-analysis of published trials suggests that clonidine is less efficacious than stimulants, and that side-effects may be significant (Connor *et al*. 1999). Although clonidine is not effective in treating inattention *per se*, it may be used alone to treat behavioural symptoms in children with tics (Steingard *et al*. 1993) or in those where stimulants are ineffective or not tolerated. When discontinuing clonidine, the dosage should be reduced gradually to avoid a *withdrawal syndrome* consisting of increased motor restlessness, headaches, agitation, elevated blood pressure and pulse rate and possible exacerbation of tics reported in patients with symptoms of Tourette syndrome and ADHD (Leckman *et al*. 1986). Depression and impaired glucose tolerance are side-effects that can occur in susceptible patients.

Open trials suggest that clonidine may be useful in combination with a stimulant for the treatment of ADHD, when the stimulant alone is ineffective or when the dose is limited by side-effects. Recently, there has been concern about the use of clonidine in combination with stimulant medication (Swanson *et al*. 1995), based on the cases of four children who died suddenly. The evidence derived from these cases is hard to interpret because of special circumstances and inadequate detail (Wilens & Spencer 1999). Recommendations are conflicting: Swanson *et al*. (1999) believe that the use of the combination is ill-advised until controlled studies can be conducted to evaluate efficacy and side-effects. Most practitioners appear to be taking the line of cautious use rather than a complete ban, and including ECG monitoring in their evaluations.

Clonidine has also been used in Tourette syndrome in both open and double-blind trials. Positive studies suggest that about 40% of patients with Tourette syndrome benefit from its use (Leckman *et al*. 1991), but there are at least as many negative

Table 59.5 Basic pharmacology of anxiolytics, sedatives and miscellaneous drugs used in child psychiatry.

Drug	Mechanism of action	Actions	Side-effects	Pharmacokinetics
Benzodiazepines: Lorazepam Oxazepam Alprazolam Temazepam Nitrazepam Diazepam Chlordiazepoxide Flurazepam Clonazepam	Enhancement of inhibitory effect of GABA acting on GABA-A receptors	Sedative Anxiolytic Anticonvulsant Reduces muscle spasm	Confusion Amnesia Impaired co-ordination Tolerance and dependence	Most are well absorbed orally Inactivated by hepatic metabolism Half-lives vary from 6–12 h (e.g. lorazepam) to over 48 h (e.g. diazepam). Active metabolites prolong effect of many benzodiazepines
Valproate	Uncertain Weak GABA-enhancing and Na-channel blocking actions	Mainly antiepileptic Also has sedative/antimanic action	Nausea Somnolence Hepatotoxicity Weight gain	Well absorbed orally Half-life 12–15 h
Carbamazepine	Block of Na channels	Mainly antiepileptic, with weak stimulant activity. Used in trigeminal neuralgia	Nausea Dizziness May cause tics Occasionally causes emotional lability, aggressive behaviour Leucopenia and hepatotoxicity at high plasma levels	Well absorbed Plasma half-life varies from 12 to 60 h, tending to decrease because of induction of metabolizing enzymes Monitoring of plasma level is advisable to keep below 10 mg/L
Clonidine	Partial agonist at α_2 adrenoceptor Inhibits noradrenaline release in brain	Sedation Reduced sympathetic activity, causing lowering of blood pressure	Hypotension Sedation Dry mouth Dangerous in overdose (bradycardia, hypotension)	Well absorbed by mouth Can be given as skin patch to provide sustained action Plasma half-life is about 12 h, but pharmacological effect is briefer (2–4 h)
Naltrexone	Antagonist at μ- opioid receptors	Little effect in absence of opiates Inhibits opiate effects, and can precipitate withdrawal syndrome in addicts	Drowsiness Nausea Headache	Well absorbed orally Plasma half-life about 4 h Action prolonged by formation of active metabolite
Antihistamines: Promethazine Diphenhydramine	Antagonists at histamine H_1 receptors	Sedation Antiemetic	Drowsiness and confusion Anticholinergic effects	Well absorbed orally Plasma half-life approx. 12 h (6 h for diphenhydramine)

studies (reviewed by Riddle *et al.* 1999). In addition to reducing the simple motor and phonic symptoms in Tourette syndrome, clonidine seems useful in reducing hyperactivity and ameliorating complex motor and phonic symptoms. Clonidine tends to have a slower onset of action than antipsychotic drugs. Tolerance to clonidine does not appear to develop. Its major side-effect is sedation, which commonly appears early in the course of treatment, but tends to abate after several weeks.

Clonidine has been shown in double-blind placebo-controlled trials to improve hyperactivity, irritability and oppositional behaviour in autism, a clinical group in whom stimulants may be contraindicated because of a tendency to increase rigidity or stereotypies (Fankhauser *et al.* 1992).

Guanfacine hydrochloride

Guanfacine hydrochloride is a long-acting α_2-agonist and has a more favourable side-effect profile than clonidine. It has recently been used as monotherapy for children with ADHD and Tourette syndrome, whose tics may become worse with the use of stimulants (for a review see Scahill *et al.* 2000). It has also been used in combination with a stimulant in the treatment of children with ADHD who cannot tolerate the sedative or rebound side-effects of clonidine. As yet only open trials have been published (Hunt *et al.* 1995), and this drug is not licensed in the UK.

Benzodiazepines

Benzodiazepines may be used on a short-term basis (few weeks) for anxiety symptoms in rare circumstances. Despite their anxiolytic properties, benzodiazepines have significant dependence-producing potential in adults and should be used with caution in children, although there have been no studies of dependence in young people. In general, pharmacological management has a relatively minor role in the treatment of anxiety disorders in children and adolescents (Labellarte *et al.* 1999). Case reports and several studies indicate that alprazolam is useful in treating anxiety symptoms in children and adolescents. In an open label trial, small doses of alprazolam were found to be effective for anticipatory and acute situational anxiety in paediatric oncology patients undergoing bone marrow aspirations and spinal taps (Pfefferbaum *et al.* 1987). However, a double-blind placebo-controlled study of 30 children and adolescents with avoidant or overanxious disorders failed to show any statistically significant difference between alprazolam and placebo (Simeon *et al.* 1992), as did another small double-blind cross-over study of 15 children with anxiety disorders comparing clonazepam with placebo (Graae *et al.* 1994). Adolescents with panic disorder treated with clonazepam experienced a decrease in the frequency and level of anxiety symptoms after 2 weeks of treatment (Kutcher & MacKenzie 1988).

Buspirone

Buspirone is a full 5-HT$_{1A}$ agonist at the somatodendritic autoreceptor and a partial agonist at the post-synaptic 5-HT$_{1A}$ receptors, acting therefore on the noradrenergic, serotonergic and dopaminergic systems. Side-effects are uncommon and usually very mild and include nausea, headaches, daytime tiredness and weight gain. Buspirone has been reported to improve hyperactivity, anxiety, stereotypy, irritability and global behaviour in open trials (Buitelarr *et al.* 1998), but there have been no controlled studies in children or adolescents. Recently, an open trial showed buspirone to produce global improvement in symptoms of ADHD (Malhotra & Santosh 1998). Case reports suggest that buspirone is effective in treating adolescents with overanxious disorder and school refusal (Kranzler 1989), social phobia and mixed personality disorder (Zwier & Rao 1994). Riddle *et*

al. (1999) review the general case-report studies on the use of buspirone in children and adolescents, some of which suggest improvements in oppositionality, anxiety and school refusal.

Anticonvulsant drugs

Both sodium valproate and carbamazepine have an established role in the management of adult bipolar disorder, and are probably effective as mood stabilizers in early onset forms of this illness (for a review see Ryan *et al.* 1999). As yet there is very little controlled trial evidence for their efficacy in young people, although there have been some promising open studies of sodium valproate in mania (Papatheodorou *et al.* 1995).

There have also been trials of carbamazepine in children with behavioural problems, or high activity levels. Studies from the early 1970s suggested benefit over placebo, but more recent studies in children with aggression showed no advantage over placebo (Cueva *et al.* 1996). A meta-analysis of 10 studies suggests that carbamazepine may be beneficial in ADHD (Silva *et al.* 1996), but methodological limitations make this uncertain and the far from benign side-effect profile make this drug an alternative only for highly resistant cases.

Naltrexone

Naltrexone, an opioid antagonist, has been used in autism, on the hypothetical basis that opioid dysfunction may occur in this condition. The results have been inconsistent but have shown a mild improvement in hyperactivity, impulsivity, restlessness and self-injury (Koleman *et al.* 1995).

In spite of a lack of a sound evidence basis, it is reasonable in certain circumstances, such as in autism, to try one of the medications for which positive claims are being made. In such circumstances it is sometimes illuminating to carry out a double-blind placebo-controlled case study. Many psychotropic agents have been used in autism, and the consensus is that any trials of medication should be part of an overall treatment plan that includes psychosocial, behavioural and language interventions. Despite SSRIs, risperidone and clonidine being reported to increase social relatedness, there is very little evidence that treatment can change the core features of autism. However, pharmacotherapy may decrease the severity of some of the autistic features, help control harmful or dangerous behaviours and may improve the patient's accessibility to psychosocial and language interventions. The first-choice medication is usually determined by the target symptoms that need to be controlled. Thus, if hyperactivity is a target, methylphenidate or clonidine may be chosen; if rituals, self-injurious behaviour or stereotypies are a target, an SSRI such as fluvoxamine or sertraline may be a reasonable choice while clonidine, risperidone, haloperidol or buspirone may be appropriate for treating irritability and aggression (Santosh & Baird 1999). Subjects with anxiety may respond to buspirone, propranolol or clonazepam. At the present time, there is no clear-cut evidence that opiate antagonists are of value in the promotion of social behaviour. There is currently no convincing evidence to suggest any positive therapeutic effect of megavitamin therapy or dietary manipulation in autism.

Melatonin

Melatonin, a hormone secreted under adrenergic control by the pineal gland, has been the subject of case study and small trials for the treatment of severe sleep disorders. The evidence is weak, but some studies suggest that it is effective in correcting disturbed sleep patterns (Jan *et al.* 1999).

Secretin

Secretin has been advocated as treatment for the maladaptive behaviours of autism, but there is no objective evidence to support this (Volkmar 1999).

Electroconvulsive therapy

The use of ECT presents particular dilemmas in children and adolescents, as there are only limited numbers of case reports or studies on ECT in this population (Rey & Walter 1997). ECT continues to be used in adolescents in many countries despite the various advances in pharmacotherapy, because some patients continue to be drug-resistant. The current practice estimate of ECT use in adolescents is 0.5–1 treatment per million people (Cohen *et al.* 2000).

A cautious recommendation of indications for the use of ECT in adolescents would be to limit its use to treat catatonia, severe resistant mood disorders and intractable acute psychotic disorders. Other rare indications include its use in managing neuroleptic malignant syndrome and status epilepticus. Apart from the diagnoses, the urgency for the need for rapid response, the danger of suicidal or homicidal behaviours, the severity of the psychiatric disorder, the number and adequacy of previous treatments need to be taken into account. ECT can be ethically justified in cases where there is a risk of death or suicide, sometimes even without the patient's consent—using consent from carer, or a second medical opinion (Reiter-Theil 1992). In rare cases, court petition may be necessary when parents' and children's interests are opposed. Although the benefits of ECT are often impressive, the secondary effects—in particular cognitive impairment—need to be considered, as an adequate risk–benefit analysis is currently difficult as studies on cognitive consequences of ECT are unavailable in young people.

Cohen *et al.* (2000) have outlined the various complications of ECT in adolescents as the following.

1 Complications of the anaesthetic time: lip-biting, teeth chattering, agitated awakening, face flush and prolonged seizures.

2 Early secondary effects are quite frequent but usually only entail moderate discomfort: headache, post-ECT asthenia, nausea, muscular pain and post-ECT confusion.

3 Infrequent complications: disinhibition and spontaneous seizures.

4 Cognitive secondary effects have not been prospectively studied in the adolescent population.

There have been no deaths with ECT in children or adolescents reported, probably because of fewer anaesthetic complications in the young.

Despite views of certain organizations and professionals that ECT should be banned for youth (Baker 1995)—based on the ethics of uninformed consent, possible risk of brain damage and misapplication, and inadequate knowledge and equipment—a balanced view dictates that ECT could be used in the rare instances detailed above. There is an obvious need for controlled short-term and follow-up studies on ECT use in adolescents, including its possible effects on cognitive functioning. Techniques such as transcranial magnetic stimulation (TMS) might ultimately replace ECT; TMS is currently only available in research centres but is producing encouraging results in adult mood disorders (Hallett 2000), apparently with fewer side-effects.

Dietary treatments

Exclusion diets are the key to management of certain rare metabolic disorders, such as phenylketonuria (see Skuse & Kuntsi, Chapter 13). More controversially, a variety of diets for supposed metabolic disorders have been proposed without empirical support. In particular, Feingold's hypothesis—of a toxic action of salicylates, and cross-reacting synthetic dyes and preservatives, as a main cause of hyperactivity, autism and mental retardation—has been tested and found not to be correct (Conners 1980; Committee on Toxicity of Food 2000). A weaker hypothesis—that food dyes can worsen the behaviour of certain predisposed children—has had inconclusive evaluation.

However, there is preliminary evidence for an idiosyncratic effect of diet upon the behaviour of certain predisposed individuals (reviewed by the Committee on Toxicity of Food 2000). Two challenge studies have selected children with ADHD; identified suspect foods by trying their effect, one at a time, while the diet is otherwise highly restricted; and then given the suspect foods in a placebo-controlled random-allocation cross-over design. Both found that suspect foods produced more behaviour problems than placebo. Two experimental diet studies have used random-allocation trial designs to compare a control diet with one that eliminates the most common suspect foods identified in the challenge studies. Both found fewer behavioural problems in children with ADHD taking the elimination diet than the control.

There are reservations about these promising findings. They are based on small-scale trials, and highly selected series of children. The foods involved vary from child to child and include 'natural' foods such as eggs, wheat flour and citrus fruit as well as 'artificial' ones such as food dyes. The action appears to be on irritable and non-compliant behaviours rather than specifically on ADHD, and the mechanism of action is unknown. The diets are difficult to prepare, unwelcome to children, and usually infeasible for older children and adolescents. It is not clear how to select children for a trial of diet—except for the finding that response was more probable when parents had themselves noted a suspect food (Carter *et al.* 1993).

One can conclude only that parents who have noticed that diet affects their children's behaviour are, probably, sometimes right. Prescription of the diet is not yet justified. However, families who wish to explore the possibility further should be supported—either by assistance in keeping a food diary to identify suspect foods, or by referral to a paediatric dietician for a diagnostic trial of a 'few-food' diet, to identify the specific foods that could be eliminated in the longer term.

Surgery

There have been no controlled studies of the effects of epilepsy surgery on psychiatric symptoms in young people. Descriptive investigations have all shown that positive behavioural outcomes are highly correlated with reduction in severity of seizures. For example, 22 children (all except two had mental retardation) were followed at 19 months post-corpus callosotomy for intractable seizures (Yang *et al.* 1996). Half were reported to have improved attention span and social skills, and reduced hyperactivity. Parents' reports of satisfaction with quality of life was significantly correlated with good seizure outcome. Nonresective surgery (multiple pial transections) has also been reported to improve language and social skills temporarily, in a group of children with epilepsy-related autistic features (Nass *et al.* 1999).

Positive behavioural outcomes have also been reported for resective surgery. Eight individuals followed by Lindsay *et al.* (1987), who underwent hemispherectomy for severe epilepsy, were said to have excellent relief from behavioural disorder. Several earlier studies reported similar findings (reviewed by Goodman 1986) although, by contemporary standards, all of these studies are impaired by lack of systematic behavioural measures.

Temporal lobectomy is the most common surgical procedure for intractable seizures but, once again, behavioural outcomes have been little studied in children. One series (Davidson & Falconer 1975) reported that the underlying pathology is related to positive seizure and behavioural outcome, in this case mesial temporal sclerosis being positively associated. A more recent study of nine children reported no change in neuropsychological measures following temporal lobectomy, and suggested improvement in emotional disturbance and social interaction (Williams *et al.* 1998). Psychosurgery, other than as used in the treatment of epilepsy, has no place in child psychiatry.

Conclusions

Prescribing habits in child and adolescent psychiatry continue to be determined as much by dogma as by evidence. For many interventions there is a lack of objective evidence to support clinical decisions, but in other areas there are increasingly robust clinical trial data to guide rational prescribing. Treatment decisions can only be made on the basis of rigorous assessment and diagnostic evaluation, and child psychiatry is no different from any other part of medicine in this respect. However, emotions continue to run high in the debate 'for' and 'against' drug treatments in child psychiatry, with ideologies determining treatment in some cases. Worrying findings continue to emerge, e.g. the dramatic increase in the rates of prescribing of psychotropic medication in preschool-age children in the USA (Zito *et al.* 2000), despite there being little evidence for safety or efficacy. Perhaps as the stigma associated with mental illness declines, we will move towards more rational prescribing for children with psychiatric disorders. Routes into mental disorder can be developmental, genetic or environmental (and most likely a combination of these) but aetiology does not generally determine treatment in psychiatry. Clearly, the final common pathway to behavioural, emotional or cognition dysfunction is through alteration in brain function, and an effective part of treatment may be to use drugs which act on the brain. Psychological as well as pharmacological interventions can produce measurable effects on brain chemistry, and all of these powerful tools which are employed in the treatment of children must be carefully evaluated to ensure we do good, not harm.

References

Baker, T. (1995) ECT and young minds. *Lancet*, 345, 65.

Ballenger, J.C., Carek, D.J., Steele, J.J. & Cornish-McTighe, D. (1989) Three cases of panic disorder with agoraphobia in children. *American Journal of Psychiatry*, 146, 922–924.

Barkley, R.A., McMurray, M.B., Edelbrock, C.S. & Robbins, K. (1990) Side effects of methylphenidate in children with attention deficit hyperactivity disorder: a systemic, placebo-controlled evaluation. *Pediatrics*, 86, 184–192.

Barkley, A., DuPaul, G. & Connor, D. (1999) Stimulants. In: *Practitioner's Guide to Psychoactive Drugs for Children and Adolescents* (eds J. Werry & M. Aman), pp. 213–241. Plenum, New York.

Barrickman, L.L., Perry, P.J., Allen, A.J. *et al.* (1995) Bupropion versus methylphenidate in the treatment of attention-deficit hyperactivity disorder. *Journal of the American Academy of Child and Adolescent Psychiatry*, 34, 649–657.

Berkovitch, M., Pope, E., Phillips, J. & Koren, G. (1995) Pemoline-associated fulminant liver failure: testing the evidence for causation. *Clinical Pharmacology and Therapeutics*, 57, 696–698.

Berney, T., Kolvin, I., Bhate, S.R. *et al.* (1981) School phobia: a therapeutic trial with clomipramine and short-term outcome. *British Journal of Psychiatry*, 138, 110–118.

Bernstein, G.A., Garfinkel, B.D. & Borchardt, C.M. (1990) Comparative studies of pharmacotherapy for school refusal. *Journal of the American Academy of Child and Adolescent Psychiatry*, 29, 773–781.

Biederman, J. (1991) Sudden death in children treated with a tricyclic antidepressant. *Journal of the American Academy of Child and Adolescent Psychiatry*, 30, 495–498.

Biederman, J., Baldessarini, R.J., Wright, V., Knee, D. & Harmatz, J.S. (1989) A double-blind placebo-controlled study of desipramine in the treatment of ADD. I. Efficacy. *Journal of the American Academy of Child and Adolescent Psychiatry*, 28, 777–784.

Birmaher, B., Waterman, G.S., Ryan, N. *et al.* (1994) Fluoxetine for childhood anxiety disorders. *Journal of the American Academy of Child and Adolescent Psychiatry*, 33, 993–999.

Black, B. & Robbins, D.R. (1990) Panic disorder in children and adolescents. *Journal of the American Academy of Child and Adolescent Psychiatry*, **29**, 36–44.

Black, B. & Uhde, T.W. (1995) Psychiatric characteristics of children with selective mutism: a pilot study. *Journal of the American Academy of Child and Adolescent Psychiatry*, **33**, 1000–1006.

Bourin, M. & Couetoux du Tertre, A. (1992) Pharmacokinetics of psychotropic drugs in children. *Clinical Neuropharmacology*, **159** (Suppl. 1), 224A–225A.

Bradley, C. (1937) The behaviour of children receiving benzedrine. *American Journal of Psychiatry*, **94**, 577–585.

Brylewski, J. & Duggan, L. (1999) Antipsychotic medication for challenging behaviour in people with intellectual disability: a systematic review of randomized controlled trials. *Journal of Intellectual Disability Research*, **43**, 360–371.

Buitelarr, J.K., van der Gaag, R.J. & van der Hoeven, J. (1998) Buspirone in the management of anxiety and irritability in children with pervasive developmental disorders: results of an open-label study. *Journal of Clinical Psychiatry*, **59**, 56–59.

Campbell, M. (1992) The pharmacological treatment of conduct disorders and rage outbursts. *Psychiatric Clinics of North America*, **15**, 69–85.

Campbell, M., Silva, R.R., Kafantaris, V. *et al.* (1991) Predictors of side effects associated with lithium administration in children. *Psychopharmacology Bulletin*, **27**, 373–380.

Campbell, M., Adams, P.B., Small, A.M. *et al.* (1995) Lithium in hospitalized aggressive children with conduct disorder: a double-blind and placebo-controlled study. *Journal of the American Academy of Child and Adolescent Psychiatry*, **34**, 445–453.

Campbell, M., Armenteros, J.L., Malone, R.P., Adams, P.B., Eisenberg, Z.W. & Overall, J.E. (1997) Neuroleptic-related dyskinesias in autistic children: a prospective, longitudinal study. *Journal of the American Academy of Child and Adolescent Psychiatry*, **36**, 835–843.

Campbell, M., Rapoport, J.L. & Simpson, G.M. (1999) Antipsychotics in children and adolescents. *Journal of the American Academy of Child and Adolescent Psychiatry*, **38**, 537–545.

Carlson, G.A., Rapport, M.D., Pataki, C.S. & Kelly, K.L. (1992) Lithium in hospitalized children at 4 and 8 weeks: mood, behavior and cognitive effects. *Journal of Child Psychology and Psychiatry*, **33**, 411–425.

Carlson, G.A., Rapport, M.D., Kelly, K.L. & Pataki, C.S. (1995) Methylphenidate and desipramine in hospitalized children with comorbid behaviour and mood disorders: separate and combined effects on behaviour and mood. *Journal of Child and Adolescent Psychopharmacology*, **5**, 191–204.

Carter, C.M., Urbanowicz, M., Hemsley, R. *et al.* (1993) Effects of a food diet in attention deficit disorder. *Archives of Disease in Childhood*, **69**, 564–568.

Castellanos, F.X. (1999) Stimulants and tic disorders: from dogma to data [Comment]. *Archives of General Psychiatry*, **56**, 337–338.

Cohen, D., Flament, M., Taieb, O., Thompson, C. & Basquin, M. (2000) Electroconvulsive therapy in adolescence. *European Child and Adolescent Psychiatry*, **9**, 1–6.

Committee on Toxicity of Food (2000) Adverse reactions to food and food ingredients. Department of Health, London.

Connell, P.H. (1958) *Amphetamine Psychosis*. Maudsley Monographs 5. Chapman & Hall, London.

Conners, C.K., Casat, C.D., Gualtieri, C.T. *et al.* (1996) Bupropion hydrochloride in attention deficit disorder with hyperactivity. *Journal of the American Academy of Child and Adolescent Psychiatry*, **35**, 1314–1321.

Conners, K. (1980) *Food Additives and Hyperactive Children*. Plenum, New York.

Connor, D.F., Fletcher, K.E. & Swanson, J.M. (1999) A meta-analysis of clonidine for symptoms of attention-deficit hyperactivity disorder. *Journal of the American Academy of Child and Adolescent Psychiatry*, **38**, 1551–1559.

Cook, E.H. Jr, Rowlett, R., Jaselskis, C. & Leventhal, B.L. (1992) Fluoxetine treatment of children and adults with autistic disorder and mental retardation. *Journal of the American Academy of Child and Adolescent Psychiatry*, **31**, 739–745.

Crumrine, P.K., Feldman, H.M., Teodori, J., Handen, B.L. & Alvin, R.M. (1987) The use of methylphenidate in children with seizures and attention deficit disorder. *Annals of Neurology*, **22**, 441–442.

Cueva, J.E., Overall, J.E., Small, A.M., Armenteros, J.L., Perry, R. & Campbell, M. (1996) Carbamazepine in aggressive children with conduct disorder: a double-blind and placebo-controlled study. *Journal of the American Academy of Child and Adolescent Psychiatry*, **35**, 480–490.

Davidson, S. & Falconer, M.A. (1975) Outcome of surgery in 40 children with temporal-lobe epilepsy. *Lancet*, i, 1260–1263.

DeLong, G.R. & Aldershof, A.L. (1987) Long-term experience with lithium treatment in childhood: correlation with clinical diagnosis. *Journal of the American Academy of Child and Adolescent Psychiatry*, **26**, 389–394.

Demb, H.B. & Nguyen, K.T. (1999) Movement disorders in children with developmental disabilities taking risperidone. *Journal of the American Academy of Child and Adolescent Psychiatry*, **38**, 5–6.

DeVeaugh-Geiss, J., Moroz, G., Biederman, J. *et al.* (1992) Clomipramine hydrochloride in childhood and adolescent obsessive-compulsive disorder: a multicenter trial. *Journal of the American Academy of Child and Adolescent Psychiatry*, **31**, 45–49.

Dummit, S.E., Klein, R.G., Tancer, N.K., Asche, B. & Martin, J. (1996) Fluoxetine treatment of children with selective mutism: an open trial. *Journal of the American Academy of Child and Adolescent Psychiatry*, **35**, 615–621.

Elia, J., Borcherding, B.G., Rapoport, J.L. & Keysor, C.S. (1991) Methylphenidate and dextroamphetamine treatments of hyperactivity: are there true non-responders? *Psychiatry Research*, **36**, 141–155.

Emslie, G.J., Rush, A.J., Weinberg, W.A. *et al.* (1997) A double-blind, randomized, placebo-controlled trial of fluoxetine in children and adolescents with depression. *Journal of Clinical Psychiatry*, **58**, 14–29; discussion 30–1.

Emslie, G.J., Walkup, J.T., Pliszka, S.R. & Ernst, M. (1999) Nontricyclic antidepressants: current trends in children and adolescents. *Journal of the American Academy of Child and Adolescent Psychiatry*, **38**, 517–528.

Ernst, M., Malone, R.P., Rowan, A.B., George, R., Gonzalez, N.M. & Silva, R.R. (1999) Antipsychotics. In: *Practitioner's Guide to Psychoactive Drugs for Children and Adolescents*. (eds J. Werry & M. Aman) pp. 297–320. Plenum, New York.

Fankhauser, M.P., Karumanchi, V.C., German, M.L., Yates, A. & Karumanchi, S.D. (1992) A double-blind, placebo-controlled study of the efficacy of transdermal clonidine in autism. *Journal of Clinical Psychiatry*, **53**, 77–82.

Faraone, S.V. & Biederman, J. (1998) Neurobiology of attention-deficit hyperactivity disorder. *Biological Psychiatry*, **44**, 951–958.

Frazer, A. (1997) Pharmacology of antidepressants. *Journal of Clinical Psychopharmacology*, **17** (Suppl. 1), 2–18.

Frazier, J.A., Gordon, C.T., McKenna, K., Lenane, M.C., Jih, D. & Rapoport, J.L. (1994) An open trial of clozapine in 11 adolescents with childhood-onset schizophrenia. *Journal of the American Academy of Child and Adolescent Psychiatry*, **33**, 658–663.

Furlanut, M., Benetello, P., Baraldo, M., Zara, G., Montanari, G. & Donzelli, F. (1990) Chlorpromazine disposition in relation to age in children. *Clinical Pharmacokinetics*, **18**, 329–331.

Gadow, K.D., Sverd, J., Sprafkin, J., Nolan, E.E. & Grossman, S. (1999) Long-term methylphenidate therapy in children with comorbid attention-deficit hyperactivity disorder and chronic multiple tic disorder. *Archives of General Psychiatry*, **56**, 330–336.

Geller, B., Cooper, T.B., Sun, K. *et al.* (1998) Double-blind and placebo-controlled study of lithium for adolescent bipolar disorders with secondary substance dependency. *Journal of the American Academy of Child and Adolescent Psychiatry*, **37**, 171–178.

Geller, B., Reising, D., Leonard, H.L., Riddle, M.A. & Walsh, B.T. (1999) Critical review of tricyclic antidepressant use in children and adolescents. *Journal of the American Academy of Child and Adolescent Psychiatry*, **38**, 513–516.

Gillberg, C., Melander, H., von Knorring, A.L. *et al.* (1997) Long-term stimulant treatment of children with attention-deficit hyperactivity disorder symptoms: a randomized, double-blind, placebo-controlled trial. *Archives of General Psychiatry*, **54**, 857–864.

Gittelman-Klein, R. & Klein, D.F. (1971) Controlled imipramine treatment of school phobia. *Archives of General Psychiatry*, **25**, 204–207.

Gittelman-Klein, R. & Klein, D.F. (1973) School phobia: diagnostic considerations in the light of imipramine effects. *Journal of Nervous and Mental Disease*, **156**, 199–215.

Gittelman-Klein, R., Klein, D.F., Katz, S., Saraf, K. & Pollack, E. (1976) Comparative effects of methylphenidate and thioridazine in hyperkinetic children. I. Clinical results. *Archives of General Psychiatry*, **33**, 1217–1231.

Goodman, R. (1986) Hemispherectomy and its alternatives in the treatment of intractable epilepsy in patients with infantile hemiplegia. *Developmental Medicine and Child Neurology*, **28**, 251–258.

Graae, F., Milner, J., Rizzotto, L. & Klein, R.G. (1994) Clonazepam in childhood anxiety disorders. *Journal of the American Academy of Child and Adolescent Psychiatry*, **33**, 372–376.

Grados, M., Scahill, L. & Riddle, M.A. (1999) Pharmacotherapy in children and adolescents with obsessive-compulsive disorder. *Child and Adolescent Psychiatric Clinics of North America*, **8**, 617–634.

Green, W.H. (1995) The treatment of attention-deficit hyperactivity disorder with nonstimulant medications. *Child and Adolescent Psychiatric Clinics of North America*, **4**, 169–195.

Greenhill, L.L., Halperin, J.M. & Abikoff, H. (1999) Stimulant medications. *Journal of the American Academy of Child and Adolescent Psychiatry*, **38**, 503–512.

Grob, C.S. & Coyle, J.T. (1986) Suspected adverse methylphenidate–imipramine interactions in children. *Journal of Developmental and Behavioural Pediatrics*, **7**, 265–267.

Gualtieri, C.T., Quade, D., Hicks, R.E. *et al.* (1984) Tardive dyskinesia and other clinical consequences of neuroleptic treatment in children and adolescents. *American Journal of Psychiatry*, **141**, 20–23.

Hagino, O.R., Weller, E.B., Weller, R.A., Washing, D., Fristad, M.A. & Kontras, S.B. (1995) Untoward effects of lithium treatment in children aged four through six years. *Journal of the American Academy of Child and Adolescent Psychiatry*, **34**, 1584–1590.

Hallett, M. (2000) Transcranial magnetic stimulation and the human brain *Nature*, **406**, 147–150.

Hazell, P., Heathcote, D.O.C., Robertson, J. & Henry, D. (1995) Efficacy of tricyclic drugs in treating child and adolescent depression: a meta-analysis. *British Medical Journal*, **310**, 897–901.

Hunt, R.D., Arnsten, A.F.T. & Asbell, M.D. (1995) An open trial of guanfacine in the treatment of attention-deficit hyperactivity disorder. *Journal of the American Academy of Child and Adolescent Psychiatry*, **34**, 50–54.

January, J.E., Freeman, R.D. & Fast, D.K. (1999) Melatonin treatment of sleep–wake cycle disorders in children and adolescents. *Developmental Medicine and Child Neurology*, **41**, 491–500.

Jensen, P.S., Bhatara, V.S., Vitiello, B., Hoagwood, K., Feil, M. & Burke, L.B. (1999) Psychoactive medication prescribing practices for US children: gaps between research and clinical practice. *Journal of the American Academy of Child and Adolescent Psychiatry*, **38**, 557–565.

Keepers, G.A., Clappison, V.J. & Casey, D.E. (1983) Initial anticholinergic prophylaxis for neuroleptic-induced extrapyramidal syndromes. *Archives of General Psychiatry*, **40**, 1113–1117.

Klein, R.G., Landa, B., Mattes, J.A. & Klein, D.F. (1988) Methylphenidate and growth in hyperactive children: a controlled withdrawal study. *Archives of General Psychiatry*, **45**, 1127–1130.

Klein, R.G., Koplewicz, H.S. & Kanner, A. (1992) Imipramine treatment of children with separation anxiety disorder. *Journal of the American Academy of Child and Adolescent Psychiatry*, **31**, 21–28.

Koleman, B.K., Feldman, H.M., Handen, B.L. & Janosky, J.E. (1995) Naltrexone in young autistic children: a double blind, placebo-controlled crossover study. *Journal of the American Academy of Child and Adolescent Psychiatry*, **34**, 223–231.

Kranzler, H.R. (1989) Buspirone in an adolescent with overanxious disorder. *Journal of the American Academy of Child and Adolescent Psychiatry*, **50**, 382–384.

Kumra, S., Frazier, J.A., Jacobsen, L.K. *et al.* (1996) Childhood-onset schizophrenia: a double-blind clozapine–haloperidol comparison. *Archives of General Psychiatry*, **53**, 1090–1097.

Kumra, S., Jacobsen, L.K., Lenane, M. *et al.* (1998) Childhood-onset schizophrenia: an open-label study of olanzapine in adolescents. *Journal of the American Academy of Child and Adolescent Psychiatry*, **37**, 377–385.

Kutcher, S. (1997) *Child and Adolescent Psychopharmacology*. W.B. Saunders, Philadelphia, PA.

Kutcher, S.P. & MacKenzie, S. (1988) Successful clonazepam treatment of adolescents with panic disorder. *Journal of Clinical Psychopharmacology*, **8**, 299–301.

Kutcher, S., Boulos, C., Ward, B. *et al.* (1994) Response to desipramine treatment in adolescent depression: a fixed dose, placebo controlled trial. *Journal of the American Academy of Child and Adolescent Psychiatry*, **33**, 689–694.

Labellarte, M.J., Ginsburg, G.S., Walkup, J.T. & Riddle, M.A. (1999) The treatment of anxiety disorders in children and adolescents. *Biological Psychiatry*, **46**, 1567–1578.

Law, S.F. & Schachar, R.J. (1999) Do typical clinical doses of methylphenidate cause tics in children treated for attention-deficit hyperactivity disorder? *Journal of the American Academy of Child and Adolescent Psychiatry*; **38**, 944–951.

Leckman, J.F., Ort, S. & Caruso, K.A. (1986) Rebound phenomena in Tourette's syndrome after abrupt withdrawal of clonidine. *Archives of General Psychiatry*, **43**, 1168–1176.

Leckman, J.F., Hardin, M.T., Riddle, M.A., Stevenson, J., Ort, S.I. & Cohen, D.J. (1991) Clonidine treatment of Gilles de la Tourette's syndrome. *Archives of General Psychiatry*, **48**, 324–328.

Leonard, H.L., Swedo, S.E., Lenane, M.C. *et al.* (1991) A double-blind desipramine substitution during long-term clomipramine treatment in children and adolescents with obsessive-compulsive disorder. *Archives of General Psychiatry*, **48**, 922–927.

Leonard, H.L., Swedo, S.E., Lenane, M.C. *et al.* (1993) A 2- to 7-year follow-up study of 54 obsessive-compulsive children and adolescents. *Archives of General Psychiatry*, **50**, 429–439.

Lindsay, J., Ounsted, C. & Richards, P. (1987) Hemispherectomy for childhood epilepsy: a 36-year study. *Developmental Medicine and Child Neurology*, **29**, 592–600.

Livingston, R.L., Dykman, R.A. & Ackerman, P.T. (1992) Psychiatric comorbidity and response to two doses of methylphenidate in children with attention deficit disorder. *Journal of Child and Adolescent Psychopharmacology*, 2, 115–122.

Malhotra, S. & Santosh, P.J. (1998) An open clinical trial of buspirone in children with AD/HD. *Journal of the American Academy of Child and Adolescent Psychiatry*, 37, 364–371.

Mandoki, M.W., Tapia, M.R., Tapia, M.A., Sumner, G.S. & Parker, J.L. (1997) Venlafaxine in the treatment of children and adolescents with major depression. *Journal of the American Academy of Child and Adolescent Psychiatry*, 36, 725–736.

March, J.S. & Vitiello, B. (2001) Advances in paediatric neuropsychopharmacology: an overview. *International Journal of Neuropsychopharmacology*, 4, 141–147.

March, J.S., Biederman, J., Wolkow, R. *et al.* (1998) Sertraline in children and adolescents with obsessive-compulsive disorder: a multicenter randomized controlled trial. *Journal of the American Medical Association*, 280, 1752–1756.

McDougle, C.J., Naylor, R.N., Cohen, D.J., Volkmar, F.R., Heniger, G.R. & Price, L.H. (1996) A double-blind placebo-controlled study of fluvoxamine in adults with autistic disorder. *Archives of General Psychiatry*, 53, l001–1008.

McDougle, C.J., Holmes, J.P., Bronson, M.K. *et al.* (1997) Risperidone treatment of children and adolescents with PDD: a prospective open-label study. *Journal of the American Academy of Child and Adolescent Psychiatry*, 36, 685–693.

McDougle, C.J., Holmes, J.P., Carlson, D.C. *et al.* (1998) A double-blind, placebo-controlled study of risperidone in adults with autistic disorder and other pervasive developmental disorders. *Archives of General Psychiatry*, 55, 633–641.

Mezzacappa, E., Steingard, R., Kindlon, D., Saul, P. & Earls, F. (1998) Tricyclic antidepressants and cardiac autonomic control in children and adolescents *Journal of the American Academy of Child and Adolescent Psychiatry*, 37, 52–59.

MTA Cooperative Group (1999) A 14-month randomized clinical trial of treatment strategies for attention-deficit/hyperactivity disorder. The MTA Cooperative Group Multimodal Treatment Study of Children with ADHD. *Archives of General Psychiatry*, 56, 1073–1086.

Nass, R., Gross, A., Wisoff, J. & Devinsky, O. (1999) Outcome of multiple subpial transections for autistic epileptiform regression. *Pediatric Neurology*, 21, 464–470.

Nestler, E.J. (1998) Antidepressant treatment in the 21st century. *Biological Psychiatry*, 44, 526–533.

Olvera, R.L., Pliszka, S.R., Luh, J. & Tatum, R. (1996) An open trial of venlafaxine in the treatment of attention-deficit/hyperactivity disorder in children and adolescents. *Journal of Child and Adolescent Psychopharmacology*, 6, 241–250.

Papatheodorou, G., Kutcher, S.P., Katic, M. & Szalai, J.P. (1995) The efficacy and safety of divalproex sodium in the treatment of acute mania in adolescents and young adults: an open clinical trial. *Journal of Clinical Psychopharmacology*, 15, 110–116.

Pelham, W.E. Jr (1999) The NIMH multimodal treatment study for attention-deficit hyperactivity disorder: just say yes to drugs alone? *Canadian Journal of Psychiatry*, 44, 981–990.

Peterson, B.S. & Leckman, J.F. (1998) The temporal dynamics of tics in Gilles de la Tourette syndrome. *Biological Psychiatry*, 44, 1337–1348.

Pfefferbaum, B., Overall, J.E., Boren, H.A., Frankel, L.S., Sullivan, M.P. & Johnson, K. (1987) Alprazolam in the treatment of anticipatory and acute situational anxiety in children with cancer. *Journal of the American Academy of Child and Adolescent Psychiatry*, 26, 532–535.

Pliska, S.R. (1989) Effect of anxiety on cognition, behaviour, and stimulant response in ADHD. *Journal of the American Academy of Child and Adolescent Psychiatry*, 28, 882–887.

Pliska, S.R., Greenhill, L., Crimson, M.L. *et al.* (2000) The Texas Children's Medication Algorithm Project. Report of the Texas Consensus Conference Panel on Medication Treatment of Childhood AD/HD. Part I. *Journal of the American Academy of Child and Adolescent Psychiatry*, 39, 908–919.

Popper, C.W. (1998) Antidepressants in the treatment of attention-deficit/hyperactivity disorder. *Journal of the American Academy of Child and Adolescent Psychiatry*, 37, 52–59.

Potenza, M.N., Holmes, J.P., Kanes, S.J. & McDougle, C.J. (1999) Olanzapine treatment of children, adolescents, and adults with pervasive developmental disorders: an open-label pilot study. *Journal of Clinical Psychopharmacology*, 19, 37–44.

Quintana, H., Birmaher, B., Stedge, D. *et al.* (1995) Use of methylphenidate in the treatment of children with autistic disorder. *Journal of Autism and Developmental Disorder*, 25, 283–294.

Rapoport, J.L. (1998) Child psychopharmacology comes of age. *Journal of the American Medical Association*, 280, 1785.

Rapoport, J.L., Buchsbaum, M.S., Weingartner, H., Zahn, T.P., Ludlow, C. & Mikkelslen, E.J. (1980a) Dextroamphetamine: its cognitive and behavioral effects in normal and hyperactive boys and men. *Archives of General Psychiatry*, 37, 933–943.

Rapoport, J.L., Mikkelsen, E.J., Zaradil, A. *et al.* (1980b) Childhood enuresis. II. Psychopathology, tricyclic concentration in plasma, and antienuretic effect. *Archives of General Psychiatry*, 37, 1146–1152.

Rapport, M.D., Denney, C., DuPaul, G. & Gardner, M.J. (1994) Attention deficit disorder and methylphenidate: normalization rates, clinical effectiveness, and response prediction in 76 children. *Journal of the American Academy of Child and Adolescent Psychiatry*, 33, 882–893.

Realmuto, G.M., Erikson, W.D., Yellin, A.M., Hopwood, J.H. & Greenberg, L.M. (1984) Clinical comparison of thiothixene and thioridazine in schizophrenic adolescents. *American Journal of Psychiatry*, 141, 440–442.

Reiter-Theil, S. (1992) Autonomy and beneficience: ethical issues in electro-convulsive therapy. *Convulsive Therapy*, 8, 237–244.

Rey, J.M. & Walter, G. (1997) Half a century of ECT use in young people. *American Journal of Psychiatry*, 154, 595–602.

Riddle, M.A., Hardin, M.T., King, R., Scahill, L. & Woolston, J.L. (1990) Fluoxetine treatment of children and adolescents with Tourette's and obsessive compulsive disorders: preliminary clinical experience. *Journal of the American Academy of Child and Adolescent Psychiatry*, 29, 45–48.

Riddle, M.A., Bernstein, G.A., Cook, E.H., Leonard, H.L., March, J.S. & Swanson, J.M. (1999) Anxiolytics, adrenergic agents, and naltrexone. *Journal of the American Academy of Child and Adolescent Psychiatry*, 38, 546–556.

Riddle, M.A., Kastelic, E.A. & Frosch, E. (2001) Pediatric psychopharmacology. *Journal of Child Psychology and Psychiatry*, 42, 73–90.

Rifkin, A., Karajgi, B., Dicker, R. *et al.* (1997) Lithium treatment of conduct disorders in adolescents. *American Journal of Psychiatry*, 154, 554–555.

Ryan, N.D., Puig-Antich, J., Rabinovich, H. *et al.* (1988) MAOIs in adolescent major depression unresponsive to tricyclic antidepressants. *Journal of the American Academy of Child and Adolescent Psychiatry*, 27, 755–758.

Ryan, N.D., Bhatara, V.S. & Perel, J.M. (1999) Mood stabilizers in children and adolescents. *Journal of the American Academy of Child and Adolescent Psychiatry*, 38, 529–536.

Safer, D.J. & Allen, R.P. (1989) Absence of tolerance to the behavioral effects of methylphenidate in hyperactive and inattentive children. *Journal of Pediatrics*, 115, 1003–1008.

Sallee, F.R., Nesbitt, L., Jackson, C., Sine, L. & Sethuraman, G. (1997) Relative efficacy of haloperidol and pimozide in children and adolescents with Tourette's disorder [see comments]. *American Journal of Psychiatry*, **154**, 1057–1062.

Sallee, F.R., Kurlan, R., Goetz, C.G. *et al.* (2000) Ziprasidone treatment of children and adolescents with Tourette's syndrome: a pilot study. *Journal of the American Academy of Child and Adolescent Psychiatry*, **39**, 292–299.

Santosh, P.J. & Baird, G. (1999) Psychopharmacotherapy in children and adults with intellectual disability. *Lancet*, **354**, 233–242.

Santosh, P.J. & Taylor, E. (2000) Stimulant drugs. *European Child and Adolscent Psychiatry*, **9** (Suppl. 1), I27–43.

Scahill, L., Chappell, P.B., King, R.A. & Leckman, J.F. (2000) Pharmacologic treatment of tic disorders. *Child and Adolescent Psychiatric Clinics of North America*, **9**, 99–117.

Seeman, P., Lee, T., Chau-Wong, M. & Wong, K. (1976) Antipsychotic drug doses and neuroleptic/dopamine receptors. *Nature*, **261**, 717–719.

Shapiro, E., Shapiro, A.K., Fulop, G. *et al.* (1989) Controlled study of haloperidol, pimozide and placebo for the treatment of Gilles de la Tourette's syndrome. *Archives of General Psychiatry*, **46**, 722–730.

Silva, R.R., Munoz, D.M. & Alpert, M. (1996) Carbamazepine use in children and adolescents with features of attention-deficit hyperactivity disorder: a meta-analysis. *Journal of the American Academy of Child and Adolescent Psychiatry*, **35**, 352–358.

Silva, R.R., Munoz, D.M., Alpert, M., Perlmutter, I.R. & Diaz, J. (1999) Neuroleptic malignant syndrome in children and adolescents. *Journal of the American Academy of Child and Adolescent Psychiatry*, **38**, 187–194.

Simeon, J.G., Knott, V.J., Thatte, S., Dubois, C.D., Wiggins, D.M. & Geraets, I. (1992) Pharmacotherapy of childhood anxiety disorders. *Pediatric Psychopharmacology*, **15** (Suppl. 1), 229A–230A.

Solanto, M.V. (1998) Neuropsychopharmacological mechanisms of stimulant drug action in attention-deficit hyperactivity disorder: a review and integration. *Behavioural Brain Research*, **94**, 127–152.

Spencer, E.K. & Campbell, M. (1994) Children with schizophrenia: diagnosis, phenomenology, and pharmacotherapy. *Schizophrenia Bulletin*, **20**, 713–725.

Spencer, E.K., Kafantaris, V., Padron-Gayol, M.V., Rosenberg, C. & Campbell, M. (1992) Haloperidol in schizophrenic children: early findings from a study in progress. *Psychopharmacology Bulletin*, **28**, 183–186.

Spencer, T.J., Biederman, J., Harding, M., Faraone, S.V. & Wilens, T.E. (1996a) Growth deficits in ADHD children revisited: evidence for disorder-associated growth delays? *Journal of the American Academy of Child and Adolescent Psychiatry*, **35**, 1460–1469.

Spencer, T., Biederman, J., Wilens, T., Harding, M., O'Donnell, D. & Griffin, S. (1996b) Pharmacotherapy of attention-deficit hyperactivity disorder across the life cycle. *Journal of the American Academy of Child and Adolescent Psychiatry*, **35**, 409–432.

Steingard, R., Biederman, J., Spencer, T., Wilens, T. & Gonzalez, A. (1993) Comparison of clonidine response in the treatment of attention-deficit hyperactivity disorder with and without comorbid tic disorders. *Journal of the American Academy of Child and Adolescent Psychiatry*, **32**, 350–353.

Steingard, R.J., Zimnitzky, B., De Maso, D.R., Bauman, M.L. & Bucci, J.P. (1997) Sertraline treatment of transition-associated anxiety and agitation in children with autistic disorder. *Journal of Child and Adolescent Psychopharmacology*, **7**, 9–15.

Sternbach, H. (1991) The serotonin syndrome. *American Journal of Psychiatry*, **148**, 705–713.

Strober, M., Morrell, W., Lampert, C. & Burroughs, J. (1990) Relapse following discontinuation of lithium maintenance therapy in adoles-

cents with bipolar I illness: a naturalistic study. *American Journal of Psychiatry*, **147**, 457–461.

Swanson, J.M., Flockhart, D., Udrea, D., Cantwell, D., Conner, D. & Williams, L. (1995) Clonidine in the treatment of ADHD: questions about safety and efficacy. *Journal of Child and Adolescent Psychopharmacology*, **5**, 301–304.

Swanson, J.M., Connor, D.F. & Cantwell, D. (1999) Combining methylphenidate and clonidine: ill-advised. *Journal of the American Academy of Child and Adolescent Psychiatry*, **38**, 617–619.

Tannock, R., Ickowicz, A. & Schachar, R. (1995) Differential effects of methylphenidate on working memory in ADHD children with and without comorbid anxiety. *Journal of the American Academy of Child and Adolescent Psychiatry*, **7**, 886–896.

Taylor, E. (1999) Development of clinical services for attention-deficit/hyperactivity disorder. *Archives of General Psychiatry*, **56**, 1097–1099.

Taylor, E., Schachar, R., Thorley, G., Wieselberg, H.M., Everitt, B. & Rutter, M. (1987) Which boys respond to stimulant medication? A controlled trial of methylphenidate in boys with disruptive behaviour. *Psychological Medicine*, **17**, 121–143.

The Research Unit on Pediatric Psychopharmacology Anxiety Study Group (2001) Fluvoxamine for the treatment of anxiety disorders in children and adolescents. *New England Journal of Medicine*, **344**, 1279–1285.

Thomsen, P.H. (1997) Child and adolescent obsessive-compulsive disorder treated with citalopram: findings from an open trial of 23 cases. *Journal of Child and Adolescent Psychopharmacology*, **7**, 157–166.

Tosyali, M.C. & Greenhill, L.L. (1998) Child and adolescent psychopharmacology: important developmental issues. *Pediatric Clinics of North America*, **45**, 1021–1035.

Tueth, M.J., Murphy, T.K. & Evans, D.L. (1998) Special considerations: use of lithium in children, adolescents, and elderly populations. *Journal of Clinical Psychiatry*, **59**, 66–73.

Vincent, J., Varley, C.K. & Leger, P. (1990) Effects of methylphenidate on early adolescent growth. *American Journal of Psychiatry*, **147**, 501–502.

Vitiello, B., Behar, D., Malone, R., Delaney, M.A., Ryan, P.J. & Simpson, G.M. (1988) Pharmacokinetics of lithium carbonate in children. *Journal of Clinical Psychopharmacology*, **8**, 355–359.

Volkmar, F.R. (1999) Lessons from secretin. *New England Journal of Medicine*, **341**, 1842–1844.

Volkow, N.D., Wang, G.J., Fowler, J.S. *et al.* (1998) Dopamine transporter occupancies in the human brain induced by therapeutic doses of oral methylphenidate. *American Journal of Psychiatry*, **155**, 1325–1331.

Wahlbeck, K., Cheine, M., Essali, A. & Adams, C. (1999) Evidence of clozapine's effectiveness in schizophrenia: a systematic review and meta-analysis of randomized trials. *American Journal of Psychiatry*, **156**, 990–999.

Walsh, B.T. (1998) *Child Psychopharmacology*. American Psychiatric Press, Washington D.C.

Werry, J. & Aman, M. (1999) *Practitioner's Guide to Psychoactive Drugs for Children and Adolescents*. Plenum, New York.

Wilens, T.E. & Spencer, T.J. (1999) Combining methylphenidate and clonidine: a clinically sound medication option. *Journal of the American Academy of Child and Adolescent Psychiatry*, **38**, 614–616.

Wilens, T.E., Biederman, J., Baldessarini, R.J., Puopolo, P.R. & Flood, J.G. (1992) Developmental changes in serum concentrations of desipramine and 2-hydroxydesipramine during treatment with desipramine. *Journal of the American Academy of Child and Adolescent Psychiatry*, **31**, 691–698.

Wilens, T.E., Biederman, J., Geist, D.E., Steingard, R. & Spender, T. (1993) Nortriptyline in the treatment of ADHD: a chart review of 58 cases. *Journal of the American Academy of Child and Adolescent Psychiatry*, 32, 343–349.

Wilens, T.E., Spencer, T.J., Biederman, J. & Schleifer, D. (1997) Case study: nefazodone for juvenile mood disorders. *Journal of the American Academy of Child and Adolescent Psychiatry*, 36, 481–485.

Williams, J., Griebel, M.L., Sharp, G.B. & Boop, F.A. (1998) Cognition and behavior after temporal lobectomy in pediatric patients with intractable epilepsy. *Pediatric Neurology*, 19, 189–194.

Wright, H.H., Cuccaro, M.L., Leonnardt, T.V., Kendall, D.F. & Anderson, J.H. (1995) Case study: fluoxetine in the multimodel treatment of a preschool child with selective mutism. *Journal of the American Academy of Child and Adolescent Psychiatry*, 34, 857–862.

Yang, T.F., Wong, T.T., Kwan, S.Y., Chang, K.P., Lee, Y.C. & Hsu, T.C. (1996) Quality of life and life satisfaction in families after a child has undergone corpus callostomy. *Epilepsia*, 37, 76–80.

Zametkin, A.J. & Liotta, W. (1998) The neurobiology of attention-deficit/hyperactivity disorder. *Journal of Clinical Psychiatry*, 59 (Suppl. 7), 17–23.

Zito, J.M., Safer, D.J., DosReis, S. & Riddle, M.A. (1998) Racial disparity in psychotropic medications prescribed for youths with Medicaid insurance in Maryland. *Journal of the American Academy of Child and Adolescent Psychiatry*, 37, 179–184.

Zito, J.M., Safer, D.J., dosReis, S., Gardner, J.F., Boles, M. & Lynch, F. (2000) Trends in the prescribing of psychotropic medications to preschoolers. *Journal of the American Medical Association*, 283, 1025–1030.

Zwier, K.J. & Rao, U. (1994) Buspirone use in an adolescent with social phobia and mixed personality disorder (cluster A type). *Journal of the American Academy of Child and Adolescent Psychiatry*, 33, 1007–1011.

60 Treatment of Delinquents

Sue Bailey

Introduction

Delinquency, conduct problems and aggression all refer to anti-social behaviours that reflect a failure of the individual to conform his or her behaviour to the expectations of some authority figure, to societal norms, or to respect the rights of other people. The 'behaviours' can range from mild conflicts with authority figures, to major violation of societal norms, to serious violations of the rights of others (Frick 1998). The term 'delinquency' implies that the acts could result in conviction, although most do not do so. The term 'juvenile' usually applies to the age range, extending from a lower age set by age of criminal responsibility to an upper age when a young person can be dealt with in courts for adult crimes. These ages vary between, and indeed within, countries and are not the same for all offences (Justice 1996; Cavadino & Allen 2000).

This chapter sets out to review the historical context of the justice, welfare, treatment, punishment, issues of definition, size of the problem, assessment, range of interventions and the evidence base for efficacy of treatment and outcomes. Of particular interest is the role of mental health practitioners in assessment and treatment of young delinquents, their role in court proceedings, risk and needs assessment and service delivery and the interplay between offending and mental disorder (Bailey 1996).

Historical context

The need to control a small group of very persistent recalcitrant children is perennial. Specific methods have been available since at least the eighteenth century (Hagell *et al.* 2000). In the eighteenth and nineteenth centuries children were seldom distinguished from adults and were placed with adults in prison. In the England of 1823, boys as young as 9 years were held in solitary confinement for their own protection in ships retired from the Battle of Trafalgar. In the nineteenth century, legislation regarding Children's Rights was tied into the need for labour. There have been periodic reactions against convicting, imprisoning and punishing young people. The pioneers who sought to rescue both young offenders and those children offended against provided the beginnings of youth justice, care and child protection. Both community and secure residential innovations in youth justice have been characterized by a pattern of reforming zeal, followed by gradual disappointment fuelled by the results of research evaluations.

Throughout the twentieth century, concerns about levels of juvenile offending increasingly absorbed the attention of public, politicians, practitioners and researchers (Burt 1925; Glover 1960; Rutter & Giller 1983; Rutter *et al.* 1998). Throughout the Western world (Junger-Tas 1994) there has been a growing widespread perception that juvenile crime is inevitable, a fact of life in an increasingly violent society (Shepherd & Farrington 1993). The necessity to curb the spread of serious juvenile crime has clearly acquired a new urgency. A hundred years ago, the conception of juvenile justice in the USA had as its purpose, through the juvenile court, the creation of a whole new system of law for responding to youthful offending based on the developmental premise that young people were still malleable and could be saved from a life of crime. This philosophy held its ground for 90 years until the USA experienced a high tide of youth violence that began in the late 1980s (Zimring 1998). Grisso (1996) commented that in its wake the 'rehabilitative approach to juvenile justice has all but disappeared in the USA in an avalanche of massive legislative efforts to transform it'. These changes are echoed in the overhaul of the Youth Justice System in England and Wales (Bailey 1999a).

Size and nature of the problem

In describing young offenders, the terms 'frequent', 'persistent', 'serious' and 'chronic' have been used to indicate a perceived extreme end of a continuum of juvenile offending. Identifying and providing successful treatment for 'persistent' young offenders is a practical imperative but there is considerable variation in how 'persistence' in offending has been defined (Wolfgang *et al.* 1987; Hagell & Newburn 1994; Farrington 1995; Graham & Bowling 1995).

A picture of 'persistent' offenders emerges that show them to be broadly similar to other offenders but that they show their characteristics to a much greater degree (Farrington & West 1993). They are more likely to be male and have started offending at a young age (Junger-Tas & Block 1988) but the profile of offences does not differ strikingly from that of other young offenders (Weitekamp *et al.* 1996). The focus on frequency over severity of offending raises the possibility of overemphasizing the dangerousness of persistent juvenile offenders. Of relevance to multiagency treatment responses is the emerging pattern of persistent offenders displaying more educational problems, a lack of social integration, more disruptive family backgrounds, experience of institutional care (Hagell & Newburn 1994) and a group that are more likely to have more developmental difficulties including hyperactivity (Magnusson *et al.* 1994). The proportion of 'persistent' young offenders is likely to be about 3–6% of males in the general adolescent population and this group have been estimated to account for between one-quarter and one-half of juvenile crime. The increased recognition of the heterogeneity of serious antisocial behaviour is leading to the development of possible key differentiations that should in turn inform the direction and development of treatment programmes for a group of young offenders who commit particular crimes (Rutter & Smith 1995; Rutter *et al.* 1998).

Longitudinal research suggests that at least two main groups can be delineated. The more common group involves 'adolescent limited' antisocial behaviour involving one-quarter or more of the general population (Moffit 1993). 'Life-course-persistent' antisocial behaviour is different in having both an unusually early age of onset and a tendency to persist into adult life. This occurs in some 6% of the population (Stattin & Magnusson 1991, 1996; Moffit *et al.* 1996; Kratzer & Hodgins 1997). This incidence is comparable to that for antisocial personality disorder in adult males (Robins & Price 1991).

Reviews have reported a rise in antisocial behaviour over recent decades in both Europe and North America (Smith 1995; Elliott *et al.* 1998; Rutter *et al.* 1998). Most juvenile crime is theft related (Junger-Tas & Block 1988; Wikstrom 1990; Snyder *et al.* 1996). Rutter *et al.* (1998) illustrated this with figures showing a fivefold increase in recorded offences in the UK over the period 1950–90; the great majority of such offences will have been committed by those under 25. Elliott *et al.* (1998) reported a steady rise in crime in those under 18 in the USA, noting a particular rise in violent crime in this age group. Smith (1995) reported similar trends in European countries.

The greater male involvement in crime is a universal finding that applies across cultures over time and is evident on all types of measure. However, over the last 40 years the sex ratio for crime has fallen from about 11 : 1 to 4 : 1, with the peak age of offending being 18 for young men and 15 for young women. Rates differ by country and by type. Violent crimes form a small proportion of known offending by young people—about 10%—but most very frequent offenders will have a violent offence on their record. Crimes involving the use of a gun by young people are 15 times higher in the USA than in Europe.

Ethnic minorities are overrepresented in official statistics but do not appear to be more antisocial on self-reports, as noted by both Krisberg *et al.* (1987) in the USA and Graham & Bowling (1995) in the UK. This discrepancy between official statistics and self-report data leads to questions about how law enforcement agencies deal with young people from diverse cultural and ethnic backgrounds (Lockman & Wayland 1994).

Self-report procedures (Huizinga & Elliot 1986; Graham & Bowling 1995) have shown high levels of self-reported offending behaviour, with a strong connection between self-report and official records when more serious offences are considered (Huizinga & Jacob-Chien 1998; Farrington 2000).

Findings from a second sweep of the Youth Lifestyle Survey (YLS; Home Office 2000; Flood-Page *et al.* 2000) provides a recent snapshot of admissions of offending among 12–30 year olds confirming previous findings. One-quarter of young men and one in 10 young women had offended, but the majority reported only one or two minor offences (criminal damage, buying stolen goods). Nevertheless, 12% of men and 4% of women were persistent offenders, and 2% of the whole sample (10% of offenders) were responsible for nearly half the crimes admitted. One-quarter of the young people aged 12–17 who were persistent offenders had been cautioned or taken to court. Other key findings were a rise over time in male violence by 14–17 year olds. The YLS study showed that poor parental supervision, having delinquent friends and acquaintances, persistent truanting and exclusion from school were all predictive of offending. It also showed the importance of lifestyle factors as a link to higher offending rates for males. Drug use was highly predictive across the full 12–30-year-old age range and heavy drinking was predictive for 18–30 year olds.

Risk assessment and management

The adult literature

Predicting the future risk of violent behaviour has a long and difficult history (Dolan & Doyle 2000). There has been a gradual and helpful shift from dangerousness as a subjective concept to risk as a quantitative concept of factors that predict violence, although not in themselves direct indicators of violence. The combination of factors that makes up risk will fluctuate over time and may be modified and managed. Violence risk assessment and management are key components of clinical practice (Monahan 1992).

Clinicians have traditionally assessed risk on an individual basis, using case formulation ('unaided clinical judgement'). Adult research has focused on the accuracy of risk prediction variables in large heterogeneous populations using relatively static actuarial predictions. The debate about clinical vs. actuarial risk prediction has led to the development of violence prediction instruments that combine the importance of static actuarial variables and clinical/risk management items that clinicians take into account in risk assessment of individuals.

The MacArthur Violence Risk Assessment Study (Monahan & Appelbaum 2000) highlighted the significance of clinical factors in the prediction of violent outcomes among non-forensic psychiatric patients discharged from hospital (Steadman *et al.* 1994, 1998). Domains in the MacArthur Risk Assessment Study were grouped under:

1 dispositional factors;
2 historical factors;
3 contextual factors; and
4 clinical factors.

Structured clinical judgements are a composite of empirical knowledge and clinical professional expertise. Webster *et al.* (1997) developed the Historical/Clinical Risk Management 20-item (HCR-20) Scale to assess risk of violence in clinical contexts. This and other similar instruments (Douglas & Cox 1999) emphasize the importance in risk assessment of the following.

1 Use of well-defined published schema.

2 Good agreement among assessors, obtained through training and experience.

3 Prediction for a defined type of violent behaviour over a specified period.

4 Violent acts predicted should be detectable and recorded.

5 All relevant information should be available and substantiated.

6 Actuarial estimates should be adjusted only if there is sufficient justification.

Putting systematic risk assessment into practice, Gardner *et al.* (1996) developed a 'regression tree' (structured sequences of yes/no answers that lead to classification of cases as high or low risk, employing a two-stage screening process). Monahan & Applebaum (2000) also developed an iterative classification tree (ICT). These methods appear to be a useful means for violence risk assessments in large populations with relatively low base rates of violence. In smaller samples of high-risk patients or offenders, more in-depth batteries of relevant tools, such as HCR-20, are required to assess future risk of violent recidivism.

Risk assessment in young people

The literature on specific needs and risk assessment in adolescents who offend and/or have mental health problems is developing. The issue of assessment is closely linked to the issues of both prevention and treatment.

Reviewing both prospective and retrospective research, Boswell (1997) suggested that victimization and family breakdown at an early age are associated with an increased risk of later physical abuse and violence. Stiffman *et al.* (1996), in their US longitudinal study, found that a combination of personal variables (gender, substance misuse) and environmental variables (history of child abuse, stressful and traumatic events, rates of unemployment) predicted almost one-third of the variance in adolescent violent behaviour.

Studies of associations between violent behaviour in adolescents and psychosis are rare (Clare *et al.* 2000). Inamder *et al.* (1982) discussed the impact of adolescent developmental crises and how sociocultural factors may mediate the expression of both violence and psychosis. Developmental aspects of violence, criminality and illness are critical considerations.

General principles in managing risk in adolescents include the following.

• Gathering of information from several sources.

• Acceptance that risk cannot be eliminated or guaranteed, but is dynamic and so must be frequently reviewed.

Table 60.1 Approach to risk assessment in young people (Sheldrick 1999).

Index offence
Seriousness
Nature and quality
Victim characteristics
Intention and motive
Role in offence
Behaviour
Attitude to offence
Victim empathy
Compassion for others

Past offences
Juvenile record
Number of previous arrests
Convictions for violence
Cautions
Self-reported offending

Past behavioural problems
Violence
Self-harm
Fire setting
Cruelty to animals
Cruelty to children

• Who does what part in multidisciplinary and multiagency teams. Decisions should not be made by one person alone.

• Some risks are general and others specific, with particular victims.

• Outcomes must be shared but within the boundaries of 'needs to know' and level of confidentiality expected.

Sheldrick (1999) suggested the approach to risk assessment in young people in Table 60.1. Attention should be paid to predisposing situations, triggers, frequency, severity and trends over time. The assessment of empathy with the victim must take into account the emotional and developmental status of a young person and with an understanding of the protective mechanisms of amnesia and clinical denial following a violent offence (see section on juvenile homicide below). Risk escalates when there is failed multiagency risk assessment and management, which in turn includes failure to respond to reported episodes of violence, poor record-keeping and communication, and taking a cross-sectional rather than long-term view of the young person and their behaviour.

More specific needs and risk assessment tools are being developed for young people. The HCR-20 now has a version for boys aged 12 and under (EARL-20B; Augimeri *et al.* 1998). Work is also underway on an adolescent HCR-20. Hare's adult psychopathy checklist (PCL-R) has been used with adolescent offenders (Gretton *et al.* 1997). The Psychopathy Screening Device has been developed for children, and is rated by parent and teachers (Frick 1996). A second instrument derived from the PCL-R (PCL:YV) is designed to measure psychopathy amongst adolescents (Forth 1995; Forth *et al.* in press).

Any risk assessment should be accompanied by a comprehensive needs assessment. The Salford Needs Assessment Schedule for Adolescents (Kroll *et al.* 1999) identifies 21 areas of potential need, assesses the significance of each need in young people and how each may be met by services. Areas covered include material, familial, social education and psychiatric problems including aggression and self-harm.

Young people are often referred for the assessment of anger and aggressive acts. Attention needs to be paid to *where* the behaviour takes place (home, school, shops, on public transport, in recreational areas) and whether drugs, alcohol or solvents are involved. *Who* else is involved (mother, father, siblings, friends, strangers, neighbours), together with their *reaction*, should be determined. *Frequency*, *intensity*, *duration*, form of expression, effect on relationships, effect on school work and the effect on health should all be brought into the risk equation. Once assessment has been made, the practitioner needs to state the risk as specifically as possible and each risk should be stated separately. Risk should only be predicted for the immediate/short-term future. Whatever type of risk assessment is used by the clinician, the multiagency team needs to know the situational factors. Will the behaviour occur in the public/domestic domain, with/without provocation, in the immediate or extended vicinity? Will the victim(s) be perceived by the young person as vulnerable? Will the young person hold hostile attributions to the victim? Will the victim elicit certain meanings for the young person (e.g. authority abuser, bully)? Will the victim be in the immediate or in an extended vicinity? Always list who are potential victims. Finally, does the young person lack an adequate concept of emotion, lack skills (e.g. thinking or non-aggressive coping strategies), abuse substances, engage in other high-risk behaviour and is he or she easily provoked? Risk assessment and management in young delinquents must be informed by those with expertise in developmental understanding of young people. Mental health practitioners have an important role, a role that is likely to increase and which will have particular importance when the young delinquent has 'special needs' and mental health problems.

Interventions

Although current early preventative initiatives, well established in the USA and underway in Europe, have shown promising results with generally disadvantaged children (Olweus 1993; see also Offord & Bennett, Chapter 52), many early intervention programmes with pre-adolescents have been found to be least effective with individuals whose antisocial behaviour is severe and chronic and also for individuals with comorbid conditions (Kazdin 1996, 1997; Le Blanc 1998). This has been confirmed by results from both peer, school and community interventions (Brewer *et al.* 1995).

Andrews *et al.* (1986) put forward the 'risk principle' for those with established antisocial behaviours. Intervention is most effective when the young person being treated has appreciable risk of an adverse outcome. Little & Mount (1999) concluded that the further down the various pathways and psychological problems a child goes, the more predictable his or her behaviour becomes. Results from the Cambridge study of working class boys showed one-third of 8 year olds followed up had been convicted by the time they were 25, but up to 60% of those convicted in adolescence were convicted again in adulthood (Farrington 1995).

In dealing with high-risk individuals, both obtaining their engagement and innovation in intervention is needed. Tolan & Gorman-Smith (1997) concluded that the choice of group to intervene with is a practical trade-off between the likely responsiveness to treatment and the predictability of risk and seriousness of offending. In designing interventions, consideration has to be given to the size of the target population, the choice of risk factors to be tackled and the need for early or late intervention. Multiple interventions at multiple points throughout the life course are required to overcome the problems of those at higher risk, beginning with broad community-based interventions and progressing to highly specific interventions for a small group who require more intensive input.

Multimodal treatments are more like to tackle the multiple causes of severe behavioural problems as well as providing a sufficient 'dosage' to impact on severe and chronic antisocial behaviour (Kazdin 1996). To date, interventions with adolescents show limited results. There is no conclusive evidence regarding the effectiveness of any single intervention. This reflects the inadequacy of evaluations as much as any inherent inadequacy of the intervention itself (McGuire & Priestley 1995). Any intervention has to be theory based, addressing known causal factors, building on a young person's strength as well as tackling antisocial behaviour and antecedent risk factors. Regardless of the treatment setting, the interventions should be carried out in a manner consistent to their original design; treatment integrity affects results. Interventions should address comorbid conditions, such as substance misuse and depression, that aggravate behavioural problems. These features have yet to be incorporated into an evaluation study without methodological flaws. However, multimodal well-structured intensive lengthy programmes that are cognitive-behavioural in orientation are required to provide a sufficient 'dosage' to impact on adolescents with marked levels of antisocial behaviour. Interventions closely tailored to the characteristics of the individual may be more successful than broader population-based strategies. Interventions will need to be lengthy and/or repeated to sustain improved functioning in those at highest risk.

In the long run, multimodal interventions that are well organized, structured and intensive for adolescents at highest risk of offending and adult personality disorder, although initially more costly, may prove more effective (McGuire 1996; Lipsey & Wilson 1998).

Early interventions

There are four types of prevention and early intervention that can reduce juvenile offending (Tonry & Farrington 1995).

1 *Criminal justice prevention*: deterrence, incapacitation and rehabilitation strategies operated by law enforcement and criminal justice agencies.

2 *Situational prevention*: designed to reduce the opportunities for antisocial behaviour and to increase the risk and difficulty of committing antisocial acts.

3 *Community prevention*: interventions designed to change social conditions and social institutions that influence antisocial behaviour in communities.

4 *Developmental prevention*: interventions designed to inhibit the development of antisocial behaviour in individuals by targeting risk and protective factors that influence human development.

Successful early interventions for juvenile offending depend on the efficacy of parent training (Bank *et al.* 1991; Webster-Stratton 1994; Smith 1996; Byng-Hall & Putman 1998; see also Offord & Bennett, Chapter 52; and Scott, Chapter 56) and preschool programmes (Schweinhart *et al.* 1993) that enable young people to understand more readily the consequences of their behaviour for self and peers, critically helping them to make safe choices and teach safe autonomy in adolescence. Lipsey (1995) suggested the importance of three strategies:

1 primary population-based preventative intervention;

2 secondary interventions focused on high-risk groups; and

3 programmes centred on tertiary treatment.

'Communities that care' (Joseph Rowntree Foundation 1997) is now established in the UK, modelled on the US programmes (Hawkins & Catalano 1992) and on other UK preventative public health campaigns. A risk-focused prevention programme tailored to the needs of each community targets five main behaviours that are damaging to the lives of adolescents and the communities where they live: youth crime, drug abuse, school-age pregnancy, sexually transmitted disease and school failure.

Treatment qualities

Since the early 1920s, accounts of residential settings for disturbed and delinquent adolescents have focused on theoretical considerations and treatment models but there are core general factors that cut across both theoretical orientations in both residential and community treatment programmes. These are:

1 good leadership;

2 good discipline, firmness;

3 special education;

4 work programme;

5 recreation programme;

6 adolescent–adolescent relations;

7 staff–adolescent relations;

8 staff–staff relations;

9 milieu—warmth and harmony; and

10 milieu—organization, practicality, high expectations.

Adolescent–adolescent and staff–adolescent relationships should be fostered, seeking to encourage positive rather than negative features. Staff–staff relationships require attention, communication, working co-operatively, and being work orientated, together with no avoidance of conflicts, rivalries and negative attitudes that could undermine the operation and morale of the programme (Harris *et al.* 1987).

Social skills interventions have focused on microskills, such as eye contact, body posture and tone of voice, and macro skills, such as techniques to walk away from physical confrontation. These have led to changes in institutional performance but with less certainty about a reduction in future offending. More promising are the changes that can be brought about by cognitive-behavioural programmes, in particular multimodal programmes incorporating elements of self-control, self-instruction, anger control, role taking, social problem-solving and programmes derived to increase the young offender's moral reasoning ability, during and after detention in secure facilities (see Brent *et al.*, Chapter 54; Compas *et al.*, Chapter 55).

Overall factors influencing successful outcomes of community or institutional programmes include the following.

1 Avoidance of indiscriminate choice of treatment foci.

2 The use of more structured and focused treatments.

3 The inclusion of a cognitive component that includes tackling the attitudes, values and beliefs that support antisocial behaviour.

4 Interventions that are conducted in the community; residential programmes, however, can be effective when structurally linked with community-based interventions (Hollin 1993).

Specific treatment

Cognitive-behavioural therapy

Cognitive-behavioural therapy (CBT) involves strategies with roots in behavioural, social learning and cognitive theories. There is an explicit emphasis on learning, and on personal and situational influences on learning. Personal factors include both biological and developmental features (Kendall 1993). Offending is shaped by the social environment extending across family, peers, neighbourhood and culture. The young offender has failed to acquire or to use certain skills, or has learnt inappropriate ways of behaving. A strength of CBT should be its ability to bridge the gap between behaviour modification and traditional insight-orientated therapies (Hollin 1990; Wilde 1996).

Specific measures, e.g. Adolescent Cognition Scale (Hunter *et al.* 1991) and the Multi-phasic Sex Inventory (Nichols & Molinder 1984), are used to assess beliefs, attitudes and cognitions in adolescent sexual abusers. Establishment of a baseline, with respect to the overall level and fluctuations in frequency and intensity, enables intervention effects to be determined more clearly. Functional analysis (see Herbert, Chapter 53) can be used across a range of situations to assess factors that foster or inhibit antisocial behaviour in each individual. Combined with regular reviews of programme effectiveness, this creates a needs- and risk-driven therapeutic culture that should shape clinical decision-making (Epps 1997).

The 1990s saw the expansion of CBT from institutional to community settings, following a succession of reviews of the effectiveness of CBT in reducing recidivism in young offenders (Hollin 1993; Lipsey 1995; Losel 1995; Home Office 1997). The dual goals are:

1 to increase and strengthen self-control; and
2 to develop the capacity of the young offender to understand the perspective of others.

The most commonly employed CBT intervention is that of Anger Management Training (Novaco 1994), designed to reduce angry arousal and to improve coping strategies. Comparisons across programmes are difficult when they have been employed across a wide variety of settings, and when terms such as 'violence', 'aggression' and 'sexual force' are used interchangeably. Core to such programmes (Feindler & Ecton 1986; McGuire 1996) are:

• helping the young person to recognize feelings of anger and its associated physiological and cognitive sequelae;
• challenging beliefs that support triggers for aggression, in order to foster techniques for self-control;
• aiding relaxation;
• increasing motivation to avoid angry aggression; and
• understanding negative consequences of angry aggression for self and others.

It has long been recognized that young offenders are poor at, and inflexible in their approach to, solving interpersonal problems, lacking skills and strategies taken for granted by others (Bandura 1973). Poverty of thought and poor verbal reasoning skills can be present in spite of an average overall IQ. There are five steps for individual practice (D'Zurilla & Godfried 1971).

1 Development of a general orientation or set to recognize the problem.
2 Definition of the problem specifics and what needs to be done.
3 Generalization of alternative courses of action.
4 Exploration of the consequences, benefits and risks of the alternative courses of action.
5 Checking that chosen alternatives are achieving the desired outcome.

Self-instructional training

Self-instructional training, whereby children regulate their behaviour through overt and then covert speech (what they say to themselves), has been applied successfully to problems such as aggression and impulsivity (Kendall 1993). The ability to delay gratification is impaired in delinquents. Failures in the components for self-control, goal-setting, self-monitoring, self-education and self-reinforcement undermine self-control. Lacking confidence in achieving conventional goals, delinquents choose antisocial goals and are more likely to have an external locus of control, believing they have little control over events.

Self-management training for delinquents

This focuses on educational, vocational and interpersonal skills. Deficits in perspective taking are prominent among delinquents, and role-play may be a useful treatment technique. Teaching offenders to identify the emotional state of others (affect identification), to understand the other person's point of view (perspective taking), and to experience within themselves the emotions felt by others (emotional responsiveness). Empathy skill training is particularly important in treatment with delinquents at high risk of adult antisocial personality disorder (McGuire 1996; Feshbach & Feshbach 1982).

Aggression replacement therapy

This has been used with violent young offenders in institutional secure facilities and community settings (Goldstein & Soriano 1994). This approach brings together social skills training, self-instructional and anger control training and moral reasoning enhancement (Goldstein & Glick 1987) and may be useful for a wide range of problems (McGuire 1996).

Multimodal interventions

These combine a range of behavioural and cognitive components.

Reasoning and rehabilitation programmes

The programme used in the Correctional Services of Canada (Ross & Ross 1995) has also been employed in the UK, including the Thinking Skills programme in Young Offender Institutions and the Straight Thinking Probation (STOP) programme (Knott 1995).

Whereas these interventions reduce the risk of re-offending among 'ordinary' young offenders, current programmes do not provide an adequate means to address the needs of or risks presented by young people exhibiting serious antisocial behaviour or who have complex mental health problems.

• Outcomes are related to crime more than to antisocial behaviour *per se*.
• Both prevention and intervention programmes are geared to the common antisocial features rather than to serious antisocial behaviour (see Earls & Mezzacappa, Chapter 26).
• Programmes are largely directed towards males.
• Programmes use techniques that are primarily risk focused rather than taking a holistic approach, addressing quality of life and current mental health needs.
• The overall approaches do not always encompass individual development and psychopathology.
• There remains a need for specialist treatment and care for the group exhibiting serious antisocial behaviour.

Multisystemic therapy

Multisystemic therapy (MST) was developed in the USA by Henggeler *et al.* (1998) and Henggeler (1999) and offers intensive and comprehensive input designed to overcome the limitations of traditional interventions for young people with behavioural and mental health problems. At the core of MST is directing the intervention not just at the young person but towards the social contexts in which he or she lives. The range of treatment approaches are therefore directed at the young person, family, school peer group and local community. Problem behaviour is viewed as a function of difficulty within and at the interface between each of these systems. MST involves nine key principles. Interventions should:

1 provide an assessment designed to understand the fit between the identified problems and their broader systemic context;

2 emphasize the positive and use systemic strengths as levers of change;

3 be designed to promote responsible behaviour and to decrease irresponsible behaviour among family members;

4 be present-focused and action-orientated, targeting specific and well-defined problems;

5 target sequences of behaviour within or between multiple systems that maintain identified problems;

6 be appropriate to the developmental needs of the young people;

7 be designed to require daily or weekly effort by family;

8 include continuous evaluation of effectiveness from multiple perspectives, with providers assuming accountability for overcoming barriers to successful outcomes; and

9 be designed to promote treatment generalization and long-term maintenance of therapeutic change by empowering caregivers to address the needs of family members across multiple systemic contexts, with specific implementation guidelines.

Service delivery characteristics include:

- low case loads (five families per clinician);
- delivery of service in community settings;
- time limited treatment (4–6 months);
- 24 h a day access to therapists to enable crisis intervention;
- provision of comprehensive services.

Strict adherence to the MST principles and guidelines demonstrate positive long-term outcomes; poor adherence predicts high risk of re-arrest and incarceration (Henggeler *et al.* 1997).

Efficacy of interventions

Given the range of treatments and interventions available, is offender treatment of practical significance? McGuire (2000) set this important question in the context of other 'medical' treatments. The key point is that many well-established medical interventions (such as the use of aspirin to prevent heart attacks or chemotherapy for breast cancer) have smaller effects than those for delinquency. Between 1985 and 2000, 18 meta-analytic reviews were published. Cumulatively they incorporate more than 2000 'primary studies'. The majority deal with offenders in the age range 12–20 and, although modest, the 'mean effect size' is positive in the 0.10–0.29 range.

Custodial approaches

Official reconviction rates show that custody is relatively ineffectual in reducing offending. Home Office figures in England and Wales 1997 (Home Office 1999) showed that 88% of 14–16-year-old males, and 82% of 17 year olds, were reconvicted within 2 years of release from prison; Kershaw *et al.*'s (1999) findings were similar. Reconviction rates are highest for younger male offenders and for crimes most commonly linked with youth (theft and burglary).

During the 1990s several meta-analyses showed that correctional treatments could be effective if they supported clinically relevant and psychologically informed principles of human service, risk, need and general responsivity. These apply to female as well as male offenders and are effective in reducing both general and violent recidivism (Dowden & Andrews 1999). Their meta-analysis of 134 primary studies of correctional treatment largely concerned male offenders. The overall mean effect size for the studies was 0.09 with a 95% confidence interval of 0.07–0.12 suggesting that the effects of correctional interventions were positive but small. The introduction of human service within a justice context was associated with substantial reductions in the re-offending levels of young offenders (effect size of 0.13 for 175 studies). Programmes that used a 'fear of official punishment' yielded a significant negative relationship (effect size of −0.2 for 54 studies).

The way in which an institution is run affects outcomes for young people. Rutter *et al.* (1998) found that whereas the deterrent and incapacitation effects of incarceration were negligible, beneficial effects derived from:

- education and training that could open up new opportunities on release from custody;
- help with drug abuse/misuse, with no access to drugs during custody;
- the maintenance of a prosocial ethos with good relationships and models for behaviour;
- enhancement of self-efficacy; and
- encouragement of strong regular links with families.

Family participation in the residential experience (Sinclair & Gibbs 1998) and co-operation with community agencies are important factors in successful outcomes.

Delinquency and mental illness

Prevalence of mental disorders in juvenile justice populations

Cocozza (1992) noted the very limited evidence on the prevalence of mental disorders among delinquents in either community or residential settings. In a recent review, Kazdin (2000) noted that most studies did not use standard diagnostic interviews, samples were small and usually restricted to just one location. Although some data derived from epidemiological studies using diagnostic interviews, comparisons were difficult because of variations in criteria, informants used, ages and ethnicity of subjects and geographical location.

Kazdin (2000), putting together evidence from a range of studies, concluded that mental disorders of all kinds were several times as frequent in delinquents than in the general population. Some one in five children and adolescents in the general population suffer significant developmental, emotional or behavioural problems. The proportion of 'incarcerated adolescents' with some form of psychiatric disorder in North American studies has been found to be much higher—about four out of five. A comprehensive study of over 1200 delinquents (aged 10–17) in juvenile detention centres, using the Diagnostic Interview Schedule for Children, found that some 80% had at least one mental disorder (Teplin *et al.* 1998). Systematic standardized mental health screening for young offenders is still not readily available (Kurtz *et al.* 1998). Nevertheless, studies of juveniles presenting to juvenile courts in North America and Europe have all shown high levels of psychiatric disorder, family psychopathology and inadequate resources to deal with these problems (Doob *et al.* 1995; Dolan *et al.* 1999; Doreleijers *et al.* 2000; Vermeiren *et al.* 2000). Nicol *et al.* (2000) found marked similarity in the level of need in adolescents whether in penal or welfare establishments. Studies of incarcerated adolescents in England and Wales (Maden *et al.* 1995; Lader *et al.* 2000) have all demonstrated high rates of psychiatric disorder, particularly in those facing the stress of incarceration while awaiting trial. Studies have highlighted the particular needs of adolescents from diverse ethnic groups (Lockman & Wayland 1994) and of the difficulties faced and posed by adolescent female offenders (Jasper *et al.* 1998; Lenssen *et al.* 2000). Caution needs to be exercised in interpreting these various figures because rates of disorder will be influenced by numerous aspects of delinquents' backgrounds and by definitions of disorder. Thus, for example, the figures on drug abuse will be affected by how abuse is conceptualized and by the range of substances included (Weinberg *et al.* 1998). What is clear, however, is that the overall rate of psychopathology in delinquents is substantially raised. Its clinical implications will depend, amongst other things, on the extent and type of comorbidity (Kazdin 1996; Rutter 1997; Ulzen & Hamilton 1998), the degree of chronicity, and developmental impact.

Relevance of specific disorders to juvenile offending

Hyperactivity and attention disorders predispose to both antisocial behaviour in childhood/adolescence and antisocial personality disorder in adult life (Barkley 1990, 1997). It seems that disinhibition, poor impulse control and educational difficulties are all implicated in this risk. Some youths respond by seeking acceptance and feelings of mastery by joining delinquent groups. Affective disorders play some part in youth violence

(Pliszka *et al.* 2000). Depression in adolescence can manifest itself as anger, which in turn is correlated with aggression. Anxiety and post-traumatic stress disorders show raised rates in delinquent populations (Boswell 1995, 1997). Part of the pattern of stress reactions includes a heightened sensitivity to potential threat, which can in turn involve the risk of a young person acting explosively or unexpectedly. Psychotic disorders occur only infrequently (Clare *et al.* 2000; Kazdin 2000). Pre-psychotic problems in the form of borderline and schizoid personality disorders may be important because their difficulties with interpersonal relationship have a role in their delinquencies. Neurodevelopmental dysfunction may be relevant, through leading to impairments in the youths' ability to adapt to stress, to recognize the consequences of their actions, and to exercise impulse control. Serious mental disorders may have similar effects.

Although there has been progress in other aspects of youth justice, there are continuing difficulties in recognizing and providing treatment for mental health problems. Juvenile justice facilities are not clinical facilities. There has been a noticeable lack of standardized screening tools for young offenders that can assist non-clinical staff to collect information speedily to inform decision-making with respect to referral to mental health professionals. The Massachusetts Youth Screening Instrument (MAYSI2) was developed for routine use in juvenile justice facilities (Grisso 1999). It focuses on symptoms covering a range of mental disorders. The identification of youths with potential health needs may lead on to the use of more in-depth evaluation, such as the Minnesota Multiphasic Personality Inventory Adolescent (Butcher *et al.* 1994), the Millon Adolescent Clinical Inventory (Millon 1993) and the continuing refinements of the Child Behaviour Checklist (Achenbach 1991). Needs assessment tools, such as the Salford Needs Assessment Schedule for Adolescents (SNASA) (Kroll *et al.* 1999), can assist multiagency planning and service delivery as a young offender with greater or lesser degrees of mental health problems moves within and between systems.

Treatment interventions for young offenders with psychiatric disorders

Affective disorders

Depression is commonly present in delinquents. Clinic attenders with conduct disorder have rates of depression of between 15 and 31% (Goodyer *et al.* 1997; Kovacs & Devlin 1998). As antisocial youths are generally viewed as difficult and disruptive, the risk is that depression will go unrecognized by non-mental health agencies. Where depression and conduct disorder coexist, the risk of substance (especially alcohol) misuse is high in female offenders. Young offenders with comorbidity for depression and conduct disorder are particularly vulnerable to suicide attempts (Shaffer *et al.* 1996).

Treatment of depression, as in any young person, will depend on its severity, the person's psychosocial circumstances and the capacity and ability of the system to engage him or her. Use of interpersonal therapy (IPT) may be of benefit as an acute intervention. In addition to CBT approaches geared to reduce offending behaviour, CBT can be used to challenge and restructure the distorted negative cognitions that depressed adolescent offenders hold about themselves. Where young offenders have severe depression with persistent symptoms, medication may be indicated. When depression is severe, a combination of pharmacological and psychological interventions is called for, with continuation for 6–12 months (Harrington *et al.* 1998; see also Harrington, Chapter 29). Mental health screening in the young offender population may also be important to ensure the early detection of subthreshold cases of mania where there can be chronic and rapidly fluctuating symptoms of irritability, emotional liability, increased energy and reckless behaviours (American Academy of Child and Adolescent Psychiatry Official Action 1997).

Early onset psychosis

A prodromal phase of non-psychotic behavioural disturbance occurs in about half of early onset cases of schizophrenia, and can last between 1 and 7 years (Maziade *et al.* 1996). It includes externalizing behaviours, attention deficit disorder and conduct disorder. Mental health screening should include a focus on changes in social functioning (often from an already chaotic baseline level) to a state including perceptual distortion, ideas of reference, and delusional mood. As in adult life (Taylor & Gunn 1999), most young people with schizophrenia are non-delinquent and non-violent. Nevertheless, there may be an increased risk of violence to others when they have active symptoms, especially when there is abuse of drugs or alcohol. The risk of violent acts is related to subjective feelings of tension, ideas of violence, delusional symptoms that incorporate named persons known to the individual, persecutory delusions, fear of imminent attack, feelings of sustained anger and fear, passivity experiences reducing their sense of self-control and command hallucinations. Protective factors are responding to and compliance with physical and psychosocial treatments, good social networks, a valued home environment, no interest in or knowledge of weapons as the means of violence, good insight into the psychiatric illness and any previous violent aggressive behaviour and a fear of their own potential for violence. These features require particular attention but the best predictors of future offending in mentally disordered young people are much the same as in the general population (Clare *et al.* 2000).

Autistic spectrum disorders

These are being increasingly recognized but are often overlooked in forensic groups (see Lord & Bailey, Chapter 38). Their identification is critical to the understanding of offending, especially in adolescents with a learning disability. This is par-

ticularly so when an offence or assault is 'bizarre' in nature, the degree or nature of aggression is unaccountable and when there is a stereotypic pattern of offending. Howlin (1997) proposed that offending and aggression in autistic persons can arise by four means.

1 Their social *naïveté* may allow them to be led into criminal acts by others.
2 Aggression may arise from a disruption of routines.
3 Antisocial behaviour may stem from a lack of understanding or misinterpretation of social cues.
4 Crimes may reflect obsessions, especially when these involve morbid fascination with violence. There are similarities with the intense and obsessional nature of fantasies described in some adult sadists (MacCulloch *et al.* 1983).

Learning disability

Surprisingly little is known about criminal behaviour in individuals with a learning disability (Lyall *et al.* 1995; Holland 1997). The clinical issues that arise concern the additional care needed in interviewing and at assessment, as much as the possible special implications with respect to antisocial risk that arise from their cognitive level or profile. Associated psychopathology, life experiences and personal background should constitute part of the assessment. Treatment programmes often need to be carried out over a long time period, balancing inherent vulnerability with continued level of risk to others (O'Brien 1996).

'Prodromal' personality disorder

Models used to describe severe personality disorder in adults (Royal College of Psychiatrists 1999) may also be applied to young people (see J. Hill, Chapter 43). Hare (1993) differentiated between 'psychopathic personality', characterized by an unemotional and callous interpersonal style, and 'antisocial personality disorder' in which the key elements are poor impulse control and antisocial behaviour. O'Brien & Frick (1996) argued that these two groups have a different aetiology. Christian *et al.* (1997) described a group of children with a callous unemotional interpersonal style, who lacked guilt and who did not show empathy or emotions. The pathway to their serious antisocial behaviour (Zoccolillo *et al.* 1992) and interpersonal violence was thought to lie in family features, evolving personality and situational context. A parallel may be drawn with reactive attachment disorder (Fahlberg 1994; Delaney 1995; but see O'Connor, Chapter 46 for a discussion of the lack of precision in this diagnostic concept). Individual psychotherapy may be needed alongside traditional multimodal interventions, and long-term support to multiagency services may constitute a key role for emerging specialist forensic psychotherapy services (Bailey 2000d). Bailey (1997) and Bailey *et al.* (2001) have summarized the features involved in the pathways to serious antisocial behaviour under three headings: family features, personality features and situational features.

Family features

Parental antisocial personality disorder.
Violence witnessed.
Abuse, neglect, rejection.

Personality features

Callous unemotional interpersonal style.
Evolution of violent and sadistic fantasy.
People viewed as objects.
Morbid identity.
Paranoid ideation.
Hostile attribution.

Situational features

Repeated loss and rejection in relationships.
Threats to self-harm.
Crescendo of hopelessness and helplessness.
Social disinhibition in group settings.
Substance misuse.
Changes in mental state over time.

Medicolegal assessment

There are common core principles that should be applied to medicolegal assessments of juveniles. Key questions concern the young person's 'fitness to plead' and capacity to 'effectively participate in the proceedings' (Grisso & Schwartz 2000). The European Court of Human Rights has made explicit that the right of an accused to a fair trial has to include children. Two key suggestions for practice emerge from a review of international practice.

1 All young defendants, including those charged with serious offences, should be tried in youth courts (with permission for adult sanctions for older youths if certain conditions are met). This should enable a mode of trial for young defendants to be subject to safeguards that can enhance understanding and participation.

2 The maturity of young defendants' cognitive and emotional capacities should be assessed before a decision is taken about venue and mode of trial.

One fundamental distinction in the criminal law is between conditions that negate criminal liability and those that might mitigate the punishment deserved under particular circumstances. Very young children and the profoundly mentally ill may lack the minimum capacity necessary to justify punishment. Those exhibiting less profound impairments of the same kind may qualify for a lesser level of deserved punishment even though they meet the minimum conditions for some punishment. Immaturity, like mental disorder, can serve both as an excuse and as mitigation in the determination of just punishment. Capacity is sometimes thought of as a generic skill that a person

either has or lacks; however, that is not so. To begin with, it is multifaceted, with four key elements.

1 *Understanding*: the capacity to understand information relevant to the specific decision at issue.

2 *Appreciation*: the capacity to appreciate one's situation as the defendant is confronted with a specific legal decision.

3 *Reasoning*: the capacity to think rationally about alternative courses of action.

4 *Choice*: the capacity to express a choice among alternatives.

The second key point is that capacity is a feature that is both situation-specific and open to influence—as brought out in discussions of the assessment in relation to children's consent to treatment (British Medical Association 2001), participation in research (Royal College of Psychiatrists 2001) and criminal responsibility (Justice 1996). Young children may well appreciate the difference between right and wrong but yet not understand the seriousness of some forms of irresponsible behaviour. With respect to their ability to understand legal procedures (as distinct from their crime), much can be done to aid their understanding (Ashford & Chard 2000).

Any evaluation of competence (Grisso 1997) should include assessment of possibly relevant psychopathology, emotional understanding as well as cognitive level, the child's experiences and appreciation of situations comparable to the one relevant to the crime and to the trial, and any particular features that may be pertinent in this individual and this set of circumstances. The clinician should also be alert to possible treatment needs, and should be aware of how these might be met for this individual, given the forensic situation. Before the evaluation it is important to be sure that the rules and limits of confidentiality for the evaluation are clear and that the child and the family understand them (Bailey 2000a). The appropriate level of clinical thoroughness and detail will vary with the intrinsic clinical complexity of the case, with the specific legal context and with the consultant's role in the legal system. The general principles to be used in the assessment are broadly comparable to those employed in any clinical evaluation (see Rutter & Taylor, Chapter 2). However, particular attention needs to be paid to developmental background, emotional and cognitive maturity, trauma exposure and substance misuse. The likely appropriate sources for obtaining clinical data relevant to assessment of a juvenile's competence to stand trial will include a variety of historical records, a range of interviews and other observations and, in some cases, specialized tests.

Records of the child's school functioning, past clinical assessment, treatment history and previous legal involvements need to be obtained. In coming to an overall formulation, there should be a particular focus on how both developmental and psychopathological features may be relevant to the forensic issues that have to be addressed.

Evaluation of functional capacities

Here the main focus is on the youth's ability to understand and cope with the legal process. This comes from three sources:

direct questioning of the defendant, inferences from functioning in other areas and direct observation of the defendant's behaviour and interaction with others. It is useful to enquire about the youth's expectations about what the consequences of the court involvement might prove to be. Because the course of juvenile proceedings can vary so widely, with consequences ranging from the extremely aversive to extremely beneficial, rational understanding will necessarily involve a high degree of uncertainty.

Potentially relevant problems include: inattention, depression, disorganization of thought processes that interferes with the ability to consider alternatives; hopelessness, such that the decision is felt not to matter; delusions or other fixed beliefs that distort the understanding of options (or their likely outcomes); maturity of judgement; and the developmental challenges of adolescence.

Gudjonsson (1992) and Gudjonsson & Singh (1984) found that adolescents were more prone than adults to offer inaccurate information to persons in authority when they were pressured. Younger adolescents were significantly more likely to change their stories to give answers that were less accurate than their original descriptions. This has practical implications for interviewing by police and lawyers. The ability to take another person's perspective is important for effective communication, an ability that has matured by middle adolescence but is less reliably found in early adolescence.

Concerns about a youth's conduct may sometimes be raised as potentially significant to his or her competence (Barnum 2000). A youth may be impulsive, loud, angry or disruptive during trial and it may be suggested that these tendencies may undermine the formality or integrity of the proceedings. In addressing this question, it is important to be clear about the general clinical basis for any expected functional problems and even more important to be clear about specific implications of potential disruptiveness for the relevant features of competence. If a youth's impulsiveness may be expected to interfere with his or her attention to the proceedings in the courtroom and if this attention to those proceedings actually matters to his or her understanding and effective collaboration with council then it will be important to characterize these expectations or implications. For instance if the youth is so angry and disruptive that he or she seems unable to sit and confer with council this may have important implications for his or her ability to understand the issues and respond helpfully to them. The clinician therefore needs to attend to these issues and show how they stem or do not stem from clinical disorder or developmental deficit.

In providing information to the court, written reports have the advantage of a standard format that helps the consultant to be sure that he or she has considered all the relevant questions; it also provides a familiar structure for readers. In essence, for the sake of consistency and clarity, competence reports need to cover the following areas.

1 Identifying information and referral questions.
2 The description of the structure of the evaluation including sources and a notation of the confidentiality expectations.

3 The provision of clinical and forensic data.
4 Discussion and presentations of opinions.

The assessment of competence to stand trial presents challenging questions. Consultants need to appreciate the systems implications of competence questions and must be able to provide opinions and recommendations that match the legal and systems circumstances of individual cases. This area is full of uncertainty and the complexity of these challenges can sometimes seem overwhelming. However, in responding carefully and thoughtfully to questions posed, consultants can contribute to the development of a potentially important aspect of legal and clinical practice (Zimring 2000).

Treatment and special crimes

Violence and juvenile homicide

Violent behaviour often involves a loss of sense of personal identity and of personal value. A young person may engage in actions without concern for future consequences or past commitments. Loeber & Hay (1994) described four groups of young people:
1 those who desist from aggression;
2 those whose aggression is stable and continues at the same level;
3 those who escalate in the severity of their aggression and make the transition into violence; and
4 those who show a stable pattern of aggression.

Violence denotes the 'forceful infliction of physical injury' (Blackburn 1993). Aggression involves harmful, threatening or antagonistic behaviour (Berkowitz 1993). Longitudinal studies are invaluable in mapping out the range of factors and processes that contribute to the development of aggressive behaviour and in showing how they are causally related (Farrington 1995). However, in attempting to work with any individual who has committed a violent act, the question to be answered is 'Why has this individual behaved in this unique fashion on this occasion?' (Lipsey 1995).

Studies show that children and adolescents who murder share a constellation of psychological, cognitive, neuropsychiatric, educational and family system disturbance (Cornell *et al.* 1987; Myers *et al.* 1995; Myers & Scott 1998). In the UK, young people who commit grave sadistic crimes including juvenile homicide are liable to periods of lengthy incarceration. Detention itself can provide time for further neurodevelopmental, cognitive and emotional growth. Irrespective of treatment models, the provisions of education, vocational training, consistent role models and continued family contact are of critical importance.

The majority of young persons who have killed initially dissociate themselves from the reality of their act, but gradually experience a progression of reactions and feelings akin to a grief reaction. The young person, while facing a still adversarial and public pretrial and trial process, has to move safely through the process of disbelief, denial, loss, grief and anger/blame. Post-traumatic stress disorder arising from the participation in the sadistic act (either directly or observing the actions of codefendants) has to be treated, as does trauma arising from their own past personal emotional, physical and/or sexual abuse.

A combination of verbal and non-verbal therapies are effective, but qualities such as previous frequent and severe aggression, low intelligence and a poor capacity for insight weigh against a safe outcome (Myers *et al.* 1995; Bailey 1996; Myers & Scott 1998). In understanding the role of violence and sadism in a young person's life, one has to understand the depth of their sensitivity and reaction to perceived threat and their past maladaptive behaviours aimed at allowing them to feel in control of their lives. In coming to terms with their internal rage, addressing victim empathy saying sorry and reattribution of blame, expression of anger and distress within sessions is expected and is often sexualized in both form and content. This can spill outside sessions when the young person and carers can become collusively dismissive and rejecting of therapists. Heide (1999) and Bailey (2000c) emphasized the importance of intensive work to prepare the young person for transition from long-term incarceration and re-entry into the community together with extended aftercare.

Delinquents who sexually offend

Sexually inappropriate behaviour in children and adolescents constitutes a substantial health and social problem (James & Neil 1996). Most, but not all, abusers are male, often come from disadvantaged backgrounds with a history of victimization, sexual and physical abuse (Skuse *et al.* 1998) and show high rates of psychopathology (Dolan *et al.* 1996; Graves *et al.* 1996; Hummel *et al.* 2000; see also Glaser, Chapter 21, and Emery & Laumann Billings, Chapter 20). Of particular concern are a significant subgroup with mild learning disability whose treatment programmes have to be tailored to their level of development and cognitive ability. Young abusers come within the criminal justice system but should also be considered in their own right within the child protection framework. Most adult sexual abusers of children started their abuse when adolescents and yet neither ICD-10 nor DSM-IV has a diagnostic category for paedophilia in those under 16. Vizard *et al.* (1996) suggested the creation of a new disorder 'sexual arousal disorder of childhood' to help identify this vulnerable group who in turn place vulnerable others at risk. Langstrom *et al.* (2000) advocated the development of empirically based typologies for this offender group.

A structured carefully planned multiagency approach is required when working with sexually aggressive younger children and sexually abusive adolescents. The three stages of assessment of juvenile sexual offenders (O'Callaghan & Print 1994; Vizard *et al.* 1996; Becker 1998) are:
1 clarification and rapport building;
2 mapping the abuse: the fantasies, strategies and behaviours; and
3 the future, placement treatment and personal change.

Increasing awareness of the existence of young sexual abusers has been accompanied by a proliferation of treatment programmes (Becker 1990). Treatment can include work with the individual, group work, work with the family and support for the professional network. A review of treatment approaches (Sirles *et al.* 1997) concluded that 'multiple theoretical approaches and treatment modalities have been found useful for intervention but all programmes reviewed contained a cognitive behavioural approach to assessment (Calder 1997). With respect to family treatment, Bentovim & Williams (1998) emphasized the importance of 'assessment of potential to engage in treatment', describing the treatment processes in terms of:
1 the crisis of disclosure;
2 family assessment;
3 therapeutic work in a protective context for the victim; and
4 reconstruction and reunification of the family.
The 'family' (Bentovim 1998) in this context may include foster carers or long-term residential carers.

Firesetting/arson

Arson can have a devastating impact on the victim and the wider society. Juvenile arsonists are not a homogeneous group, with a wide range of familial (Fineman 1980), social (Patterson 1982), developmental interpersonal (Vreeland & Levin 1980), clinical and 'legal' needs. Kolko & Kazdin (1992) highlighted the importance of attraction to fire, heightened arousal, impulsivity and limited social competence. As with other forms of serious antisocial behaviours, no single standard treatment approach will be appropriate for all individuals (Repo & Virkunnen 1997). In addition to the general assessment of antisocial behaviour, the specific domains to be considered include:
• history of fireplay;
• history of hoax telephone calls;
• social context of firesetting (whether alone or with peers);
• where the fires were set;
• previous threats/targets;
• type of fire, single/multiple seats of firesetting;
• motivation (anger resolution, boredom, rejection, cry for help, thrill-seeking, fire fighting, crime concealment, no motivation, curiosity and peer pressure).

For recidivistic firesetters therapy may include:
• psychotherapy to increase the understanding of the behaviour, including antecedents defining the problem behaviour, and establishing the behavioural reinforcers;
• skills training to promote adaptive coping mechanisms;
• understanding environmental factors to manage or self-trigger solutions;
• counselling to reduce psychological distress;
• behavioural techniques to extinguish the behaviour;
• education to promote understanding of cause and effect; and
• supervision for the staff caring for the adolescent.
Early modelling experiences and early exposure to related phenomena militate against a good outcome.

Approaches to service delivery

Forensic mental health includes the assessment and treatment of those who are mentally disordered and whose behaviour has led or could lead to offending. Defining forensic psychiatry in terms of the assessment and treatment of the mentally abnormal offender delineates an area of concern that could potentially engulf much of mental health. Making available mental health expertise to address the mental health component of social problems should not conflict with tradition and medical practice if the aim is to identify and relieve disorder primarily to benefit patients but also, through their more adequate care and management, to benefit those they potentially threaten. Public health policy has long recognized the government's obligation to attend to the basic health needs of prisoners and the importance of meeting the health and mental health needs of children. Traditionally, child and adolescent mental health practitioners have continued to work as generalists. Within their specialism they may include forensic work, not only child care proceedings, but also direct forensic medicolegal work where the young children are the alleged perpetrators rather then the victims.

Child psychiatrists need to be closely involved with developing specialist community and inpatient resources, including secure facilities for children and adolescents who may be:

• mentally disordered offenders;
• sex offenders and abusers;
• severely suicidal and self-harming adolescents;
• very severely mentally ill adolescents;
• adolescents who need to begin psychiatric rehabilitation in secure circumstances; and
• brain injured adolescents and those with severe organic disorders.

Weaving together local generic and more regional specialist services allows for multidimensional concepts of problems encountered by these young people to be tackled by the local mental health services in conjunction with other agencies (Bailey 2000b). Local specialist child and adolescent mental health services can be augmented by advice and training offered by an identified peripatetic outreach team that is based in, and works from, specialized centres of expertise in forensic child and mental health. The primary responsibility would remain with the staff of local services and the role of the outreach services would be supportive and consultative. Very specialized peripatetic services would be outreach services in which the young people are seen directly by members of an outreach service.

There has to be a seamless delivery of service between general child and adolescent services and specialist forensic provision, with solutions tailored to local need. Services delivered directly to patients and their families by centres of specialist expertise in forensic child and adolescent mental health would include specialist community assessment and treatment services providing input not only to other child and mental health services but working with secure social care units, young offender institutions/correctional institutions and juvenile justice services in the community.

A range of inpatient provision is required including medium-secure inpatient psychiatric units for adolescents with early onset psychosis and serious risk to others. There may well be a small need for an adolescent forensic inpatient unit offering maximum security (Bailey & Farnworth 1998).

For services to develop successfully there needs to be:

• staff wanting to and suited to working in this field;
• systems in place to offer comprehensive appropriate training programmes;
• such programmes and interventions have to be evidence-based; and
• adolescent forensic mental health research and development networks nationally and internationally should be established to ensure that what is learnt from research is put promptly into practice.

Farrant (2001) (Prison Reform Trust), representing the view of agencies outside health, stressed the importance of an approach to young offenders that is not dependent on adult mental health services, together with an emphasis on delivering mental health training to non-mental health professionals. The latter will improve the ability of non-health professionals to identify early indicators of mental health vulnerability in high-risk young people. Interagency training is the best way of ensuring a balance is struck between overloading child and adolescent mental health services with inappropriate referrals and vulnerable young people being missed in the system who then present with severe mental health problems in crisis and late in their offending career.

Gender-specific issues

Any national strategic framework offering treatment for young offenders must consider appropriate provision for the special needs of young females who constitute an important minority of offenders (Zoccolillo 1993; Miller *et al.* 1995; Bailey 2000e). The thinking patterns of violent girls are similar to those of violent boys (Jasper *et al.* 1998; Lenssen *et al.* 2000). Specific consideration should be given to sexual and reproductive health, including education, contraceptive advice, information about help for sexually transmitted diseases, appropriate support for problems around menstruation, support and access to relevant resources in the event of a pregnancy. When the adolescent female is ready to engage in it, post-abuse counselling from an appropriate adult should take into account the gender of the therapist. Medical and psychiatric assessment followed by appropriate treatment of parasuicidal behaviour, remembering the distraction and attention provided by the emergency may be an important component in reinforcing the use of this behaviour as a coping strategy. Different leisure pursuits in girls, and a recognition that eating problems are far more common in girls (see Steinhausen, Chapter 34) may be relevant.

Substance misuse

Drug abuse among young people has increased rapidly over the past 10 years (Weinberg *et al.* 1998). The interaction between offending or high-risk antisocial behaviour and substance abuse is complex and has bidirectional influence, with possible connections among substance use, including alcohol abuse, executive cognitive functioning, aggressivity and impulsivity (Giancola *et al.* 1997; Myers & Scott 1998). Intensive forms of intervention for drug users with complex care needs may require specialist residential (as well as community) services and the involvement of mental health teams, following the principles such as those applied in MST.

Key principles

Because young offenders vary greatly, flexibility in service response is essential. Nevertheless, a strategic, comprehensive and integrated interagency approach to their mental well-being is needed (Kurtz *et al.* 1998). Service delivery has to recognize the high geographical mobility of delinquents, their poor planning, and the changing and diverse nature of their needs.

Youth justice services and mental health services, even in the era of 'joined-up working', have to face the fact that each may not have the same shared purpose. Youth justice services has at its heart the reduction of offending, whereas mental health services focus on fostering the mental health of young people. Bridging that gap may pose real challenges.

This can only be achieved with a shared common language when working with a client group whose needs do not conform to usual academic or administrative boundaries. They fuse together and often coalesce to produce new needs, which in turn impact on risk. Disagreement remains among practitioners and policymakers about definitions used in the development of a common language. Evidence-based research has to place 'evidence' in the wider context of legal, moral, pragmatic and consumer concerns when dealing with young offenders (Dartington Social Research Unit 1998; Little & Mount 1999).

A better understanding of the process of moral development through childhood and adolescence will inform interventions with young offenders. Risk and offence reduction is most likely to be achieved through a comprehensive needs assessment (Kroll *et al.* 1999) linked into an integrated standardized review of prosocial and antisocial behaviour that includes the internal attributional thinking of the young person.

Multiagency research in this field will best inform treatment interventions by integrating qualitative and quantitative methods in the study of developmental psychopathology (Sullivan 1998). Developmental understanding has to underpin treatment programmes for young offenders.

Young offenders have a right to a full range of mental health services. The right of 'children' to be involved in decisions about their own treatment for either physical or mental illness is set within complex child care, mental health, criminal and European human rights legislation. Governments will continue to demand cost-effective youth justice services.

Prevention and early intervention programmes to reduce rates of offending in young people may take a minimum of 10 years to demonstrate direct results. Denying mental health and social services benefits to children and adolescents today to save money will only ensure that the future prison population will grow (Bailey 1999b).

Conclusions

The major challenge of altering the trajectories of persistent young offenders has to be met in the context of satisfying public demands for retribution, together with welfare and civil liberties considerations.

Treatment of delinquents in institutional settings has to meet the sometimes contradictory need to control young people, to remove their liberty and to maintain good order in the institution, at the same time as offering education and training to foster future prosocial participation in society and meeting their welfare needs. At least in England and Wales, the recent legislative overhaul of youth justice (Crime & Disorder Act 1998) has mandated practitioners to bridge the gap between residential and community treatments and to involve families using youth offending teams (YOTs) to meet this complex mix of needs.

Over the last 30 years there has been a gradual shift in opinion regarding effectiveness of intervention with delinquents, from the 'nothing works' approach to a 'what works' approach. The jury is still out for 'what works' in the long term but the evidence base that can be placed before the jury is growing. In practice, the pressure from politicians and public will remain, for a quick fix solution to problems that span cultures, countries and generations. The most important childhood predictors of adolescent violence include troublesome and antisocial behaviour, daring and hyperactivity, low IQ and attainment, antisocial parents, poor child-rearing, harsh and erratic discipline, poor supervision, parental conflict, broken families, low family income and large family size (Farrington 1999). Important policy implications are that home visiting programmes, parent training and skills training programmes singly and in combination should be implemented at an early stage to prevent adolescent high-risk behaviour and offending. The best knowledge about risk factors has been obtained in longitudinal studies and the best knowledge of effective programmes has been obtained in randomized experiments.

The apparent adversity of the current response to young delinquents should be seen as an opportunity to take advantage by combining experimental methods with preventive experiments in longitudinal studies. Provision of appropriately designed programmes can significantly reduce recidivism amongst persistent offenders. The mode and style of delivery is important; high-quality staff and staff training are required together with a system for 'monitoring integrity'. Where comparisons are possible, effect sizes are higher for community-based than institution-based programmes. In prison settings, the strongest effects are obtained when programmes are integrated into the institutional regimes.

Our knowledge of true prevalence rates of mental disorders in a young offending population has to be developed further (Kazdin 2000) so that mental health issues can be addressed. Child and adolescent mental health practitioners have the skills to set the understanding of delinquency in a developmental context (Moran & Hagell 2000) and to assess and treat those young offenders with mental disorders.

References

Achenbach, T. (1991) *Integrative Guide for the 1991 BCL/4–18, YSR and TFR Profiles*. University of Vermont, Department of Psychiatry, Burlington, VT.

American Academy of Child and Adolescent Psychiatry Official Action (1997) Practice parameters for the assessment and treatment of children and adolescents with bipolar disorder. *Journal of American Academy of Child and Adolescent Psychiatry*, 36, 138–157.

Andrews, D.A., Kiessling, J.J., Robinson, D. & Mickus, S. (1986) The risk principle of case classification: an outcome evaluation with young adult probationers. *Canadian Journal of Criminology*, 28, 377–396.

Ashford, M. & Chard, A. (2000) *Defending Young People in the Criminal Justice System*, 2nd edn. Legal Action Groups, Glasgow.

Augimeri, L.K., Webster, C.D., Keogh, C.J. & Levene, K.S. (1998) *Early Assessment Risk List for Boys*, Version 1 consultation edition. Earls Court Child and Family Centre, Ontario, Toronto.

Bailey, S. (1996) Current perspectives on young offenders: aliens or alienated? *Journal of Clinical Forensic Medicine*, 3, 1–7.

Bailey, S. (1997) Sadistic and violent acts in the young. *Child Psychology and Psychiatry Review*, 2, 92–102.

Bailey, S. (1999a) Serious antisocial behaviour. In: *Young People and Mental Health* (eds P. Aggleton, J. Harry & I. Warwick), pp. 91–110. Wiley, Chichester.

Bailey, S. (1999b) The interface between mental health, criminal justice and forensic mental health services for children and adolescents. *Current Opinion in Psychiatry*, 12, 425–432.

Bailey, S. (2000a) Confidentiality Myths and Realities. In: *Confidentiality and Mental Health* (ed. C. Cordess), pp. 71–85. Jessica Kingsley, London.

Bailey, S. (2000b) European perspectives on young offenders and mental health. *Journal of Adolescence*, 23, 237–241.

Bailey, S. (2000c) Juvenile Homicide. *Criminal Behaviour and Mental Health*, 10, 149–154.

Bailey, S. (2000d) Sadistic, sexual and violent acts in the young: contributing and causal factors. In: *Home Truths About Child Sexual Abuse* (ed. C. Itzin), pp. 119–221. Routledge, London.

Bailey, S. (2000e) Violent adolescent female offenders. In: *Violent Children and Adolescents: Asking the Question Why* (ed. G. Boswell), pp. 104–120. Whurr, London.

Bailey, S. & Farnworth, P. (1998) Forensic mental health services. *Young Minds*, 34, 12–13.

Bailey, S., Smith, C. & Dolan, M. (2001) The social background and nature of 'children' who perpetrate violent crimes: a UK perspective. *Journal of Community Psychology*, 29, 305–317.

Bandura, A. (1973) *Aggression: a Social Learning Analysis*. Prentice Hall, Englewood Cliffs, NJ.

Bank, L., Marlowe, J.H., Reed, J.B., Patterson, G.R. & Weinvat, M.R. (1991) Comparative evaluation of parent training interventions for families of chronic delinquents. *Journal of Abnormal Child Psychology*, 19, 15–23.

Barkley, R.A. (1990) *Attention Deficit Hyperactivity Disorder. A Handbook for Diagnosis and Treatment*. Guilford Press, New York.

Barkley, R.A. (1997) *Defiant Children: A Clinician's Manual for Assess-*

ment and Parent Training, 2nd edn. Guilford Press, New York.

Barnum, R. (2000) Clinical and forensic evaluation of competence to stand trial in juvenile defendants. In: *Youth on Trial: a Developmental Perspective in Juvenile Justice* (eds T. Grisso & R. G. Schwartz), pp. 193–224. University of Chicago Press, Chicago.

Becker, J.V. (1990) Treating adolescent sex offenders. *Professional Psychology: Research and Practice*, 21, 362–365.

Becker, J.V. (1998) The assessment of adolescent perpetrators of childhood sexual abuse. *Irish Journal of Psychology*, 19, 68–81.

Bentovim, A. (1998) Family systemic approach to work with young sex offenders. *Irish Journal of Psychology*, 19, 119–135.

Bentovim, A. & Williams, B. (1998) Children and adolescents: victims who become perpetrators. *Advances in Psychiatric Treatment*, 4, 101–107.

Berkowitz, L. (1993) *Aggression: its Causes, Consequences and Control*. McGraw-Hill, New York.

Blackburn, R. (1993) *The Psychology of Criminal Conduct*. John Wiley, Chichester.

Boswell, G. (1995) Violent victims: the prevalence of abuse and loss in the lives of Section 53 offenders. The Prince's Trust, London.

Boswell, G. (1997) The background of violent young offenders, the present picture. In: *Violence in Children and Adolescents* (ed. V.Varmci), pp. 23–36. Jessica Kingsley, London.

Brewer, D.D., Hawkins, J.D., Catalano, R.F. & Neckeman, J.J. (1995) Preventing serious, violent and chronic juvenile offending: a review of evaluations of selected strategies in childhood, adolescence, and the community. In: *Serious, Violent and Chronic Juvenile Offenders* (eds J.C. Howell, B. Krisberg, J.D. Hawkins & J.J. Wilson), pp. 61–141. Sage, London.

British Medical Association (2001) *Consent, Rights and Choices in Health Care for Children and Young People*. BMJ Books, London.

Burt, C. (1925) *The Young Delinquent*. University of London Press.

Butcher, J., William, C., Graham, J. *et al.* (1994) *Manual for administration scoring and interpretation: MMPI-A*. University of Minnesota Press, Minneapolis, MN.

Byng-Hall, J. & Putman, F.S. (1998) *Rewriting Family Scripts*. Guilford Press, New York.

Calder, M.C. (1997) Assessing juveniles who sexually abuse: a framework. In: *Juveniles and Children Who Sexually Abuse: a Guide to Risk Assessment* (ed. M.C. Calder), pp. 50–98. Russell House, UK.

Cavadino, P. & Allen, R. (2000) Children who kill: trends, reasons and procedures in violent children and adolescents. In: *Asking the Question Why* (ed. G. Boswell), pp. 1–18. Whurr, London.

Christian, R.E., Frick, P.J., Hill, N.L., Tyler, L. & Frazer, D.R. (1997) Psychopathy and conduct problems in children: implications for subtyping children with conduct problems. *Journal of the American Academy of Child and Adolescent Psychiatry*, 36, 233–241.

Clare, P., Bailey, S. & Clark, A. (2000) Relationship between psychotic disorders in adolescence and criminally violent behaviour. *British Journal of Psychiatry*, 177, 275–279.

Cocozza, J., ed. (1992) *Responding to mental health needs of youth in the juvenile justice system*. National Coalition for the Mentally Ill in the Criminal Justice System, Seattle.

Cornell, D.G., Benedek, E.P. & Benedek, B.A. (1987) Juvenile homicide: prior adjustment and a proposed typology. *American Journal of Orthopsychiatry*, 57, 383–393.

D'Zurilla, T.J. & Godfried, M.R. (1971) Problem solving and behaviour modification. *Journal of Abnormal Psychology*, 78, 107–126.

Dartington Social Research Unit (1998) *Background Paper 2: Towards a Common Language*. Ashgate, Aldershot.

Delaney, R.J. (1995) *Fostering Changes: Treating Attachment Disordered Children*. Waller J. Corbet, Fort Collins, USA.

Dolan, M. & Doyle, M. (2000) Violence. Risk Prediction. Clinical and actuarial measures and the role of the psychiatrist. *British Journal of Psychiatry*, **177**, 303–311.

Dolan, M., Holloway, J., Bailey, S. & Kroll, L. (1996) The psychosocial characteristics of juvenile sex offenders. *Medicine, Science and the Law*, **36**, 343–352.

Dolan, M., Holloway, J. & Bailey, S. (1999) Health status of juvenile offenders: a survey of young offenders appearing before the juvenile courts. *Journal of Adolescence*, **22**, 137–144.

Doob, A.N., Manners, V. & Varma, K.N. (1995) *Youth Crime and the Youth Justice System in Canada: a research perspective*. Centre of Criminology, University of Toronto.

Doreleijers, T.A.H., Moser, F., Thijs, P., Van England, H. & Beyaert, F.H.L. (2000) Forensic assessment of juvenile delinquents: prevalence of psychopathology and decision-making at court in the Netherlands. *Journal of Adolescence*, **23**, 263–275.

Douglas, K.S. & Cox, D.N. (1999) Violence risk assessment: science and practice. *Legal and Criminology Psychologist*, **4**, 149–184.

Dowden, C. & Andrews, D.A. (1999) What works in young offender treatment: a meta analysis. *Forum on Corrections Research*, **11**, 21–24.

Elliott, D.S., Hamburg, B. & Williams, K.R. (1998) *Violence in American Schools: A New Perspective*, pp. 3–28. Cambridge University Press, New York.

Epps, K.J. (1997) Looking after children in secure settings: recent theories. *Educational and Child Psychology*, **14**, 42–52.

Fahlberg, V. (1994) *A Child's Journey Through Placement*. BAAF, London.

Farrant, F. (2001) *Troubled Inside: Responding to the Mental Health Needs of Children and Young People in Prison*. Prison Reform Trust, London.

Farrington, D.P. (1995) The Twelfth Jack Tizard Memorial Lecture. The development of offenders and antisocial behaviour from childhood: key findings from the Cambridge study in delinquent development. *Journal of Child Psychology and Psychiatry*, **36**, 929–964.

Farrington, D.P. (1999) The psychosocial milieu of the offender. In: *Forensic Psychiatry: Clinicial, Legal and Ethical Issues* (eds J. Gunn & P.J. Taylor), pp. 252–285. Butterworth-Heinemann, Oxford.

Farrington, D.P. (2000) Adolescent violence: findings and implications from the Cambridge study in violent children and adolescents. In: *Asking the Question Why* (ed. G. Boswell), pp. 19–35. Whurr, London.

Farrington, D.P. & West, D.J. (1993) Criminal, penal and life histories of chronic offenders: risk and protective factors and early identification. *Criminal Behaviour and Mental Health*, **3**, 492–523.

Feindler, E.L. & Ecton, R.B. (1986) *Adolescent Anger Control: Cognitive-Behavioural Techniques*. Pergamon Press, New York.

Feshbach, N.D. & Feshbach, S. (1982) Empathy training and the regulation of aggression. Potentialities and limitations. *Academic Bulletin*, **4**, 399–413.

Fineman, K.R. (1980) Firesetting in childhood and adolescence. *Psychiatric Clinics of North America*, **3**, 48, 3–500.

Flood-Page, C., Campbell, S., Harrington, V. & Miller, J. (2000) *Youth crime: findings from the 1998/99 youth lifestyle survey*. Home Office Research Study 209. Home Office, London.

Forth, A.E. (1995) *Psychopathy and young offenders: prevalence, family background and violence*. Unpublished report, Carleton University, Ottawa, Ontario.

Forth, A.E., Kosson, D. & Hare, R.D. (in press) *The Hare Psychopathy Checklist Youth Version*. Multi Health Systems, Toronto, Canada.

Frick, P.J. (1996) Callous unemotional traits and conduct problems: a two-factor model of psychopathy in children. In: *International Perspectives on Psychopathy Issues in Criminological and Legal Psychology* (eds D.J. Cooke, A.E. Forth, J.P. Newman & R.D. Hare), **24**, pp. 47–51. British Psychological Society, Leicester.

Frick, P.J. (1998) *Conduct Disorders and Severe Antisocial Behaviour*, pp. 9–20. Plenum Press, New York.

Gardner, W., Lidz, C.W., Mulvey, E.P. & Shaw, E.C. (1996) A comparison of actuarial methods for identifying repetitively violent patients with mental illnesses. *Law and Human Behaviour*, **20**, 35–48.

Giancola, P.R., Messick, A.C. & Tarter, R.F. (1997) Disruptive, delinquent and aggressive behaviour in female adolescents with a psychoactive substance use disorder relation to executive cognitive functioning. *Journal of Studies on Alcohol*, **59**, 560–567.

Glover, E. (1960) *The Roots of Crime*. International University Press, New York.

Goldstein & Soriano (1994) Juvenile gangs. In: *Reason to Fight: a Psychological Perspective on Violence and Youth* (eds L.D. Eron, J.H. Gentry & P. Schlegel). American Psychological Association, Washington D.C.

Goldstein, A.P. & Glick, B. (1987) *Aggression Replacement Training. A Comprehensive Intervention for Aggressive Youth*. Research Press, Champaign, IL.

Goodyer, I.M., Herbert, J. & Secker, S.M. (1997) Short term outcome of major depression. I. Comorbidity and severity at presentation as predictors of persistent disorder. *Journal of the American Academy of Child and Adolescent Psychiatry*, **36**, 179–187.

Graham, J. & Bowling, B. (1995) *Young People and Crime (Home Office Research Study No 145)*. HMSO, London.

Graves, R.B., Openshaw, D.K., Aaone, F.R. & Erikson, S.L. (1996) Demographic and parental characteristics of youthful sexual offenders. *International Journal of Offender Therapy and Comparative Criminology*, **40**, 300–317.

Gretton, H.M., McBridge, H.L., O'Shaughnessy, R. & Hare, R.D. (1997) *Sex offender or generalised offender? Psychopathy as a risk marker for violence in adolescent offenders*. Paper presented at the 5th International Congress on the Disorders of Personality, Vancouver, British Columbia.

Grisso, T. (1996) Society's retributive response to juvenile violence: a developmental perspective. *Law and Human Behaviour*, **20**, 229–247.

Grisso, T. (1997) The competence of adolescents as trial defendants. *Psychology, Public Policy and Law*, **3**, 3–32.

Grisso, T. (1999) Juvenile offenders and mental illness. *Psychiatry, Psychology and the Law*, **2**, 143–151.

Grisso, T. & Schwartz, R.G. (2000) *Youth on Trial: A Developmental Perspective on Juvenile Justice*. University of Chicago Press, Chicago.

Gudjonsson, G. (1992) *The Psychology of Interrogations: Confessions and Testimony*. John Wiley, New York.

Gudjonsson, G. & Singh, K. (1984) Interrogative suggestibility and delinquent boys: an empirical validation study personality and individual differences. *Journal of Adolescence*, **5**, 425–430.

Hagell, A. & Newburn, T. (1994) *Persistent Young Offenders*. Policy Studies Institute, London.

Hagell, A., Hazel, N. & Shaw, C. (2000) *Evaluation of Medway Secure Training Centre*, **1**, 1–13. Home Office, London.

Hare, R.D. (1993) *Without Conscience: The Distorting World of the Psychopaths Among Us*. Pocket Books, New York.

Harrington, R., Whittaker, J. & Shoebridge, P. (1998) Psychological treatment of depression in children and adolescents: a review of treatment research. *British Journal of Psychiatry*, **173**, 291–298.

Harris, D.P., Cole, J.E. & Vipond, E.M. (1987) Residential treatment of disturbed delinquents. Description of a centre and identification of therapeutic factors. *Canadian Journal of Psychiatry*, **32**, 579–583.

Hawkins, J.P. & Catalano, R.F. (1992) *Communities That Care*. Jossey-Bass, San Francisco, CA.

Heide, K.M. (1999) *Treating Young Killers in Young Killers: The Challenge of Juvenile Homicide*, pp. 219–238. Sage, Thousand Oaks, CA.

Henggeler, S.W. (1999) Multisystemic therapy: an overview of clinical procedures, outcomes and police implications. *Child Psychology and Psychiatry Review*, **4**, 2–10.

Henggeler, S.W., Melton, G.B., Brondino, M.J., Schever, D.G. & Hanley, J.H. (1997) Multisystemic therapy with violent and chronic juvenile offenders and their families: the role of treatment fidelity in successful dissemination. *Journal of Consulting and Clinical Psychology*, **65**, 821–833.

Henggeler, S.W., Schoenwaid, S.K., Borduin, C.M., Rowland, M.D. & Cunningham, P.B. (1998) *Multisystemic Treatment of Antisocial Behaviour in Children and Adolescents*. Guilford Press, New York.

Holland, A. (1997) Forensic psychiatry and learning disability. In: *Seminar in the Psychiatry of Learning Disabilities* (ed. O. Russell), pp. 259–273. Gaskell, London.

Hollin, C.R. (1990) *Cognitive-behavioural Interventions with Young Offenders*. Pergamon Press, Oxford.

Hollin, C.R. (1993) Advances in the psychological treatment of delinquent behaviour. *Criminal Behaviour and Mental Health*, **3**, 142–157.

Home Office (1997) *Changing Offenders' Attitudes and Behaviour. What Works?* Research Study 171. Home Office, London.

Home Office (1999) *Aspects of Crime. Young Offenders 1997* Crime and Criminal Justice Unit, Research, Development and Statistics Directorate, Home Office, London.

Home Office (2000) *Findings from the Youth Lifestyle Survey – 2nd Sweep*. Home Office, London.

Howlin, P. (1997) *'Autism' Preparing for Adulthood*. Routledge, London.

Huizinga, D. & Elliot, D.P. (1986) Reassessing the reliability and validity of self report delinquency measures. *Journal of Quantitative Criminology*, **24**, 293–327.

Huizinga, D. & Jacob-Chien, C. (1998) The contemporaneous co-occurrence of serious and violent juvenile offending and other problems. In: *Serious and Violent Juvenile Risk Factors and Successful Interventions Offenders* (eds R.L. Loeber & D.P. Farrington), pp. 47–67. Sage, Thousand Oaks, CA.

Hummel, P., Thomke, V., Oldenburger, H.A. & Specht, F. (2000) Male adolescent sex offenders against children: similarities and differences between those offenders with and those without a history of sexual abuse. *Journal of Adolescence*, **23**, 305–317.

Hunter, J.A., Becker, J.V. & Goodwin, D.W. (1991) The reliability and discriminative utility of the Adolescent Cognition Scale for juvenile sexual offences. *Annals of Sex Research*, **4**, 281–286.

Inamder, S.C., Lewis, D.O., Siomopoulos, G. *et al.* (1982) Violent and suicidal behaviour in psychotic adolescents. *American Journal of Psychiatry*, **139**, 932–935.

James, A.C. & Neil, P. (1996) Juvenile sexual offending: one year prevalence study within Oxfordshire. *Child Abuse and Neglect*, **13**, 477–485.

Jasper, A., Smith, C. & Bailey, S. (1998) One hundred girls in care referred to an adolescent forensic mental health service. *Journal of Adolescence*, **21**, 555–568.

Joseph Rowntree Foundation (1997) Communities that care (UK): a new kind of prevention programme—a guide. Joseph Rowntree Foundation, York.

Junger-Tas, J. (1994) *Delinquent Behaviour Among Young People in the Western World*. Kugler, Amsterdam.

Junger-Tas, J. & Block, R. (1988) *Juvenile Delinquency in the Netherlands*. Kugler, Amsterdam.

Justice (1996) *Children and Homicide: Appropriate Procedures for Juveniles in Murder and Manslaughter Cases*. Justice, London.

Kazdin, A. (1996) Combined and multimodal treatments in child and adolescent psychotherapy: issues, challenges and research directions. *Clinical Psychology, Science and Practice*, **3**, 69–100.

Kazdin, A.E. (1997) Practitioner review: psychological treatments for conduct disorder in children. *Journal of Child Psychology and Psychiatry*, **38**, 161–178.

Kazdin, A.E. (2000) Adolescent development, mental disorders, and decision making of delinquent youths. In: *Youth on Trial, a Developmental Perspective on Juvenile Justice* (eds T. Grisso & R.G. Schwartz), pp. 33–65. University of Chicago Press, Chicago.

Kendall, P.C. (1993) Cognitive-behavioural therapies with youth, guiding theory, current status and emerging developments. *Journal of Consulting and Clinical Psychology*, **61**, 235–247.

Kershaw, C., Goodman, J. & White, S. (1999) Reconvictions of offenders sentenced or discharged from prison in 1995, England and Wales. *Home Office Statistical Bulletin*, Issue 19/99. Home Office, London.

Knott, C. (1995) The STOP Programme: reasoning and rehabilitation in a British setting. In: *What Works? Reducing Re-offending* (ed. J. McGuire), pp. 115–126. John Wiley, Chichester.

Kolko, D.J. & Kazdin, A.E. (1992) The emergence and re-occurrence of child firesetting: a one year prospective study. *Journal of Abnormal Child Psychology*, **201**, 17–37.

Kovacs, M. & Devlin, B. (1998) Internalising disorders in childhood. *Journal of Child Psychology and Psychiatry*, **39**, 47–63.

Kratzer, L. & Hodgins, S. (1997) Adult outcomes of child conduct problems: a cohort study. *Journal of Abnormal Child Psychology*, **25**, 65–81.

Krisberg, B., Schwartz, I., Fishman, G., Eisikovits, Z., Guttman, E. & Joe, K. (1987) The incarceration of minority youth. *Crime and Delinquency*, **33**, 173–205.

Kroll, L., Woodham, A., Rothwell, J. *et al.* (1999) Reliability of the Salford Needs Assessment Schedule for Adolescents. *Psychological Medicine*, **29**, 891–902.

Kurtz, Z., Thornes, R. & Bailey, S. (1998) Children in the criminal justice and secure care systems: how their mental health needs are met. *Journal of Adolescence*, **21**, 543–553.

Lader, D., Singleton, N. & Meltzer, H. (2000) *Psychiatric Morbidity Among Young Offenders in England and Wales*. Office for National Statistics, London.

Langstrom, N., Grann, M. & Lindblad, F. (2000) A preliminary typology of young sex offenders. *Journal of Adolescence*, **23**, 319–329.

Le Blanc, M. (1998) Screening of serious and violent juvenile offenders: identification, classification and prediction. In: *Serious and Violent Juvenile Offenders: Risk Factors and Successful Intervention* (eds R. Loeber & D.P. Farrington), pp. 167–193. Sage, CA.

Lenssen, S.A.M., Doreleijers, T.A.H., Van Dijk, M.E. & Hartman, C.A. (2000) Girls in detention: what are their characteristics? A project to explore and document the character of this target group and the significant ways in which it differs from one consisting of boys. *Journal of Adolescence*, **23**, 287–303.

Lipsey, M.W. (1995) What do we learn from 400 research studies on the effectiveness of treatment with juvenile delinquents? In: *What Works: Reducing Offending* (ed. J. McGuire). John Wiley, Chichester.

Lipsey, M.W. & Wilson, D.B. (1998) Effective intervention for serious juvenile offenders: a synthesis of research. In: *Serious and Violent Juvenile Offenders: Risk Factors and Successful Interventions* (eds R. Loeber & D.P. Farrington), pp. 313–345. Sage, CA.

Little, M. & Mount, K. (1999) *Prevention and early intervention with children in need*. Ashgate Publishing Company, Aldershot.

Lockman, J.E. & Wayland, K.K. (1994) Aggression, social acceptance and race as predictors of negative adolescent outcomes. *Journal of the American Academy of Child and Adolescent Psychiatry*, **33**, 1026–1035.

Loeber, R. & Hay, D.F. (1994) Developmental approaches to aggression and conduct problems. In: *Development Through Life: a Handbook for Clinicians* (eds M. Rutter & D. Hay). Blackwell Science, Oxford.

Lösel, F. (1995) Increasing consensus in the evaluation of offender rehabilitation: lessons from recent research syntheses. *Psychology, Crime and Law*, **2**, 19–39.

Lyall, I., Holland, A. & Collins, S. (1995) Offending by adults with learning disabilities and the attitudes of staff to offending behaviour: implications for service development. *Journal of Intellectual Disability Research*, **39**, 501–508.

MacCulloch, M.J., Snowden, P.R., Wood, P.J.W. & Mills, H.E. (1983) Sadistic fantasy: sadistic behaviour and offending. *British Journal of Psychiatry*, **143**, 2–9.

Maden, A., Taylor, C., Brooke, D. & Gunn, J. (1995) *Mental Disorder in Remand Prisoners*. Institute of Psychiatry and Home Office, London.

Magnusson, D., Klintebert, B. & Stattin, H. (1994) Juvenile and persistent offenders: behavioural and physiological characteristics. In: *Adolescent Problem Behaviours: Issues and Research* (eds R.D. Ketterlinus & M.E. Lamb), pp. 81–91. Erlbaum, Hillsdale, NJ.

Maziade, M., Bouchard, S., Gingras, N. & Charson, L. (1996) Long term stability of diagnosis and symptom dimensions in a systematic sample of patients with onset of schizophrenia in childhood and early adolescence. I. Positive/negative distinction and childhood predictors of adult outcome. *British Journal of Psychiatry*, **169**, 371–378.

McGuire, J. (1996) Psycho-social approaches to the understanding and reduction of violence in young people. In: *Violence in Children and Adolescents* (ed. V. Varma), pp. 65–83. Jessica Kingsley, London.

McGuire, J. (2000) *Working with young offenders in secure settings*. Paper presented at University of Sheffield, Sheffield.

McGuire, J. & Priestley, P. (1995) Reviewing 'What Works': past, present and future. In: *What Works: Reducing Reoffending* (ed. J. McGuire), pp. 3–34. John Wiley, Chichester.

Miller, D., Tropani, C., Fejes-Mencloza, K., Eggleston, C. & Dwiggins, D. (1995) Adolescent female offenders: unique consideration. *Adolescence*, **30**, 429–435.

Millon, T. (1993) *Millon Adolescent Clinical Inventory*. National Computer Systems, Manual, Minneapolis, MN.

Moffitt, T.E. (1993) Adolescence limited and life course persistent antisocial behaviour: a developmental taxonomy. *Psychological Review*, **100**, 674–701.

Moffitt, T.E., Caspi, A., Dickson, N., Silva, P. & Stanton, W. (1996) Childhood onset versus adolescent onset antisocial conduct problems in males: natural history from ages 3–18 years. *Development and Psychopathology*, **9**, 399–424.

Monahan, J. (1992) Mental disorder and violent behaviour. *American Psychologist*, **47**, 511–521.

Monahan, J. & Appelbaum, P.S. (2000) Developing a clinically useful actuarial tool for assessing violence risk. *British Journal of Psychiatry*, **176**, 313–320.

Moran, P. & Hagell, A. (2000) *Intervening to Prevent Antisocial Personality Disorder: a Scoping Review*. Policy Research Bureau Final Report to Home Office, November 2000.

Myers, W.C. & Scott, K. (1998) Psychotic and conduct disorder symptoms in juvenile murderers. *Journal of Homicide Studies*, **2**, 160–175.

Myers, W.C., Scott, K., Burgess, A.W. & Burgess, A.G. (1995) Psychopathology, biopsychosocial factors, crime statistics and classification of 25 homicidal youths. *Journal of the American Academy of Child and Adolescent Psychiatry*, **34**, 1483–1489.

Nichols, H.R. & Molinder, I. (1984) *Multiphasic Sex Inventory*. Tacoma, WA.

Nicol, R., Stretch, D., Whitney, I. *et al.* (2000) Mental health needs and services for severely troubled and troubling young offenders in an NHS region. *Journal of Adolescence*, **23**, 243–261.

Novaco, R.W. (1994) Anger as a risk factor for violence among the mentally disturbed. In: *Violence and Mental Disorder* (eds J. Monaghan & H. Steadman), pp. 21–59. University of Chicago Press, Chicago.

O'Brien, B.S. & Frick, P.J. (1996) Reward dominance associations with anxiety conduct problems and psychopathy in children. *Journal of Abnormal Child Psychology*, **24**, 223–240.

O'Brien, G. (1996) The psychiatric management of adult autism. *Advances in Psychiatric Treatment*, **2**, 173–177.

O'Callaghan, D. & Print, B. (1994) Adolescent sexual abusers research: assessment and treatment. In: *Sexual Offending Against Children: Assessment and Treatment of Male Abusers* (eds T. Morrison, M. Erooga & R.C. Beckett), pp. 146–177. Routledge, London.

Olweus, D. (1993) *Bullying at School: What We Know and What We Can Do*. Blackwell Publishers, Oxford.

Patterson, G.R. (1982) *Coercive Family Process*. Castalia, Eugene, OR.

Pliszka, S., Stienman, J., Barrow, V. & Frick, S. (2000) Affective disorders in juvenile offenders: a preliminary study. *American Journal of Psychiatry*, **157**, 130–132.

Repo, E. & Virkunnen, M. (1997) Young arsonists, history of conduct disorder, psychiatric diagnosis, and criminal recidivism. *Journal of Forensic Psychiatry*, **8**, 311–320.

Robins, L.N. & Price, R.K. (1991) Adult disorders predicted by child conduct problems: results from the NIMIT Epidemiological Catchment Area project. *Psychiatry*, **54**, 116–132.

Ross, R.R. & Ross, R.D. (1995) *Thinking Straight: the Reasoning and Rehabilitation Programme for Delinquency. Prevention and Offender Rehabilitation*. Air Training and Publications, Ottawa, Canada.

Royal College of Psychiatrists (1999) *Offenders with Personality Disorders*, Council Report CR 71. Gaskell, London.

Royal College of Psychiatrists (2001) *Guidelines for researchers and for research ethics committees on psychiatric research involving human participants*, Council Report CR 82. Gaskell, London.

Rutter, M. (1997) Antisocial behaviour: developmental psychopathology perspectives. In: *Handbook of Antisocial Behaviour* (eds D.M. Stoff, J. Brieling & J.D. Maser), pp. 115–124. John Wiley, Chichester.

Rutter, M. & Giller, H. (1983) *Juvenile Delinquency Trends and Perspectives*. Penguin, London.

Rutter, M. & Smith, D.J. (1995) *Psychosocial Disorders in Young People: Time Trends and Their Causes*. John Wiley, Chichester.

Rutter, M., Giller, H. & Hagell, A. (1998) *Antisocial Behaviour by Young People*. Cambridge University Press, Cambridge.

Shaffer, D., Gould, M. & Fisher, P. (1996) Psychiatric diagnosis in child and adolescent suicide. *Archives of General Psychiatry*, **53**, 339–348.

Schweinhart, L.J., Barnes, H.O. & Weikart, D.P. (1993) *Significant benefits the High/Scope Perry Preschool Study through age 27*. High/Scope, Ypsilank, MI.

Sheldrick, C. (1999) Practitioner review: the assessment and management of risk in adolescents. *Journal of Child Psychology and Psychiatry*, **40**, 507–518.

Shepherd, J.P. & Farrington, D.P. (1993) Assault as a public health problem. *Journal of the Royal Society of Medicine*, **6**, 89–92.

Sinclair, I. & Gibbs, I. (1998) *Children's Homes: A Study in Diversity*. John Wiley, Chichester.

Sirles, E.A., Araji, S. & Bosek, R. (1997) Redirecting children's sexually abusive and sexually aggressive behaviours: programs and practices. In: *Sexually Aggressive Children: Coming to Understand Them* (ed. S.K. Araji), pp. 161–192. Sage, CA.

Skuse, D., Bentovim, A., Hodges, J. *et al.* (1998) Risk factors for development of sexually abusive behaviour. Sexually victimised adolescent boys: cross sectional study. *British Medical Journal*, **317**, 175–179.

Smith, C. (1996) *Developing Parenting Programmes.* Joseph Rowntree Foundation, York/National Children's Bureau, London.

Smith, D. (1995) Youth crime and conduct disorders: trends, patterns and causal explanations. In: *Psychosocial Disorders in Young People: Time Trends and Their Causes* (eds M. Rutter & D.J. Smith), pp. 393–489. John Wiley, Chichester.

Snyder, H.N., Sickmund, M. & Peo-Yamagata, E. (1996) *Juvenile Offenders and Victims: 1996. Update on violence.* Office of Juvenile Justice and Delinquency Prevention, Washington D.C.

Stattin, H. & Magnusson, D. (1991) Stability and change in criminal behaviour up to age 30. *British Journal of Criminology*, **31**, 327–346.

Stattin, H. & Magnusson, D. (1996) Antisocial development: a holistic approach. *Development and Psychopathology*, **8**, 617–645.

Steadman, H.J., Monahan, J., Appelbaum, P.S. *et al.* (1994) Designing a new generation of risk assessment research in violence and mental disorder. In: *Developments in Risk Assessment* (eds J. Monahan & H.J. Steadman), pp. 297–318. University of Chicago Press, Chicago.

Steadman, H.J., Mulvey, E.P., Monahan, J. *et al.* (1998) Violence by people discharged from acute psychiatric inpatient facilities and by others on the same neighbourhood. *Archives of General Psychiatry*, **55**, 393–401.

Stiffman, A.R. & Dorep, Cunningham, R.M. (1996) Violent behaviour in adolescents and young adults: a person and environmental model. *Journal of Child and Family Studies*, **5**, 407–450.

Sullivan, M.L. (1998) Integrating qualitative methods un the study of developmental psychopathology in context. *Development Psychopathology*, **10**, 377–393.

Taylor, P.J. & Gunn, J. (1999) Homicides by people with mental illness: myth and reality. *British Journal of Psychiatry*, **174**, 9–14.

Teplin, L.A., Abram, K.M. & McClelland, G.M. (1998) Psychiatric disorders among juvenile detainees. Paper Presented at the Annual Conference on Criminal Justice Research and Evaluation (July, 1998) Bureau of Justice Assistance. Office of Juvenile Justice and Delinquency Prevention, Washington D.C.

Tolan, P.H. & Gorman-Smith, D. (1997) Treatment of juvenile delinquency between punishment and therapy. In: *Handbook of Antisocial Behaviour* (eds D.M. Stoff, J. Breiling & J.D. Maser), pp. 405–415. John Wiley, Chichester.

Tonry, M. & Farrington, D.P. (1995) Strategic approaches to crime prevention. In: *Building a Safer Society: Strategic Approaches to Crime Prevention* (eds M. Tonry & D.P. Farrington), pp. 1–20. University of Chicago Press, Chicago.

Ulzen, T. & Hamilton, H. (1998) The nature and characteristics of psychiatric co-morbidity in incarcerated adolescents. *Canadian Journal of Psychiatry*, **43**, 57–63.

Vermeiren, R., De Clippele, A. & Deboutte, D. (2000) A descriptive survey of Flemish delinquent adolescents, *Journal of Adolescence*, **23**, 277–285.

Vizard, E., Wynick, S., Hawkes, C., Woods, J. & Jenkins, J. (1996) Juvenile sexual offenders. *British Journal of Psychiatry*, **168**, 259–262.

Vreeland, R.G. & Levin, B.M. (1980) Psychological aspects of firesetting. In: *Fires and Human Behaviour* (ed. D. Canter), pp. 31–61. John Wiley, New York.

Webster, C.D., Douglas, K.S., Eaves, D. & Hart, S.D. (1997) *HCR-20 Assessing Risk of Violence* (Version 2). Vancouver Mental Health Law and Policy Institute, Simon Fraser University.

Webster-Stratton, H.M. (1994) *Troubled Families: Problem Children.* John Wiley, Chichester.

Weinberg, N.Z., Rahdert, E., Colliver, J.D. & Glantz, M.D. (1998) Adolescent substance abuse: a review of the past ten years. *Journal of the American Academy of Child and Adolescent Psychiatry*, **37**, 479–485.

Weitekamp, E., Kerner, H.J., Schubert, A. & Schindler, V. (1996) Multiple and habitual offending among young males: criminology and criminal policy lessons from a re-analysis of the Philadelphia Birth Cohort Studies. *International Annals of Criminology*, **12**, 9–52.

Wikstrom, P.O.H. (1990) Age and crime in a Stockholm cohort. *Journal of Quantitative Criminology*, **6**, 61–83.

Wilde, J. (1996) *Treating anger, anxiety, and depression in children and adolescents: a cognitive-behavioural perspective.* Accelerated Development, Washington D.C.

Wolfgang, M.E., Thornberry, T.P. & Figlio, R.M. (1987) *From Boys to Men: from Delinquency to Crime.* University of Chicago Press, Chicago.

Zimring, F. (1998) *The Challenge of Youth Violence.* Cambridge University Press, Cambridge.

Zimring, F.E. (2000) Penal proportionality for the young offender: notes on immaturity, capacity and diminished responsbility. In: *Youth on Trial: a Developmental Perspective on Juvenile Justice* (eds T. Grisso & R.G. Schwartz) Vol. 10, pp. 271–288. University of Chicago Press, Chicago.

Zoccolillo, M. (1993) Gender and the development of conduct disorder. *Development and Psychopathology*, **5**, 65–78.

Zoccolillo, M., Pickles, A., Quinton, D. & Rutter, M. (1992) The outcome of childhood conduct disorder: implications for defining adult personality disorder and conduct disorder. *Psychological Medicine*, **22**, 971–986.

Provision of Intensive Treatment: Inpatient Units, Day Units and Intensive Outreach

Jonathan Green

Introduction

The last decade has seen a rapid evolution in the structure and delivery of mental health services in many countries. The use of inpatient beds has declined in many systems and there is an increasing interest in evaluating other models of service delivery, such as day provision or intensive outreach, as well as modified models of inpatient care. In parallel, the context within which children's mental health disorders are seen has progressively widened to encompass the context of the family, school and wider community. A stage emphasis in personality and social development, which provided a rationale for intensive episodic interventions, has been complemented with a new appreciation of chronicity and long-term pathways in the evolution of many disorders. Acute episodes of intensive treatment have therefore to be considered now in the current contexts of both family and local environment as well as in the longitudinal context of what is known about the natural history of particular disorders. This chapter reviews new developments in current practice and the evidence base for intensive treatments in the light of these considerations, before suggesting prospects for the future.

Inpatient treatment

Historical roots

Two broad forms of residential mental health care for young people emerged in the early twentieth century. The first was based on the idea that a self-contained social environment could act as a 'therapeutic milieu', effecting personality and behaviour change (Kennard 1983). Examples in the UK were Homer Lane's 'Little Commonwealth' (Bazeley 1928) and residential therapeutic schools, such as the Mulberry Bush and the Cotswold Community; in the USA, the work of Bettelheim (1955). A second historical root was the adaptations made for children within the asylums of the nineteenth century (Parry Jones 1998) and the accelerated development of specialized medically based psychiatric units for children following the encephalitis epidemic in the USA in the 1920s (Beskind 1962). Such hospital units developed to provide a comprehensive approach to assessment and treatment based on a biopsychosocial model (Cameron 1949). Here the hospital environment is the *location* for assessment and treatment rather than its *primary agent*.

The decades after the Second World War saw a rapid expansion of inpatient units, usually combining elements of both models. Recent years have seen a plateauing or reduction in numbers and increasing specialization alongside an awareness of the potential negative effects of residential treatment (Wolkind 1974). However, the two historical themes remain a useful way of conceptualizing inpatient treatment process.

The ward as a therapeutic environment

The 'therapeutic milieu' is a term subject to numerous reinterpretations but little empirical research (Green & Burke 1998). Early psychodynamic formulations (Bettelheim 1955) contained an assumption that the milieu substituted for a lack in the child's previous experience—particularly, sensitive parental type care. This model emphasized a total environment and intense efforts of care staff over long treatments. Later systemic models (Woolston 1989) have emphasized the ward's 'open system' character and its potentially mediating role in improving the 'goodness of fit' between young people and their environment. The focus here is on collaboration with other agencies and the family; parents often take an active part in the ward caregiving.

Other models have emphasized the ward environment as a corrective emotional experience with high levels of warm staff communication, peer contact and active behavioural control (Cotton 1993), while a few specialized developments have involved admitting whole families (Lynch *et al.* 1975). Five-day residential patterns have become common (Green & Jacobs 1998). Recent developments—notably driven by managed care in the USA (Nurcombe 1989; Harper 1989)—have in contrast reduced the ward environment to its most minimal form. The emphasis here is on symptom stabilization and 'minimum necessary change' before rapid discharge. Stays are often under 2 weeks: a radically different form of milieu from the 3-year or more stays described by earlier writers. In this recent model, the therapeutic milieu as historically understood has essentially disappeared and inpatient care has returned to its root in acute hospital practice.

While adult psychiatric research has addressed the character and effect of different forms of residential milieu, there has been virtually no equivalent work in child and adolescent psychiatry. A Ward Atmosphere Scale (WAS) identified six styles of treatment environment in 144 adult psychiatry units in the USA (Price & Moos 1977) which can be associated with differential outcomes (Moos *et al.* 1973). Just one published study (Steiner *et al.* 1991) has reported on an adaptation of the WAS for an adolescent setting. Systematic research into the efficacy of different milieu solutions for children and adolescents is long overdue and has been identified as a priority in a number of reviews (Pfeiffer & Strzelecki 1990; Pottick *et al.* 1993).

Social functioning and education

Admission can have value as a removal from external difficulty as well as an exposure to an active treatment environment. By the time of admission, a young person's social adaptation in their community has often broken down, sometimes in all areas of school, family and community life. Widespread social difficulties were found in 58 consecutive general admissions in New Zealand, including a moderate to severe language handicap in 40% of cases (Paterson *et al.* 1997). A study of 126 hospitalized children and adolescents in the USA (Luthar *et al.* 1995) similarly found severe impairments in the Vineland social competency scores of inpatients admitted with externalizing and mixed internalizing/externalizing disorders. Social competency here was associated with specific reading scores rather than broad IQ. These findings have practical implications. The traditional therapeutic milieu contains elements of group living, peer relationships and intensive staff–patient contact. Removal from social difficulties in the external environment and exposure to such a milieu can produce rapid gains in functioning and self-esteem. However, children with significant social impairments may not be able to make effective use of such a socially orientated therapeutic environment. Assessing and targeting social difficulties more precisely and defining the effective milieu characteristics for different problems is an important task for future developments in milieu treatment.

Similarly, many inpatients have a history of school failure or acute school breakdown. The individualized assessment and intensive educational input possible within the inpatient unit can make a radical impact (French & Tate 1998). Green *et al.* (2001) found a rapid reduction in teacher ratings of behavioural disturbance in the classroom from pre-admission to 1 month post-admission in a consecutive sample of 55 child admissions, persisting when reassessed at 6-month follow-up.

Such rapid gains in socialization and academic achievement represent two of the potential therapeutic strengths of residential treatment. They can be used as a platform from which to reintegrate patients into their own communities with enhanced resilience, as long as there is good linkage into aftercare. However, such targeted interventions take time and are not compatible with ultra-short inpatient stays.

Admission practice

Admission rates into inpatient care differ greatly between countries. A national survey of young people receiving mental health treatment in the USA during 1986 (Pottick *et al.* 1993) found that 5% of the children (6–12 years) and 30% of the adolescents (13–18 years) were being treated in inpatient facilities (com-

bined proportion 20%). In the UK, admission rates are much lower, estimated at around 1% of the clinical pool of children under 12 in one area (Maskey 1998), a fifth of the US rates. Current recommended provision in the UK is for two to four child and four to six adolescent beds per district of 250 000 population, to be provided in subregional units of 15 beds for children and 25 for adolescents (Royal College of Psychiatrists 1997).

Studies have addressed the criteria for admission. Costello *et al.* (1991) studied 389 children between 2 and 12 years referred for inpatient evaluation in the USA. Factors leading to admission included deterioration despite outpatient treatment; increasing aggressiveness; difficulties with assessment or diagnosis; family difficulties in the context of psychiatric disorder making treatment impossible; and the need for 24-h observation or nursing care. Two UK-based studies of children (Garralda 1986; Wolkind & Gent 1987) formulated similar criteria. A prospective study of 276 admissions to adolescent units (Wrate *et al.* 1994) characterized diagnostic formulations accounting for most admissions. However, Pottick *et al.* (1995) found that the strongest influence on admission in the USA was the presence of insurance cover: a cut in insurance benefit between 1978 and 1983 also coincided with a significant drop in US inpatient usage (Patrick *et al.* 1993). Proximity to a specialist centre increases referral rates (Gutterman *et al.* 1993) and Blanz & Schmidt (2000) describe how devolution of inpatient care to smaller local units in Germany reduced admission times and changed admission practice.

A pragmatic model of the process of admission (Bruggen & O'Brien 1987) describes common practice—a negotiation between referrer, family and admitting unit around which specific needs of each party could be met by admission. In the future it is to be hoped that an increasing part of such decision-making will be the empirical evidence regarding the effectiveness of inpatient treatments in particular situations and for particular disorders (see below). Whereas the inpatient resource is rightly held in reserve for the most complex and severe cases, referral should not be overdelayed: a well-timed intensive treatment may often prevent further deterioration in an acute disorder.

Admissions generally fall into a number of broad categories.

1 The need for detailed assessment in complex cases when the formulation is unclear. The combination of the medical setting with the range of health professionals makes the ward particularly well able to address the interaction of biological, psychological and social aspects of disorders.

2 When it is useful for assessment or treatment to take place away from the family. This can be crucial when the role of family in a presentation may be unclear, e.g. when fabricated or induced illness is suspected, or when complex symptoms seem confined to home.

3 When psychiatric symptomatology is escalating, despite the most intensive outpatient treatment available, the ward gives access to intensive nursing in a controlled environment. This will include acute risk management of self-harm or family disruption associated with psychiatric disorder.

4 For controlled trials of specific interventions.

Pre-admission evaluation is thus a crucial area. The admission must be seen within the context of a continuum of service use and the developmental trajectory of the child, because it will be a brief episode in both these areas. Many of the key predictors of inpatient outcome lie in details of previous family adaptation, child social functioning and child symptomatology (see below): assessment should thus focus on these aspects as well as the needs and motivation of patient and family. Pre-admission evaluation may lead to a decision not to admit. Many children with social and behavioural difficulties, for instance, may be more appropriately cared for within the social care system with psychiatric input.

Emergency admission

Studies of referrer attitudes emphasize the high priority given to the specialist unit's responsiveness and capacity to admit emergencies (Gowers & Kushlick 1992). Good and responsive consultation around the emergency may meet the need without admission (Cotgrove 1997), and Dimond & Golberg (1999) gave a helpful perspective on this from a referring team. However, provision of acute beds is likely to be an increasing priority and will shape service provision. The use of acute admission to paediatric and adult psychiatry beds is often used as an alternative in this area, and is beyond the remit of this chapter—but forms an important aspect of health care planning.

Discharge and aftercare

Discharge planning should receive equal attention to admission planning. Many studies point to the crucial role of aftercare in the maintenance of treatment gains made during admission (Pfeiffer & Strzelecki 1990). In a minority of cases admission may prove to be a stepping stone towards longer term alternative care or residential schooling. Because of the multifaceted nature of inpatient problems the team will need to liaise with a wide variety of local services in education, social services and mental health. In adolescents a 'care programme approach' may be used along lines developed in adult mental health as an aid to transition into adult services. A recent study of service use (Hoagwood 2000) showed that a limited period of intensive specialist treatment resulted in a more effective use of other services thereafter and may explain some 'sleeper' effects. It is to be hoped that inpatient treatment could catalyse similar improvements in service usage during aftercare—presuming such services are available.

Unwanted effects of inpatient treatment

There is little systematic research in this area. Potential unwanted effects can usefully be grouped into those consequent on:
1 loss of support from the child's local environment;
2 presence of adverse effects within the inpatient environment; and
3 the effects of admission on family life (Green & Jones 1998).

Losses consequent on admission

Reporting bias towards acute problems during pre-admission assessment can obscure hidden sources of support and resilience in the local environment—within the extended family, peers or school. Pre-admission assessment should therefore actively focus on strengths as well as difficulties and identify key areas of individual resilience. Admission may also result in the loss of important local professional input, which should be ameliorated by good communication between unit, referring teams and local services. These factors need particular attention from inpatient clinicians because they may be less obvious than active effects from within the inpatient environment itself.

Impact of the inpatient environment

Some young people may enter the ward with a profound sense of relief but others may find it at least initially frightening and bewildering. Patient ratings after inpatient psychiatric care (usually collected by the units themselves) generally show positive evaluation of the treatment. However, parents are often concerned that their child may be negatively affected ('contaminated') by other patients' problems. Units must be constantly vigilant to the possibility of peer abuse. To counter such potential problems, Newbold & Jones (1998) suggested a proactive emphasis on child welfare and rights throughout a unit, embodied in the appointment of a 'welfare co-ordinator', with a role to investigate any complaints. This is performed in the context of procedural agreements with local child protection agencies and a continuing programme of awareness training and education of staff.

There have been no specific studies into institutionalization in child or adolescent psychiatry units, but attitudes may be influenced by studies of non-medical residential care, even though these environments may be very different. Colton (1988) found residential children's homes performing extremely badly on measures of staff relationships, physical environment and community involvement in comparison with children in foster care. Well-publicized episodes of abuse in residential social care environments (Levy & Kahan 1991) may also be generalized into attitudes towards residential psychiatry treatments by families, although it is to be hoped that the intensity of monitoring and supervision in the latter makes such disasters less likely.

Effect on families

Much professional concern has focused on the disruptive effect of admission on family dynamics, e.g. the reinforcement of 'scapegoating'. This may indeed be a contraindication to admission, although equally a scapegoated child has a right to the best possible assessment and care—and this may involve admission. As the child engages with the ward there can also be a danger that the parents feel deskilled (Green 1994). Good family contracting pre-admission and sustained family work can counteract these negative effects. A family's commitment to intensive treatments can be disruptive and expensive and on occasion threaten employment. It is essential to anticipate this by building support for family travel into the contracting around the case and actively to support the family in relation to employers.

Given the powerful intervention and therapeutic potential of inpatient treatment, some associated unwanted effects are likely. There is a need for their systematic study—rather than reliance on purely theoretical concerns or anecdote. Along with general standards of good practice, systematic procedures of anticipation, prevention, recognition and repair should minimize unwanted effects (Green & Jones 1998)—but again this needs to be studied.

Characteristics of day units

The concept of psychiatric day care emerged from the therapeutic elaboration of school provision for young children (Zimnet & Farley 1985) and psychiatrically orientated day hospital units have grown up as an intermediate form of treatment between outpatient and residential work (Connell 1961). Relieved of the need to provide residential aspects of care, day unit environments have been able to evolve in a host of different directions. These have ranged from specific day programmes for young children with developmental problems, as an adjunct to specialist school provision, to intensive 5-day-a-week treatment interventions with whole families. The range is now too great to summarize neatly. Of UK day hospital units, 46% are now associated with inpatient residential units (Bailey, V., personal communication). This combination has the advantages of sharing staff and expertise and allowing a flexible use of day care as a transition out of and into residential care. The advantages of independent day units relate to flexibility in the use of staff. The reduced need for a shift system to cover nights allows ward staff to work predictable hours and be available regularly for liaison sessions and outreach work. Partial attendance also means that staff can have days free for supervision and continuing education.

Amid the variety of day unit functioning, a number of broad themes may be distinguished.

1 Day units for the treatment of disruptive behaviour. A number of programmes have been developed in this area. They usually use multimodal treatment packages with a combination of individual family and liaison intervention together with psychopharmacology. Grizenko (1997) and Rey *et al.* (1998) have reported outcomes of such programmes.

2 Some units have specialized in the management of younger children with developmental disorders such as autism, speech and language disorders or neuropsychiatric disorder. These provide centres for comprehensive assessment and initiation of treatment management involving family and school liaison.

3 Units whose prime aim is to influence family functioning in situations of family breakdown or child maltreatment. A number of influential programmes of this kind have been described (Asen *et al.* 1982).

The partial milieu of the day unit shares care with family or local school to a greater extent than residential units. Thus liaison takes up correspondingly more time and contact with parents may be more frequent. The day unit has the opportunity to generate treatment programmes that link very closely with parental care. The emphasis on education means that the academic focus of the milieu in day care can be fully exploited. Educationally, therefore, inpatient and day unit treatment can be identical.

Disadvantages of the day unit milieu mirror these advantages. Many day units may not have the facility to mount a full educational programme and make do with sessional teacher inputs. This may not in itself be enough to achieve the key academic goals necessary for a child failing in school. Secondly, if the school provision is complete then there is little time left during the day for other kinds of therapeutic programming, which might take place in the evening on the inpatient unit. The day unit will have to achieve a balance between adequate intense academic input on the one hand and the socialization and therapeutic experience on the other. They may find that they have insufficient time to do both properly with complex children. The child may have to make multiple adaptations to different environments during the week and in many areas the daily transport to and from the unit can be complex and tiring. The opportunities for completeness and intensity of treatment and observation are less.

The milieu on the day unit can be investigated in precisely the same way to that of the inpatient unit. As it does not contain the total residential care element it tends to focus on specific adaptive behavioural issues. The focus is likely to be less on the relationship between the child and the institution and more on the relationship between child, family and school of origin. The provision of staff can be flexible and draw on sessional input from a wide range of professionals. There is less need for a core nursing provision. In many units the parents are engaged in providing much of the shared care in the unit.

Common aspects of day unit and inpatient treatment

Therapeutic alliance

Therapeutic alliance is poorly researched in child psychiatry when compared to adult mental health treatments (Hougaard 1994), yet proxy measures of therapeutic alliance such as 'parental co-operation' commonly provide the most significant predictor of inpatient and day patient outcome (Sourander *et al.* 1996; Grizenko 1997). Kroll & Green (1997) reviewed the complexity of the therapeutic alliance in inpatient and day patient care. Alliances form between child and parents separately and members of a complex inpatient team. The team itself acts in a number of different roles, ranging from a quasi-parenting role in relation to a child's basic needs to a therapeutic role while undertaking specific programmes; from a 'collaborative' role with parents to a 'patient' status for adults within family therapy. Adult studies find that therapeutic alliance relates to pretreatment social adaptation (Hougaard 1994) and social competency is found to be a key variable predicting adaptation into an adolescent inpatient treatment environment (Luthar *et al.* 1995). Such findings emphasize the importance of preadmission work for building a therapeutic alliance. Techniques for maximizing alliance independently with both child and parent need consideration. In a prospective study of 55 patients in inpatient and day patient care (Green *et al.*, 2001), child and parental alliance were independent of each other and it was the alliance with the child that predicted health gain during admission, including good outcome in externalizing disorder.

Assessment strategies

The ward environment creates opportunities for detailed assessment of biological and psychological aspects of disorder. Covert causes of behavioural difficulties can be elucidated, e.g. a study of unselected adolescent admissions (Szabo & Magnus 1999) revealed 4% of patients with undiagnosed complex partial seizures. Wards need ready access to the full range of biological investigations, including scanning, EEG and clinical chemistry; a range of developmental assessments such as detailed speech pathology, occupational therapy and psychometric evaluation; and the opportunity for paediatric and neurological liaison. There are unique opportunities for observational studies in settings ranging from highly structured individual assessments to naturalistic observations during ward and school activities. Making best use of these opportunities requires good planning because important observations are often made by the least experienced staff and multiple assessments have to be integrated into a whole. One solution is to have structured assessment protocols for particular problems in which different staff have defined tasks towards a common end (Green 1996). Assessments performed in this way are always challenging—initial assumptions based on limited information can be examined critically in the light of different staff perspectives; this is one of the strengths of multidisciplinary working in the ward environment. Staff will use specific skills from their core profession as well as skills developed within the team to serve these tasks. The team thus needs a programme of generic skill development to meet the priorities of the unit.

Planning treatment goals

The concept of treatment goal planning was elegantly outlined by Shaw (1998) and has many attractive features. It acts to organize thinking and focus treatment in complex cases and counters therapeutic drift. However, it is deceptively simple and depends on significant assessment and engagement with the family. Shaw suggested that treatment goals should be understandable, ideally framed in the child's own words, achievable and measurable: they are distinguished from the *staff hypothesis*

(a professional formulation of the case) and the *treatment plan* established by the staff group on the basis of this hypothesis. Rothery *et al.* (1995) made an audit of treatment goals in admissions to four adolescent units. They found that the majority of treatment goals reflected relationship and maturational aims rather than symptom change alone. Improvement across such goals was noted during treatment. Goals should be flexible enough to be able to evolve in potentially unexpected directions when necessary during treatment.

Adapting treatments to the inpatient and day patient setting

In addition to individualized treatments, there remain generic aspects of ward management. Behavioural management on any unit is a key area, requiring ward policies on the management of aggression, use of seclusion or restraint, bullying and runaway behaviour (American Academy of Child and Adolescent Psychiatry 2000). Minimization of problems begins with thorough initial risk assessment and treatment planning, but equal emphasis needs to be placed on the overall culture of the unit, staff behaviour and the ongoing use of social skills and anger management programmes (Cotton 1993; Higgins & Burke 1998). The American Academy of Child and Adolescent Psychiatry review commented that the trend to brief treatment stays can undermine such a culture. Luisielli *et al.* (1998) applied a behavioural analysis to incidents of mechanical restraint in a US unit and concluded that such extreme measures were often the result of a failure of preplanning, unit policy or staff awareness. Antecedents to restraint were commonly an escalation of conflict initiated by staff behaviour rather than child behaviour and based on unrealistic staff expectations of child compliance. The authors advocated a comprehensive functional assessment, proactive treatment planning and the use of short time-out procedures in which the child has control as to duration. When prevention fails, crisis intervention techniques can range from de-escalation strategies and seclusion to brief carefully trained physical holding. More controversial techniques include use of medication and mechanical restraint (papoose boards or holding blankets) and are contraindicated for younger ages and where there is previous trauma related to confinement (American Academy of Child and Adolescent Psychiatry 2000). There are no comparative studies of the relative value of these techniques and the whole area is relatively underresearched and subject to clinical fashion (Angold & Pickles 1993). However, careful reviews of available evidence and explicit clinical guidelines, such as those from the American Academy of Child and Adolescent Psychiatry, form the best current safeguard for patients and professionals alike.

Individual treatments, such as cognitive-behavioural therapy (CBT) and individual psychotherapy, are incorporated into individualized treatment planning. The trend towards shorter treatment stays favours brief and focal treatments, such as CBT. The detailed assessments provided by individual psychotherapy have continuing value but there are particular challenges in adapting psychotherapeutic treatment techniques to the modern treatment milieu when stays are relatively short (Leibenluft *et al.* 1993; Magagna 1998).

The challenge of mounting family therapy in the context of a busy inpatient unit was reviewed by Lask & Maynerd (1998). Pre-admission family functioning has been found to be a predictor of health gain during treatment in a number of studies (Pfeiffer & Strzelecki 1990) but Green *et al.* (2001) found that family functioning did not improve during admission in their study. An option may be for the formal family therapy to take place at the local site of referral in partnership with the inpatient team. The ward staff provide a form of psychological care which inevitably has elements of substitute parenting, especially for younger children, and has the opportunity to pioneer the development of specialized forms of care for extreme difficulties. In wards taking multiple diagnostic groups, flexibility and thoughtfulness is needed; the management of a behaviourally disturbed child with attachment disorder will be very different to superficially similar behaviours in a child with pervasive developmental disorder or obsessive-compulsive disorder (OCD).

Consent and motivation

The United Nations Convention on the Rights of the Child (UNICEF 1995) and national legislation with regard to children (e.g. the UK Children Act, White *et al.* 1990) have significant implications for practice. The trend is for consent to be increasingly explicit, treatment-specific and involving of the child. Developmental issues around competency have been reviewed (Shaw 1998). Within residential units, the social and linguistic impairments of patients, described elsewhere in this chapter, need to be carefully considered. In a useful study of competency in a consecutive series of 25 psychiatric child inpatients, Billick *et al.* (1998) found that 'legal competency' (the ability to understand legal rights and the principle of consent) was associated with the achievement of a 5th or 6th grade (12 years' equivalent) reading level.

Another principle of consent should be collaboration with parents. A generic consent to treatment can be obtained early in admission in conjunction with treatment goal planning, based on what is likely to happen within a particular programme of care. Such an approach combines the best principles of both consent and treatment goal planning. In the case of enforced treatment there is debate as to whether various aspects of children's legislation or adult-orientated mental health legislation is best used in particular circumstances (Cotgrove & Gowers 1999).

The staff team

As treatment approaches become more sophisticated, the staff team in both inpatient and day patient care have increasingly complex tasks to perform. In many countries, nurses with mental health and/or children's qualifications form the main ward staff group, but play specialists, trainee psychologists and vol-

Table 61.1 Factors indicating the need for higher shift ratios. (Adapted with permission from Cotton 1993.)

1 *Patient heterogeneity*
   Greater number of patients
   Broader range of ages
   Variation in levels of developmental functioning and diagnosis (e.g. combining cognitively impaired or psychotic children with brighter behaviourally disordered children)
2 *Case severity*
   Greater severity and pervasiveness of impairments
   Severity of symptoms, such as suicidality, aggressiveness, sexualization
3 *Lack of family or support systems outside the hospital*
4 *Poor therapeutic alliance* (e.g. families with statutory orders or referred from courts)
5 *Frequent staff turnover*
6 *Shorter lengths of stay* (more acute admissions and an inability to develop routines and relationships)

unteers can also usefully add to the skill mix. Guidance from both the USA (American Academy of the Child and Adolescent Psychiatry 1990) and the UK (Royal College of Psychiatrists 1999) emphasizes the wide variety of professionals that should be represented in well-running inpatient or day patient units. These will include consultant child and adolescent psychiatrists, social workers, psychologists, speech and language therapists, occupational therapists, family therapists and psychotherapists. Attempts to operate with too few staff are a recipe for stress, burn-out and institutional decay. Staff numbers are best discussed in 'shift ratios' (number of staff per shift) or in sessional terms because this allows application to diverse unit functioning. For nursing staff, factors influencing the shift ratio include skill mix, the task demands of a particular shift (from low-intensity observation at night to high-intensity active therapy) and patient dependency (Table 61.1). Furlong & Ward (1997) have piloted a dependency measure that shows predictable weekly fluctuations and interactions with staffing levels and quality of care. American and UK guidelines (Furlong & Ward 1997) recommend nursing shift ratios of 1:3 for low-intensity activities rising to 1:2 for active treatment and 1:1 for intensive care. Recommendations for other staff include one whole time equivalent (WTE) consultant per 10–12 bedded unit, up to one WTE in clinical psychology and up to 0.5 WTE sessional inputs from social work, psychotherapy, family therapy and occupational therapy. The UK recommendation for specialized teaching is one teacher to four students per lesson.

Models of team management and functioning will vary with the style of the unit. A popular current style is a model of 'matrix management', which combines different disciplines with multiple tasks in a flat hierarchy with task-focused 'mini teams' (Maskey 1998). Whatever the organization, responsive and adequate staff supervision is vital.

Effectiveness of inpatient and day patient treatment

Generic outcomes

Inpatient and day units are considered as a single entity for the purposes of administrative planning and therapeutic organization and many studies have investigated generic outcomes across a range of disorders. Pfeiffer & Strzelecki (1990) reported an important meta-analysis of 34 such inpatient outcome studies and there have been subsequent reviews (Curry 1991; Pottick *et al.* 1993) and individual reports. These studies point to the overall efficacy of inpatient care and have been able to identify quite robust predictors of outcome. However, the reviews have also highlighted significant methodological limitations. Few early studies included control groups or standardized outcome measures and sample sizes have often been insufficient to overcome problems of patient heterogeneity. Pottick *et al.* (1993) argued for more experimental designs to investigate the value of the residential component of care against other components and prospective randomized trials of inpatient vs. other forms of treatment for particular disorders are now beginning to appear (see below).

Outcome measurement is also becoming more sophisticated with 'triangulation' methods to measure multiple perspectives on outcome (Jensen *et al.* 1996). Use of change-sensitive common methodologies in future studies will greatly help progress. It will also be necessary to be creative in the variables measured: markers such as social competency may be more relevant for treatment and outcome than diagnostic groupings *per se*.

Predictors of outcome

Pfeiffer & Strzelecki (1990) identified a number of robust predictors of inpatient outcome, which have received support and extension in subsequent studies. High levels of aggressive antisocial behaviour and 'organicity' of *symptoms*, as in schizophrenia, predict poor outcome; emotional disorders do better. *Well-organized treatment*, *positive alliance* and *good aftercare* are common positive predictors. *Intelligence* measured as IQ shows a moderately positive effect, but the study of Luthar *et al.* (1995) suggested that functional achievement may be the more critical variable. Pretreatment *family functioning* is a strong predictor of outcome, but the effects may be complex and disorder-specific. In a study of anorexia nervosa, North *et al.* (1997) found that the child's perception of family functioning was prognostic but parents' perception was not. *Gender*, *age* and *emergency or elective admission* were found to have little predictive value.

Length of stay (LOS) had only a modest association with outcome in Pfeiffer & Strzelecki's (1990) review. However, interest in treatment lengths has been increased by the rapid progress in the USA and elsewhere towards managed care and very short hospital stays. Influences on LOS are complex. A retrospective case note study of pre-admission variables in 100 children in one private US unit (Gold *et al.* 1993) found that longer LOS was predicted by greater global impairment, post-traumatic symptoms and psychosocial stressors; diagnosis of adjustment disorder predicted shorter stays. In contrast, Christ *et al.* (1989) found that LOS was predicted by funding constraints or unit philosophy rather than diagnosis. Mossman *et al.* (1990) achieved significant overall LOS reduction managerially by setting a discharge date early in admission and actively engaging community services regarding aftercare, but they did not study the therapeutic effectiveness of this approach. The clinical lore that symptoms often decline rapidly early in an admission and then worsen—the 'honeymoon' effect—was supported by LaBarbera & Dozier (1985) who showed symptom increase from early to late in admission. No measure of pre-admission symptomatology was made here, but the authors argued that shortening admissions beyond a certain limit might well produce spurious health gains based on symptom inhibition early in admission. Alternatively, the fact of admission may relieve contextual causes of symptoms in the young person's environment and the early symptom reduction may be a valid effect—but the work needed to maintain these positive changes into discharge will take longer. Green *et al.* (2001) showed considerable symptom reduction from pre-admission to 1 month; there was some rise by discharge although not to pre-admission levels. Length of stay in this study did not predict outcome nor was it associated with pre-admission variables.

Further studies of treatment effects through admission should identify better process variables for prediction than the gross length of stay. However, the drive for maximal efficiency of treatment and the financial pressure of managed care will make the issue of LOS of continuing relevance in treatment studies and policy decisions.

Outcome for specific disorders

Eating disorders

There is unresolved debate on the value of inpatient treatment for eating disorders (see Steinhausen, Chapter 34). The anxiety that these disorders induce, the issues around control and the significant mortality often combine to produce a desire for admission as a safe option. Adolescents themselves, however, often resist admission and some of the extreme behavioural methods previously used on units to promote eating continue to cause anger when patients recount their experiences (Shelley 1997). On the other hand, the removal from considerable family difficulties, the group cohesion achieved in many more specialist units and the quality of supervision available can make the residential experience therapeutically powerful.

Studies of the outcome of inpatient treatment show widely differing results. Steinhausen & Seidel (1993) followed 50 patients over 5 years and found a 68% recovery rate with 14% still diagnosable with eating disorder. Saccomani *et al.* (1998) followed 81 children over 9 years and found a 53% good outcome.

But comparisons between outpatient and inpatient treatment (Crisp *et al.* 1991; Gowers *et al.* 2000) have shown little additional benefit from inpatient care. Indeed, the 21 inpatients treated in the latter study did particularly badly, with only 14% having good outcome and a regression analysis of the whole cohort of 72 cases showed that inpatient treatment was a predictor of poor outcome, independent of presenting severity. This was not a randomized study and may have been affected by selection bias because the service reserved admission for the most intractable cases. Potentially mediating variables, such as motivation, family context and therapeutic alliance, were not measured. Others have argued that these latter factors are likely to be more important than severity scores in deciding on admission and predicting its outcome (Wood & Flowers 2000). This issue will only be resolved by well-designed randomized controlled treatment studies and at least one of these is currently underway.

Depression and suicidality

Admission practice following suicide attempts shows great regional variation. A recent large study found that, for similar presentations, 39% of cases in the USA were admitted compared with 12% in Europe (Safer 1996). There are no studies directly comparing hospitalization with other forms of post-overdose care, although a recent UK evidence-based review (Hawton *et al.* 1998) recommended that psychiatric admission should *not* be the intervention of first choice for self-harm.

A number of recent uncontrolled studies have investigated suicide risk following inpatient treatment of depression or suicidality. Twenty per cent of 111 emergency admissions remained depressed and suicidal at 2–4 year follow-up (Ivarsson *et al.* 1998), 18% of 100 patients admitted with depression reported suicidal behaviour at 6-month follow-up (King *et al.* 1995) and 25% of 180 similar admissions attempted suicide within 5 years of discharge (Goldston *et al.* 1999). Predictors of ongoing symptoms were suicide attempts prior to hospitalization, high levels of depressive symptomatology and family dysfunction at inpatient assessment.

Psychosis

Adolescents with first onset psychotic illness will commonly be admitted but there are no studies comparing admission with alternative forms of treatment at this stage. One study of 58 adolescents admitted with psychotic disorder showed that 78% at follow-up after 2 years were continuously ill (Cawthron *et al.* 1994).

Conduct disorder

The presence of unsocialized aggressive or externalizing behaviours at presentation is a consistent predictor of poor outcome for inpatient treatment (Pfeiffer & Strzelecki 1990). However, this reflects the general prognosis for these disorders. Conduct disorder was a specific exclusion criterion in some units but accounted for 25% of child admissions overall in a study of UK child psychiatry units (Green & Jacobs 1998) and 15% of children and adolescents referred to Finnish inpatient units in 1990 and 1993 (Sourander & Turunen 1999).

Current evidence suggests that the management of conduct disorder is best seen in terms of long-term maintenance rather than episodes of care and the contextual basis of much of the symptomatology supports community intervention as a first choice treatment (Henggeler *et al.* 1999). In spite of these arguments and the often disruptive effect of such children on the milieu, there is good indication for admitting selected patients.
1 For assessment when there are concerns about covert underlying comorbidity relevant to treatment, such as attention deficit, emotional disorder, pervasive developmental disorder, specific learning disability or subclinical seizures (Jacobs 1998).
2 When a trial of treatment is needed within a controlled setting.

Children with externalizing disorders receiving a multimodal day programme showed improvements in adjustment at 5-year follow-up (Grizenko 1997). Another multimodal day programme (Rey *et al.* 1998) also showed improvement over matched controls who had received other treatments; however, both groups showed poor outcome. In a study of inpatient treatment of adolescents with emotional and conduct disorder, patients who completed the treatment showed more progress 1 month post-discharge than patients who were early drop-outs, but these differences had become insignificant at 1- and 2-year follow-up (Wells & Faragher 1993).

Substance misuse

A number of inpatient and day patient addiction programmes have been evaluated. Of 280 adolescents treated in a substance abuse inpatient programme (Dobkin *et al.* 1998), 67 subjects completed 1 month follow-up questionnaires; 19 had improved and 48 had not. The improvers tended to be older with better motivation for social adjustment and less emotional symptomatology; those who did worse were distinguished by more mental state abnormalities at admission. Cornwall & Blood (1998) compared inpatient and day patient programmes in this area and found they showed similar outcomes. A random allocation trial comparing inpatient and intensive community treatment of adolescents with substance misuse and juvenile offending (Schoenwald *et al.* 1996) showed additional benefits for the community treatment. Friedman *et al.* (1993) report a matched study comparing long-term outpatient treatment with short-term inpatient treatment and found benefits in the longer term outpatient treatment.

Obsessive-compulsive disorder

In a prospective naturalistic study (Wever & Rey 1997) examined the effectiveness of combined CBT and psychopharmacology in a group of 57 children and adolescents first diagnosed with OCD, 20% of whom received inpatient treatment. Factors leading to admission included the severity and type of OCD symptoms, the failure of past therapy, comorbidity, family factors and geographical isolation. The inpatient group had double the rate of comorbid diagnoses compared to outpatient group and they showed a poorer outcome.

Intensive home-based care and outreach services

Recent developments in the USA have seen the increasing use of intensive forms of community support, such as the 'wraparound' model (Vandenberg & Grealish 1996). These programmes address mental health problems but often exclude mental health personnel. At the same time, new research in developmental psychopathology emphasizes the social context of much child psychopathology. Woolston *et al.* (1998) described a synthesis of these developments in an intensive home-based model of psychiatric care. The service is brought to the family home and individualized to the family's needs. Assessments are made at the level of child and family, the immediate community and the wider environment. The primary outreach team works to identify the smallest possible change in these systems that will create improved and stable functioning and then links with the wider network within the child's environment to sustain this change. A similar model of multisystemic therapy (MST) has been described by Henggeler *et al.* (1994).

The theoretical paradigm behind these approaches is not new — it is a recasting of the biopsychosocial model that implicitly informs much child psychiatry practice. Indeed, Woolston has argued that, in an age of severely restricted inpatient stays, this model is the best way of preserving the holistic and in-depth approach that characterized the best inpatient tradition. What is new is the platform of delivery of the service and the intensity of the outreach provision. There is, in addition, an underlying rationale — albeit untested — that a small change accomplished with the young person in their own social ecology will be more beneficial than a possibly larger change in a removed setting (Woolston, personal communication; Henggeler *et al.* 1999).

These intensive outreach models need much skilled professional time. Between three and five professional teams, consisting of two senior clinicians or counsellors, provide the home-based assessment and therapeutic input. They are backed up by a multidisciplinary infrastructure described in Woolston's model as a programme director and medical director, a child psychiatrist, a clinical programme co-ordinator, two senior clinicians and an administrator. This staffing is quoted as sufficient for a caseload of 25 patients. (The seniority and experience of the majority of the professionals is notable). The intensity of the involvement can vary according to need and expense but a 24-h 7-day on-call crisis intervention service is provided throughout the duration of the input. In one study of MST (Schoenwald *et al.* 1996), the average duration of treatment was 130 days (SD 32 days) during which there was an average of 40 direct contact hours between professionals and family (range 12–187 h, SD 28 h). In Woolston's report the length of provision had a mean of 13 weeks with a range of 1–40 weeks. Woolston emphasized that the intensive home-based services are considered as supplementary to an array or more traditional services, including inpatient and day patient hospitalization and outpatient programmes.

Henggeler *et al.* have conducted a number of experimentally based studies comparing MST with other forms of intervention. These provide some of the first randomized controlled treatment trials in this area of child and adolescent psychiatry, including the first specifically to include cost analysis. Schoenwald *et al.* (1996) randomized MST against service as usual for adolescent substance misusers. The MST treatment resulted in a 46% decrease in the need for residential care at 1-year follow-up and succeeded in reducing dramatically the rate of imprisonment for substance abuse and abuse-related inpatient stays. The cost savings made through this almost compensated for the increased cost of the MST treatment. A recent randomized trial (Henggeler *et al.* 1999) compared MST vs. brief hospitalization for a diverse group of adolescent psychiatric emergencies in a relatively disadvantaged population. MST was given for 4 months while hospitalization was for 2 weeks (only) followed by standard community aftercare. The MST condition involved a mean of 97.1 h of therapy contact time during the study and 24-h 7-day per week availability of staff. Staff had a caseload of three cases each and there was high-frequency psychiatric supervision. By comparison, the hospitalization condition had a mean contact time of 8.5 h subsequent to the admission period. Nearly half of the young people in the MST condition needed psychiatric admission in the initial period and MST only had the effect of reducing out-of-home placement by 50% through the whole study. Given these methodological qualifications, the MST had a significantly greater effect than hospitalization on externalizing symptoms and targeted social outcomes, such as enhanced family cohesion, structure and school attendance. Family and youth satisfaction was also higher. The hospital condition showed a significantly greater impact on youth self-esteem — a result that may reflect the individually orientated treatment model in the hospital group. No follow-up data beyond 4 months are reported. The study concluded that even this highly intense form of ecologically focused care does not substitute for the need for inpatient provision — but it can reduce the need, and results in enhanced outcomes over treatment as usual. It was unfortunate for the design of the study that there was such an imbalance between the treatment intensity in the two conditions. The study — important as it is — does not yet address the question of the added value of the residential component *per se*.

Future directions

A number of contemporary themes and future directions may be summarized. The trend for shorter inpatient stays and the development of intensive care alternatives to residential treatment is likely to continue but there may well also emerge a reactive emphasis on the value of longer intensive residential treatment experience for selected conditions. The demand for adolescent units to respond to acute emergencies is likely to continue to grow as the severity of presenting psychopathology moves down the age range. In well-provided health services there may be increasing growth of specialist environments, such as specialized eating disorder or forensic units. Referral to intensive care facilities is often thought to follow a bimodal pattern: high when there are relatively few outpatient services, lower as outpatient services are more developed, and higher again when outpatient provision becomes still better and more complex need is identified. This should not imply that the potential demand for inpatient services is endless: epidemiological surveys of children with complex needs suggest that the pool of these problems in communities is finite and measurable (Kurtz *et al.* 1998).

At the complex end of the spectrum, young people are likely to be involved with multiple agencies (Kurtz *et al.* 1998). This implies another necessary development; a more sophisticated integration between mental health care, education and social services to form complementary and mutually supporting provision. Some children who now are admitted to inpatient psychiatric units may be better placed in residential social care institutions with psychiatric input or in specialist residential schools; some children in these other institutions may be better placed in primarily mental health facilities.

It is to be hoped that there will be a burgeoning of randomized controlled trials comparing residential, intensive day and outreach alternatives for particular groups or severity of problems. Along with this we can hope for an increasing delineation of methodologies to measure inpatient and day patient unit process. The result of these two developments may be further clarification of the specific value of residential treatment. The current evidence suggests that the residential milieu has a particular ability to provide stabilization and rapid reduction of symptomatology and risk. In medium-term treatments it provides an environment where treatment and rehabilitation can occur outside the demands of the home environment—this is the historical function of respite. Notwithstanding the efforts that have been made in recent years to engage effectively with families, the residential unit is inevitably largely focused on the individual and individual pathology. This can prove highly advantageous in situations where assessment or treatment of complex individual psychopathology is at a premium but needs to be complemented by an emphasis on the environmental context during pre-admission and follow-up. Reduction in the length of inpatient stays beyond a certain minimum negates any value of the inpatient milieu as a treatment in its own right, but the very fact of removal from a noxious mental environment in the community of origin may still result in temporary benefit.

Intensive outreach programmes are at an early stage of development but have already generated high levels of rigorous treatment programming and evaluation. The face validity of this theory of intervention is strong and in keeping with recent research in the developmental psychopathology of a number of disorders. The emphasis on changing presumed maintaining factors in the young person's environment may result in longer stabilization of treatment gains—although this has not yet been tested. On the other hand, it should be quite apparent that these outreach solutions are no easy option, either financially or in terms of professional expertise. The first randomized trial including costing shows that the extra cost of the service only approaches being met if non-health cost savings are taken into account and there is evidence that the efficacy of the intervention drops if the intensity of the intervention is not strictly adhered to (Henggeler *et al.* 1994). Nevertheless, the early studies of the effectiveness of MST are impressive and deserve replication outside the developing centre. They suggest that this intensive outreach model does not replace the need for the inpatient option but can reduce its usage. The emphasis in this treatment on the social context of psychopathology is a strength and complementary to inpatient care but runs the risk of overlooking intrinsic problems in the patient.

Day unit care may seem to be a compromise between these two extremes and may often usefully be so. For the most severe problems, however, it may fall between the two and offer insufficient containment for safety or intensive outreach for effectiveness. The great strength of the day unit resource is its flexibility to adapt to different disorders and circumstances. It is unrealistic to believe that the day unit provision can substitute for other intensive treatment modalities.

Thus, in an ideal future, there would be a set of flexible and complementary platforms for the delivery of intensive care for acute and complex disorders. Service providers would identify themselves as 'serious disorder' or 'intensive care' services offering a variety of different modes of delivery. In practice, organization and financial constraints will often lead health services to have to make preferred choices. There is now a greater likelihood that in the future an increased evidence base may inform such decisions.

Acknowledgements

The author would like to thank Dr Andy Clarke, Dr Tony Jaffa and Dr Tony James for helpful advice in the preparation of this chapter.

References

American Academy of Child and Adolescent Psychiatry (1990) *Model for minimum staffing patterns for hospitals providing acute inpatient treatment for children and adolescents with psychiatric illnesses.* American Academy of Child and Adolescent Psychiatry, Washington D.C.

American Academy of Child and Adolescent Psychiatry (2000) *Practice parameter for the prevention and management of aggressive behaviour in child and adolescent psychiatric institutions with special reference to seclusion and restraint.* Draft 9. American Academy of Child and Adolescent Psychiatry, Washington D.C.

Angold, A. & Pickles, A. (1993) Seclusion on an adolescent unit. *Journal of Child Psychology and Psychiatry*, **34**, 975–990.

Asen, K., Stein, R., Stevens, A., McHugh, B., Greenwood, J. & Cooklin, A. (1982) A day unit for families. *Journal of Family Therapy*, **4**, 345–358.

Bazeley, E.T. (1928) *Homer Lane and the Little Commonwealth*. George, Allen & Unwin. London.

Beskind, H. (1962) Psychiatric inpatient treatment of adolescents: a review of clinical experience. *Comprehensive Psychiatry*, **3**, 354–369.

Bettelheim, B. (1955) *Truants from Life*. Free Press, New York.

Billick, S.B., Edwards, J.L., Burget, W., Serlen, J.R. & Bruni, M.S. (1998) A clinical study of competency in child psychiatric patients. *Journal of American Academy of Psychiatry and Law*, **26**, 587–594.

Blanz, *B.* & Schmidt, *M.H.* (2000) Practitioner review: preconditions and outcome of inpatient treatment in child and adolescent psychiatry. *Journal of Child Psychology and Psychiatry*, **41**, 703–712.

Bruggen, P. & O'Brien, C. (1987) *Helping Families: Systems, Residential and Agency Responsibility*. Faber & Faber, London.

Cameron, K.A. (1949) A psychiatric inpatient department for children. *Journal of Mental Science*, **95**, 560–566.

Cawthron, P., James, A., Dell, D. & Seagroatt, V. (1994) Adolescent onset psychosis: a clinical and outcome study. *Journal of Child Psychology and Psychiatry*, **35**, 1321–1332.

Christ, A., Tsernberis, S. & Andrew, H. (1989) Fiscal implications of a childhood disorder DRG. *Journal of the American Academy of Child and Adolescent Psychiatry*, **28**, 729–733.

Colton, M. (1988) Dimensions of foster and residential care practice. *Journal of Child Psychology and Psychiatry*, **29**, 589–600.

Connell, P.H. (1961) The day hospital approach to child psychiatry. *Journal of Mental Science*, **107**, 969–977.

Cornwall, A. & Blood, L. (1998) Inpatient versus day treatment for substance abusing adolescents. *Journal of Nervous and Mental Disease*, **186**, 580–582.

Costello, A.J., Dulcan, M.K. & Kalas, R. (1991) A checklist of hospitalisation criteria for use with children. *Hospital and Community Psychiatry*, **42**, 823–828.

Cotgrove, A. (1997) Emergency admissions to a regional adolescent unit: piloting a new service. *Psychiatric Bulletin*, **21**, 604–608.

Cotgrove, A.J. & Gowers, S.G. (1999) Use of an adolescent in-patient unit. *Advances in Psychiatric Treatment*, **5**, 192–201.

Cotton, N.S. (1993) *Lessons from the Lions Den: Therapeutic Management of Children in Psychiatric Hospitals and Treatment Centres*. Jossey-Bass, San Francisco, CA.

Crisp, A.H., Norton, K., Gowers, S. *et al.* (1991) A controlled study of the effects of therapies aimed at adolescent and family psychopathology in anorexia nervosa. *British Journal of Psychiatry*, **159**, 325–333.

Curry, J.E. (1991) Outcome research on residential treatment: implications and suggested directions. *American Journal of Psychiatry*, **621**, 348–357.

Dimond, C. & Golberg, D. (1999) On admitting psychotic adolescents to hospital: time to review the admission process. *Child Psychology and Psychiatry Review*, **4**, 16–19.

Dobkin, P.L., Chabot, L., Maliantovitch, K. & Craig, W. (1998) Predictors of outcome in drug treatment of adolescent inpatients. *Psychological Reports*, **83**, 175–186.

French, W. & Tate, A. (1998) Educational management. In: *Inpatient Child Psychiatry. Modern Practice Research and the Future* (eds J.M. Green & B.W. Jacobs), pp. 143–155. Routledge, London.

Friedman, A.S., Garnick, S., Kreisher, C. & Terras, A. (1993) Matching adolescents who abuse drugs to treatment. *American Journal of Addictions*, **2**, 232–237.

Furlong, S. & Ward, M. (1997) Assessing patient dependency and staff skill mix. *Nursing Standard*, **11**, 33–38.

Garralda, E. (1986) Inpatient treatment of children: a psychiatric perspective. In: *Current Issues in Clinical Psychology* (ed. G. Edwards), Vol. 4, Plenum Press, New York.

Gold, J., Shera, D. & Clarkson, B. (1993) Private psychiatric hospitalisation of children: predictors of length of stay. *Journal of the American Academy of Child and Adolescent Psychiatry*, **32**, 135–144.

Goldston, D.B., Sergent-Daniel, S., Reboussin, D.M., Reboussin, B.A., Frazier, P.H. & Kelley, A.E. (1999) Suicide attempts among formerly hospitalised adolescents: a prospective naturalistic study of risk during the first 5 years. *Journal of the American Academy of Child and Adolescent Psychiatry*, **38**, 660–671.

Gowers, S.G. & Kushlick, A. (1992) Customer satisfaction in adolescent psychiatry. *Journal of Mental Health*, **1**, 353–362.

Gowers, S.G., Weetman, J., Shore, A., Hossain, F. & Elvins, R. (2000) Impact of hospitalisation on the outcome of adolescent anorexia nervosa. *British Journal of Psychiatry*, **176**, 138–141.

Green, J.M. (1994) Child in-patient treatment and family relationships. *Psychiatric Bulletin*, **18**, 744–747.

Green, J.M. (1996) A structured assessment of parenting based on attachment theory: theoretical background, description and initial clinical experience. *European Journal of Child and Adolescent Psychiatry*, **5**, 133–138.

Green, J.M. & Burke, M. (1998) The ward as a therapeutic agent. In: *Inpatient Child Psychiatry. Modern Practice Research and the Future* (eds J.M. Green & B.W. Jacobs), pp. 93–110. Routledge, London.

Green, J.M. & Jacobs, B.W. (1998) Current practice: a questionnaire survey of inpatient child psychiatry in the UK. In: *Inpatient Child Psychiatry. Modern Practice Research and the Future* (eds J.M. Green & B.W. Jacobs), pp. 9–22. Routledge, London.

Green, J.M. & Jones, D. (1998) Unwanted effects of inpatient treatment: anticipation, prevention, repair. In: *Inpatient Child Psychiatry. Modern Practice Research and the Future* (eds J.M. Green & B.W. Jacobs), pp. 212–220. Routledge, London.

Green, J.M., Kroll, L., Imrie, D., Begum, K., Frances, F.M. & Anson, R. (2001) Health gain and predictors of outcome in inpatient and related day patient child and adolescent psychiatry treatment. *Journal of the American Academy of Child and Adolescent Psychiatry*, **40**, 325–332.

Grizenko, N. (1997) Outcome of multimodal day treatment for children with severe behavior problems: a five-year follow up. *Journal of the American Academy of Child and Adolescent Psychiatry*, **36**, 989–997.

Gutterman, E.N., Markovitz, J.S., LoConte, J.S. & Beier, J. (1993) Determinants for hospitalisation from an emergency mental heath service. *Journal of the American Academy of Child and Adolescent Psychiatry*, **32**, 114–122.

Harper, G. (1989) Focal inpatient treatment planning. *Journal of the American Academy of Child and Adolescent Psychiatry*, **28**, 38–47.

Hawton, K., Arensman, E. & Townsend, E. (1998) Deliberate self-harm: a systematic review of efficacy of psychosocial and pharmacological treatments in preventing repetition. *British Medical Journal*, **317**, 441–447.

Henggeler, S.W., Schoenwald, S.K., Pickrel, S.G., Brondino, M.J., Borduin, C.M. & Hall, A.A. (1994) *Treatment manual for family preservation using multisystematic therapy*. State of Columbia Health and Human Services Finance Commission, Columbia, SC.

Henggeler, S.W., Rowland, M.D., Randall, J. *et al.* (1999) Home based multisystemic therapy as an alternative to the hospitalisation of youths in psychiatric crisis: clinical outcomes. *Journal of the American Academy of Child and Adolescent Psychiatry*, **38**, 1331–1339.

Higgins, I. & Burke, M. (1998) Managing oppositional and aggressive behaviour. In: *Inpatient Child Psychiatry. Modern Practice Research and the Future* (eds J.M. Green & B.W. Jacobs), pp. 189–201. Routledge, London.

Hoagwood, K. (2000) *Service use in the MTA study*. Presentation at the American Academy of Child and Adolescent Psychiatry, October 2000, New York.

Hougaard, E. (1994) The therapeutic alliance: a conceptual analysis. *Scandinavian Journal of Psychology*, **35**, 67–85.

Ivarsson, T., Larsson, B. & Gillberg, C. (1998) A 2–4 year follow up of depressive symptoms, suicidal ideation, and suicide attempts among adolescent psychiatric inpatients. *European Child and Adolescent Psychiatry*, **7**, 96–104.

Jacobs, B.W. (1998) Externalising disorders: conduct disorder and hyperkinetic disorder. In: *Inpatient Child Psychiatry. Modern Practice Research and the Future* (eds J.M. Green & B.W. Jacobs), pp. 220–232. Routledge, London.

Jensen, P.S., Hoagwood, K. & Petti, T. (1996) Outcomes of mental health care for children and adolescents. II. Literature review and application of a comprehensive model. *Journal of the American Academy of Child and Adolescent Psychiatry*, **35**, 1064–1077.

Kennard, D. (1983) *An Introduction to Therapeutic Communities*. Routledge & Kegan Paul, London.

King, C.A., Segal, H., Kaminski, K. & Naylor, M.W. (1995) A prospective study of adolescent suicidal behaviour following hospitalisation. *Suicide and Life Threatening Behaviour*, **25**, 327–338.

Kroll, L. & Green, J.M. (1997) Therapeutic alliance in inpatient child psychiatry: development and initial validation of the family engagement questionnaire. *Clinical Child Psychology and Psychiatry*, **2**, 431–447.

Kurtz, Z., Thornes, R. & Bailey, S. (1998) Children in criminal justice and secure care systems: how their mental health needs are met. *Journal of Adolescence*, **2**, 543–553.

LaBarbera, J.D. & Dozier, J.E. (1985) A honeymoon effect in child psychiatric hospitalisation: a research note. *Journal of Child Psychology and Psychiatry*, **26**, 479–483.

Lask, J. & Maynerd, C. (1998) Engaging and working with the family. In: *Inpatient Child Psychiatry: Modern Practice Research and the Future* (eds J.M. Green & B.W. Jacobs), pp. 75–93. Routledge, London.

Leibenluft, E., Tasman, A. & Green, S.A., eds (1993) *Less Time to Do More: Psychotherapy on the Short-term Inpatient Unit*. American Psychiatric Press, Washington D.C.

Levy, A. & Kahan, B. (1991) *The Pindown Experience and the Protection of Children: Report of the Staffordshire Child Care Inquiry*. Staffordshire County Council.

Luisielli, J.K., Bastien, J.S. & Putnam, R.F. (1998) Behavioral assessment and analysis of mechanical restraint utilization on a psychiatric, child and adolescent inpatient setting. *Behavioral Interventions*, **13**, 147–155.

Luthar, S.S., Woolston, J.L., Sparrow, S.S. & Zimmerman. L.D. (1995) Adaptive behaviours among psychiatrically hospitalised children: the role of intelligence and related attributes. *Journal of Clinical Child Psychology*, **24**, 98–108.

Lynch, M., Steinberg, D. & Ounsted, C. (1975) A family unit in a childrens psychiatric hospital. *British Medical Journal*, **2**, 127–129.

Magagna, J. (1998) Psychodynamic psychotherapy. In: *Inpatient Child Psychiatry: Modern Practice Research and the Future* (eds J.M. Green & B.W. Jacobs), pp. 124–143. Routledge, London.

Maskey, S. (1998) The process of admission. In: *Inpatient Child Psychiatry: Modern Practice Research and the Future* (eds J.M. Green & B.W. Jacobs), pp. 39–50. Routledge, London.

Moos, R., Shelton, R. & Petty, C. (1973) Perceived ward climate and treatment outcome. *Journal of Abnormal Psychology*, **82**, 291–298.

Mossman, D., Macaulay, K., Johnson, E. & Baker, D. (1990) Improving state funded child psychiatric care: reducing protracted hospitalisation through changes in treatment planning. *Quality Review Bulletin*, **16**, 20–24.

Newbold, C. & Jones, D. (1998) Child maltreatment and inpatient unit. In: *Inpatient Child Psychiatry: Modern Practice Research and the Future* (eds J.M. Green & B.W. Jacobs), pp. 201–211. Routledge, London.

North, C., Gowers, S. & Byram, V. (1997) Family functioning and life events in the outcome of adolescent anorexia nervosa. *British Journal of Psychiatry*, **171**, 545–549.

Nurcombe, B. (1989) Gold directed treatment planning in the principles of brief hospitalisation. *Journal of the American Academy of Child and Adolescent Psychiatry*, **28**, 26–30.

Parry-Jones, W. (1998) Historical themes. In: *Inpatient Child Psychiatry: Modern Practice Research and the Future* (eds J.M. Green & B.W. Jacobs), pp. 22–36. Routledge, London.

Paterson, R., Bauer, P., McDonald, C.A. & McDermott, B. (1997) A profile of children and adolescents in a psychiatric unit: multidomain impairment and research implications. *Australian and New Zealand Journal of Psychiatry*, **31**, 682–690.

Patrick, C., Padgett, D.K., Burns, B.J., Schlesinger, H.J. & Cohen, J. (1993) Use of inpatient services by a national population: do benefits make a difference? *Journal of the American Academy of Child and Adolescent Psychiatry*, **32**, 144–152.

Pfeiffer, S.I. & Strzelecki, S.C. (1990) Inpatient psychiatric treatment of children and adolescents: a review of outcome studies. *Journal of the American Academy of Child and Adolescent Psychiatry*, **29**, 847–853.

Pottick, K., Hansell, S., Gaboda, D. & Gutterman, E. (1993) Child and adolescent outcomes of inpatient psychiatric services: a research agenda. *Children and Youth Services Review*, **15**, 371–384.

Pottick, K., Hansell, S., Gutterman, E. & White, R.H. (1995) Factors associated with in patient and out patient treatment for children and adolescents with serious mental illness. *Journal of the American Academy of Child and Adolescent Psychiatry*, **34**, 425–433.

Price, R.H. & Moos, R.H. (1977) Towards the taxonomy of inpatient treatment environments. *Journal of Abnormal Psychology*, **84**, 181–188.

Rey, J.M., Denshire, E., Wever, C. & Apollonov, I. (1998) Three-year outcome of disruptive adolescents treated in a day program. *European Child and Adolescent Psychiatry*, **7**, 42–48.

Rothery, D., Wrate, R., McCabe, R. & Aspin, J. (1995) Treatment goal planning: outcome findings of a British prospective multi-centre study of adolescent inpatient units. *European Child and Adolescent Psychiatry*, **4**, 209–220.

Royal College of Psychiatrists (1997) *Model Consultant Job Description in Child and Adolescent Psychiatry*. Occasional paper 39. Royal College of Psychiatrists, London.

Royal College of Psychiatrists (1999) *Guidance for the Staffing of Child and Adolescent Inpatient Units*. Council Report 62. Royal College of Psychiatrists, London.

Saccomani, L., Savoini, M., Cirrincione, M., Vercellino, F. & Ravera, G. (1998) Long-term outcome of children and adolescents with anorexia nervosa: study of comorbidity. *Journal of Psychosomatic Research*, **44**, 565–571.

Safer, D.J. (1996) A comparison of studies from the United States and Western Europe on psychiatric hospitalisation referrals for youths exhibiting suicidal behaviour. *Annals of Clinical Psychiatry*, **8**, 161–168.

Schoenwald, S.K., Ward, D.M., Henggeler, S.W. & Pickrel, S.G. (1996) Multisystemic therapy treatment of substance abusing or dependent adolescent offenders: costs of reducing incarceration, inpatient, and residential placement. *Journal of Child and Family Studies*, **5**, 431–444.

Shaw, M. (1998) Childhood mental health and the law. In: *Inpatient Child Psychiatry: Modern Practice Research and the Future* (eds J.M. Green & B.W. Jacobs), pp. 349–362. Routledge, London.

Shelley, R. (1997) *Anorexics on Anorexia*. Jessica Kingsley, London.

Sourander, A. & Turunen, M.M. (1999) Psychiatric hospital care among children and adolescents in Finland: a nationwide register study. *Social Psychiatry and Psychiatric Epidemiology*, **34**, 105–110.

Sourander, A., Helenius, H., Leijala, H., Heikkila, T., Bergroth, L. & Piha, J. (1996) Predictors of outcome of short-term child psychiatric inpatient treatment. *European Child and Adolescent Psychiatry*, **5**, 75–82.

Steiner, H., Marx, L. & Walton, C. (1991) The ward atmosphere of a child's psychosomatic unit: ten year follow up. *General Hospital Psychiatry*, **13**, 246–252.

Steinhausen, H.C. & Seidel, R. (1993) Outcome in adolescent eating disorders. *International Journal of Eating Disorders*, **14**, 487–496.

Szabo, C.P. & Magnus, C. (1999) Complex partial seizures in an adolescent psychiatric inpatient setting. *Journal of the American Academy of Child and Adolescent Psychiatry*, **38**, 477–479.

United Nations Childrens Fund (UNICEF) (1995) *The Convention on the Rights of the Child*. UNICEF, London.

Vandenberg, J.E. & Grealish, E.M. (1996) Individualising services and supports through the wrap-around process: philosophy and procedures. *Journal of Child and Family Study*, **5**, 7–22.

Wells, P. & Faragher, B. (1993) Inpatient treatment of 165 adolescents with emotional and conduct disorders: a study of outcome. *British Journal of Psychiatry*, **162**, 345–352.

Wever, C. & Rey, J. (1997) Outcome of a combined treatment in juvenile obsessive compulsive disorder. *Australia and New Zealand Journal of Psychiatry*, **31**, 105–113.

White, R., Carr, P. & Lowe, N. (1990) *A Guide to the Children Act 1989*. Routledge, London.

Wolkind, S.N. (1974) The components of affectionless psychopathy in institutionalised children. *Journal of Child Psychology and Psychiatry*, **15**, 215–220.

Wolkind, S. & Gent, M. (1987) Children's psychiatric inpatient units: present functions and future directions. *Special Issue: Residential Provision. Maladjustment and Therapeutic Education*, **5**, 54–56.

Wood, D. & Flowers, P. (2000) Correspondence. *British Journal of Psychiatry*, **177**, 179.

Woolston, J.L. (1989) Transactional risk model for short and intermediate term psychiatric inpatient treatment of children. *Journal of the American Academy of Child and Adolescent Psychiatry*, **28**, 38–41.

Woolston, J.L., Berkowitz, S.J., Schaefer, M.C. & Adnopoz, J.A. (1998) Intensive, integrated in home psychiatric services: the catalyst to enhancing outpatient intervention. *Child and Adolescent Psychiatric Clinics of North America*, **7**, 615–633.

Wrate, R.M., Rothery, D.J., McCabe, R.J.R. & Aspin, J. (1994) A prospective multi-centre study of admissions to adolescent inpatient units. *Journal of Adolescence*, **17**, 221–237.

Zimnet, S.G. & Farley, G.K. (1985) Day treatment of children in the United States. *Journal of the American Academy of Child Psychiatry*, **24**, 732–738.

Paediatric Consultation

Paula K. Rauch and Michael S. Jellinek

Introduction

The child mental health consultant must assess the psychiatric status of an ill child in a hospital environment. Nature, nurture, development, illness, pain and anxiety add complexity. Every consultation requires respect for the power of biology, the mediating influence of family and community, and the primacy of personal meaning in defining an experience as bearable or traumatizing (Eisenberg 1995). Assessments involve:

1 children with psychiatric disorders leading to medical complications, such as a depressed adolescent admitted for an overdose, or a teenager with anorexia nervosa who is bradycardic and hypothermic; and

2 psychiatric manifestations of medical illnesses or treatments, such as central nervous system symptoms associated with HIV, disinhibition following traumatic brain injury or hallucinations secondary to morphine use following lung transplantation.

Children may need to be helped to cope with a chronic medical illness or painful procedures. This may involve working with anxious or difficult parents who complicate the care of their ill child by refusing to consent to necessary procedures or by causing dissension among the team of caregivers. The consultant also supports ward staff, as in helping a treatment team understand divisive dynamics or facilitating as staff voice feelings about a traumatic abuse case or painful death. He or she is an educator, sometimes offering didactic lectures for house staff or parents. The consultant is also an advocate for children working with hospital leadership to develop more psychologically attuned standard practices, such as routine presurgical visits for young children. The consultant can be a researcher asking and answering key questions about efficacy, outcome, quality of life and cost-effectiveness.

Consultations are occurring in a fast-paced ever-changing medical climate with shorter hospital stays, an ever-expanding array of new drugs, new diagnostic tests, treatments and technologies. Yet, in spite of all that is new, the inner world of children remains essentially unchanged. The child mental health consultant often articulates the child's inner world, and echoes the experience of seasoned clinicians who understand that a child and family will need time to build relationships with caregivers, and time to accommodate to the challenges presented by a medical illness. The consultant's challenge is to integrate the distinct and overlapping needs of the child, family, team and hospital setting to the benefit of the patient.

History

Historically, adult consultation psychiatry arose in general hospitals during the 1930s, with a recognition that a mind–body dichotomy was inadequate. Best practice demanded that attention be paid to the psychological issues that impact on medical illness and treatment (Ortiz 1997). As the integral role of psychological factors was established in adult medical care, similar attention was focused on the needs of children.

Although a role for psychiatry with the medically ill child dates back to the 1930s (Work 1989; Lask 1994), even today consultation psychiatry is not available in every paediatric medical and surgical setting. Nevertheless, throughout the world the benefits of collaboration between child psychiatrists and paediatricians are noted (Unger-Koppel *et al.* 1992; Tsai *et al.* 1995; Chan 1996), with encouragement to establish and use consultation services.

Consultation services must be supported financially. In the USA, the National Institue for Mental Health (NIMH) provided grant money in the 1970s to support interdisciplinary paediatric and psychiatric clinical collaborations, thus increasing the number of consultation services nationwide. This seed money supported unreimbursed activities such as comprehensive evaluation and interdisciplinary team meetings. As this support ended in the 1980s, consultation services were forced to decrease the range of activities and services offered (Wright *et al.* 1987).

Clinically, there has been a shift away from looking at the mother–child dyad as the source of psychopathology and towards appreciating the impact of paediatric illness on the entire family. Research has focused on measuring functional adaptation and positive coping skills, while identifying both protective factors and risk factors across multiple diseases, as opposed to chronicling the presence of negative symptoms associated with specific illnesses (Knapp & Harris 1998).

The care of children, like that of adults, is moving toward shorter hospital stays and greater use of outpatient settings for treatment of chronic and life-threatening illness. For example, outpatient oncology chemotherapy units and in-home intravenous antibiotic treatment for cystic fibrosis patients used to be inpatient interventions.

Psychological distress in the paediatric population

Some one-third to two-thirds of inpatient paediatric patients have to cope with psychological issues (Stocking *et al.* 1972; Burket & Hodgin 1993). Existing data on psychological morbidity is difficult to compare as the studies utilize different measurement tools, represent small sample sizes and use a combination of patient, parent and paediatrician reports to assess emotional distress (Shugart 1991). Nevertheless, it is difficult to imagine hospitalization in which some stress and challenges to coping are not a factor for the child and family.

Lewis & Vitulano (1988) estimated that about 12% of outpatient children with chronic illnesses had DSM-IV diagnoses and 8–10% of paediatric outpatients had psychosomatic symptoms. Using screening tools, such as the Paediatric Symptom Checklist (Jellinek *et al.* 1999), in routine (well) outpatient clinics suggests that the proportions of psychologically symptomatic children range from a high of 34% in lower socioeconomic status high-risk populations (Murphy & Jellinek 1988) to a low of 8% in more affluent communities with approximately 20% of children with chronic illness noted to be symptomatic (Jellinek *et al.* 1988).

Paediatricians and child psychiatrists: collaboration and conflict

In spite of recognizing high levels of psychological distress in their hospitalized patients, paediatricians often do not refer to the child psychiatry consultants. In one study, paediatricians identified 64% of their inpatients as having emotional issues warranting psychiatric consultation, yet referred only 11% of these children (Stocking *et al.* 1972). Paediatricians often prefer to look to their paediatric colleagues for consultation on difficult cases rather than consulting child psychiatrists. They see their paediatric colleagues as uniquely equipped to understand the demands of paediatric practice and thus able to provide more relevant practical advice. Paediatricians who sought child psychiatry consultations during their house staff training years are much more likely to continue to seek consultation compared to colleagues who had not had this experience during their training years, suggesting that approaches to patient care are best developed early (Bergman & Fritz 1985). It is essential that child psychiatry consultants be integrated into paediatric training programmes in order to facilitate appropriate long-term utilization, a goal very dependent on financial support.

Key to paediatrician satisfaction with psychiatric consultation is quality timely communication. Paediatricians' perceptions of child psychiatrists are overwhelmingly positive, but tensions do exist. Dissatisfaction with consultations is linked to a perception that the child psychiatrist was not available quickly enough, did not communicate findings, or that findings were not tailored to the needs and realities of the referring paediatrician (Burkit & Hodgin 1993).

Child psychiatrists complain that paediatricians often consult too late in the course of the hospital stay, presenting the consultant as a last resort instead of seeking the psychiatric assessment as an integral part of the routine work-up and introducing the psychiatrist at the outset as a member of the treatment team (Fritz *et al.* 1987). This is especially problematic when coupled with completion of diagnostic tests that have not produced a definitive diagnosis or when routine treatment has not been effective. The timing may suggest to the patient and family that the medical team has completed their evaluation, possibly failed, and now are deferring to the child mental health consultant to define a purely psychological origin of the symptoms or treatment failure.

Barriers to requesting consultation

There are several common barriers to child mental health consultation. The consulting paediatrician may be uncomfortable talking to the patient and family about psychiatric consultation. Frequently, senior paediatricians and house officers worry that consulting a psychiatrist will be experienced as an insult by the patient or family. They may think that the family will assume the paediatrician thinks the child or parent is 'crazy' or does not believe the child's symptom is legitimate. By reviewing least threatening ways to introduce consultations to families such as, 'Dr X is the psychiatrist on our team and we like to have her see all our patients' either 'with diagnosis Y' or 'hospitalized for X days' or 'Y times', the consultant can help alleviate some of the paediatrician's anxiety or perceived stigma. When paediatricians wait until the end of the diagnostic period to invite the consultation, they maximize the likelihood of getting a negative response from the patient and family.

In some settings, child mental health consultants are not available at all or not in a timely fashion, a critical issue with decreasing length of hospital stay. There may be only a day or two in which to accomplish multiple goals for the admission. Short stays may push paediatricians to focus on essential, sometimes high-technology procedures and defer attention to psychological issues. When patients come to the hospital from distant locations, it may be the staff's perception that psychological issues other than of a life-and-death nature can be taken up by the primary care providers in the child's own community. Unfortunately, the child may be returning to a setting in which psychiatric support is not available or the clinicians in the community may be uncomfortable in addressing emotional issues.

In the USA, the type of insurance a patient uses may present a barrier to consultation, as some insurers 'carve out' mental health care. Patients and families may be eligible for reimbursement for medical care at a given institution, but not care from mental health providers at the same institution. Insurers will sometimes make an exception to their exclusionary practice, if time-consuming appeals are made by the consultant. If the patient stays in the hospital long enough for an appeal to be completed, the demand on the consultants' time of lengthy phone contacts and extra paperwork becomes a barrier to providing care.

Consultation models

Consultation services are organized to meet the demands created by the size of the patient population, specific higher risk treatment populations, and the availability of different child mental health consultants (child psychiatrists, child psychologists, psychiatric nurse clinicians, social workers). The service will develop in response to the perceived need of the paediatricians and patterns of consultation. Child mental health consultants, particularly child psychiatrists and child psychologists, are often available only for a limited number of hours. When this is the case, the paediatricians and child mental health consultants must work together to establish a set of practice priorities. These may include using some of the consultant time to supervise nurse clinicians and social workers, who do more of the direct service, and some consultant time to see the most challenging cases. In many paediatric settings, child psychologists are the primary child mental health consultants, with child psychiatrists acting as paediatric psychopharmacologists. Child psychologists, and child psychiatrists with limited paediatric training, will need to educate themselves in the medical disease process to maximize their effectiveness as consultants. Child psychiatrists are often less well trained in behavioural interventions, such as desensitization, hypnotherapy and behaviour modification, and will need to complement their training if behaviourally trained child psychologists are not available.

Consultations can be initiated on a case-by-case basis or by protocol. In the case-by-case model, the paediatrician requests a consultation after assessing an individual patient. Consultation by protocol systematizes psychiatric consultation for children with certain diagnoses or risk factors. Common examples are cancer, inflammatory bowel disease, overdoses, eating disorders, recurrent abdominal pain, severe asthma or organ transplantation. Protocols recognize the conditions under which a psychiatric assessment is an essential part of routine good quality care. In the setting of short hospital stays, protocols for high-risk diagnoses facilitate early identification and minimize wasted time. Protocols can also specify routine consultation for any child who is hospitalized for more than 2 weeks or in an intensive care unit (ICU), has more than two hospitalizations in a year or has more than three subspecialists consulting to the paediatrician. These protocols acknowledge the emotional impact of extended or repeated hospital stays on children, and the additional stress on the family and the treatment team when multiple specialists are involved. If possible, the same consultant should follow a child over multiple hospitalizations or from inpatient to an outpatient specialty clinic.

The child mental health consultant's role will vary depending on the parameters established by the consultation service as well as by the demands of an individual patient and family. The consultant may carry out a complete assessment of the child and family or may assess the ill child while a social worker assesses the family. A child psychologist may undertake psychological assessment and the child psychiatrist may assess whether psychotropic drugs are indicated. Often the child psychiatrist will have a leadership role in the multidisciplinary team, facilitating discussions of strategies for improving communication and compliance, or allowing staff to voice frustrations or sadness. This latter function is sometimes referred to as liaison and it may be the sole purpose of the consultation or be in conjunction with direct service.

One study of several hundred consultations ascribed one-third of the consultation requests to staff-related conflict (Hengeveld & Rooysman 1983). Not surprisingly, some would argue that no consultation on an inpatient can be performed effectively without the integral 'liaison' piece of understanding the child's condition in the context of the concerns arising from the members of the treatment team (Tarnow & Gutstein 1982; Hengeveld & Rooysman 1983).

Working in a paediatric setting necessitates understanding not only the disease process, but also the care delivered by a complex medical team. It is key to respect the roles of each member of the multidisciplinary treatment team and to understand how the chain of command works within each discipline. The child psychiatrist is likely to work with a wide range of hospital workers, spanning surgeons, social workers, nurse specialists and occupational therapists.

Part of respecting differing professional roles is understanding the value of each member's contribution to care, as well as being sensitized to particular challenges inherent in each discipline's treatment demands. For example, the paediatric house officer in the ICU may feel most stressed by decision-making, whereas the nurses at the bedside may feel most stressed by observing suffering (Jellinek et al. 1996).

Work with medically ill children is enormously rewarding but it can also arouse powerful feelings of sadness, frustration and helplessness. When these shared painful feelings are addressed in the setting of a multidisciplinary team, it can help provide the staff support necessary to care for the ill child and emotionally recharge staff members so they can continue to reinvest in new patients and not act on hostile feelings at work or at home.

Some team members will inevitably face personal or professional challenges that interfere with their ability to provide quality care and will come to the psychiatric consultant for assistance. The consultant may have a key role in facilitating referral to psychiatric treatment for troubled team members seeking help. The consultant should not personally provide psychotherapy treatment to a team member as this would be crossing an essential boundary in a long-term working relationship. Concerned colleagues may approach the consultant for direction on how to help a troubling member of the team who seems unaware of the problem themselves. The consultant will encourage the concerned colleague to share observations with the appropriate supervisor of the impaired individual and may meet separately with the supervisor or director to share observations of his or her own. Behaviours that put patients at risk may be mandated to be reported to the appropriate overseeing body, such as the chief of service or hospital-based board. Concern for the mental health and vulnerable state of an impaired colleague while recognizing the responsibility to protect patient care stirs up powerful feelings in the reporter, including feeling punitive, having betrayed a friend, or feeling vulnerable to being targeted him or herself.

Approach to consultation requests

The first task for the consultant is to understand what concerns have led to the consultation request. He or she must speak with the consulting paediatrician or staff member, listening to the expressed concerns and asking for elaboration about concerns that seem to be lurking beneath the surface. It is helpful to work together to establish realistic goals for the initial consultation, with a plan to set additional goals after the initial meetings with the child and parents. The consultant should seek any supporting information that is available from other members of the treatment team and from the hospital chart. It is useful to gather the observations from several individuals as the child may be behaving differently in different settings, or may have established warmer relationships with some team members than with others.

Although the consultant will gather data from many sources, a basic tenet of consultation work is being clear about the person receiving the consultation. Ultimately, the goal is to facilitate the child receiving optimum care, but the consultant may be serving the primary paediatrician, a subspecialist, or a subspecialty team. Usually what serves the child best is helpful to many team members and to the family, but there can be conflicts. For example, the consultant to the paediatrician may recommend that an aggressively interventionist gastroenterologist chosen by the family may not be the best choice for a somatizing child with recurrent abdominal pain, or a consultant to a lung transplant team may recommend outpatient psychotherapy and a more rigorous exercise programme as a way of assessing an adolescent with questionable pretransplant compliance before accepting the paediatric pulmonologist's patient into the transplant programme.

In order for a child to be seen, a parent must give permission. In the specific situation of an older adolescent who is living or functioning independently from parents, it may be possible to consult without parental permission. It is best if the paediatrician or subspecialist, with whom the family already has a relationship, informs them of the decision to obtain a psychiatric consultation. When the paediatrician tells the family that psychiatric consultation is routine, as it is when consultation is part of the diagnostic protocol, parents are usually receptive to this additional helpful input. A psychiatric consultation can be presented as a way to help the team understand how the child is feeling and to help the child cope with the difficult circumstance of hospitalization. Some parents and children will be uncomfortable with the idea of psychiatric consultation, but will warm up

to the intervention upon finding the child mental health consultant respectful, knowledgeable and attuned to the needs of the child and family. Other parents will be resistant, but reluctantly agree under some pressure from the referring paediatrician. A small number of parents will adamantly refuse consultation under any circumstance. In this uncommon group who refuse all consultation, the consultant may meet with the team in a liaison capacity and assist the team without directly interviewing the child. In the other situations, the child mental health consultant will meet with the child and the parent(s) after receiving permission from the parents to do so.

Depending on the child's age and circumstances, the consultant will decide whether to meet with the parents first, the child first or both together. It is usually helpful to have a chance at some point to meet older children without a parent present. Even young children will often not want to say some things in front of parents. However, many children under 6 will be more comfortable meeting the consultant with a parent. As the goal is to facilitate the child being most forthcoming in talk and play, it is important to respond to the child's preferences for the initial interview.

The parents of young children are likely to want time alone with the consultant to share observations and concerns that are not appropriate to share in the child's presence. Similarly, many parents of older children will find it easier to be candid about their worries in the absence of the child. Older children may be uncomfortable knowing that parents are talking to the consultant without knowing what is being said. Nevertheless, it remains key to the initial assessment to provide an interview setting that facilitates child and parent independently being able to express feelings freely.

Assessing the child

Premorbid functioning of the child and family

When assessing a hospitalized or ill child, the consultant is seeing only 'a snapshot' of a stressful moment in the child's life. Some families will be confronting a new diagnosis or change in the prognosis, whereas others may have had time to develop an ongoing coping strategy in the face of a chronic illness or a lengthy treatment protocol. It is often startling to see how well a child and family cope, once the shock of the bad news passes and a treatment plan is underway.

A biopsychosocial model may help. Under the 'bio' heading, the consultant will want to understand the particular challenges presented by the child's medical condition and interplay of medications. Under the 'psych' heading, the consultant will want to learn about depression and anxiety preceding the medical condition as well as psychological strengths and resiliency. What successful coping strategies have the child and the family drawn upon in the past that may serve them well in the adjustment to the medical condition and current hospital stay? What are the stressors the family is experiencing, parents and siblings, related to and unrelated to the child's medical illness? For example, the child's illness may be occurring as a parent has just lost his or her job, or the maternal grandmother's recent death. In the 'social' arena, the consultant wants to know about the child's relationship with peers and his or her functioning at school. It is easier for children with good friends and solid academic skills to continue in their pre-illness activities in spite of the disruptions caused by hospitalizations and medical treatments.

To gather this information, consultants will want to look to many sources—including the referring physician, the primary paediatrician and multiple members of the treatment team. They will want to read the current hospital chart, and records on past admissions when available. With permission from the parents or guardian, the consultant will want to speak with the outpatient psychotherapist, school professionals or members of other involved social agencies, or the court system.

Developmental perspective

Development is the lens through which a childhood medical illness can best be seen. The challenges of living with leukaemia are different for a 1 year old and his or her family than for a 16 year old and his or her family and friends. A full review of the interplay of development and medical illness is well beyond the scope of this chapter, but a few key developmental points will be highlighted to illustrate common issues.

Infants and toddlers cannot understand the gravity of a given diagnosis. They live in the moment, experiencing the medical condition and treatment according to the physical limitations and discomforts imposed. Infants rely on key caregivers to hold and soothe them and to make the hospital environment feel safe. It is important for the hospital staff to support the infant–parent attachment, and not allow treatments and technologies to interfere with this key emotional milestone. The paediatric unit can provide a milieu that supports breastfeeding mothers, and allows rooming by parents. A parent who wants to be present during procedures, and can play a soothing part in supporting the infant, should be allowed to do so. Parents may be encouraged to be physically close, touching the infant or toddler if the procedure permits, but restraining a fighting older infant or toddler is usually upsetting to both parent and child and is frequently inadequate for safety during procedures.

Preschool-aged children (3–6 year olds) are egocentric: they understand all events as occurring in relation to them. They have associative logic, which means that for them any two unrelated things can be understood as if one is causing or explaining the other. The combination of egocentricity and associative logic leads to magical thinking. Magical thinking is the weaving together of fantasy and logic to explain how the preschool-age child caused something to happen. In the medical setting, it is frequently the preschool-age child's misconception that having a 'bad illness' means he or she did something wrong and the disease is punishment. It is helpful to get young children (and older children as well) to elaborate their understanding of the aeti-

ology of their medical conditions to uncover self-blaming misconceptions and correct them. When preschool-age children have a life-threatening illness, parents often wonder if the child is worrying about dying. Preschool-age children do not yet have the cognitive capacity to comprehend forever and envision death as a reversible event. The preschool-age child is likely to demonstrate the most affect around separations, such as having anxiety about going to sleep at night in his or her own bed, or wanting a parent to promise to be there when he or she wakes up from surgery.

Furthermore, preschool-age children cannot localize a medical condition to a specific body part, so they feel particularly physically vulnerable when ill. Faced with needle sticks, intravenous medication and surgical procedures, they are like little knights without any armour. They rely on parents and medical staff to prepare them for procedures, so they are not on high alert anticipating surprise medical attacks at any moment.

Children aged 7 to 12 can understand simple functional explanations of medical conditions. Many will pride themselves on mastering the names of medicines, illness-related terminology and how to use hospital paraphernalia just as they pride themselves on learning words at school and mastering ball-handling on the sports field. Children of this age look for simple cause and effect aetiologies for illnesses. They can understand viral illnesses being caused by 'germs', but are perplexed when there is no clear cause and effect explanation, e.g. why they have cancer without having smoked cigarettes. It is important to explain illness and treatment to the school-age child. In the context of understanding why a treatment plan is being initiated, the medical staff should seek the child's assent to procedures and treatments. In this age group, 'rules rule' and it is troubling to the child that so often medical illness does not follow the rules; the child does all his or her treatments and the cancer relapses or he or she avoids asthma triggers and has an asthmatic attack anyway. One of the challenges of working with younger children is to capitalize on their pride in trying hard and their wish for competency, while keeping them from becoming too disappointed by setbacks that occur in spite of their own best efforts.

Adolescents have abstract thinking, and thus are able to understand the chance luck of having an uncommon life-threatening or chronic illness with the same cognitive complexity of an adult. Education is a prerequisite for behavioural change, but on its own is not sufficient. Commonly, teenagers do not have the maturity to incorporate the consistently health-promoting behaviours they know they should engage in into appropriate changes in lifestyle. Turning cognitive understanding into behavioural change is the common battleground of adolescent and authority figure—parent or physician. Assent for medical treatments is sought from the younger child, whereas consent is sought from adolescents who have the cognitive ability to comprehend the purpose of treatment and the ramifications of refusing treatment (British Medical Association 2001). Although some physicians may view seeking consent from an adolescent for treatments and procedures as time-consuming and burdensome while knowing that parents must give legal consent to proceed, these discussions foster trust and build a valuable alliance between patient and clinician.

Adolescence is a self-conscious time, with the emergence of sexual interests and heightened reliance on peer group norms for style and status. Medical illnesses or treatments that affect appearance are particularly difficult, such as becoming cushingoid on steroids, bald with chemotherapy or remaining very short with renal failure. The medical staff is challenged to find ways to respect the teenager's appropriate wish to be more independent in the face of illness that so often increases dependency.

As children with chronic illnesses live into adulthood, the transition to young adulthood and understanding of associated issues becomes relevant. Young adults are negotiating intimate relationships, career decisions, independence from parents, and sometimes relocation or parenthood. One isue is whether to transfer care from a paediatric into an adult setting, with a new treatment team. Some patients, e.g. with cystic fibrosis or congenital heart disease, may prefer to be on an adult ward or in a waiting room with other adults, but yet find it difficult to leave lifelong caregivers behind.

Specific challenges associated with a given medical condition

Each medical condition carries its own specific challenges. When the consultant is familiar with common frustrations or limitations imposed by a particular illness, this can provide credibility in the process of acquiring the family's trust as they relate what is hardest for them. Routine consultation to the same paediatric unit enables the consultant to become familiar with technology, treatment protocols and terminology, so making it easier for the family to feel understood. Many families describe how tiring it is to try to explain the medical experience to friends who are medically naive or therapists who are so saddened by the illness that they seem unable to get to the key nuances of the child's or family's experiences. The combination of psychological and medical knowledge is key to the consultant's expertise.

Mental status examination

Hospitalized children have many reasons to have an altered mental status, including delirium, central nervous system changes secondary to medical conditions, effects of medications, and trauma. A formal mental status examination should be part of the medical record, including observations of appearance, gross and fine motor function, speech, mood, affect, thought, suicidal ideation, memory and cognition. Many consultants have had the experience of carrying out a mental status assessment only to discover significant mental impairment that has gone undetected despite multiple specialists seeing the child.

It is common for medically ill children to be developmentally delayed and sometimes emotionally immature. Coping is a function of cognitive capacity and complex defence mechanisms

that may result in temporary or long-term regression in some developmentally appropriate behaviours and adaptation in others (Freud 1969). It is helpful for the consultant to integrate the information from the mental status examination and premorbid school and developmental information to assist the medical team in understanding the child's ability to comprehend medical information. For example, a child may be 11 years old, have the cognitive skills of a 7 year old, and behave like a preschool-age child faced with the anxiety of a painful procedure. On the other hand, there are teenagers who appear several years younger than their chronological age and feel patronized by medical staff who forget their actual ages and capacities because of their appearance and interact with them as if they are much younger.

The family

No child can be understood independently of his or her family. In the initial evaluation, it is key to assess the family's level of functioning and their ability to support the child through the anticipated treatment and outcome. Every hospitalization is a family crisis. During hospitalization, parents are coping with new and anxiety-provoking information, sometimes hourly. Frequently, it is conflicting information presented by multiple caregivers. Seemingly small inconsistencies in the presentation of information—one person being more optimistic, another more pessimistic, one person emphasizing a particular laboratory value and another devaluing its importance—can leave the parents feeling they are on an emotional roller coaster riding up or down in response to each new piece of information. There is little or no privacy for the family to regroup after hearing upsetting news. Many parents identify the continuous uncertainty as the hardest aspect of adapting to the child's illness. Some parents will derive support from other parents on the paediatric unit while others will report feeling further traumatized by witnessing other families in crisis. Parental anxiety negatively impacts on the child's capacity to cope (Awad & Pozanski 1975; Kashani et al. 1994; Wright 1994), yet it is hard to imagine how parents could be other than anxious.

Asking parents to share the history of the current illness, from the first symptoms through to the present hospital stay, allows the consultant to form an impression of the extent to which parents felt responded to or ignored in the process of diagnosis and treatment. For example, did the parent have to tell the primary care doctor repeatedly that something was wrong before the concerns were taken seriously or did the first physician act immediately? Do they trust the medical professionals as a group, or are they generally mistrustful except for faith in one particular caregiver? Do one or both parents feel guilty about the illness or condition or about not getting the child to care fast enough? Sometimes parents feel guilty because of a genetically transmitted illness for which one or both parents are carriers, or for an injury that occurred while the child was in the parent's care. Even when there is no apparent reason, parents may still feel profoundly guilty about having been unable to protect the child from the pain and uncertainty of illness. Commonly, parents will voice the wish that they could switch places with their child, and be the sick one in the child's stead. Other times, a child's illness will fuel parental discord and even divorce.

Parental guilt sometimes occurs in the context of depression. An assessment of the family should include history-taking about present and past psychiatric history (including use of substances) to determine whether certain family members are particularly vulnerable. It is helpful to ask questions about neurovegetative symptoms for each parent and the siblings. In especially stressful circumstances, parents may increase their own risk-taking behaviour including use of alcohol, driving with less care, etc. Many parents who do not meet criteria for depression will benefit from being reminded of the importance of eating and sleeping so that they do not compromise their own health during what may be a long period in which the sick child will need additional care.

The family's experience is affected by past experiences with illness, and loss. The consultant wants to know if any other family members have had the same or similar illnesses, what the experience was of their care and the outcome. For example, a mother of a 3-year-old girl with cystic fibrosis whose brother died of cystic fibrosis in his teens may indulge her daughter as if she is about to die instead of likely to live well into adulthood. Helping the parent differentiate the current medical situation from past experiences helps the parent be more attuned to the child's actual needs.

Siblings are often the forgotten sufferers (Spinetta *et al.* 1999). The sick child is usually the object of everyone's attention and recipient of a multitude of gifts, whereas the siblings at home are coping with an absent parent(s), sometimes depressed parents, and a disrupted schedule. If the siblings voice feelings of envy or resentment toward the ill child, parents may become angry at their insensitivity to the ill child's situation. The consultant and social worker can model important empathy for the plight of the siblings, by talking about the ways the sick child is lucky and the ways he or she is unlucky; the sick child is lucky to get so many stuffed animals and have special time with Mom, but unlucky to have so many blood tests, medicines to swallow and uncomfortable procedures.

Frequently, paediatric hospital staff have a harder time working with the family than with the designated patient. By understanding the parents' concerns and their experience of the hospital care, the consultant can help the team understand the family better and feel more empathy for difficult behaviours that may seem callous, unappreciative or interfere with care. Difficult parents often cannot bear the feelings of helplessness, and vent their anger and frustration on hospital staff by being critical and devaluing (Groves & Beresin 1999).

Understanding the experience of the treatment team

Together with different professional roles, treatment team members are likely to focus on different stresses associated with caring for sick children. The neonatal ICU (NICU), a high stress environment, serves as a good illustration of this principle. Senior paediatricians in the NICU are most stressed by the long hours in the hospital and the conflict this creates with the demands of their personal lives (Oates & Oates 1995). Advanced trainees held in high regard by juniors for their technical skills must cope with their sense of helplessness when they are unable to live up to this image and cannot save the young lives in their care (Jellinek *et al.* 1993). Nurses in the NICU identify overcrowded units without privacy, doctor–nurse tensions, and inadequate pain relief for the neonates as their key concerns (Oates & Oates 1996).

Recommendations

After meeting the child and family for the initial assessment, the consultant will share observations and recommendations with the referring paediatrician and available team members and write a note on the hospital chart. The preliminary formulation and recommendations should avoid the use of psychiatric jargon. Clear practical recommendations to improve coping, address behavioural problems, treat primary psychiatric disorders and maintain safety are key. Hospital records are permanent documents and should not be used for private or informal communications between physicians. One should assume that patients and parents will read the record, as can hospital staff and insurers. No one should write pejorative comments about other clinicians, patients or families in the hospital record. The consultant should be thoughtful about including personal information about the patient or family members, avoiding what is not germane to the care of the patient, such as a past history of parental substance abuse, marital infidelity or sexual abuse.

When presenting recommendations, safety must be addressed first. For example, one-to-one observation will be necessary for an acutely suicidal teenager and behaviours that prevent a child from receiving urgent medical care must also be addressed immediately. Both in the initial contact with the referring paediatrician and in the presentation of recommendations, an understanding of the urgency and time frame in which the referring doctor needs assistance must be attended to by the consultant.

Sharing an understanding of motivations that may underlie maladaptive behaviours can increase empathy for the child and family, but the consultant must work with the team to come up with concrete suggestions that can be implemented. For example, the consultant could recommend that all procedures for a fearful child occur in a treatment room, so that over time the child will come to feel safer in his or her room and in the playroom. The primary nurse might resist this idea if he or she was responsible for getting a potentially thrashing child to the treatment room on his or her own. Perhaps premedicating the child with an antianxiety medication, and getting the paediatric house officer and the parents to walk the child to the treatment room will help the nurse feel respected and able to endorse the plan. Similarly, a paediatric team would need specific recommendations to help them deal with angry demanding parents. Regular meeting times with the senior paediatrician in which the important information of the day is communicated may help decrease the parents' anxiety and therefore their anger, but a regular check-in time with the paediatrician may be hard for him or her to achieve in person. Perhaps the consultant could commit to a regular time for a phone contact, during which he or she could tell the parents approximately when he or she would be on the unit that day.

Emergency consultations

The most common emergency consultations relate to the suicidal or self-abusive child admitted after an overdose or other act leading to self-harm, such as jumping off a high place or lacerations from wrist-slashing. The consultant's first recommendations focus on the child's immediate safety in the hospital setting. Hospital units are not designed with the safety of a self-injurious child in mind. There is potentially dangerous medical equipment throughout the unit, including sharp objects and flammable substances (oxygen). It is therefore necessary to assess carefully the child's risk for self-harm in the hospital. After having made an impulsive suicide attempt or gesture that is serious enough to require medical hospitalization, many children are frightened, regret their actions, feel supported by their families and may be assessed as being at low risk to hurt themselves while hospitalized on the medical unit. Others only regret that the suicide attempt was unsuccessful, or are uncommunicative, and leave the consultant unsure of their mental state. When unsure, one must err on the side of safety, providing one-to-one observation of these children on the paediatric unit. Once safety has been assured, the consultant will assess the precipitants for the acts of self-harm and recommend an appropriate treatment for the hospital and disposition.

Another common urgent consultation is for behaviour that disrupts essential medical treatment. This behaviour is sometimes driven by extreme anxiety, as in the frightened preschool-age child who kicks, screams and bites when approached; at other times it is agitation in the setting of delirium; disinhibition following head injury; or angry threatening behaviour in a child with a clear sensorium, but who views the essential medical treatment as an unnecessary assault. Medical treatment of the cause of delirium, reassessment of medications affecting the central nervous system, antianxiety medication, antipsychotic medication, behavioural treatment plans, and sensitive education may be appropriate interventions depending on the aetiology of the difficult behaviour.

Parental behaviour may be the reason for an urgent consultation. Parents may be refusing essential medical treatment for the child or acting bizarrely. The reason for the parental actions may be unclear or may represent cultural beliefs at odds with standard medical practice, mistrust of the hospital staff, psychiatric illness in the parent, or extreme anxiety. Hostile parents making physical or litigious threats may interfere with critical care by frightening the medical staff. Paediatric staff often underestimate the danger of an angry teenager or parent and the consultant's sensitivity may facilitate the appropriate use of hospital security personnel.

The consultant may be asked to interact directly with the parent to help the referring physician work with the family or to recommend further assessment, including social services or court interventions. Often parents who are obstructing essential care for their child are doing so because they are themselves overwhelmed with helplessness and are trying to control what they see as uncontrollable. They mistakenly choose a counterproductive stance to achieve the feeling of being a powerful agent in the treatment decisions for the child. By helping the parent to feel that he or she is an essential member of the decision-making process and thus has some control in productive ways, many parents will step out of a combative stance and into a more collaborative one. There are specific legal interventions that are implemented when parents prevent a life-sustaining treatment, such as a blood transfusion for a child with life-threatening blood loss. These interventions include emergency assessment of guardianship by a judge to determine what is in the best interest of the child, and may lead to custody shifting to the hospital acutely, followed by temporary and permanent custody decisions occurring after the emergency medical situation is resolved or stabilized.

Primary psychiatric illnesses

Depression

Depression is common in the hospitalized child. It may be a secondary response to the stress of acute or chronic illness, or it may be primarily presenting as psychosomatic illness or behavioural problems including self-harm. Recognition of depression in childhood is a relatively recent phenomenon and the treatment of depression with psychotropic drugs is still viewed as controversial by some clinicians. One barrier to the appropriate treatment of depression in hospitalized children is the misconception that depressed mood and neurovegetative symptoms are an appropriate response to serious illness and thus should not be identified as depression nor treated. Individual and family therapy, play therapy, behavioural therapy and medication are useful modalities in the hospital setting. Our clinical experience supports the use of antidepressants in the depressed ill school-aged child or adolescent. Selective serotonin reuptake inhibitors (SSRIs) have become the antidepressant of choice as they are generally well tolerated, have limited interactions with other medications, and present a lower risk of intentional or accidental overdose (see Harrington, Chapter 29).

Anxiety

Anxiety can be secondary to the stresses of the medical condition and treatment or pre-existing. Children with pre-existing generalized anxiety or specific fear of doctors, needles and injections are likely to have more difficulty adjusting to medical assessment and treatment. In addition to the obvious discomfort severe anxiety causes the child and parents, anxiety can interfere with procedures and complicate history-taking and symptom assessment.

Age-appropriate explanation of medical interventions for older children, and medical play with explanation for younger children, can decrease anxiety. Children from around 6 years of age can learn a variety of coping techniques to help them with anxiety-provoking procedures. Many children will respond to distraction, breathing exercises, visualization or hypnotherapy (Jay et al. 1983, 1985; Kuttner 1987; Kuttner et al., 1988).

Clinicians must pay attention to minimizing pain for every child (Schechter et al. 1993). The use of anaesthetic creams before procedures, reducing the number of times bloods are drawn, and treating chronic and acute pain with analgesics should be standard practice. For young children, all painful procedures should occur in a treatment room and not in the child's bed nor in the playroom. Protecting the child's bed and the playroom as safe havens will eventually help the young child relax in these settings.

With quality pain management, relaxation techniques and preparation for procedures, some children will continue to be too anxious to comply with treatment and may suffer sleepless nights, be nauseated, or frantic during the hospital stay or in anticipation of visits to the hospital. Benzodiazepines may be helpful adjuncts to lessen debilitating anxiety. In young children, one must be aware of the potential for benzodiazepines to disinhibit children and thus worsen coping difficulties.

Anorexia nervosa

Anorexia nervosa is characterized by significant weight loss or the absence of appropriate weight gain for age and height in the setting of distorted body image and fear of gaining weight (see Steinhausen, Chapter 34). Paediatric hospitalization usually occurs when there has been rapid or profound weight loss, cardiovascular abnormalities, electrolyte imbalance and hypothermia. The goal of paediatric hospitalization is medical stabilization with nutritional assessment and treatment, psychological assessment of the child and family, and recommendation for level of psychiatric intervention after medical stabilization (Andersen et al. 1997). If the anorexic patient has been in outpatient psychotherapy, it will be key to seek input from the outpatient therapist. Medical hospitalization may represent a failure of outpatient psychotherapy.

It is often helpful to institute a detailed anorexia protocol, because the care of the anorexic teenager differs from the care of younger medically ill children. The protocol begins with very restricted activity, including bed rest, observation during and directly after meal times, bathroom privileges only after weight gain has begun, and limited phone contact and visitation with family. As the child demonstrates that he or she is able to meet nutritional goals, privileges are added.

Once the child is medically stable, recommendations about disposition can be initiated. The consultant will consider:
1 the anorexic patient's motivation to change;
2 inpatient eating behaviour;
3 the family's commitment to psychotherapy;
4 their ability to put the child's health as a top priority;
5 the input from the outpatient psychotherapist and primary paediatrician.
The child may need to be transferred to an inpatient psychiatric hospital or may return home with outpatient psychotherapy, and weights and vital signs monitored by the paediatrician.

Paediatric and nursing staff often feel frustrated and angry at anorexia patients, whom they see as making themselves ill. This is in stark contrast to other children on the paediatric unit who are viewed as struggling to overcome 'real' illnesses. Some staff members engage in frustrating arguments with the anorexic patient believing that a logical interchange should convince him or her that he or she is not fat. Many anorexic patients will present as sweet and compliant, but a few days into the hospital stay be discovered in secretive behaviours such as hiding food, or faking weight gain by water loading. When these behaviours are revealed, staff may feel manipulated and deceived. Team meetings provide an opportunity for staff members to voice the feelings engendered by the patient, to ensure that the protocol is being instituted consistently, and that the team is unified in providing high-quality compassionate care.

Psychosomatic illness

Some children will be admitted to paediatric departments with intense persistent somatic complaints, such as headaches, abdominal pains, bowel complaints, neurological symptoms or fatigue. Paediatricians may suspect that the intensity of the symptoms or the combination of complaints exceeds what would be explained by a medical condition and reflects underlying emotional factors and thus may seek a consultation. The paediatrician's assessment that psychological factors are influencing the somatic presentation is at odds with the child and parents' understanding of the aetiology of the condition. In psychosomatic illness, the somatic complaints are an unconscious expression of emotional issues. Additionally, some families are overly invested in an exhaustive medical work-up to prove a purely medical aetiology. Although this may appropriately arouse paediatric concern, the family believe that the child is seriously ill and therefore do not view the medical tests as unnecessary or risky. Typically, psychiatric consultation is resisted, treating the recommendation for assessment as an insult, and evidence that the medical team either does not believe the symptoms or medical condition to be 'real' or is unwilling to investigate fully all the medical possibilities.

The term 'psychosomatic illness' spans a range of illnesses, conditions and presentations that include not only symptoms with no clear medical aetiology, but also those that have a medical basis, such as chronic pancreatitis or kidney disease with chronic stone production, in which the child's somatic complaints may reflect a flare of the baseline illness or may be an expression of emotional distress, or a combination of both factors. Also encompassed under the term 'psychosomatic' are medical conditions that generate debate in the medical community, such as chronic fatigue syndrome (ME) and Lyme disease, in which a family may find substantially different responses to the child's condition in different treatment centres, reflecting the differing opinions of medical specialists. In the absence of clear medical knowledge or consensus about an illness, the potential for conflict between family and medical staff is heightened.

It is common for the family to seek multiple medical opinions about the child's somatic complaints, and sometimes to choose the most aggressive specialists, e.g. those who do the most diagnostic testing or prescribe the most medications. All too often the child is maintained on multiple medications in spite of little or no improvement in symptoms. The same diagnostic tests may be repeated to satisfy parental demands for action or in an attempt to decrease persistent patient and parental anxiety about undetected serious illness. In some cases, the parents may cling to insignificant positive findings from the diagnostic work-ups to vindicate their belief that a yet undiscovered medical aetiology exists. For these families, the relentless pursuit of a medical explanation overshadows their concern about the morbidity associated with invasive tests.

The best approach to treatment is a joint medical and psychiatric one. The psychiatric consultant must be willing to listen to the somatic symptoms and associated medical hypotheses in order to establish an alliance with the patient and family. Presenting the consultant's role as one of helping the child cope with chronic symptoms that are interfering with school, peer activities or family life is less threatening to the family than suggesting that the consultant has been sought because the symptom intensity reflects psychological issues. The child and family must be reassured that the presence of the child mental health consultant will not be associated with reduced access to the medical team, but is truly an adjunct to ongoing medical care. The paediatrician has the important role of re-examining the child regularly, reassuring the patient and family that no worrying new findings exist and not acquiescing to unnecessary testing.

The medical team may recommend a graded re-entry plan to work toward getting the child back to age-appropriate activities. The child and the parents are often very anxious about the child's return to normal activities and a stepwise re-entry plan addresses some of this anxiety. The child may benefit from a face-saving explanation for his or her physical symptoms that includes reasons why he or she is now able to work toward successful reengagement in normal activities. The parents will need support to endorse the child bearing some amount of anxiety and discomfort during this time. If the parent insists on withdrawing the child from any activity at the onset of somatic complaints, the child is unlikely to be motivated to cope with his or her symptoms or to find another medium for expression of emotional distress.

Initially, the consultant is likely to hear that everything was going well for the child and family until the onset of the somatic symptoms, but over several meetings the pre-existing emotional issues may begin to surface. The consultant might discover, for example, a learning disability that interferes with school adjustment, parental discord, depression or the recent death of an important family member.

Commonly, the child's somatic symptom stabilizes the family system, which is organized around the illness being the designated family problem. The symptom becomes a solution to avoid more provocative and difficult feelings. Family therapy or parent guidance therapy will often be required to address the issues that the illness has served to mask, while the child's individual therapy will address underlying psychiatric illness as well as communication skills that allow the child to express feelings with words instead of somatic symptoms, and thus help improve self-esteem.

Non-compliance

Non-compliance with medical treatment is estimated at 50%. It varies according to illness and in some illnesses may be as high as 88%. Surprisingly, confidence in the efficacy and importance of the treatment does not necessarily translate into improved compliance rates (Van Sciver et al. 1995). Indeed, illness-related compliance rates are likely to reflect a complex array of factors including the convenience of treatment, impact on age-appropriate activities, effect on appearance, chronicity of treatment demands, discomfort caused by illness exacerbation, and degree of correlation between single acts of non-compliance and negative consequences. The impact of non-compliance ranges from essentially harmless, in the case of a child with otitis media who misses a single dose of antibiotic, to life-threatening for a brittle diabetic who ignores his or her insulin needs and precipitates an episode of ketoacidosis. When consultation is sought for non-compliance, usually it is because of risk to the child's health, escalating conflict in the family, or frustration with inappropriate use of medical resources, as with the asthmatic who does not take maintenance medication and therefore is seen repeatedly in the emergency room.

Medical non-compliance is multidetermined, associated with medical education, active vs. passive coping style, pride vs. embarrassment with respect to self-care, impulsivity, family support, peer support, relationship with medical providers and underlying psychiatric disorder.

The consultant's task is to understand why the child is non-compliant and to work with the team to modify aspects of treatments that trouble the child where possible, while working to help the child and family adopt strategies that support clinically important treatments. If there are treatable psychiatric disorders, such as attention deficit hyperactivity disorder, these need to be identified and addressed. Treatment promoting supports, including disease-specific support groups, more frequent meetings with clinicians and psychoeducation groups, can be helpful.

Child abuse

Possible physical abuse, neglect (see Emery & Laumann Billings, Chapter 20) and sexual abuse (see Glaser, Chapter 21) may need to be considered. Without educated suspicion, abuse will often go undetected. Injuries to body surfaces that do not commonly bear the brunt of an accidental fall, multiple broken bones or bruises in various stages of healing, bruises that resemble finger marks, belts or cords are highly suspicious. Implausible or inconsistent stories from caregivers, and inappropriate delay in bringing a child for medical care should raise suspicion, as should caregivers who ascribe the injury to siblings or self-inflicted injuries.

Suspicion of abuse must be reported to the appropriate social agency. When abuse is suspected, the child should be fully examined for other physical signs. It is important to notify authorities of other children known to be in a potentially unsafe home. The paediatric unit may serve as a safe haven for a child while allegations are being investigated.

Sexual abuse is believed to be seriously underreported. The prevalence has been estimated at around 15% for boys and as high as 38% for girls under the age of 18 (Crewdson 1988). Three common presentations of sexual abuse on a paediatric unit are:

1 a child with traumatic injury to genitalia or a sexually transmitted infection;

2 a child who reveals that sexual abuse has occurred without physical evidence; and

3 a child who has physical symptoms suggestive of sexual abuse, but who has not disclosed any abuse or a perpetrator (Sugarman 1990).

Münchausen by proxy

Münchausen by proxy syndrome is a form of child abuse that is particular to the paediatric setting (see Emery & Laumann Billings, Chapter 20). A parent, usually a mother, consciously distorts or fabricates medical symptoms attributed to her child, including acting to create symptoms of medical illness in the child, and then seeks paediatric hospitalization and interventions for the child. The understanding of the aetiology of this syndrome consists of a character-disordered parent who finds the support of the hospital staff and/or the drama of the child's purported illness so personally gratifying that the morbidity associated with unnecessary tests and even the death of her child becomes secondary to her need to keep the child in the sick role. These parents may ultimately kill their children, e.g. by injecting faeces into an intravenous line to cause sepsis, or suffocating a child in an attempt to create a documented cardiac or pulmonary arrest. They may use their own blood to add to a child's urine sample or vomitus in order to maintain the heightened concern of the medical team.

There is no exact profile of a Münchausen by proxy parent, but some perpetrators have worked in medical settings. The parent is unlikely to disclose her own psychiatric history, but many have documented psychiatric illness, including suicide attempts, in the past (Souid et al. 1998). Usually the mother stays at the bedside with her child, typically an infant or very young child, but at times an older socially isolated child with his or her own reasons to maintain the sick role imposed by the parent.

The mother is often seen as nurturant toward her child and ingratiating with the nursing staff, until it is suggested that the child is well or the medical findings seem spurious. At this juncture, the mother usually becomes irate and threatens to or does take the child out of the hospital unless the medical team supports her demands for continued medical interventions. The parent rarely has had long-term relationships with medical caregivers and often the child has had multiple paediatricians, multiple subspecialists and hospital stays in different facilities, each ending with the same angry response to withdrawal of acute care (Schreier & Libow 1993).

This is a difficult diagnosis to prove unless the parent is observed hurting her child, or diagnostic work demonstrates the parent's role such as typing the blood in the child's urine and having it match the mother's blood type, not the child's own. The risk of morbidity and mortality is high (Samuels & Southall 1992) forcing paediatric providers to be aware of the potential for this form of abuse. Suspicion should be aroused when the medical condition does not follow an expected course, the symptoms are inconsistent and puzzling to seasoned clinicians, the symptoms are only observed by the mother or can be traced to an intentional aetiological agent. When suspected, the caregivers should notify the hospital legal team for assistance. All caregivers should be particularly vigilant observing the parent's behaviour, especially when she is unaware. In some settings, the parent has been videotaped thus revealing the abusive actions.

It should also be noted here that, occasionally, when a child has a difficult to diagnose illness or a persistent less likable parent, a member of the medical team will raise the spectre of Münchausen by proxy as an expression of frustration. Just as it is a form of abuse that should not be regarded as trivial, it is also important not to ascribe uncertainty of diagnosis and parental anxiety to this serious form of abuse. Once suspicion of this diagnosis is written in the permanent hospital record, the parent will be viewed with suspicion by every provider to follow.

Coping with chronic illness

Chronically ill children demonstrate the enormous resiliency of childhood. These children are not defined by their illnesses: there is no typical diabetic or classic asthmatic. To the contrary, chronically ill children have the same range of personalities and coping styles seen in healthy children, and are engaged in mastering the developmental milestones and challenges they share with their peers (Perrin & Thyen 1999).

Estimates of psychological morbidity associated with chronic illnesses in childhood range from 10 to 30% (Bauman et al. 1997), which is only slightly higher than the general paediatric population. Greater morbidity is associated with multiple hospitalizations admissions (Geist 1977). Other documented risk factors for adaptation to chronic illness include physical disability and brain dysfunction, pain frequency, younger age, poverty, single-parent family, and increased psychological symptoms in the parents (Knapp & Harris 1998).

Specific illnesses may present particular challenges (Horner *et al.* 2000), such as the dietary restrictions in diabetes or the decreased exercise endurance in advancing cystic fibrosis. Many factors influence how problematic a disease-specific challenge is for an individual child. It is the consultant's job to understand the unique meaning of the illness to the child and family, and to assist in the process of adaptation.

The consultant will need to ask many questions to elucidate the child's subjective experience of the illness. What is the hardest aspect of the illness or treatment from the child's perspective? How does it affect the child's image of him or herself now, and has it changed? Does the child have worries about the future? How do the illness and treatment impact on peer interactions, and favourite activities? When and how does the child tell others about the illness and why? Are there areas of conflict between the child and parent or the child and physician in relation to the illness? What is the child's perception of the parents' worries? Variations of the same questions can be asked of the parents and the siblings.

Chronic illness requires adjustment on the part of the child, the family, and perhaps the school, friends and organizers of activities. The extent to which the child is able to continue with age-appropriate activities and special interests is central to good adaptation. Children with personal strengths, whether in academics, sports, music or interpersonal skills, are likely to have an easier time accommodating to the limits of their illness and treatment because they can rely on their strengths to maintain self-esteem and build important relationships. Temperament is also a factor, with more flexible and outgoing children likely to adapt more easily to the uncertainty and limitations imposed on their lifestyles. Parental support, warmth and attitude toward the illness and the child's adaptive style is key. Parental anxiety, anger, sadness, guilt or blame can impede adjustment.

A number of chronic illnesses have been the focus of particular interest. Strategies are being sought to understand the disease-specific challenges and to illuminate common areas of stress, models for improving compliance, and recommendations for improving quality of life. In addition, improved coping may result in reduced medical costs for emergency visits and potentially unnecessary admissions.

Asthma

Asthma is a common illness of childhood with a paediatric population prevalence of 5–10% and a mortality rate of 1–2% among severe asthmatics (Godding *et al.* 1997; see also Mrazek, Chapter 48). Although overall mortality rates are noted to be declining, the mortality rates among adolescents and young adults are unchanged as is the morbidity of the disease (Conway

1998). Recent studies have sought to understand the factors that affect adherence and compliance, delineate common psychosocial stresses that may act as triggers for asthma attacks, and devise psychoeducational programmes, combined medical and psychological treatment strategies, and teach stress management skills to improve compliance and decrease morbidity (Sadler 1982; Perrin *et al.* 1992; Godding *et al.* 1997; Conway 1998; Rutishauser *et al.* 1998; Randolph & Fraser 1999). Educational programmes should offer clear guidelines on when to call the paediatrician for appropriate timely guidance, while seeking input from the family to ascertain whether there are barriers to these contacts. The impact of triggers in the home should be addressed realistically and empathically. Common triggers, such as smoking and pets, require a major commitment from the family to alter. School-related issues need to be explored from the perspective of the child and the school, such as access to inhalers in the classroom or embarrassment about going to the school nurse. Strategies to improve parent and child anxiety, and to address parent–child conflicts around compliance are valuable.

Diabetes

Adaptation to insulin-dependent diabetes presents special challenges associated with the need for tight control of blood sugar, the intimate relationship between the primary role of food as a source of nurturance and soothing, the meaning of a child's relationship with eating and the parent's role of providing or limiting access to desirable foods, and the mode of monitoring blood sugars and delivering insulin involving needle sticks and thus pain (see Mrazek, Chapter 48). The acute consequences of blood sugar abnormalities include symptomatic hypoglycaemia, hyperglycaemia and ketoacidosis, and the long-term sequelae include effects on vision, renal function and neuropathy. Symptoms associated with hypoglycaemia are often difficult for parents to differentiate from common irritability in young children or for older children to recognize as different from anxiety in themselves. This leads either to more frequent blood testing or a tendency to keep the blood sugars at a higher level than the physician would recommend. Some children will have considerable anxiety about hypoglycaemia, either in response to an actual episode or arising independently. It is key to treat anxiety disorders and concurrent eating disorders in order to improve compliance (Jacobson 1996; Strauss 1996; Burroughs *et al.* 1997).

Parents of children with diabetes may benefit from the support of the child mental health consultant as well as parent support groups to help achieve a healthy family attitude toward eating. Concrete ways to minimize the child's experience of being deprived of age-appropriate food treats, such as having sugar-free desserts at school and at home, altering insulin to accommodate special events, and supporting the child's understanding of how insulin helps him or her grow bigger and stronger are useful.

When patterns of conflict arise between parent and child

around non-compliance, such as lying about foods eaten, hiding sweets and refusing blood monitoring, psychotherapeutic input should be initiated early. Children who enter adolescence with pre-existing parent–child conflict around health maintenance can be expected to have greater difficulty during their teenage years. Non-compliance in insulin-dependent diabetes can be life-threatening, so the full range of psychotherapeutic, educational and family supports should be utilized.

Cancer

Childhood cancer presents numerous challenges to adaptation and development, but does not lead to serious psychopathology in adulthood (Roberts *et al.* 1998). There are predictable high stress points in the course of the illness including diagnosis, onset of treatment, treatment completion, and sometimes recurrence, renewed treatment and end of life care. Psychological support for the child and parents is particularly beneficial at these critical points (see Mrazek, Chapter 48). The siblings too will benefit from support at the transitions in the course of the illness (Murray 1999; Spinetta *et al.* 1999). Diagnosis of a life-threatening illness is understandably frightening to parents and older children, creating a family crisis. Although not commonly the case, some children and parents may respond to diagnosis and aspects of treatment with symptoms seen in post-traumatic stress syndrome (Stuber *et al.* 1998).

Although cancer is rare in children, it is a common medical condition in older adults. Frequently, children and families will face the child's cancer diagnosis with past experiences of cancer in a family member or close friend colouring their understanding of what lies ahead for their child (Hoekstra-Weebers *et al.* 1999). Exploring the child's understanding of cancer with attention to the role of development, as well as the understanding of the parents and the other siblings, is important and offers an opportunity to differentiate the child's situation from that of others, while potentially uncovering misconceptions about the illness.

Challenges to psychological adaptation include persistent pain whether as a result of the cancer or of the procedures (Ljungman *et al.* 1999), persistent debilitating side-effects of treatment such as nausea, alteration in body image, school disruptions, compromised peer relationships, interference with ability to engage in favourite activities, and conflicts in the family. Adolescents may worry about future health status, sexual function and reproductive capacities, and future career choices (Kasak & Meadows 1989; Roberts *et al.* 1998).

During the course of cancer treatment, many children develop strong positive relationships with members of the medical team, experience a special closeness with supportive parents, and maintain key pre-existing peer friendships while acquiring new friends in the hospital. Many children will report feeling a special sense of purpose for living as a result of the cancer diagnosis and most will be treated with special status as a result of the illness. Resiliency and positive life change are also part of the cancer experience (Woodgate 1999).

Organ transplantation

Liver, kidney and lung transplantation are current realities for the paediatric population. Transplantation centres in the USA are required to include psychological assessment as part of the work-up in order to receive accreditation. Data on criteria for approval of candidacy for transplant are vague. The serious disease process leading up to transplantation, the risks of surgery, the long-term medical management of organ rejection post-transplantation, the threat to survival, and the vast array of medical personnel involved should place these children in the highest of high-risk populations. It is noteworthy therefore that the data on adjustment to liver transplantation suggests that overall these children view themselves as healthy and competent (Mastroyannopoulou *et al.* 1998; Tornquist *et al.* 1999). Not surprisingly, some children and parents are vulnerable to anxiety, and there is broad acceptance in transplant centres of the role of emotional support (Ullrich *et al.* 1997; Walker *et al.* 1999).

Dying in the hospital

The death of a child is an enormous tragedy that affects every member of the child's family. There is no way to protect a child or family from the unique pain of the loss of a child but sensitive care at this difficult time may serve to lessen regrets and support the impending process of bereavement. Careful attention to the child's quality of life in these last days or hours is essential. Attending to pain, anxiety and privacy/dignity needs is key. Adapting the medical setting to allow parents to nurture the dying child within the limitations of the setting, or facilitating a child's return home to die, can play a significant part in the family's experience of the death and the subsequent bereavement (American Academy of Pediatrics 2000).

The emotional impact on the medical team also requires careful attention in order to best preserve each team member's ability to continue to deliver quality care into the future. The medical staff need recognition of their grieving process. Some units will have staff meetings including the child mental health consultant or other facilitator after every death or after those deaths that are most troubling to staff members, such as favourite patients, trauma-related deaths or unanticipated deaths.

A common misconception is that a family's attachment to a child increases with age, thus making the death of an infant less difficult. Many of the hospital-based paediatric deaths occur in NICUs or during infancy. The death of an infant is both the loss of the unique child, whom the family is coming to know, and the loss of possibilities for who he or she could have become. Key to supporting the family of a dying infant is respecting the infant's full status as a loved child. This may include facilitating religious ceremonies such as a naming or christening, creating mementoes such as photographs, footprints or a lock of hair, and creating the most loving situation possible for the moment of dying such as providing a private room and allowing a parent to hold the infant at the time life support is disconnected.

From age 3 years onwards, the child's personal experience of impending death should be considered. The child should be offered developmentally appropriate opportunities to express thoughts and fears associated with dying either with words, drawings or through play. It is not uncommon for even 2 and 3-year-olds to verbalize explicit thoughts of joining dead grandparents and seeing angels, but it is also common for dying children to focus only on wanting parents with them at all times, and exhibiting a shift in behaviour with more resistance to medical treatment, loss of interest in activities and food, but without any explicit verbalization of an awareness of dying.

Children of all ages, but especially younger children, are likely to take their cues about whether explicit discussion of death is permissible from parents and caregivers. When parents invite this dialogue it is common for it to occur. When parents signal that such discussion would be unbearable, the child is likely either not to speak about dying or to talk with a medical staff member when the parent is not present.

Child mental health consultants may help prepare parents for discussions with their dying child. Asking the parents for observations about shifts in the child's behaviour may help the parents recognize that they would not be introducing a new scary idea to the child in talking about death, but would rather be accompanying the child in the thoughts that he or she is already engaged in. Asking open-ended questions about worries, enquiring whether the child has questions that he or she is afraid to say aloud, or asking if he or she thinks about peers from the hospital who have died, may serve as invitations to begin the dialogue. Reminding children that articulating worries does not make them happen may free some children who are worrying silently to speak. Many parents will feel more comfortable embarking on end of life conversations with a child if they are told that they can welcome the child's questions warmly without having specific answers. 'I am interested in your ideas', 'What got you wondering about that?', 'Your good questions deserve good answers', 'I want to think about that or talk to our minister or the doctor' are examples of reasonable responses to a child's existential or medical questions. In the role of child mental health consultant, one of the most useful comments in response to questions about death is to tell a child 'I don't know what it is like to be dead, because I have never been dead. But, I am always interested to hear children's ideas about it.'

Children from age 7 onward may talk about the life experiences that they will not get to enjoy. These discussions challenge a parent's or professional's ability to bear the sadness of facing an untimely death. The child may talk about not getting to attend the next school year, never being able to drive a car, not having the chance to ride on the biggest roller coaster at the amusement park or not growing up to be a doctor or a teacher. It is often the specificity of the opportunities lost in the words of a child that is so evocative. There is a sense of privilege that one experiences in listening to children as they face the end of their lives that is as special as it is sad.

Often children will talk about being tired of the fight against the disease and will look to parents for permission to give up.

When the surviving family members can support each other in the painful process of letting go of the beloved child, believing that everything that could be done was done, and that further treatment would be unfair to the child, the final phase of dying seems more peaceful. In the setting of a long battle against an illness, it is easier to get to this difficult emotional state. In the setting of an acute event with little time for adjustment, or when parental discord interferes with the parents' ability to grieve together, such peace is harder to achieve.

The consultant should encourage subspecialists to follow up parents 6 months to 1 year after the death of a child. These calls can assess the parents' grieving and need for referral as well as help the subspecialist grieve and come to closure.

Conclusions

Child mental health consultants must stay attuned to the changes in the field of paediatrics. Advances in pharmacology, genomics and technology offer new hope and new challenges to psychosocial adaptation. Patterns of access to consultation will need to reflect shorter hospital stays and utilization of outpatient venues. New technology, such as telemedicine, may offer novel access to consultative expertise. Research in compliance outcomes, efficacy and quality of life become increasingly important as the financial pressures of modern medicine force the consultant to justify the value of the work.

However, many of the key features of quality consultation will remain unchanged. The consultant will continue to bring to the multidisciplinary medical team the combined expertise of psychodynamic understanding, psychopharmacology, a developmental perspective on the meaning of illness, adaptation to trauma, knowledge of psychiatric conditions, behavioural interventions, and central nervous system influences in medical illness and as a result of medical treatment. The goal will remain to answer the consultation request in a thoughtful timely fashion that respects the needs of the child, the family and the treatment team and facilitates quality of care and quality of life.

References

American Academy of Pediatrics, Committee on Bioethics and Committee on Hospital Care (2000) Palliative care for children. *Pediatrics* 106, 351–357.

Andersen, A., Bowers, W. & Evans, K. (1997) Inpatient treatment of anorexia nervosa. In: *Handbook of Treatment for Eating Disorders* (eds D.M. Garner & P.E. Garfinkel), 2nd edn, pp. 327–353. Guilford Press, New York.

Awad, G. & Pozanski, E. (1975) Psychiatric consultation to a pediatric hospital. *American Journal of Psychiatry*, 132, 915–918.

Bauman, L., Drotar, D., Leventhal, J., Perrin, E. & Pless, I. (1997) A review of psychosocial interventions for children with chronic health conditions. *Pediatrics*, 100, 244–251.

Bergman, A. & Fritz, G. (1985) Pediatricians and mental health professionals. Patterns of collaboration and utilization. *American Journal of Diseases in Children*, 139, 155–159.

British Medical Association (2001) *Consent, Rights and Choices in Health Care for Children and Young People.* BMJ Books, London.

Burkit, R. & Hodgin, J. (1993) Pediatrician's perceptions of child psychiatry consultations. *Psychosomatics,* **34,** 402–408.

Burroughs, T., Harris, M., Pontius, S. & Santiago, J. (1997) Research of social support in adolescents with IDDM: a critical review. *Diabetes Educator,* **23,** 438–448.

Chan, S. (1996) Child psychiatric consultation and liaison in paediatrics. *Singapore Medical Journal,* **37,** 194–196.

Conway, A. (1998) Adherence and compliance in the management of asthma. *British Journal of Nursing,* **7,** 1313–1315.

Crewdson, J. (1988) *By Silence Betrayed: Sexual Abuse of Children in America.* Little Brown, Boston.

Eisenberg, L. (1995) The social construction of the human brain. *American Journal of Psychiatry,* **152,** 1563–1575.

Freud, A. (1969) The role of bodily illness in the child. *Psychoanalytic Study of the Child,* **7,** 69–81.

Fritz, G., Pumariega, A. & Fishoff, J. (1987) Child psychiatrists' perceptions of timing and frequency of consultation requests. *Journal of the American Academy of Child and Adolescent Psychiatry,* **26,** 42.

Geist, R. (1977) Consultation to a pediatric surgical ward: creating an empathic climate. *American Journal of Orthopsychiatry,* **47,** 432–444.

Godding, V., Kruth, M. & Jamart, J. (1997) Joint consultation for high-risk asthmatic children and their families, with pediatrician and child psychiatrist as co-therapists: model and evaluation. *Family Process,* **36,** 265–280.

Groves, J. & Beresin, E. (1999) Difficult patients, difficult families. *New Horizons,* **6,** 331–343.

Hengeveld, M. & Rooysman, H. (1983) The relevance of a staff-oriented approach in consultation psychiatry: a preliminary study. *General Hospital Psychiatry,* **5,** 259–264.

Hoekstra-Weebers, J., Jaspers, J., Kamps, W. & Klip, E. (1999) Risk factors for psychological maladjustment of parents of children with cancer. *Journal of the American Academy of Child and Adolescent Psychiatry,* **38,** 1526–1535.

Horner, T., Liberthson, R. & Jellinek, M. (2000) Psychosocial profile of adults with complex congenital heart disease. *Mayo Clinic Proceedings,* **75,** 31–36.

Jacobson, A. (1996) The psychological care of patients with insulin-dependent diabetes mellitus. *New England Journal of Medicine,* **334,** 1249–1253.

Jay, S., Ozolins, M., Elliott, C. & Caldwell, S. (1983) Assessment of children's distress during painful medical procedures. *Health Psychology,* **2,** 133–147.

Jay, S., Elliot, C., Ozolins, M., Olson, R. & Pruitt, S. (1985) Behavioral management of children's distress during painful medical procedures. *Behavior Research and Therapy,* **23,** 513–520.

Jellinek, M.S., Murphy, J.M., Robinson, J., Feins, A., Lamb, S. & Fenton, T. (1988) The pediatric symptom checklist: screening school age children for psychosocial dysfunction. *Journal of Pediatrics,* **112,** 201–209.

Jellinek, M., Todres, I.D., Catlin, E., Cassem, E.M. & Salzman, A. (1993) Pediatric intensive care training: confronting the dark side. *Critical Care Medicine,* **21,** 775–779.

Jellinek, M., Herzog, D. & Todres, I. (1996) Psychiatric aspects of pediatric intensive care. In: *Critical Care of Infants and Children* (eds I. Todres & J. Fugate), pp. 684–687. Little Brown, Boston.

Jellinek, M.S., Murphy, J.M., Pagano, M.E., Comer, D. & Kelleher, K. (1999) Use of the pediatric symptom checklist (PSC) to screen for psychosocial problems in pediatric primary care: a national feasibility study. *Archives of Pediatric and Adolescent Medicine,* **153,** 254–260.

Kasak, A. & Meadows, A. (1989) Families of young adolescents who have survived cancer: social-emotional adjustment, adaptability, and social support. *Journal of Pediatric Psychology,* **14,** 175–191.

Kashani, J., Canfield, L., Borduin, C. *et al.* (1994) Perceived family and social support: impact on children. *Journal of the American Academy of Child and Adolescent Psychiatry,* **33,** 819–823.

Knapp, P. & Harris, E. (1998) Consultation-liaison in child psychiatry: a review of the past 10 years. *Journal of the American Academy of Child and Adolescent Psychiatry,* **37,** 139–146.

Kuttner, L. (1987) *No Fears, No Tears* [Videotape]. Canadian Cancer Society, BC/Yukon Div., 955 W. Broadway, Vancouver B.C., Canada.

Kuttner, L., Bowman, M. & Teasdale, M. (1988) Psychological treatment of distress, pain and anxiety for young children with cancer. *Journal of Developmental and Behavioral Pediatrics,* **9,** 374–381.

Lask, B. (1994) Paediatric liaison work. In: *Child and Adolescent Psychiatry: Modern Approaches* (eds M. Rutter, E. Taylor & L. Hersov), 3rd edn, pp. 996–1005. Blackwell Science, Oxford.

Lewis, M. & Vitulano, L. (1988) Child and adolescent psychiatry consultation-liaison services in pediatrics: what messages are being conveyed? *Journal of Development & Behavioral Pediatrics,* **9,** 388–390.

Ljungman, G., Gordh, T., Sorensen, S. & Kreuger, A. (1999) Pain in paediatric oncology: interviews with children, adolescents and their parents. *Acta Paediatrica Scandinavica,* **88,** 623–630.

Mastroyannopoulou, K., Sclare, I., Baker, A. & Mowat, A. (1998) Psychological effects of liver disease and transplantation. *European Journal of Pediatrics,* **157,** 856–860.

Murphy, J.M. & Jellinek, M.S. (1988) Screening for psychosocial dysfunction in economically disadvantaged and minority group children: further validation of the pediatric symptom checklist. *American Journal of Orthopsychiatry,* **58,** 450–456.

Murray, J. (1999) Siblings of children with cancer: a review of the literature. *Journal of Pediatric Oncology Nursing,* **16,** 25–34.

Oates, P. & Oates, R. (1996) Stress and work relationships in the neonatal intensive care unit: are they worse than the wards? *Journal of Paediatric Child Health,* **32,** 57–59.

Oates, R. & Oates, P. (1995) Stress and mental health in neonatal intensive care units. *Archives of Disease in Childhood, Fetal Neonatal Edition,* **72,** F107–F110.

Ortiz, P. (1997) General principles in child liaison consultation services: a literature review. *European Child and Adolescent Psychiatry,* **6,** 1–6.

Perrin, E., MacLean, W., Gortmacher, S. & Asher, K. (1992) Improving the psychological status of children with asthma: a randomized controlled trial. *Journal of Developmental and Behavioral Pediatrics,* **13,** 241–227.

Perrin, J. & Thyen, U. (1999) Chronic illness and its impact on development and behavior. In: *Developmental Behavioral Pediatrics* (eds M. Levine, W. Carey & A. Crocker), 3rd edn, pp. 335–345. W.B. Saunders, Philadelphia, PA.

Randolph, C. & Fraser, B. (1999) Stressors and concerns in teen asthma. *Current Problems in Pediatrics,* **29,** 82–93.

Roberts, C., Turney, M. & Knowles, A. (1998) Psychosocial issues of adolescents with cancer. *Social Work Healthcare,* **27,** 3–18.

Rutishauser, C., Sawyer, S. & Bowes, G. (1998) Quality-of-life assessment in children and adolescents with asthma. *European Respiratory Journal,* **12,** 486–494.

Sadler, J. (1982) Childhood asthma from the point of view of the liaison child psychiatrist. *Psychiatric Clinics of North America,* **5,** 333–343.

Samuels, M. & Southall, D. (1992) Munchausen-syndrome-by-proxy. *British Journal of Hospital Medicine,* **47,** 759–762.

Schechter, N., Berde, C. & Yaster, M. (1993) *Pain in Infants, Children, and Adolescents.* Williams & Wilkins, Baltimore.

Schreier, H. & Libow, J. (1993) *Hurting for Love: Munchausen's Proxy Syndrome.* Guilford Press, New York.

Shugart, M. (1991) Child psychiatry consultations to pediatric inpatients: a literature review. *General Hospital Psychiatry*, 13, 325–336.

Souid, A., Keith, D. & Cunningham, A. (1998) Munchausen syndrome by proxy. *Clinical Pediatrics*, 37, 497–503.

Spinetta, J., Jankovic, M., Eden, T. *et al.* (1999) Guidelines for the assistance to siblings of children with cancer: report of the SIOP Working Committee on Psychosocial Issues in Pediatric Oncology. *Medical Pediatric Oncology*, 33, 395–398.

Stocking, M., Rothney, W., Grasser, G. *et al.* (1972) Psychopathology in the pediatric hospital: implications for the pediatrician. *Psychiatry and Medicine*, 1, 329–338.

Strauss, G. (1996) Psychological factors in intensive management of insulin-dependent diabetes mellitus. *Nursing Clinics of North America*, 31, 737–745.

Stuber, M., Kazak, A., Meeske, K. & Baraket, L. (1998) Is post traumatic stress a viable model for understanding response to childhood cancer? *Child and Adolescent Psychiatric Clinics of North America*, 7, 169–182.

Sugarman, M. (1990) Emergency ward evaluation and inpatient management of sexual abuse. In: *Psychiatric Aspects of General Hospital Pediatrics* (eds M.S. Jellinek & D.B. Herzog), pp. 315–323. Year Book Medical, Chicago.

Tarnow, J. & Gutstein, S. (1982) Systemic consultation in a general hospital. *International Journal of Psychiatry and Medicine*, 12, 161–186.

Tornquist, J., Van Broeck, N., Finkenauer, C. *et al.* (1999) Long-term psychosocial adjustment following pediatric liver transplantation. *Pediatric Transplantation*, 3, 115–125.

Tsai, S., Lee, Y., Chang, K. & Sim, C. (1995) Psychiatric consultations in pediatric inpatients. *Chung-Hua Min Kuo Hsiao Erh Ko I Hsueh Hui Tsa Chih*, 36, 411–414.

Ulrich, G., Meyke, A., Haase, H. *et al.* (1997) Psychological support of children undergoing liver transplantation. *Pediatric Rehabilitation*, 1, 19–24.

Unger-Koppel, J., Nussli, R. & Stauffer, U. (1992) Liaison psychiatry in pediatric surgery: a promising approach. *European Journal of Pediatric Surgery*, 2, 188–190.

Van Sciver, M., D'Angelo, E., Rapport, L. & Woolf, A. (1995) Pediatric compliance and the roles of distinct treatment characteristics, treatment attitudes, and family stress: a preliminary report. *Journal of Behavioral Pediatrics*, 16, 350–358.

Walker, A., Harris, G., Baker, A., Kelly, D. & Houghton, J. (1999) Post-traumatic stress response following liver transplantation in older children. *Journal of Child Psychology and Psychiatry*, 40, 363–374.

Woodgate, R. (1999) A review of the literature on resilience in the adolescent with cancer: parts I & II. *Journal of Pediatric Oncology Nursing*, 16, 35–43; 78–89.

Work, H. (1989) The 'menace of psychiatry' revisited: the evolving relationship between pediatrics and child psychiatry. *Psychosomatics*, 30, 86–93.

Wright, H., Eaton, J., Butterfield, P., Snellgrove, N., Hanna, K. & Cole, E. (1987) Financing of child psychiatry pediatric consultation-liaison programs. *Journal of Developmental and Behavioral Pediatrics*, 8, 221–228.

Wright, M. (1994) Behavioral effects of hospitalization in children. *Journal of Pediatric Child Health*, 31, 165–167.

63 Local Specialist Child and Adolescent Mental Health Services

Peter Hill

Introduction

The term 'mental health' refers to a broad concept. Correspondingly, a concept of 'child and adolescent mental health problems' covers a wider range than does 'child and adolescent psychiatric disorders'. It includes problems and difficulties in emotions, behaviours, relationships and development that may not be captured by orthodox psychiatric classification systems and which may be equally well or better addressed by non-psychiatrists. A service for mental health problems therefore implies a multi-professional approach, including non-psychiatric specialists in child and adolescent mental health such as psychologists, social workers and behavioural paediatricians.

Whenever child and adolescent mental health professionals see a child for assessment and treatment they are offering a professional service to that child. In one sense therefore the concept of a child and adolescent mental health service is a personal one. In many countries, provision for mental health assessment and treatment is organized so that one can talk about services in a more civic sense; planned and organized for local groups of people. Such services may be funded by individual families directly, or through health insurance schemes which may be funded privately, or through employers of family breadwinners. Alternatively, there may be provision funded by the state and available free or at reduced cost to a local population when they use it. Not uncommonly, there is a mix of various mechanisms. The thrust of this chapter is to raise issues that are predominantly to do with specialist mental health services that are planned and organized for a local population of children and adolescents, irrespective of the source of funding.

Concept of health gain

Children (a term used here to include school-age teenagers) can experience or manifest a range of problematic emotions, behaviours, developmental asynchronies and personal relationships. These can be conceptualized as mental health needs in that they merit alleviation. Such alleviation is a goal for mental health services and can be referred to as one instance of health gain. The need for such services depends upon how much the population they serve can benefit in terms of the health gain that results from their activity. How health gain is understood will vary somewhat according to what the purpose of a service is.

One view of the objectives of a health service is that it is there to solve problems. Children present or are presented to it with a mental health problem, which is then addressed and resolved. By and large such a service will be reactive, except to the extent that it takes steps to educate potential referrers to it. In order to describe how well it works in terms of health gain, it would refer to a classification of mental health problems such as a list of diagnoses and the extent to which children seen as patients have these diagnoses and recover from them as a result of treatment.

Alternatively, a service may be seen as promoting mental health in which case it will do more than assess and treat those referred to it. It will include a proactive component and include preventive measures. It would refer to an informing principle, such as social participation or a notion of ideal mental health, as well as a list of diagnoses. This is necessarily a broader approach so that health gain in such a context includes the population's capacity to benefit from prevention and rehabilitation as well as from improvement in symptoms or impairments as a result of treatment.

It is not self-evident that one approach is superior to the other. A service funded predominantly by private health insurance will tend to favour a problem-solving approach because the costing is more straightforward when a child can be considered to have or not have a condition that requires or has benefited from treatment. Social funding is a little more likely to be sympathetic to a mental health promotion approach because most child mental health promotion schemes have been rooted in local populations at risk rather than individuals (see Offord and Bennett, Chapter 52) or because insurance companies often exclude cover for chronic conditions even though these might benefit from tertiary prevention or rehabilitation approaches.

The distinction between each approach has implications for the definition of disorder. Some well-recognized diagnoses, such as attention deficit hyperactivity disorder (ADHD), are essentially defined in the language that parents and teachers use to complain about the child. Similarly, conduct disorder is recognized in terms of the problems an affected child causes other people. A tendency is evident for the condition to be recognized simply by the fact that it is a problem rather than referring to a fundamental explanatory biological or psychological dysfunction.

On the other hand, notions of ideal mental health that underpin a broader approach to child mental health services can promote medicalization of deviance or underperformance if this is responsive to professional intervention. For example, some

Table 63.1 Definition of child and adolescent mental health according to Hill (1995).

Mental health in children and adolescents is indicated by:
- a capacity to enter into and sustain mutually satisfying personal relationships
- continuing progression of development
- an ability to play and learn so that attainments are appropriate for age and intellectual level
- a developing moral sense of right and wrong
- the degree of psychological distress and maladaptive behaviour being within normal limits for the child's age and context

children who do not have the ADHD condition will nevertheless improve their concentration when given stimulants (Rapoport *et al.* 1978) and psychiatrists may therefore be asked to prescribe stimulants for them so that they can improve their school grades.

What becomes apparent is that health gain is a slippery concept. In part this reflects the fact that health is a complex concept, itself susceptible to social influence. Earlier definitions of mental health in childhood and adolescence derived from the World Health Organization's approach (Table 63.1) which promotes an idealistic view, more specifically a model of ideal psychosocial development without referring to how that development might progress.

An alternative approach is to consider mental health as a commodity; something which one has enough of in order to master particular challenges. This is pragmatic rather than ideal and allies mental health conceptually with coping and mastery. This suggests that mental health is something that can be increased by preventive interventions that tutor coping strategies. Impaired functioning becomes a matter of insufficient or poorly selected coping strategies.

There is a third approach to health which neither of the above cover, and that is the issue of the child who contains the seeds of future morbidity or mortality. By physical analogy we would regard someone as unhealthy if within their body there were an as yet undetected carcinoma, even if their ability to develop or cope was impeccable. As our understanding of genetic causation progresses, such a model of health will become more important and it will be necessary to include it in any notion of health gain or health need.

With this in mind, it may be preferable to split our understanding of health into three dimensions that could be measured.

Health 1: the absence of symptoms or signs of a recognized psychiatric disorder.

Health 2: adequate functioning so that challenges can be mastered.

Health 3: the absence of vulnerabilities to future disorder.

It is against such measures that the need for, and the performance of, a mental health service for children can potentially be assessed.

Ascertaining mental health needs

Epidemiological studies have generally confirmed quite high prevalence rates for children's psychiatric disorders: 20% or more for phenomenologically defined syndromes, about 10% if impairment is also included as a necessary condition for diagnosis (Simonoff *et al.* 1997; Meltzer *et al.* 2000). Impairment is not a single threshold but varies and can be quantified, as in the levels of personal psychological functioning described for instance in the Children's Global Assessment Scale (C-GAS) (Shaffer *et al.* 1983) or the Global Assessment of Psychosocial Disability, which is Axis VI of the multiaxial classification of child and adolescent disorders in ICD-10 (World Health Organization 1996). The degree of impairment does not covary precisely with the severity of the psychiatric disorder: in the population study by Harrington's group some children with only a few symptoms of depression were more handicapped than others with numerous symptoms (Harrington & Clark 1998).

Impairment is known to be a key variable in determining referral to specialist services (Garralda & Bailey 1988; Goodman 1999). Furthermore, many children are impaired by their psychological difficulties without these being sufficiently severe to be classified as disorders—as many as half of all children attending clinics in the Great Smoky Mountains study (Angold *et al.* 1999). In the latter study, the fact of a child's problem being below threshold for DSM-IV caseness did not stop physicians treating it.

Most children with identifiable mental health needs according to diagnosis will not be seen in specialist child mental health services (for recent studies in the UK, the USA and France see Gasquet *et al.* 1999; Laitinen-Krispijn *et al.* 1999; Wu *et al.* 1999; Meltzer *et al.* 2000). Clearly, factors other than diagnosis operate in determining who is seen.

In the group of children that might be defined as having sufficient impairment to be regarded as cases according to major classification systems, the actual diagnosis has some effect in determining whether they are referred and how they are treated, although different studies provide different estimates of its power and some find a negligible effect (John *et al.* 1995). The power of diagnosis in determining clinical engagement probably varies with what is provided within a range of services. For instance, diagnostic category had less impact in predicting admission to hospital at the well-provisioned demonstration site in the Fort Bragg study than in the comparison site (Bickman *et al.* 1996). Clinical diagnosis alone is a poor indicator of level of service needed (Harrington *et al.* 1999), as is level of intellectual disability for children with general learning disability (Haveman *et al.* 1997).

A third variable to be considered in predicting whether a child will be referred to a mental health service is the burden their problem places upon their family. It is usually the case that the agents of a child's referral to a health service are the parents so it is not surprising that in studies of service utilization, burden emerges as a key element in determining referral to specialist services (Angold *et al.* 1998; Wu *et al.* 1999; Rawlinson & Williams

Table 63.2 Proxies for estimating local child and adolescent mental health need.

Perinatal mortality rate
Infant mortality rate
Under-16 pregnancy rate
Proportion of lone-parent families
Number of children in temporary housing
Number of children on the child protection register
Number of children looked after by the local authority
Number of children with a statement of special educational needs
Number of children on the disability register
Number of children accommodated with private fostering agencies
Number of children absent from school without authority
Number of children excluded from school
Number of young carers
Number of refugee children
Number of young people involved with the police

2000). This relates interactively with service provision, so that stress among caregivers for emotionally disordered children increased with poor co-ordination of services (Yatchmenoff *et al.* 1998).

In order to measure the extent of mental health need in a population, a direct epidemiological approach would assess all children (for instance in a particular school) or a sample of such children in one or more stages. Even the latter may be prohibitively expensive if the population is large. With this in mind, a number of proxy measures or indicators have been suggested, using particularly statistics that have been collected for other means (see Table 63.2).

Such attempts to quantify need do not predict absolute levels of required health care; rather, they indicate how resources might be allocated relatively within a population.

Targeting and focusing

Given the common nature of child mental health problems, it is unlikely that any society would ever be able to allocate specialist child and adolescent mental health care to all affected children. Nor would this necessarily be appropriate. Mental health problems are likely to coexist with social privations, physical health problems, educational difficulties and wider family or peer group relationship problems. Some of these are primary in terms of a chain of causal factors and the mental health complications will resolve when the primary conditions are addressed in their own right.

Furthermore, some childhood mental health problems are milder than others. Some authorities have used different descriptive categories for different levels of severity (Health Committee 1997) and imply a hierarchy. Thus, sleep-settling problems or breath-holding episodes in preschool-age children,

enuresis in middle childhood and private hypochondriacal anxieties in teenagers are generally mild and may be termed *mental health problems*. Persisting and severe extremes of emotion or behaviour which are significantly impairing and associated with considerable suffering are *psychiatric disorders* and are listed in formal psychiatric classification systems as diagnoses. Among these, children's disorders that are similar in form to serious adult disorders, such as bipolar disorder or schizophrenia, are *mental illnesses*.

There is a terminological problem with such an approach because the term for the milder conditions ('problem') is also that commonly used to encompass all psychological morbidity. Nevertheless, there is value in drawing attention to an apparent hierarchy of severity, particularly when detection is considered, because some adult inventories predominantly pick up the relatively less common cases of mental illness whereas these may well be missed by some epidemiological screening instruments for child psychiatric disorder. However, this framework of terms cannot consistently predict which diagnoses belong to which group and breaks down when conditions classified within a list of psychiatric disorders can be mild or severe yet true to type in form. Unipolar depression, Tourette syndrome and obsessive-compulsive disorder can all present at varying degrees of severity: from that associated with the terminology of mental health problem at one extreme to devastating and crippling severity at the other. Nor does such an approach work well with developmental disorders, such as autism, for similar reasons. As it covers the whole field and allows a multiprofessional and multiagency approach, it is worth retaining for service planning reasons but no more.

Mild psychological problems can usually be dealt with by health professionals who are not specialists in child mental health, so long as they have had some training. Advice and information for parents and teachers of young children, and for teenagers in their own right, straightforward advisory or simple behaviour programmes can be implemented without the need for specialist input.

Some professionals concerned with children, such as paediatricians, educational psychologists, therapists or teachers, have a significant yet not encompassing knowledge of child mental health. Without being specialists in child mental health they can make a significant contribution to assessment and treatment, especially of mild and moderate problems. Indeed, in many settings they see more disturbed and disturbing children than mental health services do (Kurtz *et al.* 1994).

Child mental health specialists will see a number of children while working solo and this will overlap with the activities of this group although extend the range of problems that can be managed. The work may be directly with children and their families or be consultative to other agencies or parts of a service.

More complex cases, those with severe, entrenched and co-morbid patterns or with multiagency involvement, will need a team approach, traditionally from a multidisciplinary group operating in an outpatient or day patient setting. Cases that cannot be assessed or managed at this level will require highly specialized services such as day units, inpatient units or highly specialized outpatient clinics.

This differentiated approach represents a spectrum of resource that attempts to correlate resource or spend with clinical severity and complexity (extent of mental health need). It also makes the best use of rare or costly specialist expertise while acknowledging the contribution that less specialized professionals or services make to child mental health work. It assumes a gradient of severity and complexity rather than a single threshold of caseness. In the UK, it is referred to as a tiered service model and attempts have been made to link it across agencies to form a matrix but, although it is a recommended pattern for child mental health services, it has not yet been either fully developed or evaluated. The approximate equivalent in the USA is the continuum of care approach, evaluated, for instance, in the Fort Bragg experiment (Bickman *et al*. 1996).

Community and hospital services

In a number of countries there has been a parallel evolution of child mental health services in the community on one hand (child guidance clinics/child and family consultation centres, etc.) and the hospital or university clinic on the other. The community care approach, fashionable in general adult psychiatry, is often extended in an unthinking way to child and adolescent mental health so that hospital-based clinics, which are nevertheless community-focused, may be seen as undesirable on ideological grounds. Coupled with this is the relatively low demand by child mental health for hospital services such as inpatient beds, investigative imaging or chemical pathology. This, together with the expense of hospital premises, has provided further impetus for child mental health activity often to be situated away from hospitals.

Where this has happened there seems to have been greater separation from paediatrics and sometimes from adult psychiatric practice although this can be obviated by establishing community polyclinics. The opportunity to move mental health services to where the children predominantly are (schools) has not usually been taken, although there are arguments that this would be logical (Kestenbaum 2000) and there have been valiant efforts to provide this, especially in the USA (Adelson 1999).

The risk of community-based practice is that of professional isolation from colleagues, libraries and regular academic meetings. Cross-cover, so that colleagues can attend distant academic and professional meetings, is harder to obtain than in a hospital setting. There are other potential impediments to the development of a service. Innovations are apparently adopted more slowly if there is no colleague of the same profession with whom to discuss methods. Training posts are harder to establish if there is a relative lack of academic support. Community clinics sited in small buildings are harder to expand physically.

Nor is it the case that community-based provision is necessarily cheaper. Harrington *et al*. (2000) found no significant dif-

ferences in cost or outcome to service or family when hospital-based outpatient and community clinic services for young children with behaviour problems were compared. Ideology seems a poor basis for blanket service provision and there are options for adopting a flexible approach, especially when interface with primary care systems is the focus. For instance, the use of non-specialist community-based health visitor services, supported by mental health training and supervision, can be shown to be effective (Davis & Spurr 1998).

The above remarks are relevant for developed countries with established systems for child and adolescent mental health promotion and care. Models more feasible for developing countries might need to be based on existing primary mental health care systems (Nikapota 1991; De Jong 1996; Khoja & Adlaim 1997; Rahman *et al*. 2000).

Generalist or specialist?

As a general rule in medicine, specialist centres achieve better results than generic services. This has to be offset against expense and inconvenience to patients who have to travel further. A point of balance needs to be established for a specialty that is predominantly community-orientated and outpatient in nature. A truly generalist service will have to make compromises. Premises suitable for preschool-age children are not necessarily judged favourably by middle or late teenagers. Inpatient units that admit teenagers with conduct disorders as well as those with anorexia nervosa are not viewed favourably by parents (Health Committee 1997). Staff with expertise in managing self-injurious behaviour in a child with general learning disability are not necessarily able to cope with borderline personality disorder. Heroin dependency and epilepsy have different nursing needs.

On the other hand, specialized services make exclusions, by definition. A well-planned service that provides broad coverage can allow for this but, even so, comorbidity can result in some children being hard to place, e.g. a 17 year old with both brittle diabetes and self-harming behaviour.

It is sometimes assumed that specialized services are for rare conditions, e.g. gender identity disorders. On the other hand, common conditions such as ADHD may best be managed in a clinic devoted to it (Taylor & Hemsley 1995). The arguments in favour include the use of routines for procedures such as questionnaire completion, the availability of electrocardiography (ECG) services, the presence of particular professionals or provision of parents' groups on a specified day, and a setting that allows informal educational contact between concerned professionals on one hand and between affected families on the other.

In achieving some sort of balance, a common trend has been to separate some features of services for children and for adolescents. In Finland, for instance, these are two separate mental health services (Piha & Almqvist 1999). In many countries, inpatient services for these two developmental epochs are differentiated, not uncommonly with a tendency for children's units to be close to paediatric nursing resources and adolescents to be near adult psychiatric facilities.

Contextual issues

A child mental health service rarely exists in isolation because children with mental health problems often have other exceptional needs to be met: educational, physical, forensic, etc. Children who can no longer be looked after by their families and who enter some form of charitable or public residential or substitute family care are known to have a high rate of mental health problems (McCann *et al.* 1996; Dimigen *et al.* 1999), as do recidivist young offenders (Kurtz *et al.* 1998), the homeless (Vostanis *et al.* 1998) and children with chronic physical conditions (Eiser 1990). In each case there will be non-mental health care professionals involved in the management of such children who can potentially contribute to their mental health and assist in the resolution of mental health problems. Their ability to do this will be assisted by consultation arrangements with local child mental health services, and although it has been hard to evaluate the contribution of such input there is little doubt that it is well received (see Nicol, Chapter 64).

If the resource spectrum (tiered service) which can be established within a health service is expanded to social, educational or criminal justice systems, a matrix can be drawn that resembles a pyramid (Williams & Richardson 1995). A relatively small number of children or teenagers will be known to several agencies and is likely to consume a considerable slice of their budgets. Such an arrangement is an obviously sensible move where agencies duplicate each other's service inputs, yet interagency communication is notoriously ineffective (Health Committee 1997). Establishing a matrix of concern and provision for child and adolescent mental health enables a contextual approach and sharing rather than duplication of resources.

Coverage

There are common uncertainties about the boundaries of a child and adolescent mental health service. Part of the reason for this is the tendency for some children to be clients of several social agencies because of their general distortion of social or psychological maturation. However, there are further administrative confusions that are shared by other areas of children's medicine, especially the single-organ specialties.

One is the upper age limit. In most countries, paediatrics is preoccupied numerically with babies and preschool-age children. Adolescents with physical disorders are often seen by adult physicians and surgeons. Child and adolescent psychiatry cannot reliably take its cue from other aspects of children's medicine in such circumstances. Other social guidelines do not help. There is no clear-cut boundary between childhood and adolescence and a variety of age thresholds separate the two. Boundaries defined by biological, social, or educational considerations rarely coincide.

Not surprisingly therefore different countries and different services set different upper age limits for the age range served by a child and adolescent mental health service. This would not matter particularly if there was consistent dialogue between adult and child services but this cannot be guaranteed. Children with ADHD, conduct disorder or specific developmental disorders who have been managed by the health services as adolescents can easily find no adult service willing to take them on. The mental health needs of the children of adult psychiatric patients are often, it is said, overlooked by the psychiatrist who is seeing the parent (Poole 1996).

Children with a measure of general learning disability are at increased risk for psychiatric disorder yet may, in some countries, also be excluded from mainstream child mental health services. Their needs may be addressed by developmental paediatrics or by all-age mental handicap services instead.

Access to mainstream child mental health services may also be difficult for children who do not have a conventional family and are looked after by charitable or statutory agencies, for refugee children whose families have other priorities or do not understand the system, and for ethnic and linguistic minorities (Vostanis *et al.* 1998).

Duplication

There has been a recurring problem of duplicated and competing child and adolescent mental health provision, particularly between clinical psychology, child and adolescent psychiatry, and community paediatrics. A child with recurrent enuresis, for instance, might be seen in any service. To an extent this has been reduced in some places by the adoption of a tiered service structure but there persists a relative failure to differentiate what might best be treated by medical specialists, what by psychologists, and what by combinations of both. Child psychiatrists prefer, it would seem, to work in teams, but to what extent this is efficient is untested. Their medical responsibilities to examine bodies and mental states, to prescribe and to seek the application of special laws are universal but it seems to be the case that many would welcome a wider brief.

Components of a child and adolescent mental health service

The coverage of a specialist child and adolescent mental health service can only be decided by referring to its context and the contributions (or deficiencies) of other adjacent services, such as education or social care. Doubtless, the roots of a service will be in primary health care of some sort (see Garralda, Chapter 65) where the greatest number of children would be seen by any health service. Specialist services might be directly accessible for families but are more likely to be referred to by some form of gatekeeper within the health service (family doctor or paediatrician) or from an adjacent service (such as a special educational needs teacher). It would be rational to anticipate that initial contact with a referred child would be provided by only one or two professionals in order to use resources efficiently. Most children's problems might be dealt with at that level but some will require more detailed assessment by a specialist outpatient clinic, multidisciplinary team, or local day unit. Relatively few children require inpatient management so that an inpatient psychiatric unit appropriate to their age might be more remote if there is an insufficient number of children needing admission in a particular locality. A service would need access to such a unit but it might not be a managed part of the local service.

In order to facilitate other agencies, there needs to be liaison arrangements with, for instance, paediatrics, special education resources, and social care or voluntary agencies.

A generally replicated finding that low-income families are relatively high users of child mental health services (see, for example, the Ontario Child Health Study; John *et al.* 1995) has led a number of authors to suggest that the design of such services should make them accessible to the poor.

The structure of a service needs consideration yet is not necessarily a key feature in producing health gain, as was demonstrated in the Fort Bragg experiment in which an ambitious programme of continuum-of-care at one US army base could not be shown to yield better mental health outcomes than more traditional service models at two comparison bases (Bickman *et al.* 1995, 2000). The content of what is provided in terms of clinical skills and knowledge is more important. Although the scientific evidence base for child and adolescent mental health practice is rather limited and there is still considerable reliance on expert testimony and open trials (Graham 2000), remarkable consensus is emerging as to what skills are required for a comprehensive service. Systematic reviews, practice parameters and official guidelines exist for most child mental health problems encountered and there is good agreement between them.

All child and adolescent services need easy access to a psychiatric contribution, not just because of the occasional need for mental state and physical examination, medical diagnostic skill or medication prescription, but because of the advocacy potential of senior medical figures within health systems.

Although not restricted to psychological practitioners in many countries, the skills of formal psychometric and neuropsychological assessment are best developed by psychologists. It is also the case that cognitive-behavioural approaches are usually delivered by them.

Dynamic psychotherapies, individual, group and family, may be offered by any trained professional and there seems little a priori reason for assuming them to be restricted to any particular health professional.

The care of children and adolescents within residential treatment settings is generally in the hands of nurses but focused training for them seems rather unusual. Rather similarly, the contributions of occupational therapists, speech and language therapists (speech pathologists) and creative therapists do not

often stem from a body of professional knowledge and skills specifically tailored to child and adolescent mental health. Commonly, they derive on an individual basis from paediatric or adult mental health practice. An exception is the tradition of pedagogy in some European countries in which therapeutic education, particularly for children with learning disabilities, has been established for decades.

The evidence base is strongest for medication and cognitive-behaviour therapy (CBT), less so for family and multisystemic therapies, and weak for individual and group dynamic therapies (Kazdin & Weisz 1998; Graham 2000). Indeed, recent trials of individual psychotherapy in real-life settings have indicated that it is usually ineffective compared with placebo (Weiss *et al.* 1999) or shows no dose–effect relationship (Salzer *et al.* 1999). Nevertheless, dynamic approaches have informed much thinking about developmental deviance and distorted family functioning and have informed therapeutic interviewing and nursing care so that they are still remarkably influential in the child and adolescent mental health systems of most developed countries (Remschmidt & van Engeland 1999).

It is no longer possible to assume that one form of therapy or conceptual framework will provide demonstrable effectiveness for all cases and all modern systems have adopted a more or less differentiated approach on eclectic lines: the preferred treatment for a particular child being based on rational assessment and available evidence. The place of consumer choice within this is less clear, especially when it is unclear who the consumer might be.

The last point merits some consideration. In some countries, referrals to a child mental health service may be made or prompted by a variety of people: parents, teenagers themselves, paediatricians, GPs, teachers, social workers and so on. A child with a mental health problem is likely to be known to several of these and they may have differing ideas of what constitutes improvement. They may also have differing explanatory models for the child's problem or condition. Essentially, medical approaches of diagnosis and treatment 'are of secondary importance for the benefit of other missions, such as educational, protectional, and/or legal' (Matot *et al.* 1999). Indeed, there may be competition between different frameworks, with misconceptions about a reputedly reductionist 'medical model' and difficulties arising from perceived stigmatization. This can have secondary difficulties for the language used to describe children's difficulties. Although the major classification systems are widely used by psychiatrists internationally, non-medical staff in a service are sometimes less ready to do so or are even openly hostile, which makes for problems in documentation and communication.

Contact with a specialist child and adolescent mental health service

It is apparent that there is some uncertainty as to what constitutes an appropriate referral to a specialist service. On the basis of a study of referral pathways, Leff & Bennett (1998) argued for written guidelines for potential referrers. In a large national UK study (Audit Commission 1999), 25% of referrals to specialist outpatient/community child mental health services were from non-medical sources.

Given the historical recency of much child and adolescent mental health service provision, it is not surprising that in a number of countries there are waiting lists for specialist opinion. It is recognized that this is an important factor in determining whether a referred child will be brought to the service, long waiting times correlating with higher non-attendance rates for first appointments (Rawlinson & Williams 2000). This is a perversity in that wasted first appointment times further increase waiting times so that pressure on specialist services increases even without an increase in demand. It has proved impossible to identify any single factor predicting non-attendance and attempts to alleviate the problem by preliminary telephone contact have met with varying results (contrast Mathai & Markantonakis 1990 with Burgoyne et al. 1983). What may be better is to reduce the amount of clinical resource devoted to first contact in order to limit waste and place first-contact evaluation at a point in a spectrum of resources or tiered structure.

Priorities within a service

There are huge variations among countries in psychiatric provision for children. Within Europe, Remschmidt & van Engeland (1999) were able to show that the ratio of senior specialists in child and adolescent psychiatry to child population (age < 20 years) varied from 1:5300 (Switzerland) to 1:45000 (Hungary). The figures for the UK and Ireland were intermediate, 1:27500 and 1:31500, respectively. It is not surprising that a number of countries have services with long waiting lists for first appointments. This sharpens the need for prioritization and various indices of priority have been developed by local services. These are often complex and difficult to 'sell' to referring agencies who, it is said anecdotally, will find ways round them in order to gain preference for their own referrals.

In such a setting, developing prevention strategies (see Offord & Bennett, Chapter 52) becomes politically difficult because it takes clinical resources away from reactive services that are already not coping with demand. Considerable courage is required to mount prevention programmes in such a setting and in spite of the logical claim for prevention, comparative costing does not always show benefit for primary prevention over later treatment (Harrington & Clark 1998). In an attempt to resolve this dilemma, concepts of early intervention have been promoted although their impact outside pilot programmes is largely untested.

Issues of health economics

As Knapp & Henderson (1999) pointed out, economics con-

tributes importantly to decisions about resource allocation and 'is concerned with how resources can be transformed into improved outcomes for the users of services, their families and wider society' and that 'the underlying prompt for economics—scarcity—is as prevalent and constraining in [child and adolescent mental health] as it is elsewhere'. This applies both to the policymakers of publicly funded services and to health insurance companies who wish to operate managed care.

The cost to society of mental health problems in the young is not confined to a health service. Indeed, major costs, particularly of disruptive behaviour, can be charged to social services, special education and property in childhood as well as having secondary costs to parents (loss of earnings because of increased supervision and care requirements, etc.). Because these separate services or households have individual budgets, the cost saved by treatment in a health service goes unrecognized (Light & Bailey 1993). In a small study of the costs of conduct disorder in 10 children, Knapp et al. (1999) found that the average annual cost to the health service (£2457) was about half that to local education services (£4754) and the annual cost to social services (£991) nearly half that to the health service. Average direct and indirect costs to the family of a child with conduct disorder (loss of employment, additional home repairs, etc.) were estimated at £13109 per annum. Attempting to derive cost–benefit figures simply from health service costs misses the point.

Nevertheless, there is value in applying microeconomic analyses to specific interventions or groups in order to illustrate or compare. The extraordinary expense of the Lovaas programme for young children with autism demonstrated by Gresham & Macmillan (1998) is an instance of illustration. Comparison of two alternative approaches to dealing with adolescent deliberate self-harm: routine care and routine care plus four sessions of home-based family intervention (Byford et al. 1999; Harrington et al. 1998) found, surprisingly, no difference in cost or outcome between the two but greater parental satisfaction for the intervention that included home-based sessions. This suggests greater benefit from the latter at no increased cost.

Quality assurance

The performance of a service requires relevant information to be collected and, for instance, the degree of adherence to particular administrative and clinical procedures to be ascertained by this. It has become popular to use peer audit to examine the performance of clinical services and a number of strategies have been developed for child mental health services (Hardman & Joughin 1998). However, the final stage of the audit cycle, closing the loop, may cost extra resources and these have not always been forthcoming. Audit is a useful tool for improving clinicians' adherence to care or administrative procedures but cannot of itself improve clinical outcome unless there is sound evidence for effectiveness of a procedure or, better, direct measurement of outcome.

Outcome evaluation

Outcome measures for research studies do not easily transfer across to services. Research studies usually aim for homogeneous populations and select their patients, excluding comorbidity, standardizing treatments, and admitting only consenting volunteers. Services, however, deal with heterogeneous groups of children with problems of varying severity and complexity and operate in a wider context of non-health agencies whose own contribution may or may not be helpful. In order to measure the outcome of processes within a child mental health service, allowance has to be made for all this.

Several parameters have been suggested (adapted from British Psychological Society 1993):
- clinical symptom/sign improvement;
- achievement of mutually agreed goals for change;
- acquisition of new skills
- improved functioning;
- reduced duration of inpatient stay/school exclusion, etc.; and
- improved self-management of ill-health/disability.

To these may be added:
- improved quality of life;
- improved mental health; and
- improved social participation.

Rather similarly, Hoagwood et al. (1996) and Jensen et al. (1996) suggested five outcome domains to be considered in their SFCES model.
- Symptoms/diagnoses
- Functioning
- Consumer perspectives
- Environmental contexts
- Systems.

The common denominator is thus a recognition that optimal outcome measurement is complex, perhaps too complex for routine evaluation in the field. Even in research studies, hardly any work is sufficiently comprehensive as to tap all criteria; Jensen et al. (1996) found only two studies assessing all domains of the SFCES model. There seem to be three major areas in which more usable frameworks are being developed. Symptomatic improvement is generally popular in research studies but many symptom scales are intended primarily for epidemiology. The Health of the Nation Outcome Scales for Children and Adolescent Mental Health (HONOSCA) have been developed in the UK with the intention of being acceptable to a wide range of professionals, only requiring a few minutes to complete and being sufficiently sensitive. Initial experience in field trials (Gowers et al. 1999) and a large national survey (Audit Commission 1999) has been promising.

A second area is to evaluate functioning rather than clinical change, as instanced by the SumOne for Kids system (Beck et al. 1998). Thirdly, a rather more cumbersome but arguably relev-

ant method of identifying agreed outcomes as a result of negotiation with key stakeholders or families and assessing criterion referenced change accordingly has been advocated by Berger et al. (1993) and Hernandez et al. (1998). This third approach has the advantage in bridging the poor agreement between clinicians' and families' views of a child's problems (Yates et al. 1999).

There is also the dimension of service performance that hinges upon activity indicators: number of cases seen, wait for first appointment, consumer or referrer satisfaction, etc. These are easier measures to obtain and can be taken as indices of service quality but are arguably less fundamental measures than clinical change.

It is clear that no single scale will tap all aspects of change thought to follow an intervention. To a certain extent, what is selected will depend upon what the goals of the service are in terms of health promotion or problem-solving (see above). One way through is to use the agreed goals approach coupled with Likert scaling (Berger et al. 1993). However, this depends upon goals negotiated by therapist, parent(s) and child which may not agree with goals that would have been set by other agencies. Ratings of clinical outcome in an unpublished pilot of such an approach (Spender, Byrne & Hill, unpublished data) showed good agreement between parent and therapist but poor correlations with school and GP opinion. The matter might be improved by adding one of the various scales of functioning, such as the C-GAS (Shaffer et al. 1983), but even so there will be aspects of service provision such as expert report drafting, liaison consultation and child protection intervention which would not be well served by such an approach.

It is also the case that attempts to offer treatment are thwarted by poor attendance, failure to complete homework tasks or take medication and a judgement about compliance needs to be made by the treating clinician. Similarly, the extent to which schools, housing, poverty, peer group and so forth support or hinder treatments must be made explicit. Once again, the context in which a child mental health service, a child psychiatry or psychology service, or an individual clinic operates has to be considered.

Looking ahead

Two contrasting forces currently operate in developed societies. On the one hand, the impact of evidence-based practice means that children are being treated better than ever before. Differentiated practice with an eclectic basis and a focus on specified treatment goals is now widely accepted. The days of protracted psychotherapy for (nearly) all and lengthy inpatient stays have gone. On the other hand, economic pressures can mean less state or insurance funding available for child mental health with adverse consequences for clinical practice. The advent of managed care in the USA has, it is argued, led to a disruption of 'attaching, trusting and caring' and a diffusion of the full benefit of the skills of child and adolescent psychiatrists because psychiatrists have found their role narrowed to 'using structured questionnaires, conducting symptom-based interviewing, and prescribing medication all in an hour or less' (Jellinek 1999). Similar statements could be made about specialist practice in state-funded health care when finances become scarce.

Constrained resources, funding by separate agencies, and political pressures to reduce waiting times seem likely to encourage a focus on symptom relief where this can be demonstrated. In terms of the earlier definitions of health gain this supports a focus on Health 1 approaches and a tendency to concentrate on episodes of care rather than a longer view. Because it is cheaper and faster in producing symptom relief, psychopharmacology might thus be favoured by a reimbursing or funding body over, say, CBT in the treatment of obsessive-compulsive disorder, because the latter takes longer to produce benefit and requires more clinician time. Yet, given the rate of relapse following discontinuation of medication it would appear that, in this example, medication functions as water-wings compared with the swimming lessons of CBT. The longer view could therefore indicate different economic benefits when the two treatment approaches are compared although, in order to demonstrate this, research findings are required. There is then the comparable problem of how to obtain research funding for longer term evaluation, rather than the short project with definable goals. In parallel with this there is often a need for breadth in interdisciplinary or interagency study so that the effect of specialist treatment can be assessed across a variety of social and personal domains. Fortunately, there are signs that this is beginning to happen.

References

Adelson, S.L. (1999) Psychiatric public health opportunities in school-based health opportunities in school-based health centers. In: *Adolescent Psychiatry* (ed. A.H. Esman), pp. 75–89. The Analytical Press, Hillsdale, NJ.

Angold, A., Messer, S.C., Stangl, D. *et al.* (1998) Perceived parental burden and service use for child and adolescent psychiatric disorders. *American Journal of Public Health*, 88, 75–80.

Angold, A., Costello, E., Farmer, E. *et al.* (1999) Impaired but undiagnosed. *Journal of the American Academy of Child and Adolescent Psychiatry*, 38, 129–137.

Audit Commission (1999) *Children in Mind*. Audit Commission, London.

Beck, S.A., Meadowcroft, P., Mason, M. & Kiely, E.S. (1998) Multiagency outcome evaluation of children's services. *Journal of Behavioural Health Services Research*, 25, 163–175.

Berger, M., Hill, P. & Walk (1993) A suggested framework for outcomes in child and adolescent mental health services. In: *A Proposed Core Data Set for Child and Adolescent Psychology and Psychiatry Services* (eds M. Berger, P. Hill, E. Sein, M. Thompson & C. Verduyn), pp. 99–110. Association for Child Psychology and Psychiatry, London.

Bickman, L., Guthrie, P.R., Foster, E.M. *et al.* (1995) *Evaluating Managed Mental Health Services: the Fort Bragg Experiment*. Plenum Press, New York.

Bickman, L., Foster, E.M. & Lambert, E.W. (1996) Who gets hospitalised in a continuum of care? *Journal of the American Academy of Child and Adolescent Psychiatry*, 35, 74–80.

Bickman, L., Lambert, E.W., Andrade, A.R. & Penaloza, R.V. (2000) The Fort Bragg continuum of care for children and adolescents: mental health outcomes over 5 years. *Journal of Consulting and Clinical Psychology*, 68, 710–716.

British Psychological Society (1993) *Purchasing clinical psychology services: services for children, young people and their families*. Briefing Paper 1. British Psychological Society, Leicester.

Burgoyne, R., Acosta, F. & Yamamoto, J. (1983) Telephone prompting to increase attendance at a psychiatric outpatient clinic. *American Journal of Psychiatry*, 140, 345–347.

Byford, S., Harrington, R., Torgerson, D. *et al.* (1999) Cost-effectiveness analysis of a home-based social work intervention for children and adolescents who have deliberately poisoned themselves. *British Journal of Psychiatry*, 174, 56–62.

Davis, H. & Spurr, P. (1998) Parent counselling: an evaluation of a community child mental health service. *Journal of Child Psychology and Psychiatry*, 39, 365–376.

De Jong. J.T.V.M. (1996) A comprehensive public mental health programme in Guinea-Bissau: a useful model for African, Asian and Latin American countries. *Psychological Medicine*, 26, 97–108.

Dimigen, G., Del Priore, C., Butler, S., Evans, S., Ferguson, L. & Swan, M. (1999) Psychiatric disorder among children at time of entering local authority care: questionnaire survey. *British Medical Journal*, 319, 675.

Eiser, C. (1990) *Chronic Childhood Disease*. Cambridge University Press, Cambridge.

Garralda, M.E. & Bailey, D. (1988) Child and family factors associated with referral to child psychiatrists. *British Journal of Psychiatry*, 153, 81–89.

Gasquet, I., Ledoux, S., Chavance, M. & Choquet, M. (1999) Consultation of mental health professionals by French adolescents with probable psychiatric problems. *Acta Psychiatrica Scandinavica*, 99, 144–150.

Goodman, R. (1999) The extended version of the strengths and difficulties questionnaire as a guide to child psychiatric caseness and consequent burden. *Journal of Child Psychology and Psychiatry*, 40, 791–799.

Gowers, S.G., Harrington, R.C., Whitton, A., Lelliott, P., Wing, J. & Beevor, A. (1999) A brief scale for measuring the outcomes of emotional and behavioural disorders in children: HONOSCA. *British Journal of Psychiatry*, 174, 413–416.

Graham, P. (2000) Treatment interventions and findings from research: bridging the chasm in child psychiatry. *British Journal of Psychiatry*, 176, 414–419.

Gresham, F.M. & Macmillan. D.L. (1998) Early intervention project: can its claims be substantiated and its effects replicated? *Journal of Autism and Developmental Disorders*, 28, 5–13.

Hardman, E. & Joughin, C. (1998) *FOCUS on Clinical Audit in Child and Adolescent Mental Health Services*. Royal College of Psychiatrists' Research Unit, London.

Harrington, R. & Clark, A. (1998) Prevention and early intervention for depression in adolescence and early adult life. *European Archives of Psychiatry and Clinical Neuroscience*, 248, 32–45.

Harrington, R., Kerfoot, M., Dyer, E. *et al.* (1998) Randomized trial of home-based family intervention for children who have deliberately poisoned themselves. *Journal of the American Academy of Child and Adolescent Psychiatry*, 37, 512–518.

Harrington, R., Kerfoot, M. & Verduyn, C. (1999) Developing needs-led child and adolescent mental health services: Issues and prospects. *European Child and Adolescent Psychiatry*, 8, 1–10.

Harrington, R., Peters, S., Green, J., Byford, S., Woods, J. & McGowan, R. (2000) Randomised comparison of the effectiveness and costs of community and hospital based mental health services for children with behavioural disorders. *British Medical Journal*, 321, 1047–1050.

Haveman, M., Van Berkum, G., Reijnders, R. & Heller, T. (1997) Differences in service use, time demands and caregiving burden among parents of persons with mental retardation across the life cycle. *Journal of Applied Family Studies*, **46**, 417–525.

Health Committee (of the House of Commons) (1997) *Child and Adolescent Mental Health Services*. The Stationery Office, London.

Hernadez, M., Hodges, S. & Cascardi, M. (1998) The ecology of outcomes: system accountability in children's mental health. *Journal of Behavioural Health Services Research*, **25**, 136–150.

Hill, P. (1995) Cited in *Together We Stand* (eds R. Williams & G. Richardson), p. 15. Health Advisory Service, HMSO, London.

Hoagwood, K., Jensen, P.S., Petti, T. & Burns, B. (1996) Outcomes of mental health care for children and adolescents. I. A conceptual model. *Journal of the American Academy of Child and Adolescent Psychiatry*, **35**, 1055–1063.

Jellinek, M.S. (1999) Changes in the practice of child and adolescent psychiatry: are our patients better served? *Journal of the American Academy of Child and Adolescent Psychiatry*, **38**, 115–117.

Jensen, P., Hoagwood, K. & Petti, T. (1996) Outcomes of mental health care for children and adolescents. II. Literature review and application of a comprehensive model. *Journal of the American Academy of Child and Adolescent Psychiatry*, **35**, 1064–1077.

John, L.H., Offord, D.R., Boyle, M.H. & Racine, Y.A. (1995) Factors predicting use of mental health and social services by children 6–16 years old: findings from the Ontario Child Health Study. *American Journal of Orthopsychiatry*, **65**, 76–86.

Kazdin, A.E. & Weisz, J.R. (1998) Identifying and developing empirically supported child and adolescent treatments. *Journal of Consulting and Clinical Psychology*, **66**, 19–36.

Kestenbaum, C.J. (2000) How shall we treat the children in the 21st century? *Journal of the American Academy of Child and Adolescent Psychiatry*, **39**, 1–10.

Khoja, T.A.M. & Adlaim, F.A. (1997) *National Manual for Primary Mental Health Care*. Ministry of Health, Riyadh, Saudi Arabia.

Knapp, M. & Henderson, J. (1999) Health economics perspectives and evaluation of child and adolescent mental health services. *Current Opinion in Psychiatry*, **12**, 393–397.

Knapp, M., Scott, S. & Davies, J. (1999) Antisocial behaviour in younger children. *Clinical Child Psychology and Psychiatry*, **4**, 457–473.

Kurtz, Z., Thornes, R. & Wolkind, S. (1994) *Services for the Mental Health of Young People in England: a National Review*. Maudsley Hospital and South Thames (West) Regional Health Authority, London.

Kurtz, Z., Thornes, R. & Bailey, S. (1998) Children in the criminal justice and secure care system: how their mental health needs are met. *Journal of Adolescence*, **21**, 543–553.

Laitinen-Krispijn, S., Van der Ende, J., Wierdsma, A. & Verhulst, F. (1999) Predicting adolescent mental health service use in a prospective record linkage study. *Journal of the American Academy of Child and Adolescent Psychiatry*, **38**, 1081–1090.

Leff, S. & Bennett, J. (1998) Developing guidelines for community child health staff and examining the referral pathways and outcomes of care in support of emotionally and behaviourally disturbed children. *Public Health*, **112**, 237–241.

Light, D. & Bailey, V. (1993) Pound foolish. *Health Services Journal*, **103** (5339), 16–18.

Mathai, M. & Markantonakis, A. (1990) Improving initial attendance to a child and family psychiatric clinic. *Psychiatric Bulletin*, **14**, 151–152.

Matot, J.-P., Verbeeck, B. & Hayez, J.-Y. (1999) Child and adolescent psychiatry in Belgium. In: *Child and Adolescent Psychiatry in Europe* (eds H. Remschmidt & H. van Engeland), p. 11. Steinkopff, Darmstadt & Springer, New York.

McCann, J., James, A., Wilson, S. & Dunn, G. (1996) Prevalence of psychiatric disorders in young people in the care system. *British Medical Journal*, **313**, 1529–1530.

Meltzer, H., Gatward, R., Goodman, R. & Ford, T. (2000) *Mental Health of Children and Adolescents in Great Britain*. The Stationery Office, London.

Nikapota, A.D. (1991) Child psychiatry in developing countries. *British Journal of Psychiatry*, **158**, 743–751.

Piha, J. & Almqvist, F. (1999) Child and adolescent psychiatry in Finland. In: *Child and Adolescent Psychiatry in Europe* (eds H. Remschmidt & H. van Engeland), pp. 93–103. Steinkopff, Darmstadt & Springer, New York.

Poole, R. (1996) General adult psychiatrists and their patients' children. In: *Parental Psychiatric Disorder* (eds M. Göpfert, J. Webster & M. Seeman), pp. 3–6. Cambridge University Press, Cambridge.

Rahman, A., Mubbashar, M., Harrington, R. & Gater. R. (2000) Developing child mental health services in developing countries. *Journal of Child Psychology and Psychiatry*, **41**, 539–546.

Rapoport, J.L., Buchsbaum, M.S., Zahn, T.P., Weingartner, H., Ludlow, C. & Mikkelson, E. (1978) Dextroamphetamine: cognitive and behavioural effects in normal prepubertal boys. *Science*, **199**, 560–562.

Rawlinson, S. & Williams, R. (2000) The primary/secondary care interface in child and adolescent mental health services: the relevance of burden. *Current Opinion in Psychiatry*, **13**, 389–395.

Remschmidt, H. & van Engeland, H., eds (1999) *Child and Adolescent Psychiatry in Europe*. Steinkopff, Darmstadt & Springer, New York.

Salzer, M.S., Bickman, L. & Lambert, E.W. (1999) Dose–effect relationship in children's psychotherapy services. *Journal of Consulting and Clinical Psychology*, **67**, 228–238.

Shaffer, D., Gould, M.S., Brasic, J. *et al.* (1983) A Children's Global Assessment Scale (CGAS). *Archives of General Psychiatry*, **40**, 1228–1231.

Simonoff, E., Pickles, A., Meyer, J.M. *et al.* (1997) The Virginia twin study of adolescent behavioral development: influences of age, gender and impairment on rates of disorder. *Archives of General Psychiatry*, **54**, 801–808.

Taylor, E. & Hemsley, R. (1995) Treating hyperkinetic disorders in childhood. *British Medical Journal*, **310**, 1617–1618.

Vostanis, P., Grattan, E. & Cumella, S. (1998) Mental health problems of homeless children and families: longitudinal study. *British Medical Journal*, **316**, 899–902.

Weiss, B., Catron, T., Harris, V. & Phung, T.M. (1999) The effectiveness of traditional child psychotherapy. *Journal of Consulting and Clinical Psychology*, **67**, 82–94.

Williams, R. & Richardson, G. (1995) *Child and Adolescent Mental Health Services: Together We Stand*. HMSO, London.

World Health Organization (1996) *ICD-10 Classification of Mental and Behavioural Disorders. Multiaxial Classification of Child and Adolescent Psychiatric Disorders*. Cambridge University Press, Cambridge.

Wu, P., Hoven, C., Bird, H. *et al.* (1999) Depressive and disruptive disorders and mental health service utilisation in children and adolescents. *Journal of the American Academy of Child and Adolescent Psychiatry*, **38**, 1081–1090.

Yatchmenoff, D.K., Koren, P.E., Friesen, B.J., Gordon, L.J. & Kinney, R.F. (1998) Enrichment and stress in families caring for a child with a serious mental disorder. *Journal of Child and Family Studies*, **7**, 129–145.

Yates, P., Garralda, M.E. & Higginson, I. (1999) Paddington complexity scale and health of the nation outcome scales for children and adolescents. *British Journal of Psychiatry*, **174**, 417–423.

Practice in Non-medical Settings

Rory Nicol

Introduction

Child and adolescent mental health services led the way in developing multidisciplinary work in the early part of the last century. Even at that time, the boundary between medical and non-medical settings seemed arbitrary. Many clinics were sited outside mainstream medical settings and referral policies were designed to offer services directly to social service and educational departments as well as health services. Attempts to channel all referrals through health agencies alone have occurred from time to time, usually in order to limit access to overloaded services or to satisfy some bureaucratic dogma. Such an arrangement simply results in a perception of the service as remote and inefficient.

Most clinicians work in non-medical settings as part of their duties; indeed, many of the other chapters of this book refer to such a role, if only implicitly. In the previous edition a list of eight advantages offered by this flexible approach were listed (Nicol 1994). These included:

1 the reluctance of many families to attend a formal clinic;
2 the possibility of rapid response to straightforward problems;
3 avoidance of the administrative complexities of referral;
4 encouragement of interagency collaboration as a result of a mental health service presence in the community;
5 taking the treatment to the environment where the problem is manifest, as a way of dealing with situational influences; and
6 opportunities for primary and secondary prevention.

Relevant non-medical settings and the children's problems they contain

A brief review of non-medical settings illustrates the relevance of practice outside the clinic and hospital.

The mainsteam school

There are a variety of political views about the aims and priorities of schooling but few deny that good quality schooling is an experience from which all children learn more than the formal curriculum, e.g. how to cope with a wide variety of human relationships including competition, co-operation, coping with authority, friendships, enemies and love relationships. Children's psychopathology will also be evident in the school setting. Influences at school can modify the behaviour of the students (Maughan 1994; Mortimore 1995).

Young people's prisons

The aim of this setting may be punishment and rehabilitation but this does not alter the fact that mental health problems among young prisoners are extremely common. Maden *et al.*'s (1995) study of British remand prisoners (with 206 male young offenders) showed an overall prevalence of 'psychiatric disorder' of 19% (including a few with psychosis). In the USA, Yates *et al.* (1983) assessed 339 young offenders aged 18–19 who were remanded in a secure facility. Three had schizophrenia and two an organic disorder; the overall rate of psychiatric disorder was extremely high.

Suicide and attempted suicide in prison constitutes a substantial problem (Liebling 1992). This includes a few instances in children between the ages of 15 and 16 (Garfield 1998, personal communication), although the rate is higher in older teenagers and young adults. Use of alcohol and drugs in the populations of young offender institutions is a persistent and growing problem. A survey by McMurren (1989) of 100 sentenced British young offenders revealed that 43% were heavy drinkers, consuming over 50 units per week. In Maden *et al.*'s study of remand prisoners, nearly one-quarter of male remand prisoners used drugs of dependence. Obviously, the young people who end up in prison bring their emotional and behavioural problems with them, but the contrast between behaviour in prison and in well-run (but much more expensive and non-punitive) facilities with similar populations suggests that the setting is a crucial influence.

Children's homes

In recent years there has been great concern in the UK about the state of children's homes. With a recognition, some 20–30 years ago, that even quite small group homes did not offer a satisfactory long-term alternative to family life, there has been a major movement towards fostering of children in public care (see Rushton & Minnis, Chapter 22). Group homes have therefore changed in an attempt to accommodate those whose behaviour is so difficult that fostering is not an option. The provision of children's home accommodation has shrunk and now stands at around 10 500 places in England, accommodating some 7000, mostly adolescents (Utting 1997); around 400 of these offer secure provision. Much is known about the qualities of effective children's homes. These include a clear statement of purpose and orientation; a degree of self-determination, as opposed to an extension of local authority bureaucracy; manageable size; and agreement among the staff about how the establishment should be run. The negative reputation that children's home have suffered needs to be balanced by the fact that, in a recent survey, local authority homes for adolescents were seen by the residents as more helpful than among a comparable group in young people's prisons (Nicol *et al.* 2000).

A survey of the mental health of young people in the children's homes and foster care of one local authority showed that nearly all manifested some form of psychopathology (McCann *et al.* 1996). Disorders involving major depression, anxiety or conduct disturbance were particularly common. Berridge & Brodie (1998) found that there was little or no contact or other link between health service provision of mental health services and the child care sector or social services departments. Nicol *et al.* (2000) found that in both care and penal settings there were gross shortages of mental health services.

As with prisons, children in children's homes bring many problems with them. With recent problems of widespread child abuse in such institutions, it is more than ever clear that the experience in the setting itself can add to their difficulties.

Foster care

A higher proportion of children in public care are now in foster placements than used to be the case, although the absolute number has changed little over the last 30 or so years. Foster care includes so-called shared care, used particularly with disabled children, and also emergency or short-term placements. The therapeutic potential of foster care is recognized in many pioneering schemes (Hazel 1981) and has led to specialist foster care programmes for children with particularly severe emotional and behavioural problems.

Among the homeless

This is the ultimate failure of all the social settings mentioned above and is common among young people leaving care. British census figures in 1991 showed that of the 2650 people sleeping rough only 35 were under 18. On the other hand, the best UK study, where a representative sample of young London homeless were interviewed, suggested that the majority of older teenagers actually started their street career when they were under 18 (Craig *et al.* 1996). Of this sample, 85% had their first episode of homelessness before the age of 18, and the same proportion had run away from home before the age of 16.

The reason for the homelessness in this sample was also important. Disagreements with parents was the major cause, including a substantial minority where violence had been involved. Leaving care or prison together made up 17% of the group. Material poverty, housing or occupational reasons were given as the cause in only 9% of the sample. These figures tell a story of social and relationship problems being the leading cause of the vast majority of homelessness at the outset and the homeless group scored higher than a comparison group on all measures of social adversity, including physical and sexual abuse. Conduct disorder from an early age, and attempted suicide at any age, was much more common in the homeless group; substance dependency/abuse was also common. Many had contact with the homeless primary care service, although not with family doctors. The authors argued that the provision of a specific psychiatric service would make a substantial difference to their care.

Similar studies in other countries, e.g. Shaffer & Caron (1984) in New York and Reilly *et al.* (1994) in Australia, have revealed a similar picture.

Intervention in non-medical settings

The mainstream school

Dewey (1916) traced the school as arising from apprenticeship situations where skills were commonly passed down the family. According to this interpretation of history, the child's development was originally given over entirely to the local family and community. As society became more complex with industrialization, this was no longer possible. The school environment is one where the child spends a large proportion of his or her waking life and where he or she has to learn to cope with many challenges, not only in the sphere of learning but also of coping with relationship issues such as co-operation and sharing, competition and authority—all challenges and growth points for the child and opportunities for the perceptive teacher. The learning situation is full of challenges: the management of students' anxiety, rebelliousness, discouragement and unhappiness are essential to good teaching (Galloway 1985).

The influence of schooling on pupil behaviour, attendance and attainment has been examined in a range of studies using the same basic strategy designed to differentiate between outcome differences caused only by variations in the characteristics of children at the time of school entry and differences that derive from school influences on the children (Rutter 1983; Maughan 1994; Mortimore 1995). Intake variations are assessed through measures of children's behaviour, educational attainments, and social background prior to starting at the schools to be studied. Longitudinal data are then used to determine the same features after some years at those schools, or at school leaving. The test is provided by determining whether pupil outcomes vary among schools, after taking into account schools' intake characteristics, and whether the outcome variation is a function of measured school characteristics. There has been a consistent finding of large differences among schools that cannot simply be put down to the characteristics of the children, and which are systematically associated with variations in school qualities (Rutter 1983). Positive leadership from the head teacher is associated with better adjustment and progress of pupils. This leadership style involves staff in decision-making, provides active curriculum planning and staff training, and includes effective monitoring of pupils' progress. This was associated with a staff consensus on key values, low staff turnover, and good communication among teachers taking the same class. At the class level, a degree of lesson structure, together with a teaching pace and style that challenged the children intellectually is associated with good pupil progress. A work-centred environment that concentrated on one or two themes at a time, even if at different levels for different children, seemed to be the key to success. High levels of communication in the shape of good teacher record-keeping and links with children and parents are key ingredients. What results is an accent on rewards and praise, and an atmosphere of direction and orderliness that makes the school a comfortable and facilitating place to be. Most of the studies have used a rather limited set of measures to assess pupil outcomes, but those studies that have considered a wider range of indicators of quality have, on the whole, showed a reasonable degree of correlation among them (Mortimore *et al.* 1989).

Clinical implications

Sensitive visitors quickly recognize the well-run school. However, greater expertise is needed to recognize the particular qualities that matter at school and classroom levels and in the individual interactions of staff and pupils. Collaboration with educational psychologists and school advisors are needed to help teachers bring about change in the classroom. Does the influence of being in a particular social environment, such as the school, affect subsequent adjustment? A follow-up of children attending 12 schools in London suggests some interesting possibilities. The schools showed quite wide variation in truancy and behaviour (Rutter *et al.* 1979) but also variation in post-school adjustment (Gray *et al.* 1981). The latter seemed to be caused entirely by the fact that children in the less successful schools dropped out earlier and failed to attend school consistently. This illustrates the importance of indirect chain effects in developmental processes: a depriving experience in one period of life, be it difficult circumstances in the early years, poor school experiences or an early pregnancy, may put the child at a disadvantage at subsequent life stages, not because of direct effects on personality structure but because it sets in motion a chain of risk experiences (see also Rutter, Chapter 19). The clinician with a perspective that extends beyond the clinic has many opportunities to observe the unfolding of transactional processes.

Interventions that use the environment: the example of bullying

An example of marshalling the resources of the non-medical setting for intervention is provided by the case of bullying.

Bullying has always occurred but over recent decades its extent and destructiveness has become apparent as a result of some well-publicized suicides by children and of some seminal research (Olweus 1993, 1994; Rigby & Slee 1993; Smith & Sharp 1994). There is also an issue concerning the right of all children to feel free and comfortable in environments and activities that they have to attend by law. Studies show that as many as 15% of children are involved in any one school either as bullies or as victims (Olweus 1993). A special helpline that was set up in the UK in 1990 was besieged by several thousand calls in 3 months (La Fontaine 1991). Bullying does not come readily to the attention of the school staff and, when it does, it is all too easy to deny its importance and gravity—or even side with the bully. Because it is so closely linked to the school setting, it can only be handled within the school with the active co-operation of the school staff.

Many studies have attempted to characterize the bully and the victim. The most important studies have been by the Scandinavian psychologist, Dan Olweus, and this account is heavily dependent on his findings. His main method of investigation has been survey techniques using the anonymous questionnaire developed by him.

Olweus defined bullying as negative actions directed at one individual and repeated over time. Bullying may be direct with unprovoked attacks, or indirect with schemes to undermine the self-confidence of the victim using social isolation, humiliation, malicious rumours and name-calling. Indirect methods are just as destructive but are more difficult to detect and deal with. Olweus found the problem to be just as grave in small village schools in Norway as in large city schools but was more prevalent in junior schools than secondary schools.

Typically, the bully emerges as relatively socially competent and confident, from a background where discipline and child-rearing is inconsistent and chaotic, aggression is condoned and interactions are along a power-assertive dimension and, in some 40% of cases, with other seriously antisocial and offending behaviour. Most bullies are boys. Girl bullies have not been studied in such depth but seem more likely to use indirect bullying methods.

The victim is more likely to be shy, anxious and socially isolated. Apart from being physically weaker than bullies, victims are commonly younger. Characteristics of the victim's family are also sharply different from those of the bully. Family relationships are close, particularly with the mother and the family atmosphere is non-violent. All these aspects of the relationship mean that the bully can attack with little fear of retaliation. Victims have not been found, as some have suggested, to have an excess of physical stigmata. The effects of the bullying were described in the UK study of Smith & Sharp (1994) as sleeplessness, severe loss of self-esteem, social withdrawal and depression. These symptoms can long outlive the experience of bullying at school.

According to Olweus, the bully quickly identifies a potential victim. It is not difficult for him or her to recruit a few assistants to perpetrate the torment that then gets underway. The bullies (characteristically two or three in number) can then justify their behaviour by isolating the victim in the class and the school by humiliation and ridicule. In this way, the confidence of the initially insecure and shy youngster is further undermined, thus encouraging further attacks.

The group dynamics within the school are of great importance in understanding bullying. Olweus found that most bully-ing happens in the school grounds, not, as some have suggested, on the way to and from school. Poorly supervised breaks and lunch times are a fertile breeding ground for bullying, as is a cul-ture of staff detachment from the social life of the children. The culture of group identity possible in school offers a tempting environment for the bully and his or her lieutenants, offering a weakening of inhibitions to misbehaviour, social support for misbehaviour and reduction of the probability of being caught.

Treatment of bullying should start with a study of the size of the problem in the particular school involved (using anonymous questionnaires). Comparison of the findings with those of other studies gives a firm starting point from which to tackle the prob-lem with school staff, governors, parents and students. The intervention itself can best be understood at three levels:

1 the whole school level;
2 the classroom; and
3 the individual child.

Whole school level

There should be an explicit policy that bullying is unacceptable and must not be allowed to happen. This should be accepted by all staff, governors, parents and pupils, using the regular con-sulting structure of the school to ensure that this happens. Stu-dents must be included because the target of the whole school component of the programme is the entire student body, not just those children who are suspected of being involved in bully/ victim problems. Pupil opinions should be canvassed at an early stage of planning.

Bullying flourishes in isolated and unsupervised changing rooms and corridors, out of the sight of supervising staff; this needs to be borne in mind in building design and alterations. Se-cluded paths and bus stops in the vicinity of the school offer other vulnerable points. However, the key considerations con-cern the attitudes of staff and their willingness to take part in the antibullying programme, which may impinge on their relaxa-tion time over lunch and coffee breaks. It is at these times that vulnerable areas should be supervised. If a staff member detects suspicious group activity, intervention should be immediate and questioning assertive. Better to be overvigilant, writes Olweus, than allow bullies to benefit or be seen to get away with their be-haviour. In Smith & Sharp's (1994) British study, a whole school approach of this kind was encouraged and monitored. There was a moderate correlation between school commitment, and the intensity of the school's intervention, and a good outcome.

Attention to the ethos of the school is crucial to the manage-ment of bullying. There should be an atmosphere of autonomy in the context of support, with an overall sense of the school as a community where each is responsible for the self and others. Stu-dents need to be told that they have the right to attend school without fear of being bullied.

All these issues point up the central importance of staff morale in the management of bullying. A contented and dedicated staff group means punctuality, good supervision, a well-structured

curriculum and attention to the children's needs. Cases of bully-ing identified early can be quickly discouraged; conversely, neglect of warning signs can be taken as permission to continue by the potential bully. Pastoral staff or heads of house can iden-tify and so support isolated children who are likely to be vulner-able. A special group of interested staff can be appointed to take the question of bullying in the school forward and develop an antibullying plan. It may be possible to involve more senior and mature children to offer support in the form of peer counselling.

Classroom level

A similar clear and explicit set of principles is needed at the class-room level. Olweus (1993) recommends the following three rules as a starting point:

1 not to bully other students;
2 try to help other students who are being bullied; and
3 make a point of including students who become easily left out.

It is very important to describe what types of behaviour con-stitute bullying (including indirect bullying). Techniques to in-crease student empathy with victims of bullying include the use of story material, and role-play in the classroom, followed by classroom discussion. It is particularly important to address the issue of the passive onlooker or follower. Such students are in a very good position to blow the whistle on bullying. Students should be praised when improved behaviour is shown—not just to the passive student who has taken on a more active role, but to a potential aggressive bully who has shown evidence of re-straint, respect for agreed rules, and victim empathy. Progress can be formally checked in regular class, year or tutorial group meetings.

Individual level

Bullying requires sanctions on occasions. These may consist of confronting bullies with regard to their behaviour and depriving them of privileges when appropriate. As in all such cases, it is im-portant that the sanction does not put the staff member to more inconvenience than the culprit! Care must be taken to avoid an overpunitive stance that will simply model yet again the vindic-tive attitude that led to the problem in the first place. The young bully is likely to have serious problems of his or her own in the shape of a developing antisocial tendency. Mentoring and super-vision may be needed and parental co-operation should be sought as well as attempts to guide the student towards proso-cial behaviours.

Not everything can be achieved by ameliorating the school en-vironment. Bullying is a serious, secretive and malignant process and must ultimately be met head-on and dealt with without delay (Rigby & Slee 1993; Smith & Sharp 1994). For this to hap-pen, the bullies must be confronted and interviewed to make crystal clear that their behaviour will not be tolerated. Equally, the victim must be interviewed and counselled. The immediate task here is to offer protection against further attacks by the bullies. Any protective move should be done with the knowledge and preferably the consent of the victim. Victims will often pressurize their parents not to take steps to stop the persecution. Beyond this, steps can be taken to assist in the building of the self-confidence of the child by building on latent abilities and encouraging mixing with appropriate peers.

Effectiveness

A major evaluation of a nationwide campaign against bullying which involved the whole school system has been carried out in Norway and included training for both teachers and parents. The research design was to measure change between two time points: before and after the introduction of the programme. While this is a relatively weak research design, the results showed a spectacular 50% reduction in bullying problems (Olweus 1993, 1994). The programme was particularly effective for direct attacks, and seemed to become more effective over the 2 years of the evaluation. It was not simply that the bullying shifted to other settings. There was no increase in bullying outside the school grounds. New bullying problems were also reduced. In a large study in Sheffield (Smith & Sharp 1994), encouraging results were also found, although the improvements were not quite as spectacular as in Norway.

The school as an environment to support treatment

Therapeutic success in one setting does not necessarily, or even often, extend to another environment because situational influences are important. The implications are well appreciated by researchers who have evaluated therapy in schools, e.g. behaviour modification programmes to encourage on-task behaviour (O'Leary & O'Leary 1976); special teaching/therapeutic sessions outside the classroom; social problem-solving training/social skills training; or crisis intervention (Maher & Zins 1987).

One particularly comprehensive study illustrates some of the key features. This controlled comparison of interventions with 7- and 11-year-old children gave pointers regarding the most effective approaches (Kolvin et al. 1981) and some tentative leads about the effects of the environment. The interventions for 7 year olds were parent counselling–teacher consultation, nurture work (a teacher aid support) and playgroup therapy, using the technique developed by Axline (1947). Compared with a no-treatment control group, the playgroup therapy had the greatest impact on the children's problems, followed by the nurture work. The consultation programme was only marginally effective. For the 11 year olds, the programmes were group counselling using a Rogerian technique (Rogers 1951), behaviour modification in the classroom and, again, a parent counselling–teacher consultation approach. The most effective interventions in this case were group therapy and behaviour modification. In short, direct intervention of skilled and

trained professionals with the children was associated with effective intervention. The theoretical framework underlying the treatment approach seemed less important.

Follow-up, at 18 months and 3 years, showed that the therapeutic effects of the study persisted, with continuing differences from the control group. Possibly, these reflected therapeutic qualities present in the school. There was also some evidence of generalization, in that the children who had the more successful interventions also showed changes in home-based measures.

Skills that can be used in non-medical settings

The skills needed in non-medical settings are similar to those used in health-service-based settings but there are some special considerations. Professional isolation could be a problem but it is easily overcome. In practice, working in high-risk community settings requires an awareness of possible street violence. A little 'street wisdom' is a valuable asset. In family homes, it is necessary to make clear that you have come to do a job of work rather than to visit as a guest. If the television is interfering, ask for it to be turned off; if there are neighbours in the home, politely ask that they be invited to leave.

A particularly successful example of work in non-medical settings is multisystemic therapy (Henggeler et al. 1998). This technique is governed by careful assessment of all the settings and relationships that make up the life of the young person. Great care is taken in developing a treatment hypothesis that governs the development of intervention across a number of environments. Perhaps the boldest innovations are the intensity of the therapy (the clients and their families are seen every day) and the commitment of the therapy team. Each family is taken on by one therapist whatever the intervention style — be it individual therapy, family work or school consultation. Some other principles of the work are an emphasis on positive behaviours, avoidance of an 'illness' model that absolves the client and family from responsibility for their actions, an emphasis on responsible behaviour, encouragement of appropriate discipline and sanctions (but not inappropriate or unenforceable discipline) and positive reinforcement for positive behaviours. What is striking is that none of these components of the programme are particularly new. It is probable that the degree of rigour, the intensity and the commitment in application contribute to the success of the project. Case loads of individual therapists are very low but the severity of the problem behaviour that is tackled by this team is correspondingly high.

This programme has been carefully evaluated since the outset in the late 1970s. Early modestly funded evaluations using quasi-experimental designs yielded promising results but, by the mid-1990s, results of larger designs using random allocation began to appear. These involved the treatment of chronic delinquency, sexual offences and substance misuse, with findings indicating useful improvement over a period of 1–2 years, as compared with controls who had either routine management or a comparison treatment.

If this intervention can make inroads into the negative and expensive 'revolving door' treatment of the recidivist young offender, it could provide the beginning of a revolution in the management of serious and persistent offenders. The authors commented that it may be applied from a base in a variety of different agencies, including mental health agencies.

Roles for the general child mental health worker

Programmes like the 'Help Starts Here' project or Multisystemic Treatment for Antisocial Behaviour may ultimately contribute to more effective routine clinical practice but, at present, the intensity and focus required for these special programmes puts them outside the range of resources available in most services. One attempt to solve this problem has been through the concept of mental health consultation. In the USA, this became extremely popular in the 1960s and 1970s. In the UK, it has failed to achieve the same full-hearted support and training structures. However, as demands for the services of the child and adolescent services grow, it is surely time to re-examine these techniques in a much more professional way than has been carried out so far to assess their effectiveness.

Mental health consultation

This set of techniques consists of the mental health professional working collaboratively with another professional who is in regular contact with the client but who lacks the skills in the assessment and management of children or young people with mental health problems. This could be the staff of the organizations described above: schools, children's homes, prisons, foster carers or the staff of shelters for the homeless. The approach originates from a psychoanalytic tradition associated with Caplan (1970).

Varieties of consultation

There are now a variety of theoretical underpinnings of consultation, including:
1 traditional consultation from the medical tradition;
2 Caplan-style mental health consultation;
3 behavioural consultation; and
4 social systems consultation.

The traditional approach

This is traditional in the sense that consultants use their expertise to carry out their own assessment of the child, the family and their problems (Mattison 2000). After this, they may join with other staff to develop further assessment or treatment. The prac-

tice is common but is seen by some as conservative, paternalistic and likely to promote dependency. On the other hand, many of the problems seen in non-medical situations today are extremely complex and need the most skilled evaluation available. It is not helpful to sustain a false image that the consultees are more expert than they actually are and can undertake specialized diagnoses and treatment that is beyond their experience and training. However, it may be entirely appropriate for the staff of an institution to take on the treatment or management of a problem, once questions about diagnosis and treatment recommendations have been clarified. Alternatively, a member of staff at a residential setting may work collaboratively with a consultant. This can be the essence of a good creative partnership.

Caplan-style mental health consultation

Caplan (1970) has had an enormous influence on the field of consultation, and his book remains required reading for anyone wanting to enter the field, even if some of his ideas now seem questionable. One of the central ideas is that the difficulties encountered in relationships between consultees and their clients arises from distortions in perception related to stereotypes held by consultees related to their own cultural traditions and childhood or other experiences. Caplan saw this as the most common reason for misunderstandings of client's behaviour and certainly the most important. He strongly emphasized that his method of consultation was not a form of therapy for the consultee. He was also strong in his belief that responsibility for the conduct of the relationship between consultee and client should remain with the consultee and that to take this over both emasculated the consultee and encouraged dependency. The consultant's responsibility, wrote Caplan, should be to the mental health of the children in general in the institution or the district. It is difficult to see how this position could be sustained today in many of the settings where there have been major problems of abuse. Another of Caplan's recommendations which remains fresh today is the care with which the arrangements for consultation should be developed, including with the institution itself and with the administrative or local government bodies responsible. Some of his ideas have been incorporated in the section below on setting up consultation.

Behavioural approach to consultation

Many attempts have been made to develop a behavioural approach to consultation, the best developed being that of Bergan & Kratochwill (1990), which centres on the principle of operant conditioning, and that of Brown et al. (1998), which centres on social learning theory. The behavioural principles have tended to follow those of other applications (see Herbert, Chapter 53).

The principles and precision of behaviour modification programmes are their strength and an aid to clarity at all levels. Nevertheless, the detail and the relatively structured approach does add to the demands placed on busy consultees, who may have a misleadingly simplified idea that all that is necessary is the giving of gold stars and sweets. For this reason, the groundwork may have to be carried out with considerable rigour. Considerable training in the basic approach is needed which may raise doubt about whether the true spirit of consultation as the specialist assisting the non-specialist is being followed. Maybe the non-specialist has simply had to become a specialist!

In addition, the ethical issues have to be discussed. Some people's first reaction may be to suspect bribery or dehumanization of the client. Studies of consultation sessions in school psychology have shown that, in fact, consultation in school environments are far from 'an equal collaborative partnership' and that consultees judge consultants who adopt a leadership role to be more effective than those who remain more tentative (Erchul & Martens 1997). Behavioural consultation, in schools at least, does not seem to be very popular. Erchul & Martens (1997) reported a study showing that consultation was considered one of the most complicated and least effective ways of responding to children's learning difficulties and behaviour problems. Ysseldyke et al. (1983) reported that consultation came low in the list of priorities about what to do for school problems. Happé (1982) reported that only half the plans that consultees agreed to implement may be actually completed. Erchul and Martens (1997) emphasized that, apart from problem-solving, two other components must be present if behavioural consultation is to be successful. The first is social influence within the school; the authors discussed several mechanisms by which this could be achieved. Although the claim is that the techniques that might be used are not coercive, the impression is that the consultant would have to move quite a long way from Caplan's (1970) original principle that the advice of the consultant is something that the consultee can take or leave. The second added component is psychological and material support. This can consist of any way in which the consultant can put the teacher in touch with services that may be of help in their work. Instruction in class craft or other aspects of skill development could be included and modelling or coaching of a variety of skills. The same principle is true of residential care. Consultation will always be an adjunct to training in managing groups and individuals in residential situations, group work and counselling, planning programmes and activities associated with regular routines and administrative issues. It will have to be very useful if it is to win friends among potential consultees. It is important to note that behavioural approaches have been used primarily for secondary prevention and for study problems rather than major psychopathology.

Social systems approaches

School differences research suggests that benefits could come from modifying the social systems in schools. Efforts have been made in this direction but mostly to improve academic achievement. Silence surrounds any results from recent policies of appointing 'superheads', 'naming and shaming' of schools or privatization. More serious attempts to help schools in a general way have proved difficult, although the successful attempts to reduce bullying show that, given a clear focus, much can be achieved.

General points

A number of principles are relevant to all types of consultation. In the problem-solving process, workers do not wait for professional guidance before starting to problem-solve; they attempt their own solutions before thinking of consulting a professional outsider. This has been confirmed in the school work of Ysseldyke et al. (1983). In many cases their own attempts succeed and no more is heard about the matter. It is essential that the consultant find out about, and show respect for, these preconsultation methods. This dimension is taken into account in Bergan and Kratochwill's system under the heading of 'plan' (planning of treatment package).

Setting up consultation

The consultant must be aware that an approach to an institution is likely to be treated with suspicion rather than unalloyed enthusiasm. Approaches must be carefully planned to negotiate with the leaders and to tap usefully into the communication network of the institution. Some may feel that the consultant is usurping their role. This requires sensitive clarification and negotiation. Staff may harbour negative feelings about a newcomer driven by previous experiences or the general reputation of mental health professionals. Genuine and non-patronizing respect for the difficult work carried out by the staff, courtesy, consideration and humour are essential. A lecture seminar at which the consultant exposes his or her skills and a non-threatening approach may be a help. It is the consultant's responsibility to understand the language of the consultee's profession and of the consultee institution. The ground rules of how the consultant can help and how he or she can be approached have to be established and essential aspects of the institution understood.

It is essential to gain the support of higher levels of management in the agency that employs the potential consultees and of the consultant's own agency. This should preferably be in the form of a written contract.

Is the climate right for consultation?

It is particularly important at an early stage for the consultant to decide whether the organization is suitable for consultation. Relevant questions might include how the consultant is handled by the organization, e.g. how do referrals come forward? Are they really not problems at all but success stories to reassure the consultant that all is well? Is time allocated for the consultation process? Does the director of the organization really see the point of consultation or is he or she merely going along with something that has been imposed?

Worrying signs include inadequate line management, minimal

direct management contact with children and staff, unsatisfactory or absent placement policies and processes, inadequate recruitment processes and staff training, reluctance to use secure provision and more specialized alternative services, inadequate or no external expert advice and the presence of a 'macho' or bullying culture. Unusual and untested 'therapy', or the taking over of the running or control of the home by a group of senior boys who are imposing a reign of terror on younger and weaker children, should set alarm bells ringing (Berridge & Brodie 1998).

Relationship building and intervention

Having dealt with the organizational issues, we must now turn to the practical matter of consultant–consultee interaction. The starting point must be the problem that is troubling the consultee about the client. With this in mind, the consultant must encourage the consultee to tell the story. Often this will start with something like, 'What do you do with a child who shouts "knickers" in class all the time?' or, 'What do you do with children who keep running away?' or, 'What do you do with a mother who threatens to beat up the headmaster?' These are the openings of professionals who on the one hand may be feeling a bit worried and defensive, and on the other want to test the mettle of the consultant. Gentle encouragement to move towards describing concrete examples is the best response at this stage. Once this is achieved, the consultant should become quite active, asking for details about the setting, others typically present when the behaviour occurs, and more details about the child and family. A good start is to ask the consultee to describe a typical day.

Where? It is helpful to ask about the setting in which the behaviour manifests. Is it in one place or several? If more than one, what do they have in common? Is it to do with an audience? Is it a setting, such as a classroom, where the child may feel unable to cope?

What else has happened? How does the behaviour relate to possibly significant life events? For example, a home visit or the admission of a new child to the class or foster placement?

Towards or against whom? One of the stressful aspects of front line work in non-clinical settings is the intensity with which children develop feelings about members of staff which relate to their experience of parenting and family life (called transference feelings in individual therapy; see Jacobs, Chapter 58). A common example is the child who behaves particularly badly towards a foster carer or house parent, in place of their own mother. These relationships can also have all the agonizing ambivalence of any disturbed relationship. Examples are children who test limits to the extent that they elicit the rejection that they most fear, or children who seem to develop a relationship of being 'too good' but at the same time show their underlying rage by stealing from the foster family.

What is the pace and intensity? Behaviour can be diverted into more adaptive channels if these take account of the level of intensity. It is no good asking a hyperactive child to sit quietly reading a book but an opportunity to let off steam in a more constructive way is more likely to help.

Executive skills. It is essential not only that the consultant be active but also that they have clinical skills and techniques relevant to the problem under discussion. The details will differ according to the theoretical orientation of the consultant and the trick is to select areas from one's own experience that may be relevant and simple enough to be applied by someone whose skills are less specialized. As in all clinical work, it is important, according to orientation, to arrive at a behavioural hypothesis or dynamic formulation (see Herbert, Chapter 53; Rutter & Taylor, Chapter 2). This can be shared in simple jargon-free language with the consultee. In the normal way, it should inform further work. It is very important to be optimistic. In behavioural terms, the consultant's main contribution can often be as a reinforcer of the consultee's efforts, which are often not acknowledged by authoritarian and bureaucratic management structures. A common put-down for the enthusiastic consultant is 'it's been tried before'—it is essential not to be put off by this. A final word of warning: some professionals take on the consultation mode of practice as an exclusive way of working, abandoning face-to-face clinical work almost entirely. This is a mistake. The consultant should be respected as having high-level skills in direct clinical work.

Other aspects of practice in non-medical settings

The enthusiastic clinician, keen to move out of the clinic to where the action is, may be bewildered and discouraged when, instead of an equally enthusiastic response, he or she meets polite resistance and even sabotage of carefully prepared ideas. These road-blocks can be negotiated and two themes come to mind: communication difficulties and legitimacy.

Communication

Community workers may be categorized into those who have almost continuous contact with the child, such as foster parents; those who have long periods of contact, such as teachers, nursing staff and care workers; and those with relatively fleeting contact, such as a field social worker. All these professionals will meet with a lot of child disturbance, although it is not their sole or even main concern.

Psychiatric terminology may have little currency outside clinic confines. The move from the clinic can be experienced as a liberation, but it has its frightening aspects. Models of behaviour based on descriptive psychiatry are unlikely to be received with sympathy. Although systems, behavioural or psychodynamic theories may provide points of contact, there may be differences in terminology, perception and level of training that can become very apparent in community settings. However, there may be other explanatory models, more or less well formulated and explicit, that form the basis for the management of problems. In the search for points of contact it is vital to try to detect the frame of reference of the other professionals in the field, a process that can only be achieved by listening, by asking tactful questions and by an attitude of humility.

There are several reasons why subtle detective work may be needed. The community worker may not be fully aware, and therefore may not easily be able to report their own set of assumptions. The clinician may be part of the assumptive system, viewed in a less than complimentary light. For example, the mental health worker may be seen as an unwelcome agent of social control on the part of the 'powers that be'. The worker may be reluctant to reveal a working model that they fear may be criticized or ridiculed by the mental health worker. Crucially, the mental health worker may find it difficult to cope with the assumptions of others because of different underlying political assumptions or because the assumptions of the other worker seem to cast him or her in an unfair light. Similarly, the mental health worker may be dismissive of the model and belief systems of others and unable to accept that they may have usefulness and validity.

Practice in non-clinic settings is a collaborative exercise. Not to accept the need for this detective work is to run the high risk of blocks in communication that are certain to derail co-operation. For this reason, it is worth citing some of the concepts that are commonly found among community workers in child care and education. Differences and disagreements about assumptions are best resolved around clinical case work. What the child or parents say is always the important first step to a solution to practical problems.

Labelling theory

The idea here is that each child is an individual, and that the application of labels (such as those contained in ICD-10) is damaging as it tends to depersonalize, to rob individual children of responsibility for their actions and to push them into a deviant role. Few would deny the importance of all these considerations but empirical evidence for labelling is much more limited than the claims of some professionals would suggest (Rutter & Giller 1983). Two areas provide examples. First, there are the effects of court appearance on delinquent boys. In a major longitudinal study, Farrington (1977) compared boys who appeared before the court with a group who had similar self-report delinquency scores but no court appearance. In the years after the court appearance, the self-report scores of the convicted boys increased whereas those of the non-convicted controls decreased. On the other hand, these differences were not sustained at further follow-up.

The second example comes from research in the classroom. A great deal of research has been carried out about the effect of teachers' preconceptions of children's abilities on academic progress (for a brief review see Rutter & Madge 1976). Some studies have used an experimental approach, giving teachers false information and assessing the effect on the progress of children in their classes. This approach has yielded mixed results, possibly because the attempt to prejudice teachers was unsuccessful (teachers make up their own minds). The second strategy has been to find naturalistic differences in teachers' attitudes. For example, teachers' assessments of ability can be compared with those gained from objective tests, or children whose older siblings are known to the teachers can be compared according to whether those siblings were high or low achievers. These studies have been more consistent in showing that teacher expectations can, in some circumstances, have effects on pupil progress (Pilling & Kelmer Pringle 1978). With some children, in some situations, labelling effects can be important.

Although this is true, to fail to analyse and classify also leads to problems in that without a common language of diagnosis and management, which to some would mean labelling, co-operative progress becomes extremely difficult. A wide variety of ideologically driven practices will be found in non-clinic settings. These may impinge on the work of the psychiatrist in many ways. For example, it is not uncommon for institutions to be operating a total ban on the use of psychotropic drugs, on the grounds that they imply an illness label. To avoid stigmatization is a sensible principle, but should not be a pretext to avoid effective treatment.

Challenging behaviour

'Challenging behaviour' is a common modern but somewhat ambiguous term used in practical situations. It may reflect the fact that the individual child's challenging behaviour disrupts the well-ordered setting of the school or youth club, or it may be that the child's behaviour is a challenge to the professional skills of those who care for him or her. It is perhaps typical of a number of such terms in that its usage seems to implicitly reject a deeper understanding of behaviour, including any notion of diagnosis or interpretation. It is a further indication of the deep distrust abroad of any suspicion of labelling or categorization of children. That it is behaviour and emotional problems that need to be categorized is not in dispute; the children should be valued as unique people.

Single-problem agencies

There are currently many agencies that have a central focus on one type of problem. For example, rape crisis centres are geared towards the victims of rape and the National Society for the Prevention of Cruelty to Children is directed principally at that aim. It would be extremely unfair to say that such organizations cannot have a broader focus, but collaboration with a mental health service may be both mutually beneficial and serve the needs of children by offering a broad choice of frameworks and approaches.

Panic behaviour

A panic response can occur. This often takes the form of an assumption that there is a 'cut-off' point where troublesome problems are seen to change in quality by community workers and become a 'mental illness' that they are incompetent to handle. This assumption may be linked to perplexity in the face of disturbed behaviour, to ingrained attitudes in the leadership or to relationship problems in the establishment concerned. The result is a helpless call for 'experts', a belief that drug therapy is needed and that the current environment is unsuitable for the child's needs. Often an undercurrent of hostility hampers collaboration. The clinician who is comfortable in work outside medical settings can at least detect this phenomenon, even if, at this stage, a helpful response is often difficult. Mental illnesses such as schizophrenia certainly present in non-medical settings, particularly in work related to the youth justice system, but the same attitude of partnership and collaboration is needed as with other problems, although the details of management will be different from the variety of other problems that may be encountered.

Legitimacy

Recent years has seen a massive extension of managerial control over the delivery of services. This trend is not limited to medical services; indeed, line management is far more evident in other major agencies. This means that informal working relationships on the ground are increasingly hard to sustain unless supported by senior management. Resistance to obvious need may be because of the fact that contractual arrangements have not been negotiated at a higher level of management. It is not possible for fieldworkers on the ground to respond unless this homework has been carried out.

Networking

Enormous numbers of professional workers can become involved in situations of family difficulty. In a recent study of a random sample of teenagers with severe learning difficulties, and who did not necessarily have special behavioural difficulties, Dossetor & Nicol (1991) found an average of six professionals visiting any given family, and this was in a district without lavish resources! Co-ordination of effort is needed if criminal waste of scarce resources is to be avoided. A variety of devices can be useful. These include:

1 the case conference;
2 regular network meetings;
3 information gathering;
4 parent organizations; and
5 knowledge of community agencies.

The case conference

This has been the main vehicle for co-ordination of effort in net-work situations. It was developed in a major way in relation to work in child abuse, where co-ordination is of vital importance. It is also the cornerstone of work with other client groups. A new edition of the guide *Working Together to Safeguard Children* was published in 1999 by the Home Office and Departments of Health and Education (1999). This is compulsory reading for the mental health professional in non-medical settings.

Regular network meetings

The fact that professionals serving the same child population are employed in different agencies and management structures does not mean that they cannot collaborate closely. Regular meetings to discuss individual problems can be of great benefit.

Information gathering

This includes telephone calls, letters and case notes reviews. Collection of information from as many sources as possible can put assessment work on a different basis. The present author, together with most clinicians, can remember situations where co-ordination and simple review of voluminous notes from a variety of agencies could have prevented a disaster.

The life table

This technique was developed by Adolf Meyer in relation to life events and illness to plot the relationship between the two. It can be of great help in organizing and making sense of historical information where time relationships are complex. The process is very simple. A large sheet of paper is taken and a series of columns are drawn up. Each column is designed to chart the progress of a particular problem area for the child and family. For example, one column could be times the father was out of work and another could be a record of the child's change of school. The development of such a chart from old and not very legible records is extremely laborious but it does clarify the course of events and can pay big dividends in terms of understanding.

Life story book (Ryan & Walker 1985)

A somewhat similar technique can be used diagnostically and therapeutically involving the child or young person. A good quality scrapbook or album is used as a life story book. Information from the notes can be gathered, old photographs can be brought into play, and memories evoked to recall people and places which have figured in the child's life. Places which have a key emotional meaning or which are important in the development of the child's identity can be visited. Access to the case notes is now within the child's rights and this also can play a part. This work can be undertaken by the child's key worker with back-up consultation. Such consultation can be important in helping the key worker to use the opportunities which such an exercise affords for counselling and also in identifying points at which the material is likely to put the child under stress.

Geneograms

The geneogram (Leiberman 1979) is another technique that can be very useful in helping a child to make sense of their experience.

Review and follow-up

The need to follow-up and review difficult situations is also a crucial part of the process of networking. A common finding in the tragedy of child abuse cases that have come before the courts and judicial inquiries is that follow-up has been sloppy and inadequate.

Parent and family organizations

Recent decades has seen the growth of a large number of organizations for different sorts of problems in children: examples in the mental health field are Mencap, for people with learning difficulties, the Autistic Society and the Schizophrenia Fellowship. It would be difficult to overestimate the importance of these organizations as a source of mutual support and in the struggle for adequate resources for children with difficulties. Compared to families of children with disabilities of physical origin, such organizations are relatively sparse in the field of mental health and there can be little doubt that further development in this area would be a powerful force against stigma and in favour of a voice for children with emotional difficulties and their families—never forget parent power.

Knowledge of community agencies

The vast panoply of statutory and voluntary agencies that now exist and the fact that they are of potential help to children and families in difficulties is evidence of the health, vigour and altruism of modern society. It is important that the clinician knows of their existence in the relevant area.

There are several other techniques that are common in network situations. It is important that the clinician has some knowledge of them.

Organization of a service in non-medical settings

The organization of services varies from country to country. However, when clinicians are attached to a clinic that is capable of providing a wide range of services to the local community, sometimes in medical and sometimes in non-medical settings, several basic principles apply.

First, there needs to be an agreement that, as part of the clinic's operational policy, work in non-medical settings is important. It is best if the service as a whole has a statement of aims. This can include direct work in the clinic, in other medical settings such as the paediatric ward, special care baby unit or the child development centre, and in non-medical settings such as the special school and residential home. In addition, there should be agreement that consultation is important and appropriate. Teaching activity is another area that should be accepted as part of the clinic's task. A teaching commitment to non-medical professionals in the local community, either on courses developed by the clinic or as a visiting speaker or tutor, may be one of the most effective ways of helping them to help children.

What are the needs of the community? Calculations can be made from epidemiological findings that give some guidance but do not by themselves identify the wish for services by families and workers in primary care settings. Some attempts have been made to estimate need, e.g. in a recent large survey in England and Wales by Meltzer & Gatwood (2000). One of the problems is that need is likely to be much greater than the supply of expertise available from the clinic. The simple conclusion must be that the major problems of child unhappiness and maladjustment will not be helped by one profession or in one setting alone so collaboration with other agencies and professionals is essential. Providers of services are likely to be the only people who can identify gaps in the service and they have a duty to identify these and bring them to the attention of those responsible for funding.

One way to identify gaps is to draw up a 'district profile'. This can include all the settings where service should be being provided. Against this list of settings a second column can be filled in, stating whether the need in each setting is being met. In completing this second column it is important to consider other agencies that may be fulfilling the role. It could be that there are areas where collaboration could mean that relatively little input from the child psychiatry service can make a great difference.

Effectiveness of interventions

Child mental health services have been notoriously short on research into their effectiveness. Examples of evaluation have been given in relation to the treatment of maladjustment in schools (Kolvin *et al.* 1981); to the reduction of bullying in school (Olweus 1993; Smith & Sharp 1994); and to delinquency (Henggeler *et al.* 1998). The more general theme of consultation is a particularly difficult area because it contains so many components and variables. Nevertheless, beginnings have been made (Mannino & Shore 1975; Kenney 1986). Most of the work is on consultation within education, with a strong emphasis on school work rather than emotional and behaviour problems. Medway *et al.* conducted a meta-analysis of school-based consultation and reported evidence of effectiveness, particularly in behavioural methods (Medway & Updyke 1985). Apart from the area of school consultation, where there is some evidence of effectiveness, these have mainly been small-scale studies lacking power to demonstrate useful changes on outcome. However, in the large-scale Newcastle study, a pro-gramme of teacher consultation and parent supportive coun-selling came out with a disappointing result when compared with more direct approaches to treatment, such as playgroups and behaviour modification (Kolvin *et al.* 1981). The verdict therefore has to be 'not proven'.

The simple question 'Is consultation effective?' is, as with so many other similar questions, not likely to be productive. What is needed is to define the context much more carefully. It seems likely that consultation in mainstream schools has more in com-mon with other school effectiveness research than it does with, say, consultation with disturbed delinquent adolescents in res-idential care. Consultation in this area may be a useful adjunct to the multisystemic approaches to young delinquents which is currently showing such promise (Henggeler *et al.* 1998) and could, where conditions such as a very scattered population sug-gest it, be included in such a programme. New legislation in the UK criminal justice system gives rise to multidisciplinary teams (youth offender teams) that will have resources to offer a variety of management programmes. This gives ample opportunity for mental health consultation if the will, energy and initiative can be found among mental health workers to respond. The development of court diversion schemes offer opportunities to develop assessment and treatment programmes without the complex administration and time taken for a special referral to mental health clinics.

References

Axline, V. (1947) *Play Therapy.* Houghton Mifflin, Boston.

Bergan, J.R. & Kratochwill, T.R. (1990) *Behavioral Consultation and Therapy.* Plenum Press, New York.

Berridge, D. & Brodie, I. (1998) *Children's Homes Revisited.* Jessica Kingsley, London.

Brown, D., Pryzwansky, W.B. & Schulte, A.C. (1998) *Psychological Consultation. Introduction to Theory and Practice,* 4th edn. Allyn and Bacon, Boston.

Caplan, G. (1970) *Principles of Mental Health Consultation.* Tavistock, London.

Craig, T.K.J., Woodward, S., Hodson, S. & Richardson, S. (1996) *Off to a Bad Start.* Mental Health Foundation, London.

Dewey, J. (1916) *Democracy and Education.* Macmillan, New York.

Dossetor, D. & Nicol, A.R. (1991) Community care of adolescents with developmental retardation: problems and proposals. *Health Trends,* 4, 148–151.

Erchul, W.P. & Martens, B.K. (1997) *School consultation. Conceptual and Empirical Bases in Practice.* Plenum, New York.

Farrington, D.P. (1977) The effects of public labelling. *British Journal of Criminology,* 17, 112–125.

Galloway, D. (1985) Pastoral care and school effectiveness. In: *Studying School Effectiveness* (ed. D. Reynolds), pp. 25–88. Falmer Press, Lewes.

Garfield, P. (1999) *Psychiatric Disorder among Juvenile Offenders in Prison.* Dissertation for Master of Sciences Degree, University of Leicester Medical School.

Gray, G., Smith, A. & Rutter, M. (1981) School attendance and the first year of employment. In: *Out of School: Modern Perspectives on Tru-*

ancy and School Refusal (eds L. Hersov & I. Berg), pp. 343–370. Wiley, Chichester.

Happé, D. (1982) Behavioural intervention: it doesn't do any good in your briefcase. In: *Psychological Approaches to Problems of Children and Adolescents* (ed. J. Grimes), pp. 15–41. Department of Public In-struction, De Moines, IA.

Hazel, N. (1981) *A Bridge to Independence.* Blackwell Publishers, Oxford.

Henggeler, S.W., Schoenwald, S.K., Borduin, C.M., Rowland, M.D. & Cunningham, P.B. (1998) *Multisystemic Treatment of Antisocial Behavior in Children and Adolescents.* Guilford Press, New York.

Home Office, Department of Health and Education (1999) *Working Together to Safeguard Children: A Guide to Inter-agency Working to Safeguard and Promote the Welfare of Children.* HMSO, London.

Kenney, K.C. (1986) Research in Mental Health Consultation: Emerg-ing Trends Issues and Problems. In: *Handbook of Mental Health Consultation* (eds F.W. Mannino, E.J. Trickett, M.F. Shore, M.G. Kidder & G. Levin), pp. 435–469. U.S. Government Printing Office, Washington D.C.

Kolvin, I., Garside, R., Nicol, A.R., Macmillan. A., Wolstenholme, F. & Lieitch, I. (1981) *Help Starts Here.* Tavistock, London.

La Fontaine, J. (1991) *Bullying: The Child's View.* Calouste Gulbenkian Foundation, London.

Leiberman, S. (1979) *Transgenerational Family Therapy.* Croom-Helm, London.

Liebling, A. (1992) *Suicide in Prison.* Routledge, London.

Maden, A., Taylor, C.J.A., Brooke, D. & Gunn, J. (1995) *Mental Dis-order in Remand Prisoners.* Home Office, Research and Statistics Directorate Information Section, London.

Maher, C.A. & Zins, J.E., eds (1987) *Psychoeducational Interventions in the Schools.* Pergamon, New York.

Mannino, F.V. & Shore, M.F. (1975) Effecting change through con-sultation. In: *The Practice of Mental Health Consultation* (eds F.V. Mannino, B.W. MacLennan & M.F. Shore), pp. 25–44. Gardner Press, New York.

Mattison, R.E. (2000) School consultation: a review of research on issues relevant to the school environment. *Journal of the American Academy of Child and Adolescent Psychiatry,* 39, 402–413.

Maughan, B. (1994) School influences. In: *Development Through Life: a Handbook for Clinicians* (eds M. Rutter & D.F. Hay), pp. 134–158. Blackwell Scientific, Oxford.

McCann, J.B., James, A., Wilson, S. & Dunn, G. (1996) Prevalence of psychiatric disorder in young people in the care system. *British Medical Journal,* 313, 1529–1530.

McMurren, M. (1995) Substance use and delinquency. In: *Clinical Approaches to Working with Young Offenders* (eds C.R. Hollin & K. Howells), pp. 209–235. Wiley, Chichester.

Medway, F.J. & Updyke, J.F. (1985) Meta-analysis of consultation outcome studies. *American Journal of Community Psychology,* 13, 489–505.

Meltzer, H. & Gatwood, R. (2000) *Mental Health of Children and Ado-lescents in Great Britain.* HMSO, London.

Mortimore, P. (1995) The positive effects of schooling. In: *Psychosocial Disturbance in Young People: Challenges for Prevention* (ed. M. Rutter), pp. 333–363. Cambridge University Press, New York.

Mortimore, P., Sammons, P., Stoll, L., Lewis, D. & Ecob, R. (1989) *School Matters: The Junior Years.* Open Books, London.

Nicol, A.R. (1994) Practice in nonmedical settings. In: *Child and Adolescent Psychiatry: Modern Approaches* (eds M. Rutter, E. Taylor & L. Hersov), 3rd edn, pp. 1040–1053. Blackwell Scientific, Oxford.

Nicol, A.R., Stretch, D., Whitney, I. *et al.* (2000) Mental health needs of people with difficult behaviour including young offenders in an NHS region. *Journal of Adolescence*, **23**, 244–261.

O'Leary, S.G. & O'Leary, K.D. (1976) Behaviour modification in the school. In: *Handbook of Behaviour Modification* (ed. H. Leitenberg), pp. 475–515. Prentice Hall, Englewood Cliffs, NJ.

Olweus, D. (1993) *Bullying at School: What We Know and What We Can Do.* Blackwell Publishers, Oxford.

Olweus, D. (1994) Bullying at school: basic facts and effects of a school based intervention program. *Journal of Child Psychology and Psychiatry*, **35**, 1171–1190.

Pilling, D. & Kelmer Pringle, M. (1978) *Controversial Issues in Child Development.* National Children's Bureau/Paul Elek, London.

Reilly, J., Herman, H.E., Clerle, D.M., Neil, C.C. & McNamara, C.L. (1994) Psychiatric disorders in and service use by young homeless people. *Medical Journal of Australia*, **161**, 429–431.

Rigby, K. & Slee, P. (1993) Dimensions of interpersonal relating among Australian school children and their implications for psychological well being. *Journal of Social Psychology*, **133**, 33–42.

Rogers, C. (1951) *Client Centred Therapy.* Houghton Mifflin, Boston, MA.

Rutter, M. (1983) School effects on pupil progress: research findings and policy implications. *Child Development*, **54**, 1–29.

Rutter, M. & Giller, H. (1983) *Juvenile Delinquency: Trends and Perspectives.* Penguin, Harmondsworth, Middlesex.

Rutter, M. & Madge, N. (1976) *Cycles of Disadvantage: a Review of Research.* Heinemann Educational, London.

Rutter, M., Maughan, B., Mortimore, P. & Ouston, J. (1979) *Fifteen Thousand Hours: Secondary Schools and Their Effects on Children.* Open Books, London.

Ryan, T. & Walker, R. (1985) *Making Life Story Books.* British Association of Adoption and Fostering, London.

Shaffer, D. & Caron, C.L.M. (1984) *Runaway and Homeless Children in New York City: A Report of the Ittleston Foundation.* New York State Psychiatric Institute, New York.

Smith, P.K. & Sharp, S. (1994) *School Bullying: Insights and Perspectives.* Routledge, London.

Utting, W. (1997) *People Like Us: The Report of the Review of the Safeguards For Children Living Away From Home.* Department of Health and the Welsh Office, The Stationery Office, London.

Yates, A., Beutler, L.E. & Crago, M. (1983) Characteristics of young, violent offenders. *Journal of Psychiatry and the Law*, **11**, 137–149.

Ysseldyke, J.E., Pianta, B., Christenson, S., Wang, J. & Algozzine, B. (1983) An analysis of pre-referral interventions. *Psychology in the Schools*, **20**, 184–190.

65 Primary Health Care Psychiatry

M. Elena Garralda

Introduction

Contact with primary health care—also called general practice or family doctor service—is a common experience in childhood. Over the course of 1 year most parents take their children to primary care health services, and work with children has been estimated to occupy about one-quarter of the doctor's time. There are age trends reflecting the differential experience of illness, with young preschool-age children being seen more often than older children. Thus, over 90% of preschool-age children but about two-thirds of 5–14 year olds will consult at least once a year, and the average annual number of consultations—over four a year—is also higher in preschool-age children (OPCS 1995).

The majority of children's consultations are for physical health problems but a small proportion are for psychological or developmental problems, and responding to psychological and social issues is one of the tasks of the primary care practitioner.

Families often trust general practitioners (GPs) as providers of information, support and advice. Regular contact with children and adolescents with psychiatric disorders provides primary care doctors with a potential opportunity for early identification and treatment of disorder. Primary care interventions have the advantage that GPs often have knowledge of families' circumstances over time, that general practice is less stigmatizing than psychiatric services, and patients tend to prefer this option.

This chapter reviews the organization of primary care services and research on the contribution of psychiatric disorder to primary care work. Specific issues that are addressed include the following. How much does psychiatric disorder feature amongst children attending general practice clinics? How much of it presents somatically? To what extent is it recognized? What happens after recognition? What determines referral of children by GPs to child psychiatrists?

Consideration is given to working models for psychiatric and primary care liaison, and to attempts that have been made at evaluating professional interventions in this setting. Work aimed at improving detection of psychiatric cases, the provision of psychiatric management within primary care, the public health education role of primary care and simple interventions for high-risk groups are outlined. Future directions for clinical practice and research are discussed.

Primary care services

Primary care services are delivered to children through three main avenues: first, through GPs, family practitioners or general paediatricians; second, by child health clinics, which often have a preschool as well as school medical service component; and, third, through hospital casualty departments, particularly in big cities.

The organization of services varies from country to country. Continuity of care is not universal and in some countries primary care doctors work in restricted settings such as emergency departments. Graham (1982) reviewed variations as they apply to paediatric services in European countries. These variations involve:
1 the degree to which primary services are delivered by family doctors and GPs rather than primary care paediatricians;
2 the extent to which preventive work is linked to general practice illness services;
3 the proportion of services which is delivered privately, on an insurance basis, or as part of centrally organized and funded national or regional health service;
4 the level of surveillance service provided; and
5 the degree of compulsion or inducement attached to preventive services.

In the UK, GPs provide primary care services for the whole population. Their services are free; they are family services in that they attend to both children and adults; they are involved in assessment and in treatment and also in the prevention of ill health, including mental health. A GP will attend to the needs of about 2000 patients in the local general population but some doctors work together with other doctors in health practices with correspondingly larger populations and with more opportunities for providing a number of primary care services, including the appointment of paramedical staff. Many general practices have nurses attached with a special commitment to supervise the development and health of under 5 year olds (paediatric nurses or health visitors). Some practices also employ psychiatric nurses, counsellors or psychologists.

Primary care doctors are the major referring source to many secondary or hospital medical services, including child psychiatric clinics. In the UK, about 10% of attendances for all types of medical consultation will result in a referral (OPCS 1995). Some children with emotional or behavioural problems are referred by family doctors to community or hospital paediatric services who will often investigate possible associated somatic problems and then refer on to child psychiatry. However, in countries where there is no such sharp differentiation between primary and secondary paediatric care, many paediatricians provide both. This review, although primarily emphasizing primary care work, will also consider the psychiatric problems of children who present to general paediatric clinics.

Child psychiatric morbidity in primary care

Behavioural and emotional problems are the main reason for consultation in many children presenting to general paediatric and hospital outpatient paediatric clinics but, in addition to this, they also constitute an associated problem in a considerably larger proportion of children presenting with somatic symptoms.

Presentation to primary care with emotional or behaviour problems

A number of surveys in various countries have documented that some 2–5% of children and adolescents who attend primary care or general paediatric clinics present with psychological problems (e.g. anxiety, behavioural problems, overactivity) (Goldberg et al. 1979, 1984; Jacobson et al. 1980; Starfield et al. 1980; Garralda & Bailey 1986a,b, 1989; Kramer & Garralda l998). Educational and social problems also feature as reasons for consultation.

Frequency of associated child and adolescent psychiatric disorders amongst attenders

There is evidence that psychiatric disorders are present in a considerably higher number of children attending primary care than may be supposed from the overt presenting complaint. Independent psychiatric research interviews carried out with children and their parents following primary care contact have found psychiatric disorders in about one-tenth to one-quarter of children across different countries (Giel et al. 1981; Garralda & Bailey 1986b; Costello et al. 1988; Gureje et al. 1994). The rates are probably higher in adolescents attending primary care (over 30%; Kramer & Garralda 1998) and amongst schoolchildren attending general hospital outpatient paediatric services (28%; Garralda & Bailey 1989).

Most children with psychiatric disorders present at the surgery with somatic symptoms. Do the high levels of psychopathology simply reflect general population rates? Are they relevant to the somatic presentations? Although there is no unequivocal answer to these questions, there are some indications that child and adolescent psychiatric disorder may contribute to consultations by increasing the likelihood of attendance for somatic symptoms. This is suggested:

1 by the comparatively high rates of disturbance among con-

sulting children in relation to general population prevalence (Garralda & Bailey 1986a,b; Kramer & Garralda 1998);

2 by the associations found amongst preschool-age children between behavioural/emotional symptoms and increased primary care use (Lavigne et al. 1998);

3 by the particularly high levels of psychopathology amongst *frequent* surgery attenders (Bowman & Garralda 1993); and

4 by findings from general population studies of high levels of medical service use by children and adolescents with psychiatric disorders (Richman et al. 1982; Offord et al. 1987; Monck et al. 1994).

Interestingly, there is tentative evidence that children with psychiatric disorders may be comparatively more likely to attend primary care with somatic symptoms and less likely to attend mental health services in areas with low levels of psychosocial disadvantage (Garralda & Bailey 1986a).

Are there specific associations between psychiatric disorders and physical presentations or symptoms amongst primary care attenders?

This is a pertinent question, because most children with psychiatric disorders present in primary care with somatic symptoms, but in older children and in adolescents there seems to be little specificity in the range of physical symptoms presented at consultation by children with psychiatric disorders (Garralda & Bailey 1986a,b; Kramer & Garralda 1998).

A more indirect link between physical symptoms and psychopathology is suggested by findings that mothers of primary care frequent attenders—when compared with mothers of other frequent attenders without psychiatric disorder—are more likely to view their children as lethargic, in poorer general health and more handicapped by their symptoms (Garralda et al. 1999). In a study of children attending general paediatric clinics, parents of those who were found to have psychiatric disorders were particularly likely to report tiredness and lethargy in the child (8/36 or 22% vs. 2/90 or 2% of non-disordered attenders); this meant that 8/10 attenders reported as tired and lethargic had an associated psychiatric disorder (Garralda & Bailey 1989). In adolescents attending primary care, psychiatric disorders have been found to be associated with high levels and intensity of, and more impairment from, physical symptoms (Kramer & Garralda 1998). These findings suggest poorer general physical well-being in attenders with psychiatric disorders in spite of the lack of specificity in the presenting symptomatology.

The nature of psychopathology amongst primary care attenders

There may be more specificity in the type of psychiatric problems identified in children attending medical settings. Although the range of common psychiatric disorders is seen, in contrast with general population findings, surveys of schoolchildren and adolescents in primary care tend to find more emotional than conduct disorders (Garralda & Bailey 1986b, 1989; Costello *et al.* 1988; Kramer & Garralda l998). This suggests that enquiry about the presence of and expertise in the management of associated emotional symptoms is specially appropriate if primary care is to have an enhanced role in the identification and management of child psychiatric disorders.

Family stress and the consultations of children with psychopathology

It has long been recognized that family stress and maternal neurotic problems are related to both an increased tendency to consult for children's physical symptoms (Roghmann & Haggerty 1972; Woodward *et al.* 1988) and to childhood psychiatric disorder. On both accounts it seems highly likely that family stresses will contribute to the consultations of children with psychiatric disorders.

Bailey & Garralda (1987) documented an excess of recent (in the previous 3 months) undesirable life events—including family arguments and changes in parental financial and work status—in schoolchildren with psychiatric disorders attending primary care when compared with attenders without disorder. Mothers of schoolchildren with psychiatric disorders who are frequent general practice attenders report reduced maternal well-being, an increase in marital problems and maternal health attitudes characterized by overemphasis on the ill-health implications of symptoms and a tendency to affective inhibition from negative feelings (Garralda *et al.* 1999). Children are usually taken to health services by their mothers, and maternal stress and health attitudes may contribute to disordered children consultations by undermining their mothers' sense of confidence in parenting in relation to both the somatic and behavioural problems.

Psychosomatic problems

The presence of psychiatric disorder—defined as handicapping abnormalities of emotions, behaviour or relationships—is not sufficient to explain the range of problems presenting to GPs and paediatricians where psychosocial factors have a significant part to play. A useful complementary concept is that of psychosomatic presentations. These can be defined in either a broad or narrow sense.

The *narrow definition* implies that certain somatic symptoms (e.g. abdominal pains, headaches) are often an expression of the somatization of distress. Starfield *et al.* (1980) found psychosomatic problems so defined (e.g. children presenting with insomnia, headache, asthma, abdominal pain or other abdominal symptoms) in 8–10% of children attending various primary care facilities in the USA. Campo *et al.* (1999) reported aches and pains with no organic diagnosis in 2% of 11–15-year-old paediatric primary care attenders. There is suggestive evidence that these presentations are found in excess at psychosocial transitional periods: during the early elementary school years (particularly in boys) and in early adolescence (especially in

girls), perhaps reflecting the stress of early learning performance for boys and of puberty in girls (Schor 1986), and the possibility that some of these symptoms represent a response to life stresses.

Defined in a broad way, psychosomatic problems would apply to any physical presentations where the doctor makes a clinical judgement that psychological or social factors are contributing in significant way, e.g. aggravating the symptom. This broad definition is in keeping with the commonly held view amongst medical practitioners which assumes that psychological events can be relevant in the aetiology or in the maintenance of virtually any physical condition.

When doctors are asked to note any physical presentations with associated or contributing psychological factors, e.g. asthma exacerbated by stress, such presentations are recorded for about one-fifth of schoolchildren attending primary care and for as many as half in outpatient paediatric clinics, indicating a high degree of sensitivity and vigilance by many clinicians to these issues (Bailey *et al.* 1978; Garralda & Bailey 1987, 1990). Presenting symptoms in these cases tend to be those regarded traditionally as having psychosomatic components (e.g. aches and pains, incontinence, asthma and blackouts) but virtually any physical complaint is featured. These children do have an excess of emotional and behavioural symptoms, with mood changes and relationship problems. However, most do not suffer from psychiatric disorders. A special stress by mothers over parenting and concerns over schooling have particularly been noted in primary care settings, suggesting the relevance of high academic and behavioural expectations.

Addressing the psychosocial concerns of families with children with psychosomatic presentations may have substantial consequences for medical service use. These children come from families with a high tendency to focus on health issues, as shown by the fact that they are high users of primary care and that the children themselves are given more hospital appointments, more referrals to specialist clinics and more follow-up appointments at the surgery than children with purely physical presentations (Garralda & Bailey 1987; Campo *et al.* 1999).

Recognition of psychiatric disorders and psychosomatic problems in primary care

The recognition of child psychiatric disorders by physicians is obviously a prerequisite if primary care and paediatric services are to become fully involved in attending to the mental health of children and adolescents, but the evidence indicates that recognition is often quite limited. The adult literature shows that while between one-quarter and one-half of primary care patients have psychiatric morbidity, doctor recognition is only 40–50% of the actual rates (Upton *et al.* 1999). Doctor recognition of child and adolescent psychiatric disturbance in primary care settings is similarly reduced (Garralda & Bailey 1986a; Chang *et al.* 1988; Kramer & Garralda 1998). Although doctors identify psychological problems associated with somatic presentations in a considerable percentage of children, this cannot be equated with recognition of psychiatric disorder because the majority of these children fail to show psychiatric disturbance from research interviews, and conversely many disturbed children are not identified as such by doctors.

As in adult studies there is wide variation between doctors, with some not identifying any disturbed children at all. Doctors' assessments tend to be highly specific but only moderately sensitive: they identify few non-disturbed children and adolescents as disturbed but they miss a considerable percentage of disturbed children. Recognition is higher when children have severe, as opposed to milder, problems and accordingly the more severely affected children are more likely to be referred to psychiatric services (Costello & Edelbrock 1985; Kramer & Garralda 1998). As well as severity, recognition may partly be linked to the child's age (more 7–14 year olds), social circumstances and stresses (being on welfare, broken homes) and to presenting symptoms (chronic conditions, digestive problems and ill-defined problems) (Goldberg et al. 1979; Kramer & Garralda 1998).

Interventions by primary care doctors for child mental health problems

What sort of interventions are provided by the primary care doctors and teams once child psychiatric disorders have been identified? Goldberg et al. (1984) asked primary care paediatricians in the USA to indicate the treatment provided by them to 7–14 year olds attending with diagnoses of mental health problems. Doctors reported providing some treatment for the majority of detected disturbed children and for nearly one-third this was the only known source of care for the problem. Most frequently provided by paediatricians were supportive therapy or counselling (81%) and suggestions for environmental change (half of the presentations).

There is very little knowledge on the exact nature of the supportive and psychotherapeutic interventions provided by doctors in primary care. The relative importance given by them to reflective or behavioural approaches has not been systematically scrutinized, nor have the benefits in terms of parent satisfaction of symptom reduction. However, there is some evidence that the style of the intervention affects parent satisfaction. Work with young mothers in health clinics has documented the superiority of statements by doctors reflecting empathy and encouragement over the simple expression of support (Wasserman et al. 1984).

In the survey by Goldberg et al. (1984), of children attending primary care with mental health problems, drugs were prescribed for 11% of affected children (amphetamines in 4%). However, there are indications that drug prescribing for behavioural and emotional problems in primary care has increased since this study was carried out. A diagnosis of attention deficit disorder in some primary care clinics in the USA virtually predicted the use of methylphenidate and the lack of use of other treatment forms a decade ago (Wolraich et al. 1990). There is

now alarm at the trend for a marked increase in the use and range of psychotropic medication in ambulatory care organizations, even for preschool-age children (Zito et al. 2000).

Referrals to child psychiatry by primary care workers and paediatricians

Referral to child psychiatry remains the most frequent interface between primary care and child psychiatrists. A significant proportion of children seen in psychiatric clinics are referred by GPs (Garralda et al. 2000). However, each GP refers few children and the factors that determine referrals are not well understood. Whilst doctors' recognition of disturbance is obviously important, so are parental and doctor attitudes. Length of time the patient is known to the doctor is probably relevant (Goldberg et al. 1979) as is a maternal request for referral in many cases (Bailey & Garralda 1989), the GP's role in the process being often rather passive. This may be accounted for by differences in GPs' and parental perceptions of problems such as hyperactivity. GPs appear more unsure than parents whether hyperactivity is a medical disorder warranting a diagnosis and specific treatment, more often seeing it as a passing phase related to family stresses (Klasen & Goodman 2000).

Once children are referred to child psychiatry clinics by GPs, the majority are found to be disturbed, whether from research interviews, GPs' estimates, or both (Garralda & Bailey 1988; Bailey & Garralda 1989; Garralda et al. 2000). The factors associated with referral by GPs in this age group are comparable to those that determine referral for the majority of children attending clinics and are therefore probably not specific. A study sought to clarify this by comparing non-referred children with psychiatric disorders attending primary care with disordered children who were referred by GPs to psychiatric clinics. Referred children had higher severity levels of disturbance, more appreciation by parents of the child's disturbance, more male sex, antisocial symptoms and psychosocial disadvantage (Garralda & Bailey 1988). Higher severity and male sex are consistently found in other surveys (Laclave & Campbell 1986; Lavigne et al. 1998).

An interesting minority of children referred by GPs to child psychiatry clinics is found not to be sufficiently disturbed to be considered as having psychiatric disorders. When compared with non-referred non-disordered children attending general practice, parents of referred children, contrary to expectations, do not regard their children as disturbed more frequently, nor is the referral a 'ticket' for help with psychiatric morbidity in the parents. It seems likely from this work that, quite specifically, for a number of parents the difficulty they experience in controlling and coping with exuberant activity in somewhat rebellious children in the context of difficult economic and housing circumstances and perhaps a family history of serious antisocial behaviour contributes to help-seeking (Garralda & Bailey 1988). However, the fact that all these features are common in the general population, and that referrals of non-disordered children are few, indicates that additional unknown factors must determine referrals.

On the basis of the little audit work which has been carried out in this area, most parents appear to be satisfied with the part played by the primary care doctor in the referral process (Bailey & Garralda 1989). However, this only applies to children who have been referred, and there may be many non-referred children whose parents' attitudes toward GPs' helpfulness are more jaundiced.

Child psychiatry and primary care liaison

Adult psychiatrists have been actively involved in primary care liaison work for several decades and the models proposed by them provide useful guidance for the little documented area of liaison schemes between child psychiatric and primary care teams.

Gask et al. (1997) summarized the purpose of the common current consultation-liaison approach as:
• to help GPs identify psychiatric morbidity in the practice;
• to assist them to deal directly with cases within their competence and skill;
• to help define the best time for specialist referral;
• for the specialist to take on the assessment and to initiate the joint care of referral patients and their relatives; and
• to share with the primary care team the continuing burden of chronically sick patients, to explore the limits both of the doctor–family relationship and that of GP and specialist in the setting of general practice.

The history of these developments in adult psychiatry was comprehensively outlined by Mitchell (1985). Balint pioneered the field through GP seminars focused on the relationship between the doctor and the patient using a psychodynamic perspective as the primary diagnostic and management tool. By the 1980s one in five British psychiatric consultants surveyed indicated that they or their junior staff spent more time in a general practice setting (Strathdee & Williams 1984) and other members of the psychiatric team have similarly reported attachment liaison schemes in general practice. Subotsky & Brown (1990) described a child psychiatric clinic in general practice.

A number of different ways of working together were discussed by Mitchell (1985) within the attachment-liaison style.
1 Regular and co-ordinated home visits.
2 Shift of psychiatric clinics to health centres or surgeries.
3 Visits to health centres or surgeries by psychiatrists to see selected patients.
4 Regular group discussions at the health centre or surgery.
5 Conjoint consultations in the health care centre or surgery to be used with highly selected prepared patients.
In child psychiatry this would involve members of the psychiatric and the general practice multidisciplinary teams, including health visitors, community child psychiatric nurses and psychologists or counsellors.

The different options within the attachment-liaison model are not exclusive and have several elements in common which may be important for its success. They include regular and readily available face-to-face contacts between professions, time for the growth of understanding of what each wants from the other, a common and acceptable meeting ground, and openness of communication based on mutual respect and trust. In addition, an important way to promote liaison between child psychiatrists and primary care doctors is the participation of child psychiatrists in the postgraduate training of GPs, in order that basic information on assessment, handling and counselling skills can be taught.

Currently, there is active interest in the UK in the development of primary care child and adolescent mental health workers to help take on some of these attachment-liaison tasks. As in adult psychiatry, however, practical considerations limit the value of liaison schemes. The ratio of child psychiatric teams to primary care units is low, and only a minority of GPs in a health district could be involved and benefit. Moreover, child psychiatric teams also consult with other services, such as education and social services. In any case, consultation-liaison interventions must be closely monitored and evaluated to help determine provision, and different professionals from both services should be involved. These schemes will be shown to be worth carrying out if more children with psychiatric disorders are identified and successfully helped in the general practice setting and if it results in more efficient referrals to specialist clinics. They should be shown to have an impact on referral patterns, changes in the primary care workers' ability to detect and manage cases that are not referred, and be cost-effective (Gask et al. 1997).

Improving the detection of cases for specialist treatment in primary care

The prospects of receiving treatment for actual psychiatric disturbance are currently limited by low rates of detection within primary care. Simple, quick, easy-to-complete questionnaires have been developed or adapted to screen children and young people with behaviour problems, depression and parent–teenager conflict in primary care and paediatric settings (Jellinek et al. 1986; Campo et al. 1999). They have proved efficient but the impersonal nature of questionnaires begs the question of how useful they will turn out to be for face-to-face interventions in paediatric consultations. It seems probable that the use of open questions during the consultation about existing emotional or behavioural problems in the children will similarly prove useful as an aid in the identification of psychiatric disorders (Costello et al. 1988). Exploration of the actual rather than the ostensible reason for seeking paediatric attention may also reveal family stresses, possibly related to child psychopathology (Bass & Cohen 1982).

Training primary care workers in the identification of child psychiatric disorders

The World Health Organization has sponsored interesting initiatives to explore the potential of primary care to respond to mental health problems in children. Giel *et al.* (1988) showed that, with the use of a small set of simple questions, it was possible to identify probably disturbed children and to increase awareness on the part of family care workers in various developing countries. Brief training sessions led to improved identification by the carers of severe psychiatric problems (e.g. emergencies such as suicidal behaviour, depression or psychosis), neuropsychiatric problems (epilepsy and mental retardation) and in improved attitudes by them towards the management of cases.

Bernard *et al.* (1999) developed a training package on child and adolescent mental health problems for primary doctors in training. This included preparatory reading (Hughes *et al.* 1995) and teaching sessions with problem exercises, role-play and video-vignettes. Evaluation demonstrated enhanced detection of child and psychiatric disorder as well as improved self-perceived competence and knowledge amongst GP trainees. My colleagues and I (Gledhill *et al.*, unpublished) developed and tested a package to train GPs in the identification and management of adolescent depression opportunistically during routine consultations for any kind of presentation. Its use resulted in improved detection of adolescent depression by GPs and in positive feedback by doctors and adolescents.

The screening role is far from exclusive to doctors working in primary care. The contribution of nurses is particularly important for young preschool-age children, and the appointment of counsellors, psychologists and psychiatrically trained nurses offers the opportunity to develop dedicated screening clinics. The motivation of clinicians to recognize psychiatric problems will be enhanced by the existence of appropriate and effective therapeutic strategies in primary care and in paediatric clinics.

Interventions for children with psychiatric disorders

Studies within adult mental health have shown that primary care interventions are feasible and can be effective, but comparatively little is known about the treatment available for psychiatrically disturbed children in primary care or paediatric settings. Controlled studies of interventions are methodologically difficult to implement but there is growing interest in this area.

Bower *et al.* (2001) carried out a systematic review of interventions for child and adolescent mental health problems in primary care. Studies can be divided into those describing treatments carried out by the primary health care team, management delivered by specialist mental health professionals, and consultation-liaison models. Most work on children and adolescents with actual psychiatric disorders falls within the first category

and involves treatment in primary care by mental health specialists. Most interventions described are brief (6–12 sessions) but they include a variety of techniques from behaviour-cognitive to family therapy, non-directive counselling, dynamic therapy, psychiatric evaluation and guidance, parent education and counselling, group work and child education. Study designs tend to consist of simple before-and-after studies without control groups and there are often important gaps in the description of details of the process of treatment delivery. Problems in the statistical analysis include lack of power analysis, the treatment of losses to follow-up and the presentation of differences between groups. Results can therefore only be regarded as tentative and pointing the way to further work. Examples will be considered here briefly.

Earlier attempts at screening children for psychological problems as part of a paediatric evaluation and at providing interventions in this setting resulted in poor uptake (Metz *et al.* 1976). Subsequently, Finney *et al.* (1991) showed that it was possible for mental health professionals to offer short interventions (one to six visits) in primary care to parents of children and adolescents with behavioural and mental health problems. Individualized treatments were offered, guided by problem-specific protocols. Parent outcome and behaviour checklist ratings showed improvement or resolution in 74% of cases with high satisfaction. Use of medical services in the following year, especially primary care visits, showed a decrease when compared with a matched control group having routine care. Finney *et al.* (1989) also described a psychological intervention for children with recurrent abdominal pains referred to a primary-care-based paediatric psychology service. The treatment involved a self-monitoring of pain, limiting the attention given to the symptom, use of relaxation and dietary fibre supplementation and encouraging the child to participate in routine activities. The results indicated improvements in pain symptoms and reduced school absences. More complex approaches have been implemented and monitored. In an example of a 'shifted outpatient clinic', family therapy clinics based on systemic ideas within a large group general practice in London were found helpful by many families (Graham *et al.* 1992).

Child psychiatrists have successfully developed and piloted short interventions, which may be adapted for use by primary care workers. Coverly *et al.* (1995) provided a protocol-guided single psychiatric consultation in primary care to mothers of frequently attending schoolchildren found from psychiatric interviews to be psychiatrically disturbed. The intervention aimed to boost parental confidence in dealing with difficult behaviour through clarification of the problems, empathic and encouraging remarks, and succinct advice on management. Most mothers attended for the intervention of which two-thirds reported it had been markedly helpful at short-term (3-month) and longer-term (18–24 month) follow-up. Westman & Garralda (1996) piloted a brief psychotherapeutic intervention (four to six sessions) for adolescents with depressive and anxiety disorders attending a health promotion clinic in primary care. Less than half the adolescents offered the intervention attended, but the majority of these attenders felt subjectively improved. It was noted that most youngsters with mood disorders had attended their GP in the previous year and that more of these youngsters could be reached if the intervention was provided by the GPs themselves.

My colleagues and I (Gledhill et al., unpublished) therefore developed a treatment package incorporating cognitive and interpersonal behavioural principles, suitable for delivery by GPs opportunistically during adolescent consultations. The study showed the feasibility of training GPs in its use because most GPs applied the therapy techniques in the majority of youngsters identified by them as depressed. Their intervention was associated with reductions in depression-related functional impairment. The key question is how much it is possible to generalize these interventions and how to document any possible benefits rigorously.

Primary care as a resource for public child mental health education and simple intervention for high-risk groups

The virtually universal attendance of young children at primary care and child health paediatric clinics is an opportunity to provide parents and children with general information aimed at promoting child and adolescent mental health. This is an extension of the well-recognized role by primary care paediatric services in the dissemination of information about health, child development and behaviour.

Mothers of young children value and make use of general health advice provided during general practice consultations to manage health problems in their children (Cunningham-Burley & Irvine 1987). They also rely on health care professions for advice about child-rearing and psychosocial issues (McCune et al. 1984). However, different professionals (e.g. GPs, clinical medical officers and community paediatricians) can give conflicting advice (Jewel & Bain 1985), probably reflecting insufficient emphasis in training. It seems important therefore that serious attention is given to education in this area for primary care workers.

Some reports have documented the effects of educative/supportive interventions in primary care for parents of young children. In an early controlled study, Gutelius et al. (1977) described an intensive child health supervision programme started by a project nurse during pregnancy and continued by the nurse and by a paediatrician at well-being clinics over several years. The emphasis was on counselling and anticipatory guidance for mothers of normal first-born black infants from low-income families and on group sessions where mothers were given direct advice about their personal life. When compared with a control group there were behavioural benefits during the first 6 years of life, with positive effects also found in diet and eating habits, toilet training and in child-rearing practices.

Since then a variety of community programmes have been developed and shown to be effective in the prevention of behavioural problems in young children and in the support of positive parenting (Cox 1993; Olds et al. 1997; Webster-Stratton 1998). However, these programmes require specifically trained staff and a great deal of input to access and maintain the co-operation of mothers and children. How realistic, feasible and appropriate is it for generic health services such as primary care or paediatric health surveillance clinics to develop this degree of therapeutic sophistication for emotional and behavioural problems?

Promotion of young children's mental health by GPs

The study by Cullen (1976) is of interest because it involved an intervention by a single GP and because of the long-term follow-up. The author, a GP in a rural community in Australia, arranged to see the mothers of 124 children for a series of interventions spaced at intervals of 3 months in the first year and at 6 months in the succeeding 4 years of the child's life. Child-rearing concepts and attitudes were explored. When compared with a control non-intervention group of children, those in the index group showed fewer behavioural problems at 6 years of age from mothers' reports and the children themselves expressed more positive feelings towards their mothers. However, a greater number were late for school and boys were more excitable and hard to control. The author wondered whether the confidence of the boys' mothers in the intervention group might have been affected by too cautious an approach to disciplining problems. Follow-up of these children 20 years later (Cullen & Cullen 1996) suggested long-lasting favourable effects for the girls in the experimental group, who reported fewer neurotic symptoms. A larger proportion had also attained a university degree or diploma, and fewer were overweight.

The study demonstrated that mental health promotion interventions can be carried out systematically by GPs and that, through regular supervision, doctors may be able to influence parental actions and have some long-lasting effects on their children's behaviour. It seems unlikely, however, that the majority of primary care doctors or even paediatricians would regard this area as one for priority development and one in which they would be prepared to invest such a degree of time and effort.

Attempts at training primary care community nurses or health visitors and doctors to promote parenting in order to reduce behavioural problems in young children have reported positive but also often inconsistent or equivocal results and remain an area requiring further exploration (Cox 1993; Bower et al. 2001). It is important to establish and evaluate what is the minimum intervention that may be taught, is realistically used by primary care staff and results in worthwhile mental health gains for children.

There have been more focused pilot interventions for specific problems; these deserve further evaluation. For example, group therapy sessions have been set up for mothers who are frequent attenders to primary care and been followed by reduced consultation rates suggesting better coping strategies with concerns over children's health problems (Benson & Turk 1988). General counselling by paediatricians for parents on consistent and effective management of childhood behaviour may be helpful for young children with combined physical and behavioural problems.

Work with adolescents

The primary care setting may prove a resource for promoting mental health in adolescents. In a preliminary investigation, a GP invited youngsters registered at the practice to attend his surgery for a general health discussion. Following a single-letter approach, over half the youngsters attended, and this resulted in consultations found by the doctor to be both enjoyable and productive, with effective discussion of general health issues and also of personal problems (Donovan & McCarthy 1988). Westman & Garralda (1996) investigated the feasibility of inviting 14–15 year olds to a health promotion clinic to explore mental and physical health and to identify those at high risk of depression. Although overall attendance rates were low (22%) a high proportion of attenders had psychiatric disorders and the authors calculated that the clinic had probably attracted all adolescents with depression registered at the surgery. Specific training for GPs has been shown to have beneficial effects on the quality of medical consultations with adolescents and to achieve improvements in knowledge, skill and self-perceived competence (Sanci *et al.* 2000). These are basic requirements for the development of more specific mental health promotion initiatives in primary care.

Work with parents of children with psychiatric disorders

Adult psychiatric services now have several decades of experience in developing links with primary care. Controlled trials of patients with mood disorders have documented beneficial effects of interventions in primary care techniques, such as anxiety management, intensive patient education, medication adherence counselling, behavioural treatments to improve coping strategies and problem-solving (Kendrick 2000). Parental mastery in dealing with mood disorders could influence children's mental health and their own ability to manage mood changes. Supportive care by social workers attached to general practice can result in valuable clinical and social benefits to patients with neurotic disorders (Corney 1987). In so far as psychiatric disorders in parents influence childhood disturbance, these interventions could have beneficial effects on the children's mental health.

This is more directly the case for disorders starting in the puerperium. Counselling mothers with postnatal depression by health visitors or nurses in general practice can lead to substantial clinical improvement. This may be expected to have implications for the mother's ability to respond to the child and to promote child health and psychological development (Wickberg & Hwang 1996).

It can be concluded that, generally, educational or therapeutic interventions—not necessarily focused on any particular treatment modality but involving ongoing support, advice and guidance with child-rearing in well-being clinics—can be instituted in general practice and may lead to favourable behavioural outcomes in young children. The challenge lies in how much these interventions can incorporate more sophisticated psychotherapeutic components, be generalized across services and evaluated rigorously.

Future directions

The main mental health task for primary care remains attention to children and adolescents presenting with primary behavioural, emotional and psychosomatic problems. Secondary to this is the screening for associated psychiatric disorders amongst children presenting with somatic symptoms, and the promotion of child adolescent mental health. All of these tasks have organizational and service development, educational and research components.

Attention to children and adolescents presenting in primary care with behavioural, emotional and psychosomatic problems

Nature of presenting problem

As for any presenting problem, the primary care doctor needs to make a well-informed judgement as to whether:
1 the presenting complaint is a mild short-lived problem, understandable on the basis of environmental changes and intrinsic vulnerabilities, and likely to resolve spontaneously;
2 whether it is causing handicap and therefore requires attention in its own right, whatever its origins and transient nature; and
3 whether adequate attention can be provided at the surgery or whether it requires specialist referral.

Knowledge on the nature of the common and severe psychiatric disorders will form the basis of these decisions. Increased teaching on these basic concepts in medical and nursing school and in postgraduate general practice training programmes should facilitate this task. There is an ongoing need for academic institutions to develop, update and document the quality, breadth and reach of teaching and training programmes to ensure universal coverage.

Information and advice

A wealth of information is now available to families on a variety of child mental health problems. GPs and primary care teams are in a good position to draw parents' and youngster's attention to suitable written and electronic information and to complement this with clarification of the meaning of the symptoms presented and basic advice about its management. Although there are existing guidelines specifically designed to help family doctors identify and manage child mental health problems, these need further development and evaluation. It is important to find ways of distilling the main knowledge on management principles of child psychiatric disorders in a way that can be conveyed in an authoritative and empathic manner by a generalist medical service during a brief intervention.

Referral to specialist services

For clearly diagnosable psychiatric problems in children who are not already under the care of mental health services, the primary care clinician needs to make a decision about whether and how to refer. Existing research indicates that psychiatric referrals by primary care doctors are generally appropriate (children with the more severe problems and associated psychosocial complexity). However, increasing awareness of child and adolescent psychiatric problems by parents and primary care teams alike is likely to result in more referrals than specialist services can possibly accommodate. Protocols refining the criteria for severity, psychosocial complexity and likely response to treatments will need to be developed and audited jointly by child and adolescent mental health and primary care services. This is where the development of consultation-liaison activities or of primary care mental health worker posts may be specially helpful and should be monitored against measures of success of the referral process.

Primary care interventions for the milder/moderate psychiatric problems

Most reports on primary care interventions for children and adolescents with mental health problems have been based on the 'shifted' outpatient clinics in primary care by mental health professionals or counsellors. This may have the advantage of destigmatizing, facilitating attendance and accessing more children with milder problems who would not normally be referred to specialist services. At the same time, and given the limited resources available generally for child and adolescent mental health, shifted outpatient clinics run the risk of providing sophisticated interventions for problems that do not require them at the expense of treating more severe disorders in the specialist setting.

An alternative approach is that of adapting more complex specialist interventions for the primary care setting for primary care doctors and their staff to deliver opportunistically during consultations. This strategy has the advantage of being more primary care syntonic, it may be more realistic and less demanding of resources. By giving primary care doctors/paediatricians confidence in the management of psychiatric disorders, it might also reduce the use of psychotropic medication in primary paediatric care and halt the recent alarming increase. However, it calls for a serious effort to improve the training of GPs and paediatricians in psychiatric diagnosis and in the use of psychosocial management techniques.

The two approaches ('shifted' outpatient specialist clinic vs. more child mental health care by primary care staff) are not incompatible and are likely to be developed varyingly across services depending on local demand and professional attitudes. It seems important that both are researched in relation to clinical outcomes.

Screening for psychiatric disorders amongst children presenting with somatic complaints

The high levels of psychiatric disorders amongst schoolchildren and adolescents attending primary care with somatic complaints and the willingness by parents to take up treatment at the surgery when disorders are identified suggest that screening for psychopathology during consultations is appropriate. Given the comparative high frequency of emotional disorders, psychosomatic concerns, associated stressful psychosocial circumstances and high primary care attendance rates amongst those with disorders, it would seem appropriate to target these problems and situations in screening and for management. Screening questionnaires or open questioning by clinicians may be used varyingly in different settings. Their relative advantages and disadvantages can easily be audited.

Screening children at high risk in primary care

Health screening is one of the roles of primary care and paediatric health clinics, of health visitors and school nurses and doctors. It would seem logical for child mental health to be part of this screening, particularly but not exclusively in work with young preschool-age children. Future research can helpfully investigate the potential of these services to inform parents and children on child and adolescent psychiatric problems, their role in prevention and at the interface with the community parenting support programmes which are being developed for young children at risk.

Primary care psychiatry is slowly beginning to emerge as a child and adolescent mental health service. New clinical initiatives need to be developed and evaluated rigorously for short- and long-term effects and for user attitudes.

References

Bailey, D. & Garralda, M.E. (1987) Children attending general practice: a study of recent life events. *Journal of the American Academy of Child and Adolescent Psychiatry*, 26, 858–864.

Bailey, D. & & Garralda, M.E. (1989) Referral to child psychiatry: parent and doctor motives and expectations. *Journal of Child Psychology and Psychiatry*, 30, 449–458.

Bailey, V., Graham, P. & Boniface, D. (1978) How much child psychiatry does a general practitioner do? *Journal of the Royal College of General Practitioners*, 28, 621–626.

Bass, L.W. & Cohen, R.L. (1982) Ostensible versus actual reasons for seeking pediatric attention: another look at the parental ticket of admission. *Pediatrics*, 70, 870–874.

Benson, P. & Turk, T. (1988) Group therapy in a general practice setting for frequent attenders: a controlled study of mothers with pre-school children. *Journal of the Royal College of General Practitioners*, 38, 539–541.

Bernard, P., Garralda, E., Hughes, T. & Tyle, A. (1999) Evaluation of a teaching package in adolescent psychiatry for general practitioners. *Education for General Practice*, **10**, 21–28.

Bower, P., Garralda, E., Kramer, T., Harrington, R.C. & Sibbald, B. (2001) The treatment of child and adolescent mental health problems in primary care: a systematic review. *Family Practice*, **18**, 373–382.

Bowman, F.M. & Garralda, M.E. (1993) Psychiatric morbidity among children who are frequent attenders in general practice. *British Journal of General Practice*, **43**, 6–9.

Campo, J.V., Jansen-McWilliams, L., Comer, D.M. & Kelleher, K.J. (1999) Somatization in pediatric primary care: association with psychopathology, functional impairment, and use of services. *Journal of the American Academy of Child and Adolescent Psychiatry*, **38**, 1093–1101.

Chang, G., Warner, V. & Weissman, M.M. (1988) Physicians' recognition of psychiatric disorders in children and adolescents. *American Journal of Diseases of Children*, **142**, 736–739.

Corney, R.H. (1987) Marital problems and treatment outcome in depressed women: a clinical trial of social work intervention. *British Journal of Psychiatry*, **151**, 652–659.

Costello, E.J. & Edelbrock, C.S. (1985) Detection of psychiatric disorders in pediatric primary care: a preliminary report. *Journal of the American Academy of Child Psychiatry*, **24**, 771–777.

Costello, E.J., Costello, A.J., Edelbrock, C. et al. (1988) DSM-III disorders in pediatric primary care: prevalence and risk factors. *Archives of General Psychiatry*, **45**, 1105–1116.

Coverly, C.M., Garralda, M.E. & Bowman, F.M. (1995) Psychiatric intervention in primary care for mothers whose school children have psychiatric disorder. *British Journal of General Practice*, **45**, 235–237.

Cox, A. (1993) Preventative aspects of child psychiatry. In: *Managing Children with Psychiatric Problems* (ed. E. Garralda), pp. 179–207. British Medical Journal Publishing, London.

Cullen, K.J. (1976) A six-year controlled trial of prevention of children's behaviour disorders. *Journal of Pediatrics*, **88**, 662–666.

Cullen, K.J. & Cullen, A.M. (1996) Long-term follow-up of the Busselton six year controlled trial of prevention of children's behaviour disorders. *Journal of Pediatrics*, **129**, 136–139.

Cunningham-Burley, S. & Irvine, S. (1987) Practice research: 'And have you done anything so far?' An examination of lay treatment of children's symptoms. *British Medical Journal*, **295**, 700–702.

Donovan, C.F. & McCarthy, S. (1988) Is there a place for adolescent screening in general practice? *Health Trends*, **20**, 64–66.

Finney, J.W., Lemanek, K.L., Cataldo, M.F., Katz, H.P. & Fuqua, R.W. (1989) Paediatric psychology in primary care: brief targeted therapy for recurrent abdominal pain. *Behaviour Therapy*, **20**, 283–291.

Finney, J.W., Riley, A.W. & Cataldo, M.F. (1991) Psychology in primary health care: effects of brief targeted therapy on children's medical care utilisation. *Journal of Paediatric Psychology*, **16**, 447–461.

Garralda, M.E. & Bailey, D. (1986a) Psychological deviance in children attending general practice. *Psychological Medicine*, **16**, 423–429.

Garralda, M.E. & Bailey, D. (1986b) Children with psychiatric disorders in primary care. *Journal of Child Psychology and Psychiatry*, **27**, 611–624.

Garralda, M.E. & Bailey, D. (1987) Psychosomatic aspects of children's consultations in primary care. *European Archives of Psychiatry and Neurological Sciences*, **236**, 319–322.

Garralda, M.E. & Bailey, D. (1988) Child and parental factors related to the referral of children to child psychiatry. *British Journal of Psychiatry*, **153**, 81–89.

Garralda, M.E. & Bailey, D. (1989) Psychiatric disorders in general paediatric referrals. *Archives of Disease in Childhood*, **64**, 1727–1733.

Garralda, M.E. & Bailey, D. (1990) Paediatric identification of psychological factors associated with general paediatric consultations. *Journal of Psychosomatic Research*, **34**, 303–312.

Garralda, M.E., Bowman, F.M. & Mandalia, S. (1999) Children with psychiatric disorders who are frequent attenders to primary care. *European Child and Adolescent Psychiatry*, **8**, 33–44.

Garralda, M.E., Yates, P. & Higginson, I. (2000) Child and adolescent mental health service use: HONOSCA as an outcome measure. *British Journal of Psychiatry*, **177**, 52–58.

Gask, L., Sibbald, B. & Creed, F. (1997) Evaluating models of working at the interface between mental health services and primary care. *British Journal of Psychiatry*, **170**, 6–11.

Giel, R., de Arango, M.V., Climent, C.E. et al. (1981) Childhood mental disorders in primary health care: results of observations in 4 developing countries. *Pediatrics* **68**, 677–683.

Giel, R., Harding, T.W., ten Horn, G.M.H.H. et al. (1988) The detection of childhood mental disorders in primary care in some developing countries. In: *Handbook of Studies on Social Psychiatry* (eds A.S. Henderson & G.D. Burrows), pp. 233–244. Elsevier, Amsterdam.

Goldberg, I.D., Regier, D.A., McInerny, T.K., Pless, I.B. & Roughmann, K.J. (1979) The role of the pediatrician in the delivery of mental services to children. *Pediatrics*, **63**, 898–909.

Goldberg, I.D., Roughmann, K.J., McInerny, T.K. & Burke, J.D. (1984) Mental health problems among children seen in pediatric practice: prevalence and management. *Pediatrics*, **73**, 278–292.

Graham, H., Senior, R., Lazarus, M. et al. (1992) Family therapy in general practice: views of referrers and clients. *British Journal of General Practice*, **42**, 25–28.

Graham, P. (1982) Child psychiatry in relation to primary health care. *Social Psychiatry*, **17**, 109–116.

Gureje, O., Omigbodun, O.O., Gater, R., Acha, R.A., Ikuesan, B.A. & Morris, J. (1994) Psychiatric disorders in a paediatric primary care clinic. *British Journal of Psychiatry*, **165**, 530–533.

Gutelius, M.F., Kirsch, A.D., MacDonald, S., Brooks, M.R. & McErlean, T. (1977) Controlled study of child health supervision: behavioural results. *Pediatrics*, **60**, 294–304.

Hughes, T., Garralda, M.E. & Tylee, A. (1995) *Child Mental Health Problems*. St. Mary's Hospital Medical School, London.

Jacobson, A.M., Irving, D.G., Goldberg, I.D. et al. (1980) Diagnosed mental health disorder in children and use of health services in four organized health care settings. *American Journal of Psychiatry*, **137**, 559–565.

Jellinek, M.S., Murphy, J.M. & Burn, B.J. (1986) Brief psychosocial screening in outpatient pediatric practice. *Journal of Pediatrics*, **109**, 371–378.

Jewell, D. & Bain, J. (1985) Common childhood problems, variations in management. *British Medical Journal*, **291**, 941–944.

Kendrick, T. (2000) Depression management clinics in general practice? Some aspects lend themselves to the mini-clinic approach. *British Medical Journal*, **320**, 527–528.

Klasen, H. & Goodman, R. (2000) Parents and GPs at cross-purposes over hyperactivity: a qualitative study of possible barriers to treatment. *British Journal of General Practice*, **50**, 199–202.

Kramer, T. & Garralda, M.E. (1998) Psychiatric disorders in adolescents in primary care. *British Journal of Psychiatry*, **173**, 508–513.

Laclave, L.J. & Campbell, J.L. (1986) Psychiatric intervention in children: sex differences in referral rates. *Journal of the American Academy of Child Psychiatry*, **24**, 430–432.

Lavigne, J.V., Arend, R., Rosenbaum, D. et al. (1998) Mental health service use among young children receiving pediatric primary care. *Journal of the American Academy of Child and Adolescent Psychiatry*, **37**, 1175–1183.

McCune, Y., Richardson, M.M. & Powell, J.A. (1984) Psychological health issues in pediatric practices: parents' knowledge and concerns. *Pediatrics*, **74**, 183–190.

Metz, J.R., Allen, C.M., Barr, G. & Shinefield, H. (1976) A pediatric screening examination for psychosocial problems. *Pediatrics*, **58**, 595–606.

Mitchell, A.K.R. (1985) Psychiatrists in primary health care settings. *British Journal of Psychiatry*, **147**, 371–379.

Monck, E., Graham, P., Richman, N. & Dobbs, R. (1994) Adolescent girls. I. Self-reported disturbance in a community population. *British Journal of Psychiatry*, **165**, 760–769.

Offord, D.R., Boyle, M.H., Szatmari, P. *et al.* (1987) Ontario Child Health Study. II. Six-month prevalence of disorder and rates of service utilization. *Archives of General Psychiatry*, **44**, 832–836.

Olds, D.L., Eckenrade, J., Henderson, C.R. *et al.* (1997) Long-term effects of home visitation on maternal life course and child abuse and neglect. *Journal of the American Medical Association*, **278**, 637–643.

OPCS (1995) *Morbidity Statistics from General Practice*. HMSO, London.

Richman, N., Stevenson, J. & Graham, P.J. (1982) *Pre-school to School: A Behavioural Study*. Academic Press, London.

Roghmann, K.J. & Haggerty, R.J. (1972) Family stress and the use of health services. *International Journal of Epidemiology*, **1**, 279–286.

Sanci, L.A., Coffey, C.M.M., Veit, F.C.M. *et al.* (2000) Evaluation of the effectiveness of an educational intervention for general practitioners in adolescent health care: randomised controlled trial. *British Medical Journal*, **320**, 224–229.

Schor, E.L. (1986) Use of health care services by children and diagnoses received during presumably stressful life transitions. *Pediatrics*, **77**, 834–841.

Starfield, B., Gross, E., Wood, M. *et al.* (1980) Psychosocial and psychosomatic diagnoses in primary care of children. *Pediatrics*, **66**, 159–167.

Strathdee, G. & Williams, P. (1984) A survey of psychiatrists in primary care: the silent growth of a new service. *Journal of the Royal College of General Practitioners*, **34**, 615–618.

Subotsky, F. & Brown, R.M. (1990) Working alongside the general practitioner: a child psychiatric clinic in the general practice setting. *Child Health Care Development*, **16**, 189–196.

Upton, M.W.M., Evans, M., Goldberg, D.P. & Sharp, D.J. (1999) Evaluation of ICD-10 PHC mental health guidelines in detecting and managing depression within primary care. *British Journal of Psychiatry*, **175**, 476–482.

Wasserman, R.C., Barriatua, R.D., Carter, W.B. & Lippincott. B.A. (1984) Pediatric clinician's support for parents makes a difference: an outcome based on analysis of clinician parent interaction. *Pediatrics*, **74**, 1047–1063.

Webster-Stratton, C. (1998) Preventing conduct problems in Head Start children: strengthening parenting competencies. *Journal of Consulting and Clinical Psychology*, **66**, 715–730.

Westman, A. & Garralda, M.E. (1996) Mental health promotion for young adolescents in primary care: a feasibility study. *British Journal of General Practice*, **46**, 317.

Wickberg, B. & Hwang, P.C. (1996) Counselling of postnatal depression: a controlled study on a population based Swedish sample. *Journal of Affective Disorders*, **39**, 209–216.

Wolraich, M.L., Lindgren, S., Stromquist, A., Milich, R., Davis, C. & Watson, D. (1990) Stimulant medication use by primary care physicians in the treatment of attention deficit hyperactivity disorder. *Pediatrics*, **86**–101.

Woodward, C.A., Boyle, M.H., Offord, D.R. *et al.* (1988) Ontario Child Health Study: patterns of ambulatory medical care utilization and their correlates. *Pediatrics*, **82**, 425–434.

Zito, J.M., Safer, D.J., dosReis, S., Gardner, J.F., Boles, M. & Lynch, F. (2000) Trends in the prescribing of psychotropic medications to preschoolers. *Journal of the American Medical Association*, **283**, 1025–1030.

66 Genetic Counselling

Emily Simonoff

Genetic counselling and the role of the genetic counsellor

Genetic counselling is distinctive from other topics discussed in this book. The nature of the clinical contact could not be described as treatment, although at times it may be therapeutic. Other consultations focus on the diagnosis and treatment of a health problem, or upon surveillance to ensure a health problem does not occur. In genetic counselling, by contrast, whether or not the client is affected, the contact centres on the sharing of information in order to allow the client to make fully informed decisions. Genetic counselling focuses on providing clients with a range of information that will allow them to make informed decisions with regard to family planning (Kelly 1986). A range of areas may require coverage to achieve this. First, a discussion of the nature of the disorder is important so that the clients have a clear conception of the potential range and severity of the disorder, the impact on the quality of life and the treatment options open. Secondly, it is necessary to ensure that clients appreciate the mode of transmission of the disorder and how this influences the risk of being affected. Thirdly, the options for determining whether particular individuals are at risk either of being carriers or affected require discussion, together with the potential implications when this is detected. Finally, genetic counselling may consider the choices available to couples considering prenatal planning to reduce the likelihood of having an affected child.

Genetic counselling is an educational and consultative, rather than a prescriptive service. People presenting for genetic counselling often do not have a health problem at the time of presentation. Because the goals for genetic counselling are primarily educational, the counselling process tends to be driven more by the patient or client than would be the case in many medical or psychiatric consultations. Although the term 'counselling' is used, the type and extent of this process is rather different in genetic than in mental health counselling. Most consultations will extend from one to three visits only and, where there is more than one consultation, many of the additional visits are information-gathering rather than 'counselling'. Unlike mental health counselling, where an objective may be to enhance understanding of one's emotional state and explore alternative ways of managing difficult situations, genetic counselling rarely takes on such an introspective dialogue but rather focuses on communication of information necessary to help clients make informed choices.

Changes in genetic counselling over time

The recognition of familial transmission of some diseases and a desire to influence marriage and family planning dates back as far as the Talmud, when the nature of haemophilia was recognized (Walker 1996). Key shifts in genetic counselling have followed from an understanding of genetic mechanisms. The earliest phase occurred in the post-Mendelian era, when there was an appreciation of the modes of single gene inheritance, but where there was no ability to determine whether presymptomatic individuals carried the gene or not. In that period, diagnosis of the medical disorder and determination of the mode of inheritance were key features of the counselling process, which was generally led by a medical geneticist. Problems occurred when diagnosis was uncertain, when the relationship between diagnosis and mode of inheritance was variable, or when non-Mendelian inheritance occurred. The information given to families was limited information based on the mode of transmission and their place in the pedigree. There were also serious abuses of the limited scientific information during the eugenics movement. Inaccurate conclusions were drawn about the inheritance of mental retardation and psychiatric disorders in one generation and the probability of their occurrence in subsequent generations. A coercive approach to family planning, including forced sterilization, was taken in a number of countries. Despite a radical change in the 1940s with respect to the role of the genetic counsellor and government in relation to reproductive choices, genetic counselling remained limited by scientific knowledge.

Genetic counselling changed with the advent of accurate biological markers of disease and especially molecular genetic techniques. The advance here was to identify *within* affected families those individuals who will develop or pass on the disorder. A number of new activities developed at this point. For autosomal recessive and X-linked disorders, this involved the detection of carrier states. For autosomal dominant disorders of late onset, early diagnosis, with all its complexities, became possible. Prenatal diagnosis was feasible for a range of serious disorders, allowing couples at risk selectively to terminate pregnancies of affected fetuses. As other medical advances have occurred, preimplantation diagnosis has allowed couples to select unaffected embryos for implantation and avoid the distress of therapeutic abortion. These genetic advances opened the possibility of population-based screening programmes.

Further developments have occurred when advances in genetics have provided an explanation to patterns of inheritance that had previously proved puzzling. One such breakthrough occurred with fragile X, where the elucidation of the expanding trinucleotide repeats explained the 'Sherman paradox' (Sherman *et al.* 1985) in which males appeared normal although their position in a pedigree indicated they must carry the disease gene and, under the expectations of X-linked inheritance, should have expressed the disorder. The determination that fragile X represented a *dynamic mutation* that changed over generations not only explained the puzzling inheritance pattern but also allowed more accurate information to be given to family members (although in some cases there is also greater uncertainty). The accuracy of prediction of risk and disease severity has improved for other dynamic mutations, including Huntington disease and myotonic dystrophy. Similar advances occurred with respect to *imprinting* (see Skuse & Kuntsi, Chapter 13), in which parent of origin for the mutation may affect the phenotype, and *mitochondrial inheritance* (Clarke 2000) in which DNA is almost exclusively inherited from the mother.

A further stage in genetic counselling is just beginning, with two key advances. One is in the detection of *susceptibility genes*, or genes of minor effect. Unlike the genes of major effect that account for Mendelian disorders, susceptibility genes increase the risk of disease but they are neither necessary nor sufficient for its development. Other factors, genetic and/or environmental, must be present for disease expression. Most common diseases, including the bulk of psychiatric disorders, are ones in which the genetic contribution is of this type. Furthermore, the variants of genes influencing risk of the disorder occur at high frequencies in the general population, unlike the rare mutations in Mendelian disorders. The role of the dopamine D_4 receptor (DRD4) in attention deficit hyperactivity disorder (ADHD) provides such an example. A number of studies confirm that the presence of a set of allelic variants, present in some 15–20% of the population, increases the risk of ADHD by a factor of 1.5 (Thapar *et al.* 1999). However, many individuals with ADHD may not have the high-risk DRD4 allele and others who do have it do not have ADHD.

Current developments in genetic counselling are also influenced by the advances in techniques that detect smaller chromosomal abnormalities (see Skuse & Kuntsi, Chapter 13). Cytogenetic screening for major chromosomal abnormalities in people presenting with a range of physical and psychological abnormalities has been performed for several decades, but now new cytogenetic and molecular techniques can detect more subtle variations where the distinction between normality and abnormality is less clear. Counselling families with respect to such findings can be difficult as it may be unclear whether to consider the finding as aetiologically relevant. Even when an aetiological link seems likely, the range of the phenotype associated with a new abnormality may not be defined, making it difficult to give useful genetic counselling.

Tasks of the genetic counsellor

A range of professionals are involved in genetic counselling. Clinical geneticists are medically trained with advanced training in genetics. Much of genetic counselling is carried out by other medical doctors who diagnose and treat genetic disorders, and by obstetricians in relation to prenatal screening. Genetic counsellors come from a variety of non-medical backgrounds, including nursing and social work, but have developed specialist knowledge of genetics and counselling. Professionals with a more pure scientific background have a key role in developing and interpreting diagnostic tests. If the anticipated demands for genetic testing in the future are made, it may be that primary health care providers will need training to deliver information regarding testing and risks (Reynolds & Benkendorf 1999). Within this chapter, the terms 'genetic counsellor' and 'geneticist' are used interchangeably to refer to all these individuals. Because genetic counselling deals with a wide range of situations, the tasks for the counsellor may vary, as summarized in Table 66.1. For any one clinical situation, aspects of the clinical problem may overlap (e.g. making a diagnosis if a genetic disorder in one child may lead to pre-conception counselling in relation to future children). Nevertheless, because each clinical problem requires slightly different tasks from the geneticist, they are considered separately.

Diagnosis of genetic disorders

Geneticists may be called upon to help make a diagnosis of a genetic disorder, either prenatally or later. A range of medical skills is required for the task and diagnosis may be based on a characteristic history, physical examination for congenital anomalies and dysmorphic features, and laboratory investigations, including genetic tests. Although it is increasingly possible to detect mutations, most diagnoses of Mendelian disorders are initially made on the basis of other features, although molecular testing may be used to confirm clinical opinion. Diagnostic issues with respect to chromosomal anomalies are somewhat different. When the observed chromosomal anomaly has been previously linked to the phenotype observed, cytogenetics is often the definitive diagnostic tool. Determining whether there is a risk for other family members usually involves parental chromosomal analysis to determine whether the abnormality has arisen *de novo* (in which case the risk to other family members is small) or whether one parent carries a balanced translocation or even the same abnormality (in which case the risk may be substantial). The wider family is unlikely to be at risk.

Once a diagnosis is confirmed, the geneticist needs ample time to discuss it with the affected person and/or their family, bearing in mind that the information may represent a double tragedy: confirmation that something is seriously wrong and also that other family members are at risk. This may be a time when the family needs considerable extra support. While it is appropriate that the genetic counsellor is available, the potential benefit of

Table 66.1 Tasks undertaken as part of genetic counselling.

Type of clinical problem	Tasks to be undertaken
1 Diagnosis of genetic disorder	Use of appropriate physical examination and medical/genetic investigations to determine presence of genetic disorder
	Advise individual and/or family of nature and impact of disorder
	Counsel family on implications of disorder for affected individual and support family in adjusting to diagnosis
	Consider risk for wider family and determine method of communication
2 Preconception counselling for couples at risk	Confirm nature of couple's risk (diagnosis of disorder and mode of inheritance)
	Explanation of degree of risk and nature of disorder
	Consider appropriateness of medical/genetic tests on couple (carrier testing)
	Consider prenatal diagnosis
3 Prenatal diagnosis	Counsel couple on prenatal diagnostic strategies
	Counsel couple with positive screening result
	Counsel couple with definite fetal abnormality
4 Presymptomatic testing	Discuss utility of results for screening and treatment of affected individuals
	Consider financial and psychological drawbacks of identification
	Consider impact on wider family
	Specific considerations attached to testing of children
5 Carrier determination	Education about risks to client and offspring
	Determination of appropriateness of carrier testing
6 Population screening for:	Advise on practical feasibility, sensitivity and specificity of population screening
Disorders where early diagnosis and treatment is possible	Advise/manage characteristics distinguishing genetic from other screening programmes
Moderately rare disorders with significant impact on quality of life and/or longevity	Complete or shared management of screening programmes
Common, usually genetically complex disorders	Monitor effectiveness of screening in relation to enhanced population understanding of individual risk and altered reproductive behaviour

lay support groups for the disorder should be considered. The geneticist should have a clear plan about informing families of the potential risk to other family members. It is often tempting when families are distressed to postpone discussion of the genetic basis of the disorder. While this may be appropriate in the acute phase of adjusting to the diagnosis, the risk of delay is that the family could move on to other professionals for further treatment without being apprised of the genetic aspects of the disorder. Risk also needs to be discussed in the context of the wider family and a plan made for how others will be contacted. This may be a particularly sensitive topic when there has been little communication between braches of the family or if there has been a rift. In some cases, this is expedited if communication is initiated from doctor to doctor. Going against the wishes of the patient to inform other family members is undesirable because of the violation of confidentiality and requires careful weighing up of the conflicting ethical issues.

Pre-conception counselling for couples at risk

Couples present for genetic counselling because they believe themselves to be at risk of having an affected child. A necessary first step is confirmation of the putative diagnosis and its mode of inheritance. Although this may prove difficult, it is essential to obtain as clear a picture as possible, as basing information on an incorrect diagnosis can lead to highly inaccurate risks. Family history for both sides is important to clarify that the risk is not compounded, as well as to reduce guilt and blame. As for all tasks in genetic counselling, it is important to ensure that the couple have a full and accurate understanding of the disorder under consideration. Where the affected relative was distant, they may have no direct experience of the disorder. On the other hand, first-hand experience may be biased with respect to severity or management of the disease in the relative, and the couple may have a distorted view. The discussion of the disorder should take into account both the impact of the disorder on the child and family and also the types of treatment that are currently available. Some consideration of treatments likely to be available in the future is also helpful.

Depending upon the disorder and its mode of inheritance, it may be possible to define the couple's risk more accurately with genetic tests. On Mendelian principles, a normal sibling of someone affected with an autosomal recessive disorder (such as phenylketonuria) has a two in three chance of being a heterozygote carrier and a one in three chance of not carrying the gene. Similarly, a person whose parent has a late onset autosomal dominant disorder (such as Huntington disease) has a one in two chance of inheriting the disorder and a similar chance of being normal. For many disorders, molecular tests can indicate who carries the mutation.

The issues surrounding this testing in relation to the individuals are discussed under carrier detection and presymptomatic testing, respectively. Although there are other important considerations, it should be borne in mind that test results could define a couple's risk more precisely. Finally, should the couple decide they wish to have children, the options for prenatal diagnosis should be discussed.

Prenatal diagnosis

The aim of prenatal diagnosis is to detect severe abnormalities (both genetic and otherwise) at an early stage of fetal development. In most cases, this is to allow parental choice on whether to continue with the pregnancy; in rare cases, it is to allow prenatal intervention. A number of features should be in place before considering prenatal diagnosis with a view to potential termination (Harper 1998).

1 The disorder must be sufficiently severe to warrant termination of pregnancy.
2 The treatment options should be absent or unsatisfactory.
3 Termination of an affected pregnancy should be acceptable to the couple considering prenatal diagnosis.
4 An accurate prenatal diagnostic test must be available.
5 There should be a reasonable chance that the pregnancy is affected.

In relation to child psychiatry, prenatal diagnosis currently is only available for disorders associated with mental retardation, such as fragile X and Down syndrome. However, this is likely to change in the next decade as susceptibility genes for severely disabling disorders such as autism are identified.

Three main clinical situations arise in relation to prenatal diagnosis. As indicated above, a couple who present for preconception genetic counselling may choose to take up a prenatal diagnostic test. In such cases, the geneticist will have been involved from an early stage and have ensured that the criteria outlined above are met. Second, and more commonly, a couple may have a positive result from a routine prenatal screening, either by blood tests (the most common being for Down syndrome and neural tube defects) or by fetal ultrasound. This is discussed in more detail below, under Population Screening. Finally, geneticists may be called in when a prenatal diagnostic test arranged by the obstetrician is abnormal. The role of the geneticist will be to clarify the effects of the abnormality and to support the couple in making a decision whether to proceed with the pregnancy and in adjusting to that decision.

Prenatal diagnosis is possible for chromosomal abnormalities and for many Mendelian disorders. The most commonly used techniques are amniocentesis and chorionic villous sampling (CVS; Wilson 2000). Amniocentesis is the first choice for low-risk pregnancies where cytogenetic abnormalities are in question. Although it is the safer technique, a potential drawback is

timing: sampling is best performed at 15–16 weeks' gestation and a result is often not available before 18 weeks. CVS, which usually takes place at 10–12 weeks, provides good samples for molecular and enzymatic analysis but has a higher complication rate. The technique of isolating for genetic analysis fetal blood cells that are normally present in the maternal circulation is still under evaluation; the technique appeals because of its lack of invasiveness, but circulating fetal cells are rare and its reliability in detecting fetal abnormalities has not yet been adequately demonstrated (Goldberg 1997).

Presymptomatic testing

Molecular genetic tests allowing detection of genetic mutations that will subsequently lead to a disorder in currently healthy persons, or presymptomatic testing, is frequently considered in families with later onset disorders, but raises many difficult issues. Presymptomatic testing should be differentiated according to whether there are any therapeutic implications of a positive test result. In some conditions, including the hereditary cancers (both early onset, such as familial adenomatous polyposis, and later onset, such as breast/ovarian cancer as a result of *BRCA1* and *BRCA2*), a positive presymptomatic result has direct implications for screening and surveillance of individuals carrying the mutation, whereas a negative test result obviates the need for such time-consuming, expensive and sometimes uncomfortable investigations. For other conditions, such as Huntington disease, there are at present no therapeutic consequences of a positive result and the reasons for requesting testing are more complex. The uptake of presymptomatic testing has, not surprisingly, varied according to treatment implications of a positive result. Uptake for Huntington disease has been around 10–20% (Crauford *et al.* 1989; Quaid & Morris 1993), compared with about 50% for hereditary breast cancer, where early treatment is uncertain, and 80% for familial adenomatous polyposis, for which early surgical intervention has a significant health impact (Harper 1998).

The emphasis will vary depending upon the extent to which genetic status has therapeutic implications, but in all cases pre- and post-test counselling should discuss several issues, as well as the potential medical benefits. Pre-test counselling should explore the impact on family relationships. The test results of one family member have implications for the risk of others. If a grandchild of a person affected with Huntington disease tests positive, this implies that his or her parent also carries the gene, and that parent usually gains knowledge of this, even if he or she did not wish to be tested. Impact on reproductive plans should be raised and the extent of family support in relation to both positive and negative results, especially if a number of family members are being tested. Counselling should also consider the potential effect of a positive result on employment and health insurance. Although the studies are limited (Braidstock *et al.*, 2000) and individual responses vary widely (Wahlin *et al.* 1997), follow-up studies of Huntington disease where careful pre- and post-test counselling is given do not indicate that there is greater long-standing emotional distress following test results and, furthermore, that emotional status is not predicted by whether the test is positive or negative (Braidstock *et al.*, 2000).

With regard to presymptomatic testing of children, there is agreement amongst geneticists that children should not be tested for disorders for which there are no therapeutic consequences until they are of an age to give consent themselves (Clarke *et al.* 1994). A survey indicated that non-geneticists were more likely to offer presymptomatic and carrier testing of children at parental request; one commonly stated reason for testing was to reduce parental anxiety (Clarke *et al.* 1994). Although the impact has not been examined in children, it is noteworthy that the adult studies did not find reduction in anxiety to be a long-term effect of testing (Braidstock *et al.*, 2000). In relation to diseases such as cancers in which a positive test result may alter the screening practice, it has been proposed that genetic testing should be permitted at an age no sooner than the earliest age of onset of first cancer (Kodish 1999). Such a policy has the advantage of delaying testing in some cases until an age at which children can participate in the consent process while not jeopardizing the child's health.

Carrier detection

A carrier is someone who carries a single copy of a genetic mutation (and also a single copy of a normal gene, making them *heterozygous*) and is healthy at the time of study. Some individuals, by their position in the pedigree, are potential or obligate carriers. With the exception of carriers of late onset dominant disorders, carrier status is therefore of importance only for subsequent generations. The risk that offspring of a carrier will be affected will vary, depending upon the mode of inheritance. Under autosomal recessive inheritance, if both parents are carriers, on average one in four offspring will be affected and two in four carriers. With autosomal dominant transmission, 50% of children on average will inherit the gene (and disorder). Because many autosomal dominant disorders have variable expression or reduced penetrance, where the disease apparently skips a generation, a one-to-one correspondence between genotype and phenotype cannot be assumed, and specific tests to determine carrier status may be appropriate. Under X-linked inheritance, where the mutation is passed on by a female carrier, 50% of all males will develop the disorder and 50% of female offspring will be carriers. Where the mutation is passed on by an affected father, all female offspring will be carriers whereas all males will be normal. Female carriers will vary in phenotype, depending upon X inactivation. Advances in molecular genetics have revolutionized carrier detection and either molecular or other biological markers are available for many disorders. When the gene responsible for the disorder has been identified, carrier testing can be virtually 100% accurate. When there is only rough gene location from linkage strategies, genetic status will be less certain.

The first task for the genetic counsellor is to ensure that the client understands the mode of transmission and chances that their children will be affected. For autosomal recessive disorders, the partner must also be a carrier for the offspring to be affected. For a rare recessive disorder with a general population prevalence of 1 in 40 000, the risk of a partner also being a carrier is 1 in 100 and the risk of an offspring being affected 1 in 400. However, if the carrier is from a special population in which the prevalence is higher, and is also likely to marry within that population, as with Tay–Sachs disease and Ashkenazi Jews, the risks of a partner also being a carrier may be substantially greater. For autosomal dominant and X-linked disorders, it is generally not important to consider the partner's genotype, but the chances of offspring being affected are very much greater. There are no clear thresholds of recurrence risk for deciding when carrier detection should be carried out and risk to offspring should be considered along with ease of carrier detection and the wishes of the client.

Although parents with one affected child may press to have other children tested for carrier status, this should be resisted until the children themselves are of an age to give informed consent (Clarke *et al.* 1994). In cystic fibrosis where genetic carrier testing has been available for some years, uptake amongst siblings of affected people has been poor. A number of reasons have been identified, including the difficulty their parents have discussing genetic issues and feeling that affected siblings would have difficulty accepting their decision to be tested (Fanos & Johnson 1995a). The finding that beliefs about carrier status were not influenced by educational or income level suggests that emotional issues play an important part in attitudes about screening (Fanos & Johnson 1995b).

Population screening

Population screening involves identifying those with genetic disorders or at risk of having offspring with genetic disorders amongst the general population or large subgroups of the general population. The two main aims of population screening are detecting diseases for which early treatment improves prognosis and the identification of severe disorders in fetuses, or a genetic risk of such disorders, to allow couples to make informed reproductive decisions. There is a potential conflict between the public health aim of reducing disease and the genetic counsellor's desire to maximize individual choices. Population screening may occur at four time points.

1 Prenatal screening to detect fetal abnormalities and diseases for which termination, or treatment, would be considered is routinely conducted through ultrasound for structural abnormalities and maternal blood testing (for Down syndrome and neural tube defects).

2 Newborn screening detects treatable disorders, such as phenylketonuria and sickle cell anaemia. The possibility of using newborn screening to identify severe but untreatable disorders, such as Duchenne muscular dystrophy, so that parents are aware of the genetic risk prior to the birth of a sibling, has been more controversial.

3 Population screening in adult life for common carrier states, such as cystic fibrosis and beta thalassaemia, has been implemented in a limited fashion.

4 Population screening has started for common genetic variants that may influence disease, both in a Mendelian pattern, such as hypercholesterolaemia associated with low density lipoprotein (LDL) receptor abnormalities, and as a susceptibility allele, such as apolipoprotein (Apo) E4 in late onset Alzheimer's disease. Cascade screening is an intermediate strategy involving systematic contact of more distant at-risk family members with the offer of testing.

Genetic population screening differs from other forms of population screening not by the nature of the test (indeed, many of the screens do not look directly for mutations) but rather because it detects disease of genetic origin, for which there may be implications for other family members. A general criticism of many of the genetic screening programmes is their failure to evaluate the wider family impact of screening. Many of the principles of population screening have emanated from screening of family members of affected individuals; however, it is not clear that this extrapolation is appropriate in relation to informed decision-making or the psychological consequences of screening (Marteau & Croyle 1998).

Unlike individual genetic testing regarding a disorder that has occurred in the family, in population screening clients may have little knowledge of the disorder. There is a general concern about the extent to which informed consent is obtained for screening. In relation to screening for Down syndrome, although the findings suggest that all women wish to be given the choice whether or not to participate in such screening, the policies in many centres may not be presented as voluntary and women may not be given sufficient information to make informed decisions (Al-Jader *et al.* 2000). Furthermore, screening tests such as the triple marker serum test for Down syndrome have a high false-positive rate and moderate specificity (Piggott *et al.* 1994). A lack or misinterpretation of information subsequent to a positive serum result (indicative of significant but still low risk) is common (Gekas *et al.* 1999) and some of the associated distress of a positive screening result might be avoidable with better pre-test information (Hall *et al.* 2000).

The finding that the higher the rate of participation in testing, the poorer the quality of information is of considerable concern (Marteau & Croyle 1998). Those who take part in population screening usually perceive themselves at low risk and expectations of a negative result may lead to higher levels of distress when a positive one is received. The problem of potential false reassurance has been highlighted in cystic fibrosis, where negative test results may exclude only some of the cystic fibrosis mutations but may lead test participants to believe they are definitely not carriers (Axworthy *et al.* 1996; Clausen *et al.* 1996b). Being informed of carrier status may have impact on one's self-perception. Although cystic fibrosis carrier status has no impact on health of carriers, there is variation in reports with some suggesting that those informed of carrier status can have a more negative perception of their own health (Axworthy *et al.* 1996; Clausen *et al.* 1996a).

There has been considerable debate over the merits of population screening for fragile X. As the most commonly inherited form of mental retardation, detection with genetic counselling has the potential to promote greater reproductive choice. A cascade system was evaluated in Australia, with detection of fragile X from those presenting with developmental delay/mental retardation followed by genetic testing of all relatives at risk for the disorder or carrier status (Turner *et al.* 1997). Uptake of testing amongst relatives was high, with a substantial reduction in the rate of children born with fragile X. However, the recommendations from the American College of Medical Genetics are that population screening for the carrier state should not be conducted at present because of concerns about whether consent to such testing and its wider implications could be reliably informed (Park *et al.* 1994).

There are further concerns about informed consent and decision-making with respect to 'multiplex' genetic testing, which is likely to be increasingly available from primary care doctors. Multiplex tests assess a person's genotype for a range of different genes, much in the way current laboratory tests determine a range of blood chemistries. However, current testing kits are not organized to assess genetic risk for a particular condition, e.g. to examine a range of risk genotypes for atherosclerotic disease. Because the use of such tests may provide the simplest and least expensive way to assess risk for one condition, there is concern that unwanted genetic information in relation to a different gene may be acquired, and without fully informed consent (Council on Ethical and Judicial Affairs 1998).

Practical aspects of genetic counselling

Referral for genetic counselling

It is useful to consider at the referral stage whether a request for genetic counselling is appropriate. Almost all child psychiatric disorders show some degree of genetic risk (Rutter *et al.* 1999; see also McGuffin & Rutter, Chapter 12), but this does not mean genetic counselling is necessarily appropriate. The quality and precision of the evidence in favour of genetic factors requires consideration. Table 66.2 presents a summary of disorders that may present in childhood in which it is thought that genetic factors have a significant role. Heritability refers to the proportion of variance explained by genetic factors in discriminating between those affected and those not, and it is important in determining the extent to which familial aggregation results from genetic vs. environmental factors. The sibling recurrence risk is helpful to families in giving practical information about the probability of having another affected child. This recurrence risk will include both genetic and environmental causes of recurrence. There is an absence of firm data for either statistic for several of the disorders, including obsessive-compulsive disorder and anorexia nervosa, where it is commonly believed that genetic factors are important. Without such data, it is not possible to provide genetic counselling. A related consideration is the

Table 66.2 Psychiatric disorders with childhood onset and probable significant genetic aetiology*.

Disorder	Heritability	Sibling recurrence risk
Autism	>90% (Bailey *et al.* 1995)	5% (Bolton *et al.* 1994; Smalley *et al.* 1988), broader phenotype up to 30% in males, 10% in females (Bailey *et al.* 1998)
Idiopathic mental retardation	Unknown[†]	Mild retardation, no family history: 5–35%, higher when male index case positive family history in first-degree relative: 37–39% Severe retardation, no family history: 3–10% positive family history: 5–15% (Bundey & Carter 1974)
Attention deficit hyperactivity disorder	60–90% (Thapar *et al.* 1999)	Uncertain, perhaps as high as 25% (Biederman *et al.* 1986; Faraone *et al.* 1991)
Tourette syndrome	Unknown[†]	9% for Tourette, 17% for chronic tics, 11% for obsessive-compulsive disorder[§] (Pauls *et al.* 1991)
Bipolar disorder	~80% (McGuffin *et al.* 1994)	15–20% risk of severe affective disorder[§] (McGuffin & Katz 1986)
Obsessive-compulsive disorder	Unknown[†] (Pauls & Alsobrook 1999)	Variable from no increased risk to 17%, 10% best estimate[§] (Pauls & Alsobrook 1999)
Schizophrenia	60–70% (McGuffin *et al.* 1984)	10% if no first-degree relative affected; up to 45% if both parents affected; up to 45% if both parents affected (McGuffin *et al.* 1994)
Anorexia nervosa	Uncertain[‡] (Bulik *et al.* 2000)	Uncertain: 0–10% (Kipman *et al.* 1999)

*Includes only disorders where inheritance thought to be multifactorial.
†Indicates absence of studies with sufficient data to determine heritability/recurrence.
‡Indicates wide variability amongst currently available heritability/recurrence estimates.
§Risk is for first-degree relatives; no evidence of differential risk for parents and siblings.

consistency of the findings across studies for the role of genetic factors. For example, heritabilities of oppositional and conduct disorder vary from 7 to 74% without any clear explanation (Simonoff 2001), there is similar inconsistency for depressive symptoms (Simonoff 1995) and inadequate data on childhood anxiety disorders. It should be noted that many of the data on heritability involve symptoms rather than disorders and it remains to be demonstrated that genetic factors operate in the same way for symptoms and disorders.

A second consideration is the extent of impairment or disability caused by the problem. For example, traits such as emotionality and sociability are strongly genetic but infrequently impairing in their own right. Although professionals should not impose their view as to which traits or disorders are sufficiently undesirable to warrant genetic counselling, issues of severity, impairment and treatability should be considered by families and professionals alike.

The childhood disorder for which there is the strongest case for formal genetic counselling is autism (see Lord & Bailey, Chapter 38). Twin studies indicate a high heritability (Bailey *et al.* 1995) and several family studies concur that the sibling recurrence risk is 5–6% for autism and pervasive developmental disorder (Rutter *et al.* 1997). The disorder is lifelong, essentially untreatable, severely impairing and creates a heavy burden on families. Although individual genes are not yet isolated, there are replicated linkage findings from several groups and it is a

matter of time until individual genes are identified (International Molecular Genetic Study of Autism Consortium 1998; Barrett *et al.* 1999). As with almost all other genetically mediated child psychiatric disorders, the genetic influence appears to involve a number of susceptibility genes. At present, there is more systematic experience of genetic counselling in autism than any other child psychiatric disorder, bar mental retardation. Although formal genetic counselling may not be appropriate for some other child psychiatric disorders, it might be helpful for parents to know that genetic influences may play a part in their child's difficulties. This might particularly be the case if parents have inappropriately blamed themselves, but research is required.

When and by whom genetic counselling is delivered will vary. The clinicians diagnosing and caring for an affected child should alert the family to a genetic component. Whereas families may need to adjust to the diagnosis before genetic counselling is undertaken, it is important that they have access to genetic counselling before planning further children. If genetic counselling is to be offered by the clinician looking after affected family members, such counselling is best undertaken in an appointment specifically designated for this purpose.

Particular issues may arise when a child is being considered for adoption and there is a family history of a serious disorder. Genetic counselling may be sought from the social worker/adoption agency or prospective family. It is expected that adoption agencies discuss with prospective parents factors from the child's background, whether these are genetic risk, adverse experiences or known health problems, that might have an impact on child-rearing. Mental disorder in the birth parents may contribute to children being put up for adoption but many of these disorders will not be evident until adult life. For disorders such as Huntington disease, presymptomatic testing may be requested. In considering the child's best interests, there is a tension between ensuring that children placed for adoption will not subsequently be rejected, and protecting the child's right to choose whether or not to be tested at an age when they are able to consent independently. Although there are no firm guidelines at present, these are needed (Nuffield Council on Bioethics 1998); most practitioners consider that testing should be undertaken only in exceptional circumstances. In other instances, adoption agencies and prospective parents may request information about recurrence risk. It is generally good practice to provide interested parties with information about recurrence and also the nature of the disorder. Limitations may occur in gaining accurate information regarding both biological parents. The latter is important because of the evidence for strong assortative mating for severe psychiatric disorder (Mednick 1978). It has been suggested that adopted children might be informed about known genetic risks from their birth parents at age 18, when they are able to request knowledge of the identity of their birth parents; otherwise, adopted children are at a disadvantage with respect to knowledge of their potential genetic risks (Nuffield Council on Bioethics 1998).

Assessment

A first step in genetic counselling is confirming the diagnosis in the proband. In some cases the referral may contain sufficient information, in others it may be necessary to obtain additional medical records or to examine the proband personally. The latter two are relatively straightforward when the couple seeking counselling are the parents of the proband. In other circumstances, the couple seeking counselling may feel uncomfortable about discussing this with other family members, particularly the parents of the proband. Further complications may occur for disorders like autism, where a developmental history is paramount for diagnosis and when the affected individual is now adult. Despite these challenges, every effort should be made to clarify the correct diagnosis. Table 66.2 demonstrates that the recurrence risks for autism and mental retardation may be very different, and these two disorders are easily confused with a sketchy retrospective history. The same would apply to autism and Rett syndrome, in which a gene on the X chromosome has been shown to cause at least some cases (Amir *et al.* 1999; Wan *et al.* 1999).

In taking a history and examining the proband, it is important to consider the possibility of identifiable medical/genetic causes of the disorder and also that of phenocopies. In relation to autism, 5–10% of cases may be caused by a recognized medical disorder, the most common of which will be tuberous sclerosis

and fragile X (Rutter *et al.* 1997). In such instances, the genetics of autism will be the genetics of the medical disorder; for both of the above disorders, this is substantially different from idiopathic autism. The term 'phenocopy' refers to a disorder that appears identical to the genetically mediated disorder but where the aetiological factors are very different. For practical purposes, this is usually where an environmental cause for the disorder can be identified. In autism, congenital rubella is one such cause. There has been much debate about whether the association of autism with obstetric complications (usually with milder levels of adversity) indicates a causative role (Goodman 1990); the further association of such complications with congenital anomalies suggests that abnormal development in the fetus may be responsible for the obstetric complications (Bailey *et al.* 1995; Bolton *et al.* 1997). Nevertheless, it is likely that severe perinatal adversity associated with structural brain damage could cause autism. The same applies to other causes of brain injury, including severe head injury or encephalitis. There is much debate currently about the possible ill-effects of the measles, mumps and rubella (MMR) vaccine (Wakefield *et al.* 1998), but there is a lack of scientific evidence for a causative role (Medical Controls Agency 1999; Taylor *et al.* 1999). The importance of identifying phenocopies for genetic counselling lies in the different expectations regarding recurrence risks. In such cases, the recurrence risk can be considered either as the prevalence rate in the general population or, if the environmental risk is familial, as the joint probability of recurrence of the environmental risk in a subsequent child and the chance that the environmental risk will cause the disorder. Although the latter probabilities are usually unknown, it is nevertheless useful to consider whether the relatives are at increased risk for the occurrence of a similar environmental event.

In gathering information, a systematic family history is crucial. This is aided by letting the family know prior to their appointment about the type of information required. Obtaining a family history has a range of aims. First, one is confirming that the pattern of inheritance fits with what is expected. In child psychiatric disorders that are usually multifactorial, finding a Mendelian pattern of inheritance alerts the clinician to the possibility of an alternative diagnosis or a chromosomal abnormality associated with the disorder. However, seeing a pattern consistent with Mendelian inheritance in a particular family is entirely different from inferring that Mendelian inheritance is occurring. In idiopathic autism, where there is a highly skewed sex ratio in favour of males, it would not be surprising for families to show a pattern of affected relatives consistent with X-linked inheritance. However, there is at present no evidence for susceptibility genes for autism on the X chromosome (International Molecular Genetic Study of Autism Consortium 1998) and it would be highly misleading to give the recurrence risks of X-linked disorders. When the findings in any one family differ from the characteristic picture, a number of possibilities should be considered. These include new mutations and non-paternity, as well as an absence of information or misinformation, possibly misdiagnosis, of other relatives.

Second, the occurrence of other disorders in the family history may also raise suspicions about the correct diagnosis. A history of fragile X in a maternal uncle might warrant re-examination of fragile X status in the proband. Related to this, a history of multiple miscarriages in the parents alerts suspicion to a possible chromosomal abnormality. Third, in multifactorial disorders where heavier family loading is thought to indicate greater disease liability within the family and therefore predict a higher recurrence risk for individuals (Carter 1976; Falconer 1981), such information might be used to alter the recurrence risk information given to families. In practice, there are few empirical data to vary recurrence risk dependent on family history for any of the child psychiatric disorders. One possible exception may be idiopathic mental retardation, as indicated in Table 66.2. It is not clear whether families with two autistic children should be given higher risks; 1 in 20 two-child families with an autistic child would be expected to have a second affected child. Fourth, in obtaining the family history, it is important to enquire about both sides of the family, even when it appears that risk is conferred by one side of the family only. However, the risk for the couple seeking counselling depends upon the genetic contribution of each side. The family history from the 'unaffected' side may reveal other genetically mediated problems of equal risk to the couple. Obtaining a family history from both sides has the added benefit of diffusing any possible blame of one side of the family.

Fifth, obtaining the family history often guides the clinician to the preconceived notions of the couple with regard to the cause of the disorder in their family. Quite unwarranted extrapolations about the behaviour of relatives, leading to blame of one side of the family or assumptions that the recurrence risk may be higher for their family, are not uncommon. Finally, the family history may alert one to current or past difficulties experienced by the parents that might interfere with their interpretation of information. In autism, an association with depression and other emotional disorders has been consistently described (Szatmari *et al.* 1991; Bolton *et al.* 1994; Smalley *et al.* 1995), although the cause is not understood (Bolton *et al.* 1998). Whatever the reason, depression amongst clients receiving genetic counselling could influence their perception of risk (Marteau 1999).

Communication

When families attend for genetic counselling, it is essential to clarify at the outset the questions they wish to have answered. It is helpful to find out who has sought the referral and, if not the family, how they view it. There will be a small minority of families who do not accept the diagnosis; without this preliminary, genetic counselling is unlikely to be helpful to families. Clients may have additional questions about the risk for other family members having an affected child; the usual policy is to give counselling only to the couple attending the clinic (while extending the invitation to see other family members if they wish and it is appropriate). A further question for families can be whether

there was a causal role of environmental factors. Families may wish to know whether there are any measures they can take to reduce the chances of having an affected child.

In feeding back on risk, it is important to discuss the range of severity. With autism, this includes the broader phenotype of speech and language delay, literacy problems and social eccentricities. Whereas these are substantially more common, they are also much less impairing and this is important to emphasize to families (Rutter *et al.* 1997). Similarly, the couple may be preoccupied with the risk of the disorder present in their family and it can be helpful to remind them of the risks that apply to all couples, which are roughly 1 in 50 of having a child with a significant mental or physical handicap.

There is a general view that genetic counselling should be non-directive, making information available to families but not advising them on how to proceed. In practice, this may be difficult to achieve. For example, in counselling families with regard to autism, giving a sibling recurrence risk of 5% may sound less than 1 in 20. Similarly, placing the emphasis on the 95% probability that a sibling will be unaffected sounds more positive. It is easy for phrases like 'only' or 'as high as' to slip in, giving the client a view of the counsellor's perspective. The view that counselling should be non-directive developed in response to the abuses during the eugenics movement. However, Michie *et al.* (1997) found that counsellors made an average of 5.8 'advice' comments and the same number of 'evaluative' comments per counselling session, throwing into question the perception of the counselling process as non-directive. This may not be undesirable; in another study, 80% of clients at risk for having an offspring with a blinding disease reported they wished to receive an opinion from their genetic counsellor on what course of action to take (Furu *et al.* 1993) and, in another study, patients receiving non-directive counselling perceived their risk to be higher than those obtaining more directive counselling, possibly feeling in the former case that the neutral counsellor was withholding information (Shiloh & Saxe 1989).

A great deal of information is exchanged during genetic counselling and often a range of different recurrence risks are given to families. It is advisable to write directly to families following the consultation to summarize the recurrence risk (and other) information they have been given. It may be appropriate to offer follow-up sessions to the clients, particularly if there is a large difference in how each member of the couple views the information they have been given.

Problems and limitations in counselling for child psychiatric disorders

Giving information with respect to recurrence risks depends crucially on correct identification of the disorder. Despite the advances in the last 15 years with respect to operationalized diagnoses, there remain a number of cases where individuals with a severe impairing disorder fall short of diagnostic thresholds or where symptomatology crosses over diagnostic boundaries (Angold *et al.* 1999). Because the genetic evidence comes from cases meeting the strictest criteria, it is unclear to what extent the same risks are applicable to clinical variants. In autism, this arises with respect to Asperger syndrome and other disorders of the broader phenotype, and where autism coexists with profound mental retardation or ADHD. Similar issues will apply to Tourette syndrome and the lesser phenotypes of transient and chronic motor tics and obsessive-compulsive disorder (Pauls *et al.* 1991). There are situations for which genetic counselling is requested and recurrence risks cannot be given. For example, people with high-functioning autism marrying and wishing to have their own families; there are no studies to guide them as, depending on the number of genes and whether they act dominantly or not, risks could be either higher or lower than the sibling recurrence risk.

A related issue is that of genetic heterogeneity. Where information on recurrence risks is available, it is based on the aggregate risk of all families with affected probands. Genetic heterogeneity is the rule and current diagnostic categories almost certainly include cases with varying degrees and types of genetic risk. Comparison of monozygotic twins with autism suggests that clinical features are unlikely to be a good marker of genetic heterogeneity, as the within-twin pair variance was essentially as great as that between twin pairs (Le Couteur *et al.* 1996). In giving families an averaged recurrence risk, it is possible that this is highly inaccurate for individual families. One of the ambitions of molecular genetics is to be able to give families more precise risks, but large studies of families will be necessary.

Future directions

It is certain that advances in molecular genetics will have massive effects on genetic counselling for child psychiatric disorders. As susceptibility genes are discovered, it is likely that the demand for genetic testing will increase, both among families with affected relatives and the general population. However, it is unclear as yet how helpful it will be in identifying the genetic status of individuals when the genotype relative risk (the risk of developing a disorder given a particular genotype) is in the region of 1.5–2, as has been reported for ApoE4 in Alzheimer's disease (Post *et al.* 1997) and DRD4 in ADHD (Thapar *et al.* 1999). For multigenic disorders, it so far appears that knowledge of genotypic status for one susceptibility gene modifies the empirical recurrence risk only slightly (Nuffield Council on Bioethics 1998). Being able to account for more than one gene will require knowledge of interaction among the genes being evaluated. Even if all susceptibility genes are discovered, the accuracy of individual risk will not exceed the concordance rate for monozygotic twins (who share all their genes), which is around 50–60% for many psychiatric disorders.

Key steps following the identification of susceptibility genes will include understanding the structure and function of the gene as a way of elucidating disease pathogenesis; clarifying the interplay amongst a range of genetic susceptibility factors to give more precise information about individual risk; and understanding the links between genetic susceptibility and environmental factors, both for aetiology and treatment (Rutter & Plomin 1997). Although a major long-term aim of the human genome project has been the identification of genes to allow more effective treatment of human disease, this has not yet been forthcoming, with developments in gene therapy being particularly disappointing (Li & Huang 2000). Treatments providing more specific environmental interventions may prove more effective. Discovery of susceptibility genes may also help to identify which environmental risks are sufficiently severe to cause disorder in the absence of genetic risk.

Implications for genetic counselling are potentially huge. With multiple susceptibility alleles, risk information for families is likely to be more complex and novel modalities for helping families to understand the information will be important. However, if the demand for genetic counselling increases, there may be a greater expectation that primary care will provide information (Reynolds & Benkendorf 1999). The anticipated demand for susceptibility gene testing will also need to be evaluated in relation to the potential diversion of health care resources from other activities. Furthermore, considerable effort is being put into identifying susceptibility genes for disorders where the magnitude of genetic risk factors and the phenotype they affect remain uncertain, such as anorexia nervosa. Although molecular genetic knowledge may help to answer these questions, it is possible that requests for counselling will precede sufficient knowledge for its delivery.

A related concern is that genes conferring susceptibility in a particular situation may be protective or beneficial in another. For example, the long repeat variant of the DRD4 allele has now been replicated in a number of studies as a risk allele for ADHD; however, a (unreplicated) study suggested that the alternative short repeat allele was a risk factor for Tourette syndrome (Grigorenko *et al.* 1997). Although this finding has not been replicated, it highlights the potential complexities that a genotype could increase risk for one disorder but be protective for another, or have selective advantage either in the heterozygous state or in combination with other genes or environments.

As susceptibility genes for multifactorial disorders are identified, research examining the interplay between genetic susceptibility and environmental risk will be considerably more fruitful. A key question will be whether knowledge of the genotype is helpful in developing prevention and treatment programmes, or whether these are more effectively applied to a wider population without knowledge of genotype. In part, this will depend on the extent to which genotypes have specific and powerful effects on the outcome of intervention; in further part, it will depend on the extent to which knowledge of genotype alters behaviour and compliance with treatment. It will be important to understand how genotypic information may influence people's perception and motivation (Marteau 1999). One experimental study suggested that giving genetic risk information as genetic rather than non-specific risk reduced people's perception of the disease as potentially preventable (Senior *et al.* 2000). In another study, smokers who were told they were genetically predisposed to develop lung cancer were not more likely to quit smoking, but were more fearful about the effects (Lerman *et al.* 1997). On the other hand, the finding that high-risk status, such as pregnancy and heart disease, may enhance success in quitting smoking highlights the importance of how risk and possibilities for change are presented (Law & Tang 1995). Much more knowledge is required about the impact of genetic testing on self-perception and health behaviour. With the identification of susceptibility genes for child psychiatric disorder, new pressures for testing children are likely to occur. As with Mendelian disorders, it will be important to weigh up the clear disadvantages of testing at an age when the child cannot give informed consent with the potential benefit.

The possibility that genotyping could be used for diagnostic purposes in child psychiatry has been raised. For Mendelian disorders, there has been a close correspondence between genetic mutation and diagnosis, although many disorders have more than one genetic cause. However, genotyping is often not used for diagnosis but rather for counselling family members. Although the present evidence is limited, susceptibility genes may affect more than one disorder; it has been suggested (but not yet confirmed in subsequent studies) that the same variant of DRD4 that increases susceptibility to ADHD is also associated with attachment disorders (Lakatos *et al.* 2000). It is unclear to what extent genotyping may help with planning treatment or determining prognosis, but current evidence suggests that pairs of monozygotic cotwins can vary enormously in phenotype (Le Couteur *et al.* 1996). It is as yet unclear what clinically useful information genotypic profiling will add to a careful consideration of the phenotype, and it is unlikely to replace the latter.

It is hoped that identification of susceptibility genes and individual gene testing will lead to more effective interventions. Pharmacogenetics is one area that may benefit, because variation in drug-metabolizing enzymes and receptor pharmacology is genetically influenced. Such analysis could detect variation indicating that drugs are less likely to be effective, may be most effective in different doses or in conjunction with another drug, or could produce more side-effects (Catalano 1999). On first sight, such testing would appear wholly beneficial, helping to target and specify treatment. However, the issues surrounding genotyping becomes more complicated if the variation that predicts drug response is also associated with other clinical characteristics, e.g. with worse prognosis, or probability of recurrence. It has been suggested that identification of susceptibility alleles will allow early detection of individuals at risk (Rutter & Plomin 1997), but it remains to be seen whether this will be viable, with regard both to the size and cost of the testing programmes, the accuracy and precision of the results, and the potential benefits of treatment in the absence of any symptoms. With regard to ADHD, it may be cheaper, more accurate and equally effective to base early intervention programmes on reports of hyperactivity symptoms, regardless of DRD4 genotype. The use of genetic testing will become the preferred alternative only when the health benefits of this form of screening are clearly demonstrated, and it is shown that they outweigh the potential drawbacks of genetic testing.

Pre-implantation diagnosis of fertilized embryos will lead to important changes in prenatal genetic testing. Where it has been implemented with respect to Huntington disease, it has two potential benefits. By selecting for implantation only those embryos without the mutation, it not only removes the need for termination of pregnancy but also, where genotype of the parent at risk has not been confirmed, it may avoid disclosure of parental genotype where this is not wanted (Maat-Kievit *et al.* 1999). However, there may be practical difficulties as well as legal barriers to maintaining confidentiality of embryonic status (Braude *et al.* 1998). If pre-implantation selection becomes generally available, it may have wider influences on fetal selection. Although there has been general agreement that prenatal diagnosis with a view to selective abortion should occur only for disorders that are severe and for which there is no treatment, it might be that lower thresholds would be applied to pre-implantation methods. This could raise questions about selecting against susceptibility genes associated with some psychiatric disorders and also in favour of genes associated with beneficial traits, such as intelligence, or in favour of a particular sex (Wertz & Fletcher 1993).

Concern continues about the way in which insurance companies may discriminate against people who have participated in genetic testing (Harper 1995). The possible conflict between obtaining genetic information to improve one's lifestyle and modify health risks and the threat of not being eligible for insurance is a real one. It is unclear to what extent regulation of insurance companies will be possible. It is possible that similar issues might be taken up by employers as a method for controlling the future health status of employees. If genetic testing were to be enforced as part of occupational health screening, this could well be discriminatory and a breach of human rights (Nuffield Council on Bioethics 1998).

The future for genetic testing and counselling is exciting, important in improving health, but also filled with possible pitfalls and abuses. Involvement of the wider community is essential in developing new policies. More important than testing *per se* will be the development of interventions that make best use of genotype information. Planned research is needed to determine whether genotype information results in health improvement.

Acknowledgement

Thanks to Professor Theresa Marteau for reading an early draft and making invaluable suggestions.

References

Al-Jader, L.N., Parry-Langdon, N. & Smith, R.J. (2000) Survey of attitudes of pregnant women towards Down syndrome screening. *Prenatal Diagnosis*, 20, 23–29.

Amir, R.E., Van den Veyver, I.B., Wan, M., Tran, C.Q., Francke, U. & Zoghbi, H.Y. (1999) Rett syndrome is caused by mutations in X-linked MECP2, encoding methyl-CpG-binding protein 2. *Nature Genetics*, **23**, 185–188.

Angold, A., Costello, E.J., Farmer, E.M., Burns, B.J. & Erkanli, A. (1999) Impaired but undiagnosed. *Journal of the American Academy of Child and Adolescent Psychiatry*, **38**, 129–137.

Axworthy, D., Brock, D.J., Bobrow, M. & Marteau, T.M. (1996) Psychological impact of population-based carrier testing for cystic fibrosis: 3-year follow-up. UK Cystic Fibrosis Follow-Up Study Group. *Lancet*, **347**, 1443–1446.

Bailey, A.J., Le Couteur, A., Gottesman, I.I., Bolton, P., Simonoff, E. & Rutter, M. (1995) Autism is a strongly genetic disorder: evidence from a British twin study. *Psychological Medicine*, **25**, 63–78.

Bailey, A.J., Le Couteur, A., Palferman, S. & Heavey, L. (1998) Autism: the phenotype in relatives. *Journal of Autism and Developmental Disorders*, **28**, 269–392.

Barrett, S., Beck, J.C., Bernier, R. *et al.* (1999) An autosomal genomic screen for autism: collaborative linkage study of autism. *American Journal of Medical Genetics*, **88**, 609–615.

Biederman, J., Munir, K., Knee, D. *et al.* (1986) A family study of patients with attention deficit disorder and normal controls. *Journal of Psychiatric Research*, **20**, 263–274.

Bolton, P., Macdonald, H., Pickles, A. *et al.* (1994) A case–control family history study of autism. *Journal of Child Psychology and Psychiatry*, **35**, 877–900.

Bolton, P.F., Murphy, M., Macdonald, H., Whitlock, B., Pickles, A. & Rutter, M. (1997) Obstetric complications in autism: consequences or causes of the condition. *Journal of the American Academy of Child and Adolescent Psychiatry*, **36**, 272–281.

Bolton, P.F., Pickles, A., Murphy, M. & Rutter, M. (1998) Autism, affective and other psychiatric disorders: patterns of familial aggregation. *Psychological Medicine*, **28**, 385–395.

Braidstock, M., Michie, S. & Marteau, T. (2000) Psychological consequences of predictive genetic testing: a systematic review. *European Journal of Human Genetics*, **88**, 731–738.

Braude, P.R., De Wert, G.M., Evers-Kiebooms, G., Pettigrew, R.A. & Geraedts, J.P. (1998) Non-disclosure preimplantation genetic diagnosis for Huntington's disease: practical and ethical dilemmas. *Prenatal Diagnosis*, **18**, 1422–1426.

Bulik, C.M., Sullivan, P.F., Wade, T.D. & Kendler, K.S. (2000) Twin studies of eating disorders: a review. *International Journal of Eating Disorders*, **27**, 1–20.

Bundey, S. & Carter, C.O. (1974) Recurrence risks in severe undiagnosed mental deficiency. *Journal of Mental Deficiency Research*, **18**, 115–134.

Carter, C.O. (1976) Genetics of common single malformations. *British Medical Bulletin*, **32**, 21–26.

Catalano, M. (1999) The challenges of psychopharmacogenetics. *American Journal of Human Genetics*, **65**, 606–610.

Clarke, A. (2000) The biology of mitochondrial disease. *Archives of Disease in Childhood*, **82**, 339–340.

Clarke, A., Fielding, D., Kerzin-Storrer, L. *et al.* (1994) The genetic testing of children: report of a Working Party of the Clinical Genetics Society. *Journal of Medical Genetics*, **31**, 785–797.

Clausen, H., Brandt, N.J., Schwartz, M. & Skovby, F. (1996a) Psychological and social impact of carrier screening for cystic fibrosis among pregnant woman: a pilot study. *Clinical Genetics*, **49**, 200–205.

Clausen, H., Brandt, N.J., Schwartz, M. & Skovby, F. (1996b) Psychological impact of carrier screening for cystic fibrosis among pregnant women. *European Journal of Human Genetics*, **4**, 120–123.

Council on Ethical and Judicial Affairs, American Medical Association (1998) Multiplex genetic testing. *Hastings Center Report*, **28**, 15–21.

Crauford, D., Dodge, A., Kersin-Storrar, L. & Harris, R. (1989) Uptake of presymptomatic testing for Huntington's disease. *Lancet*, **ii**, 603–605.

Falconer, D.S. (1981) *Introduction to Quantitative Genetics*. Longman, London.

Fanos, J.H. & Johnson, J.P. (1995a) Barriers to carrier testing for adult cystic fibrosis sibs: the importance of not knowing. *American Journal of Medical Genetics*, **59**, 85–91.

Fanos, J.H. & Johnson, J.P. (1995b) Perception of carrier status by cystic fibrosis siblings. *American Journal of Human Genetics*, **57**, 431–438.

Faraone, S.V., Biederman, J., Keenan, K. & Tsuang, M.T. (1991) A family-genetic study of girls with DSM-III attention deficit disorder. *American Journal of Psychiatry*, **148**, 112–117.

Furu, T., Kaaruaunen, H., Sankila, E.M. & Norio, R. (1993) Attitudes towards prenatal diagnosis and selective abortion among patients with retinitis pigmentosa or choroideremia as well as among their relatives. *Clinical Genetics*, **43**, 160–165.

Gekas, J., Gondry, J., Mazur, S., Cesbron, P. & Thepot, F. (1999) Informed consent to serum screening for Down syndrome: are women given adequate information? *Prenatal Diagnosis*, **19**, 1–7.

Goldberg, J.D. (1997) Fetal cells in maternal circulation: progress in analysis of a rare event [Editorial]. *American Journal of Human Genetics*, **61**, 806–809.

Goodman, R. (1990) Technical note: are perinatal complications causes or consequences of autism? *Journal of Child Psychology and Psychiatry*, **31**, 809–812.

Grigorenko, E.L., Wood, F.B., Meyer, M.S. *et al.* (1997) Susceptibility loci for distinct components of developmental dyslexia on chromosomes 6 and 15. *American Journal of Human Genetics*, **60**, 27–39.

Hall, S., Bobrow, M. & Marteau, T.M. (2000) Psychological consequences for parents of false negative results on prenatal screening for Down's syndrome: retrospective interview study. *British Medical Journal*, **320**, 407–412.

Harper, P. (1995) Science and Technology Committee's report on genetics [Editorial]. *British Medical Journal*, **311**, 275–276.

Harper, P.S. (1998) *Practical Genetic Counselling*, 4th edn. Butterworth-Heinemann, Oxford.

International Molecular Genetic Study of Autism Consortium (1998) A full genome screen for autism with evidence for linkage to a region on chromosome 7q. *Human Molecular Genetics*, **7**, 571–578.

Kelly, T.E. (1986) *Clinical Genetics and Genetic Counselling*. Year Book, Chicago.

Kipman, A., Gorwood, P., Mouren-Simeoni, M.C. & Ades, J. (1999) Genetic factors in anorexia nervosa. *European Psychiatry*, **14**, 189–198.

Kodish, E.D. (1999) Testing children for cancer genes: the rule of earliest onset. *Journal of Pediatrics*, **135**, 390–395.

Lakatos, K., Toth, I., Nemoda, Z., Ney, K., Sasvari-Szekely, M. & Gervai, J. (2000) Dopamine D4 receptor (DRD4) gene polymorphism is associated with attachment disorganization in infants. *Molecular Psychiatry*, **5**, 633–637.

Law, M. & Tang, J.L. (1995) An analysis of the effectiveness of interventions to help people stop smoking. *Archives of Internal Medicine*, **155**, 1933–1941.

Le Couteur, A., Bailey, A., Goode, S. *et al.* (1996) A broader phenotype of autism: the clinical spectrum in twins. *Journal of Child Psychology and Psychiatry*, **37**, 785–801.

Lerman, C., Gold, K., Audrain, J. *et al.* (1997) Incorporating biomarkers of exposure and genetic susceptibility into smoking cessation treatment: effects on smoking-related cognitions, emotions, and behavior change. *Health Psychology*, **16**, 87–99.

Li, S. & Huang, L. (2000) Nonviral gene therapy: promises and challenges. *Gene Therapy*, 7, 31–34.

Maat-Kievit, A., Vegter-van der Vlis, M., Zoeteweij, M. *et al.* (1999) Experience in prenatal testing for Huntington's disease in the Netherlands: procedures, results and guidelines (1987–97). *Prenatal Diagnosis*, 19, 450–457.

Marteau, T.M. (1999) Communicating genetic risk information. *British Medical Bulletin*, 55, 414–428.

Marteau, T.M. & Croyle, R.T. (1998) The new genetics: psychological responses to genetic testing. *British Medical Journal*, 316, 693–696.

McGuffin, P. & Katz, R. (1986) Nature, nurture and affective disorder. In: *The Biology of Depression* (ed. J.F.W. Deakin), pp. 26–52. Gaskell/RCP, London.

McGuffin, P., Farmer, A.E., Gottesman, I.I., Murray, R.M. & Reveley, A.M. (1984) Twin concordance for operationally defined schizophrenia: confirmation of familialty and heritability. *Archives of General Psychiatry*, 41, 541–545.

McGuffin, P., Owen, M.J., O'Donovan, M.C., Thapar, A. & Gottesman, I.I. (1994) *Psychiatric Genetics*. Gaskell, London.

Medical Controls Agency (1999) Current problems in pharmacovigilance. *Current Problems*, 25, 1–3.

Mednick, S.A. (1978) Berkson's fallacy and high-risk research. In: *The Nature of Schizophrenia: New Approaches to Research and Treatment* (eds L.C. Wynne, R.L. Cromwell & S. Matthysse), pp. 442–452. Wiley, New York.

Michie, S., Bron, F., Bobrow, M. & Marteau, T.M. (1997) Nondirectiveness in genetic counselling: an empirical study. *American Journal of Human Genetics*, 60, 40–47.

Nuffield Council on Bioethics (1998) *Mental Disorders and Genetics: the Ethical Context*. Nuffield Foundation, Oxford.

Park, V., Howard-Peebles, P., Sherman, S., Taylor, A. & Wulfsberg, E. (1994) Fragile X syndrome: diagnostic and carrier testing. *American Journal of Medical Genetics*, 53, 380–381.

Pauls, D.L. & Alsobrook, J.P. (1999) The inheritance of obsessive-compulsive disorder. *Child and Adolescent Psychiatric Clinics of North America*, 8, 481–496.

Pauls, D.L., Raymond, C.L., Stevenson, J.M. & Leckman, J.F. (1991) A family study of Gilles de la Tourette Syndrome. *American Journal of Human Genetics*, 48, 154–163.

Piggott, M., Wilkinson, P. & Bennett, J. (1994) Implementation of an antenatal serum screening programme for Down's syndrome in two districts (Brighton and Eastbourne). The Brighton and Eastbourne Down's Syndrome Screening Group. *Journal of Medical Screening*, 1, 45–49.

Post, S.G., Whitehouse, P.J., Binstock, R.H. *et al.* (1997) The clinical introduction of genetic testing for Alzheimer disease: an ethical perspective. *Journal of the American Medical Association*, 277, 832–836.

Quaid, K.A. & Morris, M. (1993) Reluctance to undergo predictive testing: the case of Huntington disease. *American Journal of Medical Genetics*, 43, 41–45.

Reynolds, P.P. & Benkendorf, J.L. (1999) Genes and generalists: why we need professionals with added competencies. *Western Journal of Medicine*, 171, 375–379.

Rutter, M. & Plomin, R. (1997) Opportunities for psychiatry from genetic findings. *British Journal of Psychiatry*, 171, 209–219.

Rutter, M., Bailey, A., Simonoff, E. & Pickles, A. (1997) Genetic influences and autism. In: *Autism and Pervasive Developmental Disorders* (eds D.J. Cohen & F.R. Volkmar), pp. 370–387. Wiley, New York.

Rutter, M., Silberg, J., O'Connor, T. & Simonoff, E. (1999) Genetics and child psychiatry. II. Empirical research findings. *Journal of Child Psychology and Psychiatry*, 40, 19–55.

Senior, V., Marteau, T.M. & Weinman, J. (2000) Impact of genetic testing on causal models of heart disease and arthritis: an analogue study. *Psychology and Health*, 14, 1077–1088.

Sherman, S.L., Jacobs, P.A., Morton, N.E. *et al.* (1985) Further segregation analysis of the fragile X syndrome with special reference to transmitting males. *Human Genetics*, 69, 289–299.

Shiloh, S. & Saxe, L. (1989) Perception of risk in genetic counselling. *Psychology and Health*, 3, 45–61.

Simonoff, E. (1995) Genetic influences on depressive symptoms and disorders. *Childhood Depression, Occasional Paper, Association for Child Psychology and Psychiatry*, 1, 29–44.

Simonoff, E. (2001) Genetic influences on conduct disorder. In: *Cambridge Monographs in Child and Adolescent Psychiatry: Conduct Disorder* (eds J. Hill & B. Maughan), pp. 202–234. Cambridge University Press, Cambridge.

Smalley, S.L., Asarnow, R.F. & Spence, A. (1988) Autism and genetics: a decade of research. *Archives of General Psychiatry*, 45, 953–961.

Smalley, S., McCracken, J. & Tanguay, P. (1995) Autism, affective disorders, and social phobia. *American Journal of Medical Genetics (Neuropsychiatric Genetics)*, 60, 19–26.

Szatmari, P., Boyle, M.H. & Offord, D.R. (1991) Familial aggregation of emotional and behavioural problems of childhood in the general population. *American Journal of Psychiatry*, 150, 1398–1403.

Taylor, B., Miller, E., Farrington, C.P. *et al.* (1999) Autism and measles, mumps, and rubella vaccine: no epidemiological evidence for a causal association. *Lancet*, 353, 2026–2029.

Thapar, A., Holmes, J., Poulton, K. & Harrington, R. (1999) Genetic basis of attention deficit and hyperactivity. *British Journal of Psychiatry*, 174, 105–111.

Turner, G., Robinson, H., Wake, S., Laing, S. & Partington, M. (1997) Case finding for the fragile X syndrome and its consequences. *British Medical Journal*, 315, 1223–1226.

Wahlin, T.B., Lundin, A., Backman, L. *et al.* (1997) Reactions to predictive testing in Huntington disease: case reports of coping with a new genetic status. *American Journal of Medical Genetics*, 73, 356–365.

Wakefield, A.J., Murch, S.H., Anthony, A. *et al.* (1998) Ileal-lymphoid-nodular hyperplasia, non-specific colitis, and pervasive development disorder in children. *Lancet*, 351, 637–641.

Walker, A.P. (1996) Genetic counseling. In: *Emery and Rimoin's Principles and Practices of Medical Genetics* (eds D.L. Rimoin, J.M. Connor & R.E. Pyeritz), pp. 595–619. Churchill Livingstone, New York.

Wan, M., Lee, S.S., Zhang, X. *et al.* (1999) Rett syndrome and beyond: recurrent spontaneous and familial MECP2 mutations at CpG hotspots. *American Journal of Human Genetics*, 65, 1520–1529.

Wertz, D.C. & Fletcher, J.C. (1993) Prenatal diagnosis and sex selection in 19 nations. *Social Science and Medicine*, 37, 1359–1366.

Wilson, R.D. (2000) Amniocentesis and chorionic villus sampling. *Current Opinion in Obstetrics and Gynecology*, 12, 81–86.

# Services for Children and Adolescents with Severe Learning Disabilities (Mental Retardation)

Sarah H. Bernard

Introduction

It is widely recognized that children and adolescents with severe learning disabilities are at risk of developing behavioural or emotional problems and have an increased likelihood of physical and sensory disabilities, epilepsy and physical injury as compared to the general population (Rutter *et al.* 1970; Bregman 1991; Dunne *et al.* 1993; Borthwick-Duffy 1994). These young people are dependent on others for the acquisition of their basic needs and have problems compounded by social stigmatization (Goffman 1963; Gibbons 1985). Their parents, siblings and extended family also have their own needs (Friedrich *et al.* 1985), and while recognizing that it is the child who is the patient, frequently it is the whole family that is in need of a service (Robards 1994). Generic child and adolescent mental health services are unable to meet these multiple and complex needs in a comprehensive manner; accordingly, specialist but integrated multidisciplinary services are required. These should be able to offer flexibility in the light of changing and multiple needs. Service providers have to take into account the age of the child, the level of the child's learning disability, physical disability, the structure and ethnicity of the family and the many other variables which influence how the child's behavioural or mental health problems might best be assessed and managed (Bernard 1999). As the difficulties posed by having a severe learning disability continue into adulthood, service provision has to do likewise.

The twentieth century witnessed great changes in the provision of care for people with learning disabilities (Ryan & Thomas 1987; Blunden 1990; Hassiotis *et al.* 2000). In the UK, the move away from institutionalized care began in the 1960s with public attention drawn to the plight of those in the asylums (Ryan & Thomas 1987). In 1971, the government White Paper 'Better Services for the Mentally Handicapped' paved the way to the development of individualized care in the community with the subsequent closure of the large asylums.

Other factors that have influenced these changes include the normalization principle, which emphasizes that people with a learning disability 'should have access to patterns of life and conditions of everyday living which are as close as possible to the regular circumstances and ways of life of society' (Nirje 1970). Service provision continues to strive to achieve this goal, with the acknowledgement that people with a learning disability are entitled to a valued role in society (Wolfensberger 1983). O'Brien described five key accomplishments for people with learning disabilities, these being a community presence, relationships, competence, respect and choice (O'Brien 1987). All should be considered when planning services.

Despite massive moves forward in service provision, children and adolescents with severe learning disabilities remain relatively poorly provided for (Fraser & Murti Rao 1991; Royal College of Psychiatrists 1998). Where services do exist they tend to be fragmented and lack co-ordination (Richardson *et al.* 1986; Slatter & Black 1986) although some groups of children and adolescents with specific disorders appear to be better served than others, e.g. those with Down syndrome (Byrne *et al.* 1988). The various agencies involved (including health, education, social services and the voluntary sector), recognizing this gap in service provision, have now begun to address how services might be better developed to meet the needs of these young people (Audit Commission 1994; NHS Executive 1998).

This chapter focuses on the prevalence of various needs and how services may meet them, with particular reference to families' needs for preventative services, accurate diagnosis, specialist mental health services (to include assessment, treatment and management) residential services, education, family support, help in the transition to adult life, and a helpful legal framework

Terminology and classification

The terms used to refer to people with learning disabilities have changed over time, reflecting changing attitudes. Currently, in the UK, the term 'learning disability' is the most widely accepted term used to refer to people who have a level of intellectual functioning significantly below the average. This, statistically, is at least 2 SD below the mean IQ of 100, giving a measured IQ of 70 or less. Low IQ alone cannot be used to define learning disability. The individual has impairments in other areas, including the development of adaptive skills, self-care, social skills, communication, academia, leisure and employment (see Volkmar & Dykens, Chapter 41). It is also recognized that to have learning disabilities, the impairments should have been evident prior to 18 years of age. Whereas 'learning disability' is the terminology recognized in the UK, this is not the situation internationally. In the USA, this term refers to children with specific educational problems, with 'mental retardation' being the term used to define people with a global impairment. Other terms used include 'intellectual disability', 'developmental disability' and 'mental handicap' (Russell 1997).

Historically, other terms have been used. In the early twentieth century, 'idiocy', 'imbecility' and 'feeblemindedness' were the accepted labels of the time but, partly because of the negative connotations of such terms, the accepted terminology altered to 'mental subnormality' in 1959, 'mental handicap' in 1983 and, in the 1990s, to 'learning disabilities' (Ryan & Thomas 1987). Terminology continues to be debated because, with each change in label, the associated stigma gradually recurs. It seems to arise from society's perception of the disability, rather than from the term used as a descriptor. 'Mental retardation' remains the internationally recognized term even though it is felt by some to be derogatory. Parents are often confused by the variety of labels, especially by whether 'learning disability' refers to global or specific deficit. Some continue to prefer 'mental handicap', believing that it reflects the devastating impact.

Educational services have introduced alternative terms: in the UK, for example, 'moderate' and 'severe' learning defficulties has been the terminology since the Warnock Report of 1978.

The World Health Organization (1980) suggested a model that puts the person's disability into a social context using the terms 'impairment', 'disability' and 'handicap'.

- Impairment is defined as any loss or abnormality of psychological, physiological or anatomical structure or function that may be temporary or permanent.
- Disability is the restriction or lack (resulting from an impairment) of ability to perform an activity in the manner or within the range considered normal for a human being.
- Handicap is social disadvantage resulting from the impairment and disability. Thus, the disease, effect of the disease on the body, performance and ability to carry out a social function are accounted for, with handicap clearly defined as the result of an impairment and not the cause of it (Robards 1994).

Terminological confusion has had an impact on service provision and terms such as 'behavioural disturbance' as opposed to 'psychiatric disorder' have added to this, with the contribution of psychiatrist vs. psychologist coming into question (Fraser et al. 1986). Criteria have been suggested in an attempt to define 'problem behaviour' (Zarkowska & Clements 1988). The behaviour should be inappropriate for the person's age and level of development, dangerous to the person or to others, constitute a significant handicap, cause significant stress and be contrary to social norms. Many professionals found this term unhelpful and the term 'challenging behaviour' became accepted. This is defined as 'behaviour of such an intensity, frequency or duration that the physical safety of the person or others, is likely to be placed in serious jeopardy, or behaviour which is likely to limit seriously, or delay access to or the use of, ordinary community facilities' (Emerson et al. 1988).

There are some difficulties in using the classifications of

behavioural and emotional problems that were designed for those without a learning disability. Physical problems, for example, alter presentation: less mobile children cannot exhibit some of the symptoms of hyperactivity or conduct disorder. In spite of these difficulties, it is clear that certain disorders are more common in children with severe learning disabilities, especially pervasive developmental disorders (see below; see also Volkmar & Dykens, Chapter 41). The applicability, reliability and validity of current international systems of classification, including ICD-10 and DSM-IV, for children and adolescents with severe learning disabilities have been questioned (Einfeld & Aman 1995). Despite these difficulties, the diagnosis of psychiatric disorder serves the function of informing about the clinical condition, assisting in the evaluation of treatment outcomes, establishing causal connections between psychopathology and clinical presentation and identifying at-risk populations (Russell 1997).

Prevalence of specific needs

The prevalence of mild learning disability, as defined by an IQ of more than 2 SD below the mean, is 2–3%, but this has been shown to vary with socioeconomic circumstances. The prevalence of severe learning disability, 3 SD below the mean, is 3–4 per 1000, this figure being little influenced by socioeconomic factors and having a strong organic or genetic aetiology. There are many population studies of prevalence of learning disabilities that vary in criteria used. Total population studies include the Isle of Wight study (Rutter et al. 1970) which investigated children aged 9–10 years using an IQ criterion of under 70 and demonstrating a prevalence of 2.5%. Other studies replicated these findings also using an IQ criterion to define learning disabilities (Birch et al. 1970; Granat & Granat 1973). Studies that used the combination of IQ and impairment find a much lower prevalence, between 0.5 and 1.5% (Rutter et al. 1970; Gostason 1985).

There is an increased prevalence of certain specific disorders in people with learning disabilities. These include neurological deficits, epilepsy, sensory deficits, communication disorders and behavioural and mental health problems. The prevalence of these disorders varies with age. Epilepsy occurs in 20–50% of people with severe learning disabilities, this frequency increasing in specific conditions such as tuberous sclerosis and neurodegenerative disorders. Of people with severe learning disabilities, 15–40% have cerebral palsy, 10–30% serious visual impairments, 60–85% severe communication disorders and up to 5% have auditory deficits (Fryers & Russell 1997).

Children and adolescents with severe learning disabilities are at enhanced risk of developing mental health problems similar to those that affect their non-disabled peers; and show an even greater degree of risk of the development of certain specific disorders, including autistic spectrum disorder and attention deficit disorders (Rutter et al. 1970; Corbett 1979; Dossetor & Nicol 1981; Gilberg et al. 1986; Cormack et al. 2000). About

Table 67.1 Estimates of prevalences in very rare disorders.

Syndrome	Prevalence
Down	1 in 600 (age dependent)
Fragile X	1 in 1000–3000
Lesch–Nyhan	1 in 100 000–200 000
Phenylketonuria	1 in 4500–15 000
Rett	1 in 10 000–15 000 (females)

one-half of children, aged from 0 to 15 years, who had severe learning difficulty also showed a psychiatric disorder, according to an epidemiological study by Corbett (1979). In addition, children without a specific diagnosis are still at risk of developing behavioural problems or 'challenging behaviours' (Einfield & Tonge 1996). Studies that have looked at challenging behaviour in children with severe learning disabilities have shown 8% to have behaviours presenting severe management problems and a further 14% to show milder problems of this nature (Keirnan & Keirnan 1994).

Risk factors for the development of behavioural problems in children with severe learning disabilities include limitations in daily living skills, with one study of children aged 4–11 years finding this a better predictor than poor communication (Chadwick *et al.* 2000). This study also demonstrated that children who were ambulant had more problems, although those problem behaviours that were less dependent on walking were as common in non-ambulant children. Other studies have confirmed these findings, with the severity of physical disability having a direct relationship on ratings of behavioural and emotional problems (Cormack *et al.* 2000).

Other specific behavioural problems that are more common in those with severe learning disabilities and have service implications include severe sleep disorders (Wigg & Stores 1999), severe self-injury (Oliver 1995) and communication problems. These have been found to be associated with a skills deficit (Chadwick *et al.* 2000).

There are certain behaviours associated with specific conditions (Flint 1996; see also Skuse & Kuntsi, Chapter 13). These 'behavioural phenotypes' include overeating in Prader–Willi syndrome (Clarke *et al.* 1995), severe self-injury in Lesch–Nyhan syndrome, sleep disturbance in Smith–Magenis syndrome and social disinhibition in Williams syndrome. The diagnosis of these disorders and knowledge of the associated behavioural problems enables interventions to be planned aimed at minimizing these difficulties (Berney 1997). Despite this, it is recognized that many of these syndromes are rare, as indicated by the estimates of prevalence in Table 67.1 (Berney 1997).

Children with very rare disorders will only account for a small proportion of the caseload of a local service. This has resulted in expertise in these disorders being concentrated in a few regionally or nationally based services, allowing both clinical and research expertise to be developed. The advantage of this approach is that the needs of these small groups of children can be considered in a systematic way with individual variables ac-counted for. Obvious disadvantages are geographical, with families having to travel long distances to be seen, the child not being seen within their own environment and intensive community work not being practical. To overcome these obstacles it is vital that specialist services liaise locally and transfer the skills to those providing the local long-term services to the child and their family.

Service needs

The move away from institutionalized care to community care has had, as expected, major influences on service provision for people with learning disabilities. Children and adolescents with learning disabilities are now recognized as requiring a child-based service integrated into other services for young people (Children Act 1989). The aim of service providers is to ensure that the person's medical, emotional, cognitive, behavioural, social, educational and legal needs are being met (Turk 1997), while recognizing the prerequisite of good liaison with the multitude of professionals and agencies involved (Hall & Prendergast 1990). In the UK, various statutory bodies have attempted to ensure that the child's service needs are provided, with the passing of the Children Act (1989) in which these children are referred to as 'children in need', and the Education Act which encourages integration and access to the national curriculum for all children.

Mental health services for children and adolescents with severe learning disabilities should not be considered in isolation. This group of young people will also fall into the remit of the community paediatric services and, some believe, the psychiatrist should be a core member of this team. If this is not the case then it is essential that the two teams are able to work closely together, with the main areas of responsibility being clearly defined (Sturge 1989). When considering the role of the specialist mental health services, the Royal College of Psychiatrists (1992) outlined a model of service provision for children and adolescents with learning disabilities and mental health needs. They suggested that skills should cover the following.

- Prevention and amelioration of mental health problems.
- Diagnosis of cases with often complex and multifactorial presentations and aetiologies.
- Focused and specialist treatment interventions.
- Multi-agency liaison and collaboration with professionals involved in clinical management.
- Prevention of complications.

A subsequent report in 1998 (Royal College of Psychiatrists 1998) again emphasized the need for specialist services with the proposal that such services should be comprehensive and able to cater for children and adolescents of all ages and all levels of disability. Specialist areas of input were expanded upon, with autistic spectrum disorders, serious psychiatric disorders and hyperactivity being highlighted as major areas of service need. Behavioural disorders associated with epilepsy, emotional disorders, aggression, self-injury, eating and sleep disorders, child abuse, offending and substance abuse all need particular consideration. The types of specialist interventions need to include diagnostic services, adjustment counselling, behaviour modification approaches, family work, individual therapies and pharmacological therapies.

Generic child and adolescent mental health services are not usually able to offer the specialist provision. In one study, only 32% of child and adolescent psychiatrists offered a service to those with severe learning disabilities (Joint College Working Party 1989).

Specific areas of service need

Preventative services

Prevention may be either primary, secondary or tertiary. Primary prevention, ensuring that the condition does not occur at conception, takes the form of pre-conceptional counselling with minimization of the risk factors associated with specific conditions. Examples include dietary advice and the use of pre-conceptional folic acid to reduce the risk of neural tube defect, and immunization to prevent congenital rubella.

Recent developments in molecular genetics have allowed the identification of abnormal gene sequences in rare conditions associated with learning disabilities. As a result of this, individuals may now be screened for many more disorders than before. It is hoped that the identification of these abnormal gene sequences could also lead to specific interventions and therapies aimed at preventing the development of these disorders (Muir 2000).

Secondary prevention of specific conditions is possible as a result of prenatal screening and diagnosis, with selective termination of an affected pregnancy. Conditions that may be screened for include neural tube defect (anencephaly, encephalocele and spina bifida) and Down syndrome. Tertiary prevention aims to prevent the complications of a disorder. An example of this, for children with severe learning disability, would be the prevention of a behavioural disturbance.

Primary prevention

Primary prevention of learning disability demands a knowledge of the underlying aetiological factors contributing to the disorder. These include genetic, organic and sociocultural influences that give rise to the deficits in cognitive functioning in a multifactorial manner. In those with severe learning disabilities, the genetic and organic factors have a major role, with socioeconomic factors exerting a lesser influence (Dykens 2000; Muir 2000; see also Volkmar & Dykens, Chapter 41).

The report of the Commission of Enquiry on Mental Handicap (1965) discussed the principal preventative measures as being related to health education, better obstetric services, control of epilepsy, early identification of disorders, routine neonatal testing, genetic counselling and alleviation of cultural and environmental deficiencies. Health education must be at both a local and national level, with the importance of work being done at school level recognized.

With the rapid growth of genetic knowledge of the last three decades, thought has been given to the role of genetic counselling services. These services offer detection of risk factors, the ability to make accurate diagnoses and assist in the diagnosis of rare disorders. Genetic counselling for families who have a child with learning disabilities or are at risk of having an affected child poses practical and ethical dilemmas. In a small number of conditions there is the possibility of the reduction of risk factors, neural tube defect being an example with the use of periconceptional folate. More often, the role of the clinical geneticist, in collaboration with other disciplines, is the ability to offer accurate diagnoses, prenatal testing of pregnancies with termination being the only preventative intervention available (see also Simonoff, Chapter 66).

Secondary prevention

Diagnosis of congenital abnormalities during the antenatal period may be achieved as a result of chorionic villus sampling, amniocentesis and ultrasonography. More invasive procedures include fetoscopy. The ethical and moral considerations surrounding prenatal diagnosis have not advanced as rapidly, posing serious dilemmas for many professionals and families (West 1988; Boyd et al. 1998; Green et al. 1993). One group of disorders in which the benefits of both screening and prenatal diagnosis has been considered extensively is neural tube defect.

Defects of the neural tube include the following.
• *Anencephaly*: the most severe form of neural tube defect, resulting in exposure of the brain and spinal cord and causing abnormal development of the brain and spine.
• *Encephalocele*: a defect in the skull, usually occipitally, with protruding brain.
• *Spina bifida*: failure of closure of the spine, with protrusion of meninges through the defect and abnormal development of the spinal cord.
Anencephaly is almost always a lethal condition but encephalocele and spina bifida, while usually resulting in severe if nonlethal consequences, have a variable outcome from severe global intellectual and physical disability to minimal or no problems.

Neural tube defect was one of the first disorders in which a prenatal screening programme was developed with the identification of a biochemical marker in maternal serum. This marker, maternal serum alpha-fetoprotein (MSAFP), was found to be elevated in women carrying a fetus affected with an open neural tube defect. Unfortunately, although the marker was reasonably sensitive and specific, it could be elevated in a number of situations and was highly dependent on accurate knowledge of the gestation of the fetus. There were also situations in which false-negative results occurred. This led to questioning of the advantages and disadvantages of the screening programmes of neural tube defect, with some believing that it was only of benefit to mothers living in areas where there was a high risk of neural tube defect (Standing *et al.* 1981). It has also been commented that the screening programme was weighted towards fetuses that were, in any case, incompatible with life.

There were, subsequently, studies of women's experiences of MSAFP screening that concentrated on the anxiety created as a result of screening. One study of 179 women undergoing screening demonstrated a more positive attitude towards the pregnancy following screening. This study used the state–trait anxiety inventory to assess anxiety levels but responses were not considered in conjunction with the management of the women at the time of screening (Bennett *et al.* 1980). Other studies demonstrated a raised level of anxiety in women with both positive and negative outcomes of screening, with anxiety being reduced with good family and social support (Robinson *et al.* 1984).

Amniocentesis, a diagnostic test used to detect a number of disorders including neural tube defect and Down syndrome, creates anxieties because of both the possible serious outcome of the test, but also because the investigation itself carries risks of damage to the pregnancy whether it is normal or not (Marteau *et al.* 1993).

Ultrasonography during the antenatal period may be used as either a screening or diagnostic investigation. It is routinely used to assess gestational age and fetal growth. An obvious benefit of this procedure is the reassurance of not detecting an abnormality in an at-risk pregnancy (Tsoi *et al.* 1987), but there is a high rate of detection of false-positives leading to unnecessary anxiety for many women (Boyd *et al.* 1998).

Down syndrome is another disorder in which serum screening can now be offered, giving an estimate of the risk of an affected pregnancy. Between 36 and 76% of those affected can be detected antenatally, although take-up rates for the programme vary (Wald *et al.* 1997). Although there are concerns about the false-positive results of screening (Boyd *et al.* 1998), there are also concerns about the effects of false-negative results, with one study of 179 parents of children with Down syndrome demonstrating an adverse effect on parental adjustment when the child was born following a false-negative screening result (Hall *et al.* 2000).

Decision-making after the detection of a fetal abnormality is influenced by a number of factors including the nature of the abnormality, the counselling received, and the family's own experiences, religious and moral beliefs. Some women, despite the identification of a pregnancy affected with a congenital abnormality, will refuse termination of pregnancy (Meryash 1992). The psychological impact on families undergoing these procedures has been recognized (Berne-Fromell *et al.* 1983) and the professional support that is subsequently needed has been highlighted (Donnai 1987). There are also eugenic concerns that are particularly relevant to those with severe learning disabilities (Seller 1982; Lilford 1989; Richards 1989). While acknowledging the problems arising as a result of prenatal diagnosis, the benefits are also evident (Pueschel 1991). There has been an argument that termination of pregnancies that might result in a child being affected with a disability devalues the life of people with disability, although others believe it is the right of the fetus to be born healthy (Pueschel 1991).

A small number of conditions can be treated in the neonatal period, so neonatal screening programmes are essential if early detection is to be achieved. Examples of particular disorders are phenylketonurea and congenital hypothyroidism.

Phenylketonuria, a disorder of amino acid metabolism, has a reported incidence of 1 in 10 000 live births. There is a variable deficiency of phenylalanine hydroxylase, and the condition, if untreated, creates an accumulation of phenylalanine in the body tissues, with subsequent cellular damage including brain damage. Untreated cases that are not detected at birth have a dramatic cognitive decline in the first year of life, with treatment being unable to reverse this. Neonatal screening enables the disorder to be detected prior to a build-up of phenylalanine and the subsequent cellular destruction that ensues. Implementation of an appropriately low phenylalanine diet in the neonatal period prevents brain damage. Despite this, there are reports that, even in treated cases, there are some clinical deficits, including problems with concentration and abnormalities of visuomotor and spatial skills (Thompson *et al.* 1990).

Congenital hypothyroidism, occurring in 1 in 4000 live births, is another metabolic disorder that if treated early in the neonatal period prevents the severe developmental delay and gross retardation that results from lack of thyroxine.

Tertiary prevention

Reduction of the additional handicaps associated with learning disabilities is also important. These include sensory problems and the complications of epilepsy. Early detection of problems, to minimize these secondary handicaps, is important although the benefits of routine health screening on a regular basis have been debated (Hall 1991). It has been suggested that current health surveillance which includes a neonatal and 6-week check, monitoring of neurologically damaged children, and detection by those closely involved with the child, such as parents, health visitors and general practitioners, is adequate (Hall 1991). Concerns are that parents are not best able to monitor their child's development and that early detection of problems will not occur (Bax & Whitmore 1985). Advantages are that many disorders will be detected neonatally or at the 6-week check and further surveillance is costly, with a low detection rate.

Diagnosis

The diagnosis of the underlying cause of the child learning disability is, in general, the remit of the paediatrician, sometimes in conjunction with a clinical geneticist (for a scheme of investigation see Bailey, Chapter 10). Occasionally, the child may be referred to a mental health service because of a behavioural problem, with the nature of this problem suggesting a specific medical diagnosis, such as Lesch–Nyhan syndrome. The diagnosis of disorders such as these is dependent on a knowledge of the behavioural phenotypes associated with rare syndromes, a thorough history, careful physical examination, specialist investigations and good liaison with paediatricians and clinical geneticists.

The diagnosis of childhood psychiatric conditions in children with severe learning disability is one obvious remit of the specialist mental health service for this group of individuals. Before being able to make such diagnoses there must be a detailed assessment, including the history of the disorder, observations of the child at home and at school, and information from others involved in their care, including teachers and carers. An assessment of the child's level of functioning is invaluable in allowing appropriate behaviours for the child's cognitive level to be accounted for.

Even with detailed information there are difficulties in attaching diagnostic labels to children with severe learning disability and behavioural problems. Despite this, it remains important to identify conditions such as autism, attention deficit disorder and the other childhood psychiatric disorders that have diagnostic and treatment implications for the child and their family.

Interventions

Behavioural approaches

The most widely accepted intervention for behavioural problems in children and adolescents with severe learning disability is behavioural modification (Yule & Carr 1987). However, there is limited research evidence to support the long-term benefits of such an approach, with the prognosis remaining poor for adulthood (Oliver & Head 1990). Early interventions for cognitive or behavioural problems are often home-based. One well-studied intervention of this nature is the Portage scheme (Shearer & Shearer 1972). This involves regular visits by a trained home advisor who provides short-term goals and training methods. Initial studies of this intervention demonstrated impressive gains, but the scheme was aimed at children with mild or specific learning disabilities. Despite some criticisms, this home-based input became popular, particularly in the USA. The gains made by those families offered this service continued to be demonstrated as being greatest for those whose children had mild problems or who were disadvantaged, with the benefits questioned for those with severe learning disabilities (Clements et al. 1982; Robards 1994).

Other early interventions have also been developed. Some, it was hoped, would reduce the level of the child's disabilities and increase their level of cognitive functioning. The Infant Health and Development Programme offered enrichment for children of low birth weight but, while demonstrating improvements up until the age of 3 years, there was little evidence that this was sustained (Richmond 1990). It was also evident that those children with IQs of less than 70 were less likely to benefit from this approach.

In general, punitive forms of behavioural modification have been superseded by programmes aimed at improving skills while addressing undesirable behaviours (Zarkowska & Clements 1988). Parent training programmes, recognized as benefiting children with conduct disorders with no global developmental delay, are also reported to be of benefit in the learning disabled population (Brightman et al. 1982; Webster-Stratton 1984). Long-term follow-up of such interventions remains sparse (Baker et al. 1980). Difficulties with behavioural approaches centre on poor compliance and low rates of participation, and it is evident that families who benefit most come from a relatively well-educated background (Baker et al. 1981).

Behavioural approaches rely on a detailed assessment of environmental events that precipitate and maintain behavioural disturbances (see Herbert, Chapter 53). This type of assessment is referred to as functional analysis, and involves detailed history-taking, direct measures and observations and analysis of the situations in which problem behaviours arise. Many procedures have been identified as a means of carrying out a functional analysis, with the ultimate aims being a clear description of the problems behaviours, predictors of when the problem behaviours occur, consequences of maintenance of the problem behaviours, the development of hypotheses to account for the behaviours and supporting evidence via direct observations (O'Neill et al. 1997).

Other psychological approaches

Whereas behavioural modification and behavioural psychotherapy are the best recognized psychotherapeutic interventions for behavioural disturbance in children with learning disabilities, there are a number of other psychological approaches that have also been implemented. These include individual therapies, such as drama therapy, play therapy, art therapy and psychodynamic psychotherapy, group work, family and marital therapies. There is a lack of research evidence to support the benefits of these interventions, but anecdotally it has been argued that, in some cases, there has been a reduction of behavioural problems (Waitman & Conboy-Hill 1992; Lindsey 1997).

Medication

Historically, medication has been used to sedate and calm people with severe learning disability and severe behavioural disturbance, although good practice dictates that medication should only be indicated in cases where there is a treatable underlying psychiatric disorder. An example of one such disorder is attention deficit hyperactivity disorder. Whereas there is a lack of systematic research in the learning disabled population, stimulant medication is effective in children with mild to moderate learning disability, with the benefits decreasing as the level of learning disability increases (Gadow 1985). In the learning disabled population it has also been demonstrated that stimulant medication is more likely to create side-effects, with social withdrawal being a particular problem (Handen et al. 1990). In a survey of 100 child psychiatrists in the UK, only half of the prescribers were willing to use this medication on children with learning disability, despite it being recognized that this group of children have higher rates of attention deficit symptomatology (Bramble 1997).

With the development of a massive range of psychotropic medication, research into the benefits for children with learning disability and behavioural problems is awaited, although there is anecdotal evidence that certain classes of medication, including the selective serotonin reuptake inhibitors (SSRIs), might benefit children with severe learning disability, autistic spectrum disorder and the resultant severe behavioural problems that they experience (see Heyman & Santosh, Chapter 59). Scientific evidence remains essential if adverse effects are to be minimized without clear evidence of clinical efficacy.

Other intervention approaches

Conductive education has been advocated as a means of optimizing the level of functioning in children with developmental disabilities (Hari & Tillemans 1984). A holistic approach is used, with trained therapists stimulating the children. There is little objective measurement of outcome, but reports indicate the benefits are unlikely to be greater than conventional approaches (Bairstow *et al.* 1991). The Dolman–Delacato method of stimulation offers intensive programming exercises aimed at accelerating the child's development (Pennock 1991). It has been criticized by many leading professionals for not offering benefits substantial enough to justify the heavy demands imposed on families (Cummins 1988).

Inpatient treatment

The treatment setting is generally based in the community and aimed at offering both home- and school-based interventions. Rarely, the child presents with a problem of such complexity or severity that inpatient assessment is required. This enables investigative procedures to be performed, including detailed neuropsychiatric monitoring of conditions such as epilepsy where skilled observations are required over a period of time. Other investigative procedures are more readily offered on an inpatient basis, with video-telemetry of seizures to monitor frequency and associated behavioural problems not being possible in the community. Neuroimaging, while generally provided on an outpatient basis, frequently requires general anaesthesia in severely disturbed individuals with a learning disability and, at times, a 24-h period to ensure recovery from sedation is indicated. Intense behavioural observations can also be undertaken that would not be possible in a community setting, although moving a child from their usual setting has the disadvantage of altering the child's behaviour.

Treatments might also need to be monitored with the child in an inpatient facility. Medication, although not the first line of treatment for behavioural disturbance, does have an important role in these children. Side-effects are a concern and can be atypical so inpatient manipulation of medication may be necessary. Specific groups of young people with learning disability who require inpatient care are adolescents with a possible psychotic disorder who are presenting a danger to either themselves or others in the community; severe eating disorders in which the child's health is in danger; severe self-mutilation; and conditions associated with epilepsy or neurodegenerative disorders. Such service provision is, by nature, highly specialized and regionally or nationally based. Units can bring problems (e.g. institutionalization), but they can deliver intensive assessments and therapies (Newman & Emerson 1991). Research into inpatient treatments for children and adolescents with severe learning disabilities is extremely sparse. There are very few inpatient settings specifically aimed at addressing the needs of this group and (as in generic child and adolescent psychiatry), the treated group is heterogeneous and ill-defined (Jacobs 1993).

Other studies have looked at the adult population with learning disabilities and seriously challenging behaviour. A postal survey of 19 specialist behavioural treatment units indicated that these units were able to offer assessment, intervention and containment but, while usually underoccupied, with a mean of 12 places, were still felt to be too large. These units were able to offer one-to-one staffing but could not provide outreach facilities. There was a low turnover of occupancy. The advantages of such specialist residential units were that extreme and complex behavioural disturbances could be assessed and managed in a setting with the appropriate level of skills and staffing. Disadvantages were isolation and the problem of generalizing complex behavioural programmes back into the community (Newman & Emerson 1991). While these issues are considered for adult residential units they are applicable to children's inpatient and residential settings. Additional concerns for children include removing the child from their family, with the risk of care being offered in a less nurturing environment.

Education

The educational provision for children with severe learning disabilities has undergone a change in many countries, with the emphasis now being on integration into mainstream schooling wherever possible and ensuring that, should this not be possible, children still access as normal a curriculum as possible. In the UK, the Education Act of 1981 lacked clarity and there was wide variation in the provision of educational resources with a lack of accountability. As a result of professional and parental concerns, a code of practice was developed which emphasized the need for integration, parental involvement and the legal obligation of the local authority to provide appropriate education. The majority of children with severe learning disabilities are now educated in day school provision with additional specialist input when indicated. Rarely, children with severe learning disabilities have such disturbed behaviour or complex medical needs (e.g. epilepsy) that they require residential provision. Residential schools are able to offer the intensive and expert input required on a 24-h basis, ensuring the child's safety while addressing their educational, behavioural and long-term health needs. Educational provision is considered in more detail by Howlin (Chapter 68).

Voluntary organizations

Voluntary organizations have an important role as part of the multi-agency provision for families with a child with a severe learning disability. In the UK, these organizations provide a massive and highly varied network of information and support that is an essential part of service provision (Crombie & Coid 2000). They include organizations which address a wide variety of issues encountered by people with a learning disability (Mencap), issues for those with a specific condition (Down Syndrome Association, Fragile X Society, Debra, and many more), specific behavioural or medical problems (Challenging Behaviour Foundation, National Society for Epilepsy), specific religious groups (Ravenswood for the Jewish community), and other locally, nationally and internationally based organizations. There are difficulties in assessing the benefits offered, as the groups are so diverse (Crombie & Coid 2000), and uncertainties about the involvement of health professionals in these groups (Black 1988). Despite this, many families find this source of support informative and a valuable addition to their support network.

Statutory and legal issues

Children and adolescents with severe learning disability are a highly vulnerable group of individuals open to abuse and exploitation (Mental Health Foundation 1993). Certain factors increase the risk of abuse, including lack of knowledge of what is acceptable behaviour from others, dependency on others for meeting personal needs and the inability to speak for themselves. Those presenting with a severe behavioural disturbance may, rarely, require methods of control or restraint involving physical interventions to ensure the child's safety (Lyon 1994).

In the UK, the Children Act (1989) provides a legal framework for the provision of services for children with learning disabilities while continuing to recognize that these children are 'children first'. The Act draws upon legislation relating to children, allowing safeguards to be implemented. Particular areas that are addressed include accommodation of children with disabilities, provision of a disability register and optimization of opportunities with the reduction of disabilities. The Act aims to ensure that services are integrated and multidisciplinary. The role of parents and families are emphasized, with the understanding that there will be partnership between them and the professionals involved. Child protection issues are paramount. The Act takes into account the transition period and outlines social services departments' statutory responsibilities in this area.

The impact of the Act on issues surrounding the care, control and safety of children with learning disabilities has been questioned. The legality of physical restraint that might have to be used, although rarely, was a major issue. A lack of legal guidance became apparent, with local authorities being expected to offer their own interpretations or seek legal advice (Lyon 1994). As a result of a detailed research report into the area, guidelines were formulated for professionals, parents and carers, which gave advice to people caring for children with severe behavioural problems (Lyon 1994). Issues including restraint, locking of doors, consent and suspicions of harm are discussed using practical examples and the application of civil and criminal law. The overriding principle remains, as stated in the Children Act (1989), that the child's welfare remains paramount.

Consent in relation to children and adolescents with severe learning disability is an issue that requires careful consideration when planning interventions for those who present with severe behavioural disturbances and may require hospitalization or long-term medication. In the UK, the law reflects a strong belief in civil liberty with the right of the individual to refuse medical treatment even if doing so is not in his or her best interests (British Medical Association 2001; see also Little, Chapter 71). This right assumes that the individual is competent to make such decisions. Children and adolescents with severe learning disabilities have the same legal status as those without learning disabilities. Parents of children aged 16 years and under are able to consent to medical treatment for their child if that child lacks sufficient understanding and intelligence of the situation. For those aged between 16 and 18 years who are considered not to be competent, then the consent of the parents or legal guardian remains valid (Lyon 1994).

Impact on the family

The news that a child has a severe learning disability has major and devastating consequences for the family (Raech 1966; Althouse & Wald 1980; Wallander & Varni 1998). There is an initial period of shock and disbelief followed by confusion, blame and guilt (Drotar et al. 1975; Blacher 1984; Cunningham et al. 1984; Carr 1988). After the initial stages of shock, families move to a period of confusion and subsequently through an adjustment phase to one of acceptance (Wright 1976). How families are told of the diagnosis has important consequences, with delay causing distress and dissatisfaction (Carr 1975). Lack of information at the time of being given the diagnosis and lack of professional support has also been documented; this adds to the distress the family suffers (Walker et al. 1971). To be able to offer support at this time, professionals need adequate and appropriate training (Forrest et al. 1982; Standish 1982; Delight & Goodall 1988). A knowledge of the underlying cause of the child's learning disability serves a number of important functions, including relief from uncertainties and alleviation of guilt, assistance with the resolution of grief and the ability to plan for the future. In many cases, appropriate support groups can then be identified (Turk 1997; Black 1988). An understanding of the cause also allows accurate genetic counselling to be offered. In a few specific disorders, the diagnosis contributes to the types of treatments and interventions that may be offered (Turk 1997).

Support and respite for families

Once the early days and months following the diagnosis have passed, families frequently find that caring for their child is demanding and exhausting. The input required is continuous, with families finding that they lack support. Parental stress is increased if the child has limited self-help skills (Sloper *et al.* 1991), poor communication, a disrupted sleep pattern (Wigg & Stores 1999) or behavioural problems (Quine 1986). Socioeconomic difficulties and marital problems also add to the burden of care (Hirst 1985). Mothers have been found to experience the highest levels of stress, with one 15-year study demonstrating that whereas over one-third of families functioned well, a further third had major difficulties in coping. In this study, as in others, marital instability and behavioural problems were more likely in those families finding the situation difficult (Koller *et al.* 1992). Certain factors have been found to contribute to family functioning: social networks, problem-solving skills, general and specific beliefs, utilitarian resources and good health and morale (Frey *et al.* 1989).

Respite care is a valuable service provision for families of children with severe learning disabilities (Jawed *et al.* 1992). The burden resulting from having a child with severe learning disabilities is both an emotional and physical one. Many hours each day may be taken up with caring for the child; one study indicated a total of 7h every day of the week (Dupont 1980; Beresford 1994). Almost two-thirds of these families had stopped having holidays and contact with friends was reduced. Mothers tend to take a major proportion of the burden of care (Carr 1975). Parents have been found to benefit from home-based respite in particular, but this type of provision is relatively rare. One study of 160 families which looked at the different types of respite provision found that families receiving residentially based local authority respite were unaware of alternatives. Families from ethnic minority groups and from lower socioeconomic backgrounds were also less likely to have access to home-based provision (Stalker & Robinson 1994). The need for a flexible approach was emphasized.

There is often a delay in parents getting the respite they require. One study found that 90% of family-based respite care schemes in the UK had waiting lists, with almost 60% of families waiting over 1 year (Prewett 1999). Many families find that the amount of respite they receive is inadequate (Stalker & Robinson 1994; Treneman *et al.* 1997).

The demand for respite care has been studied, with the indication being that the use of respite is related to the child's level of disability (Geall & Host 1996; Treneman *et al.* 1997). Younger children are less likely to use respite (Halpern 1985). Family factors are also important, including the level of family distress and lack of family support (Factor *et al.* 1990).

Siblings

The needs of siblings have also been studied. There are positive as well as negative effects for siblings (Gath 1973; Eisenberg *et al.* 1998). Siblings at risk of problems include those in families where parental stress is high and where the disabled child receives a disproportionate amount of attention. Isolation and stigma also create additional risks. Further negative factors are overidentification with the child with disabilities, caregiving responsibilities, and pressure to compensate. Positive effects, such as personal growth experiences, have been described. The place of residence of the disabled child does not seem to exert much influence on the outcome of siblings; but, in those families where the child is in residential care, there may be a less warm relationship but one without conflict. In the long term, siblings may take on the responsibilities that had been the remit of the parents. Many brother–sister relationships have been found to be warm and involved (Wilson *et al.* 1992).

Transition period

The transition period from adolescence to adulthood is a time of stress for the young person with a learning disability, and also for their family (Beckman 1983; Carr 1988; Brooks & Bouras 1991). The individual is predisposed to the development of mental health problems. This area of service provision is recognized as being one with many unmet needs and, where provision does exist, it has been found to be poorly planned and often unsatisfactory (Chamberlain 1993; Hirst & Baldwin 1994). Families find that there are few opportunities for independent living, a lack of information about future services, little help with communication difficulties and little practical help (Richardson & Ritchie 1986; Quine & Pahl 1992).

Service planning should involve the active participation of the young people involved and their parents and carers (Tausig 1995). Specific resources are needed with service structures designed to cross the barriers between child and adult provision. Multi-agency collaboration, as in all services for those with learning disabilities, is essential and minority groups must be catered for (Young Adults Transition Project 1998). Some authors have emphasized the need for the young person to leave the family home by the age of 20, as sudden and unplanned moves occurring because of the breakdown of the primary carer are traumatic (Lawrenson *et al.* 1997). The need for the young person to develop their own identity is also important and attempts to move away from the family home may be hampered by parental overinvolvement and the individual's frustrations which can lead to aggression (Kymissis & Leven 1994).

Up to 35% of adolescents with learning disabilities have been found to have a psychiatric disorder (Eaton & Menolascino 1982; Ruedrich & Menolascino 1984). Low IQ in childhood is also associated with the development of emotional problems in adolescence (Douglas *et al.* 1968) but adolescents with learning disabilities and psychiatric disorders are a poorly researched group. Few professionals have specific training in this area and, possibly as a result of the complex problems with which these young people present, few choose to work in this field (Kymissis & Leven 1994).

Parents with a learning disability

The move from institutionalized care to care in the community has led to an increased number of people with learning disabilities having relationships, marrying and having children. The eugenic fears of the early twentieth century have, in general, been superseded by concerns about competency to parent and whether training can influence this (Feldman 1986). There is little systematic research in this field, with studies being hampered by biases in selection, small sample size and unclear measures (Dowdney & Skuse 1993). Problems in controlling for variables such as socioeconomic factors also raise questions about the reliability and validity of some studies. The definitions of learning disabilities and of competent parenting add to the complexity of this area of research.

The measures that have been used to investigate parenting ability fall into three groups.

1 Global measures use the physical and emotional development of the child as outcome measures of adequate parenting. These measures are relatively non-specific but have indicated positive and negative findings.

2 Direct observational assessments; an example of one such schedule is the HOME scale (Feldman 1986) which measures the quality of the home environment.

3 The least satisfactory measure is one of parental failure resulting in abuse, neglect and family breakdown (Dowdney & Skuse 1992).

There have been a number of studies that have considered factors that influence parenting. It appears that in parents whose IQ is over 55–60, IQ alone does not predict parental competency (Dowdney & Skuse 1992). Other factors that exert an influence include parental ability to plan and make judgements and a commitment to the child. The characteristics of the child also have an influence, with age, sex, temperament and the child's own disabilities being important. Family size, family relationships and the support offered by the extended family are also influential. The ability to work in partnership with professionals is another key predictor (Andron & Tymchuk 1987).

Interventions that have been attempted aim to increase parenting abilities. These address caregiving skills and play skills and some try to improve the situation in families where abuse or neglect has occurred. Some success has been documented in learning care skills, but parents have had problems in generalizing skills and the skills are not maintained over time. In general, the prognosis has been gloomy (Andron & Tymchuk 1987).

Conclusions

The twentieth century witnessed massive changes in attitudes towards people with learning disability, and with these changes came a shift from institutionalized and custodial care to individualized and community-based service provision. Many of these changes have been politically driven, rather than based on systematic research evidence. It would be hoped that, in the twenty-first century, the provision of services is formulated with a clearer knowledge and appreciation of the underlying aetiology of learning disability, consideration of psychopathological processes and a greater understanding of appropriate interventions that might optimize the functioning of this highly vulnerable group of people within society.

Specific areas that demand consideration include the prevention of primary, secondary and tertiary disabilities and handicaps associated with severe learning disability, early identification of behavioural or mental health problems and the development of appropriate diagnostic criteria that take account of the global intellectual impairment that these people have. Effective interventions, both psychological and psychopharmacological, should be based on research evidence, with an understanding of outcome both in the short and long term.

It is to be hoped that the major challenge of the provision of efficient and effective services for young people with severe learning disability will be addressed, and that services continue to develop, ensuring liaison with all involved, including researchers, clinicians, purchasers, providers, politicians and the individuals and families receiving these services.

References

Althouse, R. & Wald, N. (1980) Survival and handicap of infants with spina bifida. *Archives of Disease in Childhood*, 55, 845–850.

Andron, L. & Tymchuk, A. (1987) Parents who are mentally retarded. In: *Mental Handicap and Sexuality* (ed. A. Craft), pp. 238–262. D.J. Costello, Kent.

Audit Commission (1994) *Seen But Not Heard: Interagency Collaboration in Services for Children in Need*. HMSO, London.

Bairstow, P., Cochrane, R. & Rusk, I. (1991) Selection of children with cerebral palsy for conductive education and the characteristics of children judged suitable and unsuitable. *Developmental Medicine and Child Neurology*, 33, 984–992.

Baker, B.L., Heifetz, L.J. & Murphy, D.M. (1980) Behavioural training for parents of mentally retarded children: one-year follow-up. *American Journal of Mental Deficiency*, 85, 31–38.

Baker, B.L., Clarke, D.B. & Yasuda, P.M. (1981) Predictors of success in parent training. In: *Frontiers of Knowledge in Mental Retardation* (ed. P. Mittler). University Park Press, Baltimore.

Bax, M.C.O. & Whitmore, K. (1985) *District Handicap Teams: Structure, Function and Relationships. Report to DHSS.* Community Paediatrics Research Unit, Westminster Children's Hospital, London.

Beckman, P.J. (1983) Influences of selected child characteristics on stress in families of handicapped infants. *Journal of Mental Deficiency Research*, 88 (2), 150–156.

Bennett, M.J., Gau, G.S. & Gau, D.W. (1980) Women's attitude to screening for neural tube defects. *British Journal of Obstetrics and Gynaecology*, 87, 370–371.

Beresford, B. (1994) Resources and strategies: how parents cope with the care of a disabled child. *Journal of Child Psychology and Psychiatry*, 35, 171–209.

Bernard, S.H. (1999) Mental health services for children and adolescents with learning disabilities. *Tizard Learning Disabilities Review*, 4 (2), 43–46.

Berne-Fromell, K., Kjessler, B. & Jesefson, G. (1983) Anxiety concerning foetal malformations in women who accept or refuse alpha-fetoprotein screening in pregnancy. *Journal of Psychosomatic Obstetrics and Gynaecology*, 202, 94–97.

Berney, T. (1997) Behavioural phenotypes in seminars. In: *The Psychiatry of Learning Disabilities* (ed. O. Russell), pp. 63–80. Gaskell, London.

Birch, H.G., Richardson, S.A., Baird, D., Horobin, G. & Ilsley, R. (1970) *Mental Subnormality in the Community: A Clinical and Epidemiological Study*. Williams & Wilkins, Baltimore.

Blacher, J. (1984) Sequential stages of parental adjustment to the birth of a child with handicap: facts or artefact? *Mental Retardation*, 22, 55–68.

Black, M. (1988) Self-help groups and professionals: what is the relationship? *British Medical Journal*, 296, 1485–1486.

Blunden, R. (1990) Services for people with learning difficulties and challenging behaviour: a brief review of recent developments. *International Review of Psychiatry*, 2, 5–10.

Borthwick-Duffy, S.E. (1994) Epidemiology and prevalence of psychopathology in people with mental retardation. *Journal of Consulting and Clinical Psychology*, 62, 17–27.

Boyd, P.A., Chamberlain, P. & Hicks, N.R. (1998) Six-year experience of prenatal diagnosis in an unselected population in Oxford, UK. *British Medical Journal*, 352, 1577–1581.

Bramble, D. (1997) Psychostimulants and British child psychiatrists. *Child Psychology and Psychiatry Review*, 2 (4), 159–162.

Bregman, J.D. (1991) Current developments in the understanding of mental retardation. II. Psychopathology. *Journal of the American Academy of Child and Adolescent Psychiatry*, 30, 861–872.

Brightman, R.P., Baker, B.L., Clarke, D.B. & Ambrose, S.A. (1982) Effectiveness of alternative parents training formats. *Journal of Behaviour Therapy and Experimental Psychiatry*, 13, 113–117.

British Medical Association (2001) *Consent, Rights and Choices in Health Care for Children and Young People*. British Medical Association, London.

Brooks, D. & Bouras, N. (1991) *Assessment and services for adolescents with a mental handicap and their families*. Division of Psychiatry, UMDS, London.

Byrne, E.A., Cunningham, C.C. & Sloper, P.A. (1988) *Families and their Children with Down Syndrome: One Feature in Common*. Routledge, London.

Carr, J. (1975) *Young Children with Down Syndrome*. Butterworth, London.

Carr, J. (1988) Six weeks to twenty-one years old: a longitudinal study of children with Down syndrome and their families. *Journal of Child Psychology and Psychiatry*, 29 (4), 407–431.

Chadwick, O., Piroth, N., Walker, J., Bernard, S. & Taylor, E. (2000) Factors affecting the risk of behaviour problems in children with severe intellectual disability. *Journal of Intellectual Disability Research*, 44, 108–123.

Chamberlain, M.A. (1993) Physically handicapped school leavers. *Archives of Disease in Childhood*, 69, 399–402.

Children Act 1989 (1991) *Guidance and Regulations*, Vol. 6. *Children with Disabilities*. HMSO, London.

Clarke, D.J., Boer, H. & Webb, T. (1995) Genetic and behavioural aspects of Prader Willi syndrome. *Mental Handicap Research*, 8, 38–53.

Clements, J.C., Evans, C., Jones, C., Osbourne, K. & Upton, G. (1982) Evaluation of a home-based training programme with severely mentally handicapped children. *Behaviour Research and Therapy*, 20, 243–236.

Commission of Enquiry on Mental Handicap (1965) [As cited by Report of the Review Group on Mental Handicap Services 1990.] *Needs and Abilities: A Policy for the Intellectually Disabled*. The Stationary Office, Dublin.

Corbett, J.A. (1979) Psychiatric morbidity and mental retardation. In: *Psychiatric Illness and Mental Handicap* (eds. F.E. James & R.P. Snaith), pp. 11–25. Gaskell, London.

Cormack, K.F.M., Brown, A.C. & Hastings, R.P. (2000) Behavioural and emotional difficulties in students attending schools for children and adolescents with severe intellectual disability. *Journal of Intellectual Disability Research*, 44, 124–129.

Crombie, I.K. & Coid, D.R. (2000) Voluntary organizations: from Cinderella to White Knight? *British Medical Journal*, 320, 392–393.

Cummins, R.A. (1988) *The Neurologically Impaired Child: Doman-Delacato Techniques Reappraised*. Croom-Helm, London. [As cited by Robards, S.M.F. (1994) In: *Running a Team for Disabled Children and their Families*. MacKeith Press, Cambridge.]

Cunningham, C., Morgan, P. & McGrucken, R.B. (1984) Down syndrome: is dissatisfaction with disclosure inevitable? *Developmental Medicine and Child Neurology*, 26, 33–39.

Delight, E. & Goodall, J. (1988) Babies with spina bifida treated with surgery: parents' view on home versus hospital care. *British Medical Journal*, 297, 1230–1233.

Donnai, D. (1987) The management of the patient having foetal diagnosis. *Balliere's Clinical Obstetrics and Gynaecology*, 1, 1–9.

Dossetor, D. & Nicol, R. (1981) Community care for adolescents with developmental retardation: problems and proposals. *Health Trends*, 22, 148–151.

Douglas, T.W.B., Ross, J.M. & Simpson, H.R. (1968) *All Our Future* [As cited by Kymissis, P. & Leven, L. (1994) In: *Mental Health in Mental Retardation Recent Advances and Practices* (ed. N. Bouras). Cambridge University Press, Cambridge.]

Dowdney, L. & Skuse, D. (1993) Parenting provided by adults with mental retardation. *Journal of Child Psychology and Psychiatry*, 34, 25–47.

Drotar, D., Baskiewics, A., Irvin, N., Kennell, J.H. & Klaus, M.H. (1975) The adaptation of parents to the birth of an infant with a congenital malformation: a hypothetical model. *Pediatrics*, 56, 710–717.

Dunne, R.G., Asher, K.N. & Rivara, F.P. (1993) Injuries in young people with developmental disabilities: comparative investigation from the 1988 national health interview survey. *Mental Retardation*, 2, 83–88.

Dupont, A. (1980) A study concerning the time related and other burdens when severely handicapped children are reared at home. *Acta Psychiatrica Scandinavia*, 62 (Suppl. 285), 249–257.

Dykens, E.M. (2000) Psychopathology in children with intellectual disability [Annotation]. *Journal of Child Psychology and Psychiatry*, 41, 407–417.

Eaton, L.F. & Menolascino, F.J. (1982) Psychiatric disorders in the mentally retarded: types problems and challenges. *American Journal of Psychiatry*, 138, 1297–1303.

Einfeld, S.L. & Aman, M. (1995) Issues in taxonomy of psychopathology in mental retardation. *Journal of Autism and Developmental Disorders*, 25, 143–167.

Einfeld, S.L. & Tonge, B.J. (1996) Population prevalence of psychopathology in children and adolescents with intellectual disability. II. Epidemiological findings. *Journal of Intellectual Disability Research*, 40 (2), 99–109.

Eisenberg, L., Baker, B.L. & Blacher, J. (1998) Siblings of children with mental retardation living at home or in residential placement. *Journal of Child Psychology and Psychiatry*, 39 (3), 355–363.

Emerson, E., Cummings, R., Barnett, S., Hughes, H., McCool, C. &

Toogood, A. (1988) Challenging behaviour and community services: who are the people who challenge services? *Mental Handicap*, **16**, 16–19.

Factor, D.C., Perry, A. & Freeman, N. (1990) Stress, social support and respite care use in families with autistic children. *Journal of Autism and Developmental Disorders*, **20**, 139–146.

Feldman, M.A. (1986) Research of parenting by mentally retarded persons. *Psychiatric Clinics of North America*, **9**, 777–796.

Flint, J. (1996) Behavioural phenotypes: a window on the biology of behaviour. *Journal of Child Psychology and Psychiatry*, **37**, 355–368.

Forrest, G.C., Standish, E. & Baum, J.D. (1982) Support after perinatal death: a study of support and counselling after perinatal bereavement. *British Medical Journal*, **285**, 1475–1479.

Fraser, W.I. & Murti Rao, J. (1991) Recent studies of mentally handicapped young people's behaviour. *Journal of Child Psychology and Psychiatry*, **32**, 79–108.

Fraser, W.I., Leudar, I., Gray, J. & Campbell, I. (1986) Psychiatric and behavioural disturbance in mental handicap. *Journal of Mental Deficiency Research*, **30**, 49–57.

Frey, K.S., Greenberg, M.T. & Fewell, R.R. (1989) Stress and coping among parents of handicapped children: a multidimensional approach. *American Journal of Mental Retardation*, **94**, 240–249.

Friedrich, W.N., Witurner, L.T. & Cohen, D.S. (1985) Coping resources and parenting mentally retarded children. *American Journal of Mental Deficiency*, **90** (2), 130–139.

Fryers, T. & Russell, O. (1997) Applied epidemiology. In: *Seminars in the Psychiatry of Learning Disabilities* (ed. O. Russell), pp. 31–47. Gaskell, London.

Gadow, K. (1985) Prevalance and efficacy of psychostimulant drug use with mentally handicapped children and youth. *Psychopharmacology Bulletin*, **21**, 291–303.

Gath, A. (1973) The school age siblings of mongol children. *British Journal of Psychiatry*, **123**, 161–167.

Geall, R. & Host, N. (1996) *Sharing the Caring: Respite Care in the UK for Families and Children with Disabilities*. National Children's Homes, London.

Gibbons, F.X. (1985) Stigma perception: social comparisons among mentally retarded persons. *American Journal of Mental Deficiency*, **90**, 98–106.

Gillberg, C., Pearson, E., Grufman, M. & Themner, U. (1986) Psychiatric disorders in mildly and severely mentally retarded urban children and adolescents, epidemiological aspects. *British Journal of Psychiatry*, **149**, 68–74.

Goffman, E. (1963) *Stigma: Notes on the Management of Spoiled Identity*. Prentice Hall, Englewood Cliffs, NJ.

Gostason, R. (1985) Psychiatric illness among the mentally retarded: a Swedish population study. *Acta Psychiatrica Scandinavica*, **71** (Suppl. 381), 1–117.

Granat, K. & Granat, S. (1973) Below average intelligence and mental retardation. *American Journal of Mental Deficiency*, **78**, 27–32.

Green, J.M., Statham, H. & Snowdon, C. (1993) Women's knowledge of prenatal screening tests. I. Relationships with hospital screening policy and demographic factors. *Journal of Reproductive and Infant Psychology*, **11**, 11–20.

Hall, D.B.M. & Prendergast, M. (1990) An integrated child health service. *British Medical Journal*, **301**, 1341–1342.

Hall, S., Bobrow, M. & Marteau, T.M. (2000) Psychological consequences for parents of false negative results on prenatal screening for Down syndrome: retrospective interview study. *British Medical Journal*, **320**, 407–412.

Hall, D.M.B. (1991) *Health for all children. A programme of child health surveillance*. The report of the joint working party on child health surveillance, 2nd ed. Oxford University Press, Oxford.

Halpern, P. (1985) Respite care and family functioning in families with retarded children. *Health Social Work*, **10**, 138–150.

Handen, B.L., Breaux, A.M., Gosling, A., Ploof, D.L. & Feldman, H. (1990) Efficacy of methyl phenidate amongst mentally retarded children with attention deficit hyperactivity disorder. *Pediatrics*, **86**, 922–930.

Hari, M. & Tillemans, T. (1984) Conductive education. In: *Management of Motor Disorders of Children with Cerebral Palsy. Clinics in Developmental Medicine No 90* (ed. D. Scrutton), pp. 19–35. Spastics International Medical Publications, London.

Hassiotis, A., Barron, P. & O'Hara, J. (2000) Mental health services for people with learning disabilities. *British Medical Journal*, **321**, 583–584.

Hirst, M. (1985) Dependency and family care of young adults with disabilities. *Child: Health, Care and Development*, **11**, 241–257.

Hirst, M. & Baldwin, S. (1994) *Unequal Opportunities: Growing Up Disabled*. Social Policy Research Unit/HMSO, London.

Jacobs, B. (1993) Treatment in child and adolescent psychiatry. In: *Seminars in Child and Adolescent Psychiatry* (eds D. Black & D. Cottrell), pp. 211–212. Gaskell, London.

Jawed, S.H., Krishnan, V.H.R. & Oliver, B.E. (1992) Respite care for children with mental handicap: Service evaluation and profile of children. *British Journal of Mental Subnormality*, **74**, 15–23.

Joint College Working Party (1989) Section for the psychiatry of mental handicap and section of child and adolescent psychiatry. The training required to provide a psychiatric service for children and adolescents with mental handicap. *Psychiatric Bulletin*, **13**, 326–328.

Keirnan, C. & Keirnan, D. (1994) Challenging behaviour in schools for children with severe learning difficulties. *Mental Handicap Research*, **7**, 177–201.

Koller, H., Richardson, S.A. & Katz, M. (1992) Families of children with mental retardation: comprehensive view from an epidemiological perspective. *American Journal on Mental Retardation*, **97** (3), 315–332.

Kymissis, P. & Leven, L. (1994) In: *Mental Health in Mental Retardation: Recent Advances and Practices* (ed. N. Bouras), pp. 102–107. Cambridge University Press, Cambridge.

Lawrenson, R., Rohde, J., Bott, C., Hambleton, I. & Farmer, R. (1997) Trends in the need for services for people with learning disabilities: implications for primary health care. *Health Trends*, **29** (2), 37–41.

Lilford, R.J. (1989) In my day we just had babies. *Journal of Reproductive and Infant Psychology*, **7**, 187–191.

Lindsey, M. (1997) Disorders in children. In: *The Psychiatry of Learning Disabilities* (ed. O. Russell), pp. 81–104. Gaskell, London.

Lyon, C. (1994) *Legal Issues Arising from the Care, Control and Safety of Children with Learning Disabilities who also Present Severe Challenging Behaviour*. Mental Health Foundation, London.

Marteau, T.M., Plenicar, M. & Kidd, J. (1993) Obstetricians presenting amniocentesis to pregnant women: practice observed. *Journal of Reproductive and Infant Psychology*, **11**, 3–10.

Mental Health Foundation (1993) *Don't forget us: Children with Learning Disabilities Who Also Present Challenging Behaviour*. London.

Meryash, D.L. (1992) Characteristics of Fragile X relatives with different attitudes towards terminating an affected pregnancy. *American Journal of Mental Retardation*, **96**, 528–535.

Muir, W.J. (2000) Genetic advances and learning disability. *British Journal of Psychiatry*, **176**, 12–19.

Newman, I. & Emerson, E. (1991) Specialist treatment units for people with challenging behaviours. *Mental Handicap*, **19**, 113–119.

NHS Executive (1998) *Signposts for Success in Commissioning and Providing Health Services for People with Learning Disabilities*. Department of Health, London.

Nirje, B. (1970) The normalization principle: implications and comments. *Journal of Mental Subnormality*, 16, 62–70.

O'Brien, J. (1987) A guide to lifestyle planning. In: *A Comprehensive Guide to the Activities Catalogue: An Alternative Curriculum for Youths and Adults with Severe Learning Disabilities* (eds B. Wilcox & G.T. Bellamy). Paul H. Brookes, Baltimore.

Oliver, C. (1995) Self-injurious behaviour in children with learning disabilities: recent advances in assessment and intervention [Annotation]. *Journal of Child and Adolescent Psychology*, 30 (6), 909–927.

Oliver, C. & Head, D. (1990) Self-injurious behaviour in people with learning disabilities: recent advances in assessment and intervention. *Journal of Child Psychology and Psychiatry*, 30, 909–927.

O'Neill, R.E., Horner, R.H., Albin, R.W., Sprague, R.J., Storey, K. & Newton, J.S. (1997) *Functional Assessment and Program Development for Problem Behaviour B: a Practical Handbook*. Brooks/Cole, USA.

Pennock, K. (1991) *Brain Injured Children*. Ashgrove Press, Bath, UK.

Prewett, B. (1999) *Short-term Break, Long-term Benefit: Family-based Short-term Care for Disabled Children and Adults*. Social Service Monographs: Research in Practice. Joint Unit for Social Services Research, University of Sheffield.

Pueschel, S.M. (1991) Ethical considerations relating to the prenatal diagnosis of foetuses with Down syndrome. *Mental Retardation* 29, 185–190.

Quine, L. (1986) Behavioural problems in severely mentally handicapped children. *Psychological Medicine*, 16, 895–907.

Quine, L. & Pahl, J. (1992) Growing up with severe learning difficulties: a longitudinal study of young people and their families. *Journal of Community and Applied Social Psychology*, 2, 1–16.

Raech, H. (1966) A parent discusses initial counselling. *Mental Retardation*, 2, 25–26.

Richards, M.P.M. (1989) Social and ethical problems of foetal diagnosis and screening. *Journal of Reproductive and Infant Psychology*, 7, 171–185.

Richardson, A. & Ritchie, J. (1986) *Making the Break*. King's Fund Publishing Office, London.

Richardson, S.A., Koller, H. & Katz, H. (1986) A longitudinal study of numbers of males and females in mental retardation services by ages, IQ, and placement. *Journal of Mental Deficiency Research*, 30, 291–300.

Richmond, J. (1990) Low birth weight infants: can we enhance their development? *Journal of the American Medical Association* 263, 3069–3070.

Robards, M.F. (1994) *Running a Team for Disabled Children and Their Families*. MacKeith Press, Cambridge.

Robinson, J.O., Hibbard, B.M. & Laurence, K.M. (1984) Anxiety during a crisis: emotional effects of screening for neural tube defects. *Journal of Psychosomatic Reseach*, 28, 163–169.

Royal College of Psychiatrists (1992) Council Report CR17. *Psychiatric Services for Children and Adolescents with Mental Handicap*. RCP, London.

Royal College of Psychiatrists (1998) Council Report CR70. *Psychiatric Services for Children and Adolescents with a Learning Disability*.

Ruedrich, S. & Menolascino, F.J. (1984) Dual diagnosis of mental retardation and mental illness: an overview. In: *Handbook of Mental Illness in the Mentally Retarded* (eds F. Menolascino & J. Stark), pp. 45–81. Plenum Press, New York.

Russell, P. (1997) The code of practice; new partnerships for children with special educational needs. *British Journal of Special Educational Needs*, 21 (2), 48–52.

Rutter, M., Graham, P. & Yule, W. (1970) *A Neuropsychiatric Study in Childhood*. Heinemann/Spastics International Medical Publications, London.

Ryan, J. & Thomas, F. (1987) *The Politics of Mental Handicap*. Free Association Books, London.

Seller, M.J. (1982) Ethical aspects of genetic counselling. *Journal of Medical Ethics*, 8, 185–188.

Shearer, M. & Shearer, D.E. (1972) The portage project: a model for early childhood education. *Exceptional Children*, 36, 210–217.

Slatter, M.A. & Black, P.B. (1986) Urban rural differences in the delivery of community services: Wisconsin a case in point. *Mental Retardation*, 24, 153–161.

Sloper, P., Knussen, C., Turner, S. & Cunningham, C. (1991) Factors relating to stress and satisfaction with life in families of children with Down syndrome. *Journal of Child Psychology and Psychiatry*, 32, 655–676.

Stalker, K. & Robinson, C. (1994) Parents' views of different respite care services. *Mental Handicap Research*, 7, 97–117.

Standing, S.J., Brindle, M.J., Macdonald, A.P. & Lacey, R.W. (1981) Maternal alpha-fetoprotein screening: two years experience in a low risk district. *British Medical Journal*, 283, 705–707.

Standish, E. (1982) The loss of a baby. *Lancet*, II, 611–612.

Sturge, J.C. (1989) Joint work in paediatrics: a child psychiatry perspective. *Archives of Disease in Childhood*, 64, 155–158.

Tausig, M. (1995) Factors in family decision making about placement for developmentally disabled adults. *American Journal of Mental Deficiency*, 89, 352–361.

Thompson, A.J., Smith, I., Brenton, D. *et al.* (1990) Neurological deterioration in young adults with phenylketonuria. *Lancet*, 336, 602–605.

Treneman, M., Corkery, A., Dowdney, L. & Hammond, J. (1997) Respite care needs met and unmet: assessment of needs for children with disability. *Developmental Medicine and Child Neurology*, 39, 548–553.

Tsoi, M.M., Hunter, M., Pearce, M., Chudleigh, P. & Campbell, S. (1987) Ultrasound scanning in women with raised serum alpha fetoprotein: short term psychological effect. *Journal of Psychosomatic Research*, 31, 35–39.

Turk, J. (1997) The mental health needs of children with learning disabilities. In: *Mental Health in Learning Disabilities* (eds. N. Bouras & G. Holt), 2nd edn, pp. 131–142. Pavilion Publishing, Brighton.

Waitman, A. & Conboy-Hill, S. (1992) *Psychotherapy and Mental Handicap*. Sage Publications, London.

Wald, N.J., Kennard, A., Hackshaw, A. & McGuire, A. (1997) Antenatal screening for Down syndrome. *Journal of Medical Screening*, 4, 181–246.

Walker, J.H., Thomas, M. & Russell, I.T. (1971) Spina bifida and the parents. *Developmental Medicine and Child Neurology*, 13, 462–476.

Wallander, J.L. & Varni, J.W. (1998) Effects of paediatric chronic physical disorders on child and family adjustment. *Journal of Child Psychology and Psychiatry*, 39 (1), 29–46.

Warnock, H.M. (1978) *Special Educational Needs: Report of the Committee of Inquiry into the Education of Handicapped Children and Young People*. Command Paper 7212. HMSO, London.

Webster-Stratton, C. (1984) Randomized trial of two parent training programmes for families with conduct disordered children. *Journal of Consulting and Clinical Psychology*, 52, 666–678.

West, R. (1988) Ethical aspects of genetic disease and genetic counselling. *Journal of Medical Ethics*, 14, 194–197.

Wilson, C.J., McGillivray, J.A. & Zectlin, A.G. (1992) The relationship between attitude to disabled siblings and ratings of behavioural competency. *Journal of Disability Research*, 36, 325–336.

Wolfensberger, W. (1983) Social role valorization: a proposed new term for the principle of normalization. *Mental Retardation*, **21**, 234–239.

World Health Organization (1997) *The International Classification of Diseases*. World Health Organization, Geneva.

Wright, L.S. (1976) Chronic grief: the anguish of being an exceptional parent. *The Exceptional Child*, **23**, 160–169.

Young Adults Transition Project (1998) *Working paper 2: Profes-sionals' view of transitional planning*. Draft Final Report. Optimum Health Services NHS Trust, London.

Yule, W. & Carr, J. (1987) *Behaviour Modification for People with Mental Handicaps*, 2nd edn. Chapman & Hall, London.

Zarkowska, E. & Clements, J. (1988) *Problem Behaviour in People with Severe Learning Disabilities: A Practical Guide to the Construc-tional Approach*. Croom-Helm, Beckenham, Kent.

68 Special Educational Treatment

Patricia Howlin

Introduction

There are many reasons why children may, at some point in their school lives, experience difficulties that disrupt learning and for which they will require special educational help. As has been recognized since the late nineteenth century, there are those pupils with sensory or physical disabilities that interfere with their ability to learn or to attend school (Currey 1898). These include children with visual or hearing impairments, epilepsy, physical disabilities or chronic illness. There are children who, because of developmental delays or disorders, lack the cognitive, linguistic or social skills needed to cope with ordinary schooling. This would apply to children with intellectual disabilities, language disorders, autism or certain other genetic conditions. There are also children with more specific problems (e.g. in reading, spelling, mathematics or motor skills) who will require help in these areas if they are to gain access to the wider teaching curriculum. There are children with severe emotional and/or behavioural difficulties that make it difficult for them to be taught in ordinary classes. Finally, there are many who require special educational help because of a combination of these difficulties.

Different needs clearly have different implications for educational provision. In order to cater for pupils with sensory or severe physical disabilities, there may be a need for special facilities, such as wheelchair access, particular equipment (computers and dedicated software, communication aids, etc.), or adaptations to the modes of teaching. Access to medical treatment may also need to be available. For those with more pervasive cognitive difficulties, the educational curriculum and teaching approaches may require much more radical modification.

The extent of an individual's disabilities will also affect educational goals. Some children may be so severely disabled that they are unlikely ever to lead independent lives. For the majority, however, although their difficulties may interfere with schooling, this should not ultimately reduce their chances of having a full role in society. Scholastic attainments are obviously important, but these must be of an appropriate kind and level, and of potential *practical* value, and hence may differ greatly from one child to another. Moreover, school is a crucial social environment, and attention needs to be paid to broader aspects of children's social, emotional and behavioural development. There is a need, too, to prepare pupils for life during the years after schooling. This is not just a question of appropriate preparation for employment but also of learning to live in the broader community, developing friendships, and learning how to get along with individuals who do not share the same problems.

Historically, at least in much of North America and Europe, the main focus of education for children with special needs was on special teaching and special equipment. This resulted in the establishment of segregated schools (Gordon 1885; Lettsom 1894) whose strength lay in the development of highly specialized and disability-specific teaching methods. However, even at that time, it was recognized that the separateness of special schools had problems as well as advantages (Cole 1989) and it was evident that a *range* of facilities was needed to provide adequately for all pupils. For example, the majority of children with even quite significant physical and sensory disabilities can be well catered for within mainstream schools *if* the necessary physical aids are provided, and if teachers are adequately prepared to deal with the social and emotional difficulties these pupils also experience. For some other children, particularly those with severe cognitive or behavioural difficulties, separate provision, at least at certain stages of their education, may be needed. However, there are many permutations in between, all of which will have certain advantages as well as possible drawbacks. No one form of provision is likely to suit all, nor should choice of school be made simply on the basis of a diagnostic label. Instead, individual assessments of the child's needs, skills and disabilities are required, with decisions about placement being based on what best suits that particular child, and his or her family. It must also be recognized that as the child grows and changes, changes in educational provision are likely to be needed, so *flexibility* of placement is also crucial.

The arguments for and against inclusive education more generally are addressed in the next section. The remainder of the chapter discusses the educational options for pupils whose special educational needs stem from relatively mild, transient or specific disorders, and the role of more specialist services for those whose disability is profound, pervasive and persisting.

The movement towards inclusive education

It has been estimated that around 20% of school-aged children will require additional help within school and that for approximately 2% of pupils the extent of their problems will severely restrict access to regular educational provision (Warnock 1978). Historically, these children tended to be excluded from mainstream schools. However, in the USA, Public Law 94–142 (Education for All Handicapped Children Act 1975) stated that, for all handicapped children between 3 and 21 years, state provision was to ensure that 'special classes, separate schooling, or removal . . . from the regular education environment occurs only when the nature . . . of the handicap is such that education in regular classes with the use of supplementary aids and services cannot be achieved satisfactorily'. Pressure for integration has since steadily increased across the developed world (Meijer *et al.* 1994) and UNESCO's (1994) Salamanca Statement called for the inclusion of pupils with special educational needs into mainstream schools.

Nevertheless, there are few empirical data to support claims that 'there are strong educational and social grounds for educating children with disabilities with their peers' (Department for Education and Employment 1998). There is little agreement as to what is meant by special educational needs and limited information on which children are most likely to benefit from inclusion.

What is inclusion?

The term 'inclusion' has come to replace 'integration' within the special educational field, largely because of concerns that 'integration' had become too narrowly interpreted as simply *placement* in a mainstream setting, without any regard to the quality of that placement (Lewis 1995; Burack *et al.* 1997; Farrell 1997; Florian 1998). However, there is controversy as to what inclusion actually means. Definitions range from 'extending the scope of ordinary schools so that they can include a greater diversity of children' (Clark *et al.* 1995) to 'a set of principles which ensures that the student . . . is viewed as a valued and needed member of the community' (Uditsky 1993). In the UK, the Department for Education and Employment (1997) refers to the 'right' of pupils to be educated in mainstream schools, despite acknowledging a continuing need for special schools. A subsequent report (Department for Education and Employment 1998) notes 'inclusion is a process, not a fixed state'. It can involve 'the placement of pupils with special educational needs in mainstream schools; the participation of all pupils in the curriculum and social life of mainstream schools; the participation of all pupils in learning which leads to the highest possible level of achievement; and the participation of young people in the full range of social experiences and opportunities once they have left school'.

The human rights argument for inclusion

The Centre for the Study of Inclusive Education (CSIE 1996) states that 'segregation in education because of disability or intellectual disability is a contravention of human rights as is segregation because of race and gender'. It has even been suggested

that it is unethical to conduct research that might produce findings in favour of segregation (Booth 1996). In contrast, others argue that the aim of education should be to meet individual needs and to help *all* children to have an active role in society (Burack *et al.* 1997; Farrell 1997). For some children, education in a special setting will be required in order to achieve these aims. There is also the question of *whose* rights should take precedence because the rights of the child, the parents or other pupils may not always be compatible. The right to choose is another issue, and research indicates that parents' attitudes to inclusion are affected by many different factors (Palmer *et al.* 1998). Parents of younger children or those already in mainstream schools are more likely to prefer inclusion than parents whose children are older or in segregated placements. The nature of the disability may also be important and, for example, parents of a child with Down syndrome tend to favour integration more than those with an autistic child (Kasari *et al.* 1999).

Empirical evidence for inclusion

Despite the extensive literature for and against inclusive education, arguments on both sides are based more on opinion or notions of political correctness than hard evidence. Most of the favourable reports are descriptive accounts of children, or schools, for whom the process has appeared to be successful (Thomas *et al.* 1998; Tilstone *et al.* 1998). Empirical research is limited (Hegarty 1993; Farrell 1997) and randomized controlled trials virtually non-existent. Matched control studies are also difficult to find, because children in specialist settings tend to show more academic and behavioural problems than pupils of similar IQ integrated in mainstream schools (Madden & Slavin 1983).

The very variable profile of children with disabilities and the lack of data on their cognitive, linguistic, social and behavioural characteristics also mean that it is almost impossible to generalize from one study to another. Even terminology is a problem. Learning disability has a different meaning in the UK than in the USA, and although children may be referred to as having mild, moderate or severe intellectual impairments, the degree of cognitive delay involved is rarely defined.

Further difficulties arise from the limited focus of many outcome studies and variability across settings. Educational provision in some of the segregated settings evaluated is sometimes far from adequate and not necessarily representative of standards elsewhere (Hornby *et al.* 1997). In contrast, much integration research in the USA has been conducted in well-resourced (often university-based) nurseries (Guralnick & Groom 1988) and the successful findings have not necessarily been replicated in less advantaged settings, or with older pupils.

International trends towards inclusion

In the UK, the proportion of children in special schools has fallen steadily from around 2% in 1978 to 1.5% in 1996 (Norwich 1996). Italy has a total integration policy (although education is only compulsory between ages 6 and 13) and in Sweden less than 1% of pupils are in special schools. In the USA and Denmark the overall figure is between 1 and 2%, rising to around 4% in the Netherlands, Germany and Belgium (Meijer *et al.* 1994). However, there is wide regional variation. In the USA, the proportion of school districts pursuing a full inclusion policy varies from 100% in some states to 1% in others (Katsiyannis *et al.* 1995). In England and Wales, three-quarters of local education authorities reduced the numbers of pupils in special schools over the past two decades but the remainder reported an increase, of up to 25%, in numbers in special provision (Swann 1991).

Education for children with mild to moderate intellectual disabilities

Implications of inclusion for intellectual and personal development

Much of the research and political debate concerning integration has focused on children with mild to moderate intellectual disability and, for them, there are strong arguments in favour of inclusion. In principle at least, integration should avoid the stigma of negative labelling and, by enabling children to learn with and from their peers, should enhance academic skills, social adjustment and self-esteem. Moreover, once a child is placed in separate education he or she is likely to remain there, with chances of reintegration diminishing with age (Farrell & Tsakalidou 2000).

In an early review, Carlberg & Kavale (1980) concluded that integration led to more positive social and learning outcomes for children with mild retardation, although not for those with *specific* learning difficulties. Self-esteem was also said to be enhanced (Lakhen & Norwich 1990; Cole & Meyer 1991). However, other research indicates that, wherever these pupils are placed, their school experience is often very negative. Several studies (Zigler & Hodapp 1987; Gottlieb 1990; Bear *et al.* 1991) have found that integration resulted in lower self-esteem and increased stigmatization and rejection by peers. Many pupils with special needs in mainstream schools also prefer to be taught in separate classes, although this may depend on how they view themselves in comparison to their typically developing peers (Harter 1984). Other reviews (Danby & Cullen 1988; Lindsey 1989; Hornby 1992; Burack *et al.* 1997) have failed to find evidence of enhanced educational attainments, social skills, self-esteem, or peer acceptance within integrated settings. Indeed, Hornby *et al.* (1997) conclude that the only obvious advantage of integrated provision is its lower cost.

The few methodologically sound studies reported (Madden & Slavin 1983; Burack *et al.* 1997) suggest that although integration *can* be successful, this only occurs if mainstream teachers are appropriately trained and when teaching is adapted to children's individual needs. So-called 'maindumping' (placing children in mainstream settings without adequate support) simply results in educational deprivation and social alienation (Stainback & Stainback 1990).

Improving the curriculum and classroom structure within mainstream settings

The poor progress of many pupils in special schools may be caused not by segregation *per se*, but by the poor quality of teaching they receive there (Giangreco 1997). Over a decade ago, Bickel & Bickel (1986) suggested that rather than concentrating on the issue of integration, it would be more productive to think in terms of 'powerful effective education' for all children and to adapt what is known about good educational practice to meet special needs. More recently, Ainscow (1995) concluded that the effectiveness of special educational provision is inextricably linked with a school's effectiveness in optimizing teaching for all pupils. Research on the factors that constitute an effective school is complex (Reynolds 1991), but the findings are clearly relevant for pupils with intellectual disabilities (Hopkins *et al.* 1996; Lipsky & Gartner 1996).

To maximize the chances of success, the curriculum and teaching programmes should be appropriately individualized and structured (Deno *et al.* 1990; Center *et al.* 1991; Lewis 1995; Farrell 1997). Goals should be clear to both teachers and pupils and be modified according to children's skills and needs (Bickel & Bickel 1986; Fuchs *et al.* 1990). The use of more directive teaching methods, together with reinforcement, feedback and monitoring techniques, is associated with improved classroom behaviour (Nowacek *et al.* 1990), as is the amount of time spent on learning tasks (Rich & Ross 1989). Other studies indicate that integration is enhanced when class size is small, e.g. in the successful preschool studies of Guralnick & Groom (1988), the total number of pupils was only eight. When this is not possible, carefully structured small group teaching can play an important part in enhancing both academic and social skills (Cooper & Spence 1990; Sebba *et al.* 1993; Ware 1994; Ainscow 1995) and is said to profit pupils with intellectual disability as well as their peers. There may be a need for some individual teaching, especially when the child is acquiring a new skill, and extra assistance in the classroom is usually required for this. However, unless properly planned, pupils with special needs can become excessively dependent on the teaching assistant, and this in turn may prove a barrier to inclusion.

Alternative approaches

Because of the conflicts faced by teachers trying to cope with the demands of perhaps 30 other pupils, as well as the child with special needs, various alternatives to full-time integration have been explored.

'Resource room' model

The 'resource room' model, although poorly defined, usually means a separate classroom where children with special needs can be offered individual teaching. Studies by Rich & Ross (1989), Lingard (1994) and Marston (1996) suggest that a *combination* of resource room and regular classroom teaching results in improved educational progress. In principle (although not always in practice), the use of resource rooms had fallen out of favour until recently because of concerns that these were simply a means of excluding difficult pupils from the classroom and could lead to isolation for both students and teachers. However, government policy in the UK now appears to be moving once more in this direction.

Partial integration

This can involve children in special units spending some of the school week in mainstream classes, either on the same site or in another school close by. Despite criticisms of 'tokenism' (Hall 1996) and claims that the availability of a 'continuum' of provision is counter to the philosophy of inclusion (Booth 1994), there is clearly a need for better evaluation of these alternative procedures (Warnock 1992; Kauffman & Hallahan 1995; Borthwick-Duffy *et al.* 1996; Little & Witter 1996). The little research that does exist indicates that placement on the same site as the mainstream school and the development of programmes that can be implemented within regular classrooms are necessary in order to achieve real integration (Burack *et al.* 1997).

Specialist teaching programmes

Despite vast numbers of publications offering advice on 'the making of the inclusive school', and how to improve the curriculum, environment, support structures and general attitudes, there is virtually no empirical support in favour of one particular approach or another. Co-operative learning (groups of students working together to achieve mutual goals) has been recommended in a number of studies but there is little evidence that this is more effective than individual learning (Tateyama-Sniezek 1990). Self-evaluation and self-monitoring programmes (Sainato *et al.* 1992), the Adaptive Learning Environment Model (ALEM; Wang & Walberg 1993), Direct Instruction, Mediated Learning (Dale & Cole 1988), Instrumental Enrichment (Feuerstein *et al.* 1980), or 'creative' action planning techniques (Forest *et al.* 1996) all have their advocates, but experimental evaluations are either non-existent or equivocal (Hornby *et al.* 1997). Even within the extensive literature on the effectiveness of behavioural or cognitive behavioural approaches, the majority of reports are of single cases, or small samples without control groups (Sulzer-Azaroff & Gillat 1990; Cole *et al.* 1994; Ayres *et al.* 1995).

Improving acceptance by peers

Without specific intervention, integration is unlikely to increase social competence in children with intellectual disabilities or to improve acceptance by peers (Hall 1994; Hendrikson *et al.* 1996). Social interactions may occur more frequently in integrated settings, but children with developmental delays still remain relatively isolated; spontaneous joint play is infrequent and close friendships are rare (Saintano *et al.* 1992; Guralnick *et al.* 1995; Burack *et al.* 1997; Siperstein & Leffert 1997). Acceptance is more likely to occur if the perceived differences between the handicapped child and his or her peers are slight (Truesdell 1990). Nevertheless, programmes that have focused on training normal peers to initiate interactions or implement co-operative learning strategies have been successful in increasing the frequency and quality of social responses and in enhancing academic skills (Acton & Zarbatany 1988; Fox 1989; Topping 1990; Putnam 1993). Although caution is needed in interpreting the results of much of this research (Topping 1990), peer tutoring, at least if adequately structured, seems to be far more effective than attempts to change the attitudes of normal peers by indirect methods, such as teaching tapes, stories or simulations. Positive results, in terms of academic gains, social maturity and increased empathy, have also been reported for the peer tutors (Maheady *et al.* 1988; Hornby *et al.* 1997). 'Circles of friends' or carefully structured pairings of normally developing and disabled children are among other strategies reported to promote social inclusion but evaluations are few and generalization is often limited (Kishi & Meyer 1994; Newton *et al.* 1996).

Improving teacher training and support

While mainstream classrooms and curricula *can* be adapted to meet the needs of children with mild to moderate intellectual disabilities, this is not an easy task for most teachers who are already working under considerable pressure. A survey of pupils with special educational needs in mainstream schools found that the quality of teaching was unsatisfactory in around half of all lessons (Her Majesty's Inspectorate (HMI) 1989). Although training in special education is crucial in order to improve this situation, financial restraints mean that full-time courses have been increasingly replaced by cheaper, part-time modular courses (Deno *et al.* 1990; Nowacek *et al.* 1990). Moreover, even the best-trained teachers are unlikely to be effective unless they have adequate support.

Giangreco (1997) identified a number of common features in schools where inclusive education seemed to be thriving. These included collaborative teamwork and a shared framework for teaching, clear role relationships among professionals and effective use of support staff. 'Meaningful' individual educational plans (IEPs) for pupils and procedures for evaluating teaching effectiveness were also important. Consultation services, by specially trained professionals who can offer teachers continuing help in the classroom, may also be effective (Dyson 1990; Fuchs *et al.* 1990; Jordan 1994) although others claim that such interventions can undermine teacher status and independence (Farrell 1997). Jenkins & Heinen (1989), in a study of 337 children with special needs, found the majority preferred to receive additional help from their own teacher rather than from a specialist, because this made them feel less conspicuous. The provision of specialist support teachers (*not* untrained classroom assistants) working alongside the class teacher may be more appropriate, but support teaching often fails because of inadequate liaison and planning (Thomas 1992).

Teachers' attitudes clearly have an impact on the success or otherwise of inclusive programmes. In a recent review, Scruggs & Mastropieri (1996) found that although 65% of teachers supported the general concept of inclusion, only 40% believed this to be a realistic goal for most children. Around half indicated that they were willing to teach children with special educational needs and considered that these pupils would benefit from inclusion. However, only one-third believed that mainstream classroom teaching was the best option and 30% suggested this could have a negative impact on other students in the class. Less than one-third considered that they had the necessary teaching expertise and the majority felt that classroom sizes would need to be reduced and resources greatly improved if inclusion were to be successful. Other research has also indicated that regular education teachers have little confidence in their ability to modify their teaching procedures or the classroom environment to accommodate pupils with special needs (Schumm & Vaughan 1991; Whinnery *et al.* 1991).

Attitudes to inclusion tend to be less positive amongst teachers of older pupils (Hanrahan *et al.* 1990) and the move towards school league tables and 'payment by results' in the UK is unlikely to improve this situation. There is some evidence too (Gersten *et al.* 1988) that effective class teachers in normal schools may be *less* tolerant of children with special needs, presumably because of their higher expectations and standards. Unless calls for greater inclusion can be reconciled with the increasing demands for higher standards and the need to meet the requirements of the National Curriculum, many teachers will understandably feel that they are being faced with an impossible task. There is no evidence that exposure to pupils with special needs has any positive effects *per se*. Instead, adequate preparation and training in the skills necessary to promote progress and minimize difficulties, and a far higher level of ongoing support, are required to improve both attitudes and practice.

Parental views

Research suggests that parents will support mainstreaming, but only if they consider resources are adequate (Bailey & Winton 1987; Simpson & Myles 1992). Parents with children in mainstream schools generally express satisfaction with the placement (surveys vary from 65 to 88%; Lowenbraun *et al.* 1990; Kidd & Hornby 1993), although there is a marked preference for special units in the mainstream setting, rather than placement in regular classes. However, around 70–80% of parents with children in segregated provision are also satisfied with these placements (Meyers & Blatcher 1987; Kauffman 1991). There is little evidence to suggest that parents are either overwhelmingly for or against inclusive education (McDonnell 1987) and Hornby *et al.* (1997) suggest that this in itself reinforces the importance of maintaining a continuum of specialist placements.

Recommendations for successful inclusion

Vaughan & Schumm (1995), in a 2-year study of primary schools in large urban areas in the USA, concluded that to achieve 'responsible inclusion' there were a number of essential components.

1 *For pupils.* A continuum of services should be available, including withdrawal for small group teaching and access to special education classrooms. Alternative teaching strategies and modifications to the curriculum should be offered to meet individual needs—these pupils should not be expected to profit from the same teaching and curriculum as other students. There should also be continual monitoring of the curriculum and teaching provision in order to ensure that students' needs are met.

2 *For teachers.* They should be allowed to choose whether or not to be involved in teaching inclusive classes—it should not be imposed on everyone, regardless of attitudes or expertise. Ongoing professional development should be available to all staff and there should be adequate provision of human and physical resources. Inclusion should *not* be expected to reduce educational costs.

3 *For the community.* The inclusive models developed by individual schools should be adapted to suit the needs of the pupils, parents and local community. There should be an agreed philosophy and policy on inclusion, providing guidance to teachers, parents and colleagues. A standardized policy of inclusion should not be imposed on schools.

Education for children with 'specific' learning disabilities

Language disorders

Language impairments are among the most common of childhood disorders. In a recent study in Ontario, 19% of 5-year-old children were found to have speech and/or language difficulties (Beitchman *et al.* 1996). Of these, 49% had a diagnosable psychiatric disorder (mainly attention deficit hyperactivity disorder or anxiety/depression) and many subsequently developed other cognitive problems, especially related to reading. Although many children with early language delays eventually 'catch up' without intervention (Whitehurst & Fischel 1994; Rescorla *et al.* 1997), in a substantial proportion of cases (estimates vary from 50 to 90%) linguistic and other impairments are both persistent and pervasive (Tomblin *et al.* 1992; Beitchman *et al.* 1996; Stothard *et al.* 1998). Scholastic problems related to reading, spelling and mathematics are common and there is a significant risk of later emotional, social, behavioural and psychiatric problems (for review see Stevenson 1996). However, educational provision remains very inadequate. Despite some evidence for the effectiveness of language therapy (see meta-analyses by Nye *et al.* 1987; Swanson *et al.* 1999), such input is rarely sustained beyond the junior school stage and advice and support for regular class teachers are limited (Davison & Howlin 1997). Howlin *et al.* (2000), in a follow-up study of 20 individuals with severe developmental language impairments, found that although half were educated in specialist (often residential) placements during the primary years, by secondary school 50% were in mainstream schools with little or no additional support. One-third were in settings for children with mild retardation or learning difficulties and the remainder were in schools for children with mixed disorders. The group also experienced frequent changes of school throughout childhood. Post-school education was very limited which, in turn, adversely affected later job prospects and social opportunities.

Assessment of intervention programmes is complicated because of the heterogeneity of language impairments. On the whole 'general stimulation' programmes tend to have less impact than those utilizing more direct approaches (Nye *et al.* 1987), but comparative studies are sparse. Interventions with a focus on the *social* use of language (Rinaldi 1992) are currently popular, as are programmes involving parents as therapists. These include the Language Interaction Intervention programme of Weistuch & Lewis (1985) and Weistuch & Byers-Brown (1987) and the Hanen approach (Weitzman 1992). The use of normally developing 'peer confederates' (Goldstein *et al.* 1992) is claimed to reduce the adult prompt–dependant interaction on which children with language impairments often come to rely. More specific intervention programmes (e.g. that of the Speech Foundation of Ontario, Hayden & Pukonen 1996; or the ECLIPSE project of Schwartz *et al.* 1998) stress the need for individual assessment and involve the creation of an environment that is designed to elicit and enhance communication; the structuring of interactions with and by peers; and the use of naturalistic teaching strategies, together with specific techniques such as modelling, turn-taking, topic manipulation, conversational repair, scripts and time delay. Although single case reports indicate that these approaches can be very effective, there are no substantive group trials, nor is it possible to identify which of the various teaching components are most effective.

There are no well-designed studies of integrated vs. specialist teaching for children with developmental language disorders. The Language Acquisition Pre-school Program at the University of Kansas (Rice & Wilcox 1991) suggests that their integrated preschool model, involving parent participation and normal peers, significantly increases children's chances of remaining with their peer group in subsequent academic placements. However, in most areas preschool provision is scarce, available mainly in segregated settings and on a short-term basis only. Once spoken language appears to improve (even though many other difficulties persist) children are often transferred to mainstream school, without additional help or recognition of their needs. The history that follows is all too frequently one of educational failure, bullying by peers, school exclusion, social rejection, and low self-esteem. In adulthood, occupational levels are low and there is a high level of dependence on families (Haynes & Naidoo 1991; Howlin *et al.* 2000).

Reading and spelling difficulties

It is estimated that between 3 and 10% of school-aged children have persistent and marked reading and/or spelling disabilities (at least 2 SD below predicted levels) and the adverse effects on educational progress have been well documented (see Snowling, Chapter 40). In the UK, the Department for Education and Employment's Code of Practice (Department of Education and Employment 1994a,b) lists the learning and behavioural deficits associated with literacy problems and requires schools to keep meticulous records of children's progress and difficulties. In principle, this should lead to all such pupils, regardless of their IQ, having an IEP, to ensure that their needs are met. In practice, lack of adequate classroom support makes it difficult to provide them with the intensive help they often require. The current government strategy of insisting on a set reading period each day, in itself, will do little to help children with specific difficulties in this area (Hurry 1999). Extra tuition for children with reading and/or spelling problems still tends to be provided outside the classroom, or in privately funded centres, both of which limit opportunities for participating fully in the school curriculum.

There is also little agreement on what remedial programmes should entail. Almost any type of intervention initially seems to produce short-term gains, but these are rarely maintained (Maughan & Yule 1994). Overall, the approaches that are effective for children who are just beginning to learn to read (a combination of training in phonological awareness with explicit work on letter sound correspondence; Foorman *et al.* 1991) have been found to help children with reading delays (Hatcher *et al.* 1994). Adaptations of the Reading Recovery approach (intensive, structured, individualized reading programmes; Clay 1985) which incorporate additional phonological training (Bryant & Bradley 1985) also seem to be successful (Iverson & Tunmer 1993; Tunmer 1994; Sylva & Hurry 1995). However, Sylva & Hurry (1995) found that the improved performance of pupils receiving such intervention tended to disappear after 18–24 months. Moreover, control children, who received phonological training alone, made similar progress to pupils *in the same schools* receiving the total package. Snowling (1996) suggested that this may be because the extra support provided to the poor readers relieved the stress on their teachers, leading to improvements in the classroom situation more generally.

Research with 'dyslexic' children (those with specific reading or spelling difficulties) has also indicated that a variety of different strategies can be effective but often the improvements do not generalize to other reading problems or to new situations. Lovett *et al.* (1990), for example, found that training in word recognition significantly increased children's sight vocabularies, but they were still unable to recognize new words. Children provided with phonological training improved in their ability to read non-words (Lovett *et al.* 1994) but word identification skills did not increase. The Colorado remediation project (Wise *et al.* 1990; Olson & Wise 1992) found that computer feedback using synthesized speech could help to improve reading.

Children given segmented feedback (e.g. 'd/ish', rather than 'dish') showed particular improvements in their ability to read non-words. However, outcome also depended on the amount of direct monitoring by adults—when left to work independently children tended to skip the difficult words unless they were assured of whole word feedback. There was also an interaction between the severity of children's reading problems and response to treatment. Onset–rime feedback ('d/ish') worked less well than vowel–consonant feedback ('di/sh') for children with the most severe difficulties, while the opposite was true for the least severely disabled readers.

On the whole, a combination of direct training in reading *plus* phonological awareness is now considered to be most effective. Although there has been considerable research into the effectiveness of individualized teaching programmes (based on analysis of the child's specific pattern of deficits and skills), Snowling (1996) suggested that there is still 'no compelling evidence that dyslexic children who read in different ways should be given different kinds of remedial teaching'. Raban (1991) also noted the importance of other factors, such as teacher effectiveness, classroom organization, time spent on reading and the provision of resources. Parental participation in the programme can help to enhance outcome, but only if they are given appropriate guidance in what to do (Whitehurst *et al.* 1994). Simply encouraging them to listen to their child at home has little effect (Toomey 1993). Similarly, classroom assistants *can* have an important role, but only if they are fully trained to understand and implement the literacy programme. The use of older reading-disabled peers is also suggested as an effective means of enhancing reading in young children 'at risk' of reading failure (Juel 1994). Nevertheless, the benefits, even of the most effective programmes, tend to be short-lived, and research is needed to identify the factors required to maintain longer term progress (Snowling 1996).

Behavioural and emotional problems

The term 'emotional and behavioural disorders' covers a vast range of problems. It may include children with conduct disorders, antisocial behaviours, hyperactivity, attention deficits, psychiatric or mood disorders, or a combination of these. The causes may be genetic, environmental or constitutional. Moreover, many of these children have additional learning difficulties and hence it is not surprising that they present such a challenge to educational services. However, judgements as to whether a child has behavioural or emotional problems often depend more on the attitudes, policies and practices of the school, or the tolerance level of individual teachers than on any objective criteria. A child who shows very disruptive behaviour in one setting may not do so elsewhere (Werthamer-Larsson *et al.* 1991) and the role of schools in maintaining or minimizing disruptive behaviours has been widely investigated (Rutter 1983; Hallinger & Murphy 1986; Reynolds 1991). In some cases, transfer to a different class or a move to a school where teachers are more sensitive to the child's needs may be sufficient significantly to reduce the level of problems. In others, intervention may need to be much more complex.

Ideally, detailed assessment of the child's behavioural difficulties, family circumstances, social competence, learning strategies and academic capabilities is required in order to address the many and complex problems associated with this group of disorders. Programmes such as those of Hechtman *et al.* (1996) illustrate the many facets of therapy that may need to be included. These can involve cognitive-behavioural therapy, interpersonal problem-solving and social skills training, parent training and counselling, and play or other individual therapies. Remedial input to enhance general academic skills, memory, auditory and visual processing, and sequencing is also essential (Hechtman *et al.* 1996). Unfortunately, apart from those children enrolled in specialist multimodal programmes, few are likely to be offered anything other than relatively brief interventions, which may be home-, clinic- or school-based, but rarely all three.

Management techniques within the classroom

Although only a partial approach to the problems faced by a child with emotional and/or behavioural problems, strategies based on behavioural principles have been shown to be very effective. This approach has a number of advantages, in that it does not require removal of the child from the class and the basic techniques can be adapted to the particular needs of an individual child or classroom. On the whole, placing the focus of intervention on positive on-task behaviours is more effective than concentrating on disruptive behaviours (McNamara & Jolly 1990; Herbert 1995; Barkley 1997). Scott (1998) and Warner-Rogers (1998) provided a number of guidelines for enhancing performance in children with conduct disorders, hyperactivity and/or attention deficits. Instructions should indicate what the child *should* be doing ('Please speak quietly') rather than what he or she should *not* do ('Don't shout'). The task should be explicit ('Put the cars in the cupboard', rather than simply 'Tidy up') and single instructions are more likely to be obeyed than a string of orders. If it is necessary to stop the child before he or she completes an activity, advanced warning should be given ('You will have to get off the computer when the bell goes'). 'When–then' commands ('When you've finished that page then you can play outside') should replace vague threats ('You'll be sorry if you do that'), and all directions should be given firmly and clearly. The consequences, both positive and negative, of the child's actions should be clear, consistent and immediate and must always be followed through. Tasks should be broken down into small steps, thereby allowing greater opportunity for positive feedback and avoiding the need for prolonged attention. Positive strategies should always be in place before negative ones are employed. Although techniques such as extinction or time-out can be extremely effective (Barkley 1997), it can be very difficult to implement these consistently. Other children or staff may respond to activities that the teacher is trying to ignore, or the behaviour may escalate to such a level that ignoring is no longer an option. Time-out is all too often used as a synonym for 'removal from the classroom', which may act as anything but a deterrent for many children, and there is a danger of exclusion periods becoming increasingly lengthy.

Other behavioural approaches, such as token economies, differential reinforcement or response–cost, have been reported to be highly effective but much of this work has been conducted in specially designed or experimental classes (Carlson *et al.* 1992). The consistent use of these strategies may not be feasible for teachers coping with 30 or more pupils, although in smaller classes, or when additional help is available, it may be possible to adapt them successfully (for practical teaching guidelines see Abramowitz *et al.* 1992; Gordon & Asher 1994).

Research suggests that in order for schools to have a significant impact on severely disturbed or disruptive pupils, attention must also focus on factors outside the classroom, such as the wider school curriculum, organization and climate (Galloway & Goodwin 1987; MacAulay 1990). Nevertheless, even relatively minor changes to the classroom or timetable may have positive effects. Some children with hyperactivity and attentional problems, for example, seem to perform better on classroom activities in the morning. Brightly coloured materials may hold children's attention better, and the presentation of materials in small chunks, interspersed with brief breaks, is likely to benefit pupils with concentration problems (Warner-Rogers 1998). Modifications to classroom organization, alterations to seating arrangements or providing specially designated areas for study may also significantly reduce classroom disruption (Wheldall & Lam 1987; Ware 1994).

Strategies for *avoiding* problems can also have an important role. Remedial intervention for academic difficulties may prevent the escalation of secondary behaviour problems. Planning ahead can avoid potentially high-risk situations (those when the setting, peer group, or even a particular teacher is likely to exacerbate difficulties). Negotiating potentially difficult situations with children themselves, so that they feel part of the consultation and planning process, can also increase appropriate behaviours.

Although cognitive-behavioural approaches to therapy have little direct impact on attention problems (Abikoff 1991; Bloomquist *et al.* 1991), problem-solving and 'self-instruction' techniques can be effective in reducing impulsive reactions to frustration and enabling children to slow down and devise more effective ways of responding (Hinshaw & Melnick 1992; Petersen & Ganonii 1992). Anger management may also assist the child to recognize internal cues of anger and to develop strategies for decreasing or redirecting this (Novaco 1979). However, because many children with conduct and attentional disorders tend to have communication problems, verbally mediated techniques may need to be specially adapted (Hinshaw 1992). Training in communication and social skills may also enable these children to work more effectively and co-operatively with teachers and peers (Guevremont 1990; Cousins & Weiss 1993; Gray *et al.* 1994). (For more general texts on teaching approaches see Ayres *et al.* 1995; McNamara & Moreton 1995; Cooper & Ideus 1996; O'Brien 1998.)

Children who are excluded from mainstream school

As noted earlier, the push towards inclusion has coincided, in the UK at least, with governmental demands for a rise in classroom standards. Many teachers feel unable to meet these demands if they also have to cope with very disturbed pupils and the number of children officially excluded from school on behavioural grounds has risen sharply over recent years (from 3833 in 1991 to 12 458 in 1994–55; Department for Education 1995). Unofficial exclusions may be even higher and rates of exclusion have also risen within the special school system (Paffrey 1994). Boys are almost five times more likely to be excluded than girls, with rates being highest among African-Caribbean boys. The main reasons for exclusion are aggressive, violent or disruptive behaviours but schools (and local authorities) differ widely in both their reasons for and rates of exclusion and headteachers' attitudes and school status, policies and practices may play a greater part than a pupil's behaviour (Hornby *et al.* 1997)

The outlook for children excluded from mainstream school is bleak. Around 25% receive home tuition, although rarely for more than a few hours a week; 40% attend pupil referral units for half time or less (Young 1996). Those with very severe emotional problems may be offered temporary placements in psychiatric units but mainstream schools then tend to be even more unwilling to re-admit them (Hornby *et al.* 1997). Indeed, many mainstream schools remain reluctant to accept pupils who have been excluded from another school. These children frequently also come from disrupted homes and, without the stability that school can offer, many then simply drift into a life of delinquency and further deprivation.

Although the cost of exclusion to pupils, their families and to society more generally has been widely publicized, the question of how to deal with it remains largely unsolved. There is general agreement that effective intervention for children with complex behavioural and learning problems requires better training and resources for teachers, together with the expertise and input of a network of interagency support (Department for Education and Employment 1994b). However, many teachers tend only to use such services when the classroom situation has totally broken down, rather than at an earlier stage when there is some chance of remediation (Hanko 1993). Stainback & Stainback (1990) conclude that it should be possible to reintegrate these children with adequate help for teachers but such provision is frequently lacking. The old notion of 'contagion' (Redl 1966) has proved hard to dispel in an age of increasing classroom violence and many teachers have no wish to submit other students, or themselves, to the disruption that a very disturbed child can cause.

A range of on- and off-site provision for these children has been provided over the years in the form of resource rooms, tutorial classes, educational guidance centres, intermediate treatment units and, more recently, 'pupil referral units'. The stated goal of such facilities has been to offer individualized remedial teaching and general support to 'challenging' pupils *on a temporary basis* while maintaining links with the parent school. However, there have been many concerns about their general effectiveness, poor physical and educational standards, limited access to the normal curriculum and tenuous links with the parent school (Mortimore *et al.* 1983; Galloway & Goodwin 1987). The high proportion of pupils from disadvantaged backgrounds or those from minority ethnic groups (especially those of African-Caribbean origin) is also a cause for concern (ILEA 1981).

Despite recent calls by the Department for Education and Employment (1998) in the UK for an increase in 'pupil referral units' in order to reduce rates of exclusion from schools, past experience suggests that separate centres of this kind are expensive, discriminating and stigmatizing and do little to facilitate children's return to mainstream school (Galloway & Goodwin 1987). An alternative solution, also strongly supported by present government policy, is the provision of specialist schools for pupils with emotional and behavioural problems (formerly known as 'maladjusted schools'). However, again, relatively few children (around 20% or less) subsequently return to mainstream school and reintegration rates are even lower for pupils in boarding schools (Dawson 1980). Nevertheless, there may still be a place for residential provision for children whose difficulties are largely brought about by a severely disturbed or deprived family environment and for whom placement away from home may offer some chance of progress.

Post-school

Although children with mild to moderate intellectual disabilities, and those with more 'specific' learning difficulties, can and should profit from mainstream education, it is increasingly clear that this will not be achieved without adequate support for all involved. Unless this is forthcoming, the social exclusion experienced by these children may well extend into adult life. Drop-out rates from school are extremely high (generally between 35 and 50%; de Bettencourt *et al.* 1989) and access to *appropriate* tertiary education is limited (Bursuck *et al.* 1989). Employment rates are poor, with only around 50–60% of individuals with specific learning or behavioural problems finding work, and even higher unemployment rates (60–70%) among those with mild intellectual disability (Hasazi *et al.* 1989). Earnings, job status and stability are low (Zetlin & Murtaugh 1990) and work experience is frequently very negative (Szivos 1990). Long-term dependence on parental support is also typical (deBettencourt *et al.* 1989; Hasazi *et al.* 1989; Howlin *et al.* 2000). Although there has been an increase in vocational training programmes—Zetlin & Murtaugh (1990) report 75% participation in post-school educational programmes in the USA—few such courses are of high academic or vocational level. Thus, students may find it difficult to gain access to courses that adequately meet their needs, and drop-out rates are high (Harrison 1996). Better transition services to facilitate the move from school or college into employment are also essential.

Special education for children with physical and sensory handicaps

Physical disabilities

The desirability of integrating children with physical handicaps into normal classrooms has been recognized for well over a century (Charity Organization Society 1893, cited in Cole 1989). However, the difficulties experienced by these pupils are multiple and complex. For example, while many children with cerebral palsy are of normal IQ, they may also be incontinent or have seizures, their uncontrolled movements may upset other children, they may be unable to communicate effectively, and emotional and psychiatric problems are common (Harris 1998). Cerebral palsy is also associated with increased behavioural difficulties (McDermott *et al.* 1996), high rates of visual and hearing problems (Capute & Accardo 1991) and around 30–60% have some degree of intellectual disability (Evans *et al.* 1990). Kohn (1990) and Harris (1998) discuss the many components required for a comprehensive package of educational care but, in practice, 'integration' often involves simply the provision of physical aids, some—often inadequate—adaptations to the physical environment, and the use of support staff or classmates to assist the class teacher. Few mainstream schools have adequate access to trained nursing or physiotherapy help, and little guidance is provided on how to deal with the child's educational, social and emotional problems, particularly those related to teasing, isolation or low self-esteem. Although children with physical disabilities are a very heterogeneous group, on the whole research indicates that those of normal IQ do better, both socially and academically, in mainstream settings (Carr *et al.* 1981; Carr 1982). However, as is the case with other disabilities, tolerance among teachers and peers tends to decrease with age (Hunt 1981; Anderson *et al.* 1982) and in secondary school, when access to the normal curriculum is particularly important in terms of future academic progress, real inclusion often becomes more difficult to achieve.

Hearing impairments

One in 770 children is born with a significant hearing loss and for 1 in 2000 the loss is profound (Gregory & Hindley 1996). Around 25% will show additional intellectual, physical or sensory problems, and emotional and psychiatric difficulties are also common (Roberts & Hindley 1999). In addition to these complications, the strength of the deaf advocacy movement, particularly in the USA, has resulted in the debate over appropriate education becoming particularly contentious. The poor signing skills of many hearing parents or teachers (Gregory & Hindley 1996), and the fact that deaf children of deaf parents often make better academic and social progress than deaf children of hearing parents (Schilling & DeJesus 1993; Spencer 1993; Prendergast & McCollum 1996), has led to claims that this latter group is best educated in specialist schools (residential if necessary). Remedial interventions, such as cochlear implants, have been condemned because they deny children's right to belong to the deaf community (Balkany *et al.* 1996); and fluency in signing, with its own grammar and idiom, is considered to be a crucial educational goal. However, as Groenveld (1998) points out, this may have the result of alienating children from their families and neighbourhood. Consequently, 'bilingual education' (the combination of a formal deaf signing system with written and spoken language) has become more widely adopted, both in special schools and some mainstream placements (Hindley & Brown 1994). Nevertheless, success is at least partly dependent on the adequacy of adults' signing skills (Gregory *et al.* 1995), the degree of liaison with and amount of support offered to parents, and the effectiveness of teachers in fostering pupils' spontaneous communication (Wood *et al.* 1986). Early intervention programmes, involving a combined oral–visual approach, are suggested as being particularly important in avoiding the 'cultural divide' that may otherwise develop between hearing parents and their deaf children (Meadow-Orlans 1987; Reed & Hindley 1998)

The poor cognitive and educational attainments of many deaf children and their increasing social isolation as they grow older are well documented (Hindley & Brown 1994). Although some authors have argued strongly in favour of integration for all children with hearing impairments (Lynas 1984), others, such as Gregory *et al.* (1995), suggest their difficulties are often greatly underestimated by mainstream teachers, and hence they may do better in the more supportive atmosphere of a special school or unit. However, the choice of an appropriate placement will depend on may other factors, such as age, IQ, level of hearing disability, presence of other impairment and, most importantly, on the quality of instruction offered (Roberts & Hindley 1999). (Two useful references on general educational approaches for deaf children in mainstream and special schools are Gregory *et al.* 1995; Watson *et al.* 1999.)

Visual problems

Children with visual difficulties are also likely to suffer from a range of additional problems including cerebral palsy, epilepsy, linguistic and hearing impairments, autism, intellectual disability and emotional and psychiatric disturbance (Hindley & Brown 1994; Groenveld 1998). In the UK, the majority of such children are still educated in segregated settings, and although more (around 60%) are in mainstream placements in the USA many are still educated in resource rooms or special classes. Again, educational outcome depends on the child's cognitive level, the presence of additional impairments, the quality of teaching and the availability of resources. More able children are likely to do better in appropriately adapted mainstream provision (Arter *et al.* 1999) than children of lower IQ, although they may also succeed in specialist placements (Chapman & Stone 1988). Resource room provision (albeit with careful preparation of staff, sighted pupils and their parents beforehand) can also be successful in increasing functional integration (Hegarty *et al.* 1982a,b).

Special education for children with severe and pervasive intellectual disabilities

Most research indicates that these pupils are less likely to profit from mainstream placements than those with milder or more specific disabilities (Ispa & Matz 1978; Carlberg & Kavale 1980; Rich & Ross 1989; Deno *et al.* 1990). Moreover, acceptance by peers and teachers tends to decrease with age and, although inclusion may succeed in the infant years, relatively few studies have reported on successful integration within secondary school (Budgell 1986; although see Beveridge 1996; Booth 1996). The degree of support available also affects integration and, unless this is adequate, children with severe disabilities may receive less individualized instruction in normal classes than in segregated classes. The role of support staff is crucial here (Center *et al.* 1991; Gregory 1996; Mencap 1999) but they need to be able to plan and carry out individually tailored teaching programmes with the child, and to work collaboratively with other staff and pupils in order to ensure social integration and academic progress. Working individually with a child with special needs in the corner of the classroom (or in the library or medical room) may actually increase rather than decrease segregation. All too often, lack of adequate preparation and of systematic and on-going training for support workers, and their isolation from other teaching staff (Lopez 1994; Farrell 1996), has meant that their role tends to focus more on the minimization of behavioural difficulties, so that the child is tolerated but certainly not assimilated.

One of the strongest arguments proposed by advocates of inclusive education for children with severe intellectual disabilities is that it has a positive impact both on their social development and that of their typically developing peers. However, social interaction is unlikely to occur unless the environment, teaching materials and children's activities are appropriately structured (Steele & Mitchell 1992). Although support staff play an essential part in encouraging interactions between the child with disabilities and his or her classmates, their presence may actually interfere with social integration (Farrell 1996) and it may be more productive for them to focus on training other pupils to interact with the child with special needs. Team teaching and co-operative learning approaches are important (Ware *et al.* 1992) and the structuring of collaborative learning activities between handicapped and nonhandicapped children helps to improve classroom behaviours (Putnam 1993). There is little evidence that simple exposure to non-handicapped peers improves either language or social skills (Lewis 1995). If peers are taught to prompt, respond to or initiate social and verbal interactions this can enhance communication skills and academic and social attainments in children with intellectual disabilities, although there are problems with maintenance over time and generalization across settings (Hundert & Houghton 1992; Saintano *et al.* 1992; Stainback *et al.* 1994). Moreover, although guided contact with their disabled peers may have a positive impact on other pupils' *attitudes* (Farrell 1996), joint spontaneous interactions remain limited and close reciprocal friendships are very *unlikely* to develop (Gottlieb 1990; Saintano *et al.* 1992; Burack *et al.* 1997).

The enthusiasm for integration expressed by politicians and educational theorists is not necessarily shared by teachers. Ward *et al.* (1994) and Forlin (1995) found that teachers were much less positive about integration than administrative personnel. The most negative views were expressed by teachers who were more experienced and those working with very severely disabled children. Stress levels among class teachers were often high, and there were concerns about inadequate support and their lack of choice in decisions about the placement of a child with special needs.

There are also other practical dilemmas pertaining to the integration of this group of children. For example, whereas communication skills seem to be enhanced when therapists employ 'facilitative' teaching styles to encourage initiations and spontaneous language (Mirenda & Donnellan 1986), in mainstream classes the interactional styles of both teachers and other pupils tend to be mainly directive (Bayliss 1995).

While many children with severe intellectual disabilities respond best to structured individualized teaching programmes, this approach may limit inclusion within the classroom (Philps 1994; Rouse & Florian 1996). Achieving the correct balance between fostering social skills and encouraging individual learning can prove very difficult. Moreover, because the main educational goals for this group of pupils often concern the development of self-help and independence skills, it is difficult to incorporate these within the more academic National Curriculum. For this reason Jordan & Powell (1994) suggest that the notion of 'Curriculum principles for all' makes better educational sense than a 'curriculum for all'.

Although curricular content and teaching standards in specialist schools have been widely criticized, evaluations of good practice are limited. For example, although language training programmes and social skills training packages are becoming increasingly popular, there are no comparative studies of their effectiveness. Behavioural (and more recently cognitive-behavioural) approaches have also been widely employed and single case or small group studies suggest that these strategies can be effective in minimizing behavioural problems, increasing self-control and in improving learning skills. Harris *et al.* (1996) report on a 'whole school' approach to reduce challenging behaviour in pupils with severe intellectual disabilities. Behavioural methodologies were combined with strategies to enhance communication and social skills, and many positive behaviour changes were recorded. Nevertheless, many teachers still found the demands made of them (recording behaviours, etc.) difficult to cope with, and did not feel they had adequate support. Generalization to other settings or staff members was also limited.

Finally, it is important to recognize that the extent of help offered to children with special educational needs is extremely variable. Indeed, one of the most significant factors determining whether pupils are offered specialist provision at all (either within or outside mainstream schooling) is not related to the pupil's needs but 'the level of determination of the school or parent and whether or not the parent was represented by a lawyer or voluntary organization' (Audit Commission 1992).

Although children with severe disabilities can benefit from access to mainstream school (Hunt & Goetz 1997), Farrell (1997) concludes that 'full, functional integration . . . can never be a viable option for all . . . throughout their school lives'. He proposes that 'policymakers need urgently to review their existing provision so as to ensure maximum opportunities for integration for those children who will benefit, while providing high quality, if segregated provision for those who may not'. Properly planned resource bases or units within mainstream settings are suggested as providing the most flexible option, allowing full-time integration (with support as necessary) for some children, while providing others with the daily opportunity to mix with their mainstream peers.

'Syndrome-specific' approaches to education

Dykens (2000) noted that there are now over 750 known genetic causes of intellectual disability. Although behavioural data on most of these syndromes are sparse, there are a few conditions that have been studied more intensively, and for which research findings have important practical educational implications. Children with fragile X, for example, are relatively impaired (compared to mental age matched controls) in their visuospatial abilities, abstract reasoning, motor co-ordination and motor planning, and short-term auditory and visual memory. They have particular difficulty in processing sequential and novel information. On the other hand, they show relative strengths in vocabulary, simultaneous processing, and in learning verbally based factual material. Perceptual organization, visuospatial memory and fine motor skills are particular strengths in children with Cornelia de Lange syndrome. Short-term auditory memory deficits are typical of children with Down syndrome. Smith–Magenis syndrome is characterized by difficulties with sequential processing and in auditory, visual and motoric short-term memory. Arithmetic skills are poor while long-term memory (for facts and information) is good. Most individuals with Prader–Willi syndrome have specific deficits in arithmetic, writing, visual and auditory short-term memory and auditory attention, but are likely to do well on tasks involving visual organization and perception, long-term memory and in reading and vocabulary (for an overview of psychological functioning in many different genetic syndromes see Udwin & Dennis 1995).

Despite claims that 'the cause of mental retardation has little relevance in planning an educational program' (Blackhurst & Berdine 1993), it is increasingly evident that knowledge about the deficits associated with particular syndromes can help teachers to develop strategies to circumvent deficits and build on children's strengths, and to adapt teaching methods to suit pupils' specific profiles of skills and difficulties (Hodapp &

Fidler 1999). (For teaching guides to specific syndromes see Saunders 1999 for fragile X; Waters 1999 for Prader–Willi syndrome; Lewis & Wilson 1998 for Rett syndrome; and Lorenz 1998 for Down syndrome.)

Children with autism

Educational approaches for children with autism have been studied in particular detail, and many different educational programmes are suggested as having a significant impact on outcome (Howlin 1998; Volkmar *et al.* 1999). Although data to support most such claims are minimal, the importance of structure has been well documented over the last 25 years. Studies by Rutter & Bartak (1973) confirmed that autistic children exposed to structured task-orientated 'academic' programmes made better educational and social progress than children in less structured environments. The TEACCH (Treatment and Education of Autistic and Related Communication-handicapped Children) programme (Schopler & Mesibov 1995; Schopler 1997) provides a framework for teaching that emphasizes the need for structure, appropriate environmental organization and the use of clear visual cues to circumvent communication difficulties. The programme also takes account of developmental levels and the importance of individually based teaching, as well as incorporating behavioural and cognitive approaches. A recent controlled study by Ozonoff & Cathcart (1998) reported significant short-term gains in preschool-age children with autism following the introduction of a daily TEACCH session into their home programme, but no controlled school-based comparisons have been conducted.

Many other approaches to education, focusing specifically on strategies to overcome the fundamental impairments in autism, have been reported (Olley & Reeve 1997; Siegel 1999). Quill (1995), for example, provides detailed information on programmes designed to improve social and communication functioning. The Picture Exchange Communication System (PECS; Bondy & Frost 1996) uses symbols, pictures or objects to enhance communication skills in the classroom. Lord (1995) and Wolfberg & Schuler (1993) report on the effectiveness of using normal peers to enhance social interactions and play. Butera & Haywood (1995) describe the Bright Start Programme, which concentrates on the development of cognitive and metacognitive abilities. Jordan *et al.* (Jordan & Powell 1995; Powell & Jordan 1997; Jordan & Jones 1999) describe a variety of innovative techniques (including the use of computers) that can be used to enhance learning. Cumine *et al.* (1998, 1999) provide practical suggestions for teaching children with autism and Asperger syndrome within mainstream settings. Koegel & Koegel (1995) illustrate how traditional behavioural techniques can be successfully adapted for use in more naturalistic school settings. The success of peer tutoring (Kamps *et al.* 1994) and co-operative learning groups (Dugan *et al.* 1995) has also been demonstrated. However, there are few comparative large-scale evaluations of any of these approaches.

In summarizing developments in education for children with autism over the last two decades, Harris (1995) notes the move towards more naturalistic approaches; the use of intrinsic rather than extrinsic reinforcers; the reduction of aversive procedures; the increasing emphasis on social relationships with peers; the development of more effective communication strategies (rather than a focus on speech); and the value of functional assessments in the reduction of behavioural problems. However, she also suggests that the current emphasis on *totally* non-aversive techniques may be inappropriate for the small minority of students whose highly dangerous or disruptive behaviours cannot be brought under control by other means.

The most effective programmes appear to be those that begin early (between the ages of 2 and 4 years), and have a relatively high adult:child ratio (Rogers 1996, 1998). There needs to be a focus on the maintenance and generalization of skills, and educational provision should also be able to meet children's social and emotional needs (Volkmar *et al.* 1999). However, for more able children with autism, this latter goal can prove difficult to achieve. In special schools it is often not possible to provide them with sufficient intellectual stimulation; on the other hand, unless extra support is provided within mainstream school, teasing and bullying by other pupils and lack of understanding from teachers may often result in severe emotional stress.

One approach that has given rise to particular controversy, mainly because of claims of 'recovery from autism' is the intensive (40h per week over 2 years) behavioural programme of Lovaas *et al.* (Lovaas 1993, 1996; McEachin *et al.* 1993). However, problems in group selection and data collection complicate the interpretation of results and while Sheinkopf & Siegel (1998) concluded that while 'behavioural therapy is a *good* option for children with autism [it is still unclear] whether such a treatment approach is *better* than other treatments of similar intensity or structure'.

Arguments for and against inclusive education are as rife in the field of autism as for any other disability (Mesibov 1990; Simpson & Myles 1993; Burack *et al.* 1997). Some studies conclude that academic and social attainments are enhanced by inclusion, but the educational settings have usually been experimental in nature (Hoyson *et al.* 1984; Harris *et al.* 1991). Other research suggests that mainstreaming does not necessarily improve social, cognitive or language skills (Harris *et al.* 1990; Sigafoos *et al.* 1994; Burack *et al.* 1997). Nevertheless, for autistic children of normal IQ access to the normal school curriculum is crucial for their future academic and employment prospects. Unless their very specific needs and difficulties are adequately understood, children may become extremely isolated, lonely and rejected, and hence adequate training and support for the regular classroom teachers is essential (Jordan & Jones 1999). In the absence of such support, it may sometimes be preferable for education in the early years to be provided in specialist autistic units where major behavioural or learning difficulties can be modified. Gradual integration into more normal provision can then be undertaken.

Early prevention of learning, emotional and behavioural difficulties

The failure of many intervention approaches, particularly with older children, has led to a heightened awareness of the need to intervene in high-risk groups of children before they even enter school. One of the best known forms of early intervention is the Head Start Program (current budget $4.6 billion; Zigler 1999) although many variations also exist (Odom *et al.* 1999). The problems involved in evaluating these programmes have been widely discussed over the past two decades (Cave & Maddison 1978; Guralnick 1998; Bailey *et al.* 1999) but the short-term effects on children's cognitive, social and physical development are well established (Guralnick 1998). Early intervention of this kind also appears to bring about improvements in mother–child interaction and a reduction in problem behaviours (Webster-Stratton 1998). There is less agreement about the longer term benefits (Devaney *et al.* 1997). Barnett (1995, 1998a), in critical reviews of almost 40 studies, found that preschool programmes, including Head Start, produced persistent effects on academic achievement and social adjustment and participants were subsequently less likely to be placed in special education. However, the impact on IQ was more variable. There was little difference between Head Start and other public school, child care or home visiting programmes, although the better-funded models programmes tended to have a greater effect. Outcome also seems to be more positive if parents and teachers work together (Fantuzzo *et al.* 1997). Barnett (1998b) concluded that the long-term social and economic return from providing early education to deprived children far exceeds the cost. However, he and other authors (Ramey 1999; Ripple *et al.* 1999; Scarr 1999) also noted the very variable time span and quality of these programmes across different states, the relatively small number of children (under 1.7% of the total infant population) who gain access to them and the racial imbalance (poor blacks are significantly more likely to be enrolled than poor whites; O'Connor 1998). There remain many questions to be answered about the goals and structures of these early programmes and the types and ages of children for whom they prove most effective. Attention to wider social issues and the linking of preschool education to later schooling are also crucial (Guralnick 1998; Siegel 1999).

Amongst preschool interventions specifically for children with severe developmental delays, the Portage programme (Shearer & Shearer 1972) has probably been one of the most widely used in the USA and UK. Nevertheless, despite its widespread use, methodological problems and the lack of long-term follow-up studies mean, again, that the comparative effectiveness of this approach remains unclear (Sturmey & Crisp 1986; Cameron 1997).

Clinical recommendations

Education has a major influence on the life of any child, but for pupils with disabilities the quality of schooling they receive is likely to have an even greater and longer lasting impact. Access to appropriate education *from the earliest years* is therefore crucial. Any clinician involved in the care of children with special needs has a responsibility to liaise closely with families and educational professionals in order to ensure that the provision available will maximize opportunities for educational and social success. While it may not be appropriate to recommend specific placements, clinicians can have an important role in providing broad guidelines for a child's educational welfare. These will be based on a full understanding of the child's basic condition, knowledge of associated behavioural or cognitive impairments and, increasingly, of the particular profiles associated with underlying genetic disorders. Detailed individual assessments of the child's linguistic, cognitive, social and behavioural patterns, and information about family factors of relevance to educational placement, will also be required. Families also need advice on how to obtain information on the full range of educational provision available locally. Although these recommendations may be viewed as adding to the workload of already hard-pressed clinicians, failure to pay adequate attention to educational needs may well undermine the effects of any other forms of treatment. With such support, parents may be prevented from seeking out alternative, expensive and often unproven therapies.

Conclusions

Few educational professionals would disagree that pupils with special needs should preferably be educated on the same site as other children in their neighbourhood. However, there is little evidence to support the effectiveness of total inclusion for all children with special needs in regular classes. Current pressures on mainstream education may result in schools being both less able and less willing to cater for pupils who, almost inevitably, will demand more and achieve less (at least in academic terms). As Hornby *et al.* (1997) concluded, unless less idealistic and better considered policies for inclusion are adopted, the outcome could be far from beneficial for pupils with special needs, their families, peers and teachers. Instead, the aim should be to ensure that all children with special needs are provided with an education that enables them to make optimum academic, social and emotional progress and will offer them the best chance of integration as adults. This will require a flexible continuum of specialist provision, including special schools, resource units and special classes which, as far as possible, allow ready access to mainstream school and the normal curriculum. The perspective of the family, the teachers and other pupils should also be acknowledged and involvement with non-disabled peers fostered as early as possible. Finally, increasing knowledge about the genetic and cognitive deficits associated with intellectual disability should be harnessed in order to develop education programmes that build on children's specific strengths and minimize specific weaknesses.

References

Abikoff, H. (1991) Cognitive training in ADHD children: less to it than meets the eye. *Journal of Learning Disabilities*, **24**, 205–209.

Abramowitz, A.J., Eckstrand, D., O'Leary, S.G. & Dulcan, M.K. (1992) AHDH children's responses to stimulant medication and two intensities of a behavioural intervention. *Behaviour Modification*, **16**, 193–203.

Acton, H.M. & Zarbatany, L. (1988) Interaction and performance with co-operative groups: effects on non-handicapped students' attitudes towards their mildly retarded peers. *American Journal of Mental Retardation*, **93**, 16–23.

Ainscow, M. (1995) Special needs through school improvement: school improvement through special needs. In: *Towards Inclusive Schools?* (eds C. Clark, A. Dyson & A. Milward), pp. 63–77. David Fulton, London.

Anderson, E.M., Clarke, L. & (with Spain, B.) (1982) *Disability in Adolescence*. Methuen, London.

Arter, C., Mason, H., McCall, S., McLinden, M. & Stone, J. (1999) *Children with a Visual Impairment in Mainstream Settings: A Guide for Teachers*. David Fulton, London.

Audit Commission/Her Majesty's Inspectorate (1992) *Getting in on the Act: Provision for Pupils with Special Educational Needs: the National Picture*. HMSO, London.

Ayres, H., Clarke, D. & Murray, A. (1995) *Perspectives on Behaviour: a Practical Guide to Effective Intervention for Teachers*. David Fulton, London.

Bailey, D.B. & Winton, P.J. (1987) Stability and change in parents' expectations about mainstreaming. *Topics in Early Childhood Special Education*, **7**, 73–88.

Bailey, D.B., Aytch, L., Odom, S., Symons, F. & Wolery, M. (1999) Early intervention as we know it. *Mental Retardation and Developmental Disabilities Research Reviews*, **5**, 11–20.

Balkany, T., Hodges, A.V. & Goodman, K.W. (1996) Ethics of cochlear implantation in young children. *Otolaryngology, Head and Neck Surgery*, **114**, 748–755.

Barkley, R.A. (1997) *Defiant Children: a Clinician's Manual for Assessment and Parent Training*, 2nd edn. Guilford Press, New York.

Barnett, W.S. (1995) Long-term effects of early childhood programs on cognitive and school outcomes. In: *The Future of Children*, Vol. 5. *Long-term Outcomes of Early Childhood Programs* (ed. R.E. Behram), pp. 25–50. Center for the Future of Children, David & Lucile Packard Foundation, Los Altos, CA.

Barnett, W.S. (1998a) Long term cognitive and academic effects of early childhood education on children in poverty. *Preventive Medicine*, **27**, 204–207.

Barnett, W.S. (1998b) Long-term effects on cognitive development and school success. In: *Early Care and Education for Children in Poverty* (eds W.S. Barnett & S.S. Boocock), pp. 11–44. State University of New York Press, Albany, NY.

Bayliss, M. (1995) Integration and interpersonal relations: interactions between disabled children and their non-disabled peers. *British Journal of Special Education*, **22**, 131–140.

Bear, G.G., Clever, A. & Proctor, W.A. (1991) Self-perceptions of nonhandicapped children and children with learning disabilities in integrated classes. *Journal of Special Education*, **24**, 409–426.

Beitchman, J.H., Brownlie, E.B. & Wilson, B. (1996) Linguistic impairment and psychiatric disorder. In: *Language, Learning and Behaviour Disorders: Developmental, Biological and Clinical Perspectives* (eds J.H. Beitchman, N.J. Cohen, M.M. Konstantareas & R. Tannock), pp. 493–514. Cambridge University Press, Cambridge.

de Bettencourt, L.U., Zigmond, N. & Thornton, H. (1989) Follow up of post-secondary age rural learning disabled graduates and dropouts. *Exceptional Children*, **55**, 40–49.

Beveridge, S. (1996) Experiences of an integration link scheme: the perspectives of pupils with severe learning difficulties and their mainstream peers. *European Journal of Learning Disabilities*, **26**, 87–101.

Bickel, W.E. & Bickel, D.D. (1986) Effective schools, classrooms and instruction: implications for special education. *Exceptional Children*, **52**, 489–500.

Blackhurst, A.E. & Berdine, W.H. (1993) *An Introduction to Special Education*. Harper Collins, New York.

Bloomquist, M.L., August, G.J. & Ostrander, R. (1991) Effects of a school-based cognitive-behavioral intervention for ADHD children. *Journal of Abnormal Child Psychology*, **19**, 591–605.

Bondy, A. & Frost, L. (1996) Educational approaches in pre-school: behavior techniques in a public school setting. In: *Learning and Cognition in Autism* (eds E. Schopler & G.B. Mesibov), pp. 311–334. Plenum Press, New York.

Booth, T. (1994) Continua or chimera? *British Journal of Special Education*, **21**, 21–24.

Booth, T. (1996) A perspective on inclusion from England. *Cambridge Journal of Education*, **26**, 87–101.

Borthwick-Duffy, S.A., Palmer, D.S. & Lane, K.L. (1996) One size doesn't fit all: full inclusion and individual differences. *Journal of Behavioral Education*, **6**, 311–329.

Bryant, P. & Bradley, L. (1985) *Children's Reading Problems*. Blackwell Publishers, Oxford.

Budgell, P. (1986) Drifting towards segregation. *British Journal of Special Education*, **13**, 94–96.

Burack, J.A., Root, R. & Zigler, E. (1997) Inclusive education for children with autism: reviewing ideological, empirical and community considerations. In: *Handbook of Autism and Pervasive Developmental Disorders* (eds D. Cohen & F. Volkmar), 2nd edn, pp. 796–807. Wiley, New York.

Bursuck, W.D., Rose, E., Cowen, S. & Yahaya, M. (1989) Nationwide survey of postsecondary education services for students with learning disabilities. *Exceptional Children*, **56**, 236–245.

Butera, G. & Haywood, H.C. (1995) Cognitive education of young children with autism: an application of Bright Start. In: *Learning and Cognition in Autism* (eds E. Schopler & G. Mesibov), pp. 227–256. Plenum Press, New York.

Cameron, R.J. (1997) Early intervention for young children with developmental delay: the Portage approach. *Child: Care, Health and Development*, **23**, 11–27.

Capute, A.J. & Accardo, P.J. (1991) *Developmental Disabilities in Infancy and Childhood*. Brookes, Baltimore, MD.

Carlberg, C. & Kavale, K. (1980) The efficacy of special versus regular class placement for exceptional children: a meta-analysis. *Journal of Special Education*, **14**, 295–309.

Carlson, C.L., Pelham, W.E., Milich, R. & Dixon, J. (1992) Single and combined effectiveness of methylphenidate and behavior therapy on the classroom performance of children with attention-deficit hyperactivity disorder. *Journal of Abnormal Child Psychology*, **20**, 213–232.

Carr, J. (1982) *Social Relationships Amongst Spina Bifida Children Attending Ordinary or Special Schools*. Report to ILEA Research and Statistics Group, London Education Authority.

Carr, J., Hallwell, M. & Pearson, A. (1981) Educational attainments of spina bifida children attending ordinary or special schools. *Zeitschrift fur Kinderchirurgie*, **34**, 364–370.

Cave, C. & Maddison, P. (1978) *A Survey of Recent Research in Special Education*. NFER, Oxford.

Center, Y., Ward, J. & Ferguson, C. (1991) Towards an index to evaluate the integration of children with disabilities into regular classrooms. *Educational Psychology*, **11**, 77–95.

Centre for the Study of Inclusive Education (1996) *Developing an Inclusive Policy for Your School: A CSIE Guide*. Centre for the Study of Inclusive Education, Bristol.

Chapman, E.K. & Stone, J.M. (1988) *The Visually Handicapped Child in Your Classroom*. Cassell, London.

Clarke, C., Dyson, A., Millward, A. & Skidmore, D. (eds) (1995) *Innovatory Practice in Mainstream Schools for Special Educational Needs*. University of Newcastle upon Tyne, Newcastle upon Tyne.

Clay, M. (1985) *The Early Detection of Reading Difficulties*, 3rd edn. Heinemann, Auckland.

Cole, D. & Meyer, L. (1991) Social integration and severe disabilities: a longitudinal analysis of child outcomes. *Journal of Special Education*, **25**, 340–351.

Cole, T. (1989) *Apart or A Part? Integration and the Growth of British Special Education*. Open University Press, Milton Keynes.

Cole, T., Visser, J. & Upton, G. (1994) *Effective Schooling for Pupils with Emotional and Behavioural Difficulties*. David Fulton, London.

Cooper, D.H. & Spence, D.L. (1990) Maintaining at risk children in regular education settings: initial effects of individual differences and classroom environments. *Exceptional Children*, **56**, 117–126.

Cooper, P. & Ideus, K. (1996) *Attention Deficit/Hyperactivity Disorder: A Practical Guide for Teachers*. David Fulton, London.

Cousins, L.S. & Weiss, G. (1993) Parent training and social skills training for children with attention deficit hyperactivity disorder: how can they be combined for greater effectiveness? *Canadian Journal of Psychiatry*, **38**, 449–457.

Cumine, V., Leach, J. & Stevenson, G. (1998) *Asperger Syndrome: a Practical Guide for Teachers*. David Fulton, London.

Cumine, V., Leach, J. & Stevenson, G. (1999) *Autism in the Early Years: a Practical Guide*. David Fulton, London.

Currey, W.E. (1898) *Report of the Departmental Committee on Defective and Epileptic Children* (Sharpe Report), Vol. 2, pp. 97–99. HMSO, London.

Dale, P.S. & Cole, K.N. (1988) Comparison of academic and cognitive programs for young handicapped children. *Exceptional Children*, **54**, 439–447.

Danby, J. & Cullen, C. (1988) Integration and mainstreaming: a review of the efficacy of mainstreaming and integration for mentally handicapped pupils. *Educational Psychology*, **8**, 177–195.

Davison, F.M. & Howlin, P. (1997) A follow-up study of children attending a primary-age language unit. *European Journal of Disorders of Communication*, **32**, 19–36.

Dawson, R. (1980) *Special Provision for Disturbed People: a Survey*. MacMillan Education, London.

Deno, S., Maruyama, G., Espin, G. & Cohen, C. (1990) Educating students with mild disabilities in general education classrooms: Minnesota alternatives. *Exceptional Children*, **57**, 150–161.

Department for Education (1995) *National Survey of LEAs Policies and Procedures for the Identification of and Provision for Children who are out of School by Reason of Exclusion or Otherwise*. Department for Education, Pupils and Parents Branch, London.

Department for Education & Employment (1994a) *Code of Practice on the Identification and Assessment of Special Educational Needs*. Department for Education & Employment, London.

Department for Education & Employment (1994b) *The Organization of Special Educational Provision* (circular 6/94). Department for Education & Employment, London.

Department for Education & Employment (1997) *Excellence for All Children: Meeting Special Educational Needs*. Department for Education & Employment, London.

Department for Education & Employment (1998) *Meeting Special Educational Needs: A Programme of Action*. Department for Education & Employment, London.

Devaney, B.L., Ellwood, M.R. & Love, J.M. (1997) Programs that mitigate the effects of poverty on children. *Future of Children*, **7**, 88–112.

Dugan, E., Kamps, D., Leonard, B., Watkins, M., Rheinberger, A. & Stackhaus, J. (1995) Effects of cooperative learning groups during social studies for students with autism and fourth grade peers. *Journal of Applied Behaviour Analysis*, **28**, 175–188.

Dykens, E.M. (2000) Psychopathology in children with intellectual disability [Annotation]. *Journal of Child Psychology and Psychiatry*, **41**, 407–417.

Dyson, A. (1990) Effective learning consultancy: a future role for special needs coordinators? *Support for Learning*, **5**, 116–127.

Education for All Handicapped Children Act (1975) HMSO, London.

Evans, P.M., Evans, S.J.W. & Alberman, E. (1990) Cerebral palsy: why we must plan for survival. *Archives of Disease in Childhood*, **65**, 1329–1333.

Fantuzzo, J., Childs, S., Hampton, V., Ginsburggblock, M., Coolahan, K.C. & Debnam, D. (1997) Enhancing the quality of early childhood education: a follow-up evaluation of an experiential, collaborative training model for head start. *Early Childhood Research Quarterly*, **12**, 425–437.

Farrell, P. (1996) Integration: where do we go from here? In: *Whose Choice? Contentious Issues for Those Working with People with Learning Difficulties* (eds J. Coupe O'Kane & J. Goldbart), pp. 177–195. David Fulton, London.

Farrell, P. (1997) The integration of children with severe learning difficulties: a review of the recent literature. *Journal of Applied Research in Intellectual Disabilities*, **10**, 1–14.

Farrell, P. & Tsakalidou, K. (2000) Recent trends in the re-integration of pupils with emotional and behavioural difficulties in the United Kingdom. *School Psychology International*, **20**, 323–337.

Feuerstein, R., Rand, Y., Hoffman, N. & Miller, M. (1980) *Instrumental Enrichment: an Intervention Programme for Cognitive Modifiability*. University Park Press, Baltimore.

Florian, L. (1998) Inclusive practice: what, why and how. In: *Promoting Inclusive Practice* (eds C. Tilstone, L. Florian & R. Rose), pp. 13–26. Routledge, London.

Foorman, B.R., Rancis, D.J., Novy, D.M. & Liberman, D. (1991) How letter-sound instruction mediates progress in first-grade reading and spelling. *Journal of Educational Psychology*, **83**, 456–469.

Forest, M., Pearpoint, J. & O'Brien, J. (1996) 'MPAS': educators, parents, young people and their friends planning together. *Educational Psychology in Practice*, **11**, 35–40.

Forlin, C. (1995) Educators' beliefs about inclusive practices in Western Australia. *British Journal of Special Education*, **22**, 179–186.

Fox, C.L. (1989) Peer acceptance of learning disabled children in the regular classroom. *Exceptional Children*, **56**, 50–59.

Fuchs, D., Fuchs, L.S. & Bahr, M.W. (1990) Mainstream assistance teams: a scientific basis for the art of consultation. *Exceptional Children*, **57**, 128–134.

Galloway, D. & Goodwin, C. (1987) *The Education of Disturbing Children: Pupils with Learning and Adjustment Difficulties*. Longman, London.

Gersten, R., Walker, H. & Darch, C. (1988) Relationship between teachers' effectiveness and their tolerance for handicapped students. *Exceptional Children*, **54**, 433–438.

Giangreco, M.F. (1997) Key lessons learned about inclusive education: summary of the 1996 Schonell Memorial Lecture. *International Journal of Disability*, **44**, 193–206.

Goldstein, H., Kaczmarek, L., Pennington, R. & Schafer, K. (1992) Peer-mediated intervention: attending to, commenting on and acknowledging the behaviour of preschoolers with autism. *Journal of Applied Behavior Analysis*, **25**, 289–305.

Gordon, J.C. (1885) Deaf-mutes and the public schools from 1815 to the present day. *American Annals of the Deaf*, **40**, 137–147.

Gordon, S.B. & Asher, M. (1994) *Meeting the ADD Challenge: a Practical Guide for Teachers*. Research Press, Champaign, IL.

Gottlieb, J. (1990) Mainstreaming and quality education. *American Journal of Mental Retardation*, **95**, 16–17.

Gray, G., Miller, A. & Noakes, J. (1994) *Challenging Behaviour in Schools: Teacher Support, Practical Techniques and Policy Development*. Routledge, London.

Gregory, S.P. (1996) Inclusive education for preschool children with disabilities. *Support for Learning*, **11**, 77–83.

Gregory, S. & Hindley, P. (1996) Communication strategies for deaf children [Annotation]. *Journal of Child Psychology and Psychiatry*, **37**, 895–905.

Gregory, S., Bishop, J. & Sheldon, L. (1995) *Deaf Young People and Their Families*. Cambridge University Press, Cambridge.

Groenveld, M. (1998) Sensory difficulties. In: *Behavioural Approaches to Problems in Childhood* (ed. P. Howlin), pp. 114–135. MacKeith Press, London.

Guevremont, D. (1990) Social skills and peer relationship training. In: *Attention Deficit Hyperactivity Disorder: a Handbook for Diagnosis and Treatment* (ed. R.A. Barkley), pp. 540–572. Guilford Press, New York.

Guralnick, M.J. (1998) Effectiveness of early intervention for vulnerable children: a developmental perspective. *American Journal of Mental Retardation*, **102**, 319–345.

Guralnick, M.J. & Groom, J.M. (1988) Friendships of pre-school children in mainstreamed playgroups. *Developmental Psychology*, **24**, 595–604.

Guralnick, M.J., Connor, R.T. & Hammond, M. (1995) Parent perspectives of peer relationships and friendships in integrated and specialized programs. *American Journal of Mental Retardation*, **99**, 457–476.

Hall, J. (1996) Integration, inclusion: what does it all mean? In: *Whose Choice? Contentious Issues for Those Working with People with Learning Difficulties* (eds J. Coupe O'Kane & J. Goldbard), pp. 177–185. David Fulton, London.

Hall, L.J. (1994) A descriptive assessment of social relationships in integrated classrooms. *Journal of Association for Persons with Severe Handicaps*, **14**, 302–213.

Hallinger, P. & Murphy, J. (1986) The social context of effective schools. *American Journal of Education*, **94**, 328–355.

Hanko, G. (1993) *Special Needs in Ordinary Classrooms: from Staff Support to Staff Development*, 3rd edn. David Fulton, London.

Hanrahan, J., Goodman, W. & Rapagna, S. (1990) Preparing mentally retarded students for mainstreaming: priorities of regular class and special school teachers. *American Journal of Mental Retardation*, **94**, 470–474.

Harris, H.J., Cook, M. & Upton, G. (1996) *Pupils with Severe Learning Disabilities who Present Challenging Behaviour: A Whole School Approach to Assessment and Intervention*. BILD Publications, Clevedon.

Harris, J. (1998) Cerebral palsy. In: *Behavioural Approaches to Problems in Childhood* (ed. P. Howlin), pp. 136–151. MacKeith Press, London.

Harris, S.L. (1995) Educational strategies in autism. In: *Learning and Cognition in Autism* (eds E. Schopler & G. Mesibov), pp. 293–309. Plenum Press, New York.

Harris, S.L., Handleman, J.S., Kristoff, B., Bass, L. & Gordon, R. (1990) Changes in language development among autistic and peer children in

segregated and integrated preschool settings. *Journal of Autism and Developmental Disorders*, **20**, 23–32.

Harris, S.L., Handleman, J.S., Gordon, R., Kristoff, B., Bass, L. & Fuentes, F. (1991) Changes in cognitive and language functioning of preschool children with autism. *Journal of Autism and Developmental Disorders*, **21**, 281–290.

Harrison, J. (1996) Accessing further education: views and experiences of FE students with learning difficulties and/or disabilities. *British Journal of Special Education*, **23**, 187–196.

Harter, S. (1984) Processes underlying the construction, maintenance and enhancement of the self concept in children. In: *Psychological Perspectives on the Self*, Vol. 3 (eds J. Suls & A. Greenwald), pp. 24–58. Lawrence Erlbaum, Hillsdale, NJ.

Hasazi, S.B., Johnson, R.E., Hasazi, J.E., Gordon, L.R. & Hull, M. (1989) Employment of youth with and without handicaps following high school: outcomes and correlates. *Journal of Special Education*, **23**, 243–255.

Hatcher, P.J., Hulme, C. & Ellis, A.W. (1994) Ameliorating early reading failure by integrating the teaching of reading and phonological skills: the phonological linkage hypothesis. *Child Development*, **65**, 41–57.

Hayden, D.A. & Pukonen, M. (1996) Language intervention programming for preschool children with social and pragmatic disorders. In: *Language, Learning, and Behavior Disorders: Developmental, Biological, and Clinical Perspectives* (eds J.H. Beitchman, N.J. Cohen, M.M. Konstantareas & R. Tannoc), pp. 436–465. Cambridge University Press, Cambridge.

Haynes, C. & Naidoo, S. (1991) *Children with Specific Speech and Language Impairment*. Blackwell Scientific, Oxford.

Hechtman, L., Kouri, J. & Respitz, eds (1996) Multimodal treatment of the hyperactive child with and without learning disabilities. In: *Language, Learning, and Behaviour Disorders: Developmental, Biological and Clinical Perspectives* (eds J.H. Beitchman, N.J. Cohen, M.M. Konstantareas & R. Tannock), pp. 395–417. Cambridge University Press, Cambridge.

Hegarty, S. (1993) Reviewing the literature on integration. *European Journal of Special Needs Education*, **8**, 194–200.

Hegarty, S., Pocklington, K. & Lucas, D. (1982a) *Integration in Action: Case Studies in the Integration of Pupils with Special Needs*. NFER, Oxford.

Hegarty, S., Pocklington, K. & Lucas, D. (1982b) *Educating Pupils with Special Needs in the Ordinary School*. NFER, Oxford.

Hendrikson, J.H., Shokoohi-Yekta, M., Hamre-Nietupski, S. & Gable, R.A. (1996) Middle and high school students' perceptions on being friends with peers with severe disabilities. *Exceptional Children*, **63**, 19–28.

Herbert, M. (1995) A collaborative model of training for parents of children with disruptive behaviour disorders. *British Journal of Clinical Psychology*, **34**, 325–342.

Hindley, P.A. & Brown, R. (1994) Psychiatric aspects of sensory impairment. In: *Child and Adolescent Psychiatry: Modern Approaches* (eds M. Rutter, E. Taylor & L. Hersov), 3rd edn, pp. 720–736. Blackwell Science, Oxford.

Hinshaw, S.P. (1992) Externalizing behavioral problems and academic underachievement in childhood and adolescence: casual relationships and underlying mechanisms. *Psychological Bulletin*, **111**, 127–155.

Hinshaw, S.P. & Melnick, S. (1992) Self-management therapies and attention-deficit hyperactivity disorder: reinforced self-evaluation and anger control interventions. *Behavior Modification*, **16**, 253–273.

Her Majesty's Inspectorate (1989) *A Survey of Pupils with SEN In Ordinary Schools*. Department for Education and Science, London.

Hodapp, R.M. & Fidler, D.J. (1999) Special education and genetics:

connections for the 21st century. *Journal of Special Education*, 33, 130–137.

Hopkins, D., West, M. & Ainscow, M. (1996) *Improving the Quality of Education for All: Progress in and Challenge*. David Fulton, London.

Hornby, G. (1992) Integration of children with special educational needs: is it time for a policy review? *Support for Learning*, 7, 130–134.

Hornby, G., Atkinson, M. & Howard, J. (1997) *Controversial Issues in Special Education*. David Fulton, London.

Howlin, P. (1998) *Treating Children with Autism and Asperger Syndrome: a Guide for Parents and Professionals*. Wiley, Chichester.

Howlin, P., Mawhood, L.M. & Rutter, M. (2000) Autism and developmental receptive language disorder: a follow-up comparison in early adult life. II. Social, behavioural and psychiatric outcomes. *Journal of Child Psychology and Psychiatry*, 41, 561–578.

Hoyson, M., Jamieson, B. & Strain, P.S. (1984) Individualized group instruction of normally developing and autistic-like children. *Journal of the Division for Early Childhood*, 8, 157–172.

Hundert, J. & Houghton, A. (1992) Promoting social interaction of children with disabilities in integrated preschools: a failure to generalise. *Exceptional Children*, 58, 311–320.

Hunt, G. (1981) Spina bifida: implications for 100 children at school. *Developmental Medicine and Child Neurology*, 23, 160–172.

Hunt, P. & Goetz, L. (1997) Research on inclusive educational programs, practices, and outcomes for students with severe disabilities. *Journal of Special Education*, 31, 13–29.

Hurry, J. (1999) Annotation: children's reading levels. *Journal of Child Psychology and Psychiatry*, 40, 143–150.

Inner London Education Authority (1981) *Ethnic Census of School Support Centres and Educational Guidance Centres*. RS 784/81.

Ispa, J. & Matz, R.D. (1978) Integrating handicapped pre-school children within a cognitively-oriented program. In: *Early Intervention and the Integration of Handicapped and Non-handicapped Children* (ed. M. Guralnick), pp. 167–190. University Park Press, Baltimore.

Iverson, S. & Tunmer, W. (1993) Phonological processing skills and the reading recovery program. *Journal of Educational Psychology*, 85, 112–126.

Jenkins, J.R. & Heinen, A. (1989) Students' preferences for service delivery: pull-outs, in class or integrated models. *Exceptional Children*, 55, 516–523.

Jordan, A. (1994) *Skills in Collaborative Classroom Consultation*. Routledge, London.

Jordan, R. & Jones, G. (1999) *Meeting the Needs of Children with Autistic Spectrum Disorders*. David Fulton, London.

Jordan, R. & Powell, S. (1994) Whose curriculum? Critical notes on integration and entitlement. *European Journal of Special Needs Education*, 9, 27–39.

Jordan, R. & Powell, S. (1995) *Understanding and Teaching Children with Autism*. Wiley, Chichester.

Juel, C. (1994) At risk university students tutoring at-risk elementary school children. In: *Getting Reading Right from the Start: Effective Early Literacy Interventions* (eds E.H. Hiebert & B.M. Taylor), pp. 36–91. Allyn & Bacon, Needham, MA.

Kamps, D.M., Barbetta, P.M., Leonard, B.R. & Delquardri, J. (1994) Classwide peer tutoring: an integration strategy to improve reading skills and promote peer interactions among students and promote peer interactions among students with autism and general education peers. *Journal of Applied Behavior Analysis*, 27, 49–61.

Kasari, C., Freeman. S.F.N., Bauminger, R.N. & Alkin, M.C. (1999) Parental perspectives on inclusion: effects of autism and Down Syndrome. *Journal of Autism and Developmental Disorders*, 29, 297–305.

Katsiyannis, A., Conderman, G. & Franks, D.J. (1995) State practices on inclusion. *Remedial and Special Education*, 16, 279–287.

Kauffman, J.M. (1991) Restructuring the sociopolitical context: reservations about the effects of current reform proposals on students with disabilities. In: *A Regular Education Initiative: Alternative Perspectives on Concepts, Issues and Models* (eds J.W. Lloyd, N.N. Singh & A.C. Repp), pp. 57–66. Sycamore, Sycamore, IL.

Kauffman, J.M. & Hallahan, D.P. (1995) *The Illusion of Full Inclusion: a Comprehensive Critique of a Current Special Education Bandwagon*. Pro-Ed, Austin, TX.

Kidd, R. & Hornby, G. (1993) Transfer from special to mainstream. *British Journal of Special Education*, 20, 17–19.

Kishi, G.S. & Meyer, L.H. (1994) What children report and remember: a six-year follow-up of the effects of social contact between peers with and without severe disabilities. *Journal of Association for Persons with Severe Handicaps*, 19, 277–289.

Koegel, R.L. & Koegel, L.K. (1995) *Teaching Children with Autism: Strategies for Initiating Positive Interactions and Improving Learning Opportunities*. Brookes, Baltimore.

Kohn, J.G. (1990) Issues in the management of children with spastic cerebral palsy. *Pediatrician*, 17, 230–236.

Lakhen, Y. & Norwich, B. (1990) The self-concept and self-esteem of adolescents with physical impairments in integrated and special school settings. *European Journal of Special Needs Education*, 5, 1–12.

Lettsom, J.C. (1894) *The Blind: Hints Designed to Promote Beneficence, Temperance and Medical Science, 1801*. Reprinted by Sampson Low, London, 1894.

Lewis, A. (1995) *Primary Special Needs and the National Curriculum*, 2nd edn. Routledge, London.

Lewis, J. & Wilson, D. (1998) *Pathways to Learning in Rett Syndrome*. David Fulton, London.

Lindsey, G. (1989) Evaluating integration. *Educational Psychology in Practice*, 5, 7–16.

Lingard, T. (1994) The acquisition of literacy in secondary education. *British Journal of Special Education*, 21, 180–191.

Lipsky, D. & Gartner, A. (1996) Inclusion, school restructuring and the making of American Society. *Harvard Educational Review*, 66, 762–796.

Little, S.G. & Witter, J.M. (1996) Inclusion: considerations from social validity and functional outcome analysis. *Journal of Behavioral Education*, 6, 283–291.

Lopez, J.F.G. (1994) The integration of mentally retarded children: analysis of an experience in Spain. *European Journal of Special Needs Education*, 9, 145–151.

Lord, C. (1995) Facilitating social inclusion: examples from peer intervention programs. In: *Learning and Cognition in Autism* (eds E. Schopler & G. Mesibov), pp. 221–239. Plenum Press, New York.

Lorenz, S. (1998) *Children with Down's Syndrome: A Guide for Teachers and Learning Support Assistants in Mainstream Primary and Secondary Schools*. David Fulton, London.

Lovaas, O.I. (1993) The development of a treatment: research project for developmentally disabled and autistic children. *Journal of Applied Behavior Analysis*, 26, 617–630.

Lovaas, O.I. (1996) The UCLA young autism model of service delivery. In: *Behavioral Intervention for Young Children with Autism* (ed. C. Maurice), pp. 241–250. Pro-Ed, Austin, TX.

Lovett, M.W., Warren-Chaplin, P.M., Ransby, M.J. & Borden, S.L. (1990) Training the word recognition skills of dyslexic children: treatment and transfer effects. *Journal of Educational Psychology*, 82, 769–780.

Lovett, M.W., Borden, S.L., DeLuca, T., Lacrerenza, L., Benson, N.J. &

Brackstone, D. (1994) Treating the core deficits of developmental dyslexia: evidence of transfer of learning after phonological- and strategy-based reading training programs. *Developmental Psychology*, **30**, 805–822.

Lowenbraun, S., Madge, S. & Affleck, J. (1990) Parental satisfaction with integrated class placements of special education and general education students. *Remedial and Special Education*, **11**, 37–40.

Lynas, W. (1984) *Integrating the handicapped into ordinary schools*. Croom Helm, London.

MacAulay, D.A. (1990) Classroom environment: a literature review. *Educational Psychology*, **10**, 239–253.

Madden, N.A. & Slavin, R.F. (1983) Mainstreaming students with mild handicaps: academic and social outcomes. *Review of Education Research*, **54**, 519–589.

Maheady, L., Sacca, M.K. & Harper, G.F. (1988) Classwide peer tutoring with mildly handicapped high school students. *Exceptional Children*, **55**, 52–59.

Marston, D. (1996) A comparison of inclusion only, pull-out only, and combined service models for students with mild disabilities. *Journal of Special Education*, **30**, 121–132.

Maughan, B. & Yule, W. (1994) Reading and other intellectual disabilities. In: *Child and Adolescent Psychiatry: Modern Approaches* (eds M. Rutter, E. Taylor & L. Hersov), 3rd edn, pp. 647–665. Blackwell Science, Oxford.

McDermott, S., Coker, A.L., Mani, S. *et al.* (1996) A population-based analysis of behavior problems in children with cerebral palsy. *Journal of Pediatric Psychology*, **21**, 447–463.

McDonnell, J. (1987) The integration of students with severe handicaps into regular public schools: an analysis of parents' perceptions of potential outcomes. *Education and Training in Mental Retardation*, **22**, 98–111.

McEachin, J.J., Smith, T. & Lovaas, O.I. (1993) Long-term outcome for children with autism who received early intensive behavioral treatment. *American Journal of Mental Retardation*, **97**, 359–372.

McNamara, E. & Jolly, M. (1990) Are disruptive behaviours reduced when levels of on-task behaviours increase? An across settings study of a class of 12 and 13 year old pupils. II. *Behavioural Psychotherapy*, **18**, 239–250.

McNamara, S. & Moreton, G. (1995) *Changing Children with Emotional and Behavioural Difficulties in Primary and Secondary Classrooms*. David Fulton, London.

Meadow-Orlans, K.P. (1987) An analysis of the effectiveness of early intervention programs for hearing impaired children. In: *The Effectiveness of Early Intervention for at Risk and Handicapped Children* (eds M. Guralnick & F. Bennett), pp. 325–362. Academic Press, New York.

Meijer, C.J.W., Pijl, S.J. & Hegarty, S. (1994) *New Perspectives in Special Education: A Six-country Study of Integration*. Routledge, London.

Mencap (1999) *On a Wing and a Prayer: Inclusion and Children with Severe Learning Difficulties*. Mencap, London.

Mesibov, G.B. (1990) Normalization and its relevance today. *Journal of Autism and Developmental Disorders*, **20**, 379–390.

Meyers, C.E. & Blacher, J. (1987) Parents' perceptions of schooling for severely handicapped children: home and family variables. *Exceptional Children*, **53**, 441–449.

Mirenda, P. & Donnellan, A. (1986) Effects of adult interactional style on conversational behavior in students with severe communication problems. *Language, Speech and Hearing Services in Schools*, **17**, 126–141.

Mortimore, P., Davies, J., Varlaam, A., West, A., Devine, P. & Mazza, J. (1983) *Behaviour Problems in Schools: an Evaluation of Support Centres*. Croom-Helm, London.

Newton, C., Taylor, H. & Wilson, D. (1996) Circles of friends: an inclusive approach to meeting emotional and behavioural needs. *Educational Psychology in Practice*, **11**, 41–48.

Norwich, B. (1996) *A Trend Towards Inclusion: Statistics on Special School Placements and Pupils with Statements in Ordinary Schools in England 1992–96*. Centre for Studies on Inclusive Education, Bristol.

Novaco, R.W. (1979) The cognitive regulation of anger and stress. In: *Cognitive-behavioral Interventions: Theory, Research, and Procedures* (eds P.D. Kendall & S.D. Hollon), pp. 241–285. Academic Press, New York.

Nowacek, E.J., McKinney, J.D. & Hallahan, D.P. (1990) Instructional behaviours of more and less effective beginning regular and special educators. *Exceptional Children*, **57**, 140–147.

Nye, C., Foster, S.H. & Seaman, D. (1987) Effectiveness of language intervention with the language/learning disabled. *Journal of Speech and Hearing Disorders*, **52**, 348–357.

O'Brien, T. (1998) *Promoting Positive Behaviour*. David Fulton, London.

O'Connor, R.E. (1998) Race and head start participation: political and social determinants of enrolment success in the states. *Social Science Quarterly*, **79**, 595–606.

Odom, S.L., Horn, E.M., Marquart, J.M. & Hanson, M.J. (1999) On the forms of inclusion: organisational context and individualised service models. *Journal of Early Intervention*, **22**, 185–199.

Olley, J.G. & Reeve, C.E. (1997) Issues of curriculum and classroom structure. In: *Handbook of Autism and Pervasive Developmental Disorders* (eds D.J. Cohen & F.R. Volkmar), 2nd edn, pp. 484–508. John Wiley, New York.

Olson, R.K. & Wise, B.W. (1992) Reading on the computer with orthographic and speech feedback. *Reading and Writing*, **4**, 107–144.

Ozonoff, S. & Cathcart, C. (1998) Effectiveness of a home program intervention for young children with autism. *Journal of Autism and Developmental Disorders*, **28**, 28–32.

Paffrey, V. (1994) Exclusion: failed children or systems failure? *School Organisation*, **14**, 107–120.

Palmer, D.S., Borthwick-Duffy, S.A., Widaman, K. & Best, S.J. (1998) Influences on parent perceptions of inclusive practices for their children with mental retardation. *American Journal of Mental Retardation*, **103**, 272–287.

Petersen, L. & Ganonii, A.F. (1992) *Manual for Social Skills Training in Young People: Stop Think Do*. ACER, Camberwell, Victoria, Australia.

Philps, E. (1994) *A comparative study of the academic achievement and language development of children with Down's Syndrome placed in mainstream and special schools*. MPhil thesis, Department of Educational Research, University of Wolverhampton.

Powell, S. & Jordan, R., eds (1997) *Autism and Learning: a Guide to Good Practice*. David Fulton, London.

Prendergast, S.G. & McCollum, J.A. (1996) Let's talk: the effect of maternal hearing status on interactions with toddlers who are deaf. *American Annals of the Deaf*, **141**, 11–18.

Putnam, J. (1993) *Cooperative Learning and Strategies for Inclusion*. Paul H. Brookes, Baltimore.

Quill, K.A. (1995) *Teaching Children with Autism: Strategies to Enhance Communication Socialization*. Delmar, New York.

Raban, B. (1991) The role of schooling in initial literacy. *Educational and Child Psychology*, **8**, 41–59.

Ramey, S. (1999) Head Start and preschool education. *American Psychologist*, **54**, 344–346.

Redl, F. (1966) *When We Deal with Children*. Free Press, New York.

Reed, H. & Hindley, P. (1998) Promoting alternative thinking strategies (PATHS): mental health promotion with deaf children in school. In: *Taking Children Seriously: Applications of Counselling and Therapy in Education* (eds S. Decker, S. Kirby, A. Greenwood & D. Moore), pp. 113–132. Cassell, London.

Rescorla, L., Roberts, J. & Dahlsgaard, K. (1997) Late talkers at 2: outcome at age 3. *Journal of Speech and Hearing Research*, **40**, 556–566.

Reynolds, D. (1991) School effectiveness and school improvement in the 1990s. *Newsletter of the Association for Child Psychology and Psychiatry*, **13**, 5–9.

Rice, M.L. & Wilcox, K.A. (1991) *Language Acquisition Pre-school Curriculum: Development and Implementation.* University of Kansas, Lawrence, KS.

Rich, H.L. & Ross, S.M. (1989) Students' time on learning tasks in special education. *Exceptional Children*, **55**, 508–515.

Rinaldi, W. (1992) *Social Use of Language Programme.* NFER, Windsor.

Ripple, C.H., Gilliam, W.S., Chanana, N. & Zigler, E. (1999) Will fifty cooks spoil the broth? The debate over entrusting head start to the states. *American Psychologist*, **54**, 327–343.

Roberts, C. & Hindley, P. (1999) The assessment and treatment of deaf children with psychiatric disorders. *Journal of Child Psychology and Psychiatry*, **40**, 151–167.

Rogers, S.J. (1996) Early intervention in autism [Brief report]. *Journal of Autism and Developmental Disorders*, **26**, 243–246.

Rogers, S.J. (1998) Empirically supported comprehensive treatments for young children with autism. *Journal of Clinical Child Psychology*, **27**, 168–179.

Rouse, M. & Florian, L. (1996) Effective inclusive schools: a study in two countries. *Cambridge Journal of Education*, **26**, 71–85.

Rutter, M. (1983) School effects on pupil progress; research findings and policy implications. *Child Development*, **54**, 1–29.

Rutter, M. & Bartak, L. (1973) Special educational treatment of autistic children: a comparative study. I. Design of study and characteristics of units. *Journal of Child Psychology and Psychiatry*, **14**, 161–179.

Saintano, D., Goldstein, H. & Strain, P. (1992) Effects of self-evaluation on pre school children's use of social interaction strategies with their classmates with autism. *Journal of Applied Behavioural Analysis*, **25**, 127–141.

Saunders, S. (1999) *Fragile X Syndrome: A Guide for Teachers.* David Fulton, London.

Scarr, S. (1999) Freedom of choice for poor families. *American Psychologist*, **54**, 144–145.

Schilling, L.S. & DeJesus, E. (1993) Developmental issues in deaf children. *Journal of Pediatric Health Care*, **7**, 161–166.

Schopler, E. (1997) Implementation of TEACCH philosophy. In: *Handbook of Autism and Pervasive Developmental Disorders* (eds D.J. Cohen & F.R. Volkmar), 2nd edn, pp. 767–798. John Wiley, New York.

Schopler, E. & Mesibov, G.B., eds (1995) *Learning and Cognition in Autism.* Plenum Press, New York.

Schumm, J.S. & Vaughan, S. (1991) Making adaptations for mainstreamed students: general classroom teachers' perspectives. *Remedial and Special Education*, **12**, 18–25.

Schwartz, I.S., Garfinkle, A.N. & McBride, B.J. (1998) Communication and language disorders. In: *Behavioural Approaches to Problems in Childhood* (ed. P. Howlin), pp. 95–113. MacKeith Press, London.

Scott, S. (1998) Conduct disorders. In: *Behavioural Approaches to Problems in Childhood* (ed. P. Howlin), pp. 1–27. MacKeith Press, London.

Scruggs, T.E. & Mastropieri, M.A. (1996) Teacher perceptions of mainstreaming/inclusion, 1958–95: a research synthesis. *Exceptional Children*, **63**, 59–74.

Sebba, J., Byers, R. & Rose, R. (1993) Redefining the whole curriculum for pupils with learning difficulties. *Curriculum Journal*, **3**, 28–43.

Shearer, D. & Shearer, M. (1972) The Portage project: a model for early childhood education. *Exceptional Children*, **36**, 210–216.

Sheinkopf, S.J. & Siegel, B. (1998) Home-based behavioral treatment of young children with autism. *Journal of Autism and Developmental Disorders*, **28**, 15–23.

Siegel, B. (1999) Autistic learning disabilities and individualising treatment for autistic spectrum disorders. *Infants and Young Children*, **12**, 27–36.

Sigafoos, J., Roberts, D., Kerr, M., Couzens, D. & Baglioni, A.J. (1994) Opportunities for communication in classrooms serving children with developmental disabilities. *Journal of Autism and Developmental Disorders*, **24**, 259–280.

Simpson, R.L. & Myles, G.M. (1992) Full inclusion of students with autism in general education settings: values versus science. *Focus on Autistic Behavior*, **7**, 1–13.

Simpson, R.L. & Myles, B.S. (1993) Successful integration of children and youth with autism in mainstreamed settings. *Focus on Autistic Behavior*, **7**, 1–13.

Siperstein, G.N. & Leffert, J.S. (1997) Comparison of socially accepted and rejected children with mental retardation. *American Journal of Mental Retardation*, **101**, 339–351.

Snowling, M.J. (1996) Contemporary approaches to the teaching of reading [Annotation]. *Journal of Child Psychology and Psychiatry*, **37**, 139–148.

Spencer, P.E. (1993) The expressive communication of hearing mothers and deaf infants. *American Annals of the Deaf*, **138**, 275–283.

Stainback, W. & Stainback, S. (1990) *Support Networks for Inclusive Schooling: Interdependent Integrated Education.* Paul Brookes, Baltimore.

Stainback, S., Stainback, W. & East, K. (1994) A commentary on inclusion and the development of a positive self-identity by people with disabilities. *Exceptional Children*, **60**, 486–490.

Steele, J. & Mitchell, D. (1992) Special links with mainstream. *Special Children*, **55**, 14–16.

Stevenson, J. (1996) Developmental changes in the mechanisms linking language disabilities and behavior disorders. In: *Language, Learning and Behaviour Disorders: Developmental, Biological and Clinical Perspectives* (eds J.H. Beitchman, N.J. Cohen, M.M. Konstantareas & R. Tannock), pp. 78–100. Cambridge University Press, Cambridge.

Stothard, S.E., Snowling, M.J., Bishop, D.V.M., Chipase, B.B. & Kaplan, C. (1998) Language impaired pre-schoolers: a follow-up into adolescence. *Journal of Speech and Hearing Research*, **41**, 407–418.

Sturmey, P. & Crisp, A.C. (1986) Portage guide to early education: a review of research. *Educational Psychology*, **6**, 139–155.

Sulzer-Azaroff, B. & Gillat, A. (1990) Trends in behaviour analysis in education. *Journal of Applied Behaviour Analysis*, **23**, 491–495.

Swann, W. (1991) *Variations between LEAs in Levels of Segregation in Special Schools 1982–90: Preliminary Report.* Centre for Studies on Integration in Education, London.

Swanson, H.L., Hoskyn, M. & Lee, C. (1999) *Interventions for Students with Learning Disabilities: A Meta-analysis of Treatment Outcomes.* Guilford Press, New York.

Sylva, K. & Hurry, J. (1995) *Early intervention in children with reading difficulties: an evaluation of reading recovery and phonological training.* Report to the Schools Curriculum Assessment Authority, London.

Szivos, S.E. (1990) Attitudes to work and their relationship to self esteem and aspirations among young adults with a mild mental handicap. *British Journal of Mental Subnormality*, **36**, 108–117.

Tateyama-Sniezek, E. (1990) Co-operative learning: does it improve the academic achievement of students with handicaps? *Exceptional Children*, **56**, 426–437.

Thomas, G. (1992) *Effective Classroom Teamwork: Support or Intrusion*. Routledge, London.

Thomas, G., Walker, D. & Webb, J. (1998) *The Making of the Inclusive School*. Routledge, London.

Tilstone, C., Lacey, P., Porter, J. & Robertson, C. (1998) *Pupils with Learning Difficulties in Mainstream Schools*. David Fulton, London.

Tomblin, J.A.B., Freese, P.R. & Records, N.L. (1992) Diagnosing specific language impairment in adults for the purpose of pedigree analysis. *Journal of Speech and Hearing Research*, 35, 832–843.

Toomey, D. (1993) Parents hearing their children read: a review—rethinking the lessons of the Haringey Project. *Educational Research*, 35, 223–233.

Topping, K. (1990) An introduction to peer tutoring. *Education and Child Psychology*, 5, 6–16.

Truesdell, L.A. (1990) Behavior and achievement of mainstreamed junior high special class students. *Journal of Special Education*, 24, 234–242.

Tunmer, W.E. (1994) Phonological processing skills and reading remediation. In: *Reading Development and Dyslexia* (eds C. Hulme & M. Snowling), pp. 147–162. Whurr, London.

Uditsky, B. (1993) From integration to inclusion: the Canadian experience. In: *Is There a Desk with My Name on It? The Politics of Integration* (ed. R. Slee), pp. 103–127. Falmer Press, London.

Udwin, O. & Dennis, J. (1995) Psychological and behavioural phenotypes in genetically determined syndromes: a review of research findings. In: *Behavioural Phenotypes* (eds G. O'Brien & W. Yule), pp. 190–208. MacKeith Press, London.

United National Educational Scientific and Cultural Organization (1994) *The Salamanca Statement and Framework for Action on Special Needs Education*. UNESCO, Paris.

Vaughan, A. & Schumm, J.S. (1995) Responsible inclusion for students with learning disabilities. *Journal of Learning Disabilities*, 28, 264–270.

Volkmar, F., Cook, E.H., Pomeroy, J., Realmuto, G., Tanguay, P. & the Work Group on Quality Issues (1999) Practice parameters for the assessment and treatment of children, adolescents, and adults with autism and other pervasive developmental disorders. *Journal of the American Academy of Child and Adolescent Psychiatry*, 38, 32S–54S.

Wang, M.C. & Walberg, H.J. (1993) Adaptive instruction and classroom time. *American Educational Research Journal*, 20, 601–626.

Ward, J., Center, Y. & Bochner, S. (1994) A question of attitudes: integrating children with disabilities into regular classrooms. *British Journal of Special Education*, 21, 34–39.

Ware, J. (1994) *Educating Children with Profound and Multiple Learning Difficulties*. David Fulton, London.

Ware, J., Sharman, M., O'Connor, S. & Anderson, M. (1992) Interactions between pupils with severe learning difficulties and the mainstream peers. *British Journal of Special Education*, 19, 153–158.

Warnaco, H.M. (1978) *Special Educational Needs. Report of the Committee of Enquiry into the Education of Handicapped Children and Young People*. HMSO, London.

Warner-Rogers, J. (1998) Attention deficit-hyperactivity disorder. In: *Behavioural Approaches to Problems in Childhood* (ed. P. Howlin), pp. 28–53. MacKeith Press, London.

Warnock, M. (1992) Special case in need of reform. *Observer*, Schools report (3 October 1992), 18.

Waters, J. (1999) *Prader–Willi Syndrome: A Practical Guide*. David Fulton, London.

Watson, L., Gregory, S. & Powers, S. (1999) *Deaf and Hearing Impaired Pupils in Mainstream Schools*. David Fulton, London.

Webster-Stratton, C. (1998) Preventing conduct problems in head start children: strengthening parenting competencies. *Journal of Consulting and Clinical Psychology*, 66, 715–730.

Weistuch, L. & Byers-Brown, B. (1987) Motherese as therapy: a program and its dissemination. *Child Language Teaching and Therapy*, 3, 57–71.

Weistuch, L. & Lewis, M. (1985) The language intervention project. *Analysis and Intervention in Developmental Disabilities*, 5, 97–106.

Weitzman, E. (1992) *Learning Language and Loving It*. Hanen Centre, Toronto, Ontario.

Werthamer-Larsson, L., Kellam, S.G. & Wheeler, L. (1991) Effect of classroom environment on shy behavior, aggressive behavior, and concentration problems. *American Journal of Community Psychology*, 19, 585–602.

Wheldall, K. & Lam, Y.Y. (1987) Rows versus tables. II. The effects of classroom seating arrangements in classroom disruption rates on task behaviour and teacher behaviour in three special school classes. *Educational Psychology*, 7, 303–310.

Whinnery, K.W., Fuchs, L.S. & Fuchs, D. (1991) General, special and remedial teachers' acceptance of behavioral and instructional strategies for mainstreaming students with mild handicaps. *Remedial and Special Education*, 12, 6–13.

Whitehurst, G. & Fischel, J. (1994) Early developmental language delay: what if anything should the clinician do about it? *Journal of Child Psychology and Psychiatry*, 35, 613–648.

Whitehurst, G.J., Epstein, J.N., Angell, A.L., Payne, A.C., Crone, D.A. & Fischel, J.E. (1994) Outcomes of an emergent literacy intervention in head start. *Journal of Educational Psychology*, 86, 542–555.

Wise, B.W., Olson, R.K. & Treiinabm, R. (1990) Sub-syllabic units as aids in beginning readers' word learning: onset-time versus post-vowel segmentation. *Journal of Experimental Child Psychology*, 49, 1–19.

Wolfberg, P.J. & Schuler, A.L. (1993) Integrated play groups: a model for promoting the social and cognitive dimensions of play. *Journal of Autism and Developmental Disorders*, 23, 1–23.

Wood, D., Wood, H., Griffiths, A. & Howarth, I. (1986) *Teaching and Talking with Deaf Children*. John Wiley, Chichester.

Young, S. (1996) LEAs return to exclusion zone. *Times Educational Supplement*, 15 November 1996, 23.

Zetlin, A. & Murtaugh, M. (1990) Whatever happened to those with borderline IQs? *American Journal of Mental Retardation*, 94, 463–469.

Zigler, E. (1999) Head Start is not child care. *American Psychologist*, 54, 142–145.

Zigler, E. & Hodapp, R.M. (1987) The developmental implications of integrating autistic children within the public schools. In: *Handbook of Autism and Pervasive Developmental Disorders* (eds D. Cohen & A. Donnellan), pp. 668–674. Winston Wiley, New York.

Cultural and Ethnic Issues in Service Provision

Anula Nikapota

Cultural and ethnic issues in service provision

Increasing attention is being paid not only to the enormous cultural and ethnic diversity in most societies but also to its relevance politically, socially and for health care (Young 1994). Hence, as Rutter & Nikapota (Chapter 16) emphasize, the need to consider cultural and social contextual issues applies across the whole of mental health services and not just to those that serve ethnic minorities. However, there are some considerations that apply particularly strongly to ethnic minorities, and it is on those that this chapter mainly focuses. First, attention is paid to some of the key points that apply in any multicultural multiethnic society; to the great majority of industrialized, as well as developing, nations. Secondly, some of the features that apply particularly to special groups (such as street children or refugees) are discussed. Thirdly, there is a brief account of services in developing countries.

Ethnic diversity in industrialized societies

Numerous general population surveys have highlighted the enormous cultural and ethnic diversity in most societies and its implications for society and for services (Smith 2000)—see, for example, Modood *et al.* (1997) with respect to the UK, and the National Research Council (2001) regarding the USA. Not surprisingly, studies of clinic attenders have shown the same. Thus, Kramer *et al.* (2000), in a report on a London teaching hospital clinic, found that families had originated from 43 different countries, although the majority (over four-fifths) of the children had been born in the UK and had English as their first language; nearly half came from ethnic minorities. Findings across studies are somewhat contradictory with respect to referral and diagnostic patterns. However, it appears that ethnic differences on both are rather inconsistent, although attitudes to services and expectations of them probably show more variation by ethnicity and culture (Nikapota *et al.* 1998).

The implication is that all services need to be culture-sensitive in ways that recognize that culture is not a static variable, and that they need to incorporate variations by religion, place of rearing, and language as well as skin colour (see Rutter & Nikapota, Chapter 16).

Service organization for ethnic minority groups

Implications for services go beyond the provision of adequate interpreter facilities, although this is an essential basic requirement for the minority of families who need them. Services must consider consultation patterns, become familiar with characteristics of ethnic minority populations in the area served, the mix of refugee, recent and settled second- and third-generation immigrant populations, and the access these groups may have to information on access to health and welfare systems (Guarnaccia & Lopez 1998). At least in the past, some Asian parents—whether from the Indian subcontinent or from East Asia—have tended to be reluctant to use mental health services, so that underutilization of services has been a feature even where there were no limitations to access (Stern *et al.* 1990; Loo & Rapport 1998). Many parents express uncertainty about the ability of services to understand their cultural perspective, and there are also perceptions of racial bias (Nikapota *et al.* 1998). Services must relate not only to parents' perceptions but also to young people's needs. A simple example of how needs may not be met is the discrepancy in the use of the criteria of colour and race by which ethnicity is assigned to a young person accessing services (Hodes *et al.* 1998; Waters 2000). A respectful cross-cultural approach is indicated, rather than an assumption of what is best for a given minority group.

One of the important issues that give rise to debate is the extent to which ethnic-specific services should develop. On the one hand, there is evidence that suggests that engagement of families may be greater within such services (Krause & Miller 1995; Thomas 1995; Guarnaccia & Lopez 1998). On the other hand, although this may be so for some groups, such as recent immigrants, it may not be so for many others, including second- and third-generation immigrants. There is a danger that separate services could make access to the best tertiary care services more difficult because the provision of care for ethnic minorities could become viewed as an 'offshoot' rather than a prime responsibility of the main service. Furthermore, such ethnic-specific services might find it more difficult to respond to intracultural diversity and to transgenerational differences or cultural dualism. The basic need is to develop strategies that will contribute to culturally sensitive clinical work in all service sectors.

An integral aspect of effective child mental health services are functional links with other agencies, such as child health, education and welfare systems. Cultural sensitivity is not limited to one agency although, in the search for culturally appropriate solutions, conflicts among agencies can occur—such as in relation to policies for adoption and fostering of minority children (see below). Culturally sensitive collaborations with child health will be required not only for early intervention through parent training, but also for vulnerable groups of children with genetically transmitted illnesses (such as sickle cell disease) that are associated with particular racial groups.

The culture of school can support or create confusion for children by conflicting with the cultural values prevailing at home. Teacher attitude and problem identification may depend on the ethos of the school, physical environment of the school and perception of culture-related norms of behaviour among ethnic minorities. This has been illustrated in studies comparing teacher attitude to Asian and African-Caribbean children in the UK (Sonuga-Barke *et al.* 1993) and to Asian and Latin American refugee children in Canada (Rousseau *et al.* 1996). It was acknowledged that the better classroom behaviour reported of Asian children in a cross-ethnic Hawaiian study could, at least in part, have been a result of teacher bias as they were themselves Asian, although it seems likely that parent pressure on compliance with social norms, including respect and obedience towards adults, would have been a significant factor (Loo & Rapport 1998).

Clinical challenges

Assessment

Differences in psychosocial environments, social values governing behaviour and child-rearing patterns can result in differences in the meaning of behaviour (Rutter & Nikapota, Chapter 16). The first challenge is to appreciate the different cultural modalities for expressing distress, and the different cultural concepts of dysfunction or disorder. The second challenge is to develop strategies to facilitate culturally sensitive and clinically appropriate diagnoses. The need to recognize differences in sociocultural norms and values is acknowledged within the established classification systems, both the ICD-10 and DSM-IV, although the guidance given on how to judge differences in threshold according to different social and cultural norms is not made explicit, a point that has led to criticism (Canino *et al.* 1998). In fact, it may be extremely difficult to be explicit while at the same time avoiding the danger of stereotyping. It could be argued that what is needed is a basic framework of assessment that facilitates exploration of psychosocial factors, while at the same time allowing clinicians to be aware that there may be some aspects of the specific cultural background of the patient about which knowledge is required. One of the main strengths within established child psychiatry practice is that the basic principles of assessment do provide such a framework (see Rutter & Taylor, Chapter 2; Yule & Rutter, Chapter 7). This includes the use of multiple informants; exploration of parent perceptions of problems, parent expectations of the index child; and the assessment of risk and protective factors in the family (both nuclear and extended) and in social support networks. In addition, however, there will be instances where a clinician will have to obtain additional knowledge about a specific cultural aspect. This should be sought, just as one may have to obtain expert advice on any other clinical issue pertaining to accurate diagnosis.

In considering relationships among child, family and clinicians, there needs to be a recognition of the extent to which cultural issues may vary according to whether families are first-, second- or third-generation immigrants, and according to whether parents and children identify with the same culture. The extent to which the family may be in cultural transition, and the differences in the degree of acculturalization or cultural dualism among different members of the family, may be causes of intrafamilial difficulty (Landau 1982; Burnham & Harris 1996). Clinicians need also to be aware of the possibility of bias resulting from an identification with the family members whose values approximate most closely with that of the clinician. There are many accounts of history-taking and assessment of minority groups, such as for Asian and African-Caribbean families in the UK (Dhivedi & Varma 1996; Lau 2000), and by Canino & Guarnaccia (1997) for Hispanic families in the USA. Evidence of the impact of such guidance on diagnostic sensitivity and therapeutic efficacy in child psychiatry derives largely from case reports rather than systematic case comparisons.

An important issue for minority children and adolescents is that of racial/ethnic/cultural identity and how this may relate to self-esteem, resilience or vulnerability. Ethnic identity is not a fixed entity but politicized views may demand that ethnic minority children retain their racial identity in relation to country of origin, despite the degree to which their attitudes reflect a cultural dualism. A review of research on race and self-esteem around black identity notes that the majority of studies demonstrate similar or slightly higher scores for black young people than comparison white groups, positive scores increasing with age (Gray-Little & Hafdahl 2000). Self-esteem in this context was defined as self-regard as a result of an appraisal process depending on individual social context and direct experiences both positive and negative. The review did not address issues of vulnerability but did note a positive relationship between self-esteem and racially consonant surroundings. Cultural identity does not necessarily follow racial or ethnic identity. Cultural allegiances seem to relate as much to social class and peer group as to ethnicity of child or parent (Tizard & Phoenix 1995). The reasons for opting for one or other cultural or ethnic identity are complex and may vary according to both the culture of origin and a young person's own experience. A study looking at academically successful African-American adolescents found that, where this was achieved through moving away from their culture of origin, the cost was 'racelessness' and emotional vulnerability (Arroyo & Zigler 1995). The clinical significance of issues of identity, linked to dominance and disadvantage, are well illustrated in a study of suicidal behaviour among Hawaiian adolescents (Yuen *et al.* 2000). Vulnerability was greatest in those adolescents who had a Hawaiian cultural identity and least among those with cultural dualism that related also to the dominant 'white' culture.

Therapeutic approaches

Parent perceptions and concepts of problems that differ from those of clinicians may, if not recognized and addressed, lead to non-engagement with therapy. There is a substantial body of guidance on how mainstream therapeutic approaches may be modified for use with children and families within different cultural or ethnic minority groups, and case history evidence of apparent clinical effectiveness, but there is at times the danger that boundaries and differences between cultures are emphasized to a degree that could mask differences within a culture and similarities between some cultural groups. In a discussion of themes that govern cross-cultural family therapy, Krause & Miller (1995) pointed out that developing effective communication between therapist and family in the clinical setting is not limited to working cross-culturally, or to family therapy; rather, it applies to all clinical situations. Evidence is emerging on the cross-cultural application of some therapeutic approaches, such as parent training, and of the behavioural psychotherapies. There is little empirical evidence on comparisons of different methods within a given cultural context. The same criticisms that have been levelled at the use of research instruments and methodologies cross-culturally may be applied equally to specific therapies. Often there has been insufficient systematic consideration of what, within these approaches, are core concepts and what are influenced by the values of the cultural background within which the therapy developed. For example, individual psychodynamic child psychotherapy (see Jacobs, Chapter 58) may be a clinically effective therapeutic approach for particular problems but may not be acceptable, feasible or appropriate within some cultures. Parents may find the ethos of a therapy that creates a boundary of privacy between child and the parent unacceptable if their cultural values place the boundary elsewhere (Maitra & Miller 1996).

It could be argued that had psychodynamic child psychotherapy developed in a South Asian rather than a European context, ideas about the inner world of the child and how best to address them may have led to a different strategic approach, given the prevailing values in these cultures of collectivism rather than individualism and self-expression. Although clinical experience suggests that behaviour therapy *is* useful in all cultures, an attempt to involve parents in the use of behavioural techniques based on play and positive reinforcement in Hong Kong found that these ideas conflicted with child-rearing modes and beliefs about problems (Lieh-Mak *et al.* 1984). The influence of culture-based attitudes to behaviour and problem perception are well illustrated in data on conduct disorder in the Indian subcontinent where conduct problems are considered as a disciplinary issue to be handled by the family and not a 'medical' problem (Minde and Nikapota 1993; Rahman *et al.* 2000), despite the fact that conduct disorder has the highest prevalence of childhood disorder in community-based data from India (Hackett *et al.* 1998; Malhotra *et al.* in press). Community-based programmes that, at a primary care level, advocate the use of behavioural approaches have yet to be systematically devel-

oped and reported on. Family therapy is used or considered to be desirable in all cultures where child psychiatric services have developed (see Jacobs & Pearse, Chapter 57). Principles underlying effective cross-cultural family therapy highlight the value of obtaining information about the family and the culture, of exploring the value system of the family, and the avoidance of assumptions based on race, colour and socioeconomic context (Krause & Miller 1995), and of appreciating the cultural transitions that the family as a whole or individual members may be experiencing (Landau 1982; Burnham & Harris 1996).

Another neglected area is the development of therapeutic approaches that utilize modalities and resources arising from within a culture; nevertheless, there are some examples. Cuento therapy, which makes use of cautionary folk tales, was effective in reducing anxiety in high-risk kindergarten and primary school children in Puerto Rican and other Spanish-speaking children in New York (Constantino *et al.* 1986). Describing a programme for a similar age group and population using culture-based art as a means for coping with stress, Canino (1995) remarked that therapeutic approaches that draw on culturally derived material can be ethnically empowering and culture-sensitive.

A further challenging area is the involvement of alternative practitioners in therapeutic approaches. The potential value of this has been discussed not only in relation to non-Western cultures where systems such as Ayurveda have been established for centuries, but also in relation to ethnic minority groups (Rack 1982). A review of intercultural psychotherapy (Tseng 1999) discussed the technical adjustments, theoretical modifications and practical guidelines for developing cross-cultural approaches and involving traditional healers with professional staff. The inclusion of traditional healers or alternative health systems can become a medicopolitical issue within local contexts and will also lead to debate as to the balance between benefit and risk. Where traditional healers are perceived as an important source of help, they should be involved, but the challenge will be how to do so while allowing them to retain their role. For example, where mental retardation is considered to be because of an inauspicious astronomical influence, this can cause harm; acceptance of disability and use of appropriate learning strategies for the child can be delayed. Traditional healers may themselves be appreciative of being involved in providing support in these situations, so long as they do not feel threatened. Kapur (1995) gave a useful outline of a treatment approach for dissociative reactions for use in India, which included the use, within a standard treatment protocol, of non-injurious culturally accepted solutions such as going to a traditional healer. Traditional healers may be used to identify mental health problems (Patel *et al.* 1997), deliver ethnoculturally determined patterns of treatment (Tharp 1991) and provide support in situations of stress, such as supporting families with AIDS (Ovuga *et al.* 1999). Although this is particularly an issue for developing countries, working with alternative systems of healing is also an issue gaining increasing prominence within Western societies.

There are initiatives in the UK (such as the Intercultural

Therapy Centre) that focus on providing help specifically targeted for ethnic minority groups (Kareem & Littlewood 1992; Thomas 1995). This has developed multidisciplinary and multicultural therapeutic services for black and Asian groups that stress the need to acknowledge racism and other social phenomena when developing models of treatment for immigrant populations, and encourage the use of cultural advocates to help empower families. Cultural consultants to aid acquisition of information about ideas and values within a culture and help therapists respect a client or patient's cultural identity is one of the trends found useful in developing culture-sensitive family therapy for ethnic minorities (Krause & Miller 1995).

Intrafamilial discord and divorce

Although extended family systems may protect the impact of interparental conflict on a child, they may also give rise to conflict. Divorce can, rather than ending conflict, lead to a perpetuation of conflict centring on contact and access. Cultural factors may be implicated in this. Conflict may arise when there are significant cultural differences between parents, or when the marriage was a social contract between two families rather than between two people, with divorce resulting in disruption of the social networks of the families concerned. In the first instance, the prevailing professional view (Roll 1998) is that it is nevertheless important for the child to have access to both cultures with some evidence that indicates that children are able to cope with and adjust to these differences. In the second instance, attitudes may become so fixed that the child's emotional security within the resident family could be threatened or be perceived to be under threat if contact occurs. The situation is common in Asian communities, both immigrant and in the Indian subcontinent. Child psychiatric opinion at present rests on what may be best practice in the view of the individual clinician. There is a lack of evidence to indicate what might be the long-term outcome for these children. Thus, it is not known whether allowing them to adopt the negative attitudes of the resident parent and family network towards their non-custodial parent may lead to better adjustment, or whether an insistence on some form of contact is the more favoured option.

Maltreatment

Debate continues on whether a universal definition for maltreatment and abuse is possible (Korbin 1991; see Emery & Laumann Billings, Chapter 20). There is now sufficient knowledge about what normative capacities ought to be for children and adolescents to define some criteria that could be universally applicable about what might constitute abuse in terms of damage to potential function. This does not ignore the fact that there will be situations in which a practice may be considered appropriate in one context and abusive in another, children in employment being one such example. There could be resistance within communities and cultures to the idea that abuse can and does occur. Communities within a country may vary with regards to the extent that they are ready to accept, not only that abuse occurs, but also that action may be required to protect the rights of the child when they conflict with traditional community and family values. Difficulty may arise where issues of family loyalties lead to a reluctance to report or act on behalf of a child, or where services for child protection are developing, and appropriate alternative care arrangements are not available. The initial role of the child psychiatrist may then be advocacy and education about the established consequences for emotional development and well-being of deprivation and abuse. Therapeutic interventions for children cannot develop without provision of basic needs and a legal and welfare system needs to be in place. Where systems are emerging, it is the current reality that a child subject to sexual abuse may be removed from the family, be at risk of being socially ostracized and placed in the only alternative care available—usually an orphanage. Where family rights supersede those of the child, the child may be forced to remain within the abusive environment. Preventive education aimed at helping children become aware of the need to protect themselves from abuse may be particularly challenging in situations where sex education in itself is not considered culturally appropriate.

Where child protection services are well developed and in place, difficulties arise in different ways. Developing a framework for decision-making about abuse that also respects cultural differences can be problematic, particularly when there is cultural dissonance between clinician, child protection services and family. On the one hand, what may be regarded by the family as appropriate practice, such as physical punishment, could lead to allegations of abuse. This needs to be handled particularly sensitively, and careful assessments made about what would be the appropriate intervention for the child and how the family should be supported.

Some special issues

Children working or living on the street

Official estimates put the number of children who are a regular part of the labour force as 10 million children in Africa and 18–20 million in India. Whereas the majority of children employed are in developing countries, ethnicity and poverty place children at risk of hazardous employment in industrialized societies too (UNICEF 1997), yet there are few studies of the psychopathological effects of young children working. There are particular concerns about the risks experienced by street-based children and youth, of whom there are more than 100 million worldwide. However, a distinction needs to be drawn between those who work the streets (begging, selling goods, offering services) but who return home to their families each night, and those who live and work on the street outside the context of family support. The available evidence suggests that the risks are particularly great for the latter group (Campos et al. 1994).

In poorer countries, economic factors constitute the predominant reason for children taking to the street, or being placed in employment. However, other influences include harsh parenting, abuse within home or at work. Loss of family and displacement as a result of war has led to a sharp increase in the numbers of homeless street children (UNICEF 2000). Many families whose poverty has led them to place a child in a labour situation will not necessarily welcome their child back unless they, in turn, have access to income generation opportunities.

Subsequent outcomes for employed and for street children vary considerably according to the extent to which they become involved in peer group networks which may be socially supportive. Children may also be subject to abuse, victimization and liable to become involved in substance misuse. Examples of the situation of street children derive from studies in Ethiopia (Lalor 1999), Colombia (Aptekar 1989), Brazil (Campos *et al.* 1994, Honduras (Wright *et al.* 1993) as well as the overview of the problem provided by international agencies such as UNICEF (1997). Interventions for employed children or street children range from sociopolitical change and poverty alleviation programmes to the provision of alternative systems for supportive care and learning that build on the children's functional abilities (UNICEF 1997). Studies looking at the development of competence in adversity (Masten & Coatsworth 1998) may provide a theoretical underpinning for the development of programmes that foster competence. Systems to encourage participation of street children in informal education, providing opportunities for them to generate income for themselves but also participate in normative experiences, may constitute the priority line of intervention. These systems will be required before providing psychotherapeutic help becomes at all meaningful (Campos *et al.* 1994).

The situation for homeless youth in industrialized countries is rather different (Craig & Hudson 1998; Sleegers *et al.* 1998; Fietal *et al.* 1992). A case–control study in London showed that childhood adversity, low educational attainment and prior psychiatric disorder all predisposed to homelessness. One-fifth of the homeless had attempted suicide. A 1-year follow-up showed that two-thirds of those with psychiatric disorder remained symptomatic, over half had been involved in petty crime, and just under one-third had committed more serious offences. Two-fifths had substance abuse or dependence. Satisfactory accommodation outcomes were achieved by two-fifths; these were more frequent in those of ethnic minority status, better educational achievement, and where accommodation plans were negotiated through a resettlement agency. Successful resettlement may well depend on integrated services that address persistent substance abuse and mental disorder, as well as the immediate housing need.

Refugee and displaced children

Hodes (2000) provided a succinct review of the evidence on the psychological problems experienced by refugee children, with a particular focus on those in the UK. United Nations' figures put the figure of refugees (of all ages) worldwide as 21.5 million, with some 6 million in Europe, but far greater numbers in Africa

and Asia (United Nations High Commissioner for Refugees 1999). Until recently, most attention has focused on the situation of adults, but there is a growing literature on children. There has been an especial concern over the problems faced by refugee children who are unaccompanied by their parents. The numbers involved in the UK have risen hugely in the 1990s—from 197 in 1992 to 4405 in 1999.

Most of the systematic studies of refugee children (with or without comparison groups of various kinds) have been undertaken in North America. These have included Cambodian children who had experienced massive war trauma (Kinzie *et al.* 1986; Sack *et al.* 1994, 1997), as well as those without much direct experience of war (Tousignant *et al.* 1999). All studies have shown, not surprisingly, that the rates of psychopathology are substantially higher than in non-refugee populations. Nevertheless, it has also been evident that well over half have not shown any type of mental disorder. Moreover, the forms of disorder have been quite varied, although post-traumatic stress disorders have been a prominent feature in those exposed to severely traumatic specific experiences.

In considering service implications, it is important both to appreciate the considerable heterogeneity in the experiences of refugees and to note the operation of a complex mixture of risk and protective factors (Hodes 2000). The experiences that led to their becoming refugees are obviously relevant, with the psychopathological risks increased for those suffering violence, torture and family disruption (Williams & Westermeyer 1986; Ahearn & Athey 1991; Rousseau 1995). However, in addition there are the more long-term experiences of poverty, persecution, serious accommodation problems, lack of appropriate health care (Gosling 2000) and breakdown of community ties prior to, and after, seeking asylum. The children may also be affected by the occurrence of mental disorders in the adults looking after them. The need to learn a new language and to adapt to a new host culture constitutes a further challenge, although school attendance often makes both of these much less of a problem for children than for their parents.

Sharp distinctions are sometimes drawn between refugees or asylum-seekers who have suffered persecution, and immigrants who have moved country voluntarily in order to better their economic circumstances. However, the two groups overlap to a considerable extent in their background circumstances, their experiences in the new host country, and in their service needs, although there are also differences with respect to the frequency of their experience of severe stress and trauma (Guarnaccia & Lopez 1998; Hodes 2000). It has been suggested that the most at risk are the children who have been active combatants in war (UNICEF 2000). Clearly, this will have placed them in a situation quite inappropriate for their age, but systematic data are lacking on the extent to which this puts them at risk for mental disorder, as distinct from risks to the normal processes of growing up. Vulnerability to disorder may depend on the extent to which they are forcibly conscripted and also brutalized to ensure participation (Richman 1993).

Many refugees remain as displaced persons, either in their

own country or in neighbouring ones. Their situation is likely to be much affected by the continuing conflicts that led to their situation, by the poverty they continue to experience in developing nations with scarce resources, and by life in refugee camps (which is the case for many) or by the need to be on the move.

The situation for those coming to an industrialized country is very different in many important respects, but feelings of alienation and isolation may be experienced in spite of having reached a place of relative safety. The key sociocultural, education and legal issues have been discussed by Richman (1998) and Rutter & Jones (1998). Schools constitute an extremely valuable resource for these children, not only in providing predictability but also in offering a site for therapeutic interventions (Richman 1993; O'Shea *et al.* 2000; Yule 2000).

Families, if cohesive, are likely to constitute a protective feature but so too are community ties if they were maintained or reconstituted after arrival in the new country. In planning services and therapeutic interventions, it may be helpful to draw on cultural resources and contexts as illustrated by the positive outcome in Guatemalan refugee children in a camp in Mexico (Miller 1996). Resources there included a camp organization that retained community structure, a degree of family organization despite bereavements, and the teaching of Guatemalan history so children could understand their situation. In very different circumstances, retention of cultural context led to a better outcome for Finnish returnee children (Vuorenkoski *et al.* 2000). In the UK too, it is important to appreciate that refugee groups often include mental health professionals who may be able to provide a counselling role as well as providing a link with mental health services (Dihour & Pelosi 1989). The underlying concept—the importance of retaining cultural context while also adapting to new experience—is very relevant for programmes involving refugee children. The coping strategies developed by Sudanese refugee children included seeking companionship, wishful thinking and praying (Paardekooper *et al.* 1999); these, while indicating the despair of the children, also pointed to ways in which culture-related coping strategies may be strengthened.

The appreciation of culture-mediated forms of distress and the need to draw on local approaches to bereavement and healing are essential not only in war situations but also when dealing with any large-scale trauma or bereavement (Cairns & Dawes 1996), or with issues related to chronic or terminal illness. This need is highlighted by the pandemic of children and young people with HIV and whose families are dead or dying as a result of AIDS (Brown *et al.* 2000; see also Mellins *et al.*, Chapter 49).

Alternative care for high-risk groups

Community attitudes to the concept of fostering and adoption, as well as the resource implications for statutory and voluntary agencies, may determine service development in this area. In many societies with a functional extended family system, children who are orphaned or subject to neglect by a parent will be absorbed into the family system, and the concept of adopting a

child from outside the family will be viewed as unacceptable. In these contexts, the only alternative care available may be institutional. Within these contexts, fostering and adoption initiatives on a large scale will require public education as a way of creating a climate for change. This may be equally relevant when promoting adoption and fostering for children by ethnic minority groups. Where fostering and adoption are not part of the sociocultural climate of a country, the alternative provision will be institutional care. The limitations and inadequacies of institutional care need no repetition (see Rushton & Minnis, Chapter 22). The situation of children in Romanian orphanages reflected the impact of a state's policy on vulnerable children, whereas the progress of Romanian adoptees in the UK is an example of the considerable (although sometimes incomplete) recovery that is possible for children even after extreme deprivation, provided intervention is early (Rutter *et al.* 1998; see also O'Connor, Chapter 46). Where institutional care is the only feasible option, child mental health professionals have a role in highlighting issues that must be addressed to minimize disadvantage. The ability of residential settings to be child-centred and encourage development of emotional links with caring adults, thereby minimizing serious psychological problems, is demonstrated in an Eritrean study of war orphans (Wolff & Fesseha 1999).

Adoption and fostering of ethnic minority children is a separate and somewhat politicized issue. Flexible policies for fostering and adoption to ensure a stable early placement for children must include the consideration of transracial placements where no 'match' from a cultural or ethic point of view is possible, with training of adoptive parents on how to deal with issues of identity and culture. The majority of studies (Tizard 1991; Rushton & Minnis 1997) indicate that transracially adopted children are well adjusted, although more problems may arise with adolescence and some studies indicate that there may be more problems than in non-adopted comparison groups (see also Cohen, Chapter 23; Rushton & Minnis, Chapter 22).

The issue of transracial placement is not only one for ethnic minority groups within a majority community, it is also a live issue in many non-Western cultures, e.g. in South Asia transracial adoption is seen on the one hand as offering a better place economically for children, but it is also accompanied by fears that children may, thereby, be exposed to racism and be divorced from what would have been their culture of origin.

Organization of services in developing countries

The basic principles underlying the provision of services apply across developing and industrialized nations and across culturally and ethnically diverse societies (World Health Organization 1977). However, there are also important differences that influence organization and service delivery (Nikapota 1991; Hackett & Hackett 1999; Rahman *et al.* 2000). Thus, the extent to which physical ill-health and malnutrition affect children, together with the likelihood (or otherwise) that they will receive skilled attention, will have necessary consequences for the medical assessment of children referred for mental disorders (see A. Bailey, Chapter 10). Similarly, the overall patterns of disease in countries will have implications for different patterns of aetiology for mental retardation. The overall level of resources available will also influence the extent to which the main care has to be at the primary level, and the extent to which specialized services are provided by paediatricians or general psychiatrists rather than clinicians specifically trained to work with children. Similarly, resources will determine the extent to which care is provided by professionals or volunteers who have received just a focused training that prepares them to be skilled in delivering a limited range of well-defined services.

Nevertheless, it would be a mistake to view these considerations as specific to developing countries. Throughout the world, there has been an appreciation of the need to be concerned with primary prevention (see Offord & Bennett, Chapter 52); to develop parent training programmes (see Scott, Chapter 56); to liaise with paediatricians (see Rauch & Jellinek, Chapter 62); to practise in non-medical settings (see Nicol, Chapter 64); and to meet mental health needs in primary care services (see Garralda, Chapter 65). These developments have included focused training of nurse specialists and therapists of various kinds (Marks 1992; Gournay et al. 2000) mainly for work with adult mentally ill, but there have been some initiatives in the child mental health field such as the training of parent advisers in the UK (Davis et al. 1997), and training teacher counsellors in India (Kapur 1997). Protocols for the diagnosis and management of mental disorders and for the basic use of neuroleptics and anticonvulsants (World Health Organization 1996) have mainly been developed for the treatment of serious adult disorders but they are becoming more used with children as well. These all fit in with the World Health Organization (1977) summary of needs with respect to parent and community education about children's emotional needs and behaviour; early intervention to promote development among high-risk groups of young children; and task-orientated training of personnel in primary health care and education about the management of simple behaviour problems (World Health Organization 1977).

Accordingly, the need in developing countries is not to work with a different set of principles, but rather to use the same principles to adapt the specifics to local resources and local contexts. The same considerations apply within industrialized societies to the variations of services as required for rural communities and inner city populations, or for geographically concentrated populations (as in the Netherlands) or geographically scattered ones (as in many parts of Scandinavia). Similarly, the need to pay attention to cultural attitudes in primary prevention programmes arises in much the same way within industrialized and developing countries—as evident, for example, in views on sex education, family planning and substance abuse. In all cases, effective planning requires knowledge and responsivity to cultural acceptability, while also accepting that sometimes there may be a need to help families appreciate why certain interventions may be helpful if they are introduced and undertaken in the right way.

The location of access points within primary care will also need to be based on what is culturally appropriate. Schools are often a valuable point of contact (Hendren et al. 1994; Kapur 1997). Where education is a high priority, and concerns about children's learning trigger help-seeking behaviour, the location of primary care developments within schools may be particularly appropriate, especially if the health network is not comprehensive and used mainly for physical illness.

First-line management and parent training programmes should use strategies that derive from, or do not conflict with, prevailing cultural ideas. It may be most effective to combine traditional approaches with the introduction of new ideas. A programme in Turkey has demonstrated the effectiveness of this strategy (Kagitcibasi 1997). There are a number of initiatives to train primary care staff to deliver mental health care (Murthy 1998). Task-orientated training in primary care may also require the use of strategies that facilitate recognition of problems. Use of a clinical problem-solving approach based on the conceptual framework underpinning child psychiatric assessments can be effective across all cultures, adapted to fit the knowledge base and cultural context of the specific group of workers being trained. One such approach, developed for use with primary health care workers in Sri Lanka (Samerasinghe et al. 1997), is currently being evaluated.

Training and research

Training objectives to meet clinical and service needs should include an understanding of cultural influences on family functioning and on expressions of distress; risk and protective factors as they vary, or are the same, within and between cultural groups; skills to ensure culturally sensitive clinical approaches; knowledge about social policy and the legal framework for children within different contexts; skills for teaching, training and advocacy within primary care groups in line with current trends with regard to service delivery. Thus far, the content should not differ from well-thought-out training programmes already established. However, to ensure the further development of cross-cultural psychiatry, as well as psychiatry within different cultural contexts, some content derived from a sociological and anthropological perspective is important. Of particular importance are discussions on discrimination and racism; the impact on families of poverty and disadvantage (see Friedman & Chase-Lansdale, Chapter 15); and factors contributing to professional bias and how it may be avoided (Ridley et al. 2000) While this becomes most obvious in relation to intercultural differences, bias may equally exist among professionals working with intracultural groups, and may also occur as a result of training that creates a cultural distance between a professional and his or her culture. There is a growing body of evidence of the manner in which attitudes and confidence in racial stereotypes influences psychiatric diagnoses among ethnic minorities (Fernando 1995) and on how social factors can lead to bias (Littlewood 1992).

The importance of training in research skills cannot be

overemphasized. One of the most important ways in which knowledge on psychopathology and therapeutic approaches can develop cross-culturally is through the development of research expertise in non-Western cultures, in both quantitative and qualitative methodologies. This is an area where training alone may not be sufficient for progress because of the very significant resource implications. Research directions need to adopt approaches derived from cross-cultural as well as cultural psychiatry and psychology (see Rutter & Nikapota, Chapter 16).

Finally, it must be an objective of training to increase the confidence, as well as the knowledge, of the clinicians and researchers originating from or working within non-Western cultures. This requires an acceptance of both similarities and differences across cultures, and an acknowledgement of the current dominance of Western cultural values in much of the available empirical evidence.

Conclusions

Service implications that arise from cultural and ethnic issues relate just as much to intracultural groups as to cross-cultural situations, although the issues in the latter context are more obvious. There are service implications, some of which are relevant in all cultures, but the ways in which these are addressed will of necessity vary according to the magnitude of the problem, sociocultural context and resources available. There is a dearth of systematic evaluation of different therapeutic approaches used cross-culturally, and of the use of culturally derived therapeutic strategies.

References

Ahearn, F.L. & Athey, J.L. (Eds) (1991) *Refugee Children: Theory, research and services.* The Johns Hopkins University Press, Baltimore and London.

Aptekar, L. (1989) The psychology of Columbian street children. *International Journal of Health Services*, **19**, 295–310.

Arroyo, C.G. & Zigler, E. (1995) Racial identity, academic achievement, and the psychological well-being of economically disadvantaged adolescents. *Journal of Personality and Social Psychology*, **69**, 903–914.

Brown, L.K., Lourie, K.J. & Pao, M. (2000) Children and adolescents living with HIV and AIDS. *Journal of Child Psychology and Psychiatry*, **41**, 81–96.

Burnham, J. & Harris, Q. (1996) Emerging ethnicity. In: *Meeting the Needs of Ethnic Minority Children* (eds K.N. Dhivedi & V.P. Varma), pp. 130–156. Jessica Kingsley, London.

Cairns, E. & Dawes, A. (1996) Children: ethnic and political violence: a commentary. *Child Development*, **67**, 129–139.

Campos, R., Raffaelli, M., Ude, W. *et al.* (1994) Social networks and daily activities of street youth in Belo Horizonte, Brazil. *Child Development*, **65**, 319–330.

Canino, G. & Guarnaccia, P. (1997) Methodological challenges in the assessment of Hispanic children and adolescents. *Applied Developmental Science*, **1**, 124–134.

Canino, I. (1995) Coping with stress through art: a programme for urban minority children. In: *Racial and Ethnic Identity* (eds H.W. Harris, H.C. Blue & E.E.H. Griffiths), pp. 115–134. Routledge, New York.

Canino, I., Canino, G. & Arroyo, W. (1998) Cultural considerations for childhood disorders: how much was included in DSM-IV? *Transcultural Psychiatry*, **35**, 343–355.

Constantino, G., Malgady, R. & Rogler, R. (1986) Cuento therapy: a culturally sensitive modality. *Journal of Consulting and Clinical Psychology*, **54**, 639–645.

Craig, T.K.J. & Hudson, S. (1998) Homeless youth in London. I. Childhood antecedents and psychiatric disorder. *Psychological Medicine*, **28**, 1379–1388.

Davis, H., Spurr, P., Cox, A., Lynch, M. & Hahn, K. (1997) A description and evaluation of a community child mental health service. *Clinical Child Psychology and Psychiatry*, **2**, 221–238.

Dhivedi, K. & Varma, V.P., eds (1996) *Meeting the Needs of Ethnic Minority Children.* Jessica Kingsley, London.

Dihour, O.E. & Pelosi, A.J. (1989) The work of the Somali counselling project in the UK. *Psychiatric Bulletin*, **13**, 619–621.

Fernando, S. (1995) Social realities and mental health. In: *Mental Health in a Multi-ethnic Society* (ed. S. Fernando), pp. 11–34. Routledge, London.

Fietel, B., Matgetson, N., Chamas, J. & Lipman, C. (1992) Psychosocial background and behavioural and emotional disorders of homeless and runaway youth. *Hospital and Community Psychiatry*, **43**, 155–159.

Gosling, R. (2000) *The Needs of Young Refugees in Lambeth, Southwark and Lewisham.* Community Health South London NHS Trust, London.

Gournay, K., Denford, L., Parr, A.M. & Newell, R. (2000) British nurses in behavioural psychotherapy: a 25 year follow up. *Journal of Advances in Nursing*, **32**, 343–351.

Gray-Little, B. & Hafdahl, A.R. (2000) Factors influencing racial comparisons of self esteem: a quantitative review. *Psychological Bulletin*, **126**, 26–54.

Guarnaccia, P.J. & Lopez, S. (1998) The mental health and adjustment of immigrant and refugee children. *Child and Adolescent Psychiatric Clinics of North America*, **7**, 537–553.

Hackett, R. & Hackett, L. (1999) Child psychiatry across cultures. *International Journal of Psychiatry*, **11**, 225–235.

Hackett, R., Hackett, L., Bhakta, P. & Gowers, S. (1998) The prevalence and associations of psychiatric disorder in children in Kerala, south India. *Journal of Child Psychology and Psychiatry*, **40**, 801–807.

Hendren, R., Birrell-Weison, R. & Orley, J. (1994) *Mental Health Programmes in Schools.* Division of Mental Health, World Health Organization, Geneva.

Hodes, M. (2000) Psychologically distressed refugee children in the United Kingdom. *Child Psychology and Psychiatry Review*, **5**, 57–68.

Hodes, M., Creamer, J. & Wooley, J. (1998) Cultural meanings of ethnic categories. *Psychiatric Bulletin*, **22**, 20–24.

Kagitcibasi, C. (1997) Parent education and child development. In: *Early Child Development: Investing in Our Children's Future* (ed. M.E. Young), pp. 243–272. Elsevier, New York.

Kapur, M. (1995) *Internalizing Disorders in Mental Health of Indian Children*, pp. 186–215. Sage Publications, New Delhi.

Kapur, M. (1997) Interventions in school settings. In: *Mental Health in Indian Schools*, pp. 31–44. Sage Publications. New Delhi.

Kareem, J. & Littlewood, R. (1992) *Intercultural Therapy: Themes, Interpretations and Practice.* Blackwell Scientific, Oxford.

Kinzie, J.D., Sack, W.H., Angell, R.H., Manson, S. & Rath, B. (1986) The psychiatric effects of massive trauma on Cambodian children. I.

The children. *Journal of the American Academy of Child Psychiatry*, **25**, 370–376.

Korbin, J.E. (1991) Cross-cultural perspectives and research directions for the 21st century. *Child Abuse and Neglect*, **15** (Suppl. 1), 67–77.

Kramer, T., Evans, N. & Garralda, M.E. (2000) Ethnic diversity among child and adolescent psychiatric (CAP) clinic attenders. *Child Psychology and Psychiatry Review*, **5**, 169–175.

Krause, I.-B. & Miller, A.C. (1995) Themes in cross-cultural therapy: a framework for 'good enough' cross cultural understanding. In: *Mental Health in a Multi-ethnic Society* (ed. S. Fernando), pp. 172–179. Routledge, London.

Lalor, K.J. (1999) Street children: a comparative perspective. *Child Abuse and Neglect*, **23**, 759–770.

Landau, J. (1982) Therapy with families in cultural transition. In: *Ethnicity and Family Therapy* (eds M. Mccoldrick, J.K. Pearce & J. Giordano), pp. 552–572. Guilford Press, New York.

Lau, A., ed. (2000) *South Asian Children and Adolescents in Britain*. Whurr, London.

Lieh-Mak, F., Lee, P.W.H. & Luk, S.L. (1984) Problems encountered in teaching Chinese parents to be behaviour therapists. *Psychologia*, **27**, 56–64.

Littlewood, R. (1992) Psychiatric diagnosis and racial bias: empirical and interpretative approaches. *Social Science and Medicine*, **34**, 141–149.

Loo, S.K. & Rapport, M.D. (1998) Ethnic variations in children's problem behaviors: a cross-sectional, developmental study of Hawaii school children. *Journal of Child Psychology and Psychiatry*, **39**, 567–575.

Maitra, B. & Miller, A. (1996) Children, families and therapists: clinical considerations and ethnic minority cultures. In: *Meeting the Needs of Ethnic Minority Children* (eds N. Dhivedi & V. Varma), pp. 111–129. Jessica Kingsley, London.

Malhotra, S., Kohli, A. & Arun, P. (in press) Prevalence of psychiatric disorders in school children in India. *Indian Journal of Medical Research*,

Marks, I. (1992) Innovations in mental health care delivery. *British Journal of Psychiatry*, **160**, 589–597.

Masten, A.S. & Coatsworth, D.J. (1998) The development of competence in favourable and unfavourable environments. *American Psychologist*, **53**, 205–220.

Miller, K.E. (1996) The effects of state terrorism and exile on indigenous Guatemalan refugee children: a mental health assessment and an analysis of children's narratives. *Child Development*, **67**, 89–106.

Minde, K. & Nikapota, A.D. (1993) Child psychiatry and the developing world: recent developments. *Transcultural Psychiatric Research Review*, **30**, 315–346.

Modood, T., Berthoud, R., Lakey, J. *et al.* (1997) *Ethnic Minorities in Britain: Diversity and Disadvantage*. Policy Studies Institute, London.

Murthy, R. (1998) Application of interventions in developing countries. In: *Preventing Mental Illness* (eds R. Jenkins & T. Ustun), pp. 120–126. Wiley, Chichester.

National Research Council (2001) *America Becoming: Racial Trends and Their Consequences* (eds N.J. Smelser, W.J. Wilson & F. Mitchell). Commission on Behavioral and Social Sciences and Education, National Academy Press, Washington D.C.

Nikapota, A.D. (1991) Child psychiatry in developing countries. *British Journal of Psychiatry*, **158**, 743–751.

Nikapota, A., Cox, A.D., Sylva, K. & Rai, D. (1998) *Development of Culturally Appropriate Child Mental Health Services: Perceptions and Use of Services*. Report, Department of Health, London.

O'Shea, B., Hodes, M., Down, G. & Bramley, J. (2000) A school-based mental health service for refugee children. *Clinical Child Psychology and Psychiatry*, **5**, 189–201.

Ovuga, E., Boardman, J. & Oluka, E.G.A. (1999) Traditional healers and mental illness in Uganda. *Psychiatric Bulletin*, **23**, 276–279.

Paardekooper, B., de Jong, J.T.V.M. & Hermanns, J.M.A. (1999) The psychological impact of war and the refugee situation on South Sudanese children in refugee camps in Northern Uganda: an exploratory study. *Journal of Child Psychology and Psychiatry*, **40**, 529–536.

Patel, V., Todd, C. & Winston, M. (1997) Common mental disorders in primary care in Harare, Zimbabwe: associations and risk factors. *British Journal of Psychiatry*, **171**, 60–64.

Rack, P. (1982) *Race, Culture and Mental Disorder*. Tavistock Publications, London.

Rahman, A., Mubbashar, M., Harrington, R. & Gater, R. (2000) Developing child mental health services in developing countries. *Journal of Child Psychology and Psychiatry*, **41**, 539–546.

Renato, D. (2001) Hispanic Psychiatry: From Margin to Mainstream. *Transcultural Psychiatry*, **38**, 1, 5–25.

Richman, N. (1993) Children in situations of political violence [Annotation]. *Journal of Child Psychology and Psychiatry*, **34**, 1286–1302.

Richman, N. (1998) *In the Midst of the Whirlwind*. Trentham Books, Stoke on Trent.

Ridley, C.R., Chit, D.W. & Olivera, R.J. (2000) Training in cultural schema: an antidote to unintentional racism in clinical practice. *American Journal of Orthopsychiatry*, **70**, 65–72.

Roll, S. (1998) Cross-cultural considerations in custody and parenting plans. *Child and Adolescent Psychiatric Clinics of North America*, **7**, 445–454.

Rousseau, C. (1995) The mental health of refugee children. *Transcultural Psychiatric Research Review*, **32**, 299–331.

Rousseau, C., Drapeau, A. & Corin, E. (1996) School problems and emotional problems in refugee children. *American Journal of Orthopsychiatry*, **66**, 239–251.

Rushton, A. & Minnis, H. (1997) Transracial placements. *Journal of Child Psychology and Psychiatry*, **38**, 147–160.

Rutter, J. & Jones, C. (1998) *Refugee Education*. Trentham Books, Stoke on Trent.

Rutter, M. & the E.R.A. Study Team (1998) Developmental catch-up, and deficit, following adoption after severe global early privation. *Journal of Child Psychology and Psychiatry*, **39**, 465–476.

Sack, W.H., Mcsharry, S., Clarke, G.N., Kinney, R., Seeley, J. & Lewinsohn, P. (1994) The Khmer adolescent project. I. Epidemiological findings in two generations of Cambodian refugees. *Journal of Nervous and Mental Disease*, **182**, 387–395.

Sack, W.H., Seeley, J.R. & Clarke, G.N. (1997) Does PTSD transcend cultural barriers? A study from the Khmer adolescent refugee project. *Journal of the American Academy of Child and Adolescent Psychiatry*, **36**, 49–54.

Samerasinghe, D., Nikapota, A. & Rodrigo, K. (1997) Training manual for promoting children's health and well-being. UNICEF, Colombo.

Sleegers, J., Spijker, J., van Limbeek, J. & van Engeland, H. (1998) Mental health problems among homeless adolescents. *Acta Psychiatrica Scandinavica*, **97**, 253–259.

Smith, G.D. (2000) Learning to live with complexity-ethnicity, socioeconomic position and health in Britain and the United States. *American Journal of Public Health*, **90**, 1694–1698.

Sonuga-Barke, E.J., Minocha, K., Taylor, E.A. & Sandberg, S. (1993) Inter-ethnic bias in teachers' ratings of childhood hyperactivity. *British Journal of Developmental Psychology*, **11**, 187–200.

Stern, G., Cottrell, D. & Holmes, J. (1990) Patterns of attendance of child psychiatry out-patients with special reference to Asian families. *British Journal of Psychiatry*, **156**, 384–387.

Tharp, R.G. (1991) Cultural diversity and treatment of children. *Journal of Consulting and Clinical Psychology*, **59**, 799–812.

Thomas, L. (1995) Psychotherapy in the context of race and culture: an inter-cultural therapeutic approach. In: *Mental Health in a Multi-ethnic Society* (ed. S. Fernando), pp. 172–179. Routledge, London.

Tizard, B. (1991) Intercountry adoption: a review of the evidence. *Journal of Child Psychology and Psychiatry*, **32**, 743–756.

Tizard, B. & Phoenix, A. (1995) The identity of mixed parentage adolescents. *Journal of Child Psychology and Psychiatry*, **36**, 1399–1410.

Tousignant, M., Habimana, E., Biron, C., Malo, C., Sidoli-Leblanc, E. & Bendris, N. (1999) The Quebec adolescent refugee project: psychopathology and family variables in a sample from 35 nations. *Journal of the American Academy of Child and Adolescent Psychiatry*, **38**, 1426–1432.

Tseng, W.S. (1999) Culture and psychotherapy: review and practical guidelines. *Transcultural Psychiatry*, **36**, 131–179.

UNHCR (1999) Report on Refugees. UNHCR, Geneva.

UNICEF (1997) *State of the World's Children*. UNICEF, New York.

UNICEF (2000) *State of the World's Children*. UNICEF, New York.

Vuorenkoski, L., Kuure, O., Moilanen, I., Penninkilampi, V. & Myhrman, A. (2000) Bilingualism, school achievement and mental well being: a follow-up study of return migrant children. *Journal of Child Psychology and Psychiatry*, **41**, 261–266.

Waters, M.C. (2000) Immigration, intermarraige, and the challenge of measuring racial/ethnic identities. *American Journal of Public Health*, **90**, 1735–1737.

Williams, C.L. & Westermeyer, J. (1986) *Refugee Mental Health in Resettlement Countries*. Hemisphere, New York.

Wolff, P.H. & Fesseha, G. (1999) The orphans of Eritrea: a five-year follow-up study. *Journal of Child Psychology and Psychiatry*, **40**, 1231–1237.

World Health Organization (1977) *Child Mental Health and Psychosocial Development*. Technical Report Series 613. World Health Organization, Geneva.

World Health Organization (1992) *The ICD-10 Classification of Mental and Behavioural Disorders: Clinical Descriptions and Diagnostic Guidelines*. World Health Organization, Geneva.

World Health Organization (1996) *Diagnostic and Management Guidelines for Mental Disorders in Primary Care: ICD-10*, Chapter V, Primary Care Version. Hogrefe & Huber, Germany.

Wright, J.D., Kaminsky, D. & Wittig, M. (1993) Health and social conditions of street children in the Honduras. *American Journal of Diseases of Children*, **147**, 279–283.

Young, C. (1994) *Ethnic Diversity and Public Policy: an Overview*. Occasional paper No 8. World Summit for Social Development. UN Research Institute for Social Development, Geneva.

Yuen, N.Y.C., Nahulu, L.B., Hishinuma, E.S. & Miyamoto, R.H. (2000) Cultural identification and attempted suicide in native Hawaiian adolescents. *Journal of the American Academy of Child and Adolescent Psychiatry*, **39**, 360–367.

Yule, W. (2000) From pogroms to 'ethnic cleansing': meeting the needs of affected children. *Journal of Child Psychology and Psychiatry*, **41**, 695–702.

Introduction

The maltreatment of children continues to be an abhorrent and pervasive societal problem. In the past two decades, however, there has been a greater awareness among health professionals that physical, psychological and sexual abuse of children does occur and its identification, assessment and management must be handled sensitively and carefully by all involved. There has been much debate about what services can be delivered in order to minimize child abuse and neglect, and most conclude that a multisector interdisciplinary approach is the most effective (Hallett & Birchall 1992; Murphy 1995). This chapter aims to outline various strategies for child protection and their theoretical and evidential basis and to explore the role of community and mental health professionals.

The public health perspective

It has been suggested, both at national and international level, that child abuse and neglect be considered within the broader context of the community and the welfare of children and their families (National Commission of Inquiry in the Prevention of Child Abuse 1996; World Health Organization 1998, 1999; Department of Health 2000a). From a social welfare perspective, the UK Department of Health (2000a) advocated a comprehensive framework to identify children in need of protection. This involves an assessment of children's developmental needs, the capacities of parents or caregivers to respond appropriately to those needs and the impact of wider family and environmental factors on parenting capacity and children. From a health service perspective, the World Health Organization (1998) devised three integrated strategies for child protection in Eastern Europe.

1 *Safe motherhood and perinatal care*: this is designed to promote effective perinatal care through the use of appropriate technology for birth, neonatal care and breastfeeding. The aim is to promote paternal bonding to the child and sensitive parenting through positive birth experiences supported by family members.

2 *Integrated management of childhood illnesses*: designed to provide basic care and promote the prevention of the most common childhood illnesses causing morbidity and mortality in children under 5 years of age. The aim is to reduce child death and disability and limit the stress to parents of caring for a sick child.

3 *Child protection*: this focuses on preventive and protective strategies, with particular attention to the psychosocial determinants of health. Risk factors associated with child abuse and neglect are identified and intervention offered to those families deemed to be 'at risk'. Symptoms and signs of abuse and neglect are monitored and categorized into those requiring immediate protection and referral (red condition), those requiring further investigation and observation with home-based interventions (yellow condition) and those requiring continued availability of health and social care (green condition). The aim is to prevent pathological and coercive patterns of parenting before they become entrenched in the family.

All three components include the improvement of health professional skills (through training and information), health care systems and family and community practices. Thus, child maltreatment has become a public health issue, the prevention of which is the responsibility of all health professionals.

A holistic approach to child protection is compatible with the United Nations Convention on the Rights of the Child, which became international law in 1990 with the UK as a signatory (Save the Children UK 1997). From an international perspective, the World Health Organization has also adopted a worldwide public health strategy to prevent violence and injury and promote the physical and mental health of women and children. Indeed, spouse and child abuse are considered to be intrinsically linked (Jaffe *et al.* 1990; Carroll 1994; Browne & Hamilton 1999). The World Health Organization (1999) has defined and described violence as a 'health burden' to personal health, health systems and government finances.

Financial cost of child abuse and neglect

There are obvious financial costs in the provision of short- and long-term care of victims. However, the World Health Organization (1999) also listed hidden costs such as:
• medical care for victims (including long-term disabilities);
• mental health and substance abuse programmes for victims or offenders;
• criminal justice system expenditure on prosecution and treatment of offenders;
• legal costs for public child care and the rehabilitation of family breakdown;
• social welfare costs for social work provision and the prevention of delinquency;

• costs to the educational system in providing specialist educational provision for children who are developmentally delayed or who underperform at school.

In addition, there are social and economic multiplier effects, e.g. the impact on productivity through lost days at work from family violence and the impact on the quality of life for victims of violence in the family.

The costs of family violence, to both the individual and society, are immense. Over 10 years ago Gelles (1987), reporting figures from a National Crime Survey in the USA, noted that 192 000 incidences of family violence resulted in 21 000 hospitalizations, 99 800 days in hospital, 28 700 emergency department visits and 39 000 physician visits. For the individuals concerned 175 500 days were lost from paid work. For society $44 million were spent in direct medical costs in order to provide the necessary health care to victims of family violence.

Miller et al. (1996) took a broader perspective and were the first systematically to estimate the financial costs to society in the USA of 2 million child abuse and neglect cases. They identified the staggering costs of medical care at $570 million, mental health at $5110 million and public programmes at $3050 million. When other factors, such as loss of school achievement and future earnings, were taken into account, together with the possibility of delinquency and criminal damage, a further cost of $3680 million was added to the bill. This brought the total economic cost to $12 410 million.

Recently in England and Wales, the National Commission into the Prevention of Child Abuse (1996) reported in their publication *Childhood Matters* that the cost of child protection represented £735 million annually. Personal social services were responsible for 71% of expenditure, the Home Office 21%, the health service 6% and the welfare service 2%. It was also estimated that the consequences of maltreatment in childhood were responsible for at least 10% of the expenditure of the mental health services and the correctional prison services as a result of one in five victims becoming offenders (Falshaw et al. 1996). Hence, a further £348 million could be added to the cost of child abuse and neglect in England and Wales. Thus, the argument that more money should be spent on prevention is obvious when the abuse and neglect of children is costing the UK and USA governments over 1 billion pounds per annum. However, few child protection systems employ or resource strategies for prevention.

Child protection systems around the world

There is no consistent approach to child protection at an international level, despite the UN Convention on the Rights of the Child (United Nations 1990). International comparisons of child protection systems have many problems because of a lack of agreed definitions on what constitutes child abuse and neglect. Nevertheless, the International Society for the Prevention of Child Abuse and Neglect carries out regular surveys of volunteer informants from countries around the globe. The latest survey was prepared by the Kempe Children's Center, at the University of Colorado School of Medicine (Bross et al. 2000) and involved 58 countries representing 31% of the world's population (excluding China). The percentage of countries represented from each region was as follows: Africa 20.3%, Asia 22.9%, South America and the Caribbean 61.1%, Europe 75.6%, Australasia and Oceania 76%, and North America 100%.

In 26 countries, incidence studies and annual statistics are available from a register of cases, although these registers are not strictly comparable because of the different definitions and methodologies used. Thirty-two countries are reported to have an official government policy with regard to child protection, although less (27) had case management systems that could track cases. In 56.4% of the total sample, a mandatory system of reporting cases of child abuse and neglect was a part of the country's legislation. In the remaining countries (including those in the UK) a voluntary system of reporting existed (the influence of mandatory reporting is discussed in Emery & Laumann Billings, Chapter 20).

The responses to child abuse, where appropriate, are reported to involve criminal investigations in 89.7% of countries, treatment for the child in 70.7% of the countries, removing the child during the investigation in 69% of countries and treatment for the offender in 50% of the countries. The survey concluded that punitive responses to child abuse and neglect were more common than therapeutic approaches.

International surveys offer a broad picture of child protection awareness but provide little scientific evidence for effective child protection services. Those countries that have a legal mandate to report child abuse and neglect may not necessarily implement and act upon the law. The threshold for intervention will differ dramatically from country to country, depending on definition and operational criteria. The prevention services offered to children and families are often not universal, but depend on available resources from region to region. Finally, the treatment of sex offenders and violent offenders may be little more than mental health provision.

It is beyond the scope of the chapter to compare the variations in child protection systems. Those that are well developed, in North America, Western Europe, Australia and New Zealand, are based on similar principles, such as a multidisciplinary approach. These systems are beginning to influence other parts of the world by the development of UN sponsored guidelines (World Health Organization 1999). These guidelines identified the following principles of good practice.

• Clear policies, protocol and programmes.
• Data collection monitoring and evaluation.
• Co-ordinated and comprehensive services for victims and offenders.
• Training and provision of a child-friendly approach.
• Prevention strategies with families, parents and caregivers (e.g. home visiting).
• Community-based intervention and support.

- Interdisciplinary and multisector approaches involving policymakers.
- International collaboration and partnership.

The child protection system in England and Wales, which has been developed over the past 25 years, will be given as an example of good practice.

Child protection system in England and Wales

As with most countries, the development of a child protection system begins with legal reform. The introduction of the Children Act (Department of Health 1989) was a milestone in this process. It brought together a number of separate pieces of legislation to develop policy, practices and procedures that are in the best interests of the child (a person under 18 years of age). The Act was designed to clarify the legal situation for children within England and Wales and find a balance between the protection of children and recognizing the rights of parents and families. Nevertheless, the child's welfare is given paramount consideration (Section 1.1). A similar approach has been taken to legal reform in other parts of the world (e.g. Australia, New Zealand, Ireland, Hungary).

The Children Act (1989) sets out the statutory responsibilities of local authorities for investigations and the provision of child care (Herbert 1993). It is their primary duty to safeguard and promote the welfare of children who are 'in need' and to promote the upbringing of such children by their families. They provide a range of services appropriate to the level of need identified for the child and the family (Section 17.1). The services are offered by a number of different agencies and cover a wide range of difficulties and family support (e.g. maltreated children, disabled children, learning difficulties, parenting skills, family crises).

The criteria 'in need' is applied to children who are likely to suffer 'significant harm' through maltreatment, impairment of health and/or impairment of development, and relates to child protection work under Section 47. The emphasis in child protection is for multiagency work. Any person who has knowledge or suspicion of a child suffering some form of significant harm refers their concerns to the police or social services.

Although there is no legal mandate to report British cases of child abuse and neglect to the police and social services, there is a clear expectation that doctors 'must refer these concerns to the statutory agencies' (Department of Health 1994, p. 5). Indeed, it could be argued that withholding information about ongoing child maltreatment, even on the basis of patient confidentiality, is professional malpractice. The National Health Service Executive have stated that 'all health service staff have a duty to protect children'(Department of Health 1996, p. 15).

Referrals may come from any person involved with the child (e.g. doctors, health visitors, teachers, nursery workers, neighbours, babysitters), an agency involved with the family (e.g. community health, probation, housing) or even the child in question. Therefore, either the police or social services may be the first statutory agency to receive the referral but information is then shared between them. The division of responsibility is that social services are ultimately responsible for child care decisions while the police are responsible for criminal issues and proceedings.

Recent government proposals for interagency co-operation (Department of Health 1999, 2000b) will place child protection work within the context of wider health, welfare and social services for children in need, but continue to recognize the central role of police officers and social workers in protecting children from maltreatment.

It is the statutory duty of social services departments and police forces within each local authority jointly to investigate allegations of child maltreatment or where 'there is reasonable cause to suspect that a child is suffering, or likely to suffer, significant harm'. In consultation with other agencies, a case conference may be called under the framework published in *Working Together Under the Children Act 1989* (Home Office *et al.* 1991). The provisions of the Children Act (1989, Section 44) allow members of the police, health and social services to remove a child to a place of safety for their protection and wellbeing, after applying to court for an Emergency Protection Order.

Under the auspices of area child protection committees, who lay down multidisciplinary procedures at a local level, child protection case conferences are held; these conferences aim to make informed decisions about what action is needed to safeguard the child in question and to promote his or her welfare. Those representatives attending the case conference, which may be social workers, health professionals, teachers, police officers, local authority lawyers, parents and substitute carers, formulate proposals for a care plan and whether the child should be placed on the Child Protection Register. In doing so they may ask a court to issue a Child Assessment Order or an Exclusion Order (for the alleged offender).

It has been estimated that 1.45% of the 11 million children in England are subject to a child protection (Section 47) inquiry each year. Of these 160 000 referrals, 75% receive a family visit during a joint investigation and 1% experience an emergency separation. One-quarter of the children referred are the subject of a Case Conference, 15% are placed on the Child Protection Register and 2% are taken into public care (Department of Health 1995a, p. 56).

Categories of registration in England and Wales

The definitions of child maltreatment recommended as criteria for the purposes of registration on Child Protection Registers throughout England and Wales (Home Office 1991, pp. 48–49) classify cases into one of four separate categories, based on the most recent incident.

1 *Neglect*: the persistent or severe neglect of a child, or the failure to protect a child from exposure to any kind of danger. This includes cold and starvation or extreme failure to carry out important aspects of care that results in the significant impairment of the child's health or development, including non-organic failure to thrive.

2 *Physical injury*: actual or likely physical injury to a child, or failure to prevent physical injury (or suffering) to a child, including deliberate poisoning, suffocation and Münchausen by proxy syndrome.

3 *Sexual abuse*: actual or likely sexual exploitation of a child or adolescent. The child may be dependent and/or developmentally immature.

4 *Emotional abuse*: actual or likely severe adverse effect on the emotional and behavioural development of a child caused by persistent or severe emotional maltreatment or rejection. All abuse involves some emotional maltreatment. This category is used where it is the main or sole form of abuse.

All the above categories are used for both intrafamilial and extrafamilial maltreatment perpetrated by someone inside or outside the child's home or extended family. Mixed categories are also recorded, which register more than one type of abuse and/or neglect occurring to a child. The new guidance *Working Together to Safeguard Children* (Department of Health 1999) retains the above categorical system with the minor exception of the term 'physical injury' which has become 'physical abuse' (Department of Health 2000b).

Severity

Definitions related to the severity of maltreatment are still rare (see Table 70.1), as are those which attempt to take into account the sequential pattern of maltreatment. The severity of maltreatment, the duration, and whether inside or outside the family, will all greatly affect the traumatic consequences for the victim (Briere 1992; Davenport *et al.* 1994). For example, there are likely to be different dynamics and consequences for a child involved in 'repeat' maltreatment by the same perpetrator, compared to 're-abuse' by another perpetrator (Hamilton & Browne 1998). There may be different responses and interventions required, dependent on the child's adverse experiences and patterns of victimization (Finkelhor 1995).

Children on the Child Protection Register in England

Since 1989, the Department of Health has accurately assessed each year the number of children and young persons on the Child Protection Register in England. The estimates are based on annual statistical returns from 150 local government authorities. The overall rate was 27 children per 10 000 under 18 years of age. The highest rates were found in very young children under 1 year (71 per 10 000). The likelihood of being on the registers then decreases with age. Therefore, 70% of children on registers are aged under 10 years. Boys and girls were equally represented in all age groups. However, girls account for 60% of those registered for 'sexual abuse'.

Local authorities in England record each child on their protection register in only one of the eight categories presented in

Table 70.3, choosing the one that provides the most accurate picture of the situation.

Overall, 14 600 girls and 15 400 boys in England were considered to require protection from maltreatment on 31 March 2000 together with 300 unborn children, and nearly one in four (23%) of them were 'looked after' by local authorities (in care). Of the 7100 children in care on 31 March 2000, 70% were placed with foster parents, 7% were living in children's homes, 18% were placed with parents and 5% in other types of placement (Department of Health 2000b).

Similar registration rates for child abuse and neglect (30 in 10 000) children were reported previously by the NSPCC (Creighton & Noyes 1989; Creighton 1992). Furthermore, the NSPCC claim that their figures for reported physical and sexual abuse were not increasing (Creighton 1992). By contrast, the Department of Health claim a slight decrease in the number of registrations over the past 10 years (Department of Health 2000b).

During the year 1999–2000, 14% of registrations involved children who had been previously registered and perhaps taken off the register prematurely. This figure was less than in previous years where one in five children placed on the Child Protection Register had been previously registered at some time.

Importance of early intervention

It is evident that over two-thirds (69%) of children on the Child Protection Register are under the age of 10 and over one-third (39%) are under 5 years of age (Department of Health 2000b). Hence, the majority of abused children cannot be expected to be proactive in preventing their own abuse. While helplines are excellent for teenagers, they do not prevent the maltreatment of younger children (Browne & Griffiths 1988). Furthermore, many children will be abused before they have the opportunity of being exposed to school-based prevention programmes. Therefore, health professionals involved with families from the time of birth must be proactive rather than reactive in the protection of children. This is especially important for newborns, as children under 1 year have the highest rate of registration (71 in 10 000).

The most telling indicator that there is a need for early intervention is the level of fatal abuse and serious injury in the UK to children under 5 years of age. Home Office figures (Central Statistical Office 1994, p. 47) show that at least two children a week die as a result of non-accidental injury and a further two children per week become disabled for life as a result of the injuries they have suffered (Browne & Lynch 1994). Four out of five of these children are fatally assaulted by parents or step-parents (Browne & Lynch 1995; Wilczynski 1997) and two-thirds are already known to child protection agencies for previous physical injury or non-organic failure to thrive (Greenland 1986, 1987). Despite this knowledge, universal health visits to the homes of families with young children in England have been drastically reduced (Health Visitors' Association 1994; Leahy-Warren 1998).

Table 70.1 Severity of child maltreatment. (Adapted from Browne & Herbert 1997.)

Less severe

Minor incidents of an occasional nature with little or no long-term damage—either physical, sexual or psychological

Physical	Injuries confined in area and limited to superficial tissues, including cases of light scratch marks, small slight bruising, minute burns and small welts
Sexual	Inappropriate sexual touching, invitations and/or exhibitionism, sexualized behaviour in the child
Emotional	Occasional verbal assaults, denigration, humiliation, scapegoating, confusing atmosphere
Neglect	Occasional withholding of love and affection. Child weight paralleled to or slightly below third centile with no organic cause. Developmental delay. Unwashed skin and hair

Moderately severe

More frequent incidents and/or of a more serious nature, but unlikely to be life-threatening or have such potentially long-term effects

Physical	Surface injuries of an extensive or more serious nature and small subcutaneous injuries, including cases of extensive bruising, large welts, lacerations, small haematomas and minor burns/scalds
Sexual	Non-penetrative sexual interaction of an indecent or inappropriate nature, such as fondling, masturbation and digital penetration, sexualized behaviour in the child
Emotional	Frequent verbal assaults, denigration and humiliation, occasional rejection. Child occasionally witnesses family violence and intoxicated parent(s)
Neglect	Frequent withholding of love and affection, child non-organic failure to gain weight. Poor hygiene and cleanliness. Parent(s) occasionally depressed or mentally ill

Very severe

On-going or very frequent maltreatment and/or less frequent incidents with potentially very severe physical or psychological harm. Delay in seeking help and/or incongruent story for injuries to child

Physical	All large and deep tissue injuries and broken bones including fractures, dislocations, subdural haematomas, serious burns and damage to internal organs
Sexual	Sexual interaction involving attempted or actual oral, anal and/or vaginal penetration
	Symptoms include repeated urinary infections, vaginal discharge (STD), vaginal/anal bleeding and injury
Emotional	Frequent rejection, occasional withholding of food and drink, enforced isolation and restriction of movement. Child frequently witnesses family violence and intoxicated parent(s)
Neglect	Frequent unavailability of parent, guardian or spouse. Child sometimes left alone, non-organic failure to thrive, severe nappy rash with skin lesions. Parent(s) frequently depressed or mentally ill

Life-threatening

Long-term or severe psychological and physical harm that results in life-threatening situations (including perpetrators failing to seek help for injuries to child or child self-harming)

Physical	Deliberate or persistent injuries which have the potential of child's death or near death (e.g. poisoning or choking)
Sexual	Incest, coerced or forced penetration over a prolonged period. Underage pregnancy
Emotional	Persistent rejection, failure to nurture, frequent withholding of food and drink, enforced isolation and restriction of movement. Terrorizing and confining the child. Child witnesses psychotic episodes in parent(s)
Neglect	Persistent unavailability of parent, guardian or spouse. Child often left alone, non-organic failure to maintain weight Frequent illness and infection because of poor hygiene

---

Levels of prevention

The prevention of child maltreatment is traditionally classified into three levels.

1 *Primary prevention*: involves 'universal services' for the whole population.

2 *Secondary prevention*: involves 'targeted services' by identifying high-risk populations and offering intervention before abuse and neglect occur.

3 *Tertiary prevention*: involves 'specialist services' for treatment of families and institutions where parents and caregivers are already abusing and/or neglecting their children. At this level, intervention is offered only after abuse and/or neglect has occurred.

Examples of strategies for prevention at each of the above levels are listed in Table 70.2. However, the primary care of children and their families is limited usually by allocated resources to the health sector. Most countries offer child protection services only to those families most at risk of maltreating their children (Bross *et al.* 2000).

Primary prevention

Primary prevention techniques attempt a fundamental change across society (see MacMillan *et al.* 1994a,b), e.g. public awareness campaigns that challenge misconceptions and aim to increase people's understanding of the extent and nature of

Table 70.2 Strategies for prevention (Adapted from World Health Organization 1999).

Primary
Prenatal, perinatal and early childhood health care that improves
    pregnancy outcomes and strengthens early attachment
Promoting good parenting practices
Family support such as home visiting
Public awareness activities (through media and campaigns)
Community education programmes
Availability of social supports and community networks
School-based activities towards non-violence

Secondary
Perinatal and ongoing identification of high risk children and families
Clearly established referral system of social and health services
Substance abuse treatment programmes
Community-based family-centred support, assistance and networks
Information available about community resources and safety planning
Schools-based social services for high stress environments

Tertiary
Early diagnosis and identification
Interdisciplinary services to ensure medical treatment, care, coun-
    selling, management and support of victims/families
Reintegration in a child-friendly community/schools
Adequate child protection laws and child-friendly courts

physical and sexual violence against women and girls. Such approaches to primary prevention are far from easy. The campaigners have to balance the need for a clear message against oversimplifying the problem. For example, the claim that one in every two children will be sexually assaulted by the time they reach adulthood is based on a broad definition of maltreatment, which includes non-contact sexual abuse. Thus, individuals who think in terms of contact sexual abuse will regard the message as exaggerated. In addition, for messages to appear clear they need to be very specific. Hence, some campaigns do not consider the sexual abuse of young boys who are often equally at risk.

An equally controversial approach to the primary prevention of sexual abuse promotes changing the behaviour of the victim, through school education programmes for children (MacMillan *et al.* 1994b). Nevertheless, a New Zealand programme (Briggs & Hawkins 1994) was found to be effective because of teacher commitment, parental support and age-appropriate material. One important ingredient of the programme was the development of children's self-esteem. Research has shown that sex offenders target children with a low sense of self-worth who appear vulnerable and unsure of themselves, with a need to be cared for (Elliott *et al.* 1995). Thus, assertion training needs to go hand in hand with the development of self-esteem.

A more traditional approach in the UK is the use of community nurses to universally help parents with children under 5 years old, as part of the primary health care system (MacMillan *et al.* 1994a). Indeed, there is a need for health visitors to discourage parents from physically punishing their children. In fact, one

in five parents (*n* = 457) admit to severe physical assaults on their children; 16% of mothers and 21% of fathers (Nobes *et al.* 1999). This is not surprising when the UK government condones the use of physical punishment by caregivers to control children (see the parliamentary report *Protecting Children, Supporting Parents: A Consultation Document on the Physical Punishment of Children*, House of Commons 2000). However, the use of cognitive-behavioural techniques by community nurses to promote positive parenting skills and self-esteem in all parents and children is considered financially unrealistic, because of the need for training and small caseloads (Browne 1989; 1995b).

Evaluation of community-based approaches

Olds *et al.* (1993) showed that the cost of providing home visiting per family was $US1582 and this intervention by a nurse saved $US1762 in the first 2 years of the child's life. Hence, there was an overall net saving (dividend) of $US180 per family (in the 1980s). There was a 56% saving in family aid, 26% in food stamps, 11% in medical aid and a 3% decrease in child protection cases. There was also a 5% increase in income tax received from an increase in maternal part-time employment as a result of the professional advice given.

Home visitation approaches with mothers under 21 years of age, single parents and mothers with serious financial problems have been evaluated in the long term by Kitzman *et al.* (1997). They showed that home visits had positive benefits for the mothers as well as the children and that these benefits lasted for up to 15 years after birth of the first child. Olds *et al.* (1997) compared low-income mothers visited by nurses in the home with low-income mothers with no formal home visits. They demonstrated the following significant differences, 15 years later, for those who had been visited and offered advice and support:

- less child abuse and neglect;
- less births after the first child for unmarried women;
- less family aid received;
- fewer problems with alcohol and drugs; and
- fewer arrests by police.

Therefore, it may be argued that one way to prevent, or at least ameliorate, the above social problems is by maintaining well-resourced community-based health care services for families and children, especially those who are on low incomes (e.g. single mothers and teenage parents). In Queensland, Sanders *et al.* (in press) developed the Triple P-Positive Parenting Program, which is a multilevel family support strategy for the prevention and treatment of behaviour and emotional problems in children (e.g. eating and sleeping problems) that create parental stress and frustration. Similar approaches have been adopted in the UK (Herbert 1988) which have since been used for the prevention of family violence (Browne & Herbert 1997).

Parent-held records

Children who have experienced family violence, breakdown and/or separation are more likely to develop emotional problems and therefore could be considered to be a high-risk group, in priority for services. Therefore, managers of community health could adopt a secondary or tertiary prevention approach using information from parent-held records.

It is difficult to introduce the concept of child protection in parent-held records because of the sensitive nature of the topic (Armstrong-Esther *et al.* 1987). However, parent-held records are a potential source of information both from and for parents. Parent-held records are issued to every parent upon the birth of their child and are used to record all information about the child's physical growth, health, development, immunizations and consultations with health professionals. They also include advice and information on topics such as feeding, growth, development, general child care and sources of medical help and family support. This information could be expanded to cover the social and psychological growth, health and development of the child. Currently, this is a serious omission from parent-held records.

Secondary prevention

Secondary prevention involves professionals screening families and providing interventions aimed at giving special attention to high-risk groups before child maltreatment occurs within or outside the family. As with other problems in child health and development, the risk approach to child protection can be seen as a tool for the flexible and rational distribution of scarce resources and their maximal utilization. Therefore, community nurses now prioritize and 'target' their home visits to families on the basis of an assessment of need (Browne & Lynch 1998). They are often instructed to screen routinely for predictive characteristics in all families who come in contact with the service they are providing: counselling, home visits and clinic, health centre or hospital care.

Health and social services using this approach require the ability to identify parents and children in need of help from those characteristics (risk factors) of the child, parents, family and social environment that are associated with an increased risk of undesirable outcomes. The process requires resources from each local community to:

- develop methods for detecting risk factors;
- train health care and social workers in these methods; and
- provide intervention strategies to prevent or ameliorate undesired outcomes.

The surveillance and monitoring of child health, growth and development is regarded as good practice throughout the world (Hall 1995; World Health Organiztion 1999). However, there is a paucity of research into the specific components and methods used in various screening and assessment programmes for child maltreatment.

Predicting child maltreatment in the population

A number of articles have been written on the prediction of child abuse (Lynch & Roberts 1977; Altemeier *et al.* 1979, 1984; Starr 1982; Leventhal 1988; Ammerman & Hersen 1990; Adler *et al.* 1991; Ammerman 1993; Agathanos-Georgopoulou & Browne 1997), many of which have presented a list of characteristics common to abusing parents and to abused children (Browne & Saqi 1988a).

The Child Abuse Potential (CAP) inventory, developed in the USA, has taken a multifaceted approach (Milner 1986). Indeed, the CAP inventory is one of the few self-report questionnaires (160 item) that has been evaluated in terms of its reliability (internal consistency and temporal stability) and construct validity. However, the relevance of checklists and inventories for the prediction of child sexual abuse remains questionable, especially when the epidemiological differences between sexual and physical abuse are considered (Jason *et al.* 1982; Browne 1994). Nevertheless, certain risk factors are the same, such as poor relationship with parents, stepparenting, marital conflict, alcohol and drug abuse (Finkelhor 1980).

Community nurses have been significantly influenced in their work by such inventories, using the characteristics as 'early warning signs'. However, reviews of the relative value of these characteristics for the practical and routine monitoring of families have emphasized a need for caution (Barker 1990; Howitt 1992). The danger of predictive claims was demonstrated by Browne & Saqi (1988a), who retrospectively evaluated a typical checklist completed by community nurses around the time of birth. The checklist was developed from a number of demographic and epidemiological studies carried out in the UK, with special reference to non-accidental injury to children in Surrey, England.

In a prospective evaluation (Browne 1995a, 1995b), community nurses completed the 12-item checklist on all children born in 1985 and 1986 in three health districts of Surrey, England. In total, 14 252 births were screened for the potential of child abuse and neglect and 7% (964) were identified as 'high risk'. This population cohort was then followed up for 5 years and in 1991, 106 families had attended a case conference for suspected or actual maltreatment of their newborn child. Table 70.4 presents the percentage of abusing and non-abusing families that possessed the checklist characteristics (risk factors), in order of relative importance for prediction. In addition, it shows the percentage of families with a particular characteristic that go on to abuse and/or neglect their newborn in the first 5 years of life (conditional probability).

It was found that fully completed checklists, with the relative weighting for each factor taken into account, could correctly classify 86% of cases. The screening procedure was sensitive to 68% of abusing families and correctly specified 94% of the non-abusing families. Surprisingly, nearly one-third of the abusing families had few risk-factor characteristics of any weight and were incorrectly identified as 'low risk' around the time of birth. The most worrying aspect of the checklist is that 6% of the non-abusing families were incorrectly identified as high risk for potential child abuse because they were found to have a number of heavy-weighted risk factors.

Table 70.3 Percentages and rates of registrations by categories of child abuse by which they were recorded during the year ending 31 March 2000 (n = 29 300). (Adapted from Department of Health 2000b.)

Category of abuse	Number of children	Percentage	Rate per 10 000
Neglect, physical injury and sexual abuse	300	1	<1
Neglect and physical injury	1 900	6	2
Neglect and sexual abuse	600	2	1
Physical injury and sexual abuse	600	2	1
Neglect (alone)	10 100	35	9
Physical injury (alone)	6 700	23	6
Sexual abuse (alone)	3 600	12	3
Emotional abuse (alone)	4 800	17	4
Unknown*	700	2	1
Total	*29 300*	*100*	*26*

*Refers to categories used but not recommended by Department of Health (1991) or no category available.

Table 70.4 Relative importance of screening characteristics for child abuse as determined by discriminant function analysis (from Browne & Herbert 1997; p. 120).

Checklist characteristics n = Parents with a child under 5 (baseline)	Abusing families (%) (n = 106)	Non-abusing families (%) (n = 14 146)	Conditional probability(%)* 0.7
1 History of family violence	30.2	1.6	12.4
2 Parent indifferent, intolerant or overanxious towards child	31.1	3.1	7.0
3 Single or separated parent	48.1	6.9	5.0
4 Socioeconomic problems, such as unemployment	70.8	12.9	3.9
5 History of mental illness, drug or alcohol addiction	34.9	4.8	5.2
6 Parent abused or neglected as a child	19.8	1.8	7.6
7 Infant premature, low birth weight	21.7	6.9	2.3
8 Infant separated from mother for more than 24 h post-delivery	12.3	3.2	2.8
9 Mother <21 years old at time of birth	29.2	7.7	2.8
10 Step-parent or cohabitee present	27.4	6.2	3.2
11 Less than 18 months between birth of children	16.0	7.5	1.6
12 Infant mentally or physically handicapped	2.8	1.1	1.9

*Conditional probability refers to the percentage of families with a particular characteristic that go on to abuse and/or neglect their newborn in the first 5 years of life.

The relatively low prevalence of child maltreatment combined with even the most optimistic estimates of screening effectiveness implies that a screening programme would yield large numbers of false-positives (Daniel *et al.* 1978; Dalgliesh, 1998). The checklist detection rate would mean that for every 14 252 births screened it would be necessary to distinguish between 72 true risk cases and 892 false-positives in the 7% of cases (964) identified as high risk. This would indicate the requirement of a second screening procedure to be carried out with the high-risk families perhaps based on the significant differences found between abusing and non-abusing parent–child relationships (Browne & Saqi 1987, 1988b; see also Verhulst & van der Ende, Chapter 5). Thus, a second screening could possibly distinguish the true potential maltreatment cases from the false-positives by the use of behavioural indicators. A more difficult problem

would be to distinguish the 34 missed cases of potential child abuse from the 13 254 correctly identified non-abusers, as they would be mixed up in a population of 13 288 low-risk families.

Leventhal (1988) provided evidence from longitudinal cohort studies that suggested that prediction is feasible. However, he concluded that improvements in the assessment of high-risk families are necessary, including the further development and use of a standardized clinical assessment of the parent–child relationship.

Parent–child relationships in high-risk families

The aetiology of child abuse and neglect is complex. It is now generally acknowledged that the causes of child maltreatment are multifactorial (Belsky 1988; Ammerman & Hersen 1990, 1992; Browne & Herbert 1997), involving characteristics of the parent and child, the social system of the family and demographic and cultural situation of the community. Given a particular combination of these factors, an interactional style develops within the family and it is in the context of this interaction that maltreatment occurs.

Browne & Herbert (1997) proposed that the chance of risk factors resulting in child maltreatment and other forms of family violence are mediated by and depend on the interactive relationships within the family. A secure relationship between the parent and child will 'buffer' any effects of stress, facilitating coping strategies by the parent. In contrast, insecure or anxious relationships will not 'buffer' the parent under stress and any overload, such as an argument or a child misbehaving, may result in a physical or emotional attack.

The detection of early signs indicating a malfunction in the caregiver–infant relationship has been considered by Crittenden (1985; 1988) who discussed the role of the parents' thought processes in the distortion of interactive patterns in maltreating families. She discovered that two pattern, (i) co-operation/interference and (ii) involved/withdrawn, significantly discriminate abusing and non-abusing families. Furthermore, Stratton & Swaffer (1988, p. 201) also stated 'there are good theoretical grounds for supposing that the beliefs that abusive parents hold about their children are an important factor in determining whether, and in what ways, a child will be abused'. The results of their work show that abusing mothers attribute more control and more internal causes to their children and less to themselves in comparison with a non-abusing group of mothers of handicapped children. They went on to suggest that causal attributions held by abusive parents, both in general and with respect to their children, should be a powerful indicator of the chances of child maltreatment. The implications of this research work for intervention with maltreating families is discussed by Crittenden (1996).

Evaluating parent–child relationships

It is unlikely that health professionals who visit the family will directly witness physical assaults on children. However, pathological aspects of the parent–child relationship may be evident through observable attitudes, behaviours and interactions between the parent and the child. Indeed, Browne (1995a) and Browne & Herbert (1997) identified and reviewed five important aspects to the assessment of high-risk parent–child relationships.

1 *Parents' knowledge and attitudes to child-rearing*: those who maltreat their children often have unrealistic and distorted expectations about their child's ability and the way he or she should behave.

2 *Parents' perceptions of their child's behaviour*: those who maltreat their children have more negative thoughts about the behaviour of the child and perceive their children to be more irritable and demanding than other children. They may attribute a 'bad' disposition to the child and interpret certain age-appropriate behaviours as deliberate or intentional non-compliance.

3 *Parents' emotions and responses to stress*: those who maltreat their children are significantly more harsh in their disciplinary methods, which are applied in an inconsistent way compared to non-maltreating parents. They are more impulsive and less appropriate in the way they manage their child and the stress arising from ineffectual attempts to control their child's behaviour may often escalate into violence.

4 *Quality of parent–child interaction and behaviour*: those who maltreat their children are often described as being more aversive, negative and controlling in comparison to non-maltreating parents. They are less sensitive and responsive to their children, which results in less frequent positive interactions.

5 *Quality of child to parent attachment*: those children who are maltreated are significantly more likely to develop insecure/anxious attachments to their parent(s) as a result of the insensitive care taking they receive. Those who are rejected will often form an avoidant attachment pattern and those who receive inconsistent parenting will often form an ambivalent attachment pattern to their parent(s) (see review of 13 studies by Morton & Browne 1998).

Ethics of screening and evaluation

There are ethical issues raised by any process of assessment, especially where the intention is to screen for indicators of children 'in need', and account must be taken of parents' understanding of the function of such assessments. Nevertheless, all practices and procedures concerning child protection are based on the principle that the interests of the child are always paramount (Department of Health 1998, 1999).

Screening and assessment programmes have to be sensitive to needs of parents as well as children. Parents expect to be consulted about and participate in decisions that involve their children (Hall 1995). Indeed, the Department of Health (1995b) has issued guidelines about the essential principles for working in partnership with parents on child protection issues. It is suggested that 'working in partnership' will promote effective work with families by maintaining citizen's rights and empowering parents. It is hoped that parents will participate by providing information and becoming involved in decisions about the care and development of their children.

It needs to be made clear to the parents that a high number of risk factors for adverse outcome identifies them as a 'family in priority' for support and services. Negative labels such as 'high-risk family' should never be used. The parent/health professional joint evaluation of a child's need for protection therefore requires a personal (home visit) approach with parents, involving experienced health visitors, who are in regular contact with families and where there is no stigma attached to the home visit.

Tertiary prevention

Tertiary prevention or treatment involves professionals offering

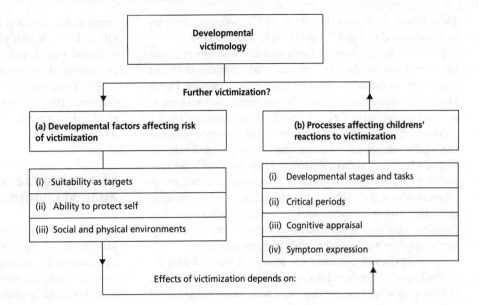

Fig. 70.1 Developmental Perspective of the victimization of children (from Browne & Hamilton 1997).

intervention only after the maltreatment has occurred. This has some limitations when recurrent and fatal abuse and neglect are considered. Physical re-abuse occurs in at least half of all cases referred for intervention (Magura 1981; Depanfilis & Zuravin 1998), and sexual abuse will recur in the majority of cases where the offender remains in the family (Bentovim 1991; Fisher & Beech 1998). There is also some evidence that services available are insufficient to provide appropriate support and therapy to abused children and their families (Browne & Falshaw 1998). In a study of 202 sexually abused children in London (Prior *et al.* 1994), 37% received no therapy; yet all these children had described contact abuse and there was a professional consensus that the abuse had occurred. It could be argued that this approach offers too little, too late.

Limitations of tertiary prevention

Finkelhor (1995) identified those factors that are likely to influence the possibility of victimization and its effects on the potential for further victimization of the individual (see Fig. 70.1). Factors associated with the initial incident of abuse and victimization (Fig. 70.1, left stem) will in turn affect the child's vulnerability to further abuse. This vulnerability will be modified to a greater or lesser degree by individual factors such as the child's reaction to a previous abusive incident. These factors can be developmental (e.g. the time of attachment formation to a primary caregiver) and cognitive (e.g. appraisal of the abusive incident). Together, developmental and cognitive factors determine the behavioural symptoms present in the child (e.g. lack of self-confidence), which may act as a signal to potential abusers that the child is an easy target. Such processes may influence the way a victim behaves which may result in increased vulnerability. For example, many children who have been sexually abused go on to develop age-inappropriate sexualized behaviour and acting out which may attract the attention of a potential abuser. The abuser

may then use the child's behaviour to justify his or her own actions and make the child feel responsible for their own further victimization. Previous literature has suggested that sexual victimization in childhood increases the risk of further sexual abuse in adulthood (Fromuth 1986; Russell 1986; Gidycz *et al.* 1993; Mayall & Gold 1995).

Browne & Hamilton (1997; 1998) claimed that, for many children, victimization occurs on more than one occasion, with the same perpetrator (repeat abuse) or different perpetrators (re-abuse). It is generally considered that repeat or re-victimization will lead to more severe trauma. Hence, memory for victimizing events may be lost from conscious memory, while those children who experience a single event may be less traumatized and details of the incident will be remembered (Terr 1991; Whitfield 1995).

Recurrent abuse of children

It is generally acknowledged that maltreatment of children frequently consists of more than one incident. In a review of 45 studies, Depanfilis & Zuravin (1998) reported repeat victimization rates of up to 50% in families followed up over a 5-year period and up to 85% for families followed for up to 10 years. This confirms other USA research, e.g. Finkelhor *et al.* (1986) who found that 40% of female sexual abuse consisted of more than one incident, with an average length of time between victimizations of 31 weeks.

In England, Hamilton & Browne (1999) studied 400 children referred to 10 child protection units in one police service area. Within the 27-month follow-up period, one in four children (*n* = 54) were subject to at least one re-referral. Once maltreated, it was found that children were more likely to be maltreated again. The majority of re-referrals (61%) occurred within 330 days of the index referral, with the greatest risk being the first 30 days.

These figures are remarkably similar to US studies of recurrent maltreatment (Fryer & Miyoshi 1994; Fluke *et al.* 1999).

Police service response in England was not significantly related to the rate or type of re-referral. A large number (64%) of index referrals led to 'no further action' police responses. This is likely to reflect the factors influencing decisions to bring charges, such as the interests of the child, insufficient evidence and the decision of the Crown Prosecution Service. In the minority of cases (13%), the referral did result in a 'caution' or 'charge' for the offender which may act as a deterrent. However, the victim may still be vulnerable to abuse by other perpetrators. Indeed, it was found that once a child has been referred on at least two occasions, their risk of re-referral over the next 27 months more than doubled. This may reflect increased vulnerability or, alternatively, vigorous monitoring by child protection agencies.

Social services involvement was also not associated with re-referral status. Therefore, the findings of Hamilton & Browne's (1999) study would suggest that the actions taken during a child protection joint investigation are not effective in preventing the recurrent maltreatment for at least one-quarter of those children referred.

The above findings provide more general evidence to alarming reports from English studies specific to the sexual abuse of children. Prior *et al.* (1997) found that only 35% of sex offenders were charged, 5% cautioned and 56% of cases resulted in no further action. Furthermore, self-reports from convicted male child sex offenders, on average, claim 6 years of undetected offending prior to their first arrest (Elliott *et al.* 1995).

Risk factors for recurrent maltreatment

Risk factors that indicate a high probability of recurrence of all forms of abuse and neglect fall into two main categories, according to recent research in the USA (Depanfilis & Zuravin 1999) and UK (Hamilton & Browne 1999).

• *Child vulnerability*: behavioural problems/conduct disorder, learning difficulties, medical problems (e.g. failure to thrive), previous referral for self or sibling.
• *Family stress*: partner abuse, drug or alcohol abuse, adult psychiatric problems, adult learning difficulties, adult criminal convictions, social support deficits.

Not surprisingly, all these risk factors are associated with fatal child abuse and neglect to children less than 5 years of age, especially when the caregivers are young and inexperienced (Greenland 1986, 1987; Strang 1992; Browne & Lynch 1995; Wilczynski 1997). Indeed, Greenland's (1986, 1987) Canadian studies in Ontario provide evidence highlighting the limitations of tertiary prevention. He found that one in five severely physically abused children had been previously assaulted prior to their hospitalization for the most recent injury. Between 10 and 16% (depending on the study reported) had brothers and sisters who had also been assaulted previously or who had died as a result of abuse and neglect.

The above evidence demonstrates the need to develop more effective strategies to prevent and detect the victimization and repeat victimization of children. The Sex Offender Act (Home Office 1997), which concentrates on convicted perpetrators of sexual assault, will only help identify and monitor a small proportion of the individuals who commit such crimes (Wyre 1997). A comparable Violent Offender Act is yet to come into existence. Hence, there is a urgent need for the prevention of child maltreatment and to ensure that all offenders receive treatment.

Managing the risk of sex offences against children

Research findings from the Home Office estimated that at least 110 000 men in the 1993 population of England and Wales had a conviction for an offence against a child (Marshall 1997). Overall, sexual assaults on children made up the majority of serious sexual offences committed by men under 40 years of age.

Disclosure of information by health professionals to warn communities (or particular sections of a community, such as educational establishments, youth clubs, etc.) about the danger posed by particular sex offenders can be seen as a way of reducing offending behaviour in a particular locality. Under the Sex Offender Act (Home Office 1997), public protection panels have been set up to act as a forum for the 'risk assessment' of offenders who have been put on probation and/or just released from prison. Most used the Thornton (1997) scale to assess risk. These panels can comprise probation, police, social services, housing services and whoever it is felt could give information or aid the assessment and prevention process.

Thus, public warning systems form part of the overall strategy for managing risk and positive steps being taken to track and control the activities of sex offenders. The limitations of current policy are that it focuses selectively on known or convicted sex offenders. It is evident that there is a larger group of sex offenders whose behaviour is hidden or suspected but not subject to criminal court proceedings (Wyre 1997).

Relationships between the perpetrator and victim affect the strategies used by the offender, as well as the frequency and duration of the abuse (Faller 1990). This will affect the chances of the sex offender being discovered. Offenders who are familiar with the victim are more likely to use psychological means of coercion (such as bribery) and maintain the child in a secret abusive relationship. By contrast, the use of physical force runs a greater risk of detection. Elliott *et al.* (1995) found that in offences in which physical force was used the offender was usually a stranger to the child. However, sex offenders do not always behave to 'type' (Fisher & Maire 1998) and the early detection of sex offences can only occur through an awareness and understanding of different types of offenders and their associated *modus operandi* (see Glaser, Chapter 21 for sex offender typologies).

It is reported that some sex offenders, especially adult males who have abused boys, have been sexually abused themselves (Browne 1994; Dobash *et al.* 1994; Elliott *et al.* 1995) but this is neither a necessary nor sufficient causal factor of sexual offending. In fact, many offenders see this as a way of denying, minimizing and distorting their behaviour. Similar denial tactics are used if alcohol consumption is involved (Allam *et al.* 1998).

Choice of victim also appears to be related to 'deviancy'. Beech (1998) found that highly deviant men were more likely to have committed offences against boys, or both boys and girls. They were also more likely to have committed both extra- and intra-familial offences. Furthermore, it has been found that those who target extrafamilial boys and those offenders who target both sexes are at higher risk of re-offending (Hanson & Bussiere 1996; Proulx *et al.* 1997; Hanson & Harris 1998).

High sexual deviancy (Hanson & Bussiere 1996) and the presence of a high number of paraphilias (Prentky *et al.* 1997) have also been known to predict sexual recidivism. More importantly, 'criminogenic needs'—those attitudes, values and beliefs that support antisocial behaviour—have been deemed to be strong predictors of sexual abuse (Andrews & Bonta 1994). A criminal lifestyle in general is a good predictor of sexual recidivism (Hanson & Harris 1998). Indeed, Browne *et al.* (1998) found that previous involvement with the police and convictions for violent offences were predictive of the 37% of sex offenders who drop out of community treatment programmes. Those men who do not complete treatment still pose a significant risk to women and children (Abel *et al.* 1988).

Treatment programmes

Sex offender treatment programmes are based on two explanatory models for sex offending that identify:

1 factors that promote a sexual assault cycle, such as distorted thinking, compensatory feelings and abusive behaviours (Wolf 1988); and
2 the preconditions for the sexual abuse of a child, such as motivation to abuse, mastering internal and external inhibitors and overcoming victim resistance (Finkelhor 1984; Finkelhor *et al.* 1986).

In a recent evaluation of the Prison Sex Offender Treatment Programme (Beech *et al.* 1998), it was found that 67% of men attending showed a treatment effect with significant changes in some or all of the main themes targeted. Long-term treatment (160 h) was more effective than short-term treatment (80 h) in creating change, especially for those offenders who showed high deviancy.

Similarly, a recent audit of a community treatment programme (Browne *et al.* 1998) showed that 81% of sex offenders showed some improvement, with all those completing a programme (63%) showing significant changes in one or more of the following six treatment modules (Allam *et al.* 1997).

1 Cycles and cognitive distortion.
2 Self-esteem, social skills and assertiveness training.
3 Sexuality.
4 Role of fantasy in offending.
5 Victim empathy.
6 Relapse prevention.

A review of seven other community treatment programmes (Beech *et al.* 1996) demonstrated that the above findings are typical. One of the few studies of treatment effectiveness (Marshall & Barbaree 1988) found that treated offenders had less re-convictions than non-treated offenders at both 2-year follow-up (5.5 and 12.5%, respectively) and 4-year follow-up (25 and 64%, respectively).

The need for comprehensive assessment and treatment of sex offenders, using cognitive-behavioural methods was emphasized by Fisher & Beech (1998). They listed 13 preconditions for a sex offender to accomplish before they consider the risk small enough for the man to be reunited with his family, even for therapy. In fact, family therapy has met with limited success in this area (Bentovim 1991). However, they also emphasized the need for work with other members of the family, especially the abused child to prevent the possibility of sibling abuse (Deblinger & Heflin 1996).

It is important to point out that the treatment programmes described above are limited to North America, Western Europe and Australasia. Few examples of such programmes exist elsewhere. Indeed, in Eastern Europe they are more likely to institutionalize the child than prosecute or treat the offender.

Child protection in Eastern Europe

The Convention on the Rights of the Child (Article 9) recognizes the right of all children to grow up in a family environment and the responsibility of states to support parents in the task of child-raising (Article 18). However, many post-communist societies have continued the practice of institutionalizing not only children who are orphaned, disabled or abandoned, but also those who come from families that are considered at risk of child abuse and neglect. In fact, the proportion of children aged 0–3 years in institutional care has actually increased in some Eastern European countries (World Health Organization 2000).

After 50 years of separate ideologies, networking between Eastern and Western Europe has led to new challenges in the theoretical understanding of children's needs. For example, most of Eastern Europe is unfamiliar with the writings of John Bowlby's (1969) attachment theory, and have developed theories based on classical conditioning much more extensively than in the West. This theoretical orientation has led to the maintenance and use of institutions to address the needs of children in adversity, rather than the development of substitute parenting (foster care and adoption).

The importance of attachment theory in highlighting the limitations and negative consequences of childhood institutionalization cannot be overestimated. It is widely recognized that the practice of institutionalization prevents children from developing to the best of their capacity. The social and emotional deprivation experienced by children in institutions can lead to physical and developmental retardation, which has lifelong implications (see O'Connor, Chapter 46).

New programmes are being formulated in order to empty the institutions of children, and either return them to their natural family or to a substitute foster family with a view to national adoption. A model of good practice from Timisoara (Romania), developed by the child psychiatrist, Dr Violeta Stan (1999), was the development of mother and baby homes and alternative family-based homes for abandoned, abused and neglected children who are taken into care as an emergency.

Mother and baby units

These small (shelter) homes give special support to parents, especially mothers who are at high risk of abandoning their children. The unit provides them with an alternative and safe living place and teaches them essential coping and parenting skills. The objective is to promote maternal bonding and child attachment, through breastfeeding, provision of adequate child and antenatal care, education on the child's developmental needs and support towards the mother's search for a stable socioeconomic living condition.

Alternative family-based care for young children and babies

These small community homes serve as an intermediate placement for abandoned babies, abused and neglected children. They are established on the principles of family-based care and attachment theory. Child-friendly furnished and equipped apartments (provided by the local authorities) are staffed with four professional caregivers that constitute the child's surrogate family; each unit can receive up to five children each. Each child has a clearly designated surrogate mother who is sensitive to the child's attachment behaviour to the primary caregiver. The child joins his or her surrogate siblings in this new home. Provision is made that a minimum of one and a maximum of two of the five children within each apartment group are physically and/or mentally handicapped, in the interest of promoting integration. The children visit the community's crèche, kindergarten and school. The local community is encouraged to help, play and care for the children. To promote infant attachment to a primary caregiver, substitute Romanian parents are found quickly, under a fostering and adoption programme located in the area. Similar approaches have been reported in the Czech Republic (Sobotkova 2000).

These approaches attempt to repair a desperate situation where abandoned, abused and neglected children were the subject of secondary abuse and neglect within large institutional settings. This is important for the future parenting behaviour of these children.

Attachment theory and child maltreatment

Despite disagreement over the degree of influence, a history of child maltreatment places an increased risk on an individual of maltreating their own children as a parent (Buchanan 1996). In their review, Morton & Browne (1998) proposed the theory of attachment (Bowlby 1969; Ainsworth et al. 1978) as one of the primary mechanisms for the intergenerational transmission of childhood maltreatment. Over time, a child develops a set of expectations based on prior experiences of interactions with their caregiver and this affects the way they see themselves (Ainsworth 1980).

Where a caregiver has consistently responded to the child in a sensitive and appropriate way, the child sees him or herself as worthy and competent in eliciting the caregiver's attention. By contrast, a maltreated child sees him or herself as unworthy and unable to elicit care, because of the unresponsive and rejecting behaviours of the parent. This early mental representation is said to be the prototype for future relationships and may be the priming process by which maltreatment continues from one generation to the next (Ricks 1985).

Indeed, studies (Boswell 1995; Falshaw & Browne 1997) have shown that three out of four young people held in secure accommodation for antisocial behaviour problems have a previous history of child abuse and neglect and should be recognized as both victims and offenders (Falshaw et al. 1996).

It is in this area that mental health professionals, child and adolescent psychiatrists can contribute to ensuring that the mental health needs of abused and orphaned children are addressed at the earliest possible opportunity in order to repair any attachment disorder. This approach would help prevent family violence from one generation to the next and its associated mental health problems. Intergenerational expression of family violence is most readily seen by the association of spouse and child abuse (Kashani & Allen 1998).

Family violence and mental health

The importance of the links between spouse abuse and child maltreatment has been recently recognized for child protection work (Browne & Hamilton 1999). Indeed, both child physical abuse and/or child sexual abuse are thought to occur in approximately half of Australian families where there is violence between the parents (Goddard & Hiller 1993). In the vast majority of cases this involves the father seriously assaulting the mother as well as the children. Where both spouse abuse and child maltreatment are occurring in the family, mental health problems, alcohol and drug dependency appear to be the most significant risk factors for violence (Browne & Hamilton 1999). In the USA, surveys of battered women typically show that 60% of their partners have an alcohol problem and 21% have a drug problem (Roberts 1987) and the majority of female victims suffer from mental health problems as a result. Some authors propose that these are the major causes of family violence (Pernanen 1991). However, it is more likely that alcohol and drug dependency relieves the man of the responsibility of his behaviour and gives the wife justification for remaining in the relationship in the hope that he will control his addiction and end his aggression. It is true that alcohol and drugs appear to exacerbate preexisting emotional problems, which increases the likelihood of violence. However, the majority of individuals who abuse drugs and alcohol admit they have been violent to their dependants while not under the influence of alcohol and drugs (Sonkin *et al.* 1985). Indeed, mental health problems, alcohol and drug dependency are not the causes of family violence but rather conditions that coexist with it, along with many other factors. Nevertheless, they are often used as excuses for violent behaviour—personally, socially and legally.

Interventions aimed at the protection of children must first address these associated factors, as individuals addicted to alcohol and drugs or suffering from mental illness can rarely benefit from social services interventions. The interagency co-operation between health and social services is a necessary prerequisite in such cases. However, adult mental health services are considered by Reder & Duncan (1999) as the missing link in the child protection system because their staff rarely contribute to the work of area child protection committees or to case conferences. This is despite the increasing evidence in the literature of a relationship between parental mental health problems, especially substance misuse, and child maltreatment (Browne & Saqi 1988a; Falkov 1996, 1997; Wilczynski 1997; Cleaver *et al.* 1998; Falkov 1998; Sanders *et al.* 1999).

Child and adolescent psychiatrists have been much more proactive in developing integrated management therapy and legal interventions for child abuse and neglect (see Furniss 1991; Bentovim 1992; Harris Hendricks *et al.* 1993; Black *et al.* 1998). Indeed, the role of the child psychiatry team in child protection has been concisely described by Davison & Nicol (1997).

A report from the NHS Advisory Service on Child and Adolescent Mental Health Services (NHS Health Advisory Service 1995) advocated collaboration in the planning and provision of services. This will ensure that interacting factors such as family discord, child abuse, socioeconomic disadvantage, discrimination, physical and learning disabilities and physical and mental health problems are considered as a whole. Without such an approach they predict a continuing spiral of child abuse, juvenile crime, family breakdown and adult mental health problems. The report recommended the development of primary or direct contact community services which, if implemented universally, could revolutionize the advice and support available to families.

Conclusions

In the past 20 years there has been debate on what services can be delivered in order to minimize the maltreatment of children. Reviews on the causes of maltreatment (Browne 1988) have emphasized a growing recognition that child abuse and neglect are products of a poor parent–child relationship. Wolfe (1991, 1993) observed that there have been promising developments in early interventions that address parental competency and family support to promote more positive parental knowledge,

attitudes, skills and behaviour. He claimed that personalized programmes such as home visits over a period of 1–3 years stand out as the most successful interventions in achieving desired outcomes in terms of fewer child injuries, emergency room visits and reports to protective agencies. Indeed, Olds *et al.* (1993, 1994) showed that home visits save on US government spending in relation to disadvantaged families in both the short and long term.

Individual counties must take a lead from the United Nations and see child abuse and neglect as a major public health problem with the same seriousness and requirement for resources as cancer, heart disease and AIDS (Merrick & Browne 1999). An international co-ordinated effort in child protection is necessary to ensure each child's right to optimal health and development. This requires an increase in the level of funding for education and training, and for prevention and treatment of child abuse and neglect on a global level.

References

Abel, G., Mittelman, M., Becker, J., Rathner, J. & Rouleau, J. (1988) Predicting child molesters response to treatment. *Annals of the New York Academy of Sciences*, **528**, 223–234.

Adler, R., Hayes, M., Nolan, M., Lewin, T. & Raphael, B. (1991) Antenatal prediction of mother–infant difficulties. *Child Abuse and Neglect* **15**, 351–361.

Agathanos-Georgopoulou, H. & Browne, K.D. (1997) The prediction of child maltreatment in Greek Families. *Child Abuse and Neglect*, **21** (8), 721–733.

Ainsworth, M.D.S. (1980) Attachment and child abuse. In: *Child Abuse: an Agenda for Action* (eds G. Gerbner, C.J. Ross & E. Zigler), pp. 35–47. Oxford University Press, New York.

Ainsworth, M.D.S., Blehar, M.C., Waters, E. & Wall, S. (1978) *Patterns of Attachment: A Psychological Study of the Strange Situation.* Erlbaum, Hillsdale, NJ.

Allam, J., Middleton, D. & Browne, K.D. (1997) Different clients, different needs? Practice issues in community-based treatment for sex offenders. *Criminal Behaviour and Mental Health*, **7**, 69–84.

Altemeier, W.A., Vietze, P., Sherrod, K.B., Sandler, H.M., Falsey, S. & O'Connor, S. (1979) Prediction of child maltreatment. *Journal of the American Academy of Child Psychiatry*, **18**, 205–218.

Altemeier, W.A., O'Connor, S., Vietze, P., Howard, S. & Sherrod, K. (1984) Prediction of child abuse: a prospective study of feasibility. *Child Abuse and Neglect*, **8**, 393–400.

Ammerman, R.T. (1993) Physical abuse and neglect. In: *Handbook of Child and Adolescent Assessment* (eds T. Ollendick & M. Hersen), pp. 439–454. Allyn and Bacon, Boston, MA.

Ammerman, R.T. & Hersen, M., eds (1990) *Treatment of Family Violence.* Wiley, New York.

Ammerman, R.T. & Hersen, M., eds (1992) *Assessment of Family Violence: a Clinical and Legal Sourcebook.* Wiley, New York.

Andrews, D.A. & Bonta, J. (1994) *The Psychology of Criminal Conduct.* Anderson, Cincinnati, OH.

Armstrong-Esther, C.A., Lacey, B., Sandilands, M. & Browne. K.D. (1987) Partnership in care. *Journal of Advanced Nursing*, **12**, 735–741.

Barker, W. (1990) Practical and ethical doubts about screening for child abuse. *Health Visitor*, **63** (1), 14–17.

Beech, A.R. (1998) A psychometric typology of child abusers.

International Journal of Offender Therapy and Comparative Criminology, **42** (4), 319–339.

Beech, A., Fisher, D., Beckett, R. & Fordham. A. (1996) Treating sex offenders in the community. *Home Office Research and Statistics Directorate: Research Bulletin*, **38**, 21–25.

Beech, A., Fisher, D., Beckett, R. & Scott-Fordham, A. (1998) An evaluation of the prison sex offender treatment programme. *Home Office Research and Statistics Directorate: Research Findings*, **79**, 1–4. Home Office, London.

Belsky, J. (1988) Child maltreatment and the emergent family system. In: *Early Prediction and Prevention of Child Abuse* (eds K. Browne, C. Davies & P. Stratton), pp. 267–287. Wiley, Chichester.

Bentovim, A. (1991) Clinical work with families in which child sexual abuse has occurred. In: *Clinical Approaches to Sex Offenders and Their Victims* (eds C. Hollin & K. Howells), pp. 179–208. Wiley, Chichester.

Bentovim, A. (1992) *Trauma Organised Systems: Physical and Sexual Abuse in Families*. Karnac, London.

Black, D., Harris-Hendriks, J. & Wolkind, S., eds (1998) *Child Psychiatry and the Law*, 3rd edn. Gaskell, London.

Boswell, G. (1995) *The prevalence of abuse and loss in the lives of Section 53 offenders*. School of Social Work, University of East Anglia.

Bowlby, J. (1969) *Attachment and Loss*, Vol. 1. *Attachment*. Hogarth Press, London.

Briere, J.N. (1992) *Child Abuse Trauma: Theory and Treatment of Lasting Effects*. Sage, Beverly Hills, CA.

Briggs, F. & Hawkins, R. (1994) Choosing between child protection programmes. *Child Abuse Review*, **3**, 272–283.

Bross, D.C., Miyoshi, T.J., Miyoshi, P.K. & Krugman, R.D. (2000) *World Perspectives on Child Abuse: The Fourth International Resource Book*. International Society for the Prevention of Child Abuse and Neglect, Chicago.

Browne, K.D. (1988) The nature of child abuse and neglect. In: *Early Prediction and Prevention of Child Abuse* (eds K.D. Browne, C. Davies & P. Stratton), pp. 15–30. Wiley, Chichester.

Browne, K.D. (1989) The health visitor's role in screening for child abuse. *Health Visitor*, **62** (9), 275–277.

Browne, K.D. (1994) Child sexual abuse. In: *Male Violence* (ed. J. Archer), pp. 210–230. Routledge, London.

Browne, K.D. (1995a) Predicting maltreatment. In: *Assessment of Parenting* (ed. P. Reder), pp. 118–135. Wiley, Chichester.

Browne, K.D. (1995b) Preventing child maltreatment through community nursing. *Journal of Advanced Nursing*, **21** (1), 57–63.

Browne, K.D. & Falshaw, L. (1998) Street children and crime in the UK: a case of abuse and neglect. *Child Abuse Review*, **7**, 241–253.

Browne, K.D. & Griffiths, P. (1988) Can telephone helplines prevent child abuse? *Changes*, **16** (4), 120–122.

Browne, K.D. & Hamilton, C.E. (1997) The repeat and revictimisation of children: possible influences on recollections for trauma. In: *Recollections of Trauma* (eds D. Read & S. Lindsay), pp. 425–433. Plenum, New York.

Browne, K.D. & Hamilton, C.E. (1998) Physical abuse between young adults and their parents: associations with a history of child maltreatment. *Journal of Family Violence*, **13** (1), 59–79.

Browne, K.D. & Hamilton, C.E. (1999) Police recognition of links between spouse abuse and child abuse. *Child Maltreatment*, **4** (5), 136–147.

Browne, K.D. & Herbert, M. (1997) *Preventing Family Violence*. Wiley, Chichester.

Browne, K.D. & Lynch, M.A. (1994) Prevention: actions speak louder then words. *Child Abuse Review*, **3** (4), 241–244.

Browne, K.D. & Lynch, M.A. (1995) The nature and extent of child homicide and fatal abuse. *Child Abuse Review*, **4** (5), 309–316.

Browne, K.D. & Lynch, M.A. (1998) Community interventions for child protection and government policy. *Child Abuse Review*, **7** (1), 1–5.

Browne, K.D. & Saqi, S. (1987) Parent–child interaction in abusing families: possible causes and consequences. In: *Child Abuse: an Educational Perspective* (ed. P. Maher), pp. 77–103. Blackwell Publishers, Oxford.

Browne, K.D. & Saqi, S. (1988a) Approaches to screening families high-risk for child abuse. In: *Early Prediction and Prevention of Child Abuse* (eds K.D. Browne, C. Davies & P. Stratton), pp. 57–86. Wiley, Chichester.

Browne, K.D. & Saqi, S. (1988b) Mother–infant interactions and attachment in physically abusing families. *Journal of Reproductive and Infant Psychology*, **6**, 163–182.

Browne, K.D., Foreman, L. & Middleton, D. (1998) Predicting treatment drop-out in sex offenders. *Child Abuse Review*, **7** (6), 402–419.

Buchanan, A. (1996) *Cycles of Child Maltreatment*. John Wiley & Sons, Chichester, UK.

Carroll, J. (1994) The protection of children exposed to marital violence. *Child Abuse Review*, **3** (1), 6–14.

Central Statistical Office (1994) *Social Focus on Children 1994*, pp. 46–47. HMSO, London.

Cleaver, H., Unell, I. & Aldgate, J. (1998) *Parents' Problems: Children's Needs: Child Protection and Parental Mental Illness, Problem Alcohol and Drug Use and Domestic Violence*. Report to the Department of Health.

Creighton, S.J. (1992) *Child Abuse Trends in England and Wales 1988–90*. NSPCC, London.

Creighton, S.J. & Noyes, P. (1989) *Child Abuse Trends in England and Wales 1983–87*. NSPCC, London.

Crittenden, P.M. (1985) Maltreated infants: vulnerability and resilience. *Journal of Child Psychology and Psychiatry*, **26** (1), 85–96.

Crittenden, P.M. (1988) Distorted patterns of relationship in maltreating families: the role of internal representational models. *Journal of Reproductive and Infant Psychology*, **6**, 183–199.

Crittenden P.M. (1996) Research on Maltreating families: Implications for Intervention. In: *The American Professional Society on the Abuse of Children (APSAC) Handbook on Child Maltreatment* (eds J. Briere, L. Berliner, J. Bulkley, C. Jenny & T. Reid). Sage, California.

Dalgleish, L.I. (1998) Risk assessment, computer learning, diagnosis and bayes: a commentary. *Child Abuse Review*, **7** (3), 189–193.

Daniel, J.H., Newberger, E.H., Reed, R.B. & Kotelchuck, M. (1978) Child abuse screening. *Child Abuse and Neglect*, **2**, 247–259.

Davenport, C., Browne, K. & Palmer, R. (1994) Opinions on the traumatizing effects of child sexual abuse: evidence for consensus. *Child Abuse and Neglect*, **18** (9), 725–738.

Davison, I. & Nicol, A.R. (1997) Role of the Child Psychiatry Team. In: *ABC of Child Abuse* (ed. R. Meadow), 3rd Ed. British Medical Journal publications, London.

Deblinger, E. & Heflin, A.H. (1996) *Treating Sexually Abused Children and Their Nonoffending Parents: A Cognitive Behavioral Approach*. Sage, California.

Depanfilis, D. & Zuravin, S.J. (1998) Rates, patterns and frequency of child maltreatment recurrences among families known to CPS. *Child Maltreatment*, **3** (1), 27–42.

Department of Health (1989) *An Introduction to the Children Act 1989: a New Framework for the Care and Upbringing of Children*. HMSO, London.

Department of Health (1995a) *Child Protection: Messages from Research*. HMSO, London.

Department of Health (1995b) *The Challenge of Partnership in Child Protection: Practice Guide*. HMSO, London.

Department of Health (1996) *Child Health in the Community: a Guide to Good Practice*. National Health Service Executive, London.

Department of Health (1998) *Responding to Families in Need*. The Stationary Office, London.

Department of Health (1999) *Working Together to Safeguard Children*. The Stationery Office, London.

Department of Health (2000a) *Framework for the Assessment of Children in Need and Their Families*. The Stationery Office, London.

Department of Health (2000b) *Children and Young People on Child Protection Registers Year Ending 31st March 2000, England (Personal Social Services and Local Authority Statistics)*. Government Statistical Service, London.

Department of Health, British Medical Association & Conference of Medical Royal Colleges (1994) *Child Protection: Medical Responsibilities (Addendum to Working Together Under the Children Act 1989*. Department of Health, London.

Dobash, R., Cranie, J. & Waterhouse, L. (1994) Child sexual abusers: recognition and response. In: *Child Abuse and Child Abusers* (ed. L. Waterhouse), pp. 113–135. Jessica Kingsley, London.

Elliott, M., Browne, K. & Kilcoyne, J. (1995) Child sexual abuse prevention: what offenders tell us. *Child Abuse and Neglect*, **19** (5), 579–594.

Falkov, A. (1996) *Study of Working Together 'Part 8' Reports: Fatal Child Abuse and Parental Psychiatric Disorder: An Analysis of 100 Area Child Protection Committee Case Reviews Conducted Under the Terms of Part 8 of Working Together under the Children Act 1989*. Department of Health, London.

Falkov, A. (1997) Adult psychiatry: a missing link in the Child Protection Network: a response to Reder and Duncan. *Child Abuse Review*, **6** (1), 41–45.

Falkov, A. (1998) *Crossing Bridges: Training Resources for Working with Mentally Ill Parents and Their Children*. Department of Health, London.

Faller, K.C. (1990) *Understanding Child Sexual Maltreatment*. Sage, Beverly Hills.

Falshaw, L. & Browne, K.D. (1997) Adverse childhood experiences and violent acts of young people in secure accommodation. *Journal of Mental Health*, **6** (5), 443–455.

Falshaw, L., Browne, K.D. & Hollin, C. (1996) Victim to offender: a review. *Aggression and Violent Behavior*, **1** (4), 389–404.

Finkelhor, D. (1980) Risk factors in the sexual victimisation of children. *Child Abuse and Neglect*, **4**, 265–273.

Finkelhor, D. (1984) *Child Sexual Abuse: New Theory and Research*. Guilford Press, New York.

Finkelhor, D. (1995) The victimisation of children: a developmental perspective. *American Journal of Orthopsychiatry*, **65** (2), 177–193.

Finkelhor, D., Araji, S., Baron, L., Brown, A., Peters, S.D. & Wyatt, G.E. (1986) *A Sourcebook on Child Sexual Abuse*. Sage, Beverly Hills, CA.

Fisher, D. & Beech, A. (1998) Reconstituting families after sexual abuse: the offender's perspective. *Child Abuse Review*, **7** (6), 420–434.

Fisher, D. & Maire, G. (1998) A review of classification systems for sex offenders. *Home Office Research and Statistics Directorate: Research Findings*, **78**, 1–4.

Fluke, J.D., Yuan, Y.T. & Edwards, M. (1999) Recurrence of maltreatment: an application of the National Child Abuse and Neglect Data System (NCANDS). *Child Abuse and Neglect*, **23** (7), 633–650.

Fromuth, M.E. (1986) The relationship of childhood sexual abuse with later psychological and sexual adjustment in a sample of college women. *Child Abuse and Neglect*, **10**, 5–15.

Fryer, G.E. & Miyoshi, T.J. (1994) A survival analysis of the revictimization of children: the case of Colorado. *Child Abuse and Neglect*, **18** (12), 1063–1071.

Furniss, T. (1991) *The Multi-professional Handbook of Child Sexual Abuse*. Routledge, London.

Gelles, R.J. (1987) *Family Violence*, 2nd edn. Sage, Beverly Hills, CA.

Gidycz, C.A., Coble, C.N., Latham, L. & Layman, M.J. (1993) Sexual assault experience in adulthood and prior victimization experiences: a prospective analysis. *Psychology of Women Quarterly*, **17** (2), 151–168.

Goddard, C. & Hiller, P. (1993) Child sexual abuse: assault in a violent context. *Australian Journal of Social Issues*, **28**, 20–33.

Greenland, C. (1986) Preventing child abuse and neglect deaths: the identification and management of high risk cases. *Health Visitor*, **59** (7), 205–211.

Greenland, C. (1987) *Preventing CAN Deaths: an International Study of Deaths Due to Child Abuse and Neglect*. Tavistock, London.

Hall, D.M.B. (1995) *Health for All Children*, 3rd edn. HMSO, London.

Hallet, C. & Birchall, E. (1992) *Co-ordination and Child Protection*. HMSO, London.

Hamilton, C.E. & Browne, K.D. (1998) The repeat victimisation of children: should the concept be revised? *Aggression and Violent Behavior*, **3**, 47–60.

Hamilton, C.E. & Browne, K.D. (1999) Recurrent maltreatment during childhood: a survey of referrals to Police Child Protection Units in England. *Child Maltreatment*, **4** (4), 275–286.

Hanson, R.K. & Bussiere, M.T. (1996) *Predictors of Sexual Offender Recidivism: a Meta-analysis*. User Report no. 1996–04. Department of the Solicitor General of Canada, Ottawa.

Hanson, R.K. & Harris, A. (1998) *Dynamic Predictors of Sexual Recidivism*. User Report no. 1998–01. Department of the Solicitor General of Canada, Ottawa.

Harris Hendriks, J., Black, D. & Kaplan, T. (1993) *When Father Kills Mother*. Routledge, London.

Health Visitors' Association (1994) *A Cause for Concern*. HVA, London.

Herbert, M. (1988) *Working with Children and Their Families*. BPS Books, Leicester.

Herbert, M. (1993) *Working with Children and the Children Act*. BPS Books, Leicester.

Home Office (1997) *The Sex Offender Act Guidelines*. Home Office, London.

Home Office, Department of Health, Department of Education, Science & Welsh Office (1991) *Working Together Under the Children Act 1989: a Guide to Arrangements for Interagency Co-operation for the Protection of Children from Abuse*. HMSO, London.

House of Commons (2000) *Protecting Children, Supporting Parents. A Consultation Document on the Physical Punishment of Children*. HMSO, London.

Howitt, D. (1992) *Child Abuse Errors: When Good Intentions Go Wrong*. Harvester Wheatsheaf, Hemel Hempstead.

Jaffe, P., Wilson, S.K. & Wolfe, D.A. (1990) *Children of Battered Women*. Sage, London.

Jason, J., Williams, S., Burton, A. & Rochat, R. (1982) Epidemiologic differences between sexual and physical child abuse. *Journal of the American Medical Association*, **247**, 3344–3348.

Kashani, J.H. & Allan, W.D. (1998) *The Impact of Family Violence on Children and Adolescents*. Sage, California.

Kitzman, H., Olds, D., Henderson, C. *et al.* (1997) Effect of prenatal and infancy home visitation by nurses on pregnancy outcomes, childhood injuries, and repeated childbearing: a randomized controlled trial. *Journal of the American Medical Association*, **278** (8), 644–680.

Leahy-Warren, P. (1998) *Community Nursing: an International Perspective*. The Stationery Office, Dublin.

Leventhal, J. (1988) Can child maltreatment be predicted during the perinatal period: evidence from longitudinal cohort studies. *Journal of Reproductive and Infant Psychology*, **6**, 139–161.

Lynch, M. & Roberts, J. (1977) Predicting child abuse. *Child Abuse and Neglect*, 1, 491–492.

MacMillan, H.L., MacMillan. J.H., Offord, D.R., Griffith, L. & MacMillan, A. (1994a) Primary prevention of child physical abuse and neglect: a critical review. I. *Journal of Child Psychology and Psychiatry*, 35, 835–856.

MacMillan, H.L., MacMillan. J.H., Offord, D.R., Griffith, L. & MacMillan, A. (1994b) Primary prevention of child sexual abuse: a critical review. II. *Journal of Child Psychology and Psychiatry*, 35, 857–876.

Magura, M. (1981) Are services to protect children effective? *Children and Youth Services Review*, 3, 193.

Marshall, P. (1997) The prevalance of convictions for sexual offending. *Home Office Research and Statistics Directorate Research Findings*, 55, 1–4.

Marshall, W.L. & Barbaree, H.E. (1988) An outpatient treatment program for child molesters. *Annals of the New York Academy of Sciences*, 528, 64–78.

Mayall, A. & Gold, S.R. (1995) Definitional issues and mediating variables in revictimization of women sexually abused as children. *Journal of Interpersonal Violence*, 10 (1), 26–42.

Merrick, J. & Browne, K.D. (1999) Child abuse and neglect: a public health concern. *Public Health Review*, 27, 279–293.

Miller, T.R., Cohen, M.A. & Wiersema, B. (1996) Victim Costs and Consequences: A new look. *Report to the National Institute of Justice (NCJ No. 155282)* (Cited in World Health Organization, 1999, p. 19).

Milner, J.S. (1986) *The Child Abuse Potential Inventory Manual*, 2nd edn. Psytec, De Kalb, IL.

Morton, N. & Browne, K.D. (1998) Theory and observation of attachment and its relation to child maltreatment: a review. *Child Abuse and Neglect*, 22 (11), 1093–1104.

Murphy, M. (1995) *Working Together in Child Protection*. Arena, Ashgate, Aldershot.

National Commission of Enquiry in the Prevention of Child Abuse (1996) *Childhood Matters*, Vol. 1 and 2. NSPCC, London.

NHS Health Advisory Service (1995) *Together We Stand: The Commissioning Role and Management of Child and Adolescent Mental Health Services*. HMSO, London.

Nobes, G., Smith, M., Upton, P. & Heverin, A. (1999) Physical punishment by mothers and fathers in British homes. *Journal of Interpersonal Violence*, 14, 887–902.

Olds, D.L., Henderson, C.R., Phelps, C., Kitzman, H. & Hanks, C. (1993) Effect of prenatal and infancy nurse home visitation on government spending. *Medical Care*, 31 (2), 155–174.

Olds, D.L., Henderson, C.R. & Kitzman, H. (1994) Does prenatal and infancy nurse home visitation have enduring effects on the qualities of parental care giving and child health at 25–50 months of life? *Pediatrics*, 93, 89–98.

Olds, D., Eckenrode, J., Henderson, C. *et al.* (1997) Long-term effects of home visitation on maternal life course and child abuse and neglect: fifteen year follow up of a randomized trial. *Journal of the American Medical Association*, 278 (8), 637–643.

Pernanen, K. (1991) *Alcohol in Human Violence*. Guilford Press, London.

Prentky, R.A., Knight, R.A. & Lee, A.F.S. (1997) Risk factors associated with recidivism among extrafamilial child molesters. *Journal of Consulting and Clinical Psychology*, 65, 141–149.

Prior, V., Lynch, M.A. & Glaser, D. (1994) *Messages from Children*. NCH Action for Children, London.

Prior, V., Glaser, D. & Lynch, M.A. (1997) Responding to child sexual abuse: the criminal justice system. *Child Abuse Review*, 6, 128–140.

Proulx, J., Pellerin, B., McKibben, A., Aubut, J. & Ouimet, M.

(1997) Static and dynamic risk predictors of recidivism in sexual offenders. *Sexual Abuse: A Journal of Research and Treatment*, 9, 7–28.

Reder, P. & Duncan, S. (1997) Adult psychiatry: a missing link in the Child Protection network. *Child Abuse Review*, 6 (1), 35–40.

Ricks, N.H. (1985) The social transmission of parental behavior: attachment across generations. *Monographs of the Society for Research in Child Development*, 50, 211–227.

Roberts, A.R. (1987) Psychosocial characteristics of batterers: a study of 234 men charged with domestic violence offences. *Journal of Family Violence*, 2, 81–94.

Russell, D.E. (1986) *The Secret Trauma: Incest in the lives of Girls and Women*. Basic Books, New York.

Sanders, M. (in press) Promoting positive parenting as an abuse prevention strategy. In: *Early Predication and Prevention of Child Abuse: A Handbook* (eds K. Browne, H. Hanks, P. Stratton & C. Hamilton). John Wiley & Sons, Chichester.

Save the Children, U.K. (1997) *United Nations Convention on the Rights of the Child Training Pack*. Save the Children, London.

Sobotkova, I. (2000) Psychological assessment of family units: the unique type of foster care in the Czech Republic. *Child Abuse Review*, 9 (3), 217–222.

Sonkin, D., Martin, D. & Walker, L. (1985) *The Male Batterer: a Treatment Approach*. Springer, New York.

Stan, V. (1999) *The House with Open Windows: A Romanian Familial Model for Temporary Child Protection, an Early Intervention*. University Department of Child Psychiatry, Timisoara, Romania.

Starr, R.H. (1982) *Child Abuse and Prediction Policy Implications*. Ballinger, Cambridge, MA.

Strang, H. (1992) *Homicides in Australia 1991–92*. Australian Institute of Criminology, Canberra.

Stratton, P. & Swaffer, A. (1988) Maternal causal beliefs for abused and handicapped children. *Journal of Reproductive and Infant Psychology*, 6, 201–216.

Terr, L.C. (1991) Childhood traumas: an outline and overview. *American Journal of Psychiatry*, 148, 10–20.

Thornton, D. (1997) Structured anchor clinical judgement risk assessment for sex offenders. *Proceedings of the NOTA Conference, Brighton, September 1997*. (Cited in Browne, Forman and Middleton, 1998.)

United Nations (1990) *Convention on the Rights of the Child*. United Nations, New York.

Whitfield, C.L. (1995) *Memory and Abuse: Remembering and Healing the Effects of Trauma*. Health Communications, FL.

Wilczynski, A. (1997) *Child Homicide*. Oxford University Press, Oxford.

Wolf, S.C. (1988) A model of sexual aggression/addiction. *Journal of Social Work and Human Sexuality*, 7(1), 131–147.

Wolfe, D. (1991) *Preventing Physical and Emotional Abuse of Children*. Guilford Press, New York.

Wolfe, D. (1993) Child abuse prevention: blending research and practice. *Child Abuse Review*, 2 (2), 153–165.

World Health Organization (1998) *First Meeting on Strategies for Child Protection*. Padua, Italy 29–31 October 1998. WHO Regional Office for Europe, Copenhagen.

World Health Organization (1999) *Report of the consultation on child abuse prevention. 29–31 March 1999*. World Health Organization, Geneva.

World Health Organization (2000) *Action Plan for Romania*. WHO Regional Office for Europe, Copenhagen.

Wyre, R. (1997) A matter of conviction. *Community Care*, 30, October 4.

71 The Law Concerning Services for Children with Social and Psychological Problems

Michael Little

Introduction

Practically everything a clinician does takes place within a legal framework. Nevertheless, the clinician is not often constrained by law. The boundaries established in professional guidance are seldom contradicted in law.

The law concerning children with social and psychological problems is closely intertwined with the development of services for those children. Many practice innovations have been enshrined in law as society seeks to rationalize its response to children's needs. At other times, legal measures have been used to compel changes in practice. There are similarities between the philosophical and theoretical underpinnings of the law and those of several of the health professions, particularly psychiatry (Nye 1980). Increasingly, decisions of law have been made in a practice context and have been used to encourage co-operation among professionals. The courts have become more reliant upon psychiatric and other expert opinion (Ash & Guyer 1986; Wald *et al.* 1988; Brophy *et al.* 2001).

Even so, the relationship between the law and services for children with problems is not always harmonious. As understanding and clinical practice improves, or when societal expectations outstrip those of the professions, it is possible for law and services to be contradictory or even to clash (Stone 1999). In some countries, the legal context can establish an atmosphere of constraint, even when there are few practical limitations on clinical decision-making. For example, when Gutheil (1995) wrote about legal issues in psychiatry, half of the chapter was devoted to legally defined malpractice.

Cutting across the relationship between law and practice are five broad themes.

1 The relationship between children's needs as defined by clinical and research experts and the rights of children and others in society as enshrined in law.
2 The need to choose between the competing rights of individuals.
3 The uneasy relationship between evidence as it is applied at the clinical case level and evidence used with respect to classes of case.
4 Understanding the way the law conveys complex social issues and what this says about clinical practice.
5 The amount of latitude the law affords services for children in need and the consequent dilemmas this can pose for practitioners.

This chapter explores these broad themes with illustrations of the intersection of law and services for children at the clinical case-by-case level, and also with regard to classes of cases. Illustrations extend beyond child psychiatry to include other professions, such as social work. As similarities and differences between legal jurisdictions are so informative, an international perspective has been taken, although illustrations tend to be limited to Europe, North America and Australasia.

The broad context

Theoretically, in most nations, it is possible for anybody to offer any service providing the recipient of that service is a willing participant. If a service is intended to make somebody do something or prevent them from doing something, or if public money is needed, then some form of legislation will be required (Eekelaar, in press). Many services for children in need have evolved from activity pioneered by voluntary organizations operating with the consent of children and families, but once activities require the dispensation of parental or children's consent, or public financial support, they must be authorized by statute. There is a close connection therefore between legal and financial frameworks. The law defines what services an agency can provide, who must pay and how much. Laws generally permit rather than guarantee expenditure.

In the context of children in need, one of two legal doctrines run through the primary legislation of most Western developed nations (Bulkley *et al.* 1996). *Parens Patriae* evolved in response to the needs of orphans but has been used to restrict parents' authority when a child's physical or mental health is jeopardized (*Prince* v. *Mass.*, 321 U.S. 158 1944 United States). Current thinking tends to put the needs of the child as paramount, so legal thinking attempts to capture the 'best interests of the child' (British Medical Association 2001). These broad doctrines have little impact on precise mechanisms for deciding whether a child's health has been jeopardized or that an action is or is not in the child's best interests. Such mechanisms vary considerably from country to country.

Crossing national boundaries are ethical principles (Rosenberg & Eth 1995) of autonomy (that patients give their informed consent to treatment), *Primum Non Nocere* (that a clinician's motivation is first to do no harm), beneficence (to prevent harm and promote well-being) and justice (to ensure some principle of equality of treatment). These lead to practical guidance of a general nature (British Medical Association 2001) or relating to specific case types (Department of Health *et al.* 1999). Providing accessible information, avoiding compulsory powers, trying to comply with the consumer's wishes, establishing collaborative trusting relationships and involving children and families in decision-making are now widely accepted as good practice.

It is rare for ethical guidance to run counter to legal statute and ethical practice will reduce and delay direct involvement of the law in clinical decision-making. For example, compulsory measures are a rarity in the treatment of eating disorders with significant mortality rates, such as anorexia nervosa. Individuals with this disorder are generally at a developmental stage that suggests competency to make valid choices about their care but poor nutrition may impair cognition and lead to refusal of treatment or accepting only ineffective treatment. However, such situations, which often appear to the lay reader to demand court oversight, are usually tackled effectively by well-managed clinical intervention. Summaries of good practice emphasize the importance of treating anorexia nervosa as a mental disorder, establishing trust with patient and parents, giving the patient sufficient information to assess the risks of treatment and its alternatives and always asking patient consent even when compulsion becomes necessary (British Medical Association 2001). Approached in this way, the requirement for clinical decisions that require legal sanction—to remove patient consent, to detain or feed by artificial means— become the exception rather than the rule (Herzog & Becker 1999).

A similar picture emerges with respect to confidentiality. In some areas of children's services (e.g. child protection) this is a thorny issue. Ethical guidance is clear. People, regardless of their age, status or mental capacity, are entitled to expect that information about them provided to, or discovered by, a professional agency is not passed to another person or agency without their consent (General Medical Council 2000). The duty of confidentiality can be breached in the public interest, e.g. to prevent or detect a serious crime or to protect another person from serious harm.

Good ethical practice can ease professional anxiety, reduce the requirement for unnecessary legal intervention and protect both the referred child and colleagues potentially at risk. It is important to explain to children not only their rights to confidentiality, but also the professional duty to prevent harm to others. In difficult cases (e.g. where the child may disclose maltreatment) giving the child time to make an informed decision and recording how this will be done will help. Where it does not put the child at risk, parents should be involved in this process. Where confidentiality is going to be breached, it is necessary to explain to the child what is happening and why (Department of Health *et al.* 1999). Such ethical guidance is rooted in the 'best interests of the child' doctrine.

Even when law is not explicit on this matter, it is generally accepted that professionals uncovering direct evidence of child maltreatment should report it. The manner in which the professional engages with the child can make a considerable difference to the way in which the principle is enacted and to outcomes for the child.

The law adapts to the vicissitudes of societal attitudes towards children and the evolving understanding of children's needs. In the last century, children gradually acquired rights of their own and there was less of an inclination to view them as property of their parents (Eekelaar 1991). The relationship between state and family and the child's position within that has been subject to sociological analysis that combines legal and social dimensions. Fox-Harding (1991) classified state intervention in family life on four dimensions: rate of separation of children from home, propensity to support children at home, respect for children's rights and acknowledgement of parent's rights. Such analysis is helpful in understanding broad social dimensions of law regarding children. Clinicians will recognize these themes in the opinions and motivations of other professionals, managers of services and consumers.

The recent acknowledgement of children's rights has probably resulted in some international convergence in laws regarding children. There are charters and constitutional treaties that cross judicial boundaries and, in the case of the US Supreme Court and the Articles of the European Convention of Human Rights, they can act as the arbiter at the final point of appeal, as well as a fundamental point of reference in legal rulings regarding children in need. Landmark rulings by the European Court carry similar weight (Fortin 1999). However, the convergence in legislation and acknowledgement of cross-border treaties probably mask marked differences in clinical practice, its organization and management.

The United Nations Convention on the Rights of the Child, ratified by 191 countries, is widely cited. Other than encouraging a general resurgence of interest in children's rights, it is difficult to assess the convention's impact on children with social and psychological problems, although in some countries, e.g. New Zealand, it is widely cited in judgements (Pipe & Seymour 1998). A country's imprimatur on the Convention cannot be taken as an indicator of effective policies or practice.

In most countries, domestic law has adapted to increasing knowledge about the complexity of children's needs by encouraging—in the European and Australasian context at least— multidisciplinary approaches and by inviting a wide range of professionals to decision-making fora. This shift has been accompanied by a move from paper to oral evidence and for a diversification in the places in which decisions are made. A clinician might typically be expected to have a rudimentary understanding of health, education and social care legislation and guidance and will find him or herself practising that understanding in administrative, quasi-legal and court settings.

Most fundamental decisions concerning a child's life, e.g. whether or not he or she is guilty of a crime, where the child should live and with whom he or she should be in contact with, are made in a court. In Europe, there has been a trend toward replacing courts with administrative procedures and conferences of professionals. New Zealand's Children and Young Persons and Their Families Act 1989 took decisions away from professionals and placed them in the community and gatherings of family members.

In most developed countries, laws distinguish between criminal matters, concerning whether a crime has been committed and what should happen to the offender, and civil matters, judging the rights of private citizens such as parents (*Lessard* v. *Schmidt* 1972; Stone 1999). The civil law also differentiates between the public domain (concerning the involvement of the state in family matters) and the private domain (dealing with relationships inside the family). The Children Act 1989 (England and Wales) is a rare example of legislation using one set of principles and orders to deal with both domains of the civil law. Although it does not have a direct impact on practice, the single framework for all children creates a helpful context for clinical practice.

For a practitioner, there is considerable overlap between criminal and civil law. When a father is accused of sexually abusing his child, the child may be asked to give evidence in the criminal case. To preserve the accuracy of testimony, the treatment of the child may be delayed until the criminal case is concluded. Civil procedures may operate in parallel, deciding where the child should live, with whom the child may have contact and whether any services are necessary, possibly requiring another decision about whether the child was maltreated using a different standard of proof.

These themes will be evident in the following discussion of the relationship between the law and practice and the way in which evidence is assembled in different legal contexts. The following evidence does not cover the detail of the law but it does address common underlying principles as they impinge on clinical practice. The evidence comes in two parts, the first dealing with decisions about individual children, the second with decisions about classes of children.

The law and professional behaviour: decisions about individual cases

A clinician's primary task is to assess the child's circumstances, make some prognosis of likely development and use this information to fashion an appropriate intervention. The law may become involved if there is parental (or other carer's) disagreement with the professional view, if the child is in disagreement or if the state has to pay for the intervention. Cutting across these issues is the child's competency to give a perspective. In certain cases this may be tested in law.

There are seven ways in which clinical practice typically interacts with the legal process and which exemplify issues of interest to practitioners. A distinction is made between civil and criminal law, although in children's issues there can be considerable overlap. In some jurisdictions, children's crimes are adjudicated in civil court. The reader will bear in mind that many of the legal decisions described below are increasingly taken in administrative or quasi-legal contexts, such as statutory meetings of professionals.

Civil issues

First are decisions to resolve disputes between relatives, most commonly separating parents, about who will look after or have contact with the child (and who should supervise contact). In some circumstances, disputes centre on aspects of the child's upbringing or elements of the parental relationship, such as domestic violence. Acrimony between adult relatives can cast doubt on the quality of evidence given by one party, such as when one parent accuses the other of maltreating the child.

Mental health professionals may be drawn into such cases to give evidence about the health of a parent or child, the likelihood of maltreatment and the benefits of treatment or restraint. Most countries have courts specializing in such cases. In New Zealand and in some parts of Australia, the USA and the UK, mediation is encouraged to help relatives resolve disputes, calling in additional professional help as necessary. There is reasonable evidence to suggest the court may have a stigmatizing effect on the participants and thus prejudice the effectiveness of any decisions made. Clearly there is less stigma to involvement in a meeting of family members to resolve family problems, but the success of alternative mechanisms is not yet known.

Second are decisions to allow the state to look after the child away from home, including the terminating of birth family rights to allow another family to adopt the child (see Rushton & Minnis, Chapter 22). Most countries have developed legislation that permits four types of separation, each type implying an increasing amount of compulsion.

1 In some jurisdictions (e.g. the UK, New Zealand and some parts of Canada) children can be looked after in state-provided placements (usually foster parents) with the agreement of relatives.

2 Some children are made subject of a court order (e.g. a residence order in England and Wales or subsidized guardianship in the USA) that permits the state to support a relative other than the parent to look after the child.

3 Small proportions of children are removed by court order for short periods and subsequently return to live with relatives.

4 An even smaller proportion is taken from birth parents into the care of the state. Most of these children return to relatives but some are subsequently adopted or remain long in state placements.

There is considerable evidence that most children separated from home eventually return home to live with relatives. The success of such reunions varies by jurisdiction (Bullock *et al.* 1998a). The pattern reflects the strength of family ties even where relationships are damaged, and the state's relative ability to provide enduring substitute care. Evidence also shows that contact during separation generally improves the chances of successful reunion, although in a minority of cases it can be damaging to the child and jeopardize the placement. Evidence on the effect of contact on child outcomes is more equivocal (Quinton *et al.* 1997; Masson 2000a). In many European countries evidence about reunion rates has influenced legislation so that there is a prescription of parental involvement and contact unless there is evidence that to do so would put the child at risk. In England and Wales, when the state assumes parental rights through a court order, responsibility for the child's upbringing is shared with parents (Ryan 1998).

Third are decisions to sanction care or treatment of the child (British Medical Association 2001). Frequently, but not always, these are taken in the context of resolving problems about domestic relations or a child's legal status. The types of issues encapsulated in this category are varied. There are questions about the medical treatment of children, e.g. when procedures known to be in the child's best interests are contrary to parents' beliefs. Related to this are questions regarding children's mental health. Most countries require a legally sanctioned medical diagnosis for intensive treatments including hospital stays. If children need to be locked up for their own safety or that of others some legal sanction is usually required, particularly if the child has not been convicted of a criminal offence. There are then questions about the length of detention or points of release for young people detained for indefinite periods following a serious crime or diagnosis of mental illness.

Legal decision-making in this area is unusual because it occurs at several points in the child's development, including the end as well as the beginning of treatment. The complexity of the decision-making usually demands a formal court setting, although specialist panels with professionals to advise a court or the executive have been tried, e.g. in decisions regarding the care of grave offenders in the UK.

In each of the categories just described, the clinician is trying to help the court or other decision-making body decide whether the child has or will suffer any developmental impairment. Each example illustrates the changing social environment in which the clinical decision is made. In the context of family disputes, there is a tendency toward allowing family members to resolve their own disputes and participate in decision-making about a child's future. In the context of decisions about a child's separation from birth relatives, there is the tendency to presume continued parental involvement in the child's upbringing and, wherever possible, to permit voluntary arrangements between relatives and a clinician acting as an agent of the state. In the context of decisions about children's care and treatment, clinical judgement is weighed against other considerations, such as the child's rights to autonomy and liberty (English 1992).

Crime

Fourth are decisions about the care or treatment of children arrested for or convicted of crime. In the case of first minor offences, clinical decision-making is generally little different than in the context of other children in need. In Europe and New Zealand, most such decisions are made outside of court. As convictions accumulate and become more serious, the court becomes increasingly important in deciding the child's future. This can considerably limit clinical focus, particularly in those cases—the majority—in which antisocial behaviour is just one aspect of the child's pathology.

All developed countries make some distinction between blame and guilt on the one hand and the child's capacity to know right from wrong—their responsibility—on the other (Rutter *et al.* 1998). Most countries (but not all US states) have a minimum age of criminal responsibility which varies between 7 (e.g. Ireland) and 18 (e.g. Belgium) years (Krisberg & Austin 1993; Pease & Tseloni 1996). Some European countries and some US states also require the prosecution to demonstrate that accused children knew the full implications of their actions, particularly when grave offences have been committed. Decisions about criminal responsibility have been the source of considerable controversy. Some research is being undertaken but, as yet, little is known about the effects of such judgement regarding either what is done to or on behalf of the child or the eventual outcomes. Important categories of children, e.g. intervention with those convicted of grave crimes prior to the age of criminal responsibility, are largely missing from the literature.

In the USA, the age at which a child can be tried in an adult court is viewed as more important than the age of criminal responsibility. A clinical perspective is not required in all such decisions. In Florida, for example, the decision to transfer can be made by a prosecuting attorney or public defender acting on the client's behalf—but where it is required the social pressures on the professional are immense. Any forensic judgement will be subject to social judgements about the child's relative well-being if tried in a juvenile or adult court.

Fifth are decisions regarding the care and treatment of children who have been victims of crime. When the accusation is serious, including possible physical and sexual abuse by parents or others, the child may be called on to give evidence (see also Ceci *et al.* Chapter 8; Emery & Laumann Billings, Chapter 20; Glaser, Chapter 21). There is much discussion about the low rate of conviction in child maltreatment cases. The implication is that the guilty are being found not guilty. However, the primary motive of the law in these criminal cases is to establish the guilt of the accused, not to protect the child (Densen-Gerber & Lothian 1985). Mental health professionals will be much more concerned with protecting the child from the additional trauma that can result from a rigorous trial and the damaging effects of a not guilty finding upon children who have given evidence against the alleged perpetrator.

There has been considerable discussion, largely inconclusive, about appropriate clinical treatment of children whose parents are being prosecuted for their maltreatment. In such cases, evidence gathered from the children as part of a diagnosis can be used by prosecution and defence at the subsequent trial. Theoretically—the empirical evidence on this matter is scant— any treatment on behalf of the child could prejudice that child's testimony in court. Furthermore, the clinician will be mindful of the potential of the trial to undermine any rehabilitation efforts. There is insufficient knowledge to draw any clear conclusions on effective practice in such contexts save to call for more research.

Sixth are civil actions for compensation by or on behalf of children who have been victims of crime. Despite their frequency, decisions about compensation for children who have been victims are poorly documented. In the USA such cases are described as a tort brought by children (or adults acting on their behalf) against individuals or institutions. Until recent rediscovery of the scope of child maltreatment, parental tort immunity existed in most US states and many still impose a time limit within which legal redress can be sought (Bulkley & Horowitz 1994). In Europe and Australasia, civil actions for wrongful acts done willingly have been relatively rare, although there has been a noticeable rise in out-of-court settlements by English and Welsh local authorities to children maltreated while in their care. In some countries, there are legally defined administrative arrangements for state compensation. The Criminal Injuries Compensation Board in the UK has varied its policy regarding financial payments to child victims, including those maltreated. Little has been written about policies in this area or effects of payments to victims.

In the three case types just given, there are evident contradictions in societies' perspectives toward children. Consequently, there are ambiguities and inconsistencies in the law and legal processes that hinder more than facilitate clinical decision-making. Whereas the civil context has emphasized parents' rights and perspectives, the criminal context brings children's rights and perspectives into relief. Herein lies some of the confusion in the law. While there has been a general acceptance that children should be accorded rights similar to adults and that the child's perspective is an essential element of effective decision-making, there is relatively little consensus about the corresponding responsibilities of children. For example, the increasingly punitive legal responses to young offenders evident in most Western developed nations sits uneasily with a clinician's knowledge about the adolescent-limited nature of much criminal behaviour. There can also be a clash between society's intention to deter criminal activity of future generations — by imposing harsh penalties on the contemporary offender — or to protect future generations from maltreatment at the hands of their parents — by facilitating the admission of child evidence in court — and a clinician's concern for the well-being of an individual client.

Decisions regarding a child's competency

Seventh, and cutting across decision-making in each of the above categories, are questions about the child's competency to give evidence, to understand procedures and proposed treatments, to recognize the consequence of his or her actions and (in some jurisdictions) to stand trial in adult court. There is also the related issue of the child's competency to participate in research (Royal College of Psychiatrists, 2001).

There is considerable variation in the way these decisions are made. When determining the admissibility of children's evidence, some US states apply policies patterned on Rule 601 of the Federal Rules of Evidence that establish a presumption of competence for all persons unless that competency is challenged. A *voir dire* hearing in court makes a ruling applying principles for the admission of evidence described below. A similar situation exists in the UK. Other US states set an age (usually between 10 and 14 years) of minimum competence. Such fixed thresholds rest uneasily with improving knowledge about children's competency (Melton 1981).

A number of principles guiding effective clinical practice can be drawn from available evidence (Rutter, 2001). Regardless of statute, a practitioner will assume that a child's evidence can be useful to clinical and legal judgement unless there is contrary evidence. A court will sometimes require a 'yes' or 'no' decision on admissibility. A clinician will work on the basis that children's evidence can be helpful in some respects but unreliable in others.

Practitioners will view children's competence in the context of their development. This has several consequences. It is not possible to say a child is competent at one stage in development but not at another. Children may display strong levels of understanding of a limited range of issues. Because children of different ages vary in cognitive and emotional development and intelligence, judgements about competence have to be taken on a case-by-case basis, taking into account the child's ability and the nature of the decision to be made. A child's competence may also change over time, an important consideration in protracted legal processes such as adoption.

Children's ability can be much influenced by the social and emotional context in which questions are asked. What is said in a protected clinical environment using appropriate methods, such as those described in the following section, may not be replicated in court or other quasi-legal settings. Children will also be strongly influenced by parents and other carers, especially when care has been inconsistent or dangerous. What a child says in the absence of parents or carers may not be repeated in their presence.

The nature of evidence in decisions about individual cases

The law makes a fundamental distinction between evidence from a lay person (who has personal knowledge of relevant facts) and that from an expert (who has special knowledge to help decision-makers understand technical, clinical and scientific issues). Professionals can find themselves in the position of being able to provide both lay and expert testimony. Myers (1996) defined as evidence 'any matter, verbal or physical, that can be used to support the existence of a factual proposition'. There are rules governing the admissibility of evidence. These vary in complexity depending on the jurisdiction and the context in which the decision is being made.

Decision-making contexts that adopt rules of court will generally distinguish between evidence reporting on what actually happened and evidence attesting to the strength or the accuracy of evidence. Experts are usually permitted to express an opinion in a way that other witnesses are not. Most expert testimony tends to be corroborative, e.g. establishing a pattern of behaviour consistent with a proposition (Lanning 1996). In cases of alleged child abuse, this might include X-rays or swabs suggesting a probability of maltreatment. In court, a further distinction is made between substantive evidence, to prove that something happened, and rehabilitative evidence, to support or challenge the competency of the witness. Experts frequently offer and can be the subject of rehabilitative evidence.

Apart from rare exceptions, mental health professionals who provide expert evidence will be guided by the best interests of the child and not by the instructions of one of the parties to the case. Myers (1996) captures the principles of expert testimony under the acronym HELP: honesty, even-handedness, limits of expertise and preparation.

There have been important judgements, mostly outside of the children's area, about the reliability of expert evidence; such judgements bear on all cases coming to court. *Fyre* v. *US* 293 F. 1013, D.C. cir. (1923) United States, for example, stated that a novel scientific principle is admissible only when that principle 'gains acceptance in the field to which it belongs'. *Daubert* v. *Merrell Dow Pharmaceuticals Inc.* 113 S. Ct. 2786 (1993) United States, sets out the criteria against which a judge can assess the reliability of expert evidence. These include:

1 whether the evidence can or has been tested;

2 whether the methods used to produce the evidence are consistent with established modes of analysis; and

3 whether the results have been published in a peer-reviewed journal.

In other words, judgements about the reliability of expert evidence in the clinical context must adhere to similar criteria about judgements about reliability in the research context.

Scientific evidence, like most clinical decisions, usually deals in probabilities. The court will often expect an absolute judgement, e.g. about whether or not the child has been maltreated. For example, half of 10-year-old children with special needs in the care of the state and placed for adoption will eventually suffer a breakdown in that placement (Thoburn 1991). The court is likely to ask: 'Is *this* case in the 50% where it does happen or the 50% where it does not?' Regular use and illustration of probabilities in expert statements is therefore desirable. The different requirements for experts and courts are not incompatible, but do require some mutual understanding. Rutter (1998) commented that, in his experience, UK courts have come to appreciate that experts need to be able to express uncertainty when that is the case.

Different criteria are used to assess the reliability of witness statements. Bulkley *et al.* (1996) noted that in considering a child's statement, the court will consider motives to lie; whether more than one person heard the statement; the character of the child; hearing the statements; spontaneity; child's performance under cross-examination; and the possibility of family reunion.

The importance of children's evidence in the prosecution of abusers and the continuing struggle to improve methods for establishing children's competence has led to some research and innovation. Melton *et al.* (1992) reported that the amount of information remembered is in proportion to the age of the child but that there is considerable variation in children's developmental progress. The type of event being remembered and information being recounted also bear on childhood memory and, as

with adults, children's competence in presenting evidence is influenced by emotion as well as intellect. Like adults, children remember salient events better than peripheral events and, although trauma has an impact on memory, it does not lead to core facts being forgotten.

Ceci *et al.* (see Chapter 8) also conclude that children generally make competent witnesses and that even very young children can provide accurate information. In laboratory conditions, and in the absence of suggestive techniques, preschool-age children provide accurate albeit sparsely detailed reports. They recommend an interviewer using a neutral tone, a limited number of misleading questions and the absence of any motive or stereotype for the child to make a false report. They also remind the reader that, although it is rare, some children will give wildly misleading occasionally bizarre accounts.

There have been important innovations in this field, including testing of cognitive interview techniques developed by psychologists to enhance the quality of children's recall (Saywitz & Goodman 1996). These require the child to reconstruct all the events surrounding the point of interest for the interviewer, including partial information which may not be directly relevant to the facts of the case. Children are encouraged to re-tell the story from differing perspectives and in different orders. Saywitz *et al.* (1993) report increased accuracy in the range of 26–45% compared to standard interview techniques. Narrative elaboration, an analogous technique, involves the coaching of children to give high amounts of detail to all stories, including who was present, what happened, how they felt and what was said (each of these diversions represented to the child by simple drawings on cards).

This evidence, like that of Ceci *et al.*, puts great emphasis on the skills of the interviewer and the context in which the interview takes place. Saywitz & Goodman (1996) concluded that the quality of children's reports reflect the ability of the interviewer to use free recall open-ended questions (such as 'What happened?'), using a language and concepts that children understand in a setting in which children feel secure. Understanding the nature of the experience being recounted by the child in the context of ordinary child development acts as a guide to the quality of information being provided. All of this speaks to the need for specialized training for professionals involved in forensic interviewing.

This need for training acts as a reminder of an important limitation of some of the techniques described by Ceci *et al.* (Chapter 8). Although they may operate effectively in experimental conditions, they are difficult to administer in court. There are considerable ethical and methodological barriers to the effective evaluation of such techniques in court.

Another class of innovations focus on helping the child manage the intimidating context in which legal decisions are made. Much can be done prior to hearings to ensure that children are not excessively interviewed so adding to the trauma of the event about which they are reporting. Video and joint interviewing are now permitted in many jurisdictions. Children are frequently prepared for court settings, e.g. with tours of the court and classes about the legal process (Plotnikoff & Woolfson 1995). In some European and a few North American jurisdictions, it is possible for the child to give the evidence out of sight of the accused, by the placement of a screen or by use of video or close-circuit television.

Most of these innovations have taken place in the context of efforts to prosecute people accused of child maltreatment, usually sexual abuse. The conviction rate is very low (2% in the UK) and has prompted creative prosecution practices in the USA, such as plea-bargaining to encourage one perpetrator to testify against another (Lanning 1996).

In summary, there have been important advances affecting the quality of evidence assembled about individual cases in the legal context (Brophy *et al.*, 1999) but such advances are unevenly applied in practice. All the evidence indicates the need for greater rigour and consistency in expert evidence. The application of scientific standards and methods can help. The ability to express opinions in terms of probabilities and to present counter evidence alongside that which supports the expert's statement will help. The ability of lawyers and administrators to use such evidence should improve with their exposure to it.

Evidence also points towards greater rigour and consistency in assembling the child's perspective. This area was viewed as largely unproblematic two or more decades ago. Subsequently, the dangers of misrepresentation produced much misunderstanding about the child's view, including questions about its usefulness, particularly for preschool-age children. The evidence summarized by Ceci *et al.* (Chapter 8) demonstrates the considerable advances made in the last decade and should leave readers in little doubt about the wisdom of listening to children. However, gathering and interpreting that evidence does require specialized skills and training.

Even a highly trained forensic interviewer will have a weather eye to the place in which that evidence will be tested. A clear view emerging from a skilled interview undertaken in a controlled environment may disintegrate in a less supportive court environment or in cross-examination. New techniques, e.g. using television or video may help, but much more work is needed to develop and evaluate new legal environments that are conducive to children giving evidence freely and ensure the accused have a fair trial.

The law and professional behaviour: decisions about classes of case

The preceding discussion has dealt with the relationship between law and clinical practice. Most professional decisions are made in a broad legal context. The law communicates important social values and expectations, and thereby has an influence on clinical decisions.

Reviews of the evolution of the law in any one jurisdiction capture this well. Eekelaar (in press) referred to several underlying themes in societal attitudes to children that have helped shape British legislation over the last five centuries. Laws have been passed to help parents maintain authority over children. Attitudes towards the poor, especially those perceived as the undeserving poor, have had a strong influence on legislation (Pinchbeck & Hewitt 1969, 1973). Society's instrumental needs have also been manifest in children's legislation, e.g. in the establishment of apprenticeship systems from the mid-1500s onwards and in the direct connection between armed services requirements for recruits and the potential supply from industrial and reform schools. Vulnerable children, such as those abandoned or orphaned, have figured strongly in legislation, as have those viewed as a threat to society. On rare occasions, e.g. the Children and Young Persons Act 1969 in England and Wales and the Children, Young Persons and Their Families Act 1989 in New Zealand, the law has made a connection between these two groups. Much law has also questioned the authority of the family, as reflected in the last century by its propensity to sanction intervention on behalf of children born outside of marriage and in this century by a willingness to protect children from maltreatment by parents.

The law is regularly used to formalize arrangements to provide services previously offered on a voluntary basis. In England and Wales, the Children Act 1948 created children's departments to assume responsibility for the administration of services pioneered (and in some cases still provided) by voluntary agencies under the guiding hand of pioneers such as Barnardo and Stephenson. Most departments worked with children separated from home. When the potential for support of children at home (as a means to preventing separation) was realized and informal experiments were underway, the law was changed to legitimize the activity (the Children and Young Persons Act 1963). The way in which voluntary and professional organizations work to, and transgress, legal limits prior to legislative change has received little attention; Barnardo was prosecuted on several occasions for testing the limits of the law.

The law is often used to recognize a social need or social psychological deficits in children receiving insufficient attention from the state. In the USA, there have been many class actions taken on behalf of specific groups of children or adults (e.g. parents or grandparents) to compel a change in patterns of state intervention or professional behaviour. Class actions generally deal with groups of individuals with similar problems, who have been dealt with unlawfully and who represent similar future cases. Dicker (1990) summarized five such cases, dealing with day care and employment rights of poor mothers, race-segregated education of children, health care of mothers, the care and treatment of children placed in secure facilities and services for children with severe behaviour disorders. This last case is particularly interesting for the mental health reader.

In the late 1970s, complaints were aired about North Carolina's failure to provide adequate services for emotionally disturbed children (Soler & Warboys 1990). One such case, an 11-year-old referred to as Willie M., and diagnosed as emotionally disturbed with unsocialized aggression and other disorders, became the first named of four plaintiffs thought to be inappropriately placed in juvenile training schools or a state psychiatric placement. At the time of the action, there were thought to be between 100 and 200 severely behaviour disordered and violent children in the class. The case was settled out of court and eventually resulted in the allocation of $30 million per annum for an estimated 1000 children, leading to a range of services from community support to secure accommodation. As with many remedies resulting from class actions, a series of targets, e.g. the proportion of class members receiving appropriate services, were established along with a review panel to monitor the implementation of the programme. Despite the optimistic review of the effects of the litigation by some commentators, little is known about the effects of class actions, as measured in terms of outcomes for the children involved or the provision of services for those outside the class.

The law also establishes the administrative and managerial structures within which services for children with social and psychological problems are provided. There is huge variation among jurisdictions. Italy, for example, has 8100 local authorities, 196 local health agencies and 98 hospital trusts compared with 150 local authorities, 105 health authorities and 451 health trusts in England and Wales. In the USA, the big cities are organized around large centralized systems focused on administrative categories of children. New York City's Administration for Children's Services deals with child protection issues for children at home and in state care, thus assuming responsibilities that 32 London local authorities discharge in co-operation with seven health authorities and 38 other provider trusts.

For the last 20 years, controlling demand for health and social care services has resulted in elaborate administrative arrangements broadly framed in legislation but delivered by bureaucrats operating in private and public agencies. These administrative arrangements are variously described as care management, managed care or quasi-markets. Because they seek to ration professional help, these arrangements are perceived to have a marked impact on clinical decision-making. Their actual impact is largely uncharted. The arrangements have been more pervasive in adults than children's services, although problems of demand, supply and spiraling budgets are at least as evident if not more evident in children's services. The arrangements have been particularly controversial in the way they have been introduced in the USA, leading Stone (1999) to devote 10% of his overview of psychiatry and the law to managed care issues. Little is known about the effect different administrative structures have on professional behaviour, but changes in those structures are frequently used by elected and career policymakers to implement developments in thinking about children's needs.

The locus of children's legislative change also varies from country to country. In the UK, laws about children's social needs have emerged from government departments of health, interior and social security, whereas elsewhere in Europe, particularly in the south of the continent, the genesis has been education. These distinctions have a considerable impact on the character of specific laws.

In addition to communicating social values, legitimizing intervention and creating the administrative structures within which these interventions are delivered, the law also changes in response to demand for greater clarity. For example, the Children Act 1989 in England and Wales emerged from a confluence of work by lawyers at the Law Commission to simplify and clarify a century of statutes regarding children and from work by central government policymakers to address weaknesses in children's services. The result was a single piece of legislation with a single set of orders for children in private and public law cases (White *et al.* 1995).

The nature of evidence in the broader context

To understand the way in which the law influences professional behaviour with respect to broad categories of cases, it is helpful to review the way in which the law is disseminated. First, there is legislation and, as has been seen, statutes can take several forms. Second, there are legal rulings requiring an authority or agency to intervene on behalf of a group of children, and for these interventions to be implemented to the satisfaction of the court. This category also includes judgements regarding individual children, setting standards (but not precise modes of intervention) for future children in similar circumstances. For example, in the case of *Gillick* v. *West Norfolk and Wisbech Health Authority* (1986) UK, the UK House of Lords ruled that a child of any age possessing sufficient understanding and intelligence could consent to medical procedures. This judgement was in response to a mother asking for assurance that her children would not be given medical treatment (specifically, be prescribed a contraceptive pill) without her agreement. Third, the law can be administered through guidance from a relevant government department or a letter from a Minister of State or senior official. This is commonly used to prescribe the actions of members of weak or new professions, e.g. social work. Fourth, where a profession is strong, as is the case with medicine, the professional body will assume some of the responsibilities of government by regulating its member's behaviour to a standard at or beyond that agreed with policymakers.

The law requires a different burden of proof in civil and criminal cases. In a criminal case, it is necessary to prove a matter beyond reasonable doubt and a court will routinely consider a greater amount of evidence admitted under stricter rules than would be necessary in a civil case. Generally speaking, the further from court a case is decided, the weaker will be the application of these rules of evidence. So, in the UK, a decision by police and youth justice professionals to administer a final warning to a young offender, while ensuring the principles of due process are adhered to, has more of the qualities of a civil than a criminal proceeding.

In all court cases, decisions must be made about the appropriate level to hear the case. In the UK, in civil public and private law cases a process known as concurrent jurisdiction is in place allowing all cases to be heard in all courts with the most complex cases being heard in a higher court. Judges and lay magistrates can pass a case to a higher or lower court if they feel it is inappropriately placed.

In criminal cases, most jurisdictions have established special children's or youth courts, excepting the most serious cases or those cases where adults and children are jointly charged. This provision has been eroded in the USA where it is of doubtful benefit because lower courts will, under public pressure, pass sentences as severe, and sometimes more severe, than those passed down by adult courts. The adult court generally has a different range of sentences from which to choose.

How do legal decisions about classes of case impinge upon clinical work? Practitioners can recognize the importance of social messages being transmitted in the law. These must never be permitted to drive clinical practice but they do provide the context in which practice decisions are made. It is not necessary for the practitioner to agree with all elements of this broader social context but understanding can help.

The mechanism used by law to communicate a social message betrays important features of that message. There is value in looking at the intention of central and local government agencies as expressed not only in legislation, but also in guidance and administrative procedure. In many developed nations, with increasing competition for parliamentary time to debate legislation, important policies are now communicated through a range of procedures in addition to legal statute.

The practitioner will want to evaluate the potential effect on the consumers of services created by the mechanism by which law is communicated. Often, a better outcome can be achieved without administrative or court hearings and, in the worst cases, the decision-making context can undermine clinical objectives. The chaining of groups of offenders by hand and ankle as they enter court is some states in North America is clearly not conducive to agnostic clinical decision-making. Finding the appropriate type and level of court in which to hear a case is also important.

Some clinical assessment will expose gaps in legislation. By highlighting the absence of effective mental health services in North Carolina, practitioners altered the balance of provision. The Willie M. decision also illustrates the limited effects of practitioner-induced legal changes. There is no evidence to suggest that the class action improved outcomes for children. The responsibilities of the advocates of change are also apparent from the case. Because there is a limit to resources allocated to children in need, increasing or improving services in one area can imply a decrease or deterioration of services in another.

Discussion

Running through the preceding description of the law are five broad themes. First is a tension between children's rights and their needs. Where the legislative framework is progressive, need tends to take precedence over rights as a guiding principle. This situation will be enhanced if the constituent professional organizations are strong and self-governing or are strongly influenced by government. Where the legislative framework is weak, or the legal power is broadly distributed, e.g. in the USA, rights have a strong bearing on judgements about individuals and client groups. The same situation is true in developing countries that have few laws governing services for children with social and psychological problems.

In some respects this relationship between needs and rights mirrors the relationship between family and state. Needs of children are determined by professionals, ideally working with parents and child. Rights are determined by the wider community and, as such, must capture the state's response to children.

Whether the guiding principle is needs or rights, problems occur. The case *T & V* v. *United Kingdom, European Court of Human Rights* (1999) dealt with two boys convicted of murder, tried in an adult court and sentenced to indefinite terms of detention (the period of detention to be decided by a Minister of State in consultation with officials and expert advisers). They were placed in secure accommodation with a reasonable standard of treatment and education. There is every reason to believe the needs of these two boys were met and there is some evidence to suggest that their treatment will produce reasonable outcomes, having taken account of their backgrounds. However, the court found that the rights of the children had been scanted. The adult court was not comprehensible to the boys, thus denying them a fair trial (Article 6), and the absence of judicial review of the period of detention was a breach of the right to liberty (Article 5). These rights will be redressed, but there is no certainty that the change will better meet children's needs.

In the UK and some other parts of Europe, attention to the needs of children has involved bypassing some aspects of due process in the law. When crimes are minor, for example, and a child admits to a crime, a final warning can be administered without a thorough test of the child's guilt. Such a procedure would be less likely and certainly less explicit in the USA where protection of legal rights results in more prosecutions, more restrictive and longer sentences which are arguably counterproductive to the meeting of children's needs.

The same dilemma can manifest itself in a different way with respect to the ethics of research. The Royal College of Psychiatrists' (2001) guidelines regarding research involving human participants start from the principle that everyone should be able to benefit from the fruits of research but that individuals should also be able to weigh up the risk and benefits of their participation in that research. The guidance searches for a balance between the needs of patients (and other recipients of services) for interventions rooted in reliable evidence and for the rights of the individual to know the consequences of taking part in research. The legal burden is considerably eased when the professional groups that comprise children's services engage in constructive dialogue about practical response to the changing social context.

A second cross-cutting theme concerns primacy when the rights of individuals compete. What is best for the child is not always acceptable to the parent. Parents' decisions are sometimes disapproved of by grandparents or other relatives. Where adoption is 'open,' meaning that birth parents have some contact with the child, it is possible for the rights of all parties to clash.

These issues are manifest in the US Supreme Court judgement the case of *Troxel* et vir v. *Granville*, Supreme Court of the United States, N99-138 (2000). Brad Troxel committed suicide, leaving a common-law wife and two daughters. His partner later married a man who legally adopted the children. Troxel's parents, unhappy with the amount of access they were allowed to their grandchildren, began a legal battle to increase it. They were supported by a powerful consumer lobby group with 38 million members which views protecting grandparents' rights as one of its roles (grandparents are the primary caregivers of 1.4 million US children). As is often the case where there are fragmented or weak legal frameworks, other interest groups filed their own petitions. In the Troxel case, these included those supporting traditional family structures and those advocating on behalf of non-traditional families, where the functional parent may have neither biological nor legal ties to the child. These diverse interest groups were looking to preserve the fundamental rights of legal parents to choose the people and ideas that may influence their children.

The case exemplifies the nature of decision-making when the law is primarily concerned with an individual's rights and not the needs of many. There are tensions between the competing rights of individuals (the children, the birth and adoptive parent and grandparents) and those of classes of individuals (grandparents, religious groups, non-traditional families).

Competing rights of individuals and groups are particularly evident in the USA (Bulkley *et al.* 1996). Parents' rights to autonomy, privacy and integrity are overridden when there are compelling state interests, e.g. to protect children from maltreatment. Because parents also have the right to due process, they must be notified about abuse inquiries regarding their child. In some states (e.g. Minnesota), parents are read their legal rights prior to a protection inquiry commencing, in much the same way that accused criminals are read their legal rights. Children in the USA always have the right to a lawyer in criminal cases and in some states in child protection cases. In addition, there are other parties with rights, e.g. unmarried non-custodial biological fathers.

A third overarching theme concerns the place of evidence in clinical and case class decision-making. Rights are not amenable to evidence because they are generally concerned with process not outcomes. It is possible to measure the proportion of cases where rights have been scanted but this will not provide a measure of the well-being or progress of children or others involved in the case. Needs are much more amenable to scientific study, although assessments of need are generally only partially dependent on research-based judgements. The same dilemma can be expressed in terms of legal and clinical requirements for certainty of judgement. A court must aspire to certainty, whereas a clinician used to research methods and findings will feel comfortable when dealing with probabilities.

The use of weighted variables can assist the court. For example, in trying to help a court decide on the wisdom of reunifi-cation in the context of a child in state care, it is known that 70% of those who go home to relatives stay at home. Log–linear analysis suggests that if the child and family are prepared for the anxieties associated with reunion, the chances of stability after reunion increase by about 2.5 : 1 (Bullock *et al.* 1998a). If a clinical assessment of family relations reveals them to be of a fairly high quality, the odds of stability are further increased by a ratio of 3.5 : 1. If the child is not an offender, the odds rise again by 1.7 : 1. In other words, if all three criteria are met, the odds of stability after reunion are eight times higher than if opposite conditions existed.

The preceding discussion presents an important challenge for researchers. There is little authoritative evidence about the efficacy of contrasting legal processes. This is because of the general lack of research interest but also because of the difficulty of undertaking robust evaluation.

In the testing of specific interventions for specified groups of children in need, methods are clear. Generally, some form of controlled trial or other quasi-experimental design will be used, notwithstanding ethical considerations that must be taken into consideration. The goal of the evaluation is always to measure the impact of the intervention on children's outcomes (Rossi *et al.* 1999). In the legal context, the evaluation must focus on the amount of change in the process and its eventual impact on child outcomes. The mechanisms mediating between process, intervention and outcome can be complex. Take, for example, family group conferences pioneered in New Zealand for bringing together family members to make decisions about a child's future, as an alternative to court and other professionally orientated decision-making fora. The primary goal of these conferences is to change the process; to encourage family members to make their own decisions. The conference encourages commitment to decisions made. These processes may result in different decisions than would have been reached in court, or they may result in the same decisions differently applied. Evaluation in these contexts demands innovative and rigorous ways of working. Similar innovation is required in testing the effects of innovation in court, because controlled experimentation is practically impossible.

A fourth cross-cutting theme concerns the way the law communicates the complexity of competing social pressures to the practice context. Sometimes it does this well, other times badly. Rigorous clinical assessment and evidence from research are among these social pressures. The law can accommodate sound diagnosis or the results of research if they are effectively communicated in the contexts in which the law is administrated and in a form that facilitates legal decision-making.

There are exceptions to the courts' requirements for certainty of judgement and they tend to occur when the law becomes ineffective in respect to both the process and the outcome. There is strong evidence that courts can hinder rather than improve chances of obtaining accurate evidence and making reliable decisions about children's future in parental separation or divorce cases. A common alternative is mediation, which takes the decision-making process out of the court and permits greater ambiguity with the intention of producing agreement (not necessarily binding) around important aspects of the child's upbringing. The use of plea-bargaining or allowing other offences to be taken into account at the sentencing stage, strategies commonly used to protect children from the rigours of the court, are other examples of legal acceptance of indefinite judgements.

Much of this discussion is relevant to the way in which the law changes. In the case of children, the weight of public opinion that has gathered periodically about their welfare, protection or about the potential threat they pose to society has led to significant shifts in legislation. Masson (2000b) charts the impact of ideology, scandals and inquiries in the context of child welfare and protection laws in England and Wales. The preceding pages highlighted a difference between legislation that has evolved in a considered way and that which has resulted from strenuous and expensive legal battles.

Several influences are evident in most legislative frameworks (Department of Health 1995; Bullock *et al.* 1998b). First are the moral sensitivities of a society, often bound up in existing legislation. Second are the pragmatic concerns of politicians, policymakers and professionals regarding their ability to deliver an agreed law, legal framework or judgement. If, for example, the moral tone of a nation demanded that all parents hitting their children were to be imprisoned, the volume of potential offenders would nevertheless make the passing of any law impracticable. Third are the perspectives of consumers of services, parents and children and the providers of services. Advocacy groups have strongly influenced children's legislation passed in the UK, Australasia and USA in recent years. Fourth is scientific evidence about children's circumstances, the aetiology of social and psychological problems and evaluations about the efficacy of different interventions. Good legislation, legal frameworks and important court judgements successfully accommodate these four dimensions.

There can be conflicts between these dimensions. A society's moral sensibilities shift. Consumers come to new perspectives and the strength of their advocacy waxes and wanes. New research results are published. The pragmatic concerns of policymakers and professionals shift over time. Effective legislation and legal frameworks must endure to accommodate such changes. Mental health professionals are both an influence on the changing legal framework but also must change their behaviour to conform to the developments.

Reliable evidence is arguably the most recent of the four influences on legislation. In the legal context it remains sparse. Building up an evidence base, encouraging innovation in research methods and a critical culture while demonstrating the practical value of research results to lawyers and colleagues with legal authority over children's lives should be a priority.

A final broad theme concerns the amount of latitude afforded by the law to practitioners working with children in need. Interventions for children are organized by health, education, social and police services. Each agency is subject to its own legislation. Children's needs cross these agency boundaries. In many cases,

professionals can choose from several legislative routes, a choice that can have profound impact on children's outcomes. For example, a child with a conduct disorder can, depending on the manifestation of the behaviour, be dealt with by mental health, special education, child welfare or youth justice agencies, each operating to a different legal framework (Bullock *et al.* 1998c). In England this could involve the Mental Health Act 1983 (providing rights to patients placed in secure facilities), Department of Education *et al.* (1994), a government health and education departments circular (setting out arrangements for children placed in residential education placements), the Children Act 1989 (providing the procedures for placing children away from home and the use of secure provision), or several pieces of youth justice legislation (dictating what should happen if a child commits a crime).

It is suggested that socioeconomic status is an important factor in determining which legislative route is taken, with wealthier children being processed through mental health and education while poorer children gravitate to child welfare and youth justice. In fact, there is little empirical evidence for this proposition, although there are many more children being processed through the mental health sector in the USA where there is no comprehensive health insurance and private policies can extend to mental health of children.

Where there is choice, the practitioner must balance the effectiveness of services designed to meet children's needs provided by each sector and attention to competing rights of people involved in the child's life. The decision will take into account predicted changes in the child's development alongside known alterations to legal rights and quality of interventions as the child gets older. Youth justice may appear a benign route for a first-time offender in England because it will permit the introduction of a range of community-based services, but a child staying in this sector for several years will eventually leave the practitioner with few choices beyond incarceration.

The dilemmas also occur within sectors and can be illustrated by the decision to remove children from their parents. Given the preceding evidence and discussion, what are the implications for practice? Wherever possible, the practitioners will want to elicit the views of and work alongside both child and family members. In several jurisdictions, separation is permitted by voluntary agreement between the child's carer and the state, and there is some evidence that this route is more likely to produce better outcomes for the child (Packman & Hall 1998). Where the child is to be removed against parents' wishes, a court hearing will be required. In England and Wales, the clinician is required to demonstrate significant impairment to the child's development or that the child is beyond parental control. Where assessments concentrate on sound evidence of impairment in all areas of the child's life and not on disputes about whether or not an abusive incident has occurred, there is some evidence of improved outcomes (Department of Health 1995). The practitioner will be mindful that, depending on the jurisdiction, up to 92% of children looked after by the state eventually go home, so keeping relatives involved in the child's life can be beneficial. By implication, at least 8% of separated children will not return, creating the dual challenge to practitioners of selecting those cases where contact and reunion will hinder the child's development and finding effective stable alternatives to the family home. In both of these areas there is a requirement for better research and development. Presently, practitioners choices are restricted not by the law, but by a lack of knowledge and effective services for the most vulnerable children.

Conclusions

The range of services available for children with social and psychological problems does not vary greatly from one country to another. However, there is considerable variation in legal frameworks and laws. In some instances these have a bearing on professional decision-making; in most they do not. There is little evidence that the age of criminal responsibility makes a great deal of difference to the treatment of young offenders, although the places in which the decision is made (juvenile or adult court) probably does. Even the court can have limited impact. In some contexts, the court is presented with cases about which there are many disputes but where the weight of professional opinion is compelling, e.g. in the UK over 90% of applications for an order to adopt a child in state care are granted (Murch *et al.* 1993; Department of Health 1999). Much work is being undertaken, but there is little evidence to date to suggest that decision-making fora outside of the court are improving outcomes for children.

There are interesting paradoxes not covered in this chapter worthy of investigation. It is noteworthy that those countries that give particular attention to the rights of specific groups are as likely, if not more likely, to take away the rights of those groups. The USA places great weight on the rights of its citizens yet it assumes rights over a greater proportion of its children than any other Western developed nation, with high rates of state care, adoption, incarceration of young people and placement in mental health facilities. The USA is particularly zealous in the assumption of parental rights of particular classes of citizens, particularly African-Americans who are greatly overrepresented in child protection, care, adoption and youth justice proceedings, and whose rights are specifically protected in that constitution.

At the clinical level, there is scope for new work to evaluate the effect of the legal process on child outcomes. To an extent this demands some attention to the way outcome as a concept applies in the study of legal process. Four examples serve to illustrate the point. First, there is a need better to understand the influence of the context in which a decision is made. Does a policeman giving an informal warning to a young offender come to a different conclusion about guilt than a court making the same decision with the same facts? Does an administrative gathering of professionals reach a different decision about a child's maltreatment than a family group conference primarily managed by the family themselves?

Second, do legal contexts achieve the objectives of those governing that context? In some jurisdictions, the court will review its own decisions, but most judges, magistrates and case conference co-ordinators know little about how their judgement is implemented. Also valuable in this context would be to clarify the relationship between decisions made in a legal context and a clinical or research diagnosis of chains of effects in children's lives.

Third, more can be learned about the impact different legal contexts have upon children's life chances. Much has been written about the damaging effect of adult court. Over the last century, much was done to move the decision-making process away from the court and nearer to the genesis of the child's problem. The sentiments behind these developments are laudable, but it is not known whether they have a great bearing on children's life chances.

Finally, there is scope to revisit the concept of legal due process as it is applied to children. It is evident from the literature underpinning this chapter that there are strengths and weaknesses in both the USA's careful protection of legal representation and due process for children and the tendency of European states to bypass these rights as a mechanism to protect the child from harm. This aspect of rights amenable to measurement and further research in this area has the potential to greatly enhance the well-being of children.

References

Ash, P. & Guyer, M. (1986) The functions of psychiatric evaluation in contested child custody and visitation cases. *Journal of the American Academy of Child Psychiatry*, 25, 554–561.

British Medical Association (2001) *Consent, Rights and Choices in Health Care for Children and Young People.* British Medical Association, London.

Brophy, J., Bates, P., Brown, L., Cohen, S., Radcliffe, P. & Wales, C.J. (1999) *Expert Evidence in Child Protection Litigation.* Stationery Office, London.

Brophy, J., Brown, L. & Cohen, S. (2001) *Child Psychiatry and Child Protection Litigation.* Gaskell Press/Royal College of Psychiatrists, London.

Bulkley, J.A. & Horowitz, M.J. (1994) Adults sexually abused as children: legal actions and issues. *Behavioural Sciences and the Law*, 12, 65–67.

Bulkley, J.A., Nusbaum Feller, J., Stern, P. & Roe, R. (1996) Child abuse and neglect laws and legal proceedings. In: *The APSAC Handbook of Child Maltreatment* (eds J. Briere, L. Berliner, J.A. Bulkley, C. Jenny & T. Reid), pp. 271–296. Sage, Thousand Oaks, CA.

Bullock, R., Gooch, D. & Little, M. (1998a) *Children Going Home: the Re-unification of Families.* Ashgate, Aldershot.

Bullock, R., Gooch, D., Little, M. & Mount, K. (1998b) *Research in Practice: Experiments in Development and Information Designs.* Ashgate, Aldershot.

Bullock, R., Little, M. & Millham, S. (1998c) *Secure Treatment Outcomes.* Ashgate, Aldershot.

Densen-Gerber, J. & Lothian, J. (1985) Emerging issues at the interface of law and medicine concerning children of the 1980s. In: *Emerging Issues in Child Psychiatry and the Law* (eds D.H. Schetky & E.P. Benedek), pp. 332–346. Brunner/Mazel, New York.

Department for Education/Department of Health (1994) *The Education of Children with Emotional and Behavioural Difficulties.* Circular 9/94-DH LAC (94), 9. Department for Education and Employment, London.

Department of Health (1995) *Child Protection: Message from Research.* HMSO, London.

Department of Health (1999) *Adoption Now: Messages from Research.* Wiley, Chichester.

Department of Health, Home Office & Department for Education & Employment (1999) *Working Together to Safeguard Children.* Stationery Office, London.

Department of Health, Welsh Office (1999) *Mental Health Act 1983 Code of Practice.* The Stationery Office, London.

Dicker, S. (1990) *Stepping Stones: Successful Advocacy for Children.* Foundation for Child Development, New York.

Eekelaar, J. (1991) Parental responsibility: state of nature or nature of the state? *Journal of Social Welfare and Family Law,* **1**, 37–50.

Eekelaar, J. (in press) Child welfare and protection in England & Wales. In: *A Century of Juvenile Justice* (ed. M. Rosenheim). University of Chicago Press, Chicago.

English, A. (1992) Legal and ethical concerns. In: *Comprehensive Adolescent Health Care* (eds S.B. Friedman, M. Fisher, S.K. Schonberg & E.M. Alderman), pp. 109–113. Mosby, St Louis.

Fortin, J. (1999) Rights brought home for children. *Modern Law Review,* **62**, 350–370.

Fox-Harding, L. (1991) *Perspectives in Child Care Policy.* Longman, London.

General Medical Council (2000) *Confidentiality: Protecting and Providing Information.* General Medical Council, London.

Gutheil, T.A. (1995) Legal issues in psychiatry. In: *Comprehensive Textbook of Psychiatry* (eds H.I. Kaplan & B.J. Sadock), 6th edn, pp. 2747–2767. Williams & Wilkins, Baltimore.

Herzog, D.B. & Becker, A.E. (1999) Eating disorders. In: *The Harvard Guide to Psychiatry* (ed. A.M. Nicholi), pp. 400–411. Harvard, Cambridge, MA.

Krisberg, B. & Austin, J.F. (1993) *Reinventing Juvenile Justice.* Sage, Newbury Park, CA.

Lanning, K. (1996) Criminal investigation of sexual victimization of children. In: *The APSAC Handbook of Child Maltreatment* (eds J. Briere, L. Berliner, J.A. Bulkley, C. Jenny & T. Reid), pp. 247–264. Sage, Thousand Oaks, CA.

Lessard *v.* Schmidt, 349, F. Supp. 1078, E. D. Wis. (1972) United States.

Masson, J. (2000a) Thinking about contact: a social or legal problem? *Child and Family Law Quarterly,* **12**, 15–30.

Masson, J. (2000b) From Curtis to Waterhouse: state care and child protection in the UK, 1945–2000. In: *Cross currents: Family Law in England and the US Since the Second World War* (eds S. Katz, J. Eekelaar & M. Macclean), pp. 564–587. Oxford University Press, Oxford.

Melton, G. (1981) Children's competency to testify. *Law and Human Behavior,* **5**, 73–85.

Melton, G., Limber, S., Jacobs, J. & Oberlander, L. (1992) *Preparing Sexually Abused Children for Testimony: Children's Perceptions of the Legal Process.* University of Nebraska Press, Lincoln, NB.

Murch, M., Lowe, N., Bovkowski, M., Copner, R. & Griew, K. (1993) *Pathways to Adoption.* HMSO, London.

Myers, J.E.B. (1996) Expert testimony. In: *The APSAC Handbook of Child Maltreatment* (eds J. Briere, L. Berliner, J.A. Bulkley, C. Jenny & T. Reid), pp. 319–340. Sage, Thousand Oaks, CA.

Nye, S.A. (1980) Legal issues in the practice of child psychiatry. In: *Child*

Psychiatry and the Law* (eds D.H. Schetky & E.P. Benedek), pp. 266–286. Brunner-Mazel, New York.

Packman, J. & Hall, C. (1998) *From Care to Accommodation.* HMSO, London.

Pease, K. & Tseloni, A. (1996) Juvenile–adult differences in criminal justice: evidence from the United Nations Crime Survey. *Howard Journal,* **35**, 40–60.

Pinchbeck, I. & Hewitt, M. (1969) *Children in English Society,* Vol. I. Routledge, London.

Pinchbeck, I. & Hewitt, M. (1973) *Children in English Society,* Vol. II. Routledge, London.

Pipe, M.E. & Seymour, F. (1998) *Psychology and Family Law.* University of Otago Press, Dunedin.

Plotnikoff, J. & Woolfson, R. (1995) *Prosecuting Child Abuse: an Evaluation of the Government's Speedy Progress Policy.* Blackstone, London.

Quinton, D., Rushton, A., Dance, C. & Mayes, D. (1997) Contact between children placed away from home and their birth parents: research issues and evidence. *Clinical Psychology and Psychiatry,* **2**, 393–413.

Rosenberg, J.E. & Eth, S. (1995) Ethics in psychiatry. In: *Comprehensive Textbook of Psychiatry* (eds H.I. Kaplan & B.J. Sadock), 6th edn, pp. 2767–2775. Williams & Wilkins, Baltimore.

Rossi, P.H., Freeman. H.E. & Lipsey, M.W. (1999) *Evaluation: A Systematic Approach,* 6th edn. Sage, Thousand Oaks, CA.

Royal College of Psychiatrists (2001) *Guidance for Researchers and for Ethics Committees on Psychiatric Research Involving Human Participants.* Council Report 82.

Rutter, M. (1998) Research and the family justice system: what has been the role of research and what should it be? *National Council for Family Proceedings Newsletter,* **15**, 2–6.

Rutter, M. (2001) Children's level of understanding of medical decisions. In: *Guidance for Researchers and for Ethics Committees on Psychiatric Research Involving Human Participants,* pp. 39–43. Royal College of Psychiatrists, Council Report 82.

Rutter, M., Giller, H. & Hagell, A. (1998) *Antisocial Behaviour by Young People.* Cambridge University Press, Cambridge.

Ryan, M. (1998) *The Children Act 1989: Putting It Into Practice.* Ashgate, Aldershot.

Saywitz, K. & Goodman, G.S. (1996) Interviewing children in and out of court. In: *The APSAC Handbook of Child Maltreatment* (eds J. Briere, L. Berliner, J.A. Bulkley, C. Jenny & T. Reid), pp. 297–318. Sage, Thousand Oaks, CA.

Saywitz, K., Nathanson, R., Snyder, L. & Lamphear, V. (1993) *Preparing Children for Investigative and Judicial Process.* Torrance, University of California, Los Angeles, CA.

Soler, M. & Warboys, L. (1990) Services for violent and severely disturbed children: the Willie M. litigation. In: *Stepping Stones: Successful Advocacy for Children* (ed. S. Dicker), pp. 61–112. Foundation for Child Development, New York.

Stone, A.A. (1999) Psychiatry and the law. In: *The Harvard Guide to Psychiatry* (ed. A.M. Nicholi), pp. 798–823. Harvard, Cambridge, MA.

Thoburn, J. (1991) Evaluating placement: an overview of 1165 placements and some methodological issues. In: *Permanent Family Placement: a Decade of Experience* (eds J. Fratter, J. Rowe, D. Sapsford & J. Thoburn), pp. 34–57. BAAF, London.

Wald, M.S., Carlsmith, J.M. & Leiderman, P.H. (1988) *Protecting Abused and Neglected Children.* Stanford University Press, Stanford.

White, R., Carr, P. & Lowe, N. (1995) *The Children Act in Practice,* 2nd edn. Butterworth, London.

Index